The Royal Society of Medicine

family health

encyclopedia

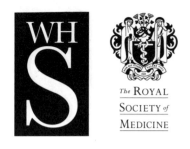

The ROYAL
SOCIETY of
MEDICINE

The Royal Society of Medicine

family health

encyclopedia

the complete A-Z medical
reference guide for every home

Dr Robert Youngson

Acknowledgements to the First Edition

In an era of such rapid scientific advance, the only way to put a book of this kind together in a reasonable time is by computer control of data. My first acknowledgement, therefore, must be to that small army of quiet geniuses who produce such brilliant software as WPCorps's *WordPerfect*, Borland's *Paradox* and Microsoft *Windows*. These wonderful products have enabled me to build, update daily, and rapidly access a computer data-base of many thousands of references from the principal medical journals and other sources. I also want to acknowledge the help I have had from the remarkable Macrex indexing program written by Hilary and Drusilla Calvert and from the indispensable Collins Electronic Dictionary.

The textbooks I have consulted are far too numerous to list but I am especially indebted to the *Oxford Textbook of Medicine* and *Scientific American Medicine* – both on CD-ROM – the latter updated four times a year by disk exchange. Other key works have been Davidson's *Principles and Practice of Medicine*, Sabiston's *Textbook of Surgery*, *Obstetrics by Ten Teachers*, *Gynaecology by Ten Teachers*, Laurence and Bennet's *Clinical Pharmacology*, *Gray's Anatomy*, Vander's *Human Physiology* and Roitt's *Immunology*. My principal sources for up-to-date detail, however, have been the *British Medical Journal*, the *Lancet*, the *New England Journal of Medicine* and the *Journal of the American Medical Association*.

After the first draft of this book was produced, the whole text was independently checked by a number of medical experts and by experienced medical editors and writers who did not hesitate to challenge me on any point which, in their view, failed to conform to current medical opinion. The review was of great value in enhancing the accuracy and completeness of the book and in curbing undue bias on my part. I am delighted to have the opportunity to acknowledge the hard work and painstaking care of the medical experts who were involved. In particular I want to pay tribute to the conscientious work of Dr Ruth Turner, who devoted many hours of patient work to the task. Other doctors who have checked and approved various parts of the text include Dr Rosalind Grant, Dr Mike Whiteside, Dr Andrea Kingston, Dr Michael Apple, Dr Kevan Thorley and Dr A.J.L. Turner. Advisers to the medical underwriters, Swiss Reinsurance Company UK Ltd., also checked the text.

On the whole, the doctors were kind. I cannot, however, say the same of my text editors. Medical editors – some of whom spend their lives checking medical facts – are often frighteningly knowledgeable people. For their unremitting efforts to ensure medical accuracy, achieving some kind of literary order in a heart-sinkingly massive manuscript, removing my many infelicities of expression and toning down the more extreme expressions of my prejudice, I am heartily grateful to Andrea Bagg, Faith Glasgow, Yvonne Lewis, Ran Lorimer and Karen Sullivan.

The excellent illustrations were drawn by Ian Foulis, Mark Walker and Ethan Danielson, working under the experienced art direction of Lydia Umney. For the highly efficient management of production I am grateful to Polly Napper and Gill Paul. The whole of the coordination of this undertaking rested in the hands of Bloomsbury's commissioning editor Rowena Gaunt.

Finally, I would like to express my grateful thanks to Mr. Howard Croft BA, the Managing Director of the Royal Society of Medicine Press Ltd., for the friendly, courteous and active interest he has shown in this publishing project.

Robert Youngson
London 1995

This edition published in 2002 exclusively for WHSmith, Greenbridge Road, Swindon SN3 3LD

First published in hardback in 2001 by
Bloomsbury Publishing Plc
38 Soho Square
London W1D 3HB

A copy of the CIP entry for this book is available from the British Library.

ISBN 0 7475 6229 6

10 9 8 7 6 5 4 3 2 1

Edited and Typeset by Book Creation Services, 21 Catherine Street, London WC2B 5JS
Printed and bound in Dubai by Oriental Press

Acknowledgements

Much has happened in medicine since the first edition of this encyclopedia was drafted and this is reflected in a different balance of content. The greatest and most far-reaching advances have been in genetics, which now overshadows the whole topic of human biology and pathology. Its influence is now so widespread that few aspects of medicine remain unaffected by it. By the time this book is published, the whole of the human genetic code will be known. This remarkable achievement will change the face of medicine and will have a notable effect on human thought and understanding. It will not be long before the intelligent lay person will be ashamed to admit ignorance of the processes by which our lives are determined by the DNA in all our cells. All the necessary information is to be found in this book, which now contains a substantially higher genetic content than the first edition.

Steady advances have also taken place in pharmacology and I have found it necessary to make a ruthless sweep of the drug entries, disposing of many drugs that have been superseded by better alternatives, introducing a whole new range of drug types and adding many more new drugs. Apart from the drug entries – of which there are over 1000 – this edition contains well over 500 new articles.

Since the first edition was published, the AIDS story has taken on a new complexion. Although there has been no reduction in the number of people infected – indeed rates of infection are higher than they have ever been – medical advances have, at last, brought new hope to sufferers and many are having their lives greatly prolonged. It is of some comfort to recognize that the AIDS disaster has led to important advances in the production of effective antiviral drugs as well as greatly increased knowledge of immunology.

The influence of the computer on medicine has received a degree of coverage which is, I hope, appropriate to its current importance. But there can be no doubt that this importance will grow, both for the practice of clinical medicine and for lay access to medical information. The Internet is both a mine and a minefield and advice is badly needed if misinformation is to be avoided. Enquire within.

The most obvious change from the first edition is the rearrangement of the entire contents in a strict A–Z format. My design principle for the first edition was that an understanding of the basic sciences underlying medicine should precede reference to what can go wrong and the book was organized accordingly with separation of the main sub-divisions of medicine. But my publishers have decided that this rather academic view is probably a mistake in a book intended for a non-medical readership. So I have been persuaded by the formidable ladies at Bloomsbury Publishing to agree to the new style. This will certainly improve accessibility. I have also added many hundreds of cross-references which will, I trust, draw the reader on to a painless extension of the initial enquiry.

My thanks to Kathy Rooney for proposing the new edition and for imposing shockingly tight deadlines which, had I not been working on the second edition almost from the date of publication of the first, would have been impossible to meet. My thanks to Nicky Thompson for her unfailing good humour and cheerful acquiescence in most of my unreasonable demands. Grateful thanks to Peter Richardson, Managing Director of the Royal Society of Medicine Press, whose energetic cooperation in this venture has been invaluable. My thanks also to Professor Aly Rashid who has kindly checked parts of the book for accuracy.

Robert Youngson
Blandford Forum, June 2000

A NOTE TO THE READER

No book of this kind, however complete, can be considered a substitute for the personal attention and professional care of a qualified doctor. Although a careful study of this book may well have a significant bearing on your health and well-being, it is not intended to replace medical consultation. If you have any reason to suspect that you might be suffering from any of the major conditions described in this book it is essential that you should consult a doctor without delay. This is especially important if you think you may have any of the diseases described as requiring urgent medical attention.

On all scientific matters this book reflects current orthodox medical thought, but does not claim to be the last word on any medical matter. On matters on which opinions differ, the views expressed in this book are those of the author.

Contents

Health and the Seven Ages Through Life

Although most diseases and disorders can affect people of any age, some occur almost exclusively within a particular age range, and many are most common at a particular stage in life. Because of this it is possible to elaborate a little on Shakespeare's idea of the Seven Ages of Man. This feature provides a general overview of the most common medical possibilities that might be encountered at each of the seven stages of life and to indicate where, in the book, a fuller account may be found. It includes many pointers for the maintenance of health at all ages. It also provides a broad account of the physical and social development of the human being. Inevitably this involves more detail in the pre-adult stages than in the later stages.

A word of warning: this feature contains such a high concentration of medical disasters and misfortunes as to suggest that every stage in life is fraught with danger. This impression is a misleading consequence of the necessary compression involved, and this feature must necessarily concentrate on the bad news. But there is plenty of good news, as a perusal of the main A–Z text will show. Living is inseparable from some danger but the fact is that modern medicine, and the spread of knowledge on healthy living among the general public, has led to a remarkable increase in life expectancy and greatly improved standards of health in all seven ages of humankind. Note that many of the most serious disorders, once present, tend to be persistent and so will also occur in later age groups.

Words and phrases in **bold** refer to articles in the main part of the book.

The Newborn Infant

A new birth is inseparable from a degree of anxiety. No matter how careful and comprehensive the antenatal care and surveillance may have been, you, the parents, will inevitably wonder whether your new baby is entirely normal and entirely healthy. This must be determined by examination, so this section devotes more detail than the others to this.

The first check after birth involves a determination of the Apgar score – a method proposed in 1953 by the American anaesthetist, Virginia Apgar (1909–74) and now in routine use all over the world. The Apgar is done a minute after birth by an experienced midwife or doctor to assess the state of well-being of the new-born baby. The figures 0, 1 or 2 are assigned to each of five variables:

Apgar score

- heart rate (over 100/minute = 2; less than 100 = 1; absent = 0);
- breathing (good = 2; gasping or irregular = 1; absent = 0);
- tension in the muscles (normal = 2; floppy = 1; limp = 0);
- response to stimulation of the foot (sharp withdrawal = 2; some movement = 1; no response = 0);
- skin colour (pink = 2; blue =1; white = 0).

The figures are then added together. A normal baby will score 8 to 10. Any baby with a score of 7 or less requires attention and a repeat of the Apgar at 5-minute intervals. At the same time, the baby is checked for visible external abnormalities.

Every baby should be thoroughly examined by a doctor within 24 hours of birth. This early check is most important, as many of the defects that may be found can be put right if diagnosed early. In some cases delay will mean that the disorder will be permanent. Quite a number of things have to be looked for. These include:

- weight, length and head circumference (see **prematurity**);
- skin colour (see **jaundice**, **rhesus factor disease**);
- abnormalities in the shape and size of the head (see **anencephaly**);
- protrusion or sinking of the fontanelles (see **fontanelle**);
- a soft, compressible swelling on the head (see **cephalhaematoma**);
- notching of the upper lip (see **cleft lip and palate**);
- ability to move the eyes to follow a moving object (see **nervous system**);
- white pupils (see **cataract**, **galactosaemia**);
- bleeding under the whites of the eyes (see **subconjunctival haemorrhage**);
- notching of the margins of the pupils or lids (see **pupil, disorders of, Treacher Collins syndrome**);
- abnormal heart sounds as heard with the stethoscope (see **heart disease, congenital**);
- distension of the tummy (see **pyloric stenosis**);
- webbing of the neck (see **Turner's syndrome**);
- state of the umbilical cord with presence of three blood vessels at the stump;
- state of the lower back (see **spina bifida**);
- clear anal canal (checked with rectal thermometer);
- presence of testicles in the scrotum in males (see **cryptorchidism, testicle, disorders of**);
- location of penile opening (see **epispadias**, **hypospadias**);
- foot deformities (see **talipes**);
- response to test for congenital dislocation of the hip (see **hip, congenital dislocation of**).

Not all of the conditions mentioned above are apparent immediately after birth, so follow-up examination is required. After the immediate post-natal period, checks at stated intervals are mandatory. Policy for dates varies but an effective routine would be examination before 1 month of age and then at 2, 4, 6, 9 and 12 months. These later examinations may reveal unexpected congenital conditions, some genetic, some acquired, that do not necessarily show themselves at birth. Some of these are remediable, some are not. The latter, or some of their effects, will persist throughout life. But even those conditions that cannot be cured can often be greatly helped by early detection and good treatment.

Conditions that may not be apparent immediately but that may be found in the first weeks or months of life include:

- cerebral palsy (see **spastic paralysis**);
- congenital syphilis (see **sexually-transmitted diseases**);
- congenital heart disorders (see **heart disease, congenital**);
- the effects of **rubella**;
- **Down's syndrome**;
- **fetal alcohol syndrome**;
- narcotic addiction (see **heroin**);
- HIV infection (see **AIDS**);
- congenital immune deficiency (see **Di George syndrome, immunodeficiency disorders**);
  congenital bowel narrowing (see **pyloric stenosis**);
- congenital **toxoplasmosis**.

There are, of course, numerous other acquired and developmentally-related disorders that can affect a baby. These include minor problems such as various respiratory infections, gastroenteritis, watering eye, conjunctivitis, umbilical hernia, squint (see **strabismus**) and deafness. Details of all of these are to be found in this book.

This catalogue of disorders may seem to imply that babyhood is a particularly dangerous period. Happily, this is no longer the case. Modern investigative and preventive medicine and the great advances in treatment that were made, mainly in the second half of the 20th century, have resulted in a remarkable improvement in baby health and a striking reduction in infant mortality.

The Toddler

This stage of life is characterized by enormous changes in the physical, mental and social development of the young human being. Toddlers, of course, vary widely in the rate of their development but for many progress is phenomenal. Everything is new and interesting, often fascinating, and during this stage the growing child acquires an immense amount of information about the world.

Most babies can sit up at 6 months and can get around by crawling, or some other individual mode of progression, by about 1 year. Some move in an upright sitting position by bottom drag, getting along by stretching out and then bending one or both legs. Some find this method of getting around so effective that they seem to have no inclination to get up on their feet and start walking. It is not unheard of for children who have developed a rapid crawling method of moving to go on using it until they are almost two years old. Other babies don't bother with crawling and proceed directly from sitting to walking. All these are entirely normal as is great variability in the age at which the child begins to walk. This has nothing to do with mental development and varies widely within the normal range of between 9 months to 17 months.

By the age of about 15 months, the child can clearly distinguish strange adults from the mother or father or other regular minder. But this ability, together with the complete physical and psychological dependence on the parents, may cause severe anxiety in the presence of a strange person. By about two years of age, however, the child has learned that there are many different people in the world and 'stranger anxiety' has usually faded.

Walking is a vital stage in development as it allows the child to explore and extend its environment thus greatly increasing the possibilities of acquiring information. At the same time, the sense of relative independence that the child experiences is an important developmental factor. At this stage you are likely to experience regular conflicts between your concern for the safety of the child and your child's quest for knowledge of the limits of what he or she can observe or control. Exploration and new experiences are important for development, and a balance is therefore necessary between over-restriction and safety. Inevitably the result will be many stormy scenes.

Once a child has learned that making a particular sound can get him or her a desired object, this connection is quickly exploited and reinforced. The average toddler of 18 months has a vocabulary of between 20 and 50 words, depending largely on how well the child is encouraged, at this stage, to talk by hearing normal speech from parents and other children. At this age infants understand many more words than they can speak – often well over 100 words. But around the end of the second year there is usually a sudden considerable increase in the power of expression and in the number of words that are understood although not spoken. Vocabulary and the ability to form sentences increase rapidly. These are rather general standards, but if the child obviously falls well behind these, you should seek professional advice. Delay in speech acquisition can be due to deafness and if you have any suspicion of this, report it at once.

At this stage parents can help children to enlarge their vocabularies by using simple normal language to refer to objects, rather than by making baby noises. Children brought up in a highly stimulating environment among people with a substantial vocabulary now rapidly develop their powers of expression and are soon prompted to enlarge their environment even more by learning to read.

Temper tantrums are common at this stage. These are the expression of frustration in a toddler who has reached the stage of wishing to demonstrate independent action but is prevented from doing so. Tantrums may be very noisy and, especially in public, embarrassing, as they seem to imply lack of parental discipline or effectiveness. The toddler soon learns to exploit the power of screaming, floor-rolling, head-banging and breath-holding and, if injudiciously handled, may come to dominate a household.

Occasional tantrums are normal and acceptable, but you must not allow a pattern to develop. Tantrums must be handled calmly, firmly and consistently with minimal necessary restraint, and the child's demands, unless reasonable, should never be met. If necessary, you may have to impose a short period of banishment to a safe cot or playpen in a separate room until the tantrum has passed. Once adequate communication by speech has been achieved, temper tantrums should settle, as the child can express his or her wishes and these can be discussed.

Another important weapon in the toddler's armoury is the breath-holding attack – a highly effective form of infantile blackmail. These are usually prompted by annoyance on the part of the child at not being allowed to have his or her own way. Although often alarming they never involve any danger to life and no treatment is needed. Breath-holding attacks affect only quite young children. They are unusual after the age of about five. Perhaps older children are able to find new and less alarming ways of manipulating their parents.

During the toddler stage, the child, who is now in contact with other children, is susceptible to many infectious diseases such as chickenpox, diphtheria, gastroenteritis, measles, meningitis, mumps, rubella, scarlet fever, thrush (see **candidiasis**), whooping cough and many others. Immunization can prevent many of these, but over-anxious parents who make strenuous attempts to avoid infections should remember that children who do not suffer various infections at this stage may be more susceptible to severe infections and other conditions later. This is not just a matter of antibodies. It appears that asthma and eczema for instance, neither of which are infections, are likely to be more severe in such children.

Among the many other disorders that can affect toddlers are:

- bow legs (see **genu varum**);
- knock knees (see **genu valgum**);
- drooping eyelid (see **eyelid, drooping**);
- **eczema**;
- infantile colic (see **colic, infantile**);
- **nappy rash**;
- **lice**;
- **fever fits**;
- **attention deficit hyperactivity disorder**;
- persistent squint (see **strabismus**);
- seborrhoeic dermatitis (see **dandruff**);
- **sickle-cell disease**;
- threadworms (see **threadworm infestation**);
- **tonsillitis**;
- twisted bowel (see **volvulus**);
- twisted neck (see **torticollis**);
- **roseola infantum**;
- narrowed penile outlet (see **phimosis**).

Experts do not, at present, think that there is any justification for amending the diets of infants under one year. During the first year of life, fats from milk are an essential source of calories and fat-soluble vitamins. Any reduction in fat intake – as, for instance, by feeding skimmed milk – might lead to a failure to thrive or even vitamin deficiency. Infants and young children need plenty of calories for energy and growth and a low-fat diet might be so unattractive that children might not eat it.

The Child up to Puberty

Most children are clean and dry by three, but many take longer to reach this stage. Undue concern is inappropriate until about half-way through the third year. By three, the average child will be anxious to avoid 'accidents' and may become anxious if for any reason access to toilet facilities is delayed. Persistent bed-wetting (see **enuresis**) after the age of five must be considered abnormal and requires attention.

During this phase of development, your anxiety may switch from concern over failure of progress in speaking to concern over the child's apparent inability to stop talking. To many healthy youngsters, the delightful ability to evoke a response from parents by speech communication, and especially by asking questions, proves irresistible. It is often apparent that questions are not being asked primarily to obtain information. Parents driven crazy by endless questioning might perhaps take comfort in this observation.

This is also the stage at which personal property and individual rights assume great importance for the growing child. Jealousy in childhood or sibling rivalry is a common result of competition, often between brother and sister. Much parental patience and diplomacy is often necessary to resolve, or at least limit, the resulting conflicts. It is always important for you to ensure that children's proprietary rights are respected by their siblings and that attempts to infringe these by siblings – a common manifestation of jealousy – are firmly repressed.

Alternatively, jealousy may be prompted by the arrival of a new baby. The usual signs are bed-wetting, a regression to a simpler and more childish mode of behaviour, temper tantrums, or sometimes evident anxiety. Children should be warned, well in advance, of an expected addition to the family and should be clearly told that time and attention will have to be given to the new baby. You must understand and tolerate the signs of jealousy and should give as much attention as possible to the older children. So far as possible, the baby should not be allowed to intrude into the older child's possessions and living area, as this will make the jealousy worse. Stuttering may develop during this stage and may require speech therapy. Fortunately, most cases recover fully.

Probably the most important health-promotion factor at this stage is good nutrition. It is during this period that faulty appetites are established and these can have a most important effect on the later health of the individual. For this reason you should be as well informed as possible on the subject of diet in childhood.

There is increasing evidence that the condition of atherosclerosis, which affects the linings of arteries, narrowing them and making them prone to obstruction, begins in childhood. Atherosclerosis is one of the two or three most serious of all diseases and is the underlying cause of heart attacks, strokes, limb gangrene and many other devastating disorders. Quite young children have obvious fatty streaks in their arteries and these are where atherosclerosis later develops. The risk of atherosclerosis is proportional to the levels of cholesterol carriers – low density lipoproteins (LDLs) – in the blood, and these relate to the amount of saturated fat consumed. Saturated fats come from animal and dairy products. Fish and vegetable fats are unsaturated. Most children get about 40 per cent of their calories from fat, and those with a regular junk food intake get over 50 per cent from fats. The average fast-food hamburger provides half its calories in fat.

The diets of children over one year should be modified to reduce the levels of total fats and LDLs. Post-toddlers who have a regular daily intake of junk foods, such as hamburgers, crisps and French fries, need to be protected from their natural appetites for high-fat food. Dairy products such as butter, high-fat cheeses, whole-cream milk, and animal fats should be avoided. Children's food should be grilled rather than fried; animal cooking fats replaced by vegetable fats; meat and dairy products replaced by fish and foods of vegetable origin; creamy milk by skimmed milk; and butter by polyunsaturated margarines. A satisfactory diet in the home will achieve little if you allow children to spend money on junk food or fat-containing sweets, or if they are having high-fat food in school lunches.

By the time they reach school age children have acquired a considerable range of personal skills – feeding and often clothing themselves, using the toilet, washing, and effectively communicating their needs and wishes to others. These skills confer a degree of independence that is usually greatly valued by the child, especially if they are clearly, and vocally, appreciated by the parents. This stage, however, brings with it new challenges and anxieties, the most significant of these being the move from an exclusively home and family environment to one that includes the school.

For most, the early experience of school involves at least a degree of separation anxiety and, at first, tears and refusal to attend are to be expected. At its worst, separation anxiety is a significant childhood disorder in which excessive and inappropriate alarm is shown whenever there is separation, or the threat of separation, from one or both parents. Security objects may become important and the child should always be indulged. It is an unwarranted cruelty to deprive a child of its security object.

It is not at all uncommon for children at the stage of starting school to show signs of real anxiety such as night terrors or complaints of various symptoms. The most popular is tummy pain. No one need be surprised at these reactions. For the whole of the child's life, he or she has had constant access to a parent; suddenly, for periods of hours at a time, this individual support is withdrawn. In the face of these child anxieties, it can be hard for parents to insist on taking children to school. But this is a statutory duty and it is rare for the anxiety to persist for more than a few days. Imaginative parents leaving their children at school have been known to ask the child to look after some small object until they return. Primary school teachers are thoroughly familiar with these problems and will almost always deal with them sympathetically and understandingly. Children are so accustomed to having, and needing, a parental figure that successful primary school teachers are often unconsciously treated by children as temporary surrogate mothers. It is commonplace for a child to address a popular teacher as 'Mummy' and then to look embarrassed or to laugh.

Because of their inherent fascination with all things new, school imposes great assimilative demands on new junior pupils. For many this huge new spectrum of experience can be exhausting and it is common for parents to find that, at first, children are apt to fall asleep as soon as they get home, or even when being driven home from school. There is no harm in this and it can be regarded with satisfaction as indicating the intensity of the child's educational experience. It is, unfortunately, a passing phase. Regrettably, few children are able to maintain the same depth of concentrated interest throughout the whole of their schooling. Those who do are usually members of a small, exceptionally gifted minority.

The period of junior school is also notable for a new and growing awareness by the child of the need for rules and regulations. Rules are important to the young child in two senses. They provide a stable framework for behaviour which permits the child to recognize the limits in which he or she may operate. Anarchy is no more comfortable in childhood than it is in adult society. And rules give the child an opportunity to become accustomed to conforming to the kind of discipline without which the child's future life is likely to be unhappy.

Many highly influential things happen to the child during the period of primary schooling. From the point of view of social and mental health, these early years are by far the most important formative period of the child's whole life. This fact has been recognized by sages throughout the centuries. The primary responsibility for the quality of the child's conditioning during this period of remarkable neurological plasticity rests, of course, with the parents, but a great deal of the responsibility devolves on the teachers who may often be perceived by the children as figures of greater authority than the parents.

In addition to the infectious diseases, a number of disorders particularly affect children at this stage in life. These include:

- **attention deficit hyperactivity disorder**;
- **autism** or Asperger's syndrome;
- bed-wetting (see **enuresis**);
- behavioural disorders (see **misbehaviour, child**);
- car sickness (see **motion sickness**);
- **dyslexia**;

- habit spasms (see **tics**);
- kidney inflammation (see **glomerulonephritis**);
- **meningitis**;
- middle ear infections (see **otitis media**);
- **nasal congestion**;
- **night terrors** and other sleep disorders;
- one-sided visual defect (see **amblyopia**);
- **streptococcal infections**;
- **stuttering**;
- styes (see **stye**).

This is the period of life in which the individual is formed and the quality of his or her future life is largely determined, and this imposes a heavy responsibility on parents, carers and primary school teachers.

The Adolescent

The initiation and principal feature of adolescence is, of course, puberty, and it is puberty that, directly or indirectly, causes most of the problems that affect adolescents. Puberty is the period of physical development during which the young person becomes sexually mature and capable of sexual intercourse and reproduction. Adolescence is the period of transition from childhood to adulthood. Puberty occurs at the start of adolescence and is a purely physical and physiological process involving body-building and sexually-maturing hormones. Adolescence involves, in addition, mental and emotional changes.

Puberty occurs at age 10–13 years in girls and 10–15 years in boys and is preceded by a striking acceleration in the rate of growth. This jumps to about 9 cm (3½ in) per year in girls and over 10 cm (4 in) per year in boys. This growth spurt often affects different parts of the body at different times so the body may appear temporarily out of proportion.

Puberty takes 3–4 years in girls and, because of the variability in age of onset, comparisons of girls of the same age may show considerable differences. Some may have reached physical sexual maturity while others may still appear childlike. This can be distressing, but by the age of 16 or 17 almost all the late starters will have caught up. Late onset of puberty has no bearing on the adequacy of future sexuality.

In girls, the first sign is usually breast budding, but sometimes pubic and underarm hair appear first. Breast buds can occur remarkably early – even as early as age 8 – and this is entirely normal. On average, however, they appear at about 11. From this point it is usually about a year before menstruation starts. By the time a girl menstruates the other changes of puberty are well established. To begin with, menstruation is often irregular, both in amount of flow and in rhythm. This irregularity commonly lasts for up to two years. During this time there may be short sequences of regular periods followed by up to several months with no menstruation. This can give rise to anxiety in sexually active young girls.

Breast growth is often rapid, and, for a time, one breast may appear larger than the other as a result of different growth rates. It is uncommon, however, for the breasts to remain of significantly different sizes. Bony changes in the pelvis cause it to widen, and the visual effect of this is emphasized by new deposits of fat laid down around the hips. The overall contours of the female body are considerably influenced by these fat deposits, which also occur under the skin of the breasts and buttocks. In girls, puberty is complete when menstruation is occurring regularly.

By the end of puberty in girls, all the female reproductive organs have matured to the stage at which normal sexual activity, conception and childbirth are possible. Many girls at this stage are, however, still mentally and socially immature. Ideally, for most, the full expression of sexuality should be deferred until late in adolescence or early adult life. Nowadays, however, the attainment of such an ideal seems to be the exception rather than the rule.

In boys, puberty usually takes about two and a half years, so it may not be complete until after the age of 17. Most boys have reached about 80 per cent of their adult height as a result of the prepubertal growth spurt, but there is nearly always considerable growth also during puberty. The physical changes of male puberty are caused by the male sex hormone testosterone. This is an anabolic steroid (growth-promoting hormone) produced in the testicles by cells lying between the sperm-producing tubules. Sperm production starts early in puberty, and thereafter sperm production is active and rapid. Very large numbers of sperms are produced – about 300–600 per gram (10,000–20,000 per oz) of testicle every second. Sperms are, of course, modified body cells.

Testosterone has an important range of growth and developmental effects. Roughly in the order in which they occur, these include:

- enlargement of the testicles, scrotum and penis;
- sperm production;
- enlargement of the sperm-carrying ducts and seminal vesicles;
- enlargement of the prostate gland and production of prostate fluid;
- enlargement of the voice box (larynx);
- lengthening of the vocal cords so that the voice deepens;
- growth of pubic and underarm hair and of the beard;
- sometimes growth of hair on the chest and abdomen;
- further acceleration of general body growth and muscular development.

The most obvious psychological consequence of puberty is the growth of sexual interest and sexual drive. Both boys and girls quickly become sensitized to, and acutely aware of, the physical differences between the sexes. The result is an intense interest in the opposite sex, and there is often a new and uncharacteristic interest in personal appearance and clothes. Adolescents may become increasingly anxious to conform to current fashions in dress.

Adolescence is a difficult time for many young people and may be equally or even more difficult for their parents. As their knowledge of the world grows and their confidence increases, some adolescents become arrogant and contemptuous of the opinions of older and more experienced people. Adult ways and views are often rejected by adolescents and they may be extremely impatient with imposed rules and regulations. There is a growing recognition of the importance of success, and if they fail to achieve this, as it is defined by adults in terms of good school reports, for instance, adolescents may then seek alternative goals and may, in particular, attempt to achieve success in the eyes of their peers. This commonly leads to juvenile delinquency, but, fortunately, this is usually only a temporary phase.

A proportion of adolescents never reach the fully adult (formal) way of thinking, in which abstract reasoning predominates. In these, thinking continues to be concerned with the particular rather than with the general, and the concrete rather than the conceptual. Thinking often remains egocentric so that the person concerned is unable to see something from another person's point of view. Some adolescents pass into adult life without ever being able to appreciate the relationship between present actions and their future consequences.

The principal medical problems of adolescence are a mixture of physical and psychological disorders. They include:

- **acne**;
- **anorexia nervosa**;
- **blushing**;
- breast problems;
- **bulimia**;
- excess sweating (see **hyperhidrosis**);
- fractures (see **fracture, bone, Colles' fracture**);
- **glandular fever**;
- **hay fever**;
- herpes simplex (see **herpes**);
- **menstrual disorders**;
- **sexually-transmitted diseases**;
- smoking (see **health maintenance, tobacco advertising**);
- substance abuse (see **solvent abuse**);
- type I diabetes (see **diabetes mellitus**);
- unwanted **pregnancy**;
- wet dreams (see **nocturnal emission**).

Adolescence, ideally, should be a period of intense interest, discovery and mind expansion, devoted largely to education in the best and widest sense of the word, under the wise but restrained guidance of older people. Regrettably, in the context of today's defective social values and preoccupation with materialistic rather than humanistic and high cultural aims, this ideal is enjoyed only by a privileged minority.

The Young Adult

The young adult is now a fully developed human being at the peak of physical and mental power. Some body growth may continue up to the age of about 25 but, thereafter, the skeleton is fully mature and fixed and, from a structural point of view, only degenerative changes can occur. Muscle power is maximal, but for about two more decades can readily be increased by hard physical work. Intellectual power, mental flexibility and inventiveness are also at their best in this stage, but the general usefulness of the individual may be limited by lack of knowledge or practical experience.

For most, a feature of this stage in life is hopeful optimism, tinged with a measure of anxiety as to the ability to achieve success. This is largely a consequence of lack of life experience, but it may be a good thing that each new generation is unaware of the difficulties and probable disappointments that may lie ahead.

In men, this stage in life is often characterized by a quality of competitive machismo and sexual display that may drive them to physical excesses or danger. When, for instance, deliberate artificial body-building is a feature of this phenomenon, the long-term effect is likely to be detrimental to health, especially if anabolic steroids are used. Machismo, however, has a much wider damaging effect as it is incompatible with the establishment of mature, equitable, mutually-respectful and stable relationships with women.

This is the stage in life in which sexual impulses can exert a dominant influence. Whether these impulses are directed to marriage or long-term partnership and family creation, or to a policy of sustained sexual promiscuity, may have a considerable bearing on health. In Britain today, more cases of AIDS are acquired by heterosexual than by male homosexual intercourse, so both forms of promiscuity offer serious dangers. Apart from AIDS, the prevalence of other sexually-transmitted diseases is at a long-time high and it is now almost impossible to engage in regular sexual promiscuity without becoming infected with at least one of these diseases. AIDS and genital herpes are still, unfortunately, incurable.

Marriage, too, imposes stresses and problems on young adults. These have always been present but, in the past, have been partly concealed by male domination and restriction of women's rights. With growth in respect for sexual and economic equality, and a decline in respect for earlier conventions, the true picture of marital breakdown is being revealed by the present very high incidence of divorce. For the young adult, this is another major factor affecting health in its widest sense – which includes happiness. Ability to sustain comfortable and satisfying relationships can be influenced by upbringing and social values. Poor ethical and philosophical standards lead to a culture of selfishness and disregard of the rights of others. Unfortunately, one of the now principal influences on young adults – the news and advertising media – strongly promotes these poor values.

Medical problems of young adults commonly relate to increasing activity of all kinds, and to stress, violence and human interaction. They include:

- **AIDS**;
- **anxiety**;
- **candidiasis**;
- **depression**;
- **dyspepsia**;
- **epilepsy**;
- exertional heat disorder (see **heat disorders** in *First Aid*);
- fractures (see **fracture, bone**);
- gun-shot injuries (see **firearms deaths**);
- **haemorrhoids**;
- **irritable bowel syndrome**;
- loneliness;
- migraine (see **headache**);
- **multiple sclerosis**;
- narcotic abuse (see **drug abuse**);
- **pregnancy** and its problems;
- **schizophrenia**;
- **sexually-transmitted diseases**;
- **slipped disc**;
- soft tissue injuries;
- **tuberculosis**;
- urinary tract infection (see **cystitis, pyelonephritis**);
- **vaginal discharge**;
- **whiplash injury**.

Early adult life should be a ideally period of health, happiness and great satisfaction. Due attention to the rules of healthy living can, in the great majority of cases, ensure that it is so.

Middle Age

The definition of this stage of humankind has never been officially established because human beings vary so much in all their characteristics. But, as an arbitrary average, it can be taken to extend roughly from the ages of 40 to about 60. The latter figure is the one that excites most controversy because of the growing number of mature people who, quite rightly, refuse to be classified as 'old' at a mere 60. Middle age, however, features a number of structural and physiological characteristics that are found in most people – although by no means all – within this age range.

The combination of increasing affluence and reducing physical exertion usually means that eating patterns that were appropriate to the energy expenditure of the young adult continue into middle age. So, since the calorie intake remains the same, there is a net balance of fuel intake that has to be stored. All nutritional intake surplus to requirement is converted into fat, which is the most chemically efficient form of energy storage. This fat is deposited in a layer under the skin called the superficial fascia, but in the abdominal region there is also a substantial fat store in a membrane called the omentum that hangs down on the inside of the front abdominal wall. Fat is also stored around the kidneys on the inside of the back wall of the abdomen. This, together with couch-potato laxity of the abdominal wall muscles, is the basis of the well-recognized 'middle-age spread' – a phenomenon far more common than is apparent, because of the concealing effect of clothes.

Middle-age spread is not simply a cosmetic disadvantage. It is an indication of the existence of a process which, unless sternly checked, is likely to proceed to a pathological state of obesity that will inevitable damage health (see **health maintenence**). And it is for this reason that so many people in the middle age of life suffer from:

- high blood pressure (see **hypertension**);
- diabetes of the maturity-onset variety (see **diabetes mellitus**);
- an increased incidence in women of breast cancer, womb cancer (see **uterus, cancer of**), ovarian cancer (see **ovary, cancer of**) and **gall-bladder cancer**;
- an increased incidence in men in cancer of the colon and rectum (see **colon, cancer of**) and prostate gland (see **prostate gland, disorders of**);
- orthopaedic problems, such as **osteoarthritis** of the knee joints and foot trouble;
- **depression**.

An even more important consequence of faulty eating habits is the high intake of saturated fats, mainly in animal and dairy products, and a low intake of high-fibre vegetables and fruit. This is one of the main risk factors for the development of the dangerous arterial disease atherosclerosis – a condition that prejudices an adequate blood supply to the brain, the heart, the limbs and most of the organs, laying the groundwork for stroke, heart attack, gangrene of the legs, kidney failure and other disasters.

Middle age is also the period in which degenerative diseases, cancers and stress-related conditions begin to become more common. Conditions most characteristic of middle age include:

- alcoholism (see **health maintenance**);
- angina (see **angina pectoris**);
- arthritis (see **osteoarthritis, rheumatoid arthritis**);
- **breast cancer**;
- chronic **bronchitis**;
- colon or rectal cancer (see **colon, cancer of**);
- **emphysema**;
- **gallstones**;

- **heart attack**;
- high blood pressure (see **hypertension**);
- **impotence**;
- **lung cancer**;
- maturity-onset (type 2) diabetes (see **diabetes mellitus**);
- menopausal disorders (see **menopause**);
- stomach or duodenal ulcer (see **peptic ulcer**);
- close vision problems (see **presbyopia**);
- prostate enlargement (see **prostate gland, disorders of**);
- prostate cancer (see **prostate gland, disorders of**);
- **varicose veins**.

It would be misleading and unduly pessimistic to leave the account at that. The fact is that all of these conditions – or their worst effects – can nearly always be avoided by knowledge which is acted upon intelligently or can be effectively treated. This knowledge is to be found in this book.

Old Age

In the last of the seven ages, health is dominated by a decline in function of most of the systems of the body. Ageing is a very variable phenomenon. The stereotype of the old as being incapable of anything is damaging and may be self-fulfilling. Undeniably, physical strength has declined markedly in old age and there are usually age-related deficiencies in the functioning of some of the sense organs – especially the ears and the eyes (see **cataract**, **glaucoma**, **presbyacusis**, **presbyopia** and **macular degeneration**). But so far as the function of the most important capacity of the human being – the intellect – is concerned, there is no reason to believe that, in the absence of actual disease of the brain, there should be any significant reduction.

In considering mental function in old age, in those free from Alzheimer's disease or other cause of dementia, there is a tendency to make the wrong comparisons. The old are compared with their young contemporaries. It is not widely known that, if the mental performance of old people is compared with their own performance when young, the difference is often negligible. This is the only fair basis of comparison, and when this basis is used it is found that mental functioning declines much less than most people suppose. Many old people, who happen to have maintained, throughout life, an active interest in any subject, including technology and its applications, will be found to perform well above average even when compared with young people.

Unfortunately, age-related bodily changes can conspire to damage, or even destroy, intellectual function. Alzheimer's disease is common, as is dementia from repeated ministrokes (multi-infarct dementia) or general deficiency of blood supply to the brain as a result of atherosclerosis. Another major hazard of old age is abnormally high blood pressure (see **hypertension**). There is a very clear association between high blood pressure and premature death. Indeed, the risk of dying rises faster than the proportionate rise in blood pressure. Regular checks and, if necessary, treatment are essential.

Osteoporosis is a reduction in the density of the collagen protein scaffolding of the bones and of the calcium salts deposited on the protein. Osteoporosis is age related and is often a serious matter, causing severe bowing of the spine or leading to fracture of the hip bone, or other bones, on minor physical stress. Some women lose bone strength rapidly and these are especially at risk of the worst effects, while others seem to lose bone mass only at about the normal rate associated with ageing in both sexes.

In general, the prevalence of cancer increases with age, and this group is more susceptible than the others. Cancers of the colon and prostate and of the womb are fairly common in the elderly. At the same time, it must be said that there is a tendency for many cancers in old people to proceed very slowly and many never cause any trouble. A surprising proportion of men are found, after death, to have an unsuspected prostate cancer. Even so, knowledge and alertness to the cancer risk are important.

Most cancers of the colon or rectum – which are among the commonest of all – start off as harmless polyps and grow slowly. They are usually well advanced before they produce symptoms. The first sign is often an alteration in the normal bowel habit, with constipation followed by frequent bowel motions. Pain is not a feature of cancer of the colon until a very advanced stage with spread to other nearby organs. The diagnosis ought to have been made well before that stage.

The prostate gland in men enlarges progressively from about the age of 30 onwards under the influence of the male sex hormone testosterone. This enlargement is due to the production of additional cells and has little effect until later in life. But about a quarter of all men over 65 have moderate to severe symptoms from the enlargement as a result of its tendency to narrow and partially block the urine outlet tube (see **prostate gland, disorders of**).

Elderly women often suffer severely from the effect of oestrogen deficiency in the vagina and surrounding area. This may become atrophied, dry and susceptible to infection. Indeed cystitis in elderly women commonly arises from this cause and can be cured by oestrogen cream applications. This, together with osteoporosis and its consequences, emphasizes the importance of restoring the normal state by hormone replacement therapy.

In addition to those mentioned, the most important medical conditions and events of old age include:

- age-associated skin changes (see **ultraviolet light, wrinkle**);
- **bedsores**;
- **constipation**;
- deep vein thrombosis (see **thrombophlebitis**);
- dizziness (see **vertigo**);
- faecal incontinence (see **incontinence, faecal**);
- falls and accidents (see **health maintenance**);
- **heart failure**;
- hypothermia (see **health maintenance**);
- **lung cancer**;
- lymphoma (see **lymphoma, non-Hodgkin's**);
- **malignant melanoma**;
- Parkinson's disease (see **Parkinsonism**);
- piles (see **haemorrhoids**);
- **stroke**;
- thyroid disorders (see **thyroid gland, disorders of**);
- urinary incontinence (see **incontinence, urinary**).

The situation is not all gloom and doom. Cataract surgery restores normal vision in a high proportion of cases, and adequate vision in almost all. Reading glasses will restore near vision, and modern hearing aids can often effectively relieve deafness. Knee joint replacement surgery is an under-used but highly effective remedy for knee osteoarthritis. The risk of hip fracture can be minimized by treatment for osteoporosis, and hip replacement surgery is highly effective in most cases. Much can be done to relieve incontinence, which is now far better understood than formerly. Early diagnosis and effective treatment can cure the commonest cancers of old age.

First Aid

What to do in a medical emergency.

The basic principles of first aid

The immediate assistance given to an injured person by someone who happens to be present is often more important than expert medical care given later. In some cases it is only the person on the spot who can save a life or prevent serious long-term disability. There is, of course, no legal responsibility on anyone to do anything, but common humanity demands that every responsible person should be ready to help. Whether this help is useful or not depends on whether the helper knows what to do. The possession of a few basic facts and a little vital knowledge about procedure can make the difference between saving a life and standing around watching a fellow human being die.

So it is necessary to learn about the priorities and how to act accordingly. There are only a few really essential points and these should be known by everyone. Apart from these, most of the detail contained in first-aid manuals is unimportant and may even direct attention away from what really matters. Most accidents occur in the home and far more deaths and serious disability occur from home accidents than from car or other accidents away from home. So it is up to all of us to know what to do.

In all cases, get medical help as soon as possible, but if action is urgently needed to ensure the person is breathing, this has priority. If necessary, send someone else to phone for an ambulance. Never delay arranging to call an ambulance, however. Ambulance paramedics are highly trained and experienced in all measures necessary to save lives in emergencies, and they carry all the necessary equipment. They can pass tracheal tubes to maintain an airway; can carry out cardiac compression and defibrillation in cases of cardiac arrest; can start a transfusion when required; and they have the equipment and skills to control serious bleeding.

> **If in any doubt as to the nature or severity of a person's injuries, seek professional medical advice immediately.**

> Words or phrases in the main text in **bold** type are cross-references to entries, under the same heading, in the A–Z or in the *First Aid* section. This is to avoid duplication of explanations.

The air supply

Successful first aid in critical situations depends on understanding and applying priorities. The first and most urgent requirement is for air, so that the brain can get its oxygen supply. It usually takes a long time to bleed to death, but total deprivation of air for even a few minutes is fatal or can cause brain damage. A person who cannot breathe for whatever reason, or whose airway is obstructed, is dying, and everything else is secondary to the critical requirement of restoring the supply of air. Brain damage from partial deprivation of air is usually more serious than any other kind of injury.

Obstruction to the airway can occur in many ways. In an unconscious person the tongue may fall back and block the air passage. Blood, vomited food, even collected saliva can block the airway. The victim may have choked on a large piece of food accidentally inhaled into the voice box in the neck (see **Choking** on page 27). Whatever the cause, the situation is critical and the obstruction must be relieved at once.

> Few people have a real grasp of the essentials and, in trying to help, often do more harm than good.
>
> - Do not delay getting seriously injured people to hospital or waste time on any trivial injuries or fancy bandaging.
> - Do not heap an injured person with blankets and clothes simply because they are shivering. This can precipitate a state of deadly surgical shock.
> - NEVER apply a tourniquet to control minor bleeding. Healthy limbs can become gangrenous.
> - REMEMBER it is vital to check that the injured person can breathe properly. Often the airway is ignored while pressure points are searched for to control relatively unimportant bleeding from small arteries.

> The Priorities
> **Remember ABC**
> AIRWAY, BREATHING and CIRCULATION.

Artificial respiration

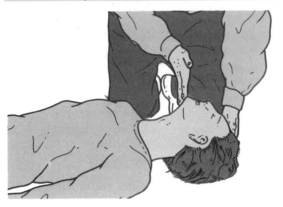

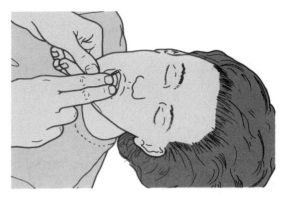

Sometimes breathing is obstructed by vomited material in the mouth or throat. This must be removed at once.

This position will allow free and safe breathing in most unconscious subjects by pulling the relaxed tongue forward off the back of the throat. It is still vital to check that the airway is clear.

Warning: Do not tilt the head back if there is any possibility that the neck is broken.

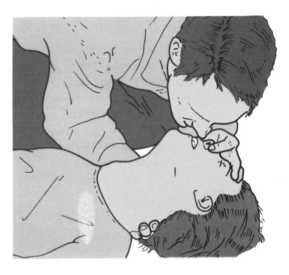

Keep the head in the extended position. Pinch the subject's nostrils before blowing into the open mouth. Check that the chest rises and listen for the air coming out again.

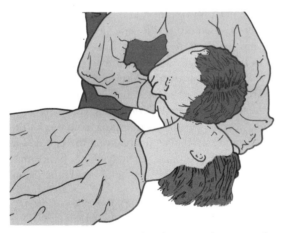

The first priority is to ensure that the unconscious person is breathing.

Clear the mouth with your finger. Remove loose dentures and all foreign material. Mop out the mouth with a handkerchief. Bend the head as far back as possible and push the lower jaw upward until the teeth are clenched. Check for breathing. If occurring, and the victim is unconscious, maintain the position of the head. If there is no breathing, start mouth-to-mouth respiration.

Mouth-to-mouth artificial respiration

The 'kiss of life' (mouth-to-mouth respiration) can be done by a single rescuer, but is much easier if there are two or more people.

The victim is turned on his or her back on the floor or ground and the clearness of the airway ensured (see above). In an unconscious person the tongue will often have fallen back to obstruct the airway and this must be overcome by tilting the head backwards and elevating the chin.

With the head kept in the extended position by one hand under the chin, the other hand pinches the nose. The rescuer now applies his or her wide open lips to the mouth of the victim, making a good seal around the victim's mouth. Regular full breaths are now blown in hard, at first as quickly as possible, then at a rate of 16–20 blows a minute. If done properly, the victim's chest will rise well with each blow, and between blows the air will come out.

It is important to ensure that air is actually going in and out and that the chest is rising and falling. If there are no chest movements there may be obstruction in the larynx – see **Choking** on page 27.

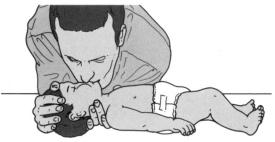

When giving artificial respiration to babies and small children it is often best to blow into both nose and mouth simultaneously.

Unconsciousness and the recovery position

A casualty who is unconscious but breathing may vomit and obstruct his or her airway. The tongue may fall back and do the same. To prevent obstruction, such a person should be placed in the recovery position while you wait for help. The recovery position keeps the victim still, makes the jaw and tongue fall forward so that breathing is free, and allows vomit or secretions to drain easily from the mouth.

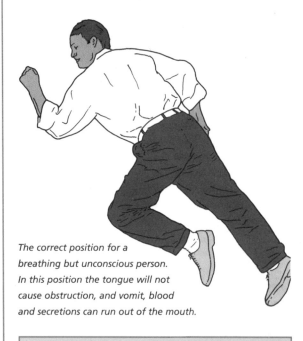

The correct position for a breathing but unconscious person. In this position the tongue will not cause obstruction, and vomit, blood and secretions can run out of the mouth.

Warning: If the injury was such that a fracture of the spine is probable, there is danger in turning the victim that further damage may be done to the spinal cord, causing permanent paralysis or even death. In such cases, any movement, except under professional supervision, is dangerous.

THE RECOVERY POSITION

Here is what to do:

- Turn the unconscious person face down, head turned to one side, and one leg bent to prevent rolling.
- Check at frequent intervals that breathing is continuing.
- If breathing stops, turn the victim over and start mouth-to-mouth respiration (see page 23).

Heart stopped (cardiac arrest)

Oxygen to the brain is the vital requirement for life, and it is essential that the blood, which carries the oxygen, is circulating properly. If the heart stops beating (cardiac arrest), the blood stops circulating, so the heart must be started again, or must be squeezed repeatedly so that the blood is circulated. A **heart attack** may stop the heart. Often the heart is not severely damaged — the arteries supplying the heart (the coronary arteries) may simply have gone into spasm — but if nothing is done then the person will die. A knowledge of cardiopulmonary resuscitation will save a life in such a case and may restore a person to normal function. Out of hospital, there is never time to summon medical assistance as delay may result in death.

Cardiac arrest does not necessarily mean that the heart has stopped contracting completely. In cardiac arrest, the lower pumping chambers (the ventricles) are no longer maintaining the circulation of the blood around the body. The heart may be stopped or it may be in a state of rapid, ineffectual

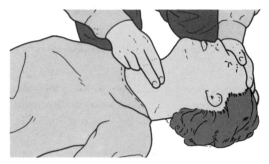

Check circulation by feeling for a pulse in the neck. Press firmly backwards with the fingertips in the hollow between the Adam's apple and the muscle beside it.

The Priorities
Remember ABC
AIRWAY, BREATHING and CIRCULATION.

EMERGENCY: CARDIAC ARREST

Here is what to do:

- If there is someone else around, send him or her to call an ambulance or get medical help.
- Check if the subject is conscious. If so, the heart has not stopped.
- Check for breathing. Tilt the head back by pushing the chin upward and lift the jaw forward. Put your ear close to the subject's mouth and watch the chest for breathing movements. If you hear or feel the breath or see the chest moving, the heart has not stopped.
- Get the patient flat on his or her back on the floor.
- Clear the mouth and throat with your finger. Make sure there is no obstruction and that the tongue is well forward.
- If there is no breathing, pinch the subject's nostrils closed with the fingers, seal your mouth tightly around the mouth, and blow until the subject's chest rises well. Remove your mouth and listen for the air coming out again. Repeat this steadily, using full breaths and allowing the lungs to deflate completely between each breath. With small children, it may be best to seal the mouth around both the child's mouth and nose, and blow into both.
- Do this 5 times and feel for a pulse in the subject's neck. If there is a pulse, carry on with mouth-to-mouth respiration, at a rate of 16–20 blows a minute, until the subject breathes spontaneously.

- If there is no pulse, place the heel of one hand over the lower part of the breastbone a hand-breadth above the angle of the ribs. Put your other hand on top. Keep your arms straight and use the weight of your body to press down firmly so that the subject's heart is compressed about 5 cm (2 in) between the breastbone and the backbone. In children much less force is needed. Do this, evenly and smoothly, 15 times in 10 seconds, and then give two full mouth-to-mouth ventilations.

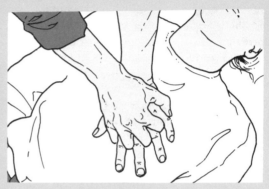

This shows the correct attitude for heart compression. The arms must be kept straight.

- Continue alternating cardiac compression with respiration in this way until the patient's heart starts or help arrives. If you have someone to help you, one of you should perform the cardiac compression and the other the mouth-to-mouth respiration.

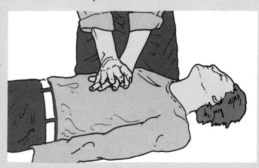

Keep the arms straight so that the weight of the body is used to depress the breastbone about 5 cm. Do this 15 times in 10 seconds then give two full mouth-to-mouth blows. Continue until help arrives or the subject recovers.

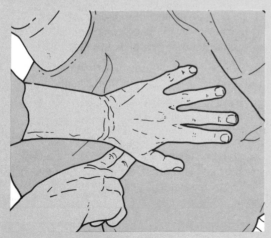

Heart compression is done over the lower half of the breastbone, centrally. Place the centre of the hand two finger-breadths above the angle of the ribs.

The Priorities
Remember ABC
AIRWAY, BREATHING and CIRCULATION.

twitching, called ventricular fibrillation. In either case, no pumping action is occurring and, unless something is done within two or three minutes, death is inevitable from failure of the oxygen and sugar supply to the brain. This is the ultimate medical emergency and is almost the only circumstance which will cause doctors and nurses to break into a run indoors.

Within seconds of a cardiac arrest, consciousness is lost, the person's breathing becomes rapid and shallow and soon stops. No pulse can be felt and the heart sounds are absent. Within minutes, the pupils of the eyes become very wide (dilated), and the skin turns bluish (**cyanosis**). To save the person's life, immediate artificial respiration and cardiac massage are needed (cardiopulmonary resuscitation).

Bleeding

After ensuring an air supply and a circulation, the next priority is the control of severe bleeding. This, too, is largely in the interests of a continued supply of oxygen to the brain. If there is not enough blood, insufficient oxygen will be carried to the brain. External bleeding is easily controlled, as will be seen. Internal bleeding requires surgical intervention, so urgency in getting the injured person to hospital is the keyword.

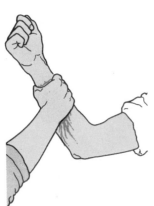

The correct method of controlling bleeding is to apply immediate, direct, firm pressure to the bleeding area. Apply pressure first and then look for a pad. Elevating the part can help.

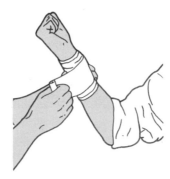

Maintain control of bleeding with a clean pad firmly bound in place.

Forget about pressure points and never use tourniquets. These can lead to gangrene. Severe injury often leads to a dangerous condition in which the blood, instead of circulating normally through tight arteries and veins, forms useless pools or depots in widely dilated vessels in the skin, digestive system and legs. This is called surgical shock and it has nothing to do with fright. Shock is another way in which the brain can be deprived of oxygen, and the prevention of shock is the next priority.

EMERGENCY: OBVIOUS EXTERNAL BLEEDING

Direct pressure, properly maintained, will stop almost any bleeding. Here is what to do:

1 Apply direct pressure to the bleeding area and maintain it. Use your hand until you have time to think.

2 Look for something with which to make a pad. Apply it firmly and fix it in place, using an encircling tie.

3 Try to elevate the bleeding part and to keep it at rest, so that a clot can form.

4 Make sure you can see what is happening and that continued bleeding is not just seeping into the clothes.

HOW TO PREVENT SHOCK

Prevention of shock is simple. It is essential for the victim to make the fullest use of the blood available and this must not be wasted by flushing the skin or filling the legs.

1 Do not pile up the injured person with blankets. Shivering and complaints of cold do not matter. Use one blanket only.

2 Elevate the legs, if possible, to improve the blood return to the heart and brain.

3 **DO NOT GIVE ANYTHING BY MOUTH**, unless the injury is limited to minor burns.

Note: A person in surgical shock desperately needs more fluid in the circulation and a drip, even of saline solution, can be life-saving. Ambulance paramedics can give this.

The Priorities
Remember ABC
AIRWAY, BREATHING and CIRCULATION.

Burns

EMERGENCY: BURNS

Here is what to do:

- Put the fire out and cool the burned area as quickly as possible.
- Chemical burns need prolonged washing. You cannot overdo this.
- Do not burst blisters.
- Do not apply any medication, grease, oil or anything else to a severe burn.
- Burns rapidly lead to loss of fluid from the blood and this has to be replaced.
- A moderately burned conscious person is the only kind of casualty who should be given plenty of fluids by mouth.

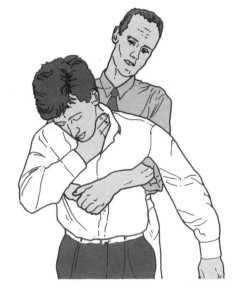

By suddenly compressing the air in the chest in the Heimlich manoeuvre it is often possible to blow out a foreign body causing obstruction.

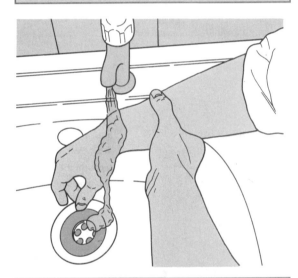

Heat destroys tissue and immediate cooling is the only measure that can help. So get the burned part under the cold tap and keep it there. This can greatly reduce the degree of injury.

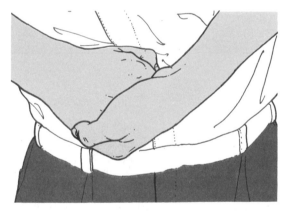

The thrust should be inward and upward and must be vigorous.

Choking

Anyone present when choking occurs is hardly likely to be unaware of what has happened. The affected person is obviously distressed, cannot speak, turns blue and often clutches the throat. A person having a heart attack can speak; a choking person cannot.

The Heimlich manoeuvre aims to dislodge the obstruction from the larynx by a sudden increase in air pressure in the upper respiratory tubes below the obstruction, so that it is forced up and out. Victims

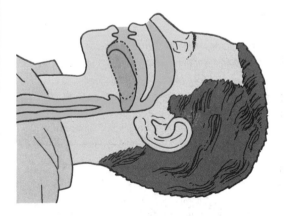

In the unconscious person the relaxed tongue and neck muscles fail to bring the tongue forward into the normal position and it may completely obstruct the airway.

can sometimes do this for themselves by forceful coughing or by sudden inward and upward compression of the upper abdomen in the 'V' below the ribs.

EMERGENCY: CHOKING

Here is what to do:

1 Get behind the victim and put your arms around him or her, just above the waist.

2 Make a fist with one hand and grasp it with the other.

3 Position the hands, with the thumb pressing inward, just below the point of the 'V' of the ribs.

4 Give a powerful, sudden, upward thrust or hug. Repeat, as necessary.

Note:

- If the victim is unconscious and lying on the ground, turn him on his back and give double-handed thrusts from the front.
- If breathing stops, begin mouth-to-mouth artificial respiration (see page 23).

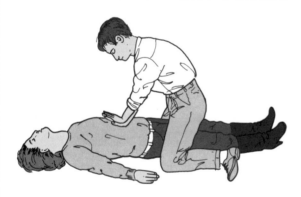

The same effect as the Heimlich manoeuvre can be achieved by an inward and upward double-handed thrust.

The recommended first aid in choking is the abdominal thrust. This is also called the Heimlich manoeuvre. Slapping the back is of little value.

Remember that a person in this situation is dying. Mere details like bruised or torn muscles are of no concern by comparison with the overriding necessity to restore the airway.

Corrosives in the eyes

Although there is no danger to life, this does call for urgent action if damage to vision is to be avoided. The accidental contamination of the eyes with corrosive chemicals such as lime or other alkalis or strong acids calls for immediate, vigorous, and prolonged washing with a large quantity of water, so that the chemical can be diluted and washed off before it has time to cause permanent damage to the transparency of the corneas.

Ideally, a water-tap should be run on to the open eye or eyes, or a hand-shower directed on to them, for 10 minutes or longer. The longer the interval between the accident and the start of the wash, the longer it should be continued. If water is not available, any bland fluid, including urine, should be used.

Electric shock

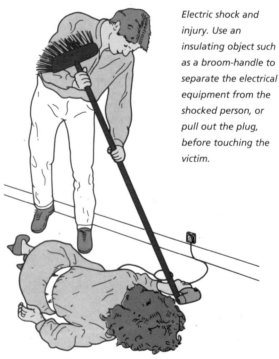

Electric shock and injury. Use an insulating object such as a broom-handle to separate the electrical equipment from the shocked person, or pull out the plug, before touching the victim.

The Priorities
Remember ABC
AIRWAY, BREATHING and CIRCULATION.

EMERGENCY: ELECTRIC SHOCK

Here is what to do:

- Switch off the current if possible because electric injuries are made worse by a continuing flow of current.
- **DO NOT TOUCH THE VICTIM** until the current is off or the contact broken.
- Move the victim from the current source with a broom-handle, a wooden chair, a dry cloth or a plastic garment.
- If breathing has stopped, start mouth-to-mouth artificial respiration (see page 23).
- If the victim is breathing, place him or her in the recovery position (see page 24).

Fainting

This is a temporary loss of consciousness due to a drop in the blood pressure so that the brain is deprived of an adequate supply of fuel (glucose) and oxygen. The drop in blood pressure results either from a reduction in the rate of pumping of blood by the heart or from an extensive widening of the arteries of the body.

Common faints usually occur from simultaneous slowing of the heart and widening of the arteries, often after prolonged standing, especially in hot conditions, when the return of blood to the heart by the veins is impeded. A severe fright or shock may cause sudden slowing of the heart, by way of the nerve which controls the heart rate (the vagus nerve). Fainting is also more likely when the volume of the blood is reduced·as in fluid loss from prolonged **diarrhoea** or excessive sweating. Low blood pressure is normally desirable, but an abnormally low degree, as in **Addison's disease** or from over-enthusiastic treatment for high blood pressure, can be dangerous. Fainting on taking exercise suggests heart disease.

A fainting person should never be raised. Elevate the feet and loosen the clothing, then leave matters to nature.

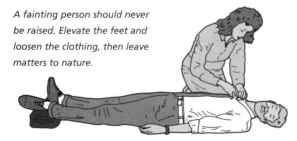

In a faint, the vision becomes misty, the ears ring, the skin becomes pale and the pulse slow. The resultant fall is exactly what is required to restore the flow of blood to the brain, and this can be encouraged by raising the legs.

Epileptic fits or convulsions are not faints and call for urgent medical attention if they do not stop within a few minutes. A prolonged series of fits is dangerous. Try to arrange the victim's surroundings so that he cannot hurt himself. Do not use a gag.

For **fever fits** (febrile convulsions) see page 296.

Convulsions or even brain damage can result if the fainting person is unadvisedly kept upright. Call an ambulance if unconsciousness lasts for more than a few minutes.

Foreign body in eye

This is a fairly common hazard, especially in industrial environments. The danger depends largely on the velocity with which the foreign body strikes the eye and a penetrating foreign body must always be suspected if the activity at the time was such as to produce high-speed fragments. Especially dangerous activities are grinding, turning, milling and hammering metal. The cold chisel with the mushroomed head is a prolific cause of serious eye injury. X-ray examination is mandatory in all such cases as a retained metallic intra-ocular foreign body will usually do serious harm to the eye – often after many months.

Most foreign bodies do not penetrate the eye, but lodge on the membrane covering the white of the eye (the conjunctiva) or behind the lids. Foreign bodies on the transparent front lens (the cornea) cause exquisite pain and intense awareness and induce an uncontrollable tendency to squeeze the lids – an activity guaranteed to increase the pain. Unless sharp and on the centre of the cornea, however, superficial foreign bodies are unlikely to do much harm.

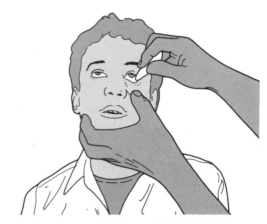

Foreign bodies in the eye can often be safely removed on the point of a folded piece of stiff paper.

29

Fractures/Heat disorders

- A foreign body behind the upper lid may sometimes be dislodged by grasping the lashes and pulling it down over the lower lid so that the lower lashes can brush it off.
- Eversion of the upper lid (turning it inside out), to examine its underside, may be very easy or very difficult depending on whether or not the affected person trusts the operator. A cotton bud, or even a matchstick, will help. Extreme care must be exercised.
- Get the victim to look down, pull the upper lid lashes downward, press the tip of the bud against the skin, 1 cm (½ in) above the lid margin, and pull on the lashes, outward and then upward. The whole thing can be done quite gently and painlessly so long as the victim refrains from squeezing and continues to look down.
- Superficial foreign bodies may safely be removed from the conjunctiva using a piece of paper folded to a point.

> Attempts to remove corneal foreign bodies may cause further damage and if the foreign body is central, permanent visual loss may result. A wash with an eyebath may occasionally be successful, but specialist advice will usually be necessary.

Fractures

Broken bones call for immobilization. Unnecessary movement may cause increased loss of blood and may precipitate surgical shock. Effective emergency splints always need to be longer than might be expected.

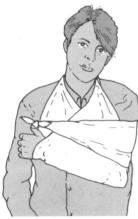

Adequate first aid immobilization of an upper arm fracture can be achieved with two squares of cloth, each folded to form a triangular bandage.

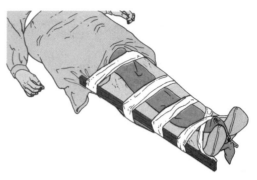

Improvised splints can be very effective in an emergency. The sound leg can also act as a splint. Good padding is important.

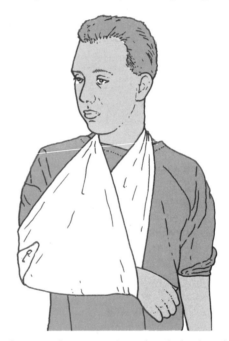

A lower arm fracture requires only a single triangular bandage sling.

- Almost any firm, elongated object may be used as a splint. Plenty of padding, of any kind, is needed and splints must be securely tied in place.
- It is often helpful, in leg fractures, to tie the legs together. Arms may be tied to the side for upper arm fractures. A sling is usually sufficient support for a lower arm fracture.

Heat disorders

The body produces considerable heat when fuel (glucose and fatty acids) is slowly burned (oxidized) to provide biochemical energy. During strenuous exercise, there is a large increase in heat production from this source and from muscle action. Heat is also gained from the environment when the external temperature exceeds that of the body.

If the external temperature is low, the body conserves heat by shutting down the blood vessels in the skin, and if additional heat is needed, the muscles shiver. If the body temperature rises too much, the skin vessels open up, causing the skin to flush so that heat is lost. In addition, the evaporation of sweat from the surface has a highly efficient cooling effect by drawing the latent heat of evaporation from the body.

These mechanisms are controlled by temperature-regulating centres in the area of the brain called the hypothalamus, which lies just above the pituitary gland. The temperature-regulating centres monitor blood heat and respond to changes. In fever, from disease, abnormal substances in the blood reset the thermostat in the hypothalamus at a higher level and the body responds by regarding the normal temperature as too low and turning on more heat production. There are various disorders of heat regulation.

HEAT CRAMPS

These are due to abnormal loss of sodium from excessive sweating and inadequate replacement. They usually occur after strenuous exercise in conditions of high ambient temperature. The onset is often sudden and incapacitating with hard spasm of the leg, arm or abdominal muscles. Heat cramps are usually rapidly relieved by drinking plenty of fluid containing a little salt. Prevention is easy, if the danger is understood and a good fluid and salt intake ensured.

HEAT EXHAUSTION

This is simply due to excessive loss of water from the body, so that there is insufficient fluid to maintain the circulation. It is a form of shock and the signs are similar to those of severe blood loss. There is:

- weakness;
- fatigue;
- collapse;
- pale, clammy skin;
- a slow, very weak pulse;
- abnormally low blood pressure;
- sometimes unconsciousness;
- generally a below-normal temperature.

Heat exhaustion occurs when fluid loss from sweating substantially exceeds the intake. The idea that one can be trained to manage on low water intake is as dangerous as it is naïve, and there has been a regular annual death rate, in military circles, from the efforts of officers and NCOs acting on this mistaken belief.

> The treatment of heat exhaustion is urgent replacement of fluid, by mouth, if possible, or by intravenous infusion if the subject is in a coma.

HEAT STROKE

Heat **hyperpyrexia**, or heat stroke, is the most dangerous of all the heat disorders. It occurs when the temperature-regulating centres are unable to cope with excessive heat production, as may occur from excessive exertion in very hot conditions, or when, as a result of disease or other causes, they fail altogether to control the temperature of the body. The temperature rises rapidly and the situation quickly becomes critical. Initially, there may be warning indications in the form of faintness, dizziness, headache, dry skin, absence of sweating, thirst and nausea. Later there may be lethargy and confusion or agitation progressing to epileptic-like fits, coma and death.

EMERGENCY: HEAT STROKE

Heat stroke is a medical emergency. The rising temperature causes brain damage which worsens with duration and level and, if the victim survives, this damage is often irreversible. A rectal temperature of 41°C (106°F) is a sign of grave danger.

- The treatment is to get the temperature down by any available means.
- The whole body should be immersed in cold water and ice-packs and fans used to supplement the cooling.
- The temperature must be monitored continuously and not allowed to drop below 38°C (101°F) as excess cooling may convert hyperthermia to hypothermia.

Near-drowning

EMERGENCY: NEAR-DROWNING

Here is what to do:

- Mouth-to-mouth artificial respiration must be started at once (see page 23), even before the victim is out of the water, if this is possible.
- If the abdomen is distended with water, the victim should be placed face down and then lifted with the hands under the midriff.
- Clear the Airway, check for Breathing and Circulation. If no pulse is felt, begin cardiopulmonary resuscitation (see **Heart stopped**, page 24).
- Survival is possible after long periods of immersion in cold water because the lowered temperature reduces the body's requirements for oxygen and brain fuel.

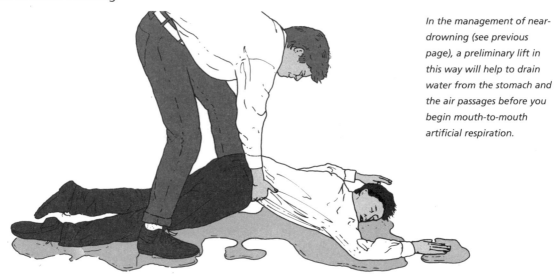

In the management of near-drowning (see previous page), a preliminary lift in this way will help to drain water from the stomach and the air passages before you begin mouth-to-mouth artificial respiration.

Near-drowning is another important cause of oxygen deprivation and, again, urgency is of the essence.

Nose bleeds

This very common event usually results from minor injury, such as nose-picking or a blow to the nose, but may also result from infection of the mucous membrane, local drying and crusting. Frequent nose bleeds are also associated with high alcohol intake.

Nose bleeding should not be considered a sign of high blood pressure, although it is fairly common in people with arterial disease who may have hypertension. It can, however, be serious, and may even be life-threatening, especially in the elderly. Occasionally, nose bleed is an indication of general disease, such as **atherosclerosis**, a blood-clotting disorder, **leukaemia** or **haemophilia**, and it may sometimes be an indication of local disease, such as **cancer** (nasopharyngeal carcinoma).

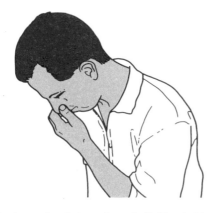

Nose bleeds can almost always be controlled by pinching the nostrils firmly for several minutes. The subject should lean forward to prevent blood running down the back of the nose.

- Nose bleeds can almost always be controlled by pinching the nostrils firmly together for 5 minutes and breathing through the mouth.
- Pressure maintained for this length of time will allow the blood to clot and the bleeding is unlikely to recur unless the site is disturbed.
- Failure to control bleeding by this method may call for medical attention – the bleeding area can be cauterized by touching with a tiny wool swab moistened with a corrosive chemical, or the nose may be firmly packed with ribbon gauze.

Rarely, the bleeding vessel is so far back in the nose, or so difficult to compress, that more major surgery is required. It is sometimes necessary to tie off the main artery from which the bleeding branch arises.

Bleeding in children, arising from persistent crusting of the insides of the nostrils, is best treated by the use of a softening ointment such as petroleum jelly.

Poisoning

There is no first aid for poisoning, unless the victim is unconscious. In this case put him or her in the recovery position (see page 24) and get to hospital, together with all available evidence of the type of poisoning – empty bottles, syringes, samples of vomit, tablets, plants or berries – as soon as possible.

ABOUT POISONS

Poisons are substances which can injure or kill living organisms when taken in small dosage. The matter of dosage is important because the great majority of substances, even some of those taken as nutrients, are poisons if taken in sufficient amounts. We commonly take very small quantities of very poisonous substances and suffer little or no ill effects. It is a mistake to believe that most, or even many, poisons accumulate

DRUG OVERDOSE

This occurs most commonly as a suicide attempt or by people seeking to modify their state of mind. Most drug overdoses occur as a result of 'recreational' use. Occasionally, drug overdose occurs by accident. The most common drugs to be taken in overdose, with brief notes on their effects, include:

DRUG	EFFECTS
heroin and morphine	vomiting, depressed breathing, pinpoint pupils
cocaine (crack cocaine)	excitement, euphoria, restlessness, feelings of power, tremor, wide pupils, fast pulse, overbreathing, cardiac arrest
amphetamines (Benzedrine, Dexedrine)	jumpiness, excitement, confusion, aggression, hallucinations
barbiturates (Amytal, Luminal, Seconal)	drowsiness, coma, hypothermia, slow and shallow breathing
benzodiazepines (Valium, Librium)	staggering, dizziness, drowsiness, shallow breathing
beta-blockers (Sectral, Visken, Angilol)	very slow pulse, collapse, drowsiness, delirium, seizures, cardiac arrest, nausea, vomiting
digoxin (Lanoxin)	diarrhoea, yellow vision, slow irregular pulse
iron (Ferrocap, Ferromyn)	abdominal pain, nausea, vomiting, rapid pulse, black stools
lithium (Camcolit, Priadel)	nausea, vomiting, apathy, tremor, muscle twitching, convulsions
NSAIDs (Brufen, Ebufac, Nurofen)	nausea, vomiting, abdominal pain, headache, rapid breathing, disorientation, jerking eyes, seizures, drowsiness, coma, cardiac arrest
paracetamol (Panadol)	nausea and vomiting. After 36 hours, acute liver failure which is often fatal
salicylates (Aspirin)	deafness, ringing in the ears, blurring of vision, profuse sweating, cardiac arrest. Coma in children
tricyclic antidepressants (Tofranil, Tryptizol)	dry mouth, wide pupils, inability to urinate, hallucinations, twitching, loss of consciousness

in the body until dangerous levels are reached. The level in the body is almost always determined by the average intake and reaches a stable state depending on the intake. Usually this level is much too low to do any harm.

Almost all drugs are poisonous if taken in excess, but are safe if taken in correct dosage under medical supervision. Adult doses may be poisonous to children. Some drugs are especially dangerous in excess and have to be used with special care. Drugs used in the treatment of cancer are capable of destroying living cells, but can be used because their effect on cancer cells is greater than on healthy cells. Nevertheless, they are very toxic.

It is impossible to list all the poisonous substances with which one might come in contact. Some substances, however, are commonly accessible and are particularly toxic and dangerous. Here are some of these, arranged under categories.

POISONS IN THE HOME
- ammonia
- liquid bleach
- toilet-bowl cleaning powder or liquid
- fungus-killing liquids
- oven-cleaning liquids and sprays
- corrosive agents, such as acids, alkalis, bleaches and disinfectants

EMERGENCY: POISONING

Here is what to do:

- Do not make the victim vomit.
- Do not give anything by mouth.
- Just get him or her to hospital by any means, with the minimum delay.
- Inform the ambulance people that it is a poisoning case and state whether or not the victim is conscious.
- If going by car, get someone to telephone the hospital casualty department and warn them.

Poisoning

- rust removers
- paint strippers
- spot removers, especially if inhaled
- sterilizing fluids such as phenols or cresol
- various liquid glues, if inhaled
- coumarin and warfarin rat and mouse poisons
- methylated spirits
- rubbing alcohol
- antifreeze
- drugs (see panel on page 33)

POISONS IN THE GARDEN AND COUNTRYSIDE
- organophosphate weedkillers, such as paraquat
- insecticides, such as Parathion and Malathion
- laburnum berries

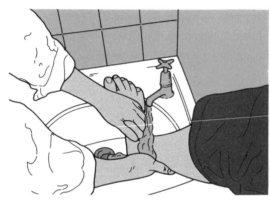

Animal bites and abrasions should be washed thoroughly under running water to remove as much bacterial contamination as possible.

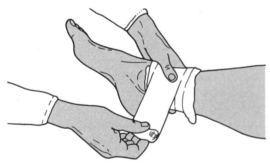

Once cleaned, wounds should be covered with a clean dressing.

- yew
- deadly nightshade
- common inkcap mushroom
- deathcap mushroom
- 'magic' mushrooms
- deadly agaric mushroom

POISONOUS ANIMALS

A few animals, insects and marine creatures produce toxins harmful to man in the doses normally acquired. These include:

- sea snakes
- ciguatera (an alga eaten by fish in the Pacific and Caribbean)
- certain shellfish contaminated by toxic protozoa
- puffer fish
- stingrays
- scorpion fish
- cone shell molluscs
- jellyfish
- land scorpions
- centipedes
- a few tropical spiders

INDUSTRIAL POISONS

Many inorganic compounds are poisonous, notably:

- the salts of the heavy metals, such as lead, iron, arsenic, gold, silver and mercury;
- strong acids and alkalis, mainly by exerting severe corrosive effects on tissues;
- hundreds of synthetic organic substances;
- many solvents;
- most of the highly reactive gases such as chlorine, bromine, ammonia, hydrogen sulphide and hydrocyanic acid.

Industrial first aid centres are familiar with the relevant toxic substances and with their particular dangers. In some cases antidotes are available.

> **The Priorities**
> **Remember ABC**
> AIRWAY, BREATHING and CIRCULATION.

a-z

of disorders, drugs and medical terms

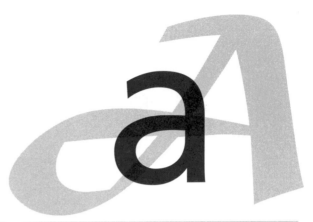

a-

Prefix meaning 'not, without', as in apyrexial (without fever).

ab-

Prefix meaning 'from', as in abnormal, (from normal).

abacavir

A nucleoside **reverse transcriptase inhibitor**. A brand name is Ziagen

abciximab

A drug that inhibits the platelet glycoprotein IIb/IIIa receptor and is used as an adjunct to heparin and aspirin (see **analgesic drugs**) in patients undergoing coronary angioplasty. The drug has been found valuable in coronary stenting. A brand name is Reopro.

abdominal breathing

Respiration in which most of the work is done by the muscles of the front wall of the abdomen rather than by the **diaphragm** and the muscles between the ribs (intercostal muscles). When the abdominal muscles tighten they compress the intestines which are forced upwards, pushing up the diaphragm so as to compress the lungs and drive out air. Deliberately employed, the method can be helpful in patients with breathing difficulties.

abdominal gestation

A type of out of location (ectopic) **pregnancy** in which a fetus develops outside the womb but in the abdominal cavity. This is a dangerous state of affairs, because the fetus will usually have established its own blood supply by forming a placenta attached to one of the abdominal organs. This is liable to lead to profuse internal bleeding, and calls for urgent specialist attention. Very rarely, an abdominal gestation has gone to full term.

abdominal pain

See **stomach, disorders of**.

Abelcet

A brand name for the antifungal drug amphotericin B. It is given by injection.

aberrant

Deviating from the normal. The term may be applied to variations in the fine detail of body structure, such as the size and position of small arteries, or to modes of behaviour not generally considered acceptable.

Abidec

A brand name for a multivitamin preparation for children containing vitamin A, calciferol, thiamine, riboflavine, pyridoxine, nicotinamide and vitamin C.

-able

Suffix meaning 'able to be' as in durable (able to last).

abnormal dryness

See **dehydration**.

abortifacient

A drug used to cause **abortion**. Many substances have been popularly reputed to cause abortion and many have been tried in an attempt to procure abortion illegally, mostly without effect. In clinical practice the drug chiefly used to induce abortion is one of the prostaglandins. Other drugs, such as oxytocin, are also used to induce labour.

The most recent effective abortifacient is the drug RU486, or mifepristone, known as the 'abortion pill'. This drug acts by blocking the action of progesterone which is essential to maintain pregnancy. A second drug, one of the prostaglandins, has to be taken within forty-eight hours to complete the expulsion of the fertilized egg.

The method is said to be 95 per cent effective.

abortion and miscarriage

The first of these terms is commonly misunderstood outside medical circles. In general terms, the word 'abortion' simply means the failure of something to reach fulfilment or maturity. Medically, abortion means loss of the fetus, for any reason, before it is able to survive outside the womb. The term covers accidental or spontaneous ending, or miscarriage, of pregnancy as well as deliberate termination. The terms 'spontaneous abortion' and 'miscarriage' are synonymous and are defined as loss of the fetus before the twenty-eighth week of pregnancy. This definition implies a legal perception of the age at which a fetus can survive out of the womb. With great advances in recent years in the ability to keep very premature babies alive, this definition is in need of revision.

At least one in ten pregnancies ends in abortion, nearly all of these being spontaneous and occurring at an early stage. In many of these cases, the woman concerned is never aware that she is pregnant. All that happens is a rather late, and perhaps unusually severe, period. Some authorities state that 10 to 15 per cent of all pregnancies diagnosed after a missed period end in abortion.

Spontaneous abortion is often necessary as it may be caused by abnormal chromosomes so that a fetus, which would have grown to be an abnormal baby, is discarded. Other possible causes are that:

- the embryo may have implanted at an unsuitable site in the womb;
- the embryo may have implanted outside the womb (see above);
- the womb may be abnormal;
- the neck of the womb may be open (incompetent cervix);
- the mother may be producing insufficient hormones (especially progesterone) to maintain the pregnancy;
- there may be infection of the reproductive organs.

Often, abortion occurs for no discoverable cause.

The unmistakable sign of threatened abortion is bleeding, or a dark brown discharge, from the vagina. Often there is a slight pain, like a period pain, in the lower abdomen. Obvious and severe lower abdominal pain suggests a possible **ectopic pregnancy**.

One in four women with bleeding and pain has an ectopic pregnancy. In threatened abortion, although the fetus remains alive, with the placenta still attached to the inner wall of the womb, the bleeding indicates that there is a risk of separation.

About a quarter go on to abortion, but most settle down after a few days' bed rest, and the pregnancy continues to full term with delivery of a healthy, normal baby. Continuation of the pregnancy can be confirmed by an ultrasound scan. In such cases, threatened abortion does not imply that there is anything wrong with the baby.

If infection of the womb occurs – and this is encouraged by the presence of blood clots that form excellent culture media for organisms – the condition is called septic abortion. This is potentially dangerous and can progress to widespread pelvic infection and infection of the abdominal cavity (peritonitis). In cases of septic abortion, the patient must be taken to hospital for urgent treatment to clear the womb, control the infection and prevent surgical shock.

If the bleeding gets worse, however, and the pain becomes more severe, cramping and rhythmical, there comes a point when it must be recognized that abortion is inevitable. Inevitable abortion means that the fetus has died and is being expelled by contractions of the womb. The cervix will now be open, and blood clots and membranes, enclosing the fetus, will pass into the vagina. Sometimes bleeding is so severe as to require blood transfusion. Often the expulsion is incomplete and a minor operation, under general anaesthesia, may be needed. This is called evacuation of retained products of conception (ERPC). The womb is emptied by suction, and the lining is carefully scraped with a sharp-edged spoon called a curette. A drug is then given to cause the womb to contract, and antibiotics may also be necessary. The patient is usually able to go home the next day.

Sometimes the fetus dies but is retained in the womb. This is called missed abortion. In this case there is usually a history of threatened abortion that has apparently settled. But later, the signs of pregnancy – morning sickness, breast enlargement and tenderness – disappear. A brownish discharge may occur. Suspicion can be confirmed by use of an ultrasound scan, which will no longer show a fetal heartbeat. In the end there is usually spontaneous expulsion of the remaining material, but an ERPC is often necessary.

Later miscarriage is less common and is often associated with abnormalities of the womb or with inability of the cervix to remain closed (**cervical incompetence**). Some women abort repeatedly and are described as 'habitual aborters'. Full gynaecological investigation will reveal the cause of this in about 40 per cent of cases. Deliberate termination of pregnancy is called induced abortion. When this is legal it is called therapeutic abortion.

If there are considered to be good reasons, abortion may be performed legally under certain circumstances and in approved hospitals or clinics. In Britain, two doctors, who have seen the patient, must agree that continuation of the pregnancy would be detrimental. The legal criteria are that the doctors concerned must be able to certify in good faith that one of the following applies:

- continuation of the pregnancy would involve a greater risk to the life of the woman than terminating it;
- continuation would involve a greater risk of injury to the physical or mental health of the woman than terminating it;
- continuation would involve risk to the physical or mental health of any children of the pregnant woman's family;
- there is a substantial risk that the child, if born, would have physical or mental abnormalities of such degree as to cause serious handicap.

The criteria are, in general, more relaxed in the United States. Following a 1973 Supreme Court decision, abortion under twelve weeks is legal if the woman wishes it and her doctor agrees. Some states have reviewed this policy and a 1989 court ruling has strengthened the position of the anti-abortion lobby. Many abortions are done for social or psychiatric reasons, the remainder because of organic medical disorders. Some forms of heart or kidney disease and some cancers – especially those of the neck of the cervix or of the breast, may be made worse by pregnancy, and almost all doctors believe that abortion is justified in such cases. Certain abnormalities in the fetus, which would lead to an abnormal baby, are also considered to justify abortion. Many of these can be diagnosed by ultrasound scan, by amniocentesis or by chorionic villus sampling.

Therapeutic abortion is safest before twelve weeks and the method varies with the stage in pregnancy. General anaesthesia is almost always used. Up to about fourteen weeks, abortion is commonly procured by dilatation of the cervix with a succession of smooth rods of increasing diameter, followed by vacuum suction through a tube or gentle scraping with a curette.

After fourteen weeks, medical methods are usual. Often, a hormone-like drug called a prostaglandin is used which, when introduced into the womb, causes the cervix to widen and the womb to contract as in a normal delivery. The procedure is always done in hospital. Prostaglandins can be injected into a vein or given in a cone of cocoa butter containing the drug (a pessary), which melts after being placed in the vagina. The patient is given drugs to control the pain of the contractions and remains awake. The procedure usually takes about twelve hours. Sometimes expulsion of the fetus is incomplete and an ERPC is necessary, but usually the patient leaves hospital twenty-four to forty-eight hours later.

The 'abortion pill' contains the drug mifepristone (RU 486). This is a progesterone antagonist that reliably interferes with early pregnancy in a dose of 600 mg. Its use is followed by the administration of a prostaglandin drug by vaginal suppository or injection to ensure expulsion of the embryo or fetus. In some cases a minor clearing operation (**D and C**) is needed. A major trial involving 2115 women, pregnant for seven weeks or less, was conducted in France and the results reported in 1990. Ninety-nine per cent of the pregnancies were terminated. This method is being increasingly used as an alternative to surgical procedures.

Criminal abortion is the termination or attempted termination of a pregnancy performed illegally or by unqualified persons. Many 'back-street' abortionists have little idea of safe practice and there is a high risk of serious injury. This may be immediate, from perforation of the womb, for instance, or from severe bleeding, or it may occur later from infection, often leading to permanent infertility. There is a close correlation between official objection to therapeutic abortion and the incidence of criminal abortion.

abortion pill

A drug, RU486 or mifepristone, that acts by blocking the action of progesterone which is essential to maintain pregnancy. A second drug, one of the prostaglandins, has to be taken within 48 hours to complete the expulsion of the fertilized egg. The method is said to be 95 per cent effective.

See also **mifepristone**.

abortion-proneness

See **Hughes' syndrome**.

abortion trauma syndrome

A good deal of media attention has been given to an allegedly common condition known as the abortion trauma syndrome. This is said to feature emotional repression, thwarted maternal instincts, intense guilt feelings, depression, thoughts of suicide, psychiatric disturbance, child neglect or abuse, and so on. Most women who undergo abortion suffer stress and emotional upset, and some will suffer severely. Studies have shown, however, that, after abortion, most women feel deeply relieved. One British series showed that psychotic breakdown occurred after normal delivery in 1.7 cases per 1000, but in only 0.3 cases per 1000 after abortion.

abrasion

Wearing away of tissue by long-sustained or unusually heavy friction between surfaces. Abrasion of the biting surfaces of teeth is common, with removal of the enamel, especially in people who use hard toothbrushes with a sawing action. Skin abrasions, in which an area is partially or wholly removed by strong mechanical friction, are among the commonest of all minor injuries. Sometimes the abrasion is deliberate, as in the cosmetic treatment of acne scars or other disfigurements. This is called **dermabrasion**.

abreaction

A process used in **psychotherapy** in which important thoughts and feelings, which have been repressed, are brought into consciousness. This often occurs in the course of catharsis – the free expression of the emotions which are associated with the repressed material. Abreaction is the result of catharsis and is most easily achieved when the trouble arises from a recent traumatic event.

abscess

A cavity full of pus surrounded by inflamed or dying tissue, or by dense fibrous tissue which cuts off blood supply to the centre. Abscesses are caused by infection and the organisms concerned often persist within them. But antibiotics are useless in the treatment of long-term abscesses, because they cannot gain access to the contents, and a walled-off abscess tends to become permanent. If it is opened surgically and the pus drained, however, healing is usual. Sometimes abscesses form a drainage track to the surface, called a sinus, and this, too, tends to be permanent unless the abscess and track are removed surgically.

Dental abscesses are common. These are collections of pus around the root of a tooth, usually due to neglect of the teeth so that decay (**caries**) allows bacteria access to the tooth pulp. Tooth abscesses cause severe aching and tenderness on chewing and sometimes track through the thin bone around the root to form a gumboil. The problem can always be solved

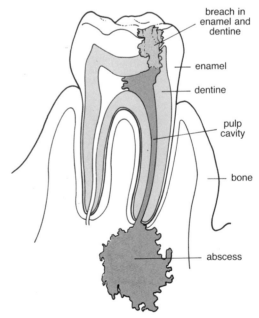

Local destruction of the enamel allows access of bacteria to the dentine and soft pulp. Infection rapidly spreads down the tooth and can reach the opening in the tip of the root to form an abscess in the surrounding bone.

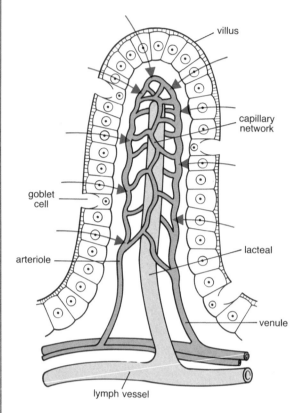

One of the millions of intestinal villi through which the absorption of digested food materials occurs. Sugars and amino acids pass into the capillary network of blood vessels, emulsified fats into the lacteals.

by extracting the affected tooth, but an attempt may be made to save it by drilling into the abscess and releasing the pus.

absence attacks

See **petit mal**.

absent testicle

See **cryptorchidism**.

absorption

The movement of liquids and of substances in dissolved form, across a membrane, from one compartment of the body to another. Thus, when food has been adequately broken down by mechanical and digestive **enzyme** action in the bowel (intestines), the wanted elements, such as sugars, fat globules, protein fractions, minerals and vitamins, pass, by absorption, through the lining of the bowel into the bloodstream. In the large bowel, reabsorption of water conserves loss and prevents constant diarrhoea; and in the kidneys, which initially filter out very large volumes of water from the blood, reabsorption of most of this water is essential to normal life.

-ac

Suffix meaning 'like, of' as in cardiac (heart-like).

acalculia

Loss of the ability to perform even simple arithmetical calculations of the type 3 + 5 = ?. This is one of the many disturbances of brain function that may occur as part of a **stroke**, or it may be one of the first signs of a disease of the nervous system such as **Alzheimer's disease**. Acalculia may exist from early childhood as a condition similar to **dyslexia**. In such cases, no amount of instruction is likely to suceed.

acamprosate

A drug used to assist in the control of alcoholism. Acamprosate has been found to be an effective and well-tolerated adjunct to the management of alcoholism. A brand name is Campral EC.

acarbose

An oral hypoglycaemic drug. A brand name is Glucobay.

accident and emergency surgeon

A general surgeon skilled in the management of accidental and other injuries of all kinds. The specialty is concerned primarily with the immediate treatment of the injured but involves a knowledge of several subspecialties.

accommodation

The automatic process by which the eyes adjust their focus when the gaze is shifted from one point to another at a different distance. Accommodation is effected by the internal crystalline lens that lies behind the pupil. This lens is naturally elastic in young people and, unless pulled outwards around its equator, assumes a near-spherical shape. The pull is provided by delicate fibres running to a circular muscle near the root of the iris. When this ring of muscle contracts, the ring becomes smaller and the pull on the fibres is less, allowing the lens to become more curved and suitable for focus on near objects. When the muscle ring relaxes, the eye is focused for distance.

Accommodation is powerful and rapid in the young but falls off progressively with advancing age. By the middle forties, most people have suffered so much loss of accommodation that, unless they are shortsighted (see **myopia**) they need reading glasses.

See also **blurred vision, presbyopia**.

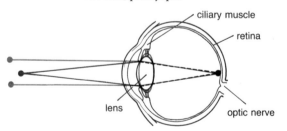

Parallel light rays from distant objects are brought to a sharp focus on the retina with relaxed accommodation and a flattened lens. Diverging rays from a near object must be more strongly bent so a more curved lens is needed. The ciliary muscle ring contracts and allows the lens to bulge more.

Accupro

A brand name for **quinapril**.

Accuretic

A brand name for **hydrochlorothiazide** formulated with an **angiotensin converting enzyme inhibitor** drug.

acebutolol

A **beta-blocker drug** commonly used to treat high blood pressure. A brand name is Sectral.

aceclofenac

A drug used in the treatment of **osteoarthritis**. A brand name is Preservex.

ACE inhibitors

See **angiotensin converting enzyme inhibitors**.

acemetacin

A drug used in the treatment of **rheumatoid arthritis**. A brand name is Emflex.

-aceous

Suffix meaning 'full of' as in pultaceous (full of pulp).

Acepril

A brand name for captopril.

acetazolamide

A drug that inhibits the enzyme carbonic anhydrase in the kidney tubules, thus acting as a diuretic. In the eye it acts similarly to reduce the rate of secretion of aqueous humour and is useful in the treatment of **glaucoma** when the intraocular pressure rise cannot be controlled with eyedrops alone. A brand name is Diamox.

acetylcysteine

A drug used to reduce the stickiness and viscosity of **mucus**. A mucolytic. It is useful for freeing sputum in **bronchitis** and in liquefying mucus in **cystic fibrosis**. It is also used to improve eye comfort in **keratoconjunctivitis** sicca. A brand name is Parvolex.

Acezide

A brand name for **hydrochlorothiazide** formulated with an **angiotensin converting enzyme inhibitor** drug.

achalasia

This is the failure of a muscle ring (sphincter) to relax when it should. Achalasia most commonly affects the sphincter at the bottom of the gullet (oesophagus). If this fails to relax during swallowing, the food cannot enter the stomach and, as a result, the oesophagus may become widely enlarged (dilated).

achlorhydria

Absence of the normal hydrochloric acid in the stomach as a result of wasting (atrophy) of the acid-secreting cells in the lining. This atrophy also leads to the absence of a factor needed for the absorption of vitamin B12, and the lack of this vitamin leads to **pernicious anaemia**. A test for achlorhydria is thus an important part of the investigation of this disease. Many people have achlorhydria without ill-effects.

achondroplasia

A defect in the growth of the cartilage at the growing sites at the end of long bones, which results in a characteristic form of dwarfism. The condition is caused by a dominant gene and 50 per cent of the offspring of an affected parent become achondroplastic dwarfs. Although the trunk and vault of the skull are of normal size, the legs and arms are very short and the face small. Most achondroplastics die in the first year, but those who survive have a good chance of a normal life span. Circus dwarfs and tumblers are usually achondroplastics. The genetic defect can be diagnosed before birth by **amniocentesis**.

achromatopsia

A severe defect of colour vision in which the world is perceived much as in a black and white television picture.

Achromycin

A brand name for **tetracycline**.

aciclovir

A drug highly active against the **herpes** simplex virus and against the closely similar varicella-zoster virus which causes chickenpox and shingles. Early treatment with the drug, taken by mouth, can greatly reduce the severity of shingles. A brand name is Zovirax.

acidosis

A serious condition in which the acidity of the blood rises. One of the commonest causes is poorly controlled **diabetes** with accumulation of acid products of abnormal sugar utilization (ketone bodies) in the blood. This can lead to coma and death. A similar condition may occur in starvation. Acidosis may also be caused by failure to eliminate carbon dioxide in lung disease, or by excess loss of alkali in **diarrhoea**. Blood acidity is normally kept within narrow limits by automatic feedback mechanisms, with acidosis occuring only during extreme or unusual circumstances.

acid reflux

The cause of the symptom of **heartburn**. The stomach is designed to tolerate strong acid, but the gullet (oesophagus) is not. So when acid regurgitates upwards into the oesophagus, there is a burning pain in the centre of the lower part of the chest. Reflux is especially common in pregnancy and obesity, because of the increased pressure in the abdomen.

-acious

Suffix meaning 'full of' as in pugnacious (full of fight).

acipimox

A drug used in the treatment of certain types of raised blood cholesterol. A brand name is Olbetam.

acitretin

A retinoid drug used by specialists in hospitals to treat severe and intractable **psoriasis**. A brand name is Neotigason.

acne

A common skin disease of adolescence and early adult life, featuring **blackheads** (comedones), **pustules** and scarring. Acne is often so severe and disfiguring as to cause great distress and misery to young people.

Acne is a disorder of the oil-secreting (sebaceous) glands of the skin in which there is excess production of their secretion (sebum) and obstruction of the outlets of the glands resulting in accumulation of sebum under the skin surface. Blackheads are not the cause of the obstruction; blackhead formation is believed to be a consequence of the sluggish flow of thickened sebum. The blackened tip is the result of oxidation of the sebum and has nothing to so with lack of cleanliness.

The secretions retained within the glands undergo chemical change to form irritating fatty acids, and the rupture of the swollen glands into the surrounding skin leads to inflammatory spots. Most acne spots are not infected, but some may become so, and pustules, or even boils, result. Pustular acne can lead to permanent scarring, but, given expert medical care, this need never happen.

Acne begins at puberty with the flare-up of hormone activity and reaches its peak in the late teens. It does, however, often persist into the twenties or even, occasionally, thirties. It mainly affects the face, shoulders, back of neck and upper trunk. Acne is not caused by eating sweets and rich, creamy, fatty foods, but these are best avoided for other reasons.

POSSIBLE CAUSES

The cause of the excess production of the sebaceous material that causes acne is still a matter of debate. The sebaceous glands are under the control of the sex hormones, the male hormone, testosterone, stimulating the glands and the female hormone, oestrogen, damping them down. Most acne sufferers do not have raised male sex hormone levels, but girls with severe acne often do.

In severe cases of acne, a doctor may prescribe the antibiotic tetracycline, to be taken by mouth, over a period of several months. This can work very well, but the drug should never be taken during pregnancy, as it will affect the baby. If these measures fail, the doctor will consider giving a female sex hormone drug, such as a high oestrogen contraceptive pill.

TREATMENT

Affected areas should be washed with ordinary soap and water, but not more often than twice a day. Blackheads should not be squeezed, as this causes the irritating material to be injected into the surrounding tissues. Courses of ultraviolet light, or sunbathing, are helpful. Antibiotic ointments are often prescribed and are useful in infected cases or to prevent infection. Many other preparations, such as ointments containing retinoic acid, benzoyl peroxide or sulphur, are recommended by dermatologists.

Tretinoin can cause fetal abnormalities if taken during pregnancy. Women using it must be on a reliable contraceptive.

Probably the most effective remedy of all is the drug tretinoin (Retin-A), a vitamin A derivative used externally as a cream or gel or, under specialist supervision, taken internally in the form of isotretinoin.

Acnecide

A brand name for benzoyl peroxide.

Acnidazil

A brand name for miconazole formulated for external use with benzoyl peroxide for the treatment of **acne**.

Acnisal

A brand name for **salicylic acid**.

acoustic trauma

See **noise, effects of**.

acrivastine

An **antihistamine** drug used in the treatment of allergies. A brand name is Semprex.

acrocyanosis

Blueness, coldness and sweating of the hands and feet in cold weather, due to spasm of small blood vessels.

See **Raynaud's disease**.

acromegaly

A serious disorder resulting from overproduction of growth hormone by the pituitary gland during adult life, usually as a result of a tumour. There is gradual enlargement of the jaw, tongue, nose, ribs, hands and feet.

Actilyse

A brand name for the **tissue plasminogen activator**, **alteplase**.

actinomycin D

An antibiotic which causes breaks in **DNA**. This side-effect renders it unsuitable as an antibacterial drug, but makes it useful as an anticancer drug. A brand name is Cosmegen Lyovac.

actinomycosis

A persistent disease caused by a bacterium whose colonies resemble those of a fungus. The organism responsible was, at one time, believed to be a fungus and was called *Actinomyces* – the golden 'sun-ray' fungus.

SYMPTOMS

The disease features multiple abscesses which discharge thin pus, containing the yellow granules of the fungus, through tracts (sinuses) leading to the surface of the skin. Actinomycosis may involve the mouth, neck, chest or abdomen and may be widespread and destructive.

TREATMENT

Fortunately, the bacterium is sensitive to penicillin and the disease usually responds to treatment if continued long enough. Surgery may also be necessary to drain deep abscesses.

Acular

A brand name for **ketorolac**.

Acupan

A brand name for nefopam.

acupressure

Acupressure is an offshoot of **acupuncture** in which finger pressure is used instead of needles. The commonest form is shiatsu, the Japanese version of the original Chinese treatment. The underlying philosophy is the same, but because the strong element of suggestion is missing, acupressure is likely to have less dramatic effects.

acupuncture

A branch of Chinese medicine based on the conception that the life force, Ch'i, flows through the body along fixed 'meridians' and that 'blockage' of one or more of these meridians causes illness. The 'unblocking' of the affected meridians, by inserting the needles and moving them with the fingers, is said to restore health. The same procedure is capable of causing anaesthesia.

HOW IT WORKS

In the most refined Chinese practice, diagnosis of the affected meridian is made by examination of the 'twelve

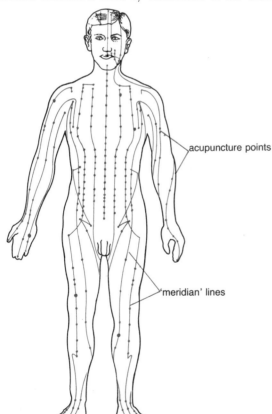

acupuncture points

'meridian' lines

The so-called 'meridians' along which energy is said to flow. The points at which needle insertion is said to 'unblock' the meridians are also shown.

pulses', six in each wrist, three deep and three superficial, each of which is said to inform about the health of an organ or part of the body. Each of the pulses is checked for twenty-seven different qualities. Often, an initial demonstration is given to show that the procedure is not especially painful. Nine different types of needle, each with a different purpose, are used and different disorders call for different angles and speed of insertion, whether the needle is twisted or pumped, and for how long it is left in place.

DOES IT WORK?

Anatomical studies do not show the meridians and it is clear that they do not exist in any normal physical form. Neither is there any discernible flow of energy, in the manner described. Moreover, Western medicine has failed to show the existence of more than one pulse at the wrist.

There is little evidence that, apart from the powerfully suggestive effect of the insertion of needles, acupuncture is of any real value in the treatment of disease. But that it has an effect as an anaesthetic is unquestionable and there is good evidence that pain pathways in the nervous system can be influenced by stimuli of the kind caused by acupuncture. The 'gate' theory of nerve impulse transmission suggests that there are nodes in the nerve pathways similar to electronic devices, such as transistors, in which a small controlling current can open or close the device to the passage of the main current flow. This effect, together with the effect of suggestion, probably accounts for the observed results.

RISKS

Acupuncture, especially in the hands of the medically unsophisticated, can be risky. Unless sterilization is scrupulous, infection of almost any kind, including **hepatitis B** and **AIDS**, may be transmitted. Sometimes a needle breaks in the tissues and becomes buried. Surgical removal may be difficult, occasionally requiring a large incision.

acute

Short, sharp and quickly over. Acute conditions usually start abruptly, last for a few days and then either settle or become persistent and longlasting (chronic). A sub-acute disorder lasts longer than an acute one but not so long as a chronic one.

-acy

Suffix meaning 'quality, state' as in celibacy (unmarried).

ad-

Prefix meaning 'to' as in adduction (drawing to).

Adalat

A brand name for **nifedipine**.

Adam's apple

The popular name for the voice box (larynx) at the upper end of the wind pipe (trachea). The larynx is larger and more protuberant in men than in women, which is why men have deeper voices.

adapalene

A drug used externally in the treatment of **acne**. A brand name is Differin.

adaptation

The adjustment of an organism, including man, in part or in whole, to changes in its environment or to external stress. Thus, the pupil of the eye adapts to darkness by enlarging and to brightness by constricting; the amount of oxygen-carrying haemoglobin in the blood increases at high altitudes where oxygen concentration is lower; bacteria adapt by natural selection to an environment containing antibiotics, so that such drugs become less effective; the muscles and their blood supply increase if persistently required to perform more work.

Adaptation is an essential feature of all living things and the likelihood of survival often depends on how effectively it operates.

Adcal-D3

A brand name for a calcium and vitamin D supplement used to treat **osteoporosis**.

Adcortyl

A brand name for **triamcinolone**.

Adcortyl in Orabase

A brand name for **triamcinolone** in an oral base formulation suitable for the treatment of mouth ulcers.

addiction

Dependence for comfort of mind or body on the repeated use of a drug such as nicotine, alcohol or heroin. In some cases, the addiction is physiological – that is, the use of the drug has led to persistent changes in the way the body functions, so that its absence causes physical symptoms (withdrawal symptoms). In others, the dependence is mental only.

A feature of addiction is the loss of control over the taking of the drug and the lengths to which the addict will go to obtain supplies. Activities such as theft or prostitution are common. People with money need not necessarily resort to such practices to maintain the habit, but would probably do so, if there were no other way.

See also **drug abuse, health maintenance**.

Addison's disease

A disorder of the adrenal glands leading to a deficient output of cortisol and aldosterone. There is weakness, tiredness and inability to cope with surgical stress.

POSSIBLE CAUSES
Addison's disease is almost always due to inflammatory damage followed by atrophy of the outer layer (cortex) of the adrenal gland. The inflammation is caused by abnormal action of the immune system in which it behaves towards the gland tissue as if this were foreign to the body. This is called auto-immune disease, and such people have antibodies to the cortex of the gland in their blood.

SYMPTOMS
The effect of adrenal cortex underaction is an inadequacy of cortisol, male sex hormone (androsterone) and the water- and salt-controlling hormone aldosterone. As a result, there is great weakness, fatigue, low blood pressure, excessive urinary output and dehydration. The pituitary gland tries to compensate by increased output of stimulating hormone and this results in the overproduction of another hormone which stimulates the pigment cells (melanocytes) in the skin. So people with Addison's disease get heavy discoloration of the skin.

TREATMENT
Treatment is by hormone replacement and this must be taken permanently. Sometimes an Addisonian crisis occurs and steroids are urgently required. In such circumstances, an injection of a steroid such as cortisone or prednisolone can save life.

adduct

To move towards the centre line of the body. Muscles that adduct are called adductors.

aden

Greek root meaning 'gland' as in adenitis (gland inflammation).

adenocarcinoma

A cancer arising from gland tissue in an epithelium (lining membrane) and usually showing the glandular features of the original tissue. Most cancers of the breast and colon (large intestine) are adenocarcinomas, and this kind of tumour can arise from many organs, including the womb (uterus), the pancreas, the kidneys, the thyroid and the salivary glands.

Adenocor

A brand name for **adenosine**.

adenoids

Gland-like tissue, present on the back wall of the nose, above the tonsils, in children, which shrivel and disappears in adolescence or early adult life.

FUNCTION
The adenoids contain white cells (lymphocytes) that are important in combating infection and are part of the body's defence system.

POTENTIAL PROBLEMS
As a result of repeated infection, the adenoids tend to enlarge and cause trouble by obstructing the airway through the nose, the drainage channels from the sinuses and the eustachian tubes from the middle ears. The result may be mouth breathing, snoring, a change in the quality of the voice, **sinusitis**, deafness and middle ear infection (**otitis media**).

TREATMENT
Enlarged adenoids are easily diagnosed and may readily be seen by the doctor. Whether or not they should be removed depends on the severity of the symptoms and the frequency with which recurrent infection and the secondary effects are interfering with schooling or the enjoyment of a normal life. Removal is often done at the time of **tonsillectomy**.

Removal of the adenoids (adenoidectomy) is performed under general anaesthesia. A sharp-edged instrument is passed through the mouth and up behind the soft palate into the cavity behind the nose so that the adenoids can be scraped off. There is usually little bleeding and the operation takes only a few minutes.

See also **hearing, defective**.

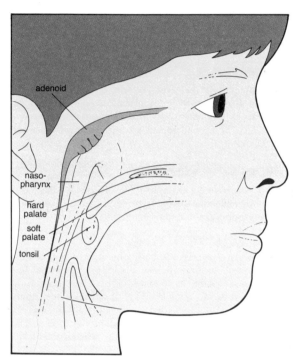

The adenoids lie high on the back wall of the naso-pharynx, above the tonsils.

adenoma

A benign (nonmalignant) tumour arising from lining tissue that contains glands. The glandular structure is retained in the tumour which may continue to secrete, and often over-produce, the original product. Commonly this is simply mucus, but adenomas from hormone-producing gland tissue may cause severe body disturbance by secreting abnormal quantities of such hormones as insulin, adrenaline or growth hormone (see **acromegaly**).

Adenomas do not spread to distant parts of the body as do malignant tumours, but, like all benign tumours, sometimes grow to a large size and may cause damage by local pressure. Occasionally they become malignant.

See also **adenocarcinoma**.

adenosine

A purine **nucleoside** consisting of one molecule of adenine and one molecule of d-ribose. It is formed in the body by the enzymatic breakdown of adenosine triphosphate (ATP). Adenosine is also a potent blocking agent for the atrioventricular node of the heart and is used by injection as a drug to correct irregularities in the action of the heart. A brand name is Adenocor.

adenosine deaminase inhibitors

Drugs that interfere with the action of the enzyme adenosine deaminase necessary for the irreversible conversion of adenosine to inosine. Failure to form inosine leads to abnormalities in purine nucleoside metabolism that are toxic to the cell concerned. This provides the opportunity to use adenosine deaminase inhibitors as anticancer drugs.

adenosis

Excessive growth of glands. The term is also used for any disease of glands.

adenovirus

One of a family of over thirty different viruses that cause colds, coughs or **gastro-enteritis**. Some of the adenoviruses (*Adenoviridae*) cause a highly infectious form of **conjunctivitis**, known as *epidemic keratoconjunctivitis* or 'shipyard conjunctivitis'. The virus commonly causes enlargement of lymph nodes and may persist in the tonsils, adenoids or other lymph tissue.

adhesion

Abnormal union between body surfaces. All body surfaces, external and internal, are covered with a 'non-stick' lining called epithelium, so that even if kept in contact for long periods, no union occurs. But if the epithelium is removed, either by disease or by surgical interference, and the bared surfaces are kept in contact, normal healing processes will ensure that adhesions form within a matter of days. Surgery on the bowels, or a penetrating injury, may, for instance, expose raw surfaces so that adhesions form between adjacent loops, to cause complications such as obstruction. Pleurisy (inflammation of the pleura – the covering of the lung) may damage the epithelium so that adhesions form between the lung pleuron and the pleuron lining the inside of the chest wall.

By their nature, adhesions are difficult to treat, since surgical removal may simply expose further raw areas and encourage recurrence.

Adie's pupil

An abnormality of the pupil of the eye affecting women. One pupil is larger than the other and does not show the normal brisk constriction on exposure to bright light or during near focusing. The condition is not of medical importance, and is no more than an interesting curiosity. But because enlarge-

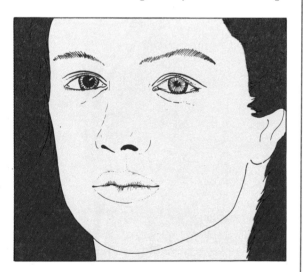

Adie's pupil. This girl's right pupil remains enlarged and the difference in pupil size is conspicuous in bright light.

ment of one pupil can be a sign of serious disorder of the nervous system, Adie's pupil often causes medical anxiety, and may prompt a full neurological investigation. Certain tests, using eyedrops, can be used to confirm the diagnosis.

Adipine MR

A brand name for **nifedipine**.

adipocere

A wax-like substance, consisting mainly of fatty acids, into which the soft tissues of a dead body, buried in moist earth, are converted. Adipocere delays the normal processes of decomposition so that the body is unnaturally preserved. It is sometimes of medico-legal importance.

adipose tissue

Human fat is liquid at body temperature and is contained in thin-walled cells, held together, in large masses, by delicate connective tissue. The whole is called adipose tissue and it forms a layer under the skin, largely responsible for the contouring and beauty of the female body. Adipose tissue acts both as an insulant and as a long-term fuel store, food in excess of requirements being converted to fat and deposited.

The characteristic shape of the woman's body is no accident. In evolutionary terms, a woman needs plenty of energy storage in the form of fat deposits in the hips and breasts so as to be able better to sustain pregnancy during which food may be harder to obtain. There is thus a good biological criterion for the 'classical' female form.

Adizem

A brand name for **diltiazem**.

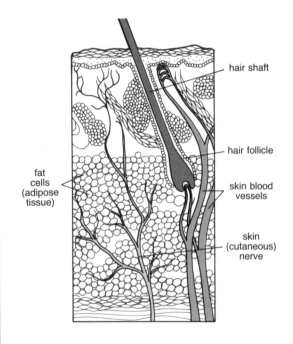

Cross-section of the skin showing the typical collection of subcutaneous fat cells (adipose tissue).

fat cells (adipose tissue)

hair shaft

hair follicle

skin blood vessels

skin (cutaneous) nerve

adjuvant

Any substance added to a drug to increase its effect.

adnexa

Adjoining parts of the body. The adnexa of the eyes are the lacrimal glands, which produce tears, the eyelids, and the lacrimal drainage system, which carries excess tears down into the nose. The uterine adnexa are the Fallopian tubes and the ovaries.

adrenal gland hyperplasia

This is an interesting example of the effects of feedback control in the **endocrine system**. Hyperplasia means enlargement of a tissue or organ due to an increase in the number of constituent cells.

POSSIBLE CAUSE

Adrenal gland hyperplasia occurs because of a genetically induced inability to synthesize certain of the normal hormones of the gland. The absence of these hormones in the blood informs the pituitary gland (feedback information) that greater output is needed and, to try to achieve this, the pituitary secretes abnormally high quantities of its adrenal cortex stimulating hormone (ACTH – adrenocorticotropic hormone). It is this overstimulation of the adrenals which causes the hyperplasia and the excessive production of those hormones which the gland *is* able to secrete – the male sex hormone and a kidney controlling hormone.

EFFECTS

These high levels cause premature masculinization (virilization) in the infant, and, in older people, hairiness, enlargement of the genitals, and serious loss of salt from the body, with low blood pressure and collapse.

adrenal glands

The adrenals are two small but important endocrine organs, sitting like triangular caps – one on top of each kidney. Each adrenal has two distinct parts, the inner core, which produces adrenaline, and an outer layer (cortex) which produces three kinds of steroid hormones – cortisol to help the body to react to stress, aldosterone to control water balance and sex hormones. Because all these hormones have such a powerful effect on the body, any disorder of the adrenals is serious.

Adrenaline is the secretion of the inner part of the adrenal glands and of certain nerve endings. It is produced when the body is required to make unusual efforts. It speeds up the heart, increases the rate and ease of breathing, raises the blood pressure, deflects the blood circulation from the digestive system to the muscles, mobilizes the fuel glucose and causes a sense of alertness and excitement. These changes allow more effective physical action, as may be needed in a situation of danger. It has been described as the hormone of 'fright, fight or flight'. One of the ways in which stress is thought to cause damage is by the over-frequent and inappropriate production of adrenaline and the resultant raising of the blood pressure with possible permanent damage to vital arteries. The natural corticosteroid hormones secreted by the cortex of the adrenal glands are cortisol, corticosterone, aldosterone and androsterone. Cortisol and corticosterone are called glucocorticoids because they are concerned with the body's usage of glucose and other nutrients. Aldosterone is called a mineralocorticoid because it is responsible for the control of blood levels of minerals such as sodium and potassium and, thereby, control of water balance. Androsterone is an androgen, a male sex hormone similar to testosterone produced in the testicles.

adrenal gland tumours

These tumours are rare but the effects can be dramatic. Tumours of the outer layer of an adrenal, whether malignant (carcinoma) or benign (adenoma), may cause an abnormally high output of adrenal cortex hormone which leads to sex changes in females – virilization, with hairiness, deep voice, upset of menstruation, enlargement of the clitoris and loss of sex drive (libido). They may also produce excess cortisol, causing muscle wasting and weakness, fat deposition in the face, trunk and lower part of the back of the neck, and abnormal elasticity of the skin with prominent stretch marks (striae). There is an increased tendency to diabetes and osteoporosis. This disorder is called **Cushing's syndrome**.

A tumour of the **adrenaline**-producing cells of the inner part of the adrenal (the medulla) can cause excess secretion of this powerful hormone. The effects are alarming, with exaggeration of all the normal responses to danger or fear. There is also a serious rise in the blood pressure.

adrenal gland underaction

See **Addison's disease**.

adrenaline

The secretion of the inner part of the adrenal glands and of certain nerve endings. Adrenaline is an important hormone which is produced when the body is required to make unusual efforts.

FUNCTION

It speeds up the heart, increases the rate and ease of breathing, raises the blood pressure, deflects the blood circulation from the digestive system to the muscles, mobilizes the fuel glucose and causes a sense of alertness and excitement. All these changes allow more effective physical action, as may be needed in a situation of danger. It has been described as the hormone of 'fright, fight or flight'.

Adrenaline is available for use as a drug. Its action in widening the bronchial tubes, and so freeing the movement of air into and out of the lungs, can be very useful in the treatment of severe asthma. But because its effects in the body are so widespread and powerful, it must be used with care.

POSSIBLE PROBLEMS

One of the ways in which stress is thought to cause damage is by the over-frequent and inappropriate production of adrenaline and the resultant raising of the blood pressure with possible permanent damage to vital arteries.

adrenaline (as a drug)

A powerful sympathomimetic drug used by injection in cases of **anaphylactic shock**. It is also used as eye drops to treat chronic simple **glaucoma**. Brand names are Epipen, Eppy and Simplene.

adrenaline cell membrane linkup site

See **beta-adrenoceptor**.

adrenaline-like drugs

See **adrenoreceptor agonists**, **sympathomimetic drugs**.

adrenergic

Having effects similar to that of adrenaline. Drugs with adrenaline-like action are called adrenergic. A nerve which releases noradrenaline (a substance closely related to adrenaline) at its endings to pass on its impulses to other nerves, or to muscle fibres, is described as an adrenergic nerve.

adrenergic-blocking drugs

Alpha-adrenergic receptors are in the muscle walls of arteries. Stimulation of these cause the arteries to narrow. Blockage will cause the arteries to widen. Beta1 (ß1) adrenergic receptors are in the heart. Stimulation causes an increase in heart rate and force. Beta2 (ß2) adrenergic receptors are in the muscles of the bronchi and of the arteries, in both of which stimulation causes relaxation. Blocking drugs that block both ß1 and ß2 slow the heart and cause constriction of the air passages and the arteries. This can be dangerous to asthmatics. Some beta-blockers are relatively selective for the heart and are less likely to constrict the air passages.

See also **alpha-adrenoceptor blocking drugs**.

adrenolytic drug therapy

The use of a drug to reduce hormonal output from the adrenal glands, in particular the 11-beta-hydroxylase inhibitor, metyrapone, to cut cortisol production in Cushing's syndrome.

adrenoreceptor agonists

An agonist is something that causes an action, usually an action similar to that of a natural body substance. Adrenoreceptor agonists are drugs with the same action as adrenaline – the natural body 'fright, fight or flight' hormone. These drugs are often very useful and can, occasionally, be life-saving. They have several effects. They can:

- widen air tubes (bronchi) tightly narrowed in asthma;
- control severe allergic reactions;
- reverse certain cases of acute heart failure;
- prevent premature labour;
- control certain kinds of glaucoma (excess internal eye pressure);
- narrow skin blood vessels to prolong the action of local anaesthetics.

Air tube widening drugs include salbutamol (Ventolin) and salmeterol (Serevent). Adrenaline itself is used in dangerous allergic reactions and to prolong the effect of local anaesthetic injections. Adrenaline drops (Eppy) are used in treating chronic simple glaucoma – the common type mainly affecting elderly, people. Heart failure may be treated with dobutamine (Dobutrex), and premature labour with salbutamol or ritodrine.

The side-effects are those that might be expected from adrenaline – jumpiness, shakiness, tremor, restlessness, anxiety, a fast pulse, a rise in blood pressure, even attacks of angina. Such effects are very rare when these drugs are used by inhalation or in eye drops or local anaesthetics.

adrenoreceptor blockers

See **adrenergic-blocking drugs**.

advancement

The surgical detachment of one end of a muscle or tendon, and its reattachment at a position in front of its normal site, so as to alter or strengthen its action. Advancement of one of the small eye-moving muscles is commonly done in the surgical correction of squint (**strabismus**). When the muscle end is moved backwards, this is called recession.

Aerobec

A brand name for **beclomethasone**.

aerobic exercises

See **health maintenance**.

Aerolin Autohaler

A brand name for a preparation of **salbutamol**.

aerophagy

The medical term for air swallowing. This is common in people with indigestion (**dyspepsia**) whose efforts to bring up wind often result in the swallowing of sufficient air to produce an eventual and satisfactory belch. The process is a common response to stress and can be cured if the mechanism is understood by the affected person. Aerophagy also accompanies the rapid gobbling of food and some of this air may be passed along the bowel to increase the normal amount of flatulence.

See also **belching**.

aerosol

A suspension of very small droplets of a liquid or particles of a solid, in air. Aerosols may be produced by causing a pressurized gas to blow across the nozzle of a tube dipping into the solution to be dispersed. Alternatively, the gas itself may be pressurized to form a liquid in which the material to be sprayed is dissolved. A range of drugs can be given in aerosol form for inhalation. Many sufferers from **asthma** rely heavily on inhalers or aerosol dispensers.

Chlorofluoromethane gases released from aerosol dispensers are believed to offer a threat to the environment by releasing chlorine that acts as a catalyst to break down the protective ozone layer in the stratosphere. It has been suggested that this effect is leading to an increase in the number of cases of skin cancer such as **malignant melanoma**, **rodent ulcer** and **squamous cell carcinoma**.

aetiology

The cause of a disease. This may involve many factors, including:

● the infective organisms;
● the susceptibility of the patient to the disease from hereditary tendency or genetic cause;
● environmental factors;
● previous related illness;
● unhealthy lifestyle;
● exposure to infective agents, and so on.

afebrile

Having a normal temperature. The term is usually applied to a patient who has been fevered, or who might be expected to be fevered.

affect

A mood or emotion. The word is often used to describe the external signs of emotion, as perceived by another person. Normal affect varies from person to person and with the factors inducing it, but will always be appropriate. An abnormal affect – either flat or excessive – may be a sign of a mental disorder.

Affective disorders are mental illnesses characterized by abnormal emotional responses. They include the very common **depression**, various rare states of excitement or euphoria (**mania**) and **manic-depressive illness** in which the mood swings between the two. Affective disorders may involve loss of contact with reality (psychotic illness) or may be neurotic (see **neurosis**) and, especially in the case of the latter, often arise in direct response to disastrous life events such as bereavement, divorce or serious injury. In some cases, organic illness may precipitate, or even cause, an affective disorder.

Recovery from affective disorders is usual within a matter of months without damage to personality or intellect, but there is a strong tendency for recurrence over the years. Treatment by drugs, behavioural therapy, and sometimes ECT (electroconvulsive therapy) is usually effective.

aflatoxin

A poison produced by the fungus *Aspergillus flavus* which grows on peanuts and grains stored in damp conditions. Aflatoxin has been proved to cause cancer in animals and is thought to be the reason for the high incidence of primary liver cancer in certain areas of the world where the fungus is a common contaminant and where hepatitis B is also common. Primary liver cancer is almost unknown in other areas, such as Europe.

Aflatoxin has also been shown to have immunosuppressive properties and some authorities have pointed out that the regular exposure of many children in parts of Africa to aflatoxins may contribute to the prevalence and virulence of the AIDS virus, HIV, among them.

Illegal heroin seized by the police has been analysed for aflatoxins. Three out of eleven samples were found to be heavily contaminated. This may help to explain the surprisingly high incidence of AIDS among intravenous drug users. The principal cause is, of course, blood infection from shared needles.

after-image

A visual impression of a bright object or light, which persists for a few seconds after the gaze is shifted or the eyes closed. A negative, or reversed after-image is common, as is one in which colours, complementary to those of the object, are seen. These are normal phenomena, due to transient photochemical changes in the retinas. The actual persistence of a fully formed image of what is seen, for a brief period after a shift of gaze, is an entirely different matter. This is called *perseveration* and may be a sign of disease of the brain.

agammaglobulinaemia

Complete absence of the normal blood gamma globulin proteins. Because the gamma globulins are immunoglobulins (antibodies) their absence leads to a dangerous susceptibility to infection – immune deficiency.

RECOGNITION AND SYMPTOMS

Agammaglobulinaemia may be present at birth (congenital) and result from a sex-linked genetic abnormality, or it may be acquired later in life, usually in the twenties or thirties. The condition features recurrent infections of the respiratory and digestive systems, the skin, the bones and other areas.

TREATMENT

Agammaglobulinaemia is treated with life-long human immune serum globulin injections. Antibiotics are frequently required.

agar

A seaweed extract, sometimes called agar-agar, much used in bacteriological laboratories because it forms a convenient gel for the suspension of culture material, such as blood or broth. It can be sterilized and melted by heat, mixed with ingredi-

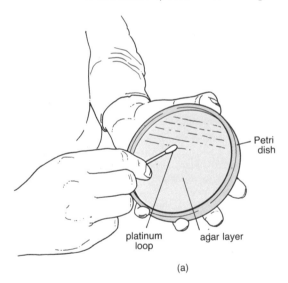

Petri dish

platinum loop

agar layer

(a)

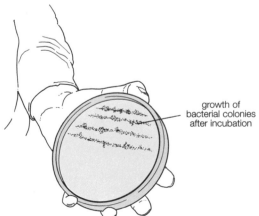

growth of bacterial colonies after incubation

ents selected to encourage growth of particular organisms, and poured into shallow glass or plastic culture plates called Petri dishes. On cooling, it solidifies and can be seeded with sample material and incubated at body temperature until satisfactory colonies grow. Agar is also sometimes use as a mild treatment for **constipation**.

ageing

The natural human life-span appears to be about 110 years and there is no evidence that this is increasing. What is happening, however, is that, with advances in medical science, more and more people are reaching the natural age limit. The bodily and mental changes associated with ageing show, in general, a phase of improvement and increasing power up to the mid-twenties and then a gradual decline. But these are broad generalizations and, in many people, both physical and mental capacity continue to increase until the end of the third decade or later.

POSSIBLE CAUSES

The causes of the physical changes associated with age – loss of muscle power, decreased efficiency of the nervous system, loss of skin elasticity, brittleness of the bones, hardening and narrowing of the arteries, and so on, are only partly understood, but what is known can be usefully applied to delay many of the obvious signs of age. Many factors, including unsuitable diet, lack of exercise of body and mind, lack of interest, smoking, use of drugs, excess alcohol and undue exposure to sunlight, are known to accelerate the process.

The latter part of life is usually associated with a progressive reduction in general capacity, but to a large extent this merely reflects cultural expectations. Surprise is commonly expressed at the achievement of the aged, but such achievement should be the norm rather than the exception. In general, the body and the mind will deliver the work output required of them, adapting, both in strength and skill, to meet the demand. It is certain that no person ever achieves his or her full potential of achievement, and the stereotype of the aged person has been that of one on whom such demands should no longer be made. Regrettably, retirement is often equated with idleness.

The problem is to provide the necessary motivation to achieve the work level needed to ensure that the body and the mind reach and maintain the optimum level of efficiency characterized as youthfulness. To the extent that this is achieved, ageing is retarded. Happily, social attitudes are changing and the central importance of work, throughout life, is gradually being understood. There is a laudable movement to recognize the work contribution that older people can make and the advantages of abandoning the concept of a statutory retirement age.

Agar is a very suitable vehicle for culture media for the growth of bacteria in an incubator. The first illustration shows the agar being inoculated with material picked up on a sterile platinum loop. The second shows many small bacterial colonies that have grown in the previous twenty-four hours in the incubator.

ageing, extreme in childhood

See **progeria**.

ageing, premature

See **Werner's syndrome**.

agenesis

Absence of an organ or part as a result of failure of development in the early stages. The drug thalidomide caused agenesis of the limbs.

agglutination

The clumping and sticking together of normally free cells or bacteria or other small particles so as to form visible aggregates. Agglutination is one of the ways in which antibodies operate. Blood serum contains antibodies that cause the red cells of a different blood group to agglutinate. This fact is used in the essential blood-grouping and cross-matching tests used before transfusion.

Agglutination is also valuable as a way of identifying bacteria, using different sera containing antibodies to known micro-organisms.

aggression

Aggression comprises feelings or acts of hostility.
POSSIBLE CAUSES
Abnormal aggression is often associated with an emotionally deprived childhood, with lack of parental affection and lack of educational and social opportunities. It may thus often be a natural manifestation of frustration and a sense of grievance and deprivation. In such people there are indications that, for want of any more mature or knowledgeable response, the tendency is to react to problems aggressively rather than constructively. In these, the threshold for aggression is low and a minor stimulus may provoke a serious outbreak. In some people, aggression appears to be part of the creative urge.

Head injury, or brain disease, such as tumour, may result in aggressive behaviour as may excessive alcohol or the use of drugs such as amphetamines. Heroin does not cause aggression, but this is common during withdrawal. Demented people often show aggression, especially when required to perform tasks beyond their mental ability, and people with **epilepsy** may show aggressive behaviour, either as a substitute for a fit, or in the confusional state after a major attack.
TREATMENT
Treatment of an aggressive tendency is as difficult as that of any other fundamental personality disorder, and is seldom entirely effective. Counselling and behaviour therapy have been tried with limited success. Happily, aggression usually becomes less common and less severe with increasing age.

See also **psychopath**.

agitation

A state of mind, usually due to anxiety or tension, which causes obvious restlessness.
RECOGNITION
The agitated person is unable to keep still and may pace up and down, wringing the hands, starting activities but not completing them, and generally indicating that the disturbed state of the mind prevents relaxation or concentration on other matters.
POSSIBLE CAUSES
Agitation, in response to a real external threat or cause of major concern, is normal, but persistent and inappropriate agitation suggests an **anxiety** disorder. Depressive illness (see **depression**) in older people often features severe agitation, and this may be misleading.

Often, too, there is an underlying physical cause such as alcohol withdrawal. Certain drugs, such as the amphetamines, the phenothiazine derivatives and some of the antidepressant drugs, may also cause agitation.

agnosia

A disorder of the *association* areas of the brain, in which the person cannot correctly interpret sense input. A person with tactile agnosia, if asked to close the eyes and handle a common object such as a dinner fork, will be unable to identify it. A person with auditory agnosia can hear but cannot perceive the sense of words uttered. In visual agnosia, vision may be normal but words read may be meaningless.

Agnosia commonly follows **stroke**, adding to the burden of disablement.

-agogue

Suffix meaning 'cause to flow' as in cholagogue (bile-flowing).

agonal

Relating to the event occurring in the last moments of life, such as the cessation of breathing or the heartbeat.

agonist

A molecule, such as a hormone, **neuro-transmitter** or drug, that attaches (binds) to a cell receptor site to produce an effect on the cell. Many drugs are agonists having an effect similar or identical to natural body agonists. Other drugs act on the receptor in a blocking role and are antagonists. An antagonist is a molecule that interferes with or prevents the action of the agonist.

agoraphobia

An abnormal fear of open spaces or of being alone or in public places.
RECOGNITION AND SYMPTOMS
Agoraphobia may be so severe that the sufferer refuses to leave his or her own home and becomes permanently housebound. It is the commonest of the phobias and is almost always associated with irrational severe anxiety that something will happen for which help will not be available. Thus it commonly occurs in connection with crowds, public transport, bridges or tunnels, and often overlaps with **claustrophobia** (fear of enclosed spaces) or social phobias such as the fear of eating in public, public speaking, or any activity that might be a cause of embarrassment or humiliation. Such fear often induces acute panic attacks.
TREATMENT
Treatment, by behaviour counselling, relaxation therapy and **desensitization**, sometimes supplemented by the use of anti-adrenaline beta-blockers, is usually successful.

agranulocytosis

A condition in which the white cells of the blood are not being produced in adequate quantity by the bone marrow. This is most commonly caused as a toxic side-effect on the bone marrow of various drugs such as the sulphonamides, the thiouracil derivatives, penicillin, chlorpromazine, chlorpropamide, phenindione, Amidopyrine and chlorothiazide. Because of the deficiency or absence of protective white cells, there is severe sore throat, fever, toxaemia and sometimes septicaemia. The condition may be fatal.

agraphia

Acquired inability to exercise the mental processes necessary for writing. There is no disorder of hand or eye function or coordination. Agraphia results from damage in the part of the brain concerned with language, usually on the left side.

ague

A burning fever with hot and cold spells and severe shivering or **rigor** when the temperature is rising, as is experienced in **malaria**.

AID

See **artificial insemination**.

AIDS

The acquired immune deficiency syndrome (AIDS) was first recognized in 1981 in groups of homosexual men in Los Angeles and New York. It was, however, at that time, present in at least four other continents. Since then AIDS has proved to be the major pandemic of the 20th and 21st centuries having been contracted by 880,000 people in Europe, 920,000 on North America, 360,00 in the Caribbean, 1.3 million in Latin America, 23.3 million in sub-Saharan Africa, 530,000 in East Asia and the Pacific and 6 million in South and South-east Asia. United Nations estimates are that, world-wide, 2.6 million people died from AIDS and AIDS-related disases in 1999. This was a larger annual total than in any year since the pandemic began. It was also estimated that during 1999, 5.6 million people became infected with AIDS. By the end of that year 32.4 millions adults and 1.2 million children were living with AIDS.

In 1999, for the first time, the number of infections acquired by heterosexual intercourse exceeded the number acquired by homosexual intercourse. At the same time, all the indications are that sexual promiscuity is being engaged in by more young people than ever before. This is being encouraged by the media, especially by television, which is actively and cynically promoting promiscuous sexual activity, both hetero- and homo-sexual, by representing it to be an acceptable and desirable norm.

AIDS is caused by the human immunodeficiency virus (HIV), which is transmitted in body fluids during sex, in blood when needles used for drug abuse are shared, and during pregnancy or delivery from mother to baby. There are also less severe but real dangers of transmission during tattooing and body piercing performed by irresponsible and ignorant practitioners of these arts. The world pandemic of AIDS is largely caused by a strain known as HIV-1, but there is a second strain, HIV-11, which is largely confined to West Africa.

The AIDS virus attacks the class of T cells (T lymphocytes) of the immune system known as the helper T cells. A severe drop in the number of these cells so interferes with the body's defence against infections that some common and relatively harmless infections become life-threatening, and other infections that are almost unknown in people with normal immune systems become florid and dangerous. In addition, because the normal surveillance exercised by the immune system over cancer development is lost, several cancers, some otherwise rare, may occur.

Some of these effects are so characteristic of AIDS that they can allow a strong presumptive diagnosis to be made even without HIV testing. These include:

- thrush (**candidiasis**) extending into the gullet and the lungs;
- herpes simplex infections likewise affecting the interior of the body (see **herpes simplex in AIDS**);
- a form of pneumonia called *Pneumocystis carinii* **pneumonia** that is almost unknown outside AIDS;
- **lymphoma** of the brain in people under 60;
- **Kaposi's sarcoma**;
- widespread **toxoplasmosis** in the brain;
- **cytomegalovirus infection**;
- **cryptococcosus infection**;
- various forms of **tuberculosis**;
- invasive cancer of the cervix;
- recurrent bacterial **pneumonia**.

There are other manifestations of the extreme immune deficiency of AIDS but these are the most important. AIDS is not the only acquired immune deficiency syndrome – immune deficiency can be acquired as a result of medical treatment to prevent graft rejection or following prolonged intensive antibiotic treatment. But these forms of immune deficiency will usually resolve when the cause is removed and their effects are much less severe than fully-developed AIDS.

The course of AIDS is characteristic. The disease has a long incubation period but about 60 per cent of people who acquire an HIV infection, and who remain untreated, will develop signs of the fully-established, invariably fatal, end-stage disease within 10 years. During that period four stages can usually be distinguished. In stage 1 there may be no signs at all or nothing more than persistently enlarged lymph nodes. Stage 2 features some loss of weight and recurrent herpes and respiratory infections, but normal life is possible. In stage 3 weight loss is more than 10 per cent, there is recurrent diarrhoea and thrush in the mouth, and there may be tuberculosis. People in this stage will be, typically, bed-ridden for an average of less than half of each day. Stage 4 is the end-stage in which any of the manifestations of the full clinical syndrome may be present.

Serial testing of the numbers of helper T cells shows that there is a close correlation between the drop in the numbers and the progression through the four stages. HIV infection is diagnosed by determining the presence of specific antibodies produced by the immune system to the protein envelope of the virus. These antibodies can be detected by a test such as the **ELISA test** within three months of infection. Antibodies to the envelope persist indefinitely. Skilled counselling is necessary both before testing and after obtaining a positive result. This is available.

Treatment of AIDS is two-fold – the treatment of the infections and cancers caused by the immune deficiency, and the specific anti-viral treatment directed against HIV. For the first, normal antibiotic, antiviral and anti-protozoal treatment is generally effective. The drug pentamidine is effective in treating *P. carinii* pneumonia. Unfortunately, all the infections and cancers encouraged by immune deficiency are liable to recur after treatment, so the second line of treatment is particularly important, as it can allow a rise in the numbers of helper T-cells and consequently an increase in the immune capacity.

Recent years have seen some remarkable advances in anti-HIV treatment, the most important development being the use of combinations of drugs that attack the virus in different ways. Anti-HIV drugs act by blocking the enzymes the virus needs for its replication. This has become much more successful since 1996 when a new class of drugs, the protease **inhibitors**, was introduced. These, used in combination with drugs from the other groups – the **reverse transcriptase inhibitors** and the **DNA polymerase inhibitors** – has revolutionized treatment, and when these are properly used the results are markedly better than with any drug used alone.

A considerable range of drugs is now used for the attack on HIV-1. In Britain, currently available nucleoside reverse transcriptase inhibitors are abacavir (Ziagen), didanosine (Videx), lamivudine (Combivir, Epivir), stavudine (Zerit), zalcitabine (Hivid) and zidovudine (Retrovir). Non-nucleoside reverse transcriptase inhibitors are nevirapine (Viramune) and efavirens (Sustiva). Protease inhibitors are indinavid (Crixivan), nelfinavir (Viracept), ritonavir (Norvir) and saquinavir (Fortovase, Invirase). DNA polymerase inhibitors are foscarnet (Foscavir), ganciclovir (Cymevene) and cidofovir (Vistide). The latter group is used to treat cytomegalovirus infections in AIDS.

Effective treatment should reduce the HIV load to one-tenth in 8 to 12 weeks.

In spite of all the advances in treatment AIDS is still a terrible disease and the consequences of acquiring an HIV infection are devastating. This is one situation in which the aphorism 'prevention is better than cure' really applies. Sexual promiscuity appears to be here to stay, but people who know the facts about AIDS and who continue to behave in this way are taking chances with their lives that many of them will regret. Sexual fidelity and belief in long-term monogamous relationships are not old-fashioned concepts; they are the way most likely to achieve happiness. And they are certainly the best way to avoid AIDS.

The probability of contracting AIDS is directly proportional to the number of a person's sexual partners. Heterosexual spread is now the commonest source in Britain. The spread of AIDS in the gay communities of New York and San Francisco was a consequence of the frantic promiscuity which was a feature of their lifestyle. Homosexual men have recognized a special duty to limit the spread of the virus and there can be few, now, who are not aware of it. The more responsible members of the London gay community have shown a readiness to acknowledge this responsibility. The Terence Higgins Trust, which is a registered charity established to inform, advise and help on AIDS, have published excellent booklets of advice on the matter and have a 'helpline', open for counselling.

Safe sex practices include:
- the avoidance of promiscuity;
- wearing a condom for all penetrative sex;
- being aware of the risks;
- avoidance of anal sex;
- avoidance of any sex act which draws blood.

The use of enemas or douches before or after anal sex, is a high-risk activity.

Medium-risk activities for homosexual men include:
- wet kissing;
- penile body contact between the thighs or buttocks;
- insertion of fingers into the anus, or of the hand into the rectum (fisting);
- the use of douches or enemas;
- oral sex – especially when prolonged to orgasm;
- sexual urination ('water sports' or 'golden showers');
- the use of shared dildos, vibrators and butt plugs.

Sexual expression should be restricted to such low-risk activities as dry kissing; general body to body contact; mutual or group masturbation; non-violent bondage, whipping or spanking, so long as the skin is not broken; the exclusive use of dildos, vibrators, enemas and douches.

Condoms, formerly a joke among gay people, have become a serious proposition as it is clear that, if intelligently used, they offer considerable protection. Like the protection against sexually transmitted disease generally, this works both ways, and offers an improvement in safety to both partners. Condom dispensing machines are ubiquitous in gay bars and restaurants.

Intravenous narcotic drug users must understand the risks of sharing needles. Unfortunately, many heroin addicts give little weight to the risks when their only preoccupation is to get a 'fix'. Derogatory attitudes are understandable but unhelpful. AIDS, generally, has attracted enough derogatory attitudes, and while many members of the public indulge their disapproval, young men and women are suffering and dying horribly. Moralistic stances may make some people feel better, but what many of the heroin addicts need is help, not condemnation. The provision of clean needles so that needles need never be shared is at least a step in the right direction. The cost is trifling compared to the medical cost of coping with AIDS, and the suggestion that to provide needles is to encourage drug abuse is naive.

People infected with HIV have to think of their blood as being potentially hazardous to others, and of their other body fluids as also being dangerous, although to a lesser degree. Any blood accidentally spilled has to be regarded as a hazard. A shaving cut, an accidental cut on the finger, a bruise with slight blood oozing, pus from a discharging boil or pimple, vomit, saliva, urine, must all be treated as possibly dangerous to others and managed accordingly. Spilt blood or other fluids should be cleaned up with a cloth soaked in household bleach, freshly diluted to one part bleach in ten parts of water.

The risks are not as great as some have suggested and we now know that only about one in 200 cases in which there is accidental skin puncture with needles contaminated with HIV positive blood results in infection. Blood contact with intact skin is very unlikely to lead to infection. Nevertheless, HIV positive people must inform doctors and dentists who are dealing with them that they are HIV positive, for the taking of blood for medical purposes or the accidental injury of a blood vessel in the course of dental treatment does involve risk to the medical or dental attendant.

See also **candidiasis, cryptococcus infection in AIDS, herpes simplex in AIDS, Kaposi's sarcoma, lymphoma in AIDS, myobacterium avium-intracellulare infection in AIDS,** *Pneumocystis carinii* **pneumonia,** and *Toxoplasma gondii* **infection in AIDS.**

AIH

See **artificial insemination.**

air embolism

Bubbles of air in the circulating blood, which cause blockage of small arteries, thereby cutting off supply to important areas, such as parts of the brain. Free air in the bloodstream is always dangerous and care is taken to ensure that no air is introduced during an intravenous injection.

INCIDENCE

Air embolism is rare. It sometimes occurs in divers who have taken in high pressure air at depth and who then surface without allowing the expanding air to escape freely. This happens if divers run out of air and hold the breath while coming to the surface. The expanding air over-inflates the lungs and air enters the veins carrying blood back to the heart, from whence it is pumped to the brain and elsewhere. The result is immediate loss of consciousness and often convulsions.

TREATMENT

The only effective treatment is immediate recompression in a suitable chamber.

See also **bends.**

air sickness

See **motion sickness.**

airway

The passages from the nose and mouth down to the air sacs in the lungs, by way of which air enters and leaves the body. A clear airway is literally vital and to ensure it is the first requirement in every case of injury or unconsciousness, from any cause. One can live for weeks without food, for days without water, but only for minutes without air.

The airway may be obstructed by the tongue falling back to block the nasopharynx; by food or other material in the nasopharynx; or, more commonly, at the level of the larynx by material or swelling. Obstruction of the trachea is less common.

> In an accident or emergency, even severe bleeding is secondary in importance to ensuring that the injured person can, and will continue to be able to, breathe freely. A face-down, head to the side, position will prevent airway obstruction from the tongue or vomit in an unconscious person, but if necessary, the tongue must be pulled forward, and blood, tissue flaps, foreign material, or any other cause of airway obstruction cleared with the fingers. See also *First Aid.*

akinesia

Loss of movement.

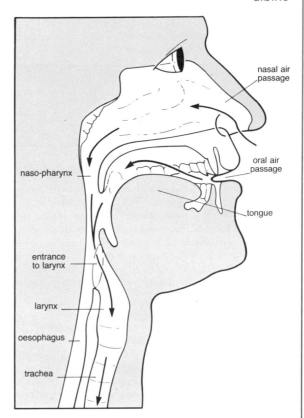

The vital airway is very narrow and may easily be blocked, especially beyond the point at which the nasal and oral air passages join.

Aknemin

A brand name for **minocycline.**

-al

Suffix meaning 'of, like' as in lateral (of the side).

ala

Latin root meaning 'wing' as in alar (wing-shaped).

albendazole

A drug used to get rid of roundworms, hookworms and other worm parasites and to treat **hydatid disease.** A brand name is Eskazole.

albino

A person with a genetic defect causing absence of the normal body pigment, melanin, which gives colour to the hair, eyes and skin. The genes responsible are recessive (see **genetics**) so can be carried by people with normal colouring. For the same reason, two albino parents need not necessarily have albino children, and the parents of albino children often have normal colouring.

POSSIBLE CAUSES

Melanin is formed from the amino acid tyrosine. If the gene pair for this is defective the person concerned will be a tyrosine-negative albino with snow-white hair, pink skin, pink eyes and severely defective vision with jerky eye movements (nystagmus). Tyrosine-positive albinos can produce some melanin pigment and the condition is much less severe.

Almost all albinos have some problems in bright light, and even mild albinos may have nystagmus, slight to moderate reduction in visual acuity, and often short sight (myopia). Unless protected from excessive sunlight, albinos may be more susceptible to various forms of skin cancer.

albumin

An important protein, soluble in water, synthesized in the liver and always present in the blood plasma. Albumin concentrates the blood and attracts water, thereby maintaining the volume. It binds, retains and transports, calcium, certain hormones and some drugs, preventing them from being lost via the kidneys. Liver disease, such as cirrhosis, can result in failure of albumin production, with serious consequences. Albumin coagulates on heating and turns white, as can be seen when eggs are boiled.

albuminuria

Albumin in the urine. Because albumin is so important to the body, it must be conserved and healthy kidneys do not allow it to pass into the urine. Albumin in the urine is thus an important finding, usually indicating kidney disease such as **glomerulonephritis** or the **nephrotic syndrome**. There are, however, exceptions. Some people have *orthostatic albuminuria*, in which some albumin is present in the urine only after they have been standing for a long time and is absent from a sample taken before rising in the morning. This is not considered dangerous. Albuminuria may also be found, in normal people, after very strenuous exercise.

Albustix

A brand name for a urine dip strip test for albumin.

alclometasone

A moderately strong corticosteroid drug used externally in the treatment of inflammatory skin disorders. A brand name is Modrasone.

alcohol abuse

See **health maintenance**.

alcohol addiction

See **health maintenance**.

Aldactide 50

A brand name for **hydroflumethiazide**.

Aldactone

A brand name for **spironolactone**.

aldesleukin

An **interleukin** 2 drug made by genetic engineering. A brand name is Proleukin.

Aldomet

A brand name for **methyldopa**.

aldosterone

One of the steroid hormones produced by the outer part (cortex) of the adrenal gland. The hormone's function is to control salt loss in the urine. In the absence of this hormone, a person might lose 35g of salt a day, with the water to dissolve it, and could die of low blood pressure from the resulting reduction in blood volume.

Alec

A brand name for **pumactant**.

alendronate

A drug used in the prevention and treatment of post-menopausal **osteoporosis**. A brand name is Fosamax.

aleukaemic leukaemia

A kind of cancer of the blood, in which the white blood cells are produced in greatly excessive numbers, but do not appear in the circulation. In this respect it differs from other **leukaemias**.

alexia

Inability to read, occurring as a result of brain damage, usually from arterial disease. Alexia is common after **stroke** affecting the left side of the brain. In some cases there is simple word blindness with normal ability to write and speak, but in others both reading and writing, and often speech, are affected.

alfacalcidol

A synthetic form of vitamin D used to treat low blood calcium and bone softening (osteomalacia) caused by kidney disease. Brand names are Alfa D and One-alpha.

AlfaD

A brand name for **alfacalcidol**.

alfentanil

A narcotic-type pain-killing drug. A brand name is Rapifen.

alfuzosin

An alpha-blocker drug used in the treatment of prostate enlargement. A brand name is Xatral.

-algia

Suffix meaning 'pain' as in myalgia (muscle pain).

Algicon

A brand name for a preparation containing **magnesium alginate**.

algid

Cold, clammy, referring to skin.

alginic acid

An **antacid** drug used in the treatment of stomach ulcer and indigestion. When supplied in combination with other drugs brand names are Algitec, Gastrocote, Gaviscon, Pyrogastrone and Topal.

algos

Greek root meaning 'pain' as in arthralgia (joint pain).

alienation

A feeling that one is separated from others or from one's 'real' self, that one's thoughts and emotions are under the control of someone else or that others have access to one's mind. It is one of the symptoms of **schizophrenia**.

alkaloids

A group of plant poisons of medical importance. The alkaloids, which include morphine, codeine, atropine (belladonna) and quinine, have powerful actions on the body.

alkalosis

An abnormal degree of alkalinity of the blood, sometimes due to excessive intake of alkaline substances such as bicarbonate of soda, but more usually due to loss of acid by prolonged vomiting or to hysterical overbreathing (hyperventilation) with abnormal loss of carbon dioxide. Alkalosis may produce muscle weakness or cramps and may even induce **tetany** with twitching and characteristic spasm of the fingers and toes.

alkaptonuria

A genetic disorder with absence of an **enzyme** needed for the normal chemical breakdown of the two **amino acids** tyrosine and phenylalanine. Because of the absence of the enzyme homogentisic acid oxidase, the process stops at the stage of homogentisic acid which accumulates to an abnormal degree causing brown discoloration of the skin and whites of the eyes and progressive damage to joints. An obvious sign is the darkening of the urine almost to blackness on standing as changes occur in the excreted homogentisic acid.

Alkeran

A brand name for **melphalan**.

alkylating agents

Drugs which interfere with **DNA** synthesis by adding an alkyl group and preventing the uncoiling of the strands. This halts DNA replication so that cells cannot reproduce, an effect useful in the treatment of cancer. Drugs in this group include nitrogen mustard, chlorambucil, **cyclophosphamide**, **busulphan** and thiotepa.

Allegron

A brand name for **nortriptyline**.

allele

Chromosomes come in near-identical pairs, both having correspondingly located sites for their genes (lengths of **DNA**). An allele, or allelomorph, is one of a pair of genes that occupy the corresponding positions on the associated (homologous) chromosomes. Each gene has two, normally identical, alleles, one on each chromosome of a pair, but it is common for one of the alleles to differ in its DNA sequence from the normal or from its normal fellow on the other chromosome. This alteration in DNA is called a mutation, and the term allele is also used for one of the ways in which a gene, at a particular location on a chromosome, may differ from its fellow. In this sense, a gene may have a dozen or more alleles, allowing many different mutations to occur.

If the corresponding chromosome sites are occupied by different alleles of a gene, the individual is said to be heterozygous for the gene. If the two alleles are both normal or are abnormal in the same way, the individual is homozygous for the error and the characteristic determined by the gene or the gene defect will be present, even if the genes are recessive (see **genetics**). Heterozygous individuals will show the features of the dominant gene. The other allele is recessive.

allergen

Any antigen causing allergy in a sensitive person. Typical allergens include animal dander, house mites, grass and tree pollens and shellfish.

allergic alveolitis

Inflammation of the small air sacs in the lungs, usually caused by inhalation of organic dusts to which the person concerned is allergic. There are various named types, including **bird** (or pigeon) **fancier's lung**, farmer's lung, mushroom worker's lung, **bagassosis**, maltworker's lung and maple bark disease. These condition are best treated by avoidance of the causal factor (allergen).

allergic rhinitis

See **rhinitis**.

allergist

A doctor concerned with the diagnosis and treatment of allergic disorders.

allergy

An abnormal response of the immune system to contact with a foreign substance (an allergen). Contact may be with the skin, the lining of any part of the respiratory system, or with the lining of the digestive system.

SIGNS
The allergic response, which cannot occur on the first exposure, may take several forms, including weals (**urticaria**), **dermatitis**, **asthma** or hay fever (**rhinitis**).

POSSIBLE CAUSES
People with an allergic tendency produce far more than the normal amounts of an antibody called immunoglobulin class E (IgE). They also produce more than the normal numbers of a particular granular cell called a **mast cell**. IgE becomes attached to mast cells and when an allergen, such as a pollen grain, links to the IgE, the membrane of the mast cell is distorted and ruptured, releasing a number of highly irritating substances, especially histamine. It is these that cause the symptoms of allergy.

allergy, basis of

See **atopy**.

allergy, life-threatening

See **anaphylaxis**.

allopathy

Conventional medicine, as taught in orthodox medical schools, based on the assumption that treatment should be directed so as to *oppose* disease processes.

allopurinol

A drug used to treat gout. Allopurinol is a xanthine oxidase inhibitor which reduces the production of uric acid from nucleic acid breakdown. A brand name is Zyloric.

alopecia

The medical term for baldness.

POSSIBLE CAUSES

The commonest form is hereditary and affects males, but baldness may also be caused by old age, disease, chemotherapy or radiation for cancer and treatment with thallium compounds, vitamin A or retinoids. In toxic alopecia, the hair loss occurs some weeks after a severe feverish illness such as scarlet fever or may occur in myxoedema, early syphilis and pregnancy. Scarring alopecia may follow burns, skin atrophy, ulceration, fungus infection (kerion) or skin tumours.

Alopecia areata is a form of patchy baldness, of unknown cause, often affecting only one or two small areas of the scalp, but sometimes affecting all the hair of the body.

TREATMENT

Baldness is of cosmetic importance only but may cause much distress, especially in women. Much interest has been shown in the possible value, in male pattern baldness, of the drug minoxidil. This is normally used to treat high blood pressure and is applied in a solution directly to the skin. Results vary considerably and when the treatment is stopped the new hair falls out. Possible dangers exist and the American Food and Drugs Administration (FDA) have resisted pressure to allow the drug to be sold without prescription.

Hair transplants from another part of the skin, or scalp reduction, may be helpful. Experimental production of a mild contact dermatitis has been used to promote hair growth in alopecia areata.

alpha-adrenoceptor blocking drugs

Drugs that cause widening of arteries (vasodilatation) by blocking the action of adrenaline-like hormones. They include **doxazosin** (Cardura), **indoramin** (Baratol), **prazosin** (Hypovase) and **terazosin** (Hytrin). Overdosage causes a drop in blood pressure, a fast pulse, nausea, vomiting and diarrhoea, a dry mouth, flushed skin, convulsions, drowsiness and coma.

alphafetoprotein

A protein synthesized in the fetal liver and intestine and present in fetal blood. Small quantities are passed into the womb fluid (amniotic fluid) and are subsequently swallowed by the fetus. Some gets into the mother's blood, by way of the placenta.

POTENTIAL PROBLEMS

The levels of alphafetoprotein rise as the pregnancy advances, and can be measured from the third month onward. If the levels are greatly raised this may indicate that the fetus has **spina bifida** or **anencephaly** and further investigation, ultrasound scanning and amniocentesis, should be offered.

Levels may also be raised in certain fetal kidney and bowel abnormalities, in multiple pregnancy, and in threatened or actual **abortion**. Confusion sometimes occurs and the levels may seem abnormally raised if there has been a mistake in the pregnancy dates.

Raised alphafetoprotein levels are also found in most people with cancer of the liver or testicle and in some with cancer of the bowel.

Alphaparin

A brand name for **certoparin**.

Alphosyl

A brand name for allantoin and coal tar, a preparation used in the treatment of psoriasis.

alprazolam

A benzodiazepine anti-anxiety drug. A brand name is Xanax.

alprostadil

A **prostaglandin** drug used by penile injection for the treatment of impotence. An erection lasting for two or three hours is commonly achieved, but sales of alprostadil may be adversely affected by the development of drugs such as Viagra. Brand names are Caverject, Muse, Prostin VR and Viridal.

Altacite Plus

A brand name for **hydrotalcite** with dimethicone.

alteplase

A **tissue plasminogen activator** drug made by recombinant NA technology. A brand name is Actilyse.

altitude sickness

Mountain sickness may occur in unadapted people who proceed to altitudes above about 3600 metres. At these heights, the reduced atmospheric pressure drives less oxygen into the blood, forcing the person to breathe more rapidly and deeply. This, in turn, causes excessive loss of carbon dioxide which reduces the stimulus to deep breathing.

RECOGNITION AND SYMPTOMS

There is a sense of fullness in the chest, headache, nausea, loss of appetite and sleeplessness. These symptoms are a warning of the danger of continuing to go higher, and a clear indication that time is needed for acclimatization. This may take only two or three days, after which the symptoms usually settle completely and cautious further ascent is possible.

If the symptoms are ignored and the affected person proceeds to higher altitudes, the condition may progress, sometimes suddenly, to a malignant and highly dangerous phase. In this, the lungs become waterlogged, so that the oxygen intake is severely restricted and blueness of the skin (**cyanosis**) may develop.

There is unsteadiness, irrational behaviour, slurred speech and other indications closely resembling intoxication, severe headache, drowsiness, coma and sometimes death.

> The symptoms of altitude sickness must not be ignored. The individual must be brought down immediately. Nothing can justify delay; it is often fatal.

altretamine

An anticancer drug used to treat advanced cancer of the ovary. A brand name is Hexalen.

Alu-cap

A brand name for **aluminium hydroxide**.

aluminium hydroxide

An antacid drug. A brand name is Alu-cap.

aluminium oxide

An abrasive preparation used externally in the treatment of **acne**. A brand name is Brasivol.

Alupent

A brand name for **orciprenaline**.

alveolectomy

A dental operation to smooth off irregular bone on the edges of tooth sockets so that a better fit may be obtained for dentures. The gum over the protuberant bone is cut and folded back and the unwanted bone nibbled off with bone-cutting forceps. The gum edges are then brought together and stitched (sutured).

alverine citrate

An antispasmodic drug used in the treatment of menstrual pain. A brand name is Spasmonal.

Alzheimer's disease

In 1907, the German neuropathologist Alois Alzheimer (1864–1915) reported the changes in the brain of a 51-year-old woman who had died after five years of progressively worsening dementia. These findings have since been confirmed and extended and we now know that the disease causes the brain substance to be severely shrunken from massive loss of nerve cells. The convolutions of the brain are narrowed and the grooves between them widened. The spaces within the brain (ventricles) are symmetrically enlarged. Microscopic examination of the nerve cells shows that they have lost many of their interconnections and that they contain tangled loops and coils of fibrous material, called amyloid protein. Changes of this degree are inevitably fatal and Alzheimer's disease almost always results in death, five to fifteen years after onset. of symptoms.

INCIDENCE

It is by far the commonest cause of loss of the higher brain functions (dementia), about three-quarters of all cases of dementia occurring in those over sixty-five being due to Alzheimer's disease. It is also alarmingly common, affecting 10 to 15 per cent of all people over sixty-five and as many as one in five of all those over eighty.

RECOGNITION AND SYMPTOMS

The disease starts with gradual, almost imperceptible, loss of brain function, usually first noticed as loss of memory, and progresses to ever more profound loss of intellectual function with disorientation and confusion and eventual grave disablement. The features vary from case to case, but three broad stages can be recognized. First there is mere forgetfulness that can be compensated for by keeping memo pads and lists. The loss of memory, however, often causes anxiety. Secondly, there is a gradual increase in the severity of the memory loss, particularly for recent events. The recollection of events in early life may be good and reminiscence will be free. Sometimes this stage includes an element of confusion and even invention (confabulation) to fill the gaps. At the same time there is progressive loss of awareness of current time or place (disorientation), with uncertainty even in familiar areas and inability to give the date or even the year. Concentration declines with inability to find the right word (dysphasia). These difficulties cause alarm and frustration, and mood may change suddenly and unpredictably.

In the final stage there is severe disorientation and confusion. There may be perception of non-existent sights, sounds and smells (hallucinations) and false ideas of persecution (paranoid delusions). These are usually worst at night. It is now that people with Alzheimer's become especially hard to live with. They become demanding, suspicious, sometimes violent. They disregard personal hygiene. Incontinence of urine and faeces is common. In the end, the burden on relatives often becomes too heavy, and institutional care becomes necessary. Once the affected person is bed-ridden, complications such as deep vein thrombosis, **bedsores**, urinary and chest infections, rapidly supervene and death from pneumonia is common.

POSSIBLE CAUSES

The cause of Alzheimer's disease remains unknown. It is a feature of **Down's syndrome** and there is a family history of Down's syndrome in 15 per cent of those with Alzheimer's disease. Recent research has concentrated on the isolation of the gene for a substance called beta-amyloid protein found in the tangled fibre masses in brains of people with Alzheimer's disease and in those of older people with Down's syndrome. This gene is on the same chromosome (chromosome 21) of which an extra copy is present in every body cell of people with Down's syndrome. It is in the region of the chromosome known to contain the gene for beta-amyloid protein. The disease is also believed to be caused by an unidentified gene on chromosome 14.

These hereditary familial forms of Alzheimer's disease start around fifty years of age and progress very rapidly. No one has been able to show any pathological or clinical difference between common Alzheimer's disease and familial Alzheimer's disease. Some workers believe that beta-amyloid protein is the cause. Some evidence has appeared in recent years as to the cause of late onset Alzheimer's disease. In 1991 it was found that there was a genetic linkage to chromosome 19 in familial groups of people with Alzheimer's disease starting after the age of sixty.

This linkage relates to a variant (e4) of a gene for a protein known as apolipoprotein E – a protein present on the surface of low density lipoprotein cholesterol carriers. These

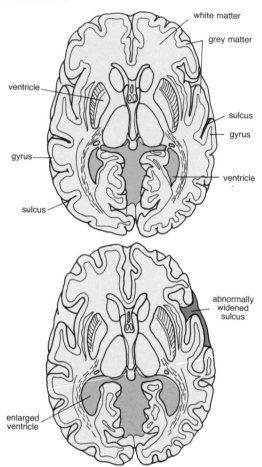

white matter

grey matter

ventricle

sulcus

gyrus

gyrus

ventricle

sulcus

abnormally
widened
sulcus

enlarged
ventricle

A normal brain, top, compared with, above, the brain of a person who died from Alzheimer's disease. Note the overall loss of brain tissue with extreme widening of the grooves (sulci) and reduction in size of the lobes (gyri). The fluid spaces inside the brain (ventricles) are enlarged.

are the cholesterol carriers associated with heart attacks and strokes (see **atherosclerosis**). This variant of the gene is present twice as often in people with Alzheimer's as in people without. Of those who do not have this gene only 2.9 per cent have Alzheimer's disease. Of those with the gene on only one of the chromosome 19 pair, 7.6 per cent have Alzheimer's; and of those with the gene on both chromosomes, 21.4 per cent have the disease. The scientists concerned in this study

> It is extremely important not to assume that every person who seems demented or seriously forgetful has Alzheimer's disease. Forgetfulness, especially for names, is a characteristic of a heavily stocked elderly mind. At least 10 per cent of people with dementia-like symptoms have a treatable disease such as thyroid underactivity (myxoedema), simple depression (pseudodementia), a brain tumour or a blood clot pressing on the brain (subdural haematoma) following a sometimes apparently minor injury. Full investigation is necessary to ensure such treatable disorders are identified. Pseudodementia, unlike Alzheimer's disease, commonly starts suddenly and the change of mental state is immediately obvious. Antidepressant drugs can often cure such cases.

state that 30 to 40 per cent of all cases of Alzheimer's disease can be attributed to this gene.

Many interesting implications follow. If these scientists are right, we will probably be able to detect those at risk from Alzheimer's disease, even before they are born. This, of course, would raise major ethical issues. But if the structure of the gene, and the way it codes for the synthesis of beta-amyloid protein, can be established it may be possible to do something positive to prevent or treat this dreadful disorder.

TREATMENT

At present, there is no effective treatment for Alzheimer's disease, but much can be done with mood-controlling drugs (tranquillizers) and other forms of medication, to reduce behaviour problems and ensure sound sleep. The burden on the family can be relieved by the use of daycare centres. The final move to the hospital or nursing home should not be delayed once awareness of the surroundings has gone.

> It is often difficult for relatives to realize the extent of the loss of functioning brain substance, and, in consequence, of mind, but it is important that they should do so, so that they can understand how little the profoundly demented person actually suffers.

amantadine

An antiviral drug, also used to treat **Alzheimer's disease** and **Parkinson's disease**. A brand name is Symmetrel.

Amaryl

A brand name for **glimepiride**.

amaurosis

An old-fashioned term for blindness. The word is still occasionally applied to blindness arising from general or toxic causes such as diabetes, nutritional deficiency, poisoning, or psychological upset, but is now normally used only in the following two special cases.

amaurosis fugax

Transient loss of vision, usually for a few seconds or minutes, caused by interference to the blood supply to parts of the brain or eye by tiny emboli. These are particles of solid matter such as cholesterol crystals or partially clotted blood which temporarily or permanently block small blood vessels. Usually they are carried up in the bloodstream from diseased neck arteries or from clots forming on the internal heart lining.

RECOGNITION AND SYMPTOMS

The symptomatic loss of vision, which is entirely painless, may be an isolated event or may occur many times a day. The more often they occur, the more seriously it must be regarded.

Amaurosis fugax is an example of a TIA (**transient ischaemic attack**).

> Amaurosis fugax must never be ignored as it is a clear warning of the risk of stroke or of coronary thrombosis. Medical investigation of the state of the heart and of the arteries is urgently indicated. About one person in twenty dies from one or other of these causes during the first year following the onset of the symptom.

amaurotic familial idiocy

An out-of-date term for a range of rare hereditary diseases, now known as the *gangliosidoses*. Progressive degeneration occurs in the brain and the retinas of the eyes, causing mental retardation and movement disorders. The commonest of the group is **Tay-Sachs disease**, which usually begins between six months and one year and is most often seen in Jewish children. There is increasing **dementia**, blindness and spastic paralysis. The conditions are incurable but, fortunately, are exceedingly uncommon. Identification before birth is possible, by **amniocentesis**, and termination of the pregnancy can be considered. Batten's disease is in the same category.

ambi-

Prefix meaning 'on both sides' as in ambidextrous (both hands right).

ambidexterity

Literally, 'both right'. The ability to use either hand with the same facility. True ambidexterity, with no bias to one side, is rare and runs in families. Surgeons, pianists and others often acquire, by long training, a degree of practical ambidexterity.

Ambisome

A brand name for **amphotericin**.

ambivalence

Having opposing feelings (such as love and hate) or attitudes (such as approval and disapproval) about a person, object or idea. The phenomenon is considered important in **psycho-analysis** and is thought to indicate an unconscious conflict of some kind.

amblyopia

For the development of normal vision it is essential that, during infancy and childhood, clear visual images should be formed on the retinas so that normal nerve impulses pass back from the eyes to the brain. Should this be prevented, normal vision will not develop. If, for instance, a baby's eye were to be covered with a patch for the first year of life, that eye would remain permanently effectively blind. Visual defect caused in this way is called amblyopia and in the majority of cases the affected eyes are structurally normal.

POSSIBLE CAUSES
Failure to form normal retinal images may result from opacity of the internal lens of the eye at birth (congenital **cataract**), uncorrected severe eyelid droop with coverage of the pupil (blepharoptosis) and severe, or unequal, focusing errors, especially **astigmatism**. But the commonest cause of amblyopia is squint (**strabismus**) in which the normal visual input to the brain, from the squinting eye, is suppressed to avoid double vision. This is why early expert treatment of squint is so important.

In general, it may be said that the maximum level of visual acuity achievable cannot exceed the highest level experienced during this developmental period. So the child who, from birth, has been able to see only a glow of light through a cataract, will never see better than this later in life.

The optic nerves run back from the eyes to two 'junction boxes' on the under side of the brain and, from these, other nerve fibres proceed to the visual part of the brain, right at the back. At these junction boxes – the lateral geniculate bodies – important neurological connections between the eyes and the brain are made, and any barrier to proper visual input interferes with this. These links can only be made before the age of eight years. Thereafter, no further development is possible and amblyopia present at that age is permanent and irremediable. This is why early diagnosis and treatment is so important and why the idea that a child will 'grow out' of a squint is so indefensible.

The term amblyopia is also applied to toxic or nutritional causes of visual defect, such as *tobacco amblyopia*.

amelogenin

A structural protein used as a drug to treat periodontitis. The drug is formulated as a gel that is placed under a flap in the gum surrounding the root of the tooth and promotes regrowth of gum tissue that has been destroyed by the inflammatory process. A brand name is Emdogain.

amenorrhoea

The absence of menstruation. This is normal before puberty and after the menopause. During the reproductive years, the commonest cause is pregnancy and **lactation** (milk secretion), but it can be caused by a number of hormonal and other disorders. Amenorrhoea is common in female athletes and is a feature of **anorexia nervosa**.

amentia

Failure of the intellectual functions to develop. **Dementia** is the state following the loss of these functions.

amethocaine

A local anaesthetic drug which is effective when in contact with surfaces as well as when given by injection. It resembles **cocaine** in its action and can readily be absorbed in dangerous amounts from mucous membranes. A brand name is Ametop.

ametropia

Any deviation from the normal relaxed focus (refraction) of the eye. Ametropia may take the form of farsightedness (**hypermetropia**), nearsightedness (**myopia**) or a meridional visual defect (**astigmatism**).

Amias

A brand name for **candesartan**.

amifostine

A drug used to reduce the side-effects of anticancer treatments, especially the dangers of infection and of damage to the kidneys. A brand name is Ethyol.

Amil-Co

A brand name for **hydrochlorothiazide** with potassium.

amiloride

A thiazide **diuretic drug** that acts by reducing reabsorption of sodium, and thus water, in the kidneys. A potassium-sparing diuretic used to treat high blood pressure, heart failure or other conditions in which excess fluid is retained in the body. Formulated in combination with other drugs under brand names such as Amil-Co, Burinex A, Fru-Co, Frumil, Kalten, Lasoride, Moducren, Moduret 25, Moduretic and Navispare.

amines

Organic compounds derived from ammonia by replacing one or more of the hydrogen atoms by a member of the paraffin series or by an aromatic group. Amines occur widely in the body, and many drugs are amines.

amino acid

The body is largely constructed of protein, and proteins are long, sometimes very long, chains of amino acids, linked together. Proteins contain hundreds or even thousands of amino acids arranged in a particular sequence. An alteration in even one amino acid can change the properties of the protein. The thousands of enzymes needed for cell function are also proteins and most of these will be inactivated or will function abnormally if the amino acid sequence is wrong as a result of a gene mutation.

Body proteins break down into 20 different amino acids. Some of these can be synthesized by the body but some can not. The latter are known as 'essential amino acids' and must be obtained from protein in the diet. Amino acids group together to form peptides. Dipeptides have two amino acids, polypeptides have many. Polypeptides join (polymerize) to form proteins. The reverse process occurs when proteins are digested by protein-splitting (proteilytic) enzymes.

amino acid error

See **missense mutation**.

amino acid selector

See **transfer RNA**.

aminobenzoic acid

A drug used in the treatment of scleroderma and **Peyronie's disease**. The action is to reduce the tendency to the formation of fibrous tissue. A brand name is Potaba.

aminoglutethimide

A drug that interferes with the synthesis of **steroids**, **oestrogens** and **androgens** by the **adrenal glands**. It does this by blocking an enzyme that allows the conversion of **cholesterol**. A brand name is Ormetan.

aminoglycoside antibiotic drugs

See **antibiotic drugs**.

aminophylline

A drug used in the control of **asthma**. In acute cases it can be given by intravenous injection but it is also effective by mouth or in a **suppository**. A brand name is Phyllocontin.

amiodarone

A drug used to treat heart rhythm irregularities such as paroxysmal atrial fibrillation. There are numerous side-effects. A brand name is Cordarone X.

amisulpride

A drug used in the treatment of **schizophrenia**. A brand name is Solian.

amitriptyline

A tricyclic antidepressant drug. Brand names are Domical, Elavil, Lentizol and Tryptizol.

amlodipine

A drug used in the treatment of **angina pectoris** and high blood pressure. A brand name is Istin.

amnesia

The loss of memory as a result of physical or mental disease or injury. Head injury often causes amnesia both for events following the injury and for a period *prior* to the injury. The latter is called *retrograde amnesia* and the length of it is, in general, a measure of the severity of the injury.

amniocentesis

This is an important method of obtaining information about a fetus and about the probability of the future development of genetic disorder. It is usually done between the 16th and 20th weeks of pregnancy. Routine amniocentesis is usually recommended for women over 35 because at that age the risk of the procedure causing miscarriage (see below) is about the same as the risk of the fetus having Down's syndrome. In other cases amniocentesis is done if there is any special reason to suspect trouble.

An area of the abdominal wall is anaesthetized with an injection of local anaesthetic. Ultrasound scanning is then used to ensure that a needle can be passed safely through the wall of the abdomen and straight through the wall of the womb into the amniotic fluid in which the fetus is floating. A sample of fluid can now be sucked out with a syringe. Because this fluid contains cells shed from the skin of the fetus and various substances secreted by the fetus, samples obtained can be of the greatest importance for diagnosis. Every fetal cell contains a complete set of the DNA of the fetus.

Amniocentesis provides information directly about the likelihood of a number of conditions, such as rhesus factor disease, congenital absence of the brain (anencephaly) and the respiratory distress syndrome. Alpha-fetoprotein levels in the amniotic fluid can give reliable information on the likelihood of congenital defects in the spinal cord and column (spina bifida). Levels in the mother's serum are also measured routinely. Cells from the amniotic fluid are grown in tissue culture so that chromosomal analysis can be done after three or four weeks. In this way, Down's syndrome, and a great range of other genetic diseases, can be diagnosed before birth. It is possible to detect cystic fibrosis, factor VIII and factor IX types of haemophilia, Duchenne muscular dystrophy, thalassaemia, sickle cell anaemia, antitrypsin deficiency and phenylketonuria.

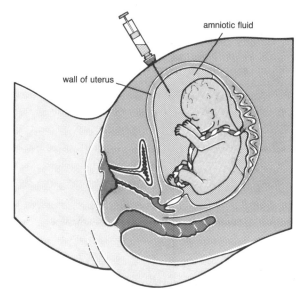

amniotic fluid

wall of uterus

By passing a needle though the wall of the abdomen, under ultrasound visualization, it is possible safely to obtain a sample of the amniotic fluid surrounding the fetus. This fluid contains cells cast off by the fetus, as well as fetal urine and various chemical substances. The sample can be used for a wide range of investigations and many conditions can be detected early.

amoebiasis

A complex of diseases caused by a dangerous amoeba, *Entamoeba histolytica*, which starts with amoebic dysentery and may proceed to cause damage to the large bowel and amoebic abscesses in the liver, lungs, brain and elsewhere.

amok

A form of homicidal mania featuring extreme agitation and the attempt to kill as many people as possible. The attack is said to be followed by loss of memory for the event. Amok was originally described as occurring among Malayan men armed with machetes (parangs). The modern form, which is far from unknown in the West, is more likely to feature a Kalashnikov automatic rifle and to be correspondingly more dangerous.

Amoram

A brand name for **amoxycillin**.

amorolfine

A drug used externally in the treatment of **tinea** infection of the skin. A brand name is Loceryl.

amotivational syndrome

An effect of prolonged heavy use of marijuana (cannabis). There is apathy, unwillingness to persist at any task and usually a gain in weight. The amotivational syndrome is one of the reasons for students to drop out of their studies or for employed persons to give up work or to be discharged.

amoxapine

A tricyclic antidepressant drug similar to **imipramine**. Overdosage may cause acute kidney failure, convulsions and coma. A brand name is Asendis.

Amoxil

A brand name for **amoxycillin**.

amoxycillin

An **ampicillin**-like penicillin antibiotic, effective in **typhoid** and many other infections. Brand names are Amoxil and Amoram.

ampakines

Drugs which act on nerve cell receptors to make them more responsive to the neurotransmitter glutamate. A few small clinical trials have suggested that ampakines can significantly improve memory in elderly people. Neuroscientists remain sceptical.

Amniocentesis is not entirely without risk and should not be done without good reason. It may cause abortion if done early. It may damage the afterbirth (placenta) or the fetus, and may cause bleeding into the amniotic fluid. The risk of fetal death from amniocentesis is as high as one per cent. Sexing of the future child is certainly not a justification for the procedure, and the practice of amniocentesis followed by abortion of a fetus of the unwanted sex, is considered reprehensible by the medical profession. The Indian government made this illegal in August 1994.

Such early methods of detection of serious or potentially serious major disorders give parents the option of an early termination of the pregnancy. They also sometimes provide the opportunity for early treatment of the disorder while the fetus remains in the uterus.

amoeba

A single-celled microscopic organism of indefinite shape commonly found in water, damp soil and as parasites of other animals. The amoeba moves by repeatedly putting out a *pseudopodium* (false foot) and then flowing into it. The most important amoeba affecting man is the *Entamoeba histolytica* which causes amoebic **dysentery** and other serious effects. Many of the white cells of the immune system, especially the phagocytes, are amoeboid.

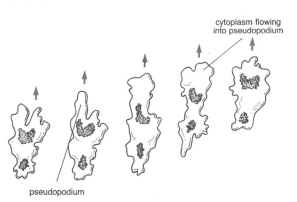

cytoplasm flowing into pseudopodium

pseudopodium

How an amoeba moves along. A 'false foot' (pseudopodium) is put out and the cytoplasm of the amoeba flows into it.

amphetamine drugs

A class of drugs formerly used widely for appetite control and to treat depression, but now considered disreputable. Amphetamines, or 'speed', cause a monoamine, called noradrenaline, which is stored in nerve endings to be released. The effect is to elevate the mood, abolish sleepiness, to appear to increase the capacity for work, and generally speed up mental action. The drug does not, however, improve performance of any kind and can be dangerous. It is used to a limited extent for a few special medical purposes but is subject to the full restrictions on controlled drugs laid down in the Misuse of Drugs Act (1971).

Amphocil

A brand name for **amphotericin**.

amphotericin

An antibiotic drug used to treat fungus infections within the body. It is moderately toxic and side-effects are common. Brand names are Abelcet, Ambisome, Fungilin and Fungizone.

ampicillin

A widely used penicillin antibiotic, effective by mouth and capable of killing many Gram-negative as well as Gram-positive organisms. About one-third of the dose is excreted unchanged in the urine. The drug precipitates a characteristic rash if given to people incubating glandular fever (infective mononucleosis). A brand name is Penbritin.

amputation

Removal, by surgery or accidental injury, of part of the body.

WHY IT'S DONE

Surgical amputation, most commonly of a foot or leg, is, nowadays, usually required because of **gangrene** (death and decay of tissues) resulting from **atherosclerosis** (disease of large arteries) and the resulting inadequacy of blood supply to the part. Amputation is also sometimes required to prevent the spread of a seriously malignant tumour of bone, such as an **osteogenic sarcoma**, or a **malignant melanoma** of the skin.

Formerly, amputation was commonly needed to save life in cases of gas gangrene after serious injury, but because of antibiotics, and a proper understanding of the principles of surgical wound management, this is now seldom necessary.

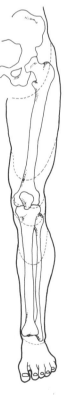

A range of possible amputation sites with the lines of the skin incisions. The latter are designed to provide optimum skin and muscle flaps to cover the cut end of the bone.

HOW IT'S DONE

Before the operation, it is necessary to decide the level of amputation. Healthy tissue, with a good blood supply, must be left, and the bone must be cut at a higher level than the skin and muscles, so as to provide the means of fashioning a well-padded and comfortable stump. In making this decision, the surgeon may be assisted by information derived from X-ray display of a radio-opaque fluid injected into the bloodstream (**angiography**).

Following amputation, stimulation of the cut ends of the limb nerves often produce the feeling that the limb is still present. This *phantom limb* effect may persist for months.

amylobarbitone

A **barbiturate** drug used for the short-term treatment of insomnia. Brand names are Amytal and Sodium Amytal.

amyloid

Any one of a range of proteins deposited in the brain in spongiform encephalopathies such as **Creutzfeldt-Jakob disease**, in other degenerative brain disorders such as **Alzheimer's disease**, and in the tissues in a wide range of long-term suppurative disorders. Amyloids are hard, waxy proteinaceous substances. There is a considerable range of amyloid proteins mainly specific for the different conditions in which amyloid is deposited.

amyotonia congenita

The 'floppy baby' syndrome, in which the new-born baby's muscles are weak and the limbs floppy. When supported across the front of its waist with one hand the baby will collapse over the hand in the form of an inverted U. In many such cases the condition is benign and recovery is complete, but some babies with amyotonia congenita are suffering from the serious condition of spinal muscular atrophy.

amyotrophic lateral sclerosis

Motor nerves are those that activate muscles so as to cause movement. Amyotrophic lateral sclerosis is a fatal condition of progressive degeneration of the motor nerve fibre tracts in the spinal cord, the brain stem and motor zone on the surface (cortex) of the brain. The effect is progressive atrophy of the disused muscles and increasing weakness. Death usually occurs within five or six years of onset. The condition is a form of motor neuron disease.

Amytal

A brand name for **amylobarbitone**, a barbiturate hypnotic drug of medium duration of action.

Anabact

A brand name for **metronidazole** formulated for external use only.

anabolic steroids

Drugs that cause an increase in body bulk by stimulating the production of protein, mainly in the muscles, but also elsewhere. They actually work inside cells, causing an acceleration of the processes by which amino acids in the cell fluid are strung together to form protein. Anabolic steroids are synthetic male sex hormone steroids such as ethyloestrenol, nandrolone, norethandrolone and stanolone.

Their use may sometimes be justified to help elderly and underweight people to gain strength and they can be valuable in women with the condition of seriously weakened bones known as osteoporosis.

Some of the anabolic steroids, being male sex hormones, cause development of male characteristics in women. This is called virilization and may feature hairiness, wasting (atrophy) of the breasts, enlargement of the clitoris, deepening of the voice and severe acne. Anabolic steroids are widely used by body-building enthusiasts and athletes to improve muscle bulk and strength. This usage has rightly been banned by sporting authorities, not only because of its unfairness to other competitors, but also because of the possible adverse effects on health. Among these are:

- virilization in women (see above);
- virilization of a female fetus;
- increased libido;
- frequent erections;
- failure of an erection to go down (priapism);
- liver damage;
- a dangerous and sometimes fatal form of heart enlargement;
- major depression;
- hallucinations;
- religious delusions and delusions of grandeur;
- aggressive or manic behaviour.

Anabolic steroids can encourage the growth of an existing cancer of the prostate gland in men.

anaemia

A reduction in the concentration of haemoglobin (the oxygen-carrying constituent of the red cells) in the blood.
RECOGNITION AND SYMPTOMS
Because a good supply of oxygen is so vital, anaemia has widespread effects, causing weakness, fatigue, tiredness and breathlessness on minor effort. The skin may appear pale and there is lowered resistance to infection.

There are several different kinds of anaemia including simple **iron-deficiency anaemia**, **haemolytic anaemia**, **pernicious anaemia**, and **aplastic anaemia**.

anaesthesia

Loss of the sensations of touch, pressure, pain and temperature in any part, or the whole of, the body. This may be due to injury or disease to the nerves carrying impulses subserving these sensations to the brain, or to damage from disease or injury to the brain itself. Hemianaesthesia (loss of sensation in one half of the body) is one of the most frequent consequences of **stroke**.
POSSIBLE CAUSES
Anaesthesia is most commonly caused by deliberate interference with the function of the brain, or by blocking the passage of nerve impulses to the brain, for the purposes of allowing surgery to be performed painlessly. In both cases, drugs are used; in the former to cause *general anaesthesia* and in the latter to achieve *local anaesthesia*. General anaesthesia is associated with loss of consciousness.

anaesthetic drugs

Modern general anaesthetic drugs are designed to keep you lightly and safely asleep, while, at the same time, causing your muscles to relax completely so as not to interfere with the surgery. They are also selected to prevent the surgery from upsetting your autonomic nervous system, and to abolish pain sensation and produce a calm, relaxed state of mind, before and after the anaesthetic. Narcotic drugs, such as morphine, Omnopon or Valium (diazepam), are used before an operation (pre-medication), to promote your confidence, relax your muscles, help you to forget the unpleasantness, and keep you comfortable afterwards. These drugs act directly on the brain, safely and temporarily interfering with the function of the nerve cells that allow sensation, consciousness and movement. The drug atropine is often given to reduce the tendency for fluid to collect in your air tubes.

So, if you are having an operation, you are likely to be wheeled to theatre in a very comfortable frame of mind, if not already asleep. If you are awake when you reach the anaesthetic room, you are unlikely to be put to sleep with a mask and anaesthetic gas or vapour. Anaesthesia is almost always induced by a small injection into a vein of a rapid-acting drug, such as the barbiturate Pentothal (thiopentone). This is very pleasant and there is hardly any awareness of what is happening. Anaesthesia is maintained, at a very light level for safety, by means of inhaled drugs such as nitrous oxide or halothane. These are often combined with a strong pain-killing **analgesic drug** because, although you are unconscious, stimuli which would otherwise be painful can still cause unwanted changes in your body. Only after you are deeply asleep will the gases, which keep you anaesthetized, be turned on. There will be none of the sense of asphyxiation which was formerly a feature of general anaesthesia.

If muscle relaxation is needed, this is now achieved by one of a number of drugs which temporarily paralyze the muscles. In this event, your breathing must be maintained artificially. Sometimes blood pressure is deliberately lowered by **antihypertensive drugs**.

anaesthetic safety aid

See **pulse oximeter**.

anaesthetist

A doctor specially trained to administer general and local anaesthetics of all kinds, to ensure the safety of patients during any form of surgery, to manage life-support systems for patients in critical conditions and, in conjunction with other specialists, to see to the efficient organization and running of intensive care facilities.

Anafranil

A brand name for **clomipramine**.

anal area, discharging

See **anal fistula**.

anal dilatation test

A test used along with other signs to help in the detection of anal sexual abuse in children. The buttocks are gently parted and the anus observed. After a short time, the anus opens (reflex dilatation). This effect, alone, provides no conclusive evidence and occurs in up to 14 per cent of children who have never been abused. Other, and more significant, signs of anal sexual abuse include anal tears (fissures), loss of sphincter control, shortening and eversion of the anal canal, vein congestion with reddening in the area and thickening of the surrounding tissues.

analeptic drugs

Drugs which stimulate the nerve centres in the brain responsible for breathing. Their action is to increase the strength of the nerve impulses going to the breathing muscles – the diaphragm and the muscles between the ribs (intercostal muscles). Analeptics, such as doxapram (Dopram) or nikethamide are used to stimulate poor or absent breathing in newborn babies and are sometimes used in cases of drug overdose when the victim is barely breathing, or to speed recovery from a general anaesthetic. The drug naloxone (Narcan), which is an antidote to narcotic drugs, while not an analeptic, is also commonly used in such cases.

Side-effects of analeptic drugs include nausea and vomiting, restlessness, dizziness, fast pulse, irregular pulse, shakiness, tremor and even convulsions. They are dangerous in people with coronary artery disease, severe high blood pressure and thyroid gland overactivity.

anal fissure

Sometimes called 'fissure-in-ano', this is a longitudinal tear in the wall of the anus, usually running directly backwards. There is inevitable infection and a swollen skin tag, called a sentinel pile, forms at the site. The main symptom is burning pain on defecation. Anal fissures usually heal spontaneously and this is helped by a high-fibre diet to maintain softness in the stools and to avoid constipation. Recurrent fissures may require anal dilatation or surgical correction although some can be treated with local vasodilators such as glyceryl trinihate paste.

anal fistula

A persistent discharging track between the anus and the exterior, opening on the skin near the anus. Fistula is usually associated with an abscess in the tissues surrounding the anal canal. Surgery to remove the lining of the fistula will allow natural healing.

analgesic drugs

This is the important group of painkilling drugs. It includes a wide range of drugs from the mild and comparatively safe (in correct dosage), such as paracetamol (Panadol), to the powerful and dangerous, such as the narcotics.

PARACETAMOL
Paracetamol works mainly by blocking the passage of the nerve impulses for pain so that they do not reach the part of the brain where pain is perceived. In general, it is a safe painkiller, but paracetamol is a serious liver poison if many tablets are taken at once. Twenty tablets can cause severe liver damage. The victim seems fine for a few days, then begins to turn yellow from the jaundice of an often fatal total liver failure. Antidotes, if given early enough, are methionine or N-acetylcysteine (Parvolex).

NSAIDS
Most of the other mild analgesics, such as the non-steroidal anti-inflammatory drugs (NSAIDs), work in a different way. When tissue cells are injured in any way they release powerful substances called prostaglandins. Prostaglandins strongly stimulate pain nerve endings and the result is the experience of pain. NSAIDs act by blocking the production of prostaglandins. Some drugs, such as morphine, act directly on the brain; others, like paracetamol, act on nerve conduction. But the aspirin-like drugs act directly on damaged cells and work solely by preventing the production of the substances which cause the pain. Aspirin has no effect on the pain of a needle-prick because this directly stimulates the pain nerve endings, nor has it any effect on the pain caused by an injection of prostaglandins.

The non-steroidal anti-inflammatory drugs include aspirin, aloxiprin (Palaprin forte), benorylate (Benoral), diflunisal (Dolobid), mefenamic acid (Ponstan), fenbufen (Lederfen), fenoprofen (Progesic), ibuprofen (Brufen), naproxen (Naprosyn), diclofenac (Voltarol), tolmetin (Tolectin), indomethacin (Indocid), phenylbutazone (Butazolidin) and piroxicam (Feldene).

NSAIDs often cause side-effects. About half of those taking them get some degree of tummy upset, with nausea and diarrhoea. They may also cause headache, sleep disturbances, allergic rashes and dizziness. Occasionally there can be interference with white blood cell production.

ASPIRIN
Aspirin can cause quite severe irritation to the lining of the stomach. If you keep a tablet of plain aspirin between your cheek and your gum for half an hour, it will turn the mucous membrane white and wrinkled and will loosen the surface. Aspirin can do the same to your stomach lining, causing congestion and bleeding around undissolved particles. Over half of all people taking aspirin have traces of blood in their faeces. So you should never use plain aspirin. Only the soluble variety, which rapidly breaks up and dissolves, is safe. If you suffer from indigestion or have a previous history of ulcer trouble you should avoid aspirin altogether.

Following a virus infection in children, aspirin can cause a serious liver and brain disorder called Reye's syndrome. Aspirin is therefore no longer given to children. Aspirin allergy is rare but may occur in people with other allergies. It can cause alarming and often dangerous reactions, including severe breathing difficulty. Aspirin and the NSAIDs interfere with blood clotting and prolong bleeding, which can be very useful in preventing heart attacks (caused by blood clotting in the coronary arteries of the heart). But it can sometimes be dangerous. People with a tendency to stroke might be saved from a cerebral thrombosis (clot), but might be at greater risk from a more serious cerebral haemorrhage. A minor eye injury with a small leak of blood into the front chamber can be turned into an eye-filling bleed by a single aspirin tablet, which doubles the bleeding time for up to a week.

INTERMEDIATE ANALGESICS
An intermediate group of analgesics consists of a mixture of these mild analgesics with the mild – and fairly safe – narcotic analgesic, codeine. There is a large range of proprietary medications consisting of various combinations of codeine, aspirin and various NSAIDs. Other moderately potent narcotic drugs, unlikely to cause addiction, are dihydrocodeine, pentazocine and dextropropoxyphene.

NARCOTIC ANALGESICS

For the relief of very severe pain, more powerful narcotic drugs may be needed. These are used only when other drugs are ineffective, and include morphine, phenazocine and methadone. The narcotic analgesics act on specific receptor sites, called opiate receptors, in the brain and spinal cord, blocking the pain sensation. The natural endorphins of the body act in the same way. These strong narcotic analgesics also produce a powerful feeling of wellbeing (euphoria) and are abused for this reason. They are strongly addictive. Heroin (diamorphine), formerly widely used in medicine, is now banned in most countries because of this danger.

anal incontinence

The inability to retain faeces voluntarily in the rectum. This is due to injury to the strong muscular ring (sphincter) around the anus, often from obstetrical tears, or to neurological or psychological disturbances, to a turning outside-in and descent (prolapse) of the rectum, to constipation with faecal impaction and hardness, or to loss of control in **dementia**.

anal intercourse

A form of sexual intercourse, usually homosexual, in which the anus performs the sexual function of the vagina. The practice is liable to lead to traumatic injury and to penile infection of the active partner.

anal stricture

An abnormal narrowing of the anus or anal canal as a result of disease.

analysis

See **psychoanalysis**.

anaphylaxis

A severe, often fatal, form of hypersensitive allergic reaction most commonly provoked by drugs such as penicillin, intravenous iron or procainamide, but also brought on by allergy to foods or food additives, peanut protein, vaccines, insect bites or snake bites and contact with latex rubber. There is always a history of a previous reaction to the **allergen**. The effects are a drop in blood pressure (hypotension), local swelling of the skin (angio-oedema) and mucous membranes, narrowing of the air tubes (bronchi), itching, vomiting and abdominal pain. The sooner the onset after exposure to the allergen, the more severe the reaction. Anaphylactic shock is a serious, widespread allergic attack which may cause death by airway obstruction from swelling of the lining of the voice box (larynx). People liable to anaphylactic attacks should carry adrenaline for immediate injection to control an attack, and may also require a large dose of steroid by injection.

anaplasia

A change in cells, so that the features which distinguish one type from another are lost. Anaplastic cells become smaller and simpler in structure and no longer combine to form recognizable tissues characteristic of particular organs. Anaplasia is a feature of cancer, and, in general, the more anaplastic the cells, the more malignant and dangerous the tumour.

anasarca

An old-fashioned term for fluid accumulation in the tissues (**oedema**).

anastomosis

A direct communication between an artery and a vein without intervening smaller vessels such as capillaries. In surgery, an anastomosis is a direct artificial connection formed between two tubular structures by stitching (suturing). For instance, if a section of bowel has to be removed for any reason, the free ends may be joined by direct anastomosis.

anastrozole

An anti-oestrogen drug used in the treatment of advanced breast cancer in post-menopausal women. A brand name is Arimidex.

Ancotil

A brand name for **flucytosine**.

ancrod

A protein-splitting enzyme occurring in the venom of the Malaysian pit viper *Agkistrodon rhodostoma*. The enzyme removes the blood clot-forming agent fibrinogen from the circulating blood without converting it to fibrin. The result is that the blood is much less likely to form clots (thromboses) or for existing clots to increase in size. Ancrod is used by Chinese doctors to treat stroke.

Andriol

A brand name for **testosterone**.

Androcur

A brand name for cyproterone acetate.

androgenic alopecia

Male-pattern baldness in a woman caused by abnormal male sex hormone output from congenital overgrowths of the adrenal glands (congenital adrenal hyperplasia) or other causes.

androgen receptor gene

Androgens are male sex hormones. The androgen receptor gene is a gene on the X chromosome which codes for the receptors for male sex hormones. Mutations in this gene have been found in men with various disorders including complete insensitivity to the male sex hormones, various motor neuron diseases, the rare condition of familial cancer of the breast, and low or absent sperm production.

androgens

Androgens are the male sex hormones. They are anabolic steroids and include testosterone and androsterone. As drugs, they are used to stimulate the development of sexual characteristics in boys when there is inadequate output from the testicles and to stimulate red cell formation in **aplastic anaemia**. See also **anabolic steroids**.

Andropatch

A brand name for **testosterone**.

Anectine

A brand name for **suxamethonium chloride**.

anencephaly

Absence of the greater part of the brain and of the bones at the rear of the skull. Anencephaly is a defect of development and although the affected fetus may survive to full term, it usually dies soon after birth.

The condition is often associated with **spina bifida** and other defects of the nervous system. It can be detected by **ultrasound** examination aided by amniocentesis and the pregnancy terminated.

aneurysm

A berry or balloon-like swelling on an artery, usually at or near a branch, and caused by localized damage or weakness to the vessel wall.

Aneurysms can also involve the heart wall after a section has been weakened by local loss of blood supply from coronary thrombosis (see **heart attack**).

Aneurysms of the blood vessels at the base of the brain may press on nerve tissue causing severe symptoms and demanding urgent treatment. Often they burst, causing serious bleeding into the fluid surrounding the brain (**subarachnoid haemorrhage**).

POSSIBLE CAUSES

Aneurysms commonly occur in the main artery of the body (the aorta). These are usually due to **atherosclerosis**, but may be due to late syphilis or to **Marfan's syndrome**.

RECOGNITION AND SYMPTOMS

The increasing swelling of an aneurysm of the aorta may press on and painfully erode the spine or may cause cough, loss of voice, and difficulty in swallowing and sometimes breathing. The wall of the artery may split and blood may be forced progressively between the layers. This is called a dissecting aneurysm.

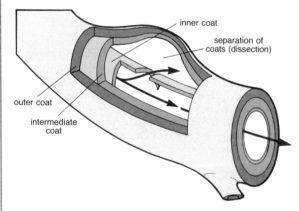

inner coat

separation of coats (dissection)

outer coat

intermediate coat

The formation of a dissecting aneurysm in an artery. Blood passes through a diseased part of the inner coat to gain access to the plane between the inner and the intermediate coat. The blood pressure forces more and more blood between the layers so that the separation tends to increase steadily.

TREATMENT

Aortic aneurysms are treated by replacing the affected segment of the artery with a graft of woven teflon or other material. Treatment of subarachnoid berry aneurysms is very difficult but they may sometimes be closed by inserting a piece of muscle so that the blood clots within them.

Anexate

A brand name for **flumazenil**.

Angel dust

A slang term for the powerful analgesic and anaesthetic phencyclidine commonly abused for recreational purposes. It is also known by the abbreviation PCP. Abuse of this drug can lead to muscle rigidity, convulsions and death.

anger

Anger is a common emotion and a major cause of unhappiness.

It has enormous individual, social and political implications. Marriages are turned to misery, wives are battered, old people mugged. Violence in the streets and in the home is, almost always, a manifestation of anger.

Anger starts with the perception of a wrong and is concerned with attempts to put it right. The perception is, of course, a very individual one, and is likely to be at odds with other people's perception of the same situation. This perception leads to the antagonistic ideas directed at the person or persons supposedly responsible for the wrong and the desire to destroy or immobilize them. A feature of this mental process is *labelling* – the uncritical identification of whole classes of people as having common and hated characteristics – the yuppies, the Trades Unions, the pro-life faction, the pro-choice faction, the Jews, the rich, the Pakis, the National Front. Anger limits clear thinking and leads to impulsive action, which is often regretted. It may give an illusory sense of being in control of a situation and lead to action which makes things worse.

People prone to anger are often people literally looking for trouble. They are very much concerned with their perception of other people's attitudes to them, take everything personally, have an often quite unrealistic idea of what the world ought to be like and feel themselves entitled to try to change it. Many such people anticipate or assume that encounters will be hostile, attributing aggressive attitudes to others. They enjoy working out punishments for others and justify themselves by dehumanizing the enemy.

> It is seldom appreciated that it is not the perceived event or apparent external stimulus that causes anger, but the nature of the perception itself – the way the person interprets what is happening to him or her. The 'internal speech' of the anger-prone is full of violent dialogue, self-justifying value judgements, and imagined successful put-downs.

RECOGNITION AND SYMPTOMS

Anger does not necessarily lead to physical aggression against others. It may be manifested by verbal abuse, by violent action against the self, dangerously risky behaviour often in a car, repression and building up of resentment, cutting off from any form of communication, running away, vandalizing property, withdrawing into apathy, overeating. Anger has important bodily effects which may be short and sharp (acute) or slow and persistent (chronic). These involve the production of adrenaline and cortisol by the adrenal glands, leading to a fast heart rate, a sense of excitement, muscle tension and other natural prerequisites for violent action. Unfortunately, some people come to enjoy these effects and learn to organize their lives to experience these 'highs' regularly.

TREATMENT

Anger-control treatment is difficult and requires the full cooperation of the subject. Predictably, few are willing to recognize that they have a problem that requires treatment and submit to it. But when anger has led to behaviour that even the aggressor recognizes as socially unacceptable, treatment is sometimes welcomed. It is a form of behavioural therapy and makes much use of acted role-playing techniques. It starts with an educational stage in which the subject is made to look critically at anger, to understand its functions and effects, to distinguish between the emotion of anger and its outward manifestations, and to recognize the kind of behaviour patterns that lead to escalation. The next stage involves learning how to analyse thoughts and feelings and identify common logical fallacies, how to deal with personal relationships and how to achieve more effective communication. The final stage is to discover, first by role-play and then in real life, how effectively these lessons have been learnt.

See also **aggression**, **violence in the home**.

angiitis

Inflammation of a blood vessel. Angiitis obliterans is one of the most serious forms. The inner layer of the artery thickens and obstruction occurs, which may lead to **gangrene**. This condition is caused by smoking, which is, incidentally, often persisted in even after both legs have been amputated.

angina pectoris

Angina is the Latin word for 'sore throat' and still persists in that sense in the name **Ludwig's angina** (an infection of the floor of the mouth). The term is now, however, used almost exclusively to refer to the severe symptom of pain in the centre of the chest which occurs when the heart is called on to do more work than the blood supply, via the coronary arteries, can support.

RECOGNITION

The pain is severe, frightening and often spreads up the neck and down the arms. It is predictably related to a given amount of exertion and comes on earlier in cold weather or after a heavy meal.

POSSIBLE CAUSE

The inadequacy of coronary blood supply is almost always caused by **atherosclerosis** of the coronary arteries – a condition which kills more people than all other diseases put together.

The pain of angina pectoris shows characteristic radiation up into the neck and jaw, through to the back and down both arms.

TREATMENT

Angina is relieved by resting or by drugs, such as nitroglycerine, which temporarily widen (dilate) the coronary arteries.

See also **heart attack**.

angiogenesis inhibitors

Substances which block the development of new blood vessels (angiogenesis) and show promise as anticancer drugs. Cancers cannot grow beyond microscopic size unless they develop new blood vessels. If this is prevented they will regress or remain dormant and harmless. Research has shown that the angiogenesis inhibitors endostatin and angiostatin are capable of eliminating cancers of the breast, colon, prostate and brain in mice and can do so without undesirable side-effects in the short term. These two drugs act in different ways and research on humans with cancer was started in mid-1998. The drugs are believed not to induce drug resistance in mice.

angiography

A special form of X-ray examination which renders the blood clearly visible in arteries and veins into which a solution opaque to X-rays has been injected (contrast medium). Angiography is much more important for arteries than for veins. Angiography does not show the vessels themselves, but outlines the shape of the blood column and this can be very revealing. Angiography shows narrowing, irregularity and obliteration of blood vessels. It detects any diseases that change the appearance of the blood vessel channel – diseases such as atherosclerosis, which causes fatty plaques to be deposited in the lining and narrow the vessel, thrombosis or embolism, which can block vessels, or weakening of the blood vessel wall with ballooning of the vessel itself (aneurysm). Angiography can also detect the development of clumps of new vessels and other abnormal patterns that suggest tumours or injury to organs.

Angiography is especially important in investigating the state of the arteries supplying the brain, the presence of abnormal arteries in and around the brain and, most of all, the state of the coronary arteries of the heart. In this case it is used to identify the sites of narrowing or blockage in arteries, so that these may be treated by balloon angioplasty or, if necessary, by a coronary artery bypass operation.

Angiography involves the insertion of a fine soft tube, called a catheter, into the blood vessel concerned. This is done under local anesthesia and the catheter is inserted either at the front of the elbow, for investigation of the neck arteries (carotid angiogram), or in the groin for a coronary angiogram. A long thin guide wire with a smooth rounded tip is first inserted and is guided, under X-ray control using a fluorescent screen or a TV image intensifier, into the vessel to be examined. When the wire is in place the catheter is slipped over it and pushed along until its tip is in the right position. The wire is now removed and the contrast fluid injected into the catheter. The image can be viewed on the screen and a video film can be made from this. Alternatively, a rapid sequence of X-ray pictures may be taken and the flow along the vessel studied by comparing these.

The solutions used are oily liquids containing iodine and rarely cause any harm unless there is pre-existing allergy to any of the constituents, from previous angiography or other exposure. Modern contrast media are safer than earlier products and the risks of allergic reactions are now small. There is a sensation of warmth when the solution is injected, felt most strongly in the area being examined.

See also **digital subtraction angiography**.

angioma

A benign (non-malignant) tumour of blood vessels.

See **haemangioma**.

angioneurotic oedema

A form of **allergy**, mostly affecting young adults, in which an insect sting or contact with certain foodstuffs, plants, drugs or pollens causes severe swelling of the lining of the nose, mouth, throat or digestive tract. These swellings are caused by a considerable accumulation of fluid in the tissues and may persist for hours or even days.

> The main danger arises when angioneurotic oedema affects the voice box (larynx). In this case the swelling can rapidly lead to complete closure of the airway, a desperate emergency often ending in death.

TREATMENT

Doctors treat danger of this sort – the closure of the airway – with massive doses of corticosteroid drugs, or with **adrenaline**. In cases in which obstruction is threatening the airway, the only hope of saving life may be a **tracheostomy** in which a cut is made through the skin and into the wind pipe (trachea) just below the Adam's apple, to allow the affected person to breathe.

Angiopine MR

A brand name for **nifedipine**.

angioplasty

A surgical procedure for opening up an artery to promote the normal flow of blood to an important part, such as the heart muscle or the brain. Various methods can be used. A common technique is *balloon angioplasty* using a fine tube, the end of which can be inflated so as to stretch the narrowed artery. This is often done in cases of coronary artery insufficiency and is surprisingly effective. Increasingly, lasers are being used, via fibre optic channels, to clear partially or wholly obstructed arteries.

See also **balloon, catheter**.

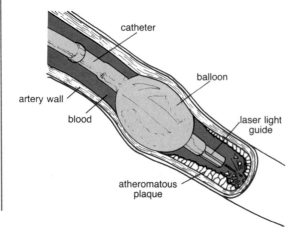

catheter

balloon

artery wall

blood

laser light guide

atheromatous plaque

angiospasm

The temporary closure or partial closure of an artery as a result of contraction of the circularly placed muscle in its wall. The early part of a true migraine attack, in which various brain functions such as vision or sensation are temporarily disturbed, is due to angiospasm.

See also **Raynaud's disease**.

angiotensin converting enzyme inhibitors

The name of this group is a real mouthful, so they are usually known as the ACE inhibitors. The kidneys produce a chemical activator (enzyme) called renin. This cuts off a piece of protein called angiotensin I from a larger blood protein. Angiotensin I doesn't do very much, but there is another enzyme in the blood called the angiotensin converting enzyme (ACE), and this converts angiotensin I to the powerfully active angiotensin II. Angiotensin II causes arteries to narrow and this raises the blood pressure. An inhibitor is something that stops something else from acting. So ACE inhibitors prevent ACE from turning the harmless angiotensin I into the active angiotensin II. They thus lower blood pressure and improve blood flow. These drugs are valuable in the management of high blood pressure and certain forms of heart failure.

ACE inhibitors include captopril (Acepril, Acezide, Capoten, Capozide) and enalapril (Vasotec, Innovace, Innozide). About 10 per cent of people taking these drugs get skin rashes and some suffer disturbances of taste sensation. Minor kidney damage can occur. About one person in 300 suffers interference with white blood cell production. In rare cases this may be very severe.

angiotensin II receptor antagonists

A new class of drugs for the treatment of high blood pressure that function by directly antagonizing the artery-constricting hormone angiotensin II at its receptor sites on smooth muscles in arterial walls. The group includes such drugs as losartan (Cozaar), candesartan (Amias), irbesartan (Aprovel) and valsartan (Diovan).

Angitil SR

A brand name for **diltiazem**.

anhidrotic

Tending to cause absence of sweating. The term is also applied to any drug or skin application which reduces or prevents sweating.

anima

Latin root meaning 'breath' as in animal (of living organisms other than plants).

animals, grafts from

See **xenograft**.

An advanced type of angioplasty catheter incorporating both a balloon and a laser light guide. The laser is used to break up atheromatous plaques obstructing the artery. The method has not yet been fully developed.

aniridia

Absence of the iris of the eye. This may be present at birth (congenital) or, more commonly, the result of injury.

anisometropia

Anisometropia is the condition in which the focus (refraction) is different in the two eyes. One eye may be normal and the other short-sighted (myopic) or long-sighted (hypermetropic), or one eye may be astigmatic (see **astigmatism**).

RECOGNITION

Anisometropia is a common cause of visual discomfort because, although eyeglasses may give clear vision in each eye, the images on the retinas will be of different sizes.

TREATMENT

There is no entirely satisfactory remedy, but contact lenses minimize the effect. Experienced optometrists will often deliberately avoid prescribing full correction in such cases, because comfort is usually to be preferred to maximal visual acuity.

A young person with one eye moderately short-sighted and the other normal or long-sighted should *not* wear glasses and should be encouraged to use one eye for close work and the other for distance. Life-long ocular contentment, without glasses, may thus be obtained.

anistreplase

A clot-dissolving drug used to try to re-establish blood flow in the heart muscle in the early treatment of heart attacks. A brand name is Eminase.

ankylosing spondylitis

A long-term (chronic) disease of the spinal column affecting mainly young adult males. Persistent inflammation of the ligaments of the spine and changes in the bones gradually lead to a stiffening and fixity so that, eventually, almost all movement is lost. The condition affects people of a particular tissue type HLA-B27 and there is a strong hereditary tendency. It is also commonly associated with an eye disorder (uveitis) in which the focusing muscle becomes inflamed.

ankylosis

Fixation of a joint by disease which has so damaged the bearing surfaces that the bone ends have been able to fuse permanently together. Sometimes ankylosis is deliberately performed, as a surgical procedure, to relief severe pain in the joint. It can be very disabling.

anodyne

Pain-relieving or relaxing. Also, a drug or other agency that relieves pain.

annexin

One of a family of over 20 **proteins** that act as binding agents for chemical molecules and were first described in 1990. They include blood vessel anticoagulant proteins, placental proteins, placental anticoagulant proteins, and other protein substances. All annexins have similar structures, usually with four domains, each of 70 **amino acids**, and all are capable of binding calcium and phospholipids (compounds of fats and phosphorus important constituents of cell membranes).

Annexins are present in a wide variety of cell types. Annexin II acts to bind plasminogen and tissue plasminogen activator to the surface of cells that line blood vessels and other structures (endothelial cells). Annexin V forms an anti-clotting shield around phospholipids that would otherwise promote blood clotting (procoagulant phospholipids).

annexinopathies

Diseases caused by abnormalities in **annexins**. An abnormally high level of Annexin II, for instance, causes a bleeding disorder with excessive breakdown of the fibrin that forms the main part of the clot (fibrinolysis). Annexin V deficiency causes accelerated blood clotting in the antiphospholipid syndrome.

See **Hughes' syndrome**.

anomaly

Anything differing from the normal.

anopheles

An important family (genus) of mosquito which transmits **malaria** from person to person when feeding on blood.

anorectic drugs

Drugs that suppress appetite and may be useful in the management of obesity. They include **amphetamine** and its derivatives, diethylpropion (Tenuate), mazindol (Teronc), phentermine (Duromine) and fenfluramine (Ponderax). These drugs have lost status since it became apparent that addiction is possible and that fenfluramine and phentermine can cause valvular heart disease.

anorexia nervosa

Anorexia simply means 'loss of appetite', something experienced by most people from time to time. But anorexia nervosa is a serious disorder of perception causing the sufferer, usually female although increasingly found in males, to believe that she is too fat, when, in fact, she may be very thin. Severe emaciation results.

INCIDENCE

Anorexia nervosa is common among those who are much concerned with the appearance of their bodies. In a minority of cases it is a symptom of a serious underlying psychiatric disorder such as severe depression or schizophrenia.

POSSIBLE CAUSES

The cause of anorexia is still a matter of debate. Many anorexics come from close-knit families, and have a particularly intimate relationship with one parent. They are often obsessional in their habits. They usually anxious to please. Some seem unwilling to grow up and appear to be trying to retain their childhood shape. Others seem to have a genuine fatness phobia with fear of eating fats or carbohydrates. It has been suggested that the disease is due to a disorder in the part of the mid-brain concerned with the linkage between the emotions and the nervous system and with such functions as hunger, thirst and sexual activity (the hypothalamus).

Social factors are probably contributory, especially the arbitrary identification of slimness with sexual attractiveness. Such influences may be powerful on girls who are deeply concerned with the effect they have on others.

RECOGNITION AND SYMPTOMS

Medically, the effects of anorexia nervosa are obvious. If calorie input is less than the energy and structural replacement needs, first the fat stores are used up and then the muscles are used for fuel. In anorexia there is extreme thinness with loss of a third or more of the body weight. There is, inevitably, extreme tiredness and weakness, and often the effects of vitamin deficiency. The skin becomes dry and the hair falls out. Early in the process there is, in almost all cases, absence of menstruation. Death from starvation, or suicide, is by no means uncommon.

TREATMENT

Anorexia nervosa demands skilled treatment in hospital under the care of those experienced in the condition. Personality problems, and the persistence of the disorder can make treatment difficult. Management depends on psychotherapy and imposed re-feeding but patients will usually make every effort to circumvent treatment, holding food in their mouths until it can be disposed of. Strict control is essential. Unless a watch is kept, food will be hidden or secretly thrown away. Often a system of rewards may be effective, in which privileges, such as visits or relative freedom, are awarded for weight gained.

Antidepressant drugs are often helpful in the early stages. Even after normal weight has been regained, girls who have had anorexia nervosa may need to remain under psychiatric care for months or years. Relapses are common and, tragically, up to 10 per cent later die from suicide or starvation.

anosmia

Loss of the sense of smell. This may occur from head injury with damage to the twigs of the nerve relating to smell (olfactory nerve) which pass down through a pair of perforated bone plates in the roof of the nose.

anovulation

Failure of the ovaries to produce normal eggs so that conception is impossible. This may result from hormonal or other disease or from natural states such as pregnancy and lactation (milk production). Anovulation is also caused by oral contraceptives.

anoxia

Local absence of oxygen, usually as a result of interference with the blood supply. This is a very serious matter as it leads, within minutes, to death of the tissues. Complete anoxia is rare, the more usual problem being a relative insufficiency, which is known as *hypoxia*.

Anquil

A brand name for **benperidol**.

Antabuse

A brand name for **disulfiram**.

antacid drugs

Drugs that reduce or neutralize excess acid in your stomach and relieve the symptoms of heartburn. Heartburn is the result of acid being pushed up from the stomach into the gullet. This is called acid reflux.

Stomach and duodenal ulcers (open sores in the inner lining) are grouped together as peptic ulcers. These are caused by the action of stomach acid and the digestive protein-splitting enzyme, pepsin, on the inner lining. Pepsin only works in the presence of acid. Your stomach lining is normally protected by a layer of mucus, produced by many cells in the lining. Any defect in this mucous layer allows the pepsin to start digesting the wall. Smoking and the over-use of irritating drugs like strong alcohol, aspirin and Brufen are among the causes of a defect in the protective mucus layer. The more acid present the more likely are you to start digesting yourself.

The part of the bowel immediately beyond your stomach is called the duodenum. This contains alkaline secretions which can neutralize normal quantities of stomach acid. So duodenal ulcers only occur if there is excess of acid and pepsin. If the acid levels can be kept low enough neither stomach nor duodenal ulcers will occur. This can be done in two ways – by preventing the acid from being produced by the use of drugs such as cimetidine or ranitidine, or by chemically neutralising the acid once it has been produced. The drugs which do the latter are called antacids.

The most popular and cheapest antacid is the alkali baking soda (sodium bicarbonate). This acts quickly and gives you rapid relief of pain. Unfortunately, the acid acts on the bicarbonate to produce volumes of carbon dioxide gas, and much belching results. The bicarbonate is also absorbed into your blood and too much of it can make your blood alkaline – which can be serious. Other antacids include magnesium oxide, magnesium hydroxide and magnesium trisilicate. These are not absorbed, but the first two act as purgatives. Magnesium trisilicate works more slowly than the oxides and you need quite large doses, but in addition to neutralizing the acid, it also inactivates the pepsin and is fairly effective. Aluminium hydroxide (Aludrox) also binds the pepsin and neutralises the acid. It, too, must be taken in large dosage for full effect. Antacids may also provide a protective coating to the lining of the stomach and duodenum.

Like the rest of the stomach contents, antacids are quickly passed out of the stomach. About half has gone in half an hour. So it is not really satisfactory to take them only when pain is felt – as most people do. Of course, the management of dyspepsia and peptic ulcers involves more than just the use of antacids. Self-treatment is not always safe.

H2 RECEPTOR ANTAGONISTS

Histamine is a powerful and important hormone found in most of your body tissues in inactivated form, mainly in cells called mast cells. Histamine is released when cells are injured, either physically or as a result of an allergic reaction. It affects other cells by way of cell receptors and has various actions. It causes the muscle in the walls of the air tubes of the lungs to tighten, it causes arteries to widen, small blood vessels (capillaries) to leak, skin to itch and the lining of the stomach to secrete acid. There are two kinds of histamine receptors – H1 and H2. H1 receptor antagonists block the effects of histamine produced as a result of allergic or other reactions and are called antihistamine drugs. The H2 receptor antagonists operate mainly in the stomach lining and to a lesser extent in the walls of the arteries.

A group of drugs known as the H2 receptor antagonists has revolutionized the treatment of stomach and duodenal ulcers. These drugs act by blocking action of histamine on the H2 receptors and thus cutting down the secretion of acid.

This important class of drugs includes cimetidine (Tagamet, Algitec, Dyspamet, Galenamet) and ranitidine (Zantac). These drugs have made a fortune for the manufacturers. They are so effective that doctors have to be very careful to ensure a correct diagnosis before using them as they can actually, for a time, relieve the symptoms of cancer of the stomach. They do not, of course, have any effect on the growth of cancer, and what may seem like successful treatment may lead to dangerous delay.

The H2 receptor antagonists are also valuable in the management of heartburn, stress ulcers in people with severe burns and the Zollinger-Ellison syndrome. This is a condition caused by a hormone-secreting tumour of the pancreas, known as a gastrinoma. This tumour produces large quantities of the hormone gastrin, which powerfully stimulates acid production in the stomach. The result is a massive outpouring of stomach acid, inevitably leading to severe ulceration of the stomach and duodenum (peptic ulceration).

The H2 receptor antagonists have few side-effects, apart from the possible concealment of stomach cancer, and these are minor. They include diarrhoea or constipation, tiredness, headache, muscle pain, and slowing of the heart. Cimetidine is mildly antagonistic to the male sex hormones and may cause enlargement of the breasts in men and, possibly, impotence. Ranitidine does not have this effect.

There is increasing evidence that the organism *Helicobacter pylori*, which is found in the bowels of a high proportion of people suffering from peptic ulceration, has a significant role to play in the causation of duodenal ulcer. Destruction of this organism with bismuth in association with amoxycillin and metronidazole is usually followed by healing of ulcers. Bismuth causes these organisms to detach from the bowel lining. The use of these drugs, especially bismuth, appears to be capable of preventing recurrence. However, bismuth can turn the inside of your mouth black, and, like iron, can also cause black faeces. Don't forget, however, that this can be caused by bleeding from the stomach.

The H2 receptor antagonists have few side-effects. Ranitidine is especially free from adverse effects.

See also **proton pump inhibitor drugs**.

antagonist drug

Any drug that opposes the action of another drug or of a natural body substance such as a hormone.

antazoline

An antihistamine drug that also has weak local anaesthetic and **anticholinergic** effects. A brand name is Otrivine-Antistin.

ante-

Prefix meaning 'before' or 'in front of' as in antepartum (before birth).

ante mortem

A term meaning before death.

ante partum

A term denoting a period of time before a baby is delivered.

anterior

An anatomical term meaning at or towards the front of the body. Contrast with *posterior* meaning 'at the back'.

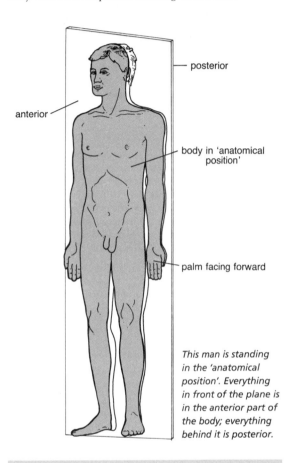

posterior

anterior

body in 'anatomical position'

palm facing forward

This man is standing in the 'anatomical position'. Everything in front of the plane is in the anterior part of the body; everything behind it is posterior.

anthelmintic drugs

Drugs used to rid the body of parasitic worms. Different kinds of drugs are used to kill or paralyse different worms and it is important to identify the type of worm before starting treatment. Paralysed worms let go of the lining of the bowel, or the tissues, and either pass out with the faeces or may, if necessary, be removed surgically from tissues. Sometimes a laxative is given with the drug to help evacuate intestinal worms.

Commonly used anthelmintic drugs include piperazine (Pripsen) for roundworms and threadworms; tetrachloroethylene or thiabendazole (Mintezol) for hookworms; niclosamide or praziquantel for tapeworms; niridazole or metronidazole (Flagyl) for guinea worm; diethylcarbamazine for filariasis; praziquantel for schistosomiasis; mebendazole (Vermox) for whipworm; and diethylcarbamazine (Banocide) or thiabendazole (Mintezol) for toxocariasis (larva migrans).

Most anthelmintic drugs can cause abdominal discomfort, nausea and vomiting. Metronidazole is remarkably free from side-effects, but long-term treatment can sometimes cause nerve problems. It reacts badly with alcohol to cause severe symptoms similar to those caused by Antabuse. From the Greek anti, against and elmins, a worm.

anthracosis

A chronic lung disease resulting from long exposure to coal dust. It can affect miners and others exposed, without adequate protection, to high levels of fine coal dust in the inspired air. Inflammation of tissues with extensive fibrous tissue formation leads to a reduction in the lung function and sometimes severe disability.

anthraquinone glycosides

An anti-inflammatory group of drug used in the treatment of mouth ulcers. A brand name is Pyralvex.

anthrax

A serious infection of the skin, intestine or lungs caused by spores from infected animals or animal products. Anthrax causes large and damaging skin boils, severe **gastroenteritis** and an often fatal **pneumonia**. Because the spores are so resistant to destruction and can cause such serious effects, anthrax has been proposed as a bacteriological weapon. The island of Gruinard off the north-west of Scotland was rendered uninhabitable for years after military trials of anthrax.

anti-

Prefix meaning 'against' as in antibiotic organisms (against living).

anti-abortion drug

See **hydroxyprogesterone hexanoate**.

anti-amoebic drugs

Drugs able to destroy or suppress amoebae of medical importance, especially the amoeba that causes amoebic dysentery, include emetine, metronidazole (Flagyl), tinidazole (Fasigyn) and chloroquine (Aclochlor, Nivaquine).

anti-androgen drugs

A group of drugs given in rare circumstances to sexually criminal men to dampen down their urges by interfering with the action of their male sex hormones. Anti-androgen drugs are also used in cases of cancer of the prostate gland. The group include cyproterone acetate (Androcur, Cyprostat), cimetidine (Tagamet) and spironolactone. Antiandrogen drugs may cause breast enlargement (gynaecomastia).

anti-angiogenic drugs

A group of currently experimental anticancer drugs that act by inhibiting the growth of the small blood vessels on which cancers depend for their growth. The group includes angiostatin, endostatin, thalidomide, squalamine, 2-methoxy-oestradiol, vitaxin and marimastat.

anti-anxiety drugs

You can't really separate severe anxiety from the physical effects that are associated with it – muscle tension, tremor, sweating and a fast heart rate. Some scientists even believe that these symptoms are actually the cause of the anxiety, rather than the effect. Certainly, any drug which controls these symptoms will relieve the level of anxiety and may even temporarily abolish it. Anti-anxiety drugs, often rather fancifully called 'anxiolytics' are, in general, minor sedatives and tranquillizers that relax muscles and slow the heart. They include beta-blockers, such as propranolol (Inderal, Betadur) and oxprenolol, and **benzodiazepine drugs**, such as diazepam (Valium) and chlordiazepoxide (Librium). **Barbiturates** are seldom used nowadays.

Anti-anxiety drugs, although useful, are not, of course, the definitive treatment for anxiety. For this, you need help to study the life problems and reactions underlying the anxiety and the benefit of the skilled counselling and advice of a wise psychotherapist. Some forms of anxiety, especially those associated with phobias, are probably best treated by behaviour therapy.

Like any other sedatives, the anti-anxiety drugs are liable to increase the effects of alcohol.

anti-arrhythmia drugs

Drugs used to control irregularities of the heartbeat. They include digitalis and quinidine, which have been in use for many decades, procainamide, **beta-blocker drugs**, **calcium channel blocker drugs** and disopyramide. These drugs act in different ways to convert irregular and inefficient contractions into steady, slower and more forceful beats, thereby improving the pumping efficiency of the heart.

antibiotic drugs

This is one of the largest groups of drugs and one of the best known. It is impossible to compute the benefits conferred on humanity by the antibiotics. Sixty years ago, medicine was dominated by bacterial infection, which was the major cause of death and was responsible for an immense amount of suffering, long-term ill-health and disability. Parents would listen with alarm to their children's coughing or contemplate with terror red streaks running up the arm from a septic area. Enlarged lymph nodes ('glands') could be a prelude to blood poisoning (septicaemia). Compound fractures of limbs often led to amputation. A squeezed pustule on the nose might cause a spreading fatal infection into the brain. Lobar pneumonia was commonplace and often fatal, and osteomyelitis (bone marrow infection) caused discharging channels (sinuses) for years. Tuberculosis sanitoria were full of people coughing up blood and sputum.

All that has changed and most people alive today have no concept of a world without antibiotics. These drugs kill germs (micro-organisms) in the body, or prevent their growth or reproduction. As a result, almost all diseases caused by infecting bacteria can now be cured by antibiotics. You should appreciate, however, that antibiotics have no effect on viruses. Antibiotics were originally derived from cultures of living organisms, such as fungi or bacteria, but, today, many can be chemically synthesized.

There are many antibiotics and the multiplication of official and brand names is bewildering, but they fall into groups, and the members of each group are related chemically, or by derivation, to each other. These groups are:

- penicillins (penicillin G, penicillin V, cloxacillin, flucloxacillin and many others);
- cephalosporins (cephaloridin, cephalothin, cefuroxime and many others);
- aminoglycosides (gentamicin, streptomycin, tobramycin, netilmicin, amikacin, neomycin and framycetin);

- tetracyclines (tetracycline, chlortetracycline – aureomycin, methacycline, oxytetracycline – terramycin and others);
- imidazoles (metronidazole – flagyl, ketoconazole, miconazole, nimorazole, mebendazole and thiabendazole).

In addition to these, there are other individual antibiotics such as chloramphenicol, erythromycin, lincomycin, clindamycin and spectinomycin.

Bacteriologists and others commonly criticize the way some doctors use antibiotics. There is some justification for the view that occasionally doctors prescribe them needlessly or for trivial infections. Sometimes, this misuse stems from pressure from patients who demand antibiotics. Sometimes it occurs because busy doctors feel they can't take chances with infections that might become serious, but which they do not have time to investigate as thoroughly as they might. Some hospital doctors, more concerned with the immediate pressing needs of their patients than with the possible future hazards to society as a whole, do sometimes prescribe powerful new drugs when safer, established, remedies would suffice. The two essential problems are the development of strains of bacteria resistant to antibiotics and the risk of undesirable side-effects.

If antibiotics are used casually and in inadequate dosage – and this is not always the doctor's fault – the bacteria which are most sensitive to the drug will be killed while those which happen to have a natural genetic resistance will survive. When the latter reproduce, new strains of resistant organisms result. This process of natural selection is accelerated by the brevity of the bacterial generation – only about 20 minutes in ideal conditions. As a result of this process many organisms are now resistant to antibiotics that formerly were effective against them. This has put heavy pressures on research workers to produce new antibiotics and keep ahead. So today, we have an on-going race between the development of resistance in bacteria, on the one hand, and the development of new antibiotics, on the other. We should be grateful to the men and women of the pharmaceutical industry who, so far, have enabled us to keep ahead in the race. You will now appreciate that, ideally, antibiotics should be used only for serious, or potentially serious infections or to prevent dangerous conditions in specially susceptible people. If you are prescribed a course of antibiotics, you should take it completely and regularly.

Powerful antibiotics often produce undesirable side-effects. These include:

- allergies, especially to penicillin, which may be serious or even fatal;
- deafness, permanent ringing or hissing in the ears (tinnitus), kidney damage or interference with normal blood production (aminoglycoside antibiotics);
- permanent staining of teeth (tetracycline antibiotics, if given to young children);
- destruction of normal, health-giving body bacteria;
- over-growth of undesirable organisms such as the candida fungus that causes thrush;
- nausea, intestinal upset and diarrhoea;
- skin rashes.

It would be naive to suppose that infections have been conquered. Many people still die from infections, and none of these side-effects will deter doctors from giving what is often life-saving therapy.

antibiotic-resistant germ

See **MRSA**, **superbug**.

antibodies

Protective, Y-shaped proteins formed by the B cells (B lymphocytes) of the immune system. Each antibody is formed by two identical, mirror-image halves. A part of each antibody is of fixed chemical structure, specific for the whole antibody class, and a part is variable and is unique to the particular antibody. The variable part makes the antibody specific so that it will only bind to a particular **antigen**. The two arms of the Y are hinged to the upright and can bend a little to assist physically in binding.

Antibodies have a range of valuable functions:

- they can bind to more than one molecule of antigen of a particular type, causing them to clump together so that their movements about the body are restricted. This is called agglutination;
- they make bacteria far more susceptible to attack and ingestion by **phagocyte** cells of the immune system;
- they make bacteria more easily broken up by complement;
- they can stop viruses from getting into cells by binding onto their protein coat;
- they can bind to the whip-like propelling flagella of bacteria so as to paralyse them and prevent the bacteria from moving.

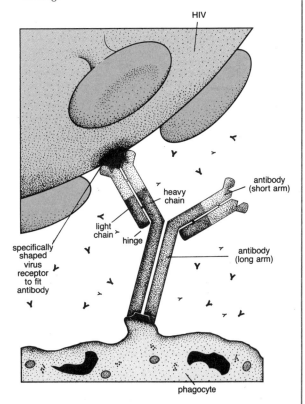

The antibody. This diagram shows how an antibody attaches to an invader which has surface features to match the antibody 'shape'. Unfortunately, in the case of HIV, natural antibodies do not have the normal neutralizing power.

cer drugs

Drugs used in the treatment of cancer. Most anticancer drugs are cytotoxic drugs – that is, drugs that destroy rapidly growing cells, but some are sex hormones or similar substances. Cytotoxic drugs are especially useful in the treatment of some forms of leukaemia, lymphomas, and cancers of the testicle and ovary. They are often used as an additional safeguard after surgery or in conjunction with radiotherapy. Cytotoxic drugs cause more damage to cancer cells than normal body cells. In most cases the drug can distinguish cancer cells from other cells by the speed with which cancer cells reproduce. Normal cells are restrained in their ability to multiply; cancer cells have lost some or all of this restraint. Cytotoxic drugs are most active against cells which are not restrained in this way. Unfortunately, the ability to distinguish between the two types is not complete and cytotoxic drugs cannot avoid causing some damage to normal cells. Consequently they always have major side-effects.

The more rapidly normal cells reproduce, the more likely they are to be damaged by cytotoxic drugs. For this reason, these drugs cause most damage to cells in the lining of the bowel, hair-producing cells, the sex glands and the blood forming tissue in the bone marrow. The typical side-effects thus include:

- nausea and vomiting;
- hair loss;
- sterility;
- anaemia and a tendency to bleeding.

People treated with these drugs always have a frequent check made of their red and white blood cell counts. Cytotoxic drugs include chlorambucil (Leukeran), cyclophosphamide (Endoxana), lomustine (CCNU), methotrexate (Maxtrex), vinblastine, vincristine, adriamycin, bleomycin and nitrogen mustard. All these substances tend to have side effects.

Some cancers are 'hormone dependent'. This means that certain hormones make them grow faster. Thus, some kinds of breast cancer are stimulated to grow by the female sex hormones known as oestrogens. This means that they can be discouraged from growing by male sex hormones – which oppose oestrogens – or by the drug tamoxifen which also has anti-oestrogenic properties. Paradoxically, the growth of some breast cancers, especially in elderly women, is discouraged by oestrogen hormones given in very high doses. In men, the common cancer of the prostate gland is male hormone dependent and can often be greatly diminished by treatment with a female sex hormone such as stilboestrol.

anticholesterol

See **hydroxymethyl glutaryl co-enzyme A reductase inhibitors**.

anticholinergic drugs

The autonomic nervous system is the collection of nerves concerned with the non-voluntary control of many body functions. The autonomic system has two generally opposing parts – the sympathetic, concerned with emergency situations (fright, fight and flight) and the parasympathetic, concerned with calm situations. Adrenaline is the sympathetic hormone and acetylcholine is the parasympathetic hormone. Acetylcholine is released at many nerve endings in the parasympathetic and has many effects. These include constriction of the pupils, contraction of the bladder wall, relaxation of controlling muscle rings (sphincters), the production of saliva, tears, sweat and respiratory secretions, slowing of the heart, narrowing of the air tubes and increasing the activity of the bowels. These acetylcholine effects are called 'cholinergic'. Anticholinergic drugs are drugs that block the receptors for acetylcholine. They have, of course, a considerable range of effects which you can work out for yourself. They cause a dry mouth, dry eyes, a dry, hot skin, widely-dilated pupils, a rapid heartbeat, relief of bowel colic and difficulty in emptying the bladder. The classic anticholinergic drug is belladonna (atropine).

Such atropine-like drugs are useful in drying up secretions prior to an operation, treating an unduly slow heart rate, and relieving the symptoms of **irritable bowel syndrome** and certain types of urinary incontinence. They are also used to treat **Parkinson's disease**, **asthma**, and **motion sickness**. Overdosage, in addition to the effects mentioned, also causes:

- difficulty in swallowing;
- retention of urine;
- blurred vision;
- anxiety;
- delirium;
- hallucinations;
- confusion and convulsions.

Apart from atropine itself, other anticholinergic drugs are hyoscine (Buscopan), scopolamine (the same as hyoscine), homatropine, banthine, propantheline (Pro-Banthine) and dibutoline.

anticoagulant drugs

Blood clotting is essential to prevent continuous loss of blood from wounds. But blood clotting within the blood vessels is very dangerous and is one of the main causes of death. Anticoagulant drugs reduce the normal tendency of blood to clot and can prevent clots forming in the circulation (thromboses). They can also prevent existing clots from getting bigger. They do not reduce the size of clots which have already formed. Anticoagulants work better in the veins than in the arteries and are most useful in the prevention and treatment of deep vein thrombosis. They are important in the prevention of clot formation on artificial heart valves or when an artificial kidney (dialysis machine) is in use. One of the most valuable uses of anticoagulant drugs is to prevent long, soft, snake-like clots forming in the deep leg veins of people immobilized after surgery or for other reasons. These loose clots are very dangerous as they can break off and be carried up through the heart to the lungs where they clog the main arteries carrying blood to the lungs. This is called pulmonary embolism and it is a common cause of death.

The most important anticoagulant drug is the body's own natural anticoagulant, heparin. This is still the most generally useful drug and is sold as Clexane, Fragmin, Hepsal, Minihep, Monoparin, etc. Heparin blocks the activity of various coagulation factors needed for the clotting of the blood. It must be given by injection at least every six hours and it begins to work within a few hours. Other anticoagulant drugs may be taken by mouth but are slow to take effect. Often these are started along with heparin, and the heparin injections stopped after three days. Oral anticoagulants include warfarin, nicoumalone, phenindione and the antiplatelet drugs protamine sulphate, dipyridamole and sulphinpyrazone.

Anticoagulant drugs must be used with great care and with constant monitoring of the blood-clotting tendency to avoid the risk of severe internal bleeding. Nevertheless, they have saved many lives. An important advance in this field is the availability of low molecular weight heparin. The side-effects of this form are less than those of the parent substance.

anticonvulsant drugs

These drugs are used to prevent epileptic seizures and must be taken continuously for long periods, usually twice a day. A single drug, rather than a combination, is usually preferred and the dose given is the least which achieves the objective. A second drug may have to be added if one fails to prevent attacks.

Anticonvulsant drugs are used in cases of established epilepsy, in certain cases of head injury in which there is a tendency to seizures, in the emergency treatment of a prolonged seizure and sometimes to prevent seizures in children with a history of fits during fevers (febrile seizures).

The choice of drug depends on the type of seizure and on the person's response. Most cases of epilepsy can be well controlled with one or other of the commonly used drugs. Phenobarbitone (Luminal), phenytoin (Dilantin), carbamazepine (Tegretol), and primidone (Mysoline) will control major fits ('grand mal') and the local twitching known as focal epilepsy. Phenobarbitone, ethosuximide (Zarontin), and methsuximide (Celontin) are effective in the repeated childhood 'switching-off' known as 'petit mal' or absence attacks. Valproic acid (Depakene) and clonazepam (Rivotril) are valuable in absence and partial seizures.

The doctor must carefully adjust the dosage to give the least necessary to prevent attacks. Sometimes a combination of two drugs gives better results than one alone. Overdosage, which can cause mental dullness, even stupefaction, must, of course, be avoided. When major attacks occur one after the other, diazepam (Valium) is given by injection until the seizures stop. This dangerous but fortunately rare complication is called status epilepticus.

anticytokine therapy

Treatment by interference with the function of **cytokines**. Tumour necrosis factor, for instance, is an inflammatory cytokine involved in the pathogenesis of **rheumatoid arthritis**. The use of a **tumour necrosis factor** antagonist has led to significant improvement in this disease.

antidepressant drugs

The treatment of **depression** involves more than just prescribing drugs, but effective treatments do exist and most affected people can be greatly helped, however severe their depression.

One of the basic facts about the nervous system is that messages (nerve impulses) are passed on from one nerve to another by means of a tiny quantity of a powerful chemical substance called a neurotransmitter. This substance floats across the gap between the two nerves and causes the second nerve to send on an impulse. There are many different neurotransmitters in the body, but among the most important are substances, similar to adrenaline, called monoamines. Depression is often caused by a shortage, or decreased effectiveness, of monoamines at the nerve endings. Too much monoamine and you get overactivity – causing elation, an exaggerated sense of well-being, even mania. Not enough, and you get black depression.

The drug **amphetamine**, or 'speed', causes a monoamine called noradrenaline, which is stored in nerve endings, to be released, speeding up mental action. In fact, amphetamine was once widely used to treat depression, until its undesirable side-effects, and the probability of its being abused, became widely known.

MONOAMINE OXIDASE INHIBITORS (MAOI)

Monoamines in the nerve endings are kept under control by a breaking-down chemical (enzyme) called monoamine oxidase. Drugs that interfere with the action of this enzyme are called monoamine oxidase inhibitors. These drugs are packaged for the treatment of depression under such names as Marplan, Marsilid, Nardil and Parnate. They are quite useful when depression is accompanied by much anxiety and phobias, but they, too, have some disadvantages and are not usually given as the first line of treatment. For instance, they interfere with the breakdown of the common monoamine (amino acid) tyramine that is found in cheese, chocolate, alcohol, yeast extracts such as Marmite, meat extracts and other foods. If you are taking monoamine oxidase inhibitors you must not eat any of these foods, because the result will be an abnormally high level of tyramine. This can dangerously raise your blood pressure.

TRICYCLIC ANTIDEPRESSANTS

When the monoamine neurotransmitters have triggered a new nerve impulse, they are not destroyed but drift away from the receptor sites and are then pumped back into their original nerve endings. This pumping action can be chemically blocked, so that more monoamine remains around – exactly what we need. The substances that do this are called tricyclic antidepressants, and this group contains the most valuable drugs for depression. They are marketed under names such as Anafranil, Aventyl, Domical, Evadyne, Lentizol, Saroten, Sinequan, Tofranil and Tryptizol. There are dozens more. It is essential for you to appreciate that all the tricyclics take from ten to fourteen days, sometimes longer, to have a worthwhile action. After that time, however, their effect may seem miraculous.

They do have side-effects, however, that you should know about. The tricyclics can cause:

- dryness of the mouth;
- difficulty with urination;
- delayed ejaculation in men;
- angle-closure glaucoma in susceptible people;
- difficulty in focusing the eyes.

They can also sometimes interfere with the action of the heart, can make epilepsy worse, and can interfere with the control of diabetes. Different members of the group have these effects to different degrees, so the doctor must choose carefully which to prescribe.

The most commonly prescribed antidepressant drugs are lithium (Camcolit), nortriptyline (Allegron), amoxapine (Asendis), citalopram (Cipramil), protriptyline

(Concordin), nefazodone (Dutonin), flupenthixol (Fluanxol), maprotiline (Ludiomil), tradozone (Molipaxin), fluphenazine (Motipress), phenelzine (Nardil), tranylcypromine (Parnate), dothiepin (Prothiaden), promazine (Sparine), thioridazine (Melleril), imipramine (Tofranil), perphenazine (Fentanyl), prochlorperazine (Stemetil), trifluoperazine (Stelazine), amitryptyline (Tryptizole), clomipramine (Anafranil), doxepin (Sinequan), isocarboxazid (Marplan), tranylcypromine (Parnate), fluoxetine (Prozac) and tryptophan (Optimax).

antidiabetic drugs

There are two kind of diabetes. Type I usually starts in childhood or adolescence and is due to destruction of the insulin-producing cells in the pancreas. Type II comes on later and is due to insufficient insulin production relative to needs. People with Type I diabetes are known as 'insulin-dependent' diabetics; those with Type II diabetes are 'non-insulin dependent', or 'maturity-onset' diabetics. Much of the food we eat is converted to the body fuel glucose (sugar). Diabetics cannot properly use this glucose and it accumulates in the blood and appears in the urine. Insulin allows muscle and other cells to use glucose normally. Too little insulin and the blood sugar level rises; too much, and it falls dangerously. The amount of insulin needed by insulin-dependent diabetics depends on the amount of food taken and the rate it is used up by exertion. The only way to be sure that the right amount of insulin is being taken is to check the blood sugar levels directly by means of a small machine.

Insulin used to be obtained from pigs and oxen, and much animal insulin is still used. But genetic engineering has now made it easy to produce genuine human insulin without involving animals at all. Human insulins, such as Humulin, are being increasingly used. Insulin has to be taken by injection and there are many preparations. Some have a quick and immediate effect, some have a more prolonged effect. Mixtures of different preparations of insulins are often used. There is a great deal more to the subject than this, and if you are a diabetic you will certainly know a great deal more than I can cover here. Diabetics cannot know too much about the condition.

Type II diabetes can often be controlled by diet alone, especially if the insulin supply is inadequate only because you are overweight. Often, however, it is necessary to go further and to take drugs of the group known as the oral hypoglycaemics. This just means that you take them by mouth and they reduce your blood sugar levels. There are two kinds of oral hypoglycaemics – the sulphonylureas and the biguanides. The sulphonureas, which include chlorpropamide and glibenclamide, act by stimulating the pancreas to produce more insulin. The biguanides are drugs such as metformin and phenformin. They work by interfering with the absorption of carbohydrates from the intestine, by reducing the production of glucose by the liver and by increasing the utilization of glucose fuel by the tissues. None of the oral hypoglycaemic drugs are any good if the pancreas is not producing any insulin. In such a case, the person concerned must have insulin injections.

antidiarrhoeal drugs

Diarrhoea nearly always serves the useful purpose of flushing out irritants from the bowel, such as infecting germs. So it is not a good idea to take a drug to check it as soon as it starts. In most cases, nature will solve the problem unaided, but if diarrhoea persists for more than two or three days, it usually needs to be treated.

Drugs to check diarrhoea may either be narcotics like codeine, which reduce the irritability of the bowel wall and cut down the rate of contraction of the bowel muscles, or substances, such as methyl cellulose or a high fibre diet, which increase the bulk and solidity of the bowel contents. Other substances, such as chalk, ispaghula husk or kaolin, can be useful. Narcotic preparations include codeine, diphenoxylate (Lomotil), loperamide (Imodium), kaolin and morphine mixture, and aromatic chalk and opium.

anti-D immunoglobulin

Human antibodies used in the management of rhesus incompatibility. A brand name is Partobulin.

antidote

A drug that neutralizes or counteracts the action or effect of a poison. There are few specific antidotes. These include naloxone for narcotic opiate poisoning, desferrioxamine for iron poisoning, cobalt edetate for cyanide poisoning, and methionine and n-acetylcysteine for paracetamol poisoning. Activated charcoal may be valuable to adsorb poisons.

All this means that for most cases of poisoning there are no antidotes, and valuable time can be wasted trying to find out about them. What is needed is professional help without delay.

anti-emetic drugs

Severe and prolonged nausea is very unpleasant. When combined with persistent vomiting it can be intolerable. Anti-emetic drugs are drugs used to relieve nausea and prevent vomiting from any cause. They are useful in the control of motion sickness, for nausea associated with various kinds of vertigo including the symptoms of Ménière's disease, and the nausea associated with medical treatment with anticancer drugs and other toxic drugs or sometimes with radiotherapy. They are valuable in the management of the nausea and vomiting of kidney failure (uraemia), widespread cancer, radiation sickness, and acute gastro-enteritis caused by viruses. Anti-emetic drugs can often be given by mouth, but if the vomiting is severe, they will have to be given by injection or by a rectal suppository.

Anti-emetic drugs should not be used to treat nausea and vomiting caused by a disease, when there is an effective remedy for the cause. The right thing to do in such a case is to treat the cause. Anti-emetic drugs are also best avoided when the cause of the vomiting is unknown as their use may conceal the cause and preclude proper treatment. They are seldom used in diseases of the intestines, for instance.

Antihistamine drugs, such as cyclizine, and **anticholinergic drugs**, such as hyoscine, can act as anti-emetics by dampening down nerve impulses from the balancing mechanisms in the inner ears. Other anti-emetics include atropine, chlorpromazine (Largactil), prochlorperazine (Stemetil), perphenazine (Fentazin), trifluoperazine (Stelazine), and ondansetron (Zofran).

antifibrinolysis

Blood clotting, which prevents bleeding, can be very important. Clots are formed mainly from a network of strands of a material called fibrin. This can sometimes be broken down so that the clot ceases to seal off a wound. Such breaking down of a clot is called fibrinolysis. Drugs that prevent the breakdown of fibrin are called antifibrinolytic drugs. The most important of these are aminocaproic acid and tranexamic acid (Cyklokapron).

These drugs are used to control undue bleeding after surgery or to prevent prolonged bleeding after dental extraction in haemophiliacs. They can, however, cause complications such as blood clotting in the kidney urine drainage tubes with possible blockage. There is a risk of thrombosis if they are used in conjunction with oral contraceptives.

anti-flu B vaccine

See **HIB vaccine**.

antifungal drugs

Drugs that act directly on the cell walls of the various fungi that infect the skin and, less commonly, the internal organs. Antifungal drugs may be applied directly to the skin or mucous membranes in the form of creams, lotions, solutions or powders, or may be taken by mouth. For very severe internal fungal infections, they may be given by injection.

Antifungal drugs are used to treat the various kinds of tinea – athlete's foot (tinea pedis), body 'ringworm' (tinea corporis), scalp tinea (tinea capitis) and jock itch (tinea cruris); they are used to control thrush (candidiasis), whether of the skin, the vagina, the mouth or the internal organs; and they are used to try to control a number of rare internal fungus infections, such as cryptococcosis or torulopsosis.

Local applications include clotrimazole (Canesten), miconazole, econazole and nystatin (Nystan). Major antifungal drugs, for internal use, include amphotericin (Fungilin), flucytosine (Alcobon) and griseofulvin (Grisovin).

Given by injection, the imidazole antifungal drugs are apt to cause vein irritation and local thrombosis. This route may also be associated with nausea, vomiting, fever and rashes. By mouth they cause little trouble, but may sometimes lead to nausea, vomiting, diarrhoea, skin itching and occasionally hepatitis. They should be stopped at once if the skin turns yellow (jaundice).

antigen

Any substance, organism or foreign material recognized by the immune system of the body as being 'non-self', and which will provoke the production of a specific **antibody**.

antihistamine drugs

Histamine is a powerful agent produced in the body by certain cells called *mast cells*, especially as an allergic response. It acts on small blood vessels, causing them to widen and allow the leakage of proteins so that these escape into the tissue fluid and cause swelling (oedema). The antihistamine group of drugs act against histamine and thus are useful in the treatment of many allergic conditions including hay fever (allergic rhinitis), asthma, urticaria, and other allergic rashes. They are commonly incorporated into cold and cough remedies because of their symptomatic effect and are valuable in the suppression of vomiting.

Side-effects are common with antihistamine drugs and include:

● sedation;
● sleepiness;
● loss of coordination;
● blurred vision;
● dizziness;
● loss of appetite;
● nausea;
● constipation;
● dry mouth and difficulty in passing urine;
● worsening of some kinds of glaucoma;
● rarely, tremor, nervousness and insomnia.

The list of antihistamines is long, but among the most important are chlorpheniramine (Piriton), terfenadine (Triludan), promethazine (Phenergan), mepyramine (Anthisan) cyproheptadine (Periactin), mequitazine (Primalan) and phenindamine (Thephorin).

anti-HIV drugs

See **HIV-protease inhibitor drugs**.

antihyperlipidaemia drugs

Drugs that reduce the levels of cholesterol and fats (triglycerides) in the blood. They include statin drugs such as **simvastatin**, **atorvastatin**, provastatin and **fluvastatin** that block the synthesis of cholesterol; bile acid sequestrants such as **cholestyramine** and **colestipol** that bind and remove from the intestine bile acids which are derived from cholesterol; fibrates such as **clofibrate**, **ciprofibrate**, benzafibrate and **gemfibrozil** that interfere with cholesterol synthesis; and nicotinic acid derivatives that interfere with the release of fats from body fat stores and increase the activity of fat-splitting enzymes.

antihypertensive drugs

Drugs used to control abnormally raised blood pressure (hypertension). They are important because untreated hypertension can lead to complications such as stroke, heart attack, heart failure and kidney damage. Unfortunately, high blood pressure produces obvious symptoms only when it is severe or has already reached a fairly advanced stage and has caused damage to the blood vessels and the heart. So it has to be looked for. Every adult should have regular blood pressure checks. Proper and effective treatment can largely eliminate the additional risk of these serious complications.

Three main classes of drugs are used to treat high blood pressure. The first, the **diuretic drugs**, act on the kidneys to cause them to pass more water and salt in the urine and reduce the volume of the blood, so bringing down the pressure. The second group, the **beta-blocker drugs**, interfere with the hormone and nervous control of the heart, slowing it and causing it to beat less forcefully, so reducing the pressure. The third group, the vasodilators, act on the arteries to widen them. This group contains drugs acting in quite different ways. They include the alpha blockers, the **calcium channel blocker drugs** and the **angiotensin-converting enzyme inhibitor drugs**.

The treatment of high blood pressure is not simply a matter of prescribing tablets. The doctor has difficult and complex decisions to make. Among others, he or she has to decide whether to use drugs at all. The body may have adapted to raised blood pressure, and reducing it may actually cause the person concerned to feel worse, rather than better. Until the body readjusts to normal pressures, there may be a sense of weakness and loss of energy, depression and a tendency to dizziness or faintness on standing up. The doctor aims to achieve control with the minimum dosage and will want to monitor the pressure regularly. Many other factors besides drugs are important in the treatment of high blood pressure. These include weight control, exercise and the avoidance of smoking.

anti-inflammatory drugs

Inflammation is the commonest effect of injury to body tissues. It occurs as a result of a wide range of injurious processes including mechanical injury, burns, radiation, infection and poisons. It is essentially a reaction of small blood vessels which widen in response to injury, giving rise to the principal features of inflammation. These are:

- redness;
- heat;
- pain;
- swelling;
- loss of function.

Inflammation is usually a protective reaction on the part of the body and it promotes effective action by the immune system and other bodily systems to combat the cause. It is not, therefore, always a good idea to combat inflammation. The correct order of procedure is to find the cause of the inflammation and, if possible, to eliminate it. There are, however, many circumstances in which inflammation, especially if unduly prolonged, does more harm than good (see **steroids**). In these cases the use of anti-inflammatory drugs may be justified. These drugs include the non-steroidal anti-inflammatory drugs (see **analgesic drugs**) and the steroid drugs.

antimetabolites

Anticancer, or cytotoxic, drugs which act by combining with essential enzymes within cancer cells so as to interfere with their growth. To be useful, antimetabolites must be significantly more toxic to cancer cells than to normal cells. See also **anticancer drugs**.

antimitotic drugs

See **anticancer drugs**.

antimonial drugs

Drugs containing antimony include sodium stibogluconate (Stibophen) and meglumine antimoniate. They are used to treat kala azar (leishmaniasis) but are rarely needed in the Western world.

anti-oestrogen drugs

Drugs that oppose the action of the female sex hormone oestrogen. The most important of these drugs is currently tamoxifen, which antagonizes the action of oestrogens at the tissue receptors. Anti-oestrogen drugs are used to assist in the treatment of breast cancer and to stimulate egg production (ovulation) in infertile women. Side-effects of anti-oestrogen drugs include hot flushes, itching of the vulva, nausea, vomiting, fluid retention and sometimes vaginal bleeding.

anti-oxidant, natural body

See **superoxide dismutase**.

anti-oxidants and vitamins

Much of the cell damage that occurs in disease is occasioned by highly destructive chemical groups known as **free radicals**. These can be combated by anti-oxidants. Fortunately, the body has its own anti-oxidants for damage limitation. One of the most effective of these is the substance tocopherol (vitamin E). This vitamin dissolves in fat and that is especially important because much of the most significant free radical damage in the body is damage to the membranes of cells and to low density lipoproteins and these are made of fat molecules. Vitamin C is also a powerful anti-oxidant, but is soluble in water, not in fat. This means, however, that it is distributed to all parts of the body. The two vitamins are both highly efficient at mopping up free radicals, and sometimes even cooperate in so doing, especially in their protective action on cell membranes.

Other natural body anti-oxidants include compounds such as cysteine, glutathione and D-penicillamine, and blood constituents such as the iron-containing molecule transferrin and the protein ceruloplasmin. These act either by preventing free radicals from being produced or by mopping them up. The body also contain a number of important anti-oxidant enzymes. The most interesting anti-oxidant enzyme is superoxide dismutase. The discovery of the function of this enzyme excited enormous interest, as it is exclusively to change the dangerous superoxide free radical to the safer hydrogen peroxide. The body has two other enzymes, catalase and glutathione peroxidase that break down hydrogen peroxide to water and oxygen.

Many large clinical trials have now shown that additional supplements of anti-oxidant vitamins – such as 2000 mg of C and 400 mg of E daily – can significantly reduce the incidence of heart attacks, strokes, cataracts and other diseases.

anti-oxidants from plants

See **flavonoids**.

anti-Parkinsonism drugs

Parkinsonism is a distressing disorder featuring tremor, poor muscle coordination, stiffness and difficulty in walking. So far there is no cure, but drugs used to control the effects include levodopa (Sinemet), amantadine (Symmetrel), bromocriptine (Parlodel) and selegilene (Eldepryl).

antiperspirants

Substances used to reduce the rate of sweating in certain areas of the body where the sweat glands produce sweat that is especially likely to cause body odour. The sweat glands that do this are called apocrine glands and occur mainly in the armpits (axillae) and groin. The sweat from apocrine glands contains not only salty water but also organic material derived from the glands themselves. This material is broken down by bacteria to form odorous substances.

Antiperspirants have an astringent action, narrowing or obstructing the outlet of the sweat glands. Used in excess they may cause skin irritation. Common antiperspirants are alum, aluminium chloride and aluminium chlorohydrate. They are often combined with perfumes.

antiphospholipid syndrome

See **Hughes' syndrome**.

antipruritic drugs

Substances that relieves itching. Calamine lotions or creams are safe and popular, but sometimes more powerful remedies are required, such as local anaesthetics or local antihistamine drugs. Both of these are liable to cause skin sensitisation and are not much approved of by dermatologists. Antihistamines are sometimes given by mouth for itching. Crotamiton (brand name – Eurax) is often prescribed.

antipsychotic drugs

Drugs used to treat the major mental illnesses such as the various forms of schizophrenia, manic depressive illness, mania and severe depression. They are also used to control the behaviour of people who are seriously agitated or aggressive. The drug treatment of psychosis has revolutionized psychiatry and has greatly reduced the number of people confined in mental hospitals.

The antipsychotic drugs include such groups as the benzamides (Amisulpride, Dolmatil, Solian); benzisoxzoles (Risperidal); butyrophenones (Anquil, Dozic, Droleptan, Haldol, Serenace); phenothiazines (Fentazin, Largactil, Melleril, Modecate, Moditen, Neulactil, Nozinan, Stelazine); and thioxanthines (Clopixol, Depixol).

These powerful drugs have side-effects, some of which are distressing. Most of them can cause:

- regular jerky movements of some part of the body (dyskinesia);
- lethargy;
- drowsiness;
- dryness of the mouth;
- blurred vision;
- difficulty in passing urine.

Lithium must be given in very carefully regulated dosage, and toxic effects are common. These include:

- tremor;
- staggering ;
- jerking of the eyes (nystagmus);
- difficulty in speaking;
- seizures.

antipyretic drugs

Drugs which lower raised body temperature. In fever, the body's thermostat is temporarily set at a higher then normal level, so you feel cold and shivering occurs to increase body heat to the required level. Antipyretic drugs work by resetting the thermostat to a normal level. The use of drugs for this purpose is now much less popular than it was prior to the introduction of antibiotics. Nowadays more attention is rightly devoted to removing the cause of the fever – usually infection. The commonest antipyretic drugs are acetylsalicylic acid (aspirin) for adults and paracetamol for children.

antirabies serum

Serum containing antibodies against rabies. It is used to try to prevent the development of the disease in those who have been bitten by a rabid animal. Antirabies serum is combined with the use of a vaccine, given in six injections on days 0, 3, 7, 14, 30 and 90 after the bite.

antirheumatic drugs

Rheumatism is a general term covering a number of joint disorders featuring inflammation, especially rheumatoid arthritis and osteoarthritis. Many drugs are used to treat rheumatism. Simple analgesic drugs are helpful in most cases but may be insufficient. The non-steroidal anti-inflammatory drugs (see **analgesic drugs**) are commonly used. Drugs such as paracetamol and the narcotic analgesic drugs may be useful in relieving pain, but have no anti-inflammatory action.

Rheumatoid arthritis and associated conditions are caused by a disorder of the body's immune system which leads it to attacks its own tissues. The most powerful antirheumatic drugs operate by interfering with the functioning of the immune system and these include the **steroids** and other **immunosuppressant drugs**. Rheumatoid arthritis is often treated with penicillamine (not to be confused with the **antibiotic drug** penicillin), gold, hydroxychloroquine and chloroquine.

All the major antirheumatic drugs may produce serious side-effects. These include:

- kidney damage (penicillamine and gold);
- loss of function of the central part of the retinas causing severe loss of vision (chloroquine);
- osteoporosis, reactivation of latent infections, reduced resistance to new infections (steroids).

Large-dosage steroids may also lead to severe shock in the event of injury or other major illness.

antiscorbutic

Tending to prevent, or able to cure, **scurvy**. The antiscorbutic substance is vitamin C (ascorbic acid).

antisense RNA

Ribonucleic acid molecules transcribed, not from **DNA** in the usual manner, but from DNA strands complementary to those that produce normal **messenger RNA**. Antisense RNA occurs in nature and acts to inhibit gene action. It can be produced synthetically and offers such therapeutic possibilities as turning off the genes of viruses so that they cannot reproduce.

antisepsis

The use of strong poisons to kill bacteria and other dangerous microorganisms. The English surgeon Joseph Lister (1827–1912) made modern surgery possible by introducing the carbolic spray to kill germs on the instruments, the skin of the patient and the hands of the operator. It soon became apparent, however, that a better method was to sterilize all instruments, cloths, etc., beforehand, so as to achieve an aseptic operating environment. Antisepsis thus became less important, but newer and less irritating antiseptics are still extensively used to clean skin and wounds and treat some persistent skin infections.

antrostomy

A surgical operation for **sinusitis**, in which an opening is made into one of the antrums (sinuses) around the nose so as to allow infected material to drain away.

antiseptics

Mildly antibacterial substances, usually applied to the skin in the form of solutions, to try to reduce the chances of infection. They are of limited value and are no substitute for thorough washing and cleansing. Alcohol, iodine, hexachlorophane (Phisohex), cetrimide (Cetavlon), allantoin and coal tar (Alphosyl), benzalkonium, thiomersal (Thimerosal) and hydrogen peroxide are among the many substances used as skin antiseptics.

antiserum

Animal blood serum, usually from a horse, which contains useful immunoglobulins (antibodies) to organisms with which the animal has been deliberately infected or to the toxins produced by these organisms (antitoxins). Such serum can be life-saving but can also cause severe reactions. It is usually given by injection into a muscle, and the danger of a severe allergic reaction (anaphylactic shock) is ever present in the mind of the doctor, who will first give a very small test dose just under the skin. Sera are used for the treatment of conditions such as diphtheria, tetanus, rabies, chickenpox and shingles, and Lassa fever.

A range of different antisera is used in medical laboratories to identify unknown organisms. Visible clumping of the organisms will occur when the right serum is added.

antispasm drugs

Spasm is a tight contraction of voluntary or involuntary (smooth) muscle in any part of the body. Smooth muscle spasm affects especially the wall of the intestine or the bladder. Antispasm drugs act by blocking the action of the nerve activator (neurotransmitter) acetylcholine, which is released from the nerve endings that stimulate the muscle contraction. They are useful in the treatment of bowel colic, as in irritable bowel syndrome, and in bladder spasm in cystitis and other conditions. Antispasmodic drugs are **anticholinergic drugs**.

antitoxin

See **antiserum**.

antitussive drugs

Drugs that prevent or relieve cough. Most of them include codeine (Benylin, Dimotane Co, Phensedyl, Terpoin), antihistamines or dextromethorphan (Actifed, Benylin, Lotussin, Sudafed). These drugs work, at a nervous system level, by actually suppressing the cough reflex to the presence of irritating material in the bronchial tubes. As this is one of the body's protective reactions, it is not always a good idea to suppress a cough. But there are some coughs that do little good and seem to go on for ever. So long as your doctor is satisfied that there is nothing seriously wrong, an antitussive medicine can be a great comfort.

antivenene

An **antiserum** containing specific antibodies to the venom of poisonous snakes, scorpions or spiders.

antivenins

A range of specific antidotes for the bites of venomous animals such as snakes, centipedes, spiders and scorpions. Antivenins are held by doctors in areas in which venomous bites are common. Identification of the animal concerned is important. They are prepared by injecting small and increasing doses of the venom into animals, such as horses, so that antibodies will be produced with specific action against the venom. Such antibodies neutralize the venoms and are called antivenins.

antiviral drugs

For many years after the introduction of the antibiotics it seemed unlikely that a comparable group of drugs with action against viruses would ever be developed. Viruses are fundamentally different from bacteria and other larger organisms in that they can only reproduce and survive within living cells. It is thus very difficult to find a drug capable of destroying viruses which is not also liable to destroy the host cell.

There have been no fundamental breakthroughs in antiviral treatment, but there have been many small advances based on the rapid growth of knowledge of the biochemistry and genetics of viruses. The most successful approaches, to date, have exploited ways of interfering with the copying (replication) of the virus's genetic material **DNA** or **RNA** (ribonucleic acid). This can be done by blocking the chemical activators (polymerase enzymes) that bring about replication. Early drugs acting on these principles were idoxuridine (Herplex), trifluridine, vidarabine and acyclovir. These drugs are all active against the herpes viruses and the latter, in particular, has had a great success. It is, at the time of writing, the most useful antiviral drug available and has saved many lives in immunocompromised people with widespread herpes infections, as well as preventing an immense amount of pain and distress in people with genital herpes infections and shingles.

The success of acyclovir has encouraged the development of similar drugs such as ganciclovir (DHPG) which is more active against the human cytomegalovirus, and zidovudine (AZT) which has some useful action in suppressing the replication of the AIDS virus, HIV. Unfortunately, AZT is toxic and affects blood production in the bone marrow. Anaemia usually appears after about six weeks of treatment, especially in people with AIDS (the acquired immune deficiency syndrome). Some patients also develop painful muscles.

Some viruses, including the AIDS virus, HIV, make use of an enzyme, reverse transcriptase, to make the necessary second strand of the double helix (RNA viruses have a single-strand genetic system). This enzyme has been closely studied by workers hoping to be able to block its action, because any drug capable of doing this would stop the reproduction of the virus concerned. The substances dideoxycytidine and phosphono-formate (foscarnet) are able to do this. Foscarnet can also inhibit the polymerases of all herpes viruses, but it too is toxic.

Ribavirin, acting in a different way, interferes with the replication of a range of viruses including many dangerous respiratory viruses for which effective drugs are badly needed. Some experimental success has been achieved, using the drug in aerosols, against some influenza strains and in serious respiratory syncytial virus infections in children and in Lassa fever. Amantadine and rimantadine are useful against Influenza A virus.

Interferons are substances produced by cells as part of the natural defence against virus infections. They do not act directly against viruses but modify other cells so that they become less capable of cooperating with viruses in achieving the assembly of their components and their replication. Genetic engineering techniques (recombinant DNA) have enabled us to produce enough interferons for clinical trials and limited clinical use, and results are encouraging. The common cold can be treated by direct application to the nose lining, but there are side-effects and the treatment is still uneconomically expensive. Genital warts and hepatitis B have been successfully treated.

We are only at the beginning of a process which, if current expectations are realised, may parallel the remarkable advances achieved in the development of the antibiotics in the last fifty years.

antisocial personality re-education

See **therapeutic community**.

antiviral drug

See **nucleoside analogue**.

anuria

Cessation of the production of urine by the kidneys. The situation is extremely serious and calls for urgent investigation and treatment.

anus, narrowing of

See **anal stricture**.

anus, split

See **anal fissure**.

anxiolytic

A drug used to treat anxiety.

anxiety

A basic biological driving force and a natural response to threat or danger, which may be real or perceived. Anxiety is unpleasant but necessary and is accompanied by certain physiological responses, mainly hormonal, which while helping to cope with the danger, also produce, to a varying degree, the symptoms described below.

Anxiety often occurs in the absence of obvious cause, and severe anxiety of this kind is abnormal and disabling. Such pathological anxiety is one of the commonest forms of psychiatric disorder. Doctors talk about *free-floating* anxiety (anxiety states or anxiety neuroses), **hypochondriasis** (psychosomatic disorder) and *situational anxiety* (**phobias**). Phobias, in turn, are divided into **agoraphobia**, social phobias and simple phobias.

SYMPTOMS

The symptoms of pathological anxiety include a rapid pulse, breathlessness, tremulousness, a dry mouth, a feeling of tightness in the chest, sweaty palms, weakness, nausea, bowel hurry with diarrhoea and abdominal colic, insomnia, fatigue, headache, and loss of appetite. There is narrowing of attention and reduced mental efficiency with disorganisation and poor performance.

POSSIBLE CAUSES

Different schools of psychological thought differ in their theories on the causation of pathological anxiety. Some psychoanalysts follow Freud's idea that anxiety originates with the child's perception of the terrible trauma of being born. Others believe it to be due to overstimulation of the early receptive mind, to which experiences come faster than it can comprehend them. Psychoanalysts also recognize a form of anxiety due to the conflict between external demands and internal drives. The proponents of learning theory see anxiety as a reaction to pain and the attempts made to avoid it or its sources. Systematic attempts to avoid events perceived as painful may, they say, lead to restricted or abnormal behaviour, as in the case of phobias. Cognitive psychologists believe that anxiety results from the way a person interprets a situation. They believe that a full explanation and reappraisal can dispel anxiety.

The reality is usually different. Anxiety often seems deeply rooted in the personality. Every doctor is familiar with patients suffering constant anxiety, depression, phobias and hypochondriasis. Many of these patients are convinced their symptoms are due to organic disease. Some suffer a purely imaginary *disordered action of the heart* (Da Costa's syndrome), others from excess sweating (hyperhidrotic syndrome), irritable bowel syndrome, and the effects of overbreathing (**hyperventilation** syndrome). The average doctor, even the average psychiatrist, may feel that he or she never has enough time to devote to these unfortunates, who often become psychologically dependent on kind doctors and on tranquillizing drugs. They seldom get effective treatment.

Anxiety may also be a symptom of various other disorders including hyperthyroidism, menopausal hormonal disturbances, drug withdrawal, **schizophrenia**, depressive illness, post-concussional syndrome, and **dementia** resulting from any organic disease such as **atherosclerosis**.

apathy

See **amotivational syndrome**.

apex

The tip of an organ with a pointed end. The apex of the heart is at the lower left side and the apex of the lung is at the top. The tooth apex is at the tip of each root.

aphakia

Absence of the internal crystalline lens of the eye. *Phakos* is the Greek word for a 'lentil' and *a-* means 'not'. Aphakia can occur either as a result of a penetrating eye injury, which causes loss or absorption of the lens, or as a result of a now largely-outmoded deliberate surgical removal for the treatment of cataract. At one time, simple removal was the only way in which cataracts could be treated. Nowadays it is unusual to leave the patient aphakic after a cataract operation and, unless there is good reason to the contrary, an artificial lens (intraocular implant) is inserted.

An aphakic person is severely long-sighted (hypermetropic) and requires a very strong lens to refocus the eye. Glasses may be used, but cause severe distortion and high magnification and are very heavy. Contact lenses are much more effective. Secondary lens implantation, some time after lens removal, is often possible but is not without risk.

aphasia

An acquired speech disorder resulting from brain damage which affects the understanding and production of language rather than the mechanical aspects of articulation. Aphasia is a common feature of **stroke** and, in all right-handed and many left-handed people, is due to damage in the left side of the brain. There are usually, but not necessarily, associated difficulties in reading and writing.

aphonia

Total or partial loss of voice, usually as a result of disorder of the voice box (larynx). Severe laryngitis, by inflaming and thickening the vocal chords, may cause temporary aphonia. Interference with one of the nerves to the laryngeal muscles commonly causes paralysis of a vocal chord and severe aphonia. In some cases, this may be the first sign of cancer of one of the structures of the neck, such as the thyroid gland.

aphrodisiac

A drug which is purported to stimulate sexual interest or excitement or to enhance performance. Man's quest for the aphrodisiac has, throughout history, been as unremitting as it has been unsuccessful. Many substances have had aphrodisiac properties attributed to them. These have included animal skin, especially that of elephants and dead human beings, goat testicle, tiger whiskers, powdered rhinoceros horn, potato, ginseng, carrot and oysters.

Unfortunately, these reputations have invariably been without foundation, but the legends persist. In truth, there is no such thing as an aphrodisiac drug, unless one counts substances like alcohol, which temporarily reduce the critical faculty, fastidiousness and common discretion and allow more primitive elements to prevail.

THE STIMULATION OF SEXUAL INTEREST

It has been discovered that **neuro-transmitters** are deficient in some parts of the brain in some people – dopamine in **Parkinsonism**, for instance – and it has been found that drugs which replace or mimic the action of dopamine tend to stim-

> An irritant poison called cantharidin, the active principle of Spanish fly (cantharides), if consumed, is excreted in the urine and causes an acute irritation of the urinary tract. This will certainly draw the unfortunate victim's attention to the area, but the discomfort is more likely to exclude than to prompt sexual desire. Cantharides is highly dangerous and people who have used it for such purposes have faced murder charges.

ulate sexual interest. Medical students' stories of old men chasing nurses down the ward were widely heard soon after dopamine treatment was introduced. Eli Lilly's shares shot up two million dollars in one day after it was announced that their new preparation LY 163502 '... may be useful in treating certain kinds of sexual dysfunction in men and women.' It was emphasized that the drug was in the preliminary stages of research, but many members of the public obviously inferred that here, at last, was the genuine aphrodisiac.

aplasia

Failure of the development of an organ or tissue.

aplastic anaemia

A serious form of anaemia in which no new blood cells are formed in the bone marrow. About 30 per cent of cases follow virus infections, especially measles, mumps and hepatitis, or are induced by drugs such as butazolidine, sulphonamides, chloramphenicol by mouth or dipyrone. Because of this risk most of these drugs are no longer prescribed. Inhalation of benzene fumes can also cause aplastic anaemia. In most cases, however, the cause remains obscure. Fortunately, the condition is rare, affecting only two to five people per million.

Because all blood cells and their products are affected, the platelets that are necessary for blood clotting are also deficient and bleeding into the skin is often the first sign of the disease. The immune system cells also cease to be produced so there is immune deficiency and a strong tendency to infections of all kinds. Careful isolation is necessary. Without treatment about half of the people affected will die within three to six months, mostly from infection or bleeding.

Blood transfusions are often necessary to maintain life. Anabolic steroids (androgens) have been found useful in prompting the bone marrow to resume cell production. Bone marrow transplants may be necessary.

apnoea

Absence of breathing for short periods. Apnoea often occurs shortly before death, and is a natural consequence of deliberate forced overbreathing (hyperventilation) which 'washes out' excess quantities of **carbon dioxide**. It occurs during swallowing and occasionally during **sleep** (sleep apnoea).

apomorphine

A morphine derivative used as an expectorant, emetic, and hypnotic. In large doses it promotes severe vomiting. Used in the treatment of Parkinson's disease. A brand name is Britaject.

apoplexy

An old-fashioned term for **stroke**.

apoptosis

An important and recently discovered aspect of cell biology. Apoptosis is cell 'suicide', a form of programmed cell death, by enzyme digestion of DNA. This is necessary to make way for new cells and apoptosis occurs constantly in the growing fetus and elsewhere. The p53 gene can induce a protective apoptosis in cells whose DNA has been dangerously damaged to the point where cancerous change is liable to occur.

The understanding of apoptosis and its roles in human biology is a growing zone in medical knowledge. As an instance, it has recently been found that the normal prion protein (PrP), which is converted to an abnormal form in diseases such as Creutzfeldt-Jakob disease, may have an essential function in preventing nerve cells from undergoing apoptosis. Because the abnormal PrP cannot do this so apoptosis causes widespread destruction of brain cells leading to loss of brain substance.

appendicectomy

Removal of the appendix. The operation for the treatment of acute **appendicitis**.

HOW IT'S DONE

An incision is made in the lower right segment of the abdomen, starting on a level with the crest of the pelvis, and sloping downward at an angle, parallel to the crease of the groin. Once through the skin, the muscles of the abdominal wall are split in layers, along the lines of the fibres, and the membrane lining the abdominal organs (the peritoneum) is reached. This is opened and the beginning of the large intestine, which bears the appendix, is carefully brought out. Care is taken not to rupture a tense and inflamed appendix.

The small blood vessels supplying the appendix are now clamped and tied off and the appendix is secured between clamps, near the bowel, firmly tied off with strong ligatures, and cut away. The stump is securely tied (ligated) and a *purse-string* suture is inserted into the wall of the bowel in a circle around the appendix stump. Before this suture is pulled tight, the stump can be pushed in and concealed.

The peritoneum is now closed with a continuous catgut suture and the abdominal muscles are, similarly, closed in layers, using absorbable sutures. Finally, the skin is closed with nylon sutures or clips.

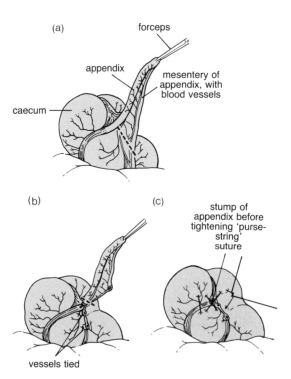

appendicitis

A disease in which an acute inflammation occurs in the blind-ended *vermiform* appendix. Obstruction to the worm-like organ is common and **gangrene** may occur.

INCIDENCE

Appendicitis is commonest in adolescents and young adults and begins with pain in the centre of the abdomen which soon moves to the lower right corner.

RECOGNITION AND SYMPTOMS

There is marked local tenderness (pain on pressure) and, because of this, bodily movement, deep breathing and coughing cause great distress. There is usually some slight fever, constipation, nausea and occasionally vomiting.

RISKS

Perforation of the appendix leads to the even more serious condition of peritonitis and this used to be a common cause of death before the period of modern surgical and antibiotic management. Often an appendix abscess forms around the leaking organ and the mass becomes walled off by fibrous tissue from the rest of the abdomen.

TREATMENT

Surgical intervention, if timely, cures the condition in almost all cases.

See **appendicectomy**.

appetite, loss of, in children

This is common in minor illnesses and need not occasion worry as it nearly always resolves when the child recovers. Loss of appetite may also accompany minor emotional upsets but, if persistent enough to lead to loss of weight, should be reported to a doctor for investigation. However poor a child's appetite may seem, if there is no loss of weight there is no cause for concern. It is common for young children to go through phases of refusing food and this often causes anxiety in parents. Even a day or two with little or no food will do no harm so long as fluid is taken. Food refusal is a normal part of child development and the child will observe, and may later cash in on, parents' obvious concern.

appetite suppressant drugs

Drugs used to reduce the urge to eat and to help in the control of obesity. On the whole, doctors are not too keen on drug treatment for obesity and usually try to persuade patients to establish new eating habits without the help of drugs. But for many, this is so difficult, and obesity is such a serious health hazard, that they eventually resort to drug treatment under close supervision. Drugs, are, however, no substitute for strict calorie counting. Amphetamine and amphetamine-like drugs have a powerful appetite-suppressant effect but are not now used for this purpose. Almost the only drug now used for this purpose is phentermine (Duromine). It is unwise to use this drug for longer than three months. People with a history of alcohol or drug abuse should avoid it. If there has not been substantial weight loss in this time, the scheme of treatment has clearly failed to reduce the food intake sufficiently. People with a severe weight problem also need plenty of sympathy.

Appendicectomy operation. Before the appendix can be removed, both it and the blood vessels supplying it must be clamped and tied off. A 'purse-string' suture allows the stumps to be infolded and covered.

apraclonidine

A drug used in the treatment of **glaucoma**. A brand name is Iopidine.

apraxia

Loss of the ability to carry out skilled movements with control and accuracy. The basic problem is in the brain, usually as a result of brain disease, often **stroke**.

Apresoline

A brand name for **hydralazine**.

Aprinox

A brand name for bendrofluazide.

aprotinin

A drug used in the treatment of bleeding resulting from the excessive breakdown of the fibrin that forms blood clots. An antifibrinolytic. A brand name is Trasylol.

Aprovel

A brand name for **irbesartan**.

Aquasept

A brand name for **triclosan**.

-ar

Suffix meaning 'of, like' as in solar (sun-like).

arachnodactyly

Having abnormally long, spider-like hands and fingers. Arachnodactyly is an almost diagnostic feature of the genetic disorder **Marfan's syndrome**.

Aramine

A brand name for **metaraminol**.

-arche

Suffix meaning 'beginning' as in menarche (start of menses).

arcus senilis

A white ring near the outer margin of the cornea. This is a normal feature of age and is of no significance. Vision is never affected. In arcus juvenilis, or *embryotoxon*, an identical appearance occurs in young people. Again, this may mean nothing, but such people may have a disorder of fat and cholesterol metabolism and should be investigated.

Aredia

A brand name for **pamidronate**.

Argyll Robertson pupil

The pupil reactions are tested with a small focusing torch, used in conditions of low illumination. Normally, both pupils constrict when light is shone into one, and open up again when the light is removed. The Argyll Robertson pupil is a small pupil that does not constrict to light or dilate in the dark, but which constricts on close focusing. This important sign is now rare, but is almost always caused by syphilis of the nervous system.

Aricept

A brand name for **donepezil**.

Arimidex

A brand name for **anastrozole**.

arm numbness and tingling

See **thoracic outlet syndrome**.

aromatase inhibitors

A group of anticancer drugs that act by preventing the enzymatic conversion of androgens to oestrogens. These drugs are used especially in postmenopausal women with breast cancers that are being encouraged by oestrogens but that fail to respond to drugs such as tamoxifen.

arousal

A state of heightened awareness and alertness caused by a strong external stimulus such as danger or sexual interest. In arousal, the nervous system is poised ready for action.

Arpicolin

A brand name for **procyclidine**.

Arpimycin

A brand name for **erythromycin**.

arrhythmia

An abnormality in the regularity of the heartbeat caused by a defect in the generation or conduction of electrical impulses in the heart. Arrhythmias include early beats, followed by a pause (extrasystoles), atrial fibrillation with fast totally irregular beats and **heart block**, with very slow irregular beats. Some arrhythmias are a sign of serious heart disease and these will usually be associated with obviously serious symptoms. But many, including most extrasystoles, do not necessarily indicate organic disease.

arteries

Arteries are elastic, muscular-walled tubes carrying blood at high pressure from the heart to any part of the body. By contrast, the veins are thin-walled, inelastic and collapsible and carry blood at low pressure back to the heart.

From the top of the heart, carrying the output from the massive left ventricle, comes the aorta – the largest artery in the body. Its first two branches are the coronary arteries. These spread, branching, over the upper surface of the heart like a crown, moving constantly as they supply the highly active heart muscle with blood. The aorta then proceeds to give off major branches to the head, the arms, the chest structures and the organs of the abdomen, and then forks to supply each leg.

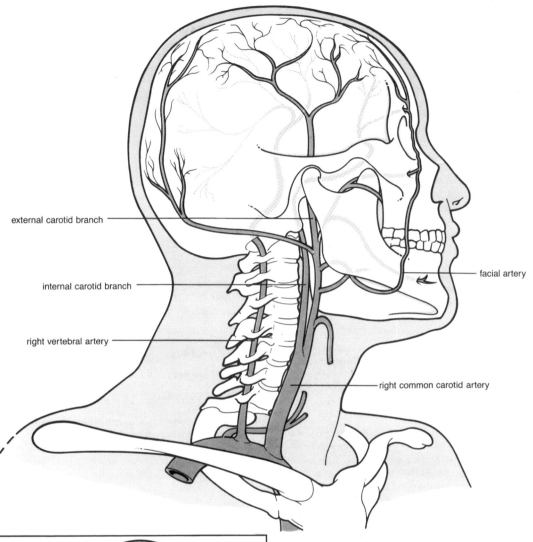

external carotid branch

internal carotid branch

right vertebral artery

facial artery

right common carotid artery

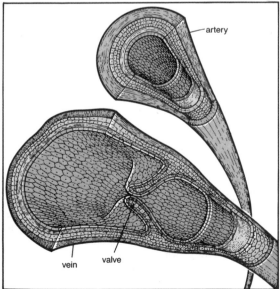

artery

vein   valve

Above: The carotid and vertebral artery supply to the head. These arteries provide the sole supply to the brain and are thus of vital importance, second only to the coronary arteries of the heart.

Left: The difference in structure between arteries and veins. The artery is thick-walled, muscular and valveless. The corresponding vein is of larger bore but has a thinner wall.

The two carotid arteries are the main routes of blood to the brain and, in conjunction with the two vertebral arteries, which course up through holes in the side processes of the neck bones (vertebrae), constitute the entire supply to the head. The carotids lie near the front of the neck, in such a position that they can be compressed between the fingers and the bodies of the vertebrae. Carotid artery disease threatens this vital blood supply to the brain and is now a principal cause of stroke and of the warning transient ischaemic attacks (TIAs), which commonly herald strokes.

In the neck, each carotid divides into an internal carotid and an external carotid. The external arteries supply the muscles of the face and scalp and the internal run through canals in the base of the skull to enter the cranium and supply the brain and the eyes. The two internal carotids link up, under the brain, with the terminations of the vertebral arteries, forming an important arterial circle from which branches run off into the brain. This is called the circle of Willis. This arrangement ensures that blockage or narrowing of one artery does not immediately cause a shut-down of the blood supply to one or other part of the brain. Such a shut-down would probably be fatal.

Near the point where the internal carotid leaves the main trunk, the arterial wall contains two collections of sensitive cells called the carotid sinus and the carotid body. The carotid sinus consists of stretch receptors which monitor blood pressure and feed back information about it to the brain. The carotid body contains chemical receptors which produce nerve impulses varying with the oxygen levels in the blood. In this way the brain is constantly provided with information which allows it to regulate the rate and depth of breathing.

The aorta gives off major branches to the arms, the chest wall and the organs of the abdomen and then divides to form a major branch for each leg.

arteriosclerosis

A term which has become so imprecise that it is falling out of use. Literally, 'hardening of the arteries', it is being replaced by the term **atherosclerosis**, which more accurately describes the common degenerative disease of arteries. It is doubtful whether arteriosclerosis ever occurs without the associated features of atherosclerosis.

arteritis

A disease of small arteries causing inflammation, with swelling tenderness and possible blockage. Giant cell arteritis involves arteries in the scalp and brain and may affect the main artery to the eye, causing blindness. There is severe scalp tenderness which may be accompanied by visible red streaks – the signs of inflammation. Urgent treatment with corticosteroids can be sight-saving.

artery closure prevention

See **stenting**.

artery constrictor

See **endothelin**.

artery inflammation

See **polyarteritis nodosa**.

artery-narrowing drugs

See **vasoconstrictor drugs**.

artery-widening drugs

See **nitrate and nitrite drugs, angiotensin converting enzyme inhibitors, calcium channel blockers drugs**.

arthralgia

Pain in a joint.

arthritis

Inflammation in a joint, usually with swelling, redness, pain and restriction of movement. The two main kinds are **osteoarthritis** and **rheumatoid arthritis** but arthritis can be caused by many other disease processes. These include **gout, Reiter's syndrome, ankylosing spondylitis, psoriasis** and a variety of infections including gonorrhoea and **tuberculosis**.

arthrodesis

The deliberate surgical fusion of the bones on either side of a joint so that no joint movement is possible. This is a procedure of last resort done only when no prospect remains of restoring pain-free movement or stability to the joint. An arthrodesis or ankylosis causes obvious disability but pain will be relieved and the postoperative state is usually greatly to be preferred to the former condition.

arthron

Greek root meaning 'joint' as in arthritis (joint inflammation).

articulus

Latin root meaning 'joint' as in articulation (connection of jointed parts).

artificial arteries

See **cultured arteries**.

artificial chromosome

The synthetic construction of a real, but simple, human chromosome has actually been achieved. The biotechnology involved is, however, still at an experimental stage. Chromosomes so far produced consist of a central constriction (centromere) of highly repetitive DNA sequences, end caps (telomeres), a marker gene and some random sequences of genomic DNA. When these ingredients were introduced into a human cell line they became coated with histone proteins and formed highly coiled structures. They also replicated and passed on copies to daughter cells through more than 200 cell divisions. The production of an artificial chromosome is a step on the way to the synthesis of a self-reproducing living organism.

artificial eye

Often inaccurately called a 'glass eye', the artificial eye, or *ocular prosthesis* is a slim plastic shell, with its front surface carefully matched to the other eye. The coloured part, the iris, which lies behind the transparent artificial cornea, may be hand painted or produced by photography.

HOW IT WORKS

It is possible to produce an eye with a pupil that changes size under changing light conditions. There is, however, no question of any visual function, and the prosthesis is worn only for cosmetic and psychological reasons. The eye fits neatly behind the eyelids within the moist cavity left when the natural eye has been removed and, unless there has been contraction of the socket by disease or delay in fitting a prosthesis, there will be no tendency for the eye to come out.

Movement of the eye adds greatly to realism and is achieved by the use of a buried plastic implant to which the eye-moving muscles are attached. This may contain a tiny ceramic magnet which will interact with another magnet in the prosthesis. Many orbital implants cause trouble and have to be removed and some surgeons have abandoned the idea. Some movement may safely be obtained by attaching the muscles to the back of the socket lining at the time of surgery.

artificial heart

A mechanical device intended to maintain the circulation of the blood.

RISKS

Unfortunately, optimistic press reports notwithstanding, in no case has an artificial heart been able to maintain a reasonable quality of life. These cumbersome external devices have been used on a small number of patients and some have been kept alive until a human heart has been obtained for transplantation. As a temporary measure, the artificial heart may have a place in the treatment of people likely to die soon from heart disease, but informed medical opinion is, at present, strongly against attempts to employ them on a permanent basis. The few patients so far given permanent artificial hearts have died from major strokes due to blood clots carried to the brain or from mechanical failure at the body/machine interface, kidney failure, infection or massive internal haemorrhage. The experience has shown the naivety of the assumption that the problems are purely mechanical and technological. Much work will have to be done before a reasonably safe artificial heart becomes available.

OTHER OPTIONS

For over twenty years, a device known as the intra-aortic balloon pump has been used to help in maintaining the circulation in those whose hearts are barely able to do so. A timer inflates the balloon automatically between heartbeats, providing an extra impetus to the blood circulation. More recently a mechanical pump that assists the action of the left ventricle – the main pumping chamber of the heart – has been widely used. This is a simple, one-way, pump connected to a tube in the ventricle and one in the aorta. The actual pump is in the abdomen and the two tubes pass through the diaphragm. The battery-driven pump takes blood from the ventricle and passes it at higher pressure to the aorta. Although this device has been used for quite long periods in some hundreds of patients, it is in no sense an artificial heart.

artificial insemination

A method of achieving pregnancy when normal sexual intercourse is impossible, or when the husband is sterile. A quantity of fresh seminal fluid donated by the husband (AIH) or by an anonymous donor (AID) is taken up in a narrow syringe or pipette and injected high into the vagina or even into the opening of the womb (uterus). The procedure is timed to coincide with the period in the menstrual cycle when egg production by the woman (ovulation) is most likely to occur. Assuming no other reasons for infertility, the success rate is high.

The procedure can be done by the couple themselves in their own home.

Artificial insemination. The vagina is held open with a speculum and the donor semen is injected into the canal of the cervix. Correct timing in the menstrual cycle is important.

artificial intelligence

The characteristics of a machine designed to perform some of the perceptual or logical functions of the human organism in a manner that appears to be beyond the merely mechanical. AI is largely a matter of computer programming, in which stored records of past experience are made to modify the program so that future responses take them into account, but it also encompasses research into humanoid methods of data acquisition, the use of fuzzy logic and of artificial neural networks. High-level programming languages, such as prologue, designed specially for AI have been developed.

artificial kidney

A somewhat misleading term, it is, in reality, a machine the size of a large television set.

HOW IT WORKS

Dialysis machines expose the patient's blood to a membrane of large surface area, on the other side of which is a fluid into which the unwanted waste materials in the blood can pass by natural diffusion. The membrane, which has a pore size that allows small molecules to pass by not large molecules, is made of cellulose acetate (cellophane), polyacrylonitrile or Cuprophan. It is in the form of hollow fibres, tubes or sheets. Such membranes are said to be semipermeable.

The process must be continued for periods of five or six hours, three times a week and during these sessions the patient's blood circulation is shunted through the machine. This necessitates a permanent line into a vein and out of an artery, and between dialysis sessions these are joined by a bypass tube.

RISKS

There are problem with infection and the maintenance of the connections.

Dialysis machines are, nevertheless, the most successful of artificial organs and can keep people alive indefinitely. The disadvantages, however, increase the attraction of kidney transplantation, if this is feasible and a suitable donor kidney available. See also **dialysis**, **haemodialysis**, **haemofiltration**.

artificial lungs

Experimental devices for maintaining the oxygenation of the blood and the removal of carbon dioxide. Research has shown that, in theory, such devices can be made small

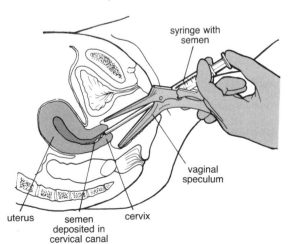

syringe with semen

vaginal speculum

uterus   semen   cervix
deposited in
cervical canal

enough for implantation into the human body. New polymer membranes, using polyimide material with added fluorine, have been developed that, compared with previous materials, increase oxygen transfer 70 times and carbon dioxide transfer 100 times.

artificial respiration

An emergency procedure urgently required to save life when normal breathing is absent or insufficient, as in partial drowning, poisoning or head injury. It is important to distinguish absent respiration from obstruction to the airway. In the latter case there will often be strenuous but ineffectual attempts to breathe and the urgent need is to clear the airway.

The most effective form of artificial respiration is the mouth-to-mouth method with the nose pinched ('kiss of life'). This should always be tried when a person is found not to be breathing and especially if a pulse can be felt.

> Artificial respiration is useless if the heart has stopped beating. In this case, it must be combined with cardiac massage.

-ary

Suffix meaning 'concerned with' as in primary (first-like).

Arythmol

A brand name for **propafenone**.

Asacol

A brand name for **mesalazine**.

asbestosis

A serious, chronic lung disease caused by inhaling asbestos dust over a period. The changes in the lung occur slowly and may take twenty years to develop. Thickening and scarring of the lung tissue occurs resulting in reduced efficiency of gas (oxygen and carbon dioxide) interchange with the blood. The result is increasing breathlessness, coughing and a feeling of tightness in the chest. Asbestosis may progress to respiratory failure in which the oxygen supply is so poor that the patient is breathless and blue (**cyanosis**) even at rest in bed. There is no effective treatment and the disease usually shortens life.

> People with asbestosis are at increased risk of developing lung cancer, especially if they smoke cigarettes.

Ascabiol

A brand name for **benzyl benzoate**.

ascariasis

Worm infestation with the roundworm *Ascaris lumbricoides* which lives, often in considerable numbers, in the small intestine. The world population of ascaris greatly exceed the number of people and in some countries almost all individuals carry the worms. The characteristic eggs are easily detected in a stool sample and effective treatment, to remove the worms, is available.

ascites

A collection of fluid in the space in the abdomen surrounding the internal organs. This space is called the peritoneal cavity and it may become distended with several gallons of fluid in any condition which causes a generalized accumulation of fluid in the tissues (**oedema**). These conditions include heart failure, the **nephrotic syndrome** (a kidney disease) or cirrhosis (fibrous scarring) of the liver. Ascites causes discomfort and difficulty in breathing, and the fluid can be drained surgically, producing great relief. A sample of the fluid should be examined, as ascites may sometimes be caused by secondary cancer. Diuretic drugs are also helpful in the treatment of ascites.

ascorbic acid

Vitamin C. A white, crystalline substance found in citrus fruits, tomatoes, potatoes, and leafy green vegetables. Small doses are needed to prevent the bleeding disease of **scurvy** and regular large doses are useful as an anti-oxidant in combatting dangerous **free radicals**. A brand name is Redoxon.

Asendis

A brand name for **amoxapine**.

asepsis

The absence of all bacteria or other microorganisms capable of causing infection. Modern surgery is performed in an environment in which the nearest possible approach to full asepsis is obtained by sterilizing all instruments, dressings and towels; by providing a sterile barrier between the patient and those working in theatre, in the form of sterile gowns, caps, gloves and masks; and by draping the whole of the patient, except the operation area, in sterile sheets.

Aserbine

A brand name for **malic acid**.

Asilone

A brand name for **aluminium hydroxide**, **magnesium oxide** and dimethicone.

Asmabec

A brand name for **beclomethasone**.

Asmasal

A brand name for **salbutamol**.

Asperger's syndrome

A condition similar to, but usually less severe than, **autism**, which affects about 1–2 persons in 1000, males more often than females. Affected people, who are normally intelligent, are physically clumsy, have unusually narrow interests, obsessional behaviour, and great difficulty in managing social relationships. Special training in social skills can be valuable.

aspermia

The absence of spermatozoa in the semen or the inability to ejaculate semen. Obstructive aspermia is due to the blockage of the vas deferens on both sides. This may be congenital or acquired from infection or injury, or from vasectomy. **Cystic fibrosis** causes aspermia as a result of failure of development of the vas or associated structures.

asphyxia

Suffocation by interference with the free airway between the atmosphere and the air sacs in the lungs. This may arise by drowning, choking, strangling, inhalation of a gas which excludes oxygen, foreign body obstruction, swelling (**oedema**) of the larynx or in other ways.

> Asphyxia is always urgent, and unless it is rapidly relieved, death is inevitable. Clearance of the airway and artificial respiration offer the only hope.

aspiration

Drawing out fluid by suction, usually by means of a syringe and needle, but sometimes by mouth or pump suction through a plastic or rubber tube.

aspirin

See **analgesic drugs**.

aspirin, action of

See **prostaglandins**.

Asprodeine

A brand name for aspirin (see **analgesic drugs**) and codeine.

asthenia

Lack or loss of strength or energy.

asthma

A disease in which the circular smooth muscles of the branching air tubes of the lungs (the bronchi) are liable to go into a state of spasm so that the bronchi are narrowed and the passage of air impeded. Often inspiration is easier than expiration so that the lungs become inflated and cannot easily be emptied. Expiratory wheeze is a common feature of an asthmatic attack.

POSSIBLE CAUSES

The bronchospasm may be induced by many stimuli, but sensitivity to an **allergy**-causing substance (**allergen**) is among the commonest. It can also be induced by infection, emotion, and in many asthmatics, exertion.

INCIDENCE

Asthma is not a trivial condition and has an annual mortality, in Britain, of at least 2000.

TREATMENT

Self-help in avoiding danger is important. This is only possible if the sufferer has knowledge of the signs of worsening of the condition and of the steps to be taken to overcome them.

> Status asthmaticus, a prolonged attack of severe asthma, is very dangerous and calls for urgent medical attention. The same applies to progressive worsening, with reduced response to simple remedies.

asthma early warning test

See **peak expiratory flow measurement**.

astigmatism

When a small spot of light (*stigma* is Greek for 'a spot') is focused by an astigmatic lens, the image formed is a smeared line instead of a sharp point.

The cornea is the main focusing lens of the eye and should, ideally, be curved like the surface of a perfect sphere. In astigmatism, although the eye is perfectly healthy, the cornea is curved like the surface of an egg, so the lens is more powerful in one meridian then in the others. A minor degree of astigmatism is normal – nearly every eye has some – and glasses are unnecessary for this. But more severe astigmatism causes blurring of objects oriented in a particular direction. A person with astigmatism might, for instance, see horizontal lines clearly while vertical lines are blurred; or the meridian of greatest blurring may be at an oblique angle.

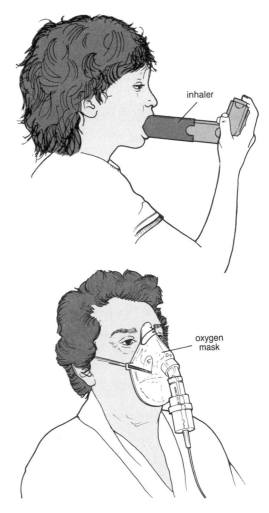

Asthma is best treated by drugs taken by inhaler so that the drug reaches the area where it is needed and the smallest dose will give the largest effect. Correct use of inhalers is vital. In severe cases it may be necessary to give oxygen.

TREATMENT

Ordinary spherical eyeglass lenses cannot correct astigmatism and lenses are needed which have more optical power in the appropriate meridian than in that at right angles. For pure astigmatism, a lens is required which has no optical power in the normal meridian but appropriate curvature in the others. These are called cylindrical lenses and must, of course, be set in the frame at exactly the correct orientation.

Hard contact lenses bridge over the anomalous corneal curve and present a perfect spherical surface for focusing. They thus give excellent vision in astigmatism. Ordinary soft lenses tend to mould to the astigmatic curve, but special *toric* soft lenses are available for astigmatism. Unfortunately, they are expensive and difficult to fit satisfactorily.

RISKS

Young children with undetected high astigmatism frequently develop a form of **amblyopia** which is confined to the out-of-focus meridia. This is called *meridional amblyopia* and, unless detected early in life and treated with accurately prescribed glasses, will be permanent and uncorrectable. High astigmatism, in one eye only, very commonly causes severe amblyopia in that eye.

See also **vision, disorders of**.

astigmatism cure

See **excimer laser refractive surgery**.

astringent

A drug that shrinks cells. Astringents precipitate protein on cell surfaces but are not intended to penetrate. If they do, they kill the cells. They have little value either in medicine or in cosmetics.

astrocytoma

A tumour derived from the star-shaped supporting tissue cells of the brain – the neural 'glue' (neuroglia) that holds the brain cells together. Astrocytomas vary widely in degree of malignancy and rate of growth, but all are serious and usually require surgical removal, the difficulty of which depends on their location. This is usually followed by radiotherapy.

astrovirus

A virus that causes diarrhoea in children and may be present in large numbers in the stools of adults without causing ill effects. Most adults have antibodies to the virus.

asymptomatic

Free of symptoms.

asystole

The form of cardiac arrest in which there is no heartbeat and the electrocardiogram tracing is straight. This is in contrast with the other form of arrest – ventricular fibrillation – in which the heart muscle is twitching rapidly without full contraction.

Atarax

A brand name for **hydroxyzine**.

ataxia

Unsteadiness in standing and walking resulting from a disorder of the control mechanisms in the brain, or from inadequate information input to the brain from the skin, muscles and joints.

The lower hind part of the brain (the cerebellum), contains the computer which coordinates the mass of information on balance, position and movement, which flows in from the eyes, the inner ear and the limbs, and any disturbance in this area will cause severe ataxia with staggering. Syphilis, **diabetes** and other diseases affecting nerves can interfere with input data from the legs, and lead to ataxia.

-ate

Suffix meaning 'possessing' as in primate (first kind).

atelectasis

Failure of the normal expansion of part or all of a lung. This occurs in various conditions, including the **respiratory distress syndrome** in babies due to **surfactant** deficiency.

atenolol

A beta adrenoceptor blocker drug that acts mostly on the heart and has a long action. It slows the heart and corrects irregularities of rhythm. It is used to treat high blood pressure and **angina pectoris**. The drug has been found to have a significant protective effect against heart attacks during the two years or so after non-cardiac surgery. Brand names are Tenormin and Tenoretic.

atheroma

Literally, this term means a lump of porridge. Atheroma is the degenerative, fatty material containing cholesterol and other fats, broken down muscle cells, blood clot, blood clotting elements (**platelets**) and fibrous tissue, which forms on the inner surface of arteries and which eventually may lead to obstruction and serious blood deprivation.

See **atherosclerosis**.

atherosclerosis

The number one killer of the Western world. Atherosclerosis is a degenerative disease of arteries in which fatty plaques (**atheroma**) develop on the inner lining of arteries so that the normal flow of blood is impeded.

Fats and cholesterol are carried around in the bloodstream in the form of tiny spherical bodies known as *lipoproteins*. There are two types: high-density lipoproteins (HDLs) with much protein and little fat; and low-density lipoproteins (LDLs) with much cholesterol and little protein. LDLs carry cholesterol to the arteries; HDLs carry it from the tissues to the liver. So LDLs are regarded as 'bad' and HDLs as 'good'. There is a very strong correlation between high levels of LDLs and a high incidence of atherosclerosis, heart attacks and strokes. High levels of HDLs are protective against these diseases. Each LDL has a small number of large molecules on its surface called *apolipoproteins*. Cells take up cholesterol by binding to these proteins.

Recent advances in the understanding of the processes by which atherosclerotic plaques develop suggest that the

Atherosclerosis. This is a progressive disease of arteries responsible for an immense amount of ill-health and mortality. The illustration shows the various stages in the progression towards near-blockage of an artery. The final blockage is often caused by blood clotting (thrombosis) on top of the plaque.

low-density lipoproteins are activated into depositing their cholesterol in the walls of the arteries by the oxidative action of **free radicals**. There is growing evidence that these can be effectively combated by regular daily doses of the anti-oxidant vitamins C and E in amounts considerably greater than are required to prevent vitamin deficiency.

INCIDENCE

Atherosclerosis affects almost all of us, the earliest signs being apparent in childhood, and the condition is, in general, steadily progressive with age. Although most arteries are affected, those in which the condition is most dangerous are the coronary arteries supplying the heart muscle with blood, and the carotid and vertebral arteries, and their branches, which supply the brain. Atherosclerosis of these two systems leads, respectively, to coronary thrombosis (see **heart attack** and **stroke**).

PREVENTION

Atherosclerosis is responsible for more deaths than any other single condition and it should be the object of everyone to delay, or halt, the progress of the disorder. This can be achieved by adopting a number of life principles.

The following basic principles will help in the fight against atherosclerosis:
- eat little more than is required to maintain a normal, low-end-of-range body weight, with avoidance of saturated fats;
- take exercise to the point of breathlessness, ideally once a day;
- on no account ever smoke cigarettes;
- drink alcohol in moderation;
- have regular blood pressure checks;
- take anti-oxidant vitamins;
- avoid undue stress.

---

athetosis

Involuntary writhing movements of the hands, arms, face and tongue caused by a form of cerebral palsy.

See **spastic paralysis**.

athlete's foot

A popular term for the unpopular fungus infection ('ringworm') commonly occurring between the toes of those insufficiently careful over personal hygiene, or unlucky in public swimming pool changing facilities. The medical term is *tinea pedis* and the fungus is encouraged by hot, sweaty conditions. Once acquired, it tends to be persistent, but responds to prolonged treatment with a suitable **antifungal** preparation. Regular careful daily washing, drying and powdering of the feet is the best preventive.

See also **tinea**.

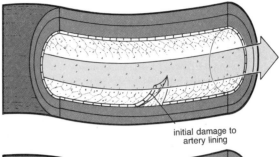

initial damage to
artery lining

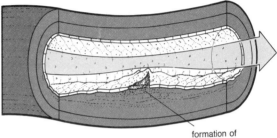

formation of
atheromatous plaque

near-blockage
by enlarging plaque

Ativan

A brand name for **lorazepam**.

atlanto-axial instability

Abnormal mobility of the articulation of the upper two vertebrae, the **atlas bone** and the **axis bone**. This is demonstrable on X-ray by a separation of more than 3 mm, at the front, between the body of the atlas and the vertical peg-like odontoid process of the axis. People with this abnormality should avoid activities that could bring about dislocation (subluxation) of the bones and serious risk to the spinal cord.

Atlanto-axial instability is found in about 20 per cent of people with Down's syndrome because of laxity in the ligaments between the skull and the spine.

atlas bone

The uppermost, or first, vertebra of the spinal column. The atlas is unique in having no body or spinous process. In head nodding, the skull moves on the atlas, but in head rotation the atlas locks with the skull and both rotate on the second vertebra, the **axis bone**.

atorvastatin

A cholesterol-lowering drug. A brand name is Lipitor.

atoms and molecules

Like everything else in nature, the human body is a chemical structure. So any account of the human body cannot avoid some reference to chemistry. Even a sketchy knowledge is helpful in understanding both the structure and the functioning of the body. Chemistry is the ultimate key to it all.

Everything is made of atoms, which are the smallest representative parts of each of the ninety-two elements that occur in nature. Elements are either metals, such as iron, copper or calcium; or non-metals such as carbon, oxygen or nitrogen. Chemistry is concerned with the way atoms link together to form molecules, which are the natural chemical units of matter. Molecules represent the smallest particle of a chemical compound which retains the characteristics and chemical properties of the compound. Pure substances, in visible quantity, consist of large collections of identical molecules of the substance.

With the rare exception of certain single atom molecules, almost all molecules consist of two or more atoms linked together. An atom of the violently active metal sodium (Na) linked to an atom of the poisonous gas chlorine (Cl), for instance, gives one molecule of common salt (NaCl) – an important body ingredient. An atom of carbon linked to four atoms of hydrogen, gives one molecule of the gas methane (CH_4). An atom of carbon linked to four atoms of chlorine, gives a molecule of the cleaning fluid carbon tetrachloride (CCl_4). In organic chemistry most molecules are much more complicated than these and consist of large collections of a few different atoms joined together in different ways. All organic molecules contain carbon atoms as a kind of central core to which other atoms are bonded. Most also contain hydrogen and oxygen atoms. Many also contain nitrogen and phosphorous.

In molecules, atoms are bound together in certain characteristic ways. They may form rings or chains, or the molecules may consist of repeating patterns of small identical groups of atoms. Sometimes these simpler groups are molecules in their own right. When many such groups are joined together they may form very long molecules. Such groups are sometimes called monomers and the large molecules formed when they join up are called polymers . 'Polythene' (polyethylene) is a polymer of many ethylene monomers. Simple sugars, like glucose, are often polymerized to form large carbohydrate molecules such as the liver storage molecule glycogen or structurally strong molecules like the cellulose of plants. **Proteins** are polymers consisting of many amino acids linked together.

The most complex molecule in the body is the molecule of **DNA** (deoxyribonucleic acid) – a molecule of enormous length (almost two metres) which, when coiled and folded up, forms a chromosome.

atopy

An inherited state giving rise to an allergy. Atopy causes an immediate hypersensitivity reaction associated with the **antibody** class immunoglobulin E (IgE) and is a maternally transmitted genetic disorder due to mutations in genes on several chromosomes including chromosome 11. These genes code for the IgE receptor on **mast cells**. Atopy causes a proneness to **asthma**, **hay fever** and **eczema** (atopic dermatitis).

Atovaquone

A drug used in the treatment of **malaria** and **toxoplasmosis**. Brand names are Wellvone and, in combination with proguanil, Malarone.

atracurium besylate

A non-depolarizing muscle relaxant drug used in anaesthesia. A brand name is Tracrium.

Atromid-S

A brand name for **clofibrate**.

atriopeptin

A recently discovered hormone which is stored in the heart and released into the blood when the blood volume increases beyond the optimum. Atriopeptin increases the rate of urine production and salt excretion.

atrophy

Wasting and loss of substance due to cell degeneration and death. This may be a natural ageing process or it may be due to simple disuse. The opposite of atrophy is *hypertrophy* and these two processes are well demonstrated by the muscles, which will soon lose bulk if unused, but may, especially in youth, be built up by regular hard work.

atropine sulphate

A powerful **anticholinergic drug** used to widen the pupils long-term and to reduce intestinal activity in some cases of diarrhoea.

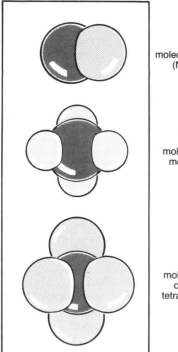

molecule of salt
(Na Cl)

molecule of methane

molecule of carbon tetrachloride

Simple molecules.

Atrovent

A brand name for **ipratropium bromide**.

attention deficit hyperactivity disorder

A childhood disorder affecting boys ten times as often as girls and featuring constant excessive physical activity, restlessness, unthinking impulsiveness, short span of attention and concentration, lack of responsiveness and unwillingness to participate with others in normal childhood activities. Only a very small proportion show objective neurological abnormality and the condition is believed to be grossly overdiagnosed. In some areas in the USA 5 per cent of boys aged 10–11 are being treated for this condition, mostly with the drug methylphenidate (Ritalin).

audiologist

A doctor or ancillary health professional specializing in the diagnosis and measurement of hearing defects. The medically qualified audiologist is an Ear, Nose and Throat specialist who has subspecialized in audiology.

audiometry

Measurement of the sensitivity, or threshold, of a person's hearing at different pitches (frequencies). Loss of the ability to hear high tones at low intensity is characteristic of age deafness (presbyacusis), noise-induced deafness or acoustic trauma (see noise, effects of) and hearing loss caused by toxic agents such as the aminoglycoside antibiotics. Audiometry can give early warning of the danger of further hearing loss at lower and more important frequencies, so that avoiding action – especially protection against noise – can be taken. It is also important in determining the suitability, and the right kind, of a hearing aid and helping in decisions about surgery.

The principle of audiometry is simple. The better the hearing, the quieter the sounds one can hear. Hearing loss is never uniform over the whole range of sounds, from low to high pitch, so it is necessary to test the hearing with sounds of different pitches.

PURE TONE AUDIOMETRY

In this test, a machine called an audiometer generates sounds which can be accurately varied in loudness, from a level too low for anyone to hear, to a level almost anyone, even the very deaf, can hear. It can do this for sounds covering the whole range of human hearing from the lowest pitch, at about 16 cycles per second (Hz) to the highest, at about 16,000 Hz.

Audiometers have switched intensities, calibrated in decibels, and switched frequencies, calibrated in cycles per second (Hz). The person being checked is usually asked to sit in a small sound-proofed box with a heavy door and a double-glazed window through which he or she can be observed by the operator. The subject is given an electric push-switch on a cord, with which to signal when any sound is heard. The ears are tested one at a time. To test air conduction – that is, how well sounds are conducted through the outer and middle ears – the subject wears a pair of padded headphones.

The operator selects a particular frequency and sets the sound level very low. He or she then presses a button which sends this sound to one of the headphones for a second or two. The subject is not able to see the operator do this. If the sound is heard, the subject presses the push-switch. If not,

the operator switches the same tone to a higher intensity and tries again. This procedure is repeated until the sound is heard and the response made. The louder the tone sent, with no response, the greater the degree of hearing loss at that frequency.

When a tone at a particular frequency is heard and the intensity noted, the operator switches the intensity down again, changes to another frequency, and proceeds as before. With each response, a mark is made on a chart, called an audiogram, to show, on the particular vertical line for the frequency concerned, the intensity in decibels needed for the sound to be heard. It would take a very long time to do this, at small frequency intervals, over the whole audible spectrum, but this is unnecessary and the test is done at only half a dozen selected frequencies, such as 64 Hz, 128 Hz, 256 Hz, 512 Hz, 1024 Hz, 2048 Hz and 4096 Hz. When all the entries have been made on the chart, the resulting graph is called an audiogram.

If there is severe hearing loss in one ear, the loud tones needed can through the skull to the good ear, so a hissing sound (white noise) is applied to the ear-piece on the good side to mask the hearing while the other ear is being tested.

It can be helpful to know how well a person can hear if the sounds are conveyed directly to the inner ear, rather than by way of the eardrum and middle ear. To do this, bone conduction is tested using a small rubber-covered device, vibrating at the same frequencies as the sound, which is applied to the bone behind and below the ear. In this way, the sound vibrations bypass the external and middle ears, and the sensitivity of the inner ear hearing mechanism can be tested at different frequencies.

If hearing by bone conduction is normal but air conduction hearing diminished, the deafness is of the conductive type. But if the tests show that both air and bone conduction hearing are diminished, then the problem is in the cochlea in the inner ear, or in the acoustic nerve connecting the ear to the brain. This is known as sensorineural deafness. Unfortunately, sensorineural deafness is very common and cannot usually be treated. Conductive deafness can often be remedied.

IMPEDANCE AUDIOMETRY

This method of testing can provide additional information, especially in cases of conductive deafness, and requires little cooperation from the subject. A special ear-piece is fitted snugly into the ear, sealing it off from the outside. This ear-piece contains three channels – a sound source, a miniature microphone and an air channel through which the air pressure on the outside of the eardrum can be varied. In conductive deafness the middle ear absorbs less sound energy and reflects more. The reflected sound is picked up by the microphone and can be measured. The effect, on this, of variations in the pressure in the ear canal, between the ear-piece and the eardrum, match changes in pressure in the middle ear, are also observed.

Impedance audiometry is especially useful in checking children suspected of being severely deaf and for investigating trouble with the eustachian tubes – which, in health, ensure that the pressure on the two sides of the eardrums remains equal.

SPEECH AUDIOMETRY

In this method a succession of two-syllable words are presented to the subject at varying levels of intensity. After each word, the subject is asked to repeat it, and a record is made of the intensity at which 50 per cent of the words are repeated correctly. This is the speech reception threshold. The operator also notes what percentage of words are correctly identified at a level much higher (40 decibels) than the speech reception threshold. This is normally 90 to 100 per cent in conductive deafness, but is reduced in sensorineural hearing loss.

OTOACOUSTIC EMISSIONS

When the cochlea is stimulated it produces its own sounds and these can be picked up by a tiny microphone in the ear canal. This fact can be used as an objective test of ear function in very young people. An otoacoustic test on a two-year-old child can be done in a few minutes. The method can also detect malingering and hysterical deafness.

auditione

Latin root meaning 'hearing' as in auditory (of hearing).

aura

The preliminary, or warning, stage before an attack of some kind. Epileptics and sufferers from migraine are usually familiar with the auras – respectively, a feeling of general coldness and the perception of sparkling lights – which herald an attack.

auranofin

A gold preparation that can be taken by mouth for the treatment of **rheumatoid arthritis**. A brand name is Ridaura.

aure

Latin root meaning 'ear' as in aural (of the ear).

Aureomycin

A brand name for the antibiotic **chlortetracycline**.

auscultation

Listening with a stethoscope to the sounds made by the heart, the lungs, blood passing through narrowed vessels (bruits), the movement of fluid or gas in the abdomen, and so on. The stethoscope is a simple tube device for conveniently coupling the sounds produced by the body to both of the doctor's ears. No amplification is involved in the ordinary stethoscope.

The chest-piece of the stethoscope can often be rotated so that the doctor has a choice of using a fairly narrow, open-ended receiver, or a wider, flatter device covered with a plastic diaphragm. The latter is more sensitive than the former, especially to high frequencies, but less directionally selective.

The 'breath sounds', as heard through the stethoscope, are produced by vibration of the vocal cords as the air passes between them, and are conducted through the lungs to the chest wall where they can be heard. Their character is, however, greatly affected by the state of the lungs through which they pass. Solid tissue conducts sound better and both the breath sounds and the sounds of the voice ('say "ninety-nine"') are heard more clearly if there is local loss of the normal spongy consistency of the lungs. Lung cavities produce a characteristic hollow sound. Disease also causes added sounds, such as wheezes, crackles and musical notes of different pitches, and these can indicate spasm of the bronchial

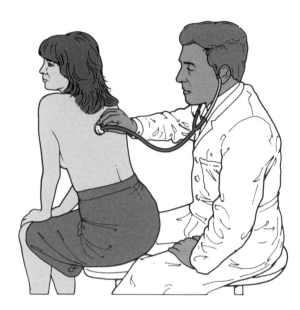

Even in this era of high-tech medicine, auscultation with the stethoscope is still a valuable diagnostic method. The stethoscope is especially useful in investigating disorders of the lungs and the heart. Expert cardiologists can derive a great deal of important information from the subtle changes in the heart sounds characteristic of various heart diseases.

tubes as in bronchitis and asthma, and fluid in the air sacs, as in pneumonia. Rubbing between the layers of the pleura (the lung linings), in pleurisy, causes a characteristic 'creaking' or 'leather-bending' sound.

See also **chest examination**, **heart examination**.

autism

A serious childhood disorder of intellectual and higher brain function which starts before the age of thirty months. Autistic children are withdrawn, self-absorbed, interested in objects but not in people and often unable to communicate by normal speech. They show stereotyped, self-centred behaviour patterns, repeating the same activity over and over again and showing rage if interrupted. The majority are, and remain, educationally subnormal and 10 to 15 per cent develop **epilepsy**.

Autism is believed by some to be a form of **schizophrenia** but does not respond to medical treatment. Some affected children respond to educational conditioning based on reward for appropriate behaviour. Parents need all the help they can possibly get.

autism variant

See **Asperger's syndrome**.

autoclave

A strong sealed chamber in which surgical instruments, towels, dressings, etc. can be sterilized by steam under raised pressure.

auto-immune disease

An important range of conditions in which destructive inflammation of various body tissues occurs. This inflammation is caused by antibodies produced because the body has ceased to regard the affected part as 'self'. The tissue affected is regarded as 'foreign' material and is attacked by the *auto-antibodies* formed in response.

autologous blood donation

Transfusion of a person's own blood. Blood may be taken some time prior to surgery, stored and then used, if necessary, during or after surgery. Alternatively, one or two units of blood may be taken immediately before surgery and replaced by a non-blood infusion. This dilutes the patient's blood so that fewer red cells are lost in bleeding. The blood is then re-transfused at the end of surgery when no further blood loss is anticipated. The method became popular among patients when concern about HIV contamination of donated blood was at its height, but interest declined when HIV antibody testing was incorporated into donor screening and stringent criteria were required for donors. Studies have shown that autologous blood transfusion is uneconomical as a routine procedure.

autonomic nervous system

This is the part of the nervous system which controls functions, such as the heartbeat, the secretion of glands and the contraction of blood vessels, that are not normally under conscious volition. Many automatic and unconscious processes are essential for health and even life, and these are controlled by the autonomic nervous system. It is subdivided into two parts, the sympathetic and the parasympathetic, and these are, in general, contrary and in balance.

The sympathetic system arises from the spinal cord in the back and lumbar region and is concerned with the automatic responses of the body to sudden stressful situations. The sympathetic system is involved in the 'fight or flight' situation and causes constriction of blood vessels in the skin and intestines and widening (dilatation) of blood vessels in the muscles. There is an increase in the heart rate, dilatation of the pupils, widening of the lung air tubes (bronchi), contraction of tiny skin muscles causing the hair to rise, relaxation of the bladder, a reduction in the activity of the bowel and promotion of ejaculation of semen. The adrenal gland is stimulated to produce adrenaline and this hormone, in turn, causes widespread similar effects.

The parasympathetic system is concerned with repose and repair activities. It constricts the pupils of the eyes, stimulates salivary secretion, decreases the heart rate, constricts the bronchi, stimulates the stomach and intestinal enzyme secretion, contracts the bladder and releases the bladder sphincter and stimulates erection of the penis.

autopsy

A post-mortem pathological examination done to determine the cause of death or assist in medical research.

autosome

Any ordinary paired chromosome other than one of the sex chromosomes. There are twenty-two pairs of autosomes and one pair of sex chromosomes. The great majority of genes are thus autosomal. The others are said to be *sex-linked*.

autosuggestion

A form of self-conditioning involving repeated internal assertion of positive and helpful propositions. The phrase had a remarkable vogue in the earlier part of the twentieth century but the procedure has not lived up to its promise.

avascular

Lacking in blood vessels. A totally avascular tissue may survive if oxygen and nutrients can be supplied by diffusion from surrounding areas, but acquired avascularity usually leads to rapid tissue death.

aversion therapy

A form of treatment for addiction or antisocial behaviour in which the undesirable activity is deliberately associated in the mind of the subject with some very unpleasant experience. The drug apomorphine which, when injected, causes distressing nausea and vomiting, has been used to try to induce an aversion to alcohol. Drinks are given and each is followed by an injection. The procedure is repeated until, purportedly, the subject prefers not to drink. Similarly, attempts have been made to treat sexual anomaly by associating the particular practice with electric shock, etc. Aversion therapy is not widely used.

avitaminosis

Any disorder caused by a deficiency of one or more vitamins.

Avloclor

A brand name for chloroquine.

Avomine

A brand name for **promethazine**.

Avonex

A brand name for **interferon beta**.

avulsion

The forcible tearing off, or separation, of part of the body usually in the course of major injury.

awareness, loss of

See **persistent vegetative state**.

Axid

A brand name for **nizatidine**.

axilla

Latin root meaning 'armpit' as in axillary (of the armpit).

axis bone

The second of the vertebrae of the spine, upon which the skull and first vertebra (**atlas bone**) can rotate. The axis bone has a short, stout vertical peg called the odontoid process around which the atlas vertebra turns.

axon

The long fibre coming from a nerve cell and forming, in bundles with many thousands of other axons, the anatomical structure known as a nerve. Although cell bodies are microscopic, axons may be relatively long – sometimes many centimetres. Axons convey nerve impulses from the cell body to a remote point, connecting with other cells or with muscle fibres or glands.

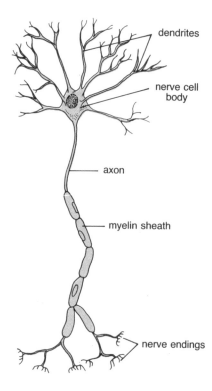

Axon. This diagram represents a nerve cell and shows the various parts. In many cases the axon is much longer than is represented. Some axons are many centimetres long. The axon is insulated by the myelin sheath.

ayurvedism

An ancient Hindu system of medicine contained in the Ayur Veda, a treatise on the art of healing and prolonging life.

Azactam

A brand name for **aztreonam**.

azapropazone

A non-steroidal anti-inflammatory (**NSAID**) drug used in the treatment of conditions such as **rheumatoid arthritis**. A brand name is Rheumox.

azatadine

An **antihistamine** and **serotonin antagonist drug** used in the treatment of allergic conditions. A brand name is Optimine.

azathioprine

A drug used to suppress the immune system so as to avoid rejection of donor transplants. Immune suppression may have serious side-effects such as the flare-up of latent infections and an increased risk of malignant tumours such as lymphomas, but azathioprine is safer than other immunosuppressive drugs. Also used to treat rheumatism. A brand name is Imuran.

azelaic acid

An antibacterial drug used externally in the form of a skin cream. A brand name is Skinoren.

azelastine

An **antihistamine drug** used in the treatment of hay fever. Brand names are Optilast and Rhinolast.

azithromycin

An **antibiotic drug** used in the treatment of a range of infections including genital Chlamydia. A brand name is Zithromax.

azlocillin

An acylureidopenicillin effective against the organism *Pseudomonas aeruginosa*, otherwise difficult to attack effectively. A brand name is Securopen.

azoospermia

Absence of spermatozoa from the seminal fluid, a circumstance causing total male sterility.

AZT

Azidothymidine or Zidovudine. A drug used in attempts to control AIDS. The drug is toxic but does seem to be able to prolong life. A short course of AZT has been shown to be capable of halving the incidence of transmission of HIV from mother to baby. AZT is now commonly used in combination with other anti-HIV drugs especially **protease inhibitors**.

aztreonam

A **beta-lactam antibiotic** effective against aerobic Gram negative organisms. A brand name is Azactam.

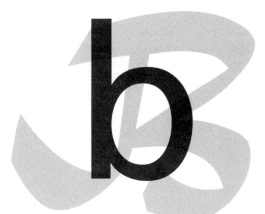

babesiosis

A rare disease caused by an organism that is spread by hard-bodied biting ticks. The causal agent behaves similarly to the malarial parasite, invading the red blood cells and causing them to rupture. This leads to fever and anaemia, but the spleen is able to cope with both the organism and the products of red cell breakdown and the condition settles in a few weeks or months. In people who, for any reason, have had the spleen removed, the haemoglobin released from the red cells colours the urine red, obstructs the kidneys and causes jaundice. In these cases, the mortality rate is very high.

Babinski's test

An important sign of serious neurological disease, first described in 1896 by the French neurologist Joseph Francois Felix Babinski (1857–1932), and still a part of every neurological examination. As in the knee-jerk, the Babinski test involves sending a strong stimulus to the spinal cord, by way of a sensory nerve, which immediately provokes an outgoing impulse to an appropriate set of muscles. In this case, when the outer side of the sole of the foot is firmly stroked longitudinally with a sharp object, the toes will, in the normal, curl downwards.

In health, the spinal reflex is kept under control by higher nerve tracts coming down the spinal cord from the brain. These *upper motor neurones* exert a dampening influence on the basic reflex, and when they are damaged, the spinal reflexes become exaggerated. The knee-jerk becomes excessively forceful and the Babinski sign becomes positive – the toes extend and fan outwards and the knee and hip bend to pull the foot away.

So Babinski's sign is an indication of neurological damage at a higher level, either in the brain or in the upper part of the spinal cord. The Babinski sign may be positive on one side, for instance, in someone who has had a stroke. When the damage is in the spinal nerves, both the knee jerk and the Babinski reflex will be absent.

baby, and mother, closeness of

See **kangaroo mother method**.

baby blues

The short-lived depression and tearfulness which assails about half of all pregnant women, especially in the first **pregnancy**. This condition must be distinguished from the much more serious and distressing condition of pathological sadness or *puerperal depression* (post-natal illness) from which some mothers suffer soon after the birth of their baby.

Puerperal depression usually starts suddenly and without warning on the second or third day after delivery and, although sometimes severe, is usually over in about two months. In most cases, the depression is minor, but in about one case in 1000 it becomes serious enough to require admission to hospital. Proper supervision and treatment of these cases are essential, for there is a real risk of suicide or murder of the baby.

baby oxygenation, life-saving

See **extracorporeal membrane oxygenation (EMCO)**.

baby spasms

See **Di George syndrome**.

baby screaming

See **colic, infantile**.

baby skin, greasy

See **vernix**.

baby skull openings under skin

See **fontanelle**.

baby stools, green

See **meconium**.

baby vomiting

See **pyloric stenosis**.

backache

See **lumbar pain**.

bacitracin

An antibiotic derived from the bacterium *Bacillus subtilis*. It acts by interfering with the formation of the bacterial cell membrane and is highly effective against many organisms especially the haemolytic streptococcus. Unfortunately, it is so liable to damage the kidneys that it must be confined to external use. Brand names are Cicatrin and Polyfax.

baclofen

A drug derived from the **neuro-transmitter GABA** that interferes with nerve transmission in the spinal cord and relaxes muscle spasm. It is used to alleviate the effects of conditions such as **stroke** and **multiple sclerosis**. A brand name is Lioresal.

bacteraemia

The presence of **bacteria** in the circulating blood. This is not necessarily serious and often happens after dental treatment, when there is a transient presence of bacteria which have originated in the mouth. There are circumstances, however, in which even these relatively harmless organisms can cause life-threatening disease.

> If a person with bacteraemia has damaged heart valves the bacteria may settle there to cause inflammation of the heart lining (bacterial endocarditis).

RISKS
Bacteraemia with disease-producing (pathogenic) organisms, commonly described as 'blood poisoning', is always serious, and there is never any doubt that the patient is gravely ill.

RECOGNITION AND SYMPTOMS
There is high fever, prostration, and a variety of effects depending on where the bacteria settle and reproduce.

TREATMENT
Early and intensive treatment with appropriate antibiotics may be the only hope of saving life.

bacteria

Single-celled, microscopic, living organisms occurring in countless numbers everywhere except in materials that have been sterilized. The bacterial population of the world exceeds, by many billions of times, the population of the visible animals and it is impossible, in normal life, to avoid them. Our bodies, and everything we come in contact with, are liberally covered with bacteria.

It is a mistake to think that all bacteria cause disease. Most of them are harmless. Many are essential in nature, causing the breakdown of dead plant and animal organic material so that the world does not become clogged up with debris, and the cycle of nature can continue. Putrefaction in animal bodies is caused by **enzymes** produced by bacteria and is an essential stage in the breakdown of complex molecules to simpler, reusable elements.

Medicine is concerned with the relatively small group of bacteria which cause infection (pathogenic bacteria). These take several forms. The cocci are spherical and usually about one thousandth of a millimetre in diameter. They may collect together in bunches, when they are called *staphylococci* (Greek *staphylos* – 'a bunch of grapes') or they may remain joined in long single strands. These are known as *streptococci* ('streptos' – 'twisted', *kokkos* – 'a berry'). Staphylococci are particularly common disease producers. *Diplococci* stay together in pairs – this group includes the organism that causes gonorrhoea. *Bacilli* are straight, rod-shaped organisms (Latin *bacillum* – 'a staff or wand'); *vibrios* are curved; and *spirilla* are wavy.

MULTIPLICATION
Bacteria reproduce very rapidly and under ideal conditions, as in the human body, have a generation about every twenty minutes. So the bacterial population can multiply eightfold in an hour and by many millions of times in a day. Compare this with the twenty-year generation in humans and two very important facts become apparent. The first is that a few bacteria can, unless opposed, quickly increase to an overwhelming infection. The second is that the normal processes of evolution by natural selection are enormously accelerated. In bacteria, these occur about half a million times faster than in humans, so it is perhaps not surprising that the misuse of antibiotics for trivial conditions and in inadequate dosage has led to the emergence of highly resistant strains.

POTENTIAL PROBLEMS
Bacteria produce their damaging effect by the production of very powerful poisons (toxins) which are among the most poisonous substances known. In some cases the toxins are released only when the bacteria die, but, in others, living bacteria can release *exotoxins* into the blood, which can circulate to all parts of the body to bind on to body cells and gravely affect their function or even survival. Fortunately, bacteria are not allowed to multiply unchecked in the body and for this advantage we are indebted to the immune system.

DEALING WITH BACTERIA
Bacteria, if accessible, are easily killed. Strong chemical poisons (disinfectants), dry or moist heat, gamma radiation, ultraviolet light, and other methods, are routinely used to sterilize instruments, dressings, drugs, operating theatre gowns, towels and sheets. The difficulty arises when the bacteria are inhabiting the human body, especially internally, and methods must be found which can kill the parasite without killing the host. Antibiotics and chemotherapeutic agents, which are able to do this, have, of course, radically altered the face of medicine.

See also **health maintenance**.

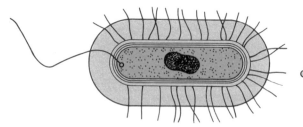

enlarged Salmonella bacillus (7 times the scale of the other examples shown)

cocci

bacilli

spirochaetes

Bacteria. This diagram shows some, but by no means all, of the varieties of infective bacteria. The actual microscopic appearance of the organisms is no longer of major importance in identifying them as many highly specific tests now exist.

back, lower, swelling on

See **spina bifida**.

back pain and bladder dysfunction

See **cauda equina syndrome**.

bactericidal

Able to kill bacteria.

bacteriology

The scientific study of bacteria. Medical bacteriology is the study of those organisms which can cause disease or which are normally present, harmlessly or beneficially, in the body.

bacteriostatic

Able to restrain or control the multiplication of bacteria, without actually killing them. When a bacteriostatic effect is achieved the organisms are more readily destroyed by the immune system.

bacteriuria

Bacteria in the urine. The urine in the bladder is normally sterile and the presence of bacteria in a specimen may be due to contamination while the urine is being passed. But the presence of 100,000 or more disease-producing (pathogenic) bacteria indicates a urinary tract infection.

Bactroban

A brand name for **mupirocin**.

Bactroban nasal

A brand name for **mupirocin**.

bagassosis

A lung disease caused by allergy to inhaled dust from sugar cane waste (bagasse). There is persistent lung inflammation (pneumonitis) with progressive replacement of functioning lung with scar tissue.

Baker's cyst

A painless swelling occurring behind the knee when there is escape of joint fluid (synovial fluid) through the capsule of the joint as a result of excessive production. Synovial fluid is secreted in excess quantity as a result of injury to the joint surfaces, usually from excessive wear (**osteoarthritis**). The fluid collects in the tissues and a new capsule condenses around it.

A Baker's cyst can be removed surgically, or the fluid can be sucked out (aspirated) with a syringe and a corticosteroid drug injected to reduce local inflammation.

balanitis

Inflammation of the bulb (glans) of the penis. Balanitis is commonest in small boys with tight foreskins (*phimosis*) or in babies left so long in wet nappies that the urea in the urine turns to ammonia.

POSSIBLE CAUSES

Balanitis in the adult is usually the result of gross neglect of personal hygiene in the uncircumcised. A white, cheesy and foul-smelling material called smegma accumulates under the foreskins of the unwashed and this eventually causes inflammation. There is some evidence that persistent balanitis from this cause may lead on to cancer of the penis. Daily washing is mandatory for men.

Other causes of balanitis include thrush (**candidiasis**) and **trichomoniasis**, both of which commonly infect the vagina. It is useless, in cases of thrush or trichomoniasis, to treat only one partner, as infection readily spreads either way. Various other **sexually transmitted diseases**, including syphilis, can cause balanitis.

baldness

See **hair loss**.

baldness, female

See **androgenic alopecia**.

balloon catheter

A fine double tube, with an expansible cylindrical portion near one end, which can be passed along an artery to an area partially blocked by disease (**atherosclerosis**) and then inflated so as to stretch and widen the vessel.

After the procedure steps must be taken to prevent blood from clotting on the roughened area left. Drugs that reduce this tendency are called anticoagulants. In many cases it is sufficient to give a small dose of aspirin each day, for an indefinite period.

WHY IT'S USED

Such blockage may, unless relieved, lead to various serious conditions including gangrene of a limb, kidney failure, and, most commonly, coronary thrombosis. Many patients with chest pain on exertion (**angina pectoris**) have been relieved of their symptom, and rendered less liable to coronary thrombosis, by this procedure. When properly performed, the success rate of balloon angioplasty, as it is called, approaches 80 per cent.

Balloon catheters have also been extensively used to treat narrowing (stenosis) of the heart valves – a common sequel to rheumatic fever and other conditions – as an alternative to major surgery.

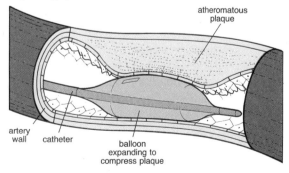

The use of a balloon catheter for angioplasty is a routine and valuable measure, especially in the treatment of narrowing of the bore of coronary arteries by atherosclerosis. The illustration shows an atheromatous plaque being compressed by the high pressure of air or fluid in the balloon.

ballottement

A physical sign produced when a solid organ or suspected mass, lying within fluid, is given a sharp push with the tips of the fingers. The mass swings quickly away and then back again to strike the fingers and confirm its presence. Ballottement may thus show either fluid or an abnormal mass.

balsalazide

A salicylate drug used in the treatment of **ulcerative colitis**. A brand name is Colazide.

base pair separation

See **helicase**.

Bambec

A brand name for **bambuterol**.

bambuterol

A selective bronchodilator (B2 agonist) drug used to treat **asthma** and other causes of bronchospasm. A brand name is Bambec.

bandage

A binder. A long strip of woven cotton, wool, plastic, rubber or other material which is wrapped firmly round any part of the body for a variety of reasons. Bandages may be non-stretch or elastic, conforming or otherwise, adhesive or plain.
USES
They can be useful as temporary fixatives for dressings or to maintain pressure over a pad in the first-aid management of bleeding. They may be used to help to immobilize an injured part and to maintain sustained pressure to support and treat **varicose veins** and varicose skin ulceration.

Nowadays, bandages are used much less often than before. It is probable that the former vogue for bandaging was inspired as much by a desire to cover up the unsightly as by any real belief in the therapeutic value of the procedure. It is certain that, in may cases, especially burns, more good would have been done by exposure.

Nevertheless, bandages still have a place in surgical practice, mainly for support and **immobilization**. Esmarch's bandage is a broad rubber strip wound tightly round a limb, from the outer to the inner end, so as to empty the blood vessels and allow short operations, such as varicose vein stripping, without bleeding. Tight bandages are also used to control the collection of fluid in a limb resulting from obstruction to the lymphatic drainage (lymphoedema).

Baratol

A brand name for **indoramin**.

barba

Latin root meaning 'beard' as in sycosis barbae ('dirty shave').

barber

The early barbers were the first surgeons and used their razors for minor operations, especially blood-letting – supposed then to have medical value, but, in fact almost always harmful and often the last straw in ensuring a fatal outcome. The symbolic barbers' pole, with its spiral of blood-stained bandages, still testifies to the activities of these enterprising tradesmen who, eventually, formed a guild of barber surgeons, setting up in opposition to the more fastidious, thoughtful and learned gentlemen – the physicians. There is some evidence that the basic differences in outlook between the two groups survives to this day. It may not be entirely coincidental that the physicians refer to themselves as 'Doctor' and refer to the surgeons as 'Mr'.

barbiturates

A range of sedative drugs, formerly used in enormous quantities, but now largely replaced by the **benzodiazepine drugs**. The best known barbiturates are phenobarbitone (Luminal), amylobarbitone (Amytal), butobarbitone (Soneryl) and thiopentone (Pentothal). Apart from phenobarbitone for epilepsy and pentothal for the induction of general anaesthesia, they have acquired the same slightly disreputable quality, in medical circles, as the once equally highly regarded **amphetamine drugs**. Much the same thing is now beginning to happen to the benzodiazepines, which are no longer considered non-addictive and entirely safe.

The origin of the term 'barbiturate' is on a par with the name of the benzodiazepine 'Mogadon' (which is said to have been tested on 'moggies'). Johann Friedrich Wilhelm Baeyer (1835–1917), the Nobel Prize winner, who was working on new derivatives of urea, a constituent of urine, is claimed to have obtained the supplies of urea from which he synthesized the new compound, from a Munich waitress called Barbara. So Barbara's uric acid became barbituric acid. The rest is history.

Barbiturates can cause arthritis, allergic reactions, liver damage and addiction. Their effect can be dangerously increased by alcohol and reduce the effects of various other drugs such as chlorpromazine (Largactil), steroids, phenytoin (Epanutin) and coumarin (see anticoagulant drugs).

barbotage

A method of pain control designed to interrupt the pain pathways in the spinal cord. 20 ml of cerebrospinal fluid are repeatedly withdrawn and reinjected from the space surrounding the cord. Most patients enjoy relief of pain for up to seven months.

bare lymphocyte syndrome

A rare recessive form of immunodeficiency caused by a gene mutation that results in the absence of the class 2 of the self-indicating 'flags' on cell surfaces, the **major histocompatibility complex** glycoprotein molecules. Children with this mutation are extremely susceptible to infection with all kinds of organisms and seldom survive for more than four years from birth.

Barker hypothesis

The proposition that the quality of a baby's nourishment while in the womb and during infancy determines the subsequent development of risk factors such as high blood pressure, blood clotting biochemistry and glucose intolerance, and is thus a major determinant of coronary heart disease later in life.

barium X-ray examination

Barium is a metal opaque to X-rays. Most barium compounds are poisonous, but barium sulphate ($BaSO_4$) is completely insoluble and forms a tasteless and harmless white chalky powder which can be made into a suspension or a smooth liquid paste. Additives improve its coating properties and reduce foaming. If some of this paste is swallowed and an X-ray taken, the limits of the barium within the gullet (oesophagus), stomach and bowel are clearly seen as a dense white outline. Barium moves freely into ulcers in the wall of the gut and these show as knobs or buttons extending out beyond the normal edge of the shadow. Should there be any mass or tumour extending into the bowel interior, the barium shadow will contain a 'hole'. This is called a *filling defect*. Any abnormal narrowing of the bowel is immediately apparent by a narrowing of the barium shadow on the X-ray.

Barium X-rays are useful in the investigation of disease or abnormality in any part of the digestive tract. They can reveal out-pouchings from the lower part of the throat, narrowing of the oesophagus, swallowing disorders, hiatus hernia, ulcers of the stomach and duodenum, tumours or polyps anywhere in the bowel but especially in the colon, abnormal pouches (diverticula), Crohn's disease (regional ileitis) and coeliac disease.

When substantial quantities of barium are taken in this way, the procedure is known as a barium meal. The progress of the barium through the stomach and down the small intestine can be followed by X-rays taken at intervals. A barium 'swallow' is used to investigate problems in the throat and oesophagus, such as pharyngeal pouch, spasm of the oesophagus, swallowing difficulties and tumours. Barium taken by mouth is dispersed and diluted by the time it reaches the large bowel (colon and rectum). Barium investigation of this part of the bowel is best achieved by giving the barium through a tube passed directly into the rectum. This is called a barium enema and can be invaluable in showing up tumours, diverticula and other disorders.

In the course of a barium examination, the subject may be given a mixture to produce gas in the bowel, and will probably be asked to roll to one side or the other, or even right over, to ensure that the lining of the bowel is properly coated. Positioning varies with different kinds of examinations. Barium liquid becomes firmer as water is withdrawn from it in the large intestine, and may even impact into a hard mass which causes constipation or is painful to pass. This problem can be overcome by taking plenty to drink and eating plenty of fibre after the examination and, if necessary, using a laxative. The stools are white for a few days after the examination.

The growth of direct observation of disease, at both ends of the intestinal tract, using fibre optic endoscopy, has somewhat reduced reliance on barium X-ray examination.

barotrauma

Injury resulting from changes in atmospheric (barometric) pressure. These mostly affect the middle ear and generally result from a failure of the mechanism that should balance the pressures on either side of the eardrum.

POSSIBLE CAUSES

If the atmospheric pressure falls, as happens in an aircraft pressurized at less than ground atmospheric pressure, the eardrum will be forced outwards by the relatively greater pressure in the middle ear space. If the external pressure rises, as in a train tunnel, the drum will be forced inwards.

Running forward, from each middle ear cavity to the back of the nose, is the Eustachian tube along which air should be able to pass in either direction. Swallowing opens the valve-like front end of the tube and this should allow the equalization of pressure and normalization of the position of the drum. But it is common for the Eustachian tube to be blocked, either by adenoids or by swelling of the mucous membrane lining, in the course of a cold or nasal **allergy**. In this case the pressures on each side of the eardrum are not equalized and the drums will be painfully displaced, and the hearing affected.

Barotrauma can occur with normal Eustachian tube function, if the pressure changes are, for any reason, extreme. The most serious forms of barotrauma result from explosive noise. When this occurs from a nearby source such as fireworks or a stun grenade, permanent damage is likely, not only to the eardrum, but much more seriously, to the cochlear hearing mechanism of the inner ear. The louder the explosion, the graver the effect. In some cases, the delicate hair-cell transducers in the middle ear are literally shaken to pieces.

Barrett's oesophagus

A gullet (oesophagus) in which long-standing inflammation (oesophagitis) has led to a change in the nature of the lining mucus membrane so that the cells assume a columnar form. An ulcer may develop (Barrett's ulcer) and lead to narrowing (stricture). The changes in the lining cells may progress to cancer.

barrier contraceptive

Any contraceptive, such as a condom or a diaphragm shield, that imposes a barrier between the spermatozoa and the ovum. Properly used, barrier contraceptives are reasonably effective.

See also **contraception**.

barrier cream

Increasing public awareness of the extent of the environmental hazards to the skin has led to a widening use of preparations designed to protect against dermatitis. Most of them are based on the water-repellent and biologically inert range of silicone compounds. Unfortunately, none of these is very effective. The requirement that they should be removable by normal washing after use, so as to avoid long-term blockage of sweat-gland pores and hair follicles, implies inefficiency. In some cases of allergy, barrier creams are more damaging to the skin than the conditions they are claimed to protect against.

In many cases it will be found that, for protection of the hands, impervious gloves offer a better alternative.

barrier nursing

See **nursing, barrier**.

Bartholin's glands

Between the back part of the vaginal orifice and the lesser lips (labia minora) on either side, lie the openings of the two Bartholin's glands, each about half an inch long and lying under the labia majora.

FUNCTION

Under the influence of sexual excitement, these glands secrete a clear mucin which lubricates the vaginal opening and facilitates coitus.

The Danish anatomist, Kaspar Bartholin (1585–1629), who first described the glands in 1679, recorded that the secretion occurred only during sexual intercourse or masturbation. This observation led to a renewal of interest in, and, eventually, a proper understanding of, the processes of reproduction.

POSSIBLE PROBLEMS

The glands sometimes become infected and may form painful abscesses requiring surgical drainage.

bartonellosis

A South American infectious disease, spread by sandflies and affecting the blood cells. The major form, *Oroya fever*, features high temperature, **anaemia**, and enlargement of the spleen and lymph nodes. The condition responds well to antibiotics.

basal cell carcinoma

See **rodent ulcer**.

basal narcosis

Premedication with narcotic drugs to reduce anxiety and post-operative shock.

base pair

Two of four small molecules that lie, linked together, between the two strands of the **DNA** double helix, like the rungs of a ladder, each linked pair forming one rung. One of the pair is in the purine chemical class and the other is in the pyrimidine class. The linkage of the base pair, which is by a relatively weak hydrogen bond between them, occurs only in a particular, complementary, way, so as to produce 'rungs' that are all the same length. Adenine links only with thymine and guanine links only with cytosine.

This is the essence of the manner in which DNA automatically reproduces itself when the linkage between the base pairs is broken and the two strands of the helix separate, leaving single bases standing out from the helical skeleton, ready to link up with the corresponding base partner from the cell fluid. RNA differs from DNA only in that the molecule uracil replaces thymine.

basiliximab

An immunosuppressant drug used to prevent organ rejection in transplantation. A brand name is Simulect.

bat ear

A minor disfigurement of childhood in which the ears are larger and more protruding than usual. Should there be a significant psychological disadvantage, the condition may easily be remedied by a simple plastic surgical procedure (see **otoplasty**).

battered baby syndrome

The clinical condition of a baby or young child who has suffered injury at the hands of parents, fosterparents or others.

RECOGNITION AND SYMPTOMS

The child is often malnourished, sometimes grossly, and there may be signs of lack of care and affection. There may be multiple bruising, evidence of old injuries, X-ray indication of old or current fractures, tearing of the central fold behind the upper lip, cigarette burns, bite marks, and sometimes indications of bleeding inside the skull or brain. Often, the cause of these signs is not immediately apparent and wilful injury is invariably denied.

INCIDENCE

Child abusers come from every social class and usually show apparent willingness to cooperate with medical staff. But there is often a delay in bringing the child to a doctor and careful examination may show signs incompatible with the claimed history. Signs of similar injury on both sides of the body are significant. There is almost always some uncertainty, but doctors are aware that the majority of battered babies discharged without supervision are again assaulted, and a high index of suspicion is always necessary in cases of inadequately explained injury.

POSSIBLE CAUSES

Many of the adults responsible have, themselves, been similarly abused in childhood. Baby battering, which is commonest in the first six months of life, and frequently involves an unwanted child, is often precipitated by excessive crying by the baby, loss of sleep, family rows, money worries, alcoholism, marital resentment, further pregnancy, unemployment and other stressful factors.

TREATMENT

Parents suspected of this form of child abuse are often young and inadequate and require much support, guidance and covert surveillance from local authority social workers and health visitors. Often, a care order is the only effective safeguard.

See also **child abuse, violence in the family**.

battle fatigue

A stress syndrome, now usually called post-traumatic stress disorder, caused by prolonged exposure to the trauma of warfare. There is repetitive reliving of the painful experience, nightmares, persistent anxiety, over-alertness, irritability, restlessness, jumpiness and insomnia.

Baxan

A brand name for **cefadroxil**.

B cell and T cell tumours

See **lymphoma**.

B cells

One of the two main classes of **lymphocytes**, white cells found in the blood, lymph nodes and tissues which, with other cells, form the immune system of the body. B lymphocytes form **clones** which manufacture **antibodies**.

BCG

Bacille Calmette-Guérin, a variant of the tubercle bacillus, obtained by repeated growing of the organism to form a culture of colonies, and then regrowing one small sample of one of these. The aim was to produce a form of the bacillus that did not cause infection but that still prompted a protective immunological response from the body. Albert Calmette (1863–1933) and his assistant Camille Guérin, working at the Pasteur Institute, Paris, started the process in 1906 and for thirteen years they patiently grew one subculture after another, until they had recultured the organism 231 times and were satisfied that the strain was safe. The vaccine, prepared from this strain, came into use in 1921.

BCG is valuable in conferring a measure of immunity on those who have not had the common, inapparent, primary infection and who are, in consequence, susceptible to the disease. It reduces the likelihood of acquiring **tuberculosis** by about 80 per cent. Before considering BCG vaccination, a simple tuberculin test, the Heaf test, is used to determine the immune state of the individual.

Bcl-2 gene

A gene involved in cancer production, of the kind known as a **proto-oncogene**. This gene is over-expressed in various tumours, especially non-Hodgkin lymphoma, resulting in resistance to **apoptosis** (programmed cell death) with encouragement of tumour growth. It has been found that clinical improvement can be achieved in these tumours by targeting BCL-2 messenger RNA with **antisense RNA** sequences to increase apoptosis.

Beclazone

A brand name for **beclomethasone**.

Becloforte

A brand name for **beclomethasone**.

beclomethasone

A corticosteroid drug used in the form of a nasal spray to relieve the symptoms of hay fever (allergic rhinitis). It is also used to treat **asthma**. Brand names are Aerobec, Asmabec, Beclazone, Becloforte, Becodisks, Beconase, Becotide, Filair, Nasobec, Qvar, and Zonivent.

Becodisks

A brand name for **beclomethasone**.

Beconase

A brand name for **beclomethasone**.

Becotide

A brand name for **beclomethasone**.

bed bath

A method of overall washing of a patient who is too weak or frail to be taken to a bathroom. A waterproof sheet is put under the patient and one side is sponged at a time, the patient being rolled carefully first on one side and then on the other. Modern views discourage this kind of patient passivity and bed baths are now performed less often than before.

bedbug

A blood-sucking insect that feeds on mammals. *Cimex lectularis* is a broad, reddish, flat parasite of man, found all over the world in human habitations, wherever low standards of hygiene and relatively high winter temperatures allow it.

It is a non-flying bug which inhabits cracks and crevices in floors and walls during the day and creeps out at night to feed on the nearest human or animal victim, leaving evidence of its activities in the form of bloodstains on the sheets or night-clothes.

The bedbug does not transmit any specific disease, but its bites cause irritation and inflammation and sometimes severe allergic reactions. Following bites on the face, extreme puffiness of the eyelids will occasionally occur, preventing vision in the mornings and arousing unwarranted alarm. Bedbug bites invariably lead to scratching, and secondary infection of the skin is common.

Residual insecticide spray is highly effective in disposing of bedbugs.

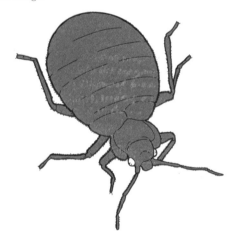

Cimex lectularis, the common bedbug, is about 5 mm long, flat and brown in colour. After a blood meal it is longer, more spherical and darker.

bedpan

A receptacle, of stainless steel, plastic or disposable moulded paper, for the excreta of those unable easily to get out of bed.

bed rest

See **rest**.

bedridden

Forced, by severity of illness, to remain permanently in bed. Some of the alleged bedridden would be better up and about.

bedsore

People who are paralysed or too debilitated to move much may, unless frequently moved, suffer sustained compression of the skin against a bed or a wheelchair in the areas taking the weight of the body. This leads to local loss of blood supply, loss of sensation and, eventually, local tissue death (**gangrene**) with ulceration.
INCIDENCE
Bedsores are especially likely to affect the buttocks, the heels, the elbows and the back of the head and are particularly common in people who have suffered loss of sensation from

neurological damage. Bedsores are especially likely in unconscious patients or in those suffering from loss of sensation, as after a stroke, or extreme weakness or paralysis.

RECOGNITION AND SYMPTOMS

The skin can remain healthy and intact only if it has a constant supply of blood, bringing oxygen, sugars and other essential nutrients. Local pressure compresses the small skin blood vessels, and this supply is cut off.

Bedsores, technically known as *decubitis ulcers*, may be very large and the ulceration may progress to complete local loss of skin with exposure of the underlying tendons or bone.

TREATMENT

Bedsores are avoided by regular changes of position and by skilled nursing to detect and deal with early signs of trouble. Diabetics, and those with compromised blood supply to the limbs from arterial disease, such as atherosclerosis, are especially liable and require special attention. Modern technology has devised all kinds of ingenious beds, which, by differential air inflation of bed segments, or movement of fluid, constantly alter the sites taking the body weight. If economics allow it, these can greatly help to reduce the risk of decubitus ulcers, but they do not eliminate the need for regular passive body movement and vigilance. The skin should be inspected daily and kept clean, dry and in good condition.

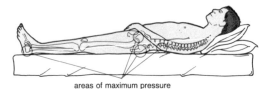

areas of maximum pressure

Bedsores may occur if patients remain for long periods in the same position so that sustained pressure on areas of skin lead to compression of small blood vessels and loss of blood supply.

bedwetting

See **enuresis**.

bee stings

See **insect and mite bites and stings**.

behaviour therapy

A way of treating neurotic disorders and modifying unacceptable patterns of behaviour that brushes aside all the theories of Freud and of later psychoanalytic schools. Behaviour therapy is based on application of *conditioned reflexes*, as described by Pavlov, and on the use of practical positive and negative reinforcement, by reward and punishment, respectively.

HOW IT WORKS

Pavlov introduced a new dimension of thought when he published an account of a classic series of experiments on dogs. Meat placed before a hungry dog induces salivation. If a bell is rung every time the meat is produced, eventually the ringing of the bell, *in the absence of the meat*, will cause salivation. The dog has developed a *conditioned* reflex response to the bell. This is an example of a large range of responses that occur automatically to a stimulus that would not normally have such an effect. Much of our learning and behaviour results from conditioned reflexes.

Behaviour therapy theory holds that neurotic disorders are conditioned responses, brought about by some earlier distressing event that has become linked – possibly accidentally – to an anxiety-producing stimulus. The neurotic disorder is not, as Freud claimed, a symptom of some hidden complex, but is, in itself, the problem. If the conditioning can be eliminated, the problem will vanish. Various methods have been used and most have achieved good results, particularly for specific **phobias**.

One method is *flooding*, in which the person under treatment is exposed, for long periods, to the stimulus which causes the conditioned response and the therapist helps the patient to face up to and overcome the resulting fears. In *modelling* the patient is shown someone, usually the therapist, who responds in an ideal and healthy way to fears and difficulties, and these responses are then compared with those of the patient. In this way, the absurdity of neurotic behaviour can be highlighted and a strong motive for modification provided.

Another method is called *desensitization* or *counterconditioning*. In this, the therapist exposes the patient to stimuli which approximate to those normally causing the problem, while ensuring that he or she remains relaxed and calm. Relaxation techniques are taught which the patient can use when faced with anxiety-provoking situations.

Behçet's syndrome

A persistent (chronic) disease of unknown cause, affecting the mouth, the genital area, the eyes, the joints and the skin.

INCIDENCE

Men are affected twice as often as women and the disease usually starts in the thirties.

RECOGNITION AND SYMPTOMS

The main features are painful, recurrent ulcers in the mouth and on the genitals, and pain and irritation in the eyes with haziness of vision from a potentially serious internal inflammation which, if not effectively treated, can lead to blindness.

The skin is particularly sensitive to minor injury, such as needle pricks, responding with severe inflammation. Small blisters, pustules and red bumps are common. Fifty per cent of patients suffer a mild form of arthritis in the large joints, but this does little harm. A smaller proportion develop problems in the leg veins with inflammation and clotting (thrombophlebitis) and, in a few, there is involvement of the brain and spinal cord. Sometimes the kidneys are also affected.

TREATMENT

Behçet's syndrome comes and goes. Periods of active disease may last for only a few weeks, or may go on for years and may require intensive treatment with steroid drugs to minimize damage from the inflammation. Immunosuppressant drugs have been used in severe cases with some success, implying that Behçet's syndrome may be due to the body's immune system reacting abnormally (autoimmune disease).

belching

The noisy expulsion of gas from the mouth. Repeated belching is due to unconscious and frequent swallowing of air which progressively distends the gullet (oesophagus) until sufficient pressure is built up to provide a satisfying belch. Gas production in the stomach is extremely rare. Air swallowing (aerophagia) is a common response to stress and a frequent feature of dyspepsia. It also occurs in greedy eating. Recurrent belching is an unnecessary affliction and can be cured by knowledge and self-discipline.

Bowel gas is quite a different matter. In the lower part of the intestine gas is certainly generated and the average person finds it necessary to fart ten to twenty times a day.

belief/action incompatibilites

See **cognitive dissonance**.

Bell's palsy

A common and distressing complaint, first described in the early nineteenth century, by the Scottish surgeon and anatomist Sir Charles Bell (1774–1842). Bell's descriptions hold good to this day. Within a matter of hours of onset, some or all of the muscles on one side of the face become paralysed so that the corner of the mouth droops, the lower eyelid falls away, and the affected side of the face becomes flattened and expressionless. Sometimes the paralysis is preceded by a pain in the bone behind the ear on the affected side.

The facial muscles, on which all facial expression depends, are caused to contract by electrical impulses passing along the two facial nerves, one on each side, which come directly from the brain, emerging from the skull by way of narrow channels through the temporal bone. Although not proved, it is believed that inflammation of one of the nerves, from virus infection or other agency, causes it to swell and become compressed within this channel so that it is no longer able to conduct nerve impulses to the muscles.

The result is a one-sided paralysis. This may be total or partial, depending on the severity. In partial paralysis, recovery always occurs, although this may take weeks or months. At least one-fifth of those with total paralysis recover fully, but the outcome is always uncertain. Sometimes, in these severe cases, the regenerating nerve fibres in the facial nerve trunk become redirected to the wrong muscles, with surprising results.

TREATMENT
Permanent facial paralysis is a grave disfigurement and affliction. Much can be done, however, by plastic surgery, to improve the lopsided appearance and to prevent secondary effects, such as eye watering. If there has been no recovery in six months, surgery should be considered. Delay leads to contracture of skin and muscle.

Bell's phenomenon

If one side of the face is paralysed, as in Bell's palsy, so that the eyelids cannot be closed, attempts to do so, or to blink, will cause the eye on the affected side to roll upwards. This is called Bell's phenomenon and it can be protective to the eye as it helps to keep the cornea moist.

belly

A common name for the abdomen. The term derives from an early Scandinavian word for a sack, but does not necessarily imply undue protuberance.

belly breathing

See **abdominal breathing**.

bends

The nautical term for **decompression sickness**. Divers at depth have to breathe air under high pressure. As a result of the high pressure, much more than the usual quantity of air becomes dissolved in the blood. The dissolved oxygen is used by the body, but the inert nitrogen is not, and remains in the blood. When the diver comes up again, the pressure is lowered and the dissolved nitrogen has to escape from the blood. If it does so quickly, as in an emergency ascent from a great depth, it will appear in the form of bubbles large enough to block off small arteries. In mild cases this simply causes pain, felt most often in or around the joints – in nautical parlance 'the bends'.

RECOGNITION AND SYMPTOMS
In more serious cases, many bubbles form throughout the body. By depriving various areas of the body of blood supply, these bubbles may cause fatigue, skin rashes, swelling (**oedema**) or marbling of the skin, pain in the abdomen or even local destruction (**necrosis**) of bone. The worst effects occur in the nervous system and include total paralysis.

> Serious decompression disease is much more common in scuba divers than in those wearing diving helmets.

TREATMENT
If the affected person is recompressed the bubbles dissolve again and the flow of blood is restored. The pressure can then be slowly released.

> The only hope for recovery in serious cases of the bends is to get the victim to a compression chamber as quickly as possible. A helicopter should be called to minimize delay.

benign

The term meaning not malignant. Not usually tending to cause death. The derivation is the Latin *bene natus*, meaning 'well born'. Although usually safe, a benign tumour may enlarge to a considerable size and may cause damage by local pressure or by displacing other tissue, especially in a confined space such as the inside of the skull. Apart from such cases, benign tumours seldom cause death. In contrast to malignant tumours, they do not seed off (metastasize) and so spread to other parts of the body.

benign familial neonatal convulsions

A rare dominant genetic disorder due to a mutated gene on the long arm of chromosome 20. The condition features brief epileptic-like seizures occurring within a few days or a week or two of birth. Longer-term follow-up, however, suggests that the condition may progress to fully established epilepsy.

benign intracranial hypertension

A syndrome of raised pressure within the skull in the absence of a brain tumour, water on the brain (hydrocephalus) or other obvious cause. The condition is only relatively benign as it often leads to visual loss from compression damage to the optic nerves. It occurs most often in women below the age of 40 and causes severe headache and nausea but no deterioration of intellect or consciousness. Obesity is a common association. Ophthalmoscopic examination shows striking swelling of the optic discs (papilloedema).

Once the diagnosis is made close surveillance is necessary to ensure that the visual function is not being prejudiced. If visual loss is noted it may be necessary to reduce the pressure within the skull by establishing a surgical shunt connection between the cerebro-spinal fluid in the lumbar region of the spinal canal (which is continuous with the fluid in the skull) and the peritoneal cavity of the abdomen.

benign positional vertigo

A very common cause of dizziness precipitated by head movements or by lying down or turning over in bed. There is a typical circular movement of the eyes (rotational nystagmus) when the head is inclined and turned to the affected side. The disorder is believed to be due to debris in the semicircular canals that moves with head movement causing a current flow in the fluid of the canals (endolymph) and stimulation of the position sense mechanism.

Benoryl

A brand name for **benorylate**.

benorylate

A drug derived from aspirin and **paracetamol** which is less irritating to the stomach than aspirin, but equally effective as a painkiller and non-steroidal anti-inflammatory drug (**NSAID**) in the treatment of arthritic pain. A brand name is Benoral.

benperidol

A drug with phenothiazine-like properties used in the treatment of socially unacceptable sexual deviant behaviour. A brand name is Anquil.

benserazide

A dopamine precursor drug used in the treatment of **Parkinson's disease**. The drug is also given in conjunction with levodopa to prevent its breakdown in the body. A brand name is Madopar.

benzhexol

An anticholinergic drug that blocks the action of acetylcholine in the nervous system. It is used to treat the symptoms of **Parkinson's disease**. A brand name is Broflex.

benzodiazepine drugs

A range of sedative and tranquillizing drugs of the Valium, Librium and Mogadon type. They were introduced in 1960 by Hoffman-LaRoche whose profits from this group alone have been astronomical. Compared with earlier sedatives, the benzodiazepines are remarkably safe and death from overdose is almost unheard of. In small doses the benzodiazepines relax muscles and relieve anxiety; in larger doses they put people to sleep. They are prescribed and consumed by the billion, about 2 per cent of the population of the Western world taking them regularly to promote sleep, reduce anxiety and relieve depression.

There is no question that they abolish much distress of mind. It is surprising, however, that so little concern has been expressed over the inevitable dependence which must occur when one relies on a drug rather than on one's own resources. Dependence of this sort is not a property of any one particular drug, and the claim that any such drugs are not habit-forming is at least dubious.

This group of drugs includes nitrazepam (Mogadon) and flurazepam (Dalmane) both of which have a prolonged action which may be cumulative; and temazepam (Euhypnos), which has a shorter action and no hangover effect; and diazepam (Valium), chlordiazepoxide (Librium), lorazepam (Ativan), medazepam (Nobrium) and clorazepate (Tranxene), all of which are widely used for the relief of mild anxiety.

benztropine

An anticholinergic drug used to control the symptoms of **Parkinson's disease**. A brand name is Cogentin.

benzydamine hydrochloride

A drug used as an embrocation in the treatment of muscle pain. A brand name is Difflam.

benzyl benzoate

An oily liquid used as a lotion for the treatment of **scabies**. A brand name is Ascabiol.

bephenium hydroxynaphthoate

An anthelmintic drug used for hookworm and roundworm. A brand name is Alcopar.

beractant

A surfactant drug used in the treatment of the **respiratory distress syndrome**. A brand name is Survanta.

bereavement

Serious loss, giving rise to a characteristic and well-recognized pattern of psychological reaction known as mourning. The strength of the reaction varies with the size of the loss.

POSSIBLE CAUSES

In most cases, the greatest loss is the loss of a loved person by death, but this is by no means the only cause of bereavement and mourning. Loss by divorce or separation, loss of physical freedom by imprisonment, loss of a loved environment, loss of a fortune, of status or reputation, even loss by burglary or theft – all can evoke the patterns of mourning.

RECOGNITION AND SYMPTOMS

The main stages are: alarm, shock, denial, mitigation (attempt at magical bargaining), anger, depression, guilt, acceptance and adjustment.

beri-beri

A deficiency disease caused by inadequate intake of vitamin B1 (thiamine). Rice contains plenty of thiamine, but this is all in the husk and a diet exclusively of highly polished rice can lead to beri-beri. Thiamine is necessary for normal nerve function and the deficiency leads to widespread nerve degeneration. *Beri* is the Indian word for 'weak'; the repetition is used for emphasis.

RECOGNITION AND SYMPTOMS

Damage occurs in the brain and the spinal cord, and the muscle fibres of the heart are also affected. The result of all this is severe fatigue, loss of memory, irritability and insomnia. The feet feel as if they are burning and the muscles develop cramps. There is severe tenderness in the calves. Eventually the legs become wasted and foot drop occurs. In very severe cases, major brain defects develop with severe confusion, paralysis, coma and death.

'Wet' beri-beri results from heart failure caused by the damage to the heart muscle. The word 'wet' refers to widespread fluid retention in the tissues (**oedema**), occurring because the heart is unable to pump blood fast enough to prevent this from happening.

berylliosis

A disease caused by contact with the highly poisonous metallic element beryllium. This is found in the light-producing phosphors in fluorescent light tubes and TV tubes, and is also used in the aerospace industry. Acute poisoning, from quite a small dose, can rapidly cause death, but more common is a form of pneumonia caused by inhaling dust or fumes containing the metal. This may show itself as long as twenty years after the exposure and can lead to a progressive loss of lung function and eventual failure to maintain a sufficient oxygen supply.

beta-adrenoceptor

One of the many receptor sites at which noradrenaline and other hormones act to cause muscle to contract or relax. Beta-adrenoceptors occur in blood vessels, in the heart, in the bronchi, in the intestines, in the bladder, in the womb and elsewhere. The effect of the hormones at these sites can be prevented by beta-blocker drugs which render the adrenoceptors insusceptible to the hormones.

beta-blocker drugs

The term 'beta-blocker' is an abbreviation of 'beta-adrenoreceptor blocking agent'. The adrenoreceptors come in two main classes, alpha and beta, and in several subclasses. The beta receptors are tiny areas scattered all over the heart, the arteries, muscles and elsewhere at which adrenaline and related hormones act. When these hormones contact the receptors their effect is to speed up the heart and constrict blood vessels, so increasing the blood pressure; to reduce the digestive processes; and to widen the airway tubes in the lungs. All this happens in moments of stress and need for action. The beta-blocker drugs have the same general chemical (molecular) shape as the adrenaline molecule and so fit into the receptor sites in the same way, effectively blocking them so that adrenaline, although present, cannot act.

If you have angina, an irregular heartbeat, high blood pressure or a tendency to overreact to stress, the result can be very advantageous. But these drugs could be disastrous for anyone with a tendency to asthma, as they can induce a severe asthmatic attack.

Many beta-blockers have been developed, some with a greater action on one part of the body than on another. Their generic names usually end in '-olol'. The most commonly used beta-blockers include propranolol (Inderal,

Beta-Prograne), atenolol (Beta-Adalat, Tenormin), labetalol (Trandate), oxprenolol (Trasicor) and acebutolol (Sectral).

One of the earliest beta-blockers, practolol, was marketed in 1970 after the most stringent tests. Four years later, after many thousands of patients had used the drug, an alert eye specialist noted that he was seeing patients with a most unusual form of dry eye, in which the outer layer of the cornea (the epithelium) was coming off in shreds. All these patients were taking practolol and some became blind. Soon it was found that the drug was also affecting the skin, the inner ear and the inner lining of the abdomen (the peritoneum). Only a small proportion of people on the drug were affected and some kind of immunological process was clearly involved. The drug was withdrawn, except for special cases, and the manufacturer accepted moral responsibility and paid compensation. Beta-blockers in current use have no such effects.

betahistine

A drug used to control the symptoms – vertigo and nausea – of **Ménière's syndrome**. A brand name is Serc.

beta-lactam antibiotics

A group of drugs that includes the penicillins and the cephalosporins. All have a 4-member beta-lactam ring as part of the basic structure. Beta-lactam antibiotics function by interfering with the growth of a layer in the cell walls of bacteria that protects them from the environment. Without this layer the bacteria burst open and are destroyed. Human cell walls do not have this layer; this is why these antibiotics are so safe. Bacteria protect themselves against these antibiotics by producing enzymes, beta-lactamases, that block this interference.

beta-lactam inhibitors

A range of drugs that block the action of the bacterial enzymes that break down the beta-lactam structure in penicillins and cephalosporins. These inhibitors, which include clavulanic acid, are used in conjunction with antibiotics. Brand names are Augmentin and Timentin.

bezoar

A ball of hair and vegetable fibres forming in the stomach or intestine. Bezoars are rare in human beings but common in ruminant animals.

bicalutamide

An anti-androgen drug used in the treatment of advanced prostate cancer. A brand name is Casodex.

bicuspid

Having two cusps, or projections, as on the biting surface of a premolar tooth. One of the valves in the heart, the mitral valve which separates the left atrium form the left ventricle, is bicuspid.

bifocal

See **spectacles**.

bifurcation

Forked, or two-pronged. Bifurcations are very common in the body, especially in blood vessels and in the bronchial 'tree' of the lungs. At a bifurcation the sum of the cross-sectional area of the two branches usually exceeds that of the parent branch. Since this happens many times, there is a progressive increase in the volume of the system. This may have important physiological consequences, as, for instance in the progressive drop in blood pressure in the arterial tree.

biguanide drugs

Drugs such as metformin and phenformin used to treat maturity-onset (Type II) diabetes. They are part of the group of oral hypoglycaemic drugs. Biguanides act by reducing the efficiency of transfer of charged dissolved substances (ions) across cell membranes thus interfering with the production of glucose by the liver and reducing the energy yield from glucose used as fuel.

bilateral

Affecting both sides. In the case of paired organs, bilateral means affecting both of them.

bile acid sequestrants

Drugs that bind to bile acids that have entered the intestine via the bile duct, so altering them that they cannot be absorbed back into the bloodstream in the usual way and are excreted in the faeces. Cholesterol is converted to bile acids by the liver. Loss of bile acids means more conversion of cholesterol and a lowering in total body cholesterol.

bile duct cancer

The bile duct passes through the head of the pancreas before entering the duodenum. Cancer of the head of the pancreas is relatively common, and the resulting blockage of the bile duct is often the first sign. Tumours originating in the bile duct itself are comparatively rare.

Unfortunately, the outlook in cases of cancer of the head of the pancreas is not usually very good. By the time obstruction has occurred, the cancer has usually spread too far to be curable by surgery. Operation is often necessary to relieve the obstruction but anticancer chemotherapy may offer the best chance.

bile duct obstruction

The great majority of cases are caused either by gallstones or by cancer – most commonly of the head of the pancreas. Whatever the cause, the effects are the same – pale stools, dark urine, progressive yellow colouring of the skin by deposition of bile pigments (jaundice), itching, loss of appetite, loss of weight, and a swollen gall-bladder which can sometimes be felt just under the ribs on the right side, in front.

Bile duct obstruction. This can occur at one of several points. The illustration shows a small stone obstructing the short duct branch leading from the gall-bladder to the common bile duct. Obstruction at the sphincter of Oddi is often due to cancer of the head of the pancreas.

bile duct X-rays

See **endoscopic retrograde cholangiopancreatography (ERCP)**.

bile-staining of brain

See **kernicterus**.

bilharziasis

A parasitic tropical disease caused by one of the blood flukes of the *Schistosoma* genus.
See **schistosomiasis**.

biliary atresia

Atresia means an abnormal narrowing or absence of a body opening or duct, present at birth (congenital). In biliary atresia the larger branches of the bile ducts are so narrowed that the bile cannot escape and the baby becomes severely jaundiced with enlargement of the liver. Unless the normal flow of bile can be established within the first two months of life, the baby suffers a severe and often fatal scarring of the liver (cirrhosis). Ultrasound scanning can usually show the narrowing of the duct and the usual associated absence of the gall-bladder. Early surgery is essential.

biliary cirrhosis

A slowly developing form of liver disease, of unknown cause, in which widespread inflammation of the small internal bile ducts gradually extends into the substance of the liver itself, replacing functioning liver with inert scar tissue. The condition appears to be surprisingly benign at first and is usually present for months or years before any trouble is suspected. Even then, the condition is often discovered by routine medical examination. Eventually, liver failure may occur and the only hope, then, rests in a liver transplant.

biliary colic

The severe pain caused by the attempts of the gall-bladder or bile duct to overcome obstruction by strong contraction of the muscle fibres in the wall. Biliary colic is often due to attempts to force a gallstone down into the bowel. The pain is felt in the upper part of the abdomen, in the centre or a lit-

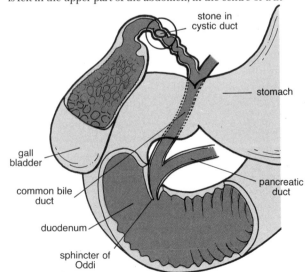

tle to the right, and usually occurs about an hour after a meal, especially if fat has been eaten. Unlike other forms of colic, which are usually spasmodic, the pain is often steady and persistent. It is commonly associated with vomiting.

Impacted stones can be shattered by extracorporeal shock-wave **lithotripsy**. The fragments will then pass easily.

biliousness

An impressive but inaccurate term for the feeling of nausea and flatulence associated with minor dyspepsia or any other mild upset of the stomach. Such symptoms have nothing to do with bile and are certainly not, as the name implies, caused by excess of bile. The term, however, gains credence from the observation that vomit is occasionally bile-stained. When one remembers that the bile enters the bowel only a few inches below the outlet of the stomach and that vomiting is essentially a reversal of the normal direction of movement of the bowel contents, this need not occasion surprise.

> Bile-stained vomit should always be reported.

binge-purge syndrome

See **bulimia**.

Binswanger's encephalopathy

A widespread brain disorder caused by severe arterial disease and high blood pressure so that multiple areas of white matter (nerve fibres) are deprived of an adequate blood supply and die. The result is progressive dementia associated with acute strokes. Deterioration is usually rapid.

bio-

A prefix which means relating to life.

bioassay

A means of measuring the potency or effectiveness of a drug or a biochemical agent by comparing its effects on animals, or other living systems such as bacteria, with those of known preparations of standard strength. Physical or chemical methods are always preferred, but are not always possible.

bioavailability

The amount of a drug that reaches the blood regardless of how it is given. After intravenous injection bioavailability is 100%, but the bioavailability of drugs given by mouth is often much less, because many drugs are broken down by the digestive enzymes and many are poorly absorbed.

biochemistry

The study of the chemical processes going on in living organisms, especially human beings. Biochemistry has been, and continues to be, one of the studies responsible for the explosive growth of biological and medical knowledge in the last thirty years or so. The patient working out of the structure of living molecules has been one of the highlights of biochemistry. This culminated in the historic breakthrough of the American biologist James Watson (b. 1928) and the British molecular biologist Francis Crick (b. 1916) when they established the double helix structure of DNA in 1953. But biochemistry is a functional as well as a structural discipline and deals with all the chemical processes underlying the functioning of the body (physiology).

Among the many subjects dealt with in biochemistry are:

- the role of enzymes, for which most of the genes code and by which almost all biochemical processes are controlled;
- the structure and function of the chemical messengers of the body (hormones);
- the chemistry of cell membranes by means of which cells communicate with one another;
- the complex chemical processes going on inside cells which govern cell survival and reproduction;
- the chemical changes underlying muscle contraction and nerve conduction;
- the processes of digestion of food and the way in which the resulting chemical substances are utilized by the body for energy and structural purposes.

biofeedback

A method of providing a person with information about the levels of activity of normally unconscious bodily processes, in the hope that some control or adjustment may be exercised.

USES

Biofeedback methods have been claimed to be effective in the control of muscle tension, headache, anxiety, panic attacks, high blood pressure, heart rate and rhythm abnormalities, poor circulation to the extremities (**Raynaud's disease**), **asthma**, **epilepsy**, **pain**, ringing in the ears (**tinnitus**) and several others. The evidence for some of these claims is flimsy, but some – particularly those in which voluntary control is possible – are feasible.

HOW IT WORKS

It is a simple matter to monitor almost any of the bodily states and to display the changing situation by one of various means. Blood pressure can be measured continuously, as can the heart rate, the respiration rate, the degree of contraction of any muscle group, the electrical conductivity of the skin (which is a measure of the amount of sweating) and the various electrical wave patterns produced by the brain. All these can be separately picked up by devices called transducers which convert the varying levels into correspondingly varying voltages. These voltages can then be amplified and used to modulate a display such as an electric meter, an expanding bar chart figure, a monitor display of some kind, or a musical sound, heard in headphones or through a loudspeaker.

> There is now general agreement that, at least in some conditions, biofeedback can be valuable. Consider the simple case of a person suffering a tension headache. An observant friend remarks 'Your forehead is all screwed up and your shoulders are hunched. Why don't you relax?' The subject does so and the headache resolves. This is an example of biofeedback. When the function concerned is capable of being voluntarily controlled, as in this example, biofeedback can work, at least at a symptomatic level.

The unresolved questions relate to whether those functions under the control of the autonomic (involuntary) nervous system can be usefully controlled. Opinions differ. But it should be remembered that all bodily functions are so intimately interrelated that it is almost impossible for a change to occur in any one without others being affected. And this most certainly applies to the relationship of the body and the mind. So there seems no fundamental reason why biofeedback should not also work for these functions too. Time will tell.

biological warfare

Happily for mankind, this has never really got off the ground, but it is clear that many countries, including Britain, have engaged in research into the possibilities. Biological warfare should be distinguished from chemical warfare using agents such as chlorine, phosgene, mustard gas, the various nerve gases and a range of hallucinogenic drugs. The essence of biological warfare is the use of living organisms to produce pandemics of disease, spread by natural means throughout whole populations.

The possibilities include **plague**, especially the very infective pneumonic form; **anthrax** of the lungs, which is deadly and exceedingly unpleasant; botulism, which kills by paralysis, leaving the mind clear to the end; and **tularaemia**, which can penetrate the unbroken skin or eye and cause extreme weakness, fever, delirium, and ulceration of the skin.

None of these horrors is likely to have deterred the average military aggressor. What has, apparently, prevented the use of such methods of persuasion, is the simple fact that countries abused in this way would be rendered inaccessible, often for years, to the conqueror. It is to be hoped that such an argument will continue to prevail.

biomedical engineering

The cooperative investigation by engineers and doctors of the possibilities of applying any branch of engineering so as to broaden the scope of medicine. Electronics, computing, robotics, hydraulics, rheology, materials science and software engineering are among the more fruitful branches from which medicine has benefited. This cooperation has thrown up the interesting fact that engineers have long been aware of ideas and principles that can provide answers to medical problems and that doctors and physiologists have knowledge that engineers can apply. Only the artificial insulation between the disciplines has, in the past, blocked this valuable interplay. It has been said that the remoter the disciplines the more fruitful the interface.

biomicroscopy

Examination of living structure using a microscope. Biomicroscopy is mainly employed, in a clinical context, by ophthalmologists using a slit lamp binocular microscope. This is the central diagnostic tool in ophthalmology.

bionic

Relating to a living or life-like system enhanced by, or constructed from, electronic or mechanical components. Bionics is the science of biological principles applied to the design of engineering systems, especially electronic systems.

biopsy

Literally 'taking a look at life'. A biopsy is the process of taking a specimen of tissue from the body for the purpose of microscopic examination so as to determine what is wrong. The term biopsy is also applied, in common medical parlance, to the specimen itself. This is a valuable and accurate method of investigation and, by establishing an important diagnosis at an early stage, is often life-saving. Biopsies, especially from the skin, may often be taken after a simple injection of local anaesthetic, the deficit being closed with a few stitches (sutures).

Breast biopsies are commonly performed to establish the nature of suspicious lumps. The 'Pap' smear test, for cancer of the neck of the womb (the cervix), is a biopsy. In the course of surgery under general anaesthesia, it is extremely common for biopsies to be taken.

The tissue obtained is soaked in molten paraffin wax, which is allowed to cool and harden into a block. A precision instrument called a microtome is used to cut exceedingly thin slices from the block and these are mounted on glass slides, the wax dissolved out with xylene, and the specimen stained to bring out the microscopic detail. A histopathologist then examines the slide under a powerful microscope and prepares a report on the findings and diagnosis.

Patients waiting for the result of a biopsy often fail to appreciate how much must be done before a report can be given. In cases of critical urgency, a report may be obtained within half an hour by freezing the tissue and cutting from the frozen block. This is known as a frozen section. It is sometimes done while the patient remains anaesthetized on the operating table. The surgeon's subsequent procedure will depend on the pathologist's findings.

biorhythms

An interesting and surprising feature of many body functions is their rhythmic or cyclical nature. The menstrual cycle is an obvious example, with a periodicity of about twenty-eight days. There is the cycle of waking and sleeping; a daily temperature cycle with a peak every twenty-four hours; there are regular cycles of change in hormone levels; spontaneous rhythmical contraction in the muscles of the bowel (peristalsis); respiration and pulse rhythms; and, at an ultimate level, ultra-high speed resonances in the atoms themselves.

HOW THEY WORK

Some of these cyclical phenomena are under the control of a central biological clock based on a 24-hour *circadian* rhythm. This has been shown to be related to the day/night cycle, but not synchronized by it. An animal kept in bright light from birth shows no circadian rhythm, but after being kept in the dark for a few hours develops a rhythm with a 24-hour cycle. The pineal gland, which secretes a hormone called melatonin, appears to be synchronized with the day/night cycle. Melatonin has been used to try to treat **jet lag**.

There is some evidence of the existence of cycles with a periodicity much greater than 28 days and much has been made of this possibility by practitioners of alternative medicine. It is claimed that multiple cycles of different periodicity exist, that the cycle length of each can be determined and that they can be plotted from birth. Coincidence of peaks and of troughs can be predicted by plotting the curves forward, and these, it is claimed, represent times when one is, respectively, best and worst able to cope with the vicissitudes of life.

RELIABILITY

There is some hard evidence to support this idea. It has been shown that in rats, the ability to survive a potentially lethal dose of a drug depends critically on when the drug is given. At present we know far too little about this to make reliable use of it, but the time may come when the method is an important element in medical treatment, especially for the timing of drug administration.

biotechnology

The use of micro-organisms or biological processes for commercial, medical or social purposes. Biotechnology, although one of the earliest technologies employed by man – such as fermentation of wines, cheese-making, etc. – is still in its infancy. It has, however, embarked on an expansion, in knowledge and application, which will rival in importance, and in its effect on society, the earlier industrial revolution and the current information technology revolution.

Staggering advances in biological engineering, including gene manipulation and synthesis, recombinant DNA techniques, enzyme chemistry, and even the possibility of biological computing systems will have an effect on our lives of a magnitude currently hard to envisage. **Genetic engineering** alone will be a major force for good (and evil) within the next decade or so, but this is but one of the many avenues opening up as a result of the explosion of knowledge derived from the interfacing of other disciplines with biology.

Biomedical engineering has, in the last ten years, become a major technology in its own right. Its applications include the development of artificial organs; the design of replacement (prosthetic) devices of all kinds; advances in the medical and biological use of lasers; the development of biological applications of ultrasound; bionics; robotics; cybernetics – the list is endless.

biperiden

An anticholinergic drug used in the treatment of **Parkinson's disease**. A brand name is Akineton.

bipolar disorder

Also called **manic-depressive illness** or psychosis, this is a severe psychiatric disorder featuring extreme alternations of mood from euphoria and hyperactivity to depression and apathy. The alternations do not usually occur quickly and there may be years between the phases.

bird-fancier's lung

A form of allergic pneumonia caused by inhaling the dust from dried bird droppings. The effects are similar to those caused by inhaling many different industrial or other dusts. There is fever, shortness of breath, tightness in the chest and cough. A few isolated attacks are unlikely to do much harm, but repeated episodes eventually lead to permanent and serious changes in the lungs.

Avoidance of the dust is the obvious course and this may involve wearing a properly protective mask.

birth control

As commonly used, this term is really a euphemism for contraception. Strictly speaking, the term 'birth control' also includes methods such as celibacy, sexual continence and abortion.

See **contraception**.

birth date, predicting

See **expected date of delivery**.

birth injury

Being born has always been dangerous, but happily it is getting safer – mainly because of the readiness with which obstetricians will now resort to Caesarean section when trouble is anticipated. Many birth injuries, in the past, resulted from attempts at difficult delivery by forceps or vacuum extraction, or from attempts to turn the baby into a better position for delivery. Such problems arose especially when the mother's pelvic outlet was narrow and the baby large.

Injuries still occur, however, and include a boggy swelling of the part of the scalp forced against the cervix (caput succedaneum); a blood clot on the scalp (**haematoma**); skull fracture; nerve injuries causing paralysis, usually temporary, of the face or arm; bleeding inside the brain; and fractures of the collar bone (clavicle), the upper arm bone (humerus) or the thigh (femur). **Spastic paralysis** (cerebral palsy) is now thought seldom to be the result of birth injury.

birthmark on face and brain

See **Sturge-Weber syndrome**.

birthmarks

They are harmless (benign) tumours or naevi of skin blood vessels, usually of cosmetic importance only, and take various forms.

INCIDENCE
Birthmarks affect about one-third of all babies and are either present at birth or appear soon after.

RECOGNITION AND SYMPTOMS
The strawberry mark is a small, bright red, raised tumour which grows to its full size during the first six months of life and then subsides. In most cases it disappears altogether by the age of five years.

The port-wine stain (capillary haemangioma) is a flat tumour of the smallest blood vessels (capillaries). It is present at birth and is permanent. It usually occurs on one side of the face and is often a conspicuous blemish.

The cavernous haemangioma is raised, lumpy and highly coloured and consists of a mass of medium-sized blood vessels and blood spaces. It, too, is permanent.

TREATMENT
Unless of small extent, neither of the latter two birthmarks is easy to treat. If small enough, the whole affected area of skin may be removed and the edges undermined and brought together with stitches. Larger haemangiomas may be removed and a skin graft applied, but it is never easy to obtain a perfect colour match, and often the bearer resorts to cosmetic coverage. Lasers and freezing have been tried, with limited success.

bisacodyl

A drug used in the treatment of constipation. A brand name is Dulcolax.

bisexuality

The inclination for sexual intercourse with either men or women. A distinction should be made between bisexual behaviour, which is common, and genuine neutrality in the choice of sex objects, which is very rare.

INCIDENCE

Bisexual behaviour is commoner than is generally supposed, and occurs in both sexes, and among those with heterosexual as well as those with homosexual preference. Often it seems to be imposed by force of circumstance, such as imprisonment, incarceration in boarding school and closed religious communities, military service, and so on.

Kinsey used a realistic scale of 0 to 6 for assessing the range of sexuality from exclusively heterosexual to exclusively homosexual. A study of the placement of his subjects on this scale suggests that about 30 per cent of the males, and about 20 per cent of the females, were capable of, or had engaged in, bisexual activity.

POSSIBLE CAUSE

Sometimes bisexual behaviour is a consequence of an apparently ungovernable appetite for orgasm, and in these cases it seems likely that the true psychosexual orientation is irrelevant.

See also **homosexuality**.

bisphosphonates

A class of drugs that resemble pyrophosphate but are not readily broken down (hydrolysed). They interfere with the action of osteoclasts and thus prevent bone reabsorption in conditions such as **Paget's disease** and **osteoporosis**.

bite

A dental term describing the relationship of the teeth of the lower jaw (mandible) to those of the upper jaw (maxilla). The dentist is primarily interested in how the teeth come together (occlusion). The grinding teeth at the back (the molars) should have their cusps fitting closely together and the lower front biters (incisors) should lie just behind the upper incisors. These relationships often become disturbed during development and orthodontic treatment may be necessary to correct them. In extreme cases of congenitally defective bite, surgery may be required.

The bite is also of much concern during the crowning of teeth and the design and construction of artificial dentures.

bites, animal

RISKS

The mouths and teeth of animals are teeming with infectious organisms, some of which are very dangerous.

> Animal bites should always be taken seriously, mainly because of the major risk of infection.

If rabies is a possibility, it is important that the biting animal should be kept under restraint for observation. If the animal remains apparently well for 10 days, the risk of rabies is eliminated. A rabid animal will die within 10 days. If the animal dies or is killed, its head should be sent, as soon as possible, to a Public Health laboratory so that the brain can be examined for signs of the characteristic rabies virus colonies found within the nerve cells.

Bites from free-ranging wild animals pose problems. If the animal can be killed, its head should be sent for examination. If it escapes, and if the area is one in which rabies has occurred in the previous 10 years, human rabies immune

globulin can be given, followed by a course of vaccination. This usually involves five injections, on days 0, 3, 7, 14 and 28. Human diploid cell vaccine is now preferred.

TREATMENT

Wounds must be thoroughly cleaned with plenty of soapy water and free bleeding encouraged. Medical attention should be sought. If surgery is necessary, it is probable that all damaged tissue will be removed. The wound may be left open for a time, as early closure can encourage infection. Antibiotics and anti-tetanus immunization will probably be given.

bites, human

RISKS

Human bites are dangerous and should be avoided, if possible. The human mouth harbours a surprising range of disease-producing (pathogenic) organisms, particularly if there is dental neglect and resulting gum disorder.

TREATMENT

Bites should be thoroughly washed with soap and water and, if possible, treated with a hydrogen peroxide soak. Antibiotics may be indicated and an anti-tetanus injection may be given.

> Medical attention should be sought without delay following any kind of penetrative bite.

biting and self-mutilation

See **Lesch-Nyhan syndrome**.

black box epidemiology

A black box is a system whose inputs and outputs are known but of which the things that go on inside are completely unknown. It is a helpful concept in some branches of science, leading to useful simplifications of otherwise very complex systems. The term 'black box epidemiology' has, however, been applied in a critical way to the growing tendency to look for associations between all sorts of factors and disease and then to assume that there must be a causal relationship. Hardly a week passes without some researcher or other suggesting, with varying degrees of plausibility, that coffee causes heart attacks, diesel fumes cause asthma, aluminium causes Alzheimer's disease, and so on.

An extreme example demonstrates how absurd such a process can be. The number of storks in a village in Transylvania has declined steadily; so has the birth rate. Therefore, the declining birth rate must be due to the declining number of storks. If, however, it was widely believed that storks brought babies, this inference would not be so absurd, although wrong. So what really matters is the quality of *additional* evidence relating the 'risk factor' with the disease. Unfortunately, all claimed relationships are not obviously ridiculous and we are apt to be influenced by factors – such as the status of the medium in which the claim is reported – which have, of course, nothing to do with the case.

Alleged links with no supporting evidence are rightly denigrated as 'black box epidemiology' and, unless highly plausible, should generally be disregarded. Some may argue that plausibility implies the existence of supporting evidence.

black death

See **plague, bubonic**.

black eye

Doctors have an impressive term for this – *periorbital haematoma* – literally 'a collection of blood released into the tissues around the eye'. The flat muscles of the eyelids and surrounding area contains many veins which bleed easily into and under the skin, causing a bluish discoloration.

The duration of the disfigurement depends on the extent of the bleeding and varies from a few days to a month. The average black eye lasts for about a fortnight and during that time undergoes an interesting series of transitions of colour, from blue to brown to yellow to a pale lemon. There is nothing to be done to accelerate the process, but cosmetics can do much to disguise the disfigurement.

TREATMENT

Raw steak has no effect, but an ice-pack applied immediately after the injury may reduce the final disfigurement.

blackheads

Technically known as comedones, these are bodies composed of compressed fatty (sebaceous) material produced in excess in the skin disorder of **acne** vulgaris. The sebaceous glands of the skin are under sex hormone control, the male hormones (androgens) causing excessive production and the female hormones (oestrogens) reducing the rate of secretion. The blackhead occurs when excess sebum cannot escape on to the surface of the skin and accumulates in the duct of the sebaceous gland. The darkened outer part of the blackhead is caused by chemical changes in the exposed sebum, not by any deficiency in cleanliness.

Other chemical changes, caused by certain resident bacteria, turn the neutral fat in the blackheads into fatty acid which is very irritant to the surrounding tissue and this is the

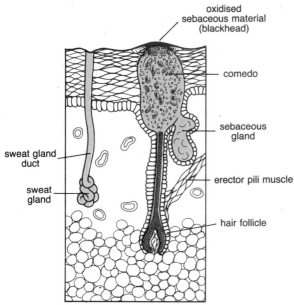

Blackheads (comedos or comedones) are formed from accumulated sebaceous secretion in a skin pore. The blackened tip is due to chemical changes in the fatty material.

main cause of the inflammation which so commonly surrounds blackheads, especially when the sebaceous gland is ruptured by squeezing. Unless very large, blackheads will not produce permanently enlarged pores.

blackout

This is not a medical term and is applied to a range of conditions varying from the trivial to the grave. In most cases it refers to a simple, harmless fainting attack or to the brief period of visual loss experienced on standing up suddenly. This is due to transient shortage of blood to the brain (cerebral ischaemia) and is of no significance.

Since the term has no medical precision, it can be applied to many conditions, including **epilepsy**, **transient ischaemic attacks**, loss of consciousness from **subdural haematoma**, hysterical loss of vision, visual loss from brain tumours, and **retinopathy** from high blood pressure or diabetes.

black stools

An appearance of tar-black faeces with various causes, the most important being the release of blood into the intestine at a high level, often into the stomach. The blood is altered by the intestinal juices and turns black. This is called melaena and may be a sign of stomach or duodenal ulcer or stomach cancer. Stools may also be blackened by dietary ingredients.

blackwater fever

A popular term for a severe form of **malaria** in which the break-down of red blood cells, by the malarial parasite, is so extensive that freed haemoglobin passes through the kidneys and darkens the urine. Black water occurs only in the most dangerous type of malaria – that caused by the parasite *Plasmodium falciparum*, and is uncommon except in those treated with quinine.

bladder cancer

INCIDENCE

This is three times as common in men as in women, possibly because some of the causal factors affect men more. Known factors include certain chemicals such as aniline dyes and some encountered in rubber manufacture, the excreted products of tobacco tars, and the presence of bladder stones.

RECOGNITION AND SYMPTOMS

Bladder cancer shows itself by the passage of blood in the urine (haematuria), pus in the urine, and a burning pain on urination. These signs are commonly an indication of other less serious conditions, but they should always be taken seriously, especially by older people, and require proper investigation. Contrast X-ray may show a mass in the bladder and this may be confirmed by direct inspection of the inside (cystoscopy) and by computerized tomography (CT) scanning or ultrasound scanning.

TREATMENT

Early cancers, confined to the inner surface of the bladder, can be destroyed by systematic burning with a hot wire (cautery) passed through a cystoscope. If the cancer has spread through the wall of the bladder the outlook is less good and major surgery and radiotherapy will be needed. The whole bladder may have to be removed and the ureters reimplanted into the lower end of the large intestine (rectum).

bladder, disorders of

See **urinary bladder, disorders of**.

-blast

Suffix meaning 'builder' as in fibroblast (fibre-maker).

-ble

Suffix meaning 'able to be' as in sensible (able to feel).

bleeding

See **haemorrhage**.

bleeding gums

This is most commonly a sign of inflammation of the gums (**gingivitis**) and is almost always due to neglect of elementary mouth hygiene. The accumulation of food residue in which bacteria multiply (plaque) as a result of failure to clean the teeth, leads to inflammation of the gum margin around the necks of the teeth with bleeding which occurs on minor injury as from toothbrushing.

POSSIBLE CAUSES
Aside from inadequate hygiene, bleeding gums may be due to vitamin C deficiency (**scurvy**), but this is rare nowadays, except in malnourished elderly people.

TREATMENT
The condition can easily be cleared up, by good dental hygiene. Regular toothbrushing and flossing after meals will remove plaque and prevent gingivitis. Adequate intake of vitamin C will promote gum health.

blennorrhoea

An inflammation of the transparent membrane covering the white of the eye (**conjunctivitis**) and of the eyelids, caused by the organism *Chlamydia trachomatis*. This organism causes **trachoma** in some developing countries and a venereal infection everywhere.

INCIDENCE
Blennorrhoea is sometimes called 'swimming pool conjunctivitis' because of the frequency with which it is acquired in this way from infected genital secretions. Direct infection, from the genitals, is also common and the condition often occurs in newborn babies.

RECOGNITION AND SYMPTOMS
The condition starts one or two weeks after exposure. The eyes become red and the conjunctivae and lids are swollen with much watering and pussy (purulent) discharge. The conjunctivae behind the upper lids usually become covered with tiny raised bumps (papillae) and these last for months.

TREATMENT
Blennorrhoea responds well to antibiotics such as tetracycline, in ointment form. The same drug is given by mouth to adults with genital infection.

blepharitis

Inflammation of the eyelids.

RECOGNITION AND SYMPTOMS
Blepharitis is very common in people of all ages and is usually mild – a little redness of the lid margins, some greasy scales on the lashes, and a constant, annoying irritation.

POSSIBLE CAUSES
It is often associated with dandruff and similar skin conditions (seborrhoeic dermatitis) and may sometimes disappear if dandruff is effectively treated. Some cases are allergic and many date from infancy as part one of the symptoms of the complex known as **atopy**.

RISKS
Severe blepharitis is distressing and disabling and may lead to ulceration of the lid margins, loss of the lashes or abnormal direction of lash growth so that the lashes rub annoyingly or painfully on the cornea. Such degrees of blepharitis seldom occur if reasonable care is given.

TREATMENT
Blepharitis is an inflammation but is not primarily an infection, although lids affected by it may become secondarily infected and develop styes and pustules. Treatment involves the control of any such secondary infection, followed, in some cases, by the use of steroid ointments which have a powerful anti-inflammatory effect.

Steroids in the eye have some potentially dangerous effects and should be used only on expert ophthalmic advice. They may cause glaucoma, may cause herpes simplex infections of the cornea to become established for life and may encourage corneal ulceration and even perforation. For these reasons steroids are often best avoided.

blepharochalasis

Baggy eyelids caused by the abnormal forward protrusion of fat from the eye sockets. The condition is readily susceptible to a cosmetic plastic surgical operation.

blepharon

Greek root meaning 'eyelid' as in blepharitis (eyelid inflammation).

blepharoplasty

Cosmetic plastic surgery for baggy eyelids. Blepharoplasty is one of the easiest of cosmetic operations and can greatly improve appearance.

HOW IT'S DONE
The skin of the lids is very thin and the surplus can readily be picked up and cut off, leaving a bare oval area which is closed with a row of hair-like stitches. The scar is in the line of a skin crease and, within a week or two, is quite invisible.

RISKS
The only thing that may possibly go wrong is the excessive removal of skin so that the eyes cannot close comfortably and the lid margins tend to turn outward. This is a serious complication and is only likely if the surgeon is careless or very inexperienced.

blepharospasm

See **tics**.

blind loop syndrome

A rare disorder featuring diarrhoea, fatty stools, abdominal pain, loss of weight, anaemia and vitamin deficiency. It is caused by stagnation of bowel contents as a result of **adhesions**, constrictions, pouches or other similar abnormalities. Bacterial changes occur and these result in defective production and absorption of vitamin B12. This can lead to **pernicious anaemia**.

blindness

See **vision, disorders of**.

blindness in childhood

See **retrolental fibroplasia**, **Tay-Sachs disease**, **glaucoma**.

blind spot

The natural blind spot is the projection into space of the head of the optic nerve (the optic disc) which consists solely of nerve fibres and has no receptor elements (rods and cones). The blind spot occurs, in the field of vision of each eye, about 15 degrees to the outer side of whatever point we are looking at. If an eye is turned outwards to align itself on the point which was previously the projection of the optic disc, the blind spot will simply move 15 degrees further out. It is mainly because of this that we are unaware of it.

It can, however, easily be demonstrated by closing the left eye, looking at a small black spot on a sheet of paper and then moving the eye slowly along, horizontally, to the left. When the image of the spot falls on the optic nerve head it will no longer be seen.

Acquired blind spots are due to damage to the retina or to the fibres passing back from it to the brain. Such spots (scotomas) can easily be plotted and their progress checked. They occur in **glaucoma**, in any form of destructive retinal disease and in any disorder affecting the conduction of nerve impulses along the optic nerve.

blisters

Fluid-filled skin swellings occurring within or just under the skin, usually as a result of heat injury or sustained, unaccustomed friction. The fluid in the blister is serum, derived from the blood, and is usually uninfected (sterile). Sometimes, as after a pinching injury, an actual blood blister may form, and occasionally an infected blister, filled with pus, may occur.

TREATMENT
Heat and friction blisters should, if possible, be kept intact, so as to avoid infection. They should be protected from further injury by padding with wool. A persistent and painful blister, or one filled with blood or pus, may require medical attention and the doctor may evacuate the blister by nicking the overlying skin with a sterile scalpel blade or needle. A sterile dressing would then be applied.

In severe burns, massive blisters, containing litres of fluid, may form. This so concentrates and reduces the blood volume that the person concerned may be in danger of dying from surgical shock (see **shock, surgical**). Transfusion of fluids, such as plasma, may be life-saving in such cases.

blockade

The use of a drug to seal, or otherwise render inoperative, a receptor for natural hormones or neuro-transmitters.

blood

The blood is a remarkable fluid vital to life. It consists of a fluid, serum, containing many dissolved substances and countless millions of cells and other microscopic bodies. As discussed earlier, the average adult has about five litres of blood and this has several major functions. It is a transport medium, especially for oxygen, which it carries in the red blood cells linked to the haemoglobin with which they are filled. Haemoglobin is an iron-containing complex protein which has the unique property of being able to combine loosely with oxygen when it is in an environment of high oxygen concentration, and to release it when it enters an environment low in oxygen. This means that when blood passes through the lungs, the red cells automatically take up oxygen and that when they are circulated to the tissues, where oxygen consumption is high, the red cells automatically give it up to the surrounding body cells. Haemoglobin linked to oxygen is called oxyhaemoglobin and is of a bright red colour. This is the characteristic of arterial blood which has just returned from the lungs. When free of oxygen, haemoglobin is a dark purplish colour, as in veins returning blood from tissues.

Each 100 ml of healthy blood contains about 500 million red cells and a total of 12 to 18 g of haemoglobin. In anaemia the amount of haemoglobin drops. In addition to red cells, the blood carries enormous numbers of uncoloured cells, called white cells, most of which are concerned in the defence of the individual against infection and cancer. These cells constitute an essential part of the immune system. The blood also transports dissolved sugars, dissolved proteins such as albumin and globulin, protein constituents (amino acids), fat-protein combinations (lipoproteins), emulsified fats (triglycerides), vitamins, minerals, waste products such as carbon dioxide, urea, lactic acid and innumerable other substances. It also carries hormones, which are chemicals produced by the endocrine glands and carried throughout the body to control many important functions.

Blood is constantly being replenished with new cells manufactured in the marrow of the flat bones such as the shoulder blades or breastbone. Red cells have a life of about 120 days after which they break down and release their haemoglobin. This is used by the liver and converted to a useful byproduct, bilirubin. Conservation of blood is so important that the circulation has an automatic self-sealing mechanism – the blood coagulation system – which operates when a blood vessel is damaged.

BLOOD CLOTTING
Blood clotting (coagulation) is an essential property of the blood to prevent dangerous loss in the event of injury to a blood vessel. In clotting, the blood at the site of the injury comes into contact with damaged tissue or some foreign substance. This contact triggers off the complex sequence of biochemical events by which the blood forms a solid mass to seal the leaking point.

Many different factors, present in the blood and tissues, are essential for coagulation. Clotting within the blood vessels is extremely dangerous, so a mechanism is required which keeps the blood fluid within the circulation, but causes it to become solid and seal off bleeding points whenever a small vein or artery is so injured as to leak blood. Such a mechanism cannot be simple and, indeed, the coagulation of the blood is one of the most complex biochemical processes in the body, involving some 30 known chemical 'factors'.

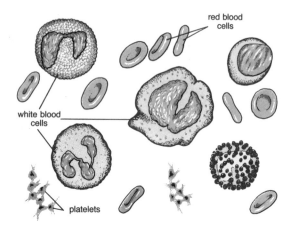

The relative size and appearance of red and white blood cells and blood platelets. The white cells are phagocytes, lymphocytes and other immune system cells. The platelets are concerned in blood clotting.

Blood vessels which seal off fully after injury are closed by an insoluble substance called fibrin, which is formed from the soluble protein fibrinogen normally present in the blood. This change is brought about by the enzyme thrombin which converts fibrinogen into long stands of insoluble fibrin. These are meshed together in a network which soon starts to contract, pulling the edges of small blood vessels together and trapping blood cells and serum. With further contraction of the forming clot, serum is squeezed out and the clot becomes more solid.

The enzyme thrombin is not present in the blood, but is formed from a precursor called prothrombin. It is in the formation of prothrombin that the main complexities lie, and a large number of different factors are involved. Some of these come from damaged tissue and some from the damaged blood vessels and this is why, in health, the blood does not clot inside the arteries and veins. People with absence, or deficiency, of any of the necessary factors, suffer from bleeding disorders, of which the best known is haemophilia A, due to absence of factor VIII. Absence of factor IX (Christmas factor) causes haemophilia B.

BLOOD GROUPS

In 1900 the Austrian bacteriologist and immunologist Karl Landsteiner (1868–1943) showed that human red blood cells fell into four groups, which he called A, B, AB and O. He also showed that the serum of the blood – the fluid part, without cells – contained antibodies to the groups not present in the red cells. Red cells clump together into useless masses (agglutinate) if brought into contact with serum containing antibodies to them. Antigens are chemical groups that stimulate the production of antibodies. The red cell antigens are genetically determined, both A and B being dominant over O.

Normally, antibodies develop as a result of exposure to foreign antigens, such as bacteria, viruses, foreign protein and so on. The case of the blood group antibodies is unique in that the serum antibodies are 'natural antibodies' produced by the body without such exposure. They are present in high concentration from early in life, and their cause is unknown.

Group A blood has A antigens in its red cells but specific antibodies, in its serum, against B red cells. Group B blood has antibodies in its serum against A cells. Group O blood is not antigenic and its serum contains both anti-A and anti-B antibodies. And group AB cells have both A and B antigens, so can have no antibodies in its serum. Group A blood, with A antigens, can safely be given to group A people, but it can also be given to group AB people, because they have no anti-red cell antibodies; group B blood, with B antigens, is safe for group B and also group AB recipients, for the same reason; Group AB blood, with both A and B antigens, can be given safely only to group AB people; but group O blood, with no antigens, can be given to anyone.

Group AB people are able to receive blood safely from anyone; they are called universal recipients. Group O people can accept neither A nor B blood and must have O blood, but they are a great asset to the community because they are universal donors and their blood can be given safely to anyone.

Blood can be grouped by mixing it on a glass slide with separate samples of the serum from A and B people. If the cells agglutinate in A serum, the blood is group B. If they agglutinate in B serum, it is group A. If in both, it is AB. If in neither, group O.

Before transfusion, blood is always cross-matched, by mixing some of the donor cells with the patient's serum, in this way, just to be sure that there is no risk of incompatibility.

blood blister on baby's head

See **cephalhaematoma**.

blood-brain barrier

The effective obstruction to the passage of certain drugs and other substances from the blood in the brain blood vessels to the brain cells and the cerebrospinal fluid. The basis of the blood-brain barrier is that the flat, lining (endothelial) cells comprising the walls of the brain capillaries are tightly joined together. In other part of the body the capillary endothelial

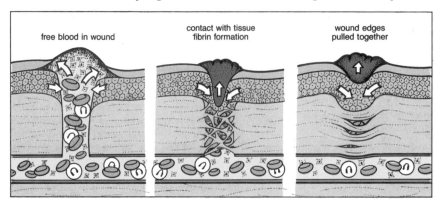

The stages in the clotting of blood and repair of a wound. The contact of the blood with raw tissue initiates a complex chain reaction ending in the formation of fibrin. The maturing fibrin pulls the edges of the wound together.

cells have gaps between them through which quite large molecules can pass. Substances in the brain blood can reach the brain cells or the cerebrospinal fluid only by passing though the cell membranes of the endothelial cells. The blood-brain barrier protects the brain against many dangers, but can interfere with attempts to treat some brain conditions.

blood clot breakdown

See **antifibrinolysis**.

blood clot-dissolving drugs

See **tissue plasminogen activators**.

blood clotting

The cascaded sequence of changes which occur when blood comes in contact with damaged tissue and which culminates in the production of a solid seal in the damaged vessel. At least 13 factors are consecutively involved in a process that culminates in the conversion of the protein fibrinogen to the fibrin that forms the main constituent of the clot. This last stage is catalyzed by the enzyme thrombin. The smooth lining of the blood vessels (the endothelium) normally prevents clotting within the circulation, but damage to this lining may allow **thrombosis** to occur.

blood clotting, prevention of

See **anticoagulant drugs**.

blood clot dissolving

See **tissue plasminogen activator**.

blood clotting component

See **platelets**.

blood clotting in vessels

See **disseminated intravascular coagulation (DIC)**.

blood clotting prevention

See **ancrod, low molecular weight heparin**.

blood clot vein filter

See **vena caval filter**.

blood contents access to brain

See **blood-brain barrier**.

blood formation failure

See **aplastic anaemia**.

blood in urine

POSSIBLE CAUSES

If the sign is associated with pain in one side of the lower back (loin), there is probably a stone in the kidney or in the tube leading down from the kidney to the bladder (the ureter). Bleeding with pain on passing urine or in the lower central part of the abdomen, suggests a severe bladder infection or a stone in the bladder.

Blood in the urine causes discoloration varying from red to brown and must never be disregarded. Blood in the urine always indicates that something at least potentially serious is going on.

Painless blood in the urine could be caused by kidney disease, such as **glomerulonephritis**, polycystic disease or **cancer**, or it could be an indication of bladder problems such as polyps, cancer, or silent stone. Other causes include **sickle-cell disease** and benign or cancerous enlargement of the prostate gland.

blood pressure

See **hypertension**.

blood pressure, anxiety-induced

See **white coat hypertension**.

blood pressure measurement

See **Korotkoff sounds**.

blood pressure, new drug for

See **angiotensin II receptor antagonists**.

blood pressure treatment

See **endothelin-receptor antagonist**.

blood sedimentation rate

More correctly, this test is known as the erythrocyte sedimentation rate (ESR). Erythrocytes are red blood cells. The rate at which red cells sediment to the bottom of a tube is an important finding. The test is more correctly called the erythrocyte sedimentation rate (ESR). Blood is drawn up into a tube, calibrated in millimetres, which is placed vertically and allowed to stand for exactly an hour. The number of millimetres of clear serum above the red cell level, after one hour, is called the sedimentation rate. This is raised in many infections, inflammations and malignancy. The sedimentation rate is not a specific test for any particular condition, but it does indicate that something, probably something serious, is going on.

Many people with inflamed, tender, forehead arteries, for instance, have been saved from blindness by urgent steroid treatment when it was found that the sedimentation rate was high. A high sedimentation rate is a feature of the condition of temporal arteritis.

blood stem cell transplant

See **placental-blood transplantation**.

blood tests

A wider range, and variety, of tests is performed on the **blood** than on any other system of the body. Only the most important can be covered in a book of this kind. Blood consists of countless millions of red blood cells floating in a fluid, which also contains hundreds of other ingredients. Tests are conducted on all the many constituents of the blood as these vary in quantity in different diseases.

Red blood cells are flat, hollowed disks consisting of a thin outer envelope filled with the complex iron-containing protein, haemoglobin. They are manufactured in the marrow of the flat bones, such as the pelvis, breast bone, shoulder blade and skull. Blood without its cells is called *plasma* and blood which has been allowed to clot, and has had the clot removed, is called *serum*.

If the tests are concerned with the red cells, the sample is prevented from clotting by being put into a tube containing an anticoagulant substance, such as heparin or EDTA. If the tests are to be done on the serum, the blood is run into a plain tube and allowed to clot. After a time, the clot separates and the yellow serum is available for testing. Blood for bacterial culture is inoculated directly into a culture medium, in which the organisms grow well, and this is put into the incubator which is kept at body temperature.

The *full blood count* is a basic screening test, routinely done in all hospital patients and many others. It includes the red cell count, an estimation of the haemoglobin level in the red cells, a count of the white cells and a breakdown of these into the percentages of each type (differential white cell count), an estimate of the number of platelets in a given volume, and a description of the appearance and shape of the cells on a blood smear (see below).

Routine blood tests on whole blood are concerned with the various kinds of anaemias and leukaemias, the demonstration of immature and abnormal red cells, the investigation of the range of abnormal haemoglobins (the haemoglobinopathies) and failure of production of red and white cells (aplastic anaemia and agranulocytosis) and as supporting evidence of infection.

THE RED CELLS

The red blood cells are very important and a range of tests is routinely done on them. In most laboratories, these red cell tests are completely automated and a print-out of the result is available in less than an hour. The total red cell count is a count of the number of cells present in one cubic millimetre of blood. This is an indication of the efficiency with which red cells which have come to the end of their natural life, of about 120 days, are replaced by the bone marrow. It can also indicate cell loss from severe bleeding.

The count is done by an electronic counter and the normal number is 4,400,000 to 6,000,000 in men and 4,200,000 to 5,400,000 in women. In iron deficiency anaemia the red cell count is normal, but the amount of haemoglobin in the cells is reduced. Pernicious anaemia is a condition in which red cell production is interfered with. In this type of anaemia, the total red cell count may be as low as 2,000,000 per cubic millimetre. After a severe haemorrhage, in which many red cells have been lost, the blood fluid volume may soon be made up by water taken by mouth, or drawn in from the tissues. But this water dilutes the remaining red cells, so the red cell count drops considerably. A blood transfusion will raise it again.

HAEMOGLOBIN

This is measured in grams per decilitre (100 ml) using a photoelectric method after converting it to a different compound cyanhaemoglobin. The normal is 13.5 to 18 g in men and 11.5 to 16.5 g in women. A typical value in iron deficiency or pernicious anaemia might be 10 grams per decilitre, but the figure can be much lower than this in severe anaemia or after severe blood loss.

If some blood is put in a tube and spun rapidly in a centrifuge, the red cells will sediment tightly and the space taken up by the compacted cells can be compared with the volume of the blood. This is called the *packed cell volume* (PCV) or haematocrit volume, and it varies in different conditions. The main value of the PCV is to enable the degree of saturation of the red cells, with haemoglobin, to be estimated.

THE BLOOD SMEAR

The features of individual red cells, as seen under the microscope, often give clues to the type of disorder. To do this, a drop of blood is allowed to fall on to a microscope slide and the edge of another slide is moved into the drop. The blood spreads along the edge and can be drawn across the slide to form a thin film. This is allowed to dry and may then be examined directly, or may be stained to bring out special features.

A normal red cell appearance is found in haemorrhage, failure of red cell production by the bone marrow and anaemias associated with long-term illness. Cells much smaller than normal suggest iron deficiency anaemia, thalassaemia, or other haemoglobin abnormalities. Irregularities of cell shape suggest anaemias of the pernicious type, myelofibrosis, or damage to the cells in their circulation. Cells of spherical shape, rather than the normal hollow disk shape indicate the condition of hereditary spherocytosis, or haemolytic anaemia, in which the red cells break up more easily than normal.

Examination of the stained blood smear may reveal organisms in the blood, such as malarial parasites, trypanosomes, Leishman-Donovan bodies, the spirochaetes causing relapsing fever or microfilarial worms.

BLOOD CLOTTING TESTS

In investigating bleeding disorders, a routine full blood count is first done. This may reveal a cause for the trouble, such as leukaemia or a low platelet count. Platelets – tiny non-nucleated bodies – are necessary for blood clotting and there are normally between 150,000 and 350,000 of them per cubic millimetre of blood. If the platelet count drops below 40,000 per cubic millimetre, spontaneous bleeding is likely. Low platelet counts cause the bleeding disorder thrombocytopenic purpura, and occur in conditions in which the bone marrow is not producing blood cells properly, such as pernicious anaemia, aplastic anaemia, acute leukaemia, drug reactions and certain autoimmune diseases. The platelet count is normal in haemophilia.

After the full blood count and platelet count, the most important preliminary tests in investigating bleeding disorders are the bleeding time, the clotting time and the prothrombin time. These can confirm that a bleeding disorder is present and can give some clues to its nature. The bleeding time is the time taken for bleeding to stop after a small puncture wound is made (normally three to five minutes). The bleeding time is prolonged in purpura, leukaemia, and severe cases of pernicious anaemia. The clotting time is the time taken for blood run into dry tubes to clot (normally four to seven minutes). Clotting takes longer in haemophilia, Christmas disease and obstructive jaundice.

In blood clotting, a substance called prothrombin is converted into thrombin. Thrombin acts on another substance, called fibrinogen, converting it into the fibrin which forms the clot. The prothrombin time is measured indirectly by the time taken for plasma to clot and this measurement is used to check the effect of anticoagulant drugs.

Some bleeding disorders are due to undue fragility in the tiny blood vessel – the capillaries. In the capillary fragility test a 6 cm circle is marked out on the front of the elbow and a blood-pressure cuff is applied well above it. The cuff is inflated to a pressure of about 50 mm of mercury and this is maintained for 15 minutes. After the pressure is released, the number of tiny blood spots seen in the circle is counted. Up to eight is normal. When there is increased capillary fragility, the number is greater.

Fibrinogen is the substance from which the fibrin clot is formed. If the amount of fibrinogen in the blood is much less than normal, clots cannot form and dangerous bleeding may occur. The fibrinogen index test measures the time taken for plasma to clot after it is added to some thrombin. Normally, this takes five to 12 seconds. In moderate fibrinogen deficiency it takes 12 to 30 seconds, and in severe deficiency it takes more than 30 seconds.

PLASMA PROTEINS

These proteins are dissolved in the liquid part of the blood – the serum – and are very important. There are several different kinds, with different functions. Albumin is essential for maintaining the ability of the blood to retain water and to prevent fluid from accumulating in the tissues as oedema. The globulin group of plasma proteins are the antibodies, or immunoglobulins, on which our defence against infection depends. Many enzymes are present in the plasma, and all are proteins. Certain plasma proteins are responsible for bringing about the clotting of the blood, and others act as transport vehicles for other substances, such as thyroid hormones, cortisol from the adrenal glands, iron, free fatty acids, bilirubin and various drugs. Changes in the levels of plasma proteins may be highly significant.

BLOOD ENZYMES

Cells contain large numbers of important substances called enzymes. When cells are damaged, enzymes are released into the blood and can be detected. The type and quantity of these can provide information about the site and degree of damage. For instance, an important laboratory test is the measurement of the enzymes which are present in the blood after a heart attack (coronary thrombosis) in which there has been damage to, or even death of, part of the heart muscle (myocardial infarction). In this case, the enzymes come from the muscle cells of the heart. The amount of muscle affected depends on the size of the artery blocked, and may be small or large. The larger the area of damage, the higher will be the levels of these enzymes in the blood. Doctors have found that measurement of the enzyme levels provides a sensitive indication of the extent of heart damage. Many different enzymes are released from damaged heart tissue and any of these could be measured, but a small group are selected because they are the easiest to estimate and can be detected in very small amounts.

Enzymes are, by their nature, very active chemical substances whose concentration in the blood is often very difficult to measure. For this reason, and because it is much easier to measure their activity than their concentration, blood enzyme estimations are usually expressed in international units of enzyme activity. The heart enzymes most commonly estimated are aspartate aminotransferase (AST), the lactate dehydrogenases (LD), and the creatine kinases (CK). One of the latter, CK-MB, is especially useful as heart muscle is the only tissue in the body containing more than about five per cent of CK-MB. One of the LDs, the heart-specific LD, is also useful in that its activity in the blood remains raised much longer than the other enzymes.

During the first three hours after a heart attack, there is no change in the levels of enzyme activity. Soon after this, they rise rapidly to a peak, subsiding over the course of the next few days at a rate which varies with the different enzymes. Later measurements are also useful to confirm that the enzyme

levels are reducing, and to confirm that further episodes are not occurring. A combination of electrocardiogram and enzyme estimation can confirm or deny the diagnosis of myocardial infarction with almost 100 per cent certainty.

Blood enzyme levels are also important in the investigation of other forms of tissue damage, especially in liver disease. Large quantities of enzymes are released in hepatitis and other forms of liver damage.

BLOOD CHOLESTEROL

Cholesterol levels vary with sex, age, diet and other factors. In people who derive most or all of their energy from carbohydrates, levels are low and there is no age-related change in cholesterol levels. Unfortunately, for most of us, the average blood cholesterol levels increase by about 1 mg per 100 ml for each year of age and this is almost certainly due to the cumulative effects of unsatisfactory and excessive diet. There is a clear correlation between the incidence of heart attacks and the levels of blood cholesterol and an especially high risk if the cholesterol consistently exceeds 235 mg per 100 ml.

The blood cholesterol, in any particular person, varies considerably from time to time, so a single reading may be seriously misleading in either direction. If there is any suggestion of a familial lipid disorder – familial hyperlipidaemia, familial hypercholesterolaemia, or familial hypertriglyceridaemia – a full study of the blood lipids is essential.

People having cholesterol estimates done must not change their normal pattern of behaviour, especially with regard to diet, alcohol and exercise, for at least two weeks before the test. The sample is taken after an overnight fast of 10 to 14 hours. Blood lipid tests can be seriously misleading if they are done within three months after a heart attack. Even a minor illness can cause a reduction in blood cholesterol, so figures taken at that time mean very little.

BLOOD ELECTROLYTES

The serum contains many simple inorganic compounds in solution. These break down in solution to form charged particles called ions and the concentration of these *ions* is critically important for normal body function. A substance like common salt (NaCl), for instance, breaks down, when dissolved, into positively charged sodium ions (Na^+) and negatively charged chlorine ions (Cl^-). Because these ions can be caused to move by the application of an electric current, they are called electrolytes. Charged ions are fundamental to much of the basic functioning of all the cells of the body. The passage of an impulse along a nerve, for instance, is a matter of the movement of charged ions from one side of the wall of the nerve fibre to the other, causing a zone of reversed charge which travels along the nerve. A reduction in the amount of calcium in the blood causes the severe disorder of tetany in which the muscles go into painful spasm.

Electrolytes, such as calcium, sodium, potassium, phosphate and chloride, must be present in the correct concentration if the body is to work properly and regulating mechanisms ensure that, in health, they do so. Many diseases, however, result in a change in the electrolyte levels and tests of these levels may be important.

OTHER BLOOD CONSTITUENTS

Chemical tests on blood serum may involve measurement of the levels of many other constituents.

These include:

- acetone and other ketones, which are raised in severe diabetes, starvation and other conditions;
- checks of levels of alcohol, usually for medico-legal reasons;

- barbiturates in poisoning;
- bilirubin in liver disease and obstructive jaundice;
- levels of calcium in various bone diseases and in disorders of the parathyroid glands;
- carbon monoxide levels in poisoning;
- carbon dioxide levels in respiratory failure;
- copper levels in Wilson's disease;
- blood fats in arterial disease;
- folic acid in malabsorption syndromes;
- globulin in immune-deficiency disorders;
- glucose in diabetes;
- iron in anaemia;
- lead and magnesium in poisoning;
- potassium and sodium in water and electrolyte imbalance;
- uric acid in gout;
- vitamin D in rickets;
- B12 in pernicious anaemia;
- vitamin C in scurvy.

Serum examination is also used to check for antibodies to a very wide range of infections and for blood grouping.

blood transfusion

The administration of blood, by instillation into a vein, to replace blood lost or to treat a failure of blood production. Before transfusion, the blood group of the recipient must be known and serum from the blood to be transfused is cross-matched with the recipient's blood cells to confirm compatibility. Sometimes the patient's own blood, collected at operation or obtained earlier, is used.

See also **autologous blood donation**.

blood vessel X-rays, high clarity

See **digital subtraction angiography**.

blood vessel formation, new

See **vascular endothelial growth factor (VEGF)**.

blood volume control

See **atriopeptin**.

blue baby

A term applied to a baby with congenital heart disease of a type in which the blood returning to the heart from the body is not wholly passed to the lungs to be reoxygenated, but is again returned to the tissues in its deoxygenated state. Blood fresh from the lungs is bright red, but after it has given up its oxygen to the body tissues it is a bluish-purple colour and gives a blue tinge to the skin through the vessels of which it is passing. This is called **cyanosis** and, when constantly present, is always an important sign of circulatory problems.

WHY IT HAPPENS

The normal heart has two sides which do not communicate with each other. The right side receives used blood from the head and body and pumps it to the lungs for reoxygenation. Freshly oxygenated blood from the lungs returns to the left side of the heart to be pumped to the whole body. In several forms of congenital heart disease, the two sides of the heart do not remain wholly separated, and

blood returning to the right side can mix with blood returning from the lungs.

The condition of 'hole in the heart' does not imply any possibility of leakage out of the heart, but refers to openings in the central wall which divides the two sides, internally. Because the pressure on the left side is usually higher than on the right, the blood is adequately oxygenated and cyanosis may not be a feature. But in some of these conditions, the right side of the heart enlarges in response to an increased load, and there is a right to left shunt, bypassing the lungs, with severe lack of oxygenation of the blood.

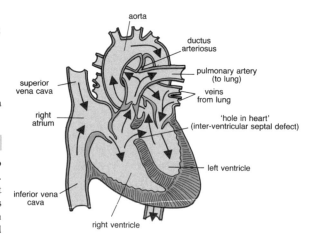

Blue baby. The 'hole in the heart' allows some of the blood to by-pass the lungs so that it returns to the general circulation without having been oxygenated. Non-oxygenated blood has a bluish colour and causes cyanosis.

blue bloater

Certain lung diseases, such as chronic bronchitis and **emphysema**, may so restrict the movement of oxygen from atmosphere to blood that the blood is inadequately oxygenated. Poorly oxygenated blood is blue, in contrast to the bright red colour of fully oxygenated blood, and imparts a bluish tinge to the skin (**cyanosis**).

At the same time, these diseases may cause a severe increase in the resistance to blood pumped through the lungs by the right side of the heart. This resistance causes the muscle of the right heart to enlarge and, for a time, this compensatory increase in pumping power may meet the need. Eventually, however, the right side of the heart may fail and it then becomes incapable of maintaining an adequate return of blood, from the rest of the body, via the veins. The result is the generalized increase of fluid in the tissues (oedema) characteristic of right heart failure.

People with cyanosis and oedema are sometimes referred to, by doctors, as *blue bloaters*.

blueness of skin

See **cyanosis**.

blunt dissection

A technique in surgery or anatomical dissection in which tissue planes are separated or opened and underlying structures exposed without cutting. Blunt dissection often involves the use of scissors in an opening, rather than a closing, mode. The closed tips are pushed into tissue and then separated so as to split or separate tissue planes.

blurred vision

See **vision, disorders of**.

blushing

A transient reddening of the face, ears and neck, often spreading to the upper part of the chest, but rarely, if ever, to more remote parts of the body. The skin contains an extensive network of small blood vessels with smooth muscle fibres in their walls. Normally, these muscles are in a state of partial contraction. Extreme contraction causes the vessels to close down so that less blood perfuses the skin and it becomes pale. Full relaxation of these muscles causes widening (dilatation), and a larger quantity of blood than normal passes through the skin causing flushing, or blushing.

POSSIBLE CAUSES

The control of these small vessel muscles (vasomotor control) is effected by the **autonomic nervous system** and this, in turn, is affected by various influences, including the emotions. Any strong tendency to blush, as in adolescence, may thus be due both to emotional instability and to undue sensitivity of the autonomic system.

Widening of blood vessels (vasodilatation) is a feature of sexual excitement and a widespread mottled flush commonly occurs. The hot flushes of the **menopause** are also caused by vasodilatation, the stimulus to the autonomic system, in this case, being a deficiency of the female sex hormone, oestrogen.

RISKS

Blushing can become a permanent problem. The disease **rosacea**, or, more correctly, acne rosacea, is a state of permanent dilatation of the blood vessels of the skin of the cheeks and nose. Happily, effective treatment exists.

body cavity lining

See **endothelium**.

body contour surgery

See **cosmetic surgery, plastic surgery**.

body fluid excess

See **oedema**.

body freezing

See **cryonics**.

body image

The mental picture of the body provided by the nerve connections in the brain between the part concerned with body sensation (the sensory cortex) and those parts concerned with vision and the other senses. Body image is distorted in various conditions, especially **anorexia nervosa**.

body, internal viewing of

See **laparoscopy**.

body odour

An unpleasant and usually socially unacceptable smell most commonly caused by the action of bacteria on the sweat produced by the apocrine sweat glands of the armpits and the groin areas and on skin debris generally. The remedy for this form of body odour is daily overall washing and, if necessary, the use of a sweat-retarding deodorant.

Body odour can also arise from inadequately washed genitalia, especially the female vulva, if there is persistent infection with the organism *gardnerella vaginalis*. This produces a characteristic fishy smell, especially when in contact with mild alkalis, as in soap.

Some volatile substances taken by mouth are excreted in the sweat in sufficient quantity to make their presence felt to others. These include alcohol, garlic and tobacco products.

body repair tissue

See **fibrous tissue**.

body shape

The outward shape of the body depends firstly on the proportions of the skeleton, then on the shape, proportion and bulk of the muscles, then on the thickness of the layer of fat covering the muscles and deposited in the abdomen and, finally, on the elasticity of the skin. The female skeleton is shaped somewhat differently from the male and this, together with the greater abundance of fat under the skin (subcutaneous fat), determines the characteristic shape of the woman's body. The appearance of the breasts depends on the state of the underlying muscles, the position and bulk of the milk-secreting glandular tissue and, to a considerable extent, on the thickness of the subcutaneous fat.

body temperature control

See **temperature regulation**.

boils

A boil is a *Staphylococcal* infection of hair follicles that has progressed to **abscess** formation.

POSSIBLE CAUSES

Boils occurring on the face or neck are usually associated with permanent colonization of the nose with staphylococci, and those on the lower part of the body with resident staphylococci in the armpit or groin.

Several factors predispose to recurrent boils. These include poor standards of personal hygiene with insufficient body washing, **scabies**, obesity, especially where there is resulting abrasion and dampness of the skin of the neck, buttocks and armpits, **diabetes** and **eczema**.

Because a boil implies a high local concentration of staphylococci, boils commonly occur in crops in the same general area. When several closely adjacent hair follicles are affected, the resulting large multiple boil is called a carbuncle. A **stye** is a small boil in an eyelash follicle.

TREATMENT

If crops are to be avoided, it must be recognized that the skin, especially in the area around the boil, is heavily contaminated with bacteria and must be treated by frequent thorough washing, preferably with a good antiseptic soap. In some cases

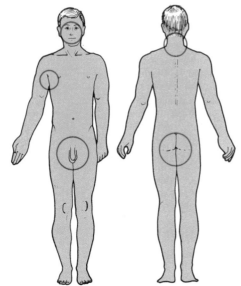

Certain areas of the body are particularly likely to harbour staphylococci and to develop boils. These areas are circled.

antibiotic treatment may be necessary, but an established boil cannot be resolved by antibiotics and must take its course.

bolus

A chewed-up quantity of food in a state ready to be swallowed. The term is also applied to a dose of a drug injected into a vein (intravenous injection) that, contrary to the normal practice, is given rapidly so that it enters the vein as undiluted as possible.

bonding

A term much used by those concerned with the science of animal behaviour (ethology) meaning the specially close and persistent relationship developing between individuals, especially those who come into close contact soon after the birth of one of them. Bonding is common between male and female birds.

The concept is now applied widely used to indicate the formation of a strong relationship, particularly that between a mother and her newborn child. Bonding is believed to be important for the future psychological wellbeing of the infant.

bonding, dental

Dentistry has not been slow to take advantage of technological advances and in recent years a wide range of new materials and methods have been adopted, especially for cosmetic purposes. Dental bonding can be used to replace or cover areas of discoloured or defective enamel with a surface so well-matched to the rest of the tooth in appearance as to be undetectable, and so hard and durable, as to be almost permanent. The surface to be bonded is first etched with a dilute acid and the material applied in a plastic form and smoothed off before it sets.

bone abscess

Bacteria carried by the blood can settle in bone and set up an infection causing local destruction and a collection of pus. This is called **osteomyelitis** and is now uncommon. In the days before antibiotics, however, such bone abscesses were exceptionally difficult to treat and usually became permanent, often with a chronically discharging opening to the exterior (a sinus). Bone infection may also follow a compound fracture, that is, a break with penetration of the skin allowing access to organisms.

bone breakdown stimulator

See **TRANCE**.

bone cancer

Secondary bone **cancer**, occurring as a remote spread (metastasis) from a primary cancer in another organ, is relatively common and indicates a major turn for the worse. Primary bone cancer, with which this article is concerned, may take several different forms, the most important being the osteogenic sarcoma which usually appears at the lower end of the thigh bone (femur). This is rare, affecting about one person in a million, but very serious. It occurs most often in young adults.

RECOGNITION AND SYMPTOMS

The first indication is bone pain, especially at night. Such pain, occurring for no obvious reason in a young adult, should never be ignored for there are few other symptoms until a late stage – at which the chances of cure are remote. Often, the next sign is cough, fever and chest pain, suggesting pneumonia, but actually caused by secondary spread of the cancer to the lungs. The tumour forms a swelling in the bone and the X-ray often shows radiating spicules of bone in the ominous 'sun-ray' pattern known to all doctors.

TREATMENT

A major advance in treatment has occurred in recent years and this has improved the five-year survival rate from one person in five to better than one in two. The drugs adriamycin and methotrexate, in conjunction with amputation and radiotherapy have greatly improved the outlook. In addition, recent immunological studies have shown that the tumour has antigenic properties which can be attacked by specific antibodies. Loss of the limb has been avoided in some cases by a bone graft from a dead donor.

bone cyst

Solitary bone cysts sometimes occur during the period of growth. They are situated near one or other growing end of the bone and are generally unsuspected until the bone suddenly and unexpectedly breaks on the application of a minor force. These cysts contain a clear fluid and may grow steadily until the outer layer of bone is reduced to a thin shell and fracture is inevitable.

POSSIBLE CAUSES

Bone cysts may be caused by tumours, especially by a tumour of the osteoclast bone cells. These are called osteoclastomas and are usually non-malignant (benign).

TREATMENT

If the cyst is discovered accidentally before the outer layer of bone is thinned until it fractures, it may be possible to stimulate new bone formation within it by an injection of a steroid drug directly into the cavity. If fracture has occurred, bone grafting is needed.

bone distortion in arthritis

See **lipping**.

bone-growth stimulators

Devices used in an attempt to promote healing of un-united fractures or fractures unduly slow to unite. They subject the fracture site to pulsed electromagnetic fields or to ultrasound. In some cases these devices appear to have a useful effect. But many different factors determine failure of normal bone healing, and not all are aided by the molecular vibration induced by such means.

bone imaging

The earliest medical X-rays revealed the bone structure of the hands and other parts and demonstrated how readily the details of the skeleton could be revealed by this new method. The dense concentration of metallic salts (calcium phosphate) in bone is far more opaque to radiation than soft tissue. Indeed bone shows up so well on X-ray examination that more recent methods of imaging, such as CT scanning and MRI, have hardly improved on long-established X-ray techniques. Bone can be a nuisance when imaging of other structures and parts is needed and methods have been developed, such as **digital subtraction angiography**, in which the bone shadows are eliminated.

Bone diseases are commonly investigated by the use of radioactive isotopes which concentrate in bone, giving off radiation that can be detected. Modern techniques of radionuclide scanning, using a gamma camera, can be more sensitive, and safer, than X-rays.

bone marrow aspiration

The removal of a small sample of bone marrow for examination. This is an important test in the investigation of leukaemia, anaemias of obscure origin or type, low white cell counts (granulocytopenia), certain infections, such as tuberculosis or leishmaniasis, lymphomas or cancer suspected of having spread to bone.

The sample is commonly taken from the crest of the pelvis, towards the back, but sometimes, especially in overweight people, it is taken from the breast bone. The skin is cleaned and sensation deadened with local anaesthetic. A stout cylindrical needle, sharpened at its free edge and reinforced by a strong inner steel stylet, is pushed through the outer layer of the bone into the marrow cavity. The inner stylet is now removed from the needle and a small quantity of liquid marrow is sucked out with a syringe. Part of the sample is used to make a smear on a microscope slide and part is injected into a tube which is sent to the laboratory for examination.

bone marrow biopsy

A valuable method of obtaining information about the state of the blood forming tissues. The sample of marrow is usually taken from the crest of the pelvis, behind, and requires a small injection of local anaesthetic. A broad needle, attached to a syringe, is passed through the outer table of the bone into the marrow and about half a millilitre sucked out. The biopsy enables an accurate diagnosis to be made of the various forms of anaemia including complete failure of red

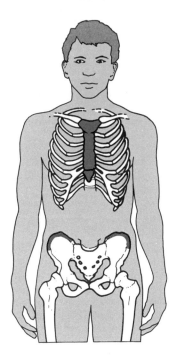

A sample of bone marrow can provide vital information about various blood diseases and certain kinds of cancers. Bone marrow is sucked out of flat bones such as the breastbone (sternum) or the crest of the pelvis (iliac crest)

cell production (**aplastic anaemia**), and of reduced white cell production (**agranulocytosis**), and the various kinds of white cell cancer (**leukaemia**).

bone marrow graft complication

See **graft-versus-host disease**.

bone marrow shutdown

See **aplastic anaemia**, **myelodysplasic syndrome**.

bone marrow transplant

A major advance in treatment which is being increasingly used to treat formerly irremediable conditions such as severe inadequacy in blood cell production (aplastic anaemia) and leukaemia. The graft provides the recipient with a new set of parent blood-forming cells (stem cells) which, all being well, may be expected to act as the source of a continuing supply of healthy new red and white blood cells.

HOW IT'S DONE

The technique of the transplant could hardly be simpler: marrow is sucked out of the marrow cavity of the pelvis or breastbone of the donor and injected into one of the recipient's veins. The marrow cells are carried, by the bloodstream, to the recipient's bone marrow where they settle and begin to produce new cell lines (clones) by normal reproduction. In some conditions the diseased bone marrow of the recipient is first destroyed by radiation. It is possible in certain forms of leukaemia, to take marrow from a person, store it, expose the person to heavy radiation and then to replace the original sample to start up the marrow function again.

booster

A dose of a vaccine, given at an interval after the primary vaccination, to boost the effect. It is a feature of the immune system of the body that once antibodies have been produced as a response to any particular infectious disease agent (antigen), the reappearance of this agent will provoke a large new production of antibodies. The B lymphocytes, which clone plasma cells to synthesize the appropriate antibodies, also produce memory cells capable of accelerating the process on the reappearance of the antigen.

Excellent protection against many infections may thus be afforded by a small booster dose of vaccine given at intervals. For some conditions, the interval may be as short as a few months, for others it may be five years or longer.

borborygmi

Bowel noises audible to others. These are caused by the gurgling of gas through the almost liquid contents of the small bowel as they are passed along in the direction of the large intestine by the process of **peristalsis**. Normally, the bowel sounds are barely audible, but any minor bowel upset or any excess gas production from dietary cause, may produce this sometimes embarrassing effect.

borderline personality disorder

The unfortunate sufferer from this condition exists on the borderline between normality and genuine psychiatric disorder. Such a person is liable to swing from a state of boredom and apathy to impulsive, often aggressive, acts, with outbursts of inappropriate **anger** and destructiveness. He or she will show sudden unexpected swings of emotion from depression to elation. There may be instability in personal relationships, inability to hold down a job, and a tendency to regard others as enemies. The disorder often leads to minor or major crime. It cannot readily be classified into any of the recognized formal patterns of psychiatric disorder.

Bornholm disease

Variously called epidemic pleurodynia, epidemic myalgia, or the Devil's grip, this infectious disorder, caused by a *coxsackie* virus, was first described after an outbreak on the Danish island of Bornholm.

RECOGNITION AND SYMPTOMS
It causes sudden attacks of pain in the central lower chest and upper abdomen, with headache, fever, sore throat and general upset. These attacks may occur repeatedly over a period of several weeks, causing much anxiety.

INCIDENCE
Bornholm disease is commonest in children and tends to occur in epidemics, during which diagnosis is easy. Isolated cases, however, often cause concern for the symptoms may be severe and may mimic more dangerous conditions. The virus can be isolated from the throat or from a stool sample.

TREATMENT
There is no specific treatment but recovery is eventually complete.

Borrelia

A genus of spiral-shaped bacteria that includes the organism *Borrelia burgdoferi* responsible for **Lyme disease** and *Borrelia recurrentis* that causes **relapsing fever**.

bottle-feeding

The popular alternative to **breastfeeding**. The subject arouses emotion and divides mothers into strongly opposing camps. There is much to be said on either side, and some important points should be made.

Formula milk cannot be made identical to human milk and the bottle-fed baby is deprived of many valuable antibodies present in the mother's milk. The risks of contamination of the feed are also greater with bottle- than with breastfeeding and care must be taken with sterilization. The special risk is of gastroenteritis and this is encouraged by the absence of antibodies, the ease with which a bottle, the teat, or the milk itself can be contaminated and the fact that milk at feeding temperature is an excellent culture medium for bacteria. This risk is, of course, greater if the milk is not used immediately but is kept warm artificially.

The advantages of bottle-feeding are obvious, especially to a working mother, and these are often socially overwhelming.

botulinum toxin

A powerful poison produced by the organism *Clostridium botulinum* which, in carefully controlled very small doses, has been found useful in the treatment of an increasing range of conditions. It is given, often with excellent effect, in:

- squint (strabismus) caused by overactive eye muscles;
- uncontrollable spasm of the eyelid muscles (blepharospasm);
- tennis elbow;
- facial spasm;
- excessive sweating of the palms;
- involuntary rejection of sexual intercourse (vaginismus);
- post-stroke spasticity;
- wry-neck (torticollis);
- writer's cramp;
- habitual tooth-grinding (bruxism);
- tics;
- swallowing difficulty (dysphagia);
- anal fissure;
- facial wrinkles.

The toxin can also be used to cause a temporary deliberate drooping of the upper lid (blepharoptosis) as an alternative to sewing the lids together (tarsorrhaphy) for the treatment of corneal ulceration and other conditions.

botulism

See **food poisoning**.

bougie

A smooth, often flexible, round-ended instrument used to detect and overcome abnormal narrowing (strictures) in a body passage. The name comes from the French word for 'candle' or 'taper'. Bougies are used to widen constrictions in the tube from the bladder to the exterior (the urethra), or to stretch a narrowed gullet (oesophagus) which is causing difficulty in swallowing.

Bournville disease

See **epiloia**.

bovine spongiform encephalopathy (BSE)

A **prion protein disease** of cattle similar to, possibly identical to, **Creutzfeldt-Jakob disease** (CJD) in human beings. The first animal cases appeared in 1985, believed to be the result of the feeding of calves in 1981–82 with meat-and-bone meal from infected animals. Only a few animals in each herd were affected and in more than one-third of these only one animal developed the disease. The question of whether new-variant CJD was acquired by eating beef products from infected animals has not been positively answered, but it now seems that there is a close connection of some kind. The abnormal prion protein causing BSE is the same as that found in the new human form.

bowel content movement

See **peristalsis**.

bowel lengthening

A surgical operation used to treat the **short bowel syndrome** in children as an alternative to bowel transplantation. The procedure involves freeing a length of intestine from the supporting membrane (the mesentery), dividing it longitudinally, converting each half into a tube and connecting these end to end. The blood supply to each half must be carefully maintained.

bowel movements, abnormal

The pattern of bowel movement varies from person to person. Anything between three times a day and three times a week is within the normal range. Some perfectly healthy people empty their bowels even less frequently. Again, no one is completely regular and occasional attacks of **diarrhoea** or **constipation** are to be expected. But each individual has an overall uniformity of bowel habit which tends not to change over the years.

> A change in the overall bowel habit must always be taken seriously, even if it has been very gradual over months. This is especially so in elderly people in whom diseases of the large intestine (colon), including cancer, are more common. Stools should always be inspected and any change in average size or shape reported. Ribbon-like stools may imply a bowel narrowing from cancer. Persistent change in colour, especially a black, tarry appearance – which denotes altered blood – or a clay-like paleness, are also significant.

bowel obstruction

See **intussusception, pyloric stenosis**.

bowel sounds

The movement of the bowel contents under the influence of peristalsis is usually almost silent, but can easily be heard using a stethoscope. Audible 'tummy rumble' is, of course, common and normal. Two major conditions affect the loudness of the bowel sounds. Any kind of blockage (intestinal obstruction), as from cancer, twisting (volvulus) or sleeve infolding (intussusception) leads to a marked increase in the

sounds as the bowel contracts vigorously and rapidly to try to overcome it. Adynamic ileus is a serious condition, usually the result of peritonitis, in which peristalsis stops and the abdomen is ominously silent.

bow legs

See **genu varum** and **rickets**.

boxing

See **brain damage**.

BP

British Pharmacopoeia. This is an official list of drugs with their properties, functions, side-effects and dosage.

brace, dental

The extent to which teeth can be moved, by applying steady pressure in one direction, is remarkable. Bone in the tooth socket actually absorbs on the side opposite to that on which pressure is applied to the tooth, and regrows on the same side, so that the new position of the tooth is permanent. This principle is the basis of orthodontics, in which a wide variety of appliances are used to apply sustained pressure in appropriate directions. Dental braces may be supplemented by an external wire structure, usually worn only at night, or may be wholly internal. Sometimes small metal anchorage points are cemented to the teeth so that pressure can most effectively be applied via attached wires.

brace, orthopaedic

Orthopaedic bracing may be used to support a leg unstable from muscle weakness. Such weakness may follow a disease like **poliomyelitis**, or severe muscle injury. Bracing may be used to prevent contracture and deformity resulting from lack of balance between muscle groups following disease, or from persisting (spastic) contraction of certain muscles in disease of the nervous system affecting motor control (see **spastic paralysis**).

Bracing is often used in children to correct deformity of the spinal column such as scoliosis, and it is sometimes used to prevent purposeless movement in conditions such as **chorea**.

bradycardia

A slow heart rate, below about 60 beats per minute. *Bradys* is Greek for 'slow'. The normal resting pulse rate lies between about 60 and 85 beats per minute. Bradycardia is often a good thing and, in healthy people, is a sign of efficiency in the heart and lung systems.

INCIDENCE

Long-distance runners almost always have bradycardia because sustained training has so increased the power and efficiency of the heart muscle that more blood is pumped by each beat. Thus, although the heart beats more slowly, the total output per minute is as high as that of a less fit person with a faster pulse. Good athletes may have a pulse rate of as low as 40 per minute. So while a person with a pulse of 80 may, on exertion, be able to double the heart output (pulse 160/minute), the athlete would quadruple the output for the same rise in rate.

POTENTIAL PROBLEMS

Bradycardia can also be a sign of disorder of the natural pacemaker of the heart (the sinoatrial node) – the sick sinus syndrome – or of heart block, in which pacemaker impulses are not properly conducted to the main pumping chambers (ventricles). It also occurs from digitalis overdosage and from the use of beta blockers and calcium antagonist drugs.

A slow pulse is a feature of thyroid underaction (myxoedema) and drug intoxication.

Braille

A method of coding information, to enable the blind to read. Groups of six raised spots, produced by embossing paper, are used, and these form a code of 63 characters, which can be read by passing a fingertip – usually of the left hand – across them. The French musician and inventor Louis Braille (1809–52), who developed the system in 1824 while a 15-year-old student at the National Institute for Blind Children in Paris, was, himself, blind from the age of three.

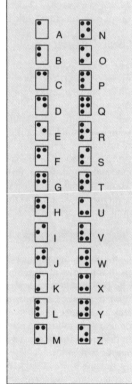

The system is logical and easy to learn, but much practice is required to achieve fluency. It is now universally used. There are special Braille codes for musical notations, mathematical symbols and for shorthand. Braille can be handwritten using a stylus and a special device called a slate. It is readily produced by electric embossing machines similar to typewriters and the electronic conversion of text into Braille, using optical character recognition software, is routine.

Blind people can acquire rapid facility with the Braille code allowing reading by touch. The main drawback is often in the supply of text converted to Braille.

brain

The brain is the seat of all personal satisfaction, of intelligence, memory and emotion and is the initiator and coordinator of all body functions. The rest of the body is the vehicle, the life-support system and the executive structure for the brain. The brain constantly receives an immense amount of data which it correlates with stored information. The result is intention and action.

But to fulfil intention, the brain must act through a system external to itself and that system must be capable of moving around, interacting with the rest of the world, obtaining and storing fuel supplies, communicating with other individuals, bringing about, for its own need and satisfaction, sensory stimulation of all kinds by way of the eyes, ears, nose, tongue, skin and sex organs.

Although this book may seem largely concerned with the body and with the means of ensuring that it does these jobs properly, that concern is, in the end, dedicated to maintaining the health of the brain and, with it, the satisfaction and comfort of the mind.

The nervous system consists of an enormous collection of interconnected neurons. Each neuron is a single nerve cell consisting of a cell body, a long nerve fibre or axon, running out of it, and one, or usually more, shorter nerve processes, known as dendrites, running into the nerve body. The cell body contains the nucleus. Neurons interconnect with each other at specialized junctions called synapses and, at most of these, activity is transmitted by release of chemical messengers called **neuro-transmitters**.

Synapses occur mainly between the end of the axon of one neuron and the cell body or the dendrites of another, but may occur between dendrites and axons. Many neurons receive up to 15,000 synapses and some more than 100,000, and the great majority are inter-neurons connecting with other nerve cells, rather than with muscles or glands. This arrangement allows for a system of transmission of nerve impulses, some excitatory, some inhibitory, which can operate similarly to electronic 'gates' in computers and by which all logical functions (AND, OR and NOT) may be performed. The same arrangement, assuming a constant circulation of nerve impulses, provides a physical basis for any form of memory, whether consciously recallable or of the form equivalent to the software in the read-only memory (ROM) of a computer.

The network of neurons is functionally, and structurally, affected by past experience and experience causes the brain to acquire greater complexity of the branching pattern of dendrites, an increase in the number of supporting cells and changes in the structure and ease of firing of synapses. The ability of the brain to change with experience is called plasticity and although plasticity in some areas, such as those concerned with vision, is lost by about the age of seven, in others it persists throughout life. Brain neuron connections which have not been challenged by experience retain simpler patterns and lower functional capacity.

The brain weighs about 1.5 kilos and contains a staggering number of nerve cells and connecting fibres. The packing density, in terms of functional elements, is still several times that of the most compact of electronic computer hardware and no present computer can challenge the capacity of the brain, weight for weight.

The neurological organization of all the millions of interconnected nerves of the brain forms a computing system broadly equivalent to many thousands of electronic microcomputers, working in parallel but with extensive interconnections. The arrangement of parallel computing is the principle difference between the brain and most present-day electronic computers, which are essentially serial and carry out only one operation at a time. It is probable that future research will show that the positive, as well as the negative, characteristics of human intelligence, memory and other functions are essentially those of a parallel computing system. As a result, we may soon need computer psychiatrists.

The brain is the information centre of the body, the seat of consciousness and pleasure. It is the physical data store (memory) and retains, in a form suitable for mass storage, all the significant individual experience and learning from birth – a unique collection of data which underlies the whole personality and capability of the individual. The brain also includes a great deal of data in the form of inherited information such as instincts, patterns of response, and so on.

It is probable that the brain cannot function unless continuously supplied with incoming stimuli. The receptors of the four main information modalities (sight, hearing, smell and taste) are connected directly to the brain by input channels in the form of short nerve tracts – the optic nerves, the auditory nerves, the olfactory nerves and the glossopharyngeal nerves. A constant barrage of data passes in by these nerves and is analysed, coordinated with existing stored data, stored and, if necessary, acted upon. In addition, a mass of sensory information comes into the brain from specialized nerve endings in the surface of the skin, in the muscles, joints and internal organs. These supply information about the environment, about the relative position of the limbs and about the state of the internal organs. Most of this incoming sensory information is relayed in the large nucleus, the thalamus, deep in the centre of the brain. Many of these data result in reflex activity, of a compensatory or adjusting kind, mediated by brain activity but mostly occurring below the level of consciousness. Many others result in conscious awareness of some bodily function or state and result in voluntary action.

The brain is the best protected of all the organs, being enclosed in a strong bony case and cushioned in a bath of water (cerebro-spinal fluid). The brain can only function properly if provided with an unceasing supply of sugar, oxygen and other nutrients by way of the bloodstream and to this end it has by far the most profuse blood supply of any organ. Two large arteries, the carotids, run up the front of the neck to the brain and two others, the vertebrals, run up through a chain of holes in the side processes of the bones of the neck (cervical vertebrae). These four vessels run into a circle of arteries at the base of the brain, from which major branches arise and run into the substance of the brain itself.

Interestingly, the word 'carotid' comes from the Greek word 'to stupefy' for it was well known that compressing these arteries could lead to unconsciousness and death. The word 'garotting' is similarly derived. Any interruption to the blood supply to the brain is dangerous. Permanent damage is done by a stoppage lasting for no more than three or four minutes, and death is inevitable if the supply is cut off, at normal temperatures, for more than about six to eight minutes.

The main mass of the brain is called the cerebrum and consists of two, almost mirror-image, cerebral hemispheres largely separated from each other but connected by a massive multi-cable junction called the corpus callosum. Tucked under the surface of the cerebrum, at the back, lies the cerebellum, or hindbrain, a smaller structure concerned mainly with unconscious and automatic functions such as balance and the control and coordination of voluntary movements.

Running down from the middle of the under side of the cerebrum, just in front of the cerebellum, is the brain stem, a thick stalk containing the roots (nuclei) of most of the 12 pairs of nerves which emerge directly from the brain. The brain stem is continuous with the spinal cord, below, and also contains the great tracts of nerve fibres running up and down, into and out of the spinal cord, which connect the brain to the rest of the body, carrying electrical impulses to cause the muscles to contract, and sensory information upwards from all regions to the brain.

The outer surface of the brain, the cortex, or grey matter, consists mainly of tightly packed nerve cell bodies interconnected by short fibres. The cortex has been accurately mapped out into areas serving known functions such as voluntary movement; sensations of touch; hearing and vision; processing and interpretation of incoming information; and many others. Destruction of these areas, by disease or injury, deprives the individual of the function concerned. The cortex is the seat of all the higher functions of humans – intellectual ability, learning, imagination, social responsibility, altruism, artistic skills, non-sexual love.

The 'association areas' of the cortex are areas which, although separate from those areas primarily concerned with these various functions, are connected to them by large

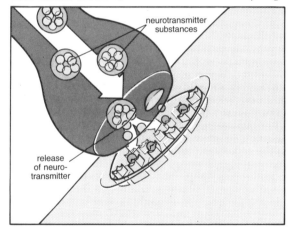

Above: Diagram of a synapse showing that there is a gap between the two neurons across which the chemical neuro-transmitter diffuses.

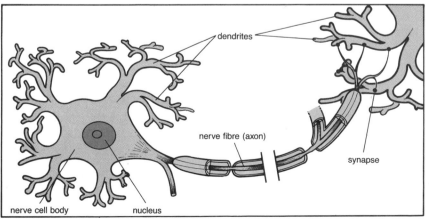

Left: A typical nerve cell (neuron). The cell body is of microscopic dimension, but in many nerve cells the axon is many centimetres in length.

numbers of nerve fibres. The association areas are concerned with the integration of input and output data with other aspects of brain function, including memory, and the elaboration of them into the complex processes underlying higher mental functions such as language, imagination and creativity. Thus, damage to the visual association area, while not in any way affecting the primary function of vision, might lead to an inability to recognize or interpret what is seen or might even produce visual hallucinations.

Under the cortex is the white matter, consisting mainly of bundles of long nerve fibres running to interconnect different parts of the cortex and to join the cortex to the cerebellum and the spinal cord. Within this white matter are several islands of grey matter. These include the basal ganglia – large collections of nerve cell bodies – and the thalamus and hypothalamus. These ganglia perform specialized computing functions in the manner of the cortex but are concerned with many unconscious and partly conscious functions.

In conjunction with the cerebellum, they exert a precise controlling and coordinating influence over all movements of the body, adjusting and balancing the nerve impulses needed to produce contraction of one set of muscles and relaxation of another, organizing the whole complex process of control which occurs, quite unconsciously, when we make voluntary movements. They control the more primitive and basic processes such as hunger, instinctual responses, sex drive, the experience of emotions, temperature control and so on. Disorders of the basal ganglia cause conditions such as Parkinson's disease or St Vitus' dance (rheumatic chorea). Understanding of the detailed function of these cell masses, and of the chemical neuro-transmitters by which they operate, is yielding rapidly to intense research and there has already been striking progress in the treatment of disorders such as Parkinson's.

The main driving (motor) system for movement is called the pyramidal system, because the great nerve fibre bundles running down from the upper surface of the brain form inverted pyramids. The basal ganglia are said to be part of the extrapyramidal system.

The extrapyramidal system is the part of the central nervous system concerned with gross movement, posture and the coordination of large muscle groups. The pyramidal system, on the other hand, which contains the main motor control pathways, is commonly involved in stroke, with resultant paralysis. In many cases, by early and determined training, it is possible to force the extrapyramidal system to take

over, to some extent, the functions of the destroyed nerve fibres of the pyramidal system and restore, for instance, the power of walking.

The limbic system, sometimes caller the visceral brain, is, developmentally, a relatively early part of the brain, centrally situated and arranged, as the name implies, in a ring. It consists of a number of interconnected nerve cell nuclei and represents much of what constitutes the brain in the lower mammals. The limbic system is greatly concerned in the coordination and regulation of that part of body function which is unconscious and automatic (autonomic nervous system function), but this function also involves associated emotional reactions, especially rage, fright and sexual interest, common to man and to the lower animals. The limbic system is also concerned with the regulation of respiration, body temperature, hunger, thirst, wakefulness, sexual activity and the link between neurological and hormonal function, controlled by the hypothalamus and the pituitary gland.

Diseases of the limbic system cause emotional disturbances, and these can include forced or spasmodic (pathological) laughing and crying, aggression, anger, violence, placidity, apathy, anxiety, fear, depression and diminished sexual interest.

The region of the brain lying near the centre of the undersurface and immediately above the pituitary gland is called the hypothalamus. It consists of three groups of collected nerve cells (brain nuclei), including the breast-like pair of mammillary bodies, most of which are connected directly, by nerve fibres, to the pituitary gland (see below), but some of which are connected to other parts of the brain.

The hypothalamus is especially important as it is the main point at which the neural and hormonal systems of the body interact. Here, electrical brain action, including that

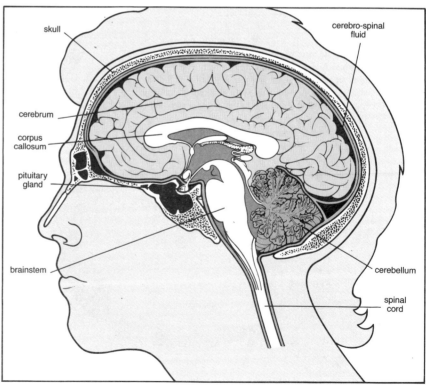

Labels on figure: skull, cerebro-spinal fluid, cerebrum, corpus callosum, pituitary gland, brainstem, cerebellum, spinal cord

The brain in relation to the skull. Note how the lower part of the brain stem passes through a large opening in the base of the skull to form the spinal cord.

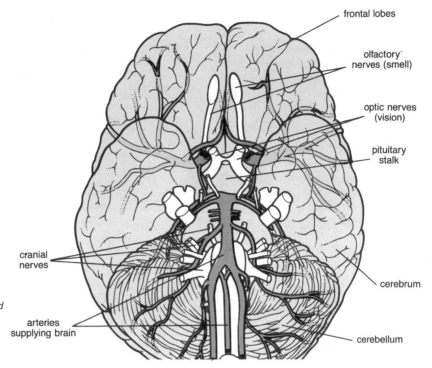

Right: Underside view of the brain, showing the emergence of the 12 pairs of cranial nerves and the profuse blood supply.

frontal lobes

olfactory nerves (smell)

optic nerves (vision)

pituitary stalk

cranial nerves

cerebrum

cerebellum

Below: The brain and spinal cord are bathed in a continuous cushion of fluid – the cerebro-spinal fluid.

arteries supplying brain

governing thought and emotion, causes changes which force the central controlling endocrine gland – the pituitary – to send out chemical messengers to any or all of the other endocrine organs and prompt them into activity. The result may be the pouring into the bloodstream of hormones such as adrenaline, cortisols, thyroid hormone, sex hormones, milk-secreting hormones and others. All these hormones are associated with changes in the state of the emotions. Baby suckling, for instance, causes the hypothalamus to prompt the pituitary to release the hormone prolactin, which causes the breasts to secrete milk. The hypothalamus, itself, releases hormones into the blood but these are carried directly to, and act mainly on, the pituitary gland.

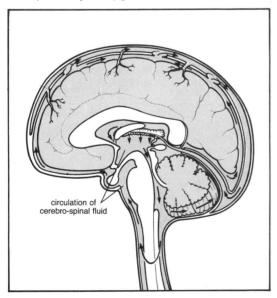

circulation of cerebro-spinal fluid

The hypothalamus constantly receives information from many parts of the body including the blood levels of the various hormones, the current state of bodily and mental stress, the requirements for physical activity and the state of the emotions. This information comes in both in neural and in hormonal form and completes the feedback loop so that adjustment to normal (homeostasis) can be achieved.

The brain is not entirely formed from nerve and supporting tissue, but contains interconnecting, fluid-filled spaces called ventricles. These also communicate with the cerebro-spinal fluid in which the whole brain and spinal cord are bathed and which fills a narrow duct, the central canal, in the spinal cord. The brain and cord are wrapped in three layers of membrane called the meninges. The inner meninx is a delicate layer, closely applied to the brain and dipping into the grooves on the surface. This is called the pia mater and the cerebro-spinal fluid lies outside it but beneath the next outermost layer, the arachnoid mater. Thus the arachnoid bridges across the grooves in the brain, and the cerebro-spinal fluid is in the space under it (the sub arachnoid space).

Outermost of all is the tough, fibrous dura mater and this is closely attached to the inside of the skull and the bony canal in the spine in which the spinal cord lies.

Many important brain arteries are also in the subarachnoid space and if one of these bleeds, the dangerous condition of subarachnoid haemorrhage exists.

Below the rear part of the cerebrum and immediately behind the stalk of the brain (brain stem) lies the cerebellum. This is the smaller subsidiary brain which operates at a totally unconscious level and is concerned with the complex task of coordinating the nerve impulses underlying all muscular activity so that smooth, balanced, purposive and effective movements can be made and the body's balance maintained in walking and in other activities. To do this, the cerebellum requires a great deal of information. It must have continuous input:

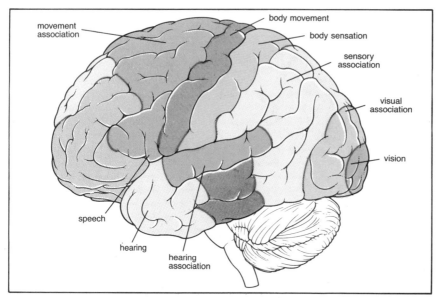

The functional areas of the brain and the association areas. The association areas are concerned with the synthesis and correlation of stored data concerned with the various functions – movement, sensation, speech, vision, hearing, etc.

- from all the muscles, so that their degree of contraction is known;
- from the eyes, informing it about the environment and the relationship of the body to it;
- from the balancing mechanisms in the inner ears, conveying information about the position of the head, relative to the different planes, and about accelerative forces experienced by the body;
- from those parts of the brain concerned with movement.

This never-ceasing input of data is passed to the cerebellum by way of large nerve tracts which join it to the brain stem and to several parts of the cerebrum. In the cerebellum the information is automatically coordinated and the complex output to all the muscles, necessary to maintain balanced posture and smooth movement, computed. This output is then passed back to the cerebrum and to the muscles.

Destructive disease of the cerebellum causes ataxia – a range of disorders of function which includes:

- staggering when walking;
- severe tremor of the hands, often worse when skilled activity is attempted;
- inability to perform rapidly repetitive movements;
- inability to judge the extent of one's movement;
- inability to perform a simple task without breaking it down into a succession of uncoordinated movements.

The study of these effects has taught us much about the function of the cerebellum.

The brain stem is the part of the brain connecting the main masses of the cerebrum and cerebellum, above, with the spinal cord, below. It consists, from above downwards, of the pons and the medulla oblongata and conveys all the large tracts of nerve fibres connecting the brain with the body. The brain stem also contains the roots (nuclei) of the cranial nerves which move the eyes, face and tongue and provide facial sensation, taste and hearing. Most important of all, it contains the net-like reticular formation which is responsible

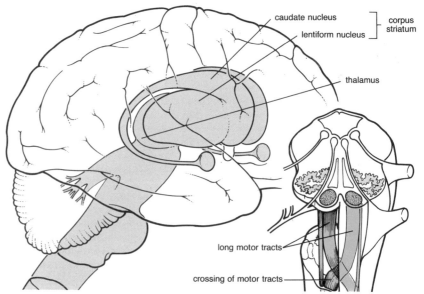

The basal ganglia of the brain – massive collections of nerve cells concerned with fine control of movement. The position of the corpus striatum, consisting of the caudate and lentiform nuclei, is shown. The thalamus is partly hidden by the lentiform nucleus. The smaller diagram shows the position, in the brainstem, of the long nerve tracts carrying impulses to the muscles of the body. Note how these tracts cross over.

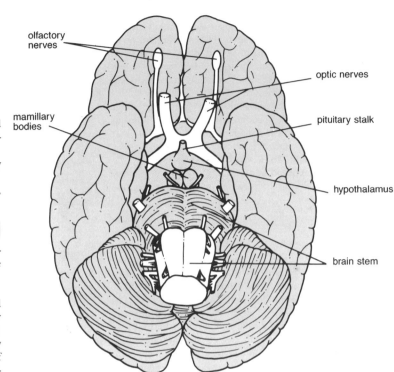

The underside of the brain showing the location of the hypothalamus with its mamillary bodies. The pituitary gland has been cut off, leaving the stalk.

olfactory nerves
mamillary bodies
optic nerves
pituitary stalk
hypothalamus
brain stem

for vital functions such as breathing and heart rate, and which controls and coordinates movement.

Brain-stem damage is always very serious and often fatal.

See also **autonomic nervous system**, **cranial nerves**, **peripheral nerves**.

brain abscess

A serious disorder occurring when pus-forming organisms gain access to the inner parts of the brain.

POSSIBLE CAUSES

The organisms may have spread through the bone following middle ear infection (**otitis media** and mastoiditis) or severe **sinusitis**, or have spread by way of the blood often as a complication of lung abscess. Brain abscess may also follow a penetrating injury of the brain by an infected object or missile.

RECOGNITION AND SYMPTOMS

The effects of a brain abscess depend on its position and on the amount of damage or local compression caused. Some abscesses cause no symptoms (silent abscesses), but most will cause some of the following effects, in order of frequency: headache, drowsiness, confusion, slowness of thinking, fits, paralysis, loss of sensation, speech disorder, visual field loss. Abscesses in the cerebellum cause loss of balance, staggering walk and a coarse jerkiness of the eyes. Brain abscesses are easily demonstrated by CT scanning or MRI.

TREATMENT

They are treated with intensive antibiotic therapy in very large dosage and, in some cases, later surgery to drain away persistent pus.

brain blood supply deficit

See **Binswanger's encephalopathy**, **vertebrobasilar insufficiency**.

brain damage

A term applied more often to the subtle, but serious, injury sustained from temporary oxygen and glucose deprivation, than to gross and obvious injury from direct violence.

POSSIBLE CAUSES

The brain has very large fuel requirements and is exceptionally sensitive to any reduction in supply, even for a few minutes. So it is often injured in the course of any misfortune that interferes with its blood supply – cardiac arrest, strangulation, massive haemorrhage – or that interferes with the oxygenation of the blood – asphyxiation, drowning, carbon monoxide poisoning, anaesthetic accidents. Birth is a dangerous time, and accidents such as interference with the blood supply from the placenta due to prolonged contractions of the uterus, or obstruction of the breathing passages by amniotic fluid or mucus may cause brain damage.

The brain is also sensitive to toxic substances, the commonest being alcohol (see **health maintenance**). Bacterial toxins released in the course of meningitis and **brain abscess** and inflammation caused by viruses (encephalitis) are also damaging. Diseases such as **multiple sclerosis** can cause brain damage.

Another avoidable and important cause of brain damage is boxing. Whatever the proponents may say to the contrary, participants in this activity are implicitly dedicated to inflicting the maximum possible brain damage on their opponents. Every successful blow to the head, with its contre-coup effect adds a quantum of damage, and the long-term result, except in the case of those few highly successful practitioners who are able to preserve their own brains at the expense of others', is commonly the pitiful state of dementia of the 'punch-drunk'.

Physical injury to the brain need not involve fracture of the skull or penetration of the brain substance. We live in an age of dangerous high speeds. It is a commonplace to see powerful cars and motorcycles driven in a manner plainly demonstrating the owners' unconsciousness of the magnitude of the forces involved, and of the horrifying physical damage to the brain when the body travelling at high speed is suddenly decelerated by striking something. In such deceleration, the brain, which is soft and almost jelly-like, continues to travel forward at the original speed and is smashed against the front of the inside of the skull. It then swings back and is smashed against the inside of the back. These are known as contre-coup injuries and their effect can be devastating.

RECOGNITION AND SYMPTOMS

Brain damage sometimes affects the areas of higher function in a patchy way with loss of certain functions and retention of others. Thus there may be paralysis and loss of sensation on one side of the body, epileptic fits, speech disturbances or loss of word comprehension (aphasia), loss of certain learned voluntary skills (apraxia), or loss of part of the field of vision.

Alternatively, brain damage may have a diffuse effect and in this case there is, in addition to focal effects, interference with the processes of conscious thought, memory and judgement. Loss of memory (amnesia) is a common feature of brain damage and this, if severe and prolonged, may be gravely disabling. A proportion of brain-damaged people end up in a state of almost complete loss of the higher mental functions (amentia).

brain death

'The time has been,' said Hamlet, 'that, when the brains were out, the man would die, and there an end.' Shakespeare could hardly have anticipated that the time would come when, as a result of artificial ventilators and artificial feeding, the body could be kept alive, indefinitely, even when the brains, in the sense of all higher mental function, were out.

The term 'brain death' is used only in cases where a cause such as deep intoxication, or the effects of paralysing drugs, can be completely ruled out; the effect of lowered body temperature (hypothermia) is eliminated; and no reflex responses above the neck, occur. In brain death, there is no spontaneous breathing and the electroencephalogram shows no sign of electrical activity.

Lay people are often misled by apparently voluntary movement in the lower part of the body in such cases. These result from purely spinal reflexes and the brain is not involved. Brain death should be distinguished from the **vegetative state**, or 'cerebral death' in which there is no awareness or mental activity, but the more primitive and less vulnerable parts of the brain are still functioning, allowing spontaneous breathing.

brain haemorrhage

See **haemorrhage, cerebral**.

brain imaging

This has now reached a high level of sophistication and the most advanced techniques of magnetic resonance imaging (MRI) almost equate, in detail, to that obtained by direct examination of slices of the brain, at autopsy. Fifth generation CT (computerized tomography) scanning also gives high resolution images, but the MRI method is inherently capable of providing higher detail. Advances in computer reconstruction of images, from data about density at all points, have been remarkable, and doctors can request print-outs of cuts at various angles. CT scanning can be made more sensitive by the use of radioactive isotopes which, given by injection just before the scan, concentrate in certain areas, such as tumours, and enhance the image. Similarly, positron emission tomography (PET scanning) can give unique information about the state of vitality (metabolic activity) of the brain using isotopes which emit short-lived positively charged electrons (positrons).

Since most brain disorders arise from interference with blood supply, brain surgeons are always greatly concerned with the state of the brain arteries. These may develop blockages from atherosclerosis and thrombosis, swellings (aneurysms) and leakage. X-ray imaging of the arteries (angiography) has long been an important method of investigation, but this has always been made difficult by thepresence of bone, which is densely opaque to X-rays. This can be overcome by **digital subtraction angiography**.

brain inflammation

See **encephalitis**.

brain, primitive

See **limbic system**.

brain tumour

Secondary spread of cancer to the brain, from a primary tumour in a remote site such as the lung, breast or prostate, is common. Primary tumours originating within the skull may arise from several different sites such as the brain coverings (meningioma), the neurological supportive tissue (glioma), the blood vessels (haemangioma), the bone (osteoma) or the pituitary gland (pituitary adenoma). Some are of congenital origin (craniopharyngioma, teratoma) and are due to abnormal development.

RECOGNITION AND SYMPTOMS

The signs and symptoms of a growing tumour within the skull are due to a progressive rise in the internal pressure, either from the growing mass or from interference with the normal circulation of the cerebrospinal fluid. The symptoms include:

- severe, persistent headache;
- vomiting which is sometimes sudden, unexpected and projectile;
- fits, either major seizures or local twitching;
- loss of part of the field of vision;
- hallucinations;
- drowsiness;
- personality changes;
- abnormal and uncharacteristic behaviour.

Headache is probably the commonest of all symptoms and only a tiny proportion of even severe headaches are due to brain tumour. But a new, persistent and severe headache without any obvious cause should certainly prompt anyone to seek medical attention. A key point in the examination, in such a case, is the inspection of the optic nerve heads within the eyes, using an ophthalmoscope. In one quarter of cases of brain tumour and in most of those with raised pressure within the head, the parts of the optic nerves visible within the eyes are obviously swollen (papilloedema).

In doubtful cases the diagnosis can usually be made by means of CT or NMR scanning.

TREATMENT

The outcome depends on the location, type and degree of malignancy of the tumour. Many common brain tumours are not malignant. Treatment is by surgical removal, often supplemented by radiotherapy.

See **astrocytoma**.

brain tumours in children

See **brain tumour**, **craniopharyngioma**.

bran

The fibrous outer coat of wheat grain normally removed in milling so that the flour will prove more attractive to many palates. Bran is undoubtedly valuable in the treatment of constipation and other disorders of the large bowel, and there is considerable statistical evidence that high-fibre diets may be protective against diverticulosis, appendicitis, piles (haemorrhoids), gallstones and other conditions.

Braxton-Hicks contractions

The common, irregular, painless and harmless contractions of the womb (uterus) which occur throughout pregnancy, increasing in intensity and frequency during the last three months.

BRCA genes

Genes that normally suppress cancers (tumour suppressor genes), but which, if suffering a mutation, can cause an inherited predisposition to breast and ovarian cancer. BRCA1 was discovered in 1990 and was found to be on the long arm of chromosome 17. It was cloned in 1994 and is involved in about 5 per cent of all breast cancers. In these cases, and in many cases of invasive breast cancer, the gene, which when normal acts to prevent cancer, is unable to function normally because of mutation. A considerable number of **frameshift mutations** or **nonsense mutations** have been found that confer high risk of cancer. Mutations of BRCA2, located on chromosome 13, are less commonly a cause of inherited breast cancer.

brittle asthma

A rare form of **asthma** affecting mainly females and featuring sudden, very severe, often life-threatening attacks. The people affected have a mild degree of immune deficiency, with poorly-controlled asthma and, in spite of substantial doses of inhaled steroids, wide swings in their **peak expiratory flow** meter readings. The term is also applied to people whose asthma is normally well controlled but who, nevertheless, suffer occasional sudden severe attacks.

breakbone fever

See **dengue**.

breakthrough bleeding

If hormone treatment to suppress the menstrual cycle, as in the use of the contraceptive pill, is continued for several months, the lining of the uterus (the endometrium) does not remain in a permanently unchanged state. From time to time, localized areas of the lining may die and be cast off, causing *breakthrough bleeding*. This can be stopped by increasing the hormone dosage, but at a later stage breakthrough bleeding may again occur. Breakthrough bleeding is not harmful.

breast

The breast is a glandular organ which secretes milk from the end of pregnancy until the continuing stimulus to further secretion ceases. The breast is a modified sweat gland, medically described as the mammary gland. Both sexes have rudimentary breasts at birth and in the male, the breast remains rudimentary. In the female, the growth of the breast after puberty, the enlargement of the nipple and the deposition of fat under the breast skin, are among the many secondary sexual characteristics which distinguish the sexes. The nipple occurs at the tip of each breast in both men and women. It is surrounded by a pigmented area, about 3.75 cm in diameter, called the areola. This enlarges and darkens in colour, and full development of the breast occurs during pregnancy.

The breast consists of a round mass of glandular tissue divided into 15 to 20 lobes, each with a milk duct leading to an opening on the nipple. The size of the breast is determined more by the amount of fat than by the amount of glandular tissue. Connective tissue strands form a kind of skeleton of the breast and these are connected to supporting strands from the underlying tissue (fascia) and the flat pectoral muscles under the breast.

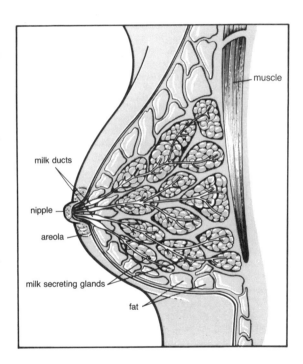

The female breast.

breast abscess

INCIDENCE

It is rare for abscesses to form in the breast except during breastfeeding. The first stage in the development of an abscess is an inflammatory process known as *mastitis*. This is common during breastfeeding because of the frequency with which the nipples suffer injury and abrasion. Germs, especially *staphylococci*, get into the breast by way of these abrasions and set up an infection.

RECOGNITION AND SYMPTOMS

At this stage, the symptoms are painful swelling of the affected breast, redness, tenderness, tension and inability to pass milk. Soon the breast becomes extremely swollen, and the mother suffers fever and general upset. The lymph nodes in the armpit swell up so that they can be felt, and become tender.

TREATMENT

If mastitis is not energetically treated with antibiotics, one or more areas of tissue softening and local tissue death (necrosis) occur, and soon a collection of pus forms, surrounded by hardened and inflamed tissue. This is an abscess which must be drained surgically. Milk production must be stopped by giving hormones or other drugs.

> General breast tenderness and tension are normal features of lactation, but any local tenderness, redness or pain must be reported at once.

breast augmentation

See **cosmetic surgery**, **plastic surgery**.

breast cancer

This is by far the commonest form of cancer in women and a very common disease affecting nearly a million women, worldwide, each year. It is estimated that about one woman in 12 in Britain will develop breast cancer.

INCIDENCE

In 1992 there were more than 15,000 deaths from breast cancer in Britain, which has the highest mortality rate from breast cancer in the world. Five per cent of all deaths in women are from breast cancer. Mortality in the age group 15 to 44 has fallen slightly but has increased in all other groups and breast cancer is the commonest cause of death in women between the ages of 35 and 54.

The condition is rare before the age of 25 and then begins to take its toll. The risk of a woman of 30 developing breast cancer is about one in 8000. In 1992, there were fewer than 300 breast cancer deaths in women of 35 or below. In the 40 to 45 year age range there were about 600 deaths; 45 to 50 about 800; 50 to 55 about 1100; 55 to 60 about 1300; 60 to 65 about 1500; 65 to 70 about 1800; in each of the three five-year groups between 70 to 85 about 2000; and over 85 about 2200 deaths. These figures are from a report published in the *British Medical Journal* in July 1994 by the Department of Public Health and Primary Care at the University of Oxford.

POSSIBLE CAUSES

There is now clear evidence that about 5 per cent of breast cancers are due to dominant genes – perhaps five different genes. The most important of these has been located on chromosome number 17 and a DNA test for this can be done if there is reason to suppose that the likelihood is high in any particular case. This is suggested by the fact of several affected relatives. Dominant genetic breast cancer tends to occur at an early age and may affect both breasts. It is also associated with other cancers, such as ovarian and colon cancers, in the same individual. About 9 per cent of breast cancers are believed to have some kind of hereditary basis.

Studies show that the risk of breast cancer is increased by about three times if the mother had it, and about three times in those who have already had it in one breast. Other risk factors are, having no children, starting menstruation early, exposure to radiation, being in a high socio-economic group,

eating a high-fat diet, taking large doses of oestrogens, and having had cancer of the ovaries or of the lining of the womb. Women with many children and those who have had their ovaries removed (oophorectomy) are less likely, than average, to get breast cancer.

RECOGNITION AND SYMPTOMS

Breast cancers are insidious and hardly ever cause pain. There may, sometimes, be a vague discomfort, but, commonly, the only sign is the finding of a slowly growing lump. There are, however, other possible signs and these should be known and looked for. They are:

- a change in the outline, shape or size of the breast;
- a new isolated lump;
- any difference between the degree of nodularity in the two breasts present early in the menstrual cycle and persisting;
- distortion of the normal breast contour by skin dimpling;
- indrawing, or alteration in direction, of the nipple;
- persistent discharge from a single duct;
- bleeding from the nipple (aside from that caused by breastfeeding);
- distortion of the area around the nipple (areola);
- orange-skin appearance (peau d'orange) of the skin of the breast;
- alteration in the position or hang of the breast compared to the other side
- rubbery, firm, easily felt glands (lymph nodes) in the armpit.

Minimal breast cancers are those confined to the milk ducts and lobes of the breast. They remain in situ for a long time before becoming invasive and spreading outside the breast and are easily curable if detected. They nearly always occur in pre-menopausal women. Unfortunately they do not produce a swelling that can be felt and are almost always detected at pathological examination for cancer suspected for other reasons – such as innocent fibrosis or cysts. Rarely, minimal cancers of this kind may become chalky (calcified) and may be detected by high-grade special X-ray examination (mammography).

The diagnosis of breast cancer is by microscopic examination, by a pathologist, of tissue from the lump. This is called a biopsy and the tissue may be obtained by sucking out some cells through a needle or by cutting into the breast and removing suspect tissue under direct inspection. The significance and probable outcome of breast cancer depend on the stage the tumour has reached when discovered. The size of the cancer is one of the most important factors. With tumours less than 2 cm across at the time of diagnosis and treatment, 60 per cent of women are free of recurrences five years later. If tumours are 2 to 5 cm across, about 45 per cent of the women are free of recurrence at five years. But for tumours more than 5 cm across, only about 20 per cent of women are free of recurrence. This highlights the importance of breast awareness and of monthly self-examination (see **breast, self-examination of**).

Several careful studies have shown that tumour size is substantially and significantly less at the time of diagnosis in women who practise regular self-examination.

Mammography as a screening method for breast cancer has greatly improved in reliability in recent years, and the dosage of radiation has been reduced. Experts now believe that mammography, if properly done, can reduce the mortality from breast cancer by one-third in women over 50.

DEVELOPMENT OF THE DISEASE

Breast cancer can spread directly, or by passing along lymph channels, to and through the lymph nodes or even by way of the bloodstream. Remote spread is usually to the lungs, bones and liver.

> The outlook in breast cancer is worsened if the cancer has spread to the lymph nodes in the armpit, and greatly worsened if there are distant outgrowths of tumour (metastases). Delay in seeking investigation and treatment is therefore most dangerous, and several studies have shown that women who delay for more than three months after finding a lump, subsequently proved to be cancer, have a substantially lower survival rate than those who report the problem within three months. This fact should be known to all women. Delays on the grounds of fright or shyness could be very dangerous.

TREATMENT

Information is available on what happens to women not treated at all. Different studies showed death rates of from 65 per cent to 95 per cent within the five-year period after diagnosis. These were, of course, unusual cases. In many cases, the reason for these not being treated was that they were old and infirm and had serious disease. Some would have died from causes other than cancer.

Conventional treatment of breast cancer has, in the past, been by radical **mastectomy**, an aggressive surgical removal of all breast tissue and connected lymph nodes together with the removal of the underlying chest muscles (pectorals). The results have not been very good. As a rough approximation, the five-year survival rate has been about 50 per cent overall. For those without lymph node involvement, the rate has been about 70 per cent and for those with lymph node cancer, about 30 per cent.

It has to be stated, however, that breast cancer can spread remotely even without involvement of the glands in the armpit (axilla). This and other factors led surgeons to pay less attention to radical and mutilating operations and more to the possibility of treatment by more limited surgery combined with various combinations of radiotherapy, anticancer chemotherapy, hormone treatment and immune system boosting.

Radical surgery is now usually restricted to total removal of the breast and lymph tissues with preservation of the muscles. This gives much improved appearance and function and makes breast reconstruction easier. In recent years there has been a trend towards even less mutilating operations and it is now common to employ a simple removal of the mass (**lumpectomy**) followed by a course of radiotherapy using linear accelerators or a cobalt 60 source.

The study of the results of such methods shows that they can be as successful as radical mastectomy and that cancerous nodes can be treated just as effectively by radiation as by operation. A great many clinical trials have been done to compare the effectiveness of various regimes of treatment for cancer that has spread beyond the breast. But the possible permutations and combinations of different methods and different groups, in terms of cancer stage, are so great that the results are difficult to interpret. Moreover, not all present methods of cancer treatment have been available long enough for the long-term outcome to be known. We do know, however, that chemotherapy substantially reduces the mortality in premenopausal women with cancer that has spread to the lymph nodes in the armpit. A review of 133 trials of such treatment has shown that a reduction of about 25 per cent in the recurrence and death rates can be achieved by the use of tamoxifen, anticancer chemotherapy and, in women under 50, the removal of the ovaries to reduce oestrogen levels. Tamoxifen has been well tried. In a series of 30,000 women taking this drug there was a reduction of 25 per cent in the annual rate of recurrence and of 17 per cent in the annual death rate. There was also a 39 per cent reduction in the risk of developing cancer in the other breast.

Hormonal therapy, such as the use of tamoxifen, has been found most useful in cases where the cancer has spread widely. Radiotherapy is no longer used after mastectomy but is used routinely after conservative treatment. New and less toxic anticancer chemotherapy drugs are being developed. The drug vinorelbine ditartrate (Navelbine) shows an excellent response when used as the initial chemotherapy. Immune system therapy is still experimental but is promising and holds out hope for the future.

A new approach to the management of breast cancer that is already widespread is exciting great medical interest in the USA and Britain. Trials are in progress in both countries. Current chemotherapy treatment, to be effective, must necessarily be toxic, and the most serious risk to life from such treatment is its effect on the bone marrow. Research has shown that if a chemotherapy treatment is quickly followed by a bone-marrow transplant, a much larger – otherwise possibly lethal – dose can be given. This greatly improves the chances of a cure. In the USA more bone marrow transplants are currently being done to treat breast cancer victims than for any other reason. The latest development in this process is to use drugs to persuade the primitive bone marrow cells from which all other blood cells are produced (the stem cells) to move out into the general circulation. These stem cells can then be easily collected, frozen, and stored for use after chemotherapy. The results of the new method are very encouraging.

This is perhaps the most promising of several lines of approach to this difficult problem. But clinical trials of every possibly worthwhile modality of treatment are in progress and the future for breast cancer therapy is optimistic.

See also **Paget's disease of the nipple**.

breast cancer, hereditary

See **BRCA genes**.

breast cancer spread detection

See **sentinel node**.

breast enlargement

The passage of female sex hormones into the fetal blood may cause enlargement of the breasts in either sex during the first ten days or so after birth. Breast enlargement in girls occurs at puberty under the influence of the sex hormones produced mainly by the ovaries. Enlargement follows a fairly consistent pattern but starts at varying ages. Budding begins around the age of 10 or 11 and breast growth progresses steadily to the age of 13 or 14. Oestrogen stimulates the growth of the ducts and progesterone the gland tissue. There is a great range of variation in the size of the normal breast and it is not uncommon for breasts to be of different sizes. Abnormal enlargement (hypertrophy) may affect one or both sides and often appears at puberty. This is due to an increase both in glandular tissue and fat, and the weight and stretching may cause great discomfort. Young girls are often gravely embarrassed by over-large breasts and surgical reduction is sometimes justified (see **plastic surgery**).

Once menstruation is established, progesterone also stimulates congestion of the glands during the second half of each menstrual cycle and breast enlargement occurs then. This settles when the next period starts.

Breast enlargement is normal during pregnancy and may be considerable. The greatest enlargement, however, occurs during milk production (lactation). This is due partly to engorgement with milk and partly to the increased flow of blood through the breasts. Most of the pregnancy enlargement usually resolves after the baby is weaned but it is common for the breasts to remain somewhat larger than before because of persistent fat deposition.

breastfeeding

The milk produced by the human breast has been evolved, over millions of years, to be the optimum source of nourishment for the newborn baby. Its chemical constitution is appropriate to the digestive capacity of the baby and the nutritional balance of its proteins, sugar and fat is exactly what is required. The immune system of the new baby is immature and has not yet had the opportunity to produce antibodies. Breast milk contains an abundance of maternal antibodies to a range of infections, so the breastfed baby acquires a valuable degree of passive immunity to cover the period before its own immune system can take over.

HOW IT WORKS

Once the placenta has been delivered, the hormone prolactin from the pituitary gland is free to exert its full effect on the breasts – which causes the secretion of milk. The stimulus of handling and touching the breasts and especially the suckling by the baby increases the production of prolactin and it is essentially this stimulus that maintains the flow. Indeed, so long as suckling continues, milk will continue to be produced. This is the basis for the protracted 'wet nursing' of former times.

Milk production is fully established two to five days after delivery, and the breasts become enlarged by about one-third in volume and are usually tender. Most of the actual synthesis of the milk occurs while the baby is suckling and the prolactin levels are at their highest.

No formula milk can compare with breast milk, which contains fat, proteins (casein, lactalbumin, lactoglobulin), sugar (lactose), vitamins (C, A and D), minerals (sodium, potassium, calcium, iron, magnesium, etc). These constituents are present in cows' milk, but in differing concentrations appropriate to the needs of calves.

The milk secreted under the influence of prolactin must move into the ducts behind the nipple before the baby can suck and squeeze it out. This movement into the ducts is called *milk let-down* and is under the influence of another pituitary hormone called oxytocin. Like prolactin, this hormone is prompted by suckling and by psychological factors. A nursing mother may find that she will leak milk on hearing her baby cry.

In about 50 per cent of cases breastfeeding prevents ovulation, but lactation should not be relied upon as a contraceptive. When nursing is discontinued for a few days, the pressure of the milk closes off the small blood vessels in the gland and, since the milk is secreted from the blood, the supply soon fails. Fat cells in the breast connective tissue increase in size and the breasts usually end up larger than before the pregnancy.

Another advantage of breastfeeding is the avoidance of intestinal infection of the newborn baby (see **bottle-feeding**).

breast lump

WHY EXAMINE YOUR BREASTS?

Women, constantly exhorted to perform breast self-examination, often find it very difficult to decide whether or not a lump is present. This difficulty may be so great as to discourage them from performing the examination and this may induce anxiety and guilt that they are not doing it. The normal feel of the breast, as of any glandular tissue, is naturally that of a lumpy structure. Moreover, the degree of lumpiness is often more marked just before a menstrual period and what may seem to be a new swelling is often felt before a period. A 'new' lump of this kind may be tender or even painful. This is not typical of a cancer, and swellings of this kind disappear after the end of menstruation. Such a swelling is most unlikely to be serious.

The secret of successful breast self-surveillance is to acquire familiarity with, and confidence in, the normal feel of the breast. The kind of lump that calls for immediate action is a firm, isolated swelling, usually painless, that is entirely unaffected in size over the course of the menstrual period and which remains present and unchanged after the period. Such a lump must be reported without delay.

About 75 per cent of breast lumps are non-cancerous and are due either to inflammation (mastitis), a breast cyst, or a benign tumour. Even so, **breast cancer** *is* very common and if there is any doubt this is a reason for reporting, not for procrastinating.

FEELING FOR LUMPS

Breast self-examination should be done every month. Cancer will not announce itself by a pain and new lumps will be inapparent unless felt or unless they have grown to a dangerously large size. The severity of the outlook, in established breast cancer, is proportional to the size of the lump. So there is every reason to carry out monthly self-examination. The trend in the surgical management of suspicious breast lumps is away from the former tendency to immediate mutilating removal of much breast and lymph node tissue. Simple sampling of the lump (biopsy) through a small incision, or even the sucking out of lump cells through a fine needle (needle biopsy), followed by rapid pathological examination is now the norm. The subsequent procedure depends on the pathologist's findings.

Women who find a lump should insist on a specialist opinion immediately.

breast implants

See **silicone and breast implants**.

breast plastic and reconstructive surgery

See **plastic surgery**.

breast pump

A device used to relieve engorged and painful breasts of excess milk, or to remove milk for later use. The pump, which can be manually or electrically operated, provides a low degree of suction and comes with a sterilizable container into which the milk flows. Milk obtained in this way can safely be fed to the baby from a sterile bottle. If refrigerated, it may be rewarmed and used up to 24 hours later. Breast milk can even be frozen and kept for up to six months.

breast, self-examination of

This should be done monthly during the week after the period. The breasts are naturally lumpy during and just before the periods and examination then is more difficult. All women should carry out this procedure. After the menopause, it should be done on a particular date each month.

HOW IT'S DONE

The following is a good routine and should be followed systematically:

1 Strip to the waist and stand straight in front of a mirror with the arms hanging loose.
2 Check that the breasts are of the usual shape, size and colour.
3 Look at the breast contours and check especially for puckering of the skin or an appearance like orange skin.
4 Check both nipples for any abnormal position, retraction or dimpling.
5 Check for bleeding from the nipples.

6 Gently squeeze around each nipple to see whether any discharge is expressed from the nipple itself.
7 Raise the arms equally above the head and check the lower parts of the breasts. Check whether the breasts move up equally.

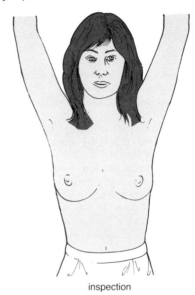

inspection

8 Lie on the back so that the muscles under the breasts are relaxed and feel both breasts for lumps. Some women find it easier if a folded towel is put behind the shoulder-blade on the side of the breast being examined. Use the right hand for the left breast and the left hand for the right. Feel only with the flat of the fingers. Do not pinch the breast tissue between the fingers and thumb – it will always feel lumpy. Work round each breast systematically checking each of the four quadrants and the tail of the breast which points up to the armpit (axillary tail). The latter part is especially important as most tumours occur here. Feel carefully for lumps in the armpit.
9 If a lump is suspected, check whether it is affected by the menstrual period.

The article on **breast lump** should be read again and the advice followed to the letter.

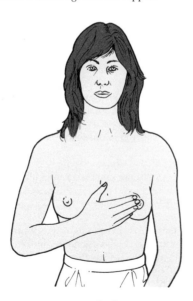

palpation

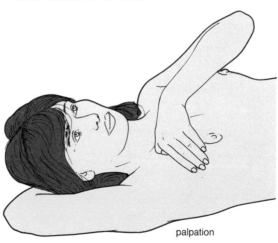

palpation

breath, character of

The character of the breath can often give a clue to disease. Local infection in the mouth, especially gum infection (gingivitis) and pyorrhoea is a common cause of an offensive breath. A septic throat will also cause an unpleasant breath as will a rare condition of degeneration of the lining of the nose, called ozena. Bronchiectasis, in which secretions in the lung stagnate in local areas of widening in the breathing tubes (bronchi) also causes bad breath.

Contrary to popular belief, indigestion does not affect the breath. It is only in cases of advanced cancer of the stomach with obstruction and fermentation of food that a digestive disorder can affect the breath.

In uncontrolled diabetes, substances called ketones are formed and these are present in the breath, causing the characteristic 'nail-varnish remover' smell of acetone. The same effect occurs in starvation and when the diet is excessively high in fats. In kidney failure, in which the waste products build up in the blood, the breath may have a urine-like smell, and in liver failure there may be a smell like musty hay. The breath of children with the genetic condition of phenylketonuria also has a musty or 'mousy' smell.

breath-holding attacks

A form of infantile blackmail imposed on indulgent parents by determined and unscrupulous babies.

INCIDENCE

Breath-holding attacks are very common and may be a source of great, but unnecessary, concern to parents. Although they may superficially resemble them, the attacks are of an essentially different nature from **epilepsy** or febrile fits and observant parents should have no difficulty in making the distinction.

Breath-holding attacks affect only quite young children. Perhaps older children are able to find new and less alarming ways of manipulating their parents.

POSSIBLE CAUSES

As many parents will be well aware, breath-holding attacks are usually prompted by annoyance on the part of the child at not being allowed to have his or her own way. Many parents will be convinced that they are manipulative in nature and will feel that the child is making use of the only major weapon at his or her disposal. Others will simply allow themselves to be dominated by the child's use of this effective strategy. Breath-holding attacks are sometimes induced by pain, but the usual causal factors are anger and frustration.

RECOGNITION

The attack starts with a period of loud crying. At the end of a long wail, during which the lungs are emptied of air, the child simply refrains from taking in a breath and soon turns blue. If his or her resolution allows it, breath-holding continues until consciousness is lost and the child goes quite rigid with arms and legs extended and back arched. Sometimes there are a few muscle twitches, but in a very short time, nature takes over and breathing starts again with rapid recovery. These episodes never involve any danger to life and no treatment is needed.

breathlessness

Breathlessness (dyspnoea) is an automatic response to changes in the levels of oxygen and of the waste gas, carbon dioxide, in the blood. These levels are constantly monitored by specialized cells in the large arteries of the neck and in the brain, and, as the levels change, altering signals are sent to the centres in the brain stem for control of breathing rate. From these, impulses are sent along nerves to the respiratory muscles to speed up or slow the rate of contraction.

POSSIBLE CAUSES

If, for any reason, the blood is not carrying enough oxygen, or is carrying too much carbon dioxide, breathlessness will result. And the degree of breathlessness will relate to the degree of deficiency of the former and of the excess of the latter.

The commonest cause of breathlessness is, of course, muscular effort requiring more oxygen than the blood is currently carrying.

> All of us should experience breathlessness every day, as a normal response to exertion, if we are to keep in reasonable condition.

But breathlessness ought to be appropriate to the level of work demanded of the body. For the man who gets breathless merely from heaving his overweight body from the dining table to the Rolls Royce, breathlessness is no cause for rejoicing, but is a sign of cardio-respiratory unfitness.

The athlete has, over many months or years, exposed his heart muscle, respiratory muscles and skeletal muscles to constant and increasing work demands, and these muscles have responded by developing a better and more profuse blood supply so that they can use fuel (glucose) and oxygen more efficiently. Thus the man in the Café Royale has a pulse rate of about 95 and gets breathless walking to his car, while the athlete has a pulse rate of 40 and can bound up four flights of stairs with a barely noticeable increase in the number of breaths he takes per minute.

So most cases of undue breathlessness are due to simple unfitness, often made worse by the additional load imposed by obesity, and merely represent a less than reasonable exercise tolerance.

MORE SERIOUS CAUSES

But breathlessness is also sometimes an important sign of disease and this may occur in several ways. Adequate access of oxygen to the red blood cells is so important that anything which even partially obstructs the airway is always serious. Conditions such as spasm of the bronchial tubes (**asthma**), collapse of the lung due to air between the lung and the chest wall (pneumothorax), acute **bronchitis**, or a breakdown of the air sacs so that the area of tissue available for oxygen passage is much reduced (**emphysema**) will always cause breathlessness.

Anaemia, in which the oxygen-carrying capacity of the blood is reduced will cause increased breathlessness on effort. Any loss of heart efficiency, from any cause, will interfere with the efficient circulation of the blood and cause breathlessness.

Smoking is a particularly interesting cause of breathlessness and does this in several ways. Cigarette smoke contains carbon monoxide, a poisonous gas that combines so stably with haemoglobin that the affected haemoglobin cannot perform its normal function. Heavy smoking is exactly equivalent, in this respect, to opening a vein and letting eight to ten per cent of the blood run away. Secondly, smoking causes a degree of obstructive airway disease from chronic bronchitis, so that access of oxygen is reduced. Thirdly, smoking reduces the ability of the heart to benefit from exercise, by its effect on the health and width of the coronary arteries. This may lead to cardiac breathlessness.

Breathlessness can sometimes be deliberate and used for social or manipulative purposes. The most common form of this is the dramatic hysterical overbreathing known as hyperventilation. This often leads to impressive spasm of the hands and feet (**tetany**) as a result of blowing off so much carbon dioxide that the blood becomes alkaline and the calcium levels drop. Tetany adds to the general chaos but is easily relieved by persuading the hyperventilator to rebreathe into a small plastic bag for a minute or so. Another form of psychogenic 'breathlessness' features deep sighing respirations frequently repeated.

TREATMENT

Undue breathlessness can always be corrected by sustained, graded exercise and by losing excess weight. As a symptom of something more critical, breathlessness must always be taken seriously and medical attention sought.

breech delivery

See **childbirth**.

bretylium tosylate

A drug used to help to restore normal heart rhythm in the form of cardiac arrest known as **ventricular fibrillation**. A brand name is Bretylate.

bridge, dental

A fixed support for false teeth which bridges the gap between surviving natural teeth. The support is almost always of metal and is securely attached to metal inlays in the natural teeth. Dentists have responded with ingenuity to the challenge to restore good cosmetic appearances and have applied a wide range of techniques and engineering skills to the problem. Titanium implants and artificial crowns are now more popular than bridgework.

Bright's disease

An old-fashioned term for **glomerulonephritis**. The English physician Richard Bright (1789–1858), working at Guy's Hospital, made important advances in the understanding of kidney disease.

brimonidine

A drug used in the form of eyedrops in the treatment of **glaucoma**. A brand name is Alphagan.

brittle bones

A popular term usually applied to bones abnormally liable to fracture because of loss of structural calcium (**osteoporosis**). This may be due to normal ageing processes or to the deficiency in sex hormones which particularly affects women after the menopause.

The term *brittle bones* is also applied to the rare condition of osteogenesis imperfecta, a hereditary disease in which fragility of bones is associated with thinning and hence blue colouring of the whites of the eyes, and sometimes deafness and dental abnormalities. The degree of fragility is variable, but some babies with the condition suffer repeated fractures and occasionally stunting of growth. **Child abuse** may be unjustifiably suspected.

broad-spectrum

A term, most commonly applied to antibiotics, that implies that the drug is effective in killing a wide range of organisms. The prolonged use of broad-spectrum antibiotics, such as **ampicillin** or the cephalosporins, will usually destroy most of the normal organisms of the bowel and these will tend to be replaced by resistant species. It is therefore considered better practice to use narrow-spectrum drugs so long as these are known to be effective against the organism concerned.

See also **MRSA**.

Broflex

A brand name for **benzhexol**.

broken veins

The proper term is *telangiectasia* and the visible appearance is due to localized widening (dilatation) of blood vessels near the surface of the skin as a result of the failure of support from loss of collagen. This is one of the natural features of the ageing skin due largely to the effect of ultraviolet light.

A condition called **rosacea**, a sort of blushing disorder, features widespread telangiectasia, which may also involve the conjunctivae of the eyes and even extend on to the corneas. The frequent use of steroid preparations on the skin also makes 'broken veins' more common and conspicuous. Apart from rosacea, the condition is of cosmetic importance only.

Some people are sufficiently distressed by telangiectasia to submit to destruction of the affected parts of the vessels by electrolysis or electrocoagulation. This may leave small scars and recurrence is likely.

bromazepam

A benzodiazepam drug used in the treatment of anxiety and insomnia. A brand name is Lexotan.

bromhidrosis

See **body odour**.

bromocriptine

An ergot derivative drug with dopamine-like effects. It is used in the treatment of **Parkinson's disease** and **acromegaly** and given to prevent **lactation** by inhibiting the secretion of the hormone prolactin by the pituitary gland. A brand name is Parlodel.

bromphenyramine

An **antihistamine** drug used in the treatment of hay fever and other allergic conditions. A brand name is Dimotane.

bronchial carcinoma

See **lung cancer**.

bronchiectasis

Permanent areas of local widening of the bronchi, usually with long-term (chronic) infection. Because of these sac-like widenings, the normal upward movement of bronchial mucus and infective material is interfered with.

RECOGNITION AND SYMPTOMS

Bronchiectasis is an unpleasant condition, causing persistent cough with much sputum, wheezing, breathlessness, bronchitis and sometimes **emphysema**. There may be coughing of blood. As the condition worsens, over the years, the amount of sputum increases and it is usually necessary to have a heavy bout of coughing every morning, in the late afternoon and again on going to bed at night. The persistent pus and putrefying secretions in the dilated areas of the bronchi may cause offensive breath.

POSSIBLE CAUSES

Bronchiectasis may, occasionally, be present from birth and result from failure of the lungs to develop properly. More often it results from damage to the walls of the bronchi by infection or inhaled irritant gases. Inhalation of industrial dusts, such as silica or talc is a predisposing factor. It commonly follows pneumonias in childhood, often complicating severe whooping cough or measles, or may result from lung infection by one of a large number of virulent organisms including viruses, staphylococci and fungi. The condition is worsened by smoking.

TREATMENT

Treatment is difficult and involves heavy antibiotic cover, physiotherapy and occasionally surgical removal of an especially severely affected lobe of the lung.

bronchitis

Inflammation of the lining of the bronchi.

POSSIBLE CAUSES

Acute bronchitis usually follows a cold, sore throat, or influenza, usually in winter, and is very common, as a winter flare-up, in people with chronic bronchitis. It may also be brought on by breathing a polluted atmosphere or by smoking.

RECOGNITION AND SYMPTOMS

There is a cough, at first dry but later with increasing production of sputum, fever for a few days, breathlessness and wheezing. There may be some pain in the chest.

TREATMENT

In most cases the condition settles within a week or two, but there is always the risk, especially in cigarette smokers, that the condition may progress to chronic bronchitis with inevitable winter flare-ups.

> Chronic bronchitis is one of the forms of obstructive lung disease and is liable to become permanent with age and lead to progressive disablement. Recurrent attacks of bronchitis should always be taken seriously and properly treated, and the cause identified and avoided. Smoking is especially dangerous in people with a persistent, productive cough.

bronchoconstrictor

A drug or other agent which causes narrowing of the air tubes (bronchoconstriction).

bronchodilatation

Widening of the bore of a bronchus by relaxation of the circular muscles in its wall. Bronchodilator drugs are used in the treatment of asthma.

bronchography

A form of X-ray examination in which the branches of the breathing tubes (bronchi) are made conspicuous by lining them with an inhaled or injected material opaque to X-rays. Well performed, the result can be a strikingly clear outline of the bronchial 'tree'. Bronchography is especially useful in the diagnosis of bronchiectasis, but is gradually giving way to less invasive methods such as refined CT or MRI scanning.

bronchopneumonia

An acute infection of the smallest air tubes and the lung substance, usually by organisms such as *streptococcus, haemophilus, klebsiella* or *legionella*. It can also be caused by the inhalation of irritant substances, especially vomit (aspiration pneumonia).

INCIDENCE

Bronchopneumonia is usually less serious than the more extensive type, known as *lobar pneumonia*, which affects a whole lobe, or even wider areas of the lung. It tends to be confined to areas of lung tissue surrounding the bronchi, but the distinction between this and more widespread involvement cannot always easily be made. In spite of antibiotics, bronchopneumonia can still be dangerous, and it claims many thousands of lives every year, especially among the old and debilitated. Although no longer high on the overall list of causes of death, pneumonia is the commonest cause of death from infection and is often the terminal event in people seriously ill from other causes, such as stroke.

RECOGNITION AND SYMPTOMS

The severity and danger varies with the type of organism. The condition often starts with a sudden fever with pain in the chest. There may be difficulty in breathing, rapid shallow breathing, cough and sputum which is sometimes rusty-coloured from blood. Temperature may rise to 40.5°C.

TREATMENT

In some cases the poisoning (toxaemia) from the infecting organisms is overwhelming. In others, the amount of lung tissue put out of action is so great that survival is impossible. The outcome depends on many factors and these include the degree of immunological resistance, the age of the person affected, the size of the dose of infecting organisms and their virulence, the speed of diagnosis and of identification of the organism and the availability of antibiotics to which the organism is sensitive. Unfortunately, many hospital staphylococci and other organisms are resistant to many commonly used antibiotics. In such cases the mortality rate may be as high as 40 per cent.

As well as intensive antibiotic treatment, oxygen, fluids by transfusion and other supportive measures may be used. Patients who recover often do so suddenly.

bronchopulmonary dysplasia

A chronic lung disorder affecting premature babies who need supplementary oxygen and artificial ventilation. There is acute and chronic lung damage with inflammation, fibrosis and structural remodelling.

bronchos

Greek root meaning 'throat' as in bronchitis (bronchial inflammation).

bronchoscopy

The procedure of direct inspection down an air passage (bronchus) into the lung. The early bronchoscopes were simple metal tubes which were pushed down the windpipe (trachea) under anaesthesia and into one or other main bronchus, affording a very limited and poorly illuminated view as far as the openings of the secondary bronchi.

Fibre optics, which allows flexibility and 'steerability', has greatly improved the method and modern bronchoscopes allow brilliant illumination along one fibre optic channel and excellent viewing along another. In addition, they allow one or more channels down which instruments can be passed. Lasers can also be used, through bronchoscopes, as surgical tools.

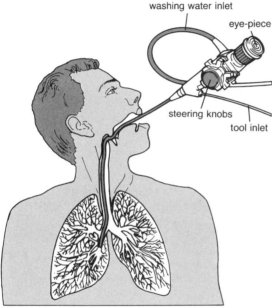

A bronchoscopy using a steerable, flexible, fibre-optic endoscope for examination of the inside of the bronchial tree.

bronchospasm

A tight contraction of the smooth, circularly placed muscles in the walls of the air tubes (bronchial tubes) in the lungs. Bronchospasm is the main feature of, and cause of the symptoms in, **asthma** and is often brought about by an allergic mechanism.

bronchus, cancer of

See **lung cancer**.

brown fat

Human body fat is an oil at normal body temperature and each fat cell contains a single large drop. This is called yellow or white fat. In many animals fat is also stored in a different physical form, as a multitude of tiny droplets held in supporting tissue. The latter gives it a brownish appearance.

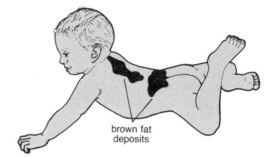

The areas in which brown fat occurs in babies.

Brown fat is more readily available for rapid conversion to heat than is white fat and it is believed that hibernating animals use their brown fat in the recovery from the winter state. Small babies have deposits of brown fat around the spine.

Soon after this discovery, there was much interest in the possibility that brown fat might have an important role in human nutrition and it was speculated that excessive food intake could be balanced by the rapid turnover of brown fat. But the excitement seems to have died down and little is heard on the subject these days.

brucellosis

An infectious disease, contracted by eating infected dairy products, or by contact with the secretions of sheep, goats and cows.

Sir David Bruce (1855–1931) is well-known in the British Army Medical Services for the pathology laboratory named after him. In 1887, while investigating the condition known as *undulant fever* or *Malta fever*, which was killing British soldiers on that island, he isolated an organism from the spleens of those who had died from the disease. This bacillus was later named *Brucella melitensis* (the Malta species of the genus named after Bruce) and was proved to be the cause. The soldiers were being infected from goats' milk.

INCIDENCE

Brucellosis is now mainly a disease of farmers, veterinary surgeons and meat packers and occurs all over the world.

RECOGNITION AND SYMPTOMS

The main feature is the tendency for the fever to last for a week or so, settle for a few days, and then return. Sometimes these recurrences persist for months or years, usually as progressively milder attacks. The fever episodes are accompanied by weakness, irritability, depression, emotional upsets, loss of appetite and weight, headache, backache and joint pain. The spleen, and often the liver, become enlarged.

TREATMENT

Antibiotics are effective, but prevention is better. This involves the avoidance of unpasteurized milk and of new cheese and the protection of those handling fresh animal products.

bruise

The effect caused by the release of blood into or under the skin, usually as a result of injury involving small blood vessels, but sometimes spontaneously in the case of bleeding disorders or disease of the blood vessels. When the cause is obvious, only patience is required. Raw steaks have no effect.

Bruising occurring without obvious cause suggests purpura and must always be reported for investigation.

bruits

A term used by doctors because the word 'noises' is insufficiently impressive. Bruits are abnormal sounds or murmurs heard in the stethoscope and usually caused by the flow of blood past some relative obstruction or narrowing. Bruits may be caused by abnormalities in the heart valves causing excessive turbulence or regurgitation of the blood flow, or they may be heard in the main arteries of the neck (carotids) if these are narrowed by atherosclerosis. The latter observation may be an important warning of impending stroke.

bruxism

Habitual grinding or clenching of the teeth, often to the point of wearing away the enamel and eroding the crowns of the teeth. The habit is often unconscious but is usually apparent to others and tends to affect both children and the elderly. It is aggravated by alcohol and may be so severe as to loosen the teeth. Bruxism is common during sleep.

A dental splint is sometimes used for protection, but the real remedy is to overcome the habit.

bryostatin-1

A drug with a unique action against cancer cells, that is being used in trials of treatment of leukaemia and malignant melanoma. Bryostatin is formed by a bacterium *Endobugula sertula* that parasitizes the boat-fouling marine animal *Bugula neritina*. The drug also shows promise as a stimulant of the immune system against breast cancer.

BSE

See **bovine spongiform encephalopathy (BSE)**.

BSE and CJD basis

See **prion protein disease**.

bubo

This word, which means a swelling in the groin, or in the armpit, has been used for 2000 years – always with a sense of grave anxiety. The bubo is, in fact, a greatly swollen lymph node, or collection of nodes, and this can occur from a wide variety of infections apart from the bubonic plague.

Enlargement of lymph nodes (wrongly called 'lymph glands' – they are not glands) commonly occurs from any severe infection in the tissues draining into the nodes. Thus a leg infection will cause groin node enlargement and an arm infection will affect those under the arm. Lymph nodes may enlarge greatly as a result of syphilis, gonorrhoea, **lymphogranuloma venereum** or **tuberculosis**.

bubonic plague

See **plague, bubonic**.

bucca

Latin root meaning 'cheek' as in buccal (of the cheek).

buccal smear

A convenient way to obtain cells for chromosomal and other studies and to obtain a sample of DNA. The inside of the cheek is gently and painlessly scraped with a spatula and the cells spread on a glass slide. Every cell thus obtained contains a copy of the whole of the person's DNA (the genome).

buck teeth

It is normal for the edges of the lower central teeth (incisors) to lie just behind those of the upper jaw, but an undue protrusion of the upper incisors is generally thought to be aesthetically undesirable and is popularly known as 'buck teeth'. The problem, if it is a problem, can readily be put right by orthodontic treatment.

Budd-Chiari syndrome

A rare condition due to clotting of the blood (thrombosis) in the large drainage veins of the liver. This may occur as a result of undue blood red cell concentration (**polycythaemia**), sickle cell disease, abdominal injury and, occasionally, pregnancy or the use of oral contraceptives. The effect is often serious, with pain, liver enlargement, yellowing of the skin (jaundice), and eventual liver failure. Less than one-third of patients survive for a year, and often a liver transplant is the only hope.

bug

One of various wingless or four-winged insects of the order *Hemiptera* and especially of the sub-order *Heteroptera*, with piercing and sucking mouth parts. The bugs of medical importance include the cone nose (*Reduviid*) 'assassin' or 'kissing' bugs which transmit South American trypanosomiasis (Chagas' disease, see **trypanosomiasis, South American**) and the bed bug, *Cimex lectularis*, which cause painful bites.

Buerger's disease

See **thromboangiitis obliterans**.

bulbar palsy

A neurological disorder causing progressive paralysis of the tongue, throat and voice box (larynx) so that swallowing and speaking become difficult or impossible. Bulbar palsy is a serious feature of various neurological diseases including **motor neuron disease**, and **poliomyelitis**.

bulimia

Bulimia is an uncontrollable, compulsive eating disorder, usually affecting intelligent young women, and causing them to eat large quantities of food in a very short period of time. Up to 15,000 calories may be taken in a few hours. In spite of this the affected girls are seldom overweight, and most of them appear normal. In many, the weight varies abnormally, fluctuating above and below the ideal. Friends and relatives often do not suspect bulimia because the 'binge eating' and the behaviour that follows are usually kept secret.

POSSIBLE CAUSES

Binge episodes are often triggered by mental or social stress. Girls with bulimia can't help themselves and regularly eat to the point of bloating and nausea.

On the psychological side, bulimia often has features in common with **anorexia nervosa**. This is so in as many as half the cases. Girls with anorexia have a distorted image of their own bodies, and in spite of the evidence of the mirror, are deeply preoccupied with becoming too fat. As a result, they starve themselves into a condition of emaciation but still seem, to themselves, to be overweight. In some cases of anorexia, the terribly limited food intake causes a constant, torturing preoccupation with food which regularly results in binge eating and, of course, this causes a major conflict. But most cases of bulimia are caused by a less serious psychological upset than anorexia, and treatment, by specialists in the disorder, is generally more successful.

RECOGNITION AND SYMPTOMS

These binges may, in mild cases, occur only once every few weeks, and, in such cases, strict dieting, in between episodes, is enough to keep the weight down. But in other cases, the cycle takes place every day or even several times a day. These unfortunate young women have to find a private place for their activities because the binges are followed by regret and a panicky concern that the result will be a gain in weight. So they deliberately cause themselves to vomit and take purgatives, to empty the bowel and undo the 'harm'. Some girls even take diuretic drugs, which cause excessive output of urine and temporary loss of weight until the resulting thirst forces them to drink and replace the deficient fluid.

The physical problems with bulimia are caused by repeated vomiting and laxative and diuretic use, which may reduce the normal acidity of the blood and upset the balance of dissolved substances even to the extent of causing muscular weakness or the state of muscular spasm called **tetany**. There may be persistently sore throat and heartburn from the vomited acid, and the salivary glands in the cheeks may be inflamed in a manner similar to mumps. Teeth may be badly damaged, even reduced to sharp stumps, by the repeated action of stomach acid and the knuckles may be scarred by the teeth during the attempts to force the fingers down the throat to induce vomiting.

TREATMENT

This is not just a matter of self-control but is a recognized medical condition which should be reported and for which medical help is badly needed.

bullet-proof vest

No wearable vest is completely bullet-proof but modern bullet-resistant vests offer considerable protection and are often life-saving. Modern protective vests are made of a nylon-like polymer called Kevlar in the molecule of which aromatic rings replace the nylon hydrocarbon structure. The difference increases the stiffness 16 times over that of earlier nylon protective vests, and a garment made from 20 fine layers of this material can prevent a 9 mm bullet moving at 366 m per second from depressing the skin more than 4 cm.

bumetanide

A quick-acting **diuretic** drug used to relieve the fluid retention (oedema) occurring in **heart failure**, kidney disease such as the **nephrotic syndrome** and liver cirrhosis. A brand name is Burinex.

bundle branch block

The heartbeat is caused by a systematic contraction of the heart muscle stimulated by electrical impulses passing along bundles of specialized muscle fibres. These impulses are conducted downwards from a biological clock (sino-atrial node)

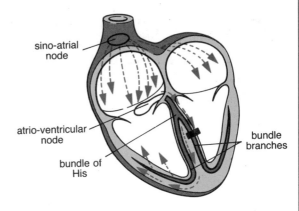

The conducting system in the heart can be interrupted by diseased areas, especially when muscle is damaged by arterial insufficiency. In bundle branch block one of the main divisions of the bundle of His is functionally severed and this seriously interferes with the timed contraction of one of the ventricles.

in the wall of the right upper chamber, by the bundle of His (Wilhelm His [1831–1904] was a German cardiologist), and this allows the correct timing of the contraction of the upper and lower chambers. The bundle of His divides into three and any disease of the heart, especially coronary thrombosis, can damage either the main trunk or one or more of the branches. As a result, there is interference with the passage of impulses to the ventricles and these may take up a spontaneous, slow, beat rate independent of the rate of the sino-atrial node. This is known as **heart block**.

The slow heart rate may lead to inadequate blood supply to the brain with sudden fainting attacks (**Stokes-Adams attacks**).

bunion

Inflammation of the protective, fluid-filled tissue bag (bursa) overlying the main joint of the big toe. This is called **bursitis** and it is due to wearing pointed shoes which lever the big toes towards the outer side of the foot, to an abnormal degree. This outward deviation of the toe is called **hallux valgus**. It is commoner in women than in men, solely because women have, in the past, been more rigorously forced by considerations of fashion, than have men, into wearing unsuitable shoes.

Pressure on the prominent toe joint leads to increased protective bone formation (exostosis) and inflammation of the overlying bursa. Treatment involves chiselling off the excessive bone. Prevention is better than cure.

buphthalmos

Literally 'ox-eye', this is the condition of enlargement of the corneas that results from an abnormally raised pressure within the eyes at birth (congenital **glaucoma**). The eyes appear large because of the greater corneal diameter.

Congenital glaucoma is due to a failure in the normal development of the internal drainage system of the eyes so that aqueous humour secreted within the eyes is unable to get out as easily as it should.

It is important that buphthalmos should be detected and treated as soon as possible so that normal vision may develop. A fairly simple operation early in life will usually ensure this.

bupivacaine

A long-acting local anaesthetic drug often used for nerve blocks, especially in epidural anaesthesia during childbirth and for the control of postoperative pain. A brand name is Marcaine.

buprenorphine

A powerful pain-killing drug that binds to the body's opioid receptors. It acts for six hours. Brand names are Subutex and Temgesic.

Burkitt's lymphoma

See **lymphoma, Burkitt's**.

burr hole

A small circular hole drilled in bone, using a burr (drill). Burr holes are often made in the skull so that a wire saw can be used to make a cut between them and raise a flap of bone so as to get access to the brain.

Drilling burr holes in the skull (trephining or trepanning) is an ancient practice, formerly performed with the laudable intention of allowing evil spirits to escape. There is little evidence to show whether the treatment was effective or not, but plenty of evidence that the practice was common.

bursitis

Inflammation of a bursa. This is a small fibrous sac lined with a membrane which secretes a lubricating fluid (synovial membrane). Bursas are efficient protective and friction-reducing structures and occur in various parts of the body, usually around joints and in areas where tendons pass over bones. Bursitis is commonly caused by excess local pressure or undue friction, but it may also result from rheumatic disease or infection. Common examples of bursitis are housemaid's knee and **bunion**.

buspirone

A non-benzodiazepine anti-anxiety drug with slow onset of effect. A brand name is Buspar.

busulphan

An anticancer drug used especially in the treatment of chronic granulocytic **leukaemia**. It is very toxic and can destroy the function of the bone marrow unless its use is carefully monitored. It can also cause widespread **fibrosis** of the lungs. A brand name is Myleran.

butyrophenone drugs

A group of **phenothiazine derivative drugs** used in the treatment of schizophrenia. They act as dopamine receptor antagonists. The group includes haloperidol, triperidol and benperidol.

bypass operations

One of the major causes of disorder in the body is partial or total blockage of a tube, such as an artery, vein, intestine, urinary passage and so on. Blockage of arteries, by the common arterial disease of **atherosclerosis**, is the major cause of death in the West. Bypass operations are designed to overcome these obstructions by shunting them with a dispensable part taken from elsewhere in the body – a length of vein or artery, a segment of intestine or a piece of plastic tubing.

Arterial bypass operations have saved many lives and relieved much distress. They are used to bypass obstructed coronary arteries in the heart, blocked carotid arteries in the neck which supply the brain, and narrowed or obstructed main arteries supplying the legs. Many hundreds of thousands of patients have enjoyed a remarkable improvement in their condition by the restoration of a good arterial blood supply by such means.

Veins, too, can be bypassed. Cirrhosis of the liver can cause severe back pressure in the blood flowing in the veins from the intestine, and this often leads to serious secondary effects, such as bleeding from varicose veins in the gullet (oesophagus). Bypass of the liver can relieve these.

Hydrocephalus is a disorder of increased pressure in the fluid surrounding the brain and spinal cord. A bypass plastic tube connecting this fluid, by way of a valve, to the cavity of the abdomen can prevent further damage to the brain.

Obstruction to the bowel is usually due to cancer and it is not always possible to remove the whole tumour and relieve the obstruction. In such cases it is common to restore the free passage of bowel contents by linking together the loops of bowel on either side of the tumour.

There was, at one time, a vogue for treating obesity by bypassing a large section of the small intestine, so that food eaten was not fully absorbed. The results were disappointing and some patients suffered serious complications. The method is now largely abandoned.

byssinosis

Another of the lung allergies, similar to **bagassosis** and **bird-fancier's lung**, caused by dust inhalation. Byssinosis is caused by the dust produced in the manufacture of cotton, flax or hemp goods. Shortness of breath, chest tightness and cough become progressively worse as the months and years of exposure pass. Eventually, the lung damage may be so severe that the body cannot obtain enough oxygen even for sedentary activities (respiratory failure) and the individual is gravely crippled.

Byssinosis is an industrial disease which can be prevented by proper control of working conditions and the use of measures such as forced-draught ventilation and protective masks. In most developed countries, employers are liable if workers are injured in this way, and, in consequence, the condition is now rare. In some developing countries, however, many thousands of workers are currently being turned into respiratory cripples.

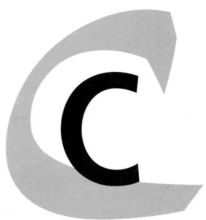

cachexia

A state of severe bodily decline occurring in the late stages of serious illnesses such as cancer. There is severe muscle wasting and weakness. Cachexia is the usual condition of those dying after long debilitating illnesses.

cadaver

A corpse. The term may correctly be applied to any corpse, but tends to be confined to corpses that are used for anatomical dissection.

cadmium

A poisonous metal sometimes encountered as an air pollutant in industrial processes. It is found in association with lead and zinc and may be released during the extraction of ores of these metals. It is used as an anticorrosive agent and extensively in nickel-cadmium batteries.

Inhaled cadmium dust can cause lung inflammation and prolonged exposure can lead to **emphysema**. Cadmium is also damaging to the kidneys and can cause softening of the bones (osteomalacia) in people with reduced intake of calcium. An epidemic of cadmium poisoning occurred in Fuchu, Japan, in the late 1940s. Known locally as *itai-itai* ('ouch-ouch') it was traced to contamination of the paddy fields by a mine extracting lead, zinc and cadmium. Many of those affected were women, and bone softening was a major feature.

CAESAR

An important trial of multiple therapy for HIV-positive people carried out in Canada, Australia, Europe and South Africa (hence the acronym). CAESAR showed conclusively that the addition of lamivudine or lamivudine plus loviride to a treatment regimen containing zidovudine can significantly reduce progression to AIDS and death. This was the most important advance in the management of the HIV-positive status since the onset of the AIDS pandemic.

café au lait patches

Milky coffee-coloured patches on the skin. These oval or leaf-shaped freckles, which may be as long as 6 to 8 cm, are usually of cosmetic significance only. But if they occur in childhood and six or more large examples are present, it is likely that the affected person has **neurofibromatosis** (von Recklinghausen's disease) and multiple skin bumps – benign

tumours of the sheaths of skin nerves – may be expected to develop in adolescence or early adult life.

café au lait spots

These look like large, oval, milky-coffee-coloured freckles and vary in size from less than 1 cm to more than 15 cm long. They may occur anywhere on the skin. If more than five of these patches are present, and especially if they extend into the armpits, there is a possibility that the person concerned may have **neurofibromatosis**. This genetic condition involves multiple, small, non-malignant tumours of the fibrous sheaths of nerves, and the possibility should be considered even if there is no known family history. Neurofibromatosis is also called von Recklinghausen's disease.

calcaneal spur syndrome

The effects of a spur of bone (exostosis), readily visible on X-ray, that forms on the inner weight-bearing surface of the heel bone (calcaneus) and extends forward horizontally into the soft tissue (plantar fascia) beneath the skin of the sole. The condition is painful in its early stages but tends to become less so as the spur enlarges. It is treated by injections of steroid mixed with a local anaesthetic.

calcific tendinitis

An inflammatory disorder of the rotator cuff tendons of the shoulder involving deposition of calcium (calcification), most commonly close to the insertion of the muscle tendon onto the larger bony protrusion (greater tuberosity) of the upper arm bone (humerus). About half of the people with this disorder suffer shoulder pain and limitation of movement at the shoulder. The condition is self-limiting, but recovery can be hastened by ultrasound treatment.

calcium channel blocker drugs

Calcium is necessary for the contraction of muscles, and charged atoms of calcium (calcium ions) must pass through special ion channels in the membrane of cells if the muscles are to contract. Calcium channel blockers block this movement and so interfere with the action of the muscle fibres, relaxing the smooth muscle in the walls of arteries so that the blood pressure is reduced and the blood flow through the arteries is improved. This is especially important in the case of the coronary arteries that supply the constantly active heart muscle with blood. Calcium channel blockers are valuable in angina pectoris and in reducing the oxygen consumption of the heart. Like many others, these drugs are broken down in the liver. Approximately four hours after a dose, half the drug has gone.

Nifedipine (Adalat) and diltiazem (Tildiem) are valuable in cases of spasm of the coronary arteries and can relieve angina. They are often used in conjunction with **beta-blocker drugs**. Verapamil (Cordilox), lidoflazine (Clinium) and prenylamine (Synadrine) are also helpful in cases of irregular heartbeat (cardiac arrhythmias). These drugs do have side-effects including headaches, flushing, fluid retention (oedema), undue slowing of the heart, heart block, and low blood pressure. Research has suggested that the risk of heart attacks in people being treated with certain calcium channel blocker drugs may be higher than with other drugs used to control high blood pressure.

calculus

A stone of any kind formed abnormally in the body. Calculi form in fluids in which high concentrations of chemical substances are dissolved. They are most commonly found in the kidneys, in the tubes leading from the kidneys to the bladder (ureters), in the bladder itself, and in the bile system of the liver, especially the gall-bladder.

See **kidney stones**, **gallstones**.

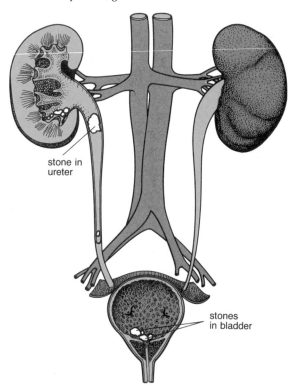

stone in
ureter

stones
in bladder

Stones (calculi) can form in any part of the urinary system. This illustration shows calculi in the tube running from the kidney to the bladder (the ureter) and stones in the bladder. Calculi can form in these sites or can be carried down to them from above.

calculus, dental

See **dental calculus**.

callosity

One of the body's protective responses; in this case, to excessive or prolonged friction or pressure on skin overlying a bony prominence. A common form of callosity is the corn on a toe caused by ill-fitting footwear or by an abnormally positioned toe. The term 'corn' derives from the name of the body's response – cornification – which is a thickening, flattening and compaction of the outer layer of skin (the **epidermis**). The degree of cornification depends on the degree of protection needed.

Callosities may occur at any point where skin pressure occurs over bone. Students may develop callosities on their elbows, guitarists on their fingertips, saints on their knees, and marathon runners on their heels. In the days of manual labour, callosities on the palm of the hands were natural to most working men.

So long as the cause persists, it is illogical and foolish to remove callosities. If the cause is removed the callosity will soon disappear.

callus, bony

A collection of new soft bone, forming around the site of a healing fracture. Callus is readily visible on X-rays, and indicates that healing is under way. It also shows, however, that the break is not yet completely healed. Over the course of weeks or months, callus is gradually replaced by normal, full-strength bone and, as this happens, the bump is slowly smoothed off and the bone is remodelled to its normal appearance.

callus, skin

See **callosity**.

caloric test

If a quantity of water, at a temperature of about 6° C above or below body temperature, is syringed on to an eardrum, the balancing mechanism of the inner ear is affected in such a way as to cause the eyes to perform a series of jerking movements to one side. This is called nystagmus and it is a normal response. If, however, there is disease of the balancing mechanism (semicircular canals), the nystagmus will be absent or much reduced in extent.

The test is thus a valuable way of finding out whether a person with a tendency to fall (vertigo) or dizziness has a defect of the inner ear, or whether the trouble is caused by something else.

calorie

In science generally, the calorie is the amount of heat needed to raise one gram of water 1° Celsius, from 15° to 16°. For nutritional purposes, this is an inconveniently small figure and the Calorie (capital C) is used. This is equal to 1000 calories and is sometimes called the kilocalorie.

The calorific value of a fuel (including food) is the number of heat units obtained by burning it completely in a closed container. This value can be expressed in calories per gram, in joules per gram or in BTU (British Thermal Units) per pound. Thus, the calorific value of protein and carbohydrate is about four Calories per gram, that of fat about nine Calories per gram and that of alcohol about seven Calories per gram. In the now widely accepted SI (Systeme

Internationale) for units, the calorie is replaced by the joule. One calorie is equal to 4.184 joules. The same relationship applies to Calories and kilojoules.

More precise values for consumables are:

	Calories	Kilojoules
Carbohydrates	3.8	16
Proteins	4.1	17
Fats	9.1	38
Alcohol	6.9	29

calvaria

Latin root meaning 'skull' as in calvarium (vault of the skull).

Campral EC

A brand name for acamprosate.

Canale-Smith syndrome

An **auto-immune disease** caused by gene mutation that leads to defective **apoptosis** in **lymphocytes**. The result is an enormous over-production of lymphocytes (a lymphoproliferative disorder) with enlarged lymph nodes, spleen enlargement, possible development of **lymphomas** and other effects including excess production of gamma globulin **antibodies**.

cancer

The word 'cancer' is one of the few layman's terms accepted and used by the medical profession. It is used because it is a convenient and comprehensive label for many different conditions varying from the almost trivial to the inevitably fatal. Cancer is not one single disease but a multitude, and some of these are so minor that they can be cured by a needle prick and ten minutes of painless surgery.

All cancers are tumours, but not all tumours are cancers. There are two broad categories of tumours, and the two groups are entirely different in their significance.

BENIGN TUMOURS

Benign tumours are not cancers, but because of their resemblances to, and differences from, cancers, are conveniently dealt with here. Benign tumours are lumps of cells which, while still closely resembling the tissue from which they have arisen – muscle, nerve, fat, blood vessel and so on – have begun to reproduce and multiply more rapidly than normal. Benign tumours remain intact and grow by expansion only. They often develop fairly strong fibrous capsules. Sometimes they grow very large and, if left, may do serious damage by pressure on, or distortion of, surrounding structures. But the cells of benign tumours never invade other tissues and they never bud off from the tumour mass to spread to remote parts of the body.

RISKS

People do very occasionally die from benign tumours, but this is usually because the diagnosis has not been made until a very late stage when severe pressure effects on vital adjacent structures have occurred. Rarely, benign tumours can arise simultaneously in many different parts of the body and this can sometimes be fatal. But, in general, they live up to their name and do not cause serious harm. The treatment is, however, almost always by surgical removal.

The majority of tumours of the breast are benign as are the great majority of tumours of the body of the womb (uterus). A great many of the tumours of the skin are benign and so are many brain tumours. Of course, because the brain is enclosed in a rigid bone casing, anything growing inside is very likely to do harm by pressing on brain structures, so benign tumours of the brain and of the membranes covering the brain (meninges) are certainly dangerous. However, if they are detected reasonably early, most of them can be completely removed.

Benign tumours can affect almost all tissues. They occur in fibrous tissue (fibromas); glandular tissue (adenomas); fat (lipomas); cartilage (chondromas); brain linings (meningiomas); bone (osteomas); joint linings (synoviomas); blood vessels (angiomas); nerves (neuromas) and muscle (myomas). All of these tumours grow by simple expansion and if properly removed will not recur. Very occasionally benign tumours change their character and become malignant – that is, turn to cancers.

MALIGNANT TUMOURS (CANCERS)

The characteristics of malignant tumours are quite different from those of benign tumours. There are two broad classes of cancers. Those which arise from surface linings are the commonest group and are called **carcinomas**. *Carcin-* means 'hard' and *-oma* means 'a lump'. Carcinomas may occur in the skin, the stomach, the colon (large bowel), the rectum (lower end of large bowel), the bronchial tubes, the ducts of the pancreas or gall-bladder, or the milk ducts of the breast. Any lining surface, anywhere in the body, can become the site of a carcinoma.

The second, and smaller, group of malignant tumours consists of those which arise from the substance of solid tissues such as muscle, bone, lymph glands, blood vessels and fibrous and other connective tissues. These are called *sarcomas*. *Sarc-* means 'flesh'.

Both carcinomas and sarcomas have the unpleasant property of invasiveness. They do not tend to form isolated, encapsulated lumps as happens with benign tumours. Instead, the cells of cancers burrow into and invade adjacent tissues and structures, becoming incorporated into them and often destroying them.

SECONDARY CANCERS

Cancers have another way of spreading. When an invading cancer encounters a small blood vessel, it can grow through the wall until it reaches the bloodstream, and small collections of cancer cells can then be carried off by the fast-flowing blood to remote parts of the body. In this way, cancer cells from the lung or colon or prostate can be transported to the brain or bones or liver, to set up a new focus and continue to grow and invade in the new site. Throughout nearly all the tissues of the body, there are thin-walled tubes, called lymphatic ducts, whose job it is to carry off excess fluid from the tissues back to the bloodstream. Lymphatics are very easily invaded by cancers, and cancer cells find this a particularly easy way to spread.

DEGREES OF MALIGNANCY

Cancers vary enormously in the speed with which they spread locally and, consequently, in the readiness with which they form new colonies elsewhere. This tendency is called *malignancy* and malignancy may be low or high. A tumour of low malignancy may take many months or even years to cause any trouble and may not spread distantly for a very long time, if ever.

Unfortunately, tumours of high malignancy will sometimes have spread widely before the victim has any idea that anything is wrong.

A pathologist can often tell, by examining a thin slice of cancer tissue under a microscope, whether it is of high or low malignancy. In the latter case, the cells quite closely resemble the parent tissue and form themselves into aggregates that are not greatly different in structure from the normal tissue from which they arise. Highly malignant cells, on the other hand, are 'primitive' simple cells with no capacity to form recognizable tissues. They are often small, all looking very much alike, and are easy to distinguish from normal cells from the same tissue. Often they will be found filling blood vessels and it is usually very difficult to say, with any particular specimen, whether or not the whole cancer has been removed.

CANCER AVOIDANCE

Thousands of people continue to develop cancers which need never happen. An example of this is cancer of the skin caused by excessive exposure to sunlight. The commonest type of skin cancer, basal cell carcinoma (**rodent ulcer**), unless neglected, is not particularly dangerous and early removal cures it. But if neglected, it may cause severe and extensive local tissue destruction and even death. More serious is the **squamous carcinoma**, and most serious of all is the **malignant melanoma**.

> Sun-worshippers should be aware that the ultraviolet component of strong sunlight is damaging to the skin and may lead to cancer.

CERVICAL CANCER

Statistical studies have shown that women whose sexual experience is limited have a very much smaller chance of getting cancer of the cervix (neck) of the uterus than women who have had many partners. Prostitutes, and others who engage in promiscuous sex, show a substantially higher incidence of cancer of the cervix than comparable groups who do not. The incidence among Jewish women is very low and the condition is almost unknown in nuns. Studies have shown that cancers, of all kinds, are less common among Mormons and Seventh Day Adventists, whose lives are closely controlled, than among equivalent groups in the general population. The probable explanation of this is that the human wart (papilloma) virus, which is spread by sexual contact, may be contributing to the danger. See also **uterus, cancer of**.

CANCER OF THE LIVER

The incidence of any particular type of cancer varies markedly in different populations. For instance, primary cancer of the liver is very rare in the Western world, but in parts of Africa and the Far East it is one of the commonest kinds of cancer. There is good reason to believe that other factors affecting the liver are the reason for this strange anomaly. Conditions such as cirrhosis or hepatitis B virus infection seem to predispose to primary liver cancer. There is also a very interesting link between liver cancer and a poison, **aflatoxin**, produced by a mould that grows on peanuts and grains in moist, warm areas. Now it is, at least theoretically, possible to reduce the incidence of each type

of cancer to that level at which it occurs in the population with the lowest incidence. If this could be done, there would be only one case of cancer for every ten that occur today.

SMOKING

By far the most important of all the opportunities we have to avoid cancer is, of course, to refrain from smoking. The whole weight of the medical profession now supports the conviction that smoking is one of the most damaging and destructive activities in which it is possible to engage. Smoking is the reason for the horrifying rise in the prevalence of cancer of the lung, and it is also the cause of a great deal of other disease.

Heavy smokers of light shag who constantly allow a jet of hot smoke to strike the same part of the tongue may develop an area of persistent soreness. This may eventually turn to a hard, whitish, thickened area, called **leukoplakia**, and leukoplakia quite frequently turns to cancer of the tongue. Cancer of the tongue is also common in certain groups who smoke cigarettes with the hot end inside the mouth – a common practice among some Indians. Betel-nut chewers show a very high incidence of mouth cancers – indeed, this is almost the commonest type of cancer in those who indulge in this habit. In others, mouth cancer is relatively uncommon.

RADIATION

There are many other known causes of cancer although these are, generally, less relevant. In the early days of X-ray technology, workers had no idea of the dangers of the newly discovered rays and made no attempt to protect themselves. Almost all of these early pioneers developed cancer, especially of the hands, and many died from it. In a similar way, before the dangers were known, girls employed to paint the dials of watches and clocks with radium or mesothorium-containing luminous paint used to point their fine paint brushes by putting them in their mouths. Scores of these girls died from cancers of the tongue and jaw.

CANCER-CAUSING SUBSTANCES

Many substances are known to cause skin cancer and these include soot, tar, creosote, pitch and various mineral oils.

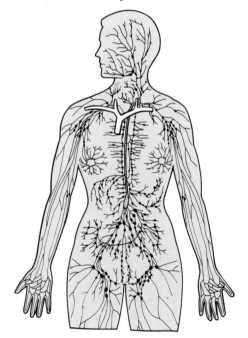

Cancer and the lymphatic system. Since the lymph vessels are thin-walled and drain all the tissues of the body, it is common for cancer cells to make their way into the lymphatics. The first sign of spread is likely to be enlargements of the lymph nodes in sites such as the armpits, the groin or the neck.

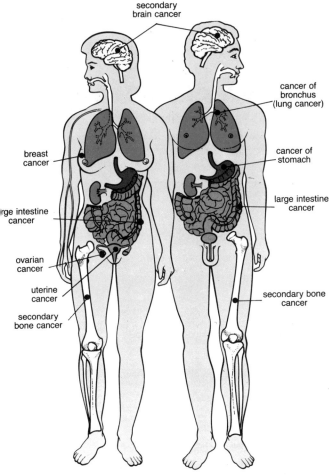

Common cancer sites. In women, cancer is common in the breast, the uterus and the ovaries. In men, cancer often attacks the prostate gland, the stomach and the bronchial tubes. In both sexes, cancer is common in the large intestine. Secondary cancer occurs in the brain, the lungs and the bones.

When shale oil was used to lubricate the high-speed spindles in the early cotton mills, a fine spray of oil used to soak the trousers of the mill workers and very large numbers of them developed skin cancer, especially of the wrinkled skin of the scrotum, where the oil tended to persist in its contact. Boys who were sent up large chimneys to sweep them were also frequent victims of skin cancer. The most dangerous group of such substances is a class of chemicals derived from benzene. These readily cause skin cancer by contact. If inhaled, they can cause lung cancer, and they can even cause breast and bladder cancer if swallowed. Injection of these substances into solid tissues, such as muscle, can cause sarcomas. Other established links are:

- alcohol (cancers of mouth, throat, gullet and liver);
- anabolic steroids (cancer of liver);
- arsenic (cancers of lung, skin and liver);
- asbestos (cancer of lung);
- chromium (cancer of lung);
- synthetic oestrogens (cancer of uterus and vagina);
- isopropyl alcohol (cancer of nasal sinuses);
- nickel dust (cancer of lung and sinuses);
- phenacetin (cancer of kidney);
- snuff-taking and tobacco chewing (cancer of mouth);
- vinyl chloride (cancer of liver);
- wood dusts (cancer of sinuses).

All the people who have developed cancers from these various substances, have been exposed to them for very long periods – in most cases for years. Many of these examples are historic relics, and nowadays few sensible people would allow foreign material, such as those mentioned, to remain for long in contact with the body.

> The explosion in synthetic chemistry has thrown up hundreds of new compounds that can cause cancer if we are exposed to them for long enough.

VIRUSES AND CANCER

Many viruses are associated with cancer. These are well-known viruses, such as the human wart virus, herpes viruses, the hepatitis B virus and HIV, that normally cause other diseases. Collectively, they are known as oncoviruses. Some viruses, the retroviruses, contain genes that can, under certain circumstances, become incorporated into the genome of normal cells and cause them to become cancerous. These are called **oncogenes**. Normal cells also contain oncogenes that can be activated by these viruses.

The Epstein-Barr virus is a herpes virus that is associated with a form of cancer known as Burkitt's lymphoma. This is a malignant tumor of the jaw that mainly affects children in certain areas of Africa. Children with Burkitt's lymphoma have antibodies to the Epstein-Barr virus and this virus can stimulate growth in B lymphocytes – the type of cell from which Burkitt's lymphoma arises. Adult T cell leukaemia, cancer of the cervix and Kaposi's sarcoma in AIDS are other forms of cancer associated with viruses.

> There is an established link between cancer of the cervix and two viruses – the human papilloma virus that causes genital warts, and the Herpes simplex virus that causes genital herpes.

CANCER DETECTION

It would be foolish to suggest that cancer can always be avoided; until the causes of all cancers are known – and we are far from that stage yet – this will be impossible. We can only hope that medical research into the causes of the other forms of cancer makes rapid progress. Since we cannot always prevent cancer, it is obviously very important that we should be sensitive to the early indications of these diseases so that we can seek treatment before too much damage is done to us, or before the condition becomes untreatable.

It would take a textbook to cover all the symptoms of all the different types of cancer, but there are some basic principles that can be adopted by all sensible people to improve their awareness of the possibility of cancer. Cancer, of course, implies that a change has occurred in the body – a change that persists – and we should always be alive to the indications of such a change.

Suppose, for instance, that a man of fifty, who had never been troubled by indigestion, begins, for no apparent reason, to have pain high in the abdomen, and, perhaps some weeks later, realizes that the pain has become persistent. Or another elderly person notices that, for a month or two, there has been a positive difference in the bowel habit – perhaps more frequent passage of much smaller or ribbon-like stools. Or a smoker may notice that a hoarseness of the voice that was taken, at first, to be no more than a mild laryngitis, is still affecting the speech after two or three months. Or there may be a painful cough that simply refuses to go away. Or a persistent, unexplained loss of weight. Or a nagging pain in the chest.

All these symptoms may have a perfectly innocent and harmless explanation. Indeed, because cancer is so much less common than the many conditions that also cause these symptoms, the probability, in any particular case, is that the symptom does have an innocent explanation. Nevertheless, one should not ignore such symptoms. To do so out of fear that one might have cancer might occasion delay during which the cancer becomes untreatable.

Advances in early diagnosis have been remarkable, even in the last ten years. The application of electronics and computer technology to medicine have made possible ways of imaging the inside of the body previously inconceivable. The still rapidly advancing technique of computerized tomography (CT scanning) has reached its 'fifth generation'. Used in conjunction with non-toxic materials which, when injected, concentrate in tumour tissue so as to 'enhance' the view, CT scanning can show up quite remarkably small tumours. But the CT scan has been overtaken by the newer technology of magnetic resonance imaging (MRI), which is capable of even higher standards of resolution. Endoscopic methods of visualization are used to inspect areas that previously could be seen only by open operation.

Various methods of screening, such as tests for hidden (occult) blood in the stools, routine mammography and Pap smear tests for early cervical cancer are now widely employed in the hope of detecting cancer at the earliest possible stage.

THE TREATMENT OF CANCER

Cancer treatment has been revolutionized in the last decade or so, and a great many kinds of cancer can now be cured, often without an operation. We now know a great deal about the biology of cancer cells and about their susceptibility to the range of new drugs now available. Drugs such as cyclophosphamide, adriamycin, methotrexate, cytosine arabinoside and 5-fluorouracil, although often causing quite severe side-effects, have the great advantage that they will attack cancer cells wherever they may lie in the body even if an unsuspected spread has occurred. They may be used alone or in conjunction with the much improved means of radiation treatment such as that afforded by the Linear accelerator, the fast neutron generator and the heavy ion linear accelerator. Many quite advanced malignancies, especially in younger people, can now often be completely eradicated. In other cases, the outcome will depend on the extent of the disease and this, of course, depends on how much delay there has been in diagnoses.

> Early cancer can, if detected, almost always be cured.

See also **cancer screening** and references to cancers of individual organs.

cancer-causing gene

See **oncogene**.

cancer gene

See **proto-oncogene**.

cancer indicator

See **tumour markers**, **tumour-specific antigens**.

cancer-killing protein

See **tumour necrosis factor**.

cancer of the breast

See **breast cancer**.

cancer of the colon

See **colon, cancer of**.

cancer of the kidney

See **kidney cancer**.

cancer of the liver

See **liver cancer**.

cancer of the lung

See **lung cancer**.

cancer of the prostate

See **prostate gland, disorders of**.

cancer of the skin

See **malignant melanoma**, **rodent ulcer**.

cancer of the womb

See **uterus, cancer of**.

cancer phobia

Most informed people have a reasonable fear of cancer, but cancer phobia has nothing to do with reason. It is a personality disorder of the phobic type (see **phobia**), with the attention of the affected person directed towards cancer.

Cancer phobia, unfortunately, does not prompt the sufferer to rational courses such as regular screening, PAP smears (Papanicolaou test), avoidance of risk factors such as smoking, and so on. Instead, it gives rise to compulsively performed rituals, especially repeated hand-washing, changing of clothes touched by others, avoidance of air breathed by others, and even avoidance of any contact with other persons. Symptoms, however minor, are interpreted as signs of cancer and panic attacks may occur. As with any other phobic disorder, cancer phobia cannot be treated by appeals to the reason. Some success has been achieved by various forms of **behaviour therapy**.

cancer-producing gene

See **Bcl-2 gene**, **oncogene**.

cancer screening

The commonest cancers are those of the lung in men, of the breast in women and of the large bowel (colon and rectum) in both sexes. Many attempts have been made, by enlightened Public Health Authorities, to provide population screening programmes for the early detection of cancer. Regrettably, screening for cancer of the lung has not been a great success. This is not because the methods are ineffective – four-monthly chest X-rays and sputum tests can detect almost 90 per cent of cases – but because the people at greatest risk (young, irresponsible smokers of the lower socio-economic groups) do not take advantage of the facility. The indications are that the money would be better spent in trying to promote measures to discourage smoking.

Much greater success has been achieved in the efforts to screen for breast cancer and the results have been most encouraging. A group of 20,000 women aged forty to sixty-four were checked by careful examination of the breasts and by a special X-ray test called **mammography**. The mortality rate was reduced by 30 per cent in comparison with an exactly equivalent group of women who were not screened. Ten years after the trial had started, there had been ninety-seven deaths from breast cancer in the screened group and 137 deaths, from the same cause, in the unscreened group. About one-third of the breast cancers detected by mammography were in the early stage before they had invaded other tissues.

> Self-examination is an important form of screening and every woman should be familiar with the signs indicating the need for immediate medical attention (see **breast, self-examination of**).

Cancers of the large bowel frequently produce very slight bleeding, not sufficient to appear as visible blood in the stools, but sufficient to be detected by a sensitive test using paper impregnated with a chemical indicator. Trials, using this method have been reported in the *Lancet* and are accepted by about half of those to whom they are offered. It is not yet quite clear whether this is a worthwhile method. Individual awareness is essential.

> Blackening of the stool, from the iron in released haemoglobin, frank blood in the stools, changes in the bowel habit, unexplained and severe constipation – indeed, almost any unusual feature – should alert one to the possibility that something serious may be wrong.

cancer stage determination

See **staging**.

cancer treatment complication

See **tumour lysis syndrome**.

cancrum oris

A disease of desperate poverty affecting seriously malnourished and neglected children. Ulceration, infection and progressive tissue destruction occurs around the mouth until large areas of both cheeks and nose are eaten away, leaving the cavities of the mouth and nose exposed. The condition is also known as *noma*.

candesartan

An **angiotensin II receptor antagonist** drug used in the treatment of high blood pressure. A brand name is Amias.

candidiasis

Commonly known as thrush, this is a fungus infection of warm, moist areas of the body with the common fungus of the genus Candida.
POSSIBLE CAUSES
Most cases are caused by the species *Candida albicans* which causes thrush of the mouth or vagina and occasionally elsewhere on the skin. Babies can develop a thrush **nappy rash**. Candida thrives best in darkness when the temperatures are right and especially when there is a good supply of carbohydrate for its nutrition. Candidiasis of the female vulva is thus particularly common if there is diabetes, in which there is sugar in the urine. A urine test is mandatory in all such cases.

Fungus infections tend to be kept in check by the presence of normal body bacteria (commensal organisms) and if these are too energetically attacked by antibiotics, fungi may get the upper hand and start to spread.

Thrush infection is encouraged by pregnancy, **diabetes**, antibiotics and immunosuppressive drugs or conditions and aggravated by sexual intercourse, tight clothing such as jeans, nylon underwear, poor hygiene, tampons, vaginal deodorants and other sprays, and bubble baths. Contrary to widespread belief, the oral contraceptive pill does not encourage thrush.
RECOGNITION AND SYMPTOMS
Vaginal thrush is easily recognized. There is persistent itching or soreness and sometimes a burning pain on contact between urine and affected areas. Inspection shows characteristic white patches, rather like soft cheese, with raw-looking inflamed areas in between. There may be a white, cheesy vaginal discharge. Vulval candidiasis is easily transmitted to a sexual partner, and men, especially if uncircumcised, often develop white patches and inflammation on the glans of the penis. This is called **balanitis** and there is constant discomfort, varying from mild to severe.
TREATMENT
Candidiasis is treated with one of a range of antifungal drugs in the form of ointments, creams or meltable pellets for insertion in the vagina (pessaries). These drugs include clotrimazole, miconazole and nystatin. An effective, one-dose, treatment is the drug fluconazole (Diflucan). Treating only one of a pair of sexual partners is a waste of time.
CANDIDIASIS IN AIDS
Candidiasis flourishes in people whose immune systems are in any way defective. In **AIDS**, candidiasis spreads widely both outside and inside the body. Freed from immunological control, the fungus spreads like wild-fire, commonly extending down from the mouth into the gullet (oesophagus), where ulceration occurs, causing severe difficulty and pain on swallowing. The whole of the genital and anal area may be covered with the white ('albicans' means 'white') fungus and the inside of the mouth thickly coated. Occasionally, systemic candidiasis may occur, in which the yeast gets into the bloodstream and is carried to any part of the body to set up a focus of infection. Most commonly involved are the eyes, the kid-

neys and the skin. Fungus infection of the inside of an eye is, of course, a serious matter and, when this happens, it is unlikely that the vision will be saved.

Candidiasis of the kidneys is also a grave development. Systemic candidiasis is fairly common in severely ill patients in hospital who have been treated with large doses of antibiotics and who are on prolonged intravenous therapy. But in AIDS, this type of spread is less common than local, inward spread from both ends of the intestinal tract.

Canesten

A brand name for the antifungal drug **clotrimazole**, effective against a wide range of fungi. It is used in the form of creams, for local application.

canine tooth

One of the four pointed 'Dracula' teeth. Counting outwards from the centre, in both upper and lower jaws, the canines are number three.

cannabis

A drug derived from the hemp plant. Marijuana is the dried leaves, flowers or stems of various species of the hemp grass *Cannabis*, especially *Cannabis sativa*, *Cannabis indica* and *Cannabis americana*. Cannabis resin contains the cannabinoid tetrahydrocannabinol which produces euphoria and an apparent heightening of all the senses, especially vision, with distortion of dimensions. There is slowing of reflexes, distortion of distance and alteration in the sense of responsibility. Driving becomes dangerous. Much valued is an illusory sense of deep philosophical insight or a conviction of omniscience. Panic attacks or acute anxiety may occur, and **schizophrenia**, **mania**, **depersonalization** or confusional psychoses have been precipitated. Persistent heavy users may become apathetic and show loss of interest and concern. Cannabis does, however, have some valuable medical uses and the former rigidity of official attitude against its therapeutic use is softening. A number of American States have approved its medical use.

cannula

A hollow tube, rigid or flexible, into which is fitted a close fitting inner stiffener. The latter is called a trocar and is usually sharp-pointed so that it can be pushed through the skin or the lining of a blood vessel or other tissue. When the trocar and cannula are in the desired position, the trocar is pulled out, leaving the cannula in place. Fluids or other materials may now be passed into or drawn out of the body. Cannulas are important in medicine and are extensively used for many purposes, both in diagnosis and treatment.

canthos

Greek root meaning 'angle' as in epicanthic (over the eye corner).

Capgras' syndrome

A rare but unusually interesting delusional disorder. People suffering from this syndrome are convinced that someone emotionally close and important to them has been replaced by an exact double. The condition affects twice as many

women as men and is commonest in middle age. Typically, the delusion starts by being applied to one member of the family, usually a spouse, and then spreads to be applied to other people. In some cases the conviction relates even to the person of the affected individual. The double is almost always deemed to have evil intentions.

POSSIBLE CAUSES

The idea of the malevolent double seems to be rooted in literature and myth and it seems likely that the disorder has affected people throughout the ages. Psychoanalysts have had a field day with Capgras' syndrome. According to some theorists, a love-hate (ambivalent) attitude to a person is resolved by creating a double who can be thoroughly and justifiably hated without promoting guilt. Others suggest that the delusion is in the nature of a split personality imposed on others or is the effect of a persistent sense of unreality coupled with the observation of small previously unnoticed physical changes in the subject. The syndrome has been found in association with an abnormal degree of sex interest (erotomania), a heavy mental burden (incubus) and the **restless legs** syndrome.

Capgras' syndrome is nearly always a sign of some underlying mental illness such as **schizophrenia**, or a mood psychosis, or of organic brain damage, such as occurs in temporal lobe epilepsy, alcohol toxicity or after physical injury.

capillaries

The smallest and most numerous of all the blood vessels. Capillaries occur in large numbers at the final stage of branching of the arteries, and form extensive networks of vessels between the system of arteries and the system of draining veins, through which blood returns to the heart. It is only in the capillary beds that interchange of oxygen, carbon dioxide and nutrients can take place with the cells and the tissues and this is because only the capillaries have walls thin enough to allow passage of these substances.

Capillary walls consist of a single layer of thin, flat cells and, except in the brain, these have small crevices at the points where they are cemented together. Through these crevices, small inorganic molecules can easily pass in and out of the blood as can some larger organic molecules. Certain white blood cells are capable of changing their shape so as to squeeze through (amoeboid action). This occurs in infections, when

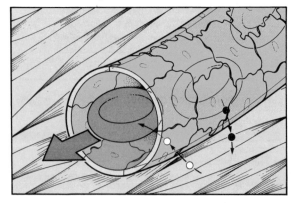

Red blood cells in capillaries. The walls of the capillaries are so thin that oxygen and carbon dioxide can diffuse through from the tissue fluids to the blood.

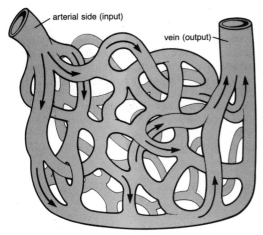

A capillary bed. Blood enters the capillary bed from the arterial side and leaves by the vein.

the white cells are needed to attack invading organisms and concentrate to form pus. In the lungs, the capillaries of the pulmonary arteries form the walls of the tiny air sacs (alveoli), thus allowing easy passage of oxygen from the atmosphere.

The brain capillaries differ from those in the rest of the body in that they do not have crevices between their wall cells. They are thus less permeable than the body capillaries. The importance of this is that certain drugs and other substances of large molecule size are unable to pass from the blood in the brain capillaries into the brain substance. This is called the blood-brain barrier.

Since capillaries provide the interface between the blood and the cells, they are of great importance. Any condition that results in failure of blood to reach the capillaries is serious.

capillo

Latin root meaning 'hair' as in capillary (hair-like).

capite

Latin root meaning 'head' as in caput (swelling on head).

capreomycin

An antibiotic drug derived from *Streptomyces capreolus* and used in the treatment of **tuberculosis** resistant to standard drugs such as **rifampicin**, **isoniazid**, ethambutol and streptomycin. A brand name is Capastat.

capsaicin

A pain-killing drug for external application used in the treatment of post-shingles pain and other painful peripheral nerve disorders. A brand name is Axsain.

capsicum oleoresin

A drug used externally with other ingredients as an embrocation for the relief of rheumatic pain, backache, fibrositis and sciatica. A brand name is Balmosa.

capsulitis

Inflammation of the capsule of a joint. See also **bursitis**.

caput

Latin for 'a head'. The term is used, as an abbreviation for *caput succedaneum*, to describe the soft boggy swelling which forms on the top of the scalp of a baby as a result of prolonged pressure of the head on the partly opened neck of the womb (cervix). The caput corresponds to the area of the scalp overlying the opening. The rest of the scalp is compressed, and congestion of veins occurs with leakage of fluid (serum) into the unsupported part, causing a swelling (oedema). Another form of caput, the *caput medusae* is the 'snakes head' of varicose veins that can form on the abdominal wall in cases of advanced cirrhosis of the liver.

carbamazepine

A drug used in the control of **epilepsy** and especially to relieve or prevent the pain of **trigeminal neuralgia**. A brand name is Tegretol.

carbenoxolone

A drug used to promote healing in stomach and duodenal ulcers. A brand name is Bioplex.

carbidopa

A drug that prevents the breakdown of the drug levodopa in the body and thus enhances its action in **Parkinson's disease**. A brand name is Sinemet.

See also **benserazide**.

carbimazole

An antithyroid drug that interferes with the production of thyroid hormone and is used in the treatment of hyperthyroidism. A brand name is Neomercazole.

carbocisteine

A drug used to disperse excess mucus or to treat glue ear in children. A brand name is Mycodyne.

carbomer

A drug used as eyedrops in the treatment of dry eyes. A brand name is Geltears.

carbon dioxide

A simple compound in which an atom of carbon is linked to two atoms of oxygen (CO_2). Carbon dioxide is a colourless, odourless gas at normal temperatures. It is one of the chief waste products of tissue metabolism and an increase in metabolic activity, as during exercise, results in increased oxygen usage and increased CO_2 production. The excess waste gas is carried to the lungs by the blood and released into the air sacs for exhalation.

FUNCTION

Carbon dioxide in the blood controls its acidity and a rise in the level is a powerful stimulant to rapid breathing by its action on the respiratory centre in the brain stem. Anaesthetists sometimes make use of this effect by adding a little carbon dioxide to the anaesthetic gases. The gas has another medical use. Persistent hiccups can be exhausting and dangerous, but in at least half of the cases it can be

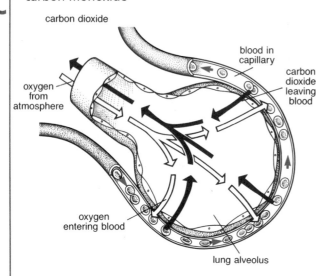

Carbon dioxide exchange in the lungs. Waste carbon dioxide is carried to the lungs in the blood and passes out into the air sacs, to be released into the atmosphere. At the same time, oxygen from the air is taken up by the red cells of the blood.

stopped by inhalation of 5 per cent carbon dioxide. Even if the hiccups continue, CO_2 inhalation will help reduce the frequency.

Carbon dioxide is easily formed into a semi-solid at a temperature of -80° C, by allowing the gas to escape into a suitable container from a high-pressure cylinder. This is called carbon dioxide snow (dry ice) and is used in medicine for destroying skin tumours and other surgical purposes (see **cryosurgery**).

PROPERTIES
Carbon dioxide is soluble in water, forming a pleasant-tasting solution that is more readily absorbed by mucous membranes than plain water. The process is usually, and inaccurately, described as *aeration* and almost any blandly flavoured water can be turned into a tempting drink by this simple expedient.

DANGERS
Carbon dioxide gas is present in low concentration in the air. It is denser than air and tends to sink downwards. Danger arises if the concentration of the gas becomes too high. In an atmosphere above about 7 per cent CO_2 there will be rapid breathing, headache, confusion, dizziness and palpitations. At a concentration of 10 per cent or more, unconsciousness and death will occur.

carbon monoxide

A colourless, odourless, tasteless, highly inflammable and poisonous gas formed when carbon is burnt in an atmosphere of limited oxygen. It is present in the exhaust of motor vehicles and may be produced by coal-burning fires or furnaces. In this compound, one atom of carbon combines with one atom of oxygen (CO) in an unsaturated, double bond linkage making a highly reactive substance.

FUNCTION
Carbon monoxide combines with the haemoglobin of the blood, forming a compound, carboxyhaemoglobin, which is much more stable than the normal loose linkage with oxygen. The carboxyhaemoglobin is very persistent and so excludes oxygen from the tissues.

DANGERS
The action of carboxyhaemoglobin is the cause of death in severe CO poisoning, which is a common mode of suicide. A concentration of 50 per cent CO in the blood is usually fatal and this may result in one hour from breathing air with only one part of CO per 1000 parts of air.

Smoking cigarettes results in a significant inhalation of carbon monoxide. Heavy smokers can achieve a blood concentration of 8 to 10 per cent. In some disorders of the heart, arteries or lungs, this loss of oxygen-carrying capacity can tip the balance against survival. In all cases, it is detrimental to health and fitness.

carboplatin

An anticancer drug. A brand name is Paraplatin.

carboxylic acids

A group of non-steroidal anti-inflammatory (**NSAID**) and **analgesic** drugs that includes aspirin, aloxiprin, mefenamic acid, fenbufen and ibuprofen.

carbuncle

A multiple-headed boil. Carbuncles, which are now rare, except in diabetics, are severe staphylococcal infections of several adjacent hair follicles and may be over five centimetres across. They occur anywhere on the skin but seem to have a preference for the back of the neck. Both surgical drainage and antibiotic treatment may be required.

The name comes from Latin and refers to a glowing, red coal. The same word is used for the red, semi-precious garnet gemstone.

carcinogen

Any substance or agency which can cause cancer.

carcinoid syndrome

A rare condition in which certain tumours of the bowel spread to other parts of the body and secrete into the bloodstream large quantities of powerful hormones and other highly active substances, including histamine, serotonin and prostaglandins.

These act on smooth muscle, especially that of the blood vessels, to cause a wide range of symptoms, including flushing, rapid alterations in skin colour, recurrent diarrhoea, cramping abdominal pain, serious damage to the heart, arthritis and asthma.

Because the tumours are multiple and widespread, treatment is difficult. Improvement can sometimes be achieved by removing particularly heavily secreting tumours or by the use of cancer chemotherapy.

carcinoma

Any cancer of a surface layer (epithelium) of the body. Carcinomas are by far the commonest form of cancer. The other large group consists of the sarcomas, which are cancers of connective tissue such as muscle, cartilage and bone. The term 'carcinoma' derives from the Greek *karkinos*, meaning 'a crab', which, in turn, came from an earlier word *karkar*, meaning 'hard'. Many carcinomas are solid, hard lumps. the ending *-oma* simply means 'a lump'.

Carcinomas can occur on any epithelium, but are especially common on the epithelial linings of the glandular tissue of the breast, on the epithelium of the skin (epidermis), the lining of the large bowel, the air tubes (bronchi) of the lungs, and the womb (uterus). Carcinomas also occur on epithelia in the pancreas, the gall-bladder, the nose, the mouth, the larynx, the bladder and the prostate gland.

The degree of malignancy – the tendency to spread rapidly and remotely – varies considerably from one tumour to another.

See also **cancer**.

carcinomatosis

The state of widespread distribution of cancer throughout the body (metastasis) occurring at a late stage in many cancers. The condition usually occurs because the disease was detected too late for effective treatment of the primary growth, but many cancers are insidious and have spread before symptoms arise.

Carcinomatosis is usually terminal, but nowadays modern cancer chemotherapy is beginning to mount an effective attack on what was once considered a hopeless situation.

cardia (gullet)

The opening of the gullet (oesophagus) into the stomach, immediately below the diaphragm. In spite of the terminological similarity, the cardia is quite unconnected with the heart, although it lies near it. 'Heartburn' is a disorder of the cardia not of the heart.

cardia (heart)

Greek root meaning 'heart' as in cardiac (of the heart).

cardiac

See **heart**.

cardiac catheterization

The passing of a fine, soft plastic tube up a vein into the right side of the heart, or up an artery into the left side. In some cases a catheter is passed from the right side of the heart through the internal wall to the left side. Cardiac catheterization may be done on people of all ages, from newborn babies to the elderly. In young children, anaesthesia is necessary, but in older children, adolescents and adults it is usually done under simple sedation. It can often provide a positive diagnosis in cases of uncertainty, in which other tests have failed.

Catheterization allows sampling of blood from the different chambers of the heart so that the blood gases can be analyzed and vital information obtained about the state of circulation. It allows fluids opaque to X-rays to be injected into the heart chambers, or directly into the coronary arteries, so that accurate pictures can be taken of the internal structures and especially of the degree of openness of the coronary arteries. The state of the heart valves can be investigated by comparing the blood pressure on either side of the valves. It is also done to obtain biopsy specimens, even of the muscle on the inside of the heart.

Catheterization enables various forms of local treatment to be undertaken, such as balloon angioplasty and dissolving of clots (thrombolysis). The procedure is especially valuable in the investigation and assessment of congenital heart disease, and has permitted major advances in understanding and in treatment. Without cardiac catheterization, heart surgery would be hazardous, and many of the major advances made in recent years would have been impossible.

Complications are uncommon, but catheterization may temporarily disturb the heart rhythm. In a normally fit person, the rhythm usually returns quickly to normal. In people with heart or bleeding disorders, there is some risk of death from disturbance of the heart action. This risk, however, is less than the risk of failing to reach a diagnosis and provide the best treatment, so it is regarded as acceptable.

cardiac neurosis

See **hypochondriasis**.

cardiologist

A physician specializing in the diagnosis and management of all disorders of the heart. Cardiologists do not perform heart surgery, but often work in close association with heart surgeons.

cardiomegaly

See **heart, enlarged**.

cardiomyopathy

Any disease of the heart muscle. The commonest is damage from an inadequate coronary blood supply, but the range includes damage from alcohol, vitamin deficiency, infections, **auto-immune disease** and sarcoidosis.

cardiomyoplasty

An experimental method of strengthening the action of the heart in cases of heart failure by wrapping the ventricles with living muscle from the back (the latissimus dorsi) and prompting this to contract in synchrony with the heartbeat by means of an artificial pacemaker.

cardiopulmonary resuscitation

A technical term for combined heart massage and the 'kiss of life'.

See *First Aid*.

cardiospasm

Tight contraction and failure to relax of the muscle ring (sphincter) at the lower end of the gullet. This causes obstruction to the passage of food.

cardiotocography

Recording the fetal heart rate and contractions of the womb during labour and late pregnancy with a microphone placed against the mother's abdominal wall or by using a fetal electrocardiograph (CTG).

cardiovascular

Relating to the heart and its connected closed circulatory system of blood vessels (arteries, arterioles, capillaries, venules and veins). Cardiovascular disease is by far the commonest cause of death and disability in the West.

cardiovascular surgeon

A surgeon who specializes in heart surgery and in the surgery of the blood vessels. He or she is also skilled in the fine microsurgery that is required to rejoin the cut ends of small arteries and veins.

cardioversion

A method of converting a dangerously rapid heartbeat to normal rhythm by applying a controlled electric shock synchronized with a particular phase in the electrocardiogram. The commonest usage is in **defibrillation** for one of the forms of heart stoppage (cardiac arrest).

carditis

See **heart, inflammation of**.

care of elderly people

Ideally, elderly people should live at home enjoying the support and loving care of a devoted family. But many are necessarily solitary or choose to live alone, and it is these who are most at risk from ill-health. It is commonly assumed that a gradual loss of capacity, both mental and physical, is an inevitable feature of old age, but this is not so. Frequently decline in health is the result of an unsuspected physical disorder, from the gradual accumulation of damage from previous illness, degenerative disease and injury. Many diseases, are, by their nature, commoner in old age. These conditions, which may seriously prejudice the quality of life, include atherosclerosis, cancer, cataract, depression, diabetes, fracture of the femur, malnutrition, especially vitamin deficiency, underaction of the thyroid gland (myxoedema), osteoarthritis, osteoporosis, pernicious anaemia and shingles. Several of these conditions may co-exist. Some are obvious, but, unfortunately, many remain concealed and, as a result, many elderly people do not receive an appropriate level of medical care.

Chronic ill-health in the elderly tends to be concealed for several reasons. Many old people expect to be frail or unwell and feel that they should not complain. Many are remarkably stoical, and the elderly often have a lowered sensitivity to pain or even a lowered level of general awareness. Most are disinclined to be a burden to others. Sometimes failure to complain is due to genuine mental impairment, but an appearance of unconcern may be the result of physical disorder and lack of stimulation. Sensory deprivation is especially important and many old people, who could be restored to self-sufficiency by a cataract operation or the provision of a hearing aid, remain sunk in lethargy and seeming indifference and require constant attention.

So it is clearly important that the elderly should have full and regular medical attention. Millions of old people suffer unnecessary invalidism, distress and disability because of remediable conditions. Gradually developing anaemia, bedsores and malnutrition may go long unnoticed and conditions such as dehydration and hypothermia may affect even those in affluent circumstances. These are only a few of the conditions which, given reasonable standards of medical and nursing care, need never occur. Self-neglect, often with serious consequences, may be the result of dementia, but it may also be due to mild confusion, forgetfulness, depression and the increasing physical difficulties imposed by organic disease. Such people should never be left unvisited for long periods. Those in greatest need of help include people recently discharged from hospital, those handicapped by poor vision and deafness, the recently bereaved and the lonely.

The nature of the person's accommodation is important. Adequate heating and a high level of artificial illumination make for comfort and safety and encourage reading, sewing and other useful activities. Accidental injury from falls remains a common danger to the elderly (see below) and for this and other obvious reasons, such people living alone should always be provided with an effective alarm system so that help can be summoned reliably and quickly. Voluntary agencies and Public Health Authorities do much to help, and full use should be made of available facilities. The Home Help service can provide more than merely domestic assistance. Home helps keep a watchful eye on their elderly charges, noting signs of difficulty and calling in professional assistance when necessary. Volunteers providing meals on wheels can also offer a valuable monitoring service. The concept of sheltered housing, in which elderly people enjoy the benefits of custom-designed accommodation while remaining under unobtrusive surveillance, is an excellent one and such housing is often preferred to a nursing or residential home.

Adequate social intercourse, mental stimulation and the encouragement of activity are essential for the elderly. These may be obtained by regular attendance at day healthcare centres, at which bathing, chiropody and launderette services are provided at workshops for the elderly, senior citizens clubs, and, when appropriate, stroke clubs and day hospitals. The latter are valuable institutions, offering full medical investigation and assessment, rehabilitative treatment and the means of health maintenance, on a daily attendance basis. Relatives are encouraged to participate in discussion of future management at home and to learn how maximal activity and independence may be achieved.

A major cause of distress to the elderly is the feeling that they no longer matter to others, that their dependence is irksome and their presence a nuisance. Such beliefs are readily fostered by the apparent neglect or unconcern of younger relatives. The refusal to allow an elderly person to participate usefully in the home is damaging, both physically and mentally. Activity of all kinds should be encouraged. Association with grandchildren is often therapeutic, especially when this promotes a sense of being valued, and, whenever possible, elderly people should be expected to take a share in the minding of children.

THE EFFECTS OF COLD

Even in the most severe winters, the number of cases of hypothermia in Britain is small. In only about twenty-five cases per year is hypothermia given on death certificates as the underlying cause of death. But the effects of cold on old people are very much more widespread and serious than this figure would suggest. We now know that cold is a major contributing factor to heart and lung disease in old people and in causing their death from these conditions.

Every year, there is an immediate rise in the death rate among old people when mean temperatures drop below freezing, and this rise continues for over a month after the extreme cold has passed. About 40,000 more people die in an average winter, in England and Wales, than during a comparable period in summer.

Body heat production is defective in old people, almost all of whom have had a marked decline in the rate at which they use up body fuel (basal metabolic rate). Even more important, shivering is less effective in producing heat, because of poor muscles.

Shivering is the most important way of raising the body temperature when this is tending to fall. Heat is normally lost by widening of skin blood vessels (vaso-dilatation) and is conserved by their constriction, so that less blood flows through the skin. Because of ageing changes in the vessel walls, elderly people's skin vessels are often unable to constrict, and so they are denied this means of conserving heat. The control of heat regulation in the brain is also less efficient in the elderly. These factors lead to a rise in the thickness (viscosity) of the blood and a rise in blood pressure. Low temperatures interfere with the efficiency of the linings of the bronchial tubes in resisting infection and can induce asthma. The net effect is a substantial increase in the death rate from serious heart and lung disorders.

Old people must be kept warm, both by effective domestic heating and by insulating their bodies in order to minimize heat loss. Multiple layers of garments are more effective than heavy material and it should be remembered that considerable heat can be lost from the top of the head. There is much to be said for woolly hats, indoors, in winter.

FALLS

Because of failing vision, unsteadiness, slower reflexes, vertigo, stiffness and muscle weakness, hazards easily avoided by younger people become significant for the elderly and falls are common. These are more dangerous than is often realized and are often fatal in their long-term consequences. Osteoporosis makes old people, especially women, particularly susceptible to fractures, even from quite minor injuries, and the resulting immobilization and decline in the level of

activity can have grave effects. Chest and urinary infections commonly follow, and these may tip the balance against survival. Delicate skin can tear and bruise easily and muscle injuries are slow to heal. Long periods of pain, discomfort and disability may follow an apparently trivial fall.

Because of these risks, every effort should be made to avoid hazards in the environment of the elderly such as loose mats on polished floors, damaged floor coverings, carelessly disposed electric cables, poorly lit stairs or corridors and icy paths. Elderly people living alone are especially at risk, and some form of alarm system which will enable the victim to summon help, even if immobilized, is mandatory.

WALKING AIDS

Walking sticks can be very helpful to those with a one-sided weakness or with a painful knee or hip joint on one side. The correct length allows an upright stance with the tip of the stick on the ground and the arm bent a little at the elbow. Walking sticks can be used in two ways. Usually the stick is held on the strong side, so that it is forward when the foot on the weak side is also forward. But if one leg is particularly weak it may be better to hold the stick close to the leg on that side so that it acts as a kind of splint. People suffering from a degree of vertigo or instability may benefit from a walking stick with a broader base consisting of three or four small feet.

For those with an even greater tendency to fall, the light alloy frame 'walker' (Zimmer frame) can be a useful aid to mobility. Progress must necessarily be slow and tedious, but a walker will often allow a person with severe weakness or disability to get around and perhaps gain strength for greater mobility.

The older arm-pit crutch design, which could injure the nerves under the head of the upper arm bone, has now been replaced by light forearm-support or elbow crutches. These can offer surprisingly good mobility to the active and can be used in several ways. For the most disabled, 'four point' walking is used in which only one foot or one crutch tip is moved forward at a time. In 'three point' walking, both crutches are moved forward together, then, while the weight is supported, one foot is moved and then the other. For the more agile, the crutches can be used to support the whole weight of the body while both legs are swung forward together.

Walking callipers are splints used to add strength to a leg weakened by muscle disorder or injury, so that standing and walking become possible. The calliper is a steel rod, usually passed through the heel of the shoe and bent upwards on each side to be held in place by a padded ring or strap, below or above the knee. In cases of foot drop, a spring can be incorporated to help keep the toe from dragging on the ground. Some callipers are hinged at the knee.

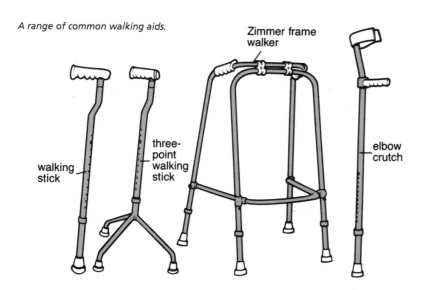

A range of common walking aids.

Zimmer frame walker

three-point walking stick

walking stick

elbow crutch

C

caries, dental

See **tooth decay**.

carisoprodol

A centrally acting muscle relaxant drug used in the treatment of muscle spasms. A brand name is Carisoma.

carmellose

A substance that can be applied to the skin or to mucous membranes to form a protective film. A brand name is Orabase.

carminative

A drug with the power to relax muscle rings (sphincters) so as to release gas and relieve flatulence.

carmustine

An alkylating agent anticancer drug. A brand name is Bicnu.

carotid artery disease

The two **carotid arteries**, together with the two vertebral arteries provide the whole blood supply to the head. Since the brain is critically dependent on a good blood supply, the carotids are, second to the coronary arteries which supply the heart, the most important arteries in the body.

For practical purposes, carotid artery disease means **atherosclerosis** – the development of fatty, obstructive plaques in the inner linings of arteries.

WHAT HAPPENS?

Atherosclerotic plaques continue to grow in size, as we continue to abuse our bodies with excessive rich food and inadequate exercise, until they are large enough to bulge far into the inner channels of the arteries. At this stage, they begin to ulcerate and break down, shedding debris into the bloodstream to cause **transient ischaemic attacks** and slowly clog up the small but vital blood vessels of the brain. Often a roughened plaque surface leads to local clotting of blood (thrombosis) on top of the plaque. This further narrows the artery and reduces the blood supply to the brain. Sometimes the thrombosis blocks off the artery altogether and, since the other carotid is usually diseased also and cannot, on its own, supply enough blood, the result will be a severe stroke.

RECOGNITION AND SYMPTOMS

Carotid artery disease often causes such narrowing of the arteries that a whooshing sound (a bruit) can be heard on listening over the arteries with a stethoscope. Such a finding is highly significant.

OUTCOME

One in five of all people with carotid bruits will suffer a major related incident within four years and one in ten will die, within that time, from the effects of arterial disease. Because carotid disease is merely a part of a generalized disease process affecting all the arteries of the body, and because the coronary arteries of the heart are much narrower and more liable to blockage than the carotids, most people who have carotid bruits die of coronary thrombosis rather than of a stroke.

carpal tunnel syndrome

The carpal tunnel is a restricted space at the front of the wrist, bounded by ligaments, through which pass the tendons that flex the fingers and wrist. This space is roofed over by a tough ligament, called the flexor retinaculum, which prevents the tendons from pulling away from the wrist when it is bent. One of the two sensory nerves to the hand, the median nerve, also passes through the carpal tunnel and there is little or no room for expansion. Any swelling in the region, from any cause, will, therefore, tend to compress the median nerve and interfere with the conduction of nerve impulses. The result is numbness and tingling, sometimes even pain, in the half of the hand – the half on the thumb side – that is supplied by the nerve.

POSSIBLE CAUSES

Carpal tunnel syndrome may be associated with excessive occupational use of the wrist. In rheumatoid arthritis, pituitary body overgrowth (acromegaly) and underaction of the thyroid gland (myxoedema), it is thickening of the overlying ligament which causes the problem. There is also a familial variety, affecting large numbers of people of Swiss origin, living in Indiana, in which a substance called amyloid is deposited in the tunnel.

ASSOCIATIONS

The syndrome often occurs for no obvious reason but is commonest in women, especially in pregnant women or those taking oral contraceptives. It is also associated with **premenstrual syndrome**.

TREATMENT

When severe, it may be relieved by a surgical operation to cut the ligament overlying the tunnel. Surgical inspection of an opened carpal tunnel often shows a deep compression mark on the median nerve.

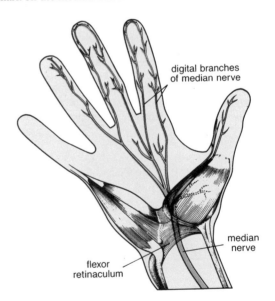

digital branches of median nerve

median nerve

flexor retinaculum

Carpal tunnel syndrome. Note the distribution of the median nerve. This is the area affected if the nerve is compressed in the tunnel under the flexor retinaculum.

carpos

Greek root meaning 'wrist' as in metacarpal (beyond the carpal bones).

carrier, bacterial

See **typhoid carrier**.

carrier, genetic

A great many inheritable diseases will be expressed only if both of the pair of corresponding genes concerned bear the defect for the condition. This is called recessive inheritance. People with one normal and one affected gene (heterozygotes) will not show the condition but will be carriers. Another form of genetic carriage occurs with sex-linked conditions.

Haemophilia is a good example. The gene is carried on the X chromosome and affects only males. Women, however, may carry the gene as a defect on one of their two X chromosomes. Males have only one X and a smaller Y chromosome, which does not neutralize the gene on the affected X chromosome. Sperms contain either X or Y chromosomes. Y chromosome sperms produce males, but do not contain the haemophilia gene. So men with haemophilia cannot pass the disease to their sons. They do, however, always pass the gene to their daughters, who will always be carriers. These female carriers pass the gene on to half their sons, and to half their daughters. All the sons who receive the gene will develop the disease, and all the daughters who receive it will be carriers.

car sickness

See **motion sickness**.

carteolol

A **beta-blocker** drug used as eyedrops in the treatment of **glaucoma**. A brand name is Teoptic.

carvedilol

A drug used in the treatment of **heart failure** and **angina pectoris**. A brand name is Eucardic.

cast

An abnormal moulded shape, corresponding to the inside of a kidney tubule or a small air tube in the lungs (bronchiole) formed when excreted material such as protein or mucus solidifies *in situ*. Such casts may also contain trapped red or white blood cells. Microscopic casts, produced in this way, are often found in the urine and indicate serious disease of the kidneys. Bronchial casts are sometimes found in sputum.

Plaster casts are used in the treatment of fractures (see **immobilization**).

castration

The Latin word '*castrare*' means to 'prune' or 'to cut off'. Castration is the removal of the testicles, or, sometimes, of all the male external genitalia. The term is also occasionally used to refer to the removal of the ovaries in women.

Castration of human beings has seldom been employed to produce sterility. Historically, the principal intention was either as a punishment for crime or to deprive the male of his chief source of sex hormones so that he would not develop adult sexual interests. The eunuchs, thus produced, could safely be left in charge of the women of the harem or could be admitted to ruling families as bodyguards or advisers.

An alternative motive was to prevent the enlargement of the Adam's apple (larynx) which occurs under the influence of male sex hormones at puberty and leads to the 'breaking' of the voice. Boys with exceptional treble singing voices could thus retain their high-pitched range into adult life. Such *castrati* became true male sopranos with powerful and often exceptionally fine voices, quite different from the falsetto or counter tenor quality. The practice, which flourished in Italy, was finally banned by Pope Leo XIII in 1878.

Castration is sometimes medically justified. Certain cancers, notably cancer of the prostate, are *hormone dependent*, and removal of the testicles (orchidectomy) can produce a remarkable resolution of the tumour, even if it has spread widely.

casualty sorting

See **triage**.

cata-

Prefix meaning 'down' as in catabolic (breaking down).

catalepsy

See **schizophrenia**.

cataplexy

The momentary paralysis, or weakness of the limbs, that sometimes affects people surprised by a powerful emotion such as anger, fear, jealousy, happiness or hilarity. The effect is often no more than a sudden arrest of movement, a sagging of the jaw, or a 'giving way at the knees', but sometimes the affected person may actually fall. Full recovery occurs within a minute or so. Many animals go into a state of immobility when suddenly frightened.

The narcolepsy-cataplexy syndrome is more serious. It features recurrent attacks of overwhelming sleepiness resulting in fifteen-minute catnaps from which the subject awakens refreshed, only to repeat the cycle from one to several hours later. Often the attacks are precipitated by boredom, but they may occur at inconvenient and inappropriate times, as when driving or when engaged in sexual intercourse. The condition can be severely disabling and usually requires treatment with amphetamine-like drugs.

cataract

Cataract has nothing to do with the cornea, nor is it a 'skin' growing over any part of the eye. It is an opacification of the internal focusing lens of the eye (the crystalline lens) due to irreversible structural changes in the orderly arrangement of the fibres from which the lens is made. The change is due to coagulation, or denaturing, of the lens fibres, in much the same way as occurs in the transparent egg albumen when it is heated. The term 'cataract' arose from the imaginative notion that the appearance of whiteness, seen in cases of dense lens opacity, was caused by a 'cataract' or waterfall descending from above.

Cataract never causes complete blindness in the sense of total absence of perception of light. People with dense cataracts can still usually distinguish an open from a closed door and will always see windows in daytime. But as the transparency of the lenses is gradually lost, image clarity slowly declines and perception of detail becomes less and less until eventually it is lost.

Contrary to popular belief, cataract is not readily visible to the external observer. Outside the professional press, most illustrations purporting to be cataract are, in fact, of white, conspicuous scars on the outer lens of the eye (the cornea) and have nothing to do with cataract. It is only the occasional and exceptionally mature cataract that is visible. The fears, commonly expressed, that cataract is going to progress to a disfiguring blemish, are quite without foundation.

WHAT HAPPENS?

Some degree of lens opacification is present in almost everyone over the age of about sixty. Usually this is patchy and worse in the edges of the lenses so that there is little effect on vision. But the process almost always progresses steadily with age and testing of people over seventy-five will usually show a drop in acuity from lens opacity. Few people in their eighties are free from appreciable visual loss from this cause. So cataract in the elderly should be considered almost normal.

POSSIBLE CAUSES

Cataract in younger people is almost always the result of a discernible cause, and there are many of these. Cataract present at birth (congenital cataract) is often caused by maternal German measles (rubella) early in pregnancy, or less often, to the effects of drugs taken by the mother during the early weeks when the eyes of the fetus were developing.

Down's syndrome is commonly associated with cataract as are various rare hereditary conditions. A number of severe skin problems, all fortunately rare, or severe childhood diabetes, with high blood sugar levels, may cause cataract. Galactosaemia is a condition in which the infant is unable to break down galactose into simpler sugars so that it accumulates in the body. Unless a galactose-free diet is given, cataract is inevitable.

People taking large doses of steroids over a long period, or those using steroid eye drops for many months, are liable to develop cataract, but are even more liable to develop **glaucoma**. Various toxic chemicals, such as naphthalene, dinitrophenol or ergot, can cause cataract. Dinitrophenol was in vogue as an aid to slimming, earlier this century, but was abandoned when it was found that many of the young women taking it developed cataracts.

Injury to the eye is an important cause of cataract. A concussive force such as that caused by a flying stone or high-speed squash ball, a sharp poke from a finger or a severe blow to the face, may cause cataract even without any external injury to the eye. Penetrating wounds of the eye are even more likely to cause cataract, especially if the lens capsule is penetrated or torn. In such cases, water immediately enters the lens substance and, within a matter of hours or days, a dense cataract will develop.

Progressive hardening of the centre of the lens (nuclear sclerosis) is common in cataract and this often leads to a special form of short sight (index myopia) in which the bending power of the lenses increases. Index myopia can progress steadily to high degrees so that many changes of glasses may be needed if correction is desired. It is the reason for the common discarding of reading glasses after years of wear, but it should be appreciated that this is a transient stage in the development of cataract and that the vision is likely to get worse. People with index myopia who can read without glasses will, of course, need spectacles for viewing objects at a distance.

RECOGNITION AND SYMPTOMS

Cataract usually causes a change in the perception of colours. Reds, yellows and orange are accentuated at the expense of blue, but, because of the very gradual nature of the change, this may remain unnoticed. Patients commonly exclaim with surprise at the brilliance of blues after cataract operations. The irregular opacification of the lenses, which is a common feature of cataract causes some rays of light entering the eye to be scattered while some are not. This may occur even at an early stage, and may be very annoying. The effect is particular noticeable when the headlights of approaching cars shine in the eyes while driving at night. Many people, otherwise barely affected, find they have to avoid night driving because of this.

TREATMENT

There is no possible way to restore transparency to a cataractous lens and it is unrealistic to imagine that cataract can be cured by any form of medication or by any means other than **cataract surgery**. Happily, this is one of the most successful operations in all areas of surgery and the expectation of an excellent result, the eye being otherwise healthy, is well over 90 per cent.

cataract emulsification

See **phakoemulsification**.

cataract surgery

The operation for cataract may be performed either under general or local anaesthesia and in neither case is there any pain. The danger to life is negligible. The operation is usually performed under microscopy using instruments of remarkable delicacy and precision.

HOW IT'S DONE

Before the operation, drops are used to dilate the pupil widely so that most of the front surface of the lens is exposed. An incision is made around the upper edge of the cornea and a small quantity of a clear gel called Healonid is injected to maintain a space between the back of the cornea and the lens. A large part of the centre of the front capsule of the lens is removed and the hard nucleus of the lens carefully squeezed out of the eye. The soft remaining parts of the lens are now cleared away by suction and washing, great care being taken to avoid damage to the back part of the capsule. It may be necessary to 'polish' the inside of the back wall of the capsule to rub off opaque matter. The artificial lens implant is now slipped into the natural lens capsule and the corneal incision sewn up with a fine nylon suture about half the diameter of a human hair.

Patients are no longer immobilized after cataract surgery and, indeed, are encouraged to move about freely as soon as possible afterwards. The corneal incision takes about a month to heal, but it will usually be about ten weeks before the corneal curvature has ceased to alter. Glasses should not be obtained until then.

In the past, patients who have had cataract operations have had to wear very strong, highly magnifying glasses, which were heavy and uncomfortable and caused much distortion at the edges of the narrowed field of vision. Such glasses are now seldom necessary because it is now almost universal practice to replace the cataractous lens with a plastic lens implant. At the worst, patients will generally require glasses similar to those used before the cataract developed. There are still, however, some patients for whom intra-ocular lens implants are unsuitable. These are mainly people with a history of eye disease. Contact lenses can offer these people excellent vision post-operatively and many elderly people are now wearing contact lenses.

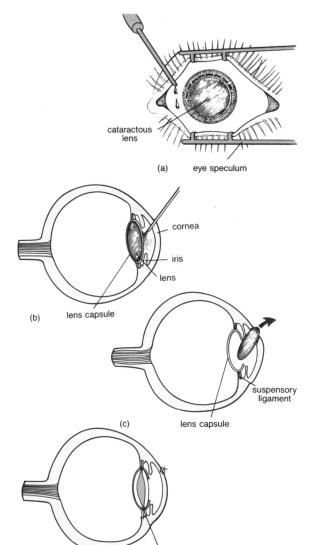

(a) eye speculum

cataractous lens

cornea

iris

lens

lens capsule

(b)

suspensory ligament

lens capsule

(c)

plastic lens implant

(d)

Above: Cataract surgery. (a) The pupil is widely dilated with drops. (b) Healonid jelly is carefully injected into the front chamber of the eye to maintain depth. (c) The front part of the capsule of the lens is removed and the lens nucleus squeezed out. (d) A clear plastic lens implant is inserted.

Right: Urinary catheter. The illustration shows a 'self-retaining' catheter with a widened section near the tip. During insertion this is stretched over a smooth metal introducer.

catatonia

See **schizophrenia**.

catharsis

Literally, 'a cleansing', which is the meaning of the Greek word *katharsis*, from *katharos*, meaning 'pure'. The term was originally used to refer to the effect of any *cathartic* or medicine calculated to purify, but later became confined to purgatives. This usage is now historic and the term has been taken over by the psychoanalysts to describe the release of anxiety and tension experienced when repressed matter, which has been 'poisoning' the mind, is brought into consciousness. There are signs that even this usage may be passing out of fashion.

catheter

A hollow, often flexible, tube, similar to a **cannula**, passed into the body to extract or introduce fluids. Catheters come in all sizes and are used for a variety of purposes. One of the oldest uses of a catheter is to empty the urinary bladder. Urinary catheters have been in use by medical men since ancient times. There are records of their use by the Indian medical genius Susruta in 3000 years BC.

Recent years have seen growing applications of catheters designed for insertion into blood vessels, both for sampling blood in otherwise inaccessible parts of the circulation – as in the heart – and for the injection of dyes opaque to X-rays. Balloon catheters have become an important means of treating partial arterial obstruction. They are widely used for balloon **angioplasty** and are increasing being used for widening abnormally narrowed areas in other body passages, such as the Fallopian tubes.

Catheters in blood vessels are also used for artificial feeding (parenteral nutrition) of those unable to take food normally. This is a necessary but hazardous procedure, causing 'blood poisoning' (**septicaemia**) in about 7 per cent of cases, often with infection with the fungus Candida.

See **catheterization, urinary**.

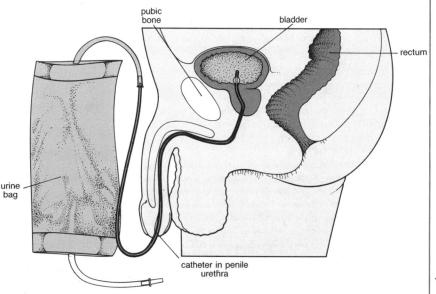

pubic bone

bladder

rectum

urine bag

catheter in penile urethra

C

catheterization, intermittent

The relief of outflow obstruction, as from prostate gland enlargement, by passage of a urinary catheter to empty the bladder on an 'as required' basis.

Men with urinary outflow difficulties can be trained to perform the procedure themselves. Current medical opinion is that, properly applied, the method is safe, effective and could, with benefit, be more widely used.

catheterization, urinary

The procedure for releasing urine from the bladder when the normal outflow channel is blocked.

WHY IT'S DONE

Neurological disturbances of urination, either temporary or permanent, are common, and often require catheterization. Blockage by enlargement of the **prostate gland**, or when normal urination cannot occur for any other reason are reasons for catheterization.

HOW IT'S DONE

Usually, the catheter is introduced through the normal urine passage (the urethra). Sometimes, however, the urethra is so narrowed (urethral stricture) due to gonorrhoea or benign or malignant enlargement of the prostate, that a catheter cannot be passed. In that event, the distended bladder is entered through the wall of the abdomen, immediately above the pubic bone, using a **cannula**, which is then replaced by a rubber or plastic catheter.

Catheterization in the female is easier than in the male because the urethra is much shorter and there is no prostate.

RISKS

There is an ever-present risk of infection, especially if the catheter has to be left in place for a long time (indwelling catheter). In spite of high standards of sterilization and aseptic technique in modern hospitals, about 10 per cent of catheterized patients acquire urinary infections.

The procedure has, through the centuries, provided enormous relief to millions, but clearly this must have been at the cost of enormous morbidity.

cathexis

The attachment of emotional energy to an idea, person or object, the investment of *libidinal* energy in something. The idea is Freud's and is part of Freudian theory. Freud used an electrical analogy and spoke of the flow of libidinal currents, charges, and so on.

cat-scratch fever

A disease of lymph nodes caused by an unknown organism transmitted by the scratch of a cat. Most cases occur in children and there is no indication that the cat is unwell.

RECOGNITION AND SYMPTOMS

A few days after a cat scratch, a small, red, crusted swelling develops at the site of the scratch. Within two weeks, the lymph nodes to which the site drains – groin for the leg, armpit for the arm – become swollen, firm and tender to pressure. By the time this is noticed the affected person feels unwell, with fever, headache and loss of appetite.

The enlarged lymph nodes then become softer and form small pus-filled abscesses which sometimes drain through to the surface of the skin and discharge. The general symptoms

soon settle, but the discharging sinuses may take several months to heal. They always do so eventually.

TREATMENT

Antibiotics can shorten the course of the disease, but sometimes surgical drainage of abscesses is necessary.

OTHER DISEASES

Other diseases caused by cats include; ringworm (tinea) – a fungus infection of the skin; **asthma** from cat skin scales; and cat flea bites, which are common and very irritating and may become infected. Mange is a mite infestation caused by mites of the same variety that cause **scabies** and there is at least a theoretical possibility that these mites may be transferred to human beings, causing scabies. **Rabies** can be contracted and transmitted by domestic cats, but in spite of the fact the disease is said to be spreading towards Britain from the continent at a rate of 30 to 50 km a year, the risk is still very small.

cats, diseases from

The most important diseases transmitted from domestic cats to human beings are two parasitic disorders of similar names but different significance – **toxoplasmosis** and **toxocariasis** – both of which are conveyed in cat faeces. The names share the common root *toxo-* (which means 'a bow' – as in *toxophilite*, a 'lover of archery') because both are bow-shaped.

TOXOPLASMOSIS

Toxoplasmosis is caused by a microscopic organism called *Toxoplasma gondii* which can infect people before they are born, gaining access to the fetus by way of the placenta during pregnancy. Toxoplasmosis can have serious effects if this occurs early in pregnancy and may cause abortion or severe congenital abnormalities. Later in the pregnancy, the fetus has more resistance, but the nervous system and the eyes are commonly infected.

Toxoplasmosis of the choroid of the eye, acquired in this way, is a possibility. The organisms tend to lie dormant for many years, but later, in adult life, often cause a flare-up of patchy **choroiditis** which may severely damage vision.

TOXOCARIASIS

Toxocariasis is caused by a small round worm, *Toxocara cati*, a similar species of which, *Toxocara canis*, is common in puppies. The infestation is acquired by children, whose fingers become contaminated by worm eggs in the anal fur or by touching cat faeces. These eggs are then transferred to the children's mouths and the cycle started. Toxocariasis causes a brief, feverish illness as the hatched worm juveniles pass around the body, but generally causes little harm unless a tiny worm happens to enter the eye. In this event a damaging reaction occurs that not only may destroy vision but may also cause a visible white mass closely resembling a malignant tumour. Many children have had an eye unnecessarily removed because of toxocariasis.

cauda

Latin root meaning 'tail' as in caudal (of the tail).

cauda equina syndrome

Pressure on the leash of nerves, in the part of the spinal canal below the end of the spinal cord, from central protrusion backwards of the pulpy inner material (nucleus pulposus) of an intervertebral disc. There is acute back pain, **sciatica** and interference with bladder function.

caudal

Pertaining to the tail, or to the tail end of the body. Although not externally visible, the human tail still exists in the shape of a short set of fused caudal spinal bones (vertebrae) forming the coccyx. The word *caudal* is generally used to denote direction in anatomy.

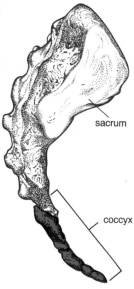

Caudal. Like most vertebrates, man has a tail. It is, however, vestigial and rigid, and is represented by a few small vertebrae fused together to form the coccyx as shown.

sacrum

coccyx

cauliflower ear

A thickening and distortion of the external ear, following repeated blunt injury which causes bleeding between the cartilage and the skin. The resulting collections of blood are called **haematomas** and these do not get the chance to reabsorb and disappear in the normal way. Instead, haematomas become invaded by cells which form fibrous tissue and become 'organized' and permanent, producing, in boxers, this conspicuous badge of self-abuse. Treatment of haematomas by surgical release of the blood has made cauliflower ear less common.

The effect is one of the least serious consequences of boxing and is trivial compared with the systematic and deliberate **brain damage** boxers inflict on one another.

causalgia

A severe burning pain in a limb caused by partial damage to a nerve trunk, usually from physical injury. The pain arises from nerve impulses stimulated in sensory nerves at the site of the injury. These pass to the brain and are interpreted as if arising further out along the limb. Nerve damage of this kind is often also associated with damage to the nerves of the autonomic nervous system which supply the small arteries. The result may be areas of red and tender skin, or cold, blue patches. Disturbance of skin and nail growth and of the ability to recover from local injury, are also common.

See also **referred pain**.

caustic

Any chemical substance that corrodes and destroys bodily tissue. Caustics have some limited use in medicine for destroying warts or removing dead skin and, occasionally, for the treatment of surface infections. Accidental or deliberate infliction of caustic burns poses serious medical and surgical problems. In particular, the swallowing of caustic solutions in suicide attempts leads to severe scarring, narrowing, and often closure of the gullet (oesophagus). Caustic burns to the eyes, as from thrown ammonia in criminal raids, have horrifying consequences in terms of blindness and suffering. The

resultant injuries to the corneas are usually followed by such severe tissue reactions and new blood vessel growth that even corneal grafting may fail to restore sight.

cauterization

The deliberate destruction of tissue by the careful local application of heat.

HOW IT'S DONE

The instrument used is known as a cautery and may take the form of a small loop of resistance wire, at the end of an insulated handle, through which a controllable direct electric current is passed. The wire loop may be bent to a point so that cauterization may be applied with some precision. More often, the direct current cautery is replaced by a high-frequency **diathermy** cautery.

The surgical cautery may be *unipolar* or *bipolar*. In the former case, a large, flexible metal contact pad is firmly strapped or bandaged to a part of the patient remote from the operation site and connected to the high-frequency generator machine by a single lead. The other lead goes to the sterilized cautery probe in its insulated handle, used by the surgeon. The probe may be applied directly to the tissues, producing a sudden sharp, crackling coagulation, often with a tiny puff of smoke, or it may be touched to a pair of metal forceps holding the tissue to be cauterized. The bipolar cautery consists of a special kind of forceps in which the two blades are insulated from one another and each connected, by a separate wire, to the machine. Any tissue held between the points of the forceps will be cauterized.

WHY IT'S DONE

High-frequency alternating currents pass more easily through human tissue and the method is invaluable in surgery, especially for coagulating and sealing off small bleeding vessels cut in the course of making incisions.

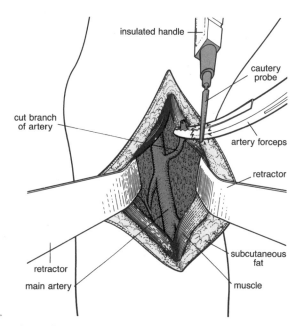

insulated handle

cautery probe

artery forceps

retractor

cut branch of artery

retractor

main artery

subcutaneous fat

muscle

The small artery branch to be sealed is gripped in artery forceps which are then touched with the tip of the electric diathermy probe. Immediately the tissues are coagulated and the blood at the site coagulated, producing a secure seal.

C

cavernous sinus thrombosis

See **thrombosis, cavernous sinus**.

cavity, dental

See **tooth decay**.

cefadroxil

A cephalosporin **antibiotic** drug. A brand name is Baxan.

cefamandole

A cephalosporin **antibiotic** drug. A brand name is Kefadol.

cefixime

A cephalosporin **antibiotic** drug. A brand name is Suprax.

cefotaxime

A third-generation cephalosporin **antibiotic** active against Gram-negative organisms but not staphylococci. A brand name is Claforan.

cefpirome

A cephalosporin **antibiotic** drug. A brand name is Cefrom.

cefpodixime

A cephalosporin **antibiotic** drug. A brand name is Orelox.

cefprozil

A new oral cephalosporin **antibiotic** drug effective against a wide range of Gram positive and Gram negative bacteria. A brand name is Cefzil.

ceftriaxone

A cephalosporin **antibiotic** drug. A brand name is Rocephin.

cefuroxime

A second-generation cephalosporin **antibiotic** active against staphylococci and some Gram negative organisms. It must be given by injection. A brand name is Zinacef.

cefuroxime axetil

A cephalosporin **antibiotic** drug. A brand name is Zinnat.

Cefzil

A brand name for the antibiotic **cefprozil**.

celiprolol

A cardio-selective **beta-blocker** drug. A brand name is Celectol.

cell

The word 'cell' derives from the Latin word *cella*, meaning a store or larder. The term was first used in 1665 by the microscopist Robert Hooke (1635–1703) to describe the spaces he observed in thin slices of cork. Hooke was actually looking at empty spaces left by cells, but the observation was important

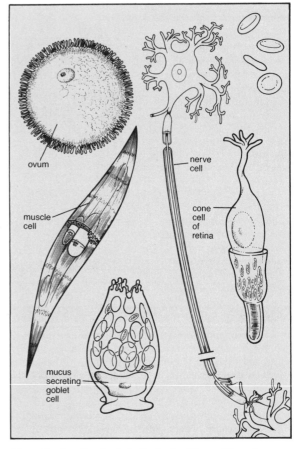

The wide diversity of cells in the body all have different functions.

and led others to search for, and find, a cellular structure in all living things and to discover that the whole of biology is based on the cell.

Although the cell has long been known to be the structural unit of the body, knowledge of the internal features of the cell and of the immensely complex biochemical processes going on in every living cell is comparatively recent. The last fifty years or so have seen an explosive growth of knowledge of cell structure and function which has revolutionized medicine and is likely to have a greater effect on the future of mankind than any other branch of scientific advance.

The body is composed entirely of countless millions of cells and their products, and may be considered to be a community of cells. Most of the cells are stuck together to form tissues but many, such as those comprising the blood and those concerned with the immune system, are separate and free to move around.

Body cells vary greatly in size, from less than a hundredth of a millimetre across, in the case of red blood cells, to about a metre long, in the case of some nerve cells with very long nerve fibres (axons). The largest cell bodies are those of the egg (ovum), which is about a tenth of a millimetre across.

Cells require fuel to provide them with energy, and oxygen with which to burn up the fuel. Without such supplies they soon die. All cells are bathed in tissue fluid and supplies reach them by diffusion through this fluid.

The central part of the cell which, in most stained sections under the microscope, appears much more densely coloured

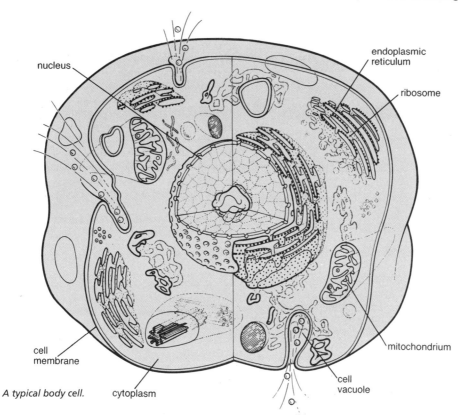

nucleus

endoplasmic
reticulum

ribosome

cell
membrane

A typical body cell.

cytoplasm

mitochondrium

cell
vacuole

than the rest of the cell, is called the nucleus and contains the chromosomes – the coiled-up lengths of DNA that form the genetic blueprint for the reproduction of the cell and for the synthesis of **proteins**. Surrounding the nucleus, within the cell, is the fluid cytoplasm. Each cell type has a different cytoplasm, but in all cells this is mainly water, sometimes up to 97 per cent. Dissolved in the water are substances such as proteins, including **enzymes**, **amino acids** (the 'building bricks' of proteins), nucleic acids, sugars (carbohydrates), sodium, potassium, calcium, magnesium, iron, copper, zinc, iodine and bromine.

Cell membranes are highly flexible structures made largely of a double layer of fat molecules, mainly **fats** (lipids) containing phosphorus (phospholipids, see below) held together by the basic forces that attract atoms to each other. They also contain cholesterol, an essential constituent of every cell, and are penetrated by many large functional protein molecules. These membranes are far more than bags for the cell constituents. They are complex and important structures containing specialized protein sites for the receipt of information from the external environment and others for the pumping of dissolved chemical substances into and out of the cell.

Our understanding of body function has been massively extended by the discovery that all cells possess such receptors, either on their surfaces, within their cytoplasm (cytosolic receptors), or on the membranes surrounding their nuclei. The chemical messengers, such as hormones or neurotransmitters are able to bind specifically to these receptors, and, in so doing, modify the function or actions of the cells. This, for instance, is how muscle cells are caused to contract and gland cells to secrete. Adrenaline receptors of three types occur on various cells and most have receptors for insulin.

Many other hormones, prostaglandins and other chemical messengers bind to surface cell receptors. Steroids and the thyroid hormones enter cells and bind to receptors on the nuclei, prompting nuclear DNA to increase the transcription of particular genes.

cell access

See **ion channels**.

cell and organism attraction or repulsion

See **tropism**.

cell controllers, external

See **cytokines**.

cell, eating

See **phagocyte**.

cell external linkers

See **integrins**.

cell interaction disrupters

See **disintegrins**.

cell junction gaps

See **connexin-26**.

cell messenger disorders

See **G protein diseases**.

cells, messengers between

See **interleukins**.

cell messengers, interior

See **G proteins**.

cell organs

The fluid in a cell (cytoplasm) contains many important structures known as organelles or 'little organs'. Permeating the whole cytoplasm is the endoplasmic reticulum, a complex network of membranes, studded all over with tiny granules called ribosomes. These are dense collections of RNA and are the sites at which proteins are formed. From the reticulum, newly made proteins are transported to other structures, known as the Golgi apparatus, named after the Italian histologist (microscopic anatomist) Camillo Golgi (1843–1926). The Golgi complexes are situated near the cell nucleus, and consist of a series of flattened, membranous sacs surrounded by a number of spherical bubbles, or vesicles. These vesicles initially form on the surface of the rough reticulum in areas not coated with ribosomes.

Proteins within the rough endoplasmic reticulum pass into these vesicles, which then travel though the cytoplasm and fuse on to the surface of the Golgi complex, transferring their contents into the Golgi sacs. Secondary transfer vesicles are now formed on the surface of the Golgi sacs, and these are 'tagged' by the addition of a carbohydrate or phosphate group to indicate where they should go. Golgi vesicles have been called the 'traffic police' of the cell as they play a key role in directing the many proteins that are formed within the cell to their required destination.

The **mitochondria** are tiny bags containing enzymes required for the building and breaking down (metabolic) processes of the cell and for the conversion of glucose and oxygen into energy. They are the power houses of the cell and contain rings of DNA of their own. This DNA is quite distinct from the DNA in the nucleus and is inherited only from the mother.

Lysosomes are little sacs (saccules) containing digestive enzymes capable of breaking down almost any organic molecule present in, or engulfed by, the cell. Lysosome enzymes act on materials taken in by cells in the process known as phagocytosis – literally 'cell eating'. They are especially conspicuous in the scavenging white cells (phagocytes) of the immune system.

See **organelle**.

cell progenitor

See **stem cell**.

cell protection against virus infection

See **virus interference**.

cell reproduction

Some body cells, once mature, never reproduce, and have to last for a lifetime. The normal cells of the central nervous system, for instance, are of this kind. Most body cells, however, reproduce frequently to allow growth and to make up for wear and tear. Rapid reproduction and replacement is necessary in the case of the cells of the skin and blood, the immune system and the lining of the digestive system. Other cells need not reproduce so often. The reproductive organs – the ovaries and the testicles – contain cells which must not only reproduce themselves, but which must also alter in a special way so as to make themselves suitable to fuse with cells from other individuals in order to reproduce the whole individual.

Cell reproduction starts with reproduction (replication) of the chromosomes which carry the genetic code or blueprint for the construction of the body. This code is represented by the genes – chemical sequences, of which there are about 100,000, strung along the chromosomes. Each human body cell contains forty-six chromosomes, arranged in twenty-three pairs. Although the chromosomes, as usually seen under the microscope, appear as short, thick bodies, this is their state only when the cell is in process of dividing. At other times, each chromosome is actually an immensely long, and very thin, strand. The term 'chromatin' is often applied to the material of which the chromosomes are made. 'Chromo' means 'coloured' and the term arose when the nuclei of cells were found to stain easily with the dye used by microscopists to make detail more easily visible. During the division phase, the chromatin strand becomes coiled.

Chromosomes are made of DNA (deoxyribonucleic acid). DNA is found in every nucleated cell in the body and is the basis of inheritance. Replication, or reproduction, of DNA is the way in which the characteristics of a cell or organism are passed on. Replication involves the separation of the two strands over a short distance, followed by the automatic formation of complementary strands on each of the separated strands. So long as the necessary sugars, phosphates and bases are present in the cytoplasm of the cell, the presence of a half ladder (separated strand) automatically leads to the formation of new DNA. Errors occur very rarely, probably fewer than one per million bases linked. If an error does occur, correction is possible, but a change (mutation) in the DNA may be perpetuated in all subsequent replications of that DNA. Errors may so alter the protein coded for by the DNA that the protein can no longer perform its normal function.

In replicating, DNA does not split along its whole length at one time. Many short loops of separated DNA form simultaneously and the replication occurs in these loops. DNA replication should not be confused with the expression of genes to form proteins – which is a similar process but with a fundamentally different purpose.

The period during which the cell is dividing to form two new daughter cells is called mitosis. First, the forty-six long strands of chromatin in the nucleus of the cell replicate,

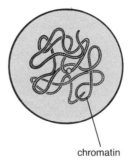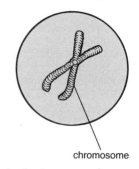

chromatin chromosome

In its resting state the DNA molecule of a chromosome forms a very long, extremely fine strand of chromatin. At the time of division the chromatin strand forms a coil and appears short and thick. In this state it is called a chromosome.

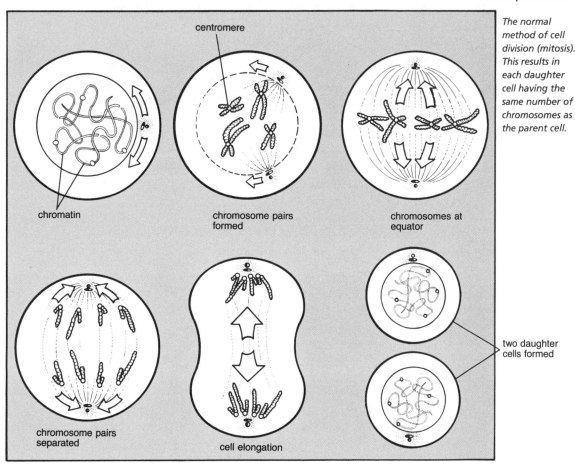

centromere

chromatin

chromosome pairs
formed

chromosomes at
equator

chromosome pairs
separated

cell elongation

two daughter
cells formed

The normal method of cell division (mitosis). This results in each daughter cell having the same number of chromosomes as the parent cell.

making ninety-two strands. These then coil up to form chromosomes, the newly formed identical pairs, resulting from DNA replication, remaining attached to one another at a central point called the centromere. The membrane surrounding the nucleus of the cell disappears and the forty-six doubled chromosomes are moved by fine strands of contractile protein to the centre of the cell and come to lie in the plane of the equator of the cell.

The centromeres now split, allowing the joined pairs of chromosomes to separate. There are now ninety-two chromosomes in the cell. One of each pair is now pulled by the protein strands to each end of the cell, so that there are forty-six at each end. The cell then elongates, narrows in the middle, and separates into two individuals, each containing forty-six chromosomes.

If a cell is examined just prior to division, it will be seen to contain twenty-two pairs of identical pairs of chromosomes and one pair of sex chromosomes. In the case of females, the sex chromosomes are fairly large and are called X chromosomes. In the case of males, there is one X chromosome and one much smaller chromosome called a Y chromosome. So females are designated XX and males XY. During the resting phase between the end of mitosis and the beginning of cell division there are twenty-three pairs of single chromosomes but these are uncoiled into long strands of chromatin which cannot be seen by a light microscope. The electron microscope can, however, readily show the chromosomes in this stage as a long apparently tangled thread. Each nucleated cell of the body contains about 2 metres of chromatin.

Cell reproduction in the case of the cells in the ovaries and testes that produce eggs and sperms is achieved in a different manner, known as meiosis. This is necessary because sperms fuse with eggs at the moment of fertilization and, if each had the normal number of 46 chromosomes, the result would be a cell containing 96 chromosomes. The process by which the halving of the number of chromosomes is achieved is called meiosis and this takes place in the testes and ovaries.

Meiosis involves a normal DNA replication, with the two strands coiling up and sticking together at the centre as in mitosis. But when the forty-six doubled chromosomes line up in the centre of the cell, they congregate in pairs, but not with any arbitrary partner. Chromosomes can be identified and are numbered. The duplicated number one chromosome that came originally from the father aligns itself with the duplicated number one that came from the mother, number two with number two, and so on for all of them. The partners in each pair of Xs now twist intimately together and become closely aligned along their entire length. While in this relationship they exchange several short corresponding segments with each other. This occurs in a random manner so that the genetic material from the father and the mother becomes thoroughly mixed and new chromosomes are formed, each with a unique blend of the genes from both parents. This is called crossing-over.

The cell now divides, but in this division the doubled chromosomes do not have their arms pulled apart as in mitosis. Instead, one of each of the pairs of the intact double chromosomes goes to each daughter cell.

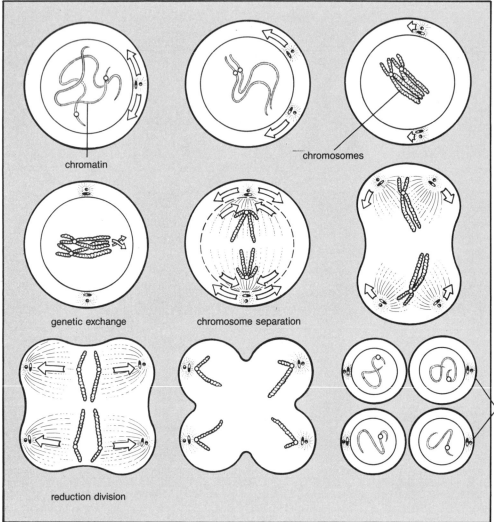

chromatin

chromosomes

genetic exchange

chromosome separation

reduction division

Cell division occurring in the sex cells (meiosis). Note that the chromosomes exchange genetic material by crossing over corresponding segments of chromosomes, but separate in such a way that the final cells contain half the number of chromosomes of the parent cell. The full number is made up when sperm unites with ovum.

cells with half the normal number of chromosomes

It is a matter of pure chance which of the pairs goes to which daughter cell. As a result, the random redistribution of genes already effected by crossing-over is further increased. Each daughter cell now has half the number of doubles. A second division then occurs but this time the halves are pulled apart by a spindle, as in mitosis, and each daughter cell receives a single chromosome from each pair. So the sperms and eggs now have half the normal number of chromosomes. This is called the haploid situation. The diploid situation is restored when a sperm fuses with an egg at fertilization.

cell suicide

See **apoptosis**.

cellular telephone dangers

These include:

- loss of vehicular control when a telephone is held in the hand during driving;
- inattention to driving, with the risk of traffic accidents;
- significant risk of interference with cardiac pacemakers;
- postulated risk to the brain from high-frequency (microwave) electromagnetic radiation.

Research suggests that the risk of pacemaker upset is significant only if the telephone is held over the pacemaker site. The jury is still out on the question of brain damage from electromagnetic radiation, but the probability of risk is believed to be small.

cellulitis

Spreading inflammation of tissue, most commonly the skin, caused by infection, often with *streptococci*. Usually, the body contains infection locally, by the formation of fibrous and other barriers around it. Thus, an infection with staphylococci typically results in a boil or pustule, which is well localized. Some organisms, however, particularly the streptococci, secrete enzymes – streptokinase, hyaluronidase and DNAse – which break down these natural defensive planes in the tissue and allow spread of infection.

RECOGNITION AND SYMPTOMS

Cellulitis starts with a contaminated scratch, prick or cut and quickly spreads to cause red, tender streaks extending along the lymph drainage channels towards the lymph nodes, which become enlarged, easily felt and tender. There is commonly fever and general upset.

TREATMENT

Cellulitis, once much feared and often a cause of death, now almost always responds readily and quickly to intensive antibiotic treatment.

cellulitis, orbital

See **orbital cellulitis**.

Celsius scale

In 1742, the Swedish professor of astronomy at Uppsala University Anders Celsius (1701–44) proposed that the temperature range between the freezing and the boiling points of water should be divided into 100 equal steps or degrees. The freezing point would be 0 degrees and the boiling point 100 degrees. Celsius called the scale *centigrade*, which means 'one hundred levels'.

The proposal was a sensible alternative to the arbitrary and illogical Fahrenheit scale, with 32^0 as freezing point and 212^0 as boiling point, and quickly caught on in Europe where the advantages of decimalization were perceived more readily than in Britain. But Britain finally fell into line. So the normal body temperature of 98.4^0 Fahrenheit became 37^0 C.

centigrade scale

Another name for the **Celsius** scale.

cephale

Greek root meaning 'head' as in cephalic (of the head).

cephalhaematoma

A collection of blood between a baby's skull and the overlying membrane (the periosteum) usually resulting from unavoidable injury sustained in the course of a difficult forceps delivery. The haematoma forms a soft, boggy swelling on the scalp which disappears over the course of the first few weeks of life.

> Cephalhaematoma appearing later in life must be accounted for, because it is an indication of a head injury, sometimes of a fractured skull. Non-accidental injury (child abuse) will have to be considered if no satisfactory explanation is forthcoming.

cephalic

Relating to the head, or in the direction of the head.

cephalosporin antibiotics

See **antibiotic drugs**.

cephazolin

A cephalosporin **antibiotic** drug. A brand name is Kefzol.

cephradine

A cephalosporin **antibiotic** drug. Brand names are Nicef and Velosef.

ceras

Greek root meaning 'horn' as in keratin (horn-like protein).

cerebral haemorrhage

See **stoke**.

cerebral palsy

See **spastic paralysis**.

cerebral thrombosis

See **thrombosis, cerebral**.

cerebrospinal fever

See **meningitis**.

cerebrovascular disease

Damage to the brain caused by disease of the arteries supplying it with blood.

POSSIBLE CAUSES

The damage is essentially caused by interference with the adequacy of the blood flow so that the supply of vital oxygen and sugar is prejudiced.

This may occur by narrowing of the large arteries, usually from the formation of plaques of fatty, degenerative material (atheroma) in the general arterial disease of **atherosclerosis**. It may also occur as a result of the blockage of smaller arteries in and around the brain by abnormal material in the bloodstream. This may comprise small blood clots that have formed in the arteries, or debris from atheromatous plaques, including crystals of cholesterol. A blockage of this kind is called **embolism**.

Blockage of cerebral arteries may also occur by the clotting of blood within them (**thrombosis**). This usually occurs on the surface of a roughened atheromatous plaque.

Less commonly, but more seriously, arterial disease causes brain damage by so weakening a brain artery that it bursts, causing a devastating cerebral haemorrhage with disruption of brain tissue.

INCIDENCE

Cerebrovascular disease is one of the commonest terminal events and we should all adjust our lifestyles so that this calamity comes on us as late as possible. Risk factors to be avoided are smoking, overeating, under-exercising and ignoring advice to have regular blood-pressure checks.

RECOGNITION AND SYMPTOMS

Insufficiency of blood supply, cerebral embolism and cerebral thrombosis all have the same effect and all are serious. In the most minor cases they cause **transient ischaemic attacks**, brief periods of interference with any of the functions of the nervous system, so that there may be a passing visual disturbance, a short episode of weakness or loss of sensation, a brief

> Transient attacks must always be taken seriously because they are warnings of the risk of stroke. In many cases they represent what is sometimes called stroke in evolution – the gradual build-up of disability. But often they herald a massive, destructive cerebral thrombosis or cerebral haemorrhage with a full-blown stroke, coma, and often death.

loss of memory or of the ability to speak or recognize the name of something, or even a passing paralysis of one side of the body. By definition, transient ischaemic attacks last for less than twenty-four hours. Recovery is apparently complete, but, in fact, there is often a small but measurable permanent loss of function.

cerebrum

Latin root meaning 'brain' as in cerebral (of the brain).

cerivastin

A drug used in the treatment of high blood cholesterol. A brand name is Lipobay.

certoparin

A heparin-like drug used to prevent the formation of blood clots in the veins. A brand name is Alphaparin.

cerumen

See **ear wax**.

cervical

Pertaining to a neck. This may be the neck of the body, as in *cervical vertebrae* – the bones of the neck part of the spine. Or it may be the neck of an organ, as in *cervical cancer*, in which the term refers to the neck of the womb (uterus). The noun, from the adjective *cervical*, is *cervix*.

cervical cancer

See **uterus, cancer of**.

cervical erosion

An inaccurate term that persists in spite of the fact that the condition it describes is in no sense an erosion or ulcer, nor is it an inflammation or the result of infection. The term refers to a raw-looking appearance of the outer part of the neck of the womb (the cervix), which is actually caused by a normal extension of the inner lining out on to the usually smooth and lighter-coloured covering membrane. The extension of this velvety red area on to the cervix is especially common during pregnancy when the high levels of oestrogen promote growth of the lining of the canal of the cervix. Some contraceptive pills produce well-marked erosions. Occasionally this extension leads to a slight blood-stained or mucus discharge. If this is caused by the Pill, an alternative method of contraception may be preferred. Erosions are seldom seen after the menopause as oestrogen levels are lower.

Formerly all kinds of symptoms were attributed to cervical erosion and many women underwent unnecessary treatment, especially cauterization. Gynaecologists now know better, and, so long as a cervical smear shows no abnormality, the condition is usually ignored.

cervical incompetence

A tendency for the inner opening of the neck of the womb to open spontaneously and prematurely during pregnancy. This affects about one pregnancy in 100 and causes repeated, painless, spontaneous miscarriages around the fourth or fifth month. The danger can be avoided by means of a temporary encircling stitch (a Shirodkar suture), but the difficulty is to know which women are likely to be affected. Women with a history of mid-term miscarriage are obvious candidates for this minor operation, which is known as cerclage. The procedure can be done as an emergency if threatened miscarriage is detected in time.

cervical osteoarthritis

A wearing-away of the cartilage surfaces of the spinal bones (vertebrae) of the neck. The disorder is commonest in middle age and runs a slow, persistent course with episodes of pain, stiffness of the neck and sometimes tenderness on pressure over the affected area. Although X-ray may show some bony extensions from the inflamed areas, it is unusual for these to involve the nerve roots or spinal cord and cause neurological effects, as in **cervical spondylosis**.

Osteoarthritis is commonly a late sequel to bone or joint injury, such as may occur from the 'whiplash' head movement suffered by the occupants of a car struck from behind by another vehicle.

cervical rib

Normally there are no ribs in the neck, but about one person in 200 has a short, floating, rudimentary rib attached to the lowest neck vertebra on one or both sides. Most people with cervical ribs are unaware of the fact, but in about 10 per cent the rib gives trouble. The opening into the chest, at the root of the neck, is very narrow and contains many important structures, including the arteries and major nerve trunks running to the arms.

RECOGNITION AND SYMPTOMS

Compression of these arteries or nerves can cause pain and tingling in the hand, arm, shoulder or neck and, occasionally, can lead to severe effects, such as partial loss of blood supply to the arm with cold, blue, numb extremities (**Raynaud's phenomenon**) or even, rarely, gangrene of the finger tips.

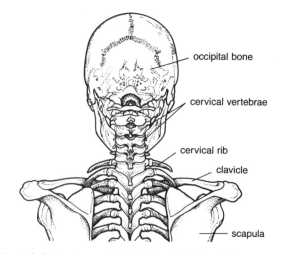

Cervical rib. An abnormal pair of ribs attached to the lowest vertebra of the neck can cause problems by leading to compression of nerves or arteries running in the confined space of the neck.

Sometimes the condition can be proved by noting that the pulse at the wrist disappears when the arm is raised and the head is turned to the opposite side.

INCIDENCE

The cervical rib syndrome, as this collection of symptoms is called, is commonest in thin, long-necked women in their forties and may occur after marked loss of weight. It has also been described in men who have developed their muscles to an unusual degree.

TREATMENT

Most cases can be controlled by physiotherapy and exercises. Surgical removal of the offending rib, or of other constricting structures in the region is sometimes needed.

cervical smear test

This important screening test has proved to be one of the most valuable ways of reducing the major problem of cancer in women. It is used to detect early cancer of the neck of the womb (cervix). The test was developed by George Nicholas Papanicolaou (1883–1962), an American pathologist of Greek origin working at Cornell Medical College, New York. If cancer of the cervix is detected at the stage at which it is still confined to the surface layer of cells, it is completely preventable. This stage is known as *carcinoma in situ* or *intraepithelial neoplasia*. All cancers start in a surface layer. In this case, cancerous change has begun, but the process has not spread below the surface.

The test is eminently worthwhile and is done on over three million women a year in Britain. As a result, there has been a striking increase in the number found to have these early changes and simple treatment can save them from the disaster of established cancer of the womb.

The 'Pap' test, as it is called in the United States, is an example of *exfoliative cytology* – a technique in which isolated cells are examined microscopically by a skilled pathologist and suspicious changes noted. Performing the Pap smear is simple; the skill lies in the interpretation of changes in the cells. A metal instrument (speculum) is gently inserted to keep the vagina open and a small, blunt-edged plastic or wooden spatula is used to scrape some cells gently from in and around the opening of the cervix. These are smeared on a microscope slide, stained, and examined.

The pathologist may find signs of inflammation from *Trichomonas vaginalis* (trichomoniasis), thrush (candidiasis), herpes and other infections, and is especially interested in the characteristic cell changes caused by the human papillomavirus – a cavity near the nucleus, or a doubling or unusually deep

staining of the nuclear (chromosomal) material. These changes are present in over 80 per cent of cases showing suspicion of malignancy. The earliest stage of possible malignant change is shown by cells with abnormal, usually enlarged, nuclei. This is called dyskaryosis.

Cytology is very difficult and can be done successfully only by experienced pathologists. Because of this difficulty, the failure to make the diagnosis (false negative rate), in the very earliest stage, is admitted to be 10 to 15 per cent. But satisfactory cytology can detect *all* cases of established carcinoma *in situ*. These facts emphasize the importance of repeated testing, especially of those with abnormal smear results. In some centres, unfortunately, the follow-up rate, following abnormal smears, is only 60 per cent.

Many experts suggest that three-yearly screening should be carried out on sexually active women over 35, women who have been pregnant three or more times and women who present for contraceptive advice. Women presenting for contraceptive advice are often advised to have a routine cervical smear test.

Those found to have abnormal smears are treated by cervical freezing, high-frequency cautery (electrodiathermy) or laser destruction of the surface layers. One treatment gives a cure rate of 95 per cent.

cervical smear test, automated

See **PAPNET**.

cervical spondylosis

A degenerative condition of the spine, in the neck region, with backward outgrowth of bone causing narrowing of the spinal canal, which contains the spinal cord. As a result, there may be compression of the cord or spinal nerve roots and sometimes serious neurological damage. Affected people may develop a stiff, scissors-like walking disorder (spastic gait) and weakness and atrophy in the arm muscles.

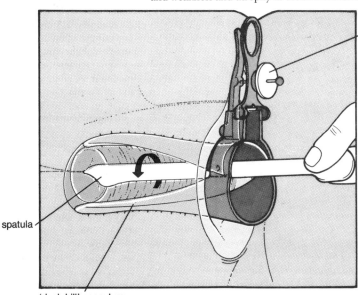

screw to keep speculum open

spatula

'duck-bill' speculum

With the vagina held open by a 'duck-billed' speculum, there is easy access to the cervix for the cervical smear test. A specially shaped wooden or plastic spatula is rotated in the mouth of the womb so as to scrape off some of the surface cells. These are then smeared on a microscope slide for examination.

In some cases, a supportive collar will relieve the symptoms, but it is often necessary to resort to surgery to relieve the pressure on the important nerve tracts in the spinal cord.

cervicitis

Inflammation of the neck of the womb (the cervix) can be an acute or a more persistent (chronic) condition.

POSSIBLE CAUSES

Most cases of acute cervicitis result from infection of the tall cells lining the canal of the cervix by germs acquired during sexual intercourse, especially *Chlamydia trachomatis*, which causes *non-specific urethritis*; the gonococcus, which causes gonorrhoea; and the *Herpes simplex* virus, type II, which causes genital herpes. Acute cervicitis may also follow childbirth or surgical widening (dilatation) of the cervix. Cervicitis seldom occurs on its own, but it usually part of a more general infection of the genital tract.

RECOGNITION AND SYMPTOMS

Surprisingly, the condition may cause no symptoms, but there may be a pussy (purulent) vaginal discharge and sometimes pain on intercourse. The organisms concerned often also cause urinary symptoms, such as frequency and a burning pain on urination.

Chronic cervicitis most commonly follows a puerperal infection of the womb lining after childbirth or abortion. The cervix becomes swollen and enlarged and contains cysts that may also become infected. There may be backache, deep pelvic pain, pain on intercourse and a persistent vaginal discharge.

TREATMENT

Both types usually respond well to antibiotics, but chronic cervicitis may require cauterization of the cervix to destroy the surface layer of cells (epithelium). Sexual partners should also be checked and treated, and intercourse should be avoided until treatment is complete.

cervix

Latin root meaning 'neck' as in cervical (of the neck).

cervix, cancer of

See **uterus, cancer of**.

cervix core removal

See **cone biopsy**.

cervix microscopic examination

See **colposcopy**.

cestodes

See **taeniasis**.

cetrimide

A detergent antiseptic and cleaning substance used in solution or as an ointment. A brand name is Cetavlon.

cetylpiridinium chloride

An antiseptic drug used in the treatment of throat and mouth infections, usually in the form of lozenges. A brand name is Merocets.

Chagas' disease

See **trypanosomiasis, South American**.

chalazion

See **meibomian cyst**.

chalky tendons

See **calcific tendinitis**.

chamomile

A drug used in ointments for the treatment of nappy rash, chapped skin or sore nipples. A brand name is Kamillosan.

chancre, hard

The painless, hard-based primary sore of syphilis, which appears on the genitals within four weeks of exposure. The chancre is a shallow ulcer with a base resembling wet chamois-leather, which oozes a clear serum that is teeming with the spirochaetes that cause the disease. A chancre must never be ignored. Healing merely means that the organisms have spread into the body where they will later cause all kinds of serious problems. Syphilis can be proved by taking a fluid sample from a chancre. Even after healing, a blood test for syphilis will always show, retrospectively, whether or not a suspicious genital sore was a chancre.

chancroid

See **sexually transmitted diseases**.

chapped skin

See **skin, chapped**.

Charcot-Marie-Tooth disease

A hereditary disorder of the nervous system causing weakness and atrophy of the muscles of the lower legs, followed later by atrophy of the small muscles of the hands. The disorder causes a characteristic 'peg-leg' deformity, with narrowing of the lower leg and foot drop. Unfortunately, there is no effective treatment. Leg braces often help.

Charcot's joints

Several conditions can affect the sensory nerves carrying sensation from the joints. The result is that pain from repeated minor injury or trauma is not felt and the normal protective responses, such as rest and avoidance of damaging activity, do not occur. Because of the absence of warning, severe damage to the joints may occur.

RECOGNITION AND SYMPTOMS

The condition may, initially, be confused with ordinary osteoarthritis, but the severity of the destructive changes soon make it apparent that a more serious process is going on. Joints become greatly swollen from fluid accumulation and internal bleeding. The breakdown of the wearing surfaces, the production of many cartilaginous loose bodies from the wearing surfaces, and the laxity of the ligaments produce weak, unstable joints from which coarse grating sounds may be heard on movement. Because of the loss of sensation, the effect is more distressing to the observer than to the victim.

POSSIBLE CAUSES

Causes of Charcot's joints include syphilis, diabetes, leprosy, tumours of the spinal cord, syringomyelia, a neurological complication of **pernicious anaemia** known as subacute combined degeneration of the cord, **Charcot-Marie-Tooth disease** and excessive steroid injections into the joints.

cheilitis

Inflammation of the lips. Cheilitis is often caused by sunlight or by thrush. The condition may also result from vitamin B_2 deficiency, streptococcal or staphylococcal infection or constant drooling at the corners of the mouth. Chronic fissuring at the angles of the mouth due to any of these causes is called perleche.

cheilos

Greek root meaning 'lip' as in cheilosis (lip disorder).

chemonucleolysis

The use of an enzyme injected into the inner pulpy centre of a disc between the bones of the spine (intervertebral disc), so as to break down and liquefy the material. This is done in cases of prolapsed disc pulp (**slipped disc**), with pressure on the nerve roots in the spinal canal, in the hope that the pressure will be relieved and the neurological damage reversed. Chemonucleolysis remains an experimental procedure and the results, so far, do not always appear to justify the early enthusiasm.

chemoprophylaxis

The use of drugs or antibacterial chemical agents to prevent the development or spread of infectious diseases.

chemotherapy

The internal use of chemical agents to treat disease, especially infections, infestations and tumours. At one time, the antibiotics were excluded from this group, as being of natural origin, but as many of these have been synthesized this distinction has become too fine. Chemotherapeutic agents include drugs used against viruses, microbes, fungi, protozoa, worms and other parasites, and cancer.

chest/abdomen partition

See **diaphragm**.

chest, central partition of

See **mediastinum**.

chest examination

This entry is concerned with the respiratory system as opposed to an examination of the heart. The examination starts with an inspection of the chest, the symmetry, range and equality of movement, and the degree of possible expansion being noted. The doctor checks the rate of breathing and observes whether there is anything unusual about the character of the chest movements. He or she would not, for instance, fail to notice if each inspiration stopped suddenly, at the same point, with a grunt of pain from the patient –

a feature of pleurisy. Deep, laboured breathing, assisted shoulder movements and the neck muscles, indicates difficulty in getting enough oxygen to meet the basic respiratory needs – a state of affairs calling for urgent action.

After inspection, the doctor feels in the central notch between the collar bones to confirm that the wind pipe (trachea) is lying centrally. Deviation to one side may indicate partial collapse of one lung – a cause of breathlessness at rest. With both hands symmetrically placed on the lower parts of the chest, the doctor will check whether the expansion is equal on the two sides.

The normal chest is partly hollow and resonant, and percussion is an important part of the examination. Fluid in the space between the lungs and the chest wall will cause a very dull note on percussion, as will the solidification of the lung substance that occurs in lobar pneumonia. On the other hand, if the pleural space is filled with air, as in a spontaneous pneumothorax, the percussion note will be very resonant.

Even in this era of MRI and CT scanning, listening to the chest with a stethoscope can provide valuable information about the state of the lungs and their linings. This is called auscultation.

chest pain

Chest pain is a major source of concern to many people, especially to middle-aged men who, aware that central chest pain may signal heart trouble, quite rightly fear that this symptom may be an intimation of mortality. Chest pain, however, has many causes and the characteristics and quality of the pain differ in these different conditions.

Angina pectoris and the pain of **heart attack** (coronary thrombosis) are the most feared, but, contrary to the general belief, these are not identical. Anginal pain is always related to exercise and usually comes on after a fixed energy expenditure, such as walking a predictable distance. It is of very variable intensity, even in the same person, and may be affected by the temperature, the state of mind and the condition of the digestion. The pain may be so mild as to be hardly a pain – more a feeling of uneasiness or pressure in the chest – or so severe as to arrest all action. It often causes breathlessness and belching. When the exertion ceases, the angina soon settles. Severe angina is very frightening. One medical sufferer commented that it was the only pain that made him fear he was going to die, or, if severe enough, that he was not going to die.

The pain of coronary thrombosis may also sometimes be mild, but is usually a crushing agony which goes on and on and is accompanied by a conviction of impending death. It often radiates up into the jaw, through to the back and down the left arm. It is associated with severe restlessness and distress and there will seldom be any doubt that something serious has happened.

Pleurisy causes a characteristic stabbing pain brought on by deep breathing. The pain is sudden and sharp and occurs at a certain point in inspiration. There is often a rubbing quality to it and it may be relieved by changing the position. There will usually be other signs of chest infection such as fever, cough and sputum.

The burning pain caused by reflux of stomach acid into the gullet (heartburn) may be felt in the centre or lower part of the chest and can be intense. It is unrelated to exercise but may be related to emotion or dietary indiscretion. It rises

then usually subsides after a few minutes.
...iated with belching.

... (see **peptic ulcer**) causes chest pain,
... between the lower ribs. This pain is
...mes on in the middle of the morning
... It is depressing in the regularity of its
..., coming on again, with characteristically accurate
timing, two or three hours after a meal. It often wakes the
sufferer at one or two o'clock in the morning. The pain of a
stomach ulcer differs in that it is caused rather than relieved
by food.

Persistent chest pain may also be due to:

- **bronchitis**;
- **lung cancer**;
- **tuberculosis**;
- **shingles**;
- chest wall injuries;
- **Bornholm disease**;
- secondary cancer, affecting the ribs.

Chest pain should always be investigated. The majority of
cases are due to innocent causes, but unless the cause is obvious, it is not a symptom which can safely be ignored.

chest pain on exertion, worsening

See **unstable angina**.

chest wall pain

See **Tietze's syndrome**.

chest X-ray

This form of examination has by no means been displaced by
more modern methods of imaging. Chest X-ray is capable of
providing invaluable information at comparatively low cost.
The risk, from radiation, of an occasional chest X-ray is
minimal and is greatly outweighed by the health benefit.
Due to its structure, the chest is uniquely suitable for X-ray
examination and a plain film of the chest gives a wider range
of information than a routine X-ray of any other part
of the body.

Routine chest X-rays are done from back to front, with the
shoulders pressed forward and the hands on the hips, so as to
get the shoulder blades (scapulae) out of the way. Side-to-side
(lateral view) X-rays are taken only if the front view reveals an
abnormality which can be better shown, or better localized,
by using the side view.

The chest film shows any abnormality, such as a fracture,
cyst or tumour, of the ribs, breast bone (sternum), mid-spine
and collar bones (clavicles). The upper points (apices) of the
lungs are well shown, as are the whole of the right lung field
and most of the field of the left lung. The roots of the two
lungs, with the lymph nodes situated there, can be well seen
especially on the right side. These areas may show mottling
from bronchopneumonia; tumour masses in lung cancer;
cavities from tuberculosis; calcified glands or lung areas from
old healed infections; disease or enlargement of lymph nodes
or areas of lung which have collapsed or become solid from
lobar pneumonia. The bases of the lungs and the curve of the
diaphragm are well revealed and evidence of lung and
pleural disease may be manifest. The state of the air tubes
(bronchial tree) can, to a limited extent, be judged from a
plain chest X-ray, but much more information can be
obtained by the simultaneous use of a substance opaque to X-
rays sprayed into the bronchi.

The heart shadow occupies much of the centre of the
chest and, while tending to obscure a part of the left lung, can
provide much information, especially about enlargement of
the left or right lower chambers (ventricles) or about abnormalities of the great vessels.

The above is a mere outline of the range of information
an experienced and knowledgeable radiologist can obtain
from a chest X-ray. The development of more refined
methods of imaging, such as the CT and MRI scans, has not
rendered the chest X-ray obsolete, and as a first step in the
investigation of chest disease of all kinds, it still remains indispensable. Imaging technology is advancing rapidly, however,
and it is probable that, in the years to come, radiation will be
replaced by other modalities of investigation.

Cheyne-Stokes respiration

This is a serious sign seldom encountered except in grave
illness and impending death. The breathing stops for a few
seconds, then resumes, at first being so shallow that it is barely
perceptible, but then increasing in depth to a maximum. It
then gradually diminishes in volume until it again stops. This
cycle repeats, and in most cases ends in permanent cessation.

chickenpox

This is an infectious disease of childhood caused by the varicella-zoster virus which also causes shingles in adults.
Chickenpox is usually a trivial disease, a minor event of
childhood which often passes almost unnoticed. It generally
occurs between the ages of two and eight, and is often
picked up at school and then passed round the other susceptible members of the family. It can be acquired from a
case of shingles, but the normal source is the dispersal of
infected droplets coughed out by another person infected
with chickenpox. Spread in this way can occur before the
skin rash appears, and is one reason for the high infectivity
of the disease. Chickenpox is one of the most highly infectious of all diseases. The skin blisters are teeming with
viruses and are also infectious, but the viruses can only live
for a few hours outside the body and this is not an important
mode of spread.

Chickenpox is most common in the winter and spring and
nearly all cases occur in epidemics, once every three years or
so. The signs appear after an incubation period of ten days to
three weeks. The trouble starts with a slight fever and a feeling of being unwell (malaise) and there may be headache
and aching in the muscles. At this stage, tiny blisters, full of
viruses, form in the mouth and throat and these ulcerate to
provide the source of infection to others.

The rash begins as tiny, flat, red spots which quickly
become small blisters (vesicles). These soon turn milky, dry to
crusts, form scabs and drop off. The sequence, from spot to
scab, takes only twelve to twenty-four hours and successive
crops occur for one to six days. Chickenpox is almost always
a very mild disease in childhood, but this is not the case if it
is acquired for the first time in adult life. It is therefore sensible not to try to protect young children from the infection, so
that they can enjoy the immunity that one attack confers.

One good reason for this is that adults with chickenpox
often suffer complications. Up to one-third suffer a persistent

form of pneumonia and this is sometimes severe. Occasionally, an adult with chickenpox develops brain inflammation (encephalitis), but this is rare. Adult chickenpox in early pregnancy can, infrequently, cause congenital malformations in the fetus.

After the chickenpox has resolved, the viruses settle in the nervous system and are kept in check by the immune system. Much later in life, with a drop in immunity, these viruses may be reactivated to cause shingles. Exposure to cases of chickenpox during adult life actually helps to reduce the likelihood of later shingles, probably by boosting the immune system, much in the manner of a vaccine.

Chief Medical Officer (CMO)

A senior doctor, appointed by the British Government, who is roughly the equivalent of the US Surgeon-General. The functions of the Chief Medical Officer (CMO) include:

- monitoring the health of the nation and and determining the factors that influence it;
- acting as a spokesperson for the medical profession;
- ensuring that all relevant government departments are kept effectively in touch with the medical profession on all matters of importance to the public welfare;
- ensuring that the United Kingdom is adequately represented internationally on medical matters.

He or she is also CMO to a range of Government departments including the Home Office, the Department of Education, the Social Security Department and the Department of Agriculture, Fisheries and Food. The CMO is also prominently involved as chairperson or as a committee member of various Health Department and national research bodies.

chiggers

The harvest mites *Trombicula*, known as chiggers, are commonly encountered in the fields in autumn. They are inconspicuous and often remain feeding on the skin for several days. The bites of these persistent little parasites will cause great irritation, a form of scabies, and sometimes a severe case of dermatitis. The remedy is avoidance and the use of insect repellents. Chiggers transmit a form of typhus, known as scrub typhus in the Far East, especially in Southeast Asia. Chiggers should not be confused with **chigoe** fleas.

chigoe

Tunga penetrans, sometimes called the 'jigger flea' or chigoe, is a parasite of man, common in tropical Africa and tropical America, which burrows under the skin, often under the big toe-nail or elsewhere on the feet. This is a favourite activity of the female flea after she has been mating and, although very small at the time of burrowing, she soon grows to the size of a pea because of the enormous swelling of her abdomen from a mass of eggs. A person may have as many as thirty of these incursions at one time.

In endemic areas, the inhabitants become adept at winkling out these gravid females, but sometimes the attempt ends in widespread infection and even death from sepsis. The chigoe can be avoided by wearing high boots and by using insect repellents.

chilblain

A raised, red, round itchy swelling of the skin of the fingers and toes occurring in cold weather. The condition, together with other related disorders, is dignified by the title of *perniosis*. The disorder is essentially due to the severe narrowing that cold can cause in the small arteries supplying the part with blood. Lack of circulation through the part leads to tissue damage from shortage of oxygen and glucose fuel. At the same time, damaging bodies such as immune complexes and bacteria accumulate at the sites. Things are made worse if garters or other constriction in clothing interfere with the blood supply. Chilblains can be avoided by keeping the extremities warm.

child abuse

This subject attracts euphemisms, and doctors usually talk about *non-accidental injury* when they mean assaults on children.

INCIDENCE

About 100 children die every year in Britain from assault and countless more lead lives of continual misery and fear. People who assault children have often had a bad start in life and many were, themselves, the victims of childhood assault. They are usually young – in their late teens or twenties – often socially inadequate and improvident and commonly have financial or emotional problems.

Unemployment, unwanted pregnancy, debt, crime, frustrated expectations and hopelessness are common features of families in which abuse occurs. But the problem is not confined to the lower socio-economic groups: child abuse occurs at every level in society. As a rule, one parent is responsible for the assaults, but the other is almost always aware of what is going on.

Child abuse may take the form of active assault or neglect, and the latter may be physical or emotional. Sustained emotional cruelty is more likely to cause life-long damage than occasional purely physical assaults in a context of reasonable affection. Certain injuries are characteristic of physical abuse (see **battered baby syndrome**).

Sexual abuse is even commoner than other forms of assault. It is estimated that one girl in ten and one boy in fifteen, under the age of sixteen, is sexually abused, usually by a father, stepfather or other resident of the house.

RECOGNITION AND SYMPTOMS

Sexually abused children show precocious awareness of sexual matters and this may be evident in their language, play and drawings. They often show sudden changes in behaviour such as loss of trust in parents and they may openly allege what has happened. Such allegations are usually true. They often have injuries of the genitalia, in girls, and of the anus, in either sex. They may have urinary infections or venereal disease. The anal dilatation test – a tendency for the anus to open when the skin is gently pulled – is only one of many factors which doctors must consider in making up their minds in suspicious cases.

Sexual abuse is often followed by serious long-term psychiatric effects and major difficulties in establishing proper sexual relationships and adjustments. Suicide is common.

TREATMENT

Public awareness of child abuse is growing and children now have a better chance of defending themselves. Greater open-

gain medical attention

...nce, encouragement to report abuse,
...d counselling centres are all helping.

ain medical attention

...drome by proxy.

...ldbed fever

See **natural childbirth**.

childbirth

By the end of the average pregnancy the pregnant woman is
carrying a considerable extra load – fetus, amniotic fluid,
placenta and a greatly enlarged womb. The prospect of childbirth and relief from all the resulting discomfort is, for most,
a welcome one. The process by which the baby is expelled
from the womb to live a relatively independent existence is
called labour and this is an appropriate term, for delivering a
baby is very hard work indeed.

The term says nothing about the pain that is almost inseparable from giving birth. In spite of this, however, to most
women, childbirth is one of the highlights of their lives and
an intensely rewarding experience.

The womb is a powerful muscular bag and it is by the contraction of the muscular wall that the baby is expelled from
the womb down through the vagina to the outside world.
Contractions squeeze the baby down, causing progressive
opening of the neck and outlet of the womb. The natural tendency of the stretched and stimulated womb is to tighten
strongly and expel its contents. This sometimes happens
before the fetus has reached full term, giving rise to a
miscarriage or to premature labour. One reason why it normally does not do so is that the womb does not increase in
size simply by passive stretching but actually grows with the
size of the fetus. Because of this, it does not normally reach
the state of tension that causes it to contract strongly enough
to expel the fetus.

Minor contractions occur from time to time during
pregnancy, but these are not strong enough to overcome the
resistance of the narrow outlet. As far as we know, it is likely
that natural body substances known as prostaglandins are the
cause of the onset of strong contractions at full term. Rupture
of the membranes that surround the fetus causes a release of
prostaglandins, as does stretching the canal of the cervix. If,
for any reason, the baby is more than about two weeks overdue, doctors can give prostaglandin drugs to get things going.

Like pregnancy, labour is divided into three stages.

The first stage lasts from the time the woman becomes
aware that the pains have started until the time the cervix is
fully opened (dilated). To begin with, the interval between
pains is usually about twenty minutes and, initially, contractions are minor and occur at irregular intervals. Soon, however,
they increase in strength and frequency until they are intense
and occurring every two or three minutes.

In the first stage the pain is mostly due to the stretching of
the cervix. During each contraction the womb can be felt to
harden. Each contraction lasts for forty to fifty seconds, during which time the pain rises to a maximum and then dies
down again. In some cases pains occur at about five-minute
intervals from the outset. As the pains become more frequent, they become more severe and also last a little longer.
It is rare, however, for a pain to last longer than a minute.

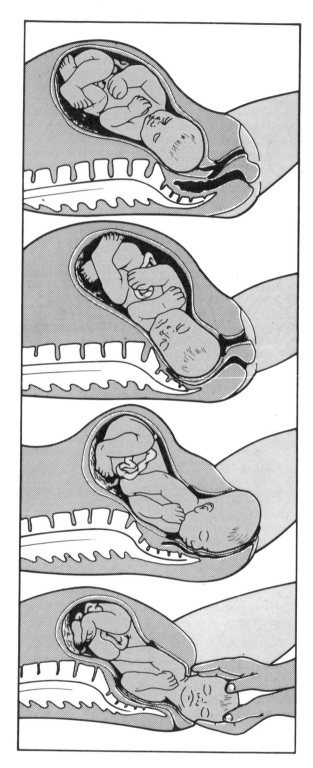

*The various stages of the descent of the baby's head, and the
stretching of the cervix of the womb, and the vagina, during
delivery.*

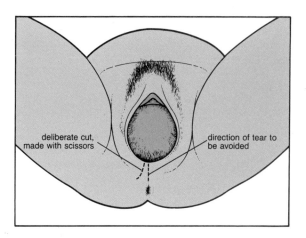

When the outlet is unusually tight and there is a risk of a tear, it is important to ensure that this occurs to one side. A tear directly backwards can weaken the muscle attachments to the floor of the pelvis and may even involve the anus.

This is just as well, as womb contractions can cut off the blood supply to the fetus.

By the end of the first stage, pains may be occurring every two or three minutes. As the canal of the cervix is widened and pulled up by the contracting wall of the womb (see illustration), the lower part of the membranes are separated from the wall of the womb. This causes a slight oozing of blood. At the same time the mucus in the cervix is squeezed out. The mixture of blood and mucus is called the show, and this is an indication that labour is getting under way. Towards the end of the first stage the fluid-filled membranes surrounding the fetus are forced down into the cervix and eventually rupture, releasing a gush of amniotic fluid. This is known as the 'breaking of the waters'.

Sometimes the membranes rupture spontaneously at an earlier stage; when they do so labour is likely to follow almost immediately. Quite often, the membranes are ruptured deliberately by the obstetrician during labour, as this allows the baby's head to descend and press on the cervix – widening it more efficiently. The results of six major trials, published in the *British Medical Journal* in August, 1994, suggest that routine rupture of the membranes offers no real advantage to mother or baby.

In a woman having her first baby (a primigravida), the first stage should not last longer than twelve hours. In subsequent pregnancies, the first stage is often much shorter. The duration of this stage depends on various factors such as the effectiveness of the contractions, the size and position of the baby, and whether the mother has had a previous delivery. A fully dilated cervix is about 10 cm in diameter.

Towards the end of the first stage, as the cervix is reaching full dilation, the pains may be very severe, frequent and distressing. Because she does not feel the cervix widening, the woman in labour has no indication, other than what she is told, that any progress is being made. She may therefore think that her pains are ineffective. However, in normal labour, severe pains almost always indicate that all is going as it should. There are many ways in which doctors and midwives can help to control pain at this stage so that mothers are not required to bear too much. But unless she is given total relief by anaesthesia, having a baby inevitably involves pain

for the mother (see below). Sometimes, dispropo between the baby's head and the pelvic opening preve progress in labour and the cervix remains only partially dilated. In such cases a Caesarean section may be necessary.

The second stage of labour is the stage of actual birth and lasts from the time of full dilation of the cervix to the completion of the delivery of the baby. By now the resistance of the cervix has been overcome so that the baby's head can descend to the muscular floor of the pelvis. For the mother to be able to expel the baby she now needs to overcome the resistance caused by the pelvic floor. She does this by pushing downward, using much the same method employed on the toilet when constipated. This is called bearing down and is partly voluntary, partly automatic.

The second stage should not last longer than an hour in a primigravida. In women who have already had babies it may be much shorter. As the baby's head is forced through the pelvis the mother may experience cramping pain in her legs from pressure on the nerves emerging from the lower part of her spinal cord. The vaginal wall is capable of being remarkably stretched, but the vaginal outlet often becomes painfully distended and is frequently in danger of tearing. To allow the outlet to stretch gradually, the advancing baby's head is often held back for a time by external pressure by the midwife's or obstetrician's hand.

Sometimes, in order to prevent the outlet tearing back into the anus or forward into the urine tube (urethra), a deliberate sideways cut is made. This is called an episiotomy and it is done when there are strong indications that tearing of the tissues in an undesirable direction is imminent. Such a tear can have undesirable long-term consequences. Episiotomy is also done to make delivery easier and may be necessary if forceps have to be used.

Once the head is born the baby's body follows quickly, either during the same or the next contraction. Until the placenta is delivered, the umbilical cord remains emerging from the vagina. Again, the times are variable and the second stage may take only a few minutes or several hours. Under proper supervision a long second stage is uncommon.

The third stage is the period from the delivery of the baby to the delivery of the after-birth (placenta). This stage usually lasts for about five minutes, but often the placenta is delivered immediately after the baby. As the baby leaves the womb the walls close down behind it and, as the area of the inner wall shrinks, the placenta is separated by the resulting shearing force. A few further contractions force the placenta downwards into the lower part of the womb or the upper part of the vagina. This causes the mother to feel the need to bear down once again and the placenta is delivered along with a small quantity of blood. Sometimes there is delay and occasionally the placenta is retained and has to be pushed out by squeezing the womb through the lax abdominal wall or even removed by putting a gloved hand into the womb (manual removal).

When the placenta has been delivered, any episiotomy incision or tear is repaired by careful suturing and the mother is checked for post-partum bleeding. Severe haemorrhage at this stage is a surgical emergency calling for urgent treatment.

Soon the womb has come down so that it lies just below the level of the navel and it can be felt as a hard muscular ball. The pituitary hormone oxytocin causes this contraction of

ocic drug can be used to assist in womb
r pituitary hormone, prolactin, promotes
the breasts, soon after delivery.

by is born it is tilted head-down so that
or mouth may drain out. If necessary,
, soft plastic tube is used to clear the
umbilical cord is tied with fine cord or clamped
and cut. The vital signs are checked – breathing, pulse, skin
colour, muscle tone and reflexes. These points are used to
determine the Apgar score – an assessment of the baby's overall general condition.

Babies are provided with two name tags, one on an ankle
and one on a wrist, which prevent the possibility of anyone
taking home the wrong baby.

The first milk to be secreted after delivery is a thick, yellowish, protein-rich, fluid called colostrum. This is produced
by the breasts for the first two or three days after the birth of
the baby. Colostrum contains large fat globules and is especially valuable for the nutrition of the newborn baby. The
immune system of the new baby has not yet had time to
mature fully, and as the baby has not yet been exposed to an
infected environment, there has not been time for the development of antibodies against infection. The mother's blood,
however, contains many antibodies and these are secreted in
considerable quantity in the colostrum. This substantial
intake of antibodies is of great value to the new baby to tide it
over the first few weeks of life, and offers invaluable control
of infection. This is one of the reasons why breastfeeding is
always to be preferred, if possible, to bottle-feeding.

As the colostrum changes to normal breast milk, its colour
changes to bluish-white.

PAIN CONTROL IN LABOUR

There is no reason why any woman in labour should suffer
excessive pain. As the pains become more severe towards the
end of the first stage, drugs such as pethidine are usually
given by injection if the woman wishes. Another commonly
used method of pain control is inhalation of the gases nitrous
oxide and oxygen, called entinox or 'gas and air'. This is
done as each pain starts. This, too, can be under the woman's
own control. Some women find **TENS** (Transcutaneous
Electrical Nerve Stimulation) helpful.

Epidural anaesthesia is popular for childbirth because,
although highly effective in the relief of pain, it has no effect
on the contractions of the womb or on the respiratory centre
of the baby. Epidural anaesthesia is safer than general
anaesthesia, especially if this has to be given urgently to an
unprepared patient who may have eaten recently and who
will be liable to vomit – a dangerous complication during full
general anaesthesia. Epidural anaesthesia is also generally
safer than a spinal anaesthetic in which the drug is injected
into the cerebrospinal fluid surrounding the spinal cord.

The spinal cord is surrounded by a tough membrane
called the dura mater. Outside the dura lies the epidural
space between the dura and the bony canal of the spine, and
it is into this space that an anaesthetic drug is injected to produce epidural anaesthesia. The needle is passed into the
space between two of the spinal bones in the small of the back
(lumbar vertebrae) and a fine plastic tube is then passed
through the needle and the end left in the epidural space so
that anaesthetic can be injected from time to time as needed.
This is a skilled procedure requiring the services of an experienced anaesthetist. It is valuable for long-term anaesthesia

but diminishes the voluntary assistance the mother-to-be can
give, and forceps have to be used more often than in deliveries without anaesthetic.

PROBLEMS IN CHILDBIRTH

During its life in the womb the fetus is wholly dependent on
its mother's blood supply for all its nutritional requirements.
The whole of the fetal growth is derived from nutrients that
pass to it from the mother's circulation. The link between the
two circulations is the umbilical cord – the irregular, varicose-
looking supply pipe which connects the fetus to the placenta.
The umbilical cord is 40 to 60 cm long, and usually arises
from the centre of the placenta. It is covered with a thin membrane and consists of a jelly-like substance through which run
two arteries and a vein. Sometimes, there is only one artery,
which may indicate an abnormality of the fetal kidneys.

During delivery, the umbilical cord may, rarely, come
down alongside the baby's head and may be compressed.
This immediately cuts off most of the blood supply to the
fetus and is an emergency, calling for an immediate
Caesarean section (see below). Quite often, the cord is found
wrapped tightly around the baby's neck. After the baby is
born the cord is tied off and cut about 2.5 cm from the
abdomen. The stump falls off within a week or two, leaving a
scar, which is known as the navel or umbilicus.

Abnormal positioning of the placenta on the inside of the
womb can give rise to problems. Its position is determined by
the point at which the very early embryo implants (see
above). Sometimes the embryo passes well down inside the
womb before it attaches and, as a result, the placenta develops in the lower part of the womb. It may even extend over
and completely occlude the outlet so that there is no possibility of the baby being delivered normally.

This misfortune is called placenta praevia. Attempts to
deliver in the presence of a placenta praevia would lead to
dangerous bleeding and risk to the baby. Fortunately, the
condition is easily detected at an early stage by ultrasound
and a Caesarean section operation arranged.

During labour, or even before it, the placenta will sometimes begin to separate from the wall of the womb. This
deprives the fetus of nutrition and delivery may become
urgently necessary. Placental separation causes pain and vaginal bleeding.

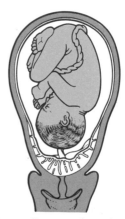

*Sometimes the placenta lies across the outlet of the uterus
(placenta praevia). This is a serious complication as the baby
cannot be delivered without first dangerously displacing the
placenta. A Caesarean section is often done.*

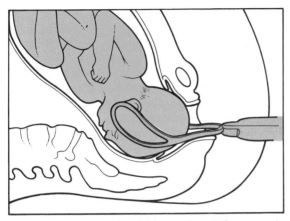

In obstructed or long-delayed delivery, obstetric forceps can be used to ease out the baby. The separate blades lock in such a way as to avoid squeezing the baby's skull, but temporary pressure marks are common.

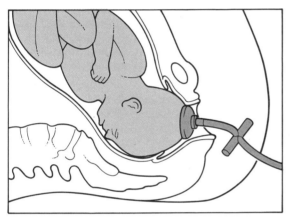

Vacuum extraction, using a suction instrument called a ventouse, is more commonly used nowadays.

Breech delivery is bottom-first birth, and it occurs, usually by chance, in about 3 per cent of labours. In most cases the baby's legs are straight but fully bent at the hips so that they lie along the body. Occasionally the knees are bent so that the buttocks and feet appear together.

Breech delivery is slightly more dangerous for the baby than normal head-first delivery, and there is a mortality of between 2 and 5 per cent in uncomplicated cases. In small premature babies, the mortality, with breech delivery, is somewhat higher. The main risk is of physical damage to the baby's brain from difficult manipulation and of brain damage from lack of oxygen caused by compression of the cord during delay in delivery. It is often necessary to deliver the head using obstetric forceps after the body has been born. Because of these risks, breech deliveries should always be conducted in hospital by an experienced obstetrician.

If detected at an early stage, a breech presentation may sometimes be turned to a normal presentation by careful external manipulation through the mother's abdominal wall. This is done after the thirty-second or thirty-fourth week and is not always free from risk. Sometimes the procedure causes separation of the placenta from the inside wall of the womb. Caesarean section (see below) is an alternative option.

Delay in delivery, with undue prolongation of the second stage, often calls for some help from the doctor. This necessary if the baby is showing signs of distress – indicating danger – or if the mother is becoming exhausted. Commonly forceps are applied to the baby's head in order to pull carefully along with the efforts of the mother. Forceps have separate blades and handles which are locked together after the blades have been placed around the baby's head.

A useful alternative to forceps delivery is vacuum extraction using an instrument called a ventouse, or vacuum extractor. A suction cup is pressed over the central part of the baby's head. This cup is connected by tubing to a vacuum pump and can be partially evacuated so that it adheres strongly to the head. A short chain with a handle is attached to the cup and by means of this, gentle traction can be applied in time with each womb contraction. In this way the baby can be safely delivered at the cost of a temporary and harmless swelling, or, at the worst, a large blood clot (cephalhaematoma), on the top of its head. The haematoma, although initially unsightly, absorbs within a month.

CAESAREAN SECTION

This is an operation, often performed in an emergency, to remove a baby from the womb of a pregnant woman through an incision in the wall of the abdomen. Contrary to popular belief, Julius Caesar was not born by Caesarean section. The origin of the term is uncertain but it may come from the Latin word *caedare*, meaning 'to cut', or from the name of the Roman law *Lex Caesarea*, which was originally enacted by Numa Pompilius (762–715 BC), and which required that any woman who died in late pregnancy should have her abdomen cut open so that the baby might be saved.

Caesarean section has become very common. About 25 per cent of babies born in the USA are delivered in this way. The operation has saved millions of babies' lives and the indications for performing it are now universally accepted.

Reasons for performing a Caesarean include:

- signs of fetal distress during labour, as judged by fetal heart monitoring and the passage of bowel contents;
- failure of normal womb contractions (uterine inertia);
- severe bleeding before delivery (antepartum haemorrhage);
- severe high blood pressure in the mother (see pre-eclampsia above);
- severe rhesus incompatibility disease;
- placenta praevia (see above);
- gross disproportion between the baby's head and the mother's pelvis, usually because the pelvic outlet is abnormally narrow;
- an unduly large baby, as in maternal diabetes;
- severe prematurity – very small babies are at risk of brain haemorrhage during normal delivery;
- the appearance of the umbilical cord before the baby's head;
- presentation of the fetal shoulder or arm, instead of the head – normal delivery is impossible and turning the baby in the womb can endanger it;
- breech (buttocks first) presentation;
- twins that have become locked together so that neither can be delivered;
- serious heart or other disease in the mother so that labour would be dangerous for her.

The modern Caesarean section is performed through an incision in the lower abdomen and a horizontal incision low in the womb. The low incision avoids unnecessary weakening of

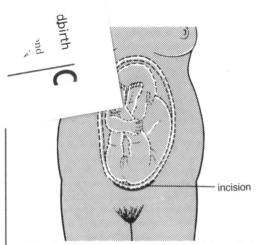

incision

When the baby cannot safely be delivered through the vagina, a Caesarean section is used. The incision is made horizontally in the lowest part of the uterus. This allows the operation to be followed by other pregnancies as damage to the uterus is minimal.

the womb muscles and allows the operation to be performed repeatedly on the same woman, if necessary. The operation is performed under general or epidural anaesthesia.

Once the abdomen is opened, the bladder is pushed down off the womb and a short transverse cut is made into the lower part of the womb and carefully deepened until the internal membranes of the womb begin to bulge through. These are kept intact and the incision enlarged sideways, by pulling with the hooked fingers, until it is wide enough to allow delivery of the baby. The membranes are now ruptured and the head delivered, followed by the body.

The placenta soon separates and is removed. The wall of the womb is closed with absorbable stitches and the abdominal wound is then closed in layers.

WOMB INFECTION

The serious and once often-fatal infection of the raw area on the lining of the womb, left after separation of the after-birth (placenta), is known as puerperal sepsis. The organism responsible is the streptococcus bacterium. Today, because of antibiotics, the condition is almost unknown, but in earlier times it took a terrible toll among women who had just given birth.

DEATH IN CHILDBIRTH

Readers of earlier literature will be aware of the tragic frequency with which women used to die giving birth to children. Indeed the fact was so common as to require no explanation and none was ever given. Happily, death in childbirth is very uncommon nowadays. Today, in the developed world, only about one woman in 10,000 dies as a result of complications of pregnancy, or diseases aggravated by pregnancy.

Puerperal sepsis (see above), once the chief cause of maternal death, has been largely eliminated by a better understanding of infection and the availability of antibiotics. Today, death from puerperal sepsis, if it occurs at all, does so because medical attention is not provided – sometimes because of the wish to conceal the birth. Womb infection can also occur after a criminal abortion, and this, too, may be a reason to avoid medical attention. Nowadays, new mothers rarely die, but when they do it is from such conditions as:

- eclampsia (see above);
- severe and uncontrolled bleeding;
- blood clots from the large veins blocking the arteries in the lungs (pulmonary embolism);
- ectopic pregnancy (see above);
- rare anaesthetic accidents;
- worsening of serious pre-existing conditions such as heart disease, diabetes and some cancers.

One of the principal reasons for routine antenatal care is to anticipate, and if possible eliminate, most of the conditions that can endanger women in and after childbirth. Obstetric knowledge, skill and experience has been remarkably successful in reducing maternal mortality, and the figures for different areas reflect this expertise and the administrative efficiency with which it is applied. Some parts of Britain have maternal mortality rates as low as 8 per 100,000 – a truly remarkable medical achievement.

child guidance

When a child develops problems such as solitariness (withdrawal), obvious anxiety or phobias, serious learning diffiiculties, late and persistent bed-wetting, sleep distubances or persistently aggressive behaviour, skilled attention is required and this is best provided under the overall guidance of a child psychiatrist who will be able to distinguish the extremes of normal behaviour from the abnormal.

HOW IT'S DONE

In some cases there is an actual physical disorder, possibly neurological, and sometimes unsuspected mental retardation. Often there are psychological problems relating to earlier emotional or physical trauma, and it must be recognized that abnormal behaviour in children is often a reflection of a psychologically unhealthy family situation.

So careful and accurate diagnosis of any possible organic disorder, or of a possible external causal factor, is a first priority. This may involve referral to other specialists such as a paediatrician or a neurologist, and the psychiatrist may wish to investigate the family setting and interview both parents and, possibly, other members of the family. A psychologist specializing in the measurement of mental performance (psychometry) may be needed.

Much may be done by attention to these factors, but in some cases psychiatric treatment may be necessary. There is comparatively little interest, in Britain, in the use of classical Freudian psychoanalysis in such cases and a greater emphasis on counselling, family discussion therapy, the judicious use of drugs and, sometimes, **behaviour therapy**.

child overactivity

See **attention deficit hyperactivity disorder**.

child psychiatrist

A doctor who has qualified as a psychiatrist and has then specialized in the psychiatric problems of young children.

child sexual abuse indication

See **anal dilatation test**.

child terror at parental absence

See **separation anxiety**.

chill

A sudden short fever causing shivering (rigor) and a feeling of coldness. This may be caused by any acute infection, not necessarily of the respiratory tract.

Chinese avian influenza

A disease which, in early 1997, caused the death of thousands of chickens in Hong Kong and later in the year a small number of human cases with a few deaths. All the poultry in Hong Kong were destroyed and a serious human epidemic avoided. The illness is caused by the H5N1 influenza virus first isolated in South Africa in the 1960s. Worryingly, the common influenza A virus exhibits genetic intermingling of avian and human strains and is capable of producing new viruses with serious pandemic potential.

Chinese malaria treatment

See **quinghaosu**.

Chinese medicine

See **medicine, Chinese**.

Chinese restaurant syndrome

This unusual disorder has been the cause of some controversy. Most medical authorities believe it to be due to monosodium glutamate, an ingredient much used by Chinese cooks. The effect is said to be proportionate to the amount eaten and to vary with different people. It is claimed not to be an allergic reaction.

RECOGNITION AND SYMPTOMS

The symptoms are headache, nausea, a tight or burning sensation in the face, head and chest and sometimes dizziness and diarrhoea. Some people get alarming chest pain. The symptoms come on one to two hours after a meal containing a large amount of monosodium glutamate, especially if this is present in a soup or other solution. Monosodium glutamate in solid food appears to be less readily absorbed. The symptoms last for an hour or so and then settle, but in some cases are more severe and persistent.

RISKS

A number of other symptoms may, more rarely, be caused by large doses of monosodium glutamate. These include mental confusion, unsteadiness of gait and asthma. In these cases, however, it is likely that an allergic element is involved and anyone who has had such a reaction should take great care to avoid any further contact with monosodium glutamate. Life-threatening asthma has been reported. The moderate doses of monosodium glutamate used in cooking, generally, offer no risk except to allergic people.

chir

Greek root meaning 'hand' as in chiropodist (hand – and foot – specialist).

chiropodist (podiatrist)

An ancillary health professional concerned with the care of the feet and the treatment of minor foot complaints such as ingrowing toenails, bunions, plantar warts, foot strain, flat feet and the care of the feet of diabetics.

chiropody

A specialty devoted to the care of the feet and the treatment of minor foot complaints. Chiropodists are concerned, among other things, with ingrowing toenails, bunions, plantar warts, foot strain, flat feet and the care of the feet of diabetics. They can be especially helpful to the elderly and the infirm, who are often unable to give their feet the attention they need. In the United States, and sometimes in Britain, chiropody is known as podiatry.

chiropractic

A form of alternative therapy based on the belief that bodily disorders spring from maladjustments of the relationships of the bones of the spine. This is said to affect the nerves and, through them, the rest of the body.

HOW IT WORKS

After a careful examination of the spine, which may include X-ray, the chiropractor decides which malalignment requires correction and then attempts to achieve this by sudden pressure on a particular spot.

DOES IT WORK?

The theory behind chiropractic has no scientific foundation and is thought by medical practitioners to be inherently incapable of accurate and reliable diagnosis.

chlamydial infections

The chlamydial organisms *Chlamydia trachomatis* and *Chlamydia psittaci* were so called because they were at first thought to be **protozoa** with cloaks, or 'mantles' (chlamydia). They were then thought to be viruses, but are now known to be bacteria like small cocci. Chlamydial organisms also cause **psittacosis**.

INCIDENCE

Chlamydia cause **trachoma**, the serious eye infection which has blinded millions throughout history and which still poses a threat to sight, unless treated. Five hundred million people currently suffer from trachoma.

Chlamydia also cause widespread infection of the genital tract, especially in women, and commonly cause inflammation of the neck of the uterus (cervicitis), inflammation and blockage of the Fallopian tubes (salpingitis), and inflammation of the glands that produce sexual lubricant mucus (Bartholinitis). These infections are usually sexually transmitted. In men, the Chlamydia cause inflammation of the urine tube (urethritis), inflammation of the tubular part of the testicle (**epididymitis**) and a serious joint and eye disorder (**Reiter's syndrome**). Chlamydia is now the commonest cause of venereal disease (**sexually transmitted disease**) in Britain and the United States.

chloasma

A mask-like area of pigmentation, involving the skin around the eyes, nose, cheeks and forehead, which often affects women during pregnancy or when taking oral contraceptives. Chloasma sometimes occurs after the menopause. It tends to be worse if the skin is exposed to sunlight and will be less conspicuous if sunscreens are used. Chloasma occasionally occurs in healthy non-pregnant women and men, but in such cases investigation of possible liver disease is called for. The pigmentation usually fades in time.

num

discoloration of the face in women,
els of certain hormones, is known as the
hloasma can also be caused by oral con-
e worse by exposure to sunlight.

betaine

A sedative drug. A brand name is Welldorm.

chloral hydrate

A bitter substance used in solution as a sedative and hypnotic. A brand name is Welldorm elixir.

chlorambucil

A nitrogen-mustard drug used in the treatment of leukaemia and lymphomas including Hodgkin's disease. A brand name is Leukeran.

chloramphenicol in premature babies

See **grey baby syndrome**.

chlordiazepoxide

Abenzodiazepine sedative and tranquillizer. Millions are dependent on this and other benzodiazepine drugs and doctors are increasingly concerned. A brand name is Librium.

chlorhexidine

A disinfectant agent widely used in surgery for preoperative skin cleansing and for sterilizing instruments by soakage. A brand name is Hibitane, but numerous commercial products contain chlorhexidine.

chlormethiazole

A sedative and anticonvulsant drug related to vitamin B1 used in the management of alcohol withdrawal syndrome and especially **delirium tremens**, in **status epilepticus**, in pre-eclampsia and eclampsia and to sedate patients unfit for general anaesthesia who are having essential surgery under local anaesthesia. A brand name is Heminevrin.

chlorosis

A greenish tinge to the skin formerly associated with severe iron-deficiency **anaemia** in malnourished young women. The condition is now almost unknown.

chloroxylenol

An antiseptic drug used as a dusting powder for external use especially in obesity with skin to skin contact. A brand name is Zeasorb.

chlorpheniramine

An antihistamine drug. A brand name is Piriton.

chlorpromazine

A drug derived from phenothiazine used as an antipsychotic, a tranquilliser and to prevent vomiting (anti-emetic). A brand name is Largactil. This was the first really effective antipsychotic drug to be widely used.

chlorquinaldol

An antibacterial and antifungal drug used externally in conjunction with a topical steroid, A brand name is Locoid C.

chlortetracycline

An antibiotic obtained from the soil bacterium *Streptomyces aureofaciens*. A brand name is Aureomycin.

chlorthalidone

A **diuretic** drug of medium potency that increases the output of urine over a period of 48 hours. A brand name is Hygroton.

choking

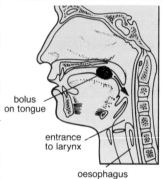
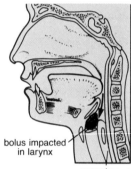

bolus on tongue

entrance to larynx

oesophagus

bolus impacted in larynx

oesophagus

Choking. A bolus of food passed over the back of the tongue normally slides straight down into the oesophagus. A sudden indrawing of breath, at the critical moment, may result in the bolus passing into the larynx. This induces a powerful coughing reflex, but if this is insufficient to expel the bolus a dangerous situation may arise.

See *First Aid*.

cholangiocarcinoma

Cancer of the bile ducts.

cholangiography

X-ray or other imaging examination of the bile ducts, usually after a fluid substance opaque to radiation has been introduced. Access may be by way of the blood-stream (*intravenous cholangiography*), by direct injection through the skin into the liver (*percutaneous, transhepatic angiography*) or, by way of an endoscope, through the bile duct opening into the duodenum (*endoscopic retrograde cholangiography*). The object of cholangiography is to show stones in the bile ducts and gall-bladder.

cholangitis

Inflammation of the bile ducts. Cholangitis usually results from obstruction of the ducts by gallstones so that infected material is unable to escape into the bowel. The result is an accumulation of pus in the gall-bladder with high fever, chills and sometimes **jaundice**. Cholangitis may lead to liver abscess or eventual cirrhosis of the liver.

chole

Greek root meaning 'bile' as in cholecystitis (gall-bladder inflammation).

cholecystectomy

Surgical removal of the gall-bladder.

cholecystitis

Inflammation of the gall-bladder.

cholecystography

X-ray of the gall-bladder, usually facilitated by the use of a contrast medium, so that gallstones can be readily seen.

cholera

A highly infectious disease caused by an organism known as the *Vibrio cholerae*.

RECOGNITION AND SYMPTOMS

Symptoms start one to three days after infection and the first sign is the abrupt onset of painless, but profuse, watery diarrhoea and vomiting. Soon there is severe dehydration from fluid loss. The cholera organism produces a toxin which damages the whole lining of the small intestine, causing inflammation so intense that some of the mucous membrane inner lining of the bowel flakes off. This produces the characteristic 'rice-water' stools by which it is often recognized. There is severe thirst, weakness, wrinkling of the skin, intense cramping muscle pain, and, in about half of untreated cases, death.

SPREAD

Cholera occurs in epidemics in areas of poor sanitation, because it is spread by contaminated water supplies or food contaminated by the excreta of people with the disease. It can easily be avoided if nothing is taken which has not been boiled. Moreover, the condition is self-limiting and recovery occurs in three to six days if the amount of fluid in the body can be kept reasonably high.

TREATMENT

Water and salt replacement is the essential element in the treatment and if this is effectively done, survival and full recovery should be assured. It is not always possible, however, to replace fluid sufficiently by mouth, and intravenous infusion may be necessary. Antibiotics, such as tetracycline, are effective against the organisms, but are no substitute for efficient fluid replacement. Cholera vaccine is effective, but regular booster injections are necessary.

cholesteatoma

A rare but serious consequence of chronic, neglected middle ear infection (**otitis media**). Cholesteatoma is a tumour-like mass of cells shed by the outer layer of the infected eardrum which sometimes invades the middle ear, through a perforation in the drum, to cause serious internal damage.

Once the process has begun, it tends to progress, slowly and relentlessly, until major complications, such as brain abscess, meningitis or paralysis of the facial muscles from nerve damage, occur.

> Because of the remote possibility of cholesteatoma, middle ear infection should never be neglected.

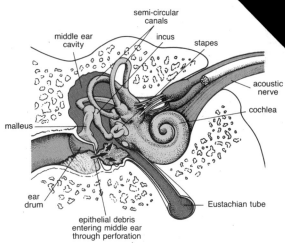

Cholesteatoma. Cells from the outside of the eardrum may continuously pass through a perforation in the drum into the middle ear where the mass may progressively expand to cause serious damage to adjacent structures.

cholesterol

Cholesterol is not, as might be thought from much that is written about it, an unmitigated menace. Cholesterol, a member of the class of compounds known as the sterols, is an essential ingredient of the body. It is found in all human cells, mainly as part of the structure of the cell membrane.

FUNCTION

Cholesterol is stored in the adrenal glands where it is converted to the essential steroid hormones, including cortisol, corticosterone, and aldosterone, and the male and female sex hormones (androgens and oestrogens). Cholesterol is also needed by the liver for the manufacture of the bile acids, from which are formed the bile salts necessary for the emulsification and absorption of fats in the diet.

Body cholesterol is derived from fatty foods but is also synthesized in the liver. If the amount obtainable from the diet is reduced, as a result of reading health advice, the liver produces more to compensate, so that the total from the two sources tends to remain constant. The rate of liver cholesterol production is under feedback control and when the dietary fat intake is high, liver cholesterol production is reduced.

POTENTIAL PROBLEMS

All dietary fats are carried first to the liver where they are processed. The liver fat output is in the form of very low density lipoprotein (VLDL) which contains cholesterol and other substances. When VLDL reaches fatty tissue, it is partially changed to low density lipoprotein (LDL) and this is the form in which cholesterol mainly moves in the blood, to and from the general tissues of the body, under the influence of various factors, including the levels of fat intake. When cholesterol moves from tissue cells back to the liver, it travels in the form of high density lipoprotein (HDL) and research has shown that high levels of HDL reduce the risk of **atherosclerosis** and heart disease. High levels of LDL, on the other hand, increase the risk.

TREATMENT

It is now believed that LDLs deposit cholesterol in the artery walls as a result of oxidation by **free radicals** and that this process can be controlled, at least to some extent, by taking antioxidants (see **anti-oxidants and vitamins**).

er feedback control, high dietary fat
to cause high blood levels of LDL and
use it is from these that cholesterol is
es of atheroma in the walls of the arter-
h reduces the levels of LDL – whether
y the use of lipid-lowering drugs – will,
duce the likelihood of developing seri-

cholesterol blood levels

See **lipid profile**.

cholesterol-control drugs

See **hydroxymethyl glutaryl co-enzyme A reductase inhibitors**.

cholesterol impunity

See **French paradox**.

cholesterol-lowering drugs

Constant high levels of fats (lipids), such as cholesterol, in the
blood are associated, among other factors, with a raised tendency to the serious arterial disease of atherosclerosis.
Atherosclerosis features raised fatty areas (plaques) inside the
arteries on which blood clots may form that can close off the
artery altogether. This is how heart attacks, strokes and gangrene of the limbs occur. Lipid-lowering drugs are given in
certain cases to reduce high levels of fats in the blood.

Most doctors now agree that there is no place for the
use of lipid-lowering drugs in people whose high blood
cholesterol levels are simply the result of an unhealthy
diet. Such drugs are no substitute for green vegetables,
fruit, fish, lean meat, skimmed milk, wholegrain bread an
fiibre. There are some people, however, for whom they ar
especially valuable. These are people whose high blood
lipid levels are a feature of a genetic disorder known as
familial hyperlipidaemia.

These drugs work in different ways. Most of the body cholesterol is synthesized in the liver, and some drugs interfere with
the chemical activators (enzymes) which do this. Others interfere with the absorption of cholesterol-containing bile salts
from the intestine. They do this by binding to the cholesterol to
form an unabsorbable compound that is lost in the faeces. Very
large amounts of cholesterol come down the bile duct into the
intestine every day but most of this is reabsorbed into the blood
with the food. Low levels of bile salts in the blood prompts the
liver to convert more cholesterol into bile. Lipid-lowering drugs
include cholestyramine (Questran A), clofibrate (Atromid-S),
probucol (Lurselle), and the statin drugs (atorvastatin, cerivastatin, fluvastatin, pravastatin and simvastatin). There is evidence
that it is harmful to lower the blood cholesterol unduly. The
side-effects of lipid-lowering drugs include diarrhoea, nausea
and an increased tendency to form gallstones.

cholesterol transport in body

See **lipoproteins**.

cholestyramine

A drug used in the treatment of **hyperlipidaemias**. It is an
anion-exchange resin that binds bile acids so that they cannot
be reabsorbed and are lost in the stools. This stimulates the
conversion of body cholesterol into more bile acids. A brand
name is Questran.

cholinesterase inhibitors

Drug or agents that block the action of cholinesterase so that
acetylcholine accumulates, often dangerously. The insecticides malathion and parathion are cholinesterase inhibitors,
as are the drugs physostigmine (eserine), neostigmine,
edrophonium, pyridostigmine, tacrine, demecarium and
ambendonium. Other cholinesterase inhibitors are the nerve
gases sarin, soman and tabun. Sarin has a lethal dose in
humans of less than 1 mg.

chondritis

Inflammation of cartilage. This is usually associated with
mechanical injury or prolonged wearing stress, as in the cartilage of a weight-bearing joint in an obese person.

chondromalacia patellae

A mild form of **osteoarthritis**, common in children and young
adolescents, affecting the cartilage on the back of the kneecap (patella) and causing pain and stiffness, especially when
climbing or descending stairs. The condition is thought to be
due to a slight displacement of the patella to one side from
an unbalanced pull by the thigh muscles, whose tendon
incorporates the bone.

Unless the patellar-bearing surface has been severely
damaged, the outlook is generally good, and exercises or
electrical stimulation of the appropriate muscles will usually
correct the problem. In severe cases the patella may have to
be removed. This flattens the knee a little but the disfigurement is minimal and the result is usually good.

chondromatosis

Multiple cartilage tumours in bone. These occur most commonly in the hands and are not malignant. A spontaneous
break (pathological fracture) may sometimes occur as a result
of thinning and weakening of bone.

chondros

Greek root meaning 'cartilage' as in chondromalacia (cartilage softening).

chondrosarcoma

A rare malignant tumour of the cartilaginous parts of bone.
It affects mainly the pelvis, ribs and breastbone (sternum)
and causes a slowly expanding swelling which may extend
inwards or outwards.

The degree of malignancy varies considerably, but the
tumour is often late-spreading and surgical removal usually
offers a favourable outlook.

chordee

Angulation of the penis, usually from a patch of scar tissue
that impedes erection at one point, as in **Peyronie's disease**,
or from the congenital deformity of **hypospadias**. Chordee
can seriously interfere with sexual intercourse.

chorea

The term derives from the Greek *choreia* meaning 'group dancing'. Chorea, sometimes known as St Vitus' dance, is an involuntary, purposeless jerky movement, repeatedly affecting especially the face, shoulders and hips. It is caused by disease of the basal ganglia of the brain. This may result from an inherited disease of the nervous system, **Huntington's chorea**, or may be the result of **rheumatic fever** in childhood, when it is known as Sydenham's chorea.

Senile chorea mainly affects the tongue and the muscles around the mouth. Chorea gravidarum is chorea occurring during pregnancy and ceasing after delivery. Those affected in this way often have a history of rheumatic fever. Women taking oral contraceptives may, rarely, be affected.

choriocarcinoma

A growth arising from the tissues which develop into the placenta (trophoblastic tissues).

The most common type of trophoblastic tumour is a benign growth called a hydatidiform mole. A malignant trophoblastic tumour that has spread outside the uterus is called a choriocarcinoma.

chorionic villus sampling

This is an alternative to **amniocentesis** and has the advantage that it can be done earlier – some eight to ten weeks after fertilization. There are, however, risks (see below). The principle is simple.

At an early stage the embryo differentiates into two parts, one becoming the future individual and the other developing into the placenta ('after-birth'). The part that forms the placenta starts out as finger-like processes called *chorionic villi* which burrow into the wall of the womb to come into close association with the mother's blood vessels. These villi are

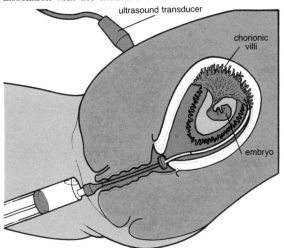

ultrasound transducer

chorionic villi

embryo

Chorionic villus sampling is a method of obtaining a tissue sample from the area of the placenta of the early embryo. Because the placental tissue comes from the same source as the tissues of the embryo it shares the embryo's genetic material and provides a sample of DNA which can be examined to detect genetic diseases. The sample is taken through a fine tube inserted under ultrasound scanning control.

formed by division of the original fertilized ovum and thus have exactly the same chromosomes, including any possible genetic abnormality, as the embryo. Any defect in one will be present in the other.

A small sample of chorionic villi can be obtained in one of two ways. It can be sucked out with a syringe through a fine flexible tube passed through the vagina and the neck of the womb (cervix) and guided to the site of the placenta under ultrasound scanning control. Or it can be obtained by passing a needle through the abdominal wall. Cells obtained in this way can be cultured and chromosome analysis done. Should abnormalities be found, many mothers find it easier to accept termination at this early stage.

Chorionic villus sampling is not entirely without risk. In about one case in 500 there is serious infection, and the rate of miscarriage (spontaneous abortion) is raised by the procedure. If performed through the cervix, the rate of fetal loss may be as high as 10 per cent. Done through the abdominal wall, fetal loss is about 6 per cent. But that may be a small price to pay for the opportunity to detect conditions such as Down's syndrome, cystic fibrosis, thalassaemia and many other conditions caused by chromosomal abnormalities in patients in high-risk groups.

choroiditis

Inflammation of the choroid coat of the eye. This invariably damages the overlying retina, usually causing localized patches of destruction. Choroiditis may be due to direct, blood-borne infection, such as syphilis, **tuberculosis, toxoplasmosis** or **histoplasmosis**, or it may be due to the presence of a parasitic worm juvenile, *Toxocara canis*, acquired from a puppy. It is often part of a general disorder, as in sarcoidosis or **Behçet's syndrome**.

> Because it is potentially so damaging, choroiditis must be treated rapidly and effectively.

In most cases there is no treatment specific to the cause and the ophthalmologist must fall back on general anti-inflammatory or immunosuppressive measures. Corticosteroid drugs are used, sometimes in large dosage, to prevent blinding spread of the disorder.

Christian Science

A religion founded in 1879 and devoted to the work of spiritual healing. Adherents believe that God and his spiritual creation are the only reality, and that the general concept of the material world is a misconception of the divine universe. Sickness provides an opportunity of demonstrating the divine power in healing and so it is impious to resort to conventional medical science, or to any material means of treatment.

This belief has posed some grave ethical problems for orthodox practitioners who are often equally convinced that the withholding of conventional medical responses, such as surgical operations or blood transfusion, may be fatal. The dilemma has never been satisfactorily resolved and legislation varies in different parts of the world. The general trend, however, is not to intervene when responsible adults take such decisions about themselves, but to provide legal protection when the probable survival of children is in issue.

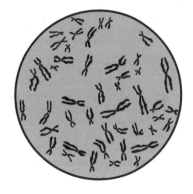

Chromosome analysis. Greatly enlarged photographs of chromosomes allow the images of the separate chromosomes to be arranged into pairs for inspection (the karyotype). This can reveal abnormalities, such as the extra chromosome 21 in Down's syndrome.

chromosome, additional

See **trisomy 13**, **trisomy 18**, **Down's syndrome**.

chromosome, additional Y

See **XYY configuration**.

chromosome analysis

It is now easy to cause human chromosomes, in cell culture, to enter a stage at which they are most widely separated and most easily visualized, stain them, photograph them and set them out in an orderly arrangement known as a *karyotype*. The matching in pairs and the inspection of the banding pattern revealed by the staining allows each one to be individually identified, so it is possible to discover whether the karyotype is normal or abnormal. This *chromosome analysis* allows ready diagnosis of a range of conditions known to be the result of gross chromosomal, rather than gene, abnormalities.

Chromosome analysis is useful in the investigation of small infants who fail to make normal progress, in those suspected of mental retardation, in those of ambiguous sex, and in those with organic disorder of a type characteristic of chromosomal abnormality. It is also useful in investigating infertile adults, women who abort repeatedly and men who wish to become sperm donors.

chromosome endings

See **telomeres**.

chromosomes, corresponding, different

See **heterozygous**.

chromosome segment displacement

See **translocation**.

chromosomes, non-sex

See **autosome**.

chronic

Lasting for a long time. The word comes from the Greek *chronos* meaning 'time', and the same root occurs in words such as 'chronometer' or 'synchronous'. A chronic disorder may be mild or severe but will usually involve some long-term or permanent organic change in the body. An *acute* disorder, on the other hand, lasts for a matter of days or for a week or two, at the most, and then either resolves or becomes chronic.

chronic obstructive lung disease

See **lung disease, chronic obstructive**.

chronic pain syndromes

Various conditions featuring persistent pain that cannot readily be attributed to any known organic disease or disorder. Also known as pain dysfunction syndromes, they include such conditions as **reflex sympathetic dystrophy** and post-traumatic pain. Repetitive strain injury was formerly included in this category but the tendency now is to use the latter term for a range of conditions in which the cause is well understood.

-cide

Suffix meaning 'killing' as in homicide (man-killer).

cidofovir

A **DNA polymerase inhibitor** drug. A brand name is Viside.

cigarette advertising

See **tobacco advertising**.

cilastatin

A drug used in combination with the beta-lactam antibiotic imipenem (carbapenem) to prevent its degradation in the kidneys, and thus prolonging its action. A brand name is Primaxin.

cilazapril

An **angiotensin converting enzyme inhibitor** used to treat **heart failure** and high blood pressure. A brand name is Vascace.

cilium

Latin root meaning 'eyelash' as in cilia (eyelashes).

cinnarizine

A drug used to treat **Ménière's syndrome**. A brand name is Stugeron.

cinoxacin

A quinolone antibiotic drug used mainly to treat urinary infections. A brand name is Cinobac.

ciprofibrate

An anti-cholesterol fibrate drug used to treat high blood lipid levels that fail to respond to dietary measures. A brand name is Modalim.

circadian rhythm

Many bodily activities, such as sleeping, eating, hormone production and menstruation are timed by biological clocks with various cycles. The circadian or diurnal rhythm is based on a 24-hour clock which is almost certainly synchronized by the day–night cycle occasioned by the rotation of the earth.

circulation

The heart is a pump and contains valves which allow blood to pass in one direction only. Blood is carried to the tissues, under pressure, via the strong, elastic-walled arteries, and returned to the heart, at low pressure, by way of the weaker, thin-walled veins. This continual rotation of blood is known as the circulation.

Phrases such as 'poor circulation' do not usually imply that the blood is being ineffectively pumped, but rather that certain areas of the body, such as the extremities, are receiving less than the optimum volume of blood, either because of active narrowing of the small arteries, as in Raynaud's phenomenon, or because of disease of the arteries, such as atherosclerosis, which permanently narrows them. Lack of blood to any part of the body is the ultimate problem for the tissues and the major cause of disease and death. Failure of the circulation to provide adequate oxygen and nutrition to the heart muscle itself, by way of the coronary arteries, and to the brain, by way of the carotid and vertebral arteries, causes more deaths than any other disease process. The immediate cause of damage, in these cases, is lack of oxygen.

Oxygen is our most urgent need. We can live without food for several weeks, without water for several days, but if we are deprived of oxygen for even a few minutes we will die. When a cardiac arrest occurs in hospital the first thing done is to check the time. A supply of oxygen to the brain must be provided within a few minutes or permanent serious damage will be done. Much of medicine is concerned with circumstances and factors which, actually or potentially, prejudice the supply of oxygen to the tissues. These include lung disorders, blood diseases, disorders of the heart and the blood vessels, many poisons, and injuries involving loss of blood and interference with air access to the lungs.

Oxygen is needed for the fundamental process of oxidation of fuel to release energy. This is a highly complex biochemical process known as oxidative phosphorylation and involving the synthesis of the universal energy carrier ATP (adenosine triphosphate) in the inner membranes of the mitochondria of the cells. In energetic terms, however, it is similar to the release of energy, as heat, which occurs when hydrogen is burned in oxygen to form hydrogen oxide, more commonly known as water (H_2O).

Around 1616, the English doctor William Harvey (1578–1657) demonstrated that blood did not ebb and flow in the veins, as was then taught, but moved in one direction only. This implied a continual circulation, and his observations, which were published in 1628 in his book *De Motu Cordis et Sanguinis in Animalibus* (*On the Motion of the Heart and Blood in Animals*), were a fundamental advance in medical understanding. Harvey's demonstration of the power of logic and common sense was also to have a major influence on the development of secure medical science.

See also illustration on following page.

circum-

Prefix meaning 'around' as in circumference (all round the edge).

circumcision

The surgical removal of the male foreskin (prepuce). The history of this practice goes back into the mists of time and it has been a major part of the ritual of many cultures. Male Jewish babies are circumcised on the eighth day after birth in accordance with Abraham's covenant with God, and all males converted to Judaism have to submit to circumcision.

Opinions on the medical and social merits of circumcision have been hotly debated for decades. The operation is widely practised in societies in which surgery has to be paid for. For years, circumcision has been the fate of almost all American boys, and in spite of the diktat of the American Academy of Pediatrics that routine circumcision was unnecessary, the practice has continued. In the 1970s, the British Medical Association came out against routine circumcision.

THE ARGUMENTS

The facts have been somewhat distorted by argument and prejudice. The foreskin is normally attached to the bulb (glans) of the penis during the early months of life, and it is normal not to be able to retract it. Failure of retraction is certainly not grounds for circumcision. The opening at the tip of the foreskin is normally quite small, but will stretch in time. A pin-point opening, so small that the foreskin is ballooned when the baby is urinating, sometimes occurs. This is called **phimosis** and can lead to later trouble, so circumcision is justified. Back-pressure of urine is undesirable and can cause urinary tract infection and kidney damage. Circumcision eliminates this risk, but the risk exists only if the outlet is extremely narrow. A study in the *American Journal of Pediatrics* that uncircumcised boys were ten times more likely to develop urinary tract infections than the circumcised was widely reported in the public press and has probably fortified the American public in its apparent conviction that nature has somehow got the human anatomy wrong.

> The foreskin should not be pulled back in infancy, but occasional attempts at gentle retraction will do little boys no harm and will help to stretch the skin. Later, it is important that the foreskin should be retracted so that the cheesy-looking and -smelling material, smegma, which collects under it, can be washed away every day. Full retraction is achieved gradually and may take months. It should certainly be possible by late adolescence. If not, circumcision should be considered.

Suggestions as to the dangers of smegma – that it can cause cancer of the penis and of the cervix in women – have

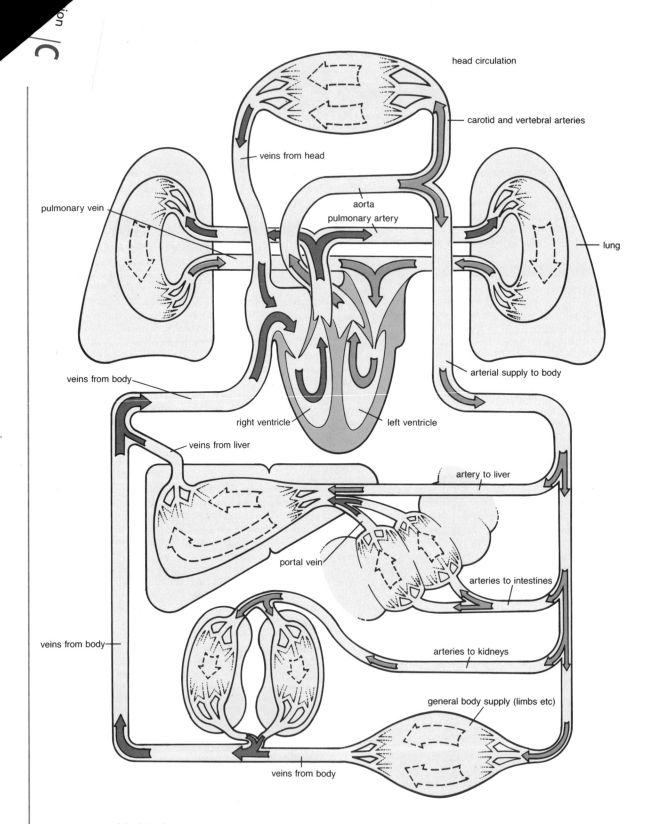

head circulation

carotid and vertebral arteries

veins from head

pulmonary vein

aorta
pulmonary artery

lung

veins from body

arterial supply to body

right ventricle

left ventricle

veins from liver

artery to liver

portal vein

arteries to intestines

veins from body

arteries to kidneys

general body supply (limbs etc)

veins from body

The circulation of the blood.

been cited as justification for circumcision. They are based on very dubious evidence involving mice and horse smegma, but, like most good stories, have been widely quoted and widely believed. At first, the evidence of the much lower incidence of cervical cancer in married Jewish women than in married Gentiles carried weight, but it was later shown that the difference could be accounted for on the basis of the virus cause of cervical cancer – the human papillomavirus – which is known to be sexually transmitted. Jewish sexual laws and family traditions, the difference in the number of sexual partners, the avoidance of sex during menstrual periods, and other factors, readily explain the reduced incidence in Jewish women.

So far as cancer of the penis is concerned, it is true that this is almost unknown in circumcised men. The reason is that penile cancer nearly always starts under the foreskin, in

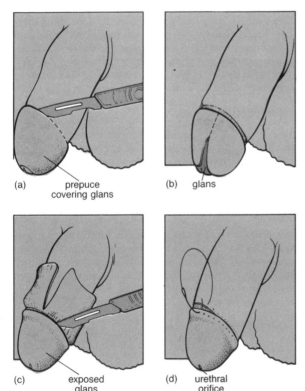

(a) prepuce
     covering glans

(b) glans

(c) exposed
     glans

(d) urethral
     orifice

Circumcision. (a) A careful cut is made around the root of the foreskin. (b) A cut is made on the back of the foreskin, from the front edge to the previous incision. (c) The foreskin is folded back and cut off. (d) The free edge of skin is now sewn to the site of the circular cut.

men with poor standards of personal hygiene. But cancer of the penis is also almost unknown in uncircumcised men – only about 100 cases occur each year in Britain – so the argument is a little disingenuous.

The latest American attack on the foreskin comes in the form of a suggestion, in a letter in the *New England Journal of Medicine*, that uncircumcised men are more likely to acquire AIDS than the circumcised. The author bemoans the declining rate of circumcision and hints that the policy may be regretted.

See also **uterus, cancer of**.

circumcision, female

Accounts of this barbaric practice appear in records dating back to before the time of Christ. The term 'female circumcision' is actually a euphemism for genital mutilation, and is a cause of pain, mutilation, infection, humiliation and distress to millions of women living in male-dominated societies throughout the world.

INCIDENCE

It is practised in over thirty countries including sub-Saharan Africa, New Guinea, the Arab world, Australia, Malaysia, Southern Europe, South America, Western Asia and India. The prevalence rates in different countries range from 5 per cent to 99 per cent. Even women in Britain are not necessarily immune. Some 10,000 are currently at risk. It is estimated that at least 100 million women and girls alive today have undergone genital mutilation.

WHY IT'S DONE

Alleged motives for this abomination vary from place to place and various claims – religious, moral, even medical – are made for the social importance of the act. Women who have not been circumcised may be rejected as marriage partners. The real basis is probably the sense of male ownership of women that cannot tolerate the thought of female infidelity. Unfortunately, this motive is potentiated by the factor of cultural identity which, for many women, is of paramount importance. For this reason, women often submit willingly to the social pressures to accept circumcision – the alternative being ostracism. None of these reasons justify this cruel practice.

HOW IT'S DONE

The procedure may involve removal of the clitoris only or may extend to radical removal of the **labia** minora and majora followed by stitching together of the raw surfaces so that they heal across and make sexual intercourse impossible. This major mutilation is called infibulation. It is done, usually between the ages of four and ten, but may be done at any age from one week to puberty.

The usual procedure, in Africa, is for the girl to be held down on her back by a young man who lies under her, while two other people grip her ankles and force her legs apart. The operation is performed using a razor blade, a sharp ceremonial or other knife or a piece of broken glass.

RISKS

No attempt is made to sterilize these implements and no anaesthetic is used. Apart from the pain and suffering, female circumcision commonly leads to severe infection, bleeding, urinary infection, kidney failure from blockage to the outflow of urine, dangerous obstructed labour from tight obstruction to the vaginal outlet, **tetanus** and death.

The practice of female circumcision has been condemned by the World Health Organization, the United Nations Human Rights Commission, Unicef, the UN Children's Fund, the International Planned Parenthood Federation, the UN Convention on the Rights of the Child and other official bodies. It is illegal in many countries, including the UK. Despite this, and despite the efforts of many enlightened women who are campaigning against it, the practice goes on. In the West, such practices are rightly regarded as criminal assault, but it must be recognized that there are still many places where, in a context of male pride and sense of property, the rights of women count for nothing.

cirrhosis of the liver

See **health maintenance**.

cisapride

A prokinetic drug that aids in stomach emptying and helps to relieve heartburn (reflux oesophagitis). A brand name is Prepulsid.

citalpram

A serotonin reuptake inhibitor drug used as an antidepressant. A brand name is Cipramil.

CJD

See **Creutzfeldt-Jakob disease**.

cladribine

An anticaner drug. A brand name is Leustat.

clap

A slang term for gonorrhoea. The origin is uncertain, but Le Clapier, the rabbit warren, was a red-light district in medieval Paris and *clapise* was a common French word for a brothel. The term appears in English literature as early as 1650 and was used by Dr Johnson in 1740.

clarithromycin

A macrolide **antibiotic** drug. A brand name is Klaricid.

-clast

Suffix meaning 'breaker' as in osteoclast (bone breaker).

claudication

See **intermittent claudication**.

claustrophobia

Fear of confined spaces. Claustrophobia is one of the **phobic** disorders and is usually associated with others such as **agoraphobia**.

clawfoot

See **talipes**.

-cle

Suffix meaning 'diminutive' as in corpuscle (little body).

cleft lip and palate

During the early development of the fetus, the face forms by the fusion of a number of processes that grow out from the front end of the primitive tube-like structure of the body. Cleft lip or cleft lip and palate is a developmental defect caused by the failure of full fusion of these processes. The cleft lip is a gap in the upper lip, which may be no more than a small notch, or which may extend right up to join one nostril. Cleft palate is a gap in the roof of the mouth, which may partially or completely divide the palate. Sometimes there are two gaps in the upper lip, extending up to both nostrils and

these may be associated with partial or complete cleft palate. Cleft palate may occur on its own, without cleft lip.

TREATMENT

The surgical management of these conditions has improved immeasurably in recent years and it is now rare to see obvious residual deformity from cleft lip ('hare lip'). Babies with cleft palate cannot breastfeed and must be fed from a bottle. Although good surgical repair is possible, usually at around one year of age, there may be a long-term problem with speech articulation, and speech therapy is often necessary.

clemastine

An **antihistamine** drug used to treat hay fever and other allergic conditions. A brand name is Tavegil.

clergyman's knee

Inflammation and swelling of the bursa in front of the knee cap (patellar **bursitis**) allegedly from excessively prolonged pressure during prayer. The condition is uncommon in these less fervent days, and probably occurs more often in cleaners than in the clergy. Happily, mechanical aids to floor cleaning are also reducing the incidence in the latter.

clergyman's throat

Hoarseness and pain on speaking due to overuse of the voice and faulty habits of voice production. The condition is due to inflammation of the vocal cords, sometimes even to the production of small polyps, and is nowadays more common in pop singers and Trades Union officials.

climacteric

The **menopause**. The time in a woman's life at which reproduction is no longer possible. This is an exclusively female phenomenon. The term 'climacteric' is, however, sometimes applied to the general decline in sexual drive and interest experienced by some men at about the same time in life as the menopause occurs in women.

clitoridectomy

See **circumcision, female**.

clitoris

The female analogue of the penis. The clitoris is the principal erectile sexual organ in women and the main erogenic centre. It lies under the pubic bone at the front junction of the inner lips (labia minora) and immediately in front of the urine outlet (urethral orifice). The front parts of the labia minora form a hood for the clitoris, which has a substantial nerve and blood supply. Recent anatomical studies in living subjects, by scanning techniques, have shown that the clitoris is substantially more extensive than was formerly thought.

clobazam

A long-acting **benzodiazepine** drug used to treat anxiety or to control epilepsy. A brand name is Frisium.

clobetasol

A powerful steroid drug used for external application in severe dermatological disorders. A brand name is Dermovate.

clofazimine

A drug used to treat leprosy. It is effective in controlling the erythema nodosum reaction. A brand name is Lamprene.

clofibrate

A fibric acid derivative drug that lowers the blood **cholesterol** levels. A brand name is Atromid-S.

clomiphene

A drug used to treat **infertility** by virtue of its ability to stimulate the production of eggs from the ovaries (ovulation). Multiple pregnancies often result. A brand name is Clomid.

clomipramine

A tricyclic antidepressant drug useful, also, in phobic anxiety and obsessive states. A brand name is Anafranil.

clonazepam

A benzodiazepine drug used to control **epilepsy** and **trigeminal neuralgia**. A brand name is Rivotril.

clone

A perfect copy, or a population of perfect copies, of any organism. Cloning occurs when an organism reproduces non-sexually, so that the genetic content (**genome**) of each is identical. The term is also used for a number of identical cells derived from a single cell by repetitive division, and for a perfect copy, or any number of copies, of any DNA sequence, such as a gene, or any other **nucleotide** sequence.

clonus

When the smoothing and controlling influence of the higher centres of the brain is removed from the more primitive spinal reflexes, the latter become over-active. In this state, even a slight stretching of a muscle may be enough to cause it to contract strongly and go into spasm. This spastic state is characteristic of certain forms of brain damage, such as occur in the development of a stroke.

'Hyper-reflexivity' of this kind can be demonstrated by exerting sustained upwards pressure on the foot to flex the ankle and stretch the calf muscles. This causes the calf muscles to contract and forcibly extend the ankle. But this in turn leads to a further stretch stimulus, and a rhythmical series of foot movements results for as long as the pressure on the foot is sustained. This repetitive contraction is called clonus and is an important physical sign of what is known as an *upper motor neurone lesion*.

clopamide

A thiazide diuretic drug. A brand name is Viskaldix.

clopidogrel

A thienopyridine drug that interferes with the aggregation of blood platelets so as to reduce the risk of thrombosis and thus strokes and heart attacks in people with arterial disease. A brand name is Plavix.

clorazepate potassium

A long-acting **benzodiazepine** drug used to treat anxiety. A brand name is Tranzene.

clot-dissolving enzyme

See **urokinase**.

clotrimazole

A drug effective against a wide range of fungi. It is used in the form of creams, for local application. A brand name is Canesten.

clozapine

An antipsychotic drug notable for its absence of side-effects such as tremors and repetitive movements (dyskinesias). It does, however, tend to affect white blood cell production and regular blood checks are necessary. Between 1 and 2 per cent of those taking the drug suffer a drop in white cell count. This returns to normal within a month of stopping the drug. Clozapine can restore people to an almost normal life after years of intractable schizophrenia. A brand name is Clozaril.

clubbing

Enlargement of the soft tissues of the end segment of the fingers or toes, with loss of the angle at the root of the nail. Clubbing is found in heart disease that causes inadequate oxygenation of the blood and consequent blueness (**cyanosis**) of the skin; in infective **endocarditis**; cancer of the lung; **bronchiectasis**; **ulcerative colitis**; and in several other conditions. Its occurrence is more of a medical curiosity than a valuable diagnostic aid, but the development of clubbing usually indicates that something serious is happening.

clubfoot

See **talipes**.

cluster B personality

The personality type of people who over-react to events, suffer frequent frustration, behave in a narcissistic and histrionic manner, are often unhappy, angry and resentful, and are inclined to blame others for their unhappiness. People with cluster B personality often seek psychotherapy but seldom derive permanent benefit from it.

CNS

The central nervous system.

co-

Prefix meaning 'together' as in co-exist (living together).

coarctation of the aorta

A congenital condition in which a short section of the main artery of the body, the aorta, is severely narrowed. The usual site for the narrowing is just beyond the point at which the arteries to the head and arms are given off. As a result, there is high blood pressure in the upper part of the body and low blood pressure in the lower parts. Babies with coarctation may suddenly develop heart failure and collapse and may require urgent supportive treatment and then surgery to open up the narrowed segment. In lesser degrees of coarctation, surgery, if necessary, may be deferred until the age of about six.

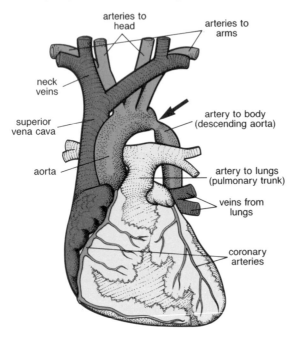

Coarctation of the aorta. The arrow shows the area of narrowing of the aorta just after the point at which the major vessels for the head and arms come off.

cobalt

An element in the vitamin B12 molecule. The radioactive isotope Cobalt-60 is a powerful emitter of lethal gamma rays and has been widely used as a source of radiation for sterilizing medical dressings, disposable syringes and other equipment. It has also been used in the radiotherapy of cancer.

cocaine

An illegal drug obtained from the leaves of the coca bush that grows in the Andes. It is supplied as a potent white powder. Cocaine is usually taken by sniffing the powder, but can also be injected.

The likelihood of severe addiction depends on the way the drug is used. People who are into 'freebasing' (smoking) or 'shooting' (injecting) are more likely to become seriously addicted than those who are only 'snorting' the drug. The trouble is that habituation and tolerance to the effect may lead snorters to want the extra 'rush' of freebasing, in which 80 per cent of the dose can get to the brain in about ten seconds. As with any other major drug, addiction, quite apart from its medical effects, may lead to serious social and financial consequences.

There is now ample medical evidence to show that cocaine is often extremely dangerous to health. The commonest serious physical effects are epileptic-type fits, loss of consciousness – 'tripping out' – unsteadiness, sore throat, running and bleeding nose, sinusitis, pain in the chest, coughing blood, pneumonia, severe itching ('the cocaine bug'), irregularity of the heart, loss of appetite and stomach upset. Some of the chest and throat problems are probably caused by the high temperature of the inhaled cocaine fumes. The nose and sinus disorders are due to the constricting effect of cocaine on the blood vessels in the nose linings. This is followed by rebound swelling, but is sometimes severe enough to destroy part of the partition between the two halves of the nose, leaving a perforation.

coccydynia

Persistent pain in the tail region of the spine, usually following an injury, such as a fall or a kick, in which a fracture of the small bones of the coccyx is sustained.

cochlear implant

A miniaturized electronic device capable of stimulating the acoustic nerve so as to produce some form of hearing in people wholly deaf from inner ear disease. There have been advances in multichannel implants, which divide the sound spectrum into several parts, but the results still cannot be said to compare with natural hearing. Cochlear implants can, however, make a substantial difference to children born deaf or becoming totally deaf before three years of age, so long as the implant is inserted before the age of five. Most of the children who receive such implants are able to develop intelligible speech.

cockroach allergy

A recently discovered unsuspected cause, or precipitant, of asthma. Research into a large group of inner-city children with asthma showed that 36.8 per cent were allergic to cockroach material, and that more of these children were allergic to cockroaches than to house dust mite droppings or to cat **dander** (scales).

codon

A sequence of three consecutive **nucleotides** (a triplet containing three **base pairs**) along a strand of DNA or RNA that specifies a particular **amino acid** or a stop signal during protein synthesis. The order of the codons along the DNA molecule determines the sequence of particular amino acids in the protein produced.

-coele

Suffix meaning 'sac, tumour' as in hydrocele (water sac).

coffee-coloured skin patches

See **café au lait patches**.

cognitive behaviour therapy

A pragmatic form of **behaviour therapy** that largely ignores psychological theory and hypothesis and concentrates on the nature, immediate motivation and effects of actual behaviour, and the individual's thoughts about them. The method is capable of achieving substantial improvement in conditions such as panic states, eating disorders, obsessive-compulsive disorder, hypochondriasis and chronic fatigue syndrome ('ME'). It has been found useful in managing attempted suicide, unexplained physical symptoms and even unemployment. Research suggests that it is a potentially useful additional treatment in cases of chronic **schizophrenia**.

cognitive dissonance

A psychological term for the conflict that results from inconsistency between beliefs and actions, as when a person professes to be honest but cheats on income tax returns.

coitus

Copulation, or the physical act of sexual intercourse. Strictly speaking, sexual intercourse is, or should be, an activity in which strong positive emotions of love or affection pass between the participants; the word 'intercourse' means 'a running between'. The term 'coitus' excludes these elements and denotes only the purely mechanical or biological aspects of sexual intercourse.

Colazide

A brand name for **balsalazide**.

cold, common

The common cold, being familiar to all, has acquired more than the usual number of medical myths. The origin of the term is not clear but it may relate to the frequency of colds in winter time, or to the feeling of chilliness at the onset of fever.

CAUSES

Colds have nothing to do with cold and are not caused by chilling the body, by getting clothes, feet or hair wet or by exposure to cold weather. Such conditions do not reduce immunity to attack from cold viruses and there is no evidence that they reactivate or encourage viruses already present. Susceptibility to colds does, however, increase in conditions of fatigue or emotional stress.

The generally accepted idea that colds are spread by inhaling air-borne droplets coughed or sneezed by other sufferers is true. But research has now shown that this is not the chief mode of spread. Most colds are acquired by close contact, mainly by direct transfer from hand to hand, and then from the hand of the recipient to his or her own nose or eyes. Transfer to the mouth is not very effective, as the mouth and stomach are very hard on viruses. The moral is that if it is impossible to avoid shaking hands with someone with a cold, one should consciously avoid touching one's own face until the hands have been thoroughly washed.

Colds are caused by more than 200 different kinds of viruses. These include influenzaviruses, parainfluenzaviruses, echoviruses, adenoviruses, myxoviruses, coronaviruses, picornaviruses and, in particular, rhinoviruses – which are responsible for up to 50 per cent of colds. It is partly because of the exceptionally large number of different causal organisms, and because of their ability to mutate, that the common cold is so difficult to treat effectively. For the same reasons, it is very hard to produce a workable vaccine.

RECOGNITION AND SYMPTOMS

The common cold comes on one to three days after infection. It is an inflammation of the lining of the nose, throat, sinuses and sometimes the voice box (larynx) and bronchial tubes. This inflammation causes:

● burning discomfort and sore throat;
● swelling of the mucous membranes, causing obstruction to air fllow;

● excessive production of watery and mucoid secretions;
● a tendency to secondary infection with pus-forming organisms so that the secretion becomes purulent.

Pus in the secretions does not necessarily imply secondary infection, but pus in the sinuses and middle ear (otitis media) does. Depending on the severity, fever may or may not be present. People with chronic bronchitis usually suffer a marked flare-up of the bronchial problems after a cold, and antibiotics may be necessary.

TREATMENT

Cold sufferers, especially those who are feverish, should stay at home and avoid donating their viruses to others. The mode of spread should be understood and behaviour should be modified accordingly. Short of repeated nasal instillation of interferon, there is no effective treatment, but a host of medicines – nasal decongestant drops, steam inhalations, throat lozenges, pain relievers, etc. – is available to relieve symptoms.

> Cold prevention seems to be possible by taking 1 to 2 grams of vitamin C every day in accordance with the advice of the Nobel Prize winning chemist Linus Pauling (1901–94). Antibiotics have no effect on viruses and are best avoided unless significant secondary chest or sinus infection occurs.

See **common cold remedies**.

cold injury

See **frostbite**.

cold preservation

See **cryopreservation**.

cold sores

A flare-up of a herpes simplex infection, featuring the familiar crops of tense, painful and crusting little blisters (vesicles) at the junction of the skin and mucous membrane of the lips and sometimes the nose.

Most of us harbour herpes viruses, but, for most of the time, they are kept in check by the activity of the immune system. When these are otherwise engaged, coping with other virus infections, such as the common cold, the resident herpes viruses are apt to get the upper hand, temporarily.

colectomy

Surgical removal of the large intestine (colon). When this is done, a new outlet must be made for the lower end of the remaining intestine, in the form of a **colostomy** or **ileostomy**.

colestipol

A **bile acid sequestrant** drug used to treat abnormally high levels of lipoproteins. A brand name is Colestid.

colic

Pain caused by stretching of a tubular structure in the body. The bowel (intestine) is very sensitive to stretching, and when the normal milking process of peristalsis, by which the contents are passed along, is impeded, segments become ballooned and stretched. The result is colicky pain which rises to a peak, as the bowel is stretched, and then passes off, as it relaxes. The same effect can be caused if the intestine contracts strongly around a hard, incompressible object, such as a lump of undigested food.

Bowel colic is usually caused by minor upsets and dietary indiscretion but may occur in genuine intestinal obstruction. In biliary and renal colic the pain is caused by contraction of the bile duct or ureter around a stone.

colic, infantile

This term is used to describe a clear-cut and distressing baby problem which probably has nothing to do with spasm of the bowel (**colic**). The affected infant is in every respect healthy and feeds well and gains weight, but seems exceptionally hungry and will suck vigorously on anything offered. The feature which can drive parents to distraction is that the child has apparently endless paroxysms of frantic crying, often at around the same times of the day or night. Such crying may cause the baby to swallow air and this may lead to distension of the abdomen and the passage of wind from either end. But there is no reason to believe that the original cause of the apparent distress is actual colic, or anything else connected with the bowels.

The essential facts are that if the crying is due to insufficient nourishment, the baby will not gain weight; if due to intestinal disorder there will be other signs, such as diarrhoea, fever, dehydration or visible movement of the bowels through the abdominal wall. In bottle-fed babies, milk intolerance may sometimes be the cause, and a change of brand may be worth trying. In breastfed babies, a milk intolerance might be exacerbated by dairy produce in the mother's diet.

Some babies are naturally hyperactive and these can then be calmed down by being firmly wrapped (swaddled) in a small sheet and turned, briefly, on the stomach.

Babies should never be left to sleep face down, because of the risk of cot death (**sudden infant death syndrome**).

Powerful crying is never harmful to the baby, however severely it may affect the unfortunate parents, and infantile colic nearly always ceases by the age of three or four months.

coliforms

See *Escherichia coli*.

colistin

An antibiotic produced by the bacterium *Bacillus colistinus* and effective against *Pseudomonas aeruginosa*. It is used to sterilize the inside of the bowel and bladder and on the skin and external ear. A brand name is Colomycin.

colitis

Inflammation of the colon.
See **ulcerative colitis**.

collar, orthopaedic

See **orthopaedic collar**.

Colles' fracture

A common fracture of the forearm bones at the wrist, usually caused by a fall on to the outstretched hand. The break results in a typical 'dinner-fork' deformity with the bones of the wrist forced backwards. Damage to the median nerve which runs down into the hand sometimes occurs. Treatment is carried out under anaesthesia. The hand is pulled strongly away from the arm and the backwardly displaced bone fragments are then forced into alignment by bending the wrist fully. When the bones are in correct alignment, a plaster is applied and checked at intervals. Six weeks in plaster is usually sufficient.

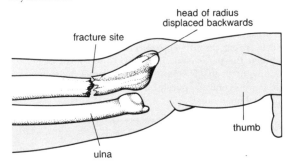

Colles' fracture. This is a fracture of the lower end of the radius bone. The lower fragment is displaced backwards, producing the typical 'dinner-fork' deformity.

colon, cancer of

INCIDENCE
Cancer of the colon is an extremely common form of cancer. After the lung, the colon is the most common site of cancer affecting both men and women, and in this group it is the second most common cause of cancer death. Cancer of the colon becomes commoner with increasing age and is rare before age forty. The peak incidence occurs in the age group sixty to seventy-five.

RECOGNITION AND SYMPTOMS
Colon cancers grow slowly and are usually well advanced before they produce symptoms. The first sign is often an alteration in the normal bowel habit, with constipation followed by frequent motions. Cancers can grow round the wall of the bowel causing partial obstruction and sometimes altering the shape of the stools into a more ribbon-like appearance. Blood in the stools is always a danger sign, but bleeding may be microscopic and detectable only by chemical tests (occult blood). Sometimes there is colicky pain or even complete obstruction.

The lower part of the colon is called the rectum, and cancer in this part is commoner in men than in women. Here, the commonest presenting sign is blood in the stools. Blood, however, arises more frequently from piles (haemorrhoids) than from cancer. Pain is not a feature of cancer of the colon until a very advanced stage with spread to other nearby organs.

The tests for occult blood in the stools are simple and are an effective method of screening. A positive result is an indication for examination, by an expert, with a viewing instrument such as a rigid tubular sigmoidoscope or a flexible, self-illuminating internal examination device (fibre optic endoscope).

TREATMENT
Cancer of the colon is treated by a wide surgical removal of the affected segment of the bowel, together with the associ-

ated lymph nodes. If the rectum has to be removed, there will have to be a permanent **colostomy**, but higher removal permits internal joining up of the cut ends. Many cases can be cured by surgery, but this depends almost entirely on the stage the cancer has reached at the time of diagnosis. If it is still confined to the internal lining of the bowel, the cure rate is 90 per cent, but if the lymph nodes are involved the outlook is much worse. The value of radiotherapy and chemotherapy in this form of cancer has not yet been fully established.

colon, irritable

See **irritable bowel syndrome**.

colonoscopy

The direct optical examination of the inside of the colon by means of a viewing device inserted through the anus and passed carefully upwards. Modern endoscopes are 'steerable' by means of rotating knobs at the control end and contain separate fibre optic viewing and illuminating channels. In addition, endoscopes allow the passage of various fine instruments, by which sample (biopsy) material can be taken, and a channel through which water or air can be passed to facilitate viewing.

colon, spastic

This is another term for **irritable bowel syndrome**.

colostomy

An operation often necessary when part of the colon has to be removed, as in the treatment of cancer. The upper open end of the bowel is brought out through an opening in the front wall of the abdomen and the edges are stitched to the margins of the opening.

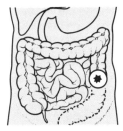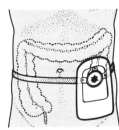

Colostomy. (a) The large intestine (colon) is cut across and the free upper end is brought out through a surgical opening in the wall of the abdomen. (b) Various forms of colostomy bag may be attached to collect the expelled bowel contents. An alternative is to wash out the bowel, once or twice a day, and cover the opening.

The cut wall of the bowel heals to the edges of the surgical incision, which is thus kept open. Bowel contents pass out through the colostomy and are collected in a waterproof bag which is sealed around the margins with special adhesive.

Colostomies are often temporary and when closed leave only a minor scar.

colour blindness

Absolute colour blindness, with no perception of any colours, is almost unknown, so the term is somewhat misleading.

INCIDENCE

Colour perception defect is common, especially in males, and involves relative insensitivity to either red, green or blue, or to some combination of these. It is almost always inherited, the defective gene being recessive and on the X chromosome. So, although almost 10 per cent of males have some degree of colour perception defect, the condition is rare in women, less than 0.5 per cent being affected. For women to show the trait, both of their X chromosomes would have to carry the defective gene.

POSSIBLE CAUSES

Aside from genetic inheritance of the condition, colour perception defect can also be acquired and is a fairly common consequence of optic nerve fibre damage from any cause, such as multiple sclerosis, diabetes or drug or chemical toxicity. In cases of one-sided damage, a comparison of the intensity of colour of an object, as viewed by each eye, will show an obvious difference.

RECOGNITION

Colour perception can be tested in various ways. The Ishihara, multi-dot test is a quick and useful screening test. People with normal colour vision see one sequence of numbers, those with colour problems see another. Colour matching is also a sensitive test of perception, as is placing in sequence a large series of discs of gradually changing colour value.

> For certain occupations, normal colour perception is needed and anyone with ambitions to join the Armed Forces should be tested well in advance. Colour perception defect is not an absolute bar to recruitment, but denies entry to certain occupations and trades. Commercial flying calls for good colour perception. Most coloured signals on the ground, such as traffic lights, can easily be interpreted by colour defective people.

colposcopy

Direct optical examination of the vagina and the neck of the womb (cervix) using a low-power binocular microscope with a long focus (colposcope), while the vagina is held open with a metal or plastic device called a speculum. Colposcopy provides an essential view of the structure of the surface lining and allows scrapings to be taken from any suspicious areas. Colposcopy is the routine next step after a cervical smear (Pap smear) has shown some abnormality. The Royal College of Obstetricians and Gynaecologists has advised that no patient with surface cervical cancer (intra-epithelial neoplasia) should be treated without prior examination by colposcopy.

In addition to accurate diagnosis, colposcopy increases the effectiveness with which local treatment can be given. The magnification provided helps to ensure that all affected areas are fully treated, using lasers or other instruments. Microsurgery of this kind has greatly advanced several of the surgical disciplines.

com-

Prefix meaning 'together' as in compare (match together).

coma

A state of deep unconsciousness from which the affected person cannot be aroused even by strong stimulation. Coma can occur in many ways, but in all cases the common cause is an interruption of the function of the higher centres of the brain.

POSSIBLE CAUSES

Coma may result from any event which cuts off the oxygen supply to the body for more than a few minutes, such as partial drowning or a period of strangulation or asphyxia. It may result from any disorder that temporarily deprives the brain of an adequate blood supply, such as **stroke**. It may follow alcoholic or other kinds of poisoning or may result from direct or indirect head injury. Other causes include liver failure, uncontrolled diabetes, excess insulin causing **hypoglycaemia** and severe alterations in the constitution of the blood.

COMPLICATIONS

A person in coma requires skilful nursing and medical attention for there are many complications that arise directly from the unconscious state itself and that will inevitably occur unless positively prevented. These include malnutrition, major ulceration over points of pressure (bed sores), severe loss of muscle bulk, contractures of the limbs into positions of flexure which cannot later be corrected, and various infections, especially of the lungs (pneumonia) and urinary system.

comedo

A **blackhead**.

commensal

A term applied to micro-organisms that live continuously in the body, but do not cause disease. Many parts of the body, especially the skin, the mouth, the nose, the large intestine and the vagina contain large numbers of organisms at all times. These do no harm and, indeed, are often valuable in that they maintain an acceptable environment from which other, more dangerous, organisms are often excluded. If commensals are killed by antibiotics, the results are sometimes unfortunate, and new organisms, including fungi such as Candida, often take over.

commode

A bedside chair with a cut-away seat under which is placed a receptacle for urine and faeces. In general, a commode, if available, is to be preferred to a bedpan which may not be easy to manage with an infirm or disabled person.

common cold remedies

If a cold is left untreated, it lasts for about a week, but if a cold 'remedy' is taken, it will last for about seven days. Jokes of this kind are merely a reflection of the fact that no practical or reasonably economical remedy exists which has any significant effect on most of the two hundred or so regularly mutating strains of viruses that cause the common cold. Some, the rhinoviruses, can probably be controlled by a large daily dose of alpha2-interferon, given as a nasal spray, but this is very expensive and causes nose bleeds.

Millions of pounds are spent every year on over-the-counter common cold remedies, but in spite of implied claims, none of these has anything but a symptomatic effect. There are drugs which stop the nose running and make it easier to breath, drugs which relieve the discomfort of the sore throat, even drugs which make you feel that a cold isn't such a bad thing after all, but these are merely covering up the symptoms.

communicable disease

A disease capable of being transmitted from one person to another; in other words, an infectious disease. Some communicable diseases are notifiable – doctors are required by law to inform a central public health authority of such conditions, so that essential statistics can be complied and steps can be taken, if necessary, to limit spread.

communication deficit

See **autism**.

community psychiatric nurse

A qualified nurse with a post-registration diploma in psychiatric nursing, whose primary function is to attend to psychiatric patients who are being cared for in the community rather than in hospital.

compartment syndrome

A condition of increased tissue pressure within a compartment of the body, usually the forearm or the lower leg, which results in compression of the veins and then the arteries so that the muscles are eventually deprived of their blood supply and become useless, shrunken and replaced by fibrous tissue. The syndrome may follow fractures, crush injuries, gunshot wounds or even drug overdose. There is pain, loss of power, paralysis and absent pulse. Urgent surgery is needed to open up the tissue planes and relieve the pressure until the swelling subsides.

compensation neurosis

A fixed preoccupation with real or imagined disability following an industrial accident or civil injury, when there is a possibility of financial compensation. The condition is especially unfortunate in that it tends to deprive the affected person of the motive to overcome the alleged disability and get on with his or her life. It tends also to prevent acknowledgement of the natural processes of recovery.

Uncompensated disability often persists for many years, but the condition often clears up soon after a satisfactory settlement.

complex

A term widely used by psychotherapists. A complex is a group of tendencies forming an emotionally charged concept which is said often to be in conflict with other behaviour tendencies. As a result it becomes repressed – with dire consequences. One of the most frequently mentioned is the Oedipus complex, which is the basis of Freudian psychoanalysis. This is said to be based on the desire of a small boy to have sex with his mother and murder his father.

The *inferiority complex* was the notion, not of Freud, but of his one-time follower, Adler. It refers to a constellation of repressed fears, arising from the natural bodily inferiority of the infant, which are said, not unreasonably, to cause a more general feeling of inferiority and negative or critical attitudes towards the self. By definition, a complex should be unconscious, so anyone aware of his or her own inferiority would be excluded. Some point out, with justice, that an inferiority complex is often manifested by aggressive dominating behaviour calculated to conceal the underlying inadequacies.

compulsive behaviour

See **obsessive-compulsive disorder**.

compulsive grunts and conduct disorder

See **Gilles de la Tourette's syndrome**.

con-

Prefix meaning 'together' as in 'conspire' (breathe together).

concussion

The *shaking-up* of the brain that occurs when a force is applied violently to the head causing an immediate brief period of unconsciousness, lasting for seconds to hours.

CAUSES

Concussion is caused by head injury, usually without skull fracture, from accelerative or decelerative forces. These cause the brain to rotate and suffer compression against the protrusions on the inside of the skull.

RECOGNITION

The injury is probably always associated with some bleeding inside the brain and it is known that in many cases actual destruction of nerve tissue occurs.

RISKS

Happily, the supply of nerve tissue is liberal and a single episode of concussion is unlikely to have observable permanent effects. But repeated episodes of concussion, such as are suffered by boxers, will inevitably cause major and irremediable **brain damage** (the 'punch-drunk' syndrome). It is for this reason that all informed and responsible medical opinion regards boxing as barbarous.

conditioning

The reports, in English, on Pavlov's celebrated work on dogs which demonstrated the conditioned reflex, contained a curious error. Pavlov showed that if, on a sufficient number of occasions, a bell was rung when food was presented to a hungry dog, then, eventually, ringing the bell alone, without producing the food, would cause the dog to salivate and secrete stomach juice. Pavlov stated that this shift of the effectiveness of the stimulus, from food to bell, was *conditional* on the procedure being repeated often. He called the response a *conditional* response. The change of terminology to 'conditioning' and 'conditioned reflex' was none of Pavlov's doing and it is questionable whether he would have approved. The term 'conditioned' has, however, become hallowed by repetition and is now beyond correction.

Clearly, the *conditioned reflex* is an important feature of the functioning of the brain, and examples of its operation abound in all human activity. For instance, favourable reactions are commonly elicited by association with someone we like. It is sufficient for someone else – perhaps a complete stranger – to resemble that person, for us to feel well disposed towards him or her. Fears are commonly conditioned by previous association of pain, for example, fear of the dentist comes from previous association of pain when sitting in a dental chair. Some children show signs of intense fear at the sight of a hypodermic syringe and needle.

Pavlov believed that all learning could be explained by conditioning, and that complex behaviour patterns could be built up from a series of simpler conditioned responses. This view has been enthusiastically endorsed by the behaviourist school who have suggested that all human behaviour can be determined in this way. The idea has not been universally popular and opposition to the suggestion that undesirable behaviour can be corrected by 'human conditioning' has been reinforced by reports of 'brainwashing'. But, like it or not, we cannot deny that conditioning is a fundamental process in all education and a major determining factor in everyday life. See also **behaviour therapy**.

condoms, ideas about

See **contraception**.

conduct disorder

A persistent pattern of behaviour which consistently violates the rights of others or the accepted norms of society. Activities typical of conduct disorder include theft, repeatedly running away from home, fire-starting, breaking and entering, destroying property, cruelty to people or animals, a tendency to initiate physical aggression and the use of a weapon in a fight.

POSSIBLE CAUSES

Conduct disorder results mainly from the defective early influence over the child by parents and others whose own problems and upbringing have prevented them from forming socially acceptable values. Many have, through a life of disappointment and frustration, developed strongly antisocial values. There is often alcoholism, and marital strife and crude machismo attitudes expressed in physical violence. Some people with conduct disorder have an unsuspected psychotic illnesses.

The affected children tend, unconsciously, to accept and act out their parents' antisocial attitudes, and this early programming becomes built in, at an almost structural level, and is very influential and very difficult to displace. Other factors known to cause conduct disorder include parental rejection, harsh institutional treatment, frequent changes of guardianship and illegitimacy. The Spanish ecclesiastic Ignatious Loyola (1491–1566), founder of the Jesuit movement, was reflecting these facts when he said: 'Give me the child until he is seven, and I care not who has him afterwards.'

TREATMENT

The treatment of conduct disorder is difficult, but a major advance resulted from the proper recognition of the fact that this is not a matter of inherent wickedness, but rather a question of defective early **conditioning**. Life experience will often, in time, bring a realization of the advantages of social conformity, and conduct disorder is less prevalent in the middle-aged and elderly than in adolescents and young adults. Psychoanalysis is of little value. Skilled and enlightened counselling can often help. But the greatest success, at least in the United States, has been achieved by group therapy based on reformed delinquent peers to whom young people with conduct disorders are willing to turn for understanding, advice and emotional support.

condyloma acuminatum

Soft **warts** on the genitals caused by the same viruses (papovaviruses) that cause all the other kinds of warts. Condylomata acuminata are pinkish, cauliflower-like growths and are spread by venereal infection.

condyloma lata

Flat, moist, highly infectious venereal **warts** occurring on the glans of the penis or on the vulva in secondary syphilis.

See also **sexually transmitted diseases**.

condylos

Greek root meaning 'knuckle' as in condyle (bump on bone).

cone biopsy

The removal of a cone-shaped or cylindrical segment of tissue from the inside of the neck of the womb to provide material for positive microscopic diagnosis. This is done under general anaesthesia when a cervical smear test suggests that cancer may be present. Even if early cancer is found, the cone biopsy will often be shown to have removed all malignant tissue, so is both diagnostic and therapeutic.

The commonest method is known as loop electrosurgical excision. This is done using a small loop of fine wire heated to incandescence by an electric current. This has the advantage over earlier methods that bleeding is less profuse and the risk of spreading cancer is less. The operation takes about five minutes. Occasionally, the procedure is complicated by late bleeding and sometimes by cervical incompetence. Microscopic examination of the specimen can show whether cancer is present and whether it has been effectively dealt with.

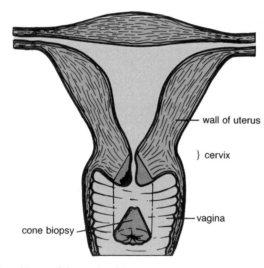

Cone biopsy of the cervix of the womb (uterus). The diagram shows the amount of tissue removed. This procedure, used when there is suspicion of local malignancy, is often curative as well as diagnostic.

confabulation

A process of filling in gaps in the memory by recounting entirely fictitious details of past events. Confabulation is a common feature of the conversation of those suffering from various forms of dementia and is most characteristic of the condition of severe brain damage, caused by persistent alcohol abuse, known as Korsakoff's syndrome. At first, the confabulation is convincing, but one soon notes that the range of invention is limited and that the same tape is being played over and over again.

confidentiality

See **ethics, medical**.

congenital

Present at birth. A congenital disorder need not be hereditary or of genetic origin, although many are. Conditions acquired during fetal life are congenital and include defects caused by infections passed on by the mother or even those acquired during the process of birth.

congestion

An abnormal collection of fluid, often blood, in an organ or body part. The condition is not a disorder in its own right, but the result of some other disease process, such as infection or interference with the normal drainage of the area. Congestion is a reactive condition which settles when the cause is removed.

congestion, nasal

See **rhinitis**.

congestive heart failure

See **heart failure**.

conjunctivitis

Inflammation of the membrane covering the white of the eye (the conjunctiva).
POSSIBLE CAUSES
It is most commonly caused by infection. Almost any organism may be responsible.

Allergic conjunctivitis is common and is occasionally dramatic. Pollen hypersensitivity (**hay fever**) can cause acute swelling of the conjunctiva, with the collection of much fluid behind it, so that the membrane bulges alarmingly forward between the lids.

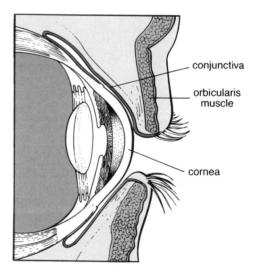

Conjunctivitis. The diagram shows the extent of the conjunctiva. In conjunctivitis this membrane becomes inflamed.

Conjunctivitis can also result from a wide spectrum of causes which includes:

- toxic influences such as contamination from dusts, liquids, gases, industrial vapours or unsuitable medication;
- radiation of various kinds, especially ultraviolet sunlight;
- rarely, irritation from mascara and eye liner.

RECOGNITION AND SYMPTOMS
The affected eye appears red or pink as a result of the widening of the tiny conjunctival blood vessels. The conjunctiva contains thousands of mucus-secreting cells (goblet cells) and many minute tear-secreting accessory lacrimal glands. Local irritation causes these to become overactive, so mucoid discharge and watering occur. In infective conjunctivitis, this discharge will often contain many inflammatory white cells from the blood (pus cells), and the mucus and pus tends to accumulate on the lashes, causing them to stick together.

> Conjunctivitis of the newborn must, by law, be notified to the Public Health Authorities. The real concern, here, is that the conjunctivitis – in this case known as ophthalmia neonatorum – might be the result of a gonorrhoea infection acquired during birth from the infected mother. Gonococcus bacteria are capable of causing blindness, by perforation of the cornea, so it is important that any newborn baby with sticky or inflamed eyes should be urgently treated. The doctor will take a swab for identification of the organism and start effective antibiotic treatment at once.

In most cases the diagnosis of conjunctivitis is fairly obvious. But there are some other causes of red eye which are not due to conjunctivitis and which are more serious.

> Pain and loss of vision should be reported urgently.

Other conditions which cause redness of the eye include:
- acute **uveitis** – infllammation of the iris and the focusin muscle;
- corneal ulceration – commonly caused by the Herpes simplex virus but may be caused by almost any organism;
- foreign body on the cornea or under a lid;
- a sudden rise in the pressure within the eye (acute **glaucoma**);
- a corneal or conjunctival foreign body;
- bleeding under the conjunctiva (sub-conjunctival haemorrhage).

The latter, although dramatic, is harmless.

TREATMENT
Infective conjunctivitis is treated with antibiotic drops or ointment. In other cases, steroid drops are sometimes prescribed, but these may be dangerous and should not be used unless the diagnosis is certain.

connexin-26

One of a number of substances known as gap junction proteins. Gap junctions between cells allow the passage of ions and small molecules from one cell to another. The gene for connexin-26 has been located and is situated on chromosome 13. A single base deletion **mutation** of this gene results in the complete absence of this connexin. This can cause a recessive form of sensorineural deafness.

Conn's syndrome

A rare condition caused by a tumour, usually benign, of an adrenal gland. The cells concerned are those which secrete the hormone aldosterone and the result is overproduction of this hormone. This causes salt and water retention with resulting excess fluid in the tissues (oedema), and high blood pressure. There may also be periods of weakness or even paralysis, and muscle spasm (**tetany**).

Treatment is by removal of the offending tumour or by the use of the drug spironolactone, which blocks the action of aldosterone.

consciousness, loss of, brief

See **Stokes-Adams attacks**.

consent

Medical or surgical treatment, or even physical examination, may be performed only with the consent of the patient, and this should, ideally, be informed – that is, the patient should know exactly what the treatment, or examination involves. In most cases the consent is implicit, in the sense that a person who consults a doctor will generally be deemed to be willing to accept that doctor's examination, advice and treatment. In the case of surgical treatment, however, implicit consent is not enough and the consent will always be recorded in writing, usually on a standard form designed for the purpose.

But it should never be forgotten that people retain their civil rights, even in a doctor's consulting room or an operating theatre, and anything done to them against their will may be deemed an assault in law.

constipation

Unduly infrequent evacuation of the bowels, with difficulty and sometimes pain on defaecation from hard stools.

INCIDENCE
Constipation is almost unknown among peoples whose diet is largely vegetable with a high fibre content. The average Western stool deposit weighs 120 to 150 grams; that of the average African or Asian on traditional diets is about 400 grams. Such people are also free from many of the colonic disorders suffered by those of us who enjoy more expensive diets.

There is a widespread belief that the failure to empty the bowels at least once a day is dangerous. This is nonsense. Many entirely healthy people defaecate only once every two or three days; some go at longer intervals. Some people have a satisfying bowel motion three times a day. All are normal. Most people defaecate once a day after breakfast, but there is no moral obligation on anyone to be so regular.

RECOGNITION AND SYMPTOMS
Constipation causes symptoms but they are not, as is alleged by some writers on alternative medicine, the result of the absorption of 'toxins' from the bowel. These symptoms, which include a sense of fullness, headache, furred tongue, loss of appetite, nausea, fatigue and depression, are mostly the result of the awareness of the constipation and of the belief that it is harmful. They can be produced by packing the rectum with sterile cotton wool.

RISKS
Constipation is as often imaginary as real, and many people, who believe that a daily bowel action is essential to health, severely abuse their lower intestines with laxatives, supposito-

ries and enemas. This response to an imaginary disorder can produce a real one. Anxious, fastidious people, especially those whose food intake is small, often feel that it is essential to get rid of 'unclean' excreta every day. Some become very anxious if there is no bowel motion. The constant use of laxatives in these circumstances can readily lead to an irritable bowel disorder. Depressed people often excrete less than average and the awareness may, in turn, make the depression worse.

TREATMENT

The way to cure constipation is to ensure adequate bulk in the stools. This is done by replacing refined carbohydrate, in the diet, with foods containing much vegetable fibre, such as fruit, vegetables and bran-containing cereals. Bran is what is left when flour is extracted from cereals. Up to half its weight is cellulose vegetable fibre which takes up large quantities of water. So plenty of fluid should be taken with the bran. It is hard to eat too much bran. This kind of regime will produce bulky, soft stools and regular motions.

See also **irritable bowel syndrome**.

contact lenses

See **lenses, contact**.

contact tracing

A public health procedure of great importance in minimizing the spread of disease, especially **sexually transmitted disease**, and conditions, such as typhoid, in which transmission by healthy carriers is notorious. Individual rights are well preserved and it is seldom necessary for the health authorities to use their legislative powers in a manner which interferes with individual liberty. See also **typhoid carrier**.

contagious

Literally, 'by touch'. A contagious disease, strictly speaking, is one in which the responsible organisms are transmitted by direct contact. The term is, however, often used simply to mean 'infectious', and this looseness of usage adds further confusion to an already confused situation as knowledge on the transmission of infectious diseases is constantly upgraded and changed.

Chickenpox, for instance, once thought to be highly contagious, in the literal sense, is now known to be transmitted by droplet spread. The common cold, on the other hand, once thought to be spread by air-borne droplets, is now known to be mainly spread by direct skin contact – to be, in fact, a contagious disease.

contentment

See **health maintenance**.

contra-

Prefix meaning 'opposite, against' as in contradict (speak against).

contraception

Contraception is not quite the same as birth control, which, for instance, includes avoidance of sexual intercourse so that contraception becomes unnecessary. But the two terms are often used interchangeably.

The aim in contraception is to avoid contact between ovum and sperm so that fertilization is impossible, but the term is also commonly used to include methods that prevent implantation of the fertilized egg into the lining of the womb. Such methods are not strictly contraceptive because conception has already taken place. The intrauterine device (IUD) mainly works in this way, although some such devices also work by releasing hormones that prevent conception. Even so, the IUD is nearly always considered as a contraceptive measure and is usually included in lists of contraceptive methods. Similarly, the 'morning-after' pill (see below) can hardly be described as a contraceptive.

Keeping sperms away from eggs can be done by putting a barrier between them, as in the case of condoms (male and female), diaphragms, cervical caps and various sterilization methods involving closure of the Fallopian tubes and male vasectomy. A more effective way of keeping the two apart is to prevent the release of the eggs from the ovary.

The discovery in the early 1950s, by the American endocrinologist Gregory Goodwin Pincus (1903–67), that this could be reliably done by a pill containing female sex hormones, sparked off a revolution in contraception and had a major effect on human sexual behaviour. The contraceptive pill was licensed and put on the market in 1957 and by 1964 more than 4,000,000 women were using it regularly.

Most women of the Western world who wish to avoid pregnancy use some form of contraception, and about one-third of them are on the Pill. Female sterilization has become easier, although not quite as simple as male sterilization by vasectomy, and in some parts of the world, such as the USA, another third of these women have been sterilized. The remainder rely on all the other forms of contraception – condoms, spermicides, withdrawal (coitus interruptus), the diaphragm, periodic abstinence (calendar, or rhythm method) and intrauterine contraceptive devices (IUDs).

There are no entirely authoritative figures for the real effectiveness of contraceptive methods because apparent failures are often due to faulty use. Many people, for instance, do not appreciate how enthusiastically sperms make for their target. If, for instance, seminal fluid is deposited on or around the vulva or even on the upper thighs, after a condom is removed, the sperms may still reach the ovum. It is possible, however, to get a useful idea of the relative reliability of the various methods, and, in general terms, contraceptive methods can be trusted in the following order, from best to worst:

- female sterilization by removal of the womb (hysterectomy);
- male sterilization by vasectomy;
- female sterilization by Fallopian tubal closure;
- the Pill and other forms of hormonal contraception such as implantation methods;
- IUD;
- diaphragm;
- condom;
- spermicides;
- withdrawal (coitus interruptus);
- 'safe period' (calendar or rhythm method).

With the exception of the first, none of these is absolutely 100 per cent reliable. Some medical papers have appeared recently showing that men who have had a vasectomy and have had a negative sperm count have still fathered a child.

Paternity in these cases has been proved by DNA fingerprinting. Such cases, however, which are believed to be due to a rejoining (recanalization) of the cut vas deferens, are exceptionally rare. For practical purposes, the first four methods of contraception in the list can be considered perfectly safe.

Oral contraceptives are by far the most generally acceptable form of contraception and, properly used, can be considered entirely effective. There are many different formulations but most contain various combinations of the oestrogens ethinyloestradiol and 3-methyl ethinyloestradiol (mestranol) and one of the five progestogens norethisterone, desogestrel, norgestimate, gestodene and levonorgestrel.

A progestogen (or progestin) is any substance having progesterone-like activity. The earlier pills contained much higher doses of hormones than modern oral contraceptives. The trend has been to ever lower dosage and those containing very small doses of oestrogens are in every way as effective as the earlier high-oestrogen pills. Some pills contain a progestogen only (POP pills). These are known as mini-pills and they are often used for women who are breastfeeding or older women whose fertility is declining as they are less effective than the combined pill.

Oral contraceptives work in different ways. Oestrogens act on the pituitary gland to prevent the production of the follicle stimulating hormone (FSH), that prompts the ovaries to produce eggs (ovulation). In the absence of FSH, ovulation does not occur. Oestrogen also interferes with the implantation of a fertilized ovum. Progesterone affects the cervical mucus, keeping it in the thickened, sticky state which obstructs the movement of sperms.

In addition to being highly effective in preventing pregnancy, oral contraceptives also have certain advantageous effects. These include a reduction in:

- blood loss in menstruation;
- anaemia;
- irregular menstrual bleeding;
- non-malignant breast disorders;
- cancer of the womb lining;
- premenstrual syndrome;
- menstrual pain;
- ovarian cysts;
- cancer of the ovaries;
- inflammation of the Fallopian tubes (salpingitis);
- post-menopausal osteoporosis.

Against these advantages are a slight increase in the risk of cancer of the cervix. There is no convincing evidence of a significantly increased risk of breast cancer for individual women, although there is a tiny effect in the population as a whole. Oral contraceptives increase the tendency for the blood to clot and may promote clotting in the deep leg veins and even in arteries.

In combination with drugs that narrow arteries, such as some ergot preparations used to treat migraine, the tendency for blood to clot can be dangerous.

Obstruction of brain arteries, leading to a form of stroke, has occurred in this way. The oral contraceptives also raise the levels of blood cholesterol. However, in one six-year study of 65,000 women using oral contraceptives and including smokers, but excluding women with high blood pressure and diabetes, no cases of coronary thrombosis occurred and there was only one case of stroke.

Other side-effects include:

- breast tenderness;
- emotional upset;
- fatigue;
- skin changes including acne;
- nausea;
- weight gain.

Oral contraceptives can sometimes reduce fertility and interfere with menstrual cycles for a time after use, but do not cause long term infertility. They have no effect on the rate of spontaneous abortion nor do they cause chromosomal abnormalities.

Short of sterilization, the Pill is by far the most effective contraceptive. Various studies have reported failure rates of from 1 women per 1000 per year to 1 women per 100 per year. For the average couple, this is really equivalent to saying that, given that the pills are taken properly, conception is almost impossible.

LONG-ACTING CONTRACEPTIVES

Long-acting hormonal contraceptives can be given by injection, by implantation under the skin or by insertion into the cavity of the womb. Commonly used examples are Depot-Provera and Noristerat, both given by a single deep intramuscular injection; Implanon (by implantation); and Mirena by womb insertion. An implantation contraceptive called Norplant consisted of six tiny progesterone-containing plastic capsules inserted under the skin by means of a syringe-like device. This caused problems and has been withdrawn.

Depo-Provera must be repeated at intervals of 12 weeks. Noristerat is intended for use up to 16 weeks and this requires two courses. Implanon has an action for two or three years and must then be removed. Mirena has to be replaced after five years. Fertility returns soon after these implants are removed.

Intrauterine devices are also long-acting contraceptives. They have a longer history than is generally appreciated: crude devices, usually made of copper, have been in use since the nineteenth century. Because of side-effects the IUD has been in and out of favour since it was first introduced. The IUD is often favoured by women for whom there is some objection to the use of oral contraceptives.

IUDs are, however, unsuitable for many women and should not be used if:

- pregnancy would be risky to health;
- the woman might possibly be pregnant;
- there is any question of infertility;
- there is a history of ectopic pregnancy;
- the womb contains fibroids;
- there is abnormal vaginal bleeding;
- there is any local infection;
- the lifestyle involves risk of sexually transmitted disease.

Some very slight risks are involved in being fitted with an IUD, and this procedure has in rare cases been associated with severe fainting, serious slowing of the heart and even epileptic seizures. Very occasionally fitting has caused perforation of the womb. IUDs are often associated with a degree of infection and there is said to be a slight increase in infertility after their use, probably as a result of infection of the Fallopian tubes (salpingitis). There is an increased risk of ectopic pregnancy. Some experts dispute that these effects are due to the IUD but opinions on this point tend to be partisan.

Some IUDs release the hormone progesterone, and these may be considered true contraceptives. Others release copper ions and probably act by causing slight but persistent inflammation of the womb lining so that implantation of the fertilized egg is prevented.

The copper-containing devices can usually be left in place for five years; the hormone-releasing devices are replaced every year. Modern IUDs such as the copper-covered T-shaped plastic device has a failure rate of 1 per 200 woman per year, i.e., a 0.5 per cent risk of pregnancy per year.

BARRIER METHODS

All the barrier methods – condoms, diaphragms and cervical caps – do also protect to some extent against sexually transmitted disease (STDs). Condoms are especially valuable in this respect, but many people dislike them. This is a pity, as they can prevent the spread of AIDS viruses, herpes and Chlamydial infections.

Male condoms are made of very thin but strong latex rubber and are in the form of a sheath that is packed and sold rolled up and is intended to be unrolled on to the erect penis before any genital contact occurs. Most have a terminal teat to accommodate ejaculated semen. If they are used only once, they seldom burst or tear, but they have to be used intelligently and with a clear understanding that their purpose is to prevent any contact between the seminal fluid and any part of the woman.

After orgasm, the penis, still within the condom, should be withdrawn before it shrinks, otherwise spillage of semen is likely. The condom should be removed and disposed of, well away from the woman's genitalia. Vaseline should not be used as a vaginal lubricant as it can damage thin rubber. K-Y jelly or a spermicidal jelly are better. Note that K-Y jelly is not a contraceptive, as is sometimes thought.

Female condoms are larger than male condoms and are intended to line the vagina. They have a large external ring. Although the idea is a good one and provides the woman with an easy way of protecting herself against both pregnancy and infection, female condoms do not seem to have caught on very widely.

A diaphragm is a shallow, soft rubber dome with a covered metal spring in the outer ring. Diaphragms come in different sizes, averaging about 7 cm in diameter, and must be properly fitted by an expert. Instruction in insertion and removal is also needed. The diaphragm covers the cervix, acts as a container for spermicide, prevents sperms from entering the womb and keeps the cervical mucus out of the vagina. This mucus is the natural channel through which sperms swim.

The diaphragm is inserted up to several hours before it is needed and must remain in place for at least six hours after intercourse. If a second act of intercourse is anticipated within six to eight hours the diaphragm should not be disturbed but extra spermicidal pessaries should be used. Between periods of use, the diaphragm should be washed and dried, inspected against a light for pinholes and stored in the container provided.

The failure rate for condoms and diaphragms is 1 to 4 per cent in women over thirty, but is much higher in women under twenty-five. Although the peripheral spring on a diaphragm is by no means strong, it can press on the bladder through the vaginal wall and this may sometimes give rise to trouble. There is evidence that women using diaphragms are more likely to suffer from urinary infection than those who do not. Possibly there may be some restriction to the outflow of urine.

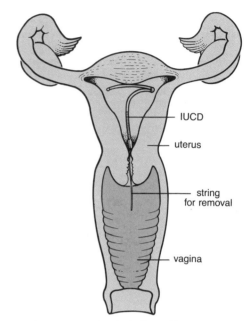

Intrauterine contraceptive device in position.

Cervical caps come in several sizes and have to be carefully fitted as they must lie snugly over the cervix, being retained in position by suction. They are more comfortable than diaphragms because they cannot press on the bladder and can be left in place for up to twenty-four hours. They, too, are used in conjunction with a spermicide and have a failure rate of around 10 per cent. They should be used only by women who have had a normal cervical smear result. Most fitting clinics recommend that all women attending should have a Pap smear test.

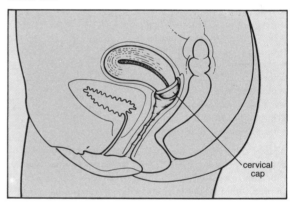

A cervical cap in position. Caps must be accurately fitted as they are retained by suction.

SPERMICIDES

Spermicides are substances that kill or, more usually, immobilize sperms. Used alone, they are not effective but are somewhat more reliable if used in the form of impregnated sponges. They are also available as vaginal creams, foams, jellies and pessaries. Sperms are readily immobilized by surfactants, that is, anything that greatly reduces surface tension – in the manner of washing-up liquid (not recommended as a contraceptive!). Most spermicides contain the surfactant nonoxynol 9. Spermicide sponges are best left *in situ* for about a day and retain their efficiency for at least this period. They should not, however, be forgotten about.

Women who have never had children are said to be as well protected by an impregnated sponge as by a diaphragm, but this is probably an unsafe generalization. On average, the failure rate is said to be twice as high as with the diaphragm. The experts argue about these assertions. It is generally believed, and is probably true, that spermicides can reduce the risks of acquiring a sexually transmitted disease. They are known to be active against viruses and it is said that women using spermicides reduce their chances of getting cancer of the cervix by one-third.

Nothing in this section should be taken to imply that spermicides, alone, are a satisfactory method of contraception. They should be regarded as an ancillary measure, to be used in conjunction with other barrier methods.

COITUS INTERRUPTUS

This widely practised attempt to frustrate the ends of nature is the responsibility of the man, as the woman seldom knows, for certain, when ejaculation is going to occur. It involves a hurried withdrawal of the penis from the vagina just at the point at which orgasm seems imminent. Predictably, the method is highly unreliable, partly because of lack of will power and partly because leakage of seminal fluid commonly occurs before the orgasm. Spermatozoa can, and do, escape into the lubricating mucus produced during coitus, and semen spilled on or around the vulva is capable of causing fertilization, by sperm migration. Couples who use the method regularly are likely to find that it lets them down in more senses than one.

Orgasms and the succeeding period of relief of tension should be enjoyed unrestrainedly in close intimacy with the partner. Coitus interruptus is incompatible with this and with the quality and naturalness of sexual intercourse. The practice has, quite rightly, been proscribed since the writer of Genesis gave us his views of the matter in the story of Onan 'who spilled his seed upon the ground' thereby incurring the wrath of the Old Testament God. This story, incidentally, seems to be the basis for theological objections to contraception.

The evil consequences of coitus interruptus, whether moral, psychological or religious, have doubtless been greatly exaggerated, and there is no reason to suppose that they include the spectrum of neurotic illness formerly claimed by psychiatry. Even so, as a regular method of contraception, the practice is not to be recommended.

SAFE PERIOD

This is the only contraceptive method sanctioned by the Roman Catholic Church. Unfortunately, even if used correctly and supplemented by the additional safeguards mentioned below, it is by far the most difficult to apply and by far the least effective. If every woman had a completely regular and reliable 28-day cycle it would be possible to predict the time of the next ovulation with reasonable accuracy by counting from the start of the last period. In such a cycle, ovulation occurs between days twelve and sixteen. There are arguments about how long sperm can survive to fertilize an ovum after deposition in the vagina, but most authorities suggest three to four days. The ovum has to be fertilized before it reaches the inner end of the Fallopian tube and this usually takes about twenty-four hours. It may take longer.

At best, therefore, the period during which fertilization can occur lasts from day eight to day seventeen. Sometimes a large part of the period from day one to day eight is taken up by the menstrual period and many people dislike intercourse during menstruation. (The idea that women are 'unclean' during this time is, of course, atavistic nonsense, but menstrual coitus can be messy.) The real trouble is that there is no way the length of the current cycle can be reliably predicted; a change commonly occurs even in women who are normally quite regular.

Uncertainty as to how long deposited sperm remain fertile is another complicating factor, and eggs can be held up in the Fallopian tubes. For all these reasons the method commonly fails. It should not be relied upon unless pregnancy is secretly wished by both parties. This method is also wide open to faulty use. The failure rate reported in some series has been about 50 for 100 women in one year, or, looked at in another way, an average of a pregnancy every two years for couples using the method.

These disappointing results can be improved upon somewhat. At the time of ovulation there is a rise in internal body temperature of about half a degree Celsius. This can only be measured reliably with a special thermometer used in the rectum, and can only be trusted if the rise persists for three days. Also, around the time of ovulation, the mucus in the cervix, normally of a thick, viscous consistency, becomes thin and watery. It is easy, however, to confuse seminal fluid with watery mucus, and intercourse in the days following menstruation can result in a misleading effect.

THE 'MORNING-AFTER' PILL

This is an emergency method that can be used after unprotected intercourse or after an accident with a condom. Some 70 per cent of unwanted pregnancies are predictable and it is in these that this method is most used. The 'Yuzpe' regimen, which can be used up to seventy-two hours after intercourse, offers a 98 per cent chance of avoiding a pregnancy. The pill has been licensed for use in Britain since 1984 and is available from most doctors and from family planning clinics. Severe nausea and vomiting are common side-effects.

OTHER METHODS

A silicone rubber ring, containing progesterone and oestrogen, and placed high in the vagina for three weeks at a time, allows regular menstruation and affords contraceptive protection as effectively as oral pills.

Breastfeeding is sometimes said to be a fairly effective contraceptive and so long as it continues (with the mother breastfeeding on demand and offering no supplementary feeds) and the periods have not started, the chances of having a baby are slight. Unfortunately, as ovulation occurs before menstruation, one cannot be sure when fertility is restored. So lactation should not be relied on as a contraceptive.

The current status of male contraceptives is uncertain, as drug manufacturers are keeping quiet, at present, about the results of their intensive research. A substance called gossypol derived from the cotton plant has undergone extensive testing, especially in China, but there are doubts about its safety. This was tried after it was noticed that many men eating food cooked in cotton-seed oil became infertile.

contraceptive drugs

Oral contraceptive pills contain sex hormones in various combinations – the oestrogens ethinyloestradiol and 3-methyl ethinyloestradiol (mestranol) and one of the five progesterone-like substances (progestogens) norethindrone, norethindrone acetate, norethynodrel, norgestrel and

contractions

laevonorgestrel. Some contain progestogen alone. The oestrogen dosage is very small these days, but the pills are just as effective as the earlier high-oestrogen formulations.

Contraceptive pills work in different ways. Oestrogens prevent ovulation but if this does occur and the egg is fertilized they also interfere with implantation. This means that their action can be, like that of IUDs, somewhat more than purely contraceptive. Progestogens, on the other hand, act on the mucus in the canal of the cervix to keep it thick and viscous and offer a barrier to sperm movement. So their action is more like that of a condom.

Contraceptive pills are highly effective. Recorded failure rates range from one pregnancy per 1000 women per year to one per 100 women per year. Either way, no one need worry and the method can be considered completely successful in preventing conception. If you forget to take a pill at the usual time you should take one as soon as you remember and you should take the next one at the normal time. But you should realize that if you are 12 hours or more late, the pill may not work and you will be at risk for seven days. If the seven days would take you past you end of the current pill pack you should start another pack straight away.

The pill has a number of benefits apart from peace of mind:

- premenstrual tension (PMT) is often reduced;
- periods become regular and less painful;
- the likelihood of fibroids of the womb and ovarian cysts and cancers is reduced;
- less blood is lost in menstruation;
- anaemia is less likely;
- the incidence of salpingitis – inflammation of the Fallopian tubes – is reduced.

Unfortunately, there is a negative side. Statistically, oral contraceptives slightly increase the chances of cancer of the cervix, but reduce the chances of cancer of the womb lining (endometrium) or of the ovaries. The risk of breast cancer is not thought to be affected. Oral contraceptives do, however, increase the blood-clotting tendency and there is a somewhat higher incidence of deep vein and arterial thrombosis. You will be at greatest risk, in this respect, if you smoke and suffer from severe migraine. Contraceptive pills can also cause:

- weight gain;
- breast tenderness;
- an increased tendency to acne;
- occasional emotional upset;
- a sense of fatigue.

They have no permanent effect on fertility.

Spermicides, in spite of the name, don't usually kill sperms; they work by making sperms tired so that they can't swim far enough to reach or penetrate the egg. They come in the form of foams, jellies, creams, pessaries and impregnated sponges. The latter can be left in place for about a day and still retain their efficiency. Spermicides actually reduce the chances of acquiring a sexually transmitted disease. They are active against some viruses and probably reduce the chances of getting cancer of the cervix.

See also **progestogen drugs**.

contractions

A term usually applied to the periodic tightening and shortening of the muscle fibres in the womb (uterus) which, as they increase in strength and frequency, gradually bring about the expulsion of the baby.

contracture

Permanent shortening of muscles and other tissues, such as tendons and skin, as a result of disuse, injury or disease. Contracture leads to the inability to straighten a joint or joints fully and to permanent deformity and often disability. Skin contractures, often following burns, lead to shortening and distortion and sometimes limitation of movement.

Muscle contracture commonly follows paralysis, as in **stroke**, and the failure to prevent this can lead to a serious reduction in the prospects of recovery of function. Patients in prolonged coma will suffer contractures unless actively managed by skilled physiotherapists.

contraindication

Anything which makes a proposed form of medical intervention undesirable or dangerous. Head injury, for instance, is a contraindication to the giving of morphine, which might depress the respiratory centres and cover up vital signs of brain damage.

contusion

A bruise.

convalescence

The period of recovery following an illness, injury or surgical operation.

conversion disorder

See **hysteria**.

convulsion

A fit or seizure. A fit may involve the whole or part of the body and may or may not be followed by loss of consciousness. In the major fit of **epilepsy** (grand mal), there is a sudden violent contraction of most of the voluntary muscles of the body (tonic contractions) followed by relaxation and then a succession of smaller jerky contractions (clonic contractions), persisting for a minute or so.

Convulsions occur in many brain conditions, of which epilepsy is only one. They are a feature of high fevers, brain tumour, **encephalitis**, head injury, **stroke** and various kinds of poisoning.

copies, perfect

See **clone**.

copolymer-1

A mixture of synthetic random polypeptides made from the amino acids alanine, glutamic acid, lysine and tyrosine that has been found to reduce the relapse rate in **multiple sclerosis**. Research suggests that the drug can reduce the relapse rate, in patients subject to relapses, from 75 per cent to 66 per cent. The drug is believed to act on helper T cells so as to promote cloning of those whose cytokines are mainly B cell antibody-stimulating (Th-2) rather than those whose **cytokines** have a mainly inflammatory and destructive effect (Th-1). A brand name is Copaxone.

copros

Greek root meaning 'dung' as in coprophilia (loving dirt).

corde

Latin root meaning 'heart' as in cor pulmonale (heart damage from lung disease).

cordotomy

A deliberate partial severing of some of the nerve tracts in the spinal cord performed for the relief of severe and otherwise uncontrollable pain. Pain sensation is transmitted up the spinal cord to the brain in certain long nerve bundles called the spinothalamic tracts. These two long tracts lie on either side of the front of the cord, and cutting those on one side abolishes the pain sensation on the opposite side of the body. This is because the sensory nerve fibres cross to the opposite side of the cord after entering.

The tracts are cut in the neck region of the cord and this is not easy to do without damaging other nerve tracts and causing other neurological deficit. So the procedure is done only in extreme cases in which all else has failed. Pain sensation often returns after a time, probably because other tracts exist which also conduct pain impulses.

corium

Latin root meaning 'skin' as in corium (true skin).

corn

The outer layer of the skin is covered with flattened, horny cells (cornified epithelium) which are protective in nature. Excessive pressure on the surface causes these horny cells to be produced more abundantly so that over areas abused in this way a thickened callosity forms. Badly fitting shoes cause pressure on prominent points, such as the toe joints or the head of the big toe, leading to the formation of dense cornified disks which the continued pressure forces painfully into the soft underlying skin.

Such increased local pressure is an added stimulus to the production of yet more cornified epithelium and soon a vicious circle is set up which will not be broken by paring corns or by use of softening solutions. Such responses are illogical attempts to interfere with a natural protective process. Unless the prime cause is removed, corns will continue to be formed.

corneal abrasion

Loss of the outer layer (epithelium) of the cornea, so that the sensory nerves are exposed to strong stimulation by every movement of the lids.

RECOGNITION AND SYMPTOMS

Even gentle blinking may be exquisitely painful. The sensation is almost indistinguishable from that of having a sharp piece of grit under an eyelid and there may be a conviction that there is a foreign body in the eye. There may be intense spasm of the lids (blepharospasm), which makes the pain worse, and copious weeping.

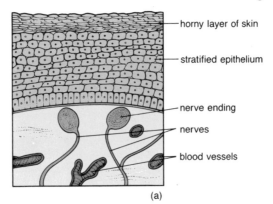

(a)

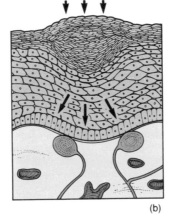

Corn. (a) Normal skin. (b) The protective thickening of the outer layer (the epidermis) which forms a dense, hard, body which is pressed down into the underlying layers of the skin, causing stimulation of pain nerve endings.

(b)

POSSIBLE CAUSES

Abrasion may be caused by any mechanical trauma, such as a scratch by a baby's fingernail, but most abrasions occur because of lack of oxygen to the cornea. The commonest cause of corneal abrasion, nowadays, is overwear of hard contact lenses.

TREATMENT

Corneal abrasions are treated by padding the eye for two or three days and the use of antibiotic drops to prevent infection. Contact lenses should be left off for two or three weeks.

> A neglected abrasion may become infected and progress to ulceration and possibly perforation with possible loss of the eye.

corneal graft

The restoration of transparency to an opaque cornea by cutting out a disc and replacing it with a disc of identical size from a healthy donor cornea. The donor cornea need not be of compatible tissue because the healthy cornea is free of blood vessels and destructive antibodies and immune system cells cannot therefore reach the graft to attack it.

HOW IT'S DONE

Corneal graft operations are almost always done under general anaesthesia, using an operating microscope. They call for great skill and steadiness. The disc is cut from the donor eye with a cylindrical cutter called a trephine and then left in place so that it does not dry up. The same instrument is used to cut a central disc from the damaged eye, thus ensuring that the donor disc will fit perfectly. When the opaque disc is removed, the clear donor disc is inserted and stitched firmly in place with a fine perlon suture – so fine that it is barely visible except under the microscope. A zig-zag 'bootlace' stitch is used. The knot is rotated so as to be buried in the cornea and the suture need not be removed. The operation takes up to an hour and healing takes about six weeks, but the patient is up and about the next day. The chances of restoration of good vision are excellent.

Corneal grafts are most likely to succeed when the affected cornea is free from active disease and when blood vessels have not grown in from the edge of the cornea. These may bring in immune cells and antibodies which may lead to loss of transparency of the graft. Results are particularly good in conical cornea or in cases of long-healed central corneal scars.

corneal injury

The commonest injury to the cornea is a scratch, or **corneal abrasion**, caused by a foreign body, a flying particle or an unexpected poke from a baby's finger. Penetrating injuries can cause scarring with loss of transparency or may cause irregularity of the corneal surface. Both can lead to defective vision.

POSSIBLE CAUSES

Ultraviolet light radiation, whether from an electric arc lamp, a sun-tan lamp or excessive sun at high altitudes, can also damage the outer layer of the cornea. This layer tends to strip off, exposing the nerve endings and causing severe pain. This may affect unprotected amateur welders, some hours after exposure. Skiers or mountaineers may suffer a similar effect and, in this case, the condition is known as 'snow blindness'.

A cornea deprived of the normal protection of the blink reflex soon becomes severely damaged. This occurs in any condition in which the lids cannot close to cover the cornea, such as **exophthalmos**, **Bell's palsy**, **ectropion**, lid scarring and failure of closure of the lids during sleep. Corneal exposure is always serious and leads to rapid drying and opacification with severe loss of vision.

Chemical injuries to the cornea can result from acid or alkali splashes. Alkali on the cornea is especially dangerous as it rapidly sinks in, causing massive and spreading tissue destruction. Many have been permanently blinded by spraying with ammonia and other alkalis. Only immediate and prolonged flushing with large volumes of water is likely to save the sight in such cases.

corneal transplant

A slightly misleading term for **corneal graft**. The whole cornea is not transplanted – only a small central disc, usually about 7 mm in diameter.

corneal ulcer

The cornea is susceptible to infection by a wide range of viruses, bacteria, fungi and some protozoa. Toxic damage by any of these may cause local tissue destruction and the formation of an ulcer. This may occur very rapidly and, defeating the body's repair processes, lead to penetration. This is a serious and sight-destroying complication.

POSSIBLE CAUSES

One of the commonest infecting organisms is the cold sore or genital herpes virus, *Herpes simplex*. This is acquired by kissing and contact and, once established in the cornea, is probably present for life. Herpes simplex causes the characteristic branching *dendritic* ulcer with pain, watering and foreign body sensation. Properly treated within a few days of onset, the condition can be cured, but if such an ulcer is treated with steroid eye ointments or drops, it may become established and cause years of distress.

Gonorrhoea can cause a dangerous corneal ulcer, especially in babies infected during birth. Perforation and blindness used to be common before antibiotics. Eye infection in the newborn is a notifiable disease.

Various fungi can cause very persistent ulcers. These are uncommon and the diagnosis may be missed unless the condition is suspected and scrapings examined. Antifungal drugs are available and are reasonably effective. Contact lens wearers sometimes develop corneal infection and ulceration from an organisms called *Acanthamoeba* which grows in contact lens solutions and containers not properly sterilized.

cornu

Latin root meaning 'horn' as in cornified (horn-like).

coronary angioplasty

A procedure, first performed in 1977, for widening coronary artery branches which have become so narrowed by **atherosclerosis** and superimposed clotting of blood (thrombosis) that the heart muscle is being deprived of an adequate blood supply. Those with this condition suffer from chest pain (**angina pectoris**), and the success rate for the operation, in relieving this pain and increasing exercise tolerance, is between 70 and 80 per cent.

HOW IT'S DONE

A fine 'steerable' guide-wire is first passed, under radiographic control, into the diseased artery. The wire is carefully pushed into and through the narrowed segment. A small-gauge tube (**catheter**) with a sausage-shaped balloon segment near one end (a **balloon catheter**) is now threaded along the wire until the balloon lies exactly in the narrowed part of the artery. The balloon is now inflated to distend the constriction. If adequate widening is not achieved, the balloon can be reinflated using higher inflation pressures. If the catheter is too large to pass through the narrowed segment, it may be exchanged without removing the guide wire. Catheters as small as 0.4 mm diameter are used with guide wires of only 0.3 mm.

The widening remains effective in most cases. The procedure works very well in those with soft clots partially blocking the coronary artery branch, but may not work at all if the plaque of atheroma is too hard and rigid to stretch or if a complete occlusion by thrombosis has been present for more than three months.

WHY IT'S DONE

In many cases, the results are dramatic. Angina is abolished and the fortunate patient is able to return to a more energetic and healthy life. In about a quarter of cases, the artery re-narrows and the angina returns within a few months. The alternative to angioplasty, **coronary artery bypass**, now carries very little risk and the results, especially when a mammary artery is used instead of a vein, are excellent. If angioplasty fails, an emergency bypass operation may be necessary and the risks may now be increased.

MEDICAL ADVANCES

The most recent advances in methods of re-opening narrowed coronary arteries include the use of catheters with high-speed rotating cylindrical cutters that shave away the atheromatous plaques and suck out the debris; catheter cutters that pulverize plaques into fragments so small that they can be safely carried away by the bloodstream to be dealt with by phagocyte cells; and laser devices that destroy the plaques. Lasers were disappointing, initially, as they tended to cause coronary artery closure and were difficult to use. But a more recent device, the excimer laser (see **myopia**) has proved more promising. Early results, from operations done since 1992, suggest a success rate of over 90 per cent.

coronary artery bypass

A highly effective form of treatment for people suffering the effects of coronary artery narrowing from **atherosclerosis**. Such people have severe chest pain (**angina pectoris**), are disabled by greatly reduced tolerance to exertion and are at risk from complete coronary artery blockage (coronary thrombosis, see **heart attack**). The outlook for bypass surgery is best in those who have not had a coronary thrombosis and whose hearts are not enlarged. In these, there is an 85 per cent chance of full recovery from all symptoms and a mortality rate, attributable to the operation, of less than 2 per cent.

HOW IT'S DONE

In the early years of bypass surgery, leg veins were used in almost all cases. The veins were connected, by microsurgery, to the coronary arteries beyond the narrowed areas and then linked to the high-pressure artery, the aorta, just above the heart. The two coronary arteries, themselves, come off the aorta. One of the coronary arteries immediately divides into two, so there are three main coronary branches. If necessary, a bypass can be done on all three (triple bypass).

Ten-year studies of the outcome of vein bypass operations showed that about one-third had blocked off and another third showed a thickening of the inner lining of the vein and clear signs of atherosclerosis – a condition previously found only in arteries. An alternative procedure, favoured by many vascular surgeons, is to connect the internal mammary artery of the chest wall to the diseased coronary artery. The mammary artery normally supplies the front wall of the chest and the diaphragm and, although delicate and difficult to dissect out, has some major advantages over veins. It shows, for instance, a surprising and unexpected immunity to atherosclerosis, and, although much narrower than the veins which were used, has the ability to enlarge to meet the requirement. Sometimes a segment of the artery is used, much in the manner of veins, as a free graft. The long-term results from internal mammary bypass surgery are usually excellent.

coronary artery disease in children

See **Kawasaki disease**.

coronary artery unblocking

See **excimer laser coronary angioplasty**.

coronary bypass advance

See **minimally invasive coronary bypass surgery**.

coronary bypass with artery

See **mammary artery grafting**.

coronary care unit

A hospital department or ward set aside for the intensive care management of people who have suffered attacks of coronary thrombosis (see **heart attack**) and are in an unstable condition. Patients in coronary care units are closely and continuously monitored by highly trained staff, using the electrocardiogram and often continuous and immediate (real-time) analysis of blood gas changes and pressure. In this way, the response to any significant alteration in the patient's condition can be almost instantaneous, and life-saving action taken. All the necessary equipment for resuscitation and the management of cardiac arrest, including electric shock defibrillators, is at hand.

Many lives have been saved in this way.

coronary thrombosis

See **heart attack**.

coroner

A coroner is a barrister, a solicitor or a doctor qualified for at least five years, appointed by the local authority in which he or she acts. The chief function of the coroner is to enquire into the cause of death in cases in which this is not immediately apparent.

A coroner may also deal with cases where death cannot be certified by an attending doctor. If satisfied that death was natural, a coroner may certify the death for the purposes of registration without holding an inquest or even without ordering a post-mortem examination (autopsy).

A coroner takes action only when a death is reported to him or her, and Registrars of Births and Deaths do so in the following circumstances:

- when the deceased has not been seen by the certifying doctor within fourteen days before the death, or after the death;
- when the cause of death is unknown or in doubt;
- when there is any reason to believe that the death was unnatural, accidental, caused by violence or neglect, or the result of poisoning or abortion;
- when there are any suspicious circumstances;
- when death occurred during a surgical operation or before recovery from an anaesthetic;
- when death appears to have been due to industrial disease or poisoning;
- when the Registrar is unable to obtain a properly completed death certificate;
- when the deceased is a baby, reported to have been born dead (a stillbirth) but the Registrar has reason to believe that the child may have been born alive.

In all such cases, preliminary enquiries are made by the coroner's officer, who is usually a serving police officer, and on the basis of his or her findings, the coroner will decide whether to order an autopsy.

In most cases the coroner has discretion as to whether or not to hold an inquest, but must do so in certain cases, including violent or unnatural death, deaths in prison, and deaths resulting from industrial disease, poisoning or injury. The inquest need not have a jury, and nowadays a jury is seldom called.

Witnesses are examined under oath, the evidence is considered, and a verdict is given. Possible verdicts include unlawful killing, self-killing, misadventure, natural causes, drug addiction, alcoholism, self-induced abortion, want of attention at birth, or an open verdict.

cor pulmonale

A heart disorder with enlargement of the main pumping chamber (ventricle) on the right side.

POSSIBLE CAUSES

This enlargement is due to a rise in the blood pressure in the lung arteries, through which the right side of the heart pumps blood, resulting from one of several lung diseases. These include long-term (chronic) **bronchitis**, **emphysema**, silicosis, widespread scarring (fibrosis) of the lung or any other of the persistent obstructive lung diseases.

RECOGNITION AND SYMPTOMS

Such disorders interfere with the free passage of blood through the tiny branches of the arterial tree in the lungs and thereby greatly increase the resistance to blood flow. They also tend to cause the small lung blood vessels to go into spasm, so that the narrowing is made even worse. The increased resistance imposes an additional load on the right side of the heart which responds by enlarging. Up to a point, the increased power of the enlarged ventricle enables the heart to compensate, but eventually the heart muscle fails and the blood returning to it from the rest of the body cannot be pumped fast enough. There is a sense of fullness in the neck and abdomen and accumulation of fluid in the tissues (oedema). The liver enlarges and the ankles swell. There is weakness, fatigue, breathlessness and blueness of the skin (**cyanosis**).

In some cases cor pulmonale is caused by disease or narrowing of the lung arteries themselves, such as may result from repeated small emboli.

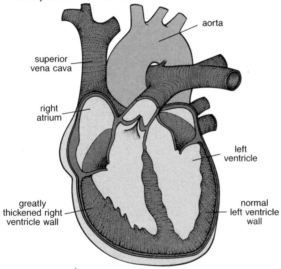

Cor pulmonale. Normally, the left lower chamber (left ventricle) is the more powerful and has the thicker wall. But in this condition, in which the right ventricle has to work much harder than usual, the right ventricle may be the stronger.

corpus

Latin root meaning 'body' as in corpse (dead body).

corresponding pair chromosomes

See **homologous chromosomes**.

corticosteroid drugs

See **steroids**.

cortisone

The first corticosteroid produced for treatment purposes. It is converted to hydrocortisone in the liver. It was used to treat rheumatoid arthritis, severe allergies, adrenal failure and other conditions but has been largely replaced by more powerful synthetic steroids. A brand name is Cortisyl.

coryza

The medical term for the common cold.
See **cold, common**.

Cosmegen Lyovac

A brand name for **actinomycin D**.

cosmetic skin improvement

See **skin peel**.

cosmetic surgery

A branch of **plastic surgery** devoted to the improvement, or alteration, of the human appearance. The most technically successful operations are those to modify the nose (**rhinoplasty**), the ears (**otoplasty**), the chin (mentoplasty) and the breasts (augmentation or reduction mammoplasty). Body contour surgery by **lipectomy**, and other major procedures to cut off the effects of years of self-indulgence, tend to have a temporary effect, as does the face lift (rhytidectomy). **Skin peel** can improve the appearance of ageing facial and other skin, but is not without risk.

WHY IT'S DONE

The desire of cosmetic surgery is often motivated by vanity. There are, however, many people whose lives are adversely affected by a conspicuous and readily remediable physical blemish. For these, cosmetic surgery may offer a legitimate and justified resource.

Some cosmetic surgeons have lost the purity of their ethical ideals and potential customers should beware those whose seem unduly to be pushing their commodity.

costa

Latin root meaning 'rib' as in costal (of rib or ribs).

costalgia

A little-used word for a seldom-experienced symptom – pain in a rib.

cot death

See **sudden infant death syndrome**.

cough

A reflex by which the lungs are able to get rid of potentially dangerous semi-solid material in the bronchial tubes, and are guarded against the entry of unwanted material.

In coughing, a deep breath is taken and the vocal cords are then pressed tightly together. The diaphragm is now forced upwards so as to compress the air in the lungs and the vocal cords are then triggered sharply apart so that a blast of air passes upwards from all parts of both lungs. This carries out any material, such as excess mucus, sputum or small foreign bodies.

Many persistent chest disorders feature regular coughing because of the production of excessive bronchial secretions.

cough, hacking

See **tracheitis**.

coughing up blood

> Coughing up blood is a sign of great importance which should never be ignored.

The medical term for coughing up blood is haemoptysis. It can be a sign of cancer of the lung, tuberculosis, lung abscess, fungus infection of the lungs, heart failure, pulmonary embolus and clotting disorders.

INCIDENCE
Blood-streaked sputum is fairly common and does not necessarily mean that something potentially fatal is happening. In about 80 per cent of cases it is a sign of bronchitis.

RECOGNITION
One should confirm that the blood is actually being coughed up and does not originate in the nose or mouth. Blood from the nose can trickle down the back of the throat and mix with secretions coughed up from the lung. Blood from tooth or gum disorders can, likewise, mix with sputum and appear to come from the lungs. A distinction should also be made between blood coughed and blood vomited. The former is bright red, the latter looks like wet coffee grounds.

Coughing of frank blood is almost always serious, especially if frequent and of more than minor quantity. This calls for urgent investigation, probably by direct visual examination of the inside of the bronchial tubes (**bronchoscopy**).

cough, smoker's

A sign of persistent bronchial irritation caused by cigarette smoke and indicating that the cells of the lining of the bronchial tubes are being progressively damaged, are losing their essential features and are possibly being changed to a type liable to develop cancerous properties.

A smoker's cough is an unequivocal indication of danger and a clear warning of the urgent necessity to give up smoking.

cowpox

A mild disease, causing skin blisters, which affects the udders and teats of cows and can be transmitted to people doing manual milking. Cowpox is caused by the vaccinia virus, which is a modified form of smallpox. It has an important place in the history of immunology as it was vaccinia which Edward Jenner used to successfully vaccinate people against smallpox. This was the first time a vaccine was used.

coxa

Latin root meaning 'hip' as in coxa (of the hip bone).

crab lice

See **lice**.

crack

Crack is a highly purified and powerful form of cocaine, volatile on heating and readily absorbed through the lungs. It acts similarly to amphetamine, causing a 'high' with a short period of intense pleasure. This feeling is strongest on the first use and is never experienced to the same intensity again. Crack quickly leads to dependence in some users and there is no way of knowing, in advance, who will become addicted and who will not. Some people seem to have little difficulty in keeping usage under control, but about 15 per cent of users go on taking larger and larger doses until they are as dependent as heroin addicts.

Crack, like amphetamine, can lead to a short-lived, acute form of mental illness. This is called a cocaine psychosis. The symptoms include severe depression, agitation, delusions, ideas of persecution, hallucinations, violent behaviour and suicidal intent. People with a cocaine psychosis often have 'lucid intervals' in which they seem normal and will often deny using the drug. Cocaine psychosis usually follows long binges or high doses. Anyone who thinks cocaine usage safe and amusing is either ignorant or extremely foolish.

cramp

A muscle disorder, usually minor, in which a single muscle, or a group of muscles, suddenly go into a state of powerful sustained contraction. This incapacitating state is quickly followed by severe pain which persists until the contraction eases off. Cramp is often caused by excess salt loss from sweating and can be prevented if lost salt is replaced by adequate drinking of fluid containing some extra salt. Salt tablets can be a convenient source, but may cause irritation of the stomach. Overdosage should be avoided.

The common problem of night cramps, which affect most people from time to time and usually involve the calf muscles, has never been satisfactorily explained, but many people have found that the cramps can be prevented by a small dose of quinine.

Swimmers' cramps can affect the abdominal or the limb muscles and sometimes lead to a panic reaction which can only make the situation worse. The best response is to tread water gently or float on the back until the spasm has passed and then to swim slowly, avoiding strenuous movements.

cramp, writer's

This condition is strange in that it affects only the activity of writing and does not occur when the same muscles are used for other purposes. Soon after starting writing, the muscles involved in holding the pen or pencil go into a state of spasm so that writing cannot continue. The implication is that there is a psychological element in the causation, possibly related to an unsuitable choice of occupation. Writer's cramp is sometimes included in the group of disorders known as *dystonia*.

Now that most writers are using word processors rather than pens, it is possible that new light may be thrown on this interesting condition.

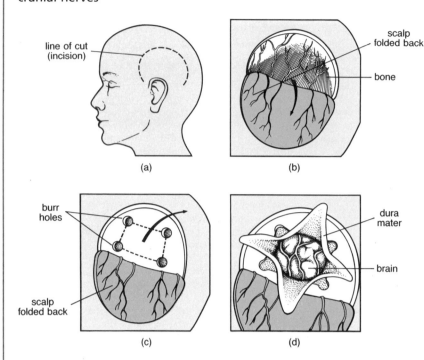

Craniotomy. The stages in gaining access to the brain for surgery. (a) A wide circular flap is cut in the skin and scalp. (b) The flap is folded back. (c) Four burr holes are drilled in the bone of the skull and these are joined by saw cuts so that the segment of bone can be removed. (d) The tough membrane covering the brain (the dura mater) is opened, exposing the surface of the brain.

cranial nerves

These are the twelve pairs of major nerves arising directly from the brain and brain stem, as distinct from the spinal nerves which emerge from the spinal cord. The cranial nerves are concerned with smell (olfactory nerves), vision (optic nerves), eye movement (oculomotor and abducent nerves), sensation in the head, secretion of tears and saliva, movement of the muscles of facial expression, hearing (acoustic nerves), tongue movement, chewing and taste. One pair, the vagus nerves, wanders out of the head and travels down as far as the bowels, supplying the heart with rate-control fibres, on the way. All but the first two pairs of the cranial nerves arise from the upper part of the broad stalk of the brain (the brain stem).

cranion

Greek root meaning 'skull' as in cranium (vault of the skull).

craniopharyngioma

A rare brain tumour affecting mainly children. The cranio-pharyngioma arises from a group of primitive cells in the region of the pituitary gland, which are present in the early embryo and which, instead of disappearing, have persisted and developed into a kind of non-malignant cyst-like swelling. Because of pressure rises within the skull and damage to the pituitary gland, the affected child may have headaches and visual loss and may show delayed physical and mental development. As the tumour grows, the neurological effects become more marked. CT or MRI scanning easily shows up this kind of tumour. The only effective treatment is surgical removal.

craniotomy

Surgical opening of the skull, usually for the purpose of operating on the brain, or to relieve dangerous pressure within the skull cavity. Craniotomy involves cutting through the scalp, folding back a flap, drilling holes through the bone of the skull (trephining), and joining these with cuts made with a fine saw. Immediately under the skull bone is a tough fibrous membrane called the dura mater and this must be cut through to expose the brain.

crepitus

The grinding or crackling sound heard when the broken ends of a fractured bone rub together. This is one of the signs of fracture that should never be deliberately produced. The term is also used for the grating sensation felt when a joint affected by arthritis is moved and dry or damaged joint surfaces rub together.

cretinism

See **thyroid gland disorders**.

Creutzfeldt-Jakob disease

A rapidly progressive transmissible disease of the nervous system affecting middle-aged and elderly people, causing death within a few months of onset. It is a spongiform encephalopathy, similar, or possibly identical, to **bovine spongiform encephalopathy** (BSE), **kuru** and scrapie in sheep and is associated with an abnormal form of a normal body protein called a prion (see **prion protein disease**). Up to 60 cases are estimated to occur each year in Britain. There is no effective treatment.

A new variant of CJD with a shorter incubation period appeared in the late 1980s and by February 1998 24 cases had been reported, 23 of them in Britain. There is clear evidence that this form is either caused by, or in some way involves, the same strain of prion as bovine spongiform encephalopathy.

Cri du chat syndrome

A genetic disorder caused by the absence of the short arm on chromosome number five. Affected babies are small with very small brains (microcephaly), have round faces with downward-sloping eyes, low and abnormally shaped ears, short necks and often heart defects. There is mental retardation but many may survive into adult life.

Babies with the 'cat cry' syndrome have a peculiar, high-pitched, mewing cry, very like that of a kitten.

crisis

A term once common but now, in the antibiotic era, seldom used. The crisis was the peak or turning-point of a disease, especially an infection like lobar pneumonia, after which one generally knew whether the patient was going to live or die. Nowadays, patients seldom reach the crisis, because infections are rapidly brought under control.

Crohn's disease

See **regional ileitis**.

Cromogen

A brand name for cromoglycate sodium.

cromoglycate, sodium

A drug used in allergies. It stabilizes the membrane of the mast cells that otherwise release histamine and other irritating substances when antibodies (IgE) and allergens (such as pollen grains) react on their surfaces. A brand name is Cromogen.

crossed eyes

See **strabismus**.

cross-eye

The popular term for **strabismus** or squint.
See also **amblyopia**.

cross matching

See **transfusion**.

crotamiton

A drug that relieves itching. An **antipruritic** drug. A brand name is Eurax.

croup

An inflammation of the main air tubes to the lungs (laryngo-tracheo-bronchitis) affecting young children and causing a partial obstruction to air flow through the voice box (larynx) so that breathing and coughing are difficult, harsh and painful. Breathing in is often more difficult than breathing out, causing the characteristic crowing sound known as inspiratory stridor. There is often a typical 'barking' cough. Croup was common in the days of **diphtheria**, but is now uncommon and is usually caused by virus infections causing inflammatory swelling of the lining of the larynx and trachea. The child may become very restless and alarmed, with a fast pulse rate, heaving of the shoulders, and even some blueness of the skin (cyanosis).

Severe croup may lead to life-threatening airway obstruction and, in such a case, it may be necessary to make an artificial opening into the trachea, just below the larynx (tracheostomy). More often, the condition requires no more than inhalation of humidified air and other general medical measures.

crus

Latin root meaning 'leg' as in crural (of the leg).

crutch palsy

Old-fashioned armpit crutches supported the weight on a part of the body through which a major network of nerves (the brachial plexus) passes. Pressure on these nerves, from the head of the crutch, would sometimes cause paralysis of some of the muscle groups in the arm supplied by the nerves. The modern elbow crutch has eliminated this danger.

cryo-

A prefix meaning relating to very low temperatures, usually artificially obtained.

cryobiology

The study of the effects of low temperatures on cells and tissues. These are normally destructive, but research has brought out methods of applying great cold to biological materials so as virtually to halt the processes of ageing and deterioration without causing serious damage.

See **cryopreservation**.

cryonics

Freezing and storing the human body soon after death to preserve it indefinitely, in the hope that future scientific advances will allow correction of the process that caused the death, so that, assuming that the damaging effects of the freezing can also be corrected, life can be restored.

cryopreservation

The prevention of destructive bacterial action and biochemical change by maintaining organic material, such as tissue for grafting, human embryos, seminal fluid, etc., at very low temperatures. Cryopreservation can be considered a kind of 'suspended animation'. Semen, deep frozen at -196°C with liquid nitrogen, can be kept indefinitely without loss of fertility.

Some people have paid large sums to have their whole bodies cryopreserved after death. This is done in the hope that future advances in medical science may allow their resuscitation and restoration to life.

cryosurgery

Controlled tissue destruction by low temperatures, usually by means of cryoprobes by which cold can be applied with precision.

Freezing has several advantages over cutting. It prevents bleeding, limits tissue destruction and can often be used without anaesthesia. It is widely used in the treatment of various skin disorders, especially warts, and in some forms of brain surgery. It has been used in the treatment of Parkinson's disease, cancer of the prostate and other organs, bone cancer, and even as a means of removing enlarged tonsils.

cryotherapy

Cryosurgical methods are routine in much ocular surgery. Cataracts can be removed by freezing the opacified lenses on to the tip of a cryoprobe, and retinal detachment is treated by using cold to cause a sterile inflammation which causes the replaced retina to adhere.

cryotherapy

The use of low temperatures in medical treatment. Temperatures of about -20°C or below are useful in surgery. They may be obtained by the use of carbon dioxide snow, liquid nitrogen, the rapid expansion of gases within a *cryoprobe* (see **cryosurgery**), or by electronic means (Peltier effect).

cryptococcus

A yeast that shows very little tendency to infect normal, healthy people, but which is particularly prone to attack those with an immune deficiency, from whatever cause.

Infection can involve the lungs, causing **chest pain**, fever, cough – sometimes with blood – and chronic illness lasting for months or years, but the chief site of cryptococcus infection is the brain and its coverings, the meninges. Cryptococcal meningitis, which occurs in 90 per cent of those severely affected, is a serious disease which is very slow in its progress and prolonged in its course. The most obvious symptom is headache, and this is associated with severe neck stiffness, fever, nausea and vomiting, marked blurring or doubling of vision, defective memory, confusion, personality changes and slowly progressive mental defect. Other parts of the body, such as the bones, the liver, the kidneys, the spleen and the lymph nodes, may be infected, but infection of these is much less common than infection of the meninges.

Happily, the effectiveness of treatment has been greatly improved in recent years, for prior to the introduction of the drug amphotericin B, the mortality in cryptococcal meningitis was 80 per cent within two years of diagnosis. Today, this mortality has been reduced to about 20 per cent. But the drug has to be given by injection into a vein, daily, or every second day, for a period of about six weeks, and may sometimes have to be combined with another drug called flucytosine. Occasionally, it may even be necessary to inject these drugs directly into the cerebrospinal fluid surrounding the brain. Both of these drugs are toxic and can cause damage to the kidneys, liver and to the production of blood elements – red and white cells – in the bone marrow.

cryptorchidism

Undescended testicle. Literally, 'a hidden testicle'. The testicles develop in the abdomen and should pass down temporary canals (the inguinal canals) into the scrotum by the time of birth. If either testicle fails to descend, or to be brought down, before puberty, the higher temperature in the abdomen inhibits normal sperm production and the testicle will be permanently sterile. Testicles retained in the abdomen are more likely to develop cancer later.

CS

A highly irritant crystalline solid, 0-chlorobenzylidene malononitrile that can be sprayed at persons from a pressurized cannister for purposes of police control. CS is used in a solution of strength 5 per cent in the UK and 1 per cent in the USA. It causes intense burning discomfort in the eyes and on the skin, profuse watering of the eyes and nose, barely controllable spasm of the eyelids, coughing, retching and a sense of constriction in the chest. The effects may last for as long as 24 hours. Corneal damage has been claimed but it is not clear whether this is due to the active ingredient or the solvent.

CTLA4-Ig

A fusion antibody protein that has been shown to be capable of persuading T cells (T lymphocytes) to recognize severely mismatched transplanted organs as 'self' even in the absence of immunosuppressive drugs. T cell activation requires two signals – a T cell-receptor-mediated signal and a co-stimulatory signal. Co-stimulation involves another receptor on the lymphocyte, the B7 receptor, for which CTLA4-Ig is specific. If this protein is attached to the B7 receptor it will block co-stimulation and prevent T cells from mounting a rejection attack.

CT scanning

A CT scanner is an advanced form of X-ray machine. Instead of using a wide beam of radiation, as in a conventional X-ray machine, the scanner sends out a succession of short-duration, very narrow, fan-shaped beams of radiation, each one passing through the body at a slightly different angle from the previous. These beams are produced by a small X-ray source which rotates around the subject on a circular arm and the radiation is picked up by a number of separate detectors arranged in an arc on the other side. With each pulse of radiation these detectors produce electrical outputs which are stored in a computer. When the beam has been right round, the process may be repeated for other 'slices' and all the information obtained is stored. The computer is then able, by solving thousands of differential equations, to reconstruct from all these data retailed images of the body. A tomogram is an X-ray taken in 'slices'; computerized tomography (CT) combines many tomograms.

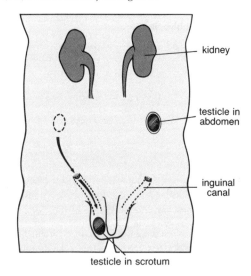

Labels: kidney; testicle in abdomen; inguinal canal; testicle in scrotum

Cryptorchidism. At around the time of birth, the testicles, which have formed in the abdomen, pass down a canal on either side into the scrotum. Cryptorchidism, or 'undescended testicle', is the condition in which one or both fail to descend.

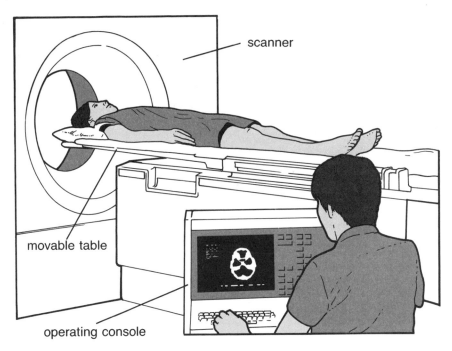

scanner

movable table

operating console

Computerized tom[...]
(CT) scanning has bec[...]
essential method of bod[...]
imaging. Initially applied [...]
only to the head, full body
scanning is now universal.
This is an X-ray method but
the radiation dosage is low.
The area to be examined is
studied in 'slices'. The
resulting information is
analysed by computer to
obtain density levels for
thousands of different
points. From these, an
internal picture is
constructed.

Ordinary X-rays can detect only a few different levels of contrast; CT scans can detect many hundreds of levels, bringing out detail impossible with conventional X-rays. In addition, the slice-like nature of the method eliminates the confusing shadows of overlying structures. The total dose of radiation is about the same as that of an equivalent standard X-ray examination, but the detail revealed is much greater.

CT scanning is especially valuable for investigating the inside of the head and the brain for possible tumours, bleeding, swellings on arteries (aneurysms) or injuries. It is also useful for studying the structures in the central, solid part of the chest which show up poorly on conventional X-rays. It is widely used to detect masses anywhere in the abdomen, including tumours and abscesses, and to reveal damage to organs in cases of severe abdominal injury. Lacerations of the spleen, kidneys or liver, such as may occur in serious automobile accidents, can be revealed by CT scan.

culdoscope

An endocope used to examine the female pelvic organs. It is passed through the vagina and then through a perforation in the cul-de-sac behind the cervix into the pouch behind the womb. Pelvic endoscopy is now more commonly performed through the abdominal wall (laparoscopy).

-cule

Suffix meaning 'diminutive' as in homunculus (little man).

-culture

Suffix meaning 'growing of' as in horticulture (garden-growing).

culture, bacterial

Bacterial culture is the cultivation of living micro-organisms, such as bacteria or viruses, in an artificial environment specially arranged to encourage growth and reproduction.

Culture media vary considerably depending on the organisms being grown and require appropriate nutritional elements and critical temperatures. Cultures are grown in an incubator in which a constant temperature is maintained. For organisms normally flourishing in the human body, or for bacteria which affect human being, the optimum temperature is that of the healthy body -37° C. Bacterial culture media commonly consist of a basis of agar heated up with a broth of meat extract or other organic nutrient. The mix must be sterilized before use and this may conveniently be done by boiling. Blood is often added before the hot mix is poured into shallow, flat, round glass or plastic dishes called Petri dishes. On cooling, the agar sets to a firm, jelly-like consistency, on to the surface of which the sample to be cultured is carefully smeared. The primary growth may be of mixed bacterial colonies, and subculture of pure growths may be achieved by picking off a small quantity of one of these colonies with a sterile platinum loop, and inoculating a fresh plate with it.

Bacteria are routinely cultured for purposes of identification and to check their sensitivity to various antibiotics. Selective culture media are often used to encourage growth of one organism and inhibit that of others. In some cases, the environment must be modified if growth is to occur, and sometimes free oxygen must be excluded – as for the growth of anaerobic organisms.

cultured arteries

The artificial production of arterial tissue by *in vitro* cell culture, in three layers, of cells taken from the proposed recipient. Such arteries would have no tendency for immunological rejection. The technology is still experimental but shows great promise.

culture, tissue

Tissue cultures are valuable for many research and diagnostic purposes, including the growth of viruses, which can only reproduce within living cells. Genetically normal body cells cannot be maintained indefinitely in tissue culture, but

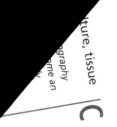

...lebrated example is the HeLa culture
...ortal and which is used in laboratories
...cells have several hundred chromo-
...nal forty-six, and so long as they are
...tion and conditions, will divide and

A long-outmoded form of treatment, mentioned for histori-cal interest. Air in a number of glass cups is heated and the cups applied firmly to the skin. As the air cools, it contracts, drawing the skin tightly up into the cups and causing an increase in the blood flow. The value of the procedure is min-imal, but it did, at least, have the merit of doing little harm.

curettage

Scraping or spooning out unwanted tissue or tissue required for examination. Curettage is performed with a spoon-shaped instrument of size appropriate to the purpose, and often with sharpened edges. It may be employed anywhere in the body, usually on the inner surface of an organ or cavity. Probably the commonest gynaecological operation is curet-tage of the lining of the womb (uterus) after enlarging the opening into the uterus by means of graded dilators (**D and C**).

curette

A spoon-shaped instrument for performing **curettage**. The curette may vary in size from a tiny 2 mm spoon for scooping out meibomian cysts in eyelids, to a 2 cm instrument for general surgical use.

curvature of the spine

See **kyphosis**, **lordosis**.

Cushing's syndrome

The bodily changes caused by excess of corticosteroid hormones.
POSSIBLE CAUSES
This may result from a tumour of the outer layer (cortex) of an adrenal gland with overproduction of cortex steroids, from a pituitary tumour with excess production of the adrenal stimulating hormone ACTH (adreno-corticotrophic) hormone, from other tumours which produce ACTH, e.g. certain forms of cancer of the lung, or the use of steroid hor-mones in high and prolonged dosage for medical purposes.
RECOGNITION AND SYMPTOMS
People with Cushing's syndrome are overweight, with fat deposits on the back of the neck and shoulders ('buffalo hump') as well as around the middle. The extremities are usually slender. The skin is thin and atrophied and wounds heal badly. There are often purplish streaks (**striae**) on the abdomen. The face is red and 'moon-shaped' and there is often male-pattern hairiness, or sometimes baldness, in women. There is weakness from wasted muscles, high blood pressure, **osteoporosis**, and often mental disturbances.
TREATMENT
The treatment is directed at the cause and this may involve removing a pituitary tumour or the use of supervoltage radi-

ation to the pituitary gland. Adrenal tumours are removed surgically and in some cases it may be necessary to remove both adrenal glands and maintain the patient on controlled doses of hormones. ACTH-secreting tumours are removed, if possible, but may have to be dealt with by drugs which antag-onize adrenal hormones.

Medically caused Cushing's syndrome is one of the prices that has to be paid for the benefits, or life-saving effect, of steroids. Doctors will always use steroids in the minimum dosage compatible with the needed effect.

cutaneous

A term meaning relating to the skin.

cutis

Latin root meaning 'skin' as in cuticle (dead outer layer of skin).

cutis verticis gyrata

An overgrowth of the skin of the forehead which, as a result, is thrown into deep vertical folds so as to resemble the surface of the brain. The condition is a feature of **acromegaly**, local inflammation and acute myeloid leukaemia. A rare primary form of the condition, which affects males only, is associated with severe learning difficulty, seizures, spastic paralysis (cerebral palsy) and eye abnormalities.

cyanoacrylate

A powerful adhesive occasionally used in surgery as a substi-tute for stitches. In many cases the results are better than with sutures. The adhesive is marketed for surgical use under the generic name enbucrilate and the trade name Histoacryl. The popular product Superglue is also a cyanoacrylate adhe-sive and is a common source of surgical problems.

cyanosis

Blueness of the skin due to the presence of blood containing insufficient oxygen. Fully oxygenated blood is a bright red colour and imparts a healthy pinkness to the skin. Blood whose oxygen has been used up is a dark reddish-blue colour and, through the skin, looks a dusky blue.

Cyanosis may occur because the blood is stagnant and is not being returned quickly enough to the lungs for re-oxygenation, or it may be due to inadequate oxygenation from asphyxia or lung disease. Cyanosis is a common feature of some forms of congenital heart disease in which blood is shunted away from the lungs. So-called 'blue babies' have cyanosis.

cyclizine

An **antihistamine** drug effective in controlling nausea and vomiting. A brand name is Valoid. Brand names of prepara-tions containing it are Diconal, Cyclimorph and Migril.

cyclo-oxygenase

The enzyme that converts arachidonic acid to prostaglandins which are commonly mediators of pain. Inhibitors of this enzyme form the large group of **NSAID** drugs.

cyclo-oxygenase-2 inhibitors

A range of drugs similar in action to non-steroidal anti-inflammatory drugs (**NSAIDs**).

cyclopenthiazide

A thiazide **diuretic** drug. A brand name is Navidrex.

cyclopentolate

A drug used to dilate the pupils of the eyes for purposes of examination of the retina and other internal parts. A brand name is Mydrilate.

cyclophosphamide

A drug that substitutes an open chain hydrocarbon radical for a hydrogen atom in a cyclic organic compound. It is an alkylating agent and is used as an anticancer drug for its alkylating action on the guanine molecule in **DNA**. The margin between the effective dose and the dangerous dose is narrow. side-effects include loss of hair, sterility, sickness and vomiting and depression of blood formation by the bone marrow. A brand name is Endoxana.

cycloplegia

Paralysis of the focusing muscle of the eye, usually temporary, as a result of deliberate medication with atropine or other similar eye drops, but occasionally permanent as a result of blunt injury to the eye. Cycloplegia makes it impossible to focus on near objects without glasses, unless the affected person happens to be short-sighted (myopic). Nearly everyone over sixty suffers from a natural form of cycloplegia and, unless myopic, must rely wholly on reading glasses for clear near vision.

cyclothymia

A personality disorder, characterized by swings of mood from elation to depression. When cyclothymia is manifested as a major mental disease, it is sometimes known as a **manic-depressive illness**.

Many perfectly normal people have cyclothymic personalities, but those with true psychiatric cyclothymia often suffer periods of severe depression which interfere seriously with social and work success. In some, the emphasis is on the manic phase and these are able to work long hours with little sleep and are often high achievers.

RECOGNITION AND SYMPTOMS

In general cyclothymia has an adverse effect on personal happiness and success. Marital discord and frequent quarrels with friends and associates, sexual promiscuity, alcohol and drug abuse and many changes of residence, occupation and religious or other affiliations are characteristic of cyclothymia.

The condition often starts gradually in adolescence or early adult life and about one-third go on to develop a major depressive illness.

TREATMENT

If treated with antidepressant drugs, such as lithium, about half suffer manic episodes. Life-long psychiatric management may be necessary. Group and family therapy is helpful.

cyproheptadine

An antihistamine and **serotonin antagonist** drug used to allergies, itching disorders and migraine. A brand name Periactin.

cyst

An abnormal walled cavity, usually non-malignant, filled with secreted fluid or semi-solid matter derived from the cyst itself. The wall may be thick or thin and the inner surface is lined with a normal body cavity non-stick lining (epithelium).

The term is also applied to the structure formed when the body reacts to the presence of a parasite by walling it off with a coat of fibrous tissue. Bacteria and other organisms may enter a protective encysted form when the environment is hostile or conditions are not conducive to reproduction. In this state they may survive dormant for long periods.

POSSIBLE CAUSES

When the outlet of normal glands becomes blocked, a retention cyst may form. Sebaceous cysts and eyelid meibomian cysts are of this type. Some cysts are of congenital origin and result from the abnormal burying, often in the skin, of collections of cells that should have been located elsewhere and that give rise to skin elements, hairs, bone and even teeth. These are called **dermoid cysts**. The ovaries are common sites for cyst formation and these often become very large but can usually be safely removed.

cystectomy

Surgical removal of the urinary bladder, usually for cancer. After cystectomy, the ureters, which constantly bring urine down from the kidneys, have to be connected elsewhere. They may be implanted into the colon so that the urine passes out with the faeces, or they may be implanted into an artificial bladder made from an isolated segment of bowel which drains out through the skin.

See illustration on following page.

cysticercosis

Infestation of muscles and other soft tissues of the body with the larval form of the tapeworm of the genus *Taenia*. Cysticercosis should be distinguished from ordinary tapeworm infestation by the adult worm, acquired by eating inadequately cooked pork (pig muscle) containing the cysts of tapeworm larvae. In this, the commoner situation, the human being has the tapeworm and the pig has cysticercosis from eating the egg-containing worm segments passed by the human being.

In human cysticercosis, the worm eggs are eaten, usually in contaminated food. When they hatch in the intestine, the larvae burrow through the bowel wall into the bloodstream and are carried all over the body to be deposited in many tissues including the muscles and the brain. These cause weakness and pain, epileptic fits, sometimes mental disorder and paralysis.

Occasionally, a person with a tapeworm may regurgitate worm segments up into the stomach, allowing hatching and the cycle of cysticercosis.

cystic fibrosis

A recessive genetic disease affecting almost all the externally secreting glandular tissue of the body. Most lining surfaces

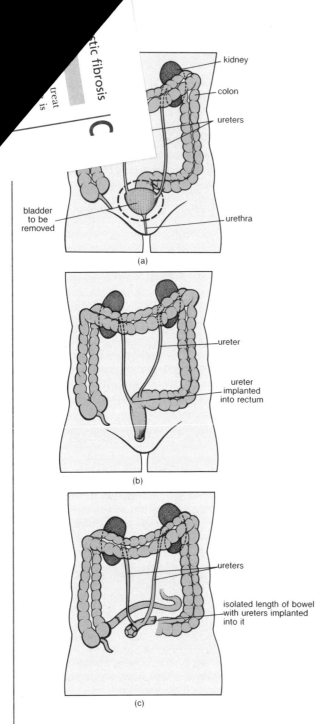

kidney

colon

ureters

bladder
to be
removed

urethra

(a)

ureter

ureter
implanted
into rectum

(b)

ureters

isolated length of bowel
with ureters implanted
into it

(c)

Post-cystectomy management. If it has been necessary to remove the urinary bladder (a), the ureters carrying urine down from the kidneys may be implanted into the rectum (b), or into an isolated segment of bowel (c), which is arranged to open on to the skin where the urine can be collected in an external bag.

contain tiny secreting glands or secreting cells and all these are affected. The result is that the salivary glands, the glands of the intestine, the pancreas, the gall-bladder, the lungs and the skin either produce excessive quantities of secretion or produce thick, sticky mucinous secretion which clogs them or obstructs the passages into which they normally discharge.

RECOGNITION AND SYMPTOMS

Babies with cystic fibrosis often get early intestinal blockage from sticky bowel contents (meconium). Others have swollen, protuberant abdomens and pass frequent oily stools. The appetite is very good but growth is slow. The sweat contains excessive salt and the skin may be powdered with dried sweat. This is a common early sign of cystic fibrosis.

About half have lung complications due to blockage of the bronchial tubes with excessive mucus secretions and plugs of thick muco-pus. There is troublesome cough, wheezing and difficulty in breathing and the chest becomes barrel-shaped from respiratory effort. Sinusitis and nasal problems are common.

Children with cystic fibrosis suffer growth retardation, delay in the onset of puberty and are unable to participate normally in games and sport because of their respiratory inefficiency.

COMPLICATIONS

The possible complications of the disease include lung collapse, secondary **heart failure**, cirrhosis of the liver, **pancreatitis**, **intussusception** and **diabetes**.

TREATMENT

Medical management involves skilled and comprehensive care and much-needed psychological support, both for the victim and the parents.

> The gene for cystic fibrosis was cloned in 1989 and over 230 mutations have been identified throughout the world. The availability of the sequenced DNA make it possible to detect carriers of the gene and this can be done early in pregnancy.
>
> If the woman tests positive, the husband can also be tested and a prenatal diagnosis can be made by chorionic villus sampling.

cystis

Greek root meaning 'bladder' as in cystitis (bladder inflammation).

cystitis

Inflammation of the urinary bladder caused by infection.

RECOGNITION AND SYMPTOMS

The symptoms are well-known, especially to women, who, mainly because of the shortness of the tube from the bladder to the exterior (the urethra), are much more prone to the disorder than men. There is an unduly frequent desire to visit the toilet, frequent passage of small quantities of urine, burning or scalding pain on passing urine, and sometimes involuntary passage of a small squirt of urine on coughing or laughing (stress incontinence). Sometimes a little blood is passed in the urine and affected people often have to get up during the night. Occasionally there may be fever, shivering, pain in the loins and general upset with nausea and a sense of illness (malaise). Cystitis in men is often associated with infection and inflammation of the prostate gland (prostatitis).

Examination of the urine, especially by **culture**, often shows that bacteria are present. These are commonly *coliform* organisms (*Escherichia coli*) which normally, and harmlessly, inhabit the bowel.

Cystitis is often due to other organisms, aside from bacteria, including those acquired during sexual intercourse such as *Chlamydia trachomatis*, *Trichomonas vaginalis*, *Haemophilus vaginalis* or *Candida albicans*.

TREATMENT

Treatment with antibiotics should be rapidly effective. If not, further investigation is called for in case the infection should be of wider extent or should be connected with some other bladder or kidney disorder.

> Cystitis can often be avoided by a frequent large fluid intake, to 'flush out' the urinary system, deliberate attempts to empty the bladder after urination seems complete ('double urination'), urination after sexual intercourse, and the avoidance of nylon underwear and vaginal deodorants. In menopausal women, cystitis may respond better to vaginal oestrogen creams than to antibiotics.

cystitis-like symptoms

See **urethral syndrome**.

cysto-

Prefix meaning relating to a bladder or cyst. Cystoscopy is the act of examining the inside the bladder with an optical instrument called a cystoscope, passed along the urethra. Cystitis is inflammation of the bladder.

cystogram, micturating

A special kind of X-ray taken while the urine contains a dye opaque to X-rays and while the subject is actually urinating. The radio-opaque fluid may be passed into the bladder via a catheter. This technique can provide information about abnormalities of the bladder and its supply and drainage passages which may not be obtainable in any other way. It is especially useful in children to investigate reflux flow of urine back up the ureters from the bladder.

cystoscopy

Examination of the inside of the urinary bladder by means of a straight, narrow, self-illuminating optical instrument which is passed in through the exit channel (the urethra). In men, a general anaesthetic is usually needed, but in women, the urethra is very short and cystoscopy can be performed with a local anaesthetic.

In examining the bladder, the doctor fills it with sterile water run in through a stopcock on the cystoscope. As this is done, the folds of the collapsed bladder are seen to flatten and smooth out and the inside of the wall can be inspected. The inspection port at the end of the instrument is at an angle, so rotating the cystoscope allows almost the whole of the inside of the bladder to be examined.

As well as allowing diagnosis of conditions such as infections, polyps, cancers and stones in the bladder, cystoscopy permits fine catheters to be passed up the tubes leading to the kidneys (ureters) through which a substance opaque to X-rays can be injected for X-ray studies (retrograde pyelography). Cystoscopy also allows biopsies to be taken and local treatment by cautery, laser and other means to be given.

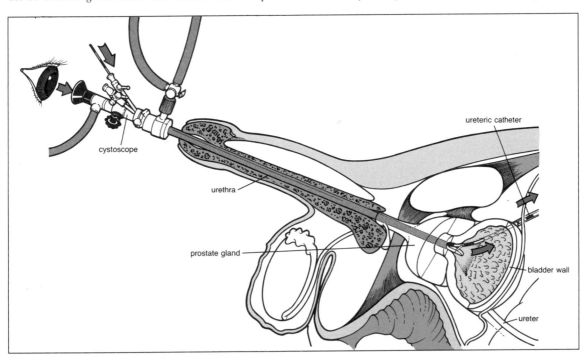

The inside of the urinary bladder can be examined by a cystoscope passed along the urine outlet tube (the urethra). The diagram also shows a ureteric catheter (striped tube) being passed up the right ureter to the kidney.

cystostomy

Cutting into a bladder. Historically, the only reason for cystostomy was to relieve the patient of the agonies of large stones in the urinary bladder. For this reason the operation was referred to as *lithotomy* or 'cutting for the stone' – a procedure which was as likely to kill the subject as cure the disorder. Nowadays cystostomy is done in a more orderly manner, by open operation under sterile conditions.

cytarabine

An antimetabolite drug used in the treatment of acute **leukaemia**. It is a purine antagonist (see purines) and acts by depriving cells of essential metabolic substances. It causes sickness and vomiting, peptic ulcers and depression of bone marrow blood formation. A brand name is Cytosar.

cytokines

A general term for a range of small proteins that exert a stimulating or inhibiting influence on the growth and spread (proliferation), change (differentiation) and function of cells of the immune system. Cytokines include **interferons**.

cytology

The study of cells. This has become a major science in its own right and there are specialists in many subdivisions of cell science. The term is often used loosely as an abbreviation of the phrase *exfoliative cytology*. This is the process of examining isolated cells, obtained from cervical smears (Pap smear test) or from sputum, to determine whether or not they are cancerous. Exfoliative cytology is performed by pathologists and calls for a high degree of expertise and care. Attempts are being made to reduce, by automation, the labour of examining hundreds of thousands of cell samples.

cytomegalovirus infection

The cytomegalovirus (CMV) is a herpes virus which does not normally cause any problems. Indeed, it is known that large numbers of perfectly healthy people carry the virus from childhood onwards. In some parts of the world, where general standards of hygiene are poor, almost everyone has the virus. But the CMV cannot be regarded so casually when there is no effective immune system to keep the virus in check. CMV is so constantly present in large numbers in AIDS patients that for a time it was suspected of being the cause of the syndrome. This error illustrates the common difficulty experienced by researchers in distinguishing cause and effect. In AIDS patients, the CMVs can be isolated from blood, urine, saliva, seminal fluid, vaginal secretions, milk and from the stools. About 60 per cent of AIDS patients show some of the effects of CMV infection. These include:

- a form of pneumonia which, in severe cases, can be fatal;
- liver inflammation with loss of liver functions and jaundice;
- fever;
- night sweating;
- damage to the retinas so that permanent visual loss may result;
- inflammation of the brain (encephalitis) which may cause permanent damage to brain function.

Cytomegalovirus is hard to attack. Most of the existing antiviral drugs have been tried; antisera have been given; steroids, even interferon, have been used, but none has been effective. Recently, however, two new drugs have been developed, both of which have shown promising results.

cytotoxic drugs

Drugs capable of damaging or killing cells. These can be used in the treatment of cancer because their effect is greatest on cells which are reproducing most rapidly. The cytotoxic drugs include alkylating agents, such as cyclophosphamide, melphalan and chlorambucil, that interfere with cell growth differentiation and function; cytotoxic antibiotics, such as dactinomycin, daunorubicin and doxorubicin, that bind to DNA blocking its transcription; antimetabolites, such as fluoruracil, cytarabine and mercaptopurine, that interfere with the action of folates; vinca alkaloids, such as vinblastine, vincristine and taxol, that block mitosis; and the topoisomerase 1 inhibitors, such as etoposide, anthracyclines and anthrapyrazoles, that interfere with nuclear enzymes required for DNA replication and the separation of daughter chromosomes.

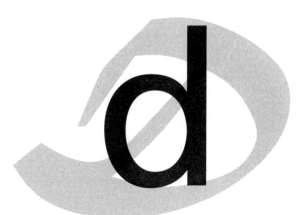

dacarbazine

An alkylating cytotoxic anticancer drug. A brand name is DTIC-Dome.

dacryocystitis

Inflammation of the lacrimal sac, the tiny bag situated in the eye socket, just inwards of the inner corner of the eye. The lacrimal sac acts as a kind of suction pump to draw tears away from the eye and pass them down the naso-lacrimal duct into the nose. Inflammation always causes problems with tear drainage and usually results in permanent blockage. Sometimes an abscess forms and this may burst externally below the inner corner of the eye.

Tear drainage can be restored by an operation, known as dacryocystorhinostomy, in which the lacrimal sac is connected to the inside of the nose by way of an artificial opening through the bone.

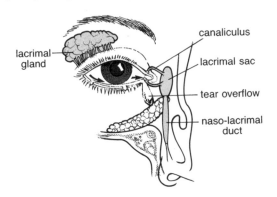

Dacryocystitis. This shows the structure of the drainage system which carries tears into the nose. In dacryocystitis, the lacrimal sac becomes inflamed and obstructed and the tears overflow the lid margin. The sac also becomes swollen causing a visible bulge near the inner corner of the eye.

dactylos

Greek root meaning 'finger' as in arachnodactyly (spider-like fingers).

dalteparin sodium

A low molecular weight **heparin** used to treat acute deep vein thrombosis. The drug is given by subcutaneous injection to adults only in a single daily dose calculated on the basis of body weight. A brand name is Fragmin.

danazole

A synthetic **progestogen** drug that inhibits secretion by the **pituitary gland** of the sex-gland stimulating hormone gonadotrophin. It is used to treat precocious puberty, breast enlargement in the male (gynaecomastia), excessive menstruation (menorrhagia) and **endometriosis**. A brand name is Danol.

D and C

Dilatation and curettage – this is a common gynaecological operation, usually done under general anaesthesia, which involves dilatation of the womb, which is then scraped clear of unwanted material.

HOW IT'S DONE

The opening into the womb (cervical canal) is gradually enlarged by pushing in a succession of ever-wider smooth metal rods (dilators), until it is able to admit a long spoon-shaped instrument (curette). This is used to scrape the inside of the womb.

WHY IT'S DONE

D and C is often used, either to treat abnormal menstrual bleeding, to remove unwanted tissue or to obtain a specimen for examination. It is also used to get rid of *retained products of conception* – a dead embryo which has not been spontaneously expelled, or to cause abortion early in pregnancy. The latter application is now used less often than before, having been replaced, in many cases, by suction curettage.

dander

Small scales from the skin, hair or feathers of animals, which commonly cause allergic effects, especially **asthma**. Dander particles may be microscopic, but still cause serious problems to sensitive individuals. In some cases, the only remedy is removal of the innocently offending animals.

dandruff

The common scaliness of the scalp from flakes of dead skin. These scales are most conspicuous when loosened and separated by combing or brushing the hair. Some loss of surface skin cells is normal, as these are constantly being pushed to the surface by the living cells beneath. Normal standards of hair care, with regular brushing, will dispose of these. Neglect will allow the exfoliated cells to accumulate. Dandruff represents either such as accumulation, or an increase in the normal rate of shedding, often because the skin is mildly inflamed and itchy from various causes. One of the commonest of these is known as seborrhoeic **dermatitis**. The cause of this condition is unknown but some dermatologists believe it may be due to a yeast fungus *Pityrosporum ovale*. It is usually worse in winter and is often so mild that little is seen except scaling. It may, however, be severe, with yellowish-red, greasy, scaly patches along the hair-line and spreading to other areas of skin such as the eyelids (**blepharitis**) or the external ears.

Dandruff responds well to the use of medicated shampoos, especially those containing selenium. Selsun shampoo is a popular remedy. Seborrhoeic dermatitis responds well to corticosteroid ointments and, in some patients, anti-yeast drugs are effective.

danger signs for health

See **health maintenance**.

dantrolene

A drug used to relieve muscle spasm. A brand name is Dantrium.

dark adaptation

The gradual acquisition of the ability to see in dim light that normally occurs in conditions of poor illumination. Dark adaptation becomes defective (night blindness) in vitamin A deficiency because this vitamin is necessary for the production of the retinal pigment visual purple, without which normal vision is impossible. Poor dark adaptation is also a feature of **retinitis pigmentosa** (tapetoretinal degeneration).

dark urine/pale stools

When red blood cells come to the end of their working life of about 120 days they are broken down and the haemoglobin from them is converted to a brownish-coloured substance called bilirubin. Normally, the bilirubin is removed from the blood by the liver and excreted, in the bile, into the small intestine. This is what gives the stools their characteristic brown colour. If there is any obstruction to the passage of bilirubin into the intestine – as from obstructive gallstones or hepatitis – the stools become pale and clay-coloured. And because the bilirubin accumulates in the blood it is excreted in the urine, giving it a dark brown colour. This combination of signs is also often associated with yellowing of the skin and of the whites of the eyes (jaundice).

dartos muscle

A thin layer of muscle lying immediately under the skin of the scrotum. The dartos tightens in the cold causing the normal skin wrinkles to deepen considerably so that the skin area is much reduced and the testes are pulled up.

day and night rhythm

See **melatonin**.

DDT

Dichloro-diphenyl-trichloroethane was the first of the widely used and highly effective insecticides. It is a nerve poison, especially effective against flies, mosquitos and lice and which quickly kills butterflies, moths and beetles. Mites and ticks are barely affected.

USES

DDT has saved millions of lives since it was first used as an insecticide in 1939. By destroying the insect carriers of many diseases, it has prevented countless cases of malaria (mosquitos), yellow fever (mosquitos), typhus (lice), plague (lice), river blindness or **onchocerciasis** (biting black flies), dysentery (house flies), sleeping sickness (tsetse flies) and **filariasis** (mosquitos). Many areas which were almost uninhabitable because of insect vectors of disease have been made safe for human habitation, and malaria has been eradicated from more than twenty countries, largely by the use of DDT. The World Health Organization sponsored many DDT spraying programmes in cooperation with local governments and these were highly successful.

RISKS

These obvious advantages were not achieved without cost, and in the 1960s it began to be apparent that bird life was suffering heavily from the effects of DDT, which, because of its chemical stability, was increasing in concentration in the animal food chain. Infertile, or fragile-shelled, eggs were being produced. In 1972 DDT was banned in the United States, being replaced by other insecticides, and since then the bird population has again increased. DDT has not been shown to be a serious toxic threat to man, which is more than can be said for its replacements, the organo-phosphorous insecticides such as Malathion, Parathion and Paraquat, but at least these break down rapidly in the soil to harmless compounds.

de-

Prefix meaning 'down from' as in decline (bend down).

deafness

See **hearing, defective**.

deafness, profound

See **cochlear implant**.

death

The cessation of the processes of living.

TISSUE DEATH

This may occur at various levels – at a tissue level, at an organ level, or at the level of the entire organism. Gangrene, for instance, is local tissue death, in which an area of dead, inert tissue is surrounded by relatively normal living skin, muscle, bone, etc. A loop of bowel, caught in a hernia, may become gangrenous and die, while the remainder of the bowel remains healthy. Part of the heart muscle may die, as a result of a coronary thrombosis, while the rest of the heart muscle carries on beating. Tissue or organ death is usually due to a major deprivation of blood supply, almost always from disease of the supplying arteries.

BODILY DEATH

Death of the whole organism (somatic death) results from a general failure of the supply of essential nutrition to the tissues, especially oxygen and sugar, or from the inability of the tissues to use them, because of poisoning or other damage. Oxygen and sugar are supplied via the blood and this is circulated by the heart and kept oxygenated by the lungs. So common causes of somatic death are stoppage of the heart or failure of the lungs to supply oxygen to the blood. The brain maintains the muscle action of breathing, so brain damage can cause somatic death if the result is a stoppage of the nerve impulses to the muscles of respiration.

It is a simple matter to maintain respiration artificially, when the brain can no longer do so, and people who would quickly have died can be kept alive indefinitely, by positive pressure respiration through a tube inserted into the wind pipe. Such people have, however, usually suffered widespread brain damage, so that many other functions, especially consciousness, are also abolished, often permanently. This gives rise to ethical dilemmas.

When the vital supplies are cut off for more than about eight minutes, widespread cell death begins, starting with the brain and at a certain point this becomes irreversible. In this case, certain changes occur in the body as a whole. The temperature begins to drop, the muscles stiffen (**rigor mortis**), the blood begins to clot in the vessels, and bacteria and enzymes in the body begin to cause chemical breakdown of the cells and connective tissue (putrefaction). These processes can be slowed by cooling the tissues and this is important if organs are required for transplantation.

> There has been much argument as to the definition of death, and this argument is far from academic in a context of the need for organs for transplantation. A widely, but not universally, agreed basis, which is often accepted for the purposes of transplantation, is that for a period of at least twelve hours there should be:
>
> ● no response, above the neck, to any stimulus;
> ● no spontaneous respiratory or other movement;
> ● widely dilated pupils with no response to light;
> ● an EEG (electroencephalogram) showing no indication of any electrical activity in the brain.

DEFINITION OF DEATH

Purely spinal refflexes, involving no brain action, ma remain. It is essential that the possibility of paralysing or anaesthetizing drugs or poisons should be ruled out. The heart may continue to beat for years after all possibility of brain function has gone (brain death).

To be absolutely sure of total somatic death, it is necessary to wait for putrefactive changes to begin. A more useful definition may be based on the fact that brain cells show death and liquefaction about fifteen minutes after the circulation of blood to the brain is cut off. Simpler organs, such as the kidneys and liver, remain functional for some hours, depending on the temperature, and muscles survive longer still.

debility

Loss or lack of strength. Debility is the common condition, although not the natural state, of old age and is due to loss of muscle bulk and of the efficiency of the heart and respiratory system (fitness) by disuse. It is the state of the chronic invalid whose life is spent in bed or in a sedentary posture.

The body adapts remarkably to the demands made on it; debility is the result of negligible demands. It is now recognized that the elderly and the infirm are more likely to be injured by rest and idleness than by exercise and work.

debridement

An important surgical principle in the management of tissue injury, the neglect of which will lead to wound infection, poor results and sometimes the dangerous muscle disorder of gas gangrene. Debridement means the radical and scrupulous cutting away of all contaminated tissue, such as the damaged edges of wounds and, especially, of all muscle suspected of being dead. Penetrating wounds must be widely opened so that proper debridement may be done. Dead or heavily contaminated tissue has already been lost to the body and its removal can only improve the situation. After effective debridement, healing and recovery are rapid.

decay, dental

See **tooth decay**.

decompression sickness

A disorder caused by sudden reduction in the pressure to which the body is exposed. It is commonest in inexperienced divers using self-contained underwater breathing apparatus (scuba). As the diver descends, the increasing pressure in the air breathed causes more and more of the oxygen and nitrogen in the air to be dissolved in the blood. If the diver comes up too quickly, these gases come out of the blood in the form of bubbles which may appear anywhere in the circulation causing blockage of small vessels with potentially serious results.

RECOGNITION AND SYMPTOMS

Pain is especially common in or near the joints, giving the common description of 'the bends'. Bone damage, which is often insidious and cumulative over a long period, may lead to serious permanent disability. 'Marbling' or swelling of the skin and an itchy skin rash may indicate early decompression sickness. Neurological effects from blockage of brain or spinal cord arteries are particularly dangerous. They include numbness, muscle weakness, vertigo, loss of bladder or bowel control, even total paralysis and death.

TREATMENT

Any signs of decompression sickness in a person who has ascended rapidly from a great depth are an indication for urgent recompression in a compression tank. If this is done,

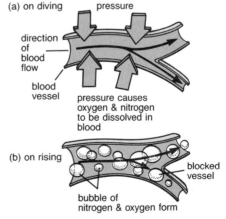

Decompression sickness. On release of pressure, nitrogen bubbles are freed into the circulation throughout the body. These do no harm until carried to a small artery, where they can obstruct blood flow. This is especially dangerous in the brain.

the bubbles re-dissolve and the blocked vessels clear. The pressure can then be slowly reduced allowing the gases to come out of solution without forming large bubbles. This can be a life-saving measure and no delay is acceptable. Divers should always be aware of the location of recompression facilities and of how to summon a helicopter, for rapid movement of the affected subject, if necessary.

See also **bends**.

decompression, spinal canal

An operation to relieve external and damaging pressure on the spinal cord or the nerve roots emerging from it.

WHY IT'S DONE

Spinal canal decompression is necessary to remove such pressure as that which occurs as a result of the pulpy material being squeezed out from the core of one of the discs between the vertebrae (see **slipped disc**). A similar problem can arise from bony outgrowths from the edges of the bodies of the vertebrae (osteophytes) or in inflammation of the spine (**spondylitis**).

Spinal cord compression occurs less commonly, but more seriously, from a tumour in the spinal canal or from a broken back (fracture of the spine). In such cases, urgent decompression may be necessary if the affected person is to be saved from permanent paralysis below the level of the pressure.

HOW IT'S DONE

Decompression is performed by open operation in which the affected area is exposed by cutting away some of the bony arches of the vertebrae and removing the material pressing on the nerve tissue.

decongestant drugs

Drugs used to shrink the congested and swollen lining of the nose and so relieve 'stuffiness'. Decongestant drugs act on the alpha adrenoreceptors (see **beta-blocker drugs**) in the small blood vessels of the nose, stimulating them to narrow the vessels supplying the mucous membrane. The result is that less fluid flows into the membrane and it becomes less swollen. You can take these drugs as drops, inhalants or sprays. Drugs used as decongestants include ephedrine (CAM, Franol), phenylephrine, tramazoline (Dexa-Rhinaspray), oxymetazoline (Afrazine) and xylometazoline (Otrivine). Most of these drugs have an adrenaline-like effect (see **sympathomimetic drugs**).

Many decongestants are highly effective in relieving nasal obstruction and reducing the thickness of the mucous membrane. Unfortunately, they have the disadvantage that this effect soon wears off and is followed by 'rebound' recongestion. Inevitably they are overused so that adrenaline- or amphetamine-like effects may be experienced – fast pulse, shakiness and physical and mental overactivity.

Friar's balsam is a long-established decongestant medication. It is a tincture of benzoin, made by dissolving crushed benzoin, aloes, tolu balsam and storax in alcohol. It is popular as an inhalant and has an impressive smell. But the ritual, although hallowed by tradition, is unsupported by evidence of any real therapeutic value.

See also **common cold remedies**.

decubitus ulcer

See **bedsores**.

defecation

This, one of our most familiar activities, is the process of emptying the bowel. It is initiated by the stretching of the wall of the terminal part of the large intestine (rectum) by the mass movement of faeces into it from the colon. This stretching causes a conscious desire to defecate, but if this is prevented by voluntary decision, the rectal wall relaxes and the desire fades until the next movement of faeces from the colon. Repeated deliberate inhibition is a common cause of constipation, as water is withdrawn from the bowel contents and they become harder.

At a convenient time, the rectum can be allowed to contract freely and the muscle rings (sphincters) at the anus be relaxed. At the same time, a deep breath is taken, the vocal cords are pressed tightly together and the abdominal muscles are contracted. This exerts pressure on the abdominal contents, including the outside of the rectum, and aids in the expulsion of the contents.

defecation, involuntary

See **anal incontinence**.

defence mechanisms

Strategies, of which there are about a dozen, used by people to avoid the anxiety or feeling of guilt that a full awareness of their own defects and shortcomings, real or imagined, would normally cause. Defence mechanisms also help to cope with anxiety caused by conflict between desires and socially approved behaviour. The mechanisms include:
- exclusion from consciousness (repression);
- denial;
- explaining away (rationalization);
- making exceptional efforts (compensation);
- transfer of unacceptable qualities to others (projection).

All human beings rely to greater or lesser extent on these strategies and some of the many troubles that may arise in relationships are the result of unwise attempts to point out and demolish one another's defence mechanisms.

defensive medicine

Medical practice that is importantly affected by fear of litigation. This fear, which has grown in parallel with the growth of legal actions against doctors, has forced many practitioners to change their working methods. Defensive medicine ranges from the decision to perform a few more tests than might strictly be necessary to a form of practice in which the first concern of the doctor is to provide his or her patients with no possible grounds for legal action. It is damaging both to doctors and to patients and is only partly due to the actions of the minority of lawyers who actively encourage law suits against doctors.

defibrillation

The attempt to restore the normal beat in a heart which is in a state of rapid, ineffectual twitching. Fibrillation of the main pumping chambers of the heart (the ventricles) is fatal within a few minutes unless reversed. The attempt to do this involves passing a strong pulse of electric current (about 300 joules) across the heart from two metal electrodes pressed to the

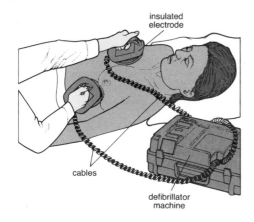

insulated
electrode

cables

defibrillator
machine

Defibrillation. This is usually an emergency measure used in an attempt to restore the normal heart beat in the form of cardiac arrest in which the main pumping chambers of the heart are not beating properly, but are merely twitching.

chest. Sometimes this succeeds in cancelling the random electrical activity in the heart and restoring the regular organized conduction which is essential for effective beating (ventricular contraction).

Fibrillation of the upper chambers of the heart (atrial fibrillation) is quite a different, and non-fatal condition, and is not normally treated by electrical means.

deficiency disease

One of a large range of conditions resulting from the lack of any of the essential nutritional elements, such as vitamins or minerals, or from the body's inability to digest, absorb or utilize these. In some cases, deficiency diseases may be due to an abnormal excretion and loss from the body of needed substances, or from an abnormal demand.

deflazcort

A corticosteroid drug. A brand name is Calcort.

degeneration

Gradual structural alteration of body tissue or organs, either from ageing or misuse, which leads to functional impairment, usually progressive. In general, degeneration causes tissues to lose their healthy, specialized properties. Structural materials, such as collagen, are chemically altered, with resultant loss of tissue elasticity; muscle cells are damaged, muscle bulk declines, specialized cells are replaced by non-functioning fibrous tissue, and many cells die.

RECOGNITION
Degenerative diseases are those characterized by a gradual wearing-away of a tissue, as in **osteoarthritis**; a gradual deterioration in the functional efficiency, as in **atherosclerosis**; or the gradual loss of structural bulk, as in **osteoporosis**.

TREATMENT
By their nature, degenerative diseases are difficult to treat. Established degeneration is irremediable, except by organ transplant or the use of artificial (prosthetic) parts, such as hip-joints. But today, as the nature and causes of the degenerative diseases gradually become clearer, more can be done to delay or arrest the processes of degeneration.

deglutition

The act, or power, of swallowing.

deglutition syncope

Fainting brought on by swallowing, especially of cold beverages. This causes inhibition of the sympathetic nervous system through stimulation of the gullet (oesophagus) in swallowing. In a severe case there may be marked slowing of the heart, widening of peripheral blood vessels and a drop in blood pressure. This may result in dangerous dizziness, confusion and fainting (syncope).

dehiscence

Splitting open. The term is usually applied to an operation wound which has failed to heal normally and which breaks down under internal pressure. This is usually the result of infection, but may be due to inadequate blood supply leading to unhealthy tissues.

dehydration

A body state in which the normal water content is reduced.
POSSIBLE CAUSES
Dehydration is usually due to excessive fluid loss which is not balanced by an appropriate increase in intake, but may be due to intake deficiency alone. It commonly results from persistent diarrhoea and vomiting and excessive sweating, as in prolonged fevers. Cholera is a classic example, in which death results solely from the extreme dehydration resulting from gross fluid loss from the bowel.

RECOGNITION AND SYMPTOMS
The signs of dehydration are a low-volume, concentrated urine, dry, flushed skin, sunken eyes, dry mouth, furred tongue, confusion and irritability.

RISKS
Dehydration leads to an alteration in the vital balance of chemical substances dissolved in the blood and tissue fluids, especially sodium and potassium. The function of many cells is critically dependent on the maintenance of correct levels of these substances, and serious and often fatal effects result from any change. The risk is especially great in babies and infants whose high mortality, from conditions such as gastroenteritis, is largely attributable to dehydration.

déjà vu

Literally, 'already seen', this term is applied to the sudden mistaken conviction that the current new experience has happened before. There is a compelling sense of familiarity, usually lasting for only a few seconds, and a persuasion, almost always disappointed, that one knows what is round the next corner.

By definition, déjà vu does not relate to actual repeat experiences or memories, so the interest lies in why the conviction occurs. One possible explanation is that the phenomenon results from a brief neurological short-circuit, with data from the current observation reaching the memory store before they reach consciousness. The conscious experience of such a memory would be very strong, as it is so recent. This suggestion gains support from the fact that déjà vu is a very common symptom of disorders resulting from brain damage, such as temporal lobe **epilepsy**.

Some experts suggest that memory is not a matter of recall of a fixed, established event, but a process of reconstruction, from stored components, which involves elaborations, distortions and omissions. Each successive recall of the event is merely the recall of the last reconstruction. The sense of recognition involves achieving a good 'match' between the present experience and our stored data, but this may now differ so much from the original event that we 'know' we have never experienced it before.

Psychologists are still arguing about déjà vu and will continue to do so until much more is known about the mechanisms of the brain.

Delhi belly

A facetious, and old-fashioned, term for the common intestinal infection suffered by travellers unaccustomed to the local bacterial contamination (usually faecal) of food or drink. The resulting diarrhoea and colic usually last only for a day or two. There is, of course, no more reason to attribute this minor misfortune to Delhi than to anywhere else.

Delhi boil

Delhi seems to have had a bad press. The Delhi boil, also known as the Aleppo, or Baghdad, boil is a form of **leishmaniasis** affecting the skin. Cutaneous leishmaniasis has now spread to Europe and is appearing in increasing frequency among sun-worshipping tourists. The condition is not a boil, and is no commoner in Delhi than in many other places.

See also **Oriental sore**.

delirium

A mental disturbance resulting from organic disorder of brain function, featuring confusion of thought, disorientation, restlessness, trembling, fearfulness and often fantasies, unwarranted conviction (**delusion**) and disorder of sensation (**hallucination**). Sometimes there is maniacal excitement.

POSSIBLE CAUSES

Delirium may be caused by high fever, head injury, drug intoxication, drug overdosage and drug withdrawal. The commonest form is probably **delirium tremens**, but the same state may be induced by **cocaine**, especially 'crack', **marijuana**, **LSD**, mescaline and other abused substances.

delirium tremens

This dramatic condition affects people on withdrawal from heavy alcohol indulgence.

SYMPTOMS

Over a period of two or three days there is irritability, restlessness, lack of concentration and insomnia or disturbed sleep with nightmares. In about a quarter of cases there is then a major epileptic-type fit.

The affected person begins to show signs of distress and perplexity. There is purposeless body movement, shakiness, tremor (hence the name), incessant and sometimes incoherent talk and an indication of constant annoyance and a sense of threat. Normal talk is misinterpreted in a paranoid manner and there are vivid hallucinations, usually of a most unpleasant nature. The affected person may see terrifying sights (visual hallucinations), smell horrifying smells (olfactory hallucinations), feel all sorts of distressing touchings (tactile hallucinations) or hear threatening or frightening sounds, including language (auditory hallucinations).

At first, there are intervals of contact with reality, but this passes and the stage is reached at which the hallucinations are continuous and the person becomes profoundly disoriented. After two or three days all these symptoms begin to settle and recovery is often sudden.

RISKS

In about 10 per cent of cases, however, the attack of delirium tremens is associated with such severe physical disorder, for example, circulatory collapse, exceptionally high fever (hyperthermia), head injury, liver failure, pneumonia or metabolic upset, that it ends fatally.

deltoid

Triangular. Literally 'like the letter D' (which, in Greek, is a triangle). The deltoid muscle is the large, triangular 'shoulder-pad' muscle which elevates the arm sideways. The deltoid ligament is the strong triangular ligament, on the inner side of the ankle, which helps to bind the foot to the leg and which may be torn if one 'goes over' one's ankle.

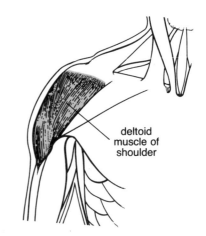

deltoid
muscle of
shoulder

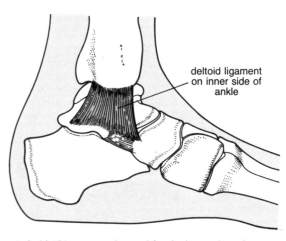

deltoid ligament
on inner side of
ankle

Deltoid. This term can be used for the large triangular 'shoulder-pad' muscle (top) and for the triangular ligament on the inner side of the ankle which helps to secure the foot to the leg (above).

delusion

A fixed belief, unassailable by reason, in something manifestly absurd or untrue. Delusions cannot always be easily distinguished from rigidly held, but generally rejected, opinions, especially if shared by a group. But most are so intrinsically improbable or so obviously based on defective perceptions or reasoning as to indicate serious mental disturbance.

Psychotic delusions fall into several categories, the commonest being delusions of persecution (paranoid delusions). Others are:

● delusions of grandeur;
● hypochondriacal delusions;
● delusions of abnormality of body shape;
● delusions of unreality or depersonalization;
● delusions of being inflluenced by others or by malignant forces;
● self-deprecatory delusions of unworthiness.

The latter are a feature of severe depression. Delusions sometimes serve useful purposes by providing an acceptable explanation for what would otherwise be too unpleasant to be borne. Systematized delusions are a characteristic feature of paranoid **schizophrenia** and these often have an inherent logic which, if one accepts the defective premises on which they are based, cannot be faulted.

demeclocycline

A tetracycline antibiotic used to treat **acne** and general infections. A brand name is Ledermycin.

dementia

A syndrome of failing memory and progressive loss of intellectual power due to continuing degenerative disease of the brain. This brain damage may occur in several different ways.

POSSIBLE CAUSES

At least 50 per cent of cases diagnosed as dementia are due to the brain shrinkage (atrophy) of **Alzheimer's disease**; about 10 per cent are due to small repeated strokes with progressive destruction of brain tissue by blood supply deprivation; 5 to 10 per cent are due to alcoholic damage from long-term over-indulgence (this figure varies with the incidence of alcoholism in the population being considered); an important 7 per cent are not dementias at all, but psychiatric conditions, such as **schizophrenia**, depression and *hysteria*, which mimic dementia and which are susceptible to treatment; about 5 per cent are caused by brain tumours and another 5 per cent by a form of 'water on the brain' (**hydrocephalus**); 3 per cent are due to long-term drug intoxication and 3 per cent to **Huntington's chorea**. Most of the remainder are either of unknown origin or are caused by one of a variety of other diseases such as liver failure, **pernicious anaemia**, syphilis, thyroid disease, **multiple sclerosis**, **Creutzfeldt-Jakob disease**, **epilepsy** or **Parkinson's disease**.

RECOGNITION AND SYMPTOMS

The early signs of dementia are subtle and are likely to be noticed only by close relatives or friends. There may be a loss of interest in work or hobbies, an increase in forgetfulness and easy distractibility. Reasonable discussion of problems becomes impossible. Later it is found that only the simplest of instructions can be followed correctly, orientation in familiar areas becomes defective and the affected person may get lost near home. Judgement is impaired. The main defect is in memory and in the use of language. Nuances of meaning are lost, vocabulary becomes simplified and limited and conversation becomes repetitive and garrulous, full of clichés and stereotyped phrases.

Sudden anger or inappropriate tearfulness is common at this stage and the mood tends towards depression and bad temper. The emotions are abnormally changeable (labile) with quick swings from laughter to weeping. Standards of personal care and hygiene decline. There is indifference to social convention and to the opinions of others. Physical deterioration is a constant feature and there is almost always eventual loss of appetite, emaciation and high susceptibility to infection.

In the end, the demented person stays in bed, inaccessible to stimuli, incontinent but indifferent to discomfort or pain, mute and mindless.

TREATMENT

It is a merciful providence of the nature of things that people in this condition are totally unaware of their vegetable state. And it is also in the nature of things that such people are often carried away by infection, usually pneumonia. To strive officiously to keep them alive, by intensive antibiotic treatment, is no part of a doctor's duty.

dementia praecox

An outdated and inaccurate term for **schizophrenia**. *Praecox* means 'premature' and this disease certainly affects the young; but it is in no sense a **dementia**.

demyelination

Nerve fibres, which carry electrical impulses in the body, are insulated from each other by a sheath of fatty tissue called myelin. This is important for the normal conduction of messages, because nerve impulses are electrical in nature. Demyelination is a disease process which causes loss of the myelin sheath, usually in a patchy manner.

INCIDENCE

Local areas of demyelination, in the form of *plaques* which extend across large numbers of nerve fibre bundles, is the hallmark for **multiple sclerosis**. It also occurs, much less commonly, in the condition of acute disseminated **encephalomyelitis**, which occasionally follows measles, chickenpox or mumps or may follow rabies or smallpox vaccination. (The latter is never now required as the disease no longer exists.)

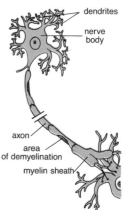

Demyelination. Nerve fibres (axons) have an insulating fatty sheath, without which they cannot operate normally. Demyelination is any process which removes or damages this sheath.

dendritic ulcer

POSSIBLE CAUSES

The cause of demyelination remains uncertain, but there is good evidence that it involves both an environmental factor, such as a virus, and an immunological disorder of the auto-immune type in which the body ceases to recognize as 'self' certain limited areas of tissue, and proceeds to attack and destroy them.

RECOGNITION AND SYMPTOMS

The effect of demyelination is to block the passage of nerve impulses along the affected nerve fibres. Thus, depending on the fibres involved, this may cause disturbance of any function involving muscle contraction (motor function), partial loss of sensation, or partial loss of the special senses such as vision. There may be partial paralysis, disturbance of bladder or bowel control, interference with the balancing mechanisms, indeed disturbance of any of the important faculties subserved by nerve conduction.

dendritic ulcer

A potentially serious condition of the cornea, caused by infection with the *Herpes simplex* virus. It may be acquired by kissing, by unknowingly rubbing the virus into the eye, or even by blowing dust out of an electric shaver. The infection causes a characteristic many-branched ulcer which, if not properly treated, will extend deeply into the cornea and may cause permanent opacification and many years, often a lifetime, of recurrent pain, discomfort and inconvenience. This outcome is greatly encouraged by the injudicious use, in the early stages, of steroid eye drops or ointments which abolish the symptoms and allow the viruses to become fully established in the cornea.

Early dendritic ulcer causes a strong 'foreign body' sensation, and sometimes slight blurring of vision. The eye is red and watering. See also **corneal ulcer**.

> It is a serious mistake to dismiss the condition as a simple conjunctivitis, for treatment by a specialist can cure it if sought early enough.

dengue

A tropical disease caused by an *arbor* (arthropod-borne) virus, maintained as a reservoir in the jungle, probably by monkeys, and transmitted to man by the mosquito *Aedes aegypti* – which also transmits yellow fever.

INCIDENCE

Dengue is commonest in Africa, India, the Caribbean and parts of the Far East.

RECOGNITION AND SYMPTOMS

It is an acute disease with sudden onset of high fever, prostration, severe headache, aches in the bones, joints and muscles, and enlargement of lymph nodes. After two to four days the symptoms settle and for about a day the affected person feels well. But the sense of recovery is illusory for a second rise of temperature then occurs accompanied by a skin rash covering most of the body but sparing the face. The palms and soles are bright red and swollen.

TREATMENT

Recovery is slow and for weeks the victim feels weak and unwell. There is no treatment for dengue, but one attack gives immunity for at least a year. Dengue can be eradicated by getting rid of *Aedes* mosquitos.

dens

Latin root meaning 'tooth' as in dental (of teeth).

dental calculus

People who don't clean their teeth properly soon develop a heavy deposit of food debris, dried saliva and bacteria around the teeth near the gum margins. This is called plaque and it is the first stage in the development of **tooth decay** (caries) and gum disease such as **gingivitis**.

RECOGNITION

The minerals calcium and phosphorous are present in the saliva and these are deposited in the plaque, gradually hardening it until a crust of chalky material forms. This is called *dental calculus* and is usually worst near the openings of the salivary glands – on the outer surfaces of the back teeth (molars) and behind the lower front teeth (incisors).

Visible calculus is yellow or white, but the material also forms underneath the gums, and the calculus, here, is black. Once started, the process of calculus formation encourages further plaque deposition and the amount and thickness of the calculus steadily increases. This means that enormous numbers of bacteria are trapped in contact with the teeth and gums and cannot be removed, even by vigorous brushing. These bacteria break down carbohydrate food particles to form acidic products and cause tooth decay. They also cause serious gum disease.

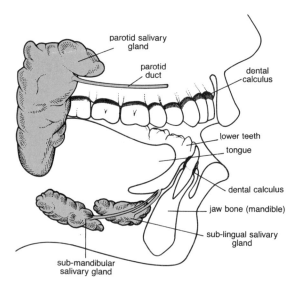

Dental calculus. This diagram shows the salivary glands which secrete the saliva from which some of the components of dental calculus (calcium and phosphorus) are derived.

TREATMENT

If progressive dental destruction is to be avoided, calculus must be removed. This can only be done by a dentist or dental technician, in the process of *scaling*. Thereafter, plaque formation is prevented by proper brushing and flossing.

dental caries

See **tooth decay**.

dental hygienist

An ancillary health professional who assists a dentist at the chair-side and provides preventive dental care, such as scaling and cleaning.

dentifrice

See **toothpaste**.

dentine

The hard tissue that makes up the bulk of the tooth. Dentine is harder than bone, but softer than the outer enamel coating and contains tubules of cells which connect the inner pulp of the tooth to the surface. These cells, the odontoblasts, are responsible for producing dentine and act to repair areas where the enamel has been worn or damaged. They also transmit temperature and pain-producing stimuli, such as tapping or pressure, to the nerves in the pulp.

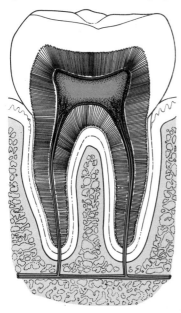

Dentine. The part of the structure of the tooth shown darkly shaded. Most of the tooth is made of dentine, which is harder than bone, but not as hard as the outer enamel.

dentist

A person concerned with prevention, diagnosis, and management of diseases of the teeth, gums and sockets and with the supply and fitting of artificial teeth. Some dentists are medically qualified, but all have specific qualifications in dentistry.

dentures

Artificial (prosthetic) replacements for missing teeth. Dentures have cosmetic and functional importance, assist in the maintenance of good nutrition and allow clear speech. To produce dentures, the dentist first takes an impression, in a quick-setting but flexible plastic, of the surfaces of the jaw and the front of the roof of the mouth. This 'negative' impression is then filled with dental plaster which makes a very precise mould of the original features of the mouth and the denture is made from this mould. Ready-made artificial teeth are selected and cemented into the denture so as to produce satisfactory facial contours and a comfortable and effective bite.

Full dentures, used when all the natural teeth are missing, are held in place by the quality of the fit and the surface tension of the film of saliva between the denture and the mouth. Partial dentures have metal hooks, or clasps, by which they are secured to natural teeth.

deodorants

The earliest deodorants were powerful perfumes which simply masked unwanted odours. Modern attempts to solve the problem of the inherent smelliness of humans rely on substances which either remove, immobilize, or chemically change odour-producing particles or prevent their production. Body deodorants contain aluminium or zinc salts and act mainly by reducing the production of sweat secretion from the glands in the armpits and groins (apocrine sweat). Apocrine sweat is broken down by skin bacteria to produce unpleasant-smelling compounds. An attack on the bacteria themselves can help, but antiseptics are not now approved of. The effective germicide hexachlorophene, once widely used in deodorants, has been restricted because of the danger of nerve toxicity. Daily washing and changing of clothes has much to commend it.

Certain substances, such as activated charcoal, Fuller's earth (aluminium silicate) or silica gel, have powerful adsorptive properties and will remove odour particles from air. Air can also be deodorized by passing it through water or other solutions to remove the particles.

deodorizing drugs

Drugs used to eliminate, mask or prevent undesirable odours. Body deodorants are often antiperspirant drugs combined with masking perfumes and have little real deodorant action. They work by reducing the amount of apocrine sweat available for bacterial breakdown – the cause of the body odour. Real deodorants are highly porous substances, such as silica gel or activated charcoal and are highly effective, but are unsuitable for general use on the body.

Antiseptics may deodorize by eliminating odour-producing organisms. Hexachlorophene, a powerful germicide, was at one time widely used in deodorants, but was found to cause nervous system damage and is no longer used for this purpose.

dependency on doctors

If doctors are not careful to prevent it happening some patients can become emotionally dependent on them.

The demands of emotional dependency soon come to exceed any reasonable share of the doctor's time. The patient attends far more often than necessary, telephones at all hours, requests private consultations. The case notes expand, tests and investigations multiply, tranquillizer and sedatives are prescribed, but all to no avail.

Such patients have often, consciously or otherwise, adopted a career of sickness. This provides a respectable basis for medical dependency and puts the ball firmly in the doctor's court. The patient provides an endless sequence of symptoms and the doctor, who is usually well aware that these have no basis in organic disease, is expected to respond by futile investigation and 'treatment'. Sooner or later, the doctor loses patience. Anger is aroused on both sides and, occasionally, the patient transfers to another list.

depersonalization

A loss of the sense of one's own reality. There is often a dream-like feeling of being detached from one's own body or there may be a feeling that one's body is unreal or strange.

INCIDENCE

Depersonalization is common, as an occasional, brief, isolated episode, and has been experienced by millions of normal people. It often occurs in children as they develop self-awareness and is, in general, commoner in young people than in the elderly.

RECOGNITION AND SYMPTOMS

The out-of-the-body experience often features a consciousness that the identity is situated at a point some feet above the physical body, which can be observed below. This is, for some people, impressive evidence of the existence of the soul. For most, however, there is clear insight into the abnormal nature of the phenomenon and awareness that it is a disturbance of the sense of reality. Depersonalization may involve size or shape distortion of parts of the body. The fingers may, for instance, feel enormously long and fat or much smaller than normal. The sense of distortion is powerful and is only temporarily dispelled by visual evidence of normality.

A depersonalization disorder is a condition in which these phenomena occur persistently or recurrently. The onset is sudden, usually in adolescence or early adult life, and, after the age of thirty, the number of episodes rapidly declines. The condition is very rare later in life.

TREATMENT

There is no effective treatment.

depilatory

A preparation or procedure for removing hair or destroying the hair-forming skin tubes (follicles).

HOW IT'S DONE

Depilatories may be chemical, thermal or mechanical. Various chemicals, such as barium sulphide or thioglycolic acid salts, can soften and dissolve hairs, so that they can be wiped off, but those that are safe do not affect the follicles, and the hair grows again. Wax depilatories merely provide a convenient way of gripping many hairs at once so that they can quickly be ripped out of the follicles. Electrolysis is a method applied to one follicle at a time. The electric current, of a few milliamps, which flows through the follicle, does not destroy it by electrolysis, but merely by heat. The electrolytic production of gas is incidental. The method can cause infection and scarring but, used knowledgeably, is a realistic way of removing a small number of prominent unwanted hairs.

Shaving is effective, but temporary. Contrary to popular belief, it does not cause the hair to thicken. This view arises from an awareness of the harsher feel of short stubble, after shaving, and from a misinterpretation of the natural thickening of the male beard as the sex hormones operate through adolescence.

depolarizing drugs

Drugs that act at the junction between a nerve fibre and a muscle fibre to cause paralysis of the muscle (neuromuscular blocking agents) may be depolarizing or non-depolarizing. Depolarizing agents so affect the electrical charges at the interface that the nerve impulse can to be passed to the muscle fibre. Non-depolarizing agents such as curare act by combing with and blocking the nicotinic cholinergic receptors at the post-junctional membrane. Polarization is the immediate cause of the formation of a nerve impulse. Nerve fibres normally carry a positive charge of some 70 millivolts on the outside of the fibre, which is balanced by an equal negative charge on the inside. When movement of potassium ions causes a local reversal of this polarization, the fibre is said to be depolarized. A zone of depolarization then passes along the fibre. This is the nerve impulse.

depot injection

A drug formulation that allows gradual absorption, over a long period, from a quantity deposited by injection under the skin or in a muscle. Many drugs and hormones can be given in this way.

depression

A mood of sustained sadness or unhappiness. The distinction between normal reactive unhappiness, which is experienced at times by all, and genuine depressive illness is important.

RECOGNITION AND SYMPTOMS

Clinical depression involves a degree of hopeless despondency, dejection, fear and irritability out of all proportion to any external cause. Often there is no apparent cause. It is associated with a general slowing down of body and mind, slow speech, poor concentration, confusion, self-reproach, self-accusation and loss of self-esteem. There may be restlessness and agitation. Insomnia, with early morning waking, is common. Sexual interest may be lost and suicide is an ever-present threat.

INCIDENCE

Depression is especially common in the elderly, and the highest incidence of first attacks occurs between fifty-five and sixty-five in men and between fifty and sixty in women.

POSSIBLE CAUSES

It is usually precipitated by a distressing major life event, such as a bereavement, retirement or loss of status. Postmenopausal depression is a reason for the higher incidence in women than in men. This is often attributed to hormonal changes but there is no positive proof of this.

The causes of depression remain speculative and this has been a fruitful field for the psychoanalytic theorists. It cannot be said that their ideas have been especially enlightening or useful as a basis for treatment. Cognitive psychologists regard depression as being the result of a negative view of oneself as being unwanted, unloved, undesirable and worthless. The depressed person, they believe, views the world as a hostile place in which failure and punishment are to be expected and suffering and deprivation inevitable. Women are particularly vulnerable, especially as their sexual attraction and energy declines, and the loss of reproductive capacity, after the menopause, adds to the sense of uselessness.

TREATMENT

The recognition of medically abnormal (pathological) depression is very important so that urgent treatment can be given. Since the condition can, in most cases, now be relieved, no time should be lost. Many depressives who could have been restored to a normal emotional and social life have committed suicide. Effective antidepressant drugs, such as lithium, the tricyclics, the monoamine oxidase inhibitors and the serotonin re-uptake inhibitors, are available. It should be noted that these drugs do not show their effect until about two weeks after starting the treatment.

dequalinium

An antibacterial and antifungal drug used as an ingredient in medicated lozenges. A brand name is Labosept.

derealization

See **depersonalization**.

derma

Greek root meaning 'skin' as in dermatology (study of skin).

dermabrasion

A technique in cosmetic plastic surgery by which rough or pitted skin is smoothed down, and its appearance improved, by sandpapering or by the use of other abrasive methods. Dermabrasion can also be useful in cases where the skin is disfigured by tattooing. So long as the abrasive effect is carefully confined to the outer layer (the epidermis), full regeneration occurs and the result can be good.

HOW IT'S DONE

Dermabrasion is done with a rapidly rotating sanding drum, disc or wire brush driven by an electric motor. The skin is frozen with a cooling spray, a small area at a time, and bleeding is controlled by pressure dressings. The abraded areas heal in about ten days leaving the skin looking rather pink. The procedure is, of course, performed under general anaesthesia or using a suitable sedative.

dermatitis

A very general term meaning inflammation of the skin from any cause. Dermatitis, or **eczema**, is not a specific disease, but any one of a considerable range of disorders in which the skin is inflamed. The appearance of many of these conditions is similar and may range in severity, with redness, blister formation, swelling, weeping and crusting. There is itching and burning and a strong impulse to scratch, which often makes the condition worse and may, in itself, keep it going. Different kinds of dermatitis may have a similar appearance, but the causes may be very diverse.

POSSIBLE CAUSES

Because the skin is the largest organ in the body and the most accessible to contact or injury, many cases of dermatitis are due to direct injury. This may be infective, from viruses, bacteria or fungi. It may be caused by tiny insects, such as the scabies mite, or lice, or it may result from chemical injury by irritants, solvents, detergents, defatting agents, and generally toxic substances. For the same reason, many are due to actual allergy in which hypersensitivity has developed to a particular substance that would not normally have any adverse effect. Allergic inflammation may occur from contact with metals, plants, cosmetics, drugs, foodstuffs or a wide range of chemical substances. Eczema, or *atopic dermatitis*, has a familial tendency and is commonly associated with **hay fever** and **asthma**.

Dermatitis commonly results from a local inadequacy in blood supply to the skin, as in varicose eczema in the region of varicose veins, especially in older people who also have arterial disease prejudicing their blood circulation. Some major forms of dermatitis may be very serious, even, rarely, fatal. In some cases, the whole surface of the skin flakes off (*exfoliative dermatitis*).

TREATMENT

The treatment of the various forms of dermatitis is often a job for an expert dermatologist who will often have to take a wide view of the problem and may find that the solution rests in the management of some general (systemic) disorder not obviously connected with the skin. Good dermatologists are often more sparing in the use of powerful drug applications, such as corticosteroids, than less experienced colleagues.

dermatitis artefacta

A self-inflicted injury to the skin, most commonly caused by deliberate and prolonged scratching, but sometimes by the application of substances that cause inflammation. Knowledge of the origins of the injuries is usually denied by the affected person, but they appear mostly on the left side, in right-handed people, and vice versa, and never involve parts that cannot be reached. Many are bizarre in shape or character and do not resemble recognized skin disorders. They heal rapidly if securely covered with occlusive plaster, but otherwise tend to persist for long periods. Great ingenuity is sometimes shown in their production.

The condition is commoner in women than in men and there is usually an underlying emotional problem. Sometimes dermatitis artefacta is resorted to in order to avoid work or obtain industrial compensation.

dermatitis herpetiformis

An uncommon skin disease causing intensely itchy blistering red spots and thought to be due to allergy to ingested wheat protein (gluten) and the formation of immune complexes. The disease comes on suddenly and affects the body symmetrically, involving especially the elbows, the shoulder-blades, the buttocks and the backs of the thighs.

These areas may all be affected within a few hours of onset and the small blisters may enlarge and join together. The itching leads to scratching and this tends to result in secondary infection and later scarring. In only a small proportion of cases does the disease resolve completely, but a gluten-free diet helps to keep it under control. The drug dapsone is usually effective in keeping the spots from recurring.

dermatoglyphics

The study of the patterns of the skin ridges on the fingers, palms, toes and soles of the feet. These ridges occur in so many combinations and permutations that each individual has a unique pattern. This offers a reliable means of identification which has been much used in forensic and criminal investigation.

dermatographia

Skin writing. A form of skin sensitivity in which a raised swollen line, surrounded by a red flare, results when the skin is scratched or firmly stroked with a blunt object. The effect is strikingly shown if the form of a word is stroked on the skin. Dermatographia permanently affects some people for no known reason, but in most cases is associated with the form of allergy known as **urticaria**. It is connected with a high level of immunoglobulin type E (IgE) and the susceptibility can be conferred by injecting serum containing IgE.

dermatologist

A doctor concerned with the study of the skin and its disorders, their diagnosis and treatment and their relationship to medical conditions in general.

dermatology

The study of the skin and the diagnosis and treatment of its disorders. Like all other organs, the skin is susceptible to a wide spectrum of injury and disease – mechanical injury; heat, cold, radiation (including sunlight) and chemical damage; infection by viruses, bacteria, fungi and protozoa; infestation by mites, various parasitic worm larvae and fly eggs; tumorous (neoplastic) changes, both malignant and benign; damage from inadequate blood supply, from disease of the skin's own blood vessels and from disease of its intrinsic nerves; congenital defects; and disturbances relating to general (systemic) disorders, including allergic reactions; **auto-immune diseases**; immunodeficiency diseases; and immune complex disorders. All these are within the province of dermatology and their management requires a comprehensive knowledge of most branches of medicine.

dermatome

This word has two meanings – a manual or electrically operated knife or cutter for taking very thin skin slices of less than full thickness (split skin) for grafting; or the area of skin from which the sensory nerves enter a single pair of nerve roots of the spinal cord. The anatomical dermatomes are paired and

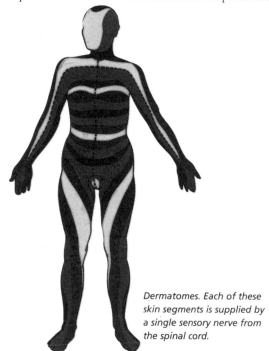

Dermatomes. Each of these skin segments is supplied by a single sensory nerve from the spinal cord.

correspond to the segments into which the body was divided at an early embryonic stage. The body surface can be mapped out in strips corresponding to the dermatomes. Conditions such as **shingles**, which usually involve a single sensory nerve root, cause skin changes affecting a single dermatome.

dermatomyositis

A general disorder affecting both the skin and the muscles, in which inflammation and degeneration of connective tissue lead to rash and progressive muscle weakness.

POSSIBLE CAUSES

The cause is unknown but is thought to be an **auto-immune** process. This is possibly induced by a virus which causes local tissue changes so that the body no longer recognizes the affected parts as 'self'. Viruses have been found in muscle and skin cells in the condition. Dermatomyositis is one of a group of similar diseases in which the muscles are seriously affected.

RECOGNITION AND SYMPTOMS

The onset tends to be sudden in children and more gradual in adults. There is muscle pain and progressive weakness so that affected people find that they cannot raise their arms above shoulder level or get up stairs. Sometimes there is even inability to rise from a sitting position. There is gradual wasting and atrophy of many muscles and the affected person may become bedridden from sheer weakness. Sometimes the heart muscle and the muscles in the bowel are affected. Even speech and swallowing may become difficult.

The skin rash affects mainly the forehead, the upper parts of the cheeks and across the bridge of the nose (butterfly area) and the V of the neckline, but may involve almost any part of the body. It is a dusky red colour and is slightly raised. In about one-third of cases the joints are also involved, but not usually severely, and without deformity. As if these problems were not enough, about 15 per cent of adults with dermatomyositis are found to have a cancer somewhere in the body. It is thought that this may be a factor in causing the trouble, probably by an immunological mechanism.

TREATMENT

The outlook in dermatomyositis is by no means hopeless. Many patients enjoy long periods of remission and some have apparently recovered. Various treatments, including corticosteroids and immunosuppressive drugs have been effective in reducing the muscle weakness. If a tumour is found and removed, the condition often settles.

dermatophytosis

Fungus infection of the skin, often called 'ringworm'. These fungi, mainly *Trichophyton*, *Microsporum* and *Epidermophyton*, affect only the surface (epidermal) layers of the skin which are already dead and are in the process of being cast off. The common medical name for these infections is **tinea** and this is qualified by reference to the site – head, usually scalp, involvement is tinea capitis; body, tinea corporis; crutch, tinea cruris; feet, tinea pedis or **athlete's foot**; nails, tinea unguium; beard area, tinea barbae.

The term 'ringworm' is simply a description of the tendency of these fungi to involve new skin while disappearing from previously affected parts. Because of this, any small patch will form a ring which expands outwards while clearing centrally. There is, of course, no question of any kind of worm being involved.

Kerion is a raised, inflamed boggy patch, often occurring on the scalp. This is due to an acute immunological reaction to the fungus and is often a sign that healing is imminent.

dermoid cyst

A usually benign tumour caused by the abnormal burying, early in embryonic life, of a small quantity of surface tissue (ectoderm) in the deeper layers of the body. Ectoderm develops into skin, hair, bones, teeth and nerve tissue and if some early ectoderm is abnormally infolded, a cyst will form which may contain any of these structures. The dermoid cyst is common on the face, around an eye, or in the ovary, and may have to be removed surgically.

When such a cyst is opened it will commonly be found to contain horny (keratinous) material, such as is produced by skin, and a tight bundle of hairs. Sometimes rudimentary teeth and spicules of bone are found. In about one case in fifty, dermoids of the ovary are found to contain a cancer.

desensitization

A means of treating allergy by the injection of very small, but gradually increasing, doses of the substance to which the affected person is allergic. Allergic hypersensitivity occurs because contact with the substance (the *allergen*), which may be pollen, a foodstuff, an insect sting, a drug, or any of a wide range of materials, stimulates the production of a quantity of antibodies of the immunoglobulin class E (IgE). The IgE molecules become attached to histamine-producing mast cells which lie just under all surfaces of the body. When a subsequent exposure to the allergen occurs, the IgE attached to the mast cells combines with the allergen and this triggers the mast cells to release histamine and other very irritating substances. These cause the allergic reaction at the site of entry of the allergen.

WHY IT'S DONE

The object of desensitization is to try to stimulate production, not of IgE, but of antibodies of different classes – IgG and IgA – so that these can take up the allergen and prevent it from reaching the mast cells. The procedure is not always very effective, and as many as fifty injections, one to three weeks apart, may be needed.

RISKS

Because of the risk of inducing severe reactions, desensitization is potentially dangerous. An average of one person a year died from this cause over a period of many years until, in the 1970s, the practice was largely abandoned. It is now, however, being used again by experts in allergy, with all suitable precautions. See also **behaviour therapy**.

desferrioxamine

An iron-chelating agent used in iron overload conditions or iron poisoning. A brand name is Desferal.

designer drugs

The lucrative market in 'recreational' drugs has prompted people, unburdened by social conscience, to exploit their chemical and pharmacological expertise for illicit gain. The chemistry of many of the drugs of addiction and stimulation is well-known, and it is not very difficult to modify other substances so as to produce seemingly new drugs not covered by existing prohibitive legislation. These 'designer drugs' are often modifications of respectable medical products and are produced in secret laboratories without regard to their obvious dangers or to the possible unknown toxic effects of modified substances. Some may cause sterility. They can often be produced very cheaply and can be sold on the street at lower prices than existing drugs. Their manufacturers and purveyors look for legal protection on the specious basis that they are new. Legislators recognize that the young, the foolish and the irresponsible, who are the prey of such people, require protection against them. The designer drug movement is already attracting some rigorous attention. Drugs such as the fentanyl analogues (e.g., 'China white') and the amphetamine derivatives (e.g., 'Ecstasy') have already been covered by legislation in the USA.

detoxification under anaesthesia

A rapid and humane method of detoxifying people who have heroin and other opioid addictions. There are several drugs, such as **naloxone**, that can effectively block the brain receptors for opioids such as heroin. If these drugs, which are called opioid antagonists, are given to heroin addicts, a very severe withdrawal reaction occurs. Detox under general anaesthesia is a procedure in which opioid antagonists are given while the patient is anaesthetized.

The method requires constant monitoring of the autonomic nervous system responses to the residual opioid, and the use of sedative drugs to control these responses. It also requires close and continuous surveillance by experienced anaesthetists. The whole process takes about 24 hours, and it can allow the addict to get through this period without awareness or distress. Detoxification, of course, does not cure addiction. It does, however, provide the addict with an opportunity to start afresh with, it is hoped, a new resolve never to touch the drug again.

Detrunorm

A brand name for **propiverine hydrochloride**.

deviant behaviour

Behaviour that contravenes accepted standards or rules in a society. These rules, or norms, are held by the majority and those who break them are condemned by the majority, but not by all. There are no absolutes in this context – behaviour that is deviant in one society may be acceptable in another. And, in any society, wide differences of opinion exist as to whether a particular pattern of conduct is to be tolerated or condemned. Disapproval by a minority has little effect, but the greater the number who disapprove, the more deviant, in the opinion of that society, is the behaviour. If disapproval reaches a sufficient level, laws are enacted and the behaviour is regarded as criminal.

deviation, sexual

See **sexual deviation**.

dexamethazone

A synthetic corticosteroid drug used for its anti-inflammatory action and for its value in reducing **oedema** of the brain. A brand name is Decadron. Brand names for preparations in

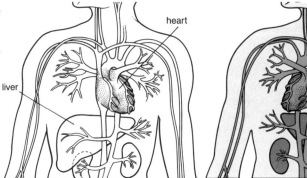

Dextrocardia. Normally, the heart is situated somewhat to the left side (a). In dextrocardia (b) the heart position is reversed so that it points to the right. There is usually an associated reversal of the position of the abdominal organs.

which this is the principal ingredient are Dexa-rhinaspray, Maxidex, Maxitrol and Otomize. Sofradex also contains antibiotics.

dexamphetamine

The dextrorotatory form of amphetamine sulphate, a drug sometimes used to treat **narcolepsy**, hyperactivity in children and as an **analeptic** in hypnotic poisoning. It is widely abused. A brand name is Dexedrine.

dextrocardia

A major, but usually harmless congenital anomaly in which the apex of the heart points to the right instead of to the left. Dextrocardia is usually discovered accidentally or on routine medical examination and is of no particular importance. It is often associated with a similar mirror-image reversal of the abdominal organs, so that the liver is on the left, the stomach and spleen on the right and the appendix on the left. This is called *situs inversus*.

dextromoramide

A powerful pain-killing drug used to treat intractable pain. A brand name is Palfium.

dextropropoxyphene

A pain-killing drug similar to **methadone**. It is also dispensed in combination with paracetamol, as Distalgesic. Overdosage is one of the commonest causes of death by poisoning, as absorption is rapid and breathing is quickly paralysed. It is not much more effective than codeine and some poisoning experts think it should be withdrawn. A brand name is Doloxene.

dextrose

Glucose.

dia-

Prefix meaning 'through' as in diarrhoea (flow through).

diabetes, bronzed

See **haemochromatosis**.

diabetes insipidus

A rare disease, not to be confused with ordinary **diabetes mellitus**, characterized by the production of excessive quantities of dilute urine and a consequent great thirst. One of the pitu-

itary hormones is the anti-diuretic hormone (ADH) or *vasopressin*. This substance acts on the kidneys to allow a massive return to the blood of water which has passed into the tubules after being filtered. In the absence of ADH this water passes out into the urine. Reduction in ADH may result from a variety of pituitary disorders including tumours, infections, blood supply deprivation, pressure from local swelling on arteries (aneurysms) and injuries in the course of skull fracture.

The affected person has to spend much of the time emptying the bladder and may pass as much as thirty litres of water a day. This leads to continual thirst and an equal quantity must be drunk if **dehydration** is to be avoided. The condition is treated with injections of ADH, or the use of an ADH-containing nasal spray, about four times a day.

Diabetes insipidus can also occur from a kidney disorder in which the kidneys are abnormally insensitive to the anti-diuretic hormone.

diabetes mellitus

The term 'diabetes' means 'a running through' and refers to the fact that the affected person passes large quantities of urine. 'Mellitus' comes from the Latin *mel*, meaning 'honey', and the sweetness of the urine has been proverbial for centuries, providing the main diagnostic feature.

DISCOVERY OF DIABETES

Nothing was known about the cause until 1788, when a post-mortem examination on a diabetic showed atrophy in the pancreas. In 1869, Paul Langerhans, a medical student, identified small islands of specialized cells in the pancreas – cells which were later shown to be source of insulin. The real breakthrough occurred in 1889 when it was noticed that a dog, whose pancreas had been removed, was passing large quantities of sweet urine. The research worker, Oscar Minkowski, was thus able to establish that removal or destruction of the pancreas caused diabetes. The final step was the isolation of insulin, in 1921, by the Canadian workers Frederick Banting (1891–1941) and Charles Best (1899–1978) and the demonstration that this hormone could relieve the symptoms of diabetes.

POSSIBLE CAUSES

It is now believed that the damage to the pancreas is in the nature of an **auto-immune** disease, probably related to a virus infection which somehow alters pancreas tissue so as to render it unrecognizable as 'self' to the immune system. There have now been several cases in which early diabetes in children has been diagnosed while the destructive process was still going on and, significantly, some of these have actually been cured by the use of immunosuppressive drugs. Once the islet cells have been destroyed, however, such treatment cannot, of course, have any useful effect.

INSULIN

Insulin is a small protein containing only fifty-one amino acids in two chains. The last few amino acids in one of the chains are especially important in determining its action. Insulin is essential for the synthesis of important large molecules such as fats, proteins and glycogen from small molecules such as glucose and amino acids. It is especially important for the utilization of glucose in muscle cells. In the absence of insulin the muscle protein cannot be built up and the muscles waste away. Body fats, likewise, cannot be formed from sugar. As a result, sugar accumulates in the blood and the kidneys are forced to excrete it. To do so, large quantities of water are needed, if the sugar is to remain in solution, and the result is massive urinary output and great thirst. Sugar in the urine is the hallmark of the disease.

INSULIN-DEPENDENT DIABETES

Type 1 or *insulin-dependency* diabetes, in which the sufferer produces little or no insulin, is an important disease, affecting 1 per cent of the population and causing untold distress. It requires lifelong treatment, constant checking of the level of sugar in the blood, either directly, or by measuring the amount of sugar passed in the urine, and a regular watch for complications. Insulin, being a protein which is digested in the bowel, cannot be given by mouth, so injection is necessary – at least once a day, often twice.

The aim of treatment is to maintain the level of sugar in the blood between certain fairly narrow limits. In diabetes, there is a constant tendency for the blood sugar levels to rise and an excessive rise is associated with the over-production of dangerous substances called ketone bodies. High levels of ketones cause coma and threaten life. Too much insulin is also dangerous because this causes a drop in the level of blood sugar to a point where brain function is threatened. Low blood sugar is called *hypoglycaemia*. A 'hypo' features strange feelings, abnormal behaviour, and a risk of lapse into coma. Hypoglycaemic coma may be fatal.

But the object of diabetic control is not simply to keep the diabetic balanced somewhere between these two kinds of coma. The blood sugar levels can swing wildly within this range without either form of coma occurring. Such poor control, however, greatly increases the risk of long-term complications and these are often serious.

MATURITY-ONSET DIABETES

Type II diabetes, often called *maturity-onset* diabetes, is usually associated with obesity and can be regarded as a condition in which the body cells do not react to insulin, or in which the amount of insulin produced by the pancreas – and this may be near normal – is insufficient to provide entry ports for the excessive tissue bulk.

Many cases of Type II diabetes can be cured simply by dieting and weight loss. This reduces the sugar intake but, possibly more important, makes lowered demands on the insulin supply. Other cases require oral anti-diabetic drugs which stimulate the pancreas to produce more insulin – at least for a time.

DIABETES IN PREGNANCY

If blood sugar control in the pregnant diabetic woman can be kept to normal, the pregnancy should proceed normally. Unfortunately, the constantly changing situation in pregnancy makes it very difficult to achieve good control. Insulin

is important to the growth of the whether natural or injected, do centa to the baby. The mother' pass through and the fetus re ducing more insulin. As a res the form of fat and protein a

Large babies can lead t through the placenta, and necessary to end the pregnan performing a Caesarean section. But increase the risk of **respiratory distress syndrome** in because the substances which allow the lung tissue to expand (surfactants) are not produced in full amounts until the baby is born. For these reasons, every attempt is made to allow the pregnancy to proceed until at least thirty-eight weeks before induction, and this can only be done safely if the mother's blood sugar control has been very good.

> Pregnant diabetic women should always be managed in hospital, or in a diabetic clinic, where close checking of blood sugar and fine tuning of insulin dosage is possible. Portable insulin pumps, with automatic monitoring of sugar levels and automatic injection of measured insulin dosage, under microprocessor control, are available and probably offer the best means of managing the pregnant diabetic. But these instruments are expensive and inconvenient and a constant connection to a vein must be maintained, so they are not popular with patients.

Gestational diabetes is the term used when diabetes, or at least impaired glucose tolerance, is first detected during pregnancy. This is treated in exactly the same way as established diabetes. After the pregnancy the state of the diabetic woman must be reassessed.

COMPLICATIONS

Poorly controlled diabetics eventually suffer damage to the blood vessels. This damage affects especially the eyes, the kidneys, the circulation to the legs, and the nervous system. Diabetic damage to the tiny blood vessels in the eyes causes much blindness in elderly people, and is a major cause of blind registration. Diabetes, by affecting the nerves to the eye muscles, is one of the commonest causes of double vision in elderly people. It is a cause of severe kidney disease which may, at a late stage, destroy kidney function altogether. Diabetes causes organic impotence in about 40 per cent of diabetic men. Diabetic disease of large blood vessels may lead to narrowing and severe interference with the blood flow.

Death from arterial disease is twice as common in diabetics as in non-diabetics. By affecting the nerves – often to the extent of producing loss of sensation – the risk of serious damage from poor blood supply is increased. So elderly diabetics more easily develop **bedsores** and even **gangrene** of a limb.

Diabetics have to understand about the risk of these complications and must be aware of the importance of meticulous control from the outset.

OTHER TREATMENT

Diabetes can be treated by a pancreas transplant but this requires lifelong immunosuppressive drugs and is really only feasible in people already on such treatment. Attempts are being made to transplant Islet cells within special capsules that allow insulin out but prevent antibodies from getting in.

...ed nurse who has undergone specialized post-...cation training in all aspects of diabetes and its ...agement. A diabetes nurse is capable of assessing the ...ical state of diabetic patients, of determining the adequacy of their treatment and of adjusting it, when necessary. He or she is also capable of recognizing the complications of diabetes.

diaeta

Greek root meaning 'diet' as in dietetics (science of diet).

dialysis

The removal of substances from a solution by using membranes through which molecules of the substance can pass. Membranes, such as cellophane, have pore sizes that allow small molecules to pass while retaining larger molecules. These are called *semipermeable membranes*. If such a membrane is used to separate two liquids, one containing the small molecules in solution and the other being plain water, the molecules will pass through into the water until the concentration is the same on both sides of the membrane.

HOW IT'S DONE

The principle is used in medicine to produce a so-called 'artificial kidney'. This takes various forms and may consist of numerous short tubes or a long, narrow tube of membrane, coiled around a drum and immersed in a watery solution. The patient's blood is directed through the tube and unwanted small molecules, such as urea and salt, pass out into the water. Large molecules, such as proteins, or large particles such as red blood cells, are retained. The solution surrounding the tube is changed constantly, so that the concentration of small molecules in it is maintained at a low level.

Patients on permanent dialysis have an external connection (shunt) made surgically between an artery and a vein in the arm. This takes the form of a short plastic tube, from the artery, connected to a tube which enters the vein. Before dialysis, the tube from the artery is connected to the machine and the vein tube is connected to the return flow of blood from the machine. A period of about six hours, twice a week, is usually sufficient to keep the level of waste substances in the blood at a low enough level for health.

diaphragm

The dome-shaped muscular and tendinous partition that separates the cavity of the chest from the cavity of the abdomen. When the muscle contracts the dome flattens, thereby increasing the volume of the chest and tending to reduce its internal pressure so that air is forced into the lungs by atmospheric pressure.

diarrhoea

The result of 'intestinal hurry' so that the normal reabsorption of water from the stools has not had time to take place and the stools are loose and liquid and often passed more frequently than normal. Conditions that interfere directly with the normal reabsorption of water or that lead to secretion of excess water into the bowel, also cause diarrhoea.

POSSIBLE CAUSES

Rapidity of bowel transit can be caused by many factors and especially by the presence of irritating or damaging sub-

stances such as bacterial toxins. Diarrhoea is a feature of **dysentery**, **food poisoning**, **cholera**, **typhoid**, **gastroenteritis**, parasitic infestation and dietary indiscretion. It is also caused by psychological factors, as in the **irritable bowel syndrome**, fear, and various psychosomatic conditions. Diarrhoea often results from the injudicious use of strong laxatives.

Diarrhoea in babies has several causes. It should be remembered that although breastfed babies are much less likely to suffer intestinal infections than those on the bottle, they normally pass very soft stools. This need cause no concern. Diarrhoea can be caused by lactose intolerance due to deficiency of lactase, the enzyme which splits disaccharide sugars. Unsplit disaccharides remain in the bowel, drawing in water from the blood, and causing diarrhoea, distention of the abdomen and bowel noises. Such babies often fail to thrive. The problem may arise if sugar is added to the feed or if fruit juices are given in excessive quantity.

Another common cause of diarrhoea in babies is the move to solid food. The unaccustomed bowel irritation may, for a time, cause intestinal hurry and diarrhoea but will soon settle. In such a situation, formulas of low lactose, easy to digest carbohydrate, with adequate electrolyte and vitamin content, may be useful for a short period. Note that these are intended for babies over four months of age. All babies with diarrhoea require careful attention and medical advice should be sought if the there is any sign of general upset.

RISKS

With the exception of cholera, adult sufferers are usually in little danger specifically from the water loss of diarrhoea. But this is not so in the case of babies and infants, in whom diarrhoea can be very dangerous. In dehydration the normal water content is reduced because of excessive fluid loss which is not balanced by an appropriate increase in fluid intake. Dehydration leads to an alteration in the balance of chemical substances dissolved in the blood and tissue fluids, especially sodium and potassium. This can lead to serious interference with the function of body cells. The signs are:

- strong urine;
- small urinary output;
- dry nappies;
- a dry, flushed skin;
- sunken eyes;
- dry mouth;
- furred tongue;
- mental confusion;
- irritability.

> Because of the ever-present risk of dehydration, diarrhoea in babies should never be taken lightly. If the faeces are very watery and runny and if there is any sign of general upset, such as fever, vomiting or failure to feed, then medical attention is urgently required. Great frequency of bowel motion is a danger sign. Babies with gastroenteritis can go downhill very rapidly and there can never be any justification for delaying definitive medical treatment while proprietary remedies are tried.

TREATMENT

The treatment of diarrhoea is the treatment of the cause. Drugs, such as codeine, which merely control the symptoms, can sometimes be dangerous as they tend to cause irritant or infective material to be retained.

diathermy

High-frequency alternating current can readily be conducted through body tissues, and, depending on the areas of the electrodes in contact with the body, may produce a diffuse warming effect (medical diathermy) or a very localized and concentrated heating or coagulating effect. The latter is the basis of surgical diathermy which may be used to cut tissue in a bloodless manner, to seal off bleeding vessels that have already been cut, or to destroy unwanted tissue, such as a tumour.

Two electrodes are necessary to complete the electrical circuit. In surgical diathermy one electrode is wide and is bandaged to the patient's leg. The other takes the form of a fine metal point, or a pair of tweezer-type forceps, at which the current is concentrated. Alternatively, both electrical connections may be made to the forceps, one to each blade, so that the high-frequency current passes between the tips of the blades and anything held in the forceps is coagulated.

Diathermy must not be used if any inflammable anaesthetic gas or liquid is in use.

diathesis

A term used to describe a greater than average tendency, in an individual or a family, to acquire a certain disease. The word, like a number of others – such as 'idiopathic' and 'essential' – is characteristic of the terminological vagueness applied, in the past, to conditions which were not understood. Now that the causation (aetiology) of many more diseases is known, these terms are gradually falling into disuse.

diazoxide

A vasodilator drug used to treat severe high blood pressure and **hypoglycaemia**. A brand name is Eudemine.

dibromomanitol

A drug used in the treatment of chronic **leukaemia**.

dibromopropamidine

An antibacterial and fungistatic agent used externally to treat conjunctivitis. A brand name is Golden Eye Ointment.

dichloralphenazone

A hypnotic drug used for short periods for the management of insomnia and sometimes to control **delirium**. A brand name is Welldorm.

dichlorphenamide

A **diuretic** drug with a short duration of action. It is also used in the treatment of **glaucoma**. A brand name is Daranide.

diclofenac

A non-steroidal painkilling and anti-inflammatory drug (**NSAID**) used to treat muscle pains, back pain and various forms of arthritis. Brand names are Dicloflex, Diclomax, Motifene, Volraman, and Voltarol.

dicyclomine hydrochloride

A brand name is Merbentyl. It is also formulated with codeine as Diarrest, and with dimethicone as Kolanticon.

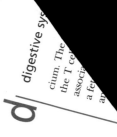

didanosine

A nucleoside analogue drug use_ brand name is Videx.

Didronel

A brand name for **etidronate**

dienoestrol

A synthetic oestrogen drug used in a cream form_ the treatment of post-menopausal vaginal atrophy. A brand name is Ortho Dienoestrol.

dietary fibre

A group of complex carbohydrates that includes plant cellulose, lignin, pectins and gums. The human body does not produce enzymes capable of breaking down these polysaccharides to absorbable sugars, so they cannot be absorbed, but remain in the intestine until excreted. Fibre bulks out the gut content and the stools and is of value in the management of constipation and diverticulitis. Some soluble fibres bind bile cholesterol and prevent it from being reabsorbed, so that blood cholesterol is lowered. High-fibre foods include bran, beans, peas, nuts, all vegetables and fruits.

diethylcarbamazine

A drug used to treat the parasitic worm diseases **filariasis** and **onchocerciasis**. The drug kills both the microfilaria and the adult worms but may provoke severe reactions when the worms die. A brand name is Banocide.

diethylstilbestrol (DES)

A synthetic female sex hormone that has fallen into disrepute because it can cause cancer in the daughters of women taking it.

dietitian

An ancillary health professional trained in the principles of nutrition and their application in the pursuit of health. The work of the dietitian includes the scientific selection of meals for people with digestive, metabolic and malnutritional disorders.

diflucortolone valerate

A powerful steroid drug used externally. A brand name is Nerisone.

diflunisal

A non-steroidal pain-killing and anti-inflammatory drug (NSAID). It is a derivative of salicylic acid and is used to control symptoms in **osteoarthritis** and other painful conditions. A brand name is Dolobid.

Di George syndrome

A disorder cause by congenital absence of the parathyroid glands and the thymus, that presents as muscle spasms in a newborn baby. The parathyroid glands control calcium levels and the spasms are due to abnormally low levels of blood cal-

thymus is necessary for the proper maturation of
s of the immune system and its absence causes an
ted T cell immune deficiency. This can be reversed by
l thymus transplant. The Di George syndrome is due to
early developmental defect involving the primitive structure in the neck from which both the parathyroid glands and
the thymus develop.

digestive system

Most of the digestive system is in the abdomen, and the
demarcation surface between the chest and the abdomen is
the diaphragm. This is an upwardly domed sheet of muscle
and tendon which forms the floor of the chest and the roof
of the abdomen. Through it pass the gullet (oesophagus), the
largest artery in the body (the aorta) and the largest vein
(inferior vena cava). Like any other working machine, the
body requires a supply of energy and this energy is supplied
in the form of chemical fuel. But the body goes one further
and incorporates a chemical processing plant which can
accept, as input, a surprising variety of different fuels. So long
as these conform to the general description of 'food', they
will be suitable, because all food is broken down in the digestive system to three simpler chemical substances, of which
one, glucose, is the basic fuel of the body.

The body needs a lot of glucose as this is constantly being
burned up (oxidized) and converted to carbon dioxide and
water, so as to release chemical energy for muscle contraction, nerve impulse production and the maintenance of body
temperature. We are accustomed to the idea of fuels, such as
petrol, being burned at high temperatures and, for non-
biological machines, fuels which oxidise at high temperatures
are most useful as they can give off their energy very quickly.
But, if certain chemical activators called enzymes are present,
oxidation can occur at much lower temperatures and that is
what happens in the body.

A shortage of glucose in the blood rapidly leads to coma,
brain damage and death. Glucose is absorbed from the intestine and stored in the liver and in the muscles as a concentrated chain of glucose molecules (a polysaccharide) called
glycogen. In a healthy body, the blood levels of glucose are
maintained within certain limits, being released from storage
as required. When stores are used up, glucose can be synthesized from protein 'building blocks' (amino acids) derived
from the muscles, from lactic acid produced by the muscles
and from glycerin in fats. Glycerol is the 'backbone' to which
fatty acids are attached in triplets to form the triglycerides of
human fat. It becomes available for glucose synthesis when
triglycerides, from the fat stores, are broken down.

The digestive system or gastrointestinal tract consists of the
mouth with its salivary glands, the teeth, the throat (pharynx),
the gullet (oesophagus), the stomach, the small intestine
(duodenum, jejunum and ileum), the large intestine (colon),
the rectum and the anus. It also includes the liver and is concerned with evacuation of waste material (**defecation**).

digital radiography

A filmless method of X-ray examination in which the image is
in a form that can be stored as a computer file and reproduced as required. In place of the film, a phosphorescent
plate is placed in a standard X-ray cassette. After exposure the
latent image on this plate is
scanned with a laser beam to
produce a succession of light
pulses. These are picked up by a
photomultiplier tube to produce a bit-mapped image file,
which can be printed or displayed
on a monitor. The phosphorescent plate can be exposed to
light and reused. Images are
available almost immediately
and can be processed to
improve contrast and detail.
Reduced X-ray dosage to
patients and a remarkable economy in storage are further
advantages. It seems inevitable
that this method, or a development of it, will become the standard in the near future.

digital subtraction angiography

A method of producing a
detailed image of blood vessels
that eliminates unwanted surrounding detail. Two digitized
images are made before and
after injecting a dye that is
opaque to X-rays and that circulates in the blood. One of these

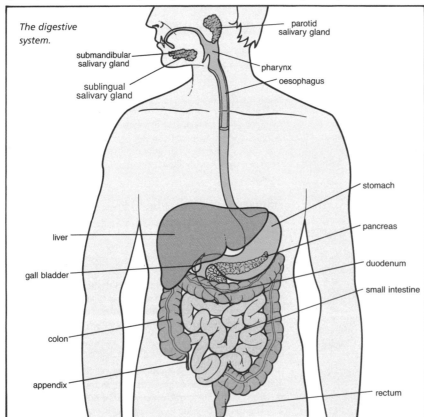

The digestive system.

submandibular salivary gland

sublingual salivary gland

parotid salivary gland

pharynx

oesophagus

stomach

pancreas

duodenum

small intestine

liver

gall bladder

colon

appendix

rectum

is then turned into a negative and the two are combined. Everything except the differences between the two have now been eliminated, so only the shape of the blood content of the vessels is visible. This provides a valuable representation of the interior of the arteries and veins.

digito

Latin root meaning 'finger' as in digital (of finger or fingers).

digoxin

A valuable heart drug derived from the white foxglove *Digitalis lanata*. It is the most widely used of the digitalis heart drugs and is a member of the group of cardiac glycosides. A brand name is Lanoxin.

dihydrofolate reductase inhibitors

A group of drugs that interfere with the conversion of folic acid to its active form in the body. The effect of this is to interfere with the synthesis of the genetic material DNA. This can be useful in the treatment of leukaemias, cancers, rheumatoid arthritis and the skin disease psoriasis. This group of drugs includes pyrimethamine, trimethoprim, triamterene and methotrexate. When such drugs are necessary, folate deficiency is treated with folinic acid rather than folic acid. Methotrexate potentiates the effects of other dihydrofolate reductase inhibitors.

dihydrotachysterol

A vitamin D analogue drug used to treat low blood calcium. A brand name is A.T. 10.

dilatation

Widening. This may be within normal limits, as when the pupil of the eye dilates in the dark, or it may imply a stretching beyond normal dimensions, either as part of a disease process or as a deliberate surgical act. Dilatation of the stomach, with retention of fluid, food and gas, may occur after an operation, or if the bowel is paralysed. Dilatation of the heart is a serious complication of heart disease. Surgical dilatation is done either with the gloved finger or with a smooth tapered instrument or a set of graded dilators, or it may be done with a balloon catheter (see **angioplasty**, **balloon catheter**).

dilatation and curettage

See **D and C**.

dilator

Any instrument used to enlarge an opening, orifice or passage. Dilators are extensively used in surgical practice.

diloxanide

A drug used to kill the amoebae that cause amoebic dysentery. A brand name is Furamide.

diltiazem

A drug used in the treatment of angina pectoris and high blood pressure. Brand names are Adizem, Angitil SR, Dilzem, Slozem, Tildiem and Viazem XL.

Dilzem

A brand name for diltiazem.

dimenhydrinate

An antihistamine drug used mainly to control motion sickness. The brand name is Dramamine.

dimethylsulfoxide

DMSO. A colourless liquid of exceptional solvent properties that readily penetrates the surface of the skin and is used as a solvent for various drugs. Under the brand name of Rimso-50 it is used as a sterile 50 per cent solution to wash out the bladder in certain cases of cystitis.

Dimetriose

A brand name for gestrinone.

Dimotane

A brand name for brompheniramine.

Dindevan

A brand name for phenindione.

dinoprostone

A prostaglandin drug used by injection into the uterus to induce labour. Brand names are Propess and Prostin E2.

Dioctyl

A brand name for docusate sodium.

Dioderm

A brand name for hydrocortisone.

dioptre

A measure of lens power. The most obvious lens parameter is the focal length – the distance from the lens to the point at which parallel rays of light, striking the lens, are brought to a focus. The focal length, however, becomes inconvenient as a measure of lens power when lenses are combined. Two lenses of focal length 10 cm have a combined focal length of 5 cm. A lens of 20 cm in combination with a lens of 10 cm produces a focal length of just below 7 cm. To calculate the focal length of the combination it is necessary to take the reciprocal of each focal length (one divided by the length), add them, and then take the reciprocal of the result.

To get round this difficulty, thin lenses, such as are used in spectacles, are graded, not by focal length, but by the reciprocal of the focal length. This is called the dioptre. The system is based on the proposition that a lens of one metre focal length has a power of one dioptre. A lens of 50 cm focal length has a power of two dioptres, and one of 20 cm focal length has a power of five dioptres. As will be seen, the dioptric power is simply obtained by dividing 100 by the focal length in centimetres.

The ability to add, to a given lens, other lenses, of plus or minus power; is indispensable to opticians when testing eyes for spectacles. Most spectacles contain lenses of between a half and five dioptres. Reading glasses, for those with normal distance vision, will start at one dioptre of plus power at the age of about forty-five, and rise to about two and a half dioptres, at the age of sixty. Four or five prescriptions should cover the whole period.

Diovan

A brand name for valsartan.

Diovol

A brand name for a preparation containing dimethicome and aluminium hydroxide.

Dipentum

A brand name for olsalazine.

diphenoxalate

A drug related to pethidine and with a codeine-like action on the bowel, used to treat diarrhoea. It is sold, mixed with a little atropine, under the brand names of Lomotil and Tropergen.

diphtheria

A serious, and highly infectious, disease, now, happily, rare in developed countries, because of immunization.

DEATH RATE

Even today, the death rate from diphtheria, in developed countries; is about 10 per cent. In underdeveloped areas it is much higher.

RECOGNITION AND SYMPTOMS

Diphtheria has one of the shortest incubation periods of all infectious diseases and the onset is very sudden. A child may become seriously ill within a day of developing the first symptoms. The disease starts one to four days after contact, with fever, sore throat, headache, difficulty in swallowing and enlarged lymph nodes in the neck. The organism causing the disease, *Corynebacterium diphtheriae*, normally attacks the throat, but may, rarely, involve the skin, especially open wounds or burns. It produces a powerful *exotoxin* which is released into the surrounding tissues, causing severe damage and the formation of a membrane-like exudate of clotted serum (fibrin), white cells, bacteria and dead surface tissue cells.

The throat membrane usually covers the tonsils and is a dirty grey colour and so firmly adherent to the surface that attempts to remove it with forceps cause bleeding. The immediate danger from the membrane is to the upper air passages, which may become obstructed, necessitating an emergency artificial opening into the windpipe (a **tracheostomy**).

The exotoxin readily gains access to the bloodstream and is carried throughout the body, where it may cause serious damage to the heart, the nervous system – causing permanent muscle weakness – or the kidneys. These effects may be severe and many children have died from severe heart damage within a few weeks of onset. Secondary damage of this kind is especially likely if there has been delay in treatment.

TREATMENT

> Treatment is always urgent and delay can be disastrous.

Diphtheria is a disease which should be prevented rather than treated, but effective measures exist and can control the damage if the diagnosis is made early. Antibiotics are available to clear the organisms and antitoxin can be given to neutralize circulating toxin.

Because of the success of the immunization programme, a generation of mothers has grown up with no knowledge of the horrors of the disease. This leads to the risk that immunization may be neglected.

Recent outbreaks in Scandinavia have shown that even if the rate of immunization in children is high, levels of immunity can fall off in adult life to a degree sufficient to allow the disease to occur. Re-immunization in adults, done every ten years, is advised by some authorities. The Schick test, in which a tiny quantity of diphtheria toxin protein is injected into the skin of the forearm, can demonstrate the status of an individual's immunity to diphtheria.

dipipanone

An antiemetic drug formulated with cyclizine under the brand name of Diconal.

dipivefrin

A sympathomimetic drug used to treat open angle glaucoma. A brand name is Propine.

diplopia

Double vision, or the perception of two images of a single object. Although we see with both eyes simultaneously, single vision is normally experienced because the brain can cause the eye-moving muscles to align the eyes accurately enough to superimpose and fuse the two images. This fusional capacity of the brain is what is meant by the phrase *binocular vision* and is the highest level of visual development. Binocularity develops in infancy and early childhood only if all is well, during that period, with the focusing and alignment capability of both eyes. Early interference with the development of binocularity, as from squint (strabismus), may eliminate binocularity altogether and many people grow up without it. Such people are incapable of experiencing double vision although they may have excellent single vision in each eye.

POSSIBLE CAUSES

Diplopia may be a normal (physiological) effect, as when a finger held in front of the eyes is seen double when we look past it into the distance. It is also common, and usually harmless, to experience double vision when turning the eyes to the extreme right or left. Some people who have had injudicious or unsuccessful orthoptic or surgical treatment for squint may have persistent diplopia, dating from the time of the treatment. This may be distressing but is not dangerous and should, if possible, be ignored.

RECOGNITION

Diplopia that appears spontaneously and that cannot be controlled, or recently acquired diplopia, occurring on looking a little to one side, is likely to be a sign of disease, either of the eye muscles or of the part of the nervous system concerned with the control of eye movement. Possible conditions include thyroid eye disease affecting the external eye muscles, disease of the arteries supplying the brain, diabetes, stroke, brain tumour or **aneurysm** on the brain arteries.

Diplopia perceived with *one* eye is rare but possible. It should be distinguished from the slight doubling of simple blurred vision, and is usually due to an internal eye problem, such as a partially dislocated crystalline lens, an unusual type of **cataract** or a glass foreign body within the eye.

> Spontaneous or uncontrolled diplopia must never be ignored and calls for full ophthalmic or neurological investigation.

Diprivan

A brand name for propofol.

Diprosone

A brand name for betamethasone in a preparation for external use.

dipyridamole

A drug used to reduce platelet stickiness and thus the risk of stroke in people having transient ischaemic attacks. Aspirin is more effective, but sometimes cannot be safely taken. A brand name is Persantin.

dirt eating

See **pica**.

dis-

Prefix meaning 'not, apart' as in dismiss (send apart).

discharge

An abnormal outflow of fluid, or of a semi-fluid substance, or an outflow of a normal fluid in abnormal quantity. Discharge is most commonly of pus mixed with normal secretions, which, as a result of inflammation, are unusually excessive. This is the case in vaginal discharge, urethral discharge or discharge from the eye or ear. Nasal discharge, due to inflammation from hay fever (allergic rhinitis), is commonly watery.

discharge, yellow, from penis

See **urethral stricture**.

disc, intervertebral, prolapse

See **slipped disc**.

disclosing agents

Stains that reveal plaque on the teeth and, it is hoped, shock the person concerned into a higher standard of dental care by regular toothbrushing and flossing.

disinfectants

See **antisepsis**.

disintegrins

A family of snake venom anticoagulants that disrupt **integrins** on the surface of **platelets** and cells, preventing their interaction with other cells and with the non-cellular tissue surrounding cells (extracellular matrix). They inhibit tumour growth and the growth of small blood vessels (angiogenesis) and may have value in the treatment of cancer.

Disipal

A brand name for orphenadrine.

dislocation, joint

The abnormal separation, or disarticulation, of the bearing surfaces of a joint with minor to major damage to the capsule of the joint and to the ligaments that hold it together. Joint dislocation may be congenital and due to an abnormal shaping of the surfaces, or it may be acquired as a result of unusual force or of disease. Once dislocation has occurred, there is usually a tendency for it to recur. Surgical repair of the soft tissues surrounding the joint will often be necessary to prevent frequent recurrent dislocation.

See also **hip, congenital dislocation of**.

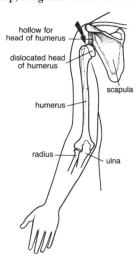

hollow for
head of humerus

dislocated head
of humerus

scapula

humerus

radius

ulna

Dislocation. This is an illustration of a common example of dislocation – in this case, dislocation of the shoulder in which the head of the upper arm bone (humerus) slips out of the shallow glenoid cavity on the side of the shoulder blade (scapula).

disopyramide

A drug used to prevent or control disturbances of heart rhythm. Brand names are Dirythmin SA and Rythmodan.

disorientation

A state of extreme bewilderment or confusion about the current state of the real world and of the affected person's relationship to it. A disoriented person may be unable to give the date, or the year, or be able to state where he or she is, or even who. Awareness of time, place and person are usually lost in that order and, on recovery, return in the reverse order.

Disorientation may be caused by drug intoxication, **dementia**, delusional disorders (see **delusion**), severe **depression**, **mania** and **schizophrenia**.

displacement activity

One of the psychological **defence mechanisms**. The emotion engendered by a person, idea or object is perceived as unacceptable and is transferred to another, more tolerable, person, idea or object. An example of this might be a young employee with a strong desire to punch his tyrannical boss,

239

who goes out at lunch time and hits a squash ball with all his pent-up fury and force.

Disprin CV

A brand name for aspirin.

Disprol paediatric

A brand name for paracetamol.

disseminated intravascular coagulation (DIC)

A serious blood clotting disorder in which widespread clotting occurs within the blood vessels. This is followed by a strong activation of the clot fibrin breakdown system (fibrinolysis) leading to a tendency to severe bleeding. DIC can be caused by extensive trauma, mismatched blood transfusion, brain injury, extensive burns, snake bite and liver disease.

dissociative disorders

A group of striking mental conditions characterized by sudden, and usually temporary, loss of a major faculty such as memory, orientation, or some aspect of self-awareness.

The dissociative disorders are not caused by organic brain disease. They include:

- loss of memory for important personal details (**amnesia**);
- a wandering away, far from home, and the assuming of a new identity and occupation, with an apparent inability to remember the past life (fugue);
- a splitting of the personality into two mutually amnesic personalities with different characteristics (multiple personality disorder);
- an alteration in the perception of self, so that the sense of one's own reality is lost (depersonalization disorder);
- the entering into trance-like states with severely reduced response to external stimuli.

POSSIBLE CAUSES

These disorders are of the nature of extreme defence mechanisms and are invariably a response to some powerfully traumatic or stressful event with which the personality of the sufferer is unable to cope. They may result from the inability to face some event in the personal life, such as an act of marital infidelity, or they may result from sexual abuse during childhood.

INCIDENCE

Dissociative disorders may be induced in anyone by sufficiently distressing circumstances. They commonly affect servicemen exposed to extreme danger or to prolonged periods of constant danger.

In the First World War they were attributed to 'lack of moral fibre' and fugue victims were shot for desertion. Some, slightly more sympathetically, were said to be suffering from 'shell shock'. In the Second World War and later, victims were described as 'psychiatric battle casualties' or, euphemistically, as suffering from 'battle fatigue'. The condition is now called *post-traumatic stress syndrome*.

TREATMENT

By the nature of their causation, these conditions usually settle in time, but a sympathetic understanding and acknowledgement of the cause and skilled psychiatric management are important in allowing affected persons to recover in the minimum time. Defective social attitudes, such as those operating in 1914 to 1918, may turn the unfortunate victim into a lifelong sufferer.

Distaclor

A brand name for cephaclor, a cephalosporin antibiotic.

distal

Situated at a point beyond, or away from, any reference point. The usual reference point is the centre of the body, so the hand is said to be distal to the forearm or to the elbow. The opposite of distal is proximal. The knee is distal to the hip, but proximal to the foot.

Distalgesic

A brand name for a mixture of paracetamol and dextropropoxyphene.

Distamine

A brand name for penicillamine.

distigmine

An anticholinesterase drug used to treat urinary retention, partial paralysis of the intestine and myasthenia gravis. A brand name is Ubretid.

district nurse

A nurse employed within the National Health Service to provide a nursing service to patients living in a particular area usually by attending them in their own homes. In the USA, a district nurse is called a Public Health nurse.

disulfiram

A drug that interferes with the normal metabolism of alcohol so that a toxic substance, acetaldehyde, accumulates. This causes flushing, sweating, nausea, vomiting, faintness, headache, chest pain and sometimes convulsions and collapse. It is sometimes used to discourage drinking, but is not without danger. The brand name is Antabuse.

dithranol

A drug used externally in the treatment of psoriasis. It is an antimitotic agent and acts to discourage overgrowth of epidermal cells. Brand names are Dithrocream, Micanol and Psorin.

Ditropan

A brand name for oxybutynin.

diuretic drugs

Various heart, kidney and liver disorders can cause water to accumulate abnormally in the tissue spaces of the body, or within some of the body cavities. Fluid in the tissues is called oedema and fluid in the cavities is called an effusion. Tissue fluid accumulation is worst in the lower parts of the body – the ankles and lower back and the lower parts of the lungs. Oedema can interfere with body function – especially in the lungs – and causes unwanted weight gain and other disadvantages. It is always an indication that something is wrong. If possible, the cause should be corrected. Usually, correction of the cause will clear up the oedema, but it is often necessary to get rid of the excess fluid in a more direct manner. This is the job of the diuretic drugs. Normally, the kidneys filter very large volumes of water out of the blood. If all this water entered the urine, we would quickly die of dehydration, so most of it is reabsorbed back into the blood. Diuretics act on certain parts of the kidneys to prevent some of this reabsorption of water and allow a proportion of it to pass out in the urine. When they do this, the blood becomes concentrated and the excess fluid in the tissues is drawn into it, thus relieving the oedema.

Diuretics are very effective. Frusemide (Lasix) or bumetanide (Burinex) acts within an hour and the effect on the kidneys lasts for about six hours. Large quantities of urine may be produced – up to 10 litres in a day. Too rapid loss of fluid may reduce the blood volume undesirably and can be dangerous. There may also be danger from the undue loss of potassium from the body, but doctors are aware of this danger and, if necessary, give potassium tablets to make up losses. Thiazide diuretics, such as bendrofluazide (Aprinox) or hydrochlorothiazide (Esidrex, Hydrosaluric) produce a smaller output of urine spread over a longer period.

Diuretics are nearly always taken by mouth, but sometimes, in an emergency, they may be given by injection. In long-term conditions causing oedema they are given in a dosage just sufficient to keep the fluid from accumulating in the tissues.

In addition to those mentioned, diuretic drugs include spironolactone (Aldactone), acetazolamide (Diamox), ethacrynic acid (Edecrine), amiloride (Moduretic, Midamor) and cyclopenthiazide (Navidrex). These drugs act in slightly different ways on the kidneys, but they all have the same useful effect.

Side-effects of diuretic drugs include:

● damage to hearing (frusemide and ethacrynic acid);
● muscle pain (bumetanide);
● stomach and duodenal ulcers (spironalactone);
● painful enlargement of the breasts in men
  (spironalactone);
● impotence (bendrofluazide, hydrochlorothiazide,
  cyclopenthiazide);
● loss of potassium (all except 'potassium-sparing' diuretics
  such as amiloride (Moduretic), triamterene, spironolactone).

Potassium loss can cause vomiting, diarrhoea, muscle stiffness, muscle weakness, drowsiness, apathy, loss of memory, excess urine production and thirst. Severe potassium loss can cause sudden stoppage of the heart (cardiac arrest). Excess of potassium is equally dangerous and this occasionally happens when a potassium-sparing diuretic is used.

Diurexan

A brand name for xipamide, a thiazide diuretic drug.

diurnal rhythm

See **circadian rhythm**.

diverticulitis

This disease presupposes the existence of diverticulosis, a disorder in which multiple small protrusions (diverticula) of the inner lining of the large intestine (colon) occur outwards through the muscular wall of the bowel. The diverticula form small flask-shaped, blind openings from the interior of the colon and these are prone to infection and readily become inflamed. This is diverticulitis.

> Infected and inflamed diverticula may perforate, causing the serious condition of peritonitis, or they may bleed, giving rise sometimes to massive haemorrhage into the bowel. Blood may be passed in the stools and there may be pain and distention of the abdomen.

Diverticulosis is due to a dietary deficiency in roughage and bulk and can be greatly helped by increasing the bran content of the diet.

Dixarit

A brand name for clonidine.

dizziness

See **benign positional vertigo**.

DMSO

See **dimethylsulfoxide**.

DNA

Deoxyribonucleic acid, a molecule some 2 metres long that is present in every living cell of the body and that winds up as a coil to form a chromosome. DNA contains the genetic code, a detailed set of instruction for the construction of the body. The molecule has a double helix outer part of alternating sugar (deoxyribose) and phosphate molecules, and between the two helices, lying like rungs in a ladder, are a succession of linked pairs of the four bases adenine, thymine, guanine and cytosine. The molecules of adenine and guanine are larger than thymine and cytosine and so, to keep the rungs of equal length, adenine links only with thymine and guanine only with cytosine. This arrangement allows automatic replication of the molecule.

The sequence of bases along the molecule, taken in groups of three (codons), is the genetic code. Each **codon** specifies a particular **amino acid** to be selected, and the sequence of these, in the polypeptides formed, determines the nature of the protein (usually an **enzyme**) which is thus synthesized. Polypeptide formation occurs indirectly by way of **messenger RNA** and transfer RNA. The periodicity of DNA is defined as the number of **base pairs** per turn of the double helix.

DNA, component of

See **nucleoside, nucleotide**.

DNA fingerprinting

A method of recording on transparent film a pattern of bands that correspond to regions in the DNA of the individual. These *core sequences* are repeated a different number of times in different people and are unique to each unrelated individuals. They contain common features in people who are closely related.

HOW IT'S DONE

To prepare a DNA 'fingerprint' a sample of DNA is obtained. Only a tiny quantity of blood, semen or any body tissue is needed. The sample is cut into fragments with restriction enzymes, and these are then separated on a sheet of gel by **electrophoresis**. The double helix fragments are then separated into single strands and blotted on to a sheet of nylon or nitrocellulose that fixes them in place. Radioactive gene probes, that bind to any fragment containing the core sequence, are now added. In this way, the core sequences become radioactive and this can be shown up by putting a photographic film in contact with the membrane. Bands are produced on the film by the action of the radiation. Banding patterns from different individuals, or from different samples from the same individual, can now be compared.

WHY IT'S DONE

DNA fingerprinting can be used as a means of positive identification or of paternity testing and has enormous forensic significance. Since no two people, apart from identical twins, have identical DNA, the test is, in theory, infallible.

RELIABILITY

Questions have been raised in court as to the validity of the methods used to conduct and interpret the method.

DNA interior shift defect

See **frameshift mutation**.

DNA polymerase inhibitors

Drugs that act against viruses by interfering with the action of the enzymes that viruses use to build up their own DNA. Examples of this class of drugs are acyclovir, ganciclovir, valaciclovir and foscarnet.

DNA, reversed

See **inversion mutation**.

DNA, RNA, transcription enzyme

See **transcriptase**.

DNA sampling

See **buccal smear**.

DNA self-copying

See **base pair, DNA**.

DNA sequence copying machine

See **polymerase chain reaction**.

DNA structure

See **Watson-Crick model**.

DNA total of individual

See **human genome**.

dobutamine

A drug used to assist in the management of heart failure. It increases the force of the contraction (inotropic agent) of the muscle of the ventricles and improves the heart output. It may be given by continuous intravenous drip. Brand names are Dobutrex and Posiject.

docetaxel

An anticancer drug related to the natural substance taxol. A brand name is Taxotere.

doctor-assisted suicide

The cooperation of a medical practitioner in bringing about the voluntary death of a patient who is suffering from a painful or distressing terminal illness. The practice is illegal in Britain but polls of doctors have shown that at least half of them agree that doctor-assisted suicide should be legalized for carefully selected cases.

In 1997 the State of Oregon in the USA passed the Death with Dignity Act, which legalized physician-assisted suicide and in 1999 33 patients received prescriptions from 22 doctors for lethal doses of medication. Twenty-seven of these died after taking the medication. The issue of the *New England Journal of Medicine* for 24 February, 2000, is largely devoted to this matter.

Doctor of Medicine

A much misunderstood title. In Britain, a doctor of medicine is a person who, having obtained a basic, registrable medical qualification (Bachelor of Medicine), proceeds to further studies, research, thesis production and examination for the degree of MD. This is equivalent to the PhD in other disciplines. The title 'doctor', universally applied to practitioners with a basic medical degree, is actually a courtesy title. So a person with a PhD is a 'real' doctor, while a person with an MB, CHB is not.

In the USA the basic qualification is Doctor of Medicine (MD), equivalent to Bachelor of Medicine in Britain. British 'doctors' who publish in the USA are liable to be embarrassed to find that what appears to be a higher degree has been conferred on them.

doctors, behaviour standards

See **ethics, medical**.

docusate sodium

A faecal softening drug used to treat **constipation**. Brand names are Dioctyl, Docusol, Fletcher's Emenette, Norgalax and Waxsol.

Docusol

A brand name for docusate sodium.

dogs, diseases from

The most common diseases transmitted to man from dogs are the parasitic worm infestations. The commonest of these is **toxocariasis** from the puppy worm *Toxocara canis*. This may, rarely, lead to blindness in one eye in children if the migrating larval stage of the worm should enter an eye. Tapeworm eggs, from dogs, can lead to **hydatid disease**. Mange, caused by a mite of the **scabies** family, can lead to scabies in man. Various other mites and ticks can cause minor problems in people.

Animal skin or hair scales (dander) commonly cause allergic asthma, and skin fungus infection in dogs (epidermophytosis or **tinea**) – commonly, but inaccurately, called ringworm – can be passed to man. In common with many mammals, dogs may, in endemic areas, be affected by **rabies** and the resulting effect on the brain (mania) makes rabid dogs especially dangerous.

Dolmatil

A brand name for sulpiride, a drug used to treat psychotic disorders.

Doloxene

A brand name for dextropropoxyphene.

dominance

Genes occur in pairs at corresponding positions (loci) on each of the paired chromosomes. Dominance is the power of a gene to exert its influence whether the other member of the gene pair is identical or dissimilar. A gene for a disorder (a mutated gene) that has its effect only if paired with an identical **allele** is said to be recessive. The effect of a dominant gene paired with a recessive gene is the same as if both genes had been identical to the dominant gene, but the recessive gene is still present in every cell in the affected person's body, including those producing sperms and eggs. Such a person is said to be heterozygous for that gene.

When the sperms and eggs are produced, only one of the pair of chromosomes is included, so there is a 50/50 chance that this will be the one with the recessive gene. Should a sperm with the recessive gene fertilize an egg which also has the recessive gene, the recessive characteristic will be expressed because there is no other genetic material for the characteristic.

dominant hemisphere

The left half of the brain in almost all right-handed people and 85 per cent of left-handed people. This is the hemisphere concerned with language and logical thought and containing the motor areas for voluntary use of the right side of the body. In 15 per cent of left-handed people, the right hemisphere is dominant and controls speech. Because of dominance it is usually more serious for a stroke to involve the left half of the brain than the right.

domiphen bromide

A quaternary ammonium disinfectant drug used in lozenges. A brand name in a preparation compounded with a local anaesthetic is Bradosol Plus lozenges.

domperidone

A drug used to control nausea and vomiting. An anti-emetic drug. It acts to close the muscle ring at the upper opening of the stomach (the cardia) and to relax the ring at the lower opening (the pylorus). A brand name is Motilium.

donepezil

A drug used in Alzheimer's disease to increase the amount of acetylcholine available for nerve transmission. A brand name is Aricept.

donor

A person, or cadaver, from whom blood, tissue or an organ is taken for transfusion or transplantation into another. The donor site, from which tissue is taken, may be part of the body of the same person who received the tissue. This commonly occurs when a very thin layer of skin (split skin) is taken from a donor site on a burn victim, for grafting to cover bare areas.

A 'universal' blood donor is a person with group O, rhesus negative, blood, which can safely be transfused into any other person.

Dopacard

A brand name for dopexamine.

dopamine receptor agonists

Drugs that have an effect on the body similar to that of dopamine, and roughly similar to that of adrenaline. They include bromocriptine and lysuride and are used to treat Parkinson's disease, acromegaly, overproduction of the hormone prolactin, and to suppress or prevent milk secretion. Possible side-effects include nausea, vomiting, constipation and unwanted fertility in women.

dopamine receptor antagonists

Drugs that compete with dopamine to occupy and block the dopamine receptor sites in the body. They include butyrophenones and thioxanthenes used to treat psychosis. Possible side-effects include those of the phenothiazine derivative drugs, especially chlorpromazine.

dopexamine

A catecholamine drug that improves the action of the heart. A brand name is Dopacard.

Dopram

A brand name for doxapram.

Doralese

A brand name for indoramin.

dornase alfa

A drug used to remove sticky and tenacious secretions from the air passages of people suffering from cystic fibrosis. A brand name is Pulmozyme.

dorsal

A term meaning 'relating to the back'.

dorso

Latin root meaning 'back' as in dorsal (of the back).

dorzolamide

A carbonic anhydrase inhibitor drug used in the form of eye-drops to treat open angle glaucoma. A brand name is Trusopt.

Dostinex

A brand name for cabergoline.

dothiepin

A tricyclic antidepressant drug. A brand name is Prothiaden.

double-blind

A trial in which neither the patient nor the persons conducting the trial know which of two identical-seeming treatments is genuine and which is a dummy.

HOW IT'S DONE

In the case of a trial of a new drug, a pharmacist makes up two sets of tablets or capsules that cannot be distinguished by appearance, taste, etc. One set contains the active ingredient and the other an inert substance. Only the pharmacist knows which is which. The medication is allocated randomly and the key as to who gets what is locked away until the end of the trial. After the results are known, the key is checked to see whether those who had the active drug did significantly better than those who took the dummy.

WHY IT'S DONE

The purpose of double-blindness is to balance out the **placebo effect** which is known to be so powerful that a single trial of a drug, of no actual medical value, will often show an apparently useful effect.

double helix separation

See **single strand binding proteins**.

double helix shaping

See **topoisomerases**.

double vision

See **diplopia**.

douche

A washing-out of a body cavity or opening by a stream of water. Vaginal douching has been popular, especially by women with vaginal discharge. Plain water from a douche bag and nozzle may be used but care should be taken to avoid the risk of infection. Antiseptics, deodorants or detergents should be avoided in douching; they are likely to do more harm than good. Some women douche routinely after sexual intercourse, but this has little or no contraceptive value.

> Excessive force may lead to the serious risk of fluid, contaminated with vaginal organisms, passing along the Fallopian tubes into the peritoneal cavity.

Used in moderation, douching may be of value, but an excessive preoccupation with the vaginal contents may lead to an alteration of the normal, and essential, bacterial population and a reinfection with undesirable strains such as the fishy-smelling *Gardnerella vaginalis*. Loss of vaginal acidity is also a possible and undesirable effect of over-douching.

Dovonex

A brand name for calcipotriol.

Down's syndrome

Formerly called 'mongolism', Down's syndrome is a major genetic disorder caused by the presence, in the maternal ovum or the fertilizing sperm, of an extra chromosome number 21 (trisomy 21). Thus the affected ovum, or sperm, as the case may be, has twenty-four chromosomes instead of the normal twenty-three, and every cell in the body of an individual with Down's syndrome has forty-seven chromosomes instead of the normal forty-six. Some cases are mosaics, with trisomy affecting only a proportion of the cells.

INCIDENCE

The incidence of the condition varies markedly with the age of the parents at the time of conception, especially with the age of the mother. For young girls, the incidence is about one in 2000. For mothers approaching menopausal age, the incidence is about one in forty. The overall incidence is about one in 700 births. In about a quarter of the cases, the extra chromosome comes from the father.

RECOGNITION AND SYMPTOMS

People with Down's syndrome have oval, down-sloping eyelid openings and a large, protruding tongue, which does not show the normal central furrow. Around the edge of the irises of the eyes, greyish-white spots are visible soon after birth, but disappear within the first year. The head is short and wide and flattened at the back and the ears are small. The nose is short and with a depressed bridge and the lips thick and everted. The hands are broad, with a single palmar crease, and short fingers, and the skin tends to be rough and dry. The stature is low and usually the genitalia remain infantile. There is slow physical development and the muscle power is weak. There is a wide gap between the first and second toes. Other congenital disorders, such as heart and inner ear defects, are common and there is a special susceptibility to leukaemia. There is always some degree of mental defect, but this need not be severe and many people with Down's syndrome are able to engage in simple employment.

OUTLOOK

Formerly, people with Down's syndrome seldom survived childhood and many were carried away by infections. Today, those without major heart problems usually survive to adult life, but the processes of ageing appear to be speeded up and most die in their forties and fifties.

Down's syndrome, partial

See **Down's syndrome**.

Down's syndrome, screening for

See **nuchal translucency test**.

doxapram

A drug that stimulates breathing and consciousness. An analeptic drug similar in its action to nikethamide. A brand name is Dopram.

doxazosin

A selective alpha-blocker drug used to treat urinary outflow difficulty. A brand name is Cardura.

doxepin

A tricyclic antidepressant drug. A brand name is Sinequan. The drug is also a powerful antihistamine and has been formulated in the form of a cream that is effective in relieving the itch of eczema. For this purpose the brand name is Xepin.

doxorubicin

An antibiotic, also known as Adriamycin, that interferes with the synthesis of DNA and is thus useful an an anticancer agent. It has many side-effects including loss of hair, sickness and vomiting, interference with blood production and heart damage. A brand name is Caelyx.

doxycycline

A tetracycline antibiotic drug, deoxytetracycline, that is well absorbed when taken by mouth, even after food. A brand name is Vibramycin.

Dozic

A brand name for haloperidol.

drainage, surgical

The provision of a route for the outflow of pus, infected or contaminated secretions, or any other unwanted fluid, from an operation site or an area of infection or disease. Drains may take the form of soft rubber tubes of varying diameter, corrugated rubber sheeting, or even just one of the fingers cut from a surgical glove.

Drainage is avoided, if possible, by meticulous cutting open all suspect areas and the removal of all dead or possibly contaminated tissue. But the accumulation of infected material, deep in a wound or cavity, is so likely to cause serious trouble, that drainage, for a few days after operation, is often unavoidable. Drainage is commonly employed in infection of body spaces, such as the pleural cavity between the outer lung lining and the inner chest wall lining. In this case, the drain requires a valve so that air cannot be sucked in during inspiration. An underwater seal for the drain is commonly used.

Dramamine

A brand name for dimenhydrinate. A drug used to control motion sickness. It may cause sleepiness.

dream analysis

Psychoanalysts, and others, have taken a close interest in dream analysis as a proposed means of access to the content of the unconscious mind. Freudian theory holds that the content of dreams is expressed at two levels: the manifest content, which the dreamer reports, and the latent content, which, being unacceptable to the ego, is repressed and concealed from the individual. Unfortunately, it is, of course, the latter which is important, and, since it is heavily disguised and expressed largely in symbols, the analyst is left with the job of symbol interpretation.

HOW IT'S DONE

Such interpretation can so readily become arbitrary that it is a matter for speculation how far it can ever be accepted as significant. In such a situation, symbolic representation tends to become standardized: every tower, pole, pencil, umbrella,

finger becomes a penis and every tunnel, hole, container, becomes a vagina. Every reference to water implies birth. The number three symbolizes the male genitalia. The ability of the penis to 'defy gravity' during erection, implies that any balloon, aircraft or bird, or any sense that one is flying, is a representation of sexual activity or desire.

Such crude and mechanical interpretation is more likely to mislead than to illuminate. But analysis based on the content of a long series of dreams, recorded honestly and unselectively immediately on wakening, and interpreted by a sensitive and intelligent analyst with a detailed knowledge of the life of the subject, can, undoubtedly, be of value.

dreaming

The subjective experience of partial consciousness during sleep. Dreaming occurs during periods of apparently light sleep, when the EEG (electroencephalogram) shows rapid waves, of a frequency almost equal to that of the awake brain, and the eyes move rapidly beneath the lids. This is called REM (rapid eye movement) sleep and in this stage, which occurs several times a night, the breathing and heart rate become irregular and males (including most of those thought to be impotent) almost always have an erection. Although people in the REM stage of sleep appear to be nearly awake, they are, in fact, harder to arouse than people at other stages, possibly because 'attention' is concentrated on the dream.

Dream thought is often irrational and often has a 'wish-fulfilment' element. Dream content is confused, mixed and repetitive. It appears to be an attempt on the part of the higher centres of the brain to make some kind of sense of a random mass of disparate packets of information arriving from the lower centres, such as the sensory nuclei and the cerebellum. Dream content relating to recent experience and preoccupations is probably used merely to structure the random signals. See also **dream analysis**.

drinking to excess

See **health maintenance**.

driving care

See **health maintenance**.

Drogenil

A brand name for flutamide.

Droleptan

A brand name for droperidol.

Dromoran

A brand name for levorphanol.

drooping eyelid

See **ptosis**.

drop attack

A tendency to fall, suddenly and without warning, and without loss of consciousness. Drop attacks are one of the forms of TIA (**transient ischaemic attack**), due to a temporary shortage of blood to the brain, and are an indication that urgent medical investigation of the state of the blood vessels is required.

> Seek medical attention immediately.

droperidol

A butyrophenone antipsychotic drug that causes emotional quietening and a state of mental detachment. It is sometimes used as a premedication before surgery. A brand name is Droleptan.

dropsy

An old-fashioned term for a collection of fluid in the tissues (**oedema**). At an earlier stage of medical understanding, oedema was believed to be a specific disease. We now know that it is not a diagnosis, but a sign of some other, underlying, condition such as heart failure, kidney disorder or cirrhosis of the liver.

drowning

Death from suffocation as a result of exclusion of air from the lungs by fluid, usually water. Drowning results most commonly from submersion in water, but any liquid, from any source, even the body itself, may likewise exclude air.

WHY IT HAPPENS

The breathing reflexes are so fundamental and powerful that when the nose and mouth are immersed in a fluid, that fluid will, eventually, in spite of the efforts of the person concerned, be inhaled into the lungs. Drowning may also occur in fluid produced within the lungs themselves (pulmonary oedema) as a result of the inhalation of irritants or of lung cancer or other disease.

PHYSICAL EFFECTS

The exclusion of air from the lungs, and, consequently, of oxygen from the blood, soon leads to brain dysfunction and loss of consciousness. Within four or five minutes, in most cases at normal temperatures, irrecoverable damage is caused to the higher centres of the brain so that, even if the affected person should be resuscitated and breathing maintained, return of normal brain function, or even of consciousness, is unlikely.

Notable exceptions to this rule have often occurred, especially in very cold conditions in which the body metabolism is slowed and the oxygen requirement is reduced. Children have been rescued and restored to apparent normality after immersion in water, under ice, for half an hour.

The so-called *diving reflex* is another protective mechanism which is believed to have saved many. The effect of this is to slow the heartbeat and constrict the arteries in the limbs, intestinal tract and other areas remote from the heart, so as to confine the circulation largely to the heart and the brain. In this way, the small amount of precious oxygen in the blood is conserved for the most vital functions and recovery is possible after a longer period under water. Eating shortly before swimming interferes with this reflex.

Inhaled fresh water is more dangerous than inhaled sea water, and often gives rise to a sharp increase in the volume of the blood with rupture and dilution of the red cells and alteration in the chemical constitution. Death may occur from this cause alone.

> In every case of apparent drowning, mouth-to-mouth artificial respiration and, if necessary, heart (cardiac) compression should be done. See also *First Aid*.

drug

The term 'drug', as used in medicine, covers every substance taken into the body, by any route, to exert some desired effect. Any chemical compound used to treat or prevent disease, relieve symptoms or even to help in the diagnosis of disease, is a drug. Today, are almost no diseases for which there is no drug treatment, either to cure or relieve symptoms.

Drugs are used to relieve pain or discomfort and to regularize and control abnormal conditions of mind and body. Some drugs act on cells within the body, often by influencing the many receptors on the cell membranes or within the cells. Others act on the various agencies which can harm the body, such as bacteria, viruses, fungi and other parasites of many kinds. Drugs are commonly used to suppress or modify normal physiological action in the body states, as in the use of oral contraceptives.

The most powerful, and hence potentially dangerous drugs can be obtained only on a doctor's prescription. Some are subject to strict regulations governing storage, recording of stocks held, methods of prescription, and so on. Nonprescription, or 'over-the-counter' drugs can be bought, without restriction, in a pharmacist's shop. They are, in general, reasonably safe even if the recommended dose is somewhat exceeded, but it should be remembered that any drug, however seemingly innocuous, can be dangerous if taken in excess.

To try to reduce the horrendous drug bill of the National Health Service, the government has progressively increased the number of drugs, formerly prescription-only, that can be bought over-the-counter. There are dangers in this as these drugs were not initially restricted without good reason. Advice on such drugs can be obtained from pharmacists.

DRUG NAMES

A generic drug is the 'official', approved, non-proprietary, and usually cheaper form of a single substance. The generic name is nearly always different from the name under which the drug is marketed (the trade or brand name), and there is often a range of different proprietary names – and prices – for the identical generic drug. Thus, 'paracetamol' is the generic name of the common painkilling drug Calpol or Medinol, also known by other names including Alvedon, Disprol paediatric and Infadrops. To make matters worse, the generic name of a drug is seldom a true chemical name. Acetaminophen, which is also paracetamol, sounds like a chemical name, but the real chemical name of paracetamol is 4'-hydroxyacetanilide.

Many proprietary preparations contain mixtures or combinations of generic drugs. Paracetamol is one of the main agents in Distalgesic, Domperamol, Fortagesic, Kapake, Midrid, Migraleve, Paradote, Paramax, Remedeine, Solpadol and Tylex. These painkilling preparations also include other drugs. Official publications, such as the *British National Formulary*, express disapproval of these compound preparations, as they tend unnecessarily to increase the cost of treatment and may make it more difficult for doctors dealing with cases of overdosage.

Almost all drugs of medical value are available in the generic form and a few doctors prescribe generic drugs only. But the advertising pressures to which doctors are constantly exposed make such behaviour as rare as it is difficult.

DRUG ADMINISTRATION

Drugs can be given in many different ways. They can be applied to the skin in the form of ointments, creams, lotions, powders or solutions. Although, in general, such drugs act only on the skin and are not absorbed in sufficient quantity to have an effect on the rest of the body, in some cases significant absorption occurs. Powdered drugs applied to large raw areas or to ulcers can be dangerously absorbed. Skin patches, from which drugs are slowly absorbed, have become popular for certain drugs. This route is used for hormone replacement therapy, for contraception and for an increasing number of other purposes.

Drugs may be given by injection into the skin, using a very fine needle (an intradermal injection), just under the skin (a subcutaneous injection), deeply into a muscle (an intramuscular injection) or into the blood flowing in a vein (an intravenous injection). Drugs given by injection usually act more quickly than drugs taken by mouth. Drugs given intravenously may act within seconds.

Injection may be necessary for a number of reasons. A drug may be so urgently required that the oral route would take too long. Many drugs, if taken by mouth, would be destroyed by the stomach acid or the digestive enzymes. Some drugs are so damaging to tissues that the only way they can safely be given is by slow intravenous injection so that they are rapidly diluted by, and carried away in, the passing blood. Deep intramuscular injections allow larger volumes to be given than can comfortably be accommodated under the skin. This allows a longer period of action. An even longer-acting effect can be achieved by formulating drugs in a vehicle such as an oil or a wax – from which absorption is particularly slow. These are called depot injections. Many different drugs and hormones may be given in depot form. They include antibiotic drugs, corticosteroid drugs, antipsychotic drugs, sex hormones and contraceptive drugs.

Injections are rarely given into arteries.

Sometimes drugs are given in the form of implants, small tablets or other formulations, which are buried under the skin through a tiny incision closed with one or two small stitches. Long-acting contraceptives are often given in this form. Injections are occasionally given into the bone marrow, into the cerebrospinal fluid surrounding the spinal cord, or into the abdominal cavity.

Drugs to be taken by mouth are formulated in various ways. These include:

- coated or uncoated tablets;
- cylindrical, two-piece capsules which are slid open to insert the drug in powder or granule form;
- sealed gelatin ovoids containing a liquid;
- soft rolled pills;
- flat cachets of rice-paper or other material.

Tablets come in all sizes and shapes, are often colour-coded, and may have manufacturer's identifying particulars impressed or printed on them. Capsules are also often colour-coded. Sometimes the two halves of capsules are differently coloured. Within capsules, individual granules may be of one or more colours. Because of the permutations of size, shape, colour and form, it is often possible for an expert to identify a drug from the appearance of the formulation. Tablet- and capsule-identification tables are available to assist doctors dealing with poisoning cases.

Oral drugs are not necessarily intended to be swallowed. Some drugs are actually absorbed more rapidly if kept in the mouth. Nitroglycerine for angina, for instance, works more quickly if the tablet is put under the tongue than if it is swallowed. Some drugs, such as aspirin and alcohol, are absorbed from the stomach, but most pass on to the small intestine, which is the normal absorption zone for food. Some drugs are less well absorbed if mixed with food and are prescribed to be taken 'on an empty stomach'. Others are irritating to the intestinal tract and are best taken immediately after a meal. In general, however, this is not a very important matter.

Drugs likely to cause severe stomach irritation are often given in a capsule made of a material which will not dissolve until it reaches the small intestine. These are called 'enteric-coated' capsules. A wide range of 'slow-release' formulations is available, usually in capsule form containing layers of the drug, or tiny spherules, each coated with a protective covering.

Many drugs may be rapidly absorbed into the circulation, or have local effect, if inhaled in aerosol or fine powder form. Nicotine from cigarette smoke, for instance, reaches the brain within a few seconds of inhalation. Inhalation from inhalers is an important route of access for drugs in such conditions as asthma, and allows drugs to reach the desired areas in high concentration, while minimizing general effects.

Other routes by which drugs may be taken depend on the fact that drugs can gain access to the circulation through any absorbent surface. Some drugs are usefully administered in the form of rectal suppositories, from which absorption is effective. These bullet-shaped medications are moulded from a substance such as cocoa butter, with which the drug is mixed, and which melts at body temperature. They are easily passed in through the anus. Similar vaginal pessaries may be administered, usually for local action against vaginal infections.

Drugs may also be absorbed from the nose lining, from the conjunctiva of the eyes, or from the inside of the bladder or urine tube (urethra). These routes, however, are not generally employed if full absorption is desired, but are normally used so that the drug can act locally.

DRUG INTERACTIONS

Many people have to take more than one drug at a time, and, regrettably, drugs are sometimes prescribed without adequate knowledge of what the patient may already be taking. Drug interactions are the effects of such simultaneous dosage, and they may be dangerous. Interaction may increase the toxicity or reduce the effectiveness.

The most familiar interaction is well-known – the additive effect of similar drugs or of drugs having similar actions – and the most familiar example is the additive effect of alcohol on any of the sedatives or tranquillizers. This can lead to a dangerous degree of sedation, and may, for instance, make driving hazardous.

Sometimes drugs combine to reduce the effect of both. One drug may interfere with the absorption of another. Drugs are commonly bound to, and carried by, proteins in the blood. One drug can sometimes displace another from its bound form, releasing it for greater activity. Much of what happens in cells is controlled by thousands of different enzymes. Drugs can interfere with enzyme action, either enhancing or interfering with it. The action of liver enzymes can be increased by barbiturates. Drugs are often broken down by enzymes, so that the duration of their action is limited. Some other drugs, by interfering with the action of these breaking-down enzymes, allow the first drug to act for much longer than normal. Some drugs prevent the action of others by blocking the receptor sites on cell membranes where drugs act.

SIDE-EFFECTS

A side-effect is any action not intended, and there are many of these. Different drugs may cause different side-effects and these include nausea, vomiting, loss of appetite, diarrhoea, constipation, drowsiness, tiredness, a dry mouth, blurring of vision, a rapid heartbeat, difficulty in urinating, even impotence. Some may lower the blood pressure and cause fainting. There may be upset of the menstrual cycle.

Drugs acting on the central nervous system, such as sedatives, narcotics and tranquillizers, commonly affect mood, judgement, memory and motivation in an adverse way, and may also disturb bodily coordination.

Drug allergy is not, strictly, a side-effect, but to those suffering allergic reactions to drugs, the distinction may seem academic. Allergy may manifest itself as a skin rash, itching, the raised, purplish swellings of urticaria, asthma, complete blockage of the airway from swelling of the lining of the voice box, intestinal upset, fainting, shock or collapse. Drug allergy is especially dangerous when the drug concerned is given by injection, and doctors are always wary of this. Usually a very small test dose is given first and then, after an interval, if nothing untoward happens, the full dose.

Allergic reactions do not occur the first time a drug is given, as the sensitivity must be acquired from a previous exposure. But allergy can be acquired from a drug with a completely different name from the drug now being given, but which happens to belong to the same group, or even to be identical. This is one of the many disadvantages of the present chaotic system of naming drugs.

RISK VERSUS BENEFIT

Drugs with powerful and valuable actions are seldom if ever free from risk. Doctors are always aware of this and do not prescribe unless the benefit is likely to outweigh the risk. In most cases, the risks are small and the doctor is in no doubt, but sometimes, especially in cases of severe illness, the risk may be only a little less than the risk of leaving the disease untreated. This can make for difficult decisions.

Anticancer drugs, for instance, are always poisonous (toxic) and usually have severe and often unpleasant side-effects. This is because they are intended to destroy cells and their damaging effect on cancer cells may not be very much greater than on normal cells. No effective anticancer drug can avoid damaging healthy cells to some extent. In such a case, however, even a small margin of benefit over risk (the therapeutic ratio) may be gladly accepted.

Doctors are often criticized for the overuse of powerful drugs, such as antibiotics, and it is probably true that the best doctors prescribe these and other drugs less often than some of their colleagues. But doctors are busy people and often have insufficient time for full examination, and a range of tests. So they may be driven by discretion to prescribe 'just in case'. GPs do not have immediate access to the facilities enjoyed by hospital doctors.

TOXICITY

Poisoning by drugs is common, usually because of excessive quantities of the drug in the body. This may be because the drug is given in excessive dosage or because, although dosage is normal, the rate of loss of the drug, by breakdown or excretion, is reduced. Kidney disease, for instance, commonly prevents normal excretion.

The liver is especially liable to drug toxicity because it is exposed to high concentrations of most drugs. Hepatitis, even liver atrophy and failure, can be caused by drugs. The kidneys, too, in their attempts to get rid of drugs, may suffer a high concentration and be exposed to toxic levels. In the days of the sulphonamides, these drugs used sometimes to occur in such high concentrations in the urine that they formed damaging crystals within the kidneys or the ureters. Drugs can cause blindness, by retinal or optic nerve toxicity, and deafness, by damage to the sensitive hair cells in the cochlea of the inner ear.

The young fetus is highly susceptible, especially in the first three months of life, to any possibly damaging agency which can gain access to it. As a result, prescribing to women in early pregnancy is now, rightly, very cautious.

Many drugs are habit-forming and this must be balanced against their advantages. 'Sleeping pills', once widely and freely prescribed, are now used with much greater caution. The same applies to sedative drugs such as the diazepams (e.g. Valium), the barbiturates and opiate drugs such as morphine and the wide range of powerful painkillers such as methadone.

Accidental or suicidal poisoning from drugs is very common and child-proof packaging methods are now routinely employed. Some drugs commonly used in suicide attempts are being combined with an antidote.

DRUGS AND OLDER PEOPLE

In general, elderly people take more drugs, and have more trouble from prescribed drugs, than younger people. Because old age commonly brings multiple disorders, there is a natural tendency to multiple prescribing – tablets for the heart, for the blood pressure, for arthritic pain, for insomnia, for swelling (oedema) of the ankles and fluid in the lungs, and for urinary infections. Many old people are taking more than four separate remedies, some as many as ten.

Elderly people tend to have faith in medicines and will often buy additional remedies from a chemist's or even take medicines recommended and given them by their friends. Some herbal remedies contain active and potentially harmful ingredients and overuse of these can add to the problem. They may even interact with prescribed medication.

Doctors concerned about this problem have made searching investigations and these have brought to light some horrifying facts – old people being seriously overdosed, suffering severe drug interactions (see above), taking medicines whose actions cancel one another, and so on. Often more than one doctor is involved and sometimes each is unaware of what the other has been prescribing. It has been found that some confusional states, diagnosed as senile dementia or Alzheimer's disease, have been due to overtreatment with tranquillizers.

It is wise for people in this situation, who are about to visit a doctor, to write down the name of everything they are taking and how many per day. If possible, the reason for the medication should also be recorded. Non-prescription drugs being taken should be included.

drug abuse

There is some general confusion as to what is meant by the term 'drug', and, in the context of drug abuse, most people think of narcotic drugs such as heroin or stimulating drugs such as cocaine. But such restriction is arbitrary. A drug is any substance, other than a food, which affects the body in any way. Thus the term includes tobacco (nicotine), alcohol (ethanol) and coffee and tea (caffeine). The great majority of the inhabitants of the world are habitual drug takers and many of them are addicted to these drugs. This kind of indulgence is not generally regarded as 'abuse'. Most heavy tea drinkers would seriously resent being described as drug abusers. So the mere regular indulgence in a drug can hardly be described as drug abuse.

There are many people who, likewise, do not consider the occasional use of substances like marijuana (cannabis) or cocaine as abuse. In many parts of the world, drugs, such as betel nut, pan or opium are used by many, habitually and in reasonable moderation, and doubtless these people would not consider themselves as abusing a drug. But no one would deny that there are many who do abuse alcohol and tobacco, to the detriment of their health. And there are millions who, with or without the tacit connivance of doctors, abuse drugs such as valium or librium (benzodiazepines), equanil (meprobamate) and many others.

So the term 'drug abuse' is unclear and unsatisfactory. One might consider that abuse exists if the drug harms the body. However, the potent drug more widely used than any other throughout the world – nicotine – appears to be almost harmless to the body. The fact that people who take nicotine by smoking cigarettes are probably engaging in the most harmful long-term activity available to them is, in this context, neither here nor there. It is the many other substances in the smoke that do the harm, and the smoker is not addicted to these. So the matter is more complicated than it first appears.

In fact, drug abuse has come to mean the use of any drug which is currently disapproved of by the majority of the members of a society. In an attempt to clarify the concept of drug abuse, the class of drugs used to alter the state of the mind for recreational or pleasure purposes is often divided into 'hard drugs' and 'soft drugs'. The distinction is somewhat arbitrary, but hard drugs are those which are liable to cause major emotional and physical dependency and thus an alteration in the social functioning of the user. This group includes heroin, morphine and pharmacologically similar natural or synthetic substances. The soft drug group includes tranquillizers, sedatives, cannabis, amphetamines, alcohol and tobacco.

The term 'drug abuse' might thus be more usefully taken to mean the use of any substance in such quantity or frequency that it leads to physical, mental or social damage to the user or to others. Such damage is not always obvious. One important element in it, which applies to all drugs and which may be the central reason why drug abuse is undesirable, is this: people who rely on seriously psychoactive drugs deprive themselves, to a greater or lesser degree, of the opportunity to solve their own problems by personal constructive effort. It is easier to take a drug than to face up to personal difficulties, analyse them, and plan and execute solutions.

DRUG ABUSE IN YOUNG PEOPLE

Without direct evidence in the form of actual drug possession or the finding of drug equipment among the young person's belongings, it is seldom that parents and others can be quite sure that a young person is abusing drugs. There are, however, several indicators that should arouse strong suspicion. Remember that the maintenance of a drug habit is expensive and that the young person must be getting the money from somewhere. Warning signs include:

- unexplained losses of money or valuables from the household;
- possession of unexplained sums of money;
- secretive behaviour;
- apparent personality changes;
- unexpected mood swings;
- deterioration in personal appearance and grooming;
- sudden reduction in school or college performance;
- loss of interest in former activities such as sport;
- acquisition of new acquaintances and rejection of old friends;
- inability to account for activities during regular periods of time;
- memory loss;
- accident prone-ness.

Many young people, unable to obtain the money they need for drugs, turn to drug-dealing. In this case, they may have more money to spend than can plausibly be accounted for. Remember, however, that most of these signs may have an innocent or alternative explanation. Schizophrenia and other psychiatric disturbances commonly develop during adolescence, and this is also a period when young people commonly have severe, but often temporary, behaviour problems. An aggressive response to these is inappropriate and unproductive and a major effort at sympathy and understanding is often required by older people. It may often be best to discuss openly the possibility of drug abuse.

drug dependence

A syndrome featuring persistent usage of a drug, difficulty in stopping and withdrawal symptoms. Drug dependent people will go to great lengths to maintain access to the drug, often resorting to crime. Drug dependence is not limited to dependence on illegal drugs.

drug idiosyncrasy

An abnormal individual response to a drug causing an effect quite different from that expected. Idiosyncrasy is inherent in the person concerned and is usually due to a genetic anomaly. It may take the form of hypersensitivity so that the normal effect is produced by a dose which is a small fraction of the standard dose.

drug, paralysing, long-term

See **botulinum toxin**.

drugs from plants

See **phytopharmaceuticals**, **phytotherapy**.

drug tolerance

A progressive reduction in the effect of a drug, following repeated exposure to it, so that it no longer has the desired effect in the original dose.

drug withdrawal aid

See **psychotropic analgesic nitrous oxide**.

dry eye

The tear film covering the front surface of the eye is more complex than is generally appreciated. It consists of three layers, an inner wetting (surfactant) layer of mucin, an intermediate layer of salt water, and an outer oily layer which slows evaporation and helps to maintain the continuity of the film. Inadequacy in any one or more of these components can cause the condition of dry eye, and one of the features of the more minor degrees of this disorder is a shortening of the interval between each blink and the time the tear film continuum is lost. This is called the *break-up time* and may be easily measured using the dye **fluorescein**.

The mucin is secreted by goblet cells in the conjunctiva, the salt water layer is secreted by many tiny accessory lacrimal glands, also in the conjunctiva, and the oil layer is secreted by the meibomian glands within the eyelids. The main lacrimal glands function during weeping or watering (lacrimation) from irritation.

POSSIBLE CAUSES

Many conditions can interfere with the component sources of the tear film and lead to dry eye. Mucin deficiency occurs in vitamin A deficiency (xerophthalmia); a very unpleasant allergic response to certain drugs, such as sulphonamides, known as the Stevens-Johnson syndrome; extensive **trachoma**; and chemical burns. Salt water secretion deficiency occurs in various connective tissue disorders such as **systemic lupus erythematosus**, scleroderma and Wegener's granulomatosis. Oil secretion abnormalities occur in chronic **blepharitis**.

TREATMENT

Tear film deficiency is treated with artificial tears or sometimes by deliberately blocking the drainage channels. This can be done, reversibly in the first instance, using gelatine plugs in the tiny openings at the inner ends of the lid margins (lacrimal puncta) into which the tears drain. If this is successful, permanent closure can easily be obtained by **cauterization**. It should be noted that the majority of those who complain of 'dry eyes' have no tear film problem and may even be producing excessive tears. A dry eye sensation is often produced by a low-grade inflammation of the conjunctiva from environmental irritation, including damage from the ultraviolet component in sunlight.

dry ice

Solid carbon dioxide. Carbon dioxide (CO_2) is a gas at normal temperatures, having a boiling point of -78°C, but solidifies at -80°C.

USES

Dry ice is widely used for its destructive action on tissue such as warts and solar **keratosis**. It also has medical applications in maintaining organs or tissue for grafting at low temperatures during transportation.

dry socket

Inflammation of the soft tissues of a tooth socket, occurring two or three days after extraction of a tooth, usually a lower molar. The condition is painful and the pain is often referred to the ear. It may persist for days or weeks.

Dry socket is usually treated by packing the socket with a little gauze soaked in a pain-relieving (analgesic) solution. This is changed daily and, in most cases, the socket heals up well. Sometimes the bone becomes involved in the inflammation and may even become severely infected (**osteomyelitis**). In this case, antibiotics are necessary.

DSM IV

The *Diagnostic and Statistical Manual of Mental Disorders*, fourth edition. This book is an attempt by the American Psychiatric Association to formalize and regularize psychiatric terminology and to provide clear descriptions of the various psychiatric entities. It is considered highly authoritative and is often regarded as the bible of American psychiatrists. There is nothing comparable in British psychiatry and DSM IV is occasionally also consulted by the British.

DTIC-Dome

A brand name for dacarbazine.

-ducent

Suffix meaning 'leading' as in adducent (leading to).

Dumicoat

A brand name for miconazole as a lacquer for dentures.

dumping syndrome

When people who have had surgical removal of part or all of the stomach (**gastrectomy**) eat a meal high in carbohydrate, the food passes quickly to the small intestine and there is a sudden rise in the blood sugar from unduly rapid absorption. This prompts normal insulin production, but the timing of this is upset and the insulin level may peak after much of the sugar has been utilized. The result is too much insulin and too little sugar (hypoglycaemia). The affected person feels weak, dizzy and nauseous and may vomit. There is excessive sweating and palpitations. This is called the dumping syndrome. It may be avoided by changing to a high-protein diet and by taking a larger number of smaller meals.

duodenal ulcer

See **peptic ulcer**.

Duovent

A brand name for fenoterol.

Duphalac

A brand name for lactulose.

Duphaston

A brand name for dydrogesterone.

Dupuytren's contracture

Local inflammation, fibrosis, thickening and shortening of a fibrous layer under the skin of the palm of the hand so that one or more fingers are pulled into a permanently bent position.

RECOGNITION AND SYMPTOMS

The ring finger is usually the first to be affected, then the little finger, the middle finger and the index finger. The right hand is affected more often than the left and the condition affects men far more often than women. It starts with a painless, nodular thickening on the palm. This gradually extends to form a thick, longitudinal irregular firm cord, to which the skin becomes adherent so that it can no longer move freely. Slow, progressive contraction occurs, with disabling bending of the finger or fingers. The rate of progress is variable.

POSSIBLE CAUSES

In the days of widespread manual labour, Dupuytren's contracture was assumed to be due to constant trauma to the palm from hand tools. This view is no longer held and the cause remains uncertain.

INCIDENCE

The condition occurs with increasing frequency after middle age and is found most often in diabetics, in people with AIDS, in those with cirrhosis of the liver and in those with tuberculosis of the lungs.

TREATMENT

The only effective treatment is careful surgical removal of the thickened, contracted tissue.

Durogesic

A brand name for fentanyl.

Duromine

A brand name for phentermine.

Duromorph

A brand name for morphine.

Dutonin

A brand name for nefazodone.

dwarfism

Abnormal shortness of stature. This may simply be the result of very short parents, but may result from serious genetic defects such as **Down's syndrome**, **cri du chat syndrome**, Trisomy 18, Turner's syndrome and Bloom's syndrome. More often, it results from glandular defects (endocrine causes) including pituitary growth hormone deficiency; defective action or response to pituitary growth hormone; primary thyroid deficiency (cretinism) or secondary thyroid underaction; premature sex hormone production with precocious puberty and early closure of the growing ends of the bones (epiphyses); **diabetes**; or adrenal gland insufficiency. Dwarfism also results from various inborn errors of metabolism, such as Hurler's syndrome, Tay-Sach's disease, Niemann-Pick disease and Gaucher's disease.

Dwarfism also occurs as a result of growth retardation in the womb (uterus) from placental insufficiency or intrauterine infection; from social and economic disadvantage during childhood; from maternal deprivation from neglect, rejection or simply from inadequate physical contact.

Achondroplasia is an inherited disorder of the growth zones (epiphyses) of the long bones. Muscular development is unaffected and intellectual ability is usually normal. Achondroplasic dwarfs often become good acrobats and tumblers, and this is the common form of dwarfism seen in circuses. They are sexually normal and fertile, but pregnant achondroplasic women can seldom deliver normally and Caesarean section is necessary.

Dyazide

A brand name for triamterene formulated with hydrochlorothiazide.

dydrogesterone

A progestogen drug used to treat menstrual disorders, endometriosis and other conditions. A brand name is Duphaston.

dying, care of the

For many, death is a taboo subject. Recent years have, however, seen the beginnings of a desirable, and, indeed, healthy, increase in interest in the psychology of dying and in the ways in which the dying can be helped to quit life with dignity and in reasonable comfort of body and mind. Dying is, in general, a process with which doctors are ill-equipped to cope, and many still find great difficulty in relating effectively to the dying. Hospital doctors, especially, often seem to find it necessary to insulate themselves from the dying and to persist in a detached course of 'therapeutic' intervention long after most lay persons would consider this appropriate. Medical attitudes and poorly understood prejudices towards the dying often prevent doctors from providing optimum care.

EXPERT CARE

The main advances in comprehensive care of the dying have come from the pioneers of the now well-established hospice movement, and the medical and nursing staff of hospices are now the inheritors of a tradition and widely agreed philosophy of patient management which, in many cases, provides a better quality of dying than that occurring in busy acute hospitals. People with the right kind of experience know that the dying fear a prolonged and painful process of dying, more than death itself. That they fear, above all, dependence, helplessness, loss of dignity before those who do not respect their dignity, and the loss of human comfort and warmth.

PAIN MANAGEMENT

These experts in caring know a great deal about pain and its nature and are well aware that the emotional component is more important than the physical. They know that if this component is dealt with, pain can be controlled with much smaller doses of drugs than otherwise, and that, in most cases, the mind need not be clouded by narcotics. They are skilled, sympathetic and effective, knowing when it is right to withhold treatment, how best to manage symptoms of all kinds by a high standard of nursing care. By these means they are able to help people through this fiina phase of life.

A HOME ENVIRONMENT

It is now universally agreed that the best place to die is at home, in the presence of one's family and friends, and that this should be arranged whenever circumstances allow. The principles of hospice care should, if possible, be provided at home, and there are many places in which good local authority organization has made this possible. But when, for medical or social reasons, this is impracticable, hospices provide the ideal alternative.

-dynia

Suffix meaning 'pain' as in coccydynia (coccyx pain).

dys-

Prefix meaning 'painful, difficult' as in dysmenorrhoea (painful periods).

dysarthria

Inability to articulate speech normally, due to loss of functional control over the muscles concerned in speech. Such defect of the muscles of the tongue, lips, cheeks or larynx usually result from neurological disorder.

dyschondroplasia

A rare progressive disease of the growing parts of bone, affecting children and causing growth retardation. Bones are abnormally, and often unequally, shortened and show nodular swellings. The arms, legs and fingers are commonly affected but the skull, spine, ribs and pelvis are usually spared. The process continues until early adult life, but by then, severe deformity may have resulted, with limbs of unequal length. Disability from finger deformity may occur.

dysentery

Inflammation of the bowel resulting from infection either with shigella organisms (bacillary dysentery or shigellosis) or with the amoeba *Entamoeba histolytica* (amoebic dysentery).

SHIGELLOSIS

Shigellosis is caused by *Shigella flexneri* or *Shigella sonnei* and is acquired by taking food contaminated with the excreta of infected people or carriers. It may be transmitted by flies. It affects children more severely than adults, and causes inflammation, swelling and superficial ulceration of the colon and the lower part of the small intestine. There is fever, nausea and diarrhoea of increasing frequency, up to twenty or more bowel actions a day being common. The stools are characteristically streaked with mucus and blood.

> In small children, the chief danger is from dehydration as a result of excessive water loss, and babies may die within a week of onset unless effective fluid replacement is achieved.

This is the most important element in the treatment of all cases and often antibiotics are unnecessary. Many strains of shigella species have become resistant to several antibiotics.

AMOEBIC DYSENTERY

Amoebic dysentery is caused by the ingestion of the cystic form of the amoeba on fruit and vegetables contaminated by human faeces. This is especially common in parts of the world where human excreta is used as fertilizer. Amoebic dysentery can also be spread by male homosexual intercourse or directly from person to person when personal hygiene is poor. The cysts turn into the active form in the intestine and the amoebae burrow into the wall of the colon to cause small abscesses, then discrete, ragged, undermined ulcers. The amoebae then enter the veins of the intestine and are carried to the liver where, if sufficiently plentiful, they may cause large abscesses full of a chocolate-brown or yellow fluid consisting of broken-down liver tissue.

Symptoms are often mild and vague, but there is persistent low-grade abdominal discomfort and malaise, mild diarrhoea with blood and mucus and sometimes tenderness over the liver. Liver abscesses may cause fever and weakness, referred pain in the right shoulder, nausea, jaundice, loss of appetite and loss of weight. Sometimes an abscess may burst through the diaphragm into the lung and the contents may be coughed up. Amoebic dysentery is more difficult to treat than shigellosis, but the drug metronidazole (Flagyl) is effective.

dyskinesia

Involuntary jerky or slow movements, often of a fixed pattern. The dyskinesias include the **tics**, **myoclonus**, **chorea** and **athetosis**.

dyslexia

An inability to achieve an average performance in reading or in comprehension of what is read, in a person of normal or high intelligence and of normal educational and sociocultural opportunity and emotional stability. Dyslexia is independent of visual or speech defect, and may vary from a very minor disadvantage to an almost total inability to read.

INCIDENCE

It is commoner in males, tends to run in families, and persists into adult life. There are clear indications of cognitive disability, with much greater than normal difficulty in the use, meaning, spelling and pronunciation of words.

RECOGNITION

In performance, there seems to be difficulty in visual perception and discrimination. Letters and words are perceived as reversed, so that 'd' becomes 'b' and 'was' becomes 'saw'. Complete mirror writing may occur. Children affected in this way seem to show an absence of cerebral dominance and are neither strongly right- nor left-handed.

It seems possible that dyslexic children are anatomically less well-equipped than others to recognize sounds presented to them in rapid succession. An interval of about 100 milliseconds is required to separate sounds. This is greater than the interval that separates the component sounds in many common syllables. Phonetic reading is the major problem for people who have dyslexia.

POSSIBLE CAUSES

In spite of major advances in psychology, neurology, brain function studies and linguistics, current views on dyslexia remain controversial. There are even those who deny the existence of dyslexia and claim that the problems are purely of educational or emotional origin.

Most authorities, however, recognize the condition and many are convinced that it is a disorder essentially of the language function. Some have suggested that, whereas language is phylogenetically early, and subserved by a distinct 'module' in the brain, reading is a later accomplishment, intimately dependent on the structural and functional normality of the language module. Any disorder or abnormality in the language module would inevitably cause reading difficulty.

Some have claimed that dyslexic people have variations in the normal brain anatomy, and show an abnormal symmetry in the size of the areas in the temporal lobes containing the auditory association areas. These are normally asymmetrical, being larger on the left side. Work published in August 1994 showed that cells in the medial geniculate nucleus of dyslexic people are smaller in the left hemisphere (the language hemisphere) than in the right. This nucleus handles auditory input. Analogous changes have been found in the layers of the lateral geniculate bodies – which handle visual input – in people with **amblyopia**.

TREATMENT

Much can be done to help dyslexic children and it is essential, for them, that the condition should be recognized as a specific difficulty and not the result of inattention or laziness.

> Parents must not add to their children's anxiety by over-emphasis on the problem, but should be ready and willing to read to the child, or to encourage the use of recorded books, long after the age at which the child would normally be able to read fluently.

Cooperation with a specialist teacher or educational psychologist can be most helpful. Some educational authorities allow dyslexic children extra time during examinations.

dysmenorrhoea

Painful menstruation. This is experienced, from time to time, by almost all women who have not had babies.

RECOGNITION AND SYMPTOMS

The symptoms occur just before, or at the beginning of the period, and consist of cramping, rhythmical pain in the lower abdomen and back, lasting usually for a few hours, but sometimes for an entire day. In severe cases they may last throughout the whole menstrual period. The pain is caused by strong contractions of the womb and with opening (dilatation) of the neck of the womb (the cervix). In effect, dysmenorrhoea is a kind of mini-labour. There may also be nausea, vomiting and diarrhoea, and cramping, colicky pain in the bowels. Some women have faintness and dizziness. About 10 per cent of women are so severely affected that they are temporarily unable to work.

TREATMENT

Dysmenorrhoea is almost always cured by having a baby, but less drastic remedies can also be effective. Drugs of the antiprostaglandin type (ibuprofen, paracetamol and aspirin) are useful, and in severe cases, menstruation can be stopped altogether by means of oral contraceptives, taken continuously. This should be done only under medical supervision.

> The condition may also result as a secondary effect of pelvic infection and other local disease, such as uterine fibroids or endometriosis and, in these cases, antibiotics for infection and surgery may be necessary.

Dyspamet

A brand name for cimetidine.

dyspareunia

Pain experienced by a woman during sexual intercourse. The word derives from the Greek *dyspareunos*, meaning 'ill-mated'.

POSSIBLE CAUSES

Pain on intercourse is usually the result of one of a range of significant gynaecological disorders that include:

- an imperforate or thick, persistent hymen;
- any inflammation of external genital area **vulvitis**);

- inflammation of the mucus-secreting glands in the labi (**bartholinitis**);
- inflammation in the urine tube **urethritis**);
- inflammation of the vagina **vaginitis**);
- old **episiotomy** scars;
- dryness of the vagina, often from oestrogen deficienc after the menopause;
- senile or post-radiational atrophy of the vagina;
- a congenital central vaginal partition (septate, or double, vagina).

This list is not comprehensive. Treatment of dyspareunia from any of these factors is the treatment of the cause.

Dyspareunia is often caused by a powerful vaginal spasm (vaginismus) of psychological origin. This may be so severe that even a finger can barely be admitted. Vaginismus is usually caused by disinclination for sexual intercourse with a particular partner or by a very real fear of sex. The spasms are reflex and uncontrollable, and may involve not only the muscles of the pelvis, but also the muscles which press the thighs together. Treatment is often difficult, and may, in some cases, be inappropriate. It involves full investigation, skilled psychotherapy and counselling, a careful explanation of the origin of the problem, training in relaxation, strong encouragement in self-familiarization with the genitals, and when appropriate, the use, by the affected woman herself, of progressively larger smooth, rounded metal or plastic vaginal dilators.

The last thing a woman with vaginismus needs is to be forced by an assertive male. This simply causes pain, and makes the whole situation worse.

dyspepsia

Any symptoms of disorder of, or abuse of, the digestive system or any symptoms attributed to digestive upset. The term usually refers to general discomfort in the upper abdomen, heartburn, a tendency to belching, nausea or a sense of bloated fullness (flatulence). Dyspepsia is not a specific condition, but may be symptomatic of several diseases including oesophagitis, gastritis, gastric or duodenal ulcer, or disorders of the gall-bladder. See also **peptic ulcer**.

dysphagia

Difficulty in swallowing. This should be distinguished from a persistent sense as of a 'lump in the throat' (see **globus hystericus**).

POSSIBLE CAUSES

Swallowing difficulty may be due to actual obstruction from a hard foreign body in the gullet (oesophagus), and in such a case there will usually be a previous history of choking. It may be due to an oesophageal or pharyngeal pouch – an outward protrusion of the inner lining through the muscle layer. Food passes into such a pouch and there is a constant sense that food eaten has not passed down. There may also be bad breath from decomposing pouch contents. Swallowing difficulty may also be caused by an actual tumour of the wall of the gullet that protrudes into the passage or by a tumour in the tissues surrounding the gullet that compresses it from outside.

One of the most common causes is a neurological disorder that affects the muscular contractions that control swallowing. This is called achalasia. Sometimes the problem arises from a localized muscular constriction ring in the gullet.

dysphasia

dysphasia

RECOGNITION

Barium-swallow X-ray may show a local narrowing, or a *filling defect*, suggesting a tumour. In motor disorders, such as achalasia, neither fluids nor solids can be swallowed, but in tumour, fluids will often pass freely.

> Real dysphagia is an emergency calling for urgent
> investigation including barium-swallow X-ray.

dysphasia

An impairment of speech or of the production or comprehension of spoken or written language, due to damage to certain parts of the brain. Dysphasia is most commonly caused by local interference with the blood supply and is a common feature of **stroke**. Dysphasia may be *motor*, in which the comprehension is normal but the execution defective; *sensory* in which there is a receptive defect; or *global*, in which both are affected. It may also be of widely varying degrees of severity. See also **aphasia**.

dysphonia

Any impairment of normal voice production, from any cause, such as acute **laryngitis**, **singer's nodes**, **clergyman's throat**, paralysis of a nerve to the larynx (recurrent laryngeal nerve palsy) or 'breaking voice' (pubertal increase in the size of the larynx).

dysplasia

An abnormal alteration in a tissue, excluding cancerous (malignant) change, due to abnormality in the function of the component cells. Dysplasias include the absence of growth, an abnormal degree of growth, and abnormalities in cell structure. Some dysplasias are regarded as a stage in the development of cancer, but many are not.

Dysplasia may affect literally any cell type in the body and is commonly described in the neck of the womb (**cervix**), in the lungs of infants, in the teeth, in the bones and in the immune system organ of childhood, the thymus.

dyspnoea

The sensation of difficult, laboured or obstructed breathing. Dyspnoea is the unpleasant experience of 'not getting enough air' and most commonly results from normal athletic or other strenuous activity. It is prompted primarily by a lowering of the oxygen content in the blood and is caused by anything which has this effect. It may thus arise from asthma or any other cause of partial obstruction or narrowing of the airway, from disorders leading to inadequate expansion of the chest, from any lung disease which interferes with the full oxygenation of the blood, from collapse of a lung, from failure of the heart to maintain an adequate circulation (heart failure), from severe anaemia, from inadequate oxygen in the inspired air, as in mountain sickness, or from psychological causes such as 'hysterical' hyperventilation.

dysrhythmia

Any irregularity or disturbance of a normal body rhythm, **arrhythmia**. The most obvious and most commonly observed dysrhythmia is that of the heartbeat, but the term may also be applied to a disturbance in the rhythm of the brain waves, as recorded by the EEG (electroencephalogram), or the rhythmical contraction of the bowel muscles (peristalsis) necessary for the onward movement of the contents.

dystonia

A group of muscular disorders featuring abnormal posture or muscle contraction, or interference with normal movement. The dystonias may affect the body generally or may be local in effect.

POSSIBLE CAUSES

One of the commonest forms of dystonia is wry-neck (**torticollis**). Other forms include writer's cramp, repetitive strong contraction of the muscles in the eyelids (blepharospasm), repetitive strain injury, and a more widespread facial disturbance, with involuntary grimacing, pursing of the mouth and chewing movements (Meige syndrome).

TREATMENT

Because the cause is often obscure, dystonias are difficult to treat, but some benefit may be gained from the use of antispasmodic or sedative drugs in large dosage. In a few cases, locally destructive operations on the brain have been tried, but the risks do not justify this approach. Some people have been helped by spinal cord stimulation and others by biofeedback. The current interest in the management of these conditions centres on the use of tiny doses of the powerful poison *Botulinum* toxin. This can be highly effective in causing temporary paralysis of muscles that go into spasm.

dystrophy

A term used for a range of conditions, of widely differing cause, in which tissues fail to grow normally, or to maintain their normal, healthy, functioning state. It is applied to several different degenerative condition of the cornea, to various retinal degenerative diseases, to a variety of other conditions involving defective growth or development and, in particular, to a large and varied group of inherited muscular disorders (**muscular dystrophies**). The term is an example of the class of descriptive words used by doctors when the cause of the problem is unknown.

dysuria

Pain on passing urine. This is most commonly due to a urinary infection and is usually associated with a temporary over-awareness of the urinary function, undue frequency in the desire to urinate, urgency and the passage, with a burning sensation, of small quantities of urine.

Dytac

A brand name for triamterene, a diuretic drug that does not lead to undue loss of potassium from the body.

Dytide

A brand name for triamterene in combination with another diuretic drug.

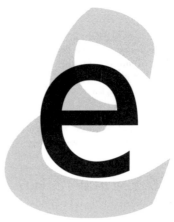

E. coli

See *Escherichia coli*.

earache

This symptom is very common in children, in whom it is usually caused by an alteration in the pressure in the middle ear due to failure of the normal pressure-equalizing mechanism. This mechanism relies on the free movement of air in and out of the middle ear, by way of the Eustachian tube. If, because of adenoids or inflammatory swelling of the nose lining, the tube becomes temporarily blocked, air cannot pass into the middle ear. When the middle ear is closed, the air within it is soon absorbed into the blood circulating in its lining walls. The higher external atmospheric pressure then forces the eardrum painfully inwards.

Earache caused in this way can be relieved by any measure that relieves Eustachian obstruction. Nasal decongestants can help, but adenoidectomy or tonsillectomy may sometimes be necessary.

Eustachian obstruction also interferes with fluid drainage of the middle ear and may lead to infection of the middle ear (**otitis media**). This is another common cause of earache resulting from pressure effects on the drum, but in this case, the drum is forced outward by the accumulation of pus and watery discharge in the middle ear. Earache also commonly

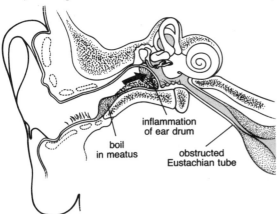

Three common causes of earache – a small boil or furuncle in the outer ear canal, inflammation of the eardrum, and blockage of the Eustachian tube leading to a rise in pressure in the middle ear from retained secretions.

results from inflammation in the external ear passage (**otitis externa**). Here, the skin is tightly bound down to the underlying tissue and there is little room for expansion. A small boil in the external passage is very painful. Infection of the skin of the passage, by viruses, bacteria or fungi, is a frequent cause of earache. Most cases of otitis externa are caused by injudicious poking with hairpins, matches or wires, so that the skin surface is damaged and infection introduced.

Paracetamol (Calpol) should be given to control the pain and medical attention sought to discover the cause.

ear, cauliflower

See **cauliflower ear**.

ear, discharging

Discharge from the ear may arise from infection of the mucous membrane lining of the middle ear (**otitis media**), and pass out through a perforation in the eardrum, or it may originate in the skin of the external ear canal (meatus) (**otitis externa**).

> A discharging ear is an indication that treatment is needed and should never be ignored.

Neglected middle ear infection may lead to deafness, mastoiditis, or even, rarely, **meningitis** and **brain abscess**. Otitis externa can nearly always be cured by skilled treatment.

eardrum opening

See **myringotomy**.

eardrum, perforated

POSSIBLE CAUSES
The commonest cause of perforation is middle ear infection (**otitis media**) in which the pressure of pus and discharge in the middle ear and the inflammation of the drum have caused destruction of a small area of drum tissue and created a hole through which the pus can drain to the exterior.

Perforation may also result from direct or indirect injury, as from an explosion, a fracture of the base of the skull, a slap on the ear or a poke from a paperclip. Sometimes perforation may result from sudden changes in the external air pressure, as in flying (**barotrauma**), or from high water pressure during diving. A perforated drum does not necessarily cause deafness, but there will always be some loss of acuity.

TREATMENT

Non-infective perforations often heal quickly without further attention, but the presence of middle ear infection, especially if there is loss of normal middle ear drainage via the Eustachian tube, tends to maintain the perforation and requires treatment. Once the cause of the perforation has been eliminated, healing may be promoted by various surgical means.

The edges of the hole may be touched with a tiny swab of caustic solution, or the hole may be covered with a small skin or muscle graft.

ear, examination of

As in every medical investigation, a careful history of the present complaint and of other possible relevant factors precedes examination. The examination starts with a look at the external ear (the pinna) and a check for tenderness on pressure on the skin and over the mastoid process of the temporal bone, just behind and below the pinna. Pressure on the bump in front of the external canal (the tragus) will reveal inflammation in the canal or middle ear. A check is also made for an enlarged lymph node in front of the pinna and in the neck below the ear.

The external canal (meatus) is now inspected with an electric auriscope or with a conical, open speculum and a perforated head mirror which reflects a bright light into the canal. Sometimes a microscope is used. The specialist will look for excess wax, discharge and foreign bodies and will examine the state of the skin. If necessary, the canal will be cleaned out so that a full view of the eardrum (tympanic membrane), situated at the inner end of the canal, can be obtained. Inspection of the drum will reveal inflammation, bulging or perforation and will show the 'handle of the malleus', the part of the outermost of the three tiny bones (ossicles) which link the drum to the inner ear.

While observing the drum, the specialist will ask the patient to pinch the nose and blow. If the Eustachian tube is working normally, the drum will balloon outwards, collapsing again when the subject swallows. Sometimes the specialist will carefully pass a fine, blunt-ended metal tube along the floor of the nose and into the opening of the appropriate eustachian tube. This Eustachian catheter can then be connected to a rubber squeeze bag and air gently blown in.

Tuning fork tests are now done to determine whether there is any difference between the acuity of the two ears and whether, on either side, bone conduction of sound is better than air conduction. More detailed and precise measurements of the hearing sensitivity, at different pitches, are made by various forms of **audiometry**. From the results of these tests, the specialist can come to an accurate diagnosis of the type and degree of any hearing loss and can determine whether the problem is essentially one of the conduction of sound vibrations (conductive deafness) or of the conversion of mechanical vibrations to nerve impulses (sensorineural deafness).

ear, foreign body in

Childhood fascination with bodily orifices inevitably leads to the introduction of anything small enough to be pushed in. Beads, pebbles, peas, beans, seeds, ball-bearings commonly become impacted. Organic objects which swell with moisture are especially troublesome. This common childhood incident is usually compounded by frantic attempts to remove the foreign body by means of various improvised instruments. Such attempts may usually be relied upon to push the foreign body further in. Contact with the drum causes pain, the perception of loud noises and a notable worsening of the situation.

A surgeon skilled in child psychology will often succeed without an anaesthetic, for the problem is not so much one of mechanical difficulty as of securing a non-moving operating field. But unfortunately, a brief general anaesthetic, or the use of a quick-acting tranquillizing drug, may be necessary. Foreign bodies can easily be removed with fine hooks, if the subject is safely still.

Early Bird

A brand name for **pyrantel**.

ear piercing

The formation of a permanent, skin-lined perforation through the earlobe, from which a decorative ring or pendant can be suspended. The only risk is infection. Contamination with pus-forming (pyogenic) organisms, such as staphylococci or streptococci, is common and small abscesses often occur. These drain when the stud or 'sleeper' are moved, and will usually soon settle. They seldom cause much trouble.

> Major risks have arisen with the spread of hepatitis B and AIDS and one should not submit to needle ear piercing without complete assurance that the needle used cannot possibly be contaminated with blood from another person. A piercing gun which 'injects' a stud is generally safe.

ear plastic surgery

See **otoplasty**.

ears, cosmetic surgery on

See **otoplasty**.

ear wax

See **wax, ear**.

eating dirt

See **pica**.

eating disorders, treatment of

See **cognitive behaviour therapy**.

Ebola virus disease

A highly dangerous infectious disease first described among laboratory workers in Marburg, West Germany, and occurring later in the Sudan and Zaire. The condition features fever, aching muscles, sore throat, diarrhoea, a widespread rash, bleeding into the bowel and damage to the brain and kidneys. If untreated, the mortality is likely to be over 90 per cent, and even in those patients given good supportive treatment about 25 per cent will die. Also known as Marburg disease.

Ebufac

A brand name for **ibuprofen**.

ecchymosis

Bleeding (haemorrhage), or bruising, in the skin or a mucous membrane, in the form of small, round spots.

ECG machine, smart

See **medical computing**.

echolalia

The regular repetition of words or phrases spoken by another person. The words repeated may be pronounced in a staccato manner, or with equal emphasis on each syllable, or may be spoken in a mocking manner. Echolalia may occur as a feature of **schizophrenia** or as part of a severe **tic** disorder.

econazole

An antifungal drug commonly used to treat skin fungal infections and thrush (**candidiasis**) of the vulva in women.

Ecostatin

A brand name for **econazole**.

Ecstasy

A popular name for the drug 3,4-methylenedioxymetamphetamine (MDMA), a hallucinogenic amphetamine with effects that are a combination of those of LSD and amphetamine. Ecstasy is widely used to promote the energy and appropriate state of mind for all-night 'rave' dance sessions, but the combination of strenuous physical exercise and the direct toxic effect of the drug has led to a number of deaths in young people.

Death can result from an uncontrolled rise in body temperature (hyperthermia), kidney failure, muscle breakdown (rhabdomyolysis) and sometimes liver failure. Urgent measures to reduce body temperature can save life. The drug can also precipitate a persistent paranoid psychosis.

ECT

See **electroconvulsive therapy**.

ectasia

Permanent distension, ballooning or widening (dilatation) of an organ or part. 'Broken veins', for instance, are small ectatic skin blood vessels.

ecto-

Prefix meaning 'outside' as in ectoderm (outside skin).

ectome

Greek root meaning 'cutting out' as in appendicectomy (appendix removal).

-ectomy

Suffix meaning 'cutting off' as in thyroidectomy (removal of thyroid).

ectoparasite

Any organism living on the outside of another organism and dependent on it for nutrition. Lice, ticks and mites may be human ectoparasites.

ectopic

Situated in a place remote from the usual location. Ectopic foci of thymus tissue, situated away from the site of the thymus gland in the upper chest, are thought to maintain thymus immunological function after the gland has atrophied. An **ectopic pregnancy** is one occurring outside the womb.

ectopic heartbeat

A heartbeat occurring prematurely so as to disturb the regular rhythm. This usually results in a compensatory pause, experienced by the subject as a 'palpitation'.

ectopic pregnancy

A dangerous complication of pregnancy in which the fertilized egg (ovum) becomes implanted in an abnormal site, such as the **Fallopian tube** or in the pelvis or abdomen, instead of in the womb lining. The great danger is severe, and sometimes life-threatening bleeding (haemorrhage). Treatment is by urgent operation to remove the growing embryo. This is mainly done by **laparoscopic surgery**. See also **abdominal gestation**.

ectropion

A common eyelid disorder, usually involving the lower lids, in which the wet, inner, conjunctival surface is exposed to view.
POSSIBLE CAUSES
Ectropion is commonest in the elderly, in whom weak and lax eyelid muscles allow the lower lid to fall away from the eye and even to turn outwards. This is called senile ectropion. Sometimes ectropion is caused by actual paralysis of the flat muscle surrounding the eye (the orbicularis oculus muscle). This is a feature of **Bell's palsy**. It may also be caused by scarring of the skin, near the lid margin, with shortening (contracture), which pulls the lid edge away from the eye. This is called cicatricial ectropion and may follow wounds or burns. This type of ectropion often affects the upper lid.
RECOGNITION AND SYMPTOMS
Ectropion carries the tear duct opening away from the tear film, so that the normal drainage of tears into the nose is prevented. The result is a permanently watering eye. In addition, because bacteria are not carried safely away, ectropion usually leads to a state of permanent low-grade infection (chronic conjunctivitis) with persistent redness, discharge and discomfort. The constant necessity to wipe the eye only makes matters worse.

> Neglected ectropion leads to skin shrinkage and turns a minor and easily remedied condition into a major surgical problem. So advice should be sought early.

TREATMENT
Procedures to tighten the lid are straightforward and effective in the early stages of ectropion. Long-neglected ectropion is much more difficult to treat effectively.

eczema

This is not a specific condition, as is commonly thought, but an effect of a number of different causes and a feature of many different skin disorders. One of the commonest types is called atopic dermatitis – a reflection of the fact that the effect occurs at a place remote from the operation of the original cause. (Greek *topos*, meaning 'a place' *a* 'not'.)

It is not contagious or infectious unless an area of eczema becomes secondarily infected.

POSSIBLE CAUSES

Eczema has a familial allergic element and often appears in the first year of life. Atopic eczema in babies is often caused by allergy to protein in wheat, milk and eggs.

In adults, the development of eczema is usually the result of contact with an allergen such as washing-up liquid, biological washing powders, nickel watch-straps or name-bracelets, or other materials to which allergy has developed. Emotional upset and stress may also precipitate the disorder. Varicose eczema is the unhealthy condition of the skin in the region of varicose veins, due to stagnation of blood and inadequate oxygenation and nutrition.

RECOGNITION AND SYMPTOMS

Eczema features itching, scaly red patches and small fluid-filled blisters which burst, releasing serum, so that the skin becomes moist, 'weeping' and crusty. Ec It commonest on the hands, ears, feet and legs, but may affect any part of the skin.

TREATMENT

The treatment of eczema involves searching for and removing the cause. Local treatment to the skin is secondary to this, but is effective in removing the irritation which so often causes uncontrollable scratching and perpetuates and complicates the condition. Steroid ointments are very effective in relieving symptoms, but have their own disadvantages. They can encourage and promote the spread of secondary bacterial or fungal infection and, if used for long periods, can be absorbed in sufficient amount to cause general effects, and can cause skin atrophy, **striae**, local loss of pigment and rebound worsening of the eczema. Experienced dermatologists use them in careful moderation and avoid them if they can. Simple, bland remedies are often preferred. In most cases, eczema clears up fully, leaving no sign.

See also **atopy**.

edentulous

Toothless.

editronate disodium

A **bisphosphonate** drug used to treat and prevent **osteoporosis** by inhibiting osteoclastic resorption of bone. A brand name of a preparation marketed with calcium in a cyclical therapy kit is Didronel PMO.

Edronax

A brand name for **reboxetine**.

Efcortelan

A brand name for **hydrocortisone** formulated for external use.

Efcortesol

A brand name for **hydrocortisone** formulated for external use.

Efexor

A brand name for **venlafaxine**.

effusion

The movement of fluid from its usual situation, to form a collection elsewhere. The collection of fluid in the abnormal site is also called an effusion. Such fluid movement can come about in several ways, the commonest being local inflammation of a membrane, such as the lining of a joint (synovial membrane) or of the lung (pleura), with the passage into the joint space, or the pleural cavity, of an excessive quantity of fluid.

Joint effusion causes obvious swelling; pleural effusion may interfere with breathing and may have to be withdrawn through a needle.

eformoterol

A selective beta agonist drug used to treat asthma. It is administered by inhaler. Brand names are Foradil, Oxis Turbohaler.

Efudix

A brand name for a preparation of fluorouracil for external application.

ego

A variously defined and arbitrary term, useful mainly in arguments between psychoanalysts. *Ego* is the Latin word for 'I' and is generally taken to mean a person's consciousness of self. The word was in use, in English, long before Freud was born. It was Freud, however, who made the concept famous, and he is well remembered for his notion that the ego is a kind of rational internal person constantly being pushed into temptation by the **id** with its instinctual, wicked (and mainly sexual) drives, but sometimes saved from disaster by the virtuous **superego**. Freud changed his definition of the ego several times.

After Freud's death and the removal of his controlling influence, the concept of the ego was extended to include most or all of the intellectual functions such as reasoning, inference-drawing and problem solving; memory; a sense of identity and uniqueness; sensory experience; and motor skills. The definition became so wide as to have little specific meaning. The term ego strength is used in behaviourist psychology to denote the useful concept of the degree of one's ability to adapt to reality, to plan and execute, and to withstand and overcome misfortune.

egomania

A preoccupation with self raised to a pathological degree. An abnormal degree of self-esteem.

Ehlers-Danlos syndrome

A genetic disorder in which the skin is abnormally elastic so that it may be stretched several centimetres, and still return to normal. Joints, too, are affected with a similar hyper-elasticity and can be extended far beyond the normal range. In addition to its elasticity, the skin is unduly fragile and gapes widely when wounded.

Scars form over the bony prominences of the knees, ankles, shins and elbows and the skin in these regions may become greatly thickened. Other tissues are affected by fragility, and hernias, flat feet, spontaneous perforation of the bowel and leakage of arteries are common. The condition is due to a widespread defect of polymerization in the basic constructional material of the body – collagen – and there is no known treatment.

People with the Ehlers-Danlos syndrome are sometimes employed in circuses or circus sideshows as 'india-rubber' men or women.

eicosapentaenoic acid

A polyunsaturated fatty acid found in fish oils which is able to reduce the tendency to blood clotting. It is believed to be protective against coronary thrombosis. It appears to act by antagonizing the formation of thromboxane A2, one of the factors in thrombus formation. A brand name is Maxepa.

Eisenmenger complex

A congenital heart anomaly featuring a 'hole in the heart' (atrial or ventricular septal defect) or a failure of closure of the fetal blood vessel which bypasses the lungs before birth (patent ductus arteriosus).

COMPLICATIONS

These defects are associated with, and may possibly cause, a serious condition of the lung blood vessels, which are exposed to higher than normal pressure (pulmonary hypertension) and offer increased resistance to the passage of blood. Once this condition – the Eisenmenger complex – has developed, the outlook is unfavourable and little can be done to help.

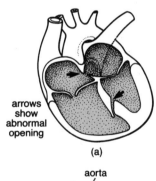

arrows show abnormal opening

(a)

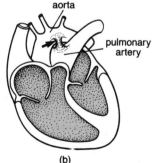

aorta

pulmonary artery

(b)

Eisenmenger complex. This serious condition of raised pressure in the lungs is the result of (a) either an abnormal opening between the two sides of the heart, or (b) a persistence of the duct between the aorta and the arterial trunk to the lungs.

In 'hole in the heart' children, or in those with a patent ductus arteriosus, some of the deoxygenated blood returning from the tissues fails to pass through the lungs but is shunted to the left side of the heart – side that pumps blood around the body – oxygen. As a result the blood haemoglobin, instead of being the bright red highly oxygenated colour, is a bluish-purple, and the affected person looks blue (cyanosed). To try to increase its oxygen carrying capacity, the blood increases its concentration of red cells and becomes thickened and more concentrated (polycythaemia).

TREATMENT

Early surgical treatment of heart holes or patent ductus arteriosus may prevent the Eisenmenger complex from developing.

ejaculation

The normal emission of semen from the penis in spasmodic spurts. Ejaculation is the usual accompaniment of the male orgasm and, once started, becomes involuntary. Ejaculation is forceful enough to ensure that, unless prevented by some barrier, semen is deposited in or about the cervix of the uterus.

DISORDERS OF EJACULATION

Most ejaculation problems, such as failure to achieve ejaculation, or to achieve it at the right time, are psycho-sexual in origin and have nothing to do with organic disease or defect. In most cases the problem lies in the nature of the relationship between the partners and it is a commonplace observation that a man may have major problems, even complete sexual failure, with one woman and none at all with another.

INCIDENCE AND CAUSES

Premature ejaculation is very common. This is the occurrence of the male orgasm at the time of penile insertion, or very soon after, or even, in extreme cases, before any physical contact has occurred.

This is a feature of early sexual experience and is a normal occurrence when the level of mental sexual excitement is high enough to trigger the orgasm.

> Premature ejaculation can often be helped by the trick of squeezing the penis tightly, just behind the bulb (glans), between the finger and thumb.

In more experienced men, premature ejaculation is often induced by **anxiety**, especially over the ability to maintain the erection. Any form of fear operates to bring the sympathetic side of the autonomic nervous system into operation. This is the 'fright and flight' mechanism and is neurologically antagonistic to the parasympathetic system, which is trying to get on with the sexual process. There is a blocking of the arousal state, a failure of the build-up of orgasmic excitement, the beginnings of erectile failure, and a premature triggering of ejaculation.

It is the fear of failure that sets up the vicious cycle and much experience has shown that when this fear is removed, the problem corrects itself. It is interesting to note that a major industry – the Masters and Johnson-based sex therapy business – has been founded on the simple observation that if you tell people that they may engage in prolonged physical intimacy but are not allowed to have sexual intercourse, male sexual problems rapidly clear up.

Absence of ejaculation is rare. It may be due to over-indulgence, in which case the problem is temporary, or to e | -el

inadequate penile stimulation from a very lax vagina, which may require manual assistance from the woman or even a tightening gynaecological operation. Another possible cause is age-related loss of penile sensitivity, in which case more manual assistance is needed. Very uncommonly, structural (anatomical) abnormality is the cause. If ejaculation can be achieved by masturbation, the latter cause is ruled out.

-el

Suffix meaning 'diminutive' as in scalpel (little knife).

Elantan

A brand name for **isosorbide mononitrate**.

elastic stockings

See **varicose veins**.

eldepryl

A brand name for **selegiline**.

Eldisine

A brand name for **vindesine**.

elective

A term relating to a medical decision in a situation not involving urgency, risk to life or to permanent health. Elective surgery, for instance, is surgery undertaken to achieve some advantage for the patient, but which is not essential to life or health. Most cosmetic surgical operations can be considered elective. In a state medical system, such as the National Health Service, elective procedures tend to have lower priority than more necessary interventions.

electrical injury

This is caused by the heating effect of a current passing through the body, by the burns caused by electrical arcs, and by the disruptive effect on nervous system and heart function. Currents passing through the body take the path of least electrical resistance and large currents tend to travel along the major arteries, causing coagulation of the blood and total blockage. Very large currents cause so much heating as to char the tissues.

> AC (alternating current) is more dangerous than DC (direct current) at the same voltage, mainly because AC causes the muscles to go into sustained contraction so that it may be difficult to let go of a conductor that has been grasped. An alternating current as low as 15 milliamps may prevent voluntary release. About 100 milliamps will produce a cardiac arrest.

Current can only flow in a circuit, but since electrical voltages exist in relation to earth potential, which is zero, a circuit occurs if the body connects earth to any point of high voltage. The value of the current that flows through the body is determined by the voltage and by the electrical resistance offered by the body. The internal resistance is low and relatively fixed, but the skin contact resistance, and the interposition of insulating material, such as plastic shoes, can make a very large

difference to the resistance – and to the outcome. Wet skin has a very low resistance – about 500 ohms – while the resistance of dry skin may be as high as 30,000 ohms. Dry footwear will offer varying resistance, depending on the material, of up to several million ohms.

DANGERS

The United Kingdom mains voltage of about 250 is quite high enough to drive a fatal current through the body, if the skin resistance, and the resistance of the path to ground, are low. If these resistances are high, a higher voltage is necessary to cause serious injury. Very high voltages occur in lightning strikes and in some industrial accidents.

> Cardiac arrest caused by electrical current flow is often reversible and no time should be wasted in getting the victim away from contact with the current, so that, if necessary, external cardiac massage and mouth to mouth ventilation can be done.

Insulating material, such as dry wood, or a plastic pipe, should be used to push the subject off the conductor, or to push the conductor away. If the current can quickly be switched off, this should be done, but time wasted in hunting for a switch may be fatal. Electrical burns are treated in the same way as other burns. Severe arterial damage in the arms or legs may necessitate amputation.

electricity cable fields, biological danger from

To get this controversial matter in perspective, some figures may be helpful. Magnetic fields are measured in gauss units. One gauss is the field strength 1 cm from a wire carrying a current of 5 amps. At 10 cm the field strength has fallen to 0.01 gauss and at 1 m to 0.0001 gauss. This is the order of field strength experienced by all of us in a domestic environment. The highest field recorded, immediately under the largest British power lines, is less than half a gauss. The earth's magnetic field varies with position, but averages about half a gauss. So it is clear, first, that the field experienced by people living near power cables is very small indeed, and, second, that a static magnetic field is unlikely to be a cause of disease.

Power lines, however, do not produce a static field. They carry alternating current so the field is increasing to a maximum in one direction, reversing and falling to zero and then increasing to a maximum in the opposite direction. This happens 50 times each second and any iron within the field will

> Studies in various places of the incidence of childhood cancers, especially leukaemia, seem to show that those most highly exposed to power lines have a slightly higher than average incidence. Various other studies showed no clear association between power lines and cancer. Perhaps significantly, studies done by electricity-generating authorities tend to produce results to show that there is no evidence of a harmful effect, while those done by environmental groups tend to suggest that there may be. This is not to imply that either side is being dishonest, but to illustrate the well-known fact that it is almost impossible wholly to eliminate the influence of personal bias in scientific studies of phenomena whose effect, if it exists, is very small.

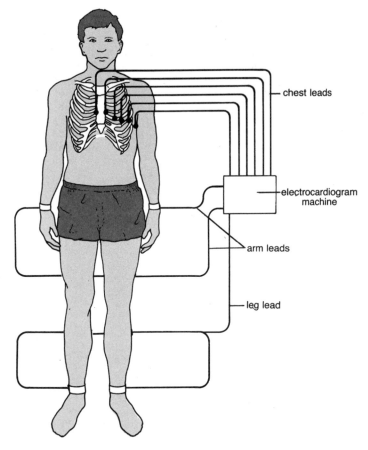

The electrocardiogram. This is a high-gain balanced amplifier feeding an electric pen device which writes a record of the electrical activity of the heart on a strip of moving paper. Different connections of the arm, leg and chest leads provide tracings from which a wide range of heart disorders can be detected.

chest leads

electrocardiogram machine

arm leads

leg lead

vibrate slightly at that frequency. Blood contains iron in the haemoglobin of the red cells.

Many studies have been done to test the effects of alternating fields. No blood changes have been detected. Vibration is not, in itself, harmful. Heat, light and sound are all mediated by vibration.

Statistics produced on the incidence of disease are very hard to interpret usefully. It is, in practice, almost impossible to isolate factors, such as alternating magnetic fields, which are directly caused by the power lines, from all the other possible effects operating on people living near power lines – or near nuclear power stations, for that matter.

electric shock treatment

See **electroconvulsive therapy**.

electrocardiogram

Heart muscle contraction is associated with rapidly varying electric currents which can be detected as varying voltage differences between different points on the surface of the body. Five connections are made to the ECG machine in the standard lead system – one from each limb and one (lead V) from various positions on the front and side of the chest. Lead I measures the potential difference between the right arm and the left arm, lead II between the right arm and the left leg, and so on. These can be switched in, in sequence, and each pair gives a different 'view' of the same basic tracing.

The voltages produced are very small and must be amplified before they can actuate a writing device, but they do provide a highly detailed record of much of what is happening in the heart as it goes through its timed sequence of contraction of both upper chambers (atria) and then both lower chambers (ventricles). Doctors have learned, by a great deal of experience, to recognize the normal range of the electrocardiogram (ECG) and the many variations caused in it by disease or defective action of the heart. The patterns are so characteristic, however, that most of them can be recognized by the machines itself, using computer comparison with stored data. Many machines will print out a suggestion as to the diagnosis. Although a computer still cannot compete with the expert in interpretation of the ECG, a good computer program will usually do better, overall, than most doctors.

The electrocardiogram is useful in diagnosing a number of abnormalities. These include:

- upsets of normal rhythm;
- abnormal rate and strength of beat;
- abnormalities of conduction of controlling impulses within the heart;
- enlargement of the chambers;
- **heart attack** (coronary thrombosis), both recent and old;
- inadequate coronary flow;
- congenital heart disorders;
- alterations in blood calcium and potassium;
- **pericarditis**;
- the effects of drugs on the heart.

To be most useful, an ECG is also taken during exercise and this will often bring to light latent abnormalities which do not show on the resting tracing. This is especially true of the common situation in which the coronary blood supply to the heart muscle is adequate for the resting state, but insufficient during exertion. If an ECG is done while the patient is running on a treadmill, this danger may be detected and appropriate treatment instituted. ECGs can also be taken while the patient is continuing with his or her normal life and the output can be transmitted to a remote receiver, in a hospital or clinic, for printout (radiotelemetry) or can be recorded on a long-running cassette recorder carried by the patient.

electrocautery

See **cauterization**.

electrocoagulation

This employs the same principle as electrocautery (see **cauterization**). High-frequency electrical heating (diathermy) is a convenient way of stopping bleeding during a surgical operation. When a small artery is cut during the operation, the spurting end is seized in artery forceps and nipped. Artery forceps have a catch on the handle so they remain closed until released. The surgeon may now get his assistant to touch the artery forceps with the tip of the coagulation electrode and press the foot switch. Immediately, the blood vessel is sealed by the current and the forceps may safely be released.

electroconvulsive therapy

ECT is a means of inducing an epileptic fit by applying a pulse of electric current to the brain. It is thought, by many who are experienced in its use, to be a valuable method of psychiatric treatment, but has aroused widespread controversy and dislike. To some extent this is an emotional judgement based on the unpleasantness of seeing a convulsion deliberately induced, but there is also a belief – based on evidence rejected by many psychiatrists – that it can cause permanent brain damage.

HOW IT'S DONE

The muscular contractions which are the most striking feature of a major fit do not now occur as ECT is done under general anaesthesia supplemented by a short-acting muscle relaxant drug. Very light anaesthesia is used. The electrodes, which resemble lightweight Walkman headphones, are padded and are damped with salty water. They are placed on the temples about 3 cm above a line joining the bump of the ear to the corner of the eye. A brief pulse of current is given and the fit, which is observable only as a twitching of the jaw and facial muscles, lasts for half to one minute.

WHY IT'S DONE

The mode of action of ECT is not fully understood, but a series of treatments raises the threshold for convulsions so that a higher level of electrical activity in the brain is necessary before a fit occurs. Brain areas that are electrically overactive before the treatment become underactive immediately after it. There is also a reduction in the effectiveness of adrenaline receptors and an increase in the production of the brain's own morphine-like substances (enkephalins).

ECT is most useful in cases of serious depression, especially in those with psychotic depression, and the great majority of patients treated in this way are depressives. The results are usually very good, the response to ECT being more rapid and associated with fewer side-effects than drug treatment. Severe, delusional or psychotic depression responds well to ECT and poorly to drugs and many lives have undoubtedly been saved in this way by preventing suicide. Some forms of acute schizophrenia, especially those featuring **catatonia** or severe emotional disturbance, also respond well to ECT. Long-established (chronic) schizophrenia does not do well with ECT and responds in only about 10 per cent of cases.

RISKS

The risk to life is the same as the mortality rate associated with a brief anaesthetic alone – about one in 10,000. Memory is nearly always impaired during the weeks following the treatment, but almost all patients are said to be back to normal by six months.

electroencephalogram

An electroencephalogram (EEG) is a multiple tracing, made by voltmeter-operated pens, of the electrical activity of the brain. The multiple readings are of the constantly varying voltage differences occurring between pairs of points on the scalp of the subject. Electro-encephalography was first described in 1929 by the German psychiatrist Hans Berger (1873–1941). Berger had hoped to show precise correlation between psychic processes and electrical brain signals, but in this he was disappointed.

The conduction of nerve impulses along nerve fibres involves the movement of electrical charges and the generation of electric currents. The associated voltages can be picked up by electrodes of thick silver wire glued to the scalp. The amplitudes are very low – of the order of 10 to 100 millionths of a volt – and powerful balanced amplifiers are needed to raise them to levels which can operate the pen movements.

In view of the many billions of nerve fibres in the brain, and their complex interconnections, especially in the outer layer of the brain, it might be expected, on statistical grounds, that this mass of electrical activity would cancel out. That it does not do so indicates that many nerve units change their electrical potentials synchronously, forming the electrical rhythms that dominate the resting state of the healthy brain. As soon as the brain's activity increases, however, these basic rhythms are disrupted and the amplitude of the regular oscillations is reduced, or they may disappear altogether, suggesting that purposeful neurological activity involves many nerve impulses moving out of step with each other.

The normal EEG is dominated by the alpha rhythm, a steady alternation at 8 to 13 cycles per second (Herz). This has its highest amplitude at the back of the head and is disrupted by visual attention. The beta rhythm is faster (of higher frequency) and of lower amplitude than the alpha rhythm. Theta and delta rhythms are very slow and, if prominent, suggest abnormal brain function. An individual's EEG remains remarkably constant throughout most of adult life and major alterations are highly significant.

The EEG is affected, characteristically, by sleep and the standard sleep pattern is strikingly disturbed during the periods of rapid eye movement (REM sleep). It is affected by hyperventilation, drugs, concussion, brain injury, brain tumours, bleeding within the brain (cerebral haemorrhage), brain inflammation (encephalitis) and various psychiatric conditions. In particular, the EEG is affected by epilepsy, and is an important means of distinguishing the various forms.

The EEG also assists in the determination of legal death and is important as an aid to making decisions about taking organs for transplantation. Repeated EEGs showing no sign of electrical activity strongly suggest that future brain activity is unlikely. It is not, however, an absolute indication and must be used in conjunction with other criteria.

electrolysis

Strictly speaking, electrolysis is the decomposition of a solution by the passage of an electric current. The decomposition of salty water into hydrogen and oxygen, by the action of an electric current, is an example of electrolysis. In popular parlance, the term is used to refer to the process by which hair follicles are destroyed by the passage of a few milliamps of current through a needle inserted in the hair pore. In fact, although some· electrolysis does occur, and bubbles of gas can be seen emerging from the pore, the main destructive effect is one of heating.

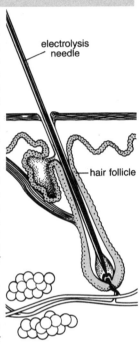

Hair removal by this means is tedious and slow, as only one hair can be dealt with at a time. The method is unsuitable for dealing with heavy growth of unwanted hair. There is some risk of scarring.

Electrolysis. A fine needle is passed down into the hair follicle until the tip lies at the root. A current of a few milliamps is passed and this destroys the hair root by heating.

electron microscopy

The magnification of light microscopes is limited to about 2000 times by the wavelength of visible or ultraviolet light; an object smaller than the wavelength of light cannot be resolved. To overcome this limitation, a medium of shorter wavelength, which can be deflected by lenses, is required. A beam of accelerated electrons admirably meets this requirement. The greater the momentum the shorter the effective wavelength. Modern instruments enable objects smaller than one nanometre (one millionth of a millimetre) to be seen. This is almost down to atomic level.

The transmission electron microscope is analogous in optical design to the light microscope. The source of electrons is a filament, similar to that in a TV tube. Because electrons are negatively charged they are easily accelerated by high positive voltages (20,000 to well over 1,000,000 volts) and are easily deflected by electric or magnetic fields obtained from charged plates or current-carrying coils, respectively. The shape of these fields is determined by the physical shape of the plates or coils and they can be arranged to have an effect, on the electron beam, identical to that of optical lenses on light. There are condenser lenses, objective, intermediate, and projector lenses, the latter producing the final image on a fluorescent screen or photographic film or plate. Because electrons are scattered by collision with air molecules, a high degree of vacuum is required within the instrument. Cooling and shielding are required because of the heat generated in the powerful deflecting coils and because accelerated electrons can prompt the emission of X-rays.

Specimens for electron microscopy must be extremely thin and must be able to withstand the effects of the vacuum and the electron bombardment. In light microscopy, chemical stains are used to bring out detail. In electron microscopy, this is done by the use of materials containing heavy atoms, such as metals. Evaporated metal, such as platinum, may be deposited on the surface of the specimen to reveal topographical features.

The scanning electron microscope operates in a manner similar to the way the electron beam in a TV tube builds up the picture by moving rapidly over the inner surface of the tube. Specimens are metal coated and a very narrow electron beam scans the surface. Reflected or transmitted electrons are picked up by a device which produces a varying current, and this is applied, as a video signal, to a TV monitor synchronized with the microscope beam deflection.

Electron microscopes are tools of the highest importance in medicine, both in research and in diagnosis. They have opened up a new world of biological detail and enormously extended our knowledge of the ultra-structure of cells and their components. Much has been learned about the nature of many disease processes, at a molecular level, and the causation of many diseases has been discovered by this means. The science of virology has been revolutionized by electron microscopy.

electronystagmography

Eye movement generates small electric currents which can be picked up by metal electrodes placed near the corners of the eyes. These currents can be amplified and used to deflect recording pens so as to produce a permanent record of the eye movements.

The method may be used to study, analyze and diagnose the various types of abnormal wobbly eye movement (nystagmus), or to record the response to caloric tests of the function of the inner ear balancing mechanism.

electrophoresis

This is the process by which charged particles in a solution (ions) are separated by the application of an electric current. Many substances ionize naturally when dissolved. For instance, a molecule of common salt (NaCl) separates into two ions, a positively charged sodium ion (Na+) and a negatively charged chlorine ion (Cl-). If an electric current is applied to the solution, the positive ions are attracted to the negative electrode and the negative ions to the positive electrode. 'Unlike' charges attract each other; 'like' charges repel.

If a solution of a particular substance, or mixture of substances is placed on the surface of a gel or a membrane or even soaked into a piece of paper and an electric current applied between separated metal plates on the surface, the ions will move. The movement occurs on the surface and the extent of the movement is dependent on the weight and the charge of the ions. Ions of low weight move more quickly than those of high weight, so separation occurs. After a time, the surface can be stained so that the characteristic patterns of separation can be recognized.

Electrophoresis is important in medicine and biochemistry and is used to separate, and measure the amount of, various substances, especially proteins, in body fluids, such as the blood. The technique is widely used in medicine to identify and measure the albumin, globulin, and fibrinogen (three kinds of plasma proteins) present in the blood and to separate the various globulin fractions constituting the different immunoglobulins. Electrophoresis is used to identify the various abnormal haemoglobins causing sickle cell anaemia and other similar conditions and is a convenient way of separating and identifying the various kinds of low and high density lipoproteins in people with abnormal blood fat (lipid) levels.

elephantiasis

A condition of enormous enlargement of a limb, the scrotum or the female genitalia.

POSSIBLE CAUSES
Elephantiasis is caused by obstruction to the lymph drainage channels by masses of parasitic microfilaria worms (mainly *Wuchereria bancrofti*) or, in the condition known as lymphogranuloma venereum, by the *Chlamydia trachomatis* organism.

INCIDENCE
Although mosquito-spread **filariasis** is common, elephantiasis is relatively rare except in communities living in primitive conditions and with poor medical facilities. It is seen most often in Africa, South-East Asia and the Pacific islands.

RECOGNITION AND SYMPTOMS
Failure of lymph drainage leads to permanent and increasing fluid collection (oedema) in the affected area. The waterlogged tissues have a high protein content and readily become infected and inflamed. The resulting ingrowth of fibrous tissue changes the oedema from a type that pits on pressure to a solid, flesh-like and irreversible form. The overlying skin becomes greatly thickened, roughened and corrugated, resembling that of the elephant.

Elephantiasis of the scrotum may lead to enlargement of such magnitude that the sufferer is forced to remain seated on an object resembling a large sack of potatoes.

TREATMENT
The remedy, for those with access to treatment, is surgical removal of the excess tissue.

ELISA test

Acronym for the enzyme-linked immunosorbent assay test – one of the most important tests used to identify antibodies in the blood. It is a commonly used screening test for **AIDS**.

The test detects the antibodies to the particular infection it is intended to look for and requires a known sample of the suspected organism (the antigen). This sample is chemically linked to an enzyme (peroxidase) which can cause a colour change in a solution. The enzyme is retained only if the specific antibody, to which the antigen attaches itself, is present. When this is so the enzyme operates and the colour changes. This is the indication of a positive result.

The ELISA test can detect antibodies to anything from specific viruses to parasitic worm proteins. Kits, for pathology laboratories, are produced to identify a very wide range of antibodies. The ELISA test for AIDS quickly attracted very

large sums of money in the United States, and, since the AIDS virus was the antigen needed for the test, a dispute over the right to use it became a matter of contention between the Pasteur Institute in Paris and the National Cancer Institute, Bethesda, Maryland, both of whom claimed to have discovered the virus. The honours were not only with the Old World but also with the female sex.

Elleste Duet

A brand name for a combination of **norethisterone** acetate and **oestradiol**.

Elleste Solo

A brand name for **oestradiol**.

Eltroxin

A brand name for **thyroxine**.

Elyzol

A brand name for **metronidazole**.

embalming

A method of temporarily preserving a dead body by removing the blood and replacing it with disinfectant and preservative fluids, such as formalin (formaldehyde), which discourage the growth of organisms responsible for putrefaction. It is of value if, for any reason, cremation or burial must be delayed. Embalming is often associated with cosmetic treatment intended to preserve, for a time, a life-like appearance.

embolectomy

The surgical opening of a large blood vessel and the removal from it of a blood clot, or other obstruction, which has been carried in the blood from elsewhere in the circulation.

> Blockage of a major artery is always an emergency, because, as soon as the blood supply is cut off, the area supplied by the vessel begins to die. Unless an alternative blood supply is available from an adjacent artery, embolectomy may be the only chance of saving a limb, of avoiding a major stroke or even of saving life. To be effective, the operation must be performed within a very short time of the onset of symptoms.

RISKS
One desperate emergency in which the procedure is occasionally successful is blockage, by a large clot from a leg vein, of the branches of the large artery carrying blood from the heart to the lungs. This is called pulmonary **embolism**. Unfortunately, in such extreme cases the mortality rate is very high. In patients becoming progressively more ill from recurrent pulmonary embolism, the operation, which involves making an incision into the artery and sucking out the clot, is much less risky than doing nothing.

See also **endarterectomy**, **balloon catheter**.

embolism

The sudden blocking of an artery by solid, semi-solid or gaseous material brought to the site of the obstruction in the bloodstream. The object, or material, causing the embolism is called an embolus (plural emboli). It is always abnormal for any non-fluid material to be present in the circulation, and because blood proceeding through arteries encounters ever smaller branches, such material will inevitably impact and cause blockage, thereby depriving a part of the body of its essential blood supply.

POSSIBLE CAUSES

Many different forms of emboli occur. Embolism is commonly caused by blood clot emboli, often arising in the veins and passing through the right side of the heart to enter the arteries carrying blood to the lungs. It may also be caused by crystals of cholesterol from plaques of **atheroma** in larger arteries; by clumps of infected material in severe injuries; by air or nitrogen in diving accidents; by bone marrow and fat in fractures of large bones; and by tumour cells and other substances.

RISKS

The chief danger in deep vein thrombosis is the formation of long, soft, snaky blood clots which may become very large before breaking loose into the bloodstream. Such clots pass quickly through the right side of the heart and impact in the main branches of the arteries to the lung. This is called pulmonary embolism and is a common cause of sudden, unexpected death. Similar, but smaller, emboli may form on the inner lining of the heart, often on the left side, after a coronary thrombosis. These are often carried upwards to cause embolism in vital brain arteries, leading to stroke. Small cholesterol emboli, arising from disease of the carotid arteries, commonly cause **transient ischaemic attacks**.

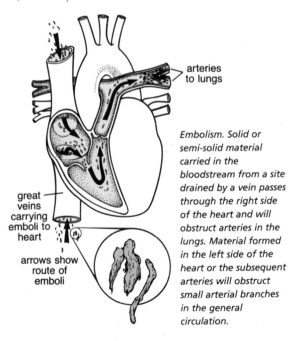

arteries to lungs

Embolism. Solid or semi-solid material carried in the bloodstream from a site drained by a vein passes through the right side of the heart and will obstruct arteries in the lungs. Material formed in the left side of the heart or the subsequent arteries will obstruct small arterial branches in the general circulation.

great veins carrying emboli to heart

arrows show route of emboli

embrocation

A lotion or other medicated liquid applied to the outside of the body, usually in the hope of relieving muscle, joint or tendon pain. Embrocations work more by faith, or by the effect of human contact, than by virtue of any effect they have on the underlying disorder, but they often smell purposeful and can impart a pleasant tingling sensation to the skin.

embryology

The study of, or the branch of science concerned with, the whole process of physical development of the body, from the time of fertilization of the ovum to the time of birth.

embryon

Greek root meaning 'fetus' as in embryo (early development stage).

embryo, research on

The use of very early human embryos for studies into such important matters as the early detection and possible correction of genetic defects, the relief of human infertility, and the use of embryonic cell grafts for medical treatment of serious disorders. Cloning experiments, the alteration of the genetic pattern and attempts at hybridization are prohibited. Early embryos of two weeks gestational age have no organs or nervous system and are incapable of any perception or consciousness. See also **ethics, medical**.

emergency opening into

See **tracheostomy**.

Emeside

A brand name for **ethosuximide**.

emesis

See **vomiting**.

emetic drugs

Drugs which induce vomiting. They are little used nowadays, but are sometimes valuable in the treatment of poisoning and in the re-conditioning treatment of alcoholism. Ipecacuanha and apomorphine are the most commonly used.

emetos

Greek root meaning 'vomit' as in emetic (causing vomiting).

Emflex

A brand name for **acemetacin**.

Eminase

A brand name for **anistreplase**.

EMI scanning

This is the same as **CT** or **CAT** (computer-assisted tomography) **scanning**. The name reflects the fact that this remarkable advance in imaging technology was developed at the EMI laboratories. Geoffrey Newbold Hounsfield (b. 1919), an EMI engineer developed the prototype scanner in 1967, thereby initiating an entirely new concept in medical diagnosis and conferring an inestimable boon on mankind. He was awarded the Nobel Prize in 1979.

Emla cream

A brand name for a mixture of lignocaine and **prilocaine** formulated as a cream for local application to allow many diagnostic and therapeutic procedures to be carried out with minimal pain or discomfort. The name is an acronym for 'Eutetic Mixture of Local Anaesthetics'.

emollient

Soothing. Also, any agent, such as a cream or ointment, that soothes or softens the skin.

emotion

A state of arousal; a mixed mental and bodily reaction to important external events or to memories of such events. Life events that evoke emotion always affect, or threaten to affect, our personal advantage or disadvantage.

There are many different emotions – fear, anger, hate, disgust, love, joy, jealousy, dread, grief, pride, shame, lust – and all can involve strong feelings, which may be pleasant or unpleasant. All are associated, to a greater or lesser degree, with physiological changes, such as a rapid heartbeat, dry mouth, sweating palms, tense stomach, pallor, flushing or trembling, and many prompt us to perform an action.

EXPRESSING EMOTION

The external expression of emotional content is technically known as *affect*. Emotions, such as fear, anger and sexual excitement are primitive, in an evolutionary sense, and are common to a wide range of animals. Smiling, frowning, sneering, and so on, are not learned activities, but are an inherent result of our genetic makeup. Blind babies, who have never seen facial expression in others, still smile, laugh, cry and show fear and distress appropriately.

HORMONAL INFLUENCES

Hormonal changes accompanying emotion are few and involve, among other changes, the secretion of adrenaline and cortisols. It is significant that an injection of adrenaline will produce either fear or pleasurable excitement depending on the external circumstances and the state of mind of the subject at the time.

EMOTIONAL CONTROL

Recent research has isolated the **limbic system** and the hypothalamus of the brain as mediators of emotional expression and feeling. The hypothalamus lies immediately above the stalk of the pituitary gland and is intimately connected with it both by many nerve fibres and by hormonal means. The pituitary is the central controlling organ of the whole hormonal system. Mental activity and interpretation of events determine the kind of emotional response, in any given situation, and it is here, at the interface between neurological and hormonal action, that thought gives rise to the hormonal bodily response (visceral arousal) which is the necessary condition for emotional experience. The hormonal effect is diffuse and general; the specific type of emotion depends on our perception of the circumstances.

emotional disorders

The disorders of mood are **depression, mania** and the bipolar or cyclothymic condition (**manic-depressive psychosis**) in which the affected person swings from an extreme of excitement to one of depression.

emphysema

A lung disease characterized by structural changes in the small air sacs (alveoli) where oxygen passes from the air into the blood and carbon dioxide passes out. As a result of disease, the walls of the alveoli break down so that larger air spaces are formed. The effect is that the surface area available for gas exchange is greatly reduced and there is diminished oxygen supply to the vital organs and a rise in the amount of carbon dioxide in the blood.

RECOGNITION AND SYMPTOMS

Bronchitis is commonly associated with emphysema and because this leads to reduction of the bore of the bronchial tubes by swelling of the lining and spasm, the passage of air is further prejudiced and there is a worsening of the situation. Air is trapped in the enlarged alveolar spaces and the lungs become over-inflated. The chest becomes barrel-shaped in appearance and there is wheezing and shortness of breath.

The deficient oxygen supply leads to a reduction in the amount of exertion possible and eventually the affected person may be able to do no more than sit up in bed. Even then, there may be breathlessness and blueness of the skin (cyanosis) requiring oxygen by mask for survival. Smoking and recurrent respiratory infections make matters worse and the state of such a respiratory cripple is indeed desperate. Death results from overwhelming infection, respiratory failure, or secondary effects on the heart.

POSSIBLE CAUSES

The primary cause of emphysema is still unclear, but smoking is the most important known factor. Inhalation of industrial pollutants can also contribute to the development of the condition. In some cases there is a strong family history, but this does not necessarily imply a genetic factor.

emphysema, surgical

The abnormal presence of air or gas in the tissues, most commonly in the neck as a result of persistent leakage from a lung. Air may also gain access to the tissues from injury to the oesophagus or from a fracture of the wall of one of the nasal sinuses.

RECOGNITION AND SYMPTOMS

Surgical emphysema produces a peculiar and characteristic crackling effect as the tissues involved are pressed with the fingers and the bubbles of air are forced through the tissue planes. The condition is not, in itself, harmful and the air will soon absorb if the leakage from the source is closed.

empirical treatment

Treatment given without knowledge, or full knowledge, of the cause or nature of the disorder; or treatment based on symptoms rather than on knowledge of the underlying disease processes (the pathology). Ideally, accurate diagnosis should always precede treatment as only thus can there be any assurance that the best treatment is being given. But there are occasions when the cause cannot be found and when the choice is to do nothing or to try something.

Sometimes the urgency for intervention makes empirical treatment mandatory – as in a severe and life-threatening infection by an organism not yet identified. In such a case a broad-spectrum antibiotic may be given empirically while the results of bacterial culture and other tests are awaited. There may also be occasions on which severe pain may call for the empirical use of powerful pain-killing drugs. This, however, is sometimes dangerous as symptoms vital to the diagnosis may be concealed.

Empirical treatment is not random treatment, but is usually based on sound general principles or clinical intuition and experience.

empyema

A collection of pus in the space between the lungs and the chest wall (the pleural cavity). This usually results from pneumonococcal pneumonia, cancer or tuberculosis of the underlying lung.

> Empyema causes lung collapse and interferes with breathing. It is serious and demands energetic treatment.

Repeated attempts are made to suck out the pus through needles, but thick, constricting membranes tend to form and it is often necessary to open the chest and drain the cavity directly. Antibiotics are also used, but are no substitute for surgery.

enalapril

An **angiotensin converting enzyme (ace) inhibitor** drug with useful action over 24 hours. A brand name is Innovace. It is also formulated in conjunction with the diuretic drug hydrochlorothiazide as Innozide.

enbucrilate

A cyanoacrylic tissue adhesive used as an alternative to stitches for minor wounds. A brand name is Histoacryl.

encephalins

See **endorphins**.

encephalitis

Inflammation of the brain.
POSSIBLE CAUSES
Most cases are caused by infection, especially by viruses. Primary encephalitis is caused by direct infection with Herpes simplex, Herpes zoster, tick-borne or mosquito-borne arboviruses, polioviruses, echoviruses or coxsackie viruses. Herpes encephalitis is rare except in the case of people whose immune systems have been compromised by natural immune deficiency, by **AIDS** or by necessary medical treatment. The other forms tend to occur in epidemics.

Cases of secondary encephalitis usually occur as a complication of viral infections and, since the viruses are seldom if ever isolated from the affected brains, are thought to be a form of allergic hypersensitivity. They may follow **mumps**, **measles**, **rubella** and **chickenpox**. In these cases, the effect on the brain is a local loss of the insulating sheaths of the nerve fibres (**demyelination**) and the condition is sometimes called acute disseminated encephalomyelitis.
RECOGNITION AND SYMPTOMS
Encephalitis causes severe headache, fever, vomiting, sickness, often a stiff neck and back, and epileptic fits, and may progress to mental confusion, coma and death. A fatal outcome may occur within hours of onset, but even gravely ill patients may make a full recovery.

TREATMENT
Drugs like acyclovir have changed the outlook in cases of Herpes simplex encephalitis.

> Long-term effects of encephalitis can be serious and may include mental retardation, epilepsy and deafness.

encephalitis lethargica

Also known as 'sleeping sickness' or 'von Economo's disease', this form of encephalitis occurred in a world-wide pandemic in the 1920s and affected millions of people, especially in Europe. No causal organism was ever found, but the features were those of a virus infection of the midbrain region. There was paralysis of the eye muscles and a striking tendency to sleepiness. A high proportion of those who survived developed **Parkinsonism** within months or years. The disease is now very rare.

The condition should not be confused with African **trypanosomiasis**, a parasitic disease spread by the tsetse fly, which is also known as 'sleeping sickness'.

encephalomyelitis

See **encephalitis**.

encephalopathy

A general term to cover any degenerative or non-inflammatory disorder affecting the brain in a widespread manner. The term was introduced when it was recognized that the term **encephalitis** should be restricted to conditions involving brain inflammation.

encephalos

Greek root meaning 'brain' as in **encephalitis** (brain inflammation).

encopresis

Faecal soiling or incontinence of faeces, not due to organic disease, but resulting from deliberate intent or psychiatric disorder.

Over 15 per cent of three-year-olds have encopresis, mainly as a result of resistance to toilet training. Children of this age have few weapons in the conflict with parents and this is one of them. Failure to perform on the potty, followed by inconvenient defaecation, is a popular ploy. In some cases there is deliberate faecal retention until control is lost. The consolation is that by four years of age the incidence of encopresis has dropped to about 1 per cent.

endarterectomy

An operation to restore full blood flow in an artery narrowed by **atherosclerosis**. Clamps are applied, an incision is made into the artery, and the whole of the diseased inner lining and any associated blood clot (thrombus) are removed. The incision is then closed with very fine stitches. The surgeon will often use an operating microscope.

Unfortunately, a person with atherosclerotic narrowing severe enough to justify this form of intervention is likely to have widespread arterial disease and the real, long-term value of this procedure has not yet been established. Even so, endarterectomy is being increasingly used as a treatment for people suffering from inadequate blood supply to the brain, or to a limb, as a result of atherosclerosis of the major supplying arteries.

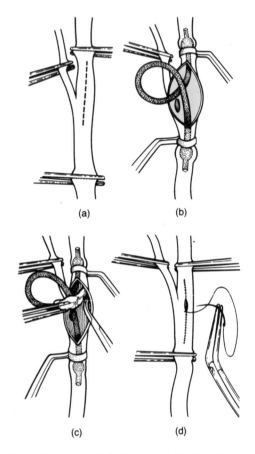

(a)　　　　(b)

(c)　　　　(d)

Endarterectomy. A surgical technique which allows the removal of an obstruction, such as a large blood clot, from an important artery. (a) The artery is clamped. (b) A shunt tube may be used to maintain the blood flow while the obstruction is being removed (c). (d) The incision in the artery is closed with fine stitches.

The procedure offers little advantage for those who have already suffered strokes, but may be of value to those having repeated **transient ischaemic attacks** and who are at risk of stroke. Emergency endarterectomy may be the only hope of saving a leg whose main blood supply is prejudiced by severe arterial narrowing and thrombus formation.

endemic

Literally, 'among the people'. An endemic disease is one which occurs continuously among the inhabitants of a particular place.

See also **epidemic** and **pandemic**.

endo-

Prefix meaning 'inside' as in endogenous (coming from inside).

endocarditis

Inflammation of the inner lining of the heart and of the heart valves, most commonly as a result of infection. The affected areas develop loose, fibrinous, infected clots (vegetations) which break off to form infected emboli, spreading infection throughout the body. These vegetations also protect the infecting organisms from the body's immune defence mechanisms so that the condition is difficult to treat. Without effective treatment infective endocarditis is usually progressive and the condition is rapidly fatal.

WHEN DOES IT HAPPEN?

A healthy heart seldom suffers endocarditis, but heart valve damage from previous rheumatic fever, congenital heart disease, the presence of artificial heart valves or damage from cardiac catheters all predispose to the condition. Intravenous drug abusers are also extremely prone to develop infective endocarditis.

Endocarditis can also be non-infective and may result from immunologically induced conditions such as **lupus erythematosus.**

RECOGNITION AND SYMPTOMS

Endocarditis often starts insidiously with low fever, sweats, loss of weight and the effects of small emboli on the brain, kidneys and elsewhere. The emboli may also cause minor or major strokes, pain in the loins with blood in the urine, coldness and loss of power in a limb from blockage of an artery, bleeding into the skin and many other effects.

TREATMENT

Treatment is by intensive and massive antibiotic therapy and sometimes by heart surgery to remove infected masses from

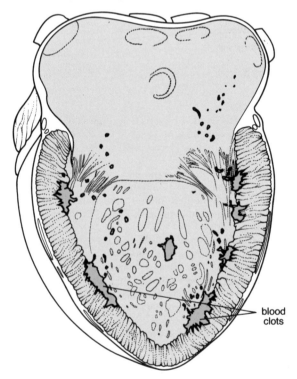

blood clots

Endocarditis. A dangerous condition in which the inner lining of the heart becomes inflamed and blood clots form on the inflamed areas. These can become infected and cause dangerous illness.

within the heart. The outcome depends on many factors, including the nature of the infecting organisms, the duration of the disease before treatment, the age of the patient and the severity of the secondary effects.

Certain procedures, such as dental treatment, result in the transient presence of bacteria in the blood. These are normally harmless except to the susceptible groups mentioned above, and it is customary, in these cases, to perform the procedure under a screen or 'umbrella' of antibiotics.

endocrine system

The hormonal system. Hormones are chemical substances produced by the various endocrine glands and released into the bloodstream to effect actions, by way of specific receptor sites, in other parts of the body. These substances control and coordinate body growth and the build-up and breakdown of body tissues (metabolism), nutrition, body temperature, the circulation of the blood, salt and water balance, the development of the secondary sexual characteristics, and reproduction.

The hormonal system of the body is under the overall combined control of psychic stimuli, external stimuli and biochemical stability mechanisms which interact and operate on the hypothalamus of the brain. The hypothalamus controls the pituitary gland, which has been described as 'the conductor of the endocrine orchestra'. This central gland releases a range of hormones which stimulates the action of the other endocrine glands.

endocrinologist

A doctor or physiological scientist specializing in the function, inter-relation and disorders of the endocrine system of

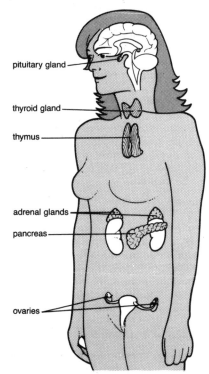

pituitary gland

thyroid gland

thymus

adrenal glands

pancreas

ovaries

Location of the endocrine glands.

the body – the group of hormone-producing glands that includes the pituitary, the pineal gland, the thyroid gland, the parathyroid glands, the islet tissue in the pancreas, the adrenal glands, the sex hormone-producing tissue in the testicles and ovaries, and the placenta during pregnancy.

endogenous

Arising without obvious external cause, and believed to result from an internal cause. For instance, a person who becomes depressed because of a succession of life calamities is said to have exogenous **depression**. If depression arises in the absence of such external reasons, it is said to be endogenous.

endometrial ablation

A surgical treatment for severe menstrual bleeding or fibroids situated near the inner surface of the womb. This involves destruction of the womb lining, which may be done by laser energy, a heated wire loop, microwave heating, or by means of hot fluid in a balloon. The treatment is an alternative to surgical removal of the womb (hysterectomy) and has largely superseded dilatation and curettage (**D and C**).

endometriosis

This is a condition involving the presence, in abnormal sites, of the tissue that is normally present only as the lining of the womb. This tissue is called endometrium.
RECOGNITION AND SYMPTOMS
In this disorder, endometrium may occur in the Fallopian tubes, on the ovaries, deep within the muscular wall of the womb itself, scattered about the interior of the pelvis, or even further away from the womb in such remote sites as anywhere in the abdominal cavity, on the lining of the nose and in the lungs.

Wherever it may be situated, endometrial tissue is affected by the hormones that control the menstrual cycle. It therefore goes through the same sequence of changes that affects the womb lining, including the monthly casting-off of blood, mucus and surface tissue. Because the blood and other material produced at these abnormal sites cannot usually escape, there is a local build-up of pressure, and pain occurs with each menstrual period.

Accumulation is especially likely with ovarian endometriosis and there is a tendency for large ovarian cysts to develop. These can attain a considerable size and sometimes persuade the affected woman that she is pregnant. When such ovarian cysts are removed they are found to be full of a dark chocolate-coloured fluid.
TREATMENT
The symptoms of endometriosis are abolished by pregnancy and by the menopause. This suggests a method of treatment and they can readily be controlled by the continuous use of oral contraceptives or by any other measure that suppresses the function of the ovaries. A complete cure, however, will usually require surgical removal of the patches of endometrial tissue wherever they might be.

endometritis

Inflammation of the inner lining of the womb, usually as a result of infection. The womb lining is normally protected from infection by the acidity of the vagina from lactic acid

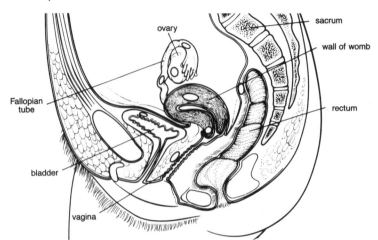

Endometriosis. This diagram shows various sites in the female pelvis in which endometrial tissue, normally present only as the lining of the womb, may occur in the condition of endometriosis. These include the wall of the womb, the ovaries, the wall of the vagina, the bladder and the tissues surrounding the colon.

and by the plug of mucus in the cervical canal. In addition, because the surface part of the endometrium is shed during each menstrual period, there is a natural clearance of any germs that might be threatening to cause infection. For these reasons, endometritis is uncommon except after delivery of a baby or after an abortion.

The most severe form of the disorder is puerperal endometritis which, even today, sometimes occurs following childbirth. Another term for this is puerperal sepsis. In this condition, the raw area formerly covered by the placenta becomes infected and the woman concerned can quickly become seriously ill.

endorphins

Drugs such as morphine act on certain receptor sites in the brain. Because these sites respond only to substances of a morphine-like chemical constitution, the question very reasonably arose whether natural substances similar to morphine might not be produced within the body. In 1975 this was proved and two compounds were isolated. Each consisted of a sequence of five amino acids (a peptide) and because they were found in the brain they were called enkephalins (*enkephalon* is Greek for 'the brain'). Subsequently, many more of these active substances were found, all with the same opioid core of five amino acids. Because of their morphine-like properties and their internal source (endogenous morphine-like substances) they have been named endorphins. They are sometimes called opioids.

Endorphins are neuro-transmitters (see above) and have a wide range of functions. They help to regulate heart action, general hormone function, the mechanisms of shock from blood loss and the perception of pain, and are believed to be involved, in some way, in controlling mood, emotion and motivation. They act on the centres of the brain concerned with the heartbeat and the control of blood pressure and on the pituitary gland. Endorphins are also believed to be involved in the mechanisms that link stress with a reduction in pain perception and this idea has given rise to the suggestion that marathon runners get hooked on their own endorphins. There is also evidence that an increase in levels of circulating endorphins occurs after taking a tablet which is believed to contain a pain-killing drug, even if it is a placebo. This, if proved, will be one more important link in the evidence of the intimate inter-relationship of mind and body.

endoscopic retrograde cholangiopancreatography (ERCP)

A widely used method of X-ray examination of the bile ducts and the duct of the pancreas. Using a steerable fibre optic endoscope, a fine catheter is passed into the common opening, in the duodenum, of the two duct systems and a dye opaque to X-rays is injected. X-rays are then taken and any abnormality, such as gallstones, bile duct disorders, pancreatitis or cancer of the pancreas, is revealed.

endoscopy

Direct visual examination of the interior of the body by means of an optical viewing instrument. The instrument may be introduced through a natural orifice – the nose, mouth, urethra or anus – or through a small purpose-made surgical incision.

Modern endoscopes are steerable, flexible, cylindrical instruments usually containing multiple channels and equipped with fibre optics for illumination and viewing. Other channels allow washing of the area under view, suction, gas inflation to ease viewing, the use of snares, cauteries, forceps and other small operating instruments, the use of lasers and the means of taking biopsy specimens.

Much use is made of endoscopes by gastroenterologists for stomach and colon examination (see colonoscopy), by gynaecologists (see laparoscopy), especially for sterilization of women by tying off the Fallopian tubes (tubal ligation) and by obstetricians for examining the fetus in the womb (fetoscopy). See also **bronchoscopy**.

endothelin

One of a range of peptide substances, containing 21 amino acids, and believed to the most powerful known constrictors of arteries. One of them, endothelin-1, derived from the inner lining (endothelium) of blood vessels, also causes constriction of the lung air passages, inhibits the release of a blood pressure-controlling substance (renin) from the kidneys, and increases the strength of the heart beat.

endothelin-receptor antagonist

Any drug that blocks the receptors for the artery-narrowing hormone **endothelin**-1 and that can thus be used as a treatment for high blood pressure.

endothelium

The single layer of flattened cells that lines the blood vessels, the heart and most of the cavities of the body, preventing such surfaces from healing together when in contact. But endothelium is no longer regarded as nothing more than a non-stick lining. It is now recognized as a physiologically and biochemically dynamic structure that, among other things, releases the hormone **nitric oxide,** which exerts a regulatory control on the tension of arteries so as to control the blood flow. Other functions of the endothelium include:

● regulation of the growth and repair of blood vessels;
● modulation of the contraction and relaxation of the heart;
● protection of blood cells from damage;
● assistance in the control of the inflammatory process;
● prevention of blood clotting within vessels;
● provision of a selectively permeable barrier to the passage through it of molecules.

The endothelium of the smallest blood vessels in the brain differs from that of blood vessels elsewhere (see **blood-brain barrier**).

endotracheal tube

A curved rubber or plastic tube, some 20–25 cm long, which a skilled anaesthetist or trained paramedic can insert through the mouth into the upper part of the wind pipe (trachea), by way of the voice box (larynx).

FUNCTION
Because of coughing and spasm of the vocal cords, this would be impossible in a fully conscious patient, so an endotracheal tube is passed after a general anaesthetic has been given or if a patient is unconscious. Even then, reflex spasm of the larynx would make the procedure very difficult so it is usual to follow induction of anaesthesia by the administration of a short-acting muscle relaxant. A laryngoscope is used to keep the tongue out of the way, to provide illumination and to allow visualization of the opening into the larynx.

Endotracheal tubes have an inflatable, balloon-like section on the outside, near the tip. After the tube is in place, a syringe is used to inject air into this balloon so that the tube is sealed firmly into the trachea. Fluid from the mouth cannot now run down into the lungs and the seal allows the anaesthetist to maintain the respiration artificially, even if the patient is completely paralysed. Often a respirator machine is used, but respiration can be maintained manually by squeezing the anaesthetic bag or using a bellows air pump.

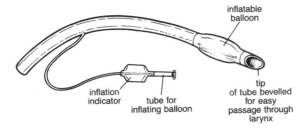

Endotracheal tube. These tubes come in a range of sizes to fit different people. Near the tip is an inflatable balloon which is blown up after the tube is inserted so as to provide a tight seal.

RISKS
Endotracheal tubes allow safe, controlled anaesthesia and are almost always used in operations on the head, or when the patient is deliberately paralysed by curare-like drugs so as to facilitate the operation and avoid deep and dangerous levels of anaesthesia. They are also used to allow maintenance of respiration in people in coma or those who are temporarily unconscious from injury or disease and who are unable to breath spontaneously.

Endoxana

A brand name for **cyclophosphamide**.

Enduron

A brand name for methyclothiazide.

enema

The introduction of watery or oily solutions or suspensions into the rectum, most commonly as a treatment for stubborn constipation when the stools have become hard and impacted. Enemas are also used in the treatment of worm infestations; for the administration of various drugs, such as sedatives; for nutritional purposes; and for X-ray examination of the rectum (barium enemas).

The patient lies on the left side with the knees drawn up and a tube with a lubricated tip is inserted gently through the anus for a distance of 7–10 cm. A funnel is attached to the other end and the liquid, at just above body temperature, is run in from a height of about 40 cm. The tube is then slowly withdrawn and the fluid retained for about half an hour, or for as long as possible before being evacuated into a toilet. Convenient, one-shot, disposable enemas are available.

engineer–doctor cooperation

See **biomedical engineering**.

enophthalmos

A slight backwards displacement of the eyeball into its bony socket so that the lids tend to come together with an obvious narrowing of the lid aperture. Enophthalmos is the opposite of **exophthalmos**. Enophthalmos is common in old age as a result of the loss of the normal volume of fat within the eye socket. Sudden enophthalmos occurs when the floor of the socket is fractured as a result of direct violence and the fat is lost downwards into the sinus (maxillary antrum). This is called a blowout fracture.

enoxaparin

A drug used to prevent blood clots forming in the veins after surgery or to treat formed clots. A brand name is Clexane.

enoximone

A **phosphidiesterase inhibitor** drug used to improve the heart's action in **heart failure**. A brand name is Perfan.

-ensis

Suffix meaning 'where found' as in sinensis (found in China).

ENT (ORL) surgeon

A surgeon specializing in the diagnosis and treatment of diseases of the ear, nose and throat. Nowadays, subspecialization is common in this discipline.

enteric fever

See **typhoid fever**.

enteric nervous system

A network of nerves and nerve connections in the wall of the intestine that can function independently of the central nervous system and has been described as the 'brain of the gut'. This system is responsible for the complex intestinal movements, including **peristalsis**, the secretory function of the intestine, the control of blood flow in the intestinal wall and the regulation of intestinal immunological and inflammatory reactions.

enteritis

Inflammation of any part of the intestine from any cause. Several different forms occur including **Crohn's disease**, **appendicitis**, **ulcerative colitis**, bacillary dysentery (**shigellosis**), amoebic dysentery and diverticulosis. **Gastroenteritis** is inflammation of the stomach and the small intestine.

enterobiasis

See **threadworm infestation**.

enteron

Greek root meaning 'gut' as in enteritis (intestinal inflammation).

enterostomy

An artificial opening, usually made through the wall of the abdomen, allowing part of the intestine to discharge to the exterior. Examples of enterostomy are **colostomy** and **ileostomy**.

entropion

A curling inwards of the margins of the eyelids so that the lashes tend to rub against the eye, or a complete inversion of the lid, so that the lashes are hidden. A harmless form of entropion, 'puppy-fat entropion', may affect fat babies. This causes little or no apparent discomfort as the lashes are very soft, and it usually disappears spontaneously within a few months.

POSSIBLE CAUSES

Spastic entropion of the lower lids is common in the elderly and is more serious because of the risk of corneal abrasion, infection and ulceration. It is caused by weakness of the flat muscle under the skin which normally keeps the lid pressed against the eye. This allows the lower edge of the fibrous lid plate to move away from the eye and the free upper edge to roll inwards so that the lashes are buried. When pressure is applied to the lower part of the lid, the lid everts into its normal position.

Surgical treatment of spastic entropion is easy and successful and the condition should be attended to before corneal damage occurs.

Entropion can also be caused by the contraction of scar tissue on the inner surface of the lid. The commonest cause of this is **trachoma** affecting the upper lids. The incurling of the lid margins leads to severe abrasion of the corneas by the lashes and the resulting ulceration and secondary infection may lead to serious loss of corneal transparency. Neglected trachoma entropion is one of the major causes of blindness in undeveloped countries.

enuresis

Bedwetting. The passage of urine during sleep. The full medical term is nocturnal enuresis. The age at which night-time control is achieved is from about two years to five years and it is common for occasional accidents to happen, thereafter, even up to the age of about ten. These, if infrequent, need not cause concern.

INCIDENCE

Genuine enuresis is commonest in boys between the ages of about five and 14. Thereafter the problem often settles spontaneously and it is uncommon for it to persist into adult life.

POSSIBLE CAUSES

Persistent bedwetting may occasionally be caused by organic disease such as **diabetes** or urinary infection, but most cases occur in physically healthy children. The causes are often obscure. Sometimes the child seems to sleep so deeply that he or she is not wakened by the desire to urinate. Often there is an emotional problem associated with the bedwetting and this may be due to over-anxious attempts by the mother to train the child to achieve control. The problem is usually made worse by punishment or obvious signs of disapproval. A very relaxed attitude, together with measures to minimize domestic labour (waterproof underblankets, drip-dry sheets) is usually eventually successful.

TREATMENT

Medical advice is helpful. Organic causes should be eliminated and sometimes drugs may be used to lighten sleep. Urine is a good conductor of electricity and an enuresis alarm, triggered by a safe, low-voltage circuit, which closes when the sheet is dampened, is sometimes effective. Fluids should be restricted in the evenings.

enzyme

These are protein molecules of fundamental importance in body chemistry (biochemistry) as they are responsible for activating and accelerating all the chemical reactions of the body. These reactions produce all the organic materials present in cells, release energy for cell function and maintain the internal environment of the cells within narrow limits. There are about 3000 different enzymes in the average cell. The name means 'in yeast' and was coined after it was discovered how yeast could convert sugars to alcohol.

An enzyme is a catalyst – a substance that promotes or speeds up a chemical reaction without itself being changed. The chemical reactions which enzymes promote in the body would not normally proceed without them, except at high temperatures or in the presence of strong acids or alkalis – conditions unsuitable for the body.

Enzymes often catalyse a long sequence of chemical reactions and if any enzyme is missing, the results can be serious. Many hereditary diseases arise because the gene which codes for a particular enzyme is defective. Most enzymes can only act in the presence of metallic atoms or substances called co-enzymes. Co-enzymes are derived from vitamins in the diet (all the B vitamins are co-enzymes) and it is the failure of enzyme action which makes vitamin or metal deficiency so serious. Many poisons act to harm the body by interfering with enzyme action.

Most enzymes operate inside cells, but some, such as the digestive enzymes, which break down the food into chemically simpler materials able to be absorbed, are released from the glands which produce them and do their work in the open.

The names of enzymes are usually descriptive of the job they do, and, to indicate that they are enzymes, the name almost always ends in '-ase'. Thus oxidases allow oxidation, or 'burning', and the release of energy at body temperature; transferases bring about the transfer of bits of complex organic molecules from one to the other; and hydrolases break down molecules by joining the $-OH$ part of the water molecule (H_2O) to one fragment and the $-H$ part to another.

enzyme replacement therapy

A treatment of genetic diseases in which the disorder is the result of biochemical dysfunction resulting from the absence of a particular enzyme. Most genes code for enzymes, and many of these can now be made by genetic engineering (recombinant DNA technology). Enzymes are proteins and must be given by intravenous injection so as to avoid digestion by protein-splitting enzymes in the intestine. The method, which is in its infancy, has been used successfully to treat Gaucher's disease, a serious disorder caused by the absence of the enzyme glucocerebrosidase.

Epanutin

A brand name for phenytoin.

ephedrine

A drug with a similar action to **adrenaline** but with a more stimulant effect on the nervous system, causing tremor, anxiety, insomnia and undue alertness. It is used to treat allergic conditions and **asthma**. Ephedrine nasal drops decongest a swollen nose lining. A brand name is CAM. Ephedrine is also formulated with other drugs under the brand names of Franol, Franol Plus and Haymine.

epi-

Prefix meaning 'upon' as in epidermis (on the skin).

epicanthus

A variant on the normal appearance of the upper eyelid. In epicanthus, the upper lid margin curves round and downwards on the inner side so as to conceal the inner corner of the eye. Epicanthus is common in babies and, if marked, may cause an appearance somewhat similar to convergent squint. In most cases, it reverts to normal as the face and nose grow. Persistent epicanthus is easily corrected by a plastic operation, should it be thought disfiguring.

Epicanthus. (a) Normal eye. (b) In epicanthus the margin of the upper lid curves down to conceal the inner corner of the eye (the canthus). Epicanthus can give an illusion of a convergent squint.

epicondylitis

See **tennis elbow**.

epidemic

The occurrence of a large number of cases of a particular disease, in a given population, simultaneously or within a comparatively short period, such as a few weeks. In an epidemic the disease spreads rapidly in a susceptible population. When spread involves multiple populations, the situation is described as a **pandemic**.

An epidemic disease is one which, for a period of months or years, may occur only sporadically, but then occurs in large numbers.

epidemiology

The study of the occurrence of diseases in populations. Although epidemics commonly involve infectious diseases, epidemiology is by no means limited to the study of these and is concerned with the whole range of conditions which affect health, such as heart disease and cancer. It includes the study of the attack rate of the various diseases and the number of people suffering from each condition at any one time. Industrial and environmental health problems are an important aspect of epidemiology.

Epidemiology is an essential factor in health administration and has contributed notably to medical research and knowledge. The relationship between cigarette smoking and lung and circulatory disorders, for instance, was elicited largely from epidemiological studies. Recent important epidemiological work has thrown much valuable light on such conditions as **AIDS**, **Lassa fever**, **Legionnaires' disease** and **hepatitis B**.

epididymitis

Inflammation of the epididymis as a result of infection, usually secondary to **urethritis**. Epididymitis is an important complication of gonorrhoea and, if both sides are affected, as is usual, may lead to sterility. Most cases are not caused by gonorrhoea. The condition causes the testicle to be hot, swollen and exquisitely tender and may lead to the development of a collection of fluid in the area (**hydrocele**) or even an abscess.

epidural anaesthesia

A form of anaesthesia, popular for childbirth because, although highly effective in the relief of pain, it has no effect on the contractions of the womb (uterus) or on the respiratory centre of the baby.

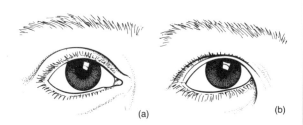

(a)   (b)

HOW IT'S DONE

The spinal cord is surrounded by a tough membrane called the dura mater. Outside the dura lies the epidural space between the dura and the bony canal of the spine, and it is into this space that an anaesthetic drug is injected to produce epidural anaesthesia. The needle is passed into the space between two of the spinal bones in the small of the back (lumbar vertebrae) and a fine plastic tube is then passed though the needle and the end left in the epidural space so that anaesthetic can be injected from time to time as needed. This is a skilled procedure requiring the services of an experienced anaesthetist.

RISKS

Epidural anaesthesia is safer than general anaesthesia, especially if this has to be given urgently to an unprepared patient who may have eaten recently and who will be liable to vomit – a dangerous complication during full general anaesthesia.

Epidural anaesthesia is also generally safer than a spinal anaesthetic in which the drug is injected into the cerebrospinal fluid surrounding the spinal cord.

It is valuable for long-term anaesthesia but diminishes the voluntary assistance the mother-to-be can give, and forceps have to be used more often than in deliveries without anaesthetic.

Epidural anaesthesia requires the continuous presence of a skilled anaesthetist able to deal with the possible complications, such as a severe drop in blood pressure, or temporary paralysis of breathing. These may occur if the anaesthetic drug accidentally gets under the dural layer. Long-term neurological damage, such as leg weakness or upset of bladder function, occur very rarely. The procedure may be followed by a headache.

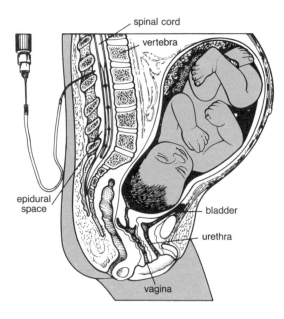

Epidural anaesthesia. A valuable and, in expert hands, safe method of anaesthesia often used in childbirth. The fetus is not affected by the anaesthetic, but the mother may not be able to push as hard as normal, and forceps or the ventouse are more often needed.

epiglottitis

Inflammation of the epiglottis. If severe, and associated with swelling, there is a grave risk of sudden urgent danger of death from obstruction of the airway and suffocation – a danger which may be circumvented only by making an emergency opening into the windpipe (**tracheostomy**).

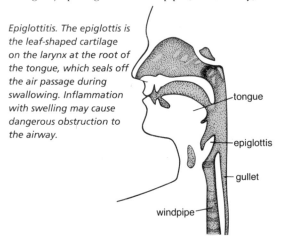

Epiglottitis. The epiglottis is the leaf-shaped cartilage on the larynx at the root of the tongue, which seals off the air passage during swallowing. Inflammation with swelling may cause dangerous obstruction to the airway.

POSSIBLE CAUSES

Epiglottitis may be a complication of severe infection of the tissues of the throat with *Haemophilus influenzae* organisms or, rarely, streptococci.

INCIDENCE

It occurs most often in children between the ages of two and five.

RECOGNITION AND SYMPTOMS

There is an acute sore throat; severe difficulty in swallowing, with drooling; rapid, laboured and very noisy breathing; restlessness and panic.

> Epiglottitis is an emergency situation calling for urgent admission to hospital for intensive antibiotic treatment and the passage of a tube to endure continuity of the airway.

Because of the suddenness with which obstruction can occur, it is often thought necessary to perform a tracheostomy, as a precaution.

epilepsy

Many different words are used to describe the epileptic attack. Words like 'convulsion', 'seizure', 'spasm', 'epileptic fit', 'ictus', 'paroxysm', 'grand mal' all mean the same thing.

Epilepsy is not a disease. It is a physical sign, an indication that something is wrong with the structure or function of a part of the brain.

INCIDENCE

About half a million people in Britain either have fits regularly, or would have them if it were not for medical treatment.

GENERALIZED EPILEPSY

Often called 'grand mal', this is the best known manifestation of epilepsy and is what most people think of when they hear the word.

THE AURA

When the grand mal attack starts there is, in about half the cases, a preliminary stage in which the discharge is beginning to have its effect but has not yet reached full intensity. This spread of discharge causes the aura and during it the person experiences one or more of several possible effects. It may consist of a feeling of fear or apprehension; a sense of nausea; the perception of a powerful smell or taste; a strong recollection of some event or place or even a formed image of some scene; an illusion of having experienced something before which is really being experienced for the first time (**déjà vu**).

The aura, if it occurs, is a part of the fit proper. It may be very brief and provide insufficient time for the sufferer to take any precautions to protect himself from the coming fit. But, in some cases, it lasts long enough for the affected person to have time to loosen tight clothing, get into a safer place, perhaps to lie down on a soft bed, or to take out false teeth which might come loose in a fit and cause damage to the mouth or even obstruct the airway. So a long aura is an obvious advantage.

THE ATTACK

This stage of the grand mal attack is caused by massive electrical discharge right across the whole of the surface of the brain on both sides. This is called the tonic stage because the affected muscles go into a state of prolonged, maximal contraction. Fortunately for the person most immediately concerned, consciousness, or at least a later awareness of what has happened, is lost early in the tonic stage. Because opposing groups of muscles are contracted simultaneously, the arms and legs will be rigid. Commonly, the legs are stiffly extended and the arms in the 'hands-up' position. The eyes and mouth tend to open wide at first and then the jaw snaps shut, sometimes biting the tongue.

There is a temporary paralysis of breathing, but before this happens, it is common for air to be forced out of the lungs and this air, as it passes between the tightened vocal cords in the voice-box (larynx), may cause a sound like a high-pitched cry or scream. This is not a real cry indicating distress but simply an involuntary sound caused by the rush of air through the voice box.

Because there is no possibility of breathing and the body is temporarily deprived of oxygen, the skin assumes a dusky bluish-grey colour. At the same time the large veins in the neck become compressed at the root of the neck and the blood, which is unable to flow, causes them to be distended. The same applies to all the veins of the face and head. So the face of the person having the grand mal attack turns blue and the veins become very prominent. The pupils of the eyes are widely dilated. The whole effect is very distressing to witness but sympathy is misplaced because the victim is quite unaware of what is happening.

CLONIC STAGE

At the end of 20 or 30 seconds the tightly knotted muscles begin to relax and air can, once again, flow into the lungs. As it does, the normal colour begins to return to the skin and the distention of the veins subsides. But now starts the third, and perhaps the most upsetting part of the fit to witness – the clonic stage. In this, all the muscles that were previously tightly contracted pass into a stage of generalized slight trembling which soon becomes a sequence of violent, repetitive, rhythmical jerky contractions.

The Greek word *clonus* means 'violent movement' and this is exactly what does happen. At first rapidly and with comparatively small contractions, but then more slowly and with greater power, the muscles tighten and relax, jerking the

limbs and head about. The muscles of the face are equally affected and this causes a series of unpleasant grimaces as if the victim were suffering great pain or distress. In this stage, also, the tongue may be bitten and the contraction of the muscles in the wall of the abdomen may squeeze the bladder or the rectum so that urine or faeces are involuntarily passed.

RETURNING TO CONSCIOUSNESS

Gradually, over the course of two or three minutes, the interval between clonic contractions becomes greater and so the fit passes off altogether. The person concerned retains no memory for any detail of the event except the aura. Sometimes, the state of mental confusion following the fit may be very prolonged and the sufferer may, for hours, remain in a kind of 'twilight' state in which he may appear to be drunk and may resist restraint with violence. Headache commonly follows an epileptic fit.

Grand mal attacks are usually single but may occur in groups of two or three.

> The most serious form of epilepsy is when the person concerned has a long series of severe grand mal attacks, one after the other, without recovery of consciousness between the attacks. This is called status epilepticus. It is very dangerous and requires urgent treatment.

PARTIAL SEIZURE EPILEPSY

This kind of epilepsy often involves the temporal lobe of the brain and is sometimes called temporal lobe epilepsy. But this is not always an accurate description because partial seizures may affect other parts of the brain. Better names are focal epilepsy or psychomotor epilepsy.

RECOGNITION

The main feature of this kind of epilepsy is that it tends to be confined to a well-localized area of the brain, and the effects usually indicate to the doctor which area is involved.

Probably the commonest types of partial seizure are the focal motor and sensory seizures. Usually, there is little or no warning and the attacks often start and end with a jerk of the arm or leg, or an area of tingling ('pins and needles') or numbness anywhere on the skin. There is no loss of consciousness and none of the confusion of mind that follows major epilepsy. Often the muscular jerking goes on rhythmically for several seconds, but the person concerned remains normally alert throughout.

Quite commonly, the part of the back of the brain concerned with vision may be the site of a partial attack and the affected person will have the illusion of flashing lights or of seeing various patterns. Another area of the brain commonly involved in simple seizures is the part of the temporal lobe responsible for the perception of sounds. In this case, noises will be heard. Similarly, powerful smells and tastes of all kinds – often quite unpleasant – are features of this kind of disorder. There may also be nausea and severe loss of balance. In all of these cases it is possible to localize, quite precisely, the area of the brain affected.

COMPLEX PARTIAL SEIZURES

Most of these begin in the temporal lobe and there is usually an aura. Typically, the affected person experiences an elaborate hallucination – perhaps a fully formed visual image or the sounds of voices or music – or he, or she, may enter a dream-like state in which some former memory comes back with striking clarity and reality.

THE ATTACK

Often there are strong sensations related to the abdomen, sensations so remote from normal experience that they cannot be adequately described. The chief emotions felt are anxiety or fear, but occasionally there is intense anger and this may lead to violent behaviour. There may be a feeling of being separated from the body so that the actions can be watched as if they are those of a stranger. This is called depersonalization. There may also be delusions of persecution and other effects so similar to schizophrenia that a mistaken diagnosis can occur.

The attack proper may consist only of a period during which the affected person is inaccessible and unresponsive. But more often the person behaves in an automatic manner, carrying out certain actions in a robot-like way and later having no recollection of having done so. At the time, however, there is a feeling of being forced to do these things – rotating the head in a particular direction, going to the sink and filling a glass with water, continuing to turn the pages of a book, sometimes even urinating or removing clothing in public. The affected person commonly makes chewing, sucking or swallowing movements and may spit repeatedly. Such features are very common in epilepsy and the reason is that, in the motor area of the brain, a disproportionately large area is devoted to the function of eating.

> During this period of automatic behaviour it is dangerous to try to restrain the person too forcibly. Usually he or she may be gently led or directed, but forcible restraint may cause an outburst of blind fury with violent results. Such outbursts are rare unless provoked by interference.

CHILDREN

In children, temporal lobe epilepsy tends to cause hyperactivity and uncontrollable rage. These effects may be the result, not of the brain defect itself, but of the child's and the parents' reaction to the experience of the epilepsy. If the child has an aura that is frightening, he or she will tend to try to dispel this fear by activity. The child may try, quite literally, to run away from the source of the fear. Again, the very natural anxiety which the diagnosis of epilepsy induces in the parents is bound to be apparent to the child who will, in turn, react with fear and restlessness.

About one child in three with temporal lobe epilepsy shows severe and uncontrollable rage. It is important for parents to understand the true nature of this rage so that they can try to respond to it in a constructive and understanding manner rather than in the instinctive way. This rage is a release of high emotional pressure arising from an overburdening of the child's brain by excess emotional stimuli. Viewed in this way, and with awareness that the expression of rage is helpful, the unpleasantness can be more readily tolerated.

Educational problems are common in children with temporal lobe epilepsy. The repeated attacks interfere with the normal functioning of the brain and will, cumulatively, add up to significant loss of educational time. Both the IQ and the ability to learn may fluctuate considerably in epileptic children. The reason for this is not apparent. Drug treatment may help or may make things worse. Although, on the whole, epilepsy tends to interfere with educational progress, many epileptic children have an outstanding scholastic performance and there have been numerous examples of high achievement.

TREATMENT

Epilepsy is treated with drugs which suppress excessive nerve activity. This must be taken long-term.

See also **petit mal** and **fever fits**.

Epilim

A brand name for **sodium valproate**.

epiloia

A rare genetic congenital disorder, also called tuberous sclerosis or Bourneville disease, in which the brain, the skin and other organs become studded with knobbly tumours derived from an abnormal overgrowth of primitive cell tissue.

INCIDENCE

Epiloia occurs either as a result of a dominant gene or as a mutation, and affects about one baby in 20,000.

RECOGNITION AND SYMPTOMS

The skin involvement takes the form of pinkish-red nodules, mainly over the nose, forehead and cheeks, known as adenoma sebaceum, as well as other abnormalities, such as white patches (**vitiligo**) and a characteristic leathery 'shagreen patch' on the small of the back.

The condition is very variable in its effect, depending on the extent of the involvement of the nervous system, but there is often mental retardation and epileptic fits are common. People mildly affected are of normal intelligence and, in these, the condition is shown only by the skin features and, occasionally, epilepsy.

RISKS

In severe cases, death must be expected during childhood or adolescence, either from severe epilepsy (status epilepticus) or other neurological effects.

The gene for epiloia can be detected by **chorionic villus sampling** or **amniocentesis** and there is the option of terminating the pregnancy at a very early stage. Because of this, genetic counselling is important if there is any family history of the condition.

epiphora

A running over of tears as a result of failure of the normal tear drainage to carry tears away into the nose. This may result from blockage of the tear duct or from **ectropion**. Treatment is by syringing with salt water to clear the obstruction, or by a surgical operation to restore normal drainage.

epiphysis, slipped

The epiphysis is the growing sector at the ends of long bones present prior to adult life. During growth, the long bones are especially susceptible to separation at the junction between the shaft of the bone and the epiphysis. This usually results from a fall or from direct violence. If there is no displacement, growth is unaffected and healing is rapid – twice as quick as fractures of bone. But if the epiphysis itself is fractured, careful reduction is necessary if growth disturbance is to be avoided. A crushing injury of the epiphyseal plate usually causes growth to cease.

See illustration (right).

epirubicin

A cytotoxic anticancer drug. A brand name is Pharmorubicin.

episcleritis

One of the least common causes of redness of the eye, episcleritis is a localized inflammation of the surface layers of the white of the eye (the sclera) caused by a disorder of the collagen fibres of which the sclera is made. The cause is unknown. The affected area is small, usually oval, and appears slightly raised and reddish-purple in colour. There is a dull, aching pain, worse at night, and bright lights usually hurt the eye (photophobia).

Steroid eye drops are very effective in suppressing the inflammation and the symptoms, but recurrence is common. Eventually, the condition will resolve spontaneously.

epispadias

A congenital abnormality of the penis, in which the urine tube (urethra) does not open at the tip, but further back on the upper surface. Sometimes the opening is right back at the root and this will lead to difficulties with urination and may affect fertility. Plastic reconstruction is possible, but is not easy and is often followed by incontinence. The outlook has been improved recently by the development of a surgical procedure using a new urethral lining derived from an artificial culture of cells taken from the patient's own urethra.

epistaxis

Nose bleed, see *First Aid*.

epithelium

The coating tissue for all surfaces of the body except the insides of blood and lymph vessels. Epithelium is a kind of non-stick surface which, in health, prevents layers from healing together. If a finger and thumb were sewn together, no healing would take place between them, however long they were left. But if the outer layers of the skin were first removed, firm fusion would occur within a few days.

Epithelium may consist of a single layer of cells, which may be squat (cuboidal) or tall (columnar), or it may be stratified and in several layers, with the cells becoming flatter and more scaly towards the surface, as in the skin. Epithelium may be covered with fine wafting hair-like structures of microscopic size (cilia) as in the respiratory tract and it may contain mucus-secreting goblet cells.

Pseudostratified epithelium may appear to be stratified, but is not. The appearance arises because the cells, which are tall and columnar, vary considerably in shape and in the position of their nuclei. It is found lining the trachea and the larger bronchi.

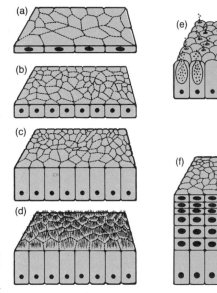

Epithelium. This diagram illustrates the different kinds of surfacing cells in the body. (a) Flat (squamous) epithelium. (b) Cuboidal cell epithelium. (c) Columnar epithelium. (d) Ciliated epithelium. The surface cells bear numerous, fine, mobile, hair-like processes. (e) Mucus-secreting glandular epithelium with 'goblet' cells. (f) Stratified epithelium.

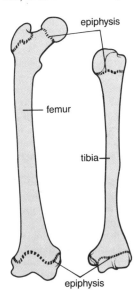

Epiphysis, slipped. The epiphysis is the growth zone in the long bone. The positions are shown by the dotted lines. During the growth period the epiphyses are vulnerable to injury and displacement. This may lead to failure of normal growth in the affected limb.

Epivir

A brand name for **lamivudine**.

epoetin

Human **erythopoietin** made by genetic engineering for use as a drug to treat severe anaemia. Brand names are Eprex and Neorecormon.

epoprostenol

Arostacyclin. A powerful inhibitor of clumping of blood platelets and thus of blood clotting. It is used with heart-lung (cardiopulmonary bypass) machines and artificial kidneys (dialysis machines) to preserve the platelets in the blood being pumped through them. Epoprostenol also widens (dilates) arteries. A brand name is Flotan.

Eppy

A brand name for **adrenaline** in the form of eye drops. Eppy is used in the treatment of chronic simple **glaucoma**.

Epstein-Barr virus

This is a member of the **herpes** family of viruses and is the cause of **glandular fever** (infectious mononucleosis) in adolescents. It is also associated with cancer of the back of the nose (nasopharyngeal carcinoma) in Chinese people and with **Burkitt's lymphoma**.

eptacog alfa

Human Factor VIIa made by genetic engineering and used to treat severe bleeding in people with **Factor VIII** or **Factor IX** deficiency (**haemophilia**) A brand name is Novoseven.

Equagesic

A brand name for a mixture of **meprobamate**, **aspirin** and **ethoheptazine citrate**.

erection

During sexual excitement, the arteries supplying the penis with blood widen and a considerable quantity of blood enters under pressure. The three columns of spongy erectile tissue are flooded with blood, and the normally small and flaccid penis become stiff and firm. This causes the veins which drain the penis to be compressed so that the blood cannot readily get out. But when the arteries constrict, more blood leaves than enters and the erection is lost.

The control of the penile arteries is much influenced by the state of their owner's mind and it is for this reason that most cases of impotence are of psychological rather than of organic origin. During orgasm, the seminal vesicles contract and expel the seminal fluid. The stimulus to erection is usually, but not exclusively, sexual interest or arousal. Erection occurs spontaneously several times every night, during the periods of rapid eye movement (REM) sleep, and can be achieved by local mechanical stimulation. Spontaneous erection, in the absence of sexual interest, is common in adolescents and may be a source of embarrassment.

erection, disorders of

See **impotence**.

ergometrine

An ergot derivative drug used to promote contractions of the muscle of the womb (uterus). This can be valuable, after the baby is born, to close off the site of separation of the afterbirth (placenta) and prevent postpartum haemorrhage. It is sometimes given when delivery of the baby is almost accomplished. A brand name is Syntometrine.

ergotamine tartrate

A drug that causes widened (dilated) arteries to narrow. It is thus useful in the treatment of migraine. Overdosage is dangerous. Brand names are Lingraine, Medihaler-ergotamine, and, formulated with other drugs, Cafergot and Migril.

eroticism

Those elements in thought, imagination, pictorial imagery, literature or the arts which tend to arouse sexual excitement or desire. The term is also used to refer to actual sexual arousal; to a greater than average disposition for sex and all its manifestations; and to sexual interest or excitement prompted by contemplation, or stimulation, of areas of the body not normally associated with sexuality.

The terms 'anal' and 'oral' eroticism are used both in a theoretical Freudian sense and in reference to adult physical sexual activity.

eruption, teeth

See **teeth**.

Erymax

A brand name for **erythromycin**.

erysipelas

An infection of the skin with streptococcal organisms, causing large, raised inflamed areas, high fever and severe illness as a result of toxicity. The lymph nodes in the area are enlarged and tender. Erysipelas is a form of **cellulitis** and most commonly affects the face, the scalp, or an arm or leg. It was once known as St Anthony's fire. Erysipelas of the leg is often the result of infection gaining access via a crack between the toes in '**athlete's foot**' (tinea pedis).

The condition responds well to antibiotics, but some people are prone to the condition and, in these, recurrences are common.

erythema

Redness of the skin or other tissue. This may result from one of a very large number of causes, but all have in common a widening (dilatation) of the small skin blood vessels. Thus erythema may result from simple blushing; **rosacea**; permanent dilatation of vessels from chronic alcoholism; inflammation from any cause including allergy and infection, undue exposure to heat, sunlight or other forms of radiation; infectious disease rashes; and many other causes.

erythema ab igne

Redness in a net-like pattern, usually of the legs, caused by excessive and over-prolonged exposure to radiant heat. The condition was much commoner in the days of open domestic fires than it is today.

erythema multiforme

A hypersensitivity disorder characterized by red, raised skin eruptions of various sizes and shapes ('multiforme') occurring symmetrically on the face, neck, forearms, backs of the hands, and legs. The condition occurs in association with drug sensitivities, allergies, many infections and pregnancy. It varies from a mild disorder to a fulminating and fatal general disease.

The most damaging form is known as the Stevens-Johnson syndrome and this often involves the mucous membranes, destroying their non-stick surfaces and allowing abnormal healing to occur between layers. The eyelids, for instance, may heal on to the globes of the eyes so that the lids cannot close, the tear glands are destroyed and the corneas are exposed and become dry and opaque. Steroids are helpful in the control of erythema multiforme and the Stevens-Johnson syndrome.

erythema nodosum

A condition in which inflammation of small blood vessels (vasculitis) causes red, raised, tender nodules to appear under the skin of both shins and sometimes elsewhere on the body. These persist for days or weeks, but eventually disappear. There may be fever, aches and pains and a general feeling of illness.

Erythema nodosum is an immunological disorder related to **tuberculosis**, sarcoidosis, streptococcal infections, drug allergies, leprosy and other conditions.

erythroblastosis foetalis

See **rhesus factor disease**.

erythrocyte

The technical term for a red blood cell. *Erythro* means 'red', and *cyte* means 'cell'.

erythromycin

An antibiotic of the macrolide class with an action similar to that of the tetracyclines. It binds to the ribosomes in bacterial cells and interferes with the synthesis of protein. Brand names are Arpimicin, Erymax, Erythrocin, Erythroped, Ilosone, Tiloryth and, formulated with other drugs for external use only, Benzamycin, Isotrexin and Zineryl.

Erythroped

A brand name for **erythromycin**.

erythropoietin

A hormone, produced mainly in the kidneys, that stimulates the bone marrow to produce more red blood cells. The amount of hormone produced is proportional to the oxygen concentration in the blood flowing through the kidneys. This blood is continuously monitored for its oxygen level.

Erythropoietin can be used as a drug to increase the production of red blood cells in anaemia or after severe blood loss. The method may sometimes be used as an alternative to blood transfusion, but this is feasible only in cases in which the patient's condition allows sufficient time for blood cell production. Erythropoietin therapy is also appropriate as a treatment for anaemia caused by kidney failure, cancer or **AIDS**.

-escent

Suffix meaning 'becoming' as in adolescent (becoming adult).

Escherichia coli

A motile, rod-shaped bacillus found in countless millions in the large intestine. *Escherichia coli* organisms are also known as 'coliforms'. The presence of *E. coli* is taken as presumptive evidence of faecal contamination.

A strain of this organism known as O 157 was first recognized as a human disease-causing agent (pathogen) in 1982, and in 1996 it caused 600 cases of food poisoning in the USA, 490 cases in Scotland and nearly 10,000 cases in Japan. In old and frail people the mortality from infection with this strain may reach 50 per cent. Coliforms have been much exploited by genetic engineers.

Eskazole

A brand name for **albendazole**.

Esmarch's bandage

A flat, wide, rubber bandage which is wound progressively and tightly round a limb, working inwards from the extremity, so as to force most of the blood back into the circulation and provide a relatively blood-free field for surgery. It is commonly used in operations for varicose veins.

eso-

Prefix meaning 'within' as in esotropia (moving in).

esotropia

Convergent squint, or 'cross-eye'. In esotropia, only one eye looks directly at the object of regard, the other being turned inwards. Esotropia in children calls for urgent treatment to avoid **amblyopia**.

ESR

Erythrocyte sedimentation rate.
See **blood sedimentation rate**.

Estelle Solo MX 40

A brand name for **oestradiol** in a transdermal patch.

Estigyn

A brand name for **ethinyloestradiol**.

Estracyt

A brand name for **estramustine**.

Estraderm MX

A brand name for **oestradiol** in a transdermal patch.

estramustine

An alkylating anticancer drug. A brand name is Estracyt.

Estring

A brand name for **oestradiol** in a vaginal ring to treat postmenopausal vaginitis.

estropipate

An oestrogen drug used for post-menopausal **hormone replacement therapy**. A brand name is Harmogen. Also formulated with a progesterone drug under the brand name of Improvera.

ethamsylate

A drug that reduces bleeding from small blood vessels and is used to treat excessive menstruation (menorrhagia). A brand name is Dicynene.

ethical problems in medicine

See **ethics, medical**.

ethics, medical

By the nature of their work, doctors enjoy unique privileges, assumed rights and considerable personal power in their relations with other people. But doctors, too, are human and are as liable as most other people to abuse privileges, rights and power for their own advantage. To help curb this tendency, the profession has, from the earliest days, recognized that a code of ethics, binding on all recognized practitioners, is necessary.

To be effective, such a code must be backed by a major sanction and doctors know that if they breach the code in any serious way, this sanction will be applied. Today, as for many years in the past, the ultimate sanction is to be deprived of the right to practice – to have one's name struck off the Medical Register. In Britain, the General Medical Council (not the British Medical Association) is the body responsible for discipline, and if a doctor steps over the line he or she may have to appear before a disciplinary committee which operates very much as a court of law.

Many of the rules of the code of ethical behaviour are clear-cut and unequivocal and every doctor knows that he or she is liable to be struck off if certain things are done. These include:

- taking advantage of the position of trust and right of access to enjoy the sexual favours of a patient;
- improperly passing on confidential information about a patient;
- operating, or otherwise practising, while drunk;
- signing fraudulent certificates;
- flagrantly advertising services;
- using his or her status to profit from the sale of a commercial product;
- trying to steal patients from another doctor;
- performing illegal abortions.

CONFIDENTIALITY

The duty of confidentiality imposes professional secrecy on a doctor, but there are five general exceptions to this. They are:

- when the patient agrees to a disclosure;
- when disclosure is in the patient's interest and it would be medically undesirable to seek the patient's consent;
- when there is an over-riding duty to society;
- when information is required for due process of law;
- when, for the purposes of medical research, approval is given by an official ethical committee.

Difficulties and dilemmas often arise over confidentiality. Minors may not wish their parents to know of some important fact discovered by the doctor, or that they are using contraceptives; a doctor may be aware that someone, such as an epileptic, continues to drive against advice; or that a male patient with a venereal disease or AIDS is likely to infect others. Whatever his or her decision, in such cases, a doctor must always be prepared to defend and justify it.

CONSENT

A doctor may not, in general, proceed with any treatment or examination, without the consent of the patient. If a doctor should touch a patient contrary to that patient's wishes, that is an assault. In most cases, of course, consent is implicit in the fact that a patient has come freely to the doctor for help, but doctors are careful not to proceed if there is any indication that consent is withheld or has been withdrawn.

Consent to perform a surgical operation is deemed to be so important that verbal consent is not considered enough and a formal signed certificate is always used. But consent must be informed, and patients sometimes complain that they are not fully aware of what the surgeon proposes to do. Consent forms usually contain a sentence authorizing the surgeon to do anything which, in the course of the operation, he or she finds necessary. This has sometimes been used by busy doctors as a substitute for a full explanation of what might possibly happen or be needed.

Patients are now becoming less willing to accept this and are, quite rightly, insisting on knowing, in detail, what may, in the worst case, be done. The total removal of a breast (radical mastectomy) is a case in point.

Medical ethics is concerned with moral decisions in medicine. With advances in medicine these have become much more complex and new dilemmas have arisen in connection with many different aspects of medicine including the possibility of prolonging life by extraordinary means, psychosurgery, organ transplantation, research on fetuses, human experimentation, the diagnosis of genetic defects at the embryonic stage, and the many possibilities of genetic engineering – such as human cloning.

LIFE PROLONGATION

Artificial breathing (ventilation) by machine and the maintenance of nutrition by tube, or even by infusing nutrients into the bloodstream, now makes it comparatively easy to maintain the body tissues in a living state. But doctors recognize that, in a sense, the body is merely a supporting vehicle for the brain, which is the essence of the individual and without which the individual can hardly be said to exist. Severe depression of the higher brain functions is common in a gravely brain-injured or seriously ill person, and it is usually impossible to say positively, at an early stage, that there is no chance of recovery of these functions.

So life-support systems are an essential means of maintaining tissue nutrition until the outcome becomes clear. These technologies are expensive and require highly trained staff. They are simply not available for everyone who might possibly benefit from them. Decisions on allocation have to be made and these are sometimes major ethical decisions. The withdrawal of life support also involves ethical decisions. Often, problems of this kind are too large for single individuals and there is a growing tendency for hospitals to form committees to consider such decisions.

The withholding of extraordinary means of life prolongation is a kind of passive euthanasia. For many years, however, doctors have taken passive euthanasia further and have felt it an important part of their responsibility to make decisions about the withholding of conventional treatment in certain cases. Faced with this situation, they have taken great comfort in the words:

> 'Thou shalt not kill, but needst not strive,
> Officiously to keep alive.'

and are able to see that in many cases, the right thing to do is to allow a suffering human being to die, especially one who is old, frail and ready. This is a very different matter from deliberately giving a lethal dose of a drug. But many doctors find themselves unable to engage in any form of passive euthanasia and go on treating, by every means in their power, at whatever cost to the patient, and without regard to the patient's wishes.

A more difficult question arises when a baby is born with a severe congenital defect of such a nature that survival, without extraordinary measures, would be unlikely or impossible. Many such infants have survived as a result of heroic medical efforts and many of them are mentally retarded and severely physically disabled. An American court has ruled that the parents of a severely defective baby had the right to refuse treatment. Later, in 1983, a presidential commission advised that treatment should not be withheld from defective infants, even if this were the parents' wishes. Society should, however, be prepared to provide humane care throughout the life of the child.

The same commission felt that a patient able to understand the nature and probable consequences of his or her illness should have the right to ask for treatment to be stopped if it was having no other effect than prolonging life. And it also felt that, in the case of a patient incapable of making such a decision, relatives should be allowed to decide.

ETHICAL PROBLEMS CONNECTED WITH THE FETUS

There are many who do sincerely believe that human life begins at the time of fertilization and that abortion, at any stage, is murder. To be consistent, this view should hold IUD contraception to be murder, because this form of birth control usually acts not by preventing fertilization, but by interfering with the implantation of the early embryo. Some forms of oral contraceptives act in the same way.

But for many, the matter becomes more than a philosophic exercise when the consequences of such beliefs are that individuals are born with grave physical and mental defects and when lives are damaged and restricted by the responsibilities imposed on parents as a result.

Abortion has been liberalized in Britain since 1967. In most parts of the civilized world, abortion is now legal when it is known that the embryo or fetus has a substantial genetic abnormality of a kind which will produce a major defect. Compliance with the law has to be carefully regulated for it is comparatively easy for doctors to agree that abortion is 'justified' if they wish to do so. Ethical questions are also involved when doctors are asked to find out the sex of a fetus at an early stage and, if female, terminate the pregnancy, as is commonplace in India and elsewhere. Indian legislation was passed concerning this in August 1994.

See also **embryo, research on, eugenics**.

ethinyloestradiol

A powerful synthetic oestrogen drug that can be taken by mouth and is widely used as a component of oral contraceptives. The drug is formulated with a **progestogen** and sold under such brand names as Binovum, Brevinor, Cilest, Eugynon 30, Femodene, Femodene ED, Femodette, Loestrin 20, Logynon, Logynon ED, Marvelon, Mercilon, Microgynon 30, Microgynon 30 ED, Minulet, Norimin, Norinyl-1, Ovran, Ovranette, Ovysmen, Schering PC4, Synphase, Tri-Minulet, Triadene, Trinordiol and Trinovum.

ethisterone

See **norethisterone**.

ethoheptazine citrate

A pain-killing drug. It is formulated with a muscle relaxant drug and with aspirin and sold under the brand name of Equagesic.

ethosuximide

An anti-epileptic drug used in the management of absence attacks (Petit mal). It has no effect against major **epilepsy** and may cause nausea and drowsiness. Brand names are Emeside and Zarontin.

ethynodiol diacetate

A **progestogen** drug used, without oestrogen, as an oral contraceptive. A brand name is Femulen.

Ethyol

A brand name for **amifostine**.

etidronate

A drug used to treat **osteoporosis** and **Paget's disease** of bone. A brand name is Didronel.

etodolac

A non-steroidal anti-inflammatory drug (**NSAID**) used to treat **rheumatoid arthritis**. A brand name is Lodine SR.

etomidate

A general anaesthetic drug. A brand name is Hypnomidate.

etoposide

An anticancer drug derived from a plant poison epipodophyllotoxin. It is used chiefly in the maintenance treatment of acute leukaemia after remission has been achieved and the bone marrow has recovered. It has been given by mouth to treat lung cancer. Brand names are Etopophos and Vepeside.

-ety

Suffix meaning 'condition' as in sobriety (state of being sober).

eu-

Prefix meaning 'good' as in eupepsia (good digestion).

Eudemine

A brand name for **diazoxide**.

eugenics

This means the control of human breeding by selective mating so as to improve the stock. The term was coined in 1883 by the English scientist Francis Galton (1822–1911) when, inspired by his cousin Charles Darwin's theory of natural selection, he saw that the improvement of species, especially the human one, need not be left to the vicissitudes of chance. Eugenics has always seemed to make sense to many people, but, in fact, it raises so many questions of human rights and the dangers inherent in the exercise of such power that, with a few exceptions, it has never been more than a theoretical consideration.

POSITIVE AND NEGATIVE EUGENICS

Hitler, whose views on 'racial purity' were based on a profound ignorance of biology and ethnology, did attempt some practical eugenics by arranging, in a limited way, for the breeding of good Aryan stock (positive eugenics). He also aimed at the widespread sterilization or elimination of those he considered genetically or racially inferior (negative eugenics). Had the Third Reich lasted, as he hoped, for a thousand years, it is likely that he might have had some influence on the genetic heritage of the German people, but there is no saying that this influence would have been good. The loss of Jewish genes would certainly have diminished the genetic richness of the race.

A personal attempt at positive eugenics seems an attractive option to some women, and many have sought and achieved artificial insemination with sperm from anonymous donors guaranteed to be of high mental or physical calibre. Some thousands of babies, sired in this way, are born each year. The frozen sperm of those Nobel Prize winners willing to participate, is stored, for this purpose, by the Repository for Germinal Choice, founded in 1979.

The eugenic implications of advances in genetic engineering and embryo selection are already raising many ethical problems.

eugeria

The state of a high quality of life in old age. Eugeria should be the normal condition of old people, but is often precluded by physical illness or injury, psychological deficit or disturbance, and unimaginative respect for the damaging cultural stereotype that old people are unemployable, sexually incapable, possibly demented and should retire from everything, including life.

Euglucon

A brand name for **glibenclamide**.

Eugynon, Eugynon 30

A brand name for an oral contraceptive containing **ethinyloestradiol** and **levonorgestrel**. See also **contraceptive drugs**.

-euma

Suffix meaning 'place for' as in museum (place for the arts).

Eumovate

A brand name for clobetasone.

eunuch

See **castration**.

euphoria

A feeling of intense well-being or happiness. Psychiatrists, perhaps with the pessimism engendered by their trade, are apt to use the word to mean an abnormally exaggerated feeling of elation.

Eurax

A brand name for **crotamiton**.

euthanasia

See **ethics, medical**.

eversion

A turning outwards.

evidence-based medicine

The use of methods of medical treatment and clinical decision-making that have been rigorously tested by properly controlled research. Before its conclusions can be adopted as a basis for practice, reports of such research must be exposed to close scrutiny and review by experts in the particular field (peer review), and must be published in respected journals for wide readership and free criticism in the correspondence columns. A journal called *Evidence-Based Medicine* is published jointly by the British Medical Association and the American College of Physicians.

evoked responses

The normal electroencephalogram is the record of the superimposed electrical signals from overall, general brain activity and shows little indication of any specific brain function. The electrical changes associated with the perception of strong sensations, however, can be detected by special electronic averaging techniques. These methods allow signals to be detected even though they are below the electrical 'noise' level. The results indicate gross function only and, so far, the method has been possible only in connection with vision and hearing.

Visual evoked brain responses may be obtained by exposing the subject to a succession of bright flashes of light or to a checkerboard pattern on a TV screen which reverses, black to white, at regular intervals. Similarly, auditory evoked responses can be detected on exposing a subject to loud noises. The methods are extremely crude compared with visual acuity testing or audiometry.

Evoked responses are important in that they provide direct, objective evidence that conduction is occurring along the nerve tracts connecting the sense organ with the brain. To some extent they provide proof, in the absence of any cooperation from the subject, that sensory experience is occurring. The method has been used in the detection of malingering, but, more usefully, in comparing the efficiency of conduction of nerve impulses in the two optic nerves.

evolution

The process by which all living organisms have developed in complexity, from a simple life form. Although roughly two million species exist today, it is estimated that this is only about one-thousandth of the total number which have existed and have died out. The development to the present stage has taken many millions of years and a record of the stages is to be found in fossilized remains, datable by their location in sedimentary rock. Some idea of the stages in the evolution of any complex creature, such as a human, are also shown in the embryological development of the individual from conception to birth. Evolutionary changes are, of course continuing, but the process is so slow as to be imperceptible in the course of the lifetime of any individual.

HOW IT OCCURS

Evolution occurs by the principle of natural selection. Spontaneous random changes in the characteristics of certain individuals in a population of living organisms alter their chances of survival. In the context of a particular environment, some have, by virtue of a particular inherited characteristic, a better chance than others of surviving to reproduce. These individuals, who are inherently better adapted to the environment, survive to pass on these characteristics to their offspring. The others die out. Characteristics acquired during life cannot be passed on genetically, because they do not affect the genes in the germ cells. Only characteristics present at birth can be passed on. Cutting off rats' tails and then breeding from them does not produce a breed of tail-less rats. But if the environmental influence consists of a mad scientist who allows only the rats with short tails to breed, in a few generations there will be a strain of short-tailed rats. This is how species change.

Evolution occurs when natural selection operates on a population of organisms containing many variations in their inheritable characteristics. The genetic heritage of a population remains constant unless changed by external influences, such as selective breeding, or by mutation. A mutation is an inheritable change in the character of a gene – a chemical alteration of the DNA (deoxyribonucleic acid) in the reproductive cells. This alters the hereditary characteristics. Mutations either occur spontaneously or are caused by an external agency, such as radiation or chemical effect. Most mutations are harmful and genetic disease, caused by an inherited mutation, usually puts the individual at a disadvantage in terms of survival. But some are advantageous and these, in the long run, may come to be the norm. The rate of mutation in humans is low.

See also **Lamarckism**.

evolutionary medicine

A paradigm for medical education and study based on the recognition of the importance of taking due account of the processes of human evolution when viewing human physiology, psychology, pathology and anatomy. Failure to do so will result in a truncated, less valid and less fruitful understanding of the whole of medicine. To quote but one of many possible instances, it should be recognized that, since throughout almost the whole of human evolution life expectancy has been no more than about 30 years, systems have evolved which are largely indifferent to conditions that do not arise until well after that age, such as **osteoporosis**, **presbyopia**, **atherosclerosis** and the **menopause**.

Evorel

A brand name for **oestradiol** in a transdermal patch.

Ewing's tumour

A highly malignant bone cancer affecting children up to the age of about 15. The tumour causes areas of bone destruction, and the body responds by surrounding these with layers of new bone, giving a characteristic 'onion skin' appearance on X-ray. The affected area is swollen, tender and painful and the child often has a fever, so the condition is apt to be confused with bone infection (**osteomyelitis**). Unfortunately, in spite of the most energetic treatment, even amputation and radiotherapy, the outlook is often unfavourable.

ex-

Prefix meaning 'out of, from' as in extract (draw out).

excimer laser

A laser used to vaporize and thin a small central area of the cornea so as to reduce or eliminate **myopia**.

HOW IT'S DONE

Laser energy can shave off very thin slices of the centre of the cornea so as to produce a less convex or even slightly concave central zone, thus neutralizing the excessive power of the myopic eye. A moving iris diaphragm in front of the laser opens and closes at a predetermined rate. Thus the central part of the laser beam falls on the cornea for longer than the peripheral part and more tissue is removed centrally than peripherally, so producing the desired effect. Hypermetropia (long sight) and astigmatism can also be corrected by a modification of the method described. Laser machines have been used to treat degrees of myopia ranging from -1 dioptre to -25 dioptres.

excimer laser coronary angioplasty

The use of a vaporizing **excimer laser** by way of an arterial catheter to cut through and remove arterial plaque in cases of **atherosclerosis** in which the blood supply to the heart, brain, other organ or limb is prejudiced by arterial narrowing. The catheter used contains over 200 individual 50- micron optical fibres surrounding a guide wire. The method is thought likely to be applicable in cases of narrowing that are unsuitable for balloon **angioplasty**.

excimer laser refractive surgery

The now widespread use of the **excimer laser** to change the curvature of the cornea, and hence its optical power, so as to alter the refraction of the eye and correct moderate degrees of short sight (myopia), long sight (hypermetropia) and astigmatism. Also known as excimer laser refractive keratectomy. Automatic machines have been developed which efficiently perform these functions.

excision

Cutting off and removing completely.

excoriation

A scratching or abrasion injury to the surface of the body.

excretory system

This system is responsible for ridding the body of unwanted substances or of excessive quantities of normal body substances. These are discharged in the urine. The system also has important blood regulatory and water control functions. Urine from each kidney is collected in a conical drain called the pelvis of the kidney and passes into a hollow tube, the ureter, which is 40–45 cm long and runs down to end in the urinary bladder. A shorter single tube, the urethra, carries urine from the bladder to the exterior.

See **urinary drainage system**.

execution by poison

See **lethal injection**.

Exelon

A brand name for **rivastigmine**.

exenteration

The total removal of all organs and other soft tissue from a bony cavity. Exenteration is a radical procedure, performed only in extreme cases of cancerous growth in which the only hope of survival is an attempt at removal of all affected tissue. In malignant tumours of the eye, for instance, it may be necessary to remove, not just the eyeball, but the eyelids, the eye muscles, the fat surrounding them, and the lining of the bony eye socket (the periosteum).

Skin grafting is then done to cover the bare bone and a surprisingly good cosmetic appearance results. Widespread tumour sometimes makes it necessary to exenterate the pelvis.

exercise, value of

See **health maintenance**.

exfoliation

Literally 'shedding leaves'. Exfoliated cells are those shed or brushed from a surface. In exfoliative dermatitis, much of the surface of the skin peels off or is shed. Exfoliative cytology is a skilled pathological technique of diagnosing cell abnormalities, such as cancer, by the examination of cells shed, brushed or scraped from a body surface.

exhibitionism

The exposure of the genitals to undesiring female observers to obtain sexual gratification. Exhibitionism is a form of vicarious sexual intercourse often engaged in by men who feel sexually inadequate or unsure of their masculinity. Sexual excitement occurs in anticipation of the exposure, but satisfaction is likely to be achieved only if the observer reacts in some way – by showing surprise, fright or disgust. Masturbation may then be used to bring about an orgasm. This is sometimes done as part of the exhibition, sometimes afterwards. Men who engage in this practice seldom, if ever, offer any physical danger to the victim.

The making of obscene telephone calls (telephone scatologia) is a common variant of exhibitionism.

exomphalos

The omphalos is the navel (umbilicus) and exomphalos is a protrusion (hernia) of some of the abdominal contents into the umbilical cord at birth.

exophthalmos

'Bugging-out' of an eyeball. Protrusion of the globe forces the eyelids apart and causes a staring appearance.
POSSIBLE CAUSES
Exophthalmos is caused by an increase in the bulk of the contents of the bony eye cavern (orbit) behind the eye. This occurs most commonly as a result of an immunological dis-

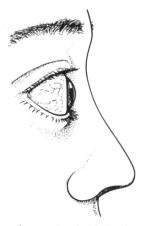

Exophthalmos. Abnormal protrusion of an eye is caused by an increase in the bulk of the tissues behind the eyeball in the bony socket. This may be due to an increase in the bulk of the eye-moving muscles as in thyroid eye disease, or to other causes such as tumour.

order associated with the thyroid gland, the protrusion being caused by enlargement of the small eye-moving muscles behind the globe as a result of the presence of antibodies (immunoglobulins) and the accumulation of white cells (lymphocytes) and fluid. Dysthyroid exophthalmos does not necessarily accompany active thyroid gland malfunction and the protrusion may occur months or years after a thyroid upset. It may, on occasion, even precede it.

Although thyroid problems are by far the most common cause of exophthalmos, even if only one eye appears to be affected, protrusion of an eyeball may be caused by the presence of other material in the orbit, such as a cancer or a mucus-filled cyst (mucocele). It should always be regarded as a potentially grave sign and should never be ignored.

TREATMENT
Persistent and disfiguring exophthalmos may be treated by removing the bony floors of the eye sockets or by reinforcing the lids with mersilene mesh implants.

exostosis

A benign (non-malignant) outgrowth from the surface of a bone, often capped by a protective capsule called a bursa. The commonest form of exostosis is the **bunion** (hallux valgus) caused by abnormal local pressure from unsuitable footwear.

exotoxin

A powerful poison, formed by certain types of bacteria, which is released by them and which may cause severe damage either locally or, if carried away by the blood, at a remote distance. The **diphtheria** organism, for instance, secretes an exotoxin which can destroy tissue lining the throat, where the organism settles, but which can also travel to damage the heart and the kidneys. Bacterial exotoxins are among the most poisonous substances known.

exotropia

Divergent squint. In exotropia only one eye is used for detailed vision, the other being directed outwards. In children, the condition is often intermittent at first but tends to become permanent. Ophthalmic attention is needed.

expected date of delivery

An estimate of the date on which a baby will be born based on an average gestation period of 266 days, counted as 280 days from the date of the first day of the last menstrual period. Since this figure is an average of a fair spread of gestation period lengths, no complete reliance can be placed on its accuracy in any particular case.

expectoration

Bringing up phlegm (sputum) and spitting it out. An expectorant is a medicine, usually in the form of a mixture, designed to assist in the removal of sticky mucoid sputum from the bronchial tubes. Cough mixtures of this kind often taste impressive and may relieve symptoms but have little medical value.

expressing milk

Artificially squeezing out milk from a breast to relieve engorgement during **breastfeeding**. The procedure is aided by the use of a breast pump.

external fixator

Surgical equipment used to immobilize a fracture of a long bone so that loss of function is minimized. A strong steel bar, of circular or square cross-section, is placed parallel to the fractured bone and securely fixed to it by a number of steel pins passed through the skin and screwed into the bone above and below the fracture site. The pins are attached to the bar by adjustable brackets.

extra-

Prefix meaning 'outside' as in extramarital (outside marriage).

extracorporeal membrane oxygenation (ECMO)

A method of maintaining the levels of vital oxygen and extracting carbon dioxide from small babies with reversible lung failure. The technology, which has been developed from adult heart-lung machines, involves the use of special silastic membranes freely permeable to oxygen and carbon dioxide but impermeable to blood. The baby is connected to the machine by cannulas in the right atrium of the heart and the right common carotid artery in the neck.

extradural haemorrhage

Bleeding between the skull and the outer layer of brain lining (the dura mater). Extradural haemorrhage results from skull fracture and is very dangerous. It is often slow and insidious in its effects at first, but, if not recognized, may be fatal because the growing blood collection can force the brain downwards and compress, and destroy, vital centres in the brainstem.

A person who is knocked unconscious, recovers consciousness, and then, later, lapses once again into coma, probably has an extradural haemorrhage and is likely to be in grave danger. An operation to open the skull, and find and tie off the bleeding vessel, may be the only hope of saving life.

extra-intracranial bypass

A surgical technique designed to reduce the risk of **stroke** in patients at risk by trying to improve the blood circulation inside the skull. The procedure involves linking a scalp artery on the outside of the skull with one inside, so as to bypass a diseased (**atherosclerotic**) artery supplying the brain.

After much initial enthusiasm a major trial was mounted to try to show whether the method was effective. This trial involved 71 neurological centres throughout the world, took eight years to complete and cost over four million pounds. The conclusions, which were published in 1985, were that the method offered no advantage and did not reduce the probability of stroke.

extravert

The personality type of the individual whose concerns are directed outward rather than inward. The extrovert is active, optimistic, gregarious, talkative, impulsive, fond of jokes and of excitement, aggressive and sometimes unreliable. The concept was invented by the Swiss psychologist and philosopher Carl Gustav Jung (1875–1961) who also described the opposite personality type, the **introvert**. No one is wholly extraverted or introverted, but most people show a fairly obvious trend in one or other of these directions.

exudation

The slow escape of fluid or cells from blood vessels, usually in the course of inflammation, and their accumulation or deposition in or on the tissues, often in the form of pus. Sometimes an exudation may be of clear serum.

eye, artificial

Although often called a 'glass eye', an ocular prosthesis is never made of glass, but usually of acrylic plastic. It is a comparatively thin, convex shell bearing a lens to simulate the cornea, behind which is a painted or photographed iris arranged to match that in the other eye. The 'white' of the eye is also matched in colour and usually shows some thread-like marks to resemble conjunctival blood vessels.

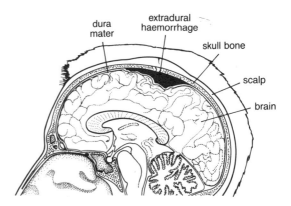

Extradural haemorrhage. After a head injury, especially when the skull is fractured, an enlarging blood clot may form between the bone and the dura mater. This can cause dangerous compression of the brain.

eye cancer in childhood

See **retinoblastoma**.

eye, examination of

As in all medical investigation, this starts with the taking of a detailed history of the complaint. The doctor then looks at the eyelids and the skin around the eyes. The conjunctivas lining the insides of the lids and covering the whites of the eyes are checked for inflammation, signs of discharge, foreign bodies, dilated blood vessels or other disorders. The lymph nodes in front of the ear are checked for swelling and tenderness.

The eye movements are checked, both slow (pursuit) and rapid following (saccade) movements. Each eye is then covered in turn as the subject looks steadily at an object (cover test). Movement of one eye as the other is covered suggests squint (strabismus). The visual acuity is now measured in each eye (see vision tests). A test of the extent of the peripheral vision (visual fields) may detect unsuspected visual field loss in glaucoma or neurological conditions. Colour vision is checked, using Ishihara plates, as it is diminished in certain disorders of the optic nerves and retina.

The main ophthalmic diagnostic instrument is the slit-lamp microscope. This is a combined low-power binocular microscope and light source, so arranged that the illumination moves with movement of the microscope. The light beam can be narrowed to an intensely bright slit which reveals every detail of the transparent front parts of the eye to the ophthalmologist, allowing examination as far back as the front part of the internal jelly of the eye (the vitreous humour).

Fluorescein is a harmless, bright yellow dye, much used in eye examination. Fluorescein solution dropped on the healthy cornea is soon washed away by the tears and dispersed, but if an ulcer is present, the dye adheres to the cornea in the area in which the surface cells are missing and the ulcer shows up conspicuously. Often a blue light is used in the examination and this causes a striking yellow fluorescence of the dye in the area of the ulcer. Under normal lighting the ulcer shows bright green.

Fluorescein is also used in a special method of examination of the retina and choroid of the eye – the important internal layers at the back of the eye. In this application, a sterilized solution of fluorescein is injected rapidly into the circulating blood and, while the dye is passing through the eye, photographs of the interior are taken using blue illuminating light. A green filter is placed in front of the film in the camera. This method provides important, and sometimes sight-saving, information about the state of the retina and the choroid.

Measurement of the pressure within the eye (applanation tonometry) is performed at the slit-lamp using a special attachment. This is an essential test for glaucoma. If the high power of the corneal lens is neutralized by strongly negative corneal contact lenses, the view through the microscope extends back as far as the retina. Other contact lenses incorporating mirrors may be used to allow examination of the eye drainage system in front of the root of the iris and the parts of the retina close behind the iris.

The retina can also be examined with an ophthalmoscope – an instrument allowing simultaneous illumination and viewing of the inside of the eye. The binocular indirect ophthalmoscope is worn on the examiner's head and provides a remarkable panoramic view of the inside of the eye. Commonly, photographs are taken of the retina and, for several important retinal and choroidal disorders, this may be done after a yellow dye, fluorescein, is injected into a vein. This method, known as fluorescein angiography, can reveal vital details not otherwise demonstrable.

eye injuries

The eye is so well protected by surrounding bone and by the rapid lid-squeeze reflex that it often escapes unharmed even when facial injury is severe and the bony socket (the orbit) has been fractured.

POSSIBLE CAUSES

The greatest danger is from small, high-speed missiles. Many children have suffered severe eye injuries by stabbing or poking with sticks, air gun pellets, catapult missiles or small stones thrown up by rotary grass cutters. Adults and children suffer injuries when the body is moving at speed. Penetrating injuries commonly arise from windscreen glass in car accidents, but the incidence of this has been greatly reduced by the use of seat belts.

Industrial accidents, too, are common especially to those using high-speed machinery such as grinders, drills, saws, lathes or milling machines without adequate eye protection. Goggles are unpopular with many workers and thousands have sacrificed vision for the want of such protection.

RISKS

The most serious injuries involve the cornea and the crystalline lens, leading to corneal scars and **cataract**. Blunt injury to the eyeball tends to be less dangerous, but, if gross, may cause rupture and collapse of the globe, loss of contents and detachment of the retina.

Lesser degrees may cause the internal lens to become opaque (concussive cataract) or may cause bleeding into the jelly of the eye (vitreous haemorrhage).

Blunt injuries, even if quite minor, may result in bleeding into the front chamber of the eye (**hyphaema**). This will affect vision for a day or two until the blood absorbs. Usually there is full recovery, but later there may be secondary **glaucoma**. Recurrent bleeding is a grave complication, tending to cause permanent visual loss.

eyelashes, disorders of

After lid injury, lashes may grow in an abnormal direction because of displacement of the roots. This may also result from severe lid infections, such as septic blepharitis and **trachoma**. Trachoma distorts the lid by scarring, leading to **trichiasis**, a condition in which the lashes turn inwards so that they rub against the cornea, causing great discomfort and even corneal ulceration. Occasionally, lashes will grow in an abnormal direction for no obvious reason. Aberrant lashes may have to be destroyed by electrolysis. A plucked lash will grow again in about six weeks. In babies, the lashes are soft and very flexible and are unlikely to cause damage to the eyes when turned inwards, as in the condition of 'puppy-fat **entropion**'.

eye, lazy

A lay term for **amblyopia**.

eyelid abscesses

See **styes**.

eyelid covering corner

See **epicanthus**.

eyelid notches

See **Treacher-Collins syndrome**.

eyelid, drooping

The technical term is blepharoptosis, often called ptosis. This may be present at birth and, if severe, calls for immediate correction if vision is to be saved. A drooping lid after the age of about eight will not damage vision, but must always be investigated. In the adult, a droop may indicate one of several serious conditions including **myasthenia gravis**, diabetic nerve damage, **Horner's syndrome** and an **aneurysm** on an artery at the base of the brain.

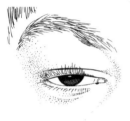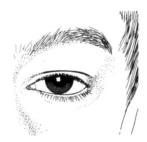

Drooping eyelid. This is often present at birth but may occur as a result of later disease or injury. If of sudden onset and for no apparent reason, the matter should be investigated at once. A drooping lid in a new-born baby may lead to severe loss of vision in the affected eye unless quickly corrected.

eyelids, baggy

A common feature of advancing age is loss of elasticity and resulting laxity of the skin of the eyelids. The youthful elasticity of skin is conferred by healthy collagen strands (fibrils) and these are gradually damaged by various factors, the most important being exposure to sunlight. The eyelid skin is very thin, highly mobile, and subjected to considerable stretching throughout life, so it is perhaps not surprising that, in many, the lid skin should become loose and redundant. Excess skin which hangs down, sometimes even over the margins of the upper lids, is called dermochalasia.

POSSIBLE CAUSES

Age is the foremost cause of baggy eyelids, but the worst cases are due to an additional factor – the protrusion forward of fat which has leaked through the tissue membrane (the orbital septum) intended to keep it back within the bony eye socket (the orbit). This is called blepharochalasia. Baggy lids also occur in thyroid underactivity (**myxoedema**) and when fluid collects in the facial tissues (**oedema**) for other reasons, including kidney inflammation (**nephritis**) and **allergy**.

TREATMENT

Dermochalasia is easily and effectively treated by a simple plastic surgery (**blepharoplasty**). Blepharochalasia is difficult to treat and tends to recur.

eye, red

See **conjunctivitis**, **glaucoma**, **corneal ulcer**, also *First Aid*.

eyes, crossed

See **strabismus**.

eyestrain

Eye specialists (ophthalmologists) do not accept the popular belief that the eyes can be damaged by being used under adverse conditions, or, except in the case of young children, by failing to wear glasses or by wearing an incorrect prescription. The term 'eyestrain' is not a medical one, but it is widely used to describe any sense of discomfort or distress related to the eyes or to seeing. In view of the central part vision plays in human psychology, it is, perhaps, not surprising that the eyes should be such a prolific source of anxiety.

'Eyestrain' is commonly complained of when focusing (refractive) errors or **presbyopia** prevent clear vision. The response to visual difficulty may be a sustained frown or a contraction of the muscles around the eyes and this may cause a sense of strain.

> The important fact is that eyes can never be damaged by being used.

eye teeth

A popular name for the long, pointed, dog-like (canine) teeth lying on either side of the four central biters (incisors).

eye tumours

Tumours of the eye itself are rare. The most important are **retinoblastoma** of infancy and **malignant melanoma** of adult life. Tumours of the eyelids are more common, especially **rodent ulcer** (basal cell carcinoma) and this is becoming increasingly common. Tumours sometimes occur in the bony eye socket (the orbit) and these cause the eye to bug outwards.

SECONDARY CANCER

Cancers elsewhere in the body can spread by **metastasis** to the eye or the orbit, where they produce effects suggestive, at first, of primary tumours.

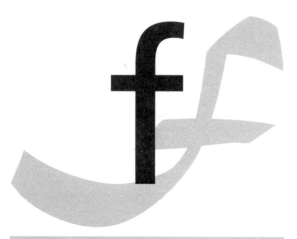

Fabahistin

A brand name for **mebhydrolin**.

face, brain-like

See **cutis verticis gyrata**.

face lift

This operation, done to ameliorate the ravages of time on the human face, is sometimes dignified with the barely serious title rhytidectomy. This, literally, means 'cutting off of wrinkles' which is not, of course, what is done.

HOW IT'S DONE

The operation is usually done under general anaesthesia, but local is possible. The skin is cut through at, or preferably just behind, the hairline, and the incision extended down in front of, and close to the ears. To conceal the upper part of the incision, some hair may be shaved to accommodate it. The only part of the incision which is exposed is cleverly located so close to the ear as to be practically invisible. Working forwards and downwards from this incision, the surgeon frees (under-

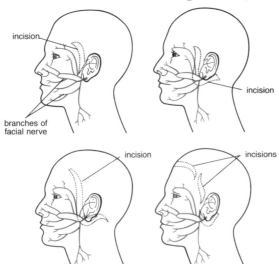

Face lift. The diagram shows various incisions which may be made to remove skin and allow tightening in various directions. The undermining must be carefully done so as to avoid damage to the extensive network of nerves shown, and to the blood vessels.

mines) the skin and then pulls it backwards and upwards so as to tighten it and get rid of the sag and the vertical lines. This produces an overlap of skin at the line of the cut.

> The undermining of the skin has to be extensive and has to be done with great care because nerves and major blood vessels must not be injured. If the operation is to succeed, the undermining must be carried forward almost to the corner of the eye and to within an inch or so of the corner of the mouth. The surgeon must exercise great care so as not to cut the skin, but must not go too deep, as to do so would risk damage to important structures, especially to the nerve twigs that supply the muscles of expression. Injury to these nerves could cause facial paralysis (**Bell's palsy**).

When the fully undermined skin is drawn back and upwards, it overlaps the ear and the line of the original incision by 1 cm to about 5 cm on each side. Having removed excess fat, the surgeon now tacks the drawn-up skin into place with two or three stitches, making sure that the tension is just right – too much tension may lead to hair loss – and then proceeds to cut off and discard the excess skin. Before completing the stitching of the new front edge of skin to the free back edge, the surgeon will probably insert a fine, tubular rubber drain on each side and these may be connected to a small pump producing gentle suction. This may be maintained for one or two days. The purpose of drains and suction is to prevent the serious complication of blood clot (**haematoma**) formation under the freed skin. Haematomas cause problems such as excessive scar formation, infection and even gangrene of the skin, and must be avoided at all costs. Some surgeons rely on pressure dressings which are kept in place for about three days.

Face lifts give an improvement for up to ten years, but, in general, the older the person, the shorter the period of 'rejuvenation'. Constant abuse of flagging collagen by sun-lamps or natural sunshine will ensure that the effect of the operation is shortened.

facial appearance and disease

Experienced doctors are able to derive much information simply from the appearance of the face. A puffy swelling round the eyes (oedema) might indicate a possible kidney problem, while a chubby, wide-cheeked, 'moon' face with high colour could be caused by an adrenal tumor with excessive corticosteroid hormone output, or by high-dose steroid medication. This is called the 'Cushingoid' appearance as it is characteristic of Cushing's syndrome. An expression of anxiety, with deep lines round the mouth, suggests dyspepsia.

Skin pallor may be natural, but might indicate anaemia. Yellowness suggests jaundice. A high flush over the cheek bones could be the malar flush of the heart valve disease mitral stenosis. Blueness of the skin (cyanosis) suggests a circulation problem, or inadequate oxygenation of the blood. Generally enlarged and coarsened features, with a massive jaw and enlarged nose and ears, suggests the growth hormone disorder acromegaly, caused by excessive output of the hormone from the pituitary gland.

A tense, staring, anxious expression, with protruding eyes, a tremulous mouth, facial sweating, lips being bitten, all suggest thyrotoxicosis – overactivity of the thyroid gland.

facial pain

See **trigeminal neuralgia**.

facial palsy

See **Bell's palsy**.

-facient

Suffix meaning 'making' as in abortifacient (making an abortion).

facies

The appearance or expression of the face, characteristic of a particular medical condition or state, which may assist a doctor in diagnosis. Typical facies are found in scores of conditions including **Down's syndrome**, enlarged **adenoids**, abdominal pain, various hereditary disorders affecting the structure of the face, various bone diseases, leprosy, **Parkinsonism**, underaction of the thyroid gland, senile **dementia** and **Alzheimer's disease**.

Factor VIII

A protein substance (globulin) necessary for the proper clotting of the blood. Thirteen main factors are needed, and the absence of Factor VIII causes **haemophilia**. The substance can be isolated from donated blood and given to haemophiliacs to control their dangerous bleeding tendency. A major disaster occurred in the early 1980s, when many haemophiliacs were inadvertently infected with **AIDS** when blood from AIDS sufferers was added to the pool from which Factor VIII was isolated.

Factor IX

One of the many factors necessary for blood clotting. Absence of Factor IX occurs as a result of an **x-linked** gene mutation and causes Christmas disease, a form of **haemophilia** almost identical to **Factor VIII** deficiency haemophilia. Human coagulation Factor IX is produced in freeze-dried form derived from donated blood under the brand names Mononine and Replenine-VF.

Factor XIII

An enzyme in the blood that catalyses cross-linking between molecules of fibrin so as to strengthen the forming blood clot. Human Factor VIII is made by genetic engineering and is sold under the brand names Kogenate and Recombinate. It is also produced in freeze-dried form from donated blood under the brand names Monoclate-P and Replenate.

faece

Latin root meaning 'stool' as in faecal (of faeces).

faeces

The common idea that faeces consist of waste material from the body is not strictly true. Faeces, or stools, consist mainly of bacteria; cast-off cells from the lining of the intestine; various secretions from the cells of the intestinal wall and from the major glands opening into the intestine; bile secretions from the liver – which produce the characteristic colour of the faeces; and a small amount of food residue, mostly cellulose.

The consistency of the faeces varies from liquid to such a state of solidity that impaction, with severe **constipation**, results. A faecalith is a hard, stone-like body formed from a small lump of faeces. It may obstruct the appendix and cause appendicitis.

> Pale faeces, resembling clay in colour, indicate the absence of bile, usually because of liver disorder or obstruction to the flow of bile into the intestine. Black faeces (melaena) result from chemical change in blood released into the stomach or upper part of the intestine and is an important indication of disease such as gastric or duodenal ulcer. Blackening may also be caused by iron tablets taken for anaemia. Blood in the faeces usually comes from piles (haemorrhoids) but may be a sign of colitis or cancer of the rectum or colon, especially in older people.

Fahrenheit scale

The temperature scale which, for many years, was used in medicine, but which has now been replaced by the **Celsius** scale. In the Fahrenheit scale, the melting point of ice is 32°, and the boiling point of water is 212°. Normal body temperature is about 98°. To convert Fahrenheit to Celsius, subtract 32 and multiply by 0.555 or 5/9.

fainting

See **vasovagal attack**. See also *First Aid*.

fainting on swallowing

See **deglutition syncope**.

faith healing

Doctors practising mechanistic scientific medicine often fail to recognize the extent to which the state of mind of the patient can influence the outcome in any attempt at treatment. They are also sometimes guilty of contributing to a negative and damaging state of the patient's mind by a cold, analytic and impersonal approach.

HOW IT WORKS

The state of the patient's mind can sometimes make the difference between success and failure, or even between life and death. A principal factor in obtaining a positive and helpful state of mind is belief, or faith, in the probability of recovery and this is not always encouraged by thoughtless doctors. People with a reputation for faith healing, on the other hand, can, and do, induce a helpful state of optimism, and, even if the effect is insufficient, can give comfort and peace of mind.

DOES IT WORK?

'Miracles', attributed to faith healing, are always due to some natural process, such as an unexpected remission, an unexplained divergence from the normal progress of a disease, or a shift of the balance of forces in favour of recovery, in the context of the intimate mind-body relationship. They do not occur by magic. Cancers do not disappear overnight. People with destroyed spinal cords do not get up and walk. People with atrophic optic nerves do not recover their sight. Heart muscle turned to fibrous scar does not recover its function.

Many disabilities result, not from organic disorder, but from psychological defensive and other processes. These are called functional disorders. Sometimes these motivational defects can be overcome by faith, so that apparently miraculous cures result, especially in seeming paralytic conditions.

> Orthodox medicine has never fully exploited the power of the mind over the body. But as the nature of the physiological links between mental and physical function becomes clearer, it may be expected that a more holistic approach will be incorporated into orthodoxy.

fallen arches

A lay term for flat foot or *pes planus*. This does not necessarily cause symptoms, but many people with fallen arches have hot, stiff, uncomfortable and painful feet, especially on prolonged standing or walking. The elastic 'heel then toe' gait is lost and, eventually, walking becomes an inelegant, awkward and painful stamping process.

POSSIBLE CAUSES

Flat foot is due, essentially to a relative weakness of the muscles of the lower leg which, by way of their tendons, support the upwardly curved arches of the bones of the feet. Insufficient upward pull on the arches throws the full strain on the ligaments of the foot and these soon stretch. Excessive muscular fatigue and overweight contribute to the problem.

TREATMENT

So long as the arches of the feet remain flexible and mobile, much can be done, by suitable footwear, exercises, arch supports, weight control and the avoidance of undue strain, to control the condition. Rigid fallen arches, with secondary damage to the joints and the bones, is irremediable, but symptoms can be reduced by deliberate surgical fusion of painful joints.

Fallopian tube

The open-ended tube along which eggs travel from the ovaries to the womb (uterus) and in which fertilization must occur if pregnancy is to result. The outer open end of each Fallopian tube has finger-like processes that sweep over the surface of the ovary at the time of ovulation, wafting the egg into the tube. Also known as a uterine tube.

Fallopian tube closure

See **Superglue sterilization, laparoscopic sterilization**.

Fallot's tetralogy

A common form of congenital heart disease in which four defects occur:

● narrowing of the main artery to the lungs;
● a hole in the wall between the two sides of the heart;
● an abnormality in the position of the main artery of the body (the aorta);
● considerable enlargement of the main pumping chamber (the ventricle) on the right side of the heart.

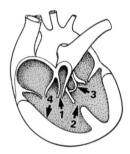

Fallot's tetralogy. This diagram shows the four defects that make up this congenital heart disorder. 1. Narrowing of the arterial trunk to the lungs. 2. A hole between the ventricles. 3. Malposition of the aorta. 4. Abnormal thickening of the right ventricle.

RECOGNITION AND SYMPTOMS

Affected children usually show bluish skin colour (**cyanosis**) and are breathless and easily tired. They often show a characteristic squatting position after exercise. They may have spells in which they are acutely cyanosed and floppy.

TREATMENT

Excellent results can be obtained by radical surgical correction of the various defects.

false memory syndrome

Alleged unearthed 'memories' of childhood sexual abuse induced by psychoanalysts and other psychotherapists with more enthusiasm for Freudian theory than insight into the nature of their own activities. Cases of flagrant invitations or suggestions by therapists to their patients to 'remember' such incidents have been reported, and some of these have led to unfounded accusations and family alienation.

famciclovir

An antiviral drug used to treat **shingles** and genital **herpes**. A brand name is Famvir.

familial

A disease or characteristic found in some families but not in others, as a result of genetic transmission and sometimes other factors. A familial disorder need not be caused by a single defective gene, nor need there be any direct chromosomal evidence that the condition is genetic. Some are thought to be due to several genes and often to the interaction of genetic and environmental influences.

familial adenomatous polyposis

A dominant genetic disorder featuring multiple benign tumours (adenomas) of the colon and rectum, benign tumours of bone (osteomas) and sebaceous cysts. The condition is caused by a mutation in a gene on the long arm of chromosome 5 and carries a strong risk of malignancy. About 12 per cent of people with the gene mutation develop a cancer of the upper intestine, usually a cancer at the point where the bile and pancreatic ducts enter the small intestine (the ampulla of Vater). The mutated gene is a tumour suppressor gene, and the mutation allows tumours to arise. In people with familial adenomatous popyposis the normal **allele** of the pair is deleted.

family therapy

Many serious behavioural and emotional problems have their roots in defective interaction within the family and many others are affected by the family relationships. Family therapy, in which the whole family participates, can therefore be more effective than therapy directed only to the person most seriously disturbed. Some of the problems dealt with by family therapy are:

- the inability of parents to agree on matters important to the children;
- marital conflict which affects the children;
- severe emotional separation between members;
- blockage of communication between members;
- lack of congruence between verbal and non-verbal communication.

The latter is particularly common, and children are highly sensitive to the real information conveyed by body language, angry looks, and lack of desired action when these conflict with what is said.

HOW IT'S DONE

It has been found that patterns of family structure, illness and behaviour tend to be repeated over many generations. One way in which a therapist can proceed is to guide the family through the construction of a *genogram*, based on the family tree, in which a picture of how the current family relates to the previous generation is built up. In eliciting the facts on which this is based, much information comes to light, not only from the answers but also from the way in which the therapist's questions are answered. Recurrent patterns of illness or undesirable behaviour, choice of type of partner, alcoholism, family secrets and other factors relevant to the present family can be brought out.

Once the therapist has established the nature of the group and has begun to see where the problems lie, it becomes possible to give all members of the family an insight into what is happening. Failure of communication is one of the commonest problems and it is one of the most important functions of the therapist to ensure that proper communication techniques are applied. As a respected moderator or chairperson, he or she is able to prevent one member from dominating, prevent two people talking at once, prevent shouting down, and so on.

Anger by one member to another must be carefully recognized, analysed and channelled, so as to avoid escalation towards worsening relationships or breaking off of the therapy. Scape-goating must be detected and discussed. Constant harping on the supposed faults of individuals is discouraged in favour of a consideration of how these faults may possibly be modified.

WHY IT'S DONE

Family therapy has been found helpful in the management of physical disorders with psychological causes or features, such as **anorexia nervosa**, **asthma** and **cancer**. It has been used effectively in cases of severe family tension, **bereavement**, truancy, defiant antisocial behaviour, deliberate soiling (**encopresis**), child neglect and sexual or other forms of **child abuse**.

Short periods of therapy – three to five sessions of less than one hour each – are often sufficient, and therapy does not call for great psychiatric expertise. Much family therapy is now conducted by general practitioners, paediatricians and other experienced counsellors.

famotidine

An **H-2 receptor antagonist** drug used to treat peptic ulcers and reflux oesophagitis (heartburn). A brand name is Pepsid.

Famvir

A brand name for **famciclovir**.

Fanconi's syndrome

A kidney disease often of genetic origin which may start in childhood or in early adult life, in which large quantities of substances normally retained in the body are excreted in the urine. There is thus a loss of essential amino acids, glucose, calcium, phosphates, sodium and potassium, and as a result there may be softening of the bones (osteomalacia), distortion of the bones (**rickets**), muscle weakness, failure to thrive, excessive output of urine, great thirst and progressive failure of the function of the kidneys.

Fanconi's syndrome can also be acquired as a result of poisoning with tetracycline antibiotic left too long on the shelf, metal salts or other substances, or as a complication of kidney transplantation, multiple myelomatosis, vitamin D deficiency and other conditions.

Fansidar

Brand name for a mixture of **pyrimethamine** and **sulfadoxine**.

Faradism

In the early part of the nineteenth century the British physicist Michael Faraday (1791–1867) showed how to produce a high-frequency, interrupted, spiky current by means of a contact breaker on an induction coil, and this kind of current was shown to cause sustained contraction if applied to muscles, an effect called Faradism. Today, Faradism is still used to maintain the health of paralysed muscles while awaiting regeneration or recovery in damaged motor nerves.

Fareston

A brand name for **toremifene**.

Farlutal

A brand name for **medroxyprogesterone**.

farmer's lung

An occupational lung disease caused by the repeated inhalation of dust containing the spores of fungus from mouldy straw, hay, grain or mushroom compost. It is not so much an infection as an allergic reaction in the tiny air sacs of the lungs. Initially, there are acute attacks of fever, nausea, breathlessness and cough a few hours after exposure. These settle, but if they are allowed to continue they may lead, after long periods of exposure, to lung damage in the form of fibrosis. Inadequate oxygen transfer to the blood (respiratory failure) – an ultimately fatal condition – may supervene.

See also **bagassosis**.

fascia

Sheets or layers of tendon-like connective tissue which lies under the skin, between the muscles and around the organs, the blood vessel and the nerves, forming sheaths and compartments throughout the body. Some fascia is dense, some delicate and much of it is bulked out by fat cells. The superficial fascia just under the skin is one of the main fat stores of the body.

See also **necrotizing fasciitis**.

fasciculation

Brief, involuntary contraction of a small group of muscle fibres, causing a visible or palpable twitch under the skin. Occasional and intermittent fasciculation of the flat muscle around the eye is common and almost always harmless. Persistent severe fasciculation may imply nerve disease and should be reported.

fasciitis

Inflammation of **fascia**. This is very rare and may be due to infection or to unknown causes. It is sometimes associated with conditions such as **ankylosing spondylitis** or **Reiter's syndrome**.

See also **necrotizing fasciitis**.

fasciotomy

Cutting fascia. This is an operation necessary to relieve severe tension in a muscle compartment or to prevent compression of arteries or nerves. Occasionally, an athlete, especially a footballer, will develop the calf or other muscles to such an extent that they outgrow the space available to them in their fascial compartments. In such a case, fasciotomy may be indicated.

Fasigyn

A brand name for **tinidazole**.

fasting

In the over-fed Western world, there is much to be said for regular refraining from food. Few of us would fail to benefit from such a practice. Unfortunately, in the wider world context, many of the people who do fast are often those least well able to sustain the reduced calorie intake. Most serious fasting is undertaken for religious, ascetic, ritualistic or politically persuasive purposes. The modest fasting of Lent, Yom Kippur or Ramadan in those who are adequately nourished is certainly as beneficial to the body as to the soul.

> So long as water is taken, most people can fast for several days with safety, living happily, if hungrily, on their excessive fat stores. If essential vitamins and minerals are taken, most people could, by fasting, safely reduce their fat stores to a very low level.

Once the fat stores are depleted, however, the necessity for a fuel supply to the brain and the heart muscle leads to consumption of the muscles, which soon become severely wasted so that the body is reduced to a skeletal state of emaciation, as witnessed in Nazi concentration camps or in hospital wards treating girls with **anorexia nervosa**.

> When the soluble proteins in the blood become depleted two important things happen. The loss of albumin reduces the ability of the blood to withdraw fluid from the tissue spaces and the body becomes water-logged (oedema). And the loss of the globulin proteins (antibodies) means that there is a degree of immune deficiency and the susceptibility to infection increases.

These are the results of fasting carried to the length of starvation. Many people have found moderate regular fasting, say for one day a week, a useful aid to health.

fatal familial insomnia

A genetically determined condition occurring between the ages of 40 and 60, involving progressively worsening insomnia, intolerance to heat, watering eyes, progressive difficulty in walking, memory deterioration, speech defect, muscle jerks, progressive physical and mental deterioration and death within 7 to 33 months of onset. The disease, which features severe loss of nerve fibres in the nerve cell clumps (thalamic nuclei) at the base of the brain, is one of the growing list of serious disorders caused by abnormal prion proteins – a list that also includes **Creutzfeldt-Jakob disease**, new variant CJD, **kuru**, and Gerstmann-Sträussler disease. Sporadic fatal insomnia is also a **prion protein disease** and is probably identical to fatal familial insomnia.

fat distribution, abnormal

See **lipodystrophy**.

fat embolism

Long bones contain considerable quantities of fat in their marrow, and following fractures, some of this is inevitably released into the blood. In most cases this causes little or no harm, but in a small proportion, relatively large quantities of fat are released to cause obstruction to vital arteries in the brain, the lungs or in the coronary arteries of the heart. In addition to obstruction, the acidic products of fat breakdown can cause permanent damage to the linings of the arteries.

This may have serious effects with delirium, coma and even death. Treatment is by intensive oxygen therapy using a chamber in which the pressure can be raised to about three times atmospheric (hyperbaric oxygen). By such means death or serious arterial damage may be prevented.

fatigue

This word has more than one meaning. It may mean the feeling of exhaustion that follows sustained physical exertion; or it may mean a feeling of extreme tiredness that is unrelated to work of any kind. Fatigue can also be caused by lack of sleep.

PHYSICAL FATIGUE

Physical fatigue is due to the accumulation in the muscles of the breakdown products of fuel consumption and energy production (metabolism). Resting for a short period will allow time for the normal blood flow through the muscles to 'wash out' these metabolites. To the extent that the affected person is aware of the symptoms caused by the metabolites, physical fatigue may be said to have a mental component.

MENTAL FATIGUE

In many cases, however, purely mental fatigue, that masquerades in most of its features as physical fatigue, can occur. While it is true that sustained, intense intellectual work can produce a sense of fatigue that urges a period of relief from the work, most cases of non-physical fatigue have nothing to do with over-use of the mental faculties. It is the result of boredom, over-long concentration on a single task, anxiety, frustration, fear or just general disinclination to perform a particular job of work. Even during periods of fatigue, the contemplation of work that is rewarding and absorbing is pleasurable, and resumption is anticipated with satisfaction.

fat removal, cosmetic

See **lipectomy, suction**.

fats

The group of substances known as lipids includes the fats, the phospholipids and the steroids. Fats form the body's main energy back-up store and are converted into fuel as required. Fat stores also insulate the body against heat loss, and act as a mechanical shock absorber and a contouring element.

Fats are of low density and, although present in considerable quantity in all cells, make up only 2–3 per cent of the weight of cells other that fat cells. Most of the body fats, however, are stored in special, thin-walled cells filled with lipids in the form of an oil that is liquid at normal body temperatures. There is almost no limit to the amount of fuel that can be stored in the form of fats, under the skin and in the abdomen. The average man has a fat store of about 14 kilos, which could support life for about two months. A fat man might carry a year's supply.

Fats are chemically known as triglycerides and these, to a large extent, give the body its outline shape. Each fat molecule consists of a kind of backbone of glycerine (glycerol) to which three fatty acids are attached – hence the term 'triglyceride'. Fat-splitting enzymes (lipases) strip off the fatty acids from the glycerol molecule freeing them for conversion to carbohydrates, for direct use as fuels, or for resynthesis of fats. If one of the fatty acids is replaced by a phosphate group and a nitrogen-containing base, we have a phospholipid. Phospholipids are the most important constituents of cell membranes and their chemical and physical properties have an important bearing on what gets in or out of the cells.

Steroids are a range of lipids which include cholesterol, the female sex hormones (oestrogens), the male sex hormones (androgens), some of the hormones from the adrenal glands (corticosteroids), and bile acids.

Most diets contain too high a proportion of fats and especially of saturated fats. Saturated fats are found in butter, milk, and other dairy products. Unsaturated fats, such as are found in vegetable and fish oils, are generally believed to be less harmful to health.

fatty acids

See **fats**.

fauces

Latin root meaning 'throat' as in fauces (space at back of mouth).

Faverin

A brand name for **fluvoxamine**.

favism

A genetically induced sensitivity to a chemical substance occurring in broad beans. Those affected develop a severe form of anaemia on eating the beans. The condition is rare except in Iran and some parts of the Mediterranean.

fear

A response to a real or imagined perception of danger. The response may be appropriate or it may be inappropriate and excessive, in which case it is deemed to be abnormal and is called a phobia. Fear is an **emotion** and is accompanied by strong physical symptoms such as an awareness of rapid heart action, tension in the muscles, a dry throat, sweating and an awareness of muscle contraction in the abdomen usually described as 'butterflies in the stomach'. These symptoms are mainly caused by release into the bloodstream of the hormone adrenaline and can, to some extent, be induced by an injection of the drug. In addition to the purely physiological effects, however, the unpleasantness of fear is compounded by the mental awareness of the danger of death, injury or loss.

febre

Latin root meaning 'fever' as in febrile (fevered).

febrile convulsions

See **fever fits**.

feeding, infant

See **breastfeeding**, **bottle-feeding**.

felbinac

A non-steroidal anti-inflammatory drug (**NSAID**) formulated in a gel for external use. A brand name is Traxam.

Feldene

A brand name for **piroxicam**.

felopidine

A calcium channel blocker drug used to treat **angina pectoris** and high blood pressure. A brand name is Plendil.

female breasts in males

See **gynaecomastia**.

female sex hormones

See **oestrogen drugs**.

female sterilization

Hysterectomy, even if the ovaries are intact, precludes any contact between the sperm and egg and is a total bar to conception. It is, of course, also a bar to implantation. The operation is not now performed simply as a contraceptive measure.

The common methods of female sterilization involve tying, cutting or clamping both Fallopian tubes by endoscopic surgery. In theory, tubes closed in this way might still allow the passage of sperm or egg, but as closure leads to healing together of the opposed surfaces, this is very unlikely. Most authorities quote a failure rate of about one in 1000.

Femara

A brand name for **letrozole**.

Fematrix 40

A brand name for **oestradiol** in a transdermal patch.

Femseven

A brand name **oestradiol** for in a transdermal patch.

Femulen

A brand name for **ethynodiol diacetate**.

femur

Latin root meaning 'thigh' as in femoral (of the thigh).

femur, fracture of

POSSIBLE CAUSES
The commonest form of femoral fracture results from **osteoporosis** and involves the short neck between the top of the bone and the near-spherical head which forms the 'ball and socket' joint with the cup in the side of the pelvis.

INCIDENCE
This kind of fracture is common in elderly women and often results in interference with the blood supply of the head of the femur and death of the free fragment (avascular necrosis). Hip-joint replacement is often the only satisfactory remedy.

RECOGNITION AND TREATMENT
Fracture of the shaft of the femur usually results from severe violence and often leads to major loss of blood into the tissues of the leg and severe surgical shock. Transfusion may be needed. In cases in which the bone does not pass out through the skin (simple fractures), effective and rapid recovery can be obtained by hammering a long steel pin down the inside of the shaft of the bone. External **fixation** may also be used.

Sometimes, open operation to secure the fracture with a steel plate and screws is required. The alternative is weeks of immobilizaion on traction or in a plaster cast. Most femoral fractures heal in about three months. See also **fracture, bone**.

Fenbid Gel

A brand name for **ibuprofen** in a preparation for external use.

Fenbid Spansule

A brand name for **ibuprofen**.

fenbufen

A non-steroidal anti-inflammatory drug (**NSAID**). A brand name is Lederfen.

fenchone

An essential oil used in a mixture with others to treat urinary stones. A brand name of such a mixture is Rowatinex.

fenclofenac

A non-steroidal anti-inflammatory drug (**NSAID**).

fenestration

A delicate operation on the inner ear, to relieve the deafness caused by the disease of **otosclerosis**. Essentially, this disease is due to the gumming-up of a vibrating window occupied by the footplate of the inner of the three tiny ossicle bones of the middle ear. Fenestration was designed to create a new window elsewhere in the wall of the inner ear so as to allow freer vibration of the fluid within. The operation gave disappointing long-term results and has now been superseded by better procedures such as **stapedectomy**.

fenofibrate

A fibrate anticholesterol drug used to treat high blood cholesterol levels that fail to respond to diet modification. A brand name is Lipantil Micro.

fenoprofen calcium

A non-steroidal anti-inflammatory drug (**NSAID**). A brand name is Fenopron.

Fenopron

A brand name for **fenoprofen calcium**.

fenoterol

A beta 2-agonist, adrenaline-like drug that is valuable in the management of asthma while having comparatively little effect on the heart. Its action is similar to that of **salbutamol**. A brand name is Berotec. It is also produced in combination with the drug **ipratropium bromide** under the brand name Duovent.

Fenox

A brand name for nasal drops containing **phenylephrine**.

fentanyl

A powerful, short-acting narcotic painkiller (analgesic). Brand names are Sublimaze and, for external use, Durogesic.

Fentazin

A brand name for **perphenazine**.

fenticonazole

An antifungal drug used to treat vaginal thrush. A brand name is Lomexin.

Feospan

A brand name for an iron preparation.

-ferent

Suffix meaning 'carry, bear' as in afferent (carrying to).

Ferfolic SV

A brand name for ferrous fumarate in conjunction with **folic acid**.

-ferous

Suffix meaning 'bearing' as in seminiferous (bearing semen).

Ferrograd

A brand name for **ferrous sulphate**.

Ferrograd Folic

A brand name for **ferrous sulphate** in conjunction with **folic acid**.

ferrous fumarate

An iron salt used to treat iron-deficiency **anaemia**. Brand names are Fersaday, Fersamal and Galfer. The drug is also formulated in conjunction with **folic acid** under the brand names Folex-350, Meterfolic and Pregaday.

ferrous gluconate

An iron compound used in the treatment of iron deficiency **anaemia**. A brand name of a formulation with **folic acid** is Ferfolic SV.

ferrous glycine sulphate

An iron compound used to treat iron-deficiency **anaemia**. A brand name is Plesmet.

ferrous sulphate

A bitter, greenish crystalline compound of iron used in the treatment of iron deficiency **anaemia**. Brand names are Ferrograd and Slow-Fe. The drug is also formulated in conjunction with **folic acid** under the brand names Ferrograd Folic and Slow-Fe Folic.

Fersaday

A brand name for **ferrous fumarate**.

Fersamal

A brand name for **ferrous fumarate**, an iron preparation used to treat **anaemia**.

fertility

See **infertility**.

fertility drugs

Drugs used to treat infertility, usually by the induction of ovulation. The drugs clomiphene, tamoxifen and cyclofenil are used to treat **infertility** due to failure to produce ova. These and other similar fertility drugs often result in multiple ovulation and multiple pregnancies may result.

fetal alcohol syndrome

Knowledge of the effects of high alcohol levels in the maternal blood on the growing fetus is not new. Doctors recorded a rise in fetal death and deformity during the gin-drinking epidemic in the early 18th century. Concern has again been raised because of the rise in alcohol consumption among young women of today.

Most of the early data came from cases of mothers who were chronic alcoholics. These women were consuming far more alcohol than the ordinary social drinker, and the effects on their babies were thought to be likely to be severe enough to consider terminating pregnancy. This proved to be an unduly pessimistic view and later studies showed that the fetal alcohol syndrome was less common than had been thought. In one study of 50,000 newborns, none of the babies were thought to have suffered obvious damage from alcohol.

RECOGNITION

The effects on the fetus of high blood alcohol include:

- poor bodily growth giving low birth weight;
- abnormally small heads (microcephaly);
- undergrowth of the upper jaw;
- receding upper teeth;
- cleft palate;
- long upper lip;
- abnormally small eyes (microphthalia);
- narrowed eyelid opening;
- hollowed breastbone (pecus excavatum);
- an increased rate of congenital heart disease;
- mental retardation, with IQs below 80 in half the cases;
- failure of development of skills requiring fine movements;
- a significant rise in the fetal death rate;
- a rise in the death rate in the period immediately after birth.

RISKS

The risk to the babies of regular but more moderate drinkers is, of course, much less than in the case of chronic alcoholics, and is hard to quantify. Even so, maternal alcohol abuse during pregnancy is now recognized as being the commonest cause of drug-induced fetal abnormality.

> Some effects on the fetus are likely in those who drink heavily throughout pregnancy, with the severity of the effects being roughly proportional to the amount of alcohol consumed. There is no known lower level of safety and the best current advice is that no alcohol should be taken at any time during pregnancy.

fetal heart monitoring

See **cardiotocography**.

fetishism

Sexual interest focused on and aroused by an object belonging to another person, or by a part of the body not normally considered of sexual significance. In fetishism, which is essentially a male disorder, the attention is often directed to articles of female clothing, especially those items in contact with the genitalia or the secondary sexual areas. But often such articles as shoes, stockings, or even handkerchiefs may become of intense sexual interest.

Some element of fetishism is probably present in all sexually mature people; the abnormality rests in the degree. In a major fetishist disorder, the affected person will prefer contact with the object to contact with the owner and will often use the object to assist in masturbation.

fetoscopy

This is a method of direct visualization of the fetus within the womb (uterus), by means of a fine fibre optic illumination and viewing system passed into the amniotic fluid, through the wall of the abdomen and uterus. In addition to examining and photographing the floating fetus, the doctor can take samples of fluid for alphafetoprotein and other estimations and can also take blood samples and biopsies.

Fetoscopy allows direct confirmation of suspected physical fetal abnormalities. It carries a slight risk of causing abortion, but in cases in which there is a high probability of inherited disease or gross physical abnormality, this risk is usually considered well worth taking.

fetuses of different ages in womb

See **superfetation**.

fever

Elevation of body temperature above the normal range of 37°–37.5°C, taken in the mouth. Rectal temperatures are a little higher.

POSSIBLE CAUSES

Fever is caused by a wide variety of infections, by many cancers, by coronary thrombosis and stroke (see **thrombosis**), by crushing injury, by blood disorders in which haemoglobin is released from blood cells (**haemolytic anaemia**), by diseases due to immunological disorder and by various acute disorders such as **gout** and **porphyria**.

WHAT HAPPENS

Body temperature is kept within the normal range by a kind of thermostat mechanism in the hypothalamus region of the brain. This monitors the blood temperature and, if it is too high, causes the skin blood vessels to widen and sweating to increase, so that heat is lost. If the temperature is too low, the muscles are induced to shiver so as to produce heat.

In fever, the thermostat is reset at a higher level and the normal blood temperature is read as being too low. Heat production is thus automatically increased. This resetting is done by a substance known as interleukin-1 which is released by certain white cells, known as macrophages and monocytes, under the influence of a range of substances called exogenous pyrogens. Interleukin-1, acting in the hypothalamus, causes the release of prostaglandins and these stimulate heat production in the muscles. Prostaglandins also cause pain.

Aspirin acts by preventing the release of prostaglandins, so it is both a pain-killer and a temperature-lowering drug (antipyretic).

> Infecting organisms reproduce best at normal body temperature and are discouraged by fever. So it is not always desirable to bring down the temperature. But temperatures above about 44.5°C usually cause fatal brain damage and, in such cases, urgent cooling, by any available means, is vital.

fever fits (febrile convulsions)

These are fits caused by a sudden rise in temperature. They are quite common in young children and may be a frightening experience for the parents, who often fear that the child is going to die. But death, in such cases, is extremely rare. The majority of children who suffer these episodes are not epilep-

tic and these fits do not occur because of any brain defect. The term febrile convulsions simply means 'fits occurring in the course of a fever'.

Between three and four children in every 100 have one or more febrile convulsion by the time they are five years old. In most cases the fits occur after the age of six months. Fits occurring earlier than that are a matter for more concern. Most febrile convulsions occur between the ages of nine months and two years and it seems likely that certain individuals have an inherited tendency to be more sensitive to fever than average. Boys are affected more often than girls.

It appears that the brains of many young children are exceptionally sensitive to a raised body temperature and that this, in itself, is enough to produce an electrical discharge.

But even children who have many fits will not necessarily become epileptic. In 19 cases out of 20, the sensitivity of the brain to fever decreases as the child grows and that is the end of the matter. As a general rule, isolated febrile convulsions may be considered unlikely to cause any permanent harm and need not occasion great anxiety.

It would be wrong, however, to suggest that febrile convulsions are unimportant. Convulsions themselves can cause brain damage – especially in the temporal lobes – which, in turn, can cause epilepsy.

The higher the fever the more likely is there to be a convulsion, and three-quarters of all convulsions occur with a temperature of more than 39.2°C. The younger the child, the more likely are the convulsions to be severe and prolonged, and the more severe the fits the more likely they are to cause permanent brain damage. Also, the probability of recurrence rises with the severity of the attack, and life-long epilepsy is much more likely if there are prolonged and severe febrile convulsions in infancy.

The implication of all this is, of course, that every effort must be made to prevent febrile convulsions. Fever, in this age group, should be controlled with paracetamol and deliberate cooling, and medical advice sought so that the cause of the fever may be treated as effectively as possible. Many childhood fevers are caused by infections which will respond rapidly to antibiotics and these are prescribed by doctors whenever necessary. Conditions commonly causing fevers include middle ear infection (otitis media), tonsillitis, kidney or urinary infection, pneumonia and any of the common infectious diseases of childhood such as measles, mumps, chickenpox and whooping cough. Many paediatricians believe it so important to avoid recurrent febrile convulsions that they view the start of any fever in a child who has already had a fever fit as a signal for immediate cooling measures. Many doctors have found that the best drug to use, for this purpose, is phenobarbitone.

Infantile convulsions have, in the past, been attributed to all sorts of alleged causes, such as teething, threadworms, constipation and so on, but there is no reason to believe that any of these minor conditions can cause fits. Modern methods of investigation will usually bring out the true cause.

Here is how to cope with a febrile convulsion: if there is preliminary warning in the form of twitching, try to prevent the fit by cool sponging. This should also be done even if the full fit occurs. Call for help. Put the child on a large polythene sheet or other waterproof surface, surround him with bath towels and sponge him down thoroughly with tepid water. If the convulsion is severe make sure that he cannot hurt himself by striking a hard object. Don't try to restrain him – just ensure that he is protected from injury. Remove all hard objects such as toys, and pad the cot sides with a folded towel or blanket, if necessary.

TREATMENT

Don't try to force open the mouth – to do so may cause the tongue to fall back and obstruct the airway. Get someone to call a doctor. Many doctors consider a febrile convulsion an indication for admission to hospital. Febrile convulsions are usually fairly brief – seldom lasting for longer than about ten minutes – and recovery is complete. But the convulsion will often resemble a full grand mal attack of epilepsy, complete with the initial massive contraction (the tonic stage) followed by the sequence of lesser, jerky contractions (the clonic stage) and then the brief period of unconsciousness. Parents inevitably become seriously alarmed and may be convinced that their child is going to be a life-long epileptic. If consciousness is lost, see to it that there is no obstruction to the breathing. Obstruction may also occur by the inhalation of vomit or saliva, so the positioning of the child is important.

As soon as the convulsion is over the child should be placed lying on his front (prone) with the face turned to one side. If the leg on the same side is drawn well up, with the knee bent, this will stabilize the position. Should there be any indication of obstruction to the breathing, clear the mouth with a finger and suck out anything in the back of the throat with some form of tubing. Continue the sponging if the fever remains. Be observant. It may be difficult to behave in a detached manner, but it can be helpful if you note down any unusual features, as this may help the doctor to decide whether or not the fit has serious significance. Note particularly:

- whether the convulsion is generalized or, if local, which parts of the body are affected;
- how long the attack lasts;
- whether there is incontinence;
- whether consciousness is lost and, if so, for how long.

Remember that almost all seizures are self-limiting and will pass. Try, however distressing the circumstances, to remain calm.

FEVERED CHILDREN AND ASPIRIN

Reye's syndrome is a disease of childhood in which swelling of the brain and a form of liver inflammation (hepatitis) occur following infection with one of several viruses including chickenpox, influenza, rubella, herpes simplex, and echovirus. Because the skull prevents the brain from expanding, swelling rapidly interferes with brain function. The liver disorder is also severe and there is some reason to believe that the effect on the brain may be secondary to the liver damage. The rise in the level of liver enzymes in the blood, which is a sign of liver damage, may be extreme. Brain swelling causes uncontrollable vomiting, delirium and disorientation and rapid onset of stupor and coma. There are indications of increasing brain damage with local or general seizures, and the disorder may progress to deepening coma. In fatal cases, the average time between admission to hospital and death is four days.

Treatment is directed at the control of brain swelling by steroids and withdrawal of fluid, from the brain, by the transfusion of strong sugar solutions into the blood. Artificial ventilation may be needed. With increasing understanding of the condition and its management the death rate from Reye's syndrome has dropped from about 50 per cent to about 10 per cent. Some children, unfortunately, suffer residual brain damage.

The condition comes on just as the child is recovering from the virus infection, and there is considerable evidence that Reye's syndrome is also connected with aspirin taking. This evidence is so strong that the medical authorities in Britain and the United States have advised that children suspected of having chickenpox or influenza should not be given aspirin. Some have gone further and have recommended that aspirin should never be given to children. The British pharmaceutical industry appears to have accepted this advice, and paracetamol has replaced aspirin in paediatric pain-killers.

There is now an absolute veto on the use of aspirin in children suffering from fevers.

fexofenadine

An **antihistamine** drug used to treat hay fever. A brand name is Telfast.

fibre optics

A branch of optics concerned with the transmission of light along optical fibres – fine, flexible rods of glass or other transparent materials.

WHY IT'S USED

Fibre optics has become increasingly important in medicine and surgery, mainly because of the growth of the technique of taking a look inside the body, through a natural orifice or through a very small artificial opening (endoscopy).

HOW IT'S USED

Optical fibres are used to guide light – both for illumination and for viewing – around complex bends or sharp corners by making use of the principle of total internal reflection. Because the glass fibre is so narrow, light rays never strike the surface at a sharp enough angle to pass out.

Fibres with a diameter of as little as 0.02 mm are arranged in tight bundles and, so long as the fibres remain in registration at both ends of the bundle, they can be bent and manoeuvred into otherwise inaccessible areas of the body. 'Steerable' endoscopes are now commonplace in routine hospital examinations.

fibric acid derivative drugs

A class of drugs capable of lowering the levels in the body of lipids (fats) including cholesterol. Fibrates can reduce low-density lipoproteins and raise high density lipoproteins. Some act by interfering with cholesterol synthesis in the liver, others by promoting the more rapid breakdown of lipoproteins. They include clofibrate, gemfibrozil, fenofibrate, ciprofibrate and benzafibrate.

fibrillation

Rapid, uncontrolled and irregular contraction of heart muscle fibres which prevents the normal pumping action. Fibrillation most commonly affects the upper chambers of the heart (the atria) but so long as the main pumping chambers (the ventricles) continue to operate normally, the blood flow continues. Atrial fibrillation, however, interferes with the conduction of normal control impulses to the ventricles and leads to a rapid and irregular pulse. It often responds well to drug treatment.

> Fibrillation of the ventricles causes death within a few minutes unless normal beating can be restored by electrical defibrillation.

Ventricular fibrillation is one of the two forms of cardiac arrest and most commonly results from a severe coronary thrombosis.

fibrin breakdown

See **fibrolase**.

fibrinolysis

The use of drugs to dissolve blood clots in the circulation. Enzymes such as streptokinase or urokinase, which break down fibrin, are used. A combination of fibrinolysis and aspirin, given soon after a coronary attack, greatly improves the chances of survival.

fibrinolytic drugs

A group of drugs capable of breaking down the protein fibrin which is the main constituent of blood clots. They are thus able to disperse dangerous blood clots (thromboses) that have formed within the circulation. They include streptokinase, alteplase, anistreplase and urokinase. Possible side-effects include headache, backache, tiny blood spots in the skin (purpura) bleeding at needle puncture sites, and allergic reactions.

fibroadenoma

A nonmalignant (benign) tumour of glandular and fibrous tissue. Fibroadenomas are the commonest cause of breast lumps in young women and are harmless. They grow slowly, taking up to a year to double in size, and usually stop growing when they are about 3 cm in diameter. Unfortunately, they are very difficult to distinguish from cancers, except by pathological examination, and they should always be removed.

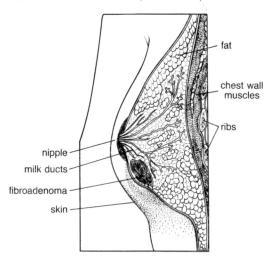

Fibrodenoma of breast. This is the commonest breast mass in young women and is quite innocent. Such benign tumours should however be removed to confirm the diagnosis and because there is a slight chance of malignant change occurring.

fibroid

A benign tumour of fibrous and muscular tissue which grows in the wall of the womb (uterus) and which may become very large. They are uncommon in women under 30.

Fibroids are often multiple and tend to cause pain and excessively heavy menstrual periods. They can cause infertility but need be removed surgically only if causing trouble. When they are very large, removal of the uterus (hysterectomy) may be the only practicable remedy.

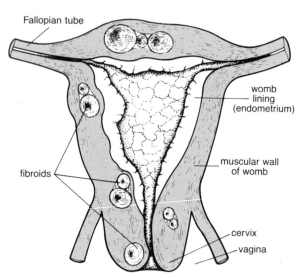

Fibroids. These very common non-malignant (benign) tumours of the womb are really tumours of muscle with a large fibrous tissue content.

fibrolase

An enzyme found in the venom of the American copperhead snake that degrades fibrin and fibrinogen directly. These substances are essential for clot formation and fibrolase is being studied as a possible treatment for occlusive disease of arteries or thrombosis in veins.

fibroma

A nonmalignant tumour of fibrous tissue.

fibromyalgia syndrome

A condition of long-persisting generalized aches and pains, fatigue, stiffness and a considerable number of different points on the body that are painful to pressure. The syndrome affects women far more often than men. The cause is unknown and investigation shows no definite objective abnormality. Some experts believe that this is a psychiatric condition but the psychological features do not resemble any such disorder.

fibrosarcoma

A malignant tumour of the cells which generate fibrous tissue (fibroblasts). Since these cells occur all over the body, almost any tissue, including bone, may be the site of origin. Fibrosarcomas usually occur in a leg or in a buttock. Those in soft tissue tend to be less malignant than those in bone. Radical surgery and possible radiotherapy will be necessary.

fibrosis

Scarring and thickening of an organ or surface by the laying down of fibrous tissue, usually following injury or inflammation. Fibrosis is the body's main healing process and the scar tissue formed is usually very strong.

fibrositis

An imaginary disease invented by doctors to provide a plausible explanation for symptoms which they cannot account for. Most cases of fibrositis are actually stress- or occupation-induced muscle or tendon pain, and careful pathological examination of the tissue at the site of the pain shows no abnormality.

General measures to improve health, such as regular exercise, postural advice, relief of anxiety and improved sleep are usually effective. In severe cases, the powerfully suggestive (placebo) effect of an injection of local anaesthetic (or even sterile water) into the trigger point may do the trick.

fibrous tissue

A simple, strong structural or repair tissue consisting of twisted stands of the protein collagen laid down by cells known as fibroblasts. These are among the commonest cells in the body and occur everywhere. Tissue damaged beyond recovery by disease is replaced by inert, blood-vessel-free fibrous tissue (scar tissue).

Fibro-vein

A brand name for **sodium tetradecyl sulphate**.

-fic

Suffix meaning 'creating' as in soporific (making sleep).

-fid

Suffix meaning 'split' as in bifid (split in two).

fifth disease

This is a comparatively rare virus infection of children caused by a parvovirus and occurring in small epidemics. The most striking feature is a rash of small red spots on the cheeks, which join to produce a general redness of the cheeks, as if the child has been slapped. After a day or two, the rash appears on the body – on the limbs more than the trunk – and at this stage there is often a mild fever. The rash has usually gone after about ten days but may recur. No specific treatment is required other than to keep the child comfortable in bed drinking plenty of fluids.

Filair

A brand name for **beclomethasone**.

filariasis

A group of parasitic tropical diseases transmitted by mosquitoes and other biting flies. The insects inject large numbers of microscopic worms (microfilariae) which survive in the blood and lymphatic vessels to grow into adult worms of from 2–50 cm in length. These worms, in turn, breed thousands of new microfilariae which spread throughout the blood circulation from whence they are taken up by insects and carried to other people. Filariasis occurs in tropical Africa, South-East Asia, the South Pacific and parts of South America.

filgrastim

Human **granulocyte stimulating factor** produced by genetic engineering and used to treat severe deficiencies of some of the white cells of the blood and the immune system. A brand name is Neupogen.

The various disease types include **onchocerciasis**, loa-loa and Calabar swellings. Repeated infection with the worms which inhabit the lymphatics causes blockage and **elephantiasis**. Onchocerciasis is also called 'river blindness', because the transmitting fly lives only near fast-flowing rivers and the microfilaria invade the eyes and destroy vision.

film badge

A precautionary measure to monitor the risks of excessive radiation dosage in staff working in X-ray and radiotherapy departments. The film badge is a small light-tight, but not X-ray proof, container for a piece of photographic film which would be fogged if exposed to radiation. All staff carry film badges, usually pinned to the clothing, and the films are regularly developed and replaced. A fogged film indicates that an accident has occurred and this can be investigated.

filmless X-rays

See **digital radiography**.

finasteride

A drug used to reduce prostate enlargement in benign prostatic hypertropy. A brand name is Proscar.

finger clubbing

This is the term given to swelling of the fingers, especially just behind the root of the nail, so that the normal depression there is replaced by a convexity. Finger clubbing is an important sign but is not specific for a particular condition. It is found in various disorders including lung cancer, bronchiectasis, congenital heart disease and cirrhosis of the liver.

firearms deaths

Happily, this is not yet a major problem in Britain, but people of influence would do well to inform themselves of the situation in the United States and be warned. History suggests that trends in the USA often manifest in the UK after some years and this is certainly one we can do without.

INCIDENCE

There are about 120,000,000 privately owned guns in the USA and about half of all the homes contain one or more firearms. Most are kept ostensibly for sporting purposes but

> Studies have shown that keeping firearms in the home carries a substantial risk of accidental injury or death and greatly increases the likelihood that domestic quarrels end in tragedy. Suicide impulses, too, are more likely to have a fatal outcome if a gun is to hand.

at least one-fifth of owners give 'self-defence' as the reason for possessing a gun.

THE STATISTICS

Almost two-thirds of gunshot deaths occur in the home and few of these involve self-protection. Less than 2 per cent of homicides are deemed legally justifiable, over 80 per cent occurring in the course of arguments or altercations. In cases of assault, people tend to reach for the most deadly weapon readily available and if this happens to be a gun, the gun is likely to be used.

> Ready access to firearms is clearly a major danger in households given to violence. In the home, handguns are about three times as often the cause of death as shotguns or rifles combined.

These facts should give us pause. The number of guns in Britain is already rising to dangerous levels and we may soon see our police routinely armed. By the time we reach the stage of owning guns 'for self-protection' the disease is already probably beyond remedy. In Britain, as in America, there are two powerful lobbies which, for all their posturing and rationalization, are unequivocally dealing in death – the tobacco and the gun lobbies. Any enlightened administration should recognize and act on these facts. There are indications that the American government is at last beginning to see that its past neglect of the gun menace is indefensible.

PREVENTING THE SPREAD

The simple truth is that the possession of any personal gun should be illegal, except for the armed forces and possibly the police. Mere possession should be visited with heavy penalties. No society can call itself civilized or mature that looks with equanimity on the existence of personal weapons.

fish oil

BENEFITS

It has been claimed that a considerable degree of protection against heart disease can be obtained by adopting a diet in which animal fats are largely replaced by fish oils. This claim is based largely on the observation that populations (such as Greenland Eskimos and mainland Danes) with a diet that is high in fish have a lower incidence of **atherosclerosis** – the arterial disease that causes more deaths than any other single condition.

Fish oils contain the polyunsaturated fatty acid eicosapentaenoic acid and there is good evidence that when this is incorporated into the blood platelets instead of the usual arachidonic acid, it alters their action in such a way as to reduce their effect in promoting blood clotting and arterial disease.

LONG-TERM EFFECTS

Unfortunately, the effect is significant only with long-term administration at large dosage and, even then, the effect is comparable only to that of taking half an aspirin tablet each day. Other workers have claimed that fish oils work by altering the levels of undesirable fats in the blood, by changing the properties of cell membranes, or by altering the function of certain of the white cells in the blood.

Whatever the explanation, it seems clear that fish oils are to be preferred to beef oils and that if we were all to live like Eskimos we would be much less likely to die from coronary thrombosis. Most of us would probably die from exposure.

fistula

An abnormal communication between two internal organs or an abnormal passage between an internal organ and the surface of the skin. Fistulas may be congenital or may arise as a result of disease processes such as abscesses or cancer.

fits

See **epilepsy**.

fixation

SURGICAL FIXATION

In surgery, the term is used to indicate any method of holding or fastening something in a fixed position, especially the holding of the broken fragments of a bone in proper alignment so that they will heal together in the correct position. Such fixation may be external, as in the use of splints or plaster casts, or internal, as in the use of metal plates with screws, or various large metal nails or screws.

An increasingly popular form of bone fixation is a combination of internal and external methods. An external stout metal bar, of square cross-section, is used, to which are attached two or more supporting pieces that have been passed in through the skin and screwed into the bone to secure the fragments.

PSYCHOLOGICAL FIXATION

The term 'fixation' is also used by psychoanalysts to imply an excessively close attachment, to an object or person, of a kind appropriate to an earlier, immature, stage of development. Thus a person may be said to have an anal fixation, a father fixation, an oral fixation, and so on. This state or condition is said to cause various neurotic reactions in the affected individuals, including the inability to form mature relationships.

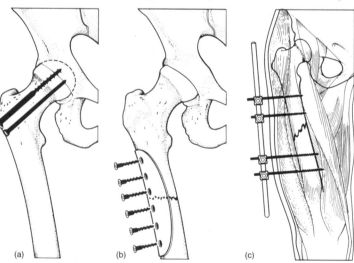

Fixation. Fractures must be immobilized if they are to heal. A plaster cast is not necessarily the best way to immobilize a fracture. Other methods include (a) simple screwing; (b) plate and screws; (c) an external fixator with threaded pins screwed through the shaft of the bone and bolted to a steel rod.

Those who believe the Freudian doctrine that the development of the personality passes through these stages and can be stopped at one or other of them, will have little difficulty in accepting the idea of emotional (affective) fixation. Others may find it hard to swallow.

FK 506

An immunosuppressive drug better known as **tacrolimus**. One of the taxoid drugs.

Flagyl

A brand name for **metronidazole**.

Flamazine

A brand name for **silver sulphadiazine**.

flat foot

See **fallen arches**.

flatulence

See **aerophagy** and **belching**.

flatus

Gas discharged from the bowel by way of the anus. The average person farts at least 20 times a day, and those who are fond of high-fibre foods such as beans and peas substantially exceed the average gas output.

Most of the gas is a mixture of nitrogen and carbon dioxide, both of which are odourless, but there are also small quantities of hydrogen and methane, both of which are inflammable (one of the lesser-known contra-indications to smoking), and hydrogen sulphide, which is very smelly indeed.

flavonoids

A range of many thousands of fat-soluble polyphenols of low molecular weight, ubiquitous in the plant kingdom. Flavonoids have a remarkable range of properties of medical value. They are antimicrobial, anti-allergic, anti-inflammatory, antithrombotic and have some anticancer power. They can modify the actions of numerous enzymes. Some are oestrogenic, some anti-thyroidal.

The principal current interest in flavonoids relates to their antioxidant and free radical-scavenging properties. These are believed to be the basis of the research findings that these compounds can reduce the risk of atherosclerosis and hence heart attacks and strokes by inhibiting the oxidation of low density **lipoproteins**, which is necessary before cholesterol can be incorporated into the atherosclerotic plaque. They also reduce platelet aggregation, which is a prerequisite for the formation of a blood clot.

The recent observation that people who eat chocolate regularly are less prone to atherosclerosis has been attributed to the flavonoid content of chocolate. The principal antioxidant vitamins, C and E, are not flavonoids.

See also **phyto-oestrogens**.

Flaxedil

A brand name for **gallamine triethiodide**.

flea

Small
Siphon...
man. ...
hindlegs ...
remarkab...
bent and ...
the fully ex...
erable dista...

INCIDENCE AN...
Fleas live in th...
and rugs. An a...
remain attache...
include the **chi**...
people walking b...
of attachment ofte...

RISKS
Most fleas are no m... ...ut the Oriental rat flea, *Xenopsylla cheop...* ...nsmitter of bubonic **plague** from rats to human beings. They do this when, having fed on plague-infected rats, their mid-guts have become blocked by the enormous proliferation of plague bacilli. 'Blocked' fleas jump restlessly from host to host trying to relieve their thirst and eventually regurgitate the bacilli into the bite puncture. Alternatively, the bacilli may be inoculated into the skin by scratching in the body of a flea. Rat fleas also transmit mouse typhus to human beings.

flecainide acetate

A drug used to treat severe heart irregularities. A brand name is Tambocor.

Fletcher's Emenette

A brand name for **docusate sodium**.

Flexin Continus

A brand name for **indomethacin**.

-flexion

Suffix meaning 'bending' as in dorsiflexion (bending back).

flies

Flies are insects with one pair of wings. They include the mosquitoes, biting midges, biting blackflies, sandflies, gadflies, blowflies, botflies, tsetse flies and the common housefly *Musca domestica*.

RECOGNITION
Sandflies cause irritating bites which may leave a spot that is troublesome for weeks. They also transmit sandfly fever, Oroya fever and both types of **leishmaniasis**. Mosquitoes also cause persistently irritating bites and transmit **malaria**, **yellow fever**, **filariasis**, and **dengue**.

Midges often attack in swarms, causing multiple skin bumps and sometimes fever and general upset. They can also transmit an unimportant form of filariasis. Blackflies cause severe bites and can so swell the eyelids as to close an eye for weeks. They transmit the form of filariasis known as river blindness (**onchocerciasis**). Female gadflies are ferocious biters: the males are rarely seen. They transmit

flipper limbs

...aremia' (loiasis). Tsetse flies tra...
...swelling' (loiasis). Tsetse flies tra...
(African **trypanosomiasis**).
The common house fly ...
bacillary dysentery (sh...
Almost any organis...
spread by the...
the blinding...
this vecto...

known as 'Calabar
...smit sleeping sickness
... a notorious vector of typhoid,
...gellosis) and amoebic dysentery.
...which can contaminate food can be
...ouse fly. In endemic areas of the world,
...disease trachoma is spread from eye to eye by
...

flipper limbs

See **phocomelia**.

floaters

Semi-transparent, cobweb-like floating shadows seen in the field of vision. Floaters move rapidly with eye movement, but drift slowly when the eyes are still. The rapid movement, often seen 'out of the corner of the eye' has given rise to the name *muscae volitantes* – flitting flies. Floaters do not affect vision.

Most floaters are shadows of developmental remnants in the jelly-like vitreous body of the eye. Some are shadows of condensed vitreous and these are especially common in people in their 60s and 70s when the vitreous body tends to shrink away from the retina. Such floaters are of no significance, and will usually disappear in time.

> Should a sudden cloud of dark floaters appear, especially if associated with bright flashes of light, the implication is that a small tear has occurred in the retina and that there is an incipient risk of retinal detachment. Such a symptom warrants immediate referral to an eye specialist. A large red floater, partly or wholly obscuring vision suggests bleeding into the vitreous (vitreous haemorrhage). This is commonest in long-term diabetics, and this, too, calls for an urgent specialist opinion.

floaters and flashes, visual

See **vitreous detachment**.

Flomax MR

A brand name for **tamsulosin**.

floppy baby

See **amyotonia congenita**, **Prader-Willi syndrome**.

floppy infant syndrome

When a normal baby is supported, face down, with a hand under the chest, the head is held back, the back is held straight, or almost so, and the arms and legs are partly bent. A floppy infant droops over the hand like an inverted U. This state is called hypotonia and it is not, in itself, a disease, but rather an indication of one of a wide variety of conditions. Investigation is needed to determine whether any of these conditions are present.

The possibilities include:

- any major debilitating disease;
- malnutrition;
- a hormonal disorder such as hypothyroidism;

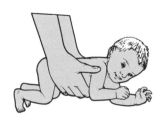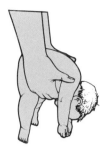

Floppy infant syndrome. Note the striking difference in the muscular response of the normal and the floppy infant.

- **Down's syndrome**;
- **Turner's syndrome**;
- a connective tissue disorder such as **Marfan's syndrome**,
- steogenesis imperfecta or the **Ehlers-Danlos syndrome**;
- a birth brain injury;
- progressive spinal muscular atrophy;
- a **muscular dystrophy** or other muscle disorder (myopathy);
- **myasthenia gravis**;
- infection with the botulinum organism (infant botulism).

Many floppy infants do not have any of these disorders, but this should not discourage investigation, for urgent treatment may be needed.

Florinef

A brand name for **fludrocortisone**.

floss, dental

A strong, often waxed thread used to remove plaque from around the gum margin areas of the teeth and discourage dental caries. The combination of effective brushing and regular flossing provides excellent protection against the formation of acids which damage the enamel.

Flotan

A brand name for **epoprostenol**.

Floxapen

A brand name for **flucloxacillin**.

flu

See **influenza**.

Fluanxol

A brand name for **flupenthixol**.

flucloxacillin

A semisynthetic **penicillin** antibiotic, readily absorbed when taken by mouth and effective against organisms that produce penicillin-destroying enzymes (beta-lactamases). Brand names are Floxapen and, formulated with ampicillin, Magnapen.

fluconazole

A triazole antifungal drug that can be taken by mouth and used to treat generalized fungus infections. Vaginal thrush can be cleared with a single dose. The drug is well tolerated, has few side-effects and is highly effective, but injudicious use may lead to the development of drug resistance. A brand name is Diflucan.

fluctuant

The property, exhibited by a swelling, of yielding to the pressure of the palpating fingers in such a way as to suggest at the swelling contains fluid. When an abscess, for instance, has fully developed, it tends to become fluctuant.

flucytosine

A drug used by hospital specialists to treat dangerous systemic fungus infections A brand name is Ancotil.

Fludara

A brand name for **fludarabine**.

fludarabine

A **cytotoxic** anticancer drug. A brand name is Fludara.

fludrocortisone

A steroid drug with a minor anti-inflammatory action but with a powerful sodium-retaining effect, similar to that of **aldosterone**. It is thus useful in the treatment of Addison's disease, to replace aldosterone. A brand name is Florinef.

fluid-removing drugs

See **diuretic drugs**.

fluid retention

See **diuretic drugs**.

flumazenil

A drug that opposes the action of **benzodiazepine** drugs and can be used to reverse their sedating effect. A brand name is Anexate.

flumethasone

A corticosteroid drug. A brand name of a preparation in which it is combined with an antibacterial drug is Locorten-Vioform.

flunisolide

A corticosteroid drug used in the form of a spray to treat hay fever. A brand name is Syntaris.

flunitrazepam

A **benzodiazepine** drug of moderate length of action used for short periods to treat insomnia. A brand name is Rohypnol.

fluocinolone

A powerful corticosteroid drug used for external applications. Brand names are Synalar, Synalar C and Synalar N.

fluocinonide

A powerful corticosteroid drug used externally to treat severe inflammatory disorders of the skin. A brand name is Metosyn.

fluocortolone

A corticosteroid drug used externally. Brand names are Ultralanum and, with a local anaesthetic to relieve symptoms of haemorrhoids, Ultraproct.

fluorescein

A green dye that fluoresces bright yellow in blue or ultraviolet light. It is used to tag (label) and thus show up **antibodies** in tissues. It is also much used by eye specialists to show up ulcers on the cornea and to delineate for photography the blood vessels of the retina. For the latter purpose, the dye is injected rapidly into the bloodstream (fluorescein angiography). Brand names are fluorescein, Minims fluorescein, Minims lignocaine (a local anaesthetic) and fluorescein, and Minims proxymetacaine (a local anaesthetic) and fluorescein.

Fluorescein

A brand name for **fluorescein**.

fluoridation

The deliberate addition of compounds of fluorine to drinking water supplies in areas deficient in fluoride. The practice is based on the knowledge that an appropriate level of fluoride – about one part per million – in water promotes stronger and healthier teeth with reduced tendency to caries. Many people have protested.

Fluorigard

A brand name for fluoride intended for use as a fluorine supplement.

fluorometholone

A corticosteroid drug in the form of eye drops used to treat inflammatory external eye disorders. A brand name is FML and, formulated with the antibiotic neomycin, FML-NEO.

Fluoroplex

A brand name for fluorouracil.

fluorosis

Long-term poisoning with the element fluorine. This may occur in workers in certain industrial processes including aluminium mining, and insecticide and phosphate fertilizer manufacture. In large dosage, fluorine gradually replaces calcium in the bones, which become soft, chalky and crumbly. Abnormal bone protrusions occur and these cause secondary pressure effects which may be serious, especially in the spinal column, where pressure on the spinal cord or nerve roots may occur.

fluoxetine

An antidepressant drug that acts by prolonging the action of the **neuro-transmitter** 5-hydroxytryptamine (5HT or serotonin). It is a **selective serotonin re-uptake inhibitor**. It is taken by mouth. This drug is currently being taken by some 10 million people, mainly in the USA, and is said to be the most popular psychoactive drug in the history of pharmacology. It has attracted a great deal of attention as a 'mood brightener' and enhancer of optimism. It is claimed to be capable of altering personality for the better.

Possible side-effects include nausea, vomiting, diarrhoea, insomnia, anxiety, outbursts of violence, fever, skin rash and convulsions. This drug can interact dangerously, even fatally, with monoamine oxidase inhibitors (MAOIs). A brand name is Prozac.

flupenthixol

A phenothiazine-like (thioxanthene) antipsychotic drug used to treat schizophrenia and other psychotic disorders. Brand names are Depixol and Fluanxol.

fluphenazine

A **phenothiazine derivative** drug used in the treatment of psychotic conditions. It can be given by injection for long-term effect. Trade names are Modecate and Moditen. The drug is also formulated with other psychoactive substances and produced under the brand names of Motipress and Motival.

flurandrenolone

A moderately powerful corticosteroid drug used externally to treat inflammatory skin disorders. A brand name is Haelan.

flurazepam

A long-acting **benzodiazepine** drug. A brand name is Dalmane.

flurbiprofen

A non-steroidal anti-inflammatory drug (**NSAID**). Brand names are Froben SR and Ocufen.

Flurets

A brand name for a fluoride preparation.

flutamide

A drug that opposes male sex hormones (androgens) and is used to treat advanced cancer of the prostate gland. Brand names are Chimax and Drogenil.

fluticasone

A corticosteroid drug used as an inhalant to treat **asthma** and hay fever. Extensive studies have shown that fluticasone is safe and effective and, in the recommended dosage, does not affect growth in childhood. Brand names are Flixonase (nasal spray), Flixotide (inhaler) and, for external use only, Cutivate.

fluvastatin

A statin drug that blocks the synthesis of cholesterol in the body and can be used to lower unduly high blood cholesterol levels. A brand name is Lescol.

fluvoxamine

A **selective serotonin re-uptake inhibitor** drug. An antidepressant drug that acts by prolonging the action of the **neuro-transmitter** 5-hydroxytryptamine (5HT). A brand name is Faverin.

FML

A brand name for **fluorometholone**.

folic acid

A vitamin of the B group originally derived from spinach leaves, hence the name (Latin *folium*, a leaf). The vitamin is necessary for the synthesis of **DNA** and red blood cells. Deficiency causes megaloblastic anaemia. Folic acid is plentiful in leafy vegetables and in liver but is also produced by bacteria in the bowel and then absorbed into the circulation. Deficiency may occur after antibiotic treatment. Folic acid taken immediately before pregnancy and during the first few weeks can virtually eliminate the risk of embryonic neural tube defects and resulting **spina bifida** or absence of the brain (**anencephaly**) in the baby. It will also reduce the risk of **cleft palate**. Normal dietary intake may not provide enough for this purpose. The drug is available under the brand name Lexpec and, in conjunction with iron salts, under the brand names Lexpec with iron, Pregaday, Ferfolic SV, Ferrograd Folic, Galfer F.A., and Slow-Fe Folic.

folie à deux

A rare delusional psychotic disorder which has developed as a result of a close relationship with another psychotic person.

Shared paranoid disorder sometimes involves more than two people and the literature contains many cases of folie à trois, à quatre, à cinq, and so on. There is a recorded case of a whole family, in which twelve people were affected (folie à douze).

OCCURRENCE

Sometimes called shared paranoid disorder, folie à deux affects women more often than men and occurs in couples relatively isolated from the rest of the community who derive mutual gain from the situation.

RECOGNITION

The dominant person is the one with the original delusional psychosis and the submissive person gains the acceptance of the other by adopting the delusions. At the same time, the dominant person retains some link with the real world through the medium of the partner. There is often a deep emotional rapport and suicide pacts occur. The delusions concerned are usually nearer to reality than in some other psychoses and are often persecutory or hypochondriacal.

TREATMENT

The most effective treatment is to separate the pair, after which the induced disorder will, with supportive management, gradually disappear. The dominant partner needs more intensive conventional treatment.

folinic acid

A drug used to treat megaloblastic anaemia that has resulted from folic deficiency. A brand name is Refolinon.

folk medicine

A system of treatments based on traditional or anecdotal methods of dealing with sickness. Folk medicine is part of the cultural tradition of all societies and has, in the past, commanded wide support for its empirical and sometimes magical claims.

DOES IT WORK?

When attempts have been made to systematize and explain the logic behind folk medicine, as has been done by the Chinese, the crudity of the reasoning has become plain. The general level has often been of the order of such propositions as: 'because this plant resembles a human womb, it must be good for labour pains'. Over the centuries, great herbals of plants with attributed properties, often based on reasoning such as this, have been written and have acquired status and veneration by age and perpetuation.

> Regrettably, the present age, for all its science and technology, is no less gullible and naive in its acceptance of asserted wisdom than any in the past. Folk medicine has become an expensively packaged and advertised commodity and whole industries are devoted to the production and sale of 'remedies' which have little therapeutic value.

folliculitis

Inflammation of multiple hair follicles in the skin, from infection, usually by *staphylococci*. The result is multiple small **boils** or **pimples**.

follitropin alpha

A gonadotrophin, a drug that promotes ovulation and is used to treat infertility resulting from absence of ovulation. A brand name is Gonal-F.

follitropin beta

A drug that stimulated the ovaries into producing eggs and is used to treat infertility. A brand name is Puregon.

fomites

Anything touched or handled by a person with an infectious disease, which thus becomes contaminated by organisms and may transmit the disease to others. Common examples are dressings, bedclothes, washing flannels, towels, eating and drinking utensils and reading material.

fontanelle

The vault of the growing skull of the baby and young infant is made of separate plates of bone which are close together except at the points where more than two meet. Towards the front of the vertex of the head, the meeting of four large plates – the two forehead (frontal) bones and the two side (parietal) bones – leaves a central gap known as the anterior fontanelle. The rear (posterior) fontanelle also lies centrally between the two parietal bones and the single rear occipital bone. The fontanelles are covered by scalp and skin and can easily be felt, as soft depressions, by gentle pressure with the fingers.

The fontanelles allow moulding of the skull during birth and allow for growth of the bone. The anterior fontanelle normally closes between 10 and 14 months of age, but the limits are wide and may extend from three to 18 months. The posterior fontanelle usually closes by two months.

food additives

Substances added to food to preserve its freshness or physical properties; to maintain or supplement its nutritional value; to improve its appearance or flavour; and to enhance its texture. Without additives, much food would soon be spoiled and wasted or would have to be consumed in a much less palatable condition.

BENEFICIAL ADDITIVES

While it is proper that public concern should be voiced about what we unwittingly eat, it is only fair to say that additives have had a strongly anti-biased press with little emphasis on the benefits.

Common additives, of unquestionable value, are B vitamins in bread and cereals; vitamin C in fruit drinks; vitamins A and D in milk and margarine; iodine in table salt; and iron in baby foods. These additives have largely eliminated vitamin and mineral deficiencies in developed countries.

RISKS

Flavourings and colourings include sugar, salt, mustard, pepper, monosodium glutamate and tartrazine. Preservatives include salt, sugar, sodium nitrite, sodium benzoate, and the antioxidants BHT (butylated hydroxytoluene) and BHA (butylated hydroxyanisole). Monosodium glutamate is believed to cause the '**Chinese restaurant syndrome**'. Tartrazine sensitivity is well-known. It causes allergic reactions such as running nose (allergic rhinitis), angioedema, urticaria and **asthma**. Sulphites can cause asthma in susceptible people. BHT and BHA are not thought to have undesirable effects, but the American Food and Drugs Administration are reviewing them for possible risks.

The case of saccharine is interesting. The FDA, in compliance with a clause in the Food, Drug and Cosmetic Act, that any substance known to be capable, in any dose, of causing cancer in man or animals should be banned, placed saccharine on the proscribed list. The result was such a public outcry that the ruling had to be reversed.

food allergy

Sensitivity to one or more of the components of normal diets. Food allergy is much less common than unscientific claims might suggest and established methods of testing, including double-blind trials, have shown that food allergy is not the basis of the many disorders commonly claimed to arise from it. Peanut allergy is rare but may be very dangerous. Monosodium glutamate can cause the '**Chinese restaurant syndrome**'. Tartrazine sensitivity is established. Other additives, such as sulphur dioxide, sulphites, azo dyes and benzoate preservatives also sometimes cause genuine allergic reactions, such as asthma. Allergy to basic foodstuffs seldom occurs.

food assimilation inadequacy

See **short bowel syndrome**.

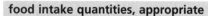

food intake quantities, appropriate

See **recommended daily amounts (RDAs)**.

food irradiation

The treatment of food by strong ionizing radiation, such as gamma rays, so as to kill bacteria and insect pests and to delay natural changes in fruit and vegetables. Irradiation does not eliminate existing toxins or viruses. If the food is tightly sealed in a container, such as a polythene bag, before irradiation, contained organisms are destroyed and further contamination does not occur.

EFFECTS

Food irradiation by gamma rays does not induce radioactivity, and the effects are chemical only. The main effect is the production of highly reactive, short-lived substances (**free radicals**) which cause cell death in living organisms. Food molecules are also affected and there may be changes in flavour and some loss of vitamins.

> A committee of the World Health Organization has expressed the view that irradiation of any food commodity, up to a dose of one million rads, would present no nutritional or bacteriological hazard to the consumer. WHO experts point out the benefits of irradiation – the destruction of disease germs, such as Salmonella in poultry, and the prolongation of shelf-life which would increase the food supply. Food irradiation is employed in nearly 40 countries, including Britain.

food poisoning

A group of disorders featuring nausea, vomiting, loss of appetite, fever, abdominal pain and diarrhoea.

POSSIBLE CAUSES

Food poisoning is caused either by living organisms present in food, which incubate and reproduce in the body until enough are present to cause illness; or by contamination of food by the toxins of organisms which have incubated outside the body. In the former case there is usually a delay of a day or two before symptoms occur; in the latter, symptoms come on within hours. Food poisoning can also be caused by inorganic or organic poisons such as metal salts or plant or animal poisons.

Bacterial toxins are very powerful and produce acute, but usually short-lived effects. A common cause of toxin contamination of food is the presence of septic spots on the skin of food-handlers. In this case the staphylococcal toxin is the cause of the illness. Living staphylococci also contaminate the food and these may incubate to produce further toxin. The commonest bacterial contamination of food is by *Salmonella typhimurium*, which is commonly found in meats and eggs. Poor standards of hygiene mean food is often contaminated by human faeces.

BOTULISM

The organism *Clostridium botulinum* can survive in canned or bottled foodstuffs. It is very occasionally found in meat pastes and other processed animal products and the great majority of cases have arisen from food prepared in the home and inadequately sterilized. The result is the dangerous condition of **botulism**, which, fortunately, is rare. This word comes from the Latin *botulus* meaning 'a sausage'. The condition, which

is grave and often fatal, was first observed in Germany and rightly attributed to eating contaminated sausage. It was many years before the contaminating organism, *Clostridium botulinum*, was isolated and the extraordinary power of its toxin appreciated. Botulinum toxin is one of the most powerful poisons known to man. It operates by interfering with the release of an essential neuro-transmitter – acetylcholine – at nerve endings. The effect of this is that nerves are unable to pass on their impulses to make muscles contract. A dose measured in thousandths of a gram is sufficient to kill.

The onset of symptoms is abrupt and occurs from four hours to a week after eating the contaminated food. The mouth becomes dry and the vision blurred and doubled; the upper lids droop; there is sickness, vomiting and diarrhoea with cramping pain in the abdomen. Soon swallowing becomes impossible and the muscles of the limbs become weak, almost paralysed. The gravest danger is that the breathing should become paralysed. In this event, death is certain unless respiration can be maintained artificially.

POISONS

Naturally occurring poisons include those in mushrooms, such as *Amanita phalloides*.

foot pain on activity

See **tarsal tunnel syndrome**.

Foradil

A brand name for **eformoterol**.

foramen

A natural hole in a bone, for the passage of some other structure such as a nerve, artery or a vein.

foreign body in eye

See *First Aid*.

forensic medicine

The application of science in the investigation of criminal cases. Forensic scientists must be experts in the science of disease processes (pathology), in the action of poisons (toxicology), in the actions and effects of firearms and other offensive weapons, in the signs of assault, including rape, in some aspects of dentistry and in the principles of determining the time of death. They are concerned with establishing the cause of death and will usually perform a post-mortem examination (autopsy) on the victim to determine signs of injury or disease that may have contributed to the death. They must be familiar with the detection of the presence of poisons or drugs found in a victim's body.

Forensic anthropology is a speciality concerned with the study of human bones and skeletal remains and, if possible, the reconstruction, from these, of an identifiable image of the deceased. Forensic dentistry applies dental evidence to the identification of human remains and is concerned with bite-mark impressions. Forensic psychiatrists study human behaviour and personality in relation to criminal conduct. They are also concerned with the difficult question of determining the degree of criminal responsibility in a malefactor, and in deciding whether an accused person is mentally fit to stand trial.

Forensic chemists and biologists, working in crime laboratories all over the world, are concerned with the evidential significance of materials such as dust, soil, skin scrapings, hair, seminal fluid, blood, natural and synthetic fibres, paint chips, fingerprints and many others. **DNA fingerprinting** has become an important means of the identification or elimination of suspects.

forensic pathologist

A doctor concerned with the application of medical science to the investigation of certain forms of crime including assault, rape, poisoning, shooting and murder. He or she is skilled in determining the time of death and in the evidential significance of such things as skin scrapings, hair, seminal fluid, blood and DNA samples.

foreskin

The skin of the penis forms a free fold, the foreskin (prepuce) which encloses the glans and is attached at the neck of the penis. This skin is normally adherent to the glans at birth, but some time before the third year should become freely retractable so that the glans may be fully exposed. The prepuce contains, on its inner surface, modified sebaceous glands and the secretion of these, together with dead cells from the skin lining, form **smegma**, a whitish, greasy material which, unless removed by regular washing, becomes cheesy and foul-smelling and may cause inflammation.

Throughout the centuries, man has been remarkably preoccupied with his foreskin. The apparent fascination with the idea of cutting off this inoffensive little bit of skin permeates the theology of half a dozen religions of mankind. More recently, circumcision has proved a lucrative source of income for mercenary surgeons. The mythology of the foreskin includes two main propositions – that uncircumcised men get cancer of the penis and that their consorts get cancer of the cervix. Both propositions are false.

foreskin problems

See **circumcision**, **foreskin**.

foreskin sebaceous secretion

See **smegma**.

forgetfulness

A natural consequence of the overburdening of a well-stocked mind with trivia. Failure to retrieve a memory becomes more likely the larger the number of similar memories that depend on the same cues. When cues prompt further cues, as in the chain of associations in an account of a subject of interest, forgetfulness is reduced. Mood, too, affects forgetfulness. Happy events are better remembered when happy, and sad events when sad. Much forgetfulness is purposive. See also **amnesia**.

> The widely believed view that, under hypnosis, every previously observed detail can be recalled with complete accuracy, is nonsense. Recollections obtained in this way are usually unreliable.

-form

Suffix meaning 'shaped' as in fusiform (spindle shaped).

formestane

An **aromatase inhibitor** drug used as an anticancer treatment for oestrogen-dependent tumours. A brand name is Lentaron.

formication

A peculiar sensation, as of many ants crawling under the skin, characteristic of a number of drug toxic effects or of certain disorders of the nervous system. The word should be pronounced with care.

formulary

A book of formulae used in the preparation of medicines, or a book of drug actions, side-effects and dosage for the use of prescribing doctors. In Britain, a popular publication is the *British National Formulary*, produced at regular intervals by the British Medical Association and the Pharmaceutical Society of Great Britain. This is an attempt to encourage rational and cost-effective prescribing by doctors.

Fortagesic

A brand name for a mixture of **paracetamol** and **pentazocine**.

Fortipine LA

A brand name for **nifedipine**.

Fortral

A brand name for **pentazocine**.

Fortum

A brand name for ceftazidime.

Fosamax

A brand name for **alendronate**.

foscarnet

A **DNA polymerase inhibitor** drug used to treat severe **herpes** infections in immunocompromised people and cytomegalovirus internal eye infections in people with **AIDS**. A brand name is Foscavir.

Foscavir

A brand name for **foscarnet**.

fosfestrol

An **oestrogen** drug used to treat cancer of the prostate. A brand name is Honvan.

fosinopril

An **angiotensin converting enzme** (ACE) **inhibitor** drug used to treat heart failure and high blood pressure. A brand name is Staril.

fracture, bone

A bone break (fracture) occurs when a force is applied which deforms the bone beyond its elastic limit. Excessive force will fracture any bone, but a bone which has been generally weakened by a disease such as **osteoporosis**, or locally weakened by a tumour or cyst, will fracture on the application of lesser force. Such a fracture is called a 'pathological fracture'.

TYPES OF FRACTURE

Fractures may be straight across the bone (transverse), oblique or spiral, or the bone may be shattered into pieces (comminuted). Transverse fractures are often harder to align and immobilize than apparently more serious oblique or spiral fractures. Young bone, subjected to bending stress, often fractures on one side but bends on the other. This is poetically described as a **greenstick fracture**.

Simple fractures are those in which the overlying soft tissue is intact and only bone is significantly injured. In compound fractures, the fractured bone is exposed and infected and the case consequently much more serious. Complicated fractures are those associated with injury to other nearby structures such as major blood vessels and nerves. Fracture-dislocations pass across a joint and involve abnormal displacement of the joint surfaces from one another.

RECOGNITION AND SYMPTOMS

Signs of a fracture include pain and swelling, abnormal angulation of the limb or part, skin discolouration, inability to move the part, and a grinding sensation (crepitation) felt in the limb on attempts at movement.

> Unless imperative, a person with a fracture should not be moved until some form of effective splint has been applied which prevents movement of the joints above and below the fracture.

TREATMENT

For a satisfactory outcome, fractures must be properly aligned. Alignment is opposed by the contraction of adjacent muscles and a general anaesthetic and strong traction is often needed to bring the fractured bone ends into alignment. Once aligned, the fracture must be secured by some form of **fixation** until the repair is strong enough for weight-bearing. This may take from a few weeks to a few months, depending on the bone involved and on the occurrence of complications such as infection or interference with the blood supply to fragments.

Healing involves the removal, by special cells called osteoclasts, of damaged bone spicules, and the formation, by other cells called osteoblasts, of a tissue called a callus, which forms a large smooth swelling around the break. In the course of time, this is nicely smoothed off and eventually the bone returns to its normal thickness.

fracture fixator, non-plaster

See **external fixator**.

fracture, partial

See **greenstick fracture**.

fragile X syndrome

Among the mentally handicapped, there are three times as many males as females. This is largely due to forms of mental defect which are transmitted by genes situated on the male X chromosome. One of the commonest of these – accounting for about one-third of the X chromosome defects – is the fragile X syndrome, so called because the chromosome has a constriction near the end of the long arm. The fragile X syndrome is second only to **Down's syndrome** as a cause of mental defect.

INCIDENCE

About one-third of the females carrying this mutation on one of their two X chromosomes are also mentally retarded. This means that for every affected female there are two unaffected carriers of the gene. About one girl in 600 carries the fragile X mutation and thus has a one in two risk that any son will be mentally retarded and a one in six chance of a mentally retarded daughter.

RECOGNITION

Men with this disorder have unusually high foreheads, large jaws, asymmetrical faces, long protuberant ears and large testicles. They have an IQ below 50 and are prone to violent outbursts and **autistic** behaviour. Their psychotic-like reactions can to some extent be controlled by giving folic acid.

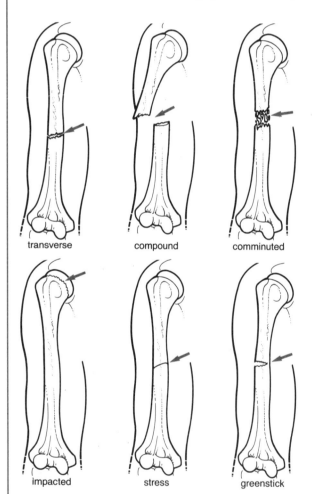

Fractures. The diagram shows some of the types of fracture. Note that a compound fracture is important solely because it is invariably infected. A twisting force will produce a longitudinal spiral fracture.

transverse   compound   comminuted

impacted   stress   greenstick

Screening for the characteristic chromosome can be done by amniocentesis or, at an even earlier stage, by chorionic villus sampling. Such screening might be offered to obviously high-risk groups such as members of families with retarded males. All mentally retarded females, especially those on the borderline who might be expected to get pregnant, should have a chromosome analysis. Sisters and aunts of affected individuals might also be checked.

Fragmin

A brand name for **dalteparin sodium**.

frameshift mutation

A genetic mutation caused by the addition or deletion of a number of DNA elements other than three. Because the genetic code consists of codons (groups of three **base pairs**), such a change shifts the reading frame for translation so all adjacent codons are changed and a completely new set is read into the messenger ribonucleic acid (mRNA).

framycetin

An **antibiotic** drug used externally for skin infections or as eye or ear drops. Brand names are Sofradex and Soframycin.

frangula

A drug for constipation. Formulated with the bulking agent sterculia, under the brand name Normacol Plus.

Franol

Trade names for **ephedrine** formulated with other drugs.

freckle

Small, yellowish or brownish skin spots due to a local accumulation of melanin, the normal skin pigment. Melanin-containing cells enlarge under the influence of sunlight, especially in the fair-skinned and, once established, are usually permanent. Their number and size can be minimized by protection from the ultraviolet in sunlight, by shading or by the use of sunscreen lotions containing para-aminobenzoic acid.

The melanin is located quite near the surface and for those desperate to be rid of their freckles there is the possibility of a chemical skin peel. But after such an assault on the skin, exposure to sunlight becomes even more dangerous, so it is better to avoid it in the first place.

free-floating anxiety

An all-pervasive, unfocused fear which is not produced by any appropriate cause or attached to any particular idea. Such anxiety is a feature of what is now called a **generalized anxiety disorder** – a state lasting for at least six months and featuring excessive or unrealistic worry about everything.

free radicals

Unstable atoms or molecules containing at least one unpaired electron (negative charge) making them highly reactive. Free radicals are produced by the body as a consequence of normal metabolism. However sometimes the body, triggered by factors such as cigarette smoke, ultraviolet light or illness, increases its free radical production, releasing more of the unstable atoms or molecules that it needs.

Some free radicals are stabilized by their peculiar structure and exist for appreciable lengths of time. But the great majority have only a very brief independent existence before either taking up an extra electron or giving one up. From the medical point of view we are interested mainly in two free radicals – the hydroxyl radical (-OH) and the superoxide radical which consists of two linked oxygen atoms (O_2) with a single, unpaired electron.

EFFECTS

When a free radical gives up an electron or captures an electron from some other molecule to make up the stable pair, the adjacent molecule affected is, itself, converted into a radical. This starts a chain reaction that can move quickly and destructively through a tissue. Fortunately, the hydroxyl free radical does not normally occur in living systems because of the strength of the bonds holding the water molecules together. But if a person is exposed to radiation, or to other disease-causing processes that promote free radicals, these bonds can be broken so that hydroxyl radicals result. This is the basis of the often fatal damage that occurs in people with radiation sickness.

If hydroxyl radicals attack DNA, chain reactions run along the DNA molecule causing damage to, and mutations in, the genetic material or even actual breakage of the DNA strands. The body does its best to repair this damage by the natural processes of DNA replication, but imperfect repair leaves altered DNA and can give rise to cancer. When strong X-ray and gamma radiation is deliberately used to destroy cancers it does so primarily by producing large numbers of hydroxyl free radicals.

RISKS

Recent research has shown that the production of free radicals is involved in many disease processes, and in the effect on the body of poisons, drugs, metals, cigarette smoke, car exhausts, heat, lack of oxygen, even sunlight. In general terms, the damage that is done by free radicals features the chemical reaction known as *oxidation* and free radical attacks on tissue is known as oxidative stress.

ANTIOXIDANTS

There is a rapidly increasing body of evidence that a class of substances known as antioxidants can 'mop up' free radicals and reduce their damaging effect on the body. In the past few years the number of medical and scientific publications on free radicals and antioxidants has grown almost exponentially. There is even a journal devoted exclusively to the subject. This is one of the growth zones in medical research.

See also **anti-oxidants and vitamins**.

French paradox

An informal term for the unexplained fact that, in spite of a national diet characterized by a high fat and cholesterol intake, the French enjoy almost the lowest incidence of coronary heart disease in Europe. Possible explanations include the antioxidant effect of **flavonoids** in red wine and the protective effect of olive oil. This hypothesis is one of the reasons for the current strength of medical interest in research showing that wine is beneficial to health. Another reason may be that doctors, like most enlightened people, enjoy drinking wine.

Freon

A brand name for the chlorofluorocarbons (CFCs) used in refrigeration and as aerosol propellants. Because of their catalytic effect on ozone in the stratosphere, freons have been strongly indicted as causes of ozone layer depletion and global warming.

frequency

This usually refers, in a colloquial kind of way, to frequency of urination – passing urine more often than usual. This may be due to the irritation of infection, to excessive fluid intake, to pregnancy, to the use of a drug which causes excessive urinary output (a diuretic) or, in men, to an enlarged prostate gland which obstructs outflow to the extent that the bladder can only be partially emptied. Frequency of urination is sometimes of psychological origin.

Freudian slip

A Freudian slip, or parapraxis as Freud called it, is any minor error, or muddle, in speech or writing – such as are inevitable in the operation of any system as complex as that of the human mind – which seems to reveal a hidden thought. Freud insisted that such slips were invariably of the highest significance as throwing light on the preoccupations, conflicts and repressed wishes of the unconscious mind. He claimed that errors always indicated the true state of the unconscious wish.

While there are numerous obvious instances in which errors may display opinions and prejudices we are trying to conceal, the insistence that every slip is of this kind is highly significant is overly dogmatic.

Freudian theory

The Austrian psychiatrist Sigmund Freud (1856–1939) was not the originator, but was certainly the best-known guru of **psychoanalysis**. His ideas have had an immense influence on 20th-century culture. To some extent, this was because of his intense preoccupation with sexual matters at a time when such subjects were considered unsuitable for polite society.

Freud was a precocious scholar who read Shakespeare at eight and steeped himself in the Latin, Greek, French and German classics. His early medical studies into neurology brought him into contact with the famous neurologist Jean Martin Charcot in Paris, who had clearly recognized the influence of the mind on physical symptoms.

FREE ASSOCIATION

Freud adopted Sir Francis Galton's method of free association and, in the repressive times in which he lived, inevitably found a strong sexual content in the half-concealed thoughts of his patients. This so impressed him that he became convinced that sex was at the basis of everything, and he gradually evolved an empirical system of thought, based on literary rather than scientific principles. Freud repeatedly insisted that his methods were scientific and, although in the context of his time they may have been, they do not now appear to be so.

THE UNCONSCIOUS MIND

Freud concentrated on the unconscious mind and its actions as motivators of behaviour. He was deeply concerned with the role of sexual symbolism in thought and dreams, and came to regard every elongated object as symbolic of the penis and every receptacle as symbolizing the vagina. He believed, rightly, that early experiences have a profound effect on later behaviour and personality and that these experiences became repressed and lay hidden under layers of subsequent mental accretion, but could be uncovered by analysis. He asserted, without proof, that the uncovering of these early experiences would disperse the psychopathology which he claimed they had caused.

He proposed arbitrary divisions of the mind into **ego**, **superego** and **id**. He asserted that infants pass though three stages – oral (birth to 18 months), anal (two to five years) and phallic (five years onward), and that the personality could be fixed at any of these stages with dire consequences, curable only by psychoanalysis. He claimed that little boys want to kill their fathers and have sexual intercourse with their mothers – the Oedipus complex – and that they fear being found out and having their penises cut off (the castration complex).

REACTIONS TO FREUDIAN THEORY

Freud's publications aroused shock and horror, especially in the orthodox medical community. But they also brought him a degree of fame, not to say notoriety, which eventually was damaging to his judgement and led him to suppose that his assertions were infallible and that anyone who doubted them was wicked. Soon the Freudian school started accepting unquestioned dogma, insisting on belief in spite of clear evidence to the contrary and persecuting heretics. Two of the best-known defectors were Adler and Jung, each of whom formed his own school of psychological thought.

VALIDITY OF FREUDIAN THEORY

There is little in Freud's voluminous and widely read literary output to support his assertion that he was a scientist. Most of his claims for psychoanalysis are essentially unverifiable but, even more damaging, are incapable of being disproved – a reliable feature, according to the philosopher Karl Popper (1902–94), of a pseudo-science.

FREUD'S CONTRIBUTION

Freud's major contribution to thought – and it is a very large one – was to draw attention to the powerful influence the unconscious mind has on behaviour and conscious thought. His school of psychoanalysis has been less successful and there is little or no evidence, apart from the assertions of its practitioners, that the application of Freudian ideas in psychoanalysis has any intrinsic value in the treatment of psychological disturbance.

Close, one-to-one relations between humans can be highly therapeutic, especially if one of them is in a position of authority and purports to be keenly interested in the mental activities and problems of the other. But the outcome is more likely to depend on the experience, maturity and human and intellectual qualities of the dominant partner than on whether the 'patient' feared castration in infancy or was prevented from playing with his or her faeces.

Friedreich's ataxia

An inherited disorder of the cerebellum and spinal cord which appears first in childhood or adolescence and which leads to unsteady gait, extremely defective movement of the upper limbs, difficulty in speaking and loss of sensation. The feet become arched (pes cavus), the spine bent sideways (**scoliosis**) and the heart muscle damaged. There is great variation in severity from case to case, but no treatment is of any avail.

frigidity

A now pejorative term, referring to a woman, and signifying loss of sexual desire or of the ability to be 'turned on' sexually. Frigidity is not the female equivalent of impotence in the male since men may fail although sexually aroused, or perform although indifferent.

POSSIBLE CAUSES

The problem may be mental or physical in origin. Often, a failure to respond sexually is merely a reflection of the very natural disinclination for sex with a disliked or unattractive man. To designate this as 'frigidity' is a face-saving reflection of male machismo and chauvinism. Other common causes are fatigue, recent childbirth with residual tenderness, pain on intercourse (**dyspareunia**), depression, fear of pregnancy, mourning following an abortion, or psychological trauma following rape. Some drugs directly or indirectly reduce libido and these include drugs for high blood pressure, for depression and for insomnia.

Many cases of lack of female sexual interest are simply due to lack of affection, or the expression of it, by the partner; lack of tenderness; lack of technique; or the habit of using sex as a means of self-gratification rather than as a vehicle for the expression of love. An intense preoccupation with the female orgasm has little to do with some of the deeper values of human relationships. Many women enjoy a satisfying sex life without even having experienced one. Some men insist on convulsive displays of sexual feeling only as a boost to their own egos.

TREATMENT

When the relationship between the partners is good, these difficulties can almost always be overcome, but counselling, or even sex therapy, may be necessary. Deliberate voluntary abstinence is often helpful.

Frisium

A brand name for **clobazam**.

Froben

A brand name for **flurbiprofen**.

fronte

Latin root meaning 'forehead' as in frontal (of the forehead).

frostbite

Freezing of tissues, usually the tips of the extremities. The damage is caused by the formation of expanding ice crystals in the tissues and the local deprivation of vital blood supply.

RECOGNITION AND SYMPTOMS

Extreme cold has an anaesthetic effect so that freezing can occur without warning, but usually, prior to onset of freezing, there is severe pain. The affected skin is white, hard and numb and blisters on thawing. Surface freezing may lead to loss of areas of skin, but deep freezing may cause **gangrene**.

TREATMENT

Surface frostbite should be treated by thawing with one's own or another person's body heat or, if available, with warm water. The part should not be exercised, as tissue nutrition is at a premium and oxygen must be conserved. Rubbing with snow is foolish and damaging.

Deep frostbite should be thawed with warm water. Because of the anaesthesia, hot water is dangerous. The whole body should, if possible, be warmed. Delay should be minimized. Recovery is often surprisingly good, but there is usually a residual numbness and a greatly increased susceptibility to further cold injury. Gangrene will usually require amputation.

frottage

Rubbing the body against another person, usually a stranger, for the purposes of sexual gratification. Frottage is a male activity usually engaged in in densely packed crowds, as in the London Underground during the rush hour. Without exposing himself, the active male rubs his genitals against a woman's buttock or thigh.

frozen shoulder

A painful, persistent stiffness of the shoulder joint which precludes normal movement. The condition may follow an injury, over-enthusiastic exercising, a stroke, a **heart attack** (myocardial infarction) or may occur for no known reason. It is uncommon in young people. The trouble is due to inflammation leading to thickening of the capsule of the joint.

A variety of treatments are used, suggesting that none is universally satisfactory. Heat lamps, cold compresses, ultrasound, manipulation under anaesthesia, even lasers have been used. Sometimes a depot injection of steroids will be helpful in controlling the inflammation and relieving the pain, but this is not entirely without risk, especially if there is any possibility of introducing infection. Most cases resolve spontaneously within two years.

frusemide

A drug that causes an increased output of urine (a diuretic) so as to relieve the body of unwanted retained water (oedema). Frusemide acts on the kidney tubules where it

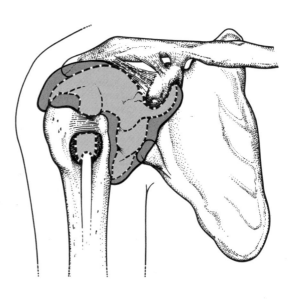

Frozen shoulder. The diagram shows the capsule of the shoulder joint which, in this condition, is inflamed and thickened. Most cases recover with or without treatment.

interferes with chloride and sodium reabsorption from the dilute filtered urine. This prevents reabsorption of water into the blood and the result is a large volume of dilute urine. A brand name is Lasix. The drug is one of the ingredients in a range of diuretic preparations such as Diumide-K Continus, Fru-Co, Frumil, Frusene, Frusol, Lasikal, Lasilactone and Lasoride.

Frusene

A brand name for **triamterene** in combination with another diuretic drug.

frustration

The emotion resulting from the blocking of aims. Some measure of frustration is inseparable from normal life, but, for various reasons, some people suffer a much higher level of frustration than others.

POSSIBLE CAUSES

Chronic frustration may occur when people attempt to achieve goals which are inherently beyond their capacity. It may also result from the wish to reach mutually incompatible, or equally attractive but mutually exclusive, goals. In the workaday world, frustration is extremely common. People must work to live, but the work is often uncongenial, and the forced submission to disliked superiors unpleasant. In this situation the conflict between the desire for money and the desire for emancipation from the hated work situation is a fruitful source of frustration.

POSSIBLE EFFECTS

Reactions to frustration vary widely. One of the commonest is **anger** which leads to aggressive attitudes to others, often to those unconnected with the source of the anger. Anger directed against the source is often dangerous, so it is displaced and directed against a safer, if inappropriate, target. Displaced anger is a common cause of marital discord. Another reaction is to return to the methods of childhood – the withdrawal into a fantasy world in which everything is exactly as it ought to be. Some people respond to frustration by a mechanism of repression – dismissing from the consciousness the awareness of the unpleasant facts. This response is liable to become a source of later trouble. Repressed problems do not go away, nor do they cease to distress. Only the effects are changed, and not always for the better.

OVERCOMING FRUSTRATION

The most mature and effective reaction to frustration is to look directly at the problem in an analytical way and try to decide what, even at the cost of some risk, must be done to correct or at least reduce it. Frustration in one area of life is commonly balanced by achievement in another, and many mature people have found adequate consolation in this way.

Fucidin

A brand name for **fusidic acid**.

Fucithalmic

A brand name for **sodium fusidate**.

-fuge

Suffix meaning 'flee' as in centrifuge (running from centre).

fugue

A rare psychological reaction in which the affected person takes on a new identity and wanders away from the old environment, apparently in a state of amnesia for the former life. Such people may take up a new occupation and, indeed, assume a completely new life. They are usually quiet, inoffensive people living a somewhat reclusive existence and avoid drawing attention to themselves.

POSSIBLE CAUSES

Fugue occurs as a response to an intolerable situation and it is likely that the 'amnesia' is a mechanism allowing the affected person to accept a course of action which would normally be considered outrageous. It is noteworthy that the amnesia is highly selective and does not preclude use of the previous general education. If there is recovery from the fugue, amnesia for the period of the fugue occurs. Deserters from military service or from nagging wives are among the ranks of the fugue 'victims'.

It is apparent that, for some, the fugue represents a reasonable and logical solution to a major life problem.

Fulcin

A brand name for **griseofulvin**.

fumigation

The use of toxic gases, vapours or volatile solids to kill bacteria, insect pests or rodents. Fumigation may be used in buildings and food stores, or in the open air if sheeting is used to confine the agents used. Poisons used include arsenic compounds, chlorine gas, organo-phosphorous compounds and cyanide. Clearly, such agents must be used under the most strictly controlled conditions and the fumigators must wear respirators or self-contained breathing apparatus. Detection devices are used to ensure that local concentrations are reduced to safe levels before public access is allowed.

Formerly, fumigation was employed in sick rooms after infectious disease. Nowadays, it is considered sufficient to remove all possible contaminated objects (**fomites**) and rely on normal standards of domestic cleanliness.

functional disorders

See **hysteria**.

fungal infections

The commonest fungal infections are known as the epidermophytoses – a term implying that it is the outer layer of the skin that is infected.

RINGWORM

The commonest group of skin fungi come from the genus *Trichophyton* and these cause the range of infections commonly called 'ringworm' – but having nothing to do with worms – which include '**athlete's foot**' (tinea pedis), body *epidermophytosis* (tinea corporis) and fungus infection of the nails (tinea unguium). **Tinea** favours the hot, moist and sometimes unwashed areas of the body and so is particularly prevalent on the feet, groin and in the armpits.

The term 'ringworm' arises from the tendency for patches of fungus infection to clear centrally and spread outwards into fresh uninfected skin. This produces the characteristic expanding ring of untreated tinea. Tinea of the nails is peculiarly persistent as the fungus becomes incorporated into the nail bed, so that even removal of the thickened, distorted infected nail is unlikely to cure the condition. Indeed, prior to the development of the drug griseofulvin, tinea of the nails, once established, was often present for life.

CANDIDA

Candidiasis is infection with the fungus *Candida albicans*, a yeast fungus which favours the mouth and the vagina. It causes 'thrush' – a distressingly irritating vaginitis which often spreads to the sexual consort, causing a similar irritation of the glans of the penis. Transmission is usually sexual. *Candida albicans* also causes mouth thrush in infants – white patches in the mouth and throat – and may occur in even the most well cared-for babies. Otherwise, the condition is most common in the debilitated and the neglected and is less prevalent today than in the past.

Widespread candidiasis in males suggests immunodeficiency and is a common feature of **AIDS** in which it tends to affect the mouth and anal region and spread inwards to involve both the intestinal tract and the respiratory system.

OPPORTUNISTIC FUNGI

Internal fungal infections are, in general, uncommon, except in immunocompromised people. Fungi which take advantage of such people are known as opportunistic fungi, and such infections tend to occur in very debilitated people, in those with widespread cancer, severe **diabetes**, or chronic infections such as **tuberculosis**. People on very heavy doses of antibiotics, those who are having to have immunosuppressive treatment and those with a long-term intravenous drip or a vein cannula are especially prone to opportunistic fungus infection. Such infections may involve any internal organ, including the heart or the eyes.

TREATMENT

Fortunately, there have been steady advances in the development of antifungal drugs and it is now often possible to control such infections.

fungicidal

Capable of killing fungi. The term is used both for drugs that can do this without, at the same time, damaging the infected person, and for agencies that can destroy fungi and their spores outside the body.

Fungilin

A brand name for **amphotericin**.

Fungizone

A brand name for **amphotericin**.

funny bone

A facetious term for that part of the elbow formed by the head of the ulna bone. The important ulnar nerve runs across this bone in a groove and, in this area, is exposed to trauma. If struck, there is severe pain, such as to evoke a

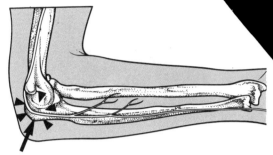

'Funny bone'. This lay term refers to the part of the elbow at which the ulnar nerve is vulnerably exposed. A blow to the point of the elbow may cause strong and painful stimulation of this nerve with an obvious reaction from the victim.

sharp physical response. There may be some humour in this, for the unsympathetic observer, but the victim is unlikely to be amused.

Furacin

A brand name for nitrofurazone.

Furadantin

A brand name for **nitrofurantoin**.

Furamide

A brand name for **diloxanide**.

furuncle

A **boil**.

fusafungine

An anti-inflammatory and antibiotic spray preparation for throat infections. A brand name is Locabiotal.

fusidic acid

A steroid antibiotic used in the form of sodium fusidate against penicillin-resistant (beta-lactamase-producing) staphylococci. It has no value against streptococci and is usually given in conjunction with another antibiotic such as **flucloxacillin**. Brand names are Fucidin and Fucithalmic.

-fy

Suffix meaning 'make, cause' as in magnify (make large).

Fybogel

A brand name for **ispaghula**.

Fybozest

A brand name for **ispaghula**.

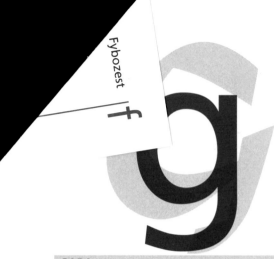

GABA

A **neuro-transmitter**.

gabapentin

An analogue of the natural **neuro-transmitter GABA** used in the management of certain types of epilepsy. A brand name is Neurontin.

Gabitril

A brand name for the anti-epilepsy drug **tiagabine**.

galactorrhoea

Literally, 'a flowing of milk'. The term is used to indicate an excessive flow, or a spontaneous production of milk at times when lactation is not normal. The milk supply can be kept up almost indefinitely if the stimulus of suckling continues, but once this is removed, lactation ceases.

INCIDENCE

Galactorrhoea can occur in both women and men, and even in babies. About 30 per cent of the cells of the front half of the pituitary gland are prolactin hormone-producing cells, and a tumour of these, a prolactinoma, will secrete large quantities of the hormone and promote a flow of milk from the breasts. Just before birth, babies are exposed to concentrations of this hormone in the maternal blood and often show some milk production – *witches' milk* – for a few days after birth (see **milk, witches'**).

> Unexplained galactorrhoea in an adult is an important sign of a possibly serious condition, such as a pituitary gland tumour, and should never be ignored.

galactosaemia

A genetic disorder in which an enzyme necessary for the breakdown of galactose, a sugar present in milk, is absent. As a result, galactose, instead of being converted to glucose, accumulates in the body and may cause mental retardation, cataracts, liver enlargement, jaundice, diarrhoea, vomiting and malnutrition. There is a great variation in severity. Early diagnosis allows the infant to be fed on a galactose-free diet and to grow up entirely normal.

The gene for the enzyme is located on chromosome 9 and it is absent in one in 150 of the population. The inheritance is recessive, so the defective gene must be present on both of the pair of corresponding chromosomes for the disease to occur. The incidence of galactosaemia in Britain is about one in 80,000 births.

Fetal antenatal screening can detect the condition before birth and, if the mother has high galactose levels, amniocentesis can demonstrate whether the fetal brain has been damaged. Unaffected heterozygote carriers of the gene can be detected by a biochemical test.

Galenphol

A brand name for **pholcodine**.

Galfer

A brand name for **ferrous fumarate**.

gallamine triethiodide

A synthetic, short-acting muscle relaxant used by anaesthetists to allow passage of an **endotracheal tube** at the beginning of anaesthesia. A brand name is Flaxedil.

gall-bladder cancer

This is rare and hardly occurs at all unless there is a history of gallstones. It is four times as common in women as in men and is, unfortunately, a very serious condition which, in most cases, is found to be inoperable at the time of diagnosis. Only those with early, well-localized tumours, treated by radical surgery, survive.

gallium

In the liver the element gallium is concentrated in tumour and inflammatory cells to a greater extent than in normal liver cells. An isotope of gallium, gallium-67 can therefore be used to produce radiological scans of the liver and reveal cancers or areas of inflammation.

gallstones

Hard round, oval, or faceted masses of stone-like material occurring in some people in the gall-bladder or the bile duct. Most gallstones are about the size of a pea or a marble, but may be multiple and very small, like fine gravel, or so large that a single stone completely fills the gall-bladder.

INCIDENCE

They are commoner in women than in men. The medical students' mnemonic is that they occur in 'fair, fat, fertile

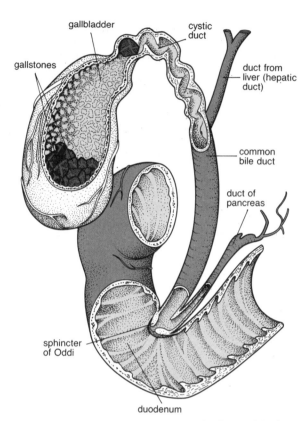

This diagram shows a collection of faceted gallstones lying in the gall-bladder. A single stone is obstructing the cystic duct. It is in the gall-bladder that the bile from the liver is concentrated before being passed down into the duodenum.

females over forty.' About a quarter of all elderly adults have gallstones.

POSSIBLE CAUSES

Most gallstones are composed of cholesterol, chalk (calcium carbonate), calcium bilirubinate, or a mixture of these. They are more likely to occur if the composition of the bile is abnormal, if there is blockage of bile outflow or local infection, or if there is a family history of gallstones. They occur when the liver produces bile with an excess of cholesterol in it. This may be caused by a relative reduction in bile salts. Excessive cholesterol may be due to factors such as:

● a high cholesterol diet;
● advancing age;
● excessive refined dietary carbohydrate;
● high oestrogen levels;
● cholesterol-reducing drugs.

In additional to a high bile cholesterol, the bile must be saturated with dissolving substances.

RECOGNITION AND SYMPTOMS

Their presence leads to inflammation of the gall-bladder (cholecystitis), and may block the bile duct leading to obstructive jaundice. The passage of a gallstone down the bile duct into the duodenum, known as biliary colic, is very painful.

TREATMENT

Treatment is by removal of the gall-bladder (cholecystectomy), by gallstone lithotripsy in which stones are shattered by concentrated sound waves, or by direct surgical removal.

Galpseud

A brand name for **pseudoephedrine**.

Gamanil

A brand name for **lofepramine**.

gambling addiction

See **gambling, pathological**.

gambling, pathological

Compulsive gambling is a disease which involves a constant preoccupation with gambling; causes the victim to become restless or irritable if unable to gamble; leads to the hazarding of money in amounts out of all proportion to what can reasonably be afforded and to the placing of ever larger bets to renew the diminishing sense of excitement. It defeats efforts to stop or to cut down even in the face of mounting debt and increasing financial problems caused by the gambling. In these respects pathological gambling resembles other forms of addiction and, like other forms of addiction, is becoming more prevalent in young people.

RECOGNITION

Like alcohol addiction, the problem is often concealed, but the secondary effects – depression, anxiety, financial difficulties, educational failure – lead one to suspect that something is wrong.

TREATMENT

The first step in trying to deal with the disease is a frank and open acknowledgement of its existence and recognition of the problem, based on unemotional discussion in a friendly and supportive atmosphere. A stern, judgmental, prohibitive moral tone is inappropriate and destructive. The discussion should include, if possible, a full and honest account of the history of the gambling behaviour and its consequences and of the victim's attitude to, and thinking on, his or her gambling.

A four-stage model for coping with the problem has been proposed. This has been found helpful in other addictions. The stages are:

● precontemplation, in which the problem is discussed but without any consideration of the need for a change in behaviour;
● contemplation, in which there is some recognition of the need, but no action;
● the action stage in which a deliberate attempt is made to modify behaviour;
● the maintenance stage, in which support is given for sustaining abstinence.

The move from each stage to the next is a short one and sets what seems to be an achievable goal.

Family counselling and the use of 'Gamblers Anonymous', which has branches in most parts of Britain, can both be very helpful.

gamma globulin

Immunoglubulins, or antibodies, are protective proteins, produced by B lymphocytes, which attach to invading organisms or foreign substances and neutralize them so that they can be destroyed by phagocytes. There are five classes of immunoglobulins, the most prevalent being immunoglobulin G, or gamma globulin. This provides the body's main defence against bacteria, viruses and toxins.

Gamma globulin is so widely effective that it is produced commercially, from pooled human plasma, and used as a means of passive protection against many infections. It is useful for protection, when the need arises, against such infections as hepatitis A and B, chickenpox, measles and poliomyelitis. It is also very useful for people who have an inherent or acquired immune deficiency, such as the condition of agammaglobulinaemia.

ganciclovir

A **DNA polymerase inhibitor** drug used to treat **cytomegalovirus infections** in people with **AIDS**. A brand name is Cymevene.

Ganda

A brand name for **guanethidine sulphate** formulated as eye-drops with adrenaline.

ganglion

A large collection of nerve-cell bodies. The term ganglion is also applied to a rubbery, tumourlike, compressible, but entirely harmless swelling occurring on tendons and other connective tissues, commonly on or around the wrist. This minor disorder used, traditionally, to be cured by slamming it with the family bible so that the capsule ruptured and the contents dispersed. More refined surgery is now usual.

gangrene

Death of tissue, usually occurring in an extremity and usually because of an inadequate blood supply.

POSSIBLE CAUSES

Gangrene is commonly caused by severe arterial disease, such as atherosclerosis, in which the blood supply able to pass through the narrowed and easily obstructed arteries is insufficient to maintain the nutrition of the remoter parts. Diabetes also increases the possibility of gangrene, mainly by its effect on the blood vessels, but also by encouraging infection. Other important causes include embolism, thrombosis, severe arterial injury and the obstructive arterial condition, Buerger's disease (thromboangiitis obliterans). The rye fungus ergot can cause gangrene by inducing prolonged occluding spasm in arteries. Mechanical obstruction to the arterial blood supply can cause gangrene, as occurs in the bowel with a strangulated hernia or a gangrenous appendix.

RECOGNITION AND SYMPTOMS

If infection is avoided, the affected part becomes dry and turns brown or black. At the interface between dead and living tissue is a zone of inflammation and sometimes this marks the plane of cleavage at which the dead part drops off. This form of dry gangrene is commonest in the smaller extremities, such as the fingers and toes.

When infection occurs, putrefaction occurs, producing the wet type of gangrene. Infection with anaerobic organisms, such as the common, gas-producing *Clostridium welchii*, which is present in most cultivated soils, causes the very dangerous gas gangrene. This features great swelling or ballooning of the tissues, especially the muscles, by gas, and a rapid spread to healthy tissue. There is discoloration, a smell of putrefaction, and severe illness with grave toxicity. Gas gangrene was a major cause of death in the First World War when so many deep wounds were contaminated by cultivated soil. The condition has nothing to do with poison gas.

Ganser's syndrome

A condition featuring fraudulent behaviour, purporting to be psychotic, but which represents the subject's idea of madness rather than any recognized psychiatric pattern. It has been described as 'the syndrome of approximate answers' because of the perversely inappropriate responses to simple questions or demands. Thus, if asked to state the sum of ten and ten, the subject might reply '21'; or if given a pencil to write with, might try to use the wrong end.

The condition indicates a personality disorder and is common among prisoners awaiting trial. The manifestations are worse when the subject believes he is being watched and are usually absent when covertly observed. Recovery is sudden and the affected person usually claims amnesia for the period of the 'illness'.

Garamycin

A brand name for **gentamicin**.

gardnerella vaginalis infection

A very common infection of the vagina which produces a thin vaginal discharge with a characteristic 'fishy' odour in the presence of a mild alkali, such as toilet soap. There are no other symptoms, but the organism, and the odour, can be sexually transmitted to the partner. The infection tends to be stubborn, but responds well to treatment with the drug metronidazole (Flagyl).

gargle

A once popular, but now almost abandoned form of treatment for sore throat. Gargling was more impressive for the noises made than for any real medical advantage.

gargoylism of face

See **Hurler's syndrome**.

gas and oxygen

In giving a general anaesthetic, an anaesthetist will commonly rely on 'gas and oxygen' as the vehicle for other, more potent, anaesthetic vapours, such as the powerful halothane, or as a basic agent to be supplemented by other drugs.

The gas is nitrous oxide which, although pleasant to inhale, has poor anaesthetic qualities. It does, however, to a useful extent, reduce pain sensation (analgesic action) and the mixture is sometimes used alone to relieve labour pains. Simple machines for self-administration of gas and oxygen are often used, under supervision, in labour. In one such machine, the patient keeps a finger on the valve and takes deep breaths when each pain starts. If unconsciousness should occur, the valve is automatically released.

Modern general anaesthesia no longer relies on deep and dangerous levels of unconsciousness to achieve muscle relaxation. The principle, today, is to rely on paralysant drugs for

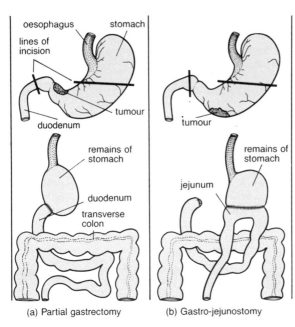

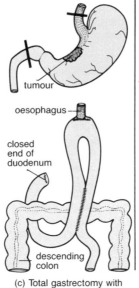

Three types of gastrectomy. After partial gastrectomy (a) and (b) the duodenum can be connected to the stomach remnant or can be closed and the stomach connected to the jejunum. After total gastrectomy (c) a loop of bowel is fashioned into an artificial stomach and the oesophagus connected to this.

(a) Partial gastrectomy

(b) Gastro-jejunostomy

(c) Total gastrectomy with formation of an artificial stomach

muscle relaxation and to keep the patient in a shallow (and safe) plane of anaesthesia by the use of minimal narcosis.

gaster

Greek root meaning 'stomach' as in gastritis (stomach inflammation).

gastrectomy

Surgical removal of the stomach, usually in part, but sometimes as a whole.

WHY IT'S DONE

Partial gastrectomy, usually combined with an operation to cut the nerves to the stomach (vagotomy), is often successful in the treatment of medically uncontrollable stomach and duodenal ulcers and for cancer of the lower part of the stomach. Removing part of the stomach reduces the amount of acid produced and so can be effective in the management of duodenal ulcers. Since the development of drugs like the histamine H2-receptor antagonists cimetidine (Tagamet) and ranitidine (Zantac), gastrectomy has been required less often.

HOW IT'S DONE

The operation is performed through a vertical incision in the upper abdomen, in the midline, or just to the left of it. Techniques for the operation vary.

gastric erosion

The most minor degree of damage to the stomach lining. Endoscopic examination, in a case of erosion, shows numerous fine red bleeding points on the surface and tests may show that the stools contain hidden (occult) blood.

Gastric erosion is caused by alcohol, aspirin, non-steroidal anti-inflammatory drugs (NSAIDs) and severe stress, including major burns and blood infection (septicaemia). If the causal factors continue to operate, the erosion may progress to frank ulceration, but if eliminated, healing is rapid.

The condition is also known as erosive gastritis.

gastric lavage

See **stomach washout**.

gastric ulcer

See **peptic ulcer**.

gastritis

See **gastric erosion**.

Gastrobid Continus

A brand name for **metoclopramide**.

gastrocneme

Greek root meaning 'calf' as in gastrocnemius (main muscle of calf).

gastroenteritis

Inflammation of the stomach and intestine, characterized by fever, abdominal pain, diarrhoea and vomiting.

INCIDENCE

Every year, ten million people, mostly babies and infants, die from acute gastroenteritis. Most of these deaths occur in tropical and developing areas and most of the children die from dehydration and malnutrition. Given adequate medical resources, all are preventable.

POSSIBLE CAUSES

Gastroenteritis is caused by bowel organisms, such as *Escherichia coli*, *Salmonella*, *Giardia lamblia*, rotaviruses, coronaviruses and other enteroviruses. In most cases, infection is the result of poor hygiene, especially in bottle-feeding; breast-fed babies are seldom affected.

TREATMENT

Most attacks clear up on their own, but if the diarrhoea and vomiting are severe, death can occur from simple loss of fluid. Babies can often be saved merely by forcing fluids by mouth but, in many cases, they are too weak to swallow and their only chance rests in rehydration by intravenous fluids. Training a barefoot doctor in the skills of inserting a scalp vein cannula and setting up a glucose-saline drip leads to the saving of hundreds of lives and great human distress.

gastroenterologist

A doctor specializing in the digestive system and its disorders and disorders of the major associated glands – the liver and the pancreas.

gastroenterostomy

An operation for duodenal ulceration in which the duodenum is separated from the outlet of the stomach and effectively by-passed by the formation of a side-to-side junction (anastomosis) between the stomach and the beginning of the small intestine. By diverting stomach acid away from the duodenum, this procedure allows the duodenal ulcer to heal.

Since the development of new and effective drugs, such as cimetidine, and new operations, such as selective vagotomy, the operation has been less often performed.

gastro-intestinal surgeon

A surgeon primarily interested in the surgical treatment of disorders of the digestive system. His or her work is con-

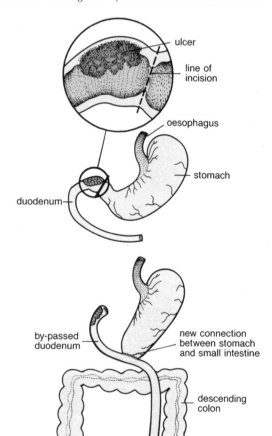

Gastroenterostomy. The outlet of the stomach is connected to the side of the jejunum so that no stomach contents enter the duodenum and the ulcer is able to heal.

cerned the oesophagus, stomach and intestines, and with the major associated glands – the liver and the pancreas. Most abdominal surgery is within the capability of the gastro-intestinal surgeon.

gastrojejunostomy

See **gastroenterostomy**.

gastric lavage

Stomach washout. This is done to remove or dilute drugs or non-corrosive poisons taken in suicide attempts. Lavage is avoided if corrosive poisons have been taken. A wide-bore soft plastic or rubber tube is pushed down the gullet (oesophagus) into the stomach, the end held high, and water run in through a funnel. The end of the tube is then lowered so that the washings drain out. This process is repeated until the returning water is clear.

Gastromax

A brand name for **metoclopramide**.

gastrostomy

Making an opening into the stomach.

gavage

Forced feeding, especially via a stomach tube. The term is also used for superalimentation – the use, for therapeutic reasons, of a very high-calorie, large-volume diet, so as to greatly increase the nutritional input.

Gaviscon

A brand name for a preparation containing sodium alginate.

gay bowel syndrome

A collection of effects on the anus, rectum and colon, related to sexual practices in homosexual men. These effects include the result of physical trauma from finger or hand insertion (fisting) or from the insertion of other objects, and from infection by a wide range of organisms. Mechanical trauma may result in fissures, fistulas, ulcers and haemorrhoids. Infection causes venereal warts, syphilis, gonorrhoea, lymphogranuloma venereum and bacillary and amoebic dysentery.

gemcitabine

A cytotoxic anticancer drug. A brand name is Gemzar.

gemfibrozil

A fibrate cholesterol-lowering drug. A brand name is Lopid.

Gemzar

A brand name for **gemcitabine**.

gender chromosomes

See **sex chromosomes**.

gender election

See **sex selection**.

gender reassignment

Gender identity is the inherent sense one has that one belongs to a particular sex. In the vast majority of cases that sex corresponds to the anatomical sex and there is no problem. But it is recognized that, for a small minority, the gender identity is for the opposite anatomical sex and most of these unfortunate people long for a sex change (gender reassignment).

The term 'sex change' is not a satisfactory one, since to the individual concerned, the real sex is obvious and it is naive to consider the purely anatomical sexual characteristics to be more important than the mental and emotional ones.

The first case in which doctors agreed to reassign the sex of an anatomical man, by hormone and surgical treatment, so that he (she) could live as a woman, occurred in Denmark 30 years ago, in the face of much criticism and opposition. Since then, the procedure has been performed many times and about 70 per cent of those so treated remain satisfied with the result. Of the others, some have requested restoration and some committed suicide. It can be inferred that this 30 per cent represent failure of the medical profession to distinguish between true gender misidentity and people with severe psychiatric or other personality disorders, misguided transvestites and homosexual people.

Guidelines have been developed for the management of trans-sexualism. The reasons for the request for the treatment must be fully and exhaustively discussed and all the implications – surgical, hormonal and emotional – must be clearly understood. Ideally, cohabitees should be fully aware of what is proposed and should agree that it is desirable. The procedure should not be performed on a whim but only if it is the only effective way of relieving genuine distress of mind for the subject and substantially improve the quality of life. The probable outcome should, if possible, be evaluated by doctors who are not members of the gender reassignment team.

The team consists of surgeons with genito-urinary, gynaecological and plastic experience; endocrinologists; dermatologists and speech therapists to help with voice amendment.

gene

See **genetic code**.

gene, alterations in

See **mutation**.

gene ascendancy

See **dominance**.

gene end marker

See **stop codon**.

gene group

See **operon**.

gene mutation, harmless

See **silent mutation**.

gene pair

See **allele**.

gene pair, identical

See **homozygous**.

gene, partially active

See **leaky mutant gene**.

general anaesthesia

Many people facing an operation are more concerned about the anaesthetic than about the surgery. Anaesthetic accidents are rightly given great publicity, but these are a tiny minority of the millions of anaesthetics given every year.

RISKS

Much attention has been given to improving the safety of general anaesthesia and the training of anaesthetists, and anaesthetics are safer today than they have ever been.

Anaesthetics are now safely given to patients who would formerly have been thought too frail or seriously ill. Monitoring equipment gives a continuous indication of the vital processes – heartbeat and breathing – and any change in these immediately prompts remedial action. One of the most important aids to safety is the pulse oximeter which continuously monitors the oxygen levels in the blood – the only really vital indication that all is well – and gives a loud signal if this drops by even a few per cent or if the equipment becomes detached. In these ways the members if the operating team, as well as the anaesthetist, are continually aware of the patient's condition and can respond to any change.

HOW IT WORKS

Modern anaesthetic methods aim to keep the patient quietly asleep, while other drugs are used to achieve loss of pain sensation, muscle relaxation and the avoidance of surgical shock. Premedication with drugs which produce a calm, relaxed state of mind, before and after the anaesthetic, is routine. It is usual for patients to wake up after their operation with no recollection of being taken to the operating theatre.

COMMON WORRIES

Many people are worried that they might speak during anaesthesia and give away private matters. Others are greatly concerned over the possibility of waking up during the operation. It is true that very lightly anaesthetized people do, rarely, mutter some meaningless sounds, but normal, recognizable speech does not occur. If a patient does make a sound, the anaesthetist at once recognizes that the level of anaesthesia is too shallow and increases the dose of the anaesthetic agent. The same applies to any slight movement during the operation. Even if a patient is wholly paralysed by muscle relaxants, any approach to consciousness causes obvious changes in physical signs which the anaesthetist is monitoring and prompt him to deepen the level a little.

Anaesthesia is seldom induced, nowadays, with a mask and anaesthetic gas or vapour. Induction, today, is almost always by the injection of a powerful drug, such as pentothal (thiopentone sodium) which acts so rapidly that the patient is barely aware that anything is happening before waking up in the recovery ward, or back in bed. Only after deep sleep is induced will the gases, which maintain anaesthesia, be turned on. There is none of the sense of asphyxiation which was once a feature of general anaesthesia.

general surgeon

A surgeon who does not limit his or her surgical activity to a particular surgical specialty but who will undertake a large range of common operations. General surgeons, however, will often refer patients to colleagues who sub-specialize.

generalized anxiety disorder

A state of inappropriate and sometimes severe anxiety, without adequate cause, which lasts for at least six months.

INCIDENCE

It affects about 2 per cent of the population, women twice as often as men, and often develops in early adult life. It can, however, start at any age. There is a definite hereditary tendency to the disorder and about 25 per cent of immediate relatives of sufferers are also affected.

POSSIBLE CAUSES

The disorder is thought to be caused by a disturbance of the functions of neuro-transmitters such as adrenaline or GABA, in the frontal lobes or the limbic system of the brain.

RECOGNITION AND SYMPTOMS

There is increased sensitivity to action of the sympathetic nervous system (which produces adrenaline) and objective indications of sleep abnormality, as shown on the electroencephalogram. REM sleep is diminished.

The chronically worried state of mind involves being constantly 'keyed up'. There is an exaggerated startle response, lack of concentration, irritability, insomnia and a tendency for the mind to 'go blank'. Closely related to these mental effects are the corresponding physical manifestations. These include muscle tension, shakiness, tooth-grinding (bruxism), trembling, restlessness, easy fatigability, breathlessness, palpitations, sweating, clammy hands, dry mouth, lightheadedness, nausea, diarrhoea, flushing, frequency of urination and a 'lump in the throat'. It is a moot point whether these symptoms result from the state of mind or cause it, or even whether both are effects of the same cause.

TREATMENT

Treatment is on pharmacological lines and is designed to counter the excessive sympathetic or neuro-transmitter effect. Beta-blockers (beta adrenergic receptor blockers) and antihistamine drugs are often very effective. The benzodiazepine drugs such as Valium and Librium were once widely used, but their disadvantages are becoming increasingly apparent and they are now being replaced by newer anxiolytic drugs, for which better things are claimed. Tricyclic and monoamine oxidase inhibiting antidepressant drugs have some part to play in the treatment of anxiety.

general paralysis of the insane

GPI, now almost unknown, was once the common effect of untreated long-term (tertiary) syphilis, affecting the nervous system. It was a form of dementia featuring grandiose delusions and mania and sometimes delusions of persecution. Prior to the discovery of penicillin, GPI used to occur ten to 20 years after the primary infection, affecting approximately 5 per cent of those in whom the syphilis involved the nervous system.

generic drugs

Drugs sold under the official medical name of the basic active substance. The generic name is chosen by the Nomenclature Committee of the British Pharmacopoeia Commission and is used in publications such as the *British National Formulary*. Doctors are encouraged to prescribe generic drugs as these are generally cheaper than the same drug under a trade or brand name.

genes determining body shape

See **homeobox genes**.

genes, jumping

See **transposons**.

genes, locating

See **mapping**.

genes, on X chromosome

See **sex-linkage, X-linkage**.

genes, position of

See **locus**.

genes, stress-activated

See **stress genes**.

genes, turning off

See **antisense RNA**.

gene therapy

This contentious subject is concerned with the treatment of hereditary disease by introducing normal genes into the body.

There are about 4000 known genetic disorders and few of them can be effectively treated. Some of these diseases are so distressing that pressures to adopt potentially effective genetic treatments have become overwhelming. Ethical committees and other authorities are now beginning to give way in some areas.

WHY IT'S DONE

Gene therapy involving somatic cells is now going ahead. The condition **severe combined immunodeficiency disorder** (SCID) is so dangerous that affected children have to be kept in plastic bubbles to insulate them from infection. The condition is caused in many cases by the absence of a gene that codes for the enzyme adenosine deaminase (ADA) necessary for the integrity of the immune system. In September 1990 scientists began to insert the gene for this enzyme into affected children.

Bone marrow transplants of genetically engineered cells are being done to treat leukaemia and other blood disorders in which new clones of blood cells can be expected to survive and give rise to healthy populations of blood cells. The gene has to be inserted in the stem cells which clone the cell populations. These are difficult to find.

HOW IT'S DONE

Genes can be introduced into cells by various methods.

- Microinjection using a fine glass pipette works very well but requires skill and is hardly practicable if many cells are to be processed.

- Electroporation involves exposure of cells to an electric shock which makes the membrane more permeable and allows material to enter the cell, but is often severely damaging.

- Perhaps the most efficient method is the use of retroviruses to carry in the new gene. Many viruses have now been engineered to serve as vectors for gene transfer. Retroviruses convert their own RNA to DNA in infected cells and insert the DNA into a chromosome. So if a retrovirus contains the required gene and is otherwise harmless, it makes an ideal delivery system. Unfortunately, retroviruses can cause cancer, especially if they are allowed to multiply in the body. This is a major problem that is being energetically tackled.

> There is a great divide in gene therapy: genes can be introduced into the general body cells (somatic cells) or they can be introduced into the germ cells – sperms, ova or early embryos. The difference is fundamental. In the first case, only the individual is affected; in the second, all that person's future offspring will be affected.
> For this reason germ cell gene therapy is currently almost universally prohibited. It simply raises too many dangerous possibilities and ethical problems.

THE FUTURE

Research is in progress to study the possibility of engineering skin cells, such as fibroblasts, to make them produce needed proteins that are normally produced in other cells. If this succeeds, implants of skin cells could correct many disorders in which a protein is absent – conditions such as haemophilia or dwarfism from growth hormone deficiency.

We are only at the beginning of a new and exciting chapter in the history of medicine. See also **genetic engineering**.

genetic abnormality detection

See **restriction fragment length polymorphism (RFLP)**.

genetic basis of asthma, hay fever and eczema

See **atopy**.

genetic cause of leukaemia

See **Philadelphia chromosome**.

genetic cell death

See **lethal mutation**.

genetic code

The sequence of chemical groups, lying along the DNA molecules in every cell, which forms the hereditary 'blueprint' of the individual. The code is represented by successions of particular trios of the chemical bases, or nucleotides – adenine, guanine, cytosine and thymine. These triplets of bases are called codons. Since each codon contains three of the four nucleotides, there are 64 possible different combinations. Most of these codons indicate one or other of the 20 different amino acids – the building bricks of protein from which the body is largely made – but others are instructions such as 'message starts here' or 'stop'. The sequence of codons in a length of DNA instructs the cell to link together particular amino acids in a particular order so as to construct a protein

molecule. The length of DNA that codes for a complete protein is called a gene. Other genes are concerned with the control of the processes of expression of the genetic code.

A row of contiguous genes on a chromosome, that operates as a unit, is called an operon. Genes in an operon are preceded by two regulatory sites in the chromosome occupied by two regulatory genes, the promoter and the operator. These are essential for the expression of the operon. Genes in an operon have related and sequential functions, so that successive steps in the synthesis of a protein or in the promotion of some biochemical event occur as they should. All the genes in the operon are turned on and off together, and their products are produced in fixed ratios of quantity. For genes to be expressed, they must first be transcribed into a piece of complementary **RNA** (ribonucleic acid) called **messenger RNA** (mRNA). All the genes in an operon are transcribed into one large segment of messenger RNA.

genetic code, conveying

See **messenger RNA**.

genetic counselling

Genetic counsellors are doctors or scientists skilled in the complex science of genetics. Some hospitals have teams that, in addition to geneticists, include a paediatrician, an obstetrician, a social worker, a nurse and, as required, special consultants who are experts in particular diseases.

HOW IT'S DONE

The counsellor will start by taking a careful family history, so it is very helpful if those seeking advice on genetic disorders find out as much as possible about previous cases of the same condition in the family.

The counsellor will then perform a full physical examination of anyone known to be suffering from, or suspected of having, the disease in question. In some cases, the physical signs of the disease are so obvious that the condition can immediately be recognized and counselling can be given. Laboratory tests will probably be arranged also. The first thing to be found out is whether or not the problem actually is genetic, and if so, how it is passed on. This is called the mode of inheritance. If the condition is hereditary, the counsellor will try to draw a family tree showing all cases in which the condition occurred. Such a tree will show the mode of inheritance.

WHY IT'S DONE

Over 3000 medical conditions are known to be caused by a single gene defect and in all of these, the chances of producing an affected baby can be mathematically determined. The gene causing the problem can be on the X chromosome, (sex-linked) or on another chromosome (autosomal). Females have two X chromosomes in every cell (XX), males have one X and one Y (XY). The male X chromosome carries genes which cause many hereditary traits. The Y chromosome is small and is concerned almost exclusively with male sex determination. Half of the sperms carry an X and half a Y. All ova, of course, contain two X chromosomes. The autosomal chromosomes consist of 22 pairs, each member of a pair being identical in size, shape and gene location. There are two, normally identical genes, for each characteristic, each one situated at corresponding locations on the pair of chromosomes. Such pairs of genes are called alleles.

HOMOZYGOUS AND HETEROZYGOUS CARRIERS

People who carry identical alleles of a particular gene are called homozygous for that gene, those with dissimilar alleles – one normal, one defective – are heterozygous. Genes which exert their effect when present on only one chromosome are dominant. Those which exert their effect only if both alleles for the defect are present are called recessive. Genetically determined defects may be single gene mutations and in these cases the mathematics of inheritance is clear. But defects may also be due to mutations involving more than one gene, which complicates matters considerably. Finally, defects may be due to complete chromosomal abnormalities or even additional chromosomes. In these cases the effects are major and are well recognized.

Autosomal dominant conditions are those non-X-linked conditions in which the gene, if present, always causes the disorder. Since genes occur in pairs (alleles), there will be a 50 per cent risk of passing on the condition if one parent carries the gene on one chromosome of the pair (is heterozygous). If both parents carry the gene on one chromosome the risk is 75 per cent. If one parent is homozygous with a dominant gene, all the offspring will have the condition because all will inherit the affected gene. Autosomal recessive conditions are those which occur only when both gene alleles carry the defect. The condition can thus arise only if both parents carry the gene. If both are heterozygous, the risk with each child is 25 per cent. If one parent has the condition (is homozygous) the risk for each child is 50 per cent. If both parents are homozygous, every child will, of course, have the disorder.

X-LINKED DOMINANT CONDITIONS

In X-linked dominant conditions, half the children of heterozygous females are affected, regardless of sex, because the affected mother has a 50 per cent chance of passing on the affected X chromosome to both daughters and sons. If the mother is homozygous, all the children will be affected. Of the children of an affected father, all the daughters and none of the sons are affected. This is simply because the father passes on his X chromosome to his daughters and his Y chromosome to his sons.

X-LINKED RECESSIVE CONDITIONS

In X-linked recessive conditions, a male with the defect will pass the gene on to his daughters but not, to his sons (who receive only the Y chromosome). A heterozygous female has the gene on only one of the chromosome pairs and is not affected. She is a carrier, and passes the gene to half her offspring. Half of her daughters become carriers and half her sons have the disorder. This is because, in males, the Y chromosome does not behave as a homologue to the X chromosome. For a daughter to inherit an X-linked recessive disorder, the father must have the condition and the mother must either have it or be a carrier. If both parents have the disorder, all the children will have the condition. If the father has it and the mother is heterozygous, the risk for daughters is 50 per cent. X-linked recessive conditions are rare in females.

GENETIC COUNSELLORS

Genetic counselling must be based on an extensive and detailed knowledge of the principles of **genetics**. But, in addition to this, it requires a great deal of knowledge of the nature of the conditions caused by gene defects. Counsellors must also be able to convey complex information to sometimes distressed parents in a form which can be understood, so that rational decisions can be made about having children.

The subject needs specialists with a high level of expertise and knowledge of recent developments that can be brought to bear effectively on these often tragic human problems.

See also **genetics**.

genetic disorder treatment

See **enzyme replacement therapy**.

genetic effect on drug action

See **pharmacogenomics**.

genetic engineering

The process of producing new hereditable characteristics in organisms, such as bacteria and fungi, by deliberately altering their DNA.

HOW IT'S DONE

Enzymes that split the molecule at predictable sites (restriction enzymes) are used to cut the DNA and other enzymes are used to splice in a gene from another organism or even a gene that has been made synthetically. The inserted gene may contain the code for the synthesis of any one of a large variety of useful proteins, and, once established, all the subsequent offspring of the organism will have the same capacity to produce this material.

WHY IT'S DONE

The method is being used to produce several proteins of great medical importance such as insulin, enzymes that dissolve blood clots, growth hormone, anti-growth hormone, blood clot-dissolving enzymes such as the tissue plasminogen activator, the valuable anti-viral agent interferon, and so on.

The same process can be used to remove from a dangerous infective organism the genes that cause it to be dangerous. Such a modified organism can then be used to make a safe vaccine against the disease the organism normally causes. In 1988, Merck, Sharp and Dohme launched the first genetically engineered vaccine against **hepatitis B**. The potential for recombinant DNA technology is enormous and this potential is being rapidly exploited. The activity is slowly but surely assuming ever greater commercial and industrial importance.

ETHICAL ISSUES

A great deal of research, and practical application, has involved the organism *Escherichia coli*, and work on this bacterium has been highly successful. This organism, which we all carry in millions in our lower intestines, is easy to grow, so innumerable offspring with the new characteristic can readily be produced in culture. In view of the ease with which bacteria can reproduce, and the possibility of creating and liberating bacteria of high virulence to humans, doubts have frequently been expressed about the dangers of 'tampering with nature' in this way.

These dangers are real. In the early stages of the work, the scientists concerned were not always as mindful of these dangers as they might have been. SV40 is a virus which causes cancer by injecting its own genetic material into the DNA of mammalian cells. One of the pioneers of genetic engineering, the American molecular biologist Paul Berg (b. 1926), was so carried away with the fascination of his work that he actually contemplated introducing this cancer-causing DNA into *E. coli* bacteria, and then cloning these organisms. *E. coli* normally inhabits the human bowel. It was only when a student of Berg's happened to mention the proposal at a workshop course that other research workers protested and the idea was abandoned.

Berg then became the leader in the movement to control such dangerous experiments, and in 1976 guidelines to restrict such research were published. Berg was awarded the 1980 Nobel prize for chemistry for his work in the field.

THE FUTURE

But all this is just a hint of what is likely in the near future. The problems of working on a manufacturing scale are much greater than implied, but advances are rapid. Hopes are rising for the large-scale production of a great range of drugs, and there is no theoretical reason why the whole range of human hormones, together with many other naturally produced substances of medical importance, should not be fabricated for us in this way.

Scores of genetically caused diseases have now been studied at DNA level and, in many, cloned copies of the genes concerned are available for use as probes in the identification of the disease in fetuses, by amniocentesis, before birth. But some of the possibilities of genetic engineering, in the hands of the irresponsible or the criminal, are horrifying. One can only hope that, as with nuclear warfare, those in a position to use such methods are so clearly aware of the consequences that they are restrained from doing so.

POTENTIAL DANGERS

It is now common for human ova to be fertilized *in vitro*, cultured for a few days, developed to an early embryo, frozen for months until a prospective mother is in a suitable state for implantation, and then thawed and placed in the womb. This procedure can lead to a normal pregnancy and, eventually, the birth of a healthy baby. In combination with what is currently possible with genetic engineering, this gives rise to astonishing possibilities. Much good may result, including the deletion of damaging genes, or even of complete chromosomes, such as the extra chromosome 21 which causes Down's syndrome, but the other side of the coin – such as the deliberate introduction of qualities and characteristics believed to be desirable, perhaps the cloning of people, and playing Frankenstein – hardly bears thinking about. Fortunately, many people have thought about it and very strict controls are imposed on such work.

Whether the risks can be contained is doubtful. For many years, codes of practice and guidelines for the conduct of research have been in existence, and, in large part, so far as can be known, adhered to. But scientists have seldom been deterred from investigating obvious possibilities, just because risk was involved. And today, when to the traditional rewards of fame and academic advance is added the incentive of huge financial profits, it seems likely that some will succumb to the temptation to take chances.

See also **gene therapy**.

genetic immune deficiency

See **bare lymphocyte syndrome, severe combined immunodeficiency disorder (SCID), thymus**.

genetic messenger

See **RNA**.

genetic prion disease

See **fatal familial insomnia**.

genetics

The study of inheritance and the units of inheritance (genes). Inheritance is the derivation of genes from the entire series of a person's forebears. The whole genome (the collection of genes) is derived from the two parents, half from each. But each of the parents derived their genes from their parents, and so on. It is thus reasonably accurate to take it that one-half of the genetic inheritance comes from the parents, one-quarter from the four grandparents, one-eighth from the eight great-grandparents and so on.

Chromosomes are divided into two groups – the pair of sex chromosomes X and Y, and the other 22 pairs known as the autosomal chromosomes, or autosomes. The male sex chromosome pair consists of an X and a Y chromosome, the latter being responsible for maleness and little else. Females have two X chromosomes, one being the father's X chromosome and the other being one of the mother's. The genes for some bodily characteristics, and at least 100 diseases, are carried on the X chromosome, but the enormous majority of genes are carried on the autosomal chromosomes.

Genes are located precisely in a particular position along the chromosome and a major preoccupation of molecular biologists is to identify the precise position of all the genes. This is a task of staggering size. There are about 100,000 genes, each one having between 2000 and 2 million base pairs. To sequence a gene, every base pair must be identified, and the start and end of each gene must also be found. The human genome project, to sequence the whole genome, reached completion during June, 2000.

DOMINANT AND RECESSIVE INHERITANCE

The 46 chromosomes exist in 23 pairs, each with corresponding sets of genes in corresponding positions. Bear in mind that nearly all genes act only by producing enzymes that catalyze biochemical reactions required at any particular body site. **Homeobox genes** determine the body shape at a very early embryonic stage.

Gene pairs on corresponding chromosomes are called **alleles**. The two genes in an allele are normally identical, but frequently are not. When they are identical, the characteristic which the gene produces, appears. If the genes are different, one of them has the full effect and the other does not. One might produce the correct enzyme; the other may be unable to do so. The gene having effect is called the dominant gene and the other the recessive gene. When a dominant gene takes effect, the result, physically, appears to be the same as if both genes had been identical to the dominant gene. But every cell in the affected person's body, including those producing sperms and eggs, contains the recessive gene. Such a person is said to be heterozygous for that gene.

When the sperms and eggs are produced only one of the pair of chromosomes is included, so there is a 50/50 chance in a person heterozygous for a gene that this will be the one with the recessive gene. Should a sperm with the recessive gene fertilize an egg which also has the recessive gene, the cells of the individual produced will contain two recessive genes and the characteristic coded for by these genes – often the failure to produce an essential enzyme – will be expressed. This is called recessive inheritance, and such an individual is said to be homozygous for that gene.

If a recessive gene is carried on an X chromosome, a special case arises. In women, the condition does not show itself because the other X chromosome is normal and will produce the normal product. Men, however, have only one X chromosome and there are, for practical purposes, no genes on the Y chromosome. So the defect coded for by the gene will show itself. But such a man cannot pass on the gene to his son because the gene is on an X chromosome and sperms with X chromosomes produce only females. A male can only acquire the condition by getting an affected X chromosome from his mother. The mother is a carrier and the son gets the disorder. This is called sex-linked, or X-linked recessive inheritance.

For a recessive condition to appear, the gene for it must be present on both of the corresponding chromosomes. If present on one only, the condition will not appear and the bearer of the gene will be a carrier. For a woman actually to develop a sex-linked recessive condition, she would have to inherit an X chromosome, with the gene, from her father, and an X chromosome, with the gene, from her carrier mother. This mating of a man, suffering from the condition, with a woman who happens to be a carrier, is, of course, highly unlikely unless the partners are close relatives in a family that often features the condition.

A female carrier of the sex-linked recessive condition has the gene on half her X chromosomes and thus has a 50/50 chance of passing the condition on to her sons. If she does so all the sons with the gene will develop the condition, because their other sex chromosome is a Y chromosome which cannot 'cancel out' the gene on the X chromosome.

Early in fetal life, one of the two X chromosomes carried by females in all their body cells is believed to be inactivated and left as a small dense mass known as a Barr body. The pair of X chromosomes found in every body cell is derived from duplication of the other X chromosome. The inactivation, however, takes place at different times in different tissues and choice of which is inactivated seems to be random. All the descendants of the body cells will have the same pattern of inactivation of the same X chromosome as the original cell in which the inactivation took place. So about half the cells thus have the X chromosomes inherited from the father in an active state and half have the maternal X chromosome in an active state.

Genetic diseases are diseases caused by abnormalities (mutations) in the genes or sometimes in the number of chromosomes. The transmission of a defective gene through generations of families may be charted in a pedigree and this is used to show how a particular trait or disease is passed on.

Disorders caused by a defect in a single gene are often called inborn errors of metabolism because single genes code for proteins the great majority of which are **enzymes**, and errors cause changes in biochemical processes. As a result of the mutation of a single gene, the enzyme or other protein is either defective, absent or present in insufficient amounts. The result is the failure of synthesis of an essential chemical or the accumulation of material which cannot be normally processed.

Some genetic disorders are caused by a defect in a number of genes or are the result of the interaction of genetic disorders and environmental factors. This is called multifactorial inheritance. Common examples include cleft lip and palate, narrowing of the outlet of the stomach (**pyloric stenosis**) and defects in the development of the vertebral column and spinal cord (**spina bifida**).

Visible abnormalities in complete chromosomes are, of course, always highly influential and serious. The commonest type is a change in the total number of chromosomes. The absence of any whole chromosome is incompatible with life. A very common result of increase in chromosomal number is **Down's syndrome**, which involves an extra chromosome number 21, making three (trisomy-21). Other trisomies occur and all cause major physical and mental defects. All human chromosome abnormalities can be detected in the developing fetus by **amniocentesis** or **chorionic villus sampling** early in pregnancy.

gene treatment

See **somatic gene therapy**.

gene, variable effect of

See **penetrance**.

-genic

Suffix meaning 'causing' as in carcinogenic (causing cancer).

Genisol

A brand name for a shampoo containing coal tar.

genital herpes

See **sexually transmitted diseases**.

genital inflammation, female

See **vulvovaginitis**.

genital warts

These are essentially the same as warts anywhere else in the body and are caused by the same virus, of the papillomavirus genus of the family of papovaviruses. They are often given the title *condylomata acuminata*, but are just ordinary warts, all the same.

Genital warts are transmitted sexually and contact with multiple sexual partners greatly increases the chances of acquiring this unpleasant condition. Because of their position, however, they are often more exuberant and extensive than warts elsewhere and may spread all round the neck of the glans of the penis or all over the labia majora. They are usually of a cauliflower-like appearance and of a pinkish colour.

Genital warts have aroused special interest because of their possible association with cancer of the cervix of the uterus. Some other factor is probably also involved. Treatment is difficult if they are extensive and sometimes local applications are insufficient and surgery under general anaesthesia is needed.

genito-urinary medicine

The speciality formerly described as venereology. Genito-urinary specialists have, in recent years come into great prominence due their expertise in all facets of the **AIDS** disaster.

See also **sexually transmitted diseases**.

genito-urinary medicine specialist

A doctor concerned with the diagnosis and treatment of sexually-transmitted diseases. Formerly know as a venereologist, the GUM specialist has, since the advent of **AIDS**, assumed a new and major importance in medicine.

genome

The complete set of chromosomes, together with the **mitochondrial DNA**. The genome is the whole of the genetic material of the cell.

genome, human, mapping

The human genome is the whole gene map of all the chromosomes, and contains all the information needed to make a human being. The information on the genome is carried in sequences of codons, each consisting of three chemical nucleotides which differ by the possession of one of four different chemical groups called bases. The genome contains about six thousand million (six billion) bases in about 100,000 genes and it is the sequence of these bases, along the length of each chromosome, which has to be determined.

THE DEVELOPMENT OF TECHNOLOGY

When the project started a research worker could decode up to about 100,000 bases a year at a cost of about 50 pence per base. So, at that time, it would have taken one worker 60,000 years to do the job. Fortunately, automated processes were developed which could sequence over 10,000 bases a day and these are being rapidly developed. The French firm Genetech, in particular, have so speeded up the process that the job is expected to be finished by the turn of the century.

There have been other problems, including the difficulty of handling the microscopic DNA and getting hold of enough to keep all the workers supplied. Cloning of DNA by genetic engineering solved this problem. Artificial yeast chromosomes were produced which could carry short sequences of inserted human DNA of up to 400,000 bases. These could be cloned to produce as many copies as required. But the real breakthrough came with the invention, in 1985, of the polymerase chain reaction system by the American molecular biologist Kary Mullis. This led to the development of machines that could clone as many copies of segments of DNA as were required, almost immediately. PCR has had many other important applications.

The recording and analysis of this immense mass of information calls for special computerized database techniques which have had to be worked out specially for this purpose, mainly at the California Institute of Technology.

A JUSTIFIABLE EXPENSE?

Altogether, this is a very expensive project, comparable, for instance, to putting a man on the moon. The moon project was mounted largely for political reasons. This one, while seemingly less spectacular, is infinitely more important for the future of mankind and will allow remarkable advances in medicine. The project is going ahead in many centres and coordination has been difficult. Critics of the expense might be reminded that, at a purely material level, informed opinion has it that, long before the project is completed, the spin-offs will, in themselves, amply justify the cost.

genome, single-X

The completion of the first draft of the human genome was announced on 26 June, 2000.

genome, triple-X

See **XXX configuration**.

Genotropin

A brand name for **somatotropin**.

gentamicin

An aminoglycoside antibiotic used mainly for the treatment of serious Gram negative infections. Otherwise, gentamicin is used topically for external infections, such as those of the eye or ear. In large dosage it can cause **tinnitus**, deafness and kidney damage. Brand names are Cidomycin, Garamycin, Genticin and Minims Gentamicin.

Genticin

A brand name for **gentamicin**.

genu

Latin root meaning 'knee' as in **genu valgum** (knock knee).

genu valgum

Commonly described as 'knock knee', this minor deformity features an abnormal increase in the distance between the ankles when the knees are touching.

POSSIBLE CAUSES

It may result from growth disturbance in rickets and is not uncommon in rheumatoid arthritis, in which the inner ligament of the knee joint may weaken. The commonest cause, however, is a natural variation of the normal in children, occurring because the line of weight-bearing falls to the outer side of the centre of the knee joint.

INCIDENCE

Over 20 per cent of all three-year-olds have at least a 5 cm gap between their ankles, while only about 1 per cent of seven-year-olds show an equivalent degree of knock knee. For this reason, moderate degrees of genu valgum in healthy children below seven may safely be ignored.

TREATMENT

In some cases it is considered worth raising the inner edge of the heel of the shoes slightly. In severe cases, walking braces or night splints may be used or even operative correction.

genu varum

Bow legs, bandy legs or genu varum, are common and normal in healthy toddlers and the condition usually comes right by about 18 months. It is not caused by bulky nappies. If the bowing is still present after this time, and particularly if it gets worse, the condition of osteochondrosis of the tibia (Blount's disease) should be suspected. Rickets, from vitamin D deficiency, is another possibility. Inspection will show that the bowing does not occur at the knees, but at the upper ends of the main bones of the lower legs, the tibias.

If treated early, bow legs can be readily straightened using night splints. Neglected genu varus, in addition to causing adult deformity, usually leads to osteoarthritis in the knee joints.

Geref

A brand name for **sermorelin**.

geriatrician

A doctor specializing in the medical aspects of old age and concerned with the practical application of the science of gerontology to the improvement of the quality of life of elderly people.

geriatric medicine

The branch of medicine concerned with the medical problems of old age. Geriatrics is steadily advancing from its former position as the Cinderella of medicine. This is mainly because of the progressive rise in life expectancy and because of new and healthier revisions of the stereotype of old age. The emphasis, today, is on a positive, striving approach to life and an optimistic determination to achieve as much as possible, regardless of age. In this light, the view that the old need not be afforded the best possible standards of medical care is no longer tenable.

THE SCIENCE OF AGEING

Gerontology is the science of ageing and is concerned with all aspects of the subject, including research into the nature and causes of ageing and how, if possible, it may be retarded. Gerontological research has also brought new and healthier attitudes to geriatrics and has been responsible for changes in the ways in which old people in institutions are treated.

AGE-RELATED CONDITIONS

Certain diseases which are, by their nature, progressive, inevitably affect the elderly more than the young. The most important of these is atherosclerosis which progressively narrows arteries and limits vital blood supplies to all parts of the body. Secondary to this are such conditions as heart disease, stroke, defective functioning of the brain, eyes and ears, and peripheral circulatory problems, sometimes leading to arterial shut-down and gangrene. Joint problems also tend to be progressive and the elderly suffer greatly from the various forms of arthritis. Diabetes is not age related, but its effects tend to worsen with age. Complications affecting the retinas, the kidneys and the arteries take their toll in old age. Cancer, too, is often age-related, many cancers increasing sharply in incidence with age.

Bone fragility increases with age, especially in women, in whom osteoporosis is such a severe problem that about one-quarter of all women over 80 suffer a fracture of the hip bone. Cataract is very common in the aged and the incidence of glaucoma rises steeply with age. Deafness and a tendency to unsteadiness, or frank vertigo are also features of age. The action of drugs is often prolonged in the old because lowered usage rates promote drug accumulation in the tissues. And sometimes the action of drugs differs in the elderly from that in younger people.

All these and many other effects special to the elderly are now receiving more attention from the medical profession, and the results are already clear in the generally improved quality of life and health of old people.

Geriplex

A brand name for a multivitamin preparation.

germ

A lay term for any infecting agent capable of producing disease. Germ plasm is living primitive tissue capable of developing into an organ or individual.

German measles

See **rubella**.

germs, very small

See **nanobacteria**.

gerontology

The study of the changes that occur in the cells and tissues of the body with age. These changes, both of structure and of function, tend gradually to limit the body's ability to respond to and adapt to changing stimuli, until, eventually, the cells cease to reproduce themselves and die.

HUMAN LIFE-SPAN

It seems to be an inherent characteristic of normal human cells that they are able to undergo a limited number of divisions. This imposes a finite maximum life-span, on the human species, of about 110 years. At about this age, regardless of how healthy they may have been, people may be expected to die. There is no evidence that anything that medicine, or improvements in public health, have achieved, have had any effect on this upper limit. Increased longevity today merely means that people are approaching ever nearer to the maximum.

TISSUE RESEARCH

Ageing is an intrinsic property of all normal living organisms. But there are tissues which seem, at first sight, to be immortal. Normal human tissue cultures in the laboratory undergo between 50 and 100 generations and then gradually lose their power of reproduction. Some cancer cells, on the other hand, go on dividing indefinitely, so long as they are kept in suitable conditions and provided with nourishment. Very large quantities of a human cancer cell culture, all derived originally from the same patient, exist throughout the world. But in any consideration of the extension of human life, the significance of this clone is probably negligible. Nevertheless, studies of human tissue cultures are being closely pursued and are an important aspect of gerontology.

ELEMENTS OF GERONTOLOGY

Other concerns of the gerontological scientist include:

- comparative studies of the biological versus the temporal age;
- cell death and the loss of structural bulk in organs;
- biochemical changes in ageing individuals;
- the age structures of different populations;
- the effects of life-style on longevity;
- the effect of physical activity on longevity;
- the changing age patterns in a given population.

The conclusions, to date, have greatly supported the view that the achievement of a worthwhile extension of life is not simply a matter of avoiding damage to the body by illness. In addition to this, it involves making life-long demands on the body and the mind so that the fullest possible degree of functional activity is maintained to the last possible moment.

Gestalt psychology

Studies made early this century showed that perception was greatly influenced, and often enhanced, by the context or configuration of the observed elements. The relationship of the various components of what is perceived may convey a sense of a whole entity when, in fact, some of the elements are missing. Thus, for instance, the observation of an oval shape may be perceived as a round soup plate if it is in the context of a dining table. A melody retains its essential features when played with different orchestration or sung, or given a different harmony.

Following this observation, that the whole might be greater than the sum of the parts, much research was done to try to determine the nature of, and conditions for, this mental extension of perception. These studies were conducted under the general designation of Gestalt psychology and were based on the premise that psychological phenomena could only be properly understood if viewed as organized structural wholes (Gestalten).

In the evolutionary and schismatic way characteristic of psychology, the title has come to be applied to various groups subscribing to bodies of views or assumptions only loosely associated with the original scientific work. These groups have given rise to schools of psychotherapy whose practitioners hold that people respond to life events in a manner that involves the mind and the body inextricably, and that the common distinction between mind and body is artificial. They hold that full awareness of the world and an accurate perception of oneself are essential. A person possessing such awareness can regulate and balance his or her experience.

If unpleasantness is deliberately avoided, the holistic response – the Gestalt – is disturbed and this has serious consequences in later life. Unfinished Gestalten are carried along and may interfere with the ability to cope with later experience. The fully aware person lives in the present and is not over-influenced by past or future events.

gestation period

The period from fertilization to birth. The human gestation period varies from 38 weeks to about 40 weeks, with an average of 40 – about nine months.

Gestone

A brand name for **progesterone**.

gestrinone

A testosterone-like drug that interferes with the release of gonadotrophic hormones and can be used in women to treat endometriosis. A brand name is Dimetriose.

giardiasis

An intestinal disease caused by the microscopic single-celled organism *Giardia lamblia*, which attaches itself, by means of a sucker, to the lining of the small intestine, and then proceeds to multiply.

RECOGNITION AND SYMPTOMS

The condition, which is usually acquired by drinking contaminated water or by sexual contact, is often symptomless but may feature diarrhoea lasting for a week or more with cramping abdominal pain, a sense of fullness and flatulence. The infection often leads to failure of normal absorption of food so that the stools are bulky and unusually malodourous.

Giardiasis can readily be diagnosed by microscopic stool examination and the finding of the parasite. In some very persistent cases, stool tests may be negative and it may be necessary to take samples of the duodenal contents by means of

a tube or by swallowing one end of a nylon string and then withdrawing it.

TREATMENT

The drug tinidazole (Fasigyn) in a single dose is effective in the treatment of giardiasis. Metronidazole (Flagyl) is also used but is less effective.

giddiness

See **vertigo**.

gigantism

When the pituitary gland secretes excessive growth hormone in childhood, before the growing ends of the bones (the epiphyses) have fused, the result is gigantism. This is rare. Much more commonly, the excess hormone production occurs after this time, producing acromegaly.

Pituitary gigantism is almost always due to a non-malignant (benign) tumour of the gland – a pituitary adenoma. The result of the excessive production of hormone is that the rate of growth of all parts – both bones and soft tissue – is uniformly increased so that the height may exceed 2.4 m. The condition often features delayed puberty and underproduction of the sex hormones, so that males may develop the features of the eunuch.

There is no practical treatment for established gigantism, but once the progressing condition has been detected the tumour responsible can be destroyed by surgery or radiotherapy, supplemented by a drug such as bromocriptine, which often has the effect of lowering growth hormone levels.

Gilles de la Tourette's syndrome

A disorder which begins in childhood with simple, involuntary, uncontrollable body movements such as shrugs, twitches, jerks or blinks (tics), but which, instead of disappearing spontaneously as these childhood tics normally do, progresses to a repertoire of ever more extensive and grotesque manifestations.

Initially, these are complex bodily movements only, but eventually the sufferer begins to emit noises, at first minor barks, grunts or coughs, but later in the form of compulsive utterances, usually of an obscene nature. Coprolalia – involuntary scatological remarks – occur in about half the cases and so the condition becomes a severe social disability.

The condition requires skilled treatment with antipsychotic drugs (neuroleptics) which cause emotional quieting, promote indifference and slow down bodily and mental overactivity. Serenace (haloperidol) is often used.

gingiva

Latin root meaning 'gum' as in **gingivitis** (gum inflammation).

gingivitis

Inflammation of the gums usually as a result of the accumulation of plaque around the necks of the teeth, but also from impacted food. Rarely, nowadays, gingivitis is caused by vitamin C deficiency (scurvy). The gums are swollen, very tender and bleed easily after eating or brushing. In severe cases areas of tissue death (necrosis) occur and there is bad breath.

Unless properly treated, gingivitis tends to progress to a stage at which the membrane securing the tooth in the bone is damaged and the tooth becomes loose. This is called periodontitis. Gingivitis can easily be prevented by routine plaque removal by brushing and flossing.

gland

A cell or organ that synthesizes or selects substances from the blood and secretes them into other bodily structures or on to surfaces, including the skin. The simplest glands are the mucus-secreting goblet cells of the intestine. The most complex are major organs such as the pancreas, which is a gland both of internal secretion (endocrine) in its production of insulin, and of 'external' secretion in its production of the intestinal juice, rich in digestive enzymes, which it passes into the small intestine.

Most of the glands of the endocrine system are pure glands of internal secretion and produce several different hormones. They include the pituitary gland, the thyroid, the parathyroids, the adrenal glands and those parts of the testes and ovaries not concerned with sperm and egg production.

The glands of external secretion (exocrine glands) discharge their products onto a surface, either directly or through ducts. They include the millions of glands in the inner lining of the intestines, the sweat glands, the tear glands, the salivary glands, the milk (mammary) glands, and the mucus glands of the genitalia that lubricate sexual intercourse.

> Note that the well-known 'glands' of the neck, groin and elsewhere, which become swollen and sometimes tender during infections, are not glands, but lymph nodes.

glanders

A rare infectious disease of horses and other equines occasionally transmitted to humans. The organism responsible is the *Pseudomonas mallei*, which may cause an acute or persistent chest infection with chills, fever and prostration, or multiple pus-filled nodules or abscesses in the skin and throughout the body.

glandular fever

Because of the inaccuracy of the title 'glandular fever' this is now known as infectious mononucleosis. It is caused by a member of the **herpes** family of viruses, the Epstein-Barr virus.
INCIDENCE
The disease occurs only in those with no previous exposure to this particular organism. Because childhood attacks are usually mild and inapparent, the overt disease is commonest in young adults. One attack confers permanent immunity.
TRANSMISSION
During the acute phase and convalescence, and indeed, intermittently afterwards, the virus is present in large numbers in the saliva. This may be why immunity is so well maintained, but it is also why infective mononucleosis is sometimes called the 'kissing disease'.
RECOGNITION AND SYMPTOMS
After an incubation period of four to seven weeks there is malaise, fever, headache, sore throat and a generalized enlargement of lymph nodes. These may be felt as rubbery swellings in the neck, armpits, elbows, groin and behind the knees. The spleen, too, is enlarged and may very occasionally rupture if struck, or too vigorously felt. Rupture of the spleen is dangerous as it usually causes severe internal bleeding.

In about 10 per cent of cases there is a rash of small, slightly raised, red spots and if this does not occur spontaneously, treatment with the antibiotic ampicillin will usually result in the appearance of the rash. The lungs may be involved, with chest pain, difficulty in breathing and cough.

Diagnosis is by blood test for antibodies. Usually there is complete recovery in less than a month, but one-tenth of affected people complain for months, or even years, of fatigue with occasional recurrences of fever and lymph-node enlargement.
TREATMENT
There is no specific treatment, but bed rest is desirable during the acute stage and strenuous exercise should be avoided as long as the spleen is enlarged.

glass eye

See **eye, artificial**.

glaucoma

One of a group of eye diseases in which the pressure of the fluid within the eyeball is too high. A certain minimum pressure is required to maintain the shape and size of the globe so that it can function efficiently as an optical instrument and not be easily indented by minor external force. But if the pressure is too high it will exceed the pressure of the blood in the small arteries inside the eye and these will be flattened and occluded. Certain arteries supplying the beginning of the optic nerve are especially susceptible to such excess pressures, and it is this region which suffers most in glaucoma.

Long-term, minor deprivation of blood to the optic nerve head gradually kills off the nerve fibres from the retina, which bundle together to form the optic nerve, and the visual capacity is gradually eroded. The disorder is insidious because the fibres first affected are those coming from the periphery of

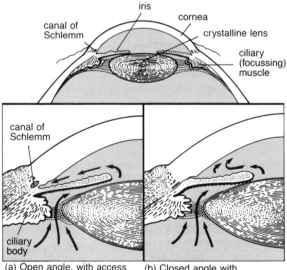

(a) Open angle, with access to canal of Schlemm

(b) Closed angle with blockage of outflow of aqueous humour

Aqueous humour is secreted by the surface cells of the ciliary body. Normally, aqueous humour leaves the eye by the canal of Schlemm via the angle between the iris and the cornea. If this angle is closed the pressure in the eye rises and acute glaucoma results.

the retina which subserve the outer parts of the fields of vision. It is a feature of visual function that one is largely unaware of the quality, or even the presence, of vision in those areas to which attention is not directed. Since we can, in general, direct attention only by looking straight at something, thus using the central retina, defects in the peripheral visual fields pass unnoticed.

> Unless looked for, glaucomatous damage is often extensive before it is detected. Chronic simple glaucoma, the commonest form, is a major cause of blindness, and visual field loss is irremediable. If detected early, the pressures can be controlled and the damage stopped.

The pressure in the eye is maintained by the continuous secretion of water (aqueous humour) inside the globe, together with its passage out of the eye by way of a circular filter, near the root of the iris, which offers resistance to outflow. The normal pressure range is maintained by a fine balance between the two. Should the resistance to outflow rise, the pressure will rise. This is what happens in chronic simple glaucoma. The process is gradual, subtle and almost entirely painless and the affected person is usually quite unaware that any harm is being suffered. The reason for the obstruction to outflow in this form of glaucoma is not fully understood.

INCIDENCE

About one person in 100 has glaucoma at the age of 40, but the incidence rises steeply with increasing age so that, by 70, about one in ten have significantly raised eye pressures.

RECOGNITION AND SYMPTOMS

Chronic simple glaucoma has a familial pattern and is more likely to occur in relatives of people with the disease. Only in the late stages will there be obvious signs and, by that time, so much peripheral visual field will have been lost that the affected person will probably be constantly bumping into others on busy pavements. Central vision is usually the last to go and one eye may be completely blinded before it is appreciated that anything is amiss.

If glaucoma is to be detected before severe damage is done, it must be looked for. One of the signs is a hollowing out (cupping) of the optic nerve head, and this can be detected during a routine eye examination. But the real test is to measure the internal pressure by a technique known as tonometry. If the pressure is found to be above the upper limit of normal, the visual fields are checked and arrangements made for follow-up. If glaucoma is diagnosed, eye drops are given to keep the pressures within normal limits. Occasionally, medical treatment fails and an operation may be needed.

In other, less common, forms of glaucoma, the outlet obstruction can be caused by mechanical or disease processes and the effects may be much more sudden and severe, with great pain and sudden loss of all vision. This is the case in acute congestive glaucoma or in glaucomas caused by inflammatory eye disease with adhesions.

The symptoms of acute glaucoma are severe. The affected eye is acutely painful, intensely red and congested, and very hard and tender to the touch. The pupil is enlarged and oval and the cornea steamy and partly opaque. The vision is grossly diminished. There is shock and sometimes pain in the abdomen. Urgent treatment to reduce the pressure is needed, so no time must be wasted.

A less severe, but commoner form, sub-acute glaucoma, causes symptoms which should be well known. These usually occur at night when the pupils are wide. There is a dull aching pain in the eye, some fogginess of vision and, characteristically, concentric, rainbow-coloured rings are seen around lights. The perception of rainbow rings around lights results from light refraction by water droplets forced into the cornea by the raised pressure.

> Such symptoms should never be ignored, for repeated sub-acute attacks can damage the eye and there is always the risk of a devastating attack of acute glaucoma. The condition can easily be prevented by the use of eyedrops and is curable by a simple operation or out-patient laser procedure.

Glaucoma present at birth (congenital glaucoma) is due to structural abnormality in the drainage angles of the eyes. This causes enlargement of the eyeballs – a condition known as buphthalmos. Operation is often necessary, but the results can be very good.

glaucoma, surgery for

See **laser trabeculoplasty**, **trabeculectomy**.

-glia

Suffix meaning 'glue' as in neuroglia (nerve glue).

glibenclamide

A **sulphonylurea** drug, similar in action and effect to chlorpropamide, and used to treat maturity onset (Type II) diabetes. Brand names are Daonil, Euglucon, and Semi-daonil.

Glibenese

A brand name for **glipizide**.

gliclazide

A **sulphonylurea** drug used to treat maturity onset (Type II) **diabetes**. A brand name is Diamicron.

glimepiride

A **sulphonylurea** drug used to treat maturity onset (Type II) **diabetes**. A brand name is Amaryl.

glioma

Gliomas are the commonest kind of brain tumour. Glial tissue is the 'glue', or neurological connective tissue, which binds nerve cells and fibres together. When glial tissue becomes malignant, the result is a glioma. A quarter of all primary brain tumours are gliomas and these vary widely in degree of malignancy and rate of growth.

The different types of gliomas are given different names, such as astrocytomas, glioblastomas, oligodendrogliomas, ependymomas and medulloblastomas, depending on their form and the type of glial tissue from which they arise. These tumours usually extend widely throughout the brain, sometimes progressing for years before causing trouble, but sometimes advancing rapidly with severe early symptoms.

Because of their nature, gliomas are very difficult to treat and can rarely be completely removed. They differ, in this respect, from the other common type of brain tumour, the meningioma, which is enclosed in a capsule and does not infiltrate into the brain substance.

glipizide

A **sulphonylurea** drug used to treat maturity onset (Type II) **diabetes**. Brand names are Glibenese and Minodiab.

gliquidone

A **sulphonylurea** drug used to treat maturity onset (Type II) **diabetes**. A brand name is Glurenorm.

globulins

One of the main groups of protein substances found in the blood, the others being the albumins and fibrinogen. The glubulins form the family of immunoglobulins, or antibodies, and are divided into five classes, each of which contains thousands of different individual and unique antibodies. The term immunoglobulin is usually abbreviated to Ig, and the five classes are IgG (gamma globulin) and IgM, which, between them, combat most bacteria and viruses; IgE, connected with allergy; IgA, which operates mainly in the intestine, lungs and urinary system and which is the main group of antibodies in milk; and IgD, whose function is still uncertain.

The globulins are produced by plasma cells which arise from selected B cells (B lymphocytes) of the immune system, following an infection or invasion of foreign matter.

globus hystericus

The sense of having a 'lump in the throat' which can neither be swallowed nor brought up. This feeling often accompanies acute anxiety, sadness or mental conflict and is due to a constriction of the circularly placed muscles around the lower part of the throat (pharynx). Globus hystericus is not caused by any organic defect and, if persistent, requires sympathetic psychiatric management after full physical investigation.

glomerulonephritis

An inflammation of the kidney caused by an immunological disorder. When bacteria, such as streptococci, invade the body, they excite an antibody response which is usually sufficient to destroy them. Sometimes, however, the quantity of antibody produced is insufficient to do this and the battle becomes a kind of stalemate, with millions of small clumps of bacteria, tightly linked to small quantities of antibody, circulating in the blood. These groups are called immune complexes and they are being increasingly recognized as an important cause of disease.

RECOGNITION AND SYMPTOMS

Glomerulonephritis is one of the major disorders caused by circulating immune complexes. These settle in the kidneys and are deposited on the walls of the filtering units (glomeruli) where they excite a severe inflammation which may be very damaging to the tissue.

The initial streptococcal infection usually involves the throat and may be very mild – sometimes passing unnoticed. One to three weeks later, the effects of kidney damage appear. The disease commonly affects children causing gen-

eralized swelling of the tissues of the body (oedema) with striking swelling of the face, fever, loss of appetite, vomiting and headache. The blood pressure is usually raised and examination of the urine shows that this is scanty and contains blood and protein – both highly abnormal constituents. In severe cases the urine may stop altogether, for a time.

After two or three days the signs and symptoms lessen, the output of urine increases and apparently full recovery occurs. There may, however, be abnormalities in the urine for weeks or months afterwards and, in some cases, the episode of glomerulonephritis is later seen to have been an episode in a prolonged course of progressive disease which may end in complete kidney failure.

There are several varieties of glomerulonephritis, some with a more serious outlook than others, and these are best distinguished by taking a small sample of kidney tissue (renal biopsy) for microscopic examination.

> Because of the danger of kidney involvement, streptococcal throat infections should be treated as early as possible with antibiotics.

glossa

Greek root meaning 'tongue' as in glossolalia ('speaking in tongues').

glossectomy

Surgical removal of the tongue. This may be total or partial and, although a major mutilation, is sometimes the only life-saving option in cancer of the tongue.

glossitis

Inflammation of the tongue, commonly resulting from nutritional inadequacy, especially iron and vitamin B deficiency. It is a feature of simple iron-deficiency anaemia. Glossitis also occurs in a number of skin and general diseases including syphilis, erythema multiforme, pemphigus, Behçet's syndrome and lichen planus.

Other causes of glossitis include:

- jagged teeth;
- repeated injury from poorly-fitting dentures;
- tongue-biting habits;
- pipe, cigarette or cigar smoking with a constantly directed jet of hot smoke to one part of the tongue;
- the excessive use of mouth washes, breath fresheners, throat lozenges;
- allergy to various substances;
- local infection.

> In the great majority of cases the condition will resolve when the cause is removed. Persistent irritation can, however, lead to cancer, and any local area of ulceration or hardness which persists should be reported without delay.

glossolalia

The production of a stream of incomprehensible and, indeed, meaningless sounds resembling words. The phenomenon is associated with a high state of religious or pseudo-religious excitement.

glossopharyngeal nerve

One of the 12 pairs of cranial nerves.

GLP-1

A glucagon-like neuropeptide claimed to be an obesity mediator. Starved rats given the drug behave as if satiated and this state is reversed if given a GLP-1 antagonist.

Glucagen

A brand name for **glucagon**.

glucagon

One of the four hormones produced by the islet cells of the pancreas, the others being insulin, somatostatin and a polypeptide of unknown function. The action of glucagon opposes that of insulin. It causes liver glycogen, a polysaccharide, to break down to glucose, thereby increasing the amount of sugar in the bloodstream. It can also mobilize fatty acids for energy purposes. A brand name is Glucagen.

Glucobay

A brand name for **acarbose**.

Glucophage

A brand name for **metformin**.

glucose tolerance test

A test used to confirm or refute the diagnosis of diabetes. In diabetes the body is unable to make normal use of the fuel, glucose, and this accumulates in abnormally large amounts in the blood. Even in health, glucose levels in the blood always rise after a meal, but they soon return to normal as the glucose is used up or stored.

In the glucose tolerance test a known quantity of glucose is given by mouth after a period of fasting and blood samples are taken half an hour, one hour, two hours and three hours later. Urine samples are also taken. In healthy people the glucose concentration rises to about twice the normal level within the first hour and returns to normal within two hours. The figures are usually plotted on a graph, which takes a characteristic shape. No glucose is excreted in the urine except sometimes in pregnancy.

In diabetes, the blood glucose rises to a much higher level than normal and the return to normal takes three hours or more. In this case, a plot of the figures on a graph shows a different shape of curve – one characteristic of diabetes. The urine test shows that a large amount of glucose is being excreted.

glucosidase inhibitor drugs

Glucosidase is a chemical activator (enzyme) that takes part in the breakdown of complex sugars such as starches and glycogen. A glucosidase inhibitor is a drug that interferes with this action so that sugars are much less easily absorbed into the body from the intestine. They are known as 'starch block-

ers' and are helpful in bringing about weight loss in people with Type II diabetes. Unfortunately, the excess of complex carbohydrates in the intestine tends to cause flatulence. The real answer, of course, is to eat less of them.

glue ear

See **otitis media**.

glue sniffing

See **solvent abuse**.

glutaraldehyde

An antiviral drug used in solution for external application to treat warts on the sole of the foot (plantar warts) and elsewhere. Brand names are Glutarol and Verucasep.

Glutarol

A brand name for a preparation of **glutaraldehyde**.

glyceryl trinitrate

Nitroglycerine, a drug highly effective in controlling the pain of **angina pectoris**. The oral preparation may be taken in a tablet that is allowed to dissolve under the tongue and the pain is usually relieved in two to three minutes. The drug is also available in patches to be applied to the skin (transdermal patches). Nitrates have a powerful action in widening (dilating) arteries, including the coronary arteries, thus improving the blood supply to the heart muscle. Sildenafil (Viagra) should not be taken by people using glyceryl trinitrate. Nitroglycerine is a well-know explosive but is formulated for medical purposes in safe dilution. Brand names are Coro-nitro, Deponit, Glytrin, Minitran, Nitro-Dur, Nitrocine, Nitrolingual, Nitromin, Nitronal, Suscard Buccal, Sustac, Percutol and Transiderm-Nitro. The latter two are for external use.

glycopyrronium bromide

An **anticholinergic** drug used by anaesthetists to dry up secretions during general anaesthesia. Brand names are Robinul and Robinul neostigmine.

glycosuria

Sugar in the urine. This is always abnormal and usually indicates diabetes. The test for sugar in the urine is a simple one and merely involves dipping a special paper or plastic strip into a sample of urine. This should be part of every reasonably comprehensive medical check-up.

Glypressin

A brand name for **terlipressin**.

Glytrin

A brand name for **glyceryl trinitrate**.

gnat bites

Gnats often attack in swarms, typically at dusk in the neighbourhood of a pool of standing water. The female of

gnathos

the species is deadlier than the male, and although they are only tiny flies, rarely more than 2 mm in length, they suck blood and can cause painful bites which leave irritating bumps, sometimes for days. Culicine midges make certain areas of the globe, especially towards the northern polar regions, almost uninhabitable. See also **flies**.

gnathos

Greek root meaning 'jaw' as in prognathous (protruding jaw).

goitre

An enlargement of the thyroid gland, which is situated across the front of the neck just below the Adam's apple (larynx). The thyroid produces hormones, the synthesis of which requires iodine. If the iodine supply is insufficient, the gland increases its activity and swells. Iodine deficiency is almost unknown in Britain, mainly because a small quantity is artificially added to table salt. Goitre was once an epidemic condition in parts of Europe.

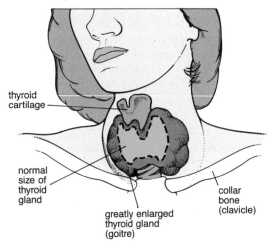

Goitre is an enlargement of the thyroid gland which lies just below the Adam's apple (thyroid cartilage). The diagram compares the normal size with an enlarged thyroid.

POSSIBLE CAUSES

Goitre occurs in the condition of Graves' disease, in which the gland is overactive and there is enlargement accompanied by excessive production of thyroid hormones. This is often associated with the staring condition of **exophthalmos**. Other conditions causing goitre include:

- Hashimoto's thyroiditis, caused by antibodies to thyroid hormone;
- sub-acute thyroiditis, which is probably a virus infection;
- dyshormonogenesis, a genetic enzyme deficiency which interferes with normal thyroid hormone synthesis;
- tumours of the thyroid gland.

Golden Eye

A brand name for eye drops containing **propamidine**.

golfer's elbow

Most of the muscles which bend the wrist have a common origin from a tendon which is attached to the bony prominence

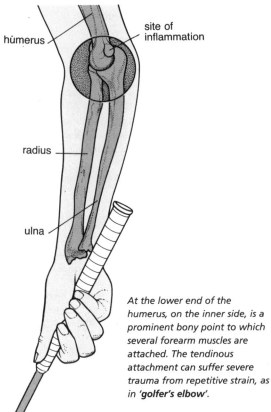

At the lower end of the humerus, on the inner side, is a prominent bony point to which several forearm muscles are attached. The tendinous attachment can suffer severe trauma from repetitive strain, as in 'golfer's elbow'.

on the inner aspect of the lower end of the upper arm bone (the humerus). Over-use of these muscles can cause partial tearing or strain in this tendon, leading to inflammation, local tenderness and disability. One must presume that one of the criteria of a 'correct' grip or swing is that it allows unlimited golf without causing this condition. The condition also affects tennis players, when it is called 'tennis elbow'.

Treatment involves rest from golf, advice from the pro, the use of pain-killing and anti-inflammatory drugs and, in extreme cases, an injection of a depot corticosteroid.

gonorrhoea

See **sexually transmitted diseases**.

Goodpasture's syndrome

A form of kidney inflammation (glomerulonephritis) most commonly affecting young adult males in the springtime, which causes acute kidney failure and often a life-threatening bleeding within the lungs. The condition is caused by antibodies to the kidney's own tissue (auto-immune disease) which attack a particular membrane in the kidneys, but also a similar membrane in the lungs.

The onset is sudden and in a day or two the damage to the kidneys may be so severe that urination almost stops. There is usually cough, often with blood-stained sputum and breathlessness.

It is essential that the diagnosis should be made quickly because urgent treatment with immunosuppressive drugs and plasma exchange transfusion can be life-saving.

Gopten

A brand name for **trandolapril**.

goserelin

A gonadotrophin-releasing hormone used as a drug to treat **endometriosis**, uterine **fibroids**, **menorrhagia** and **cancer**. A brand name is Zoladex.

gout

An acute joint disease caused by the deposition of crystals of monosodium urate monohydrate around the joints, tendons and other tissues of the body. These crystals cause severe inflammation and tissue damage. They may cause kidney structural damage and stone formation and may be deposited in the skin. Sometimes the chalky crystals break through the skin of the ear to appear on the surface (tophi).

POSSIBLE CAUSES

Crystal deposition occurs when the levels of uric acid in the body are abnormally high. The commonest cause for this is a failure of the kidneys to excrete uric acid fast enough. The reason for this is still unclear, but seems to be genetically determined. 75 per cent of cases of gout are caused in this way. In about 20 per cent of cases the cause is excessive production of uric acid. A relatively rare cause of gout is a sex-linked genetically determined error of metabolism of a group of substances found in the nuclei of cells, called purines. Uric acid is a purine and is relatively insoluble in water. Any excess, therefore, tends to lead to the formation of crystals.

RECOGNITION AND SYMPTOMS

Gout usually begins with excruciating pain and inflammation of the innermost joint of the big toe. Less often, it starts in the ankle, the knee joint, a joint in the foot, hand, wrist or, least often, an elbow. If untreated, the attack lasts for days or weeks but eventually subsides. Some people have one attack only, or attacks at intervals of years. More commonly, attacks are recurrent with increasing frequency until the condition is constantly present.

TREATMENT

Full investigation to establish the cause is important. The mainstay of treatment is non-steroidal anti-inflammatory drugs (NSAIDS), such as indomethacin or naproxen, used at the earliest possible stage and continued until the attack subsides and for a week or so afterwards. Colchicine, from crocus, is a highly effective drug but may cause side-effects. Gout can be prevented long-term by the use of a drug allopurinol which lowers the levels of uric acid in the blood. This must not be used until several weeks after an acute attack.

gouty tophi

Tophi are white, chalky nodules of crystals of uric acid salt which sometimes accumulate in the cartilage of the ear in gout and may force their way through the skin to appear externally. The appearance of tophi would prompt a check of the blood uric acid levels.

G proteins

Substances of the class known as 'second messengers'. 'First messengers' attach to receptors on the outer surface of cells and trigger off the second messengers, which move to sites inside the cells to prompt an effect. G proteins relay signals from over 1000 different cell membrane receptors to many different effectors within the cells, such as enzymes and ion channels. G proteins have three sub-units, alpha, beta and gamma, each coded for by a different gene. Their function is switched on and off by the binding and hydrolysis of guanosine triphosphate to the alpha sub-unit, which is loosely attached to the others. Binding causes the beta and gamma fragments to separate as a two-part structure (dimer) and move off to activate effectors in various parts of the cell.

G protein diseases

A group of diseases caused by abnormalities in **G proteins** so that hormonal stimulation is either reduced or is abnormally persistent. The diseases caused in this way include high blood pressure, **cholera**, **acromegaly**, night blindness, pseudohypoparathyroidism, and benign glandular tumours (adenomas) of the thyroid, adrenal and ovary.

graft-versus-host disease

A complication of bone marrow transplantation that may appear two to three weeks after a graft. The problem is caused by attacking T cells (cytotoxic T cells) present in the donated marrow, which recognize the host tissues as foreign and attack them. The effects include liver inflammation (hepatitis) with obstruction to bile flow, diarrhoea and a severe scaling skin disease called exfoliative dermatitis. Drugs such as cyclosporin and high dose steroids must be used because the condition, once fully established, has a mortality of about 30 per cent.

-gram

Suffix meaning 'scratch, write' as in electrocardiogram (heart-beat writing).

gramicidin

An antibiotic used externally in ointments and creams, often in conjunction with the antibiotics **neomycin** and **framycetin** and with corticosteroids. It is too toxic for internal use. Brand names of various combinations include Adcortyl, Graneodin, Neosporin, Sofradex, Soframycin and Tri-Adcortyl.

grand mal

A major epileptic fit.
   See **epilepsy**.

Graneodin

A brand name for an ointment containing **gramicidin** and **neomycin**.

Granisetron

A serotonin antagonist drug that blocks the nausea receptors in the small intestine and is used to control sickness and vomiting after surgery and in patients on anticancer chemotherapy. It can be used in children. A brand name is Kytril.

Granocyte

A brand name for **lenograstim**.

granulation tissue

The soft, pink, fleshy material which forms during the healing of an open wound and which provides the basis on which some regenerative inward spread of skin may occur. Granulations are rapidly budding tiny blood vessels (capillaries) surrounded by fibrils of newly generated protein material called collagen, secreted by cells called fibroblasts.

In some cases the growth of granulation tissue is so exuberant that it stands proud of the surface of the skin and may have to be deliberately discouraged. Untreated granulations usually end in firm scar tissue.

granulocyte stimulating factor

A circulating hormonal substance that controls the growth of some of the white cells of the blood. The human gene for this factor has been sequenced and the factor is produced by recombinant **DNA** techniques (genetic engineering) and sold under brand names such as Granocyte and Neupogen.

granuloma

A mass of granulation tissue forming a nodule and often stimulated by the presence of foreign material, with persistent infection and inflammation.

granuloma annulare

A common skin condition, often confused with 'ringworm', but quite unconnected with it. It usually affects the back of the feet or hands, or the back surface of the arms or legs and is seen most often in children and young adults, but may occur at any age. The appearance is of a series of deep, slightly raised bumps, arranged in a ring and usually of normal skin colour, but sometimes reddish-blue. The condition is harmless and will settle eventually without treatment, but can be got rid of by the use of steroid ointments.

granuloma inguinale

See **sexually transmitted diseases**.

Graves' disease

See **thyrotoxicosis**.

gravid

Pregnant, either of a woman or of a womb (uterus). The word comes from the Latin *gravid* meaning 'heavy', from which was derived *graviditias* meaning 'pregnancy'. A primigravida – usually contracted by midwives and obstetricians to 'prim' – is a woman pregnant for the first time. A primipara is a woman who has delivered one baby. A multigravida is a woman who has been pregnant two or more times and a multipara is one who has had two or more deliveries. A grand multipara has delivered six or more live babies or viable fetuses.

greenstick fracture

A type of long bone break common in children in which the fracture is incomplete, the bone being bent on one side and splintered on the other.

grey baby syndrome

A dangerous side-effect of the antibiotic drug chloramphenicol in premature and young babies. In such children the liver is incapable of rendering the drug safe by linking with other substances (conjugation) and high levels occur in the blood. The result is a condition of acute failure of the blood circulation. For this reason chloramphenicol is never given to premature babies.

grief

The pattern of inextricably associated physical and mental responses to major loss – usually to the loss, by death, of a loved person, but also to other losses. The pattern is the same, whatever the form of the loss, varying only with the magnitude of the deprivation.

RECOGNITION AND SYMPTOMS

The physical components of grief are caused by overaction of the sympathetic division of the autonomic nervous system and include a rapid heart rate, rapid breathing, restlessness and a tendency to move about, 'butterflies in the stomach', loss of appetite, and a 'lump in the throat' (**globus hystericus**). These symptoms are similar to those experienced in conditions of fear or rage, but, in the context of loss, are interpreted differently.

The psychological elements are complex and include feelings of guilt, anger, hostility, resentment, superimposed on an overall sense of pain, anguish and unhappiness.

> Grief follows well-marked and usually predictable stages, and there is some comfort in the knowledge that, although the practical effects of loss may persist, the severe emotional reaction to it will not. The stages include numbness, disbelief, denial, alarm, anger, guilt, consolation, adjustment and forgetting. The process may take anything from a few months to a year or two.

See also **bereavement**.

griseofulvin

An antifungal drug derived from a *Penicillium* mould that concentrates in the outer layers of the skin and in the nails and is thus useful in the treatment of 'ringworm' (tinea) infections. Skin infections settle quickly, but tinea of the nails requires treatment for months. Brand names are Fulcin and grisovin.

Grisovin

A brand name for **griseofulvin**.

grommet

A small plastic tube, narrower in the centre than at the ends, which is used to maintain drainage of the middle ear, through a tiny surgical opening in the eardrum, in cases of **otitis media**, especially of the 'secretory' type.

group therapy

A form of psychological treatment in which selected patients are brought together into a group, under the guidance of a leader or therapist, not for reasons of economy, but because most emotional disorders involve defective relationships with others and the dynamics of the group can be applied to assist the healing process. Groups may number from four to about twelve.

HOW IT'S DONE

There are many different schools of group therapy, including behaviourist conditioning therapy, Gestalt therapy, transactional analysis techniques (TA) on the principles of Eric Berne, psychodrama and group psychotherapy and family therapy, based on non-judgmental expression of feelings. Group therapy in a wider sense is also employed by many mutually supportive groups, such as Alcoholics Anonymous.

The function of the group leader or therapist is to set rules, to guide, interpret and control, but to do so as a moderator or chairperson, rather than a propounder of dogma.

WHY IT'S DONE

Some forms of group therapy have been shown to be effective, and it is clear that there are advantages in this approach. The group forms a valid microcosm – a society in miniature – in which each member has the opportunity to demonstrate, for criticism, his or her particular, and possibly aberrant, way of relating to others. It provides a forum for valuable discussion of the problems of members and a stage on which amended behaviour can be practised. And it provides a source of emotional support for members, who feel that they are not alone in their difficulties and problems.

growing pains

A medical fiction, possibly invented by doctors at a loss to account for some of the many aches and discomforts complained of by children.

> All pains have a cause, most of which are trivial, but not all of which can be explained. So long as the child is well, active, free from fever, eating and sleeping normally and gaining size, there is little likelihood that these pains are of significance.

Possible causes of vague aches and pains include overuse of muscles, tendon and ligament strain, partial dislocation of joints and hair-line fractures of bone.

But see also **bone cancer**.

growth

The size and height of an individual is genetically determined, but many factors can intervene to limit growth. These include malnutrition – lack of the essential proteins, fats, vitamins and minerals and adequate calories. Malnutrition is most influential very early in life. If it occurs during infancy there will be irreversible failure of body growth and brain development – a failure which cannot be made up later, however good the diet. Early growth is also retarded by serious illness, but this is often fully recoverable, the illness being followed by a compensatory spurt in growth.

There are two periods of maximal growth rate. The first, up to the age of two, is really an extension of the extraordinarily rapid period of fetal growth. The second period starts at puberty and progresses until the early 20s. All body growth is normally complete by age 25. Increase in body length occurs at the growing ends of the long bones of the skeleton, which have growth zones, called epiphyses, that remain active until the end of adolescence and then fuse with the rest of the bone. The pituitary growth hormone, somatotrophin, controls this process. Normal growth in bulk, as distinct from height, is essentially a matter of protein production. Growth hormone, in addition to causing elongation of the body, also promotes the synthesis of protein in many tissues other than bone. It does this by increasing the transport of amino acids – the 'building bricks' of protein – into cells and by boosting amino acid production within the cells. It also causes a major increase in the rate of cell division, and hence reproduction, which is another central element in growth.

Growth hormone is not produced continuously, but is secreted in bursts. During the day, if the individual remains sedentary, there is little growth hormone production. Exercise and stress, however, cause a burst of secretion large enough for the hormone to exert its effects. A similar outpouring of the hormone occurs an hour or two after falling asleep. Growth hormone is now being produced by genetic engineering methods, allowing greatly increased medical usage for a variety of purposes. Other hormones are indirectly important in growth. These include thyroid hormone, which controls the rate of tissue build-up, (anabolism) and breakdown (catabolism); insulin, which controls the levels of

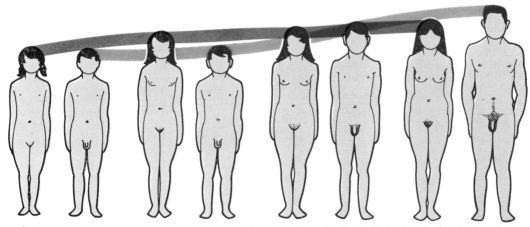

Relative growth of male and female. Growth is rapid and about equal from birth to mid childhood, when the female may grow more rapidly. The second major spurt in growth occurs after puberty and in this the male pushes ahead of the female.

fuel (glucose) in the blood and its rate of utilization; and sex hormones (androgens and oestrogens) which control the development of the male and female sexual characteristics, including body shape and bulk. Deficiency of growth hormone in children causes dwarfism. If present in excess before the epiphyses fuse, gigantism results.

guanethidine sulphate

An adrenergic receptor blocker drug used in the treatment of high blood pressure and **glaucoma**. Brand names are Ismelin and, as eyedrops with adrenaline, Ganda.

Guarem

A brand name for guar gum.

Guillain-Barré syndrome

A widespread inflammation of nerves (polyneuritis). The Guillain-Barre syndrome is a serious disorder of the nervous system caused by an immunological defect involving the fatty insulating sheaths (myelin sheaths) of the spinal nerves, and their branches. The resulting inflammation and nerve damage has the effect of preventing normal nerve conduction.

POSSIBLE CAUSES

In almost all cases, there has been a viral or bacterial infection of some kind within the four weeks prior to the onset of the disorder.

RECOGNITION AND SYMPTOMS

The disorder often starts with pain in the back and tingling and numbness in the hands and feet, spreading progressively towards the body. In other cases, the first sign is rapidly progressive muscle weakness, often involving the face.

Sometimes, within a few hours of onset, the affected person is completely paralysed, unable to move arms or legs, and in imminent danger of dying from paralysis of the muscles of respiration.

TREATMENT

An emergency tracheostomy and the insertion of a tube into the windpipe (trachea) for positive pressure artificial respiration, by machine, is necessary in such cases. When respiratory paralysis has not occurred, the affected person should, nevertheless, be closely watched, in hospital, in case of spread of the process to the respiratory muscles.

Providing effective respiration is maintained, the outlook is good and about 90 per cent of all patients recover completely within three to eight weeks. The death rate from the syndrome is about 5 per cent. About one patient in 20 is left with some permanent paralysis.

guilt

An emotional state caused by the awareness, or belief, that one has contravened early programming on standards of behaviour. Such conditioning is not normally recognized as such, but is usually interpreted as a moral, ethical or religious code to which one may or may not, in one's maturer

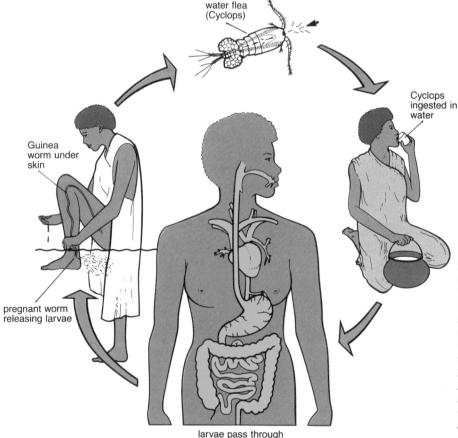

The life cycle of the Guinea worm Dracunculus medinensis. *The larvae are taken up by the water flea* Cyclops *which is swallowed if the water is drunk. Larvae pass into the blood stream and settle under the skin where the adult worms develop. The pregnant female releases larvae into water.*

water flea (Cyclops)

Cyclops ingested in water

Guinea worm under skin

pregnant worm releasing larvae

larvae pass through stomach and bowel wall into blood

judgement, subscribe. Early programming is influential throughout life, even if the precepts have been subsequently rejected on the grounds of reason, and some people experience guilt although logically convinced that their behaviour has been acceptable.

Few people are able entirely to ignore the generally accepted rules of society, and most experience some sense of guilt when contravening these rules. Severe guilt occurs when a deeply and long-accepted concept of behaviour is contravened, and this is distinguishable from any emotion aroused by the fear of punishment, and from a sense of shame in the knowledge that others are privy to one's transgression.

In psychiatric disorders, a deep, and apparently inappropriate, sense of guilt is often present, but there is usually some internal logic to this. A strong sense of guilt is often a feature of bereavement.

Guinea worm

An infestation with the parasitic worm *Dracunculus medinensis*, acquired by drinking water contaminated with the water flea *Cyclops*, containing the larvae of the worm.

When contaminated water is drunk, the larvae break through the lining of the stomach or duodenum and gain access to the blood. They settle under the skin, often in the region of the ankles, and grow to full size in about a year. The female worm is about a metre long, the male much shorter. Copulation occurs. The pregnant female worm contains about three million larvae and, in the presence of water, comes to the surface of the skin, causes a kind of boil, and then breaks through to release the larvae. These are at once taken up by *Cyclops*, usually two or three per flea.

OCCURRENCE
The condition is endemic in many parts of Africa, the Middle East, India, South America and the Caribbean.

RECOGNITION AND SYMPTOMS
While the 'boil' is forming there may be a severe general upset but this settles when it bursts. Once the larvae have been released, the worm will sometimes come out spontaneously.

TREATMENT
For centuries, Guinea worm has been treated by the trick of attaching the end of the worm to a twig and then slowly, over the course of several days, winding it out of the opening in the skin. Patience is essential as a broken worm causes a severe, and sometimes dangerous, allergic reaction. Once the worm is out, the opening soon heals over, unless there has been gross infection, in which case an abscess may form.

gula

Latin root meaning 'throat' as in gullet (swallowing tube).

Gulf war syndrome

A disorder, or group of disorders, believed by many people to be related to service in the Persian Gulf War against Iraq of early 1991. About 1500 UK troops and many more Americans are convinced that they, and even in some cases their subsequently-born children, suffered, or suffer, one or other of a wide variety of disorders as a result of this military service. Most believe these to be caused by the large range of vaccines and drugs given to them as protection against possible biological and chemical warfare, or by exposure to organophosphate insecticide agents.

The matter has been the subject of long study in the United States by a Presidential Advisory Committee, which submitted its final report in September 1997. No single cause had been found and the Committee suggested that stress was the most likely explanation for post-Gulf war symptoms experienced by military personnel. This opinion has been, and continues to be, hotly challenged by many.

gullet

The common term for the oesophagus, the part of the intestinal tract that runs vertically downwards from the throat to the stomach. In its route downwards the gullet passes through a hole in the diaphragm and then immediately enters the stomach. This area is known as the cardia.

gullet and air tube abnormal junction

See **tracheo-oesophageal fistula**.

gullet bleeding control

See **Sengstaken tube**.

gullet inflammation

See **Barrett's oesophagus**.

gullet, lower end of

See **cardia (gullet)**.

gullet, tear of

See **Mallory-Weiss syndrome**.

gumboil

An abscess of the gum and the outer lining of the bone (periosteum) of the jaw, resulting from tooth decay (dental caries) and infection.

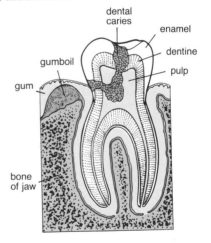

Tooth decay (dental caries) leads to infection of the periodontal membrane that binds the tooth to the bone. An abscess forms and the pus causes a swelling under the gum.

There is a local swelling with redness and great tenderness and a collection of pus under the surface of the gum, which may burst through spontaneously and leak away between the tooth and the gum, or which may have to be released by a small surgical incision. Antibiotics are sometimes necessary.

The gumboil is often an indication that a higher standard of oral hygiene, with effective brushing after meals and regular dental check-ups, is indicated.

gumma

A deep, nodule-like mass of granulation tissue, so called because the centre of the mass is of a gum-like consistency. The gumma is a feature of late (tertiary) syphilis and is now rare. It is the result of tissue destruction by a focus of the syphilis organism *Treponema pallidum* and the resulting attempt of the body to achieve healing.

Gummas can occur anywhere in the body, including the brain, the internal organs and the liver and are always associated with tissue destruction.

gut

The intestine. This is not a slang or lay term, but a normal medical expression. One of the most prestigious journals of gastro-enterology is called *Gut*.

See also **oesophagus**, **stomach**, **small intestine**, **large intestine**.

gut failure

A condition in which, for any reason, the intestinal tract cannot process enough food to maintain adequate nutrition. Permanent gut failure most commonly results from surgical removal of too great a length of the small intestine (short gut syndrome) or from **Crohn's disease** or local loss of blood supply. Other causes include failure of neurological control of intestinal motility and **diabetes**. In gut failure life must be maintained by tube feeding directly into the bloodstream (parenteral nutrition).

gynaecological surgeon

A gynaecologist who regularly performs surgical operations for the treatment of women's disorders.

gynaecologist

A doctor who specializes in the disorders of the reproductive system in women and is thus concerned, in particular, with menstrual upsets, endometriosis, pelvic infection, cancer of the uterus and adjacent organs, cysts and tumours of the ovaries, infertility, contraception and complications of childbearing including ectopic pregnancy and breast and lactation disorders. Many gynaecologists also practise **obstetrics**.

gynaecology

The term comes from the Greek *gyne* 'a woman'. Gynaecology is the province of the gynaecologist or woman specialist. The speciality is concerned with:

- malformations of the reproductive organs;
- diseases of the external genitalia (vulva), vagina, womb (uterus), fallopian tubes, ovaries and breasts;
- infection in the pelvis (pelvic inflammatory disease) which may have serious effects on the reproductive organs;
- malpositioning of the womb (which is usually harmless);
- cancer of the womb and surrounding structures (see **uterus, cancer of**);
- endometriosis;
- cysts and tumours of the ovaries;
- ectopic pregnancy and other complications of childbearing;
- infertility;
- contraception.

Cancer of the breast and the effects of sexually transmitted diseases may or may not be deemed to be within the province of gynaecology, depending on the interests of the particular gynaecologist concerned, but it is usual for breast cancer to be managed by a general surgeon.

gynaecomastia

Abnormal enlargement of one or both breasts in men or boys, so that they resemble the mature female breast. In most cases, gynaecomastia is temporary and is due to a transient hormonal imbalance, but it may be due to liver disease, such as cirrhosis, which prevents the normal liver destruction of female sex hormones; to drug therapy with steroids or oestrogens, or the diuretic spironolactone; to a tumour of the testis or pituitary gland; or to a hormone-secreting tumour of the lung, breast or other organ.

Treatment is directed to the cause, but persistent gynaecomastia, causing annoyance or embarrassment, can easily be corrected by plastic surgery.

gynaecos

Greek root meaning 'of a woman' as in gynaecology (study of female disorders).

Gyno-Daktarin

A brand name for **miconazole**.

Gyno-Pevaryl

A brand name for **econazole**.

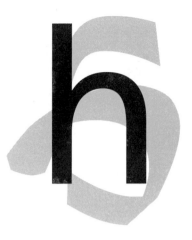

H2 receptor antagonists

A range of drugs that block the action of histamine on receptors, mainly in the stomach, and that are concerned with the secretion of acid. The most important of these drugs are cimetidine (Tagamet) and ranitidine (Zantac). Although these drugs are antihistamines, this term is normally restricted to blockers of the H-1 receptors in the blood vessels.

See also **antacid drugs**.

habit

A sequence of learned behaviour occurring in a particular context or as a response to particular events. Life without habit is inconceivable, and much of our behaviour consists in the working out of hierarchies of habit. With many people, these habit responses are largely predictable.

ROLE OF HABITS

Habits organize life, sometimes in minute detail. It is, essentially, a matter of programming – a process which is most influential early in life, but which goes on throughout life. And the obvious advantages of possessing a complex of 'good' habits illuminates the error of the unthinking reaction against the proposition that we are, at least partly, programmed beings.

ESTABLISHING A HABIT

Habits are often conditioned, are performed automatically and unconsciously, and spare us much decision-making. They start in an observation of the effect produced by behaviour. If the effect seems desirable, the behaviour is repeated. The strength and stability of a habit depends on repetition of rewards, or repeated avoidance of unpleasantness, such as punishment. These lead to reinforcement and eventual strong establishment of the habit. Once a habit is well established, it may be maintained even if the factors that began it no longer operate.

The practical importance of recognizing that habit is a matter of programming lies in the corollary that what has been programmed can always be re-programmed. This process is sometimes painful but the result can be useful. Behavioural psychology is based on the acceptance of this premise.

Haelan

A brand name for **flurandrenolone**.

haem-

A Greek-derived prefix meaning 'pertaining to blood' as in haemoglobin (blood pigment).

haemangioma

A benign tumour of blood vessels, which may occur anywhere in the body, but which often occurs in the skin. Common types include the *strawberry naevus* birthmarks, which grow for six months, remain static for two or three years and then gradually disappear; port-wine stains, which are areas of enlarged capillaries that neither grow nor diminish; cavernous haemangiomas, which consist mainly of veins, and form raised, bluish-purple masses on the skin which blanch on pressure and then refill; and cirsoid aneurysms – pulsating masses of tortuous and dilated vein-like vessels fed directly by an artery.

Small port-wine stains can be removed, along with the affected skin. Larger ones may be tattooed with skin-coloured pigment or dispersed by laser. Cavernous haemangiomas and cirsoid aneurysms can be removed surgically.

haemarthrosis

The release of blood into a joint space, either as a result of injury or disease such as scurvy or haemophilia. Haemarthrosis causes swelling, pain, a sense of warmth and muscle spasm. The blood is usually absorbed within a few days with little harm done, but repeated episodes damage the joint and lead to crippling deformity. The cause should, therefore, always be determined and, if possible, avoided.

haematemesis

Vomiting blood. The commonest causes are deep ulcers of the stomach or duodenum, gastric erosions, varicose veins in the gullet (oesophagus) – usually as a result of back pressure from cirrhosis of the liver – and the Mallory-Weiss syndrome in which excessive vomiting leads to a tearing of the lining of the stomach. Cancer of the stomach is an uncommon cause of haematemesis.

> Black stools may be the only sign of bleeding into the intestine and should never be ignored.

Vomiting blood is usually accompanied by nausea, faintness and weakness. If the blood remains for a time in the stomach before being vomited, it is altered by the acid so that it comes to resemble brown, wet coffee grounds. Blood which is not vomited, but passes down the intestine, is even more fully digested and stains the stool a tarry black colour.

haematologist

A doctor specializing in the study of the blood and blood disorders, especially the various forms of anaemia, polycythaemia, the haemoglobinopathies such as sickle-cell disease and thalassaemia, purpura, haemophilia, clotting disorders and the leukaemias. The haematologist is also concerned with all aspects of blood transfusion and its complications.

haematology

The study of the blood and the cells and tissues which generate the blood constituents, and their disorders. Haematology has become a rapidly advancing specialty of great importance in recent years, with a major, and fruitful, interface with such diverse disciplines as immunology, genetics, the science of tumours (oncology), virology and nutrition.

Among the many conditions with which it deals are those in which the blood is deficient (the anaemias); those with an excess of blood constituents (polycythaemia); those caused by an abnormality in the haemoglobin of the blood (haemoglobinopathies, sickle-cell disease and thalassaemia); those causing abnormal bleeding (purpura, haemophilia, liver disease); those causing abnormal clotting; and cancer of the blood (the leukaemias). Haematology is also concerned with blood transfusion and its complications and with the multitude of rare blood groups outside the common A,B, AB and O groups.

haematoma

An accumulation of blood in the tissues, which has partially or wholly clotted to form a semi-solid or solid mass. Haematomas are most commonly caused by injury – accidental, malicious or surgical – but may occur spontaneously as a result of bleeding disorders. They may be of fixed size or gradually increase in size. They may persist for weeks or months, and sometimes become infected to form abscesses.

The significance of a haematoma depends on its site and on whether it is enlarging. Most dangerous is the haematoma inside the skull, usually from an accelerative or decelerative head injury in which a swinging brain movement leads to arterial tearing and the release of blood under the brain linings.

> An accumulating intracranial haematoma compresses the brain and will eventually, unless treated, destroy its function. This is a common cause of death in people who engage in boxing or reckless motor cycle riding.

haematoma auris

Repeated release of blood into the tissues of the ear, usually from boxing, leading to the development of the badge of the professional pugilist – the **cauliflower ear**.

haematuria

Blood in the urine. Large amounts of blood produce a smoky, bright-red or reddish-brown appearance. Small quantities may be present without obvious change, but can be detected by simple tests. When blood appears at the start of urination and then disappears, the source is in the prostate gland or urine tube (urethra). If it is uniformly mixed with the urine, it may arise from the kidneys, the tubes carrying urine down to the bladder (the ureters) or the bladder itself.

> Haematuria is a sign of potentially serious disease and must always be investigated.

The commonest causes are:
- inflammation of the kidney (glomerulonephritis);
- injury, cancer, tuberculosis, systemic lupus erythematosus or congenital cystic disease of the kidney;
- stones in the kidney or ureter;
- benign polyps or tumours of the bladder;
- cancer or benign enlargement (hypertrophy) of the prostate;
- malignant hypertension;
- bleeding disorders.

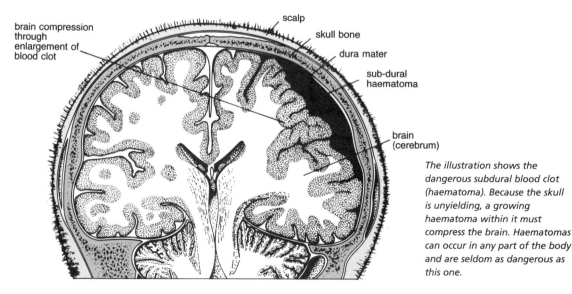

brain compression through enlargement of blood clot — scalp — skull bone — dura mater — sub-dural haematoma — brain (cerebrum)

The illustration shows the dangerous subdural blood clot (haematoma). Because the skull is unyielding, a growing haematoma within it must compress the brain. Haematomas can occur in any part of the body and are seldom as dangerous as this one.

haemochromatosis

An uncommon, genetically determined disease in which iron is absorbed and stored to an abnormal degree, so that the total body iron content rises from the usual 4 or 5 grams to as high as 60 grams. The iron is stored in various organs, especially the liver, the pancreas, the endocrine glands, the skin and the heart and the results are cirrhosis of the liver, diabetes, impotence and loss of libido, a leaden bronzing of the skin and heart failure.

INCIDENCE
Haemochromatosis is sometimes called *bronzed diabetes* and affects men ten times as often as women.

TREATMENT
It is treated by regular weekly bleeding of half a litre, to lose about 0.25 grams of iron in the form of haemoglobin. This is usually continued for about two years, until the levels of serum iron reach normal. Thereafter, occasional bleeding is done, as the need arises. Iron can also be removed by means of the drug desferrioxamine.

haemodialysis

A vital treatment in cases of kidney failure in which excessive natural waste products are removed from the blood of people whose kidneys are no longer able to perform this function. The equipment used is commonly described as an artificial kidney. Two connections are made to the patient's blood circulation, one for outflow from an artery and one for return to a vein. The blood is passed through a long, thin-walled plastic tube which is permeable to the small-molecule waste products but not to the blood cells and proteins. This tube is immersed in constantly changed water and the unwanted substances diffuse out.

haemofiltration

A technique similar to **haemodialysis** used to remove waste products from blood in cases of kidney failure. The blood is passed through a membrane filter to remove an ultrafiltrate of plasma containing many small molecules including those of the waste matter. This is replaced by an artificial solution containing the appropriate levels of the necessary small molecules (the electrolytes). Haemofiltration may be driven by the patient's own blood pressure, or by a vein to vein connection using an external pumping mechanism.

haemoglobinopathies

A group of inherited diseases in which there is an abnormality in the haemoglobin within the red cells of the blood. The group includes sickle-cell disease and the **thalassaemias.**

haemoglobinuria

Haemoglobin is the red pigment in the red blood cells. Haemoglobinuria is free haemoglobin in the urine. This is not the same as haematuria, which is whole blood in the urine. Haemoglobinuria occurs when haemoglobin has been released in large quantity from the red cells in the blood, as in the complication of severe malaria known as *blackwater fever*. In this case, the malarial parasites, which invade and multiply in the red cells, rupture the envelope of so many cells that more haemoglobin is released than the body's normal scavenging processes can deal with. The free haemoglobin pas[...] urine. Various other [...] red cell breakdown (the [...] haemoglobinuria.

haemolysis

Destruction of red blood cells by rupture of th[...] and release of the contained haemoglobin.

haemolytic anaemia

The average life of a red blood cell is 120 days. Some people's cells show increased fragility, however, and these break up sooner, causing a reduction in the available haemoglobin (anaemia). Spherocytosis is a condition in which the red cells, instead of being disc-shaped, with a hollow on each surface (bi-concave discs), are shaped like little spheres. In this heredity disorder the cell fragility leads to rapid destruction and haemolytic anaemia, which is sometimes so severe that blood transfusion is needed. Most of the breakdown of red cells occurs in the spleen, and a marked and usually permanent improvement can be effected by surgical removal of this organ.

Other causes of shortened red cell life and haemolytic anaemia are sickle-cell disease, the haemoglobinopathies, thalassaemia and malaria. Haemolysis also occurs in other conditions, such as haemolytic disease of the newborn, trauma, incompatible blood transfusions, G-6PD deficiency and vitamin K overdosage.

haemolytic disease of the newborn

See **rhesus factor disease**.

haemophilia

A condition causing a life-long tendency to excessive bleeding with very slow clotting of the blood.

CAUSE
Haemophilia is due to the absence of Factor VIII, one of the many elements necessary for normal blood coagulation. It is a recessive genetic disorder, the gene being on the X (sex) chromosome. The sons of a haemophilic man do not suffer the disease and do not pass it on to their descendants. All the daughters carry the gene on one X chromosome but, because the gene is recessive, do not suffer the disease. They are, however, carriers, and there is a 50 per cent chance that the X they transmit to their sons will be the one with the haemophilic gene. So, on average, half their sons will suffer from haemophilia. Female haemophiliacs are very rare and occur only if haemophiliacs marry carrier females.

RECOGNITION AND SYMPTOMS
In haemophilia, bleeding occurs either spontaneously or on minor trauma, most commonly into the joints, causing severe pain, swelling and spasm of the associated muscles. The blood absorbs within a few days and the symptoms settle. Repeated episodes, however, lead to damage and chronic joint disability. Bleeding may also occur into the bowel, causing symptoms which mimic other acute abdominal emergencies and problems from excessive blood loss. External bleeding, from injury, whether accidental or surgical, continues indefinitely unless special measures are taken to stop it. Dental extraction is followed by very prolonged

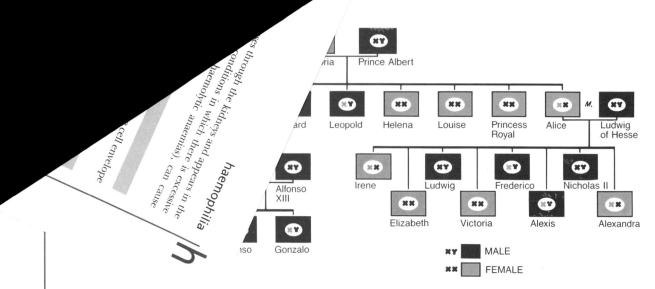

MALE XY

FEMALE XX

A typical haemophilia family. Females have two X chromosomes, males have an X and a Y. The haemophilia gene is on an X chromosome and is shown in colour. Males cannot acquire the gene from a haemophilic father as only the Y chromosome is passed on by the father. They have a fifty-fifty chance of acquiring it from a carrier mother.

bleeding. The severity of haemophilia varies with the level of Factor VIII activity in the individual and in severe cases this may be less than 2 per cent of normal.

TREATMENT

All of these troubles can be prevented by giving Factor VIII whenever bleeding occurs. The concentrate is derived from donated blood and, unfortunately, is active only for a short period, so repeated injections are necessary. Haemophiliacs are advised to try to avoid trauma, but to lead as normal lives as possible.

> Before the dangers of the AIDS epidemic were fully recognized, pooled blood containing the HIV virus was used to produce Factor VIII concentrates and many haemophiliacs acquired the disease. All concentrate is now heat-treated to kill the virus. Hepatitis B is also a problem, and many haemophiliacs contract the disease.

haemoptysis

Coughing up blood.

> Although not necessarily an indication of dangerous disease, haemoptysis is a potentially serious physical sign which must never be disregarded.

RECOGNITION AND SYMPTOMS

Coughed-up blood is bright red and can be distinguished from vomited blood, which is dark red or brown and may resemble coffee grounds. Sputum tinged with blood is a feature of bronchitis or bronchiectasis, and is often seen in the course of a bout of heavy coughing.

POSSIBLE CAUSES

Coughing of blood was once a cardinal sign of tuberculosis and this is still the cause in about 10 per cent of cases. But, today, sudden unexpected coughing-up of blood is twice as likely to be due to cancer of the lung, especially in cigarette smokers over forty.

Sometimes apparently coughed blood has its origins in the nose or mouth, or even in the stomach. Vomited blood, however, is never bright red.

haemorrhage

The escape of blood from any artery, vein, arteriole, venule or capillary. Bleeding may occur externally via a wound or from an injured blood vessel near the surface, as in nose-bleed. It may occur into the tissues, causing bruising, as in a 'black eye', or it may separate the tissues, or occur into a natural internal space, causing a larger blood collection (haematoma).

> Large blood collections often cause harm or danger by their effect on adjacent structures. Bleeding inside the skull is particularly dangerous because of the compressive effect on the brain. A person who suffers a head injury and recovers consciousness, but who later lapses again into unconsciousness, is in grave danger of dying because there is almost certainly a growing haematoma which is compressing the brain and which will, eventually, destroy the vital centres. This may occur suddenly from rupture of an internal artery (stroke). Bleeding into the potential space between the lung and the chest wall (haemothorax) forces the lung on that side to collapse.

RISKS

Major blood loss is dangerous primarily because of the loss of circulating blood volume so that there may be insufficient to provide a supply to vital parts, especially the heart muscle and the brain. This may occur even without visible external bleeding. A major fracture of the thigh bone (femur), for instance, may involve so much loss of blood from the circulation into the tissue, that the patient may die from this cause alone.

TREATMENT

The group of effects (syndrome) occurring in the body when much circulating blood is lost, is called shock, which is a technical, medical term. Shock is always serious and requires urgent treatment. An injured person suffering from shock is in urgent need of resuscitation, the most pressing necessity, after the bleeding has been stopped, being for a transfusion to restore the circulating volume of the blood. It is not even always necessary to transfuse whole blood. So long as the volume is made up with fluid of some kind – salt water (saline) or plasma – life can be saved.

haemorrhage, cerebral

See **stroke**.

haemorrhagic disorders

Because uncontrolled bleeding is so dangerous, the circulatory system has a built-in mechanism to control it. This involves a narrowing of arteries at the site of the bleeding (vasoconstriction) as an immediate reaction to injury, the plugging of small vessels by collections of tiny blood elements called platelets, the compression of the bleeding vessels by blood in the tissues, and the blood clotting (coagulation) system. The system normally works effectively to close off and seal small blood vessels, even small arteries, but sometimes goes wrong.

Blood coagulation is a very complex process involving a sequence of stages and at least seventeen different factors. Few people have a complete grasp of all that is currently known on the subject. Bleeding disorders are, however, well understood, and include such conditions as various kinds of purpura, platelet disorders, von Willebrand's disease, haemophilia, vitamin K deficiency, and certain liver diseases which interfere with clotting factor production. Most of these can be treated effectively or controlled.

haemorrhoidectomy

Surgical removal of piles (**haemorrhoids**). Most piles are not treated by haemorrhoidectomy, since injection with a sclerosing solution, such as 5 per cent carbolic acid (phenol) in almond oil, is often effective. An alternative procedure is rubber band ligation, where a tight rubber band is placed round the neck of the pile so that its blood supply is cut off and it shrivels. Destruction by freezing or with a CO_2 laser may also be used.

HOW IT'S DONE

Actual haemorrhoidectomy is reserved for those cases in which the piles are large and internally placed, and involves tying a tight string (ligature) around the base of the pile to control bleeding and cutting off the outer part. This leaves raw areas of bowel lining which gradually, over the course of three or four weeks, become covered with the normal inner surface membrane (epithelium). During this period, the stools are kept soft by the use of water-retaining agents such as methylcellulose.

RISKS

The results are generally good and only a small proportion of people operated on have recurrent symptoms. During the immediate post-operative period, however, males may find difficulty in passing urine for a time and there may be a slight tendency to incontinence.

Various methods of haemorrhoid treatment. (a) A rubber band is directed along a needle until it surrounds the pile. (b) The pile is grasped in narrow forceps and a tight constricting band forced over. Piles can be treated by injection. (c) Large piles may be tied off with ligatures and cut off with scissors.

P...
ten...
bloo...
The w...
a medi...
good me...

Haem...
Here, just...
considerable...
or so, from th...
where it joins...
become varicose...
sometimes painfu...

RECOGNITION AND S...

The varicosity can af... the anal canal, where it is k... ...cular ring (sphincter) and this cau... ...noids. Or it may affect the veins at the lo... ...e canal, just under the skin, causing external hae... ...oids. Some unfortunate people have both.

haemosiderosis

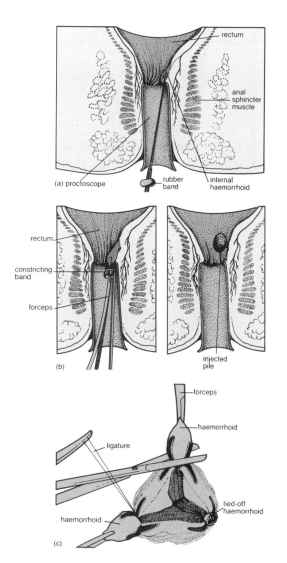

343

...bright red bleed-
...at one has not quite
...the internal pile through
...goes back spontaneously, but
...ay be needed. Eventually the pile
...Protruding piles lead to skin irritation
...and there is usually mucus discharge from the
...ous membrane.

...can become inflamed and swollen, but are seldom
...y painful, unless associated with an actual splitting
(fissure) of the anus.

POSSIBLE CAUSES

Haemorrhoids are not caused by sitting on cold, hard surfaces, prolonged standing, sedentary work and so on. These
are old wives' tales. Persistent constipation, however, with
straining to pass hard stools, can cause damage to the lining

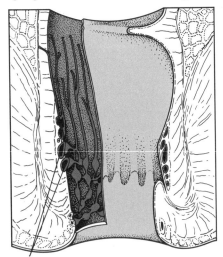

varicose
anal veins

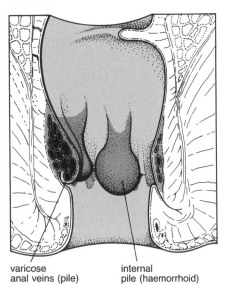

varicose   internal
anal veins (pile)   pile (haemorrhoid)

Haemorrhoids. These are varicose veins of the canal of the
anus. The anal veins drain into valveless veins and have to
sustain the weight of a long column of blood. Thus widening
and enlargement are common.

of the canal, and if this happens often enough, the veins may
lose their normal support and protection. Some people are
thought to have veins especially liable to this kind of injury.
This is probably just a matter of chance anatomical variation.

The anal veins drain into larger veins which carry the
blood through the liver and up to the heart. This part of the
system of large veins has no valves in it, and the whole weight
of the blood bears down on the lowest veins in the system
which tend to stretch. Anything restricting the free upward
flow of blood through the veins leads to an increase in pressure in them. This is why piles are so common in pregnancy.

TREATMENT

When a pile remains prolapsed, the blood flow is obstructed
and gangrene is common. This is not as serious as it sounds
and may result in a spontaneous cure. A high-fibre diet is
desirable for people with piles, as this prevents constipation
and helps to avoid the conditions which cause them.
Internal piles should be put back, if possible, by gentle pressure. This should be done while lying down. If piles will not
go back (reduce), or are causing annoying symptoms, treatment, or even surgical removal (**haemorrhoidectomy**) may be
needed. Discomfort from piles can be relieved by various
anaesthetic suppositories and ointments but such measures
are purely palliative and do not cure the condition.

haemosiderosis

A rare disorder caused by excessive deposition of iron in the
tissues and the resulting irritation and damage.

See also **haemochromatosis**.

haemostasis

The medical term for arrest of bleeding by surgical means
such as the use of ties (ligatures) around arteries, local compression and the use of various forms of cautery. Without
effective haemostasis, surgical procedures become difficult or
impossible, as the field of operation constantly becomes
obscured by blood.

The term 'haemostasis' is also applied to the natural
processes by which bleeding stops – the constriction of
small damaged arteries and the formation of a secure clot
(coagulation).

haemothorax

Free movement of the lungs during breathing is secured by
means of two layers of a smooth, wet membrane called the
pleura. One layer is firmly fixed to the inside of the chest wall
and the other is firmly fixed to the outer surface of each lung.
The two layers are normally in close contact and movement
between them is lubricated by a thin film of pleural fluid.

Haemothorax is the condition in which, usually as a result
of injury, but sometimes from disease, a quantity of blood is
released into the potential space between the two layers of the
pleura, forcing them apart and causing some degree of
collapse of the lung on the affected side. If the blood is not
removed, dense adhesions tend to occur between the two layers, causing restriction in the free movement of the lung. The
situation is made worse if the collection of blood (haematoma)
becomes infected as this leads to the collection of pus in the
pleural cavity (empyema) and much general upset.

Haemothorax is treated by securing and tying off the
bleeding vessel and draining away the blood through a tube.

hair

The hairs are threadlike filamentous growths from the hair follicles in the skin. At the base of each follicle is a growing cell mass called the papilla. This is surrounded by the bulb of the follicle, and both contain blood vessels which carry to the follicle the raw materials necessary for the synthesis of hairs. The papilla also contains nerve endings. The cells of the bulb are actively reproducing and secreting the protein from which the hairs are made. Above the bulb is the sheath of the follicle and this is lubricated by fatty sebaceous material which is secreted into it from small adjoining sebaceous glands. Outside each hair follicle is a tiny muscle attached to its side. This is called the erector pili muscle and is the one which contracts under intense emotional stimulation so as to cause the hair to 'stand on end'.

The outer layer of the hair is the cuticle, made of overlapping flat cells arranged like roof slates. Below this is the thickest layer, the cortex, consisting of cells which become horny (keratinized) as they are pushed up the sheath of the follicle. The inside of the hair is made of softer rectangular cells.

The colour of the hair, in the main hair areas, comes from pigment cells called melanocytes which are of a uniform colour, but produce the whole spectrum of hair colours, from black to blonde, merely by differences in their concentration. Very blonde people have no melanocytes. When the melanocytes die and cease to reproduce, the hair turns grey or white, but existing hair cannot suddenly lose its colour, except by external chemical applications. Much of the fine body hair is unpigmented. Curly hair has a flatter cross-section than straight hair and very curly hair comes from curved follicles.

Lanugo is the name for the normal short, soft, downy, colourless hair that covers the fetus from about the fourth month of life in the womb (uterus) up to shortly before the time of birth. A similar kind of hair may also occur in people with cancer and has been described as a side-effect of certain drugs and in anorexia nervosa.

hairball

See **bezoar**.

hair cycle

The repetitive sequence of growth and rest affecting the production of the hair follicles. The growth phase is known as *anagen* and this varies in length in different sites. The scalp anagen may last for several years. The rest phase is called the *telogen*. After about three months of telogen the hair is shed and a new anagen starts. Between these is the brief *catagen* during which the base of each hair in its follicle becomes club-shaped.

hairiness, excessive

Hairiness, or hirsutism, is one of life's little ironies. Both women and men want lots of it on the top of their heads. Young men often want plenty on their chins and upper lips, but women are horrified to find themselves so endowed. Many women like to see hair on the chests of their men, but are distressed to find it on their own.

THE GROWTH OF UNWANTED HAIR

Many men, as they get older, lose hair on the tops of their heads, only to find it growing, with unprecedented and unwanted exuberance, just about everywhere else – arms, legs, chest, back, ears, nostrils and even on the backs of their fingers. With women, excess facial hair is common and generally distressing, and this may, ironically, be associated with thinning and greying of the scalp hair. Unnatural hairiness of this kind is usually regarded as a major aesthetic blemish.

There are hair follicles everywhere in the skin except on the palms of the hands and the soles of the feet. So hair can grow almost anywhere on the surface of the body, even on the nose. Quite luxuriant growth of external nose hair is quite common, especially in men. Hair in the nostrils is, of course, normal and it serves a useful purpose. Whether hair follicles remain dormant or spring into productive life depends mainly on the sex hormones which determine the normal variations in hairiness between men and women.

Two kinds of hair are described – fine, short, lightly coloured and inconspicuous *villus* hair, and thicker, longer, coarser and heavily pigmented *terminal* hair. Some experts believe that the transition from the former to the latter is the first indication of undue male sex hormone influence in women. Unwanted hairiness in women does not necessarily imply a hormonal defect. In the great majority of cases there is no medical problem and the hirsutism is either hereditary, or ethnic, or just plain bad luck.

> Severe hirsutism is, however, a clear indication that medical investigation is required, because there may be an excess of male sex hormone, possibly caused by a hormone-secreting tumour of an ovary or an adrenal gland. In such an event, urgent treatment might be required.

POSSIBLE CAUSES

Abnormal female hirsutism is commonly associated with virilism which implies either an excess of male sex hormones or an abnormal increase in the sensitivity of the male hormones normally present. This effect may be slight or considerable. In the latter case there will be other indications in addition to hairiness – voice deepening, enlargement of the clitoris and receding hairline at the temples. Any such changes should, of course, be reported.

Drug treatment can cause hirsutism, especially steroids, phenytoin – used for epilepsy or trigeminal neuralgia – and streptomycin. These last two drugs interfere with the excretion of steroids, including the male sex hormones, by the kidneys, so that they accumulate in the bloodstream, and this may be the way in which they promote hirsutism. Hirsutism may, rarely, be due to the fact that the affected woman is actually a man to whom the wrong gender has been attributed at birth. Such a person will have a strong female gender identity and may require gender reassignment surgery.

Some races are ethnically predisposed to hairiness and there is a genetic condition in which hair follicles become sensitized to the low levels of male sex hormone normally present in the bloodstream of women. If, as is often the case, these factors cannot be controlled, we are left with the problem of what to do about the unwanted hair.

hair lip

See **cleft lip and palate**.

hair loss

INCIDENCE

Hair loss of the hereditary male-pattern type is common. The medical title *alopecia* is the correct term. This form of baldness starts as a receding at the temples or a patch on the vertex and progresses, either inexorably or in fits and starts, often leaving only a circle of hair at the sides and the back. Total loss does not occur and even the bald areas are not usually entirely hairless, but retain a fine, almost imperceptible, downy cover. The condition is genetic in origin and usually begins in the third decade, but not infrequently starts in the teens.

POSSIBLE CAUSES

Other causes of baldness are severe skin damage from infection, radiation, chemical injury, burns or scarring. Any drugs designed to kill rapidly reproducing cells, such as those used to treat cancer, can cause baldness. Depending on the severity of the effect, this may be temporary or permanent. Severe diseases with prolonged fever may lead to hair loss, as may several endocrine disorders. Sometimes women suffer a temporary increase in the rate of hair loss after pregnancy, and, rarely, women show thinning of a type similar to male-pattern loss. The effect of anxiety is difficult to assess and it is by no means certain that hair loss during a period of stress or special worry is due to that. In women especially, thinning of the hair is, in itself, a potent cause of anxiety.

Alopecia areata is a localized, patchy baldness of sudden onset which may affect any part of the head or body. The area affected varies considerably in extent. The cause is unknown and the outcome uncertain.

TREATMENT

The majority of cases of such baldness clear up completely without treatment, but some persist.

Much interest has been aroused, in recent years, in the possibility of curing male-pattern baldness with the artery-dilating drug minoxidil. This drug was introduced as a treatment for high blood pressure and worked quite well, but many patients taking it became hairier than desired, and this led to the drug being tried, as a local application, for baldness. The reports of the results of various surveys seem however to depend on whether or not the commentator had a commercial interest in the drug. It is now retailed as a solution in alcohol and propylene glycol as preparations called Regaine and Rogaine.

Minoxidil certainly encourages a fuzzy growth in those with surviving hair follicles, but it cannot cause new follicles to grow. The disinterested reports suggest that a cosmetically satisfactory result is achieved in less than 10 per cent of cases. The treatment is very expensive and must, apparently, be continued indefinitely, for there are clear indications that the new hair falls out when the treatment is stopped.

hair removal

See **depilatory**, **electrolysis**.

Halciderm

A brand name for **halcinonide**.

halcinonide

A powerful corticosteroid drug used for eternal application. A brand name is Halciderm.

Haldol

A brand name for **haloperidol**.

Halfan

A brand name for **halofantrine**.

half brain dominance

See **dominant hemisphere**.

Haliborange

A brand name for a preparation of vitamins A, D and C.

halitosis

This euphemism for bad breath is chiefly interesting for the fact that those most concerned about it usually don't have it, and those worst affected usually don't know.

POSSIBLE CAUSES

All smells, pleasant or otherwise, are caused by tiny chemical molecules floating in the air. Bad-smelling breath may acquire these odorous molecules from the mouth, nose or lungs – rarely from the stomach. Food debris in the mouth, especially around the teeth, will, unless removed by regular brushing, inevitably ferment and produce odours.

Some foodstuffs, such as garlic, are, even in the fresh state, highly efficient and persistent odour-producers and, for these, the only remedy is the passage of time. Contrary to popular belief, the odour of garlic is not, to a major extent, excreted directly from the lungs. Oil of garlic, taken in capsules, causes much less offence to others.

Smoking has been a ubiquitous cause of bad breath down the centuries. King James VI wrote in 1604:

'Herein is a great contempt, that the sweetnesse of man's breath, being a good gift of God, should be wilfully corrupted by this stinking smoke.'

Some ingested substances, including some of the ingredients of alcoholic drinks, are partially excreted in the breath, but persistent genuine odour from the lungs suggests a cause arising in the body.

Diabetes can cause an acetone-like smell; failure of the kidneys with build-up of waste products in the blood (uraemia) may give a urine-like smell to the breath; lung abscess, lung cancer, or abnormal widening of the air passages with stagnation of secretions (bronchiectasis) may cause a putrid odour; and liver failure causes a mousy smell. The state of the breath in no way reflects the condition of the digestion or the function of the bowels. Only in rare instances, such as stomach cancer with outlet blockage and food retention, will foul-smelling belching occur.

Bad breath can also be caused by:

- infection of the gums (gingivitis);
- rotten teeth;
- some degenerative conditions of the nose lining;
- sinusitis;
- tonsillitis;
- throat infections;
- other readily apparent local conditions.

TREATMENT

In these cases both the reason and the remedy are obvious. Some degree of morning breath taint is almost universal, for the self-cleaning mechanisms of the mouth are in abeyance during the night. Normal tooth brushing can be relied on to deal with this.

> The unjustified conviction that one is suffering from bad breath is common. Mostly this is simply a reflection of mild social anxiety, but it is often an indication either of depression or of a tendency to imagined illness (hypochondriasis). Hypochondriacs usually exaggerate normal body activity in their own minds. Occasionally, such a conviction may be a feature of a more serious obsessive or paranoid disorder, or may even indicate a delusion about internal putrefaction. Rarely, there may be a genuine hallucination caused by temporal lobe epilepsy.

Most cases of bad breath are easily remedied, but this should be achieved by removal of the cause rather than by trying to cover up the offence with peppermint or spearmint. Antiseptic mouthwashes and antibiotic lozenges, likewise, are unsatisfactory as they interfere with the normal bacterial content of the mouth and may encourage thrush.

Unfortunately, adaptation often renders the offender unaware, and most best friends lack the necessary moral courage to break the news.

hallex

Latin root meaning 'big toe' as in hallux valgus (bunion).

hallucination

A sense perception not caused by an external stimulus. It is thus a hallucination to see something that is not present or to hear voices which do not come from any present source of sound. Hallucinations should be distinguished from delusions – which are mistaken ideas.

INCIDENCE

Hallucinations are very common, both in health and disease, and are a feature of many psychiatric disorders. They may be visual, auditory – sometimes musical – tactile, or may relate to taste or smell (gustatory or olfactory), or to the size of things (Lilliputian). They commonly occur in normal people as they are falling asleep (hypnagogic hallucinations), or while waking from sleep (hypnopompic hallucinations).

They occur in alcoholic delirium (delirium tremens), from cocaine abuse and from the use of hallucinogenic drugs. They are a common feature of schizophrenia, temporal lobe epilepsy, depression and organic brain disease.

hallucinogenic drugs

Psychedelic drugs derived from plants have been used for centuries because of their effect on consciousness. They have featured in religious rites, have helped to elevate the status of the medicine man, or have been used simply for recreation and for a relief from the hardships of life. Among those used are the desert cactus, *Lophophora williamsii*, known in Spanish as peyote, from which mescaline is derived; 'sacred mushrooms' of the genus Psilocybe, which contain psilocybin; the leguminous plants *Piptadenia peregrina* and *Virola calophylla*, which contain dymethyltryptamine; and the seeds of the morning glory flower, which contains lysergic acid. In more recent years, many synthetically produced substances have

been employed for similar purposes but, today, in the West, the applications are almost wholly 'recreational'.

The study of hallucinogenic drugs and their action on the nervous system has been valuable in promoting knowledge of psychopharmacology. One of the important **neurotransmitters** in the brain is **serotonin** (5-HT), and it is thought that hallucinogens, some of which are chemically related to serotonin, may interfere with its normal action on brain receptor sites. Although important in research, they have found little or no application in medical treatment.

Among the drugs in common use are **lysergic acid diethylamide** (LSD), mescaline and psilocybin. A small dose of these drugs causes a sense of well-being and a heightened sensitivity to, and conviction of the significance of, all sensations and perceptions. This is followed by perceptual distortion, with vivid visual imagery and visual hallucinations. There is intensification of the emotions and modification of the emotional content so that the subject may experience anything from intense euphoria to the deepest apathy. There is an illusory, but often very strong, conviction of omniscience and of the ability to analyse and comprehend transcendental matters. Often there is a sense of expanding consciousness and a feeling of union with nature or God, accompanied by ecstasy and beatitude. Conversely, the experience may be one of terror and distress, with a sense of impending death.

The effects, of course, vary with the inclinations, stability and mental resources of the individual. Hallucinogenic drugs cannot confer data not already held and the notion that the hallucinogenic experience represents a kind of ultimate reality is nonsense. Some reactions are schizophrenic in type and these drugs may actually precipitate a frank psychotic illness in the predisposed.

hallux

The big toe.

hallux valgus

A very common deformity, caused by unsuitable footwear, in which the big toe is angled outwards away from the midline

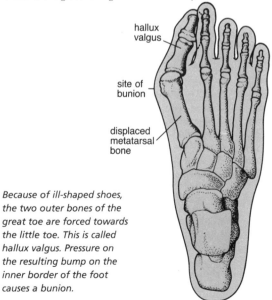

Because of ill-shaped shoes, the two outer bones of the great toe are forced towards the little toe. This is called hallux valgus. Pressure on the resulting bump on the inner border of the foot causes a bunion.

of the body (this is what *valgus* means), so that the head of the nearer toe bone forms a prominent bump on the inner edge of the foot. Sometimes the deflected toe rides over or under the other toes. Hallux valgus leads to the formation of an inflamed pressure swelling (bursitis) over the prominence – a condition known as a bunion.

halofantrine

A phenanthrene antimalarial drug used to treat both main types of malaria, those caused by *Plasmodium falciparum* and *Plasmodium vivax*. A brand name is Halfan.

haloperidol

A butyrophenone drug used in the treatment of psychiatric disorders. It is similar in its effects to the **phenothiazine derivative** drugs. Brand names are Dozic, Haldol, Haloperidol and Serenace.

halothane

A pungent, volatile, non-inflammable liquid anaesthetic agent. Halothane is a powerful drug that induces anaesthesia in a concentration of less than 1 per cent. Severe liver damage occurs very occasionally, usually after a second exposure to the drug in a sensitized subject. A brand name is Fluothane.

hamartoma

A rare, non-malignant tumour consisting of a local overgrowth of the normal constituent cells. It is a developmental abnormality, which can affect any tissue. Hamartoma in the lung may cause obstruction of one of the bronchial tubes, but, in general, these tumours do little harm.

hammer toe

A toe permanently and fixedly bent at the joint so that the outer bone points downward like the head of a hammer. The condition may affect one or more toes and is due to undue tightness of the tendons which bend the toe.

hand, intrinsic muscles of

See **lumbrical muscles**.

handedness

The preferential use of one hand, rather than the other, in voluntary actions. Ambidexterity – the ability to use either hand, indifferently, with equal skill – is very rare. About 90 per cent of people are right-handed and this correlates with the half of the brain which is dominant for speech. Some 97 per cent of right-handed people have left-hemisphere dominance for speech, and only 60 per cent of left-handed people are right-hemisphere dominant for speech.

handicap

Any disability, physical, mental or emotional, which restricts a full, normal life activity. Handicap may be present at birth (congenital) or may be acquired as a result of injury or disease. For many, the sole handicap is one of locomotion and, today, such people are greatly assisted by technological and design improvements in mechanical aids such as wheelchairs.

Many others are handicapped by severe neurological disorder, with or without mental defect, and in these cases, the purely physical shortcoming is often greatly added to by negative and unhelpful attitudes induced in others.

Public enlightenment and sympathy for those with locomotory handicap is now generally adequate and there is a strong recognition, in developed countries, of the needs and rights of handicapped people to special consideration. Physical barriers to movement and access are being progressively reconsidered so as to promote the independence of these people. But there is still a widespread suspicion, or even fear, of the mentally and emotionally handicapped and a tendency to feel that such people are best hidden tidily away in institutions. While many handicapped people need the management of those with special training and skills, many more could, with understanding and imagination, be enabled to live more satisfying lives within the community, and this is now being encouraged.

hangnail

A piece of partly separated outer skin layer at the margin of the skin at the base of the nail (the cuticle). This leaves an area of deeper skin exposed to infection and also exposes the sensitive skin nerves to undue stimulation. Loose skin should be carefully clipped off and the area protected from further trauma by a dressing or liquid plastic (collodion) seal. Infection may call for the use of an antibiotic cream.

hangover

The state of physical and mental distress experienced on waking after an evening of over-indulgence in alcohol. Ethyl alcohol (ethanol) is toxic to the brain, probably because it interferes with GABA neuro-transmitter receptors, altering the passage of nerve impulses from cell to cell in a manner which degrades the higher functions of the brain. Drinkers acquire a degree of tolerance to the effect on the GABA receptors so that when it is withdrawn the brain 'protests'. Alcohol is also irritating to the stomach lining and often causes an erosive gastritis.

SYMPTOMS

The alcohol and aldehyde congeners – secondary products of alcoholic fermentation which give character to alcoholic drinks – are believed by many to be even more toxic than pure alcohol. Congeners are present in highest concentration in drinks such as port and brandy and are lowest in purer spirits such as gin and vodka. It is thought to be the congeners, primarily, which give rise to the depression, nausea, headache, remorse, shakiness and vertigo which characterize the unhappy state of the too-indulgent reveller, after the anaesthetic effects of the ethanol have passed.

Alcohol is a diuretic – that is, it causes the kidneys to pass out more fluid than the volume drunk. This is the basis of, and often the justification for, the beer-drinker's 'thirst', but it is also one of the factors contributing to the discomfort of the hangover. Alcohol promotes diuresis by causing the pituitary gland to produce less of the antidiuretic hormone vasopressin.

The headache in hangover is due to dilatation and stretching of blood vessels in the scalp and around the brain and is of the same sort as occurs in migraine. Alcohol is a potent dilator of vessels – hence the flushed face of the drinker – but during the party it also has analgesic effects and generally reduces one's sensitivity. Dilatation persisting after much of the alcohol has left the body is also thought to be due to breakdown products such as acetaldehyde or other factors such as smoking, excessive eating, undue excitement and loss of sleep.

TREATMENT

Recovery from hangover is normally merely a matter of time, but in true alcoholics the hangover may include withdrawal symptoms and be more severe and persistent. Many suggestions have been made for the avoidance of hangover, but only those measures which reduce the total intake and rate of absorption of alcohol are likely to be of any value.

Hansen's disease

Formerly known as leprosy, this is a slow, persistent, bacterial infection of the skin and the nerves, caused by the organism *Mycobacterium leprae*. This organism is very slow in replicating, taking about two weeks to reproduce instead of the usual half an hour. The time between infection and the appearance of the disease (the incubation period) is from two to five years.

INCIDENCE

About 20 million people are suffering from Hansen's disease world-wide. If untreated, Hansen's disease may cause widespread bodily damage, including loss of fingers and toes, severe disfigurement and blindness.

Contrary to general opinion, Hansen's disease is one of the least infectious of the infectious diseases and requires prolonged close contact before it is likely to be transmitted. It is spread in droplets of nasal mucus during sneezing, but only in the early stages of the disease.

RECOGNITION AND SYMPTOMS

In former times, many unfortunates with externally disfiguring conditions were deemed to have leprosy and were shunned or confined. The leprosy of the bible must have included non-infectious conditions such as psoriasis, neurofibromatosis, vitiligo, albinism, tinea versicolor, and basal cell carcinoma, as well as many innocent skin infections.

Hansen's disease takes two main forms the lepromatous and the tuberculoid types. In lepromatous leprosy there is no bodily immune attack on the organisms and these are present in enormous numbers, mainly within cells called macrophages, in the skin and in nerves. The result is large raised lumps which may break down to form ulcers and cause widespread tissue damage and deformity. Bacteria in the nerves cause nerve thickening and loss of sensation and movement. The disease is sometimes discovered after a person realizes that a cigarette has burned down, unnoticed, between the fingers. Skin changes occur, leading to patches of whiteness. The nerve damage has major secondary effects – loss of tissue and serious deformity.

Tuberculoid leprosy occurs when the body's immune response is good and the organisms are successfully attacked. As a result, the disease is milder and probably non-infectious.

TREATMENT

Treatment is slow and long-term but effective and renders the patient unable to pass on the disease. The mainstay of treatment has long been the antibacterial drug dapsone, but resistance to this is occurring progressively and newer drugs, such as rifampicin, clofazimine and ethionamide, used in combination, are highly successfully. Thalidomide, in spite of its notorious reputation, is also a valuable drug in the management of Hansen's disease.

Lepers, who were once banished to colonies, are now managed more sympathetically. The means of eradicating Hansen's disease now exist, and this is one of the declared aims of the World Health Organization.

hantavirus disease

A disease caused by viruses of the *Hantavirus* genus that are carried by rats, field mice and bank voles and probably passed to human beings mainly by the inhalation of dried animal secretions. In Britain it can affect farm and nature conservancy workers, sewage workers and people engaged in water sports. Many cases are mild and unapparent, but severe forms feature high fever, headache, shock, nausea and vomiting and small blood spots in the skin. There is redness of the eyes, and the face, neck and shoulders are flushed. Blood pressure drops and kidney failure may occur. In 10 per cent of severe cases there is significant bleeding.

Hantavirus pulmonary syndrome is an acute respiratory illness which, after a brief period of fever, muscle pains, headache, nausea and cough, progresses to severe shock and waterlogging of the lungs (pulmonary oedema). The mortality without specific antiviral treatment is 50 to 75 per cent, but the antiviral drug ribavirin is effective. Antibiotics have no effect against viruses.

happiness drug

See **fluoxetine**.

hardening of the arteries

This long-hallowed term should now be abandoned because the hardening (sclerosis) is not, in itself, the most important thing that happens to arteries in the ubiquitous condition of **atherosclerosis**. Plaque formation (atheroma) and narrowing is the main culprit and the greatest single cause of death and disablement. The term 'arteriosclerosis', once commonly used by every doctor, is rapidly falling out of use because hardening (sclerosis) without plaque formation (atheroma) is rare.

hare lip

The appearance caused by a badly repaired cleft lip. With advances in understanding of the principles of plastic surgery and a recognition that these principles, and the appropriate skills, should always be brought to bear when congenital cleft lip is to be repaired, the condition has become relatively rare.

Harmogen

A brand name for **estropipate**.

Hashimoto's thyroiditis

A form of **goitre** – swelling of the thyroid gland – causing an ache in the neck and sometimes difficulty in swallowing. This form of thyroid gland disorder is commonest in middle-aged women and is due to the formation of antibodies to the protein produced by the gland from which the hormones are synthesized. These antibodies can be found in the blood, often in high concentration, and they return to the gland and attack it as if it were foreign tissue, causing inflammation and damage.

The condition responds well to the administration of thyroid hormone (thyroxine) and this should be continued indefinitely, as the gland will eventually become underactive. Steroids also help.

Hay-Crom

A brand name for **sodium cromoglycate**.

hay fever

The phrase *seasonal allergic rhinitis* is unlikely to catch on, but at least has the merit of being more accurate than the term 'hay fever', which is neither caused by hay nor associated with fever. Rhinitis is inflammation of the nose lining and this is not necessarily seasonal or allergic.

People who suffer from allergic rhinitis have an inherited tendency to develop hypersensitivity to substances which are harmless to 80 per cent of the population. These substances are called *allergens* and they may be eaten or inhaled and cause many problems. In hay fever the allergens are the seasonal pollens in the inhaled air. Such pollen grains enter the noses of the sufferers where they are trapped by a layer of sticky nasal mucus. Lysozyme enzymes then digest off their outer coat and release the protein allergens. Situated within and just under the epithelial lining of the nose are millions of *mast cells.*

These granule-filled cells are of fundamental importance in allergy for the granules contain a highly active substance called histamine, together with other irritating substances. Histamine has many effects when released: it contracts smooth muscle, including that in the walls of the bronchioles, increases the leakage of fluid from small veins so that membranes swell, stimulates mucus and watery secretion from the nose lining and causes local itching and burning. Between the granules, the mast cells store proteases (protein-splitting enzymes) which are thought to be capable of damaging small blood vessels.

In people with allergic rhinitis, a previous exposure to the allergen has resulted in the production of the antibody Immunoglubulin E (IgE) and the mast cell membranes already have the IgE in place. This so sensitizes the mast cells that whenever they are triggered by the same allergen they immediately start sending out not only histamine and proteases, but also prostaglandin D2 and a range of leukotrienes, which are even more potent narrowers of the air tubes (bronchoconstrictors) than histamine. All this, of course, leads to the general misery of the hay-fever victim.

POSSIBLE CAUSES

Non-seasonal allergic rhinitis is due to many causes such as house dusts, house dust mites, or animal fur or skin flakes, and commonly occurs all the year round.

The spring type of seasonal allergy is caused by air-borne tree pollens, especially elm, birch, elder, oak and maple, and the summer type is due to grass and weed pollens. In autumn, the problem is sometimes caused by air-borne fungus spores, usually in a localized geographic area.

TREATMENT

The most effective measure is to avoid the allergen, and this may even involve a change of residence, air filters, masks, closed windows and doors and avoidance of areas known to be major sources of the pollen. Desensitization injections can be helpful, especially if started after the hay-fever season and then continued all the year round. This must be done very carefully to avoid severe reactions. The injections sometimes lead to falling serum levels of IgE.

Symptomatic treatment is valuable and is the commonest response to the problem. Antihistamines block the two kinds of receptor sites for histamine and can be quite effective. Cromoglycate (cromolyn) has a more immediate effect and operates by blocking the reaction of the allergen with the mast cell membrane, but it cannot deal with symptoms due to histamine and prostaglandins already released. It is commonly used in the form of a nasal aerosol.

Alpha-adrenergic blockers have a double effect. They are useful decongestants and they can, to some extent, counteract the sleepiness caused by antihistamines. They are best given by mouth as the nasal spray preparations lead to rebound congestion. Beclomethasone-type steroids are extremely effective and, used locally (topically), do not seem to cause any of the adverse effects of steroids such as suppression of steroid production by the adrenal glands.

Haymine

A brand name for **ephedrine** formulated with other drugs.

headache

Probably the commonest of all symptoms, headache affects almost all of us from time to time and only a tiny proportion of headaches indicate serious disorder. The pain does not come from the brain – which is wholly insensitive to all the pain-causing stimuli – but from the arteries of the scalp, from some of those on the surface of the brain, and from certain areas of the membranes surrounding the brain (the meninges), especially those on the inside of the base of the skull.

Headache can conveniently be divided into three groups – tension headaches, migraine and miscellaneous. The miscellaneous group is a small proportion of the whole – perhaps 10 per cent – but contains many different causes, only a few of which are serious.

TENSION HEADACHES

Tension headaches are the commonest type and account for half or more. The pain may occur in any part of the head and is usually worse towards the end of the working day or when the stress level is especially high. These headaches are caused by the body's automatic reaction to stress – the kind of sustained contraction of muscles which can be observed on the face of any person undergoing a stressful experience. Social custom prevents us from manifesting all our stresses as facial contortions, however, and other muscles are usually involved, including those of the back of the neck and the scalp.

Tension headaches are not greatly relieved by painkillers, but do respond well to drugs which relax muscles or to other measures, such as trained relaxation, which achieve the same effect.

MIGRAINE

Migraine headaches occur at intervals of days, weeks or months. The term 'migraine' comes from the words 'hemicranial', meaning 'half-head', and it is a feature of classical migraine that the pain occurs only on one side. The condition is one-sided in a wider sense, however, as it is caused by a temporary shut-down of the blood supply to a part of one side of the brain, followed by a wide and painful dilatation of the affected arteries.

VISUAL DISTURBANCE

The preliminary spasm of these vessels often interferes seriously, but temporarily, with the function of the brain. Since it is often the arteries supplying the back of one side of the brain that are affected, the commonest result is a disturbance of vision. This usually takes the form of a small blind area with sparkling edges (a *scintillating scotoma*) which expands until a large part of the field of vision is blind, lasts for about twenty or thirty minutes and then reverts fairly quickly to normal.

RECOGNITION AND SYMPTOMS

Other parts of the brain can be similarly involved and there may be weakness or loss of sensation on the face or down one side of the body, disturbance of speech or comprehension, or other alarming effects. 'Classical' migraine of this kind is then followed by a severe headache on the opposite side of the head, with nausea, vomiting, extreme sensitivity to bright light and a strong inclination to go and lie down in a darkened room. The headache may last for up to a day or two, but eventually resolves. Some people suffer a prolonged headache which is followed by paralysis of one half of the body, gradually recovering over the course of several days.

In many cases, the preliminary stage of brain malfunction is absent and the attack starts with the headache and nausea. This type is sometimes called 'common migraine' and is less easy to distinguish from other forms of headache. Many people who claim to be migraine sufferers are actually having tension headaches.

POSSIBLE CAUSES

Migraine runs in families. It can be precipitated by many factors, including fatigue, anxiety, stress, menstruation, contraceptive pills, weather changes, fasting, cheese, chocolate and alcohol – especially red wines and brandy. Triggering foodstuffs and drinks contain the amino acid tyramine and administration of this will provoke an attack. The agent which causes the effect on the blood vessels is probably the highly reactive neuro-transmitter serotonin.

TREATMENT

The medical control of migraine calls for expert prescribing and several drugs are useful, among them ergotamine tartrate which acts to prevent or control the secondary dilatation of the blood vessels which causes the pain. Ergot should not be used by women taking oral contraceptives. Other drugs used in migraine include beta-blockers such as propranolol, antidepressants such as amitryptyline, and the serotonin antagonist methysergide.

MISCELLANEOUS GROUP

This group contains the headaches caused by disorders of structures in the face, eyes, ears, sinuses, skull and brain and includes referred headache from the teeth, the jaw joints and serious eye disease. 'Eye-strain' from uncorrected eye focusing errors is a myth but uncorrected refractive errors may cause headache from frowning and peering. Cluster headaches, usually in men, are groups of short attacks centred over one eye and causing redness and often watering. They occur in clusters, several times a day, for weeks or months, and then disappear for long periods.

The miscellaneous group also contains the following:

- headaches caused by depression;
- the toxic headaches, such as hangover and the effects of other toxic agents and drugs;
- high blood pressure (hypertension);
- inflammation of the arteries of the brain and scalp

(temporal arteritis) which causes extreme tenderness at the temples, can proceed suddenly to cause blindness and should never be neglected;
- inadequate blood supply to the brain by narrowing of the arteries from occlusive disease;
- arthritis of the spine in the neck;
- head injury leading to *post-traumatic* headache;
- a rise in the pressure within the skull from any cause;
- the neuralgias, which are not really headaches;
- the pain of meningitis, which is accompanied by severe neck stiffness, fever and general upset;
- the pain from brain tumour and from other causes of raised pressure within the skull, such as benign intracranial hypertension, both of which are rare;
- the pain of expanding aneurysms on one of the brain arteries.

> The general points to be considered in trying to decide whether or not a headache is dangerous are:
> - Duration – is the headache of recent origin, or has it been happening for years? If the latter, it is unlikely to be dangerous.
> - Associated features – are there any accompanying symptoms or signs of brain disorder such as persistent loss of visual field, double vision, projectile vomiting, hormonal changes, weakness, paralysis, vertigo or one-sided deafness.
>
> A new and persistent headache, accompanied by any such changes should certainly be investigated as a matter of urgency.

headache, sudden

See **thunderclap headache**.

Headclear

A brand name for a mixture of **paracetamol**, **pseudoephedrine** and **chlorpheniramine**.

head enlargement

See **hydrocephalus**.

head injury

Injuries to the brain and head.

INCIDENCE

Every year, one person in 500 hundred suffers a head injury serious enough to require admission to hospital. Half of these are caused by road traffic. Three-quarters of all serious head injuries are caused by cars and motorcycles. Neurological units are full of people – often young men – the quality of whose lives has been sacrificed to mindless stupidity on the roads.

WHAT HAPPENS

When a body is travelling at seventy miles an hour and its container is suddenly stopped, the body does not stop. It continues to move in the same direction and, unless restrained, strikes the inside of the vehicle at exactly this velocity. The same principle applies to a speeding brain. When its container, the skull, is suddenly stopped, the brain tries to continue in the same direction and crushes itself against the inside of the bone. Speeding bodies contains an alarming

351

amount of kinetic energy – equal to half the mass multiplied by the velocity squared. In the case of a typical driver, the velocity squared, in miles per hour, is equal to 4900, so it is little wonder that high-speed drivers commonly end up brain-damaged in wheelchairs.

EFFECTS

Primary brain damage, occurring at the time of injury, results from displacement of the brain relative to the skull and the resulting distortion and tearing of structure. Brain tissue is disrupted; arteries are torn and pump blood under pressure through soft, easily disrupted brain matter; pressure within the skull rises and the brain swells, causing further compressive damage. The swelling and compressed brain may be forced downwards and coned into the large opening in the base of the skull through which the spinal cord runs. In this case, the vital centres in the brain stem are compressed. From one or more of these effects, death is common within minutes or hours. Skull fractures can sometimes help by allowing decompression, but often bony fragments are driven into the brain to cause further damage or, in the case of survival, to lead, later, to epilepsy.

> Medical attention is necessary whenever there has been even a brief loss of consciousness, or if the blow was severe. Fracture is obvious if the bone is depressed or mobile, otherwise X-ray is needed to identify.

SURVIVING BRAIN INJURY

Those who survive serious brain injury are commonly found to have a permanent deficit in brain function causing disability, physical, mental or both, varying from the slight to the total.

See also **brain damage**.

head injury sequel

See **postconcussional syndrome**.

head-standing

A popular activity with yoga addicts, gymnasts and some people with backache, head-standing, or hanging upside-down, is generally harmless, but should not be engaged in by anyone with glaucoma or a tendency to raised pressure within the eyes. Trials have shown that gravity inversion sharply increases the intraocular pressure, often to more than twice that in the normal body position. In addition, the inverted position causes transient loss of areas of the visual fields. This was demonstrated in eleven out of nineteen eyes examined. These changes appear to be reversible, but it is exactly this kind of field loss which makes glaucoma so dangerous.

> The workers who did this research recommend that people who intend to spend much time in an inverted position should first have an eye examination and that those with a family history of glaucoma or a personal history of eye trouble should be discouraged from adopting this posture.

Heaf test

See **tuberculin test**.

healing

Healing is a property and function of the body itself and occurs automatically unless prevented by some agency such as infection, persistent injury, cancer, foreign material, radiation, medical interference or great age. Doctors do not heal. Healing is a passive process which will occur if the influences preventing it are removed. That is the function of the doctor.

health food

Concern over the possible health hazards of food additives, insecticide or fertilizer contamination, together with a growing awareness that we are made of what we eat, has led, in recent years, to widespread support for the health-food movement. The movement has been supported and encouraged by the publication of many studies suggesting possible links between certain food additives and contaminants and various diseases, including cancer. The widespread and growing concern over the protection of the environment has also promoted interest.

Definitions are loose, but 'organic foods' are generally considered to be those grown without chemical fertilizers or insecticides and natural foods are those without chemical additives.

Everything we eat is broken down in the digestive tract into a small number of common components, selectively absorbed, and then resynthesized or further broken down within the body. While it is true that an excess of certain foods, such as saturated fats, is harmful, at the present stage of knowledge, there is simply no factual basis for the view that certain foods have curative or health-enhancing properties.

This is not to say that some foods, such as those with a high-fibre or low-fat content, or possibly those containing antioxidants such as vitamins C or E may not be *protective* of health. But this remains to be seen.

Many of the recommendations of the health-food enthusiasts are based on high vitamin content and include the implicit assumption that an intake of vitamins in excess of the minimum daily requirement is somehow beneficial. This is untrue. Popular health foods, promoted on these uncertain premises, include wheat germ, dried fruit, brewer's yeast, yoghurt, bone meal, rose hips, nuts and seeds and the juices of uncooked vegetables. There is no reason to believe that these foods are, intrinsically, any more beneficial than any other normal source of energy, building materials, vitamins and minerals (although they may be richer in some nutrients). Nor is there any reason to believe that organically grown foods are in any way nutritionally superior to, or even in any way different from, foods grown using chemical fertilizers.

The health food movement has, however, helped to draw public attention to the need for constant surveillance lest commercial considerations outweigh public safety. It has also helped to reinforce the now growing appreciation that most people's diets are excessive and unsuitable. There can be no doubt that adherence to a typical 'health-food' diet would be beneficial to most of us – not because these foodstuffs have any magical properties, but because, by their nature, we would eat much less.

See also **food allergy**.

health maintenance

In the broadest sense it might be said that the whole of this book is devoted to keeping healthy. But it is possible to lay down a comparatively few basic rules. Here they are:

- try to be happy;
- try to be contented;
- keep your weight down;
- eat healthily;
- don't smoke cigarettes;
- drink only in moderation;
- take exercise every day;
- understand how infections occur;
- drive carefully;
- take note of warning signs.

It is generally true that happy people are healthier and that a positive attitude, optimism, good humour and friendliness towards one's fellow human beings promotes good health. More than 100 separate studies have established, statistically, that there is a positive correlation between a satisfactory and happy state of mind and good physical health. The claim, or assumption, that the state of mind causes the good health has, nevertheless, been sharply criticized by some who insist that there is no evidence that disease is a direct reflection of the mental state of the individual. Recent research into **psychoneuro-immunology** indicates that this criticism may be unjustified.

No one denies that good health promotes happiness and that bad health often damages it, but it is the claim that happiness promotes health that is in question. Unfortunately, this is a more difficult thing to prove. Happiness is an elusive concept and many people define it in terms of physical well-being or general satisfaction with life. People who are able to cope well with life are both happier and healthier and are often too busy looking outwards to give much time or attention to minor ailments. Pessimism and hypochondriasis go hand in hand.

None of these considerations support the proposition, but all emphasize the intimacy of the inter-relationship of mind and body and the impossibility, in the final analysis, of separating the effects of one from those of the other. It is just conceivable that fuller knowledge will enable us to abolish what may be an entirely imaginary distinction.

Behavioural psychologists have repeatedly shown that it is possible to change 'dysfunctional' behaviours and attitudes and thus to improve the state of the mental health.

CONTENTMENT

This is another elusive entity. The standard of health of people in the Western world has improved progressively from the earliest times. In the last fifty years or so there has been a dramatic improvement in life expectancy and a reduction in mortality in most of the major disease groups. In the last fifteen years there has been a considerable improvement in health due to changes in lifestyle – better diets, decline in cigarette smoking and an increase in exercising.

In spite of all this, however, there is ample evidence that people are less satisfied with the state of their health, as they perceive it, than they used to be. There is less acceptance of disease and disability, more complaint about minor disorders, more attendance on doctors, increased consumption of drugs, and less satisfaction with the quality of medical care provided by doctors. So much publicity has been given to the very real advances in medical science that many people now assume that nothing is impossible, and often resent being told that certain problems cannot be resolved. Litigation against doctors is soaring to the point at which doctors are practising **defensive medicine**, avoiding the more vulnerable specialties, and are having to pay crippling insurance premiums against damages.

Cosmetic surgery is becoming a major industry. Bodily disfigurement, real or imagined, is often regarded as a disease requiring treatment. The same applies to anomalies of behaviour, which are now being reclassified as diseases – drug addiction, alcoholic excess, wife-beating, child abuse, paedophilia. By some, these are no longer regarded as being within the province of the law, ethics, morality or religion, but rather as medical disorders calling for medical treatment. There is even a demand for medical intervention to enhance or modify normal characteristics. People demand stimulants to suppress normal fatigue, or use anabolic steroids to aid in body-building and improve athletic performance.

This lack of correspondence between health improvement and subjective satisfaction suggests that we in the materially advanced societies may have allowed our values to become defective. It may be that we are losing sight of the real elements that make for satisfaction – human relationships, love, the cultivation of the mind, hard work, creativity and humanity. In the context of achieving contentment, perhaps we need philosophers more than we need doctors.

WEIGHT CONTROL

Keeping your weight down is more important than you probably realize. Obesity is defined as the excessive storage of energy in the form of fat. This can only result from a lack of balance between food intake and energy expenditure. Whatever other factors apply, obesity cannot occur unless more food is eaten than is used. All excess of intake over expenditure is laid down as fat – a collection of thin-walled, oil-filled cells situated mostly beneath the skin.

The health implications of obesity are serious. Repeated surveys of the fate of obese people have confirmed that a significant excess of illness occurs in those whose body mass index (the weight in kilograms divided by the square of the height in metres) is greater than 27. About one-fifth of the men and about a quarter of the women in Britain have a body mass index higher than 27. Obese people suffer from:

- high blood pressure;
- diabetes of the maturity-onset variety;
- an increased incidence in women of cancers of the breast, womb, ovaries and gall-bladder;
- an increased incidence in men in cancer of the colon, rectum and prostate gland;
- orthopaedic problems, such as osteoarthritis and foot trouble;
- depression.

The stereotype of the fat, jolly person belies the truth. The connection between obesity and heart disease is complicated, but there is a connection and this is independent of the effect of high blood pressure and of smoking. The reduced expectation of life of obese people has been reflected in life insurance loading for years.

Surprisingly, most adults manage to achieve a reasonable balance between intake and energy output and remain roughly the same weight. This applies as much to very overweight people as to the underweight. Obesity is not a simple eating disorder resulting from uncontrolled greed. There is evidence that some obese people may have the same metabolic rate as underweight people, but that their energy expenditure is less. The food intake tends to be proportional to the weight so those with a low energy expenditure get heavier.

Patterns in eating may well be established early in life and it is probable that overweight mothers unconsciously encourage habits of excessive intake in their children.

This is more plausible than the suggestion that obesity – which is essentially an acquired characteristic – is hereditary. It has also been suggested that infant obesity, from excessive intake, leads to the production of an increased number of fat cells in the body and that the number of fat cells remains constant after childhood. If this is true, the obese have more cells to fill than the non-obese and are faced with an almost insuperable problem in staying slim. The idea has been disputed by some experts.

Obesity brings with it psychological problems including a sense of social disadvantage and unattractiveness. Since eating is undoubtedly a great consolation for these and other disadvantages, a vicious cycle is set up. The control of obesity must be distinguished from simply losing weight. Obese people who lose weight, by whatever means, including starvation under medical supervision, teeth wiring, bowel segment removal, and other extreme measures, almost always put it on again. There are no magic diets. Some of the fad diets are dangerous, but most of them are just silly. The commercial success of the books propagating them is a tribute to the triumph of hope over experience and to the public's insatiable appetite for miracles.

Reduced calorie intake is a far more efficient way of reducing weight than taking exercise. But regular exercise is an essential part of the process of weight reduction. Contrary to expectation, exercise helps to limit food intake. Weight cannot, however, be lost, in health, without reducing intake. So, TV adverts notwithstanding, suffering and hunger are inevitable. New, smaller, eating habits must be established. 'Crash' diets, or those involving non-nutritious food substitutes are generally pointless, as they do not get at the basic requirement of trying to amend a years-long habit of putting too much in the mouth. The only effective way to achieve permanent weight reduction must also be long-sustained. For this reason, would-be weight reducers who spend money on health farms, proprietary diets, books and magazines on dieting, and expensive exercising equipment are wasting time and money. The diet should be normal, but must be in quantities so small that they inevitably cause hunger until the body adapts. It is a miserable prospect, but better than believing in magic.

The kind of food taken is less important than the quantity, but a diet should, as well as being of small quantity, be balanced with plenty of vegetable roughage and fruit, a moderate intake of protein – preferably from fish and poultry – and low amounts of fat and dairy products.

There is a great deal of information in this book about the disease atherosclerosis. This disorder of the arteries kills more people than cancer and many other diseases put together. It is, in fact, the principal killer disease of Western civilization. It is also responsible for much ill-health in the form of heart attacks, strokes, kidney damage and limb gangrene. Although many more factors contribute to the development of atherosclerosis, not all of these are under individual control. One that you can control, however, is the kind of diet you follow.

Note that the popular idea that a high-fat, high-cholesterol diet leads directly to the deposition of cholesterol in the arteries simply does not accord with the facts. There is much more to it than that. Nevertheless, there are very good reasons – reasons related to atherosclerosis – for cutting down the amount of fat in the diet and this you should certainly do. To achieve a low-fat diet you must, in practice, necessarily increase the relative amount of fibre in the diet. Reducing dietary fat may also reduce your chances of developing cancer. The evidence for this, however, does not necessarily imply that it is the fats that cause cancer. It seems more likely that it is the absence of adequate fibre – a feature of high-fat diets – that is the cause of cancer.

Dietary fibre is not a single substance. It is a group of complex carbohydrates which includes plant cellulose, lignin, pectins and gums. The human digestive system does not have the enzymes needed to break down these polysaccharides to sugars that can be absorbed, so they remain in the intestine until excreted. Fibre bulks out the stool and is of considerable value in preventing **constipation** and **diverticulitis**.

Many nutritionists claim that high-fibre diets are valuable in the control of high blood cholesterol, are the answer to obesity, are of benefit to diabetics and prevent cancer of the colon. Most of these claims are based on observations of the absence of these disorders in races of people who have very high-fibre diets. Every day, large quantities of cholesterol pass down the bile duct into the intestine where it is reabsorbed into the blood. Soluble fibre binds cholesterol into a complex that cannot be absorbed. Thus a high-fibre diet carries away in the stools considerable quantities of cholesterol. The bulkier intestinal contents result in a more rapid transit through the bowels. Thus, if any factor causing cancer is present in the diet, it will have less time to act.

High-fibre diets are low in calories, fats and sodium and usually have a more than adequate vitamin content. They are also usually cheaper than low-fibre diets. High-fibre content occurs in bran, beans, peas, nuts, all vegetables and fruits. The richest sources are bran, beans, blackberries and prunes. High-fibre diets produce a lot of intestinal gas and over-enthusiastic indulgence has certain antisocial effects. This may also cause bloating, or even pain, but harm is unlikely. A daily intake of 50 grams is harmless and almost certainly beneficial. The proprietary breakfast cereal 'All Bran' contains 25 per cent pure fibre with an average helping providing 10 grams of fibre.

SMOKING CIGARETTES

'Smoking cigarettes is the chief, single avoidable cause of death in our society and the most important public health issue of our time.' This statement by the United States Surgeon General expresses the views of informed medical opinion world-wide. There are several reasons for this opinion and for the fact that the medical profession has, for years, waged a bitter campaign against those individuals whose purpose seems to be to persuade people to smoke cigarettes.

The lining cells of the air tubes in healthy lungs are tall (columnar) and the surfaces nearest the inside of the tube are covered with fine hairs (cilia) which move together in a manner similar to the effect of wind blowing across a field of ripe corn. The hair movement acts to carry dust and other foreign material upwards and away from the deeper parts of the lungs. This is one of the body's protective processes and, without it, a good deal of unwanted material in the air we

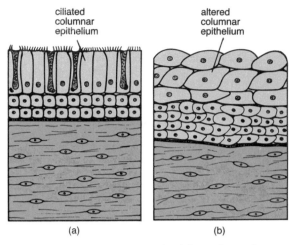

ciliated columnar epithelium

altered columnar epithelium

flattened (squamous) epithelium

(a)   (b)   (c)

This sequence shows the changes caused to the linings of the air tubes by persistent smoking. The healthy columnar epithelium (a) is replaced by simpler, more flattened cells (b) and these eventually may become more numerous and cancerous (c).

breathe in would find its way into the delicate air sacs. In people who smoke cigarettes, these important cells soon suffer three obvious changes. First, the cilia disappear, then the number of cells increases and, finally, the cells become flattened, so that the columnar lining is replaced by an abnormal atrophied, scaly layer. After a number of years, there is a tendency for these bald, flattened cells to begin to show signs of excessive multiplication. The next stage, again usually some years later, may be cancer of the lung, or, more accurately, cancer of the inner lining of the air tubes (bronchial carcinoma).

Lung cancer is now the commonest cause of cancer death in men, and is the second cause of cancer death in women, after cancer of the breast. The condition is becoming progressively commoner in women because of the considerable increase in smoking by women in the last forty years. The risk of lung cancer is about twenty times greater in smokers than in non-smokers and these figures have been shown to be true in study after study. To paraphrase an excerpt from a recent leading article in the *British Medical Journal*: '...tobacco accounts for 15 to 20 per cent of all deaths in Britain. Of every 1000 young men who smoke, 1 will be murdered, 6 will die on the roads, but 250 will be killed before their time by tobacco.'

The more cigarettes smoked, the more marked the early cell changes become. The loss of cilia and flattening of the columnar cells occur much more frequently in cigarette smokers than in those who smoke pipes or cigars. People who have given up smoking have fewer affected cells than smokers, and the number of affected cells becomes progressively less as the number of years of non-smoking increases. But the number of damaged cells never reaches the low level found in people who have never smoked cigarettes.

Ironically, smokers who inhale the smoke deeply into their lungs so that it moves quickly past the ciliated cells in the main lung tubes are slightly less liable to get cancer than those who inhale less deeply. But the deep inhalers, who carry the smoke right to the air sacs, from whence many of the 3000 or so constituents can get into the bloodstream, suffer a higher incidence of the other important effects of smoking, especially heart attack (coronary thrombosis).

Obviously, every heavy smoker does not get lung cancer. Some simply have a natural, inborn resistance to the typical changes in the cells. Others have very powerful defence mechanisms which can minimize the effects of the tiny smoke

particles on the lung tissues. But there is no way of knowing whether any particular individual will have such built-in resistance.

Apart from damaging the ciliated cells lining the bronchial tubes and eventually destroying the ciliary action altogether, chemical irritants such as cigarette smoke or other environmental or industrial pollutants also stimulate excess mucus secretion from the glands in the air passages. But because the cilia are not working properly, this mucus accumulates in the tubes. In order to clear this material from the tubes, the individual has to cough. Irritants, such as tobacco smoke, also interfere with the white blood cell mechanism which combats infection in the lungs, and the result of all this is that the stagnant material in the tubes becomes infected. This is the condition of chronic bronchitis.

People with chronic bronchitis cough up sputum, on most days, for at least three months of each year – usually the winter months. Most heavy smokers have chronic bronchitis, but refer to it simply as 'a smoker's cough'. Often the efficiency of the coughing is impeded by a tendency for the circular muscles in the wall of the bronchial tube to contract, so causing the tubes to narrow. This is called bronchospasm and it causes wheezing – another sign of chronic bronchitis. Asthma is a severe form of bronchospasm.

In the early stages, chronic bronchitis is a comparatively mild disease. But, with time and continued abuse, it is likely to progress to the very unpleasant condition called chronic obstructive airway disease (COAD), in which large numbers of the tiny lung air sacs break down to form a smaller number of larger air spaces. The trouble with this is that the total surface area now available for oxygen transfer to the blood is greatly reduced so the affected person becomes short of oxygen. In addition, the smaller bronchial tubes become inflamed, narrowed and partially blocked by mucus which cannot get out.

The end result may be a constant, exhausting and irremediable state of breathlessness in which the unhappy victim, to maintain his or her laboured breathing, is forced to use the shoulder muscles to try to increase chest movement. The skin may show an ominous blueness and, in the end, the sufferer may need to wear an oxygen mask while waiting for the inevitable eventual heart failure to supervene.

The evidence linking smoking with heart disease is slightly less direct than in the case of lung cancer. Most of the evidence comes from a series of long-term statistical studies of large population groups in which the members are examined at regular intervals. Some of these groups number over 5000 people and the studies take into account factors such as age, sex, smoking history, blood pressure, weight, amount of physical activity, blood cholesterol levels, stress, family history, the hardness of the local water, and so on. By finding out what eventually happens to these people and correlating this with the factors mentioned, it is possible to discover which factors are regularly associated with diseases.

All the studies show the same result. Cigarette smoking has invariably been found to be a major risk factor in the causation of heart attack, stroke and disease of blood vessels generally. It correlates with a raised incidence of sudden death from coronary artery blockage, and with **angina pectoris** and severe limitation of activity from disease of the blood vessels supplying the legs (peripheral vascular disease). The heavier the smoking the higher the risk. Post-mortem examination of the blood vessels of smokers shows, to a higher-than-average degree, changes in the inner layer which, instead of being perfectly smooth and even, shows irregularity and lumpiness. The lumpy areas are caused by deposition, just under the inner lining, of fatty tissue and cholesterol mixed up with degenerate muscle cells and elastic connective tissue.

This condition is called **atherosclerosis**, and the atherosclerotic plaques usually affect the larger and the medium-sized arteries. The plaques become larger with time and the inner surface of the vessel, at the site of these plaques, is so altered that blood in contact with it can actually begin to clot (thrombosis). This results in a stoppage of the supply of blood to the tissue which the vessel is feeding. The heart is a very active, hard-working, muscle and requires a substantial blood supply to keep up its considerable need for glucose fuel and oxygen. This blood supply is provided by the coronary arteries and these are usually affected, to a greater or lesser degree, by atherosclerosis. When one of these arteries becomes blocked by atherosclerosis or by blood clotting on top of an atherosclerotic plaque, the result is sudden death or, if a small branch is involved, a dangerous and disabling illness.

Smoking is not the primary cause of atherosclerosis, but there is undeniable evidence that smokers show more atherosclerosis than non-smokers and that smokers are twenty times more likely to suffer major episodes related to atherosclerosis (coronary thrombosis, angina, stroke, gangrene of the legs) than non-smokers.

The significance of nicotine is not clear. Many authorities consider that none of the risks of cigarette smoking are connected with the nicotine, but others are more wary and point out that the nicotine-induced increase in the heart rate and rise in the blood pressure, and the possible constriction of the coronary arteries, are probably contributory. But there is certainly no medical argument over the proposition that patients with coronary artery disease who continue to smoke are dicing with death.

The function of the red cells of the blood is to take up oxygen in the lungs and to carry it to all parts of the body where it is needed to oxidize fuel and release energy. The link (chemical combination) between oxygen and the haemoglobin in the red cells is a loose one, so that oxygen can easily be released when the blood reaches an area that needs it. Cigarette smoke contains a gas called carbon monoxide and this combines readily with haemoglobin. But when it does so,

the chemical bond is so strong that the carbon monoxide cannot be released and remains in the blood cells for weeks. So part of the haemoglobin of the blood is unavailable for oxygen transfer because it is converted to this stable compound, which is called carboxy-haemoglobin.

Heavy smokers have carboxy-haemoglobin levels of 5 to 8 per cent in their red cells. To compensate for the reduced availability of oxygen to the tissues, a 20 per cent increase in blood flow is necessary. Vessels narrowed by atherosclerosis may not be able to widen enough to allow this – with predictable results like thrombosis or heart attack. Carboxy-haemoglobin can tip the balance between normal tissue and gangrene, sometimes even between life and sudden death. Here is a quotation from one major textbook of medicine, in the section concerned with atherosclerosis: 'Sudden death is the most frequent clinical event associated with cigarette smoking.'

But this is not the end of the list of the harmful effects of cigarette smoking. Large-scale studies clearly demonstrate that smokers have more ulcers – both stomach and duodenal – than non-smokers. Smokers have more severe ulcers and a higher death-rate from bleeding and perforation than non-smokers. And smokers' ulcers are slower to heal on treatment, than those of non-smokers. Surprisingly, smoking does not affect the secretion of stomach acid and the digestive enzyme that helps to break down protein in the food, and there is no direct evidence that smoking causes ulcers. But the association is undeniable. It is, of course, possible that the kind of people who get ulcers are also the kind who smoke heavily. Be that as it may, the last thing needed, by anyone prone to illness of any sort, is the additional burden of insult upon the body occasioned by the dangerous activity of smoking.

The National Health Service in Britain spends hundreds of millions of pounds every year on treating, or trying to treat, tobacco-related diseases. That money is contributed by tax-paying smokers and non-smokers alike and is wasted. Society would be greatly advantaged if these large sums could be applied to purposes of health improvement for all – welfare, medical research, public health measures, preventive medicine, aids to the disabled and so on. Unfortunately, tax revenue from smoking amounts to many times the cost of the whole National Health Service, so the Government is in a dilemma. This is the reason why Government statements on such issues as tobacco advertising always sound strange.

Smoking imposes an incalculable cost on society from lost productive capacity, working time and trained expertise – which are the main source of society's wealth and prosperity. Again, all suffer. Finally, there is the terrible cost to the affected individual and the cost to families in lost income, in the health-sapping effect of having a chronic invalid in the house and in the eventual bereavement.

Smoking is a very mild form of drug addiction. A little resolution and it will be seen that the 'withdrawal symptoms' are hardly worth talking about and are over in a week or two. 'Cutting down', as a means of gradually giving up, is a pointless waste of time. Some people claim to have been helped by substitutes, like nicotine chewing gum, Nicorette dummy cigarettes, and so on. 'Group therapy', hypnosis, acupuncture, and evening classes in 'giving up' may help, but using these is often just a lack of real intention.

Here is a practical strategy for quitting:

● Get clearly in your mind the full enormity of what you are doing to your health and chances of long life. Read the above section again. Give yourself a positive motive for stopping.

- Get rid of all smoking material and associated equipment such as ashtrays.
- Tell everyone that you have stopped. Make them understand you are serious and insist on cooperation.
- Just walk away from anyone who offers you a cigarette. It is not a friendly act.
- Take regular meals but watch the tendency to eat too much.
- Dismiss from your mind the idea that smoking is an essential part of a meal.
- Eat plenty of fruit and vegetables. Take plenty of soft drinks.
- Exercise more and start a regular exercise schedule.
- Never dwell on your tensions and anxieties.
- Instead of smoking, practise relaxation.
- Above all, never, under any circumstances, have another cigarette. This is fatal. Stop, immediately, maturely and with a minimum of fuss. Join the ranks of the self-righteous. The author gave up smoking thirty years ago, and is self-righteous to this day.

ALCOHOL IN MODERATION

Alcohol has consoled and relaxed mankind since the dawn of history, and moderate usage is generally deemed to be valuable and to offer no hazard to health. But it is a blessing which, by the nature of its effects, is very easily abused. Its desired effects come from its depressant action on the higher functions of the brain which are bound up with social inhibition, anxiety, tensions and the sense of responsibility. By reducing the strength of these functions, alcohol allows the drinker to operate on a simpler, more biological, and less critical level, engaging in enjoyable activity of all kinds without the restraining effect of the normal full awareness of the consequences of his or her actions.

Under the influence of alcohol, many people will, for instance, engage in sexual activity which would be unthinkable if they were sober. Alcohol also abolishes critical awareness of its own effects and the intoxicated have little consciousness of the invariable decrease in quality of judgement and the exercise of skills.

Alcohol has other effects. The blood vessels are widened (dilated) so that the skin becomes flushed and feels warm, the appetite is stimulated so that more is eaten than is required, and the output of urine is greater than the fluid intake so that the body becomes partially dehydrated and thirst is induced which justifies further alcohol intake. This effect is especially common in beer drinkers and is one of the reasons for the often excessive quantity drunk. Dehydration contributes to the hangover.

There are the warning signs that alcohol might be becoming dangerous. 'Moderation in everything' is an excellent maxim for everyone seeking health and contentment. It is especially appropriate in relation to alcohol. The following points are a clear indication that alcohol is being used immoderately. Here are the warning signs:

- Drinking has become a central part of life, rivalling, in its importance, other major activities.
- Drinking is becoming established as a daily habit with a regular indulgence at lunchtime. (Ordinary social drinkers don't have a regular pattern of drinking.)
- Undesirable social or legal effects do not deter.
- The drinker believes he or she has a wonderful head for

drink and can carry on 'normally' after an intake that would put the next person under the table.
- About ten hours after the last drink, another one is badly needed.
- The mornings are bad. The hands shake, there is sickness, retching, gagging and depression. Ordinary sounds seem intolerably loud, there is ringing in the ears (tinnitus) and the skin itches.
- All these symptoms can be cured by a good stiff drink.

It takes, on average, ten to fifteen years to reach a stage of major addiction, but the range may be as wide as from two to twenty-five years. Alcohol consumption is rising steadily in Britain and, with it, there is a progressive rise in:

- the liver disease cirrhosis;
- alcohol-related anaemia and nutritional disease;
- the serious disease of the pancreas, chronic calcifying pancreatitis;
- alcoholic damage to the heart muscle (cardiomyopathy);
- all the social and economic damage consequent on alcohol-related loss of ability.

The unit system is useful in assessing your intake. The average heavy drinker will have a daily intake of at least 80 grams of ethyl alcohol (ethanol), or ten 'units'. One unit of drink is a half-pint of average-strength beer (about 4 per cent), or a single of 70 degree proof spirit, or one glass of wine. One unit contains 8 grams of ethanol. So someone drinking 80 grams of ethanol a day is taking about five pints of beer, or five double whiskies or a bottle of wine. The box contains some useful information about the effects of such intake. These tables should be studied in relation to the current legal levels.

The effect of alcohol on the brain is of special relevance to women – who are drinking twice as much alcohol as they did ten years ago. The greater sensitivity of women to alcohol applies as much to its effect on the brain as on other organs. CT scanning has been used to compare alcohol-induced brain changes in women and men. These changes include widespread shrinkage of brain tissue with enlargement of the normal spaces within the brain (ventricles) and widening of the grooves, and they occur after a much shorter drinking history and lower average consumption in female alcoholics than in males of the same age.

Measurements of intellectual function (psychometric testing) show that, for comparable drinking histories, women are affected significantly more than men in memory, speed of mental reaction, perception of spatial relationships, complex reasoning and abstraction ability.

Brain damage does not occur solely from the direct effect of alcohol on nerve tissue. Other factors include nutritional and vitamin (thiamine) deficiency, liver disease, hormonal factors and head injury from falls and blows. The deteriorated female alcoholic is often suffering from a true alcohol dementia. Men, too, suffer all these effects, but all of them occur earlier in women. Alcoholic dementia comes on very gradually in heavy drinkers, usually quite late in life. The patient, often female, usually around sixty, shows a definite change in personality and severe loss of memory. He or she may seem unconcerned or may be depressed but, on being tested, will be found to have suffered severe deterioration in mental powers, with poor judgement and inability to relate socially in the normal way.

She is likely to deny excessive drinking and may show cunning in keeping up her intake inconspicuously. A CT or MRI

BLOOD ALCOHOL CONCENTRATIONS, IN MILLIGRAMS PER 100 MILLILITRES			
(a) Average-sized man			
Units	At 1 hour	At 2 hours	At 3 hours
1	20	0	0
2	40	10	0
3	60	30	20
4	80	60	40
5	100	80	60
6	120	100	90
7	140	120	110
8	160	150	130
9	180	170	150
10	210	190	170
(b) Average-sized woman			
Units	At 1 hour	At 2 hours	At 3 hours
1	20	0	0
1	30	10	0
2	60	20	10
3	80	40	30
4	110	80	60
5	140	110	80
6	170	140	120
7	200	170	140
8	220	200	170
9	250	220	200
10	300	250	220

Note that the blood concentrations will vary with the weight. The lighter the person, the higher the concentration for a given input. This shows the effects of various blood alcohol concentrations on a person of average tolerance (moderate drinker).

BLOOD ALCOHOL (mg/100 ml) EFFECTS

20 Feeling good. Little or no effect on performance.

40 Able to 'let go' socially. 'Top of form'. Slightly dangerous when driving fast.

60 Feeling good. Judgement impaired. Not a time to make important decisions. Driving becoming reckless.

80 Definite loss of coordination. Unsafe at any speed. Current legal limit in Britain (liable to long-needed amendment).

100 Less sexually inhibited, if not too sleepy. Knocking over drinks.

160 Obviously drunk. Perhaps aggressive. Unmanageable. May not remember, next day, what happened.

300 Spontaneously incontinent. In coma.

500 Dead.

Memory 'blackouts' are common in heavy drinkers if the blood alcohol level gets high enough. Moderate drinkers sometimes get them if they over-indulge, but it is usually only the really hardened drinkers who can reach a high enough blood alcohol level to cause them. Such blackouts are not a sign of alcoholic dementia, but they are, nevertheless, a clear warning of danger.

DTs (delirium tremens) is a withdrawal condition occurring up to seventy-two hours after the last drink. There is clouding of consciousness, then horrifying hallucinations associated with extreme terror, violently threatening behaviour, disordered action of the heart and occasional attempts to commit suicide. The attack, unless effectively treated by injections of powerful sedatives, may go on for as long as five days and the mortality – usually from heart failure – is appreciable.

Excessive drinking can also cause mental illness indirectly by the effect on the mind of all the shattering social, sexual and economic consequences of alcohol dependency.

Cirrhosis of the liver is the replacement of part of the normal tissue of the liver by inert, non-functioning fibrous tissue. It is the end stage of a range of liver disorders which have been so damaging to the organ that the normal processes of regeneration, for which the liver is renowned, have been unable to cope. In liver cirrhosis, the whole structure of the organ is invaded by fibrous tissue, causing it to become nodular. Within large nodules, some normal liver tissue may survive, but most of the functioning liver tissue is replaced.

Almost all the blood from the intestines passes, by way of large veins, to and through the liver, so that the absorbed food material can be processed and part of it stored. One of

scan will show obvious atrophy of the outer layer (the cortex) of the brain. This is the part concerned with the higher functions of the nervous system, including intelligence.

Other effects of alcohol on the brain include the condition of Wernicke's encephalopathy, which is due to a severe deficiency of the vitamin B1 (thiamine). Its symptoms include paralysis of the movement of the eyes, severe loss of balance and gross mental confusion. It occurs only after very heavy, prolonged drinking. Treatment, by thiamine injections, is always urgently needed. If a person with Wernicke's encephalopathy does not get medical attention, the condition eventually progresses to a state, known as Korsakoff's syndrome, in which there is profound loss of memory, both for recent and remote events, so that the patient can hardly remember anything at all. There is a pitiful reaction to this in which the patient invents fictitious accounts to make up for the defect in memory (confabulation) but soon forgets what he or she has just said. Once Korsakoff's syndrome is established, treatment is almost hopeless. Only 14 per cent show any improvement, even on the best management, over a period of five years.

The alcohol unit system provides a useful guidance on consumption. Each of these – a half pint of lager, a glass of wine or sherry or a single measure of spirit – provides one unit.

the effects of the fibrosis is to compress and partly occlude these veins, with the result that the blood has to try to find an alternative route back to the heart. It can do this by way of the veins draining the upper part of the intestine, especially those in the stomach and at the lower end of the gullet (oesophagus). But, in the process, these veins become greatly enlarged and varicose, and one of the most serious complications of cirrhosis is bleeding from these varicose veins with vomiting of blood.

In addition to alcohol, cirrhosis can be caused by hepatitis B and by hepatitis non-A, non-B, by congenital syphilis, by obstruction to the bile duct and by various drugs, such as chloroform or halothane, and by toxic chemicals. But the chief cause, and the one which makes it a major menace, is long-term abuse of alcohol. In this respect as in others, women are far more sensitive to the adverse effects of excess alcohol than men. Cirrhosis is an important disease in modern society and, in the middle-aged, is the third cause of death after heart disease and cancer.

All alcohol drunk is quickly absorbed and passes in the bloodstream to the liver where the earliest observable effect is a condition known as fatty liver. This causes enlargement of the liver by the deposition of excess fat within the liver cells and is more of a warning than a danger. The various liver functions, essential to life, usually continue fairly normally. But the clinical signs of fatty liver are externally indistinguishable from those of alcoholic hepatitis and this is such a serious condition that, if a patient with a heavy drinking history has an enlarged liver, doctors will usually advise removing a small piece of liver (biopsy) for examination in order to be sure.

Alcoholic hepatitis can be diagnosed by microscopic examination of the biopsy specimen, which may reveal areas of cell death as well as patches of characteristic inflammation. Cirrhosis is insidious, and many apparently healthy and well-nourished people have it. The first signs often do not occur until a late stage in the disease. Even liver function tests may give normal results until most of the organ has been destroyed. There may be:

- some loss of weight and of appetite;
- loss of muscle power;
- itching of the skin;
- a peculiar mousy smell to the breath;
- redness of the palms of the hands;
- enlargement of the male breasts;
- loss of sex interest;
- atrophy of the testicles.

Very bad signs are vomiting of blood, the accumulation of fluid in the abdominal cavity (ascites) and yellowing of the skin (jaundice). Sometimes a network of large, knotty veins appears on the front wall of the abdomen. This is an indication that blood is being shunted through alternative vein channels and is also a grave sign.

The liver has so many functions essential to life that severe liver disease is always very serious. People with acute alcoholic hepatitis often die within two weeks of admission to hospital. They die with deep jaundice (yellow staining of the skin and eyes from retained bile), from liver coma, from bleeding into the bowel, from kidney failure or from severe, uncontrollable infection.

Treatment, as may be imagined, is not particularly effective and the only really useful measure is complete abstinence

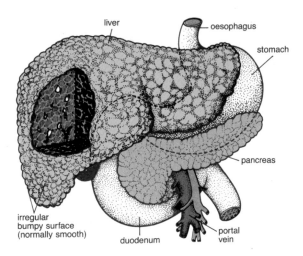

Cirrhosis of the liver is a process of generalized scarring (fibrosis) in which functional liver tissue is gradually replaced by non-functional fibrous tissue. This causes hardening (cirrhosis) and a bumpy irregularity of the surface. Eventually, if the process continues, fatal liver failure may occur.

from alcohol. One must then simply hope that sufficient liver cells have survived the onslaught of the ethanol to keep the patient alive. People who drink enough to cause this condition often eat very little, because they get enough calories from the alcohol to keep them going. Consequently, they are short of essential amino acids and vitamins and these have to be provided as part of the treatment.

Nothing can be done to cure established cirrhosis. The only hope, short of a liver transplant, is to remove the cause and allow the remaining functioning liver tissue to recover and keep one going. In such cases alcohol is deadly and should be absolutely cut out. Drugs affecting the liver should be stopped. A good balanced diet with vitamin supplements, as necessary, will help.

Alcohol does not directly affect the heart unless a great deal is drunk over a period of at least ten years. When it does, it is the heart muscle which is affected. This is called cardiomyopathy. So most of the people who develop alcoholic heart disease are chronic alcoholics. Many are employed in the liquor trade and there are fairly clear indications that the condition is caused, not only by direct alcohol damage to the heart muscle, but also by nutritional and vitamin deficiency in people who get enough calories from the alcohol and do not require to eat.

The first sign of trouble is gradually increasing breathlessness on effort and obvious awareness of the beating of the heart (palpitation). There is none of the acute chest pain of a heart attack (coronary thrombosis) or angina pectoris. If medical advice is not sought, the condition goes on to swelling of the ankles and fluid in the chest from failure of the heart to keep a sufficiently good circulation going. The heart beat becomes irregular and the pulse abnormally fast. Death may occur from severe heart failure.

The extraordinary thing about alcoholic heart muscle disease is that if the affected person can be persuaded to give up alcohol completely, even in an advanced stage of the disease, recovery is 100 per cent. Ironically, persuasion often fails and the victim goes back to drinking as soon as he or she is out of hospital. So, as with alcoholic liver disease, this is yet another way in which one can literally drink oneself to death.

Carefully conducted studies have also shown that moderate to heavy drinking – over six units a day – raises the blood pressure both in normal subjects and in those already known to have high blood pressure. These studies showed that a curtailed alcohol intake, specifically the change to low-alcohol beer, and improved blood pressure control can reduce the need for treatment. The reason for this effect has not been established, but it is well-known that many patients attending hypertension clinics are heavy drinkers and that in these, in particular, blood pressure control is poor. It is recognized that heavy drinkers may be less reliable in taking medication, but this is not thought to be the cause of the findings.

Alcohol dependence is not well-enough understood. It is sometimes thought that, as with drugs like heroin, dependence on alcohol will inevitably occur if enough is taken. This, however, does not seem to be so. It is only a comparatively small proportion of drinkers who become chronic alcoholics and, in these, the dependence seems to be psychological rather than pharmacological. Many alcoholics have a personality that is inadequate in certain respects, or have major difficulty in relating effectively to others. But the easy availability of alcohol and the encouraging social attitudes to drinking are also probably important factors.

The incidence of alcohol dependence is high in people engaged in the liquor trade and in those occupations and social groups in which regular heavy drinking is an established feature. Genetic factors may also play a part but it is very difficult to separate such effects from those of personality and the effects of early environmental influences on personality.

Because the treatment of established alcohol dependence is difficult it is important to detect the problem early and try to avoid it. Alcohol dependence is probably always related to a personality problem and it is likely that in most cases the personality problem causes the excessive drinking because of short-term gains from alcohol. Alcohol is a great consoler, and many turn to it out of a feeling of professional or business failure, frustration, repressed aggression, marital and sexual dissatisfaction, or severe social inhibition. All these, and other distressing elements, may be indicators of a liability to become permanently dependent on alcohol. People aware of any such factors and worried about drinking should see clearly that they may be gravely at risk of passing into a far worse state – that of chronic dependence.

Most experts agree that it is a waste of time to tell someone with a drinking problem to stop. It is equally futile to try to frighten him or her into stopping by recounting horror stories. To do that, without offering anything but blunt insistence on total abstinence, is cruel and pointless and will only deepen depression. The problem drinker should, of course, be as fully aware as possible of the medical consequences of his activities. He is not likely to be in any doubt about the social consequences, but vague ideas about the risk to his liver and brain are not really enough. Moreover, the drinker should never consider that the matter is out of his hands. Every drinker has some measure of control, but not every drinker wishes to exercise it, and one of the aims of treatment must be to provide strong motivation for the exercise of such control as he has.

Problem drinkers need all the help they can get, and the first step in obtaining help is to acknowledge that the problem exists, to accept it and seek help. Alcohol treatment units exist in all major towns and these are run by people whom nothing will surprise. In most of these units, the emphasis is on group therapy, along the supportive lines of 'Alcoholics Anonymous' but with, in addition, the full gamut of skilled medical and psychiatric resource. Problem drinkers attending such units receive specific treatment, not only for the alcohol dependence, but also for any associated nutritional or other secondary effects.

The use of drugs in the management of alcoholism is not generally adopted, as a primary measure, but can be valuable in some cases. The commonest drug used, disulfiram, under the brand name Antabuse, prevents the toxic substance acetaldehyde that is normally formed from alcohol, from being broken down further to harmless substances. So the acetaldehyde accumulates and this makes the subject feel very ill indeed. The effect occurs only if alcohol is taken and is so unpleasant that no one is likely to want to repeat the experience. About five minutes after taking alcohol, the skin flushes and the blood pressure falls. There is profuse sweating, breathlessness, severe headache, alarming pain in the chest, nausea and vomiting and sometimes collapse. Antabuse treatment is never used except in reasonably young fit people who are made completely aware of the effects in advance.

Another drug sometimes used is the vomit-producing apomorphine which may sometimes be helpful in what is called aversion therapy. This is a form of negative conditioning, popularly described as 'brainwashing', in which it is hoped that alcohol will become associated, in the mind of the drinker, with nausea and vomiting. It is not widely used. For the much commoner case of the immoderate drinker who has not gone too far, more positive and perhaps more effective advice can be given.

The realistic answer seems to be for a determined effort to be made to return to moderate drinking. This is, in some ways, a revolutionary idea and not every doctor agrees with it. But few doctors will deny the futility of just telling heavy drinkers to stop.

- First, the drinker must accept that the whole responsibility is his. No external factors may be used as excuses for a increase in drinking. This excuse-making must be recognized for what it is – a dangerous rationalization.
- Next, there must be an absolute and quite rigid upper limit on the number of units taken each day. This is to be regarded as a matter of central principle, involving personal honour, and a breach should be regarded as disgraceful.
- The limit should be decided upon after careful thought, having regard to the fact that too high a limit will only tend to diminish control. It should certainly not exceed six units during the day and no more than two of these should be taken before the evening.
- 'Carrying over' is prohibited.
- Drinking must be slow – small sips rather than gulps.
- It is much better to take the units in light beer or wine rather than in spirits.
- If possible, the units should be taken along with a meal so as to delay absorption.

In this battle, winning is so important that one must be ready to receive some wounds. Radical changes have to be made in lifestyle and habits. It may be necessary that certain drinking companions and, perhaps, certain pubs, should be avoided. A good use must be found for the time formerly wasted in drinking. There are plenty of activities which, in the end, will prove more rewarding than the futile endless argument and boastfulness of semi-drunken conversation.

Emotional problems must be looked at squarely and as disinterestedly as possible. Discussion with a doctor or psychiatrist can be very helpful.

EXERCISE

Fitness is a simple concept involving some very complex physiology. Essentially, the term means what it says – the ability to do something. As commonly used, however, the 'something' is a physical task, such as running a certain distance in a certain time. No one has laid down 'official' standards for fitness and these obviously vary considerably depending on the occupation or the sporting interests. For people other than athletes, a standard somewhat higher than the lifestyle would normally demand is desirable, but to go on raising this standard, in an obsessive kind of way, is, for the ordinary person, rather pointless.

The body is highly adaptable and will usually, within a matter of a few weeks, adjust its ability to perform, with reasonable ease, most physical tasks demanded of it. But this will happen only if the demand is constant and sustained. The most obvious changes which occur are in the bulk and strength of the voluntary muscles, the force and pumping efficiency of the heart muscle, and the effectiveness of the respiratory muscles. But more subtle changes also occur and these involve:

● the ability to perform more work without using up oxygen faster than the lungs and circulation can supply it (aerobic exercise);
● the speed with which the body recovers from fatigue;
● the degree of attainable tension in the muscles (plyometrics);
● the ability of the muscles to utilize the fuels glucose and fatty acids in the presence of lowered insulin level in the blood;
● the increase in the size and number of the energy-producing elements in the muscle cells (the mitochondria);
● the ability of the liver to maintain the supply of glucose to the blood, and hence to the muscles, during strenuous exercise.

All these and other factors may be involved in the changes brought about by radical alteration of the pattern of activity called 'training'. Fortunately, these subtleties need concern only the exercise physiologist. For the man and woman in the street, it is sufficient to enjoy the growing sense of physical and mental well-being and the ease with which daily physical tasks are performed.

The **evolutionary medicine** concept reminds us that during human evolution little was provided in the way of passive transportation – apart, perhaps, from floating logs or primitive boats. The use of horses came well after the present bodily form had evolved. So human beings must be considered creatures naturally dependent on their own muscular ability for movement, even survival. Exercise is natural and normal and is neglected at our peril. Much of the bodily disorder suffered by contemporary people can be attributed to the use of 'artificial' energy sources to replace the use of their own muscles. But it is a basic mistake to think that exercise is concerned only, or even primarily, with the muscles.

No muscle can contract without an adequate blood supply to bring it oxygen and fuel in the form of glucose. Nor can it continue to contract without a good blood supply to carry away the waste products of fuel consumption – the exhaust. A good blood supply requires an efficiently beating heart and a good oxygen supply requires an efficiently operating air intake system – the lungs and the muscles of respiration. These three systems – the muscles, the heart and blood vessels (cardiovascular system) and the respiratory system – are so intimately inter-related, both functionally and in terms of their physiological control mechanisms, that it is impossible to change one without changing the others.

The body, as a whole, is a uniquely responsive entity and will, within the limits of our heredity, modify itself in order to deliver what we ask of it. Athletes reach their level of performance by very hard work, demanding and obtaining a response from their bodies. The top athletes are not those with the best bodies, but those with the best motivation, character, determination. The body will also, very quickly, drop its capacity to a level appropriate to low demands. After six weeks in bed, it takes a minimum of six weeks, usually longer, of normal physical activity to return to the former level of fitness.

The changes which occur on demand are not simply changes in muscle bulk and power – they are changes in the heart, in the respiratory muscles, in the blood vessels, even in the brain. They are universal and their effect is widespread. Sustained exercise improves stamina and endurance by leading to the enlargement and growth of small blood vessels in the muscles – even in the heart – and by increasing the size and number of the energy-producing elements in the cells (the mitochondria). The efficiency of oxygen and glucose fuel usage increases and the work of which the muscles, including the heart muscle, are capable, increases. The rate at which the heart has to beat to maintain an adequate circulation drops and the pulse is slower both during exercise and rest, because the stroke volume (the amount of blood pumped with each beat) is increased. As a result, the heart has to do less work for the same level of efficiency.

These benefits are not be achieved by taking a gentle stroll once a month. Ideally, we should exercise to the point of breathlessness for a minimum of twenty minutes at least three times a week, and the exercises should involve as many muscles as possible.

If we ignore these self-evident facts and live lives of self-indulgent luxury, using our muscles only to heave our overweight bodies from bed to dining table and from table to car, it is not just our muscles that suffer. If our food intake is grossly in excess of our fuel requirements and our fuel usage rate is low, the excess is laid down in the fat storage depots of the body and some of it is laid down in the walls of our under-used and cigarette-abused arteries.

Atherosclerosis, the number one killer of the Western world, is probably the gravest consequence of this biologically disastrous way of life. It clogs or occludes the arteries, reduces the blood flow, causes coronary artery disease, and peripheral artery disease, interfering with the most fundamental of life processes and leading to an ever-worsening capacity for work of all kinds. It kills more people, often in early middle life, than any other single disease process.

Exercise is not just for the young. A well-exercised sixty year old should have a physical performance of about 60 per cent of that of a reasonably fit man of thirty. Exercise is highly beneficial, and body-altering, at every age, without exception. Well-controlled studies have shown that people in their eighties and nineties become fitter and improve their performance when they take deliberate exercise, and it is clear that much of the incapacity thought typical of old age is simply culturally induced but mistaken stereotype.

Doctors now appreciate that, apart from its general benefits, exercise under medical supervision can reduce the severity of angina pectoris, intermittent claudication, some forms of lung disease and depression.

Observance of the three golden rules – no smoking, no overeating, lots of exercise – can be relied upon to make a substantial difference to the health, happiness and capacity for work of anyone currently not complying with them, regardless of age.

In aerobic exercise, such as walking, jogging, swimming, cycling, etc., the rate of oxygen consumption is such that the supply from the lungs, via the bloodstream, is adequate to meet the need. The exercise may therefore be maintained for long periods. In intense, strenuous exercise, such as a 100-metre sprint, oxygen is used up faster than it can be supplied to the muscles. The comparatively small amount stored is rapidly consumed, and the exercise can be maintained for only a short period. Breathing is unnecessary during the ten seconds or so of the race.

By regularly engaging in jogging to the point of breathlessness, an adult of any age can increase his or her capacity for exertion, can lose weight, can lower the blood pressure, diminish the progress of arterial disease and look and feel better. The body is remarkably responsive to demands made upon it and, even in old age, will increase in efficiency and physical capability if sustained effort, in excess of the normal, is made.

But jogging is not entirely without hazard, and people beyond the first bloom of youth, and especially those who smoke or are overweight, should beware. They should remember that even a modest initial indulgence may involve demands on the power of their limb muscles, on the efficiency of their hearts and on the blood-oxygenating capacity of their lungs, in excess of what these systems can provide. So a very gradual build-up is important. Most publications on the subject recommend a full medical check-up before starting, and there may be something to be said for this, but one should not expect doctors to give a certificate of safety.

Orthopaedic injuries – sprains, torn ligaments, stress fractures of bones – are also a hazard, but the risk of these can also be minimized by a very gradual build-up and common-sense limitation of the duration of the running period, to begin with. Physical stress applied too early or too forcefully causes fatigue and injury. Most experienced runners also do warm-up exercises that include stretching the major muscle groups. A good, well-fitting, and supportive pair of running shoes is important, as the stresses on the feet and spine from pounding hard pavements can be considerable.

Physically active people live longer than sedentary people. Walking, stair-climbing and sports play relate inversely to mortality, chiefly from heart and lung diseases. Death rates decline steadily as the amount of energy expended on these activities increases, from less than 500 calories per week to 3500 calories per week. People expending 2000 calories or more per week have death rates one-quarter to one-third lower than those among the less active, of comparable age.

Walking half a mile equates to about fifty calories; climbing seventy steps to about thirty calories; light sporting activity equates to about five calories per minute and vigorous sport to about ten calories per minute. Seventy-three per cent of physically active men (over 2000 calories expended per week) of sixty survive to eighty; only 63 per cent of men of sixty survive to eighty if they are not physically active. Even after the age of eighty, over two years of extra life can, on average, be expected from earlier increased physical activity.

UNDERSTAND INFECTIONS

Infection is the entry into the body, and the subsequent reproduction and establishment within the body, of colonies of any organism capable of causing disease. Many organisms gain access to the body, but only a small proportion are able to overcome the basic defence mechanisms and cause infection.

Most swallowed organisms are destroyed by the acid in the stomach, but some, such as the Salmonella group, are able to resist this and establish themselves in the bowel. The intact skin provides a good barrier to infection, but cuts and abrasions allow access to areas where the second line of defence – the immune system – must operate. Organisms may exist in certain parts of the body without causing any harm but may become extremely harmful if they gain access to other parts. Perforation of the bowel allows organisms access to the sterile regions around the outside of organs (the peritoneal cavity) and the serious condition of peritonitis is inevitable.

When organisms gain access to normally sterile areas, the outcome depends on the balance between the number and virulence of the organisms, on the one hand, and the effectiveness of the defences, on the other. Good hygienic principles – regular washing, sanitary habits, fastidiousness about food, avoidance of obvious sources of infection, and a realistic cynicism about the standards of personal hygiene in others – help to reduce the strength of the attack. So every effort should be made to minimize the dose of infective organisms acquired.

Here are a few tips:

- Common cold viruses are spread mainly by finger contact rather than by droplet spread. Avoid shaking hands with someone with a cold and, if possible, avoid touching objects they have recently touched.
- If you do get your fingers contaminated in this way, keep them away from your face until you get a chance to wash your hands thoroughly.
- In particular, do not rub your eyes or nose. Cold viruses readily gain access via the conjunctivae of the eyes or the mucous lining of the nose.
- Look out for food-handlers with dirty hands and especially those with boils or pimples on their skin. Refuse to accept food from such people.
- Avoid eating-places where there are no obvious and adequate washing facilities.
- Assume that handles on public transport are contaminated with virulent organisms. Wear gloves when travelling, or wash before touching your face.
- Try not to inhale other people's coughed or sneezed air. Many organisms are spread in this way.
- Invite inconsiderate colleagues to cough and sneeze into handkerchiefs.
- Do not engage in casual sex. A willing partner will have been willing with others and may well have, or be incubating, a sexually transmitted disease.

Remember, also, that the pursuit of good health helps to maintain good defences.

DRIVE CAREFULLY

Road traffic accidents are a major cause of death and disablement, especially in young people. The term 'accident' is usually a misnomer, for the great majority of car crashes are not accidental but are the result of lack of imagination, foresight and knowledge. They are caused by carelessness, stupidity, aggression and ignorance. High speed is the great killer, and today's ridiculously over-powered motor vehicles allow large number of irresponsible people to use speed as a source of amusement, an expression of frustration or aggression, or a balm for a feeling of inadequacy.

In the case of those who have already had a crash, there is sometimes an element of accident-proneness believed by some psychologists to indicate deliberate, if half-conscious, intention to do themselves an injury. Accident-prone people often have an aggressive and rebellious attitude to authority and rules, which arose, initially, through rebellion against their parents. But they are also said to have a sense of guilt over their rebelliousness, which demands suffering for wrongdoing. Studies have shown that people who have had four accidents are about fourteen times as numerous as they should be by pure chance. Moreover, they tend to repeat the same type of accident.

To many, high-speed driving seems a bold, macho activity worthy of the admiration of others. It is engaged in by thousands ignorant of the most elementary idea of the forces involved – of the horrifying kinetic energy possessed by a ton of matter accelerated to seventy miles per hour. The energy built up in this way is proportional to the mass of the vehicle multiplied by the square of the velocity. Every surgeon knows, from bloody experience, what this means in practice. The ratio of deaths to injuries increases more than six times when imposed speed limits increase from thirty to sixty miles per hour. Studies in the USA have shown that death rates, from car crashes, in areas of low population density, where high speeds are possible, are more than 100 times higher than in areas of high population density, where speeds are better controlled.

Another factor determining the probable outcome of car crashes is the wearing of seat belts. Seat belts are highly effective in minimizing injury. Alcohol usage before driving is another obvious factor.

TAKE NOTE OF WARNING SIGNS

There are several well-recognized signs which should be known to all as they may give early warning of cancer or other serious disease. They should always be reported.

The warning signs are:

- a new, changed or persisting cough;
- coughing blood;
- black stools;
- any persistent change in the bowel habit;
- indigestion coming on for the first time in later life;
- difficulty in swallowing;
- vomiting blood;
- blood in the urine;
- any obvious change in a coloured skin spot, mole or wart;
- any sore that fails to heal in a month;
- hoarseness or loss of voice, without obvious cause;
- unexplained weight loss.

Any of these is an immediate indication that medical attention is required. Don't delay – wasted time could make a vital difference.

health visitor

A person, often a qualified nurse, employed by a local health authority to visit people in their homes or elsewhere in order to give needed advice and guidance on health matters. Health visitors are concerned, among other things, with the prevention of physical and emotional illness, the early detection of ill health, the prevention of spread of infection, the recognition of special needs and resources and with health teaching. They do not, however, actively engage in technical nursing procedures.

health warning signs

See **health maintenance**.

hearing

The visible part of the external ear or auricle is called the pinna. In many lower animals, this has a useful sound-collecting and direction-finding value, but it is of little functional use in the human being and its loss has little effect on hearing except in people with a degree of deafness. The ear is divided into three parts – the outer, middle and inner ears.

Sound is conveyed by rapid pressure variations in the air. These cause the eardrum to vibrate freely in sympathy. The vibrations are then transmitted across the middle ear by a chain of three tiny bones, the auditory ossicles, which act as levers matching the freedom of the drum movement to the much higher resistance to movement of an oval window in the inner ear. In this way the vibrations are conveyed to a fluid in the microphonic part (cochlea) of inner ear.

Bathed in this fluid is the basilar membrane, a spiral structure of fibres of varying length, which respond to vibrations of different frequencies, depending on their length and mass. Resting on the basilar membrane is a supporting structure for the important cells which convert vibrations into nerve impulses (hair cells) and pass these to the brain by way of the acoustic nerve. The location, along the basilar membrane, of the origin of these impulses, conveys information about the pitch (frequency) of the sound. The amplitude of movement provides information about loudness (intensity). The basilar membrane and its associated structures are known as the organ of Corti. How the information passed to the brain is converted into the subjective experience we call hearing may well remain one of life's eternal mysteries.

Hearing is most acute in childhood, when sounds of frequency from about 16 cycles per second (Hertz – abbreviated Hz) to about 20,000 Hz can be perceived. The lower limit does not alter with age, but there is a steady drop in the ability to perceive the higher pitches. Many people of seventy hear very little above about 3000 Hz. The high frequencies produce hissing sounds (sibilants) and loss of perception of these can cause difficulties in understanding speech.

The middle ear, on the inner side of the eardrum, contains air. Atmospheric pressure is constantly varying, and air in a mucous membrane-lined cavity is soon absorbed into the blood. So it is necessary to have an air inlet/outlet connection to the middle ear. This is the eustachian tube, a short passage leading backwards from the back of the nose, just above the soft palate, on either side, to the cavity of the middle ear. When we swallow, a valve-like fold of mucous membrane is opened and air is able to pass to or from the middle ear cavity, depending on whether the pressure in the middle ear is higher or lower than atmospheric. This balances the pressure on either side of the eardrum so that it can move freely in response to air vibrations. Middle ear air absorption causes the drum to be pushed inwards. On the other hand, during flying, or other rapid ascent, the external pressure drops so that the drum moves outwards. Eustachian tube action deals with both of these situations. A blocked eustachian tube, as from enlarged adenoids or infection, is a major cause of middle ear troubles. The action of the tubes can be demonstrated by pinching the nose and compressing the breath, when the movement of the eardrums will be appreciated.

The inner ear also contains the balancing mechanism, the vestibular apparatus, which includes the semicircular canals. Changes in the position of the head cause movement of fluid in these canals and the generation of nerve impulses which pass to the brain. The result is automatic reflex muscle contractions to restore balance.

hearing aids

Devices designed to improve hearing by amplifying sound. A hearing aid may be accommodated entirely within the ear, fitted behind the ear, incorporated into a stout spectacle frame, or carried on the body and be connected to the earpiece by a fine flexible wire.

HOW THEY WORK

The aid consists of a sensitive microphone, which converts sound into a varying electrical current; an amplifier, usually in the form of an integrated circuit chip; and a miniature transducer, placed within the ear canal, that converts the amplified current back into sound waves at a higher level than would have been experienced at the same point.

Mere amplification cannot relieve all cases of deafness. There are some forms which exhibit a phenomenon known as *recruitment*, in which higher sound levels are less desirable and cause discomfort or even pain, by 'blasting'. Severe sensorineural deafness, in which the elements converting sound vibrations into nerve impulses have been destroyed, will not be aided. But for many, a well-designed and selected hearing aid can be an inconspicuous and substantial asset, allowing normal conversation and avoiding much embarrassment and social isolation. Modern digital devices are capable of selective and programmable amplification of those frequencies at which the hearing loss is greatest. These can often provide real advantage to people who are not helped by the earlier analogue aids.

A valuable feature of most modern hearing aids is the inductive loop pickup facility, which can be brought in at the turn of a switch. This cuts out the microphone, so that background noise is eliminated, but allows electrical signals radiated by public telephones and in the many public buildings – churches, theatres, concert halls and conference rooms – fitted with an inductive loop to be picked up and heard.

TECHNOLOGICAL ADVANCES

The latest developments in hearing aids involve the revolutionary idea of implanting a tiny magnet onto one of the ossicle bones in the middle ear. This is then caused to move by an electromagnetic coil in the ear canal which is activated by the electrical signal from the amplifier. This method can give outstanding sound quality.

> Hearing aids should not be purchased until proper testing has shown that a real advantage would be gained. In the past, about 20 per cent of conventional aids have been abandoned within six months of supply.

See also **hearing, defective**.

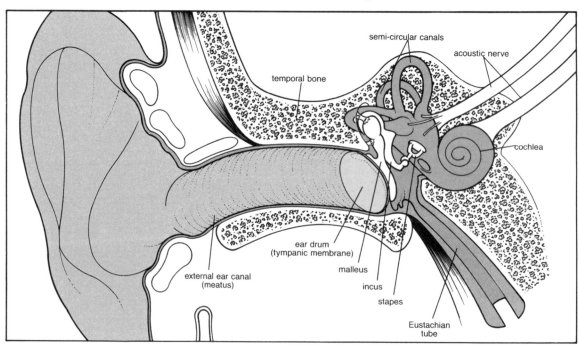

The structure of the ear.

hearing, defective

There are two kinds of deafness, conductive deafness and nerve deafness (sensorineural), and the distinction is important. Conductive deafness results from any defect of the mechanical part of the hearing system. This part is situated external to the inner ear. Nerve deafness results from defect of the innermost part of the ear in which the sound vibrations are converted into nerve impulses which are then carried to the brain.

CONDUCTIVE DEAFNESS

Conductive deafness may occur from wax blockage of the external auditory tube (meatus), through which air vibrations pass to the eardrum; from damage, such as perforation, to the drum itself; from gumming up (otitis media) of the chain of three tiny bones in the middle ear (the ossicles), which transmit the vibrations from the drum to the inner ear; or from a condition known as otosclerosis, in which the innermost of the three ossicles, the stapes, is immobilized by bone formation in the window into the inner ear, in which it should be free to vibrate.

NERVE DEAFNESS

Nerve deafness is due to damage or destruction of the delicate inner ear mechanisms in the cochlea. This contains thousands of sensitive hair cells which are stimulated by vibration to produce nerve impulses by which the brain is informed of the pitch and loudness of the sounds. Nerve cell damage is caused by prolonged exposure to loud noise; by sudden shattering sounds, as from explosions or a slap on the ear, which can literally shake the hair cell apparatus to pieces; from certain toxic chemicals and drugs, especially the aminoglycoside antibiotics in high dosage, and from the effects of ageing. Nerve deafness is commonly associated with ringing in the ears (tinnitus) and is seldom remediable. It is thus important for people to avoid the causal factors, especially loud noise, so as to minimize the long-term damage.

TREATMENT

Conductive deafness is much more readily treated than nerve deafness. Ear wax can be removed, drum perforations can be repaired, middle ear infections can be controlled and the bones sometimes freed, and otosclerosis can be treated by surgery.

See also **noise, effects of**.

hearing tests

See **audiometry**.

heart

The heart, which occupies the centre of the chest, is a controlled pump, responsive to every change in demand, and maintaining two separate, but interconnected blood circulations. It is a four-chambered organ, consisting almost entirely of muscle, and containing valves which ensure that the blood can move only in one direction. Because it must continue to operate at all times during life, the heart has a high fuel consumption and is provided with a profuse blood supply by way of the coronary arteries. These arise from the first part of the largest artery of the body – the aorta – which emerges from the top of the heart.

The two sides of the heart, each of two chambers – an upper (atrium) and a lower (ventricle) – are separated from each other by a central wall (septum). In certain congenital heart disorders this septum has an opening in it, allowing blood from one side to pass across to the other. This is what is meant by 'a hole in the heart'. In a healthy heart, however,

Cochlear implants

These are used in an attempt to restore some kind of hearing in cases of severe sensorineural deafness, but, in the present state of the art, there is no question of being able to bring back normal hearing. Electrical audio signals can be passed into the cochlea by means of electrodes, insulated except at the tips, the circuit being completed by a second electrode connected to the tissues elsewhere. The result, subjectively, is a muffled and crude reproduction of the original. Nerve fibres cannot conduct frequencies above about 500 Hz and the audio spectrum covers the range up to about 16,000 Hz.

The healthy cochlea is an amazingly sensitive discriminator of pitch, and it does so by sympathetic vibration of different parts of the resonating membrane in the cochlea (the basilar membrane). Pitch information, covering the full audible range, is conveyed to the brain by frequency-modulated signals passing along fibres of the acoustic nerve whose site of origin in the cochlea is itself an indication of frequency.

The latest 22-electrode multichannel implants allow about half of the people using them to understand speech. These implants cover a wide range of frequencies, and their multiple electrodes are placed along the basilar membrane. Anticipated problems with electrode corrosion or electrolytic effects have not been found to be serious so long as alternating currents, rather than direct currents, are used. Cochlear implants have improved remarkably in recent years and research continues apace.

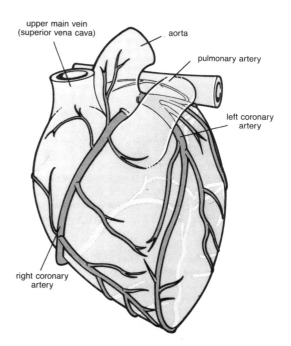

The coronary artery supply to the heart muscle. There are two coronary arteries but the left artery branches into two large trunks, effectively providing three arteries.

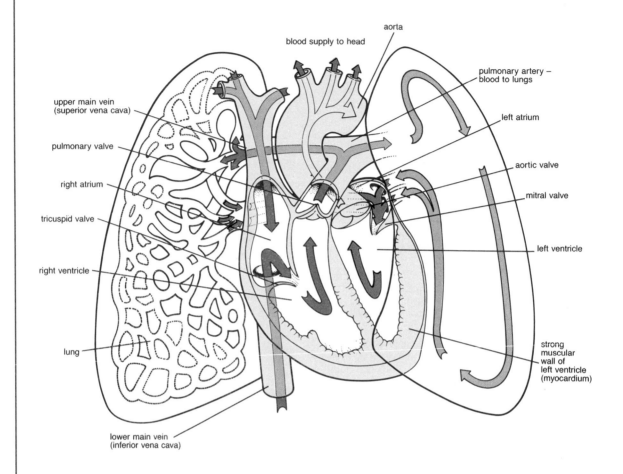

Labels on diagram:

blood supply to head
aorta
pulmonary artery – blood to lungs
upper main vein (superior vena cava)
left atrium
pulmonary valve
aortic valve
right atrium
mitral valve
tricuspid valve
left ventricle
right ventricle
strong muscular wall of left ventricle (myocardium)
lung
lower main vein (inferior vena cava)

The heart-lung circulation.

the two atria and the two larger ventricles are kept apart and blood can get from one side of the heart to the other only by way of the external circulation of arteries and veins.

Arteries carry high pressure blood from the heart, and veins bring back low pressure blood to the heart. The right side of the heart is less powerful than the left as it has only to pump blood to the nearby lungs. The left side, whose wall is three times as thick as that of the right, pumps blood to the head and all parts of the body. This blood does not return to the left side of the heart but is brought back by way of large veins to the upper chamber on the right side (the right atrium). When this chamber squeezes (contracts) the blood in it is forced down through a three-leafed valve (the tricuspid valve) into the right ventricle, whence it is pumped to the lungs by way of the pulmonary arteries.

Blood returns to the heart from the lungs by way of the pulmonary veins and enters the upper part of the left side (left atrium). From there it passes down through a two-cusped valve (the mitral valve) to the powerful left ventricle, which pumps it all around the body. It will thus be seen that the blood circulates in a 'figure of eight' manner, all blood returning from the tissues being immediately sent to the lungs for re-oxygenation, and all blood from the lungs being sent to the tissues.

At rest, each beat (contraction) of the heart moves about 70 ml of blood. This is about 5 litres per minute. During exercise, this may rise to between 20 and 35 litres per minute, depending on the degree of fitness.

The inner lining of the heart chambers is called the endocardium and this layer also lines the valves. The middle muscular layer, the myocardium, consists of a network of muscle fibres of a kind found nowhere else in the body and possessing the property of continuous, regular, rhythmical contraction at a rate of about 100 beats per minute. This natural rate is damped down to the normal 70 to 80 by nervous and hormonal control mechanisms. The outer layer, the epicardium, is surrounded by a kind of bag, the pericardium, which encloses the whole heart. Between this sac and the heart is a thin layer of lubricating fluid to allow free movement during contraction.

Immediately under the pericardium, lying on the surface of the heart, are the two coronary arteries with their many branches passing deep into the heart muscle. The coronary veins, which lie alongside the arteries, carry blood back from the heart muscle to the right atrium. The coronary arteries are critically important for the maintenance of the heart's action and, hence, life. Interference with the blood flow along the coronary arteries, by the common arterial

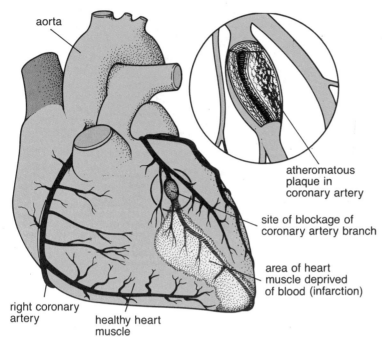

aorta

atheromatous
plaque in
coronary artery

site of blockage of
coronary artery branch

area of heart
muscle deprived
of blood (infarction)

right coronary
artery

healthy heart
muscle

What happens in a heart attack (myocardial infarction).
Obstruction to the blood flow to the heart muscle, by
blockage of a branch of a coronary artery, results in an area of
heart muscle with no blood supply. This area dies. If the
affected area is small, recovery is usual.

disease of atherosclerosis is the major cause of death in the Western world.

The heart output is an important concept in understanding fitness. Cardiac output is the volume of blood moved round the circulation each minute and, at rest, is usually about 5 litres. This is the body's minimum requirement and can be achieved by a comparatively small number of powerful, vigorous beats (slow pulse rate) or by a large number of feeble, low-volume beats (fast pulse rate). The output per beat varies with the general state of the heart muscle and is greater in fit people than in the unfit. Athletes, for instance, have an excellent output per beat and require fewer beats to achieve the same cardiac output, so good athletes usually have slow pulses. The amount of blood needed obviously varies with the state of exertion, but the greater the output per beat the less will be the increase in pulse during exertion. This is one of the important means of judging fitness. A fit person has a comparatively minor rise in heart rate during exertion and, afterwards, the rate soon drops back to normal. An unfit person's heart will race on exertion and will take a long time to get back to normal.

heart action control

See **nitric oxide**.

heart, arrest

See *First Aid*.

heart, artificial

See **artificial heart**.

heart attack

A coronary thrombosis, or heart attack, usually described by doctors as a myocardial infarction, is the result of an obstruction to blood flow in one of the branches of the two coronary arteries through which the heart muscle is supplied with blood. Because it must beat (contract) continuously, the heart has a major, and continuous, oxygen and sugar requirement. Any substantial reduction in this fuel supply to any part of the muscle interferes, not only with its ability to function, but even with its survival as a living tissue.

INCIDENCE

The arterial obstructive disease, atherosclerosis, is present, to some degree, in almost all adults in the Western world, and affects most of the arteries of the body, particularly the coronary arteries. The prevalence and degree of atherosclerosis is much worse in men than in women before the menopause and increases in both sexes with age. When these facts are considered, it need occasion no surprise that coronary thrombosis is responsible for about half of all deaths in Western countries and is generally regarded in medical circles as the major problem in preventive medicine.

RECOGNITION AND SYMPTOMS

Blockage of a main coronary artery branch (coronary thrombosis) occurs when blood, which will not normally clot within the circulation, is prompted to do so by a roughened plaque of fatty, degenerative, cholesterol-containing material called atheroma in the inner lining of the vessel. Prior to the thrombosis, these atherosclerotic plaques cause no symptoms, nor any other indication of their presence, until they narrow the artery so severely – to less than half its normal bore – that the blood flow is insufficient to permit full exertion. At rest, the person concerned seems normal, but a fixed amount of exercise – say, walking for half a mile – causes heart pain (angina pectoris).

When total blockage occurs, part of the heart muscle loses its blood supply (myocardial infarction) and dies. Depending on the size of the artery blocked, this dead area may involve the full thickness of the heart wall, or only part. The heart cannot continue to function as a pump if more than a certain proportion of the muscle is destroyed. Blockage of a major branch, with destruction of about half of the muscle in the main, left, pumping chamber, is almost always immediately fatal. Previous smaller attacks make death more likely.

Coronary thrombosis usually causes a severe pain, or sense of pressure, in the centre of the chest. The pain often spreads through to the back, up into the neck, or down either arm. There is a horrifying sense that one is about to die and often extreme restlessness. The pulse is weak, difficult to feel, and often irregular. Sometimes it is very slow. Severe pain is not always a feature. In less major cases pain may be absent and there is evidence that up to 20 per cent of mild coronaries are not recognized, as such, or even as significant illness, by those affected. This means that there are millions of people who, because of previous unrecognized attacks, are much more vulnerable than normal.

Half of those who die from a particular attack do so from heart stoppage (cardiac arrest) within three or four hours of onset, so there is always great urgency to get a person with a coronary thrombosis to hospital with minimum delay. Many who might have been saved have died because they did not recognize or believe that they had a life-threatening condition.

TREATMENT

A valuable emergency measure that can save lives is to give a drug that dissolves clots in the arteries – a *thrombolytic drug*. A small dose of aspirin is also very helpful. Regrettably, a survey published in August 1994 suggests that many general practitioners are not using thrombolysis or giving aspirin. People at risk may take a small dose of aspirin every day as protection.

PREVENTING HEART DISEASE

Factors which increase the risk of coronary thrombosis are, or should be, well-known and are dealt with, in detail, elsewhere in this book. They are smoking, lack of exercise, overeating with resultant obesity, a high-fat diet, excessive stress and parents who died of arterial disease. Only the latter factor is beyond individual control and there is now ample evidence that intelligent people able to benefit by advice are now markedly reducing their chances of coronary thrombosis by behaving accordingly. Since these facts have been widely known, the incidence of coronary thrombosis has declined significantly in certain social classes. Regrettably, all have not seen the light. In a study of 7735 middle-aged men, published in 1987, the prevalence of coronary thrombosis was found to be 44 per cent higher in manual workers than in non-manual workers. This was attributed mainly to cigarette smoking, obesity and lack of exercise in leisure time.

A strategy for the prevention of coronary artery disease, based on the concordant views of experts from nineteen countries, was published in the *Lancet* in 1987. The main points were directed to the eradication of smoking, reduced cholesterol intake with emphasis on unsaturated fat and high fibre content, and the promotion of exercise. The aim was to reduce obesity, lower blood cholesterol levels and reduce blood pressure. There was particular emphasis on encouraging social pressures against smoking.

heart attack sequel

See **reperfusion injury**.

heart beat strengthening

See **inotropic agents**.

heart block

The timing of the contraction of the chambers of the heart, necessary for the smooth directional movement of blood, is under the control of a bundle of specially conducting muscle fibres in the heart muscle called the *bundle of His*, after the German anatomist and histologist Wilhelm His (1831–1904), who discovered it. This bundle starts in a natural pacemaker (the sino-atrial node) in the wall of the right upper chamber

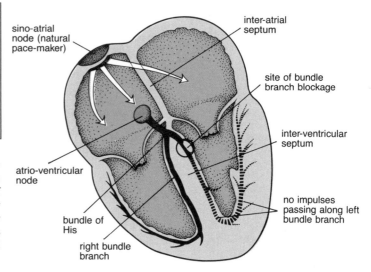

The underlying cause of heart block. Damage to the specialized muscle fibres, which conduct the coordinating impulses to cause the heart muscle to contract, leaves part of the heart muscle to beat at its own slow rate. The illustration shows interruption of the left bundle branch of the bundle of His.

(right atrium) and passes into the wall between the two halves of the heart, dividing into two and running down each side of the wall to reach the lower chambers (the ventricles). The bundle of His is the only conducting link between the upper and lower chambers of the heart.

POSSIBLE CAUSES

Heart block is the condition in which some part of the conducting bundle has been damaged so that the controlling impulses no longer pass from the upper to the lower chambers of the heart. Such damage usually occurs as a result of coronary thrombosis, but there are other causes, including drug toxicity, rheumatic fever, syphilis or tumour.

There are different kinds of block, depending on the location of the damage. There may be right bundle branch block, left bundle branch block or complete heart block, and each shows its characteristic effect in dissociating the affected chamber or chambers from the parts of the heart above the block.

RECOGNITION AND SYMPTOMS

Heart block, in general, causes the pulse to be very slow, as the lower chamber can only beat at its intrinsically low rate. Heart block is one of the major indications for the implantation of an artificial pacemaker.

heartburn

A burning or aching sensation felt behind the lower part of the breastbone (sternum) when the gullet (oesophagus) goes into spasm or when acid from the stomach regurgitates up into it.

INCIDENCE

The symptom is commonest after meals, especially after injudicious indulgence in fatty foods, and tends, for mechanical reasons, to be worse when the sufferer is lying down. Also for mechanical reasons, heartburn is common in pregnancy. It is often associated with *waterbrash* – the regurgitation of bitter-tasting stomach contents into the mouth.

POSSIBLE CAUSES

A common cause of heartburn is hiatus hernia in which part of the stomach pushes upwards, through the normal opening in the diaphragm, into the chest. A perennial concern to middle-aged and older men is whether the pain they are experiencing in the middle of the chest is due to heartburn or to heart disease. Unfortunately, cardiac pain does sometimes resemble heartburn, but a distinction can often be made on the grounds that pain from angina usually has a constant, fixed quantitative relationship to exertion. Belching will relieve both sorts of pain, but only very briefly in the case of heart disease.

In pregnancy, the increasing pressure within the abdomen from the growing uterus causes increased regurgitation into the oesophagus.

TREATMENT

Heartburn can be prevented by eating more wisely and more slowly. Any associated stomach or duodenal (peptic) ulceration should have proper medical attention. Antacids, indigestion lozenges, and so on are no substitute for self-control. Heartburn in pregnancy can be controlled by various safe medicines, available on prescription. However unpleasant, it does cease to be a problem following the birth.

See **cardiospasm**.

heart compression

See **tamponade**.

heart defects at birth

See **blue baby**, **coarctation of the aorta**, **heart disease**, **congenital**, **Eisenmenger complex**, **Fallot's tetralogy**, patent ductus arteriosus.

heart disease, congenital

This is a group of structural disorders of the heart which occur during the development of the fetus and which are present at birth. Some may not be suspected until later. Congenital heart disease affects about one live baby in 120.

POSSIBLE CAUSES

There are many different causes, including virus infections early in pregnancy, especially German measles (*rubella*); drugs, taken in the early weeks of pregnancy, such as thalidomide; diabetes or systemic lupus erythematosus in the mother; Down's syndrome and various other chromosomal defects, including trisomy 13 and trisomy 18; and Turner's syndrome.

CONGENITAL DISEASES

These diseases take several forms, of which the commonest are:

- openings in the internal wall of the heart – 'hole in the heart' (septal defects);
- a failure of a fetal blood channel to close (patent ductus arteriosus);
- narrowing of the main valves (aortic and pulmonary valve stenosis);
- a narrowing of the main artery of the body (aortic stenosis);
- a complex of four defects occurring together (Fallot's tetralogy).

Septal defects – 'hole in the heart' – are abnormal openings in the central wall of the heart so that the chambers on one side can communicate with those on the other, allowing blood which has been oxygenated in the lungs to mix with blood which has not. Septal defects may lie between the upper chambers (atrial septal defect) or between the lower (ventricular septal defects). In atrial septal defect, the

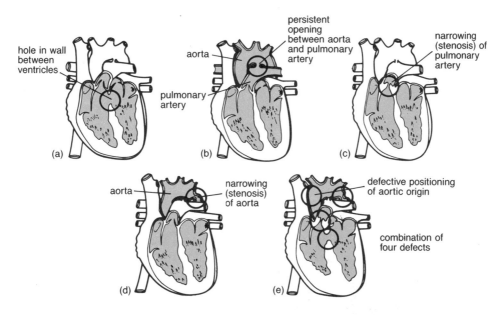

The commonest kinds of congenital heart disease.
(a) A hole in the wall between the ventricles – ventricular septal defect.
(b) Failure of closure of the connection between the main artery to the body and the artery to the lungs – patent ductus arteriosus.
(c) Narrowing of the origin of the artery to the lungs – pulmonary stenosis.
(d) Local narrowing of the main artery of the body – coarctation of the aorta.
(e) A combination of these with a misplacement of the origin of the aorta – the tetralogy of Fallot.

stronger left side tends to pump blood through the hole from the left side to the right, so an abnormal amount of blood passes through the lungs. There is a heart murmur, usually heard at about one year of age and the right side of the heart enlarges and may eventually fail. A hole between the lower chambers produces a very loud murmur as the blood is powerfully shunted from the left side to the right. The left side of the heart enlarges and, again, excess blood flows though the lungs causing respiratory distress and breathlessness.

Patent ductus arteriosus is the persistence of the connection between the main artery of the body (the aorta) and the arterial trunk to the lungs. Because the lungs do not function before birth, their arterial supply, vital after birth, must be largely bypassed. This is the function of the ductus arteriosus and this normally closes at birth. Persistence means that up to 50 per cent of the blood which should go to the body is recirculated to the lungs. This puts a heavy strain on the heart, which may eventually fail.

RECOGNITION AND SYMPTOMS

Congenital heart disorders in which there is mixing of oxygenated and non-oxygenated blood often interfere with the normal nutrition of all the tissues of the body. The effect depends on the size of the openings and on other factors. There may be blueness (cyanosis), stunting of growth and of intellectual development, thickening (clubbing) of the tips of the fingers and toes, poor tolerance of exercise, an undue tendency to respiratory and other infections, and the risk of the heart itself becoming the site of a bacterial invasion (bacterial endocarditis).

TREATMENT

Surgical correction of the congenital defect is often advised during infancy or childhood. Narrowing of the heart valves and of the aorta (aortic stenosis) may be very serious and may cause sudden heart failure and collapse. Surgery is often necessary to save life.

See also **blue baby**.

heart, enlarged

Enlargement of the heart is often a reaction to high blood pressure (hypertension) or heart valve disease, either of which forces the heart to work harder than normal so that the muscle in the walls of the lower chambers (ventricles) becomes much thicker. Heart enlargement can also occur

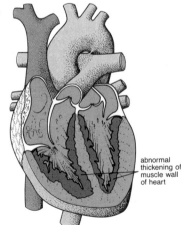

Heart enlargement. This is a common form of heart disorder and has several causes. Essentially, it is the contracting muscle – the myocardium – that becomes thickened so that the outline of the heart increases. Enlargement is usually compensatory and may prevent failure. Heart dilatation, another form of enlargement, is a kind of ballooning.

abnormal thickening of muscle wall of heart

from an increase in the volume of the chambers (dilatation). Other conditions, including various cardiomyopathies, may cause enlargement, but in several serious heart disorders, including coronary artery disease, the heart is of normal size.

heart examination

Much information can be derived from feeling the pulse at the wrist – the rate, regularity, force and nature of the pressure changes are all significant and meaningful. The pulse or beat of the heart itself is also felt and the position of the farthest out impulse (the apex beat) noted. This provides information about the strength of the contraction of the main, lower, pumping chambers (ventricles) of the heart and of any heart enlargement.

The stethoscope is then used to listen to the heart sounds. The 'lub-dub' sounds heard are caused by the blood slapping against the heart valves when they suddenly close. The 'lub' sound is caused by the closure of the valves between the upper and lower chambers of the heart (the atria and the ventricles); the 'dub' sound indicates the closing of the valves at the roots of the outlet arteries (the aorta and the pulmonary trunk).

Heart murmurs are the sound vibrations, from unusually turbulent blood flow, heard in addition to the normal heart sounds, and caused mainly by sudden acceleration or deceleration of blood movement. Murmurs do not necessarily imply disease, but any unusual sound must be regarded as an indication of possible abnormality in the blood flow. By far the most common cause of extra blood turbulence is a disorder of the heart valves, such as narrowing (stenosis) or leakage (incompetence) with regurgitation. Murmurs are also caused by:

● 'hole in the heart' (septal defect);
● failure of closure of the fetal connection between the lung and the general circulation (patent ductus arteriosus);
● loose or 'floppy' valve leaves;
● inflammation of the heart sac (pericarditis), with a pericardial 'rub';
● fever;
● other rarer conditions such as a benign tumour in a heart chamber (myxoma).

By noting the location on the chest wall at which the murmur is best heard, and the timing of the murmur in relation to the basic heart sounds, and by considering these in conjunction with other signs and symptoms, the experienced physician will usually be able to arrive at an accurate diagnosis.

See also **angiography**, **electrocardiogram**, **chest X-ray**, **heart stress test**.

heart failure

This does not mean that the heart has stopped or that it is in imminent danger of doing so. Heart failure is the condition in which, as a result of various forms of heart disease, the heart is no longer capable of producing an adequate output of blood so as to meet the needs of the body for oxygen and nutrition. In heart failure the blood flow to the tissues and to the lungs is diminished and slowed. Congestion results, with engorgement of the veins and other small blood vessels, leading to obvious signs and symptoms. Heart failure is commonly caused by coronary artery disease, high blood pressure and rheumatic heart disease, but may result from one of many different heart disorders. The features may vary considerably.

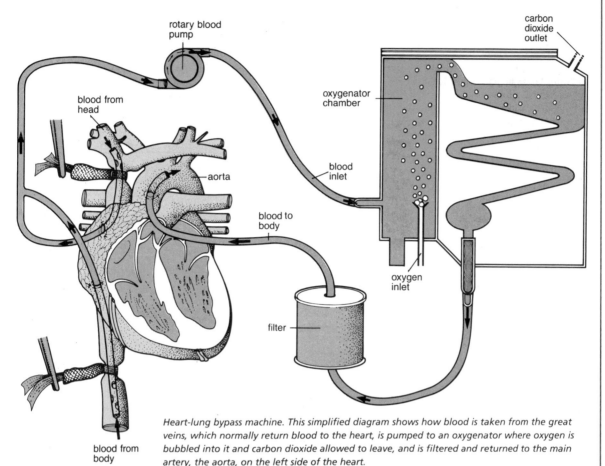

Heart-lung bypass machine. This simplified diagram shows how blood is taken from the great veins, which normally return blood to the heart, is pumped to an oxygenator where oxygen is bubbled into it and carbon dioxide allowed to leave, and is filtered and returned to the main artery, the aorta, on the left side of the heart.

RECOGNITION AND SYMPTOMS

If blood returning from the body to the right side of the heart cannot be pushed on to the lungs quickly enough, this is called right heart failure. The result is blueness (cyanosis) and the accumulation of fluid in the tissues (oedema), ankle swelling, enlargement of the liver, and, in severe cases a considerable accumulation of fluid within the abdomen (*ascites*).

When the left side of the heart is unable to clear the blood from the lungs quickly enough, causing breathlessness and fluid accumulation in the lungs, this is called left heart failure. The main symptom of left heart failure is breathlessness, which may occur on mild exertion or even when the affected person is at rest. There may be attacks of sudden breathlessness during the night. As the condition worsens, the tendency to breathlessness increases. Eventually, the degree of disability becomes extreme and the state pitiful. In both right and left heart failure there is severely restricted activity.

TREATMENT

Heart failure can usually be treated effectively, especially if the underlying cause of the heart damage is remediable. The drug digitalis is valuable in increasing the strength and effectiveness of the heartbeat (contraction) and its use often greatly improves the condition of the affected person. Fluid in the lungs and the tissues can be removed by the use of diuretic drugs, which greatly increase the urinary output. After effective treatment for heart failure, the greatly relieved patient may spend long periods in the toilet disposing of

excess water. Abdominal fluid may sometimes be removed by suction through a wide-bore needle.

heart, inflammation of

The general term is carditis, which means inflammation of any of the tissues of the heart. Endocarditis is inflammation of the inner lining (the endocardium) and this always involves the heart valves. Bacterial endocarditis is a serious disorder liable to affect people whose heart valves have been damaged by prior disease such as rheumatic fever. In such people, even a few bacteria released into the blood during a dental extraction can set up endocarditis.

Myocarditis is inflammation of the heart muscle and this is usually caused by virus infection. *Pericarditis* is inflammation of the *pericardium*, the outer covering of the heart. This occurs in most cases of heart attack (coronary thrombosis) and affects the pericardium overlying the area of muscle deprived of blood (myocardial infarction). Pericarditis also occurs from infection, usually viral, and other causes.

heart-lung machine

A device that can, for short periods, carry out the functions of the heart and the lungs, so as to allow surgery on the heart. Once the heart-lung machine has taken over the maintenance of the circulation and oxygenation of the blood, the patient's heart can be cooled and stopped so that the operation may proceed.

HOW IT WORKS

At the point at which blood would normally be returned to the heart, it is carried from the body to the machine in sterile plastic tubes. There, it is artificially oxygenated and the waste carbon dioxide removed and it is then pumped back into the body, being re-introduced at the point at which blood from the lungs would normally leave the heart. The pumps are of a special kind to minimize damage to red blood cells. The blood passing through the machine is often cooled so as to lower the patient's body temperature (*hypothermia*) and decrease the nutritional and oxygen needs of the tissues. This method of deliberate surgical hypothermia is one of the major advances in heart surgery. Anticoagulants are used to prevent the blood from clotting.

heart-lung transplant

The first successful heart and lung transplant was done at Stanford University in 1981. Since then, many advances have been made and the operation is now an accepted form of treatment for people with severe destructive lung diseases which would otherwise prove fatal. Those with healthy lungs but with a seriously diseased heart can have a heart transplant, if suitable.

> Most recipients are comparatively young, as the outlook for a transplant is poor after about fifty-five years. Diabetics, people with cancer or severe liver or kidney disease are unsuitable. The donor will, ideally, be under thirty-five, if male, or under forty, if female.

HOW IT'S DONE

The donor should, ideally, be a little smaller than the recipient, and the heart and lungs must be transplanted as soon as possible after death – preferably within four hours. The recipient heart is first removed so that the removal of the lungs is easier and the essential nerves which control the action of the respiratory muscles are not damaged. In a heart-lung transplantation it is necessary to connect up fewer blood vessels than in a pure heart transplant, but the main artery to the body and the main returning veins must be connected. In addition, the trachea of the donor lungs must be joined to the cut trachea of the recipient.

> Early failures were due to infection, breakdown at the junction in the windpipe (trachea), poor function of the transplanted organs and foreign tissue rejection. The development of the immunosuppressant drug cyclosporin has been a major advance and has reduced the need for heavy dosage of steroids. A method of flushing out the arteries of the donor lungs with a special preservative solution has allowed longer delays between the death of the donor and the transplant operation.

RISKS

With such a large bulk of donated tissue, the chances of rejection problems are increased and the procedure could not have been possible without major advances in knowledge of immunology and in the application of immunosuppressive techniques. One form the rejection reaction takes is the development of a severe inflammation of the small bronchial branches, called *obliterative bronchiolitis*. The measures taken to control rejection are, in themselves, dangerous as they deprive the body of its normal resistance to infection in much the same way as occurs in AIDS. *Pneumocystis carinii* and *Cytomegalovirus* infections of the lungs, both common features of AIDS, also sometimes occur in people who have had heart-lung transplants. In some series, *Cytomegalovirus* infections have been the major cause of death.

> The results of heart-lung transplantation are remarkable and about 70 per cent of patients are alive and well two years after the operation.

heart muscle disorders

See **cardiomyoplasty**.

heart muscle, non-functioning, recoverable

See **hybernating myocardium**.

heart muscle reduction surgery.

See **heart reduction**.

heart rate, ultra-fast

See **supraventricular tachycardia**, **Wolff-Parkinson-White syndrome**.

heart reduction

A surgical operation to reduce the volume of muscle in the left ventricle of a heart that has failed as a result of the ballooning condition known as dilated cardiomyopathy. The ballooned chamber is reduced to normal size by cutting a full-thickness segment out of the wall and stitching the edges together. This allows more effective contraction of the ventricle and improves the heart output per beat. The procedure is still experimental.

heart stress test

In an apparently fit person with an unsuspected heart problem, such as a degree of narrowing of the coronary arteries, the electrocardiogram may show a normal trace if taken at rest, but reveal abnormalities, indicating an inadequate blood supply to the heart muscle, during exertion. Since it is important to know about this, it has become common for electrocardiogram tests to be done while the subject takes exercise, such as running on a treadmill, so as to put the heart under stress. During such tests, the electrocardiogram is closely monitored so that any sign of abnormality is detected at once. Contrary to popular belief, heart attacks do not most commonly occur during exertion, when the flow through the coronary arteries is brisk, but exercise can, of course, provoke pain in people with angina pectoris.

heart transplantation

The transplantation of a donor heart into a person with damage to the heart.

WHY IT'S DONE

Most heart transplants are given to people whose hearts are damaged beyond repair by arterial disease and repeated heart attacks (coronary thrombosis) or by advanced heart failure with expansion (dilatation) and thinning of the main

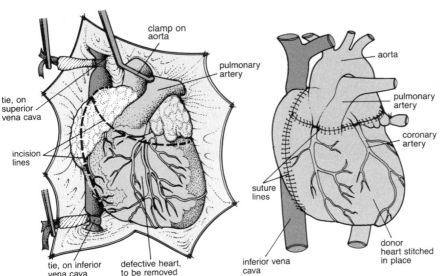

clamp on
aorta

pulmonary
artery

tie, on
superior
vena cava

incision
lines

tie, on inferior
vena cava

defective heart,
to be removed

suture
lines

inferior vena
cava

aorta

pulmonary
artery

coronary
artery

donor
heart stitched
in place

Heart transplant. Note that the upper part of the heart with all the attached blood vessels is usually left behind, thus greatly simplifying the technical problems for the surgeon. Heart disease affects the lower parts – the ventricles – much more seriously than the upper parts.

chambers. A few have to have transplants because of congenital heart disease, severe disease of the valves, inflammation of the heart muscle, ballooning of the heart after injury, widespread occlusion of the coronary arteries or heart tumours.

HOW IT'S DONE

Donor and recipient are matched for blood group and for weight within 20 per cent. Because of supply and transport problems – the heart must be implanted within four hours of removal – prospective tissue matching is impracticable. The recipient's serum is tested against the donor's white blood cells (lymphocytes) for antibodies and the donor is tested for various infections.

Removal of the donor heart is a straightforward procedure which can be done in any non-specialist hospital theatre. The heart is cooled and transported in cold salt water (saline) at 4°C. In most cases the recipient's main veins are left in place and the diseased heart cut off through the middle of the upper chambers (the atria). This makes the attachment of the donor heart easier. The other main arteries and veins must then be carefully cut through so that the cut ends may be joined up, by stitching (suturing), to those on the donor heart. Perfect suturing is essential as any leakage would be fatal.

After the operation the patient is kept under intensive care for less than a week and in hospital for less than three weeks. Deliberate immunosuppression is essential if rejection is to be avoided. This is done with immediate doses of drugs such as cyclosporin and azothioprine and the steroid prednisolone. After a day or two the patient continues on lower dosage. Cyclosporin has revolutionized the outlook in organ transplantation.

To check for rejection tendencies, tissue samples (*biopsies*) are taken at intervals from the heart lining, initially weekly, but later every three months or so. This is done under local anaesthesia, through a jugular vein, using a fine tube called a bioptome. The examination of these samples gives early warning of the need for more intensive anti-rejection treatment. Immunotherapy has the major disadvantage that the resistance to infection is greatly lowered. This is a risk that has to be taken, but it is a serious one, and the main cause of death in heart transplantation is infection.

RISKS

The results of heart transplantation are now excellent and are improving steadily. Currently, the survival rate, at two years, is over 80 per cent, and, at five years, over 60 per cent. Various complications are, however, common. These include severe kidney damage from cyclosporin, an acceleration in the severity of atherosclerosis, causing angina pectoris which the patient is not aware of because the sensory nerves have been cut, high blood pressure, cancers, especially lymphomas, and other effects of immunosuppression. Patients can die suddenly, without warning, after 'silent' angina attacks.

heart, tube into

See **Swan-Ganz catheter**.

heart valve replacement

A narrowed, leaking or distorted valve causes serious interference with the heart's efficiency and output. Narrowed valves can often be opened up by passing a finger or an inflatable balloon through them, but there are many valve disorders for which the only remedy is replacement.

The new valve may be a donated human valve, a pig heart valve or a mechanical prosthesis. Functionally, all are equally efficient, but mechanical valves tend to wear or become leaky (incompetent) after many months or years of ceaseless action and tend to cause blood clots to form unless this is prevented by the use of anticoagulants. Biological valves, whether human or porcine, present rejection problems, which must be countered by drugs (immunosuppressives). This, in turn, can cause a variety of problems. As knowledge of immunology grows, it is likely that it may be possible, in the future, to make more effective and safer use of this source.

heel bone, spur on

See **calcaneal spur syndrome**.

Hegar's sign

The softening of the neck of the womb (cervix) which is one of the confirmatory signs of pregnancy.

helicase

An enzyme that breaks the chemical linkage (hydrogen bond) between the base pairs in DNA, thus separating the two strands of the double helix so that the process of replication can proceed. Helicase works in conjunction with single-strand binding proteins that attach to the outer side of each single strand, preventing the two from rebonding, so that two rows of free-ended bases are left as templates on which new complementary strands can be formed.

Helicobacter pylori

See **peptic ulcer**.

helper T cell

A subclass of T lymphocytes (T cells) that provides essential assistance to macrophages of the immune system. When a **macrophage** has ingested an organism, **antigen** is expressed on the macrophage surface at the site of the **major histocompatibility complex** (**MHC**) surface markers. Helper T cells bind to the combination of antigen and MHC and produce the **cytokine** gamma-interferon. This diffuses to the macrophage and switches on the killing function so that the organism is destroyed.

In the absence of helper T cell assistance the protective function of the immune system is seriously undermined. The HIV attacks and kills helper T cells thus causing the acquired immune deficiency (AIDS).

hemi-

Prefix meaning 'half' as in hemiplegia (half-paralysed).

hemianopia

Loss of half of the field of vision of each eye. Depending on the cause, this may be temporary or permanent. Most commonly, the line dividing the seeing from the non-seeing areas runs vertically through the point at which the affected person is looking. Both outer halves may be lost (*bitemporal hemianopia*) or there may be loss of both right or both left halves (*homonymous hemianopia*).

POSSIBLE CAUSES

Bitemporal hemianopia almost always indicates a tumour of the pituitary gland pressing on the central crossing of the optic nerves behind the eyes. At this point fibres from the inner half of each retina cross and their destruction causes blindness in the outer halves of the field of vision. Homonymous hemianopia is usually caused by stroke in the elderly, when the blood supply to the back of one side of the brain is cut off. In young people it may be caused by migraine and is almost always transient and usually of no great significance. Homonymous hemianopia may also be due to damage to the back of the brain from other causes such as gun-shot wound or other injury, brain tumour, brain abscess or inflammation of the brain (encephalitis). Hemianopia of this kind cannot be caused by any disorder of the eyes themselves.

See also **transient ischaemic attacks**.

Heminevrin

A brand name for chlomethiazole.

hemiplegia

Paralysis of half the body. This is due to brain damage involving the main motor nerve pathways which run down through the substance of the brain to the spinal cord.

POSSIBLE CAUSES

Such damage is, in the great majority of cases, due to blood vessel disease with either obstruction (thrombosis) or rupture (haemorrhage), and hemiplegia is the hallmark of stroke. But the damage may also be caused by other disorders such as brain tumour, multiple sclerosis, brain inflammation (encephalitis) or injury.

RECOGNITION AND SYMPTOMS

In hemiplegia, the arm is usually more severely affected than the leg, and the face may or may not be involved. If it is, there is usually a down-turn of the corner of the mouth and the lower eyelid on the affected side may droop. Hemiplegia may be *spastic*, with the muscles resisting passive movement and tending to cause bending (flexion) of the joints; or it may be *flaccid*, with the muscles lying totally limp.

Hemiplegia is usually worst at onset and often improves with time.

COPING

A determination to recover function, reflected in early mobilization and maximal effort to use the paralysed parts, will usually lead to a better outcome than negative passivity.

See also **stroke**.

Henoch-Schonlein purpura

See **purpura**.

hepar

Greek root meaning 'liver' as in hepatitis (liver inflammation).

heparin

A complex polysaccharide organic acid found mainly in lung and liver tissue. Heparin is thought to bind to thrombin and antithrombin in plasma thereby assisting in their combination and interfering with the cascade of reactions that end in blood clotting (coagulation). From the Greek hepar, 'the liver'. Heparin is widely used as an anticoagulant under brand names such as Monoparin, Monoparin Ca, Multiparin and Uniparin.

See also **low molecular weight heparin**.

hepatic

Relating to the liver.

hepatitis A

Inflammation of the liver due to infection with a virus acquired by the ingestion of food contaminated with human faeces.

RECOGNITION AND SYMPTOMS

The virus is highly infectious and is appears in the stools for about two weeks before the onset of the symptoms and for about a week after onset. There is fever, severe loss of appetite (anorexia), loss of energy, slight enlargement of the liver with tenderness, yellowing of the skin (jaundice) and darkening of the urine. The stools look very pale and clay-like.

The hepatitis A virus (HAV) causes swelling of the liver and temporarily blocks the excretion into the bile of the bilirubin which is freed by the constant breakdown of red blood cells. Without bilirubin, the faeces are pale, and with too much bilirubin in the blood the skin is stained yellow (jaundice) and the urine discoloured.

> Antibodies to the virus soon develop and the liver inflammation resolves. The condition usually settles within three to six weeks and does not, as a rule, lead to permanent liver damage. Some very few cases develop liver failure and die early in the disease. Persistent (chronic) liver disorder, ending in cirrhosis of the liver, is not a feature of hepatitis A.

TREATMENT
There is no specific treatment for hepatitis A except bed rest. Often there is a marked sense of debility for two or three months after the attack. Later, a kind of hepatic hypochondriasis, called the *post-hepatitis syndrome*, which lasts for months, is common. This features loss of appetite, nausea, general malaise, and a sense of discomfort over the liver, but without any objective or biochemical evidence of liver disease.

hepatitis B

This form of hepatitis is caused by a virus, known as HBV, which is transmitted in blood, blood products or other body fluids, such as saliva, semen, vaginal secretion and urine. The disease can be spread from mother to baby at, or soon after, birth. It is commonly spread by shared intravenous needles, and is especially common among drug users. Contaminated needles are not easily sterilized and should never be used by a second person. Male homosexuals engaging in penetrative sexual intercourse are also at risk. Other modes of spread include acupuncture, tattooing and ear- and body-piercing.

Hepatitis B has been spread widely among those using pooled blood products, such as Factor VIII for haemophilia. Hospital staff at risk from needle-stick accidents are also susceptible.

RECOGNITION AND SYMPTOMS
The disease is similar to hepatitis A, but more severe, and skin rashes and joint pains often precede the main symptoms. Hepatitis B viruses vary in their virulence and there is a significant death rate from the acute stage of the disease, especially in older people. About 10 per cent of sufferers become persistent carriers after the initial stage and many of these people develop complications, including cirrhosis of the liver. Cancer of the liver is much commoner in chronic carriers than in others.

TREATMENT
Vaccination against HBV is effective and should be considered by all those at special risk including babies born to women carriers.

hepatitis C

Formerly called **hepatitis non-A, non-B**, this liver disease is caused by a small virus known as the hepatitis C virus (HCV). The disease occurs world-wide and is spread mainly by intravenous drug use, tattooing, body piercing and needle-stick injuries. Only a minority of infected people develop symptoms and the clinical course is usually mild, with jaundice in only 10 per cent. This does not, however, imply that the con-

dition is trivial. In about 80 per cent of cases the infection becomes permanent and of these about one-third end up with **cirrhosis** of the liver.

hepatitis D

See **hepatitis delta**.

hepatitis delta

A liver inflammation caused by a very small virus, hepatitis delta virus (HDV). This virus can reproduce only in the presence of the hepatitis B virus (HBV). But people with hepatitis B who also develop hepatitis delta infection are likely to suffer a considerably worsened outlook. HDV infection has caused serious epidemics and is endemic in the Mediterranean area. The method of spread is still not clearly understood.

hepatitis E

A liver inflammation caused by a single-strand, non-enveloped RNA virus known as hepatitis virus E (HEV), that is spread by the faecal-oral route. The first major outbreak, in Delhi, was spread by sewage and flooding, and caused 30,000 cases of jaundice. There is a mortality of up to 4 per cent, but the infection is much more dangerous in pregnant women in whom the mortality may be as high as 20 per cent.

hepatitis, non-A, non-B

See **hepatitis C**.

hereditary cancer

See **familial adenomatous polyposis**.

heredity

The transmission of characteristics from parent to child by the genes carried in the ova and spermatozoa and united at the moment of fertilization.

hermaphroditism

The condition in which both male and female reproductive organs are present. The term has a mythical origin. Hermaphroditos, the son of Hermes and Aphrodite, excited such passion in a young woman called Salmacis that she prayed to the Gods for total union with him. She got her wish and the two became fused into one body. The man is said to have been far from pleased.

True human hermaphroditism is rare and most of those affected have external genitalia of ambiguous character. There may be one ovary and one testis, or gonads with a combination of ovarian and testicular features. The external genitalia may be female or male or a combination of both, and some hermaphrodites are said to be capable of sexual intercourse with either sex. The cause is unknown.

Most of the affected subjects are raised as males but at the time of puberty about half of them menstruate and 80 per cent develop breasts of the female type. Often there is difficulty in deciding which sex to elect, but, in general, surgery to achieve feminization is easier and more satisfactory and should, ideally, be performed in infancy. If left until puberty or later, surgical correction must be determined by the gen-

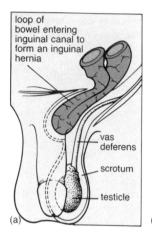

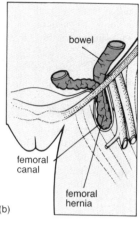

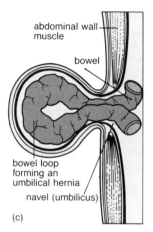

Three of the commonest kinds of hernia: (a) inguinal hernia in which a loop of bowel descends into the scrotum; (b) femoral hernia in which the loop forms a lump in the groin; (c) umbilical hernia in which a loop of bowel passes through a weakness in the abdominal wall at the navel.

der identity of the individual. This is largely determined by the sex perceived at birth by the parents.

Pseudo-hermaphroditism is much commoner and is the condition in which the genetic constitution is of one sex while the bodily appearance and behaviour are of the other. This is caused by excess male sex hormones in the female and deficiency of sex hormone in the male. These disorders are usually due to disease, but female virilization may occur from hormone therapy. Pseudo-hermaphroditism can usually be effectively treated.

hernia

An abnormal protrusion of a part of the body through an opening which is either caused, or enlarged, by the protruding part. Hernias may be present at birth, or the underlying weakness, which later allows herniation, may be present at birth. They tend to occur at points of structural weakness in the walls of body cavities, especially the abdomen, and are especially common in the groin region (*inguinal* and *femoral hernias*), at the navel (*umbilical hernia*) and at the opening in the diaphragm through which the gullet (*oesophagus*) passes to run into the stomach (hiatus hernia).

An inguinal hernia is a loop of bowel passing down the canal through which the testicle descends early in life. If not treated the hernia tends to enlarge as more and more bowel passes down into the scrotum. In femoral hernia, the loop passes forward through the canal for the large vessels and nerves to the leg and comes to lie under the skin. In hiatus hernia, part of the stomach passes up into the chest.

> A hernia which can be returned to its normal position is said to be reducible. If it cannot, it is said to be incarcerated; and if its blood supply is cut off by swelling it is said to be strangulated. A strangulated hernia leads to gangrene of the part outside the cavity, and is a surgical emergency calling for urgent operation.

TREATMENT
Surgical correction of a hernia is by repair and closure of the abnormal opening. This is not always easy and there is a tendency to recurrence, especially in inguinal hernia, in which as many as one in ten may require re-operation. This is mainly because a tunnel must be left for the spermatic cord running down to the testicle. A variety of different operations exists –

which is usually an indication that none is wholly satisfactory. The weakness may be repaired by the use of natural or synthetic materials.

heroin

Heroin is a derivative of morphine and thus of opium. Chemically, 3,6-O-diacetylmorphine hydrochloride monohydrate, or 'diamorphine', heroin is an almost white, crystalline, odourless powder with a bitter taste, which is rapidly and completely absorbed into the body after oral administration and is quickly distributed to all parts. In pregnant women it crosses the placenta to the fetus and causes respiratory depression and drug dependence in the newborn – a dependence which is subsequently increased if the woman breastfeeds as the drug is also excreted in the milk. The manufacture of heroin, even for medical purposes, is illegal in almost every part of the world, except in Britain, for the drug has no medical advantages, as a pain-killer, over safer substances, except that it is more soluble than morphine so repeated injections can be avoided in terminal-care patients. Heroin is completely converted to morphine in the body and has no medical value apart from the relief of pain of body and mind.

Heroin, considered purely as a pharmacological agent, is not particularly likely to damage health. It is, however, in other respects, extremely likely to do so. It is easy to take a dangerous or fatal dose; the associated dangers of casual intravenous use – infection with bacteria, fungi, and various viruses including those causing **AIDS** and **hepatitis B** – are obvious; and the effects on behaviour can have devastating and destructive consequences.

HEROIN ADDICTION TREATMENT
The synthetic narcotic methadone is prescribed in a clinic and is taken by mouth in orange juice, once a day. Methadone is addictive, but does not produce a heroin 'high' and blocks the brain-opiate receptors so that heroin, even if injected, has little effect. The supply of methadone is secure and is not dependent on criminal associations. The people under treatment may thus, although remaining addicted to methadone, lead a fairly normal life.

Some people come to prefer methadone to heroin and it is clear that many comply with the programme without any real intention of freeing themselves from the habit. Some use the methadone facilities only when heroin supplies are hard to get. Early reports of the success of the method were unduly sanguine and it has become increasingly clear that the solution to the heroin drug problem is not to be so easily found.

As with many other behavioural and criminal trends, the mere passage of time seems to bring improvement to the individual. The real reason for this is that drug-taking is the result of the failure to understand the factors that lead to satisfaction in life. The quality of early parental influence – which is vitally important in early programming – often leaves much to be desired, as may the later influence of school teachers. But life, itself, will often, in the end, supply the deficit, and the adolescent junky will often turn into the respectable, and disapproving, adult. See also **detoxification under anaesthesia**.

HEROIN BABIES

Heroin converts to morphine soon after entering the body and morphine in the mother's blood passes through the placenta into the blood of the fetus. Seventy-five per cent of babies born to addicted mothers show withdrawal signs and most require treatment. The signs include tremor, hyperactivity, fever, vomiting, diarrhoea, sweating, sneezing, respiratory distress and convulsions. These last for an average of about a week, but sometimes persist for three weeks.

Reports of the long-term effect on babies differ and it is difficult to separate the purely medical effects of morphine from the high level of socially disadvantageous factors in heroin addicts. In one series, for instance, only one-quarter of the mothers were married or were living in a stable relationship. Another study, from the US, showed a baby mortality rate, within a few weeks of birth, of nearly 7 per cent. This may well have been due to social rather than drug-related factors and there is also no real evidence that morphine, by itself, has a major influence on the health of these babies.

heroin detox, humane

See **detoxification under anaesthesia**.

herpes

The group of herpes viruses contains at least 80 different types, five of which affect humans – Herpes simplex virus, type 1 (HSV-1), which causes 'cold sores' around the mouth and nose; Herpes simplex virus, type 2 (HSV-2), which causes venereal Herpes (see **sexually transmitted diseases**); Herpes zoster virus, which causes chickenpox and shingles, the Epstein Barr virus, which causes glandular fever (infective mononucleosis) in adolescents and cancer of the nose and throat in the Chinese, as well as a tumour, common in Africa, called Burkitt's lymphoma; and the cytomegalovirus which can cause congenital defects and which affects people with immunodeficiency disorders.

Herpes viruses are highly contagious and few people are free from them. Most of us carry Herpes simplex viruses lying dormant in the nerves at the junction of skin and mucous membranes and Herpes zoster viruses in the sensory nerve cells near the spinal cord. Both cold sores and shingles occur in this way, from viruses that have been present for long periods, often for years.

RECOGNITION AND SYMPTOMS

Every now and then, dormant viruses become active, reproducing rapidly, moving to the skin and causing the well-known itching, tingling discomfort and spreading clusters of painful little crusting blisters.

RISKS

It is not known, for certain, why the dormant viruses flare up, but they often do so during a feverish illness, or at times of stress or emotional upset or after exposure to bright sunlight. Some people get an attack after taking certain foodstuffs or drugs. It is probable that the fighting strength of the viruses is kept under control most of the time by the immune system and that herpes only flares when the immune system is coping with demands elsewhere.

People whose immune systems are deficient, as in AIDS, have a very bad time with herpes, which often spreads to parts of the body not normally affected.

TREATMENT

One problem in trying to treat Herpes simplex infections is that, because the available drugs act to stop the viruses reproducing, it is hard to know when is the right time to start. Unfortunately, before each flare-up, viral reproduction has gone on for quite a while, so there are always plenty of viruses around before there seems to be any reason to start treatment. Short of treating all the time, the ideal is to start treatment at the earliest possible moment – at the first suggestion of a tingle.

There are several drugs with action against the herpes virus. These include virarabine (Vira-A), idoxuridine (Herpid) and acyclovir (Zovirax). Of these, acyclovir is the safest and most effective and has largely replaced the others. It works well, not only for the Herpes simplex viruses, but also for the closely similar varicella-zoster virus which causes shingles and chickenpox. There is also evidence that it may be of value in Epstein-Barr virus infections. Unfortunately, it seems to be of little value in cytomegalovirus infections. Acyclovir is a remarkable drug which remains practically inert until it contacts herpes viruses. These contain an enzyme which converts acyclovir to its active form, acyclovir triphosphate, and it is this which stops the virus from reproducing by interfering with its DNA.

Acyclovir can safely be taken by mouth and it is widely distributed throughout the body. It is excreted in the urine and about half the dose has gone in three hours. It is also available as a cream for the treatment of herpes on the lips and eyes. Genital herpes is best treated by the tablets, for the use of the cream may encourage resistant strains of the virus to emerge. The dose will be prescribed by the doctor and one should on no account try to economise. Large doses are used for primary attacks, but do not eradicate the infection. Those who suffer severe recurrent herpes can reduce the frequency and severity of the attacks by taking a tablet three times a day, but this should not be done without medical advice.

> Herpes viruses are associated with some cancers, although the nature of the relationship is not fully understood. There is a positive association between genital herpes and cancer of the neck of the womb (cervix), and between the Epstein-Barr virus and naso-pharyngeal cancer and Burkitt's lymphoma.

HERPES SIMPLEX IN AIDS

Many people worried about the possibility of developing AIDS will already be well informed on the subject of herpes. But herpes in the immune deficiency state is a very different matter from the relatively minor inconvenience of venereal herpes or cold sores around the mouth. The Epstein-Barr (EB) virus and the varicella-zoster virus are both common in

AIDS but their effects are much less serious than the common Herpes simplex virus.

The uncontrolled spread of herpes is a very painful and distressing effect of the compromised immune system. It is, essentially, an exaggeration of the kind of oral and genital herpes infection well known to many: painful, tense, opalescent blisters around the mouth or nose, or on the glans or shaft of the penis, or spreading around the skin of the vulva, anus and buttocks. These blisters come in crops, persist for several days and then ulcerate to become covered with a greyish discharge. There is fever, a feeling of illness and loss of weight and the associated lymph glands – in the neck or groin, as the case may be – become enlarged and tender. In AIDS, the effects are not confined to these sites but spread inward, both locally and remotely, to involve the inside of the mouth, the gullet and even the trachea and bronchi of the respiratory tract. At the other end, the blisters spread into the rectum and the urinary system causing severe pain, difficulty in urination or defecation and alteration in sensation around the buttocks.

Remote spread is even more serious as this often leads to involvement of the brain, causing inflammation of the brain (herpes encephalitis) and inflammation of the brain linings (herpes meningitis). These are, of course, grave complications, leading, in untreated cases, to coma and a 60 per cent mortality rate. If treatment is delayed until after the onset of coma, only 8 per cent of patients will survive without permanent brain damage.

Many trials have now been done on the control of Herpes simplex infections in immunocompromised people and these have shown, beyond any doubt, that the drug Zovirax is highly effective and safe and works well against both type 1 and type 2 herpes simplex, and against the varicella-zoster (chickenpox) virus. It can be given directly into the bloodstream without ill-effect and has a rapid action.

herpes gestationis

An uncommon skin disease affecting only pregnant women and unconnected with herpes virus infection. There are blister-like formations, each with a reddened base, anywhere on the skin, and the condition closely resembles dermatitis herpetiformis. Steroid treatment may be necessary, but the condition clears up as soon as the baby is born. Recurrences, in subsequent pregnancies, are to be expected and the problem may even recur if oral contraceptives are used. These may have to be avoided.

Herpid

A brand name for **idoxuridine**.

heterosexuality

The state of sexual orientation and attraction towards an individual of anatomical sex opposite to one's own.

heterozygous

A term describing a person who carries differing genes at the same gene position (locus) in a pair of corresponding chromosomes. This is the same as saying that the **alleles** are different. A single **dominant** gene can manifest itself in a heterozygous person. Recessive genes are only manifest if both are present (**homozygous**).

hexachlorophane

A bactericidal agent used in soaps and for skin cleansing. A chlorinated phenol. Brand names are Ster-Zac D.C., Ster-Zac Powder and, formulated with other ingredients, Dermalex.

Hexalen

A brand name for **altretamine**.

hexamine

An antibacterial drug used to assist controlling urinary tract infections. A brand name is Hiprex.

hexetidine

An antiseptic used in a weak solution as a mouthwash or gargle to treat oral ulcers, sore throat, gum inflammation (gingivitis) and bad breath. A brand name is Oraldene.

Hexopal

A brand name for **inositol nicotinate**.

hiatus hernia

The stomach lies immediately under the muscular sheet (the diaphragm) which separates the chest from the abdomen. To reach it, the gullet (oesophagus), must pass through a small opening in the diaphragm. Normally, the lower end of the oesophagus, together with its muscular controlling ring (sphincter), lies just under the diaphragm and runs, at an oblique angle, into the stomach. When the stomach is distended, pressure upwards, against the diaphragm, tends to close this sphincter and prevent the stomach contents from passing up into the oesophagus.

Sometimes the junction of the oesophagus and the stomach slides up through the oesophageal opening in the diaphragm into the chest. This is called a hiatus hernia and

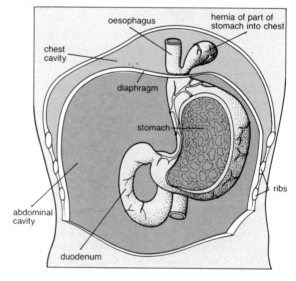

Hiatus hernia. Normally, the whole of the stomach lies in the abdominal cavity below the diaphragm. In hiatus hernia, a small part of the stomach passes up through the opening in the diaphragm for the gullet so that it lies in the chest cavity.

the main effect is that the mechanism which prevents regurgitation into the oesophagus cannot operate, so the acidified and highly irritating stomach contents are able to move up into the oesophagus, producing damage to the lining and the condition of *oesophagitis*.

INCIDENCE

Hiatus hernia is commonest in middle-aged and elderly women, especially in the obese.

RECOGNITION AND SYMPTOMS

Hiatus hernia causes severe heartburn – a deep burning pain behind the breastbone (sternum), made worse by bending forward, by straining and by lying down. The pain often disturbs sleep and may be so severe as to be mistaken for angina pectoris or a heart attack (coronary thrombosis). Hiatus hernia causes no symptoms apart from those of oesophagitis and some people have the condition without the commonly associated damage to the oesophageal lining.

RISKS

Many people suffer from severe damage to the oesophageal lining, even to the extent of having ulceration and bleeding, and anaemia may result from blood loss. Long-persistent hiatus hernia may cause dangerous changes in the cells lining the oesophagus and some authorities believe that this may progress to cancer.

TREATMENT

Oesophagitis may be prevented by:

- reducing obesity;
- taking small meals;
- avoiding fatty foods, aspirin and other non-steroidal anti-inflammatory drugs;
- avoiding too much bending from the waist;
- sleeping with the head of the bed raised;
- using H-2 receptor antagonists such as Zantac (cimetidine) or ranitidine.

If all else fails, a surgical operation can be done to restore the normal relationship of the parts.

Hibitane

A brand name for chlorhexidine.

HIB vaccine

A vaccine against *Haemophilus influenzae*, type B. This vaccine was introduced in October, 1992, following which there was a rapid reduction in the number of reported cases of this infection, especially in children under five.

hiccup

A succession of involuntary spasms of the diaphragm, each followed by sudden closure of the vocal cords, which checks the inrush of air and causes the characteristic sound. Hiccups can be caused by irritation of the nerves to the diaphragm (phrenic nerves) or by abnormal stimulation of the input nerves to the brain which supply the respiratory centres there. In most cases the cause is unknown and harmless, but hiccuping is a feature of many serious conditions, including pleurisy, pneumonia, uraemia and disorders of most of the abdominal organs. Sometimes it is so persistent as to be exhausting.

TREATMENT

The tendency to hiccup is reduced if the level of carbon dioxide in the blood is raised. This is most easily achieved by holding the breath for as long as possible or by re-breathing air in a small plastic bag. Other tricks include drinking water out of the 'wrong' side of a glass, pulling on the tongue or pressing on the eyeballs. Various sedative drugs are helpful, but if all else fails, the phrenic nerve can be temporarily prevented from transmitting impulses by injecting a small dose of local anaesthetic around it.

high blood pressure

See **hypertension**.

high-fibre diets

See **dietary fibre**.

hindbrain hernia headache

A rare form of headache caused by part of the hind-brain (*cerebellum*) passing down into the large opening for the spinal cord (the foramen magnum) in the base of the skull. The condition is brought on by coughing, straining, sneezing, laughing, exertion or certain postural changes and can be relieved by surgical enlargement of the foramen magnum.

Hioxyl

A brand name for **hydrogen peroxide**.

hip-clicking test

A method of detecting the fairly common condition of congenital dislocation of the hip, an important condition in babies, more common in girls and babies born by breech presentation. The condition is often missed, because unsuspected.

The baby is placed on her back and the hip joints are bent so that the thighs are vertical. The knees are fully bent. The doctor holds the thighs, close to the body, with his or her thumbs on the inside and the fingers over the outer side of each hip joint. The thighs are now swung apart and at the same time as the doctor's finger-tips are pressed inwards and upwards. If the hips are dislocated a sharp click or 'clunk' is heard as the head of the thigh bone (femur) slips into its socket (acetabulum) on the side of the pelvis. Some clicks may not be associated with dislocation, but clicking hips must always be followed up by an expert.

hip, congenital dislocation of

The hip joint is a ball and socket joint. Congenital dislocation, which is commoner in girl babies, implies an abnormal relationship of the ball, on the thigh bone (femur), to the socket (acetabulum) in the pelvis. This appears to be due to lax ligaments around the hip joint. Early diagnosis is important as correction (reduction) of the dislocation is easy and, once the head of the femur has been held in its acetabulum by light splinting for a few weeks, normal growth and development can occur. The splints hold the thighs apart and rotated outwards.

If congenital dislocation is not diagnosed until the child begins to walk the problem then becomes apparent. If one joint is affected there will be a limp and a lurch to the affected side. If both joints are dislocated, the gait is waddling. Delayed treatment means greater difficulty in management and usually a less satisfactory result.

See also **hip-clicking test**.

Hippocratic oath

This has been the ethical code for doctors since the times of ancient Greece. Whether the oath was drafted by the Greek physician Hippocrates is uncertain, but there are indications that it was written during the fourth century BC under the influence of the followers of the philosopher and mathematician Pythagoras.

The oath has remained an ethical inspiration to doctors through the ages and has undoubtedly been influential. Although by no means universally used in graduation ceremonies, it is still taken by the graduates of many medical schools.

In 1948 a modern version of the oath was drawn up by the World Medical Association in Geneva (see box).

The Geneva Declaration

At the time of being admitted a member of the medical profession: I solemnly pledge myself to consecrate my life to the service of humanity; I will give my teachers the respect and gratitude which is their due; I will practise my profession with conscience and with dignity. The health of my patient will be my first consideration; I will respect the secrets which are confided in me; I will maintain by all the means in my power, the honour and the noble traditions of the medical profession. My colleagues will be my brothers; I will not permit considerations of religion, nationality or race, party politics or social standing to intervene between my duty and my patient; I will maintain the utmost respect for human life from the time of conception; even under threat, I will not use my medical knowledge contrary to the laws of humanity. I make these promises solemnly, freely and upon my honour.

---

hip replacement

The hip replacement operation has come to be thought of, by many, as a routine and simple procedure. This is not so. Hip replacement is major surgery, calling for great skill and substantial surgical resources. It is expensive and time-consuming. But the results are so good that the time, trouble and cost are fully justified.

HOW IT'S DONE

Over 30,000 hip replacements are done every year in Britain. The operation is highly successful as both the natural socket (the acetabulum) and the natural ball, the head of the thigh bone (femur), are replaced. In the operation, the joint, which has been grossly damaged by arthritis or by loss of its blood supply, is completely removed and replaced by a plastic socket, which is fitted into the hollow in the pelvis, and a short, angled metal shaft, which is forced down into the hollow of the thigh bone, and which has on its upper end a smooth ball to fit into the socket.

RISKS

Complications do occur, the most important being infection – which is disastrous – and loosening of the shaft of the prosthesis in the hollow of the thigh bone. The infection rate, in spite of the most elaborate precautions is usually at least 1 per cent. Loosening, especially after a number of years, has been a major problem and this has, so far, defied the ingenuity of technology to solve it. Special bone glues are commonly used

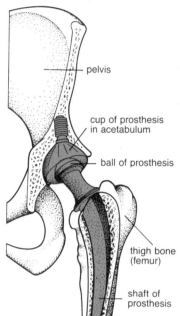

Hip replacement. The cup segment of the prosthetic hip is glued or screwed into the hollow in the side of the pelvis – the acetabulum – formerly occupied by the head of the thigh bone (femur). The segment bearing the ball head is forced down, and glued into, the hollow shaft of the femur.

pelvis

cup of prosthesis in acetabulum

ball of prosthesis

thigh bone (femur)

shaft of prosthesis

but problems of differences of elasticity between cement and bone still have to be resolved. Re-operation is often necessary in such cases.

TECHNOLOGICAL ADVANCES

Materials science plays a major part in the design of artificial hip and other joints. The early models, made of stainless steel and Teflon, eventually disintegrated and many had to be removed. High-molecular-weight polythene for the socket and titanium alloys for the shaft, and sometimes a separate ball made of an alloy of cobalt, chromium and molybdenum, are now preferred. Some have a ceramic head. Unfortunately, advances are slow because new ideas, however promising, cannot be tried out on patients unless the probability of success is very high. Some of the factors can be tested in machines which simulate many years of use in a short time, but others can only be investigated in the living subject.

Hiprex

A brand name for **hexamine**.

Hirschprung's disease

A congenital disorder in which the lower part of the large intestine has failed to develop normal nerve control of the bowel muscles. Instead of passing the contents through by the normal process of peristalsis, the affected portion of the bowel acts as if it were obstructed and the contents accumulate at a higher level, causing distension of the abdomen, pain and total constipation. These signs appear in the first weeks of life and X-ray shows the local distension. A tissue sample (biopsy) of the wall of the affected section of bowel shows absence of nerves.

The treatment for Hirschprung's disease is surgical. The affected segment is removed and the free ends are joined together to re-establish continuity.

hirsutism

See **hairiness, excessive**.

histamine

A powerful chemical substance manufactured in certain white blood and tissue cells called *mast cells* and stored in them. Histamine is released from the mast cells when antibodies attached to them come into contact with substances such as pollens. Free histamine acts on H-1 receptors on small blood vessels causing them to dilate and to become more permeable to protein. This causes the local effect we call an allergic reaction. Histamine also acts on the stomach H-2 receptors to promote the secretion of acid.

Histamine can be opposed by stabilizing the mast cells and preventing the release of histamine, as by the use of steroids or sodium chromoglycate; by using drugs, such as adrenaline, with antagonizing effects; or by preventing histamine from reaching its site of action, by the use of the H-1 receptor blockers (the great range of antihistamine drugs) or H-2 receptor antagonists such as rantidine (Zantac) or cimetidine (Tagamet).

histamine producer

See **mast cell**.

histiocytosis

See **Letterer-Siwe disease**.

Histoacryl

A brand name for **enbucrilate**.

histocompatibility antigens

Groups of proteins situated on the outer membrane of all the cells of the body which provide an identifying code unique for each individual person, except identical twins. These groups are genetically determined and are called antigens because they act to stimulate antibodies if placed in a foreign environment such as another person's body. It is the histocompatibility antigens which, unless prevented, cause rejection of grafted organs and tissues. They play a central part in immunology.

The histocompatibility antigens were first discovered on white blood cells (leukocytes) and are often called *human leukocyte associated antigens*, usually abbreviated to HLA antigens. HLA types can be classified and people fall into a finite number of HLA groups. Some of these groups are known to confer a special susceptibility to certain diseases. The HLA B27 group, for instance, is prone to ankylosing spondylitis and uveitis.

histology

The study of the microscopic structure of the body tissues. A knowledge of the normal histology is the indispensable basis for the practice of histopathology – the science of the identification of diseases. All pathologists specializing in histopathology have a detailed knowledge of histology, acquired through hundreds of hours of patient microscopic study of stained sections of all the different tissues of the body.

histopathologist

A doctor specializing in the microscopic study of disease processes in tissues and in the identification of diseases by this means.

histoplasmosis

A fungus infection of the lung caused by *Histoplasma capsulatum*. The effects are usually mild and self-limiting, but in people with immunodeficiency disorders a severe tuberculosis-like disease may develop, which is sometimes fatal. There are, however, fungicidal drugs which are effective in treatment.

Histoplasmosis is rare except in certain limited areas of the USA, such as the Ohio basin.

HIV

The human immunodeficiency virus and the cause of AIDS. HIV binds avidly to the CD4 cell surface receptors on helper T cells. Although its greatest affinity is for these cells it will also infect **macrophages**, including those of the connective tissue cells of the brain, the microglial cells, which also have CD4 receptors. HIV can be damaging to the brain.

HIV is an RNA **retrovirus** and uses the enzyme **reverse transcriptase** to convert its single strand RNA into double helix DNA, which is then incorporated into the DNA of the human cell, where it can remain latent for years. This contaminated DNA, produces more HIV RNA by using the cell's transcription mechanism, and the cell then releases large numbers of new HIVs which quickly infect other cells.

The virus was identified in 1983 by Dr Françoise Barré-Sinoussi (b. 1950) working at the Pasteur Institute in Paris. Two years later she proved that it was the cause of AIDS. She is now Head of the Retrovirus Biology Unit at the Institute and was awarded one of the French Republic's highest honours, the Chevalier de l'Ordre National de Mérite.

See also illustration on next page.

HIV drug trials

See **CAESAR**.

HIV infection avoidance

See **safe sex**.

HIV-protease inhibitor drugs

A range of drugs that interfere with the enzyme produced by the human immunodeficiency virus (HIV) that allows it to replicate itself in human cells. Recent guidelines for the early treatment of HIV infection recommend that all such patients should be given HIV-protease inhibitor drugs: Currently, these drugs are indinavir (Crixivan), nelfinavir (Viracept), ritonavir (Norvir) and saquinavir (Invirase). A further drug, amprenavir, is under investigation. These drugs, used in combination with other antiretroviral drugs, cause a sustained reduction in HIV replication and reduce morbidity and prolong life. Their side-effects include excess weight gain from fat deposition.

HIV target cells

See **helper T cell**.

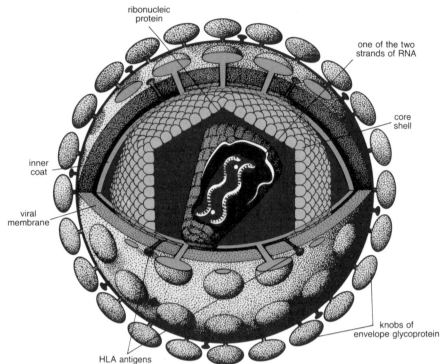

ribonucleic protein

one of the two strands of RNA

core shell

inner coat

viral membrane

knobs of envelope glycoprotein

HLA antigens

Diagrammatic representation of the human immunodeficiency virus (HIV). In spite of its complexity it is only one ten-millionth of a millimetre in diameter. The virus acts by attacking the T4 (helper) T lymphocytes, thus interfering with an essential link in the immune system and opening the way to all kinds of infections and disorders.

HLA antigens

See **histocompatibility antigens**.

HMG-CoA reductase inhibitors

Hydroxymethyl glutaryl co-enzyme A reductase inhibitors, also known as statins, are drugs that block the liver's production of cholesterol by competitive inhibition of the enzyme that catalyses the rate-limiting step of cholesterol synthesis. These drugs can lower the levels of low-density lipoproteins (LDLs) by 25–45 per cent and a number of major trials have shown their benefits in preventing heart attacks and other effects of **atherosclerosis**.

Up to 30 per cent of patients, however, have genetic variations that prevent them from responding to these drugs. The HMG Co-A reductase inhibitors include atorvastatin, cerivastatin, fluvastatin, pravastatin and simvastatin.

hoarseness

This is caused by thickening of the vocal cords, most commonly by simple inflammation (laryngitis). It may also be caused by the presence of nodules on the cords (singers' nodes), as in clergyman's throat, or by partial paralysis of the muscles which tighten the cords. The latter condition is often serious, as the commonest cause of such paralysis is damage to a nerve to the larynx, the *recurrent laryngeal nerve* in the neck, from cancer.

Hodgkin's lymphoma

A kind of cancer affecting lymphatic tissue, especially the lymph nodes. The condition usually begins in adolescence and early adult life, but can occur at any age. It affects the sexes equally.

POSSIBLE CAUSES
The cause is unknown but cancer-causing viruses are thought to be involved.

RECOGNITION AND SYMPTOMS
In Hodgkin's disease there is painless lymph-node enlargement all over the body, the nodes being rubbery, easily felt, and occasionally slightly tender to pressure. Later, the spleen and the liver enlarge, and this is part of the general involvement of lymph tissue throughout the body. Persistent but variable degrees of fever are common, as is anaemia. The pressure of the enlarging nodes on, and sometimes even the spread of the disease to, adjacent structures, causes many secondary effects, including neurological damage, obstruction to veins, difficulty in swallowing or breathing, and jaundice. Sometimes the bone marrow becomes involved, usually late in the disease. This is a serious complication.

TREATMENT
Until recent years Hodgkin's lymphoma was invariably fatal, but today early treatment with radiotherapy gives a 90 per cent chance of survival. Even in advanced disease, the outlook, in those treated skillfully with drugs such as cyclophosphamide, chlorambucil and vincristine, is good.

hole in the heart

See **heart disease, congenital**.

holistic medicine

A movement within medicine that arose as a reaction to the way the growing application of technology tends to exclude human factors and relationships. The proponents of holistic medicine rightly point out that a system which manages patients in a depersonalized way, treating them merely as machines to be modified by drugs, is neither optimum nor particularly effective.

They claim, with justice, that the doctor's function is not to treat a diseased organ but that he or she should always consider the patient as a whole person in his or her cultural and environmental context, with feelings, attitudes, fears and prejudices.

homatropine

A drug used in the form of eyedrops to widen the pupils for ophthalmic examination and temporarily to paralyse the muscles of the iris to assist in the treatment of iris inflammation (anterior uveitis). A brand name is Minims Homatropine.

homeobox genes

A family of genes that determine body shape. Homeobox genes are found in a large range of different species, including insects, and are expressed early in embryonic development. They function by dividing the early embryo into fields of cells, each of which has the potential to develop into a particular part, such as an arm, leg, tissue or organ. This is the key to the long-unexplained problem of how bodily configuration is determined by genetics. Mutations in homeobox genes cause basic, and correspondingly severe, defects in the body plan.

homeostasis

The maintenance of constant conditions in a biological system by automatic feedback mechanisms that counter trends away from the fixed limits of normality. This is a fundamental principle of modern biology and is recognized as essential to the continuation of health and life.

Self-regulating mechanisms operate at all levels of organization in the human body. These involve constant monitoring and correction of many variables, including the concentrations of a wide range of substances in the blood, the acidity (pH) of the blood, the levels of oxygen and carbon dioxide in the blood and tissues, the levels of many hormones, the body temperature, the heart rate and the blood pressure.

At the cellular level, a homeostatic mechanism called contact inhibition controls the rate of reproduction of cells in contact with each other so that cell populations do not grow larger than they should. This mechanism is lost in cancer.

Many hormones participate in the process of homeostasis. For example, an undue rise in the blood sugar is monitored by cells in the pancreas and extra insulin is secreted into the blood to increase the rate of utilization of sugar. Trends towards alteration of many bodily states lead to nerve inputs to the brain. These are reflected in changes in the output of hormones from the pituitary gland, whose actions on other endocrine glands correct the undesirable trends.

homoeopathy, or homeopathy

This system of medical practice was conceived by the German physician Christian Friedrich Hahnemann (1755–1843) and propounded in his Organon der Heilkunst of 1810. Hahnemann based his system of medicine solely on symptoms and regarded any investigation into their cause as a waste of time.

Hahnemann believed that in order to cure disease, a remedy must be given which would substitute an effect similar to the symptoms but weaker. To this end, he studied the effects of many drugs on healthy people, selecting those which produced appropriate effects. But since medicines which stimulate the symptoms of disease also aggravate them, they must, he reasoned, be used in the smallest possible doses.

Hahnemann then developed the extraordinary theory of 'potentiation' by dilution. Medicines, he insisted, gained in strength by being diluted, so long as the dilution was accompanied by vigorous shaking or pounding. On this principle, he diluted his original tinctures to one 50th; these, in turn, to one 50th; and so on for 30 consecutive dilutions. This, the 30th consecutive dilution by 50, was his favourite, to which he ascribed the highest 'potentiality'. Hahnemann's enthusiasms were matched neither by his common sense nor his knowledge of arithmetic. If a solution is diluted as he prescribed, it is impossible that it should contain even a single molecule of the original substance.

It is remarkable that the practice of homoeopathy should have persisted to this day. Notwithstanding that its principles run counter to everything science stands for, homoeopathy still enjoys a dubious respectability. In France, about a quarter of the doctors prescribe homoeopathic 'remedies'. The British public swallow millions of pounds worth of homoeopathy every year, to the satisfaction of the private pharmaceutical industry. There is a homoeopathic hospital in London, and the NHS now offers homoeopathic treatment.

homologous chromosomes

The 44 chromosomes that occur in 22 pairs and have the same set of gene positions (genetic loci), one derived from the mother and one from the father. The sex chromosomes, X and Y, are not homologous.

homologous genes

Genes from organisms of different species that code for precisely the same enzyme or other product. Homologous genes need not have exactly the same base sequences because there is some redundancy in the genetic code and a number of base triplets (**codons**) may code for the same **amino acid**.

homosexuality

A sexual preference for a person of the same anatomical sex. The term is derived from the Greek root *homos*, meaning 'same', not from the Latin *homo*, meaning 'man' or 'person'.

There is good reason to believe that the sexual preference of every person lies somewhere on a spectrum between exclusively heterosexual and exclusively homosexual. But this is too elaborate for day-to-day expression and most of us think in, and use, categorical terms. Many people experience some homosexual interest or engage in homosexual activity at some point in their lives and homosexual behaviour has been observed in most animal species.

A distinction must be made between homosexual preference and homosexual behaviour. The latter is common in conditions where heterosexual contacts are limited or absent, such as prisons, boarding schools, convents and so on, but such behaviour is often merely a substitute for heterosexual activity and is accompanied by heterosexual fantasies. There is no particular reason to believe that homosexuality is caused in this way. The experts do not believe that homosexual preferences are caused by experience, but it is clear that a pre-existing homosexual identity can be, and often is, reinforced and established by homosexual experience.

INCIDENCE

It is very difficult to arrive at reliable figures for homosexuality. Postal surveys have consistently suggested a figure of about 10 per cent for male homosexual preference, but it is likely that this figure reflects the greater willingness of homosexual men, than of others, to respond to the questionnaire. Interview methods put the figure at between 1 and 6 per cent for homosexual preference for men and up to 2 per cent for women. Many researchers believe that the frequency of exclusive homosexual preference is about 1 per cent for both sexes and that the same figure applies to bisexual preference.

POSSIBLE CAUSES

The causation of homosexuality remains obscure. Many theories have been advanced and none proven. Much work has been done on suggested hormonal differences between homosexual and heterosexual people, based on the observation in animals that adult sexual preference could be determined by doses of male or female sex hormones given at critical periods of fetal development. It has also been claimed that homosexual males produce a female type of hormonal response when given oestrogens. This work has been criticized and some studies failed to reproduce the claimed result.

It has been widely suggested that boys brought up in the absence of a father or other male figure are more prone to homosexuality, but this was refuted by a large American study.

The suggestion that there was a genetic basis for homosexuality was strongly supported in mid-1993 when an American team of researchers at the National Cancer Institute, Washington, DC, published a paper in *Science*. The research concerned a study of the families of 114 homosexual men which found that their close relatives were far more likely to be homosexual than expected from population statistics. There were also far more homosexual people on the maternal than on the paternal side. This prompted the view that homosexuality might be connected with the X chromosome. (Women are XX; men XY.) DNA was then taken from forty pairs of homosexual brothers and the X chromosome studied. Thirty-three of these forty pairs were found to have genetic markers in the same region of the chromosome. This region is called Xq28 and it is long enough to contain several hundred genes.

These findings are extremely unlikely to have arisen by chance or coincidence, and suggest that 65 per cent of the families studied were transmitting a gene that predisposes to homosexuality. The researchers believe that within a few years it will be possible to isolate the gene.

homozygous

Having identical gene pairs (**alleles**) at corresponding positions (loci) on the chromosome pairs. People who are homozygous for a quality or condition will always manifest it.

Honvan

A brand name for **fosfestrol**.

hookworm infestation

Infestation with one or both of the parasitic roundworms (nematodes) *Ancylostoma duodenale* and *Necator americanus*.

Worm eggs are deposited in the soil in excreta and hatch to release larvae which are able to penetrate the skin of the feet, causing the condition of 'ground itch'. They migrate inwards and enter small blood vessels and are then carried to the lungs in the bloodstream. In the lungs they are trapped in the small capillaries there, causing a form of lung inflammation (pneumonitis) and sometimes blood in the sputum (haemoptysis). They then break through into the air sacs, migrate up the air passages (bronchial tubes) and windpipe (trachea) to the mouth, and are swallowed. In this way the larvae reach the intestine, where they grow to adult worms in about five weeks.

INCIDENCE

These occur world-wide but present a major problem only in areas where much of the population go bare-foot. The condition is also known as ancylostomiasis.

RECOGNITION AND SYMPTOMS

The worms hook themselves into the bowel wall and derive their nourishment from blood and mucus, often causing severe anaemia, debility, abdominal pain and diarrhoea in the process. Individual worms can live for as long as ten years and the pregnant females may release several million eggs a day into the stools.

TREATMENT

Proper sanitation and hygiene, or even just the wearing of shoes, soon eliminate the threat. For those infested, effective drug treatment is available, but this is of limited value in a situation where re-infestation is inevitable.

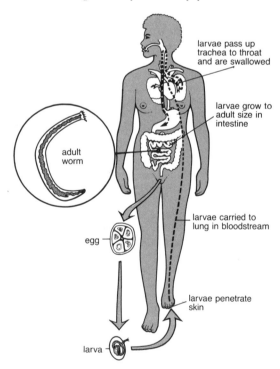

Hookworm larvae deposited on the ground can penetrate the skin and gain access to small blood vessels. They migrate via the lungs and the trachea to the intestine, where they mature, copulate and produce eggs that pass out with the faeces.

hormonal steroids

See **sex hormones**.

hormone replacement therapy

During the fertile period from the menarche (start of the periods) to the menopause (cessation of the periods), women secrete large quantities of oestrogens into their bloodstreams. These are feminizing, anabolic and, among other things, help to keep the bones strong. After the menopause, oestrogen levels drop. Males of the same age range continue to secrete sex hormones and to enjoy their anabolic effect. So women are at a disadvantage in this respect and are liable to develop osteoporosis, especially if small-boned.

WHY IT'S USED

Although it is not certain that the symptoms that commonly accompany the menopause are caused by it – hot flushes, depression, irritability, sweating, insomnia and so on – it is widely accepted that the prescription of female sex hormones (synthetic oestrogens) help to alleviate these symptoms, and few doctors would deny women the advantages of such therapy, in the short term. Similarly, vaginal dryness, and the vaginal changes that alter the bacteria present and encourage urinary infection, are readily corrected by oestrogen vaginal creams, and these are widely prescribed.

There is, however, still some controversy about the longer-term use of hormone replacement therapy to reduce osteoporosis. This is often a serious matter, causing severe bowing of the spine or leading to fracture of the hip bone on minor physical stress. Some women lose bone strength rapidly and these are especially at risk of the worst effects, while others seem to lose bone mass only at about the normal rate associated with ageing in both sexes. Osteoporosis causes hip fractures in about 26 per cent of elderly women and many of these die as a result. Women who have an early menopause are especially at risk, and hormone replacement therapy can largely eliminate the additional risk women suffer after the menopause. It is established that the chances of bone fracture can be halved by long-term hormone replacement therapy.

RISKS

The risks must, however, be understood. Oestrogens alone have been clearly shown to cause an increased risk of cancer of the breast and of the womb. Although many studies have been done, it is difficult to obtain consistent figures for the increase in the risk. Of nearly 2000 women in Kentucky who were given oestrogens after the menopause, and followed up for an average of twelve years, forty-nine developed breast cancer. The expected figure, for the general population, was thirty-nine, so ten extra cases in two thousand were, apparently, caused by the treatment. The study that showed the worst effects indicated an increase to 1.6 women with breast cancer for every one woman not on HRT. All the studies have, however, shown that the *mortality* from breast cancer is significantly reduced in women on HRT with greatly increased survival.

INCREASED SURVIVAL

One of the reasons for increased survival of women on HRT has to do with quite a different matter. Men have a much higher risk of serious, artery-blockage, heart disease than pre-menopausal women – heart attack (coronary thrombosis) is quite rare in pre-menopausal women, compared with men. This relative protection is apparently due to oestrogens and is lost after the menopause, when the incidence of atherosclerosis rises steeply in women. There seems little doubt that hormone replacement therapy allows this protective effect to continue, and this has been borne out in a number of studies.

Before the menopause, natural oestrogens are balanced by progesterone, and interest has been focused on the value of oestrogen replacement therapy combined with progesterone. The evidence suggests that this is safer, as one might expect from a regimen which closely resembles the natural state. The addition of progesterone to oestrogen HRT will, apparently, eliminate any additional risk of endometrial cancer. There is, however, the disadvantage of continuing menstruation.

Hormonin

A brand name for **oestradiol**.

horn, cutaneous

A rare condition seen in old people. It is a local overgrowth of the horny layer of the skin, forming a cylindrical protrusion which may reach 2 cm in length and about 1 cm in diameter. The cutaneous horn is easily removed, but this should be done by an expert, as the base may be cancerous.

Horner's syndrome

In the autonomic nervous system, nerve connections from the hypothalamus run down the brain stem and spinal cord to the level of the upper chest and then emerge in the spinal nerves. Some of these connections then run back up into the head in nerve plexuses in the walls of the large blood vessels and go to the eyes and elsewhere. If any part of this chain is damaged, the eye on the affected side shows characteristic signs. The upper lid droops, the globe sinks in a little, and the pupil becomes obviously smaller than the other. In addition, there will be absence of sweating on that side of the face.

This complex of signs is called Horner's syndrome, and it is an important indication that something serious is going on in the region through which these nerve fibres pass – possibly a cancer in the upper tip of a lung, or a tumour, or other disease, in the neck or spine.

hosiery, supportive

See **varicose veins**.

hospice

The archetype of the hospice movement is St Christopher's Hospice in London, founded in 1967 by Dame Cicely Saunders. This has been copied throughout the world and, in these havens of compassion and expert care, the terminally ill are provided with the physical, emotional and psychological support needed to help them to contemplate, and accept, the reality of death with dignity and in peace of mind.

A SPECIAL CALLING

The care of the dying is now a skilled specialty calling not only for high expertise, but for very special qualities of mind and personality. In hospices, teams of health-care professionals, which include doctors, nurses, psychologists, psychiatrists, ministers of religion, social workers and volunteer lay men and women, work together to help and counsel the dying and their families.

These workers are skilled in the management of the constant pain which often affects the terminally ill, and this involves as much emphasis on the reduction of fear and the other psychological components of pain, as on the pharmacological dulling of sensation. In many cases, the dosage of narcotics can, in this way, be cut so that the mind of the dying person remains clear and placid.

Emotional and psychological control, based on empathy, fosters an acceptance of the situation both by patients and relatives. After the death of a patient, bereavement counselling is given to the family. Dr Saunders has devoted her life to the fostering and development of this specialty and is known, and revered for it everywhere.

In many areas, hospice treatment is available in the dying person's own home, which is universally regarded as the best place to die. Unfortunately, for many obvious medical care reasons, this is not always feasible and in patient hospices have to be used.

hot flushes

See **menopause**.

house fly

See **flies**.

housemaid's knee

See **clergyman's knee**.

HTLV-III

The now out-dated term for the AIDS virus. HTLV-III was an abbreviation of *human T cell lymphotropic virus, type III*. The organism is now known as HIV (human immunodeficiency virus).

Hughes' syndrome

An autoimmune disorder caused by an antibody to phospholipid, which is a major constituent of cell membranes. It features recurrent clotting within the blood vessels (thromboses) causing an increased risk of strokes, heart attacks and other arterial obstruction effects. In women the condition is liable to cause recurrent spontaneous abortions during pregnancy. The syndrome is commonly secondary to systemic **lupus erythematosus** or a lupus-like disease, and commonly features an abnormally low level of blood **platelets** (thrombocytopenia).

Antiphospholipid antibodies are believed to accelerate **atherosclerosis** by interacting with low-density **lipoproteins** (LDLs). They can also occur as drug reactions or in certain infectious diseases. Also known as the antiphospholipid syndrome.

Humalog

A brand name for **insulin lispro**.

Human Actrapid

A brand name for **insulin**.

human cloning

The production of a person genetically identical to another person by the insertion of the DNA from any body cell or from an early embryo into an ovum from which the DNA has been removed. Such a clone would be the same as an identi-

cal twin of the original except for the difference in age. Human cloning is currently almost universally prohibited.

human genome

See **genome, human, mapping**.

human immunodeficiency virus

See **HIV**.

Human Insulatard

A brand name for **insulin**.

humanistic psychology

As a reaction to some of the worst absurdities of psychotherapy and the perceived acerbities of behaviourism, humanistic psychology seeks to view the individual as a person responsible for, and in control of, his or her destiny and to emphasize experience as the source of knowledge. The advocate of humanistic psychology suggests that we should try to gain insight into the inner life of another person from that person's own point of view.

In practical humanistic psychology, this is achieved by *human relations groups*, designed to help people to develop personal effectiveness and inter-personal skills, to enhance awareness of self and others and the resulting interactions, to avoid prejudice and dominance, to foster sensitivity to the emotions and desires of others, and to study the relationship of thought to word.

Human relations groups are popular and take many forms including theatrical groups, interpretive dance groups, empathy groups and self-expression, meditation, massage and transactional analysis groups. Following the success of behaviourist therapies, humanistic psychologists are beginning to incorporate behavioural methods into their therapy.

Human Mixtard

A brand name for **insulin**.

Human Monotard

A brand name for **insulin**.

human reproduction

Most biological reproduction, including that occurring constantly in our bodies, is asexual and produces clones. Single cells reproduce by duplicating their chromosomes and then elongating and splitting into two individual cells identical to the parent. This is how the countless millions of cells of our skin, intestine, blood and other tissues reproduce. This form of reproduction in which there is no change in the genetic material is called asexual reproduction. It has recently been discovered that a form of sexual reproduction occurs in many simple single-celled organisms, such as bacteria, in which exchange in genetic material occurs. This can affect their characteristics. The full implications of this have not yet been worked out and such organisms are still thought of as reproducing asexually.

Sexual reproduction traditionally refers to the production of new complex individuals, consisting of millions of cells, from specialized body cells called gametes. These, the ovum from the female and the spermatozoon from the male, contain half the full number of chromosomes. When the gametes fuse, the full complement of chromosomes is made up and fertilization is said to have occurred. A fertilized ovum starts to divide, rapidly and repeatedly, but, after the second division, the reproduced cells never separate, but stick together and continue to duplicate and specialize until a mature new individual is formed. After the first division, however, the reproduced cells may separate to form two identical twins. Sexual reproduction has the advantage that the genetic characteristics of two different individuals are combined in different ways.

EARLY HUMAN DEVELOPMENT

All the tissues of the body are derived from the single fertilized ovum and all the information necessary for planning the body is contained in the genetic code on the set of chromosomes present in each cell. Every time a cell divides and reproduces this set is copied precisely (see cell reproduction).

Following the enormous number of different instructions of the genetic code, cells differentiate to form tissues of different types and these form into organs. Although each cell carries the whole blueprint for the body, different cells use only the part of the code relevant to themselves. Genes are 'switched on' as required. The study of the development of the body, from fertilized ovum to newborn baby, is called embryology.

Development covers the period from fertilization to the stage of the sexually mature adult and involves the growth of a range of specialized tissues and organs from the single fertilized cell. Growth simply implies repeated reproduction of cells by division into two. Differentiation is the process by which cells, derived from the ovum, change their characteristics and acquire special kinds of structure and function. Muscle cells acquire the ability to contract, gland cells to secrete, nerve cells to conduct electrical impulses, and so on. The development of different cell types into organs, and their incorporation in a body structure, is called morphogenesis.

During the first few divisions, the daughter cells of the fertilized egg are smaller than the parent cell and these become packed together into a solid sphere called a morula. The cells of the morula continue to divide until it has formed into a hollow sphere, consisting of a single layer of cells, called a blastula. To begin with, every cell in the blastula has the potential of becoming any part of the future mature individual. Such cells are called totipotential. But soon, the cells at one end form a thickened layer, the innermost cells of which develop into the embryo. The other cells form a structure called the trophoblast, by which the embryo is implanted in the wall of the uterus. Particular genes, called homeobox genes divide up cells into groups which will later form a particular part of the body, such as an arm or a leg.

Once fully implanted, about two weeks after fertilization, the trophoblast produces the placenta and the yolk sac, on which the growing embryo initially feeds. Soon, the blastula begins to develop a head and a tail end and differentiates into three primary germ layers, each of which eventually develops into specific adult tissues. The outer of these germ layers is the ectoderm, the middle layer is the mesoderm, and the inner layer is the endoderm.

At this stage the developing embryo, now called a gastrula, forms a longitudinal groove into which cells from the ectoderm sink to form a sunken tube in the mesoderm. Cell migration allows distant cells to move to the correct location, to come in contact with other cells and adhere, and cells begin to communicate with each other, chemically and electrically.

The ectodermal cells which have moved inward and formed a tube develop into the spine, the central nervous system and the eyes. The ectoderm still on the surface forms the skin, the nails, the hair and the breasts. Mesodermal cells form the skeleton, muscles, heart and circulation, the kidneys and the sex organs. The endoderm forms the gut, or digestive tube, and the glands, like the salivary glands and the pancreas, which provide the intestine with digestive juice, develop as buds off the gut.

At an early stage, the cell mass forming the embryo becomes suspended within the blastocyst by a column of cells that develops into a stalk connecting it to the region of the placenta. This stalk becomes the umbilical cord (see below) and encloses the remainder of the yolk sac. Blood vessels develop within this stalk to connect the circulatory system of the embryo to the placenta and thus to the circulation of the mother.

The human organism at the stage of development between the time of implantation into the wall of the womb and the end of the seventh or eighth week of life is called an embryo. Thereafter, the developing individual is called a fetus. During the embryonic stage, growth is rapid, the main organ systems become differentiated and the external features of the body become recognizable.

The fetus has all the recognizable external characteristics of a human male or female. At ten weeks, it measures about 2.5 cm from the crown of the head to the rump. At this stage the face is formed but the eyelids are fused together. The brain is in a very primitive state. By three months, the fetus is about 5 cm long (crown to rump) and by four months it is about 10 cm long. In the sixth month, the fetus is up to 20 cm long and weighs up to 800 grams. Survival of a fetus born at this stage is unlikely. The chances of survival increase rapidly with increasing maturity and most fetuses over 1000 grams (1 kg) now do well, if properly managed in an incubator.

During pregnancy, the womb (uterus) grows with the fetus and eventually rises to a height equal to that of the abdominal cavity. The fetus is surrounded by a fluid-filled double membrane, the inner layer of which is called the amnion. The membrane normally ruptures and releases the amniotic fluid ('breaking of the waters') before the baby is born. During pregnancy, the fetus floats freely in the amniotic fluid, the volume of which, at full term, is usually about one litre. This fluid is protective and is constantly swallowed and then excreted as urine by the fetus, so it contains material from which much information about the health of the fetus can be obtained.

The placenta, at term, is a thick, disc-shaped object about 15 to 20 cm in diameter. The mother's blood enters the placenta from the uterine side and the umbilical cord comes off from the free surface. In the placenta, the maternal blood comes into close contact with, but does not mix with, the fetal blood, which is being pumped through the placenta by the fetal heart. Oxygen, carbon dioxide, sugars, amino acids, fats, vitamins, minerals, as well as many drugs, pass freely across the placental barrier. It is in this way that the fetus is provided with all necessary supplies for maintenance as well as for body growth, and is able to get rid of waste substances.

See also **menstruation** and **ovulation**.

human tissue, artificial production of

See **tissue culture**.

Human Ultratard

A brand name for **insulin**.

Human Velosulin

A brand name for **insulin**.

Humatrope

A brand name for **somatotropin**.

humerus

Latin root meaning 'shoulder' as in humerus (upper arm bone).

humours

A primitive medical theory, originating in the dawn of history, recorded in the writings attributed to Hippocrates, and officially promoted by the self-opinionated but authoritative medical writer Galen around the year AD 200. The idea became unalterable dogma, actively discouraged objective investigation and research, and held back the progress of medicine for about 1500 years. The four humours, which were said to determine a person's character, were blood, having a sanguine, or cheerful, effect; phlegm (mucus), producing a phlegmatic, or calm effect; yellow bile (choler) which produced anger; and black bile (melancholia), leading to depression. Health represented a proper balance between the four, and disease an undue preponderance of one or the other.

On the foundation of this principle, Galen developed an elaborate and arbitrary system also involving the four elements: hot, cold, wet and dry. Every known medical fact or belief was explained by this comprehensive system and no problem was without a solution. It was not until the seventeenth or eighteenth centuries that these ideas were gradually replaced by the scientific empiricism of modern medicine.

Humulin I

A brand name for human **insulin** produced by recombinant **DNA** technology.

Humulin Lente

A brand name for **insulin** produced by recombinant **DNA** technology.

Humulin M

A brand name for **insulin** produced by recombinant **DNA** technology.

Humulin S

A brand name for **insulin** produced by recombinant **DNA** technology.

Humulin Zn

A brand name for **insulin** produced by recombinant **DNA** technology.

hunchback

Angulation or extreme curvature of the spine. This may be caused by:

- a congenital disorder of the spine;
- postural defect causing curvature of the spine (kyphosis);
- angulation of the spine from an injury causing a crush fracture of a vertebra;
- spontaneous collapse of a vertebra from disease such as tuberculosis (*Potts disease*);
- severe worsening of a natural kyphosis by osteoporosis.

Huntington's chorea

A rare, dominant, hereditary brain disorder caused by a defective gene on chromosome four. It features involuntary twitching movements of the face and body (chorea), alternating periods of excitement and depression, and progressive dementia. The condition usually starts in the thirties and may progress for ten to twenty years until the patient dies. There is progressive loss of nerve cells in certain nuclei of the brain and a build-up of the neurotransmitter dopamine, which causes the chorea.

Drugs can help to suppress the movements in the early stages but there is no remedy for the intellectual deterioration. Institutional care is usually necessary.

Hurler's syndrome

Once known as *gargoylism*, this is one of the group of inherited disorders called the *mucopolysaccharidoses*. Hurler's syndrome is due to the absence of the enzyme alpha-iduronidase and features dwarfism, widespread skeletal deformity, mental retardation, heart abnormalities, opacities of the cornea and early death.

Hyalase

A brand name for **hyaluronidase**.

hyaluronidase

An enzyme that breaks down proteins holding tissue planes together. Its use assists in the dispersal of tissue fluids or injected drugs. A brand name is Hyalase.

hybernating myocardium

The myocardium is the muscle of which the heart is mainly composed. Hybernating myocardium are areas of the heart muscle that show failure of contraction (asynergy) as a result of blood deprivation from coronary artery disease, but that are capable of returning to function if an adequate blood supply is restored, as by bypass grafting. All such areas were formerly thought to have died and to have suffered irreversible change.

Hycamtin

A brand name for **topotecan**.

hydatid disease

Tapeworm can affect people in two different ways. The worm can be acquired by eating undercooked meat containing the larval stage, which hatches to release the young worm. This then attaches itself to the inside of the bowel and remains there for months or years, gradually growing longer and releasing eggs in the stools. This is the less serious form of tapeworm infestation, and is relatively easily managed by the use of anthelmintic drugs to drive out the worm.

If, on the other hand, a person, by handling dogs or pigs, or drinking contaminated water, succeeds in ingesting tapeworm *eggs*, the worm life cycle, normally occurring in the dog or pig, occurs in that person. The embryos released by the eggs get into the bloodstream from the intestines and are carried to the liver and other organs where they form slowly growing cysts. The infestation is usually acquired in childhood and the cysts take years to reach a dangerous size. They may occur in the lungs, the brain and elsewhere in the body and cause their effects by local pressure and interference with function. Brain cysts can cause epilepsy. This form of the infestation is called hydatid disease and it is difficult to treat. Large hydatid cysts may be removed surgically, with great care to avoid spillage.

The disease can be avoided if normal standards of personal hygiene are maintained and dogs regularly de-wormed.

hydatidiform mole

An abnormal pregnancy in which, instead of a fetus, the womb (uterus) is filled with a mass of grape-like cystic bodies varying in size from a pinhead to 2 cm in diameter. The name comes from its resemblance to the cysts in hydatid disease, but the condition has nothing to do with tapeworm infestation. The mole is formed from the part of the embryo which normally forms the placenta and the cysts are formed from degeneration of the finger-like processes (chorionic villi) which normally form early in the pregnancy.

INCIDENCE
Hydatidiform mole is uncommon, occurring once in about 2000 pregnancies.

POSSIBLE CAUSES
In many cases, all the chromosomal material comes from the father, suggesting that the ovum fertilized was in some way defective, possibly with a missing nucleus. Some moles contain fetus-like structures and have chromosomal patterns suggesting fertilization with two sperms or with a sperm containing the full number, instead of half the number, of chromosomes, as is normal.

> Early removal is important as about one mole in forty turns to a particularly virulent and rapidly spreading form of cancer, called choriocarcinoma, formerly invariably fatal. Modern methods of cancer chemotherapy have, however, transformed the outlook in these cases and death from choriocarcinoma is now rare.

RECOGNITION AND SYMPTOMS
There is usually bleeding before the sixteenth week of the pregnancy and the woman is often ill. The womb may be larger than the dates suggest and there is often abdominal pain. Ultrasound examination shows a 'snow-storm' appearance and no sign of a fetus.

hydralazine

A drug that causes arteries to widen (vasodilatation) and can be used as an adjunct to the treatment of high blood pressure and moderate degrees of heart failure. It is seldom used alone. A brand name is Apresoline.

Hydrea

A brand name for **hydroxyurea**.

hydrocele

An abnormal collection of fluid within the tissue capsule surrounding the testicle, resulting in a painless enlargement of the scrotum. The condition is common, especially in older men, and is usually innocent, but may occur as a response to cancer of the testicle. If the testicle cannot be felt because of the quantity of fluid, some of this should be drawn off through a needle, so that examination becomes possible. The fluid is usually straw-coloured, but if it is blood-stained, cancer may be suspected.

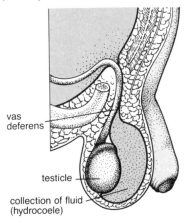

vas deferens

testicle

collection of fluid (hydrocoele)

Hydrocele. Literally a 'water hollow', a hydrocele is an abnormal collection of fluid surrounding the testicle.

> Any doubt as to the normality of the testicle justifies immediate surgical exploration to exclude cancer.

hydrocephalus

An abnormal accumulation of the normal cerebrospinal fluid within, and around, the brain. The common term is 'water on the brain'. Hydrocephalus results when the rate of production of the fluid exceeds the rate at which it can be reabsorbed, usually because of obstruction to the circulation of the fluid to its normal site of reabsorption, by a congenital abnormality or later acquired disease.

In babies or young children the pressure from accumulated fluid expands the skull, sometimes greatly, and if the cause cannot be removed it is necessary to shunt, or by-pass, the normal channels by means of a tube passed into one of the spaces in the brain (ventricle) and carried down under the skin of the neck to be inserted, by way of a jugular vein, into the heart. Alternatively, the shunt tube can be carried right down to open into the abdominal (peritoneal) cavity. In both cases, the tube contains a one-way valve so that fluid can pass out of the brain but not back in. Unfortunately, blockage of the tube is common and replacements may be required.

Unrelieved hydrocephalus causes compression of the brain, especially after the skull bones have fused together, and this leads to headache, vomiting, and damage to the cranial nerve function, including visual disturbance.

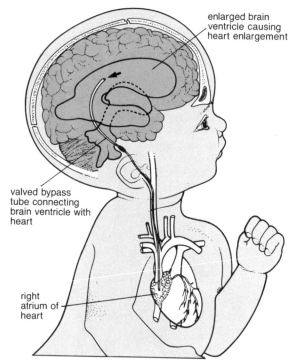

enlarged brain ventricle causing heart enlargement

valved bypass tube connecting brain ventricle with heart

right atrium of heart

'Water on the brain', or hydrocephalus, is due to the failure of reabsorption of cerebrospinal fluid. The illustration shows how compression damage to the brain can be prevented by the use of a bypass tube connecting the fluid-filled brain cavity with the heart.

hydrochlorothiazide

A drug used to increase the output of urine so as to relieve the body of surplus water. A thiazide **diuretic** drug. A brand name is Hydrosaluric. Hydrochlorothiazide is formulated in conjunction with a variety of drugs. It is available with potassium under the brand name Amil-Co; with another diuretic as Dyazide, Moduret 25, Moduretic, Triam-Co; with **angiotensin converting enzyme** (ACE) **inhibitor** drugs as Accuretic, Acezide, Capozide, Carace Plus, Innozide and Zestoretic 20; with **beta blocker** drugs as Co-Betaloc, Kalten, Moducren and Monozide 10; and with an angiotensin II antagonist drug as Cozaar-Comp.

hydrocortisone

A natural steroid hormone derived from the outer layer (cortex) of the adrenal gland. The drug **cortisone** is converted into hydrocortisone in the liver. Hydrocortisone has anti-inflammatory and sodium-retaining properties. It is widely used as a mild corticosteroid drug mainly for external use for skin disorders. Brand names are Colifoam, Dioderm, Efcortelan, Efcortesol, Hydrocortistab, Hydrocortone, Midison Lipocream. The drug is also formulated, for external use, with a variety of other drugs

such as allantoin, antibiotics, azole antifungal drugs, coal tar extracts, crotamiton (anti-itch drug), hydrating agents, local anaesthetics, zinc oxide, etc. At least 40 preparations containing hydrocortisone are available on the UK drug market.

Hydrocortistab

A brand name for **hydrocortisone**.

Hydrocortisyl

A brand name for **hydrocortisone**.

Hydrocortone

A brand name for **hydrocortisone**.

hydroflumethiazide

A thiazide diuretic drug. A brand name is Hydrenox. It is also formulated with another diuretic drug under the brand name Aldactide.

hydrogen peroxide

A powerful oxidizing and antibacterial agent. It is formulated as a cream for external use on skin infections, ulcers and pressure sores. Brand names are Crystacide and Hioxyl.

hydromorphone

A powerful narcotic painkiller drug used to relieve severe cancer pain. A brand name is Palladone.

hydronephrosis

Distension of the urine-collecting system of the kidney, and secondary changes in the kidney, due to an obstruction to the free outflow of urine down the urine tube (ureter) to the bladder. The obstruction may be at any level, but is most commonly at the point at which the wide collecting system (the pelvis) of the kidney joins the narrow ureter. Obstruction at the outlet of the bladder will cause hydronephrosis of both kidneys, because, in this case, the back pressure is applied equally to both.

POSSIBLE CAUSES

Obstruction may be from urinary stone, tumour, blood clot, inflammatory narrowing or external pressure from any cause, including an abnormally placed artery to the kidney. One of the commonest causes is enlargement of the prostate gland. Hydronephrosis can even be caused by a very tight foreskin (phimosis).

RECOGNITION AND SYMPTOMS

There is pain in the loin, sometimes made worse by drinking, and secondary infection is common, causing fever, painful urination and often blood in the urine. Occasionally the condition is silent until late symptoms arise. Hydronephrosis is damaging to the kidney and may lead to kidney failure, even absence of urination (anuria).

TREATMENT

Treatment involves the identification and removal of the cause of the obstruction, but, as an emergency measure, temporary drainage of the affected kidney through a fine tube (catheter) may save it. If one kidney only is affected and is severely damaged, it will usually be removed to prevent other serious complications.

hydrophobia

See **rabies**.

Hydrosaluric

A brand name for **hydrochlorothiazide**.

hydrotalcite

An antacid drug used to treat flatulence and dyspepsia. Brand names are Altacite and, with dimethicone, Altacite Plus.

hydroxocobalamin

Vitamin B12. This is the specific treatment for **pernicious anaemia** and is highly effective unless neurological damage has already occurred. Brand names are Cobalin-H and Neo-Cytamen.

hydroxyapatite

A calcium and phosphorus supplement used to treat **osteoporosis**, **rickets**, osteomalacia and to maintain body minerals during breast feeding. A brand name is Ossopan.

hydroxychloroquine

A drug used to reduce the activity of **rheumatoid arthritis**. A brand name is Plaquenil.

hydroxymethyl glutaryl coenzyme A reductase inhibitors

Also known as statins, these are drugs that block the liver's production of cholesterol by competitive inhibition of the enzyme that catalyses a stage in cholesterol synthesis. Statins can lower the levels of low-density **lipoproteins** (LDLs) by 25–45 per cent and a number of major trials have shown their benefits in preventing heart attacks and other effects of **atherosclerosis**. Up to 30 per cent of patients, however, have genetic variations that prevent them from responding to these drugs. The HMG Co-A reductase inhibitors include atorvastatin, cerivastatin, fluvastatin, pravastatin and simvastatin.

hydroxyprogesterone hexanoate

A **progestogen** drug used by depot injection during early pregnancy to prevent spontaneous abortion. A brand name is Proluton.

hydroxyurea

A **cytotoxic** drug used in the chemotherapy of cancer. The drug is also capable of effecting a substantial reduction in the frequency and severity of crises in **sickle-cell anaemia**. A brand name is Hydrea.

hydroxyzine

An antihistamine drug used as a sedative for anxiety and to control itching. Brand names are Atarax and Ucerax.

hygieia

Greek root meaning 'health' as in hygiene (science of health).

hygiene

The study of preventive medicine and the promotion of healthy modes of living, especially by maintaining high standards of personal cleanliness so as to avoid infection. Good hygiene can only be based on a general knowledge of the causes of disease.

The term is derived from the name of one of the two daughters of Aesculapius, the Greek God of medicine. Hygieia provided a healthy environment and Panacea provided healing. On the principle that prevention is better than cure, Hygieia was inclined to take a superior attitude to her therapeutic sister, thus promoting the first of many acrimonious medical arguments.

Hygroton

A brand name for **chlorthalidone**.

hymen

Greek root meaning 'membrane' as in hymen (membrane at vaginal orifice). This is the thin, perforated membrane that stretches over the opening of the vagina in young girls and which usually ruptures spontaneously before puberty. Sometimes the hymen is unusually thick, or it may even completely close off the vaginal orifice (imperforate hymen), and may have to be cut surgically to allow menstrual fluid to escape. The first full act of sexual intercourse is sometimes associated with a tearing of the residual parts of the hymen and there may be a little bleeding – a circumstance once much approved of by men concerned about exclusive proprietorship.

hymen reconstruction

A surgical procedure often forced on women who are the victims of a male-dominated culture, which insists on proof of virginity at the time of marriage, such as the public display of a bloody bed sheet after sexual intercourse. The procedure has been criticized on various grounds, one of which is that it involves the collusion of a surgeon in a deceitful act.

hyoscine

Scopolamine. A drug structurally related to atropine and having similar properties. It is used to treat painful menstruation and bowel colic. A brand name is Buscopan.

hyper-

A very common medical prefix covering a range of senses all of which imply an excess over the normal. It may refer to growth of a body part, for instance, indicating an abnormal increase in size, as in hypertrophy (increase in cell size) or hyperplasia (increase in cell number). It may qualify over-production of the secretion of a gland, as in hyperhidrosis (excess sweating), or the effect of excessive glandular secretion, as in hyperthyroidism. It may refer to over-sensitivity of a sense organ, as in hyperacusis (abnormally acute hearing), or over-activity of a part or of the whole organism, as in hyperactivity. It can mean an abnormal range of movement, as in hyperextension of a joint, or an abnormally high pressure, as in hypertension (high blood pressure). It is commonly used to indicate an abnormally high level of a substance in the body or in the blood, as in hypercholesterolaemia (abnormally high level of cholesterol in the blood). In almost all these senses and usages the antonym **hypo-** can also be applied.

hyperactivity

Usually applied to children, the term refers to an excessively high level of restlessness and inattentiveness and a low threshold of frustration. An alternative term is the *hyperkinetic syndrome*.

RECOGNITION AND SYMPTOMS

'Hyperactive' children are unable to concentrate, throw tantrums, are aggressive, restless, fidgety and generally infuriating to adults. They are often intelligent, but their low attention span can result in poor academic performance.

POSSIBLE CAUSES

No one knows for certain what causes 'hyperactivity', and the view that it is always caused by food additives, such as the antioxidant preservatives butylated hydroxyanisole (BHA) and butylated hydroxytoluene (BHT), is almost certainly untrue. Diets designed to eliminate all such additives have been used experimentally with inconclusive results, although some children appear to have improved.

Much is known, however, of the pharmacological methods of controlling the disorder and, paradoxically, *stimulant* drugs, such as amphetamine, have been found very helpful in some cases. Monoamine oxidase inhibitor drugs have also been found useful. These methods are, of course, only a means to the end of ensuring that such children are not deprived of the vitally important elements of proper behaviour conditioning.

There is endless evidence that children who learn early to conform to reasonable patterns of social behaviour and who have a clear idea of the rules are not only happier, but are much more likely to become effective, productive and contented adults.

See also **attention deficit hyperactivity disorder (ADHD)**.

> Widespread doubt has been expressed among experts as to whether hyperactivity is a real medical or psychological condition, and most think of it as a variety of conduct disorder or temperament. Nevertheless, there is clear evidence that children who display these characteristics do not necessarily 'grow out of it' and that almost one-third of them may continue to show them in early adult life. There is also evidence that these children are much more prone than others to later conduct disorder, including drug abuse, lying, stealing and violence.

hyperbaric oxygen treatment

A method of treatment in which the patient is placed in an airtight chamber and exposed to oxygen at pressures up to three times that of the atmosphere. Because of the high pressure, considerable quantities of oxygen dissolve in the blood serum so the oxygen-carrying capacity of the blood is greatly enhanced and the tissues of the whole body receive an excellent supply, independently of the haemoglobin transport mechanism.

The number of conditions in which such treatment has been shown to be useful is still limited, but in decompression sickness (the 'bends'), severe respiratory and circulatory disorders, recent carbon monoxide and cyanide poisoning, gas gangrene and bone damage from radiation, hyperbaric oxygen has been found highly effective.

Unfortunately, excessive oxygen is toxic to the nervous system and pressures above two and a half atmospheres will

cause epileptic-type fits if continued too long. A limit of about three hours is therefore imposed.

hyperglycaemia

An excessively high level of glucose in the blood. Hyperglycaemia is a feature of untreated or inadequately treated diabetes mellitus, and is controlled by the use of carefully judged doses of insulin, or sometimes by oral hypoglycaemic drugs or diet.

hyperhidrosis

Excessive sweating due to overactivity of the sweat glands. This may occur all over the skin, or may be confined to certain areas, such as the palms of the hands, the armpits, the groins and the feet.

In severe cases, the skin may be affected by the constant moisture, becoming soggy and macerated. Hyperhidrosis is often associated with strong body odour, caused by the bacterial breakdown of the sweat and the surface cells of the skin. This is called *bromhidrosis*.

POSSIBLE CAUSES

The condition is usually just a variant of the normal, but may be caused by thyroid gland overactivity, fever and, rarely, a disease of the nervous system. In some cases, local hyperhidrosis is due to stress reactions or other psychological causes.

TREATMENT

It can be treated by local applications to reduce the activity of the sweat glands, or even, in extreme cases, by the surgical removal of the most active groups of glands. Many people just naturally sweat a lot, and these require higher than average standards of body and clothes washing. Emotional sweating usually resolves with time and maturity.

hyperkeratosis

Thickening of the outer layer of the skin so as to produce a horny layer. Hyperkeratosis is a normal response to local pressure and produces corns or callosities, which are essentially protective. The condition may, however, occur as an inherited disorder affecting the palms and the soles, or as a general disorder, called ichthyosis, affecting most or all of the body.

hyperlipidaemias

A group of disorders characterized by an increase in the levels of fats (triglycerides) or cholesterol in the blood. This highly undesirable state may be due to conditions such as diabetes, pancreatitis or obstruction of the bile system, and the condition usually responds to the treatment of these primary causes, when this is possible. In about 5 per cent of cases these conditions are of dominant heredity and are present from birth.

RECOGNITION AND SYMPTOMS

People affected in this way have prominent white rings round the edges of their corneas (arcus juvenilis) at an early stage in life – this is normal in older people (arcus senilis) – and often have yellow plaques in the skin around the eyes (xanthelasma). Most of them develop serious heart disease, from coronary artery damage, before the age of fifty.

TREATMENT

In all such cases, stringent dietary control and correction of obesity is essential if life is to be saved. Low-calorie diets with restricted fats are necessary and, in some cases, it is also necessary to give drugs which reduce blood fat levels.

Many perfectly normal people have undesirably high levels of fats and cholesterol in their bloodstreams, but this is simply due to excessive intake.

hypermetropia

The condition in which the eyes, when in a state of relaxed focus, are unable to see clearly either distant or near objects. The greatest difficulty is experienced in viewing near objects. The term 'farsightedness' has been a cause of confusion because, even on distant viewing, people with hypermetropia must exert a focusing effort (accommodation) to see clearly. This is easy for young people, whose hypermetropia is usually concealed by an automatic and unconscious effort of accommodation. But since the power of accommodation declines steadily with age, hypermetropia sooner or later becomes manifest and glasses are needed.

The more severe the hypermetropia, the lower the age at which the difficulty appears. Initially there are problems with close work but, later, the distance vision becomes blurred also.

In hypermetropia the eye is too short for the focal length of the combined cornea and internal lens. Or, considered in another way, the lens system is insufficiently strong to focus on the retina. Hypermetropic defects are corrected by ordinary convex lenses.

hypermetropia cure

See **excimer laser refractive surgery**.

hypernephroma

A malignant tumour of the kidney, misnamed because it was originally thought to arise from tissue of the 'hyper-renal' (adrenal) gland. Hypernephroma is a cancer (carcinoma) which may be present for some years before signs become obvious. Unfortunately, the first signs of trouble may be those caused by secondary tumour in the lungs, liver or bones. In other cases the tumour shows itself by blood in the urine, pain in the loin from blood clots passing down the ureter, or fever.

The only good chance of full recovery is by early surgical removal of the affected kidney.

hyperparathyroidism

Excessive output of hormone from the parathyroid glands – the four tiny glands which control the relationship between the levels of calcium in the blood and those in the bones. The increased output is probably due to a non-malignant tumour of the hormone-producing cells, but in a very small proportion of cases is due to cancer of the gland.

RECOGNITION AND SYMPTOMS

Parathyroid hormone causes calcium to leave the bones and concentrate in the blood. When the hormone is produced in excess amounts, the effect is twofold. The loss of calcium from the bones causes osteoporosis and the excess in the blood leads to an unusual deposition of calcium in the soft tissues of the body such as the joint cartilages and tendons and even, in extreme cases, in the muscle of the heart. In an attempt to get rid of excess blood calcium, the kidneys excrete much higher than normal levels in the urine and these concentrated calcium solutions are very apt to crystal-

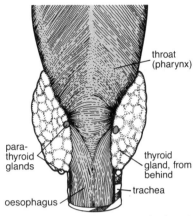

Hyperparathyroidism. This is due to overproduction of hormone from one of the four little glands lying within the substance of the thyroid gland in the neck.

lize out to form kidney stones. This occurs in about 30 per cent of cases.

TREATMENT

The treatment is to remove as much of the parathyroid tissue as is thought safe. It is common to remove three of the four glands and part of the fourth.

hyperplasia

An increase in the number of cells in a tissue or organ so that there is an increase in size. Hyperplasia is not a cancerous change and may be a normal response to increased demand. It is not the same as hypertrophy.

hyperpyrexia

An abnormally high, and dangerous, level of body temperature.

> Hyperpyrexia exists if the temperature rises above 41.1°C (106°F). At this level, urgent treatment is required to lower the temperature, if permanent brain damage is to be avoided.

hypersensitivity

A manifestation of allergy in which acute tissue reactions occur on the repeated exposure to any foreign substance to which a particular kind of antibody has been developed. 'Hay fever' is a hypersensitivity reaction.

hypertension

Abnormally high blood pressure. The circulation is a closed system in which the pressure varies constantly, rising to a peak, called the systolic pressure, soon after the contraction of the main pumping chambers of the heart (ventricles), and falling steadily to a lower level, called the diastolic pressure, which it reaches just before each heartbeat. Because of this dynamic situation, a person's blood pressure cannot be represented by a single figure, but is given as two numbers, the systolic first and then the diastolic, commonly thus: 120/80. These numbers indicate the pressure in terms of the distance in millimetres which a column of mercury would be forced up a glass tube by the pressure. This method is still widely used, in the shape of the sphygmomanometer, to measure blood pressure.

In addition to the variations within the cycle, blood pressure varies constantly with the level of physical exertion, with anxiety, stress, emotional changes, and other factors. So single measurements are not particularly meaningful and the blood pressure should be checked repeatedly under resting conditions, at different times.

Blood pressure depends on the force and volume of the heart output with each beat and on the resistance offered by the larger blood vessels. During each contraction of the heart, a quantity of blood is forced into the arterial system, but only about one-third of that volume simultaneously moves out into the capillaries. Momentarily, this extra volume has to be accommodated. If the main arteries are healthily elastic, they will give a little with each heartbeat and the systolic pressure will not be particularly high. The recoil of the arteries will then drive the remainder of the additional blood onwards. Well before the pressure has fallen to zero, another beat will occur.

RECOGNITION AND SYMPTOMS

If, however, the arteries are stiff and rigid, or abnormally narrowed, from disease, the pressure with each ventricular contraction will rise to a high peak. In addition, the diastolic pressure, just before each beat, will also be higher. Contrary to popular belief, raised blood pressure (hypertension) seldom causes symptoms until secondary complications develop in the arteries, kidneys, brain, eyes or elsewhere. Uncomplicated high blood pressure does not cause dizziness, headache, fatigue, nose bleeds or facial flushing. By the time symptoms occur, the affected person is in real trouble.

> No one can afford to ignore raised blood pressure because its complications cause more deaths and severe disability than any other group of diseases. Sustained high pressures are very damaging to the blood vessels, causing an acceleration of the ageing processes. In particular, they promote the killer arterial disease atherosclerosis, in which hardening of the arteries is associated with the deposition, in the inner lining, of plaques of cholesterol and other material. Coronary thrombosis and stroke – the two major killers of the Western world – are the major risks, but raised blood pressure can also severely damage the heart, kidneys and eyes. Hypertension has to be looked for and every adult should have regular checks. Fortunately, proper and effective treatment can largely eliminate the additional risk of these serious complications.

TREATMENT

The treatment of hypertension involves both a change in lifestyle and, if necessary, the prescription of drugs. In the case of moderately raised blood pressure in an overweight, under-exercised, middle-aged person, a change in lifestyle is the first requirement. Smoking is deadly and must be cut out – even the otherwise most effective drug treatment may fail to reduce the probability of death if smoking continues. A change in eating habits is also important. In many cases, the change to a healthy, natural lifestyle, with regular exercise, very little food, no smoking, and perhaps a reduction in salt intake, will be sufficient to get the blood pressure down to normal. Regular attendance at the doctor, for check-ups, will give confidence and help to reduce stress levels.

Three main classes of drugs are used to treat hypertension. The first, the diuretics, act on the kidneys to cause them to pass more water and salt in the urine and reduce the volume of the blood, so bringing down the pressure. The second group, the beta-blockers, interfere with the hormone and nervous control of the heart, slowing it and causing it to beat less forcefully, so reducing the pressure. The third group, the vasodilators, act on the arteries to widen them. This group contains drugs acting in quite different ways. They include the alpha-blockers, the calcium antagonists and the ACE inhibitors.

In some cases the doctor has difficult and complex decisions to make. Among others, he or she has to decide whether to use drugs at all. Because the patient's body may have adapted to raised blood pressure, reducing it may actually cause him, for a time, to feel worse, rather than better. Until readjustment to normal pressures has occurred, there may be weakness, lack of energy, depression and a tendency to dizziness or faintness on standing up. The doctor has to take these effects into account and make sure the patient does not use them as reasons for avoiding treatment. He will try to get the desired effect with the minimum possible prescription, and, in this, the patient's new lifestyle really matters. The doctor needs cooperation if he is going to be able to help the patient to live out a full life-span in safety.

hyperthermia

Exceptionally high body temperature.
See **hyperpyrexia**, **hyperthermia**, **malignant**.

hyperthermia, malignant

A rare inherited disorder due to a subtle muscle abnormality which is inapparent until the affected person is given a general anaesthetic drug such as halothane, cyclopropane or ethyl ether, or a muscle relaxant drug such as succinylcholine. The effect of these is to trigger a condition of intense muscle contraction and the production, from the muscles, of a considerable amount of heat – so much that the normal temperature-regulating mechanisms cannot cope and the body temperature rises to dangerous levels.

> Emergency treatment with ice, intravenous bicarbonate, to neutralize the rapid rise in lactic acid from the muscles, and specific drugs which reverse the abnormal muscle response, is needed to save life.

The condition runs in families but can rarely be detected before an operation. All skilled anaesthetists are thoroughly familiar with the condition.

hyperthyroidism

Overactivity of the thyroid gland.
See **thyrotoxicosis**.

hypertrichosis

See **hairiness, excessive**.

hypertrophy

An increase in the size of a tissue or organ caused by the enlargement of the individual cells rather than by an increase in the number. Hypertrophy is in no sense tumorous or malignant, but is usually a normal response to an increased demand. The increase in muscle bulk which results if increased physical work is performed is a hypertrophy.

Some conditions, such as certain types of muscle dystrophy, cause *pseudo-hypertrophy* in which the appearance of increased bulk is actually due to the deposition, in the tissue, of abnormal substances.

hyperventilation

Abnormally deep or rapid breathing, usually as a result of violent exercise. The term is often used to refer to a degree of deep breathing which is inappropriate to the physiological needs of the body and which, as a result, causes excessive loss of carbon dioxide from the blood and a consequent reduction in blood acidity. This, in turn, brings about various changes in the conductance of nerves so that certain muscle groups, such as those of the forearms and calves, may go into intense spasm causing the wrists to bend and the ankles to extend.

Hyperventilation is a common manifestation of neurotic illness, either as a panic reaction associated with a feeling of 'not getting enough air', or as a resource in those who feel that they are not getting enough attention. In this, the activity is usually highly successful, but is not without danger. If the affected person can be persuaded to re-breathe for a few minutes into a small paper bag, the blood changes will soon be reversed and the more dramatic elements abolished.

Hyperventilation can, rarely, occur as an effect of organic disease and may be a feature of brain damage from infection or injury, poisoning, fever or thyrotoxicosis.

hyphaema

Blood released into the water-filled front chamber of the eye from a small blood vessel of the iris or other nearby structure. Hyphaema is a common sequel of blunt injury to the eye, such as a poke from a finger or a blow from a squash ball. At first, vision is markedly blurred, but the released blood soon settles to the bottom of the chamber to form a conspicuous dark level, and as it does so the vision clears. In more serious cases, the whole chamber may fill with blood, causing almost total loss of vision.

In most cases the blood reabsorbs within a few days and all is well, but in a small proportion of cases secondary bleeding occurs, three to five days after the injury. This is a serious complication and patients with a hyphaema are often rested in hospital in an attempt to reduce the risk of it occurring. Absorbed hyphaema is sometimes followed by a form of secondary glaucoma.

> Aspirin should never be taken to relieve pain of an eye injury as it may increase the risk of a serious hyphaema.

Hypnomidate

A brand name for **etomidate**.

hypnosis

A state of high suggestibility and responsiveness in which instructions are closely followed, opinions and even memories are apparently modified and hallucinatory sensations experienced, as directed by the hypnotist. These effects can be extended to apply to a period after the period of hypnosis (post-hypnotic suggestion).

HOW IT WORKS
The hypnotic state is induced by asking the subject to relax and focus the attention fixedly on some object. The hypnotist then indicates, in an authoritative, but calm manner, that concentration on the object will increase, but that the eyes will become heavy and tired, the lids will droop, and the eyes will soon close. This occurs, and the subject appears to be asleep. The suggestion is now made that the eyes are so heavy that they cannot be opened. Often, this is found to be the case, and the operator may then proceed, with confidence, to make other suggestions. It may, for instance, be suggested that the subject is growing younger. In this case, the subject may begin to behave and talk as a child, relating events and experiences purporting to be those of his or her childhood.

Hypnotism is not a skill possessed by individuals. It is a function of the person hypnotized, rather than of the hypnotist, a kind of intense concentration on the suggestions made, to the exclusion of other things. The best subjects for hypnotism are those with a rich capacity for fantasy, able to become absorbed in a wholly imaginary world. The hypnotized subject may appear to be asleep, but is not so and the electroencephalographic (EEG) patterns are those of a person fully awake. The procedure becomes easier with repetition, as the subject's expectations and motivation become stronger.

DOES IT WORK?
The topic of hypnotism is full of apocryphal claims. Hypnotism is impossible without the full cooperation of the subject, but observers of the procedure have been known to fall into a hypnotic state. One cannot be hypnotized against one's will, nor can a hypnotized person be made to perform an action which would, in normal circumstances, be seriously unacceptable.

Hypnosis is not a state of trance in which the subject is under the complete control of the hypnotist. Long-forgotten memories of obscure detail are not uncovered by hypnotism. Although the subject will enthusiastically bring out detail on demand, this cannot be relied upon for accuracy. The technique has no real forensic value, although evidence obtained under hypnosis has, in the past, been admitted in some courts in the United States. The quality or reliability of evidence given by witnesses to, or victims of, a crime are not improved by hypnosis.

MEDICAL USES
Hypnosis has some value in the control of transient pain, such as that of dentistry or childbirth. This is mainly because the unpleasantness of pain is often as much a matter of fear and anticipation as of actual sensation, and these can be controlled by suggestion. Hypnosis has also been of some value in the treatment of obesity and drug abuse, in those cases in which the subject has been genuinely anxious for the treatment to succeed. It is said to be useful in the management of phobias and psychologically induced memory disorders.

> Hypnosis, itself, is no substitute for other therapeutic skills and is, at best, an adjunct. It should not be used medically except by the medically qualified who are thoroughly familiar with the nature of the conditions under treatment. Those who advertise hypnosis for such purposes should be avoided.

hypnotic drugs

Drugs that help you to sleep. They are also called sedatives or soporifics. Hypnotics damp down the action of the whole nervous system and especially that of the surface (cortex) of the brain – the seat of consciousness. Overdosage is always dangerous and causes:

- coma;
- interference with normal breathing;
- reduced blood pressure;
- a drop in body temperature;
- abolition of normal reflex activity.

Long-term use of hypnotic drugs leads to tolerance of their effects. It also leads to addiction with withdrawal symptoms. Because of this, long-term use of these drugs is now generally deprecated by doctors. Hypnotic drugs are potentially dangerous to life and are often used in suicide attempts. They include chloral hydrate, bromide salts and **barbiturates**, none of which is now commonly used, and the **benzodiazepine** drugs, which are used in great quantity. Chloral hydrate is still sometimes used to sedate sleepless children, but **antihistamine drugs**, which also have a sedative effect, are more commonly given for this purpose.

The automatic prescription of hypnotic drugs in response to a complaint of insomnia is bad medicine. It is necessary to take time to analyse the cause of the insomnia and deal with it directly. If hypnotics are used at all, they should be used sparingly and only for short periods. Millions of people are addicted to hypnotic drugs.

See also **insomnia**.

Hypnovel

A brand name for **midazolam**.

hypo-

A prefix denoting below, beneath, less than. Hypo- is the exact opposite of **hyper-** and reference to that entry will indicate the range of its uses. Almost all the hyper- entities mentioned there have their hypo- counterparts.

There is, however, one usage in which hypo- is not an exact antonym of hyper-. This is when it is used to refer to position in the body, as in hypochondrium (the abdominal area below the rib cartilages) or hypoglossal (under the tongue). In this sense, the body is to be understood as standing upright, so hypo- indicates that the entity is nearer the soles of the feet than the part it qualifies. Hypo- is also used in the sense of 'deep to' as in hypodermic (under the skin).

hypochondriasis

A defect of personality leading to a constant, but unjustified, conviction of illness. The hypochondriac is convinced that he, or she, is suffering from one or other of any number of serious organic disorders, and there is a tendency, as time passes, for the nature of the disorder to change. The derivation is complex. *Hypo-*means 'under' and *chondro* means 'cartilage'. The hypochondrium is the area of the abdomen under the lower rib cartilages. The Greeks believed that the spleen, which lies in this area on the left, was the seat of melancholy and pessimism – hence hypochondriasis.

Professor William Cullen of Edinburgh published a classic description of hypochondriasis in 1816: 'In certain persons

Hypochondriasis presents a doctor's dilemma. In the great majority of cases the complaints are entirely imaginary and to carry out repeated examinations and tests is not only to waste medical time and resources, but also to potentiate the patient's fears and make the hypochondriasis worse. The wise doctor will spend a good deal of time in careful history-taking before deciding that he or she is dealing with hypochondriasis, and will then offer a comprehensive scheme of examination and tests, with the explicit understanding that these, if negative, are to mark the end of investigation of the current complaint.

there is a state of mind distinguished by a concurrence of the following circumstances: a languor, listlessness or want of resolution and activity with respect to all undertakings; a disposition to seriousness, sadness and timidity; as to all future events, an apprehension of the worst or most unhappy state of them; and therefore, often upon slight grounds, an apprehension of great evil. Such persons are particularly attentive to the state of their own health, to every smallest change of feeling in their bodies; and from any unusual feeling, perhaps of the slightest kind, they apprehend great danger and even death itself. In respect to all these feelings and apprehensions, there is commonly the most obstinate belief and persuasion.'

RECOGNITION

The cardiac neurosis is a common form of hypochondriasis. This may take two forms. The first is an excessively high level of anxiety suffered by someone who has had a heart attack and has recovered. Symptoms such as chest pain and tightness, breathlessness and palpitations are experienced, although these are not due to recurrence of the disease, and the affected person finds great difficulty in returning to a normal working life. The second is an unjustified conviction that one is suffering from heart disease. This is notoriously persistent and difficult to treat. Often, there is a family background of heart trouble and a belief that heart disease is hereditary – which it is not. The conviction is usually fortified by various symptoms, especially harmless palpitation, and chest pain, usually arising from heartburn.

TREATMENT

Strong medical reassurance, even based on comprehensive examination and investigation, seldom succeeds in dispelling the belief and the unfortunate mental sufferer goes from doctor to doctor almost as if hoping for confirmation of the fears. There is little to be done to help such people. Logical arguments, and demonstration of the possession of physical capacity impossible to those with heart disease, do not impress. In most cases, the cardiac neurotic lives a long and medically uneventful life.

Unfortunately, the true nature of hypochondriasis remains obscure, so no logical approach to treatment is possible. It has been thought to be a form of pathological depression, but it fails to respond to antidepressive treatment. The patient has full insight and cannot, by definition, be considered psychotic. The nearest one can come to a reasonable classification is to view it as an inherent defect of personality characterized by a low threshold to fear, to sensation and to the awareness of the normal functions of the body. The hypochondriac is, essentially, a person who is constantly looking in instead of out.

hypochondriasis, treatment of

See **cognitive behaviour therapy**.

hypochondrium

The region of the abdomen immediately below the lower ribs on either side. The lower ribs are joined to the breastbone by cartilages and the term, literally, means 'below the cartilages'.

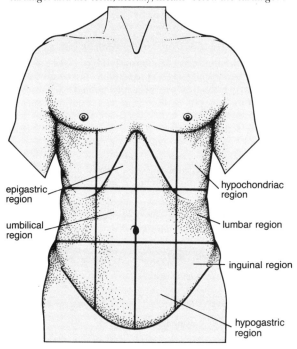

epigastric region
hypochondriac region
umbilical region
lumbar region
inguinal region
hypogastric region

The hypochondrium is one of the six anatomical regions into which each side of the abdomen is divided.

hypoglycaemia

An abnormally low level of sugar (glucose) in the blood. This is a dangerous state as the brain is critically dependent on a constant supply of fuel.

> Untreated hypoglycaemia may lead to hypoglycaemic coma which is very dangerous and requires urgent intravenous sugar if permanent brain damage is to be avoided. Diabetics undergoing surgery under general anaesthesia are at risk of hypoglycaemia and anaesthetists will usually have a glucose saline drip running throughout the operation.

RECOGNITION AND SYMPTOMS

Hypoglycaemia can cause headache, mental confusion, slurred speech, abnormal behaviour, loss of memory, numbness, double vision, temporary paralysis, fits, coma and death. The pulse is rapid, there is trembling, faintness and palpitations, and there may be profuse sweating. The behaviour is often irrational and disorderly and may be mistaken for drunkenness.

POSSIBLE CAUSES

The commonest cause of a 'hypo', as this condition is known by diabetics, is a relative overdose of insulin. The dose taken may be the same as normal but the carbohydrate intake may have been reduced or the amount of exertion been excessive so that fuel is used up faster then normal. The immediate treatment is to take sugar and this will usually end an attack. Insulin-dependent diabetics should always carry sugar lumps or glucose sweets. The drop in blood sugar can also be caused by overdosage with oral hypoglycaemic drugs, especially chlorpropamide.

hypoglycaemic drugs

Drugs used in the treatment of Type II (maturity-onset) diabetes. The term is not normally applied to insulin.

hypoglycaemics, oral

See **antidiabetic drugs**.

hypoparathyroidism

A reduced production of parathyroid gland hormone, usually from accidental surgical removal of two or three of the glands in the course of an operation on the thyroid gland. The loss of parathyroid hormone leads to a severe lowering of the level of calcium in the blood. This affects the functioning of nerves so that they may spontaneously send impulses to the muscles, leading to the condition of tetany in which certain muscle groups go into spasm. The condition is treated by giving extra calcium and vitamin D. The latter assists in the absorption of calcium from the intestine.

hypophysectomy

Surgical removal, or destruction by radiation, of the pituitary gland, or *hypophysis* (the 'growth' below the brain). This important organ may have to be removed to save life threatened by a growing pituitary tumour, to prevent the blindness caused when a tumour of the pituitary presses on the overlying crossing of the optic nerves, or to treat certain cancers of the breast, the testicle or the ovary, which are encouraged in their growth by hormones from the pituitary gland. The gland lies in an inaccessible position right underneath the centre of the brain and the usual approach is through the nose and then through the central part of the sphenoid bone in the base of the skull, in a hollow of which the pituitary lies.

As the pituitary secretes several essential hormones, these must be provided artificially for the rest of the patient's life.

hypoplasia

Underdevelopment of a tissue or organ as a result of a failure of a sufficient number of cells to be reproduced.

See also **hyperplasia**.

hypospadias

A congenital abnormality of the penis in which the tube for the urine (the urethra), instead of running the full length and opening at the tip, terminates and opens on the underside of the organ. The opening may be at the junction of the bulb (glans) and the shaft, or further back on the shaft. It may be associated with other abnormalities of the urinary system.

Hypospadias causes inconvenience in urination, but surgical correction is possible.

hypotension

Low blood pressure. In Britain, this is not regarded as a formal disease, unlike high blood pressure (hypertension). Hypotension is, however, an often dangerous, sometimes terminal, state.

POSSIBLE CAUSES

Due either to the failure of the heart to maintain the blood pressure or to a severe loss of fluid from the circulation, hypotension can occur after severe haemorrhage or burns or the excessive fluid loss of gastroenteritis, cholera or other causes of dehydration.

Hypotension is a feature of surgical shock and may occur as a result of external or internal bleeding or from a condition in which, because of widespread dilatation of peripheral blood vessels, the circulating blood volume is insufficient to maintain the supply to the brain and lungs. A mechanism of this kind, although fortunately transient and minor, is the usual cause of fainting.

RECOGNITION

Hypotension is incompatible with normal activity and claims by people going about their business that they suffer from 'low blood pressure' may be discounted. Unfortunately, the phrase is sometimes wrongly used by doctors to explain feelings of debility.

> Genuine hypotension is often life-threatening and must be treated by urgent transfusion. Unless there has been major blood loss, fluids, such as saline solutions, or plasma substitutes are sufficient.

hypothermia, surgical

All tissues of the body have a critical requirement for oxygen and fuel and without these will soon die. The requirement is, however, reduced if the temperature of the tissue is lowered and this fact is made use of to prolong the safe period for which organs may be deprived of a blood supply. The technique is especially useful in major heart surgery, which cannot be performed while the organ is performing its normal blood-pumping function. The brain is acutely sensitive to oxygen lack, and procedures, such as heart surgery, in which its blood supply may be prejudiced are made much safer by cooling the blood as it passes through the heart-lung bypass machine.

In addition, hypothermia is used to preserve the viability of the patient's heart, which is stopped by instilling a cold solution at below 10°C. Recovery to normal function occurs even after two hours. Organs taken for transplant are also kept at low temperatures while being transported.

Hypothyroidism

See **myxoedema**.

hypotonia in infants

See **floppy infant syndrome**.

Hypovase

A brand name for **prazocin**.

hypoxia

A deficiency of oxygen in the tissues. If local, this can lead to tissue death (gangrene); if general, to the death of the individual. Hypoxia is the principle immediate cause of death in the Western world, mainly as a result of occlusive diseases of the arteries (atherosclerosis). It also occurs as a result of suffocation, respiratory disease, which prevents access of oxygen to the blood, and anaemia, in which the oxygen-carrying capacity of the blood is reduced. Some poisons, such as carbon monoxide, cause hypoxia in the same way.

Hypurin Bovine Isophane

A brand name for bovine **insulin**.

Hypurin Bovine Lente

A brand name for bovine **insulin**.

Hypurin Bovine PZI

A brand name for bovine **insulin**.

Hypurin Bovine Neutral

A brand name for bovine **insulin**.

hysterectomy

Surgical removal of the womb (uterus). This may be done through the vagina, or, more easily, through a conventional incision in the front wall of the abdomen.

The operation may be 'subtotal', in which the body of the uterus is removed, but the neck of the uterus (the cervix) is left, or total, in which the upper part of the vagina is cut round and has to be sewn closed. The latter is now the more usual procedure. A Wertheim's hysterectomy for cancer involves removal of the uterus, Fallopian tubes and ovaries, the upper third of the vagina and all the lymph nodes in the region.

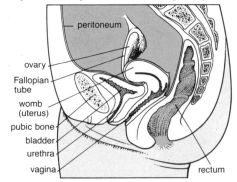
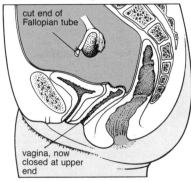

Hysterectomy, or surgical removal of the womb (uterus), involves cutting both Fallopian tubes and cutting around the vagina at the level of the cervix.

WHY IT'S DONE

Hysterectomy is done for a variety of reasons including cancer of the uterus, endometriosis, large fibroids, severely excessive menstruation (menorrhagia) and sometimes for excessive menstrual pain or sterilization.

INCIDENCE

Hysterectomy has, for various reasons, been a very common operation in the past, especially in the United States, where an estimated half a million uteruses are removed every year and where, at one time, about a quarter of all women over fifty had had the operation. In Britain, hysterectomy is performed less often.

HOW IT'S DONE

There are two possible approaches to total hysterectomy. In vaginal hysterectomy, the cervix is grasped in toothed forceps and the uterus pulled down so that the vagina is turned inside out. A cut is made around the cervix and down the front wall of the vagina, and the abdomen entered through this opening so that the attachments of the uterus to the side walls of the pelvis may be cut and the uterus removed. The floor of the pelvis is then strengthened and the opening in the vagina is stitched closed. This approach avoids a visible scar on the abdomen, but has disadvantages, as the vaginal scars are more extensive.

After abdominal hysterectomy the internal scar is confined to the upper end of the vagina, which is now a blind-ended tube. No ill-effects arise as a result of the slight shortening of the vagina, as this structure is very elastic and stretches easily. Sexual intercourse is best avoided for about six weeks after a hysterectomy, especially after vaginal hysterectomy with the additional vaginal scars. Any subsequent problems with sexual intercourse are unlikely to be caused by such mechanical problems, but may arise from hormone deficiency, if the ovaries have been removed.

RISKS

This operation is no more dangerous than any other major surgical procedure; indeed it is probably safer than most. Complications include bleeding at the time and afterwards, and damage to the bladder, bowel or ureter. Such damage is most likely if there has been pelvic infection with strong adhesions between the uterus and adjacent organs.

hysteria

Plato believed the womb (Greek *hystera*) was a rather aggressive animal lodged in the woman's body and desperate to get on with its proper function of producing children. If, he taught, the uterus was long frustrated in this desire, it became angry and caused all sorts of upsets, especially emotional instability. Out of this rather quaint, male-oriented idea arose the later concept of hysteria – a condition in which bodily upset or loss of function arises without obvious organic cause.

Hysteria is an upset of body function not caused by an organic medical condition, but resulting from purely psychological disturbance or need. The affected person is unaware of the psychological origin of the problem, nowadays, which is usually described as a *conversion disorder*. The most obvious example of the origin of hysteria is the conflict between sexual or aggressive impulse and social prohibitions. At a time – as when Freud was formulating his ideas – when such prohibitions were much stronger than they are today, hysteria was commonplace, and people like Freud were greatly impressed and influenced by it. Today, hysteria is comparatively rare, representing only about one psychiatric case in ten thousand.

The conversion of a profound psychological need or concern into a physical symptom is said to provide a means of disguising the impulse from the person concerned, so that it need not be confronted, and, at the same time, communicating to others, without actually saying anything, that there is a need for special attention. Unacceptable life situations may be changed, other people may be conveniently manipulated, responsibilities may be evaded. These effects are called secondary gains.

RECOGNITION AND SYMPTOMS

Common physical effects are loss of sensation, paralysis, tics and jerks, blindness, deafness and epileptic-like fits. Significantly, neurological disorder usually corresponds to no possible anatomical pattern – there is, for instance, no nerve disorder which could possibly cause loss of sensation affecting only the glove area of the hands. The allegedly blind do not bump into things and those having fits do not hurt themselves when they fall. In spite of gross claimed disability, people with hysteria often show a remarkable unconcern. This is known as *la belle indifférence* and is a feature of the condition.

It is dangerous for a doctor to assume hysteria and to fail to carry out a comprehensive neurological examination. Genuine neurological disease is now commoner than psychologically induced disorder, and the signs of organic disease are sometimes improbable.

TREATMENT

Once the diagnosis of hysteria is established, the affected person can safely be treated by a careful exploration of the origins of the problem. In most cases the symptoms clear abruptly after a fairly short time, but often the underlying cause remains. Further conversions, taking either the same or different forms, are common, especially in those who have much to gain.

Hytrin

A brand name for **terazosin**.

Hytrin BPH

A brand name for **terazosin**.

-ia

Suffix meaning 'disease of' as in pneumonia (lung disease).

-iasis

Suffix meaning 'disorder, like' as in elephantiasis (like an elephant).

iatrogenic

Iatros is the Greek word for a doctor. This root occurs also in the words 'geriatric' and 'paediatric'. Iatrogenic disorder is that caused by doctors in the course of treating disease. The effect may be unforeseen and due to accident, unpredictable or unusual reactions, or, rarely, to medical incompetence or carelessness. Sometimes an iatrogenic effect is an inescapable consequence, or 'side-effect', of treatment needed to save life or to relieve severe distress. Thus, loss of hair, in the course of chemotherapy for widespread cancer, is an iatrogenic effect, but is acceptable since the alternative may be loss of life. Doctors are, rightly, much concerned about iatrogenesis and cooperate wholeheartedly in official attempts to reduce it.

In Britain there is a 'yellow card' adverse drug reaction reporting scheme and one doctor in six actively cooperates in this. In the first eight years of the scheme, from 1972, no fewer than 53,685 separate reports were sent in. Non-steroidal anti-inflammatory drugs accounted for 24 per cent of the reports. Similar schemes are operated in most other developed countries.

Surgeons, too, have their share of responsibility for iatrogenic disorder, mostly as a result of surgical mishap and sheer bad luck. They are not complacent, however, and several confidential general enquiries have been set up into the causes of deaths occurring within thirty days of operations. Most surgeons – 96 per cent – have complied with these enquiries and have completed the report forms candidly and with self-criticism.

-ible

Suffix meaning 'able to be' as in edible (able to be eaten).

ibuprofen

A pain-killing (analgesic) drug with anti-inflammatory properties, useful in mild rheumatic and muscular disorders and in the relief of menstrual pain. Brand names are Brufen, Fenbid Spansule, Motrin and Nurofen. Brand names of preparations for external use include Deep Relief, Fenbid Gel, Ibugel, Ibuspray and Proflex.

Ibuspray

A brand name for **ibuprofen** in a preparation for external use.

-ic

Suffix meaning 'concerned with' as in toxic (like poison).

-ical

Suffix meaning 'relating to' as in umbilical (of the navel).

-ice

Suffix meaning 'condition of' as in jaundice (like yellow).

ice-cream headache

One of the commonest forms of headache, caused by narrowing of arteries following cooling of the back part of the hard palate. It occurs when swallowing large mouthfuls of ice cream or when eating it rapidly. The pain is felt in the forehead or temporal region, starting soon after the first mouthful, and reaches a climax within a minute. Occasionally it persists for as long as five minutes. This is a form of referred pain and there is no reason to suppose that it is harmful. It can be avoided by a more leisurely and appreciative consumption of the foodstuff.

ichthyosis

A scaly, fish-like disorder of the skin, sometimes called 'fish skin disease'. *Ichthyos* is Greek for 'a fish'. The condition is usually genetically determined and present from birth. The skin is unable to form the normal waterproof horny outer layer so that it cannot retain water and tends to dry out.

The treatment consists in soaking the skin, cleaning with aqueous cream or emulsifying ointment instead of soap, removing excessive scales by scrubbing or fine sandpapering and the use of a protective and waterproof cream. Ichthyosis is always worse in cold weather when the low atmospheric humidity encourages water loss. Sufferers fare better in warm, moist climates. The condition often improves with age.

-ics

Suffix meaning 'art or science' as in genetics (science of begetting).

icterus

A little-used medical term for **jaundice**.

-id

Suffix meaning 'state of' as in morbid (state of death).

id

That part of our nature which, according to Freud, is concerned with the single-minded pursuit of personal, mainly physical, gratification. It is the most primitive component of our being, governed entirely by the *pleasure principle*, unconcerned with reason, logic or humanity; allegedly unconscious, but concerned, nevertheless, with achieving immediate satisfaction of all animal instinctual drives. The id manifests the forces of the libido and the death wish, but is said to be the source of much of our psychic energy.

Freud was concerned to point out that his usage was not intended to denote a real entity, but was merely a useful descriptive device. The id has, however, taken on a life of its own and, in the writings of many later psychoanalysts, is apparently no longer regarded as a pure metaphor.

-idae

Suffix meaning 'name of' as in family retroviridae (retroviruses).

idarubicin

A cytotoxic anticancer drug. A brand name is Zavedos.

idiocy

Like idiopathic, this word derives from a Greek root meaning something private or personal to oneself. The idiot is the person concerned with his or her own private affairs, unaware of what is going on in the world around. The term 'idiot' is now little used in medicine, but has been defined as someone with a mental age of less than three.

idiopathic

A word useful to doctors, but to no one else, as it simply means 'of unknown cause'. *Idiopathic steatorrhoea* sounds like a diagnosis, but is not. It actually means 'I don't know why this patient has so much fat in his stools.'

idiot-savant

A feature occasionally found among autistic children, who often show great precocity in some respect such as musical ability or early reading. The idiot-savant, while severely backward in every other respect, and often with an IQ score of less than 50, displays amazing ability in mental arithmetical calculation or in the recall of a particular class of data. These abilities are, unfortunately, seldom of practical use.

See **autism**.

idoxuridine

A drug effective against herpes simplex viruses. Idoxuridine is chemically very similar to thymine, which it replaces in the viral DNA, thereby preventing replication. A brand name for a preparation for external use is Herpid.

ifosfamide

An **alkylating agent** used as an anticancer drug. A brand name is Mitoxana.

Ig

The abbreviation for immunoglobulin (antibody). This abbreviation is used because there are five classes of immunoglobulins and it is often necessary to refer to them. IgA, immunoglobulin class A, is an antibody class concerned with protection against virus and other infections in the mucous membranes of the body, especially in the respiratory and digestive systems. IgD, immunoglobulin class D, is found almost exclusively on the surface of B lymphocytes (B cells) and is thought to be concerned with the regulation of these cells. IgE, immunoglobulin class E, is the antibody class concerned with immediate hypersensitive reactions, such as in hay fever. It has an affinity for cell surfaces and is commonly found on **mast cells**. IgG, immunoglobulin class G, accounts for three-quarters of the antibodies in the blood of healthy people. It is widely distributed in the tissues and is the only immunoglobulin class that passes through the placenta to the fetus. It is concerned with protection against a wide range of infecting organisms. IgM, immunoglobulin class M, is the antibody class concerned especially with the breakdown of foreign cells and with preparing foreign material for ingestion by **phagocytes**.

Note that the term 'gamma globulin' refers to the whole class of immunoglobulins, not simply to IgG.

-ile

Suffix meaning 'of, like' as in juvenile (like the young).

ileitis, regional

See **regional ileitis**.

ileostomy

A surgical procedure in which the lower part of the small intestine (the ileum) is brought up to the front wall of the abdomen and an opening made to the exterior, so that the bowel contents can discharge externally into a suitable receptacle.

WHY IT'S DONE

Ileostomy is often a temporary necessity when there is obstruction to the bowel lower down, or when the lower bowel requires rest and freedom from the passage of food residue, to recover from disease, injury or surgical operation. Sometimes a permanent ileostomy is necessary, as when the large intestine (colon), into which the ileum empties, has had to be removed.

The *stoma* or mouth of the ileostomy is a small, nipple-like opening on one side of the wall of the abdomen. Around this, a removable plastic bag can be fixed in various ways, so as to make a water-tight seal and allow evacuation without contamination. The bowel contents are irritating to the skin, and excoriation must be avoided by the use of a well-fitting appliance and protective creams. Various plastic surgical procedures have been designed to provide a kind of artificial rectum in which faeces can be stored temporarily. This is known as a *continent ileostomy*.

ileus, adynamic

This condition, which used to be called *paralytic ileus*, is a failure, usually temporary, of the normal process of peristalsis by which the bowel contents are moved steadily onwards towards the rectum. In adynamic ileus, the muscles of the bowel wall, which carry out this onward-squeezing function, are not paralysed, but have ceased to act in a coordinated manner.

POSSIBLE CAUSES

The condition may be caused by severe infection, loss of blood, shock, abdominal injury, or from a deficiency of potassium, calcium or magnesium.

RECOGNITION AND SYMPTOMS

Because the bowel is so long – some 8 m (24 feet) – the effect of loss of peristalsis is to bring about an obstruction in a very short time. Vomiting is persistent and the abdomen becomes very distended.

TREATMENT

The stomach must be kept empty and the volume of the contents of the bowel reduced. A suction tube (naso-gastric aspiration) is inserted and as much fluid removed as possible. The cause of the condition is treated, and when this is removed the normal bowel function usually returns.

illusion

A false sense perception resulting from a misinterpretation of the incoming stimulus. Many illusions are normal and are experienced by all of us. Optical illusions are particularly well-known and popular, but similar illusions can be produced in the acoustic sphere. Much has been learned about modes of brain function from studying illusions. Illusions of a more serious nature are common in many psychiatric conditions, especially depression. They include a tendency to misinterpret the sound or meaning of actual words spoken by others so that they are taken to be adversely critical or conspiratorial. Note that such an illusion may also contain the *delusion* that one is being persecuted. **Hallucinations** are quite different from illusions.

illness, child, serious

See **serious illness in a child**.

Ilosone

A brand name for **erythromycin**.

imaginary disease

See **fibrositis**.

Imdur

A brand name for **isosorbide mononitrate**.

imidazole drugs

A class of antifungal and antibacterial drugs effective against a wide range of bacteria and fungi. The group includes **metronidazole** (Flagyl), **mebendazole**, thiabendazole, **clotrimazole** (Canesten), ketoconazole and **miconazole**.

Imigran

A brand name for **sumatripan**.

imipenem

An **antibiotic** enzyme inhibitor resistant to breakdown by most beta-lactamases. It is active against a wide range of bacteria. A brand name is Primaxin.

imipramine

A widely used tricyclic antidepressant drug. A brand name is Tofranil.

immobilization

For centuries it has been known that a closed (uninfected) fracture of bone will heal well and soundly if the broken ends are brought into reasonable apposition and then held securely in position for a number of weeks. Failure of effective immobilization results in an unstable, fibrous rather than bony, union and even the formation of a 'false joint' (pseudarthrosis) at the site of the fracture. Methods of immobilization, of increasing sophistication, have been a notable feature of orthopaedic practice.

THE HISTORY OF IMMOBILIZATION

The wooden splint, or even box, gave way to the metal splint, and this, in turn, to the plaster cast, which was later greatly improved by reinforcement with loose-woven bandage. Bandages impregnated with plaster of Paris have, for years, been the basis of the immobilization of fractures of all kinds. These are easy to apply, adaptable, strong, light and effective. If there is a danger of swelling, they may be split into longitudinal halves and then refixed with plain bandages.

TECHNOLOGICAL ADVANCES

But, today, even the ubiquitous plaster cast is beginning to give way to alternative methods of immobilization. New materials are being used in a conventional manner and old materials in an unconventional manner. High-tech has come to the orthopaedic wards with a vengeance and a whole new industry, dedicated to immobilization, has grown up. Orthopaedic units are now full of people in wheelchairs with their fractures held in place by external steel bars carrying adjustable struts which pass through the skin and are screwed into the bone. External methods of this kind are being developed rapidly and have the advantage that wounds can be inspected while the fracture is well immobilized. They have, however, by no means replaced the plaster cast.

FRACTURES

Many fractures require internal surgical immobilization by means of screws, nails or screwed-on steel plates. These are avoided if possible but are used when adequate immobilization cannot be achieved in any other way. Fractures of the neck of the thigh bone (femur) are commonly treated by means of various kinds of screws, nails or fluted pins screwed or hammered into the bone. Fractures of the shaft of the femur cannot easily be immobilized by simple plaster casts and are often treated by weight traction to keep the bones in alignment. This is applied by way of a steel pin passed though the upper end of the main lower leg bone (the tibia).

IMMOBILIZING TISSUE

Immobilization is not limited to fractures. Any diseased or injured tissue can be aided in its recovery by a limited amount of immobilization in the early stages. This must be carefully judged, however, as prolonged immobilization begins to give rise to wasting (disuse atrophy).

Immukin

A brand name for **interferon gamma**.

immune system cell messengers

See **lymphokines**.

immune system cells

See **lymphocytes**.

immunity

When, around the end of the eighteenth century, it was proved by the English physician Edward Jenner (1749–1823) that immunity against smallpox could be achieved by deliberate infection with a similar but much less serious disease (cowpox), the science of immunology was born. The term 'immunity' is now rather loosely applied to the body's ability to resist infection by means of antibodies and a complex cellular defence mechanism. Absolute immunity to infection does not exist.

To many organisms, our immunity is almost absolute, but to many others it is relative only. It is, essentially, a question of the relative strength of the opposing forces. A minor assault, by a small dose of organisms, of fairly low virulence, is easily repulsed. But a large dose of highly virulent organisms might be overwhelming. Organisms mutate and vary in the severity of their effects. The immune system also varies, both in its overall efficiency, and in its specific ability to deal quickly with a new invader.

Active immunity is the responsive process by which antibodies are produced by the body to deal with infections or are deliberately stimulated into production by medical immunization. Such active immunity may last for a lifetime or may need booster doses from time to time. Passive immunity is that conferred when antibodies from another person or animal are injected or when antibodies pass across the placenta into the bloodstream of the unborn child or are received in the breast milk after birth. Passive immunity is short-lived, but can be life-saving.

immunization

The terms 'immunization' and 'vaccination' are interchangeable. The latter term arose because the first successful application of the method involved the use of a virus modified by passage through cows. *Vacca* is Latin for 'a cow'.

Immunization against infectious disease has been highly successful and, in areas where there has been a good acceptance rate, has led to a large reduction in the incidence of diseases such as **diphtheria**, **measles**, German measles (**rubella**), **poliomyelitis** and **whooping cough** (pertussis). Smallpox enjoys the unique distinction of having been eradicated, and this was largely due to immunization.

HOW IT WORKS

The parts of the infective organisms that cause the immune reaction are not the same as those which do the harm to the infected person. Germs carry surface components (antigens) by which they are recognized by the immune system as 'foreign' and to which specific and unique defensive antibodies (immunoglobulins) are manufactured.

Fortunately, it is possible to modify samples of infective organisms so that, although no longer offering danger to the infected person, they still retain these antigenic properties. If such modified organisms are introduced into the body, the immune system reacts to them exactly as it would to the normal virulent strains and produces defensive proteins. Fluids containing such modified organisms, whether alive or dead, are called *vaccines*.

> The effect of these successes has been a major improvement in the health of the communities concerned and a substantial reduction in the incidence of early death and of congenital and acquired defects. But communities that fail to remember their histories often find them repeated; and there is anxiety among public health authorities that generations of parents, who have never known what it is to be driven to distraction by worry over diphtheria, or seen their children crippled by polio, will not have the necessary motivation to see that their children are immunized. The danger is the greater because, after a generation of freedom from such diseases as diphtheria, there is little or no natural immunity in the population and the re-introduction of the disease might lead to major epidemics.
>
> In the United States, legislation ensures compliance by prohibiting entry to schools of non-immunized children. Similar sanctions should be applied in Britain if we are to avoid future epidemics.

Immunity can be achieved in another, but quite passive, way. Immunoglobulins (antibodies) produced in another person, or in an animal, as a result of infection can be injected into someone suffering from the same infection. The immunoglobulins are fairly simple protein molecules and are not cellular organisms, so do not carry antigens. The serum in which they are found, however – the fluid forming when blood is allowed to clot – may have antigenic elements in it and care has to be taken to avoid reactions to this. Purified globulin of the class IgG (**gamma globulin**) is widely used. Human immunoglobulin is derived from pooled donated blood and contains a considerable collection of antibodies to the diseases common in the general population, including measles, mumps, hepatitis A, rubella and chickenpox (varicella). Immunoglobulins can also be taken specifically from donors who have had particular diseases. In this way, immunoglobulins are available for rarer diseases such as tetanus, rabies and hepatitis B.

TYPES OF IMMUNIZATION

There are two types of immunization – active and passive. Just as prevention is always better than cure, the former is always to be preferred to the latter. But, since it takes time for the necessary levels of antibodies to build up, passive immunization is often necessary in the treatment of acute illness. Often,

> Some children are at special risk from infectious disease and should be immunized as a matter of urgency. These include:
> - children with asthma;
> - children with congenital heart disease;
> - those with chronic lung disease;
> - those with Down's syndrome;
> - those who were premature babies and remain small for their ages;
> - children who are HIV positive.

the two are combined, passive immunization giving immediate cover while the active production of the patient's own antibodies is getting under way.

Risks

Active immunization with vaccines containing live, but modified, organisms, which is, in general, very safe in most people, can offer dangers to certain groups. These include:

- people with severe immunodeficiency disorders who might suffer severe effects even from modified organisms (but see HIV positive people, below);
- those who have shown a previous severe reaction to vaccines;
- pregnant women, since there is at least a theoretical risk of damage to the developing fetus;
- anyone suffering from any acute illness;
- anyone on high dosages of steroids or on immunosuppressive treatment;
- people suffering from cancers such as lymphomas or Hodgkin's lymphoma.

HIV

HIV-positive people, whether they have symptoms or not, should receive live vaccines for measles, mumps, rubella and polio, and inactivated vaccines for whooping cough, tetanus, polio, diphtheria, typhoid, cholera and hepatitis B.

WHAT CAN YOU IMMUNIZE AGAINST?

Immunization is readily available against diphtheria, whooping cough, tetanus, poliomyelitis, measles, tuberculosis, mumps, rubella, influenza, hepatitis A and B, rabies, cholera, typhoid, anthrax, smallpox and yellow fever. Every child should be protected against the first five of these as a matter of routine policy. In the case of tuberculosis, those who are found, on tuberculin testing, not to have already had the common, protective primary infection, should have BCG.

All girls should be vaccinated against rubella between their 10th and 14th birthdays, as should all non-pregnant women of child-bearing age who are found to be antibody negative for rubella. These should, however, be warned to use effective contraceptive measures to avoid pregnancy within three months of immunization. Vaccination should never be done in early pregnancy because, although no case of rubella damage to a fetus has been described following immunization, the theoretical risk remains. Pregnant women susceptible to rubella should be vaccinated as soon as the baby is born and before they can become pregnant again. Boys should be immunized, as if they contract the disease they could pass it to pregnant women.

SPECIAL CASES

Influenza immunization should be considered by those at special risk of serious effects from the infection, especially the elderly and infirm and those suffering from chronic diseases. Hepatitis B vaccination is usually confined to medical personnel and others at special risk, and perhaps to the close relatives and contacts of people known to be carrying the virus. It is also often given to promiscuous homosexual men, prison warders, personnel of the police and the emergency services, morticians and embalmers and long-term prisoners.

Vaccination against smallpox is no longer required and should not be done as smallpox no longer exists.

See also **rabies**, **cholera**, **typhoid fever** and **yellow fever**.

immunodeficiency disorders

An important class of diseases in which the body's immunological system of defence against infection, foreign material generally and some forms of cancer is in some way defective. The best known example of this group of disorders is, of course, the acquired immunodeficiency syndrome, AIDS, but immunodeficiency disorders were well known in medical circles long before AIDS appeared.

POSSIBLE CAUSES

Immunodeficiency disorders may be present at birth (congenital) and may be of genetic origin, or may be acquired later. The immunological mechanisms are so important for survival that major defects are seldom seen.

Some deficiency in the production of immunoglobulins is normal in the early years of life and it is not until adult life that full production occurs. This is why children are so susceptible to infections. Children depend on antibodies supplied by the mother before birth and provided in the early breast milk (colostrum) after birth. Premature babies may not, because of early birth, have received the full quota from the mother.

CONGENITAL IMMUNE DEFICIENCY

Antibodies, which are produced by the B lymphocyte system, are proteins known as immunoglobulins. Immunoglobulin deficiency is the most important immunodeficiency disorder and occurs as a sex-linked recessive trait. Although the name, *agammaglobulinaemia*, implies complete absence of the important antibody type, gamma globulin, total deficiency does not, in fact, occur. Such people have a variable degree of B cell deficiency (hypogammaglobulinaemia) and may survive for many years, although very susceptible to bacterial and other infection and requiring constant treatment. Another form of immunodeficiency disorder is a selective deficiency of the T cell group of lymphocytes. When this is present from birth the outlook is poor, but in some cases treatment by human fetal thymus gland transplantation has been effective. The most serious form of congenital immunodeficiency is the *severe combined immune deficiency* (SCID), whose victims have to become 'bubble babies' enclosed in plastic from birth to keep out infecting organisms.

ACQUIRED IMMUNE DEFICIENCY

Acquired immune deficiency may be caused by necessary medical treatment of auto-immune disease or to prevent the rejection of transplanted organs, or it may be caused by disease. Diseases causing immune deficiency include AIDS, many types of cancer, and severe dietary deficiency states, especially when the protein necessary to form antibodies is absent. Old age features a relative immune deficiency, as a consequence of a gradual consumption of the total stock of both kinds of lymphocytes. So conditions such as shingles and certain cancers, which have been kept in check by the immune system, become commoner in the elderly.

RECOGNITION AND SYMPTOMS

People with immunodeficiency disorders suffer recurrent infection, not only by the common organisms, but also by those which do not normally cause disease. These infections are known as *opportunistic* and include such conditions as *Pneumocystis carinii* pneumonia, cytomegalovirus infections and extensive Herpes simplex and thrush infections, which involve not only the skin, but also the intestinal and respiratory systems – all the features that have become so familiar in the AIDS era.

immunoglobulins

Immunoglubulins, or antibodies, are protective proteins, produced by B lymphocytes, which attach to invading organisms or foreign substances and neutralize them so that they can be destroyed by phagocytes. There are five classes of immunoglobulins, the most prevalent being immunoglobulin class G (IgG), or gamma globulin. This provides the body's main defence against bacteria, viruses and toxins.

Gamma globulin is so widely effective that it is produced commercially, from pooled human plasma, and used as a means of passive protection against many infections. It is useful for protection, when the need arises, against many infection including hepatitis A and B, chickenpox, measles and poliomyelitis. It is also very useful for people who have an inherent or acquired immune deficiency, such as the condition of agammaglobulinaemia.

immunosuppressant drugs

Drugs that act on any part of the immune system of the body so as to interfere with the normal reactions to the presence of any **antigen**. Such drugs are used to prevent graft rejection and to treat conditions caused by immune phenomena, such as immune complex disorders or autoimmune disease. They include **azathioprine**, corticosteroid drugs, cyclosporin, FK506, and the anti-lymphocyte monoclonal antibody OKT3.

immunotherapy

An experimental method of cancer treatment based on attempts to stimulate the immune system into a more vigorous attack on cancer. Substances such as BCG have been tried but without success. Tumour cells, taken from another patient with the same disease, and made harmless, have been injected, in the hope that they would stimulate the immune system into producing antibodies. Antisera containing immunoglobulins from cancer patients has also been tried, but again without success. Interferon has, however, been shown to have some useful activity against certain tumours such as non-Hodgkin's lymphoma and hairy-cell leukaemia. This substance can be linked to monoclonal antibodies produced by genetic engineering techniques.

Immunotherapy is in its infancy and, so far, seems to have been of little value on its own. It may, however, prove, in the short term, a useful supplement to other methods of treatment, such as chemotherapy. There is no saying what advances may occur in the longer term.

Imodium

A brand name for **loperamide**.

impetigo

A skin infection, commonest in children, but which affects most people, to a limited degree, in hot, moist climates.
INCIDENCE
Impetigo is now less common in western communities because of the high standards of skin cleanliness, although it is not uncommon in small children.

POSSIBLE CAUSES
Severe attacks, in temperate areas, are usually an indication of inadequate standards of personal hygiene, as the condition is normally easily controlled by regular washing and simple methods of treatment.
RECOGNITION AND SYMPTOMS
Impetigo is caused by staphylococci. The condition starts with small blisters which soon turn to golden-green crusts. It spreads rapidly by direct contact and is highly infectious to others. The face is most commonly affected, predominantly around the mouth, but in a severe case the body skin may be widely involved.
TREATMENT
The condition is treated by carefully removing the crusts with cetrimide solution, or soap and water, and applying an antibiotic ointment. Rarely, if the condition is severe, antibiotics by injection or mouth may be necessary.

implant, defibrillator

An experimental device used for patients who are liable to recurrent heart stoppage (cardiac arrest). The device senses the spontaneous high pulse rate which often precedes a common form of cardiac arrest (ventricular fibrillation), charges up its capacitors and automatically applies a 700 volt shock to electrodes permanently attached to the heart. If this fails, a second, stronger, shock is given. The shock is unpleasant, but tolerable, and the device has been shown to be lifesaving. The response time is rapid – 5 to 15 seconds to recognize the abnormal pulse and 5 to 15 seconds to charge up the capacitors from the special lithium battery used.

implant, lens

A tiny, but powerful, artificial lens, usually made of Perspex which is fixed inside the eye after removing the opaque lens, in a cataract operation. See **cataract surgery**.

impotence

Definitions differ, but impotence is generally taken to be the inability to achieve a penile erection (tumescence) of sufficient firmness to allow normal vaginal sexual intercourse.
POSSIBLE CAUSES
A very small proportion of cases of impotence are actually caused by organic disorders, and even those with an organic element, such as those caused by heart output insufficiency, hormonal changes, local arterial disorders, multiple sclerosis, spinal cord disorders or diabetic nerve damage, often have a psychological element. At the same time, some cases in which there are obvious psychological or social causal factors also have a physical element. Almost all men experience erectile failure from time to time. There are many causes.

Much apparent erectile inadequacy is actually due to fear of failure, lack of desire or unsatisfactory macho attitudes to sex. It is notorious that a man may perform better with one woman than with another. Lack of desire may simply be due to anything from boredom with the partner to active dislike of her, but may also be due to repeated past failure – a circumstance which many men find deeply humiliating and which they may become determined to avoid, even at the cost of a damaged relationship.

Psychological erectile failure is usually of fairly sudden onset and tends to be intermittent and related to one partic-

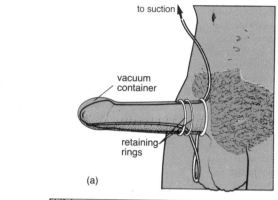

(a)

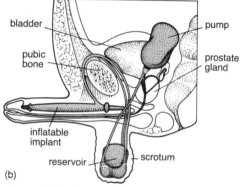

(b)

In organic impotence spontaneous erection is impossible. (a) shows a method of obtaining tumescence by temporarily sealing a vacuum chamber around the penis. (b) shows one of the various types of inflatable implant operated by a buried pump that can be manually compressed to force fluid into the implant via a releasable valve.

ular partner. A good erection is achieved during masturbation and during the periods of rapid eye movement (REM) sleep. An erection is commonly present on waking. Many factors contribute to non-organic failure. Alcohol may add to sexual desire, but, it can detract from the performance. So can several drugs, both prescribed and otherwise.

Premature ejaculation affects the man's attitude and may lead to erectile failure, but should not, in itself, be classed as a form of impotence. Although followed, like all ejaculations, by a rapid loss of erection, this is not the basic problem.

Organic impotence may be due to loss of male sex hormones, usually in the elderly, or as a result of anti-hormonal medical treatment. Other causes include diabetes and various neurological conditions. There is often total loss of interest in sex, no fantasies or erotic dreams, and sometimes loss of the male secondary sexual characteristics. Organic impotence is usually of gradual onset and erection does not occur during attempts at masturbation or during sleep. The penis tends to be small and cold. Full medical investigation is required in all such cases, unless the underlying disorder is already known.

TREATMENT

The treatment of psychological impotence depends on education, the use of methods such as the temporary prohibition of sexual intercourse, the encouragement of touching and sensual massage (sensate focus technique) and sexual counselling. Physical treatments include injections of papaverine, the use of vacuum condoms to suck the penis into a state of erection, the 'penile ring' to exert a mild compression at the base and help to sustain erections, and various implantable inflatable prosthetic devices. In some cases, due to thrombosis of a major artery, vascular surgery can effect a cure.

See also **ejaculation, disorders of, yohimbin.**

impotence pill

See **sildenafil citrate, Viagra.**

Imunovir

A brand name for **inosine pranobex.**

Imuran

A brand name for **azothiaprine.**

in-

Prefix meaning 'within' as in inject (throw in).

Inadine

A brand name for **povidone-iodine.**

incest

Sexual intercourse between close blood relatives, especially between brothers and sisters, fathers and daughters, and mothers and sons. The incest taboo is widespread, almost universal, and its origin has been a cause of much controversy. The idea that the taboo arises from a perception of the importance of avoiding the supposed ill-effects of 'in-breeding' is highly unlikely. More probably, the taboo arises from cultural factors, especially awareness of the trouble incest causes in families.

The 'degrees of prohibition' are noted for their arbitrariness and variability and there is no 'instinctive', built-in, revulsion against any particular form of incest. In some cases, the prohibition has applied to any member of the father's family; in others, to any member of the mother's.

CLASSES OF INCEST

Until recently, there were three classes of incest in Britain – criminal, such as intercourse with a daughter; illegal, but not criminal, such as intercourse with a niece; and sinful, but not illegal, such as intercourse with a deceased wife's sister. The Christian churches once held that the marriage of two godparents of the same child was as incestuous as that of a brother and sister; but, by comparison, the ruling houses of ancient Egypt had no difficulty in regarding marriages between brother and sister as not only normal, but entirely right and proper.

GENETIC IMPLICATIONS

Genetically, incest becomes undesirable only when there are recessive traits for disease in the family so that breeding carriers are more likely to produce offspring homozygous for the condition. The same genetic implication applies to marriages between first cousins, which are almost universally thought acceptable.

incidence

The frequency with which an event, such as a disease, occurs in a particular population over a given period of time. Incidence should be distinguished from prevalence, which is the number of existing instances of an event in a particular population, either at a particular point in time, or during a given period. So a statement about the number of cases of a disease occurring in Britain every year is a statement of incidence, while a statement about the number of people suffering from the disease in 1995 is a statement of prevalence.

incision

A cut made to achieve surgical access to the interior of the body or to the deeper layers of the skin. Deep surgical incisions are made in such a way that the various layers of the body wall are passed through one at a time.

The skin, the layer of tough, fibrous or fatty tissue under the skin (fascia), the muscles under the fascia and any tissue layers under the muscles, are usually treated as separate planes, to be opened sequentially, rather than in one deep cut. Often the muscle layer is split open, rather than cut, and the direction of this split is likely to be different from that of the skin incision.

The abdominal wall, which is the site of most surgical incisions, can be opened in various places, depending on the operation to be performed. Various standard incisions have evolved which allow good access but which can be securely closed without leaving the wall significantly weakened.

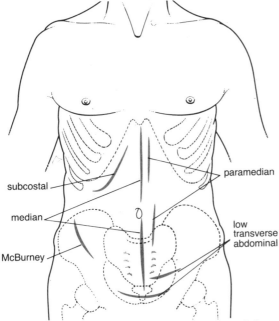

The position of various surgical incisions commonly made in the abdominal wall.

incisions, surgical, minimal

See **laparoscopic surgery**.

incisor

One of the eight, central teeth equipped with cutting edges and designed to bite pieces off the food. The canine and pre-

molar teeth, further to the side, are tearing teeth, and the molars are grinders.

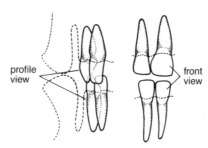

The incisor teeth are the central cutters provided with sharp edges. There are four in each jaw and they have single roots.

incontinence, faecal

The inability to maintain normal control over the passage of faeces. In health, the desire to empty the bowels is easily suppressed, even if the rectum is loaded. In involuntary faecal incontinence, this ability is lost, partly because the muscles of the floor of the pelvis and of the controlling ring (sphincter) in the anus have become weakened and partly because the awareness of distention of the rectum is diminished.

The problem is commonest in old people, especially if severely debilitated or demented, but also affects younger people if the controlling muscles have been damaged by childbirth or by various diseases. Incontinence also occurs when there is marked intestinal 'hurry' as in diarrhoea or acute gastro-enteritis. Voluntary faecal incontinence may be a feature of childhood behavioural, or adult psychotic, disturbances.

The treatment is always directed at the underlying cause.

incontinence nurse

A nurse specially trained in the problems of people suffering from urinary or faecal incontinence, whose condition cannot be corrected by medical or surgical treatment. The incontinence nurse is fully versed in the measures available for the relief and assistance of such people and is skilled in the fitting of necessary appliances.

incontinence, urinary

Involuntary urination (incontinence) is very common. It takes various forms, the most frequent in adults being *stress incontinence* in which a small quantity of urine is passed whenever the pressure within the abdomen is suddenly increased, as in coughing or laughing. This form commonly follows injury or strain, during childbirth, to the muscles forming the floor of the pelvis. These muscles support the bladder and help to keep the urethra closed. Persistent incontinence from this cause may call for surgical repair but many cases respond to pelvic floor exercises.

Incontinence may be due to damage to the nerve control of the bladder from **stroke**, local **cancer**, **tuberculosis** or **multiple sclerosis**, but most cases arise from less serious causes such as pelvic floor damage or outflow obstruction with overflow, especially in men with prostate enlargement.

In some cases of incontinence, the cause remains undiscovered. Senile dementia often features incontinence from simple loss of normal voluntary control. About 5 per cent of people over sixty-five are incontinent, and of those in institutional care, the figure is said to be about 50 per cent.

	TYPICAL AVERAGE INCUBATION PERIODS		
Virus diseases	**Incubation period**	**Bacterial diseases**	**Incubation period**
COMMON COLD	4 DAYS	FOOD POISONING	HOURS TO A FEW DAYS
INFLUENZA	5 DAYS	CHOLERA	HOURS TO A FEW DAYS
MEASLES	10 DAYS	GONORRHOEA	4 DAYS
CHICKENPOX	14 DAYS	SCARLET FEVER	5 DAYS
POLIOMYELITIS	17 DAYS	MENINGITIS	6 DAYS
RUBELLA	18 DAYS	DIPHTHERIA	6 DAYS
MUMPS	28 DAYS	WHOOPING COUGH	9 DAYS
HEPATITIS A	32 DAYS	TETANUS	10 DAYS
RABIES	30 TO 60 DAYS BUT MAY BE UP TO SEVERAL MONTHS	TYPHOID	14 DAYS

incubation period

The time interval between the entry of the infecting organisms and the first appearance of symptoms of the resulting disease. In spite of considerable variation in the size of the dose acquired and in the resistance of the host, the incubation period is a characteristic of the organism rather than of these other factors. It reflects the organism's rate of reproduction, its mode of infection and the route taken by it to reach its objective.

Incubation periods vary widely. Cholera may strike a person down within a very few hours of drinking contaminated water; rabies may start months after a bite on the foot. In the former, the organisms reach the point of attack – the bowel – almost at once; in the latter, the viruses have to make their way slowly up the immensely long journey by nerve fibre, to reach the brain. The incubation period of rabies depends on the proximity of the bite to the brain.

The table shows some typical average incubation periods.

incubator

A piece of equipment providing a closed, insulated and controllable environment so as to achieve optimum conditions for the maintenance and growth of an organism, whether bacterial, animal or human. One of the central items of equipment in the bacteriological laboratory is the incubator in which cultures of organisms are grown, usually at body temperature. This is the temperature at which organisms pathogenic to man grow best.

In the premature baby incubator, other environmental factors, besides temperature, may also be important. These include relative absence of infecting organisms, higher than normal oxygen concentration and controlled humidity of the air. The main value of the incubator is prevent hypothermia to which small infants are prone. Ports provide access for feeding and handling.

Incubators provide a micro-environment for the nurture of premature or very ill small babies. Temperature, humidity and oxygen concentration can be carefully controlled. The main value of the incubator is to prevent hypothermia to which small infants are prone. Ports provide access for feeding and handling.

indapamide

A diuretic drug used to treat high blood pressure. Brand names are Natramid and Natrilix.

indentical-product genes

See **homologous genes**.

Inderal

A brand name for **propranolol**.

Indian medicine

See **medicine, Indian**.

indigestion

See **dyspepsia**.

indinavir

A **protease inhibitor** drug used in combination with antiviral drugs to treat AIDS. A brand name is Crixivan.

Indocid

A brand name for **indomethacin**.

Indocid PDA

A brand name for **indomethacin**.

indomethacin

A non-steroidal pain-killing (analgesic) and anti-inflammatory drug (**NSAID**) of the indole acetic acid group. Brand names are Flexin Continus, Indocid, Indocid PDA and Indomod.

Indomod

A brand name for **indomethacin**.

Indoramin

A selective adrenergic alpha-blocker drug used in the treatment of high blood pressure. Brand names are Baratol and Doralese.

industrial diseases

See **occupational therapies**.

-ine

Suffix meaning 'full of' as in sanguine (full of blood).

Infacol

A brand name for dimethicone.

infant mortality

The infant mortality rate is the number of infants under the age of one year who die, for every 1000 live births. This is a sensitive index of the level of social and medical advance in a society and of the standards of public health. In 1900, in Britain, the infant mortality rate was around 150 – about one baby in seven died before reaching its first birthday. By 1950 the figure had dropped to thirty-five and by 1984 it was down to about eleven. Some regions, such as Oxford, had a mortality rate of as low as eight per thousand. It is hard to improve on figures such as these.

As the common former causes of infant mortality – respiratory and gastro-intestinal infection and malnutrition – are brought under control, the emphasis, in reducing the figures still further, swings across to the more specialized services – obstetric and neonatal care, the early identification of severe congenital disorders by antenatal diagnosis and the surgical and other treatment of congenital defects.

In underdeveloped parts of the world, babies continue to die from the many causes which are now largely conquered in the industrialized countries.

infarction

The deprivation of a part of a tissue of its blood supply so that an area of dead tissue (an *infarct*) forms. Any tissue can develop an infarct if its supplying blood vessels become blocked or too narrowed to pass sufficient blood to maintain its vital processes. The type and bulk of the tissue involved determines the gravity of the event.

A myocardial infarction is what happens when a coronary artery thrombosis occurs and this is the real cause of death or

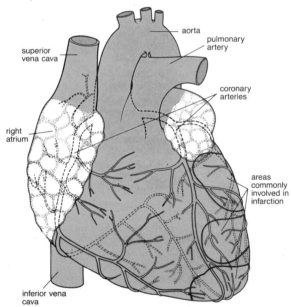

When part of the heart muscle is deprived of its blood supply by coronary artery thrombosis or spasm, it suffers an infarction – an area of tissue death (coagulative necrosis). The size and site of this area determines the seriousness.

disability. An infarction of the brain causes death or a stroke, depending on the area and the size. Infarction of the lung results from a pulmonary embolism.

infectious diseases

Diseases spread directly from person to person. Those requiring the intervention of an insect vector, such as malaria, yellow fever and leishmaniasis, are usually excluded from this group. See also **chickenpox, cholera, diphtheria, food poisoning, gastro-enteritis, glandular fever, Hansen's disease, hepatitis, influenza, measles, meningitis, mumps, plague, poliomyelitis, rubella, sexually transmitted diseases, tuberculosis, tularaemia** and **typhoid fever.**

infectious disease specialist

A doctor concerned with the epidemiology, prevention, diagnosis, management, reporting and administrative arrangements relating to infectious diseases of all kinds.

infectious mononucleosis

See **glandular fever.**

inferior

The term comes from the Latin *inferus* meaning 'below'. In medicine the word is used exclusively to refer to anything lying physically below anything else in the upright body. The bladder is inferior to the brain, but no value judgement is implied.

inferiority complex

This was originally a technical concept introduced by the Austrian psychiatrist Alfred Adler (1870–1937). Adler's initial description was of a group of fears resulting from a perception of one's own bodily defects or shortcomings, which had been repressed and had given rise to a more general sense of inferiority. In common language it became synonymous with a generally self-critical attitude. In this usage, the idea of a *complex* – which, by definition, implies some kind of unconscious mechanism – is lost, and the term simply becomes a more impressive way of referring to feelings of inferiority. Popular psychology has endowed the term with a further significance, and it is now often applied to people who, unconsciously, compensate for feelings of inferiority by behaving in a boastful, self-glorifying manner.

infertility

Most couples who engage in sexual intercourse without contraception at least twice a week can expect to achieve a pregnancy within a few months. Failure to do so after a year is usually regarded as an indication of infertility. This can be doubly distressing because of the frustration of the desire for children and also because of the implication that one or other partner is in some way abnormal. Infertility may be a cause of discord, guilt and unhappiness between partners.

INCIDENCE

In earlier times infertility was invariably attributed to the woman. We now know that in 20 to 25 per cent of cases, the failure to conceive is due to sperm problems in the male. This seems to be on the increase. A major study published in the *British Medical Journal* in September 1992, which reviewed

The labels on the diagram read:
- aorta
- pulmonary artery
- superior vena cava
- coronary arteries
- right atrium
- areas commonly involved in infarction
- inferior vena cava

sixty-one separate research reports published between 1938 and 1990, showed that there had been a genuine decline in sperm quality over the previous fifty years. There had been a decrease in volume of seminal fluid and, more importantly, a significant decrease in sperm density. In 1930, 50 per cent of men had sperm densities of 100 million per ml. By 1990, only 16 per cent had 100 million sperms per ml. The percentage with fewer than 20 million per ml was 6 per cent in 1930, but had risen to 18 per cent in 1990.

POSSIBLE CAUSES

There are, of course, many causes of failure to conceive. These include:

- lack of ovulation at the beginning of the reproductive life;
- lack of ovulation after the menopause;
- failure of ovulation during the normally reproductive years;
- absence of sperms;
- inadequate mobility of sperms;
- an excess of abnormal sperms;
- male impotence;
- ignorance of the elementary facts of life;
- tension and anxiety affecting ovulation;
- penile abnormality;
- severe female malnutrition or strenuous dieting;
- excessive athletic activity;
- anorexia nervosa;
- thyroid gland underactivity;
- poorly controlled diabetes;
- blockage of the Fallopian tubes;
- chronic alcoholism;
- womb fibroids;
- endometriosis;
- cervical mucus hostility to sperms.

INVESTIGATING INFERTILITY

Most of these problems can be overcome. The investigation of infertility begins with sperm analysis to discover if there is a low sperm count, inactive sperms or too many defective types.

The investigation of female infertility involves, among other things, tests of ovulation and of whether the Fallopian tubes are clear. Infrequent ovulation is commoner than absence of ovulation, but may still prevent conception. Irregular, unpredictable and infrequent egg production greatly reduces the chances of the egg and sperm meeting, which is, of course, necessary for fertilization. Many complex hormonal problems – involving the hypothalamus, the pituitary gland, the ovaries and the thyroid gland – can lead to infrequent ovulation or even absence of ovulation. Various tests can be carried out to establish the presence or absence of ovulation. Ovulation failure can be treated with hormones or other drugs that stimulate ovulation, or prevent its inhibition.

Blockage of the Fallopian tubes is almost always the result of infection and inflammation (salpingitis). Sexually transmitted gonorrhoea or chlamydial infection commonly lead to blockage, but infection may also follow the normal delivery of a baby or an abortion. Infection can also be the result of peritonitis from a burst inflamed appendix or of tuberculosis. Tubal blockage prevents the ova from passing along, or even from entering the tube, so that fertilization cannot occur. The state of the Fallopian tubes can be investigated by injecting a harmless dye, methylene blue, through a tube that fits tightly into the cervix. The passage of the dye through the outer open ends of the tubes can be observed through a laparoscope, if the tubes are not blocked. Laparoscopy also allows the tubes to be inspected for visible abnormalities and the ovaries for the presence of a Graafian follicle or a corpus luteum. Alternatively, a solution opaque to X-rays may be injected and an X-ray taken. This will readily show up any obstruction. Tubal blockage can sometimes be treated effectively by microsurgery.

See also **artificial insemination**, *in vitro* **fertilization**.

infestation

The condition of being attacked by parasites. In medicine, the term is usually restricted to animal parasites, such as lice, mites or ticks, on, in or just under the skin, and to worms in the intestine or the body tissues.

infibulation

See **circumcision, female**.

inflamed lid margins

See **blepharitis**.

inflammation

The response of living tissue to injury. The first-century Roman medical writer Aulus Cornelius Celsus, whose book *De Medicina* was printed in 1478, recognized, and recorded, the four 'cardinal signs' of inflammation – *rubor, calor, dolor* and *tumor* – respectively redness, heat, pain and swelling. Later Galen added the feature *functio laesa* meaning 'loss of function'. Inflammation is the commonest of all the disease processes, as is demonstrated by the number of disorders whose names end in *-itis* – a suffix meaning 'inflammation of'.

RECOGNITION AND SYMPTOMS

When a tissue suffers inflammation, its blood vessels widen and the blood flow through it increases markedly. At the same time the cells in the walls of the smallest vessels, the capillaries, separate sufficiently to allow protein molecules in the blood, including antibodies, to pass out. This leads to a protein-rich exudate in the inflamed area. White cells also emigrate from the blood vessels by squeezing through these tiny openings and proceed to investigate, and try to deal with, the cause of the inflammation. These effects account for the redness, heat and swelling. We now know that the pain is caused by the release, from damaged cells, of substances called prostaglandins, which are very strongly stimulating to pain nerve endings.

POSSIBLE CAUSES

Inflammation can be caused by many factors, of which the commonest are the toxins released by bacteria and other organisms in the course of infection. But it may result from any kind of injury, such as a blow or a cut, damage from chemical, radiational or heat energy, or even from the body's own immunological processes as in hypersensitivity reactions (allergy) or auto-immune disease.

RISKS

Inflammation is, in general, protective and leads to a return to normality. But it is not always so. It may become persistent (chronic), lasting for weeks or months, and may lead to the formation of scar tissue which may have undesirable effects.

inflammation of tip of penis

See **balanitis**.

influenza

This disease was well-known in fifteenth-century Florence when it was attributed to cosmic influences and entitled *La Influenza*. Hence the name. Influenza, popularly described as flu, is, however, caused by a virus of the *Orthomyxoviridae* family, and is spread mainly by virus-contaminated droplets coughed and sneezed by sufferers. It is highly infectious to those who are susceptible. It spreads rapidly through closed communities and in the general population, and tends to occur in epidemics during winter. Each year it causes a significant mortality, especially among the elderly and the infirm.

TYPES OF FLU

The *Orthomyxoviridae* contain three main types, distinguishable by antibody tests (serotypes) – A, B and C. Type B is the main cause of influenza. Unfortunately, a single attack does not confer complete immunity against influenza, but only against the particular serotype, and these are known to mutate in time. Type A, in particular, is very liable to mutation and is constantly producing varieties to which populations have no resistance. It is for this reason that widespread epidemics, affecting whole continents (pandemics), occur. These are caused by new strains of type A virus. Type C virus is very stable and an attack appears to confer life-long immunity. Pandemics occurred in 1890, 1918 ('Spanish flu'), 1957 ('Asian flu'), 1968 ('Hong Kong flu') and 1977 ('Russian flu').

RECOGNITION AND SYMPTOMS

Influenza is an infectious disease of the upper air passages (upper respiratory tract) featuring fever, sore throat, running nose, a dry unproductive cough, headache, backache, general muscle pains, loss of appetite, insomnia and prostration. In most cases the acute symptoms settle after about four days and then gradually disappear.

RISKS

Complications include high fever, sometimes **hyperpyrexia**, **bronchitis**, **pneumonia**, **Reye's syndrome** and sudden death.

TREATMENT

The drug amantadine has some action against influenza viruses but, in most cases, treatment is confined to general measures to alleviate symptoms and the management of complications. Antibiotics have no effect on the viruses, but may be necessary to control secondary respiratory infection, especially pneumonia.

Anti-influenza vaccines, against recent types of A and B virus, are available but are not wholly effective. The injection must be given each year, before the start of the influenza season. Vaccination is, nevertheless, highly desirable, especially for old people.

informed consent

See **ethics, medical**.

infra-

Prefix meaning 'under' as in inferior (below).

infusion, intravenous

Commonly known as a 'drip', an intravenous infusion is the introduction into the circulating blood, by way of a vein, of any fluid, for any purpose. The correction of deficiencies in the blood, whether of volume or constituent, is a major, and often life-saving element in modern medicine and there are innumerable conditions in which this is one of the primary therapeutic procedures. Intravenous infusion is used to:

- correct blood loss;
- treat surgical shock;
- replace deficiencies of substances such as sodium, chloride and potassium;
- neutralize acidity of the blood;
- maintain the blood's ability to retain fluid (osmotic pressure);
- provide nourishment and sometimes total nutrition;
- restore the clotting power of the blood.

Fluids used include saline (sodium chloride) solutions, Dextran solution, dextrose solution, lactic acid solution, potassium chloride solution, gelatin solution, bicarbonate solution and a variety of mixtures, such as Ringer's and Hartmann's solution. Various drugs, especially antibiotics, are often added to the intravenous solution for rapidity of action, and this may be the justification for setting up the infusion.

ingestion

The process of introducing food or other material into the stomach. Ingestion is followed by digestion, and then absorption and, finally, assimilation.

ingrown toenail

An inaccurate term referring to inflammation of the soft tissues surrounding the nail, following infection. This leads to much local swelling and the production of exuberant inflamed tissue which overlaps the edge of the nail causing an appearance as if the nail had grown into the tissue. In fact, the growth of the nail is quite normal.

The condition results mainly from neglect of the feet, allowing infection to occur around the edge of the nail. The infection is sometimes introduced when the skin at the corner of the nail edge is carelessly cut while the nails are being trimmed. Unsuitable footwear can also contribute by causing undue pressure on the sides of the toes.

Measures to avoid this common annoyance include improved standards of personal foot hygiene, daily washing and powdering, daily change of socks and cutting the nails straight across. If the condition has gone too far, a minor operation may be necessary, in which the edge of the nail is removed and local antibiotics applied. This will be to no avail, however, if proper standards of foot care are not also adopted.

inguinal

Relating to the groin.

inhalers

These have become increasingly important as a means of delivering medication, especially in the treatment of diseases of the bronchial tubes and lungs. *Asthma* is the principle disease treated in this way. Inhalers can produce aerosols of liquid solution or may deliver measured doses in powder form, and the contents may be propelled by gas under pres-

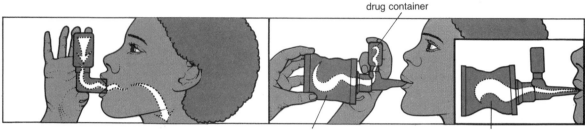

drug container

metred dose of
drug in reservoir bag

bag deflates
as drug is taken

Inhalers. Proper instruction in the use of inhalers is essential if they are to be effective. Different types need different techniques to ensure that the medication is carried into the lungs while breathing in and not simply deposited in the mouth.

sure or may be breath-activated. Drugs commonly taken in this way, include corticosteroids to combat the allergic and inflammatory responses and bronchodilators to widen the air tubes.

The use of inhalers has the notable advantage over treatment by mouth or injection that the drug is delivered directly to the point of action and that, in consequence, a much smaller dose is needed. There is then less likelihood of general side-effects.

> Studies have shown that many patients using inhalers have never been shown how to do so and merely deposit the medication in their mouths. More seriously, many asthmatics do not appreciate that failure to obtain relief from a bronchodilator inhaler means that the asthma has entered a dangerous refractory state and that more powerful treatment, such as with steroids, is urgently needed.

inheritance

See **genetics**.

injection

The introduction of medication into the body by means of a hollow needle and a syringe. Drugs given in this way are usually those which would be destroyed or rendered ineffective if acted on by the digestive system after being taken by mouth. Injections may be made into the thickness of the skin (intradermal), under the skin (subcutaneous or hypodermic), into a muscle (intramuscular) or directly into the blood in a vein (intravenous). The latter route is used if rapid action is needed or if the drug is so irritating that it would damage tissue. Irritating substances are give by very slow intravenous injection so that the flowing blood dilutes them.

injury, accidental

This is a major cause of death and disablement, especially in people below forty. In developed parts of the world, accidents, such as falls from heights, car and motorcycle crashes, burns and drowning, account for well over half of all deaths of people under twenty. In addition to the deaths, these accidents lead to an enormous amount of long-term suffering and loss of life prospect, especially in the case of head injury. Hundreds of thousands of young men owe life-long dependency, grave permanent mental loss and a wheelchair existence to unimaginative and unskilled use of motorcycles. Clearly, few of these have any idea of the dangers, to the unprotected and unsecured human body, of high speeds.

Accidents in the home, especially falls, take a major toll of the life and health of the elderly, accounting, in those over seventy-five, for about twice as many deaths as do road accidents. In many of these cases, bone fragility from **osteoporosis** leads to fractures of the hip or spine, leading to immobilization, decline in health, infection and death. Drowning, accidental poisoning and burns are other major causes of death or serious disablement.

The great majority of accidents are preventable by the exercise of foresight and by a systematic policy of risk reduction. Dangerous equipment should be repaired or replaced, slippery surfaces corrected, carpets and rugs secured, electrical devices made safe, sharp objects and poisonous substances properly stored or disposed of, fires guarded and dangerous forms of cooking over open flames avoided.

injury, psychological effects of

Major injury often has a devastating effect on the life of the victim, and sometimes on the lives of his or her relatives. This occurs with any form of injury, but is especially common after head injury, even if there has been no actual skull fracture.

Disability, real or perceived, leads to depression, bitterness and resentment. There is often a dwelling on the cause of the injury or on the person or agency perceived to have been responsible for it. Thoughts turn to compensation and then to litigation and this often becomes a central preoccupation, to the exclusion of all other considerations. It becomes impossible to take a detached and balanced view of the matter and unalterable polarization of opinion results.

There is good evidence that recovery may be severely prejudiced by failure of adequate financial compensation. Some people who might have made a good recovery and returned to normal life, have, instead, been turned into lifelong, and very unhappy, invalids by the operation of this unfortunate process. It has been shown that if the affected person fails to return to work before litigation is settled, the long-term outlook is usually poor.

ink blot test

Any of several psychological tests in which the subject is asked to interpret a random-shape pattern produced by folding a sheet of paper over a large ink-blot, revealing, thereby, it was hoped, hidden aspects of the personality. The best known is the Rorschach test.

At one time, ink-blot testing was popular and widely used and, as is characteristic of such intriguing and plausible-seeming proposals, generated a library of publications. The idea caught the lay imagination, too, and there was wide general belief that, by this means, psychologists were able to penetrate the mysteries of the human psyche.

In spite of all the learned papers, however, no real evidence was ever produced that this technique was, in itself, of any real value, except as a vehicle of interaction between patient and analyst. Like so many *psychotherapeutic* techniques, the results obtained would seem to depend on the quality of the mind of the therapist rather than in any inherent property of the process.

Innohep

A brand name for **tinzaparin**.

Innovace

A brand name for **enalapril**.

Innozide

A brand name for enalapril in conjunction with **hydrochlorothiazide**.

inoculation

Vaccination. The procedure by which the body's immune system is stimulated into producing a stock of protective antibodies to specific infective agents, such as viruses and bacteria.

See **immunization**.

inoperable

A disease, normally treated by surgery, which has progressed to the stage beyond which surgery is feasible. The term is most commonly applied to cancer which has spread so widely that its surgical removal would be likely to have fatal consequences. In such cases, treatment with radiation or chemotherapy can sometimes help.

Inosine pranobex

Isoprinosine. An antiviral drug used to treat oral and genital herpes and genital warts. The drug also enhances the efficiency of the immune system by increasing the number of T cells and enhancing the activity of natural killer cells. A brand name is Imunovir.

inositol nicotinate

A nicotinic acid derivative that is used to treat disorders such as **Raynaud's disease** that involve arterial spasm. A brand name is Hexopal.

inotropic agents

Drugs that increase the force of contraction of the heart and whose use is normally limited to cases of heart failure. They include adrenaline, noradrenaline, phosphodiesterase inhibitors, digitalis derivatives and dopamine. The safe and effective use of these drugs calls for great skill and knowledge and is generally confined to cardiologists.

insania

Latin root meaning 'madness' as in insanity (legally mad).

insanity

An imprecise term, little used in medicine. However, it has legal meaning. In ordinary speech it is equated with 'madness', 'lunacy' or 'unsoundness of mind' – all equally vague of definition. In medicine, the nearest equivalent would be psychosis, which has been defined as the inability to distinguish reality from fantasy, with impaired objective evaluation and judgement of the world outside the self, and creation of a new reality.

LEGAL INSANITY

Legal insanity is defined by the McNaughten rules. These were formulated by judges after the trial in 1843 of Daniel McNaughten, who intended to kill the Prime Minister Sir Robert Peel, but killed his private secretary Edward Drummond by mistake. McNaughten was suffering under the delusion that the government was persecuting him. The central point at issue, however, was not whether or not this was true but whether, at the time of the crime, McNaughten was responsible for his actions. The matter went to the House of Lords and the 'McNaughten Rules' were enshrined in law.

According to these rules, defendants must show that they are suffering from a 'defect of reason' arising from a 'disease of the mind', and that as a result of this they did not know what they were doing at the material time, or that, if they did know what they were doing, they did not know that it was wrong. A defendant suffering from an insane delusion is treated as if the delusion were true. If, for example, a man were to cut off another man's head under the insane belief that he was cutting through a loaf of bread, he could be acquitted of murder, since cutting a loaf of bread is a legal act. Similarly, he could be acquitted of murder if he had the insane delusion that he was acting in self-defence, as this is a defence. McNaughten was acquitted on the grounds of insanity, and, although the rules have been repeatedly criticized as inadequate, nothing better has yet been produced.

insect and mite bites and stings

Most bites from midges, mosquitoes and fleas cause little trouble apart from the annoying irritation and an occasional allergic reaction. Dog and cat fleas populate domestic areas where the animal commonly lies, and may jump on to human beings to suck blood. They usually cause bites in clusters, often in areas of skin in close contact with clothing. These can cause persistent itching. More severe reactions can arise from harvest mites and grain mites. Sandflies can cause severe and persistent skin spots, and it should be remembered that these may be due to **leishmaniasis**. The common skin mite of **scabies** burrows into the skin to lay her eggs and these hatch into larvae in a few days, causing such intense itching that the burrows are often obscured by scratching. Severe itching is also a feature of infestation with lice.

All these reactions are allergic in nature and are a response to the injection of foreign matter in the form of saliva or other material from the insect's proboscis or to insect faeces or body tissues which may be inoculated into the skin by scratching. Although scratching may seem irresistible, it should be avoided, if possible, and the itching relieved by application of a soothing lotion.

SPIDERS

Spiders are almost all harmless in Europe although, occasionally, a dangerous species is transported in a consignment of fruit. The European tarantula causes a painful, but not dangerous, bite. In some non-European countries, one may, rarely, encounter venomous spiders capable of injecting a neurotoxin which can be fatal to the infirm or the very young. These include the 'black widow' and *Atrax* species of Australia.

INSECTS

A few insects, such as bees, wasps and hornets, are capable of stinging and will do so if provoked. In these cases venom is injected into the skin from a sting sac situated at the end of the insect's abdomen. This contains intensely irritating material which causes inflammation in the surrounding skin for about two days. The risk to life is small unless a very large number of stings are received simultaneously or a sting occurs in or around the voice box (larynx) and causes such swelling that the airway is cut off. Human hypersensitivity to insect venom is fairly common and a second sting, months or years after the first, may provoke a severe and sometimes fatal reaction.

> A bee sting sac left in the skin should be carefully scraped off with a knife blade or the edge of a credit card. Grasping with tweezers or the fingernails may inject more venom from the sac. A cold local application may ease the discomfort and an analgesic drug, such as paracetamol, may be taken.

insects and disease

See **fleas**, **flies**.

insecurity

A sense of insecurity affects us all from time to time, and may involve almost any aspect of living – physical, social, spiritual or financial. Insecurity is unpleasant and induces anxiety, and this is a potent source of physical and mental disorder. Some psychologists believe that feelings of insecurity are the basic cause of all neuroses. But feelings of insecurity can also have positive effects and have often been responsible for great creative effort.

insertion mutation

A mutation caused by the insertion into a DNA sequence of one or more nucleotides.

insight

Self-awareness or self-understanding. People suffering from neurotic illnesses usually have considerable insight about their condition, although this seldom enables them to do anything about it. People suffering from psychotic illnesses are not thought to have insight. In psychoanalysis, a distinction is made between 'intellectual insight' and 'emotional insight'. The former is regarded as a form of defence mechanism, used to prevent progress to deeper and less pleasant levels of awareness; the latter is believed to be essential for effective treatment.

insomnia

Difficulty in sleeping, or disturbances of the normal sleep pattern. Insomnia is a very common complaint, but many people are unaware of the wide individual variation in sleep requirements and of the often greatly reduced sleep needs of elderly people. There is no reason to believe that shorter sleep periods are in any way harmful.

POSSIBLE CAUSES

Difficulty in falling asleep is often caused by worry or tension, while early waking, with difficulty in getting off again, tends to be a feature of depression or advancing age. A tendency to lie awake for what seems like hours, unable to relax or allow oneself to drift off to sleep, is often due to tension caused by business, personal, marital or other worries.

> Concerns of every nature are likely to seem insoluble, especially in the middle of the night, but the proper approach is to try to resolve them during waking hours and to conform to the rule that they are not to be entertained during the night. Practised, formal relaxation exercises can also be very helpful. The avoidance of high caffeine intake, in the evening, from tea or coffee, will also help.

People who fall asleep easily enough, but wake repeatedly, may be so exhausted that they go to bed too early, and then awake naturally in the early morning, having had enough sleep.

Some people sedate themselves with alcohol every night. This gets them off to sleep quite well, but, as the effect is often short-lived, they often wake early. Depression is a common cause of interrupted and restless sleep and often features early waking. Pain is another cause, as is the attempt to give up sleeping tablets to which tolerance has been acquired.

TREATMENT

When the insomnia is clearly due to any such cause, the right treatment is to deal with the cause. People who go to bed exhausted may need a short nap in the middle of the day. This can be invaluable.

Depression caused by external misfortune or bereavement will nearly always pass in time, but some depressions require skilled treatment. Pain should be fully investigated and the cause removed, if possible. If this cannot be done, the right approach is to relieve the pain with analgesic drugs, rather than to take sleeping pills.

> Sleep-inducing drugs were once prescribed in great quantity, possibly because doctors did not have time to go into the reasons for the insomnia. It is now widely recognized that they are not the real solution for problems of this kind. In selected cases, there is justification for the use of hypnotic drugs, given in the hope that the patient may, thereby, get back into the habit of normal sleeping. But taking sleeping pills over long periods is bad medicine. Addiction is likely and withdrawal problems inevitable. Tolerance soon develops and the dose will have to be increased steadily to achieve the same effect.

instinct

The American philosopher and pioneer of psychology William James (1842–1910), in his influential work *Principles of Psychology*, published in 1890, defined instinct as 'The faculty of acting in such a way as to produce certain ends without knowledge of the ends, without foresight of ends and without previous education in the performance.' Nowadays instincts are usually defined as 'fixed action patterns' or 'stereotyped complex behaviour shown by all members of a species, independently of the experience of the individual'.

The computer analogy might be helpful. The instincts could be understood as the result of the operation of the hardware (the neuro-anatomy) which is, of course, common to all members of a species, while learned behaviour could be understood as the result of the operation of the software, or programming, which is acquired after birth, via the many ports of sensory input. Instinctive responses are essential for survival and none of us could function without them, any more than a computer could operate without its operating system.

The physical basis for the instincts is hard-wired into the brain and, although much subtler in organization, is as much a part of our anatomy as the nerve tracts which subserve walking. In a sense, instincts are simply the way the nervous system operates. They are all triggered off by sensory input of one kind or another, and, because the hardware is basically the same in all of us, the effects are, broadly, the same. Instinctive responses can, of course, be inhibited by later programming, and much of social activity, consists in the complex interplay of instinctive responses modified by education.

The history of attitudes to the instincts is interesting. Theologians have equated much of instinctual behaviour with *original sin*. Freudian psychoanalysts believe in a mysterious entity known as the *id*. Modern insights into the structure and functioning of the nervous system have made it clear that all behaviour, instinctive or learned, has an organic basis.

insulin

A peptide hormone produced in the beta cells of the Islets of Langerhans in the pancreas. Insulin facilitates and accelerates the movement of glucose and amino acids across cell membranes. It also controls the activity of certain enzymes within the cells concerned with carbohydrate, fat and protein metabolism. Insulin production is regulated by constant monitoring of the blood glucose levels by the beta cells. Deficiency of insulin causes diabetes. Insulin preparations may be in the 'soluble' form for immediate action or in a 'retard' form for prolonged action or as mixtures of these. Most insulins for medical use are now produced by recombinant DNA methods (genetic engineering) and are identical to human insulin. Bovine and porcine insulins are still used. Brand names include Human Actrapid, Human Insulatard, Human Mixtard, Human Monotard, Human Ultratard, Human Velosulin, Humulin I, Humulin Lente, Humulin M, Humulin S, Humulin Zn, Hypurin Bovine Isophane, Hypurin Bovine Lente, Hypurin Bovine Neutral, Hypurin Bovine PZI, Hypurin Porcine Biphasic Isophane, Hypurin Porcione Neutral, Lentard MC, Pork Insulatard, Pork Mixtard and Pork Velosulin.

See **diabetes**.

insulin failure

See **insulin resistance syndrome**.

insulin lispro

Very rapidly acting **insulin**. A brand name is Humalog.

insulinoma

A rare tumour of the insulin-producing cells of the pancreas, which, although non-malignant, may have dangerous consequences. The insulinoma can produce quantities of insulin out of all proportion to those needed to control blood sugar, and the result is a sharp lowering of the sugar level to a point at which the brain's function is affected. This is called **hypoglycaemia**.

> If hypoglycaemia persists it may lead to severe disturbance of brain function, permanent brain damage, coma or even death. The emergency treatment is to give sugar by mouth or, in urgent cases, by injection or intravenous infusion. Definitive treatment is by surgical removal of the tumour.

insulin resistance syndrome

A state in which normal levels of insulin in the blood fail to have the normal controlling effect on the levels of blood sugar. As a result, excess insulin is produced by the normal feedback mechanism, but in spite of this the blood sugar levels may be normal or even raised. Insulin resistance is commonly associated with type II **diabetes** (non-insulin dependent diabetes mellitus), obesity and high blood pressure. It may be worsened by various drugs including corticosteroids, beta-blockers, and high dosage of thiazide diuretics.

Intal

A brand name for **sodium cromoglycate**.

integrins

A family of linked polypeptide chains, alpha and beta, that mediate interactions between cells and their immediate surrounding environment (the extracellular matrix) and between cells and other cells. Integrins are expressed on endothelial and other cells and platelets, and act as receptors for the clotting protein fibrinogen, the extracellular linking glycoprotein fibronectin, and various other extracellular clotting factors such as thrombospondin and von Willebrand factor. See also **disintegrins**.

intelligence

This has been defined in various ways. Some writers have despaired of definition and described intelligence as 'that which intelligence tests measure'. However profoundly this may comment on the supposed difficulty of defining it, the concept of intelligence is too important to be side-stepped in this way. There is considerable agreement that intelligence should be taken to consist of a group of separate, but correlated, abilities, each of which can be present to a varying degree. These abilities include memory, the speed with which relationships can be perceived, verbal skills, numerical skills and visuo-spatial perception. Few now believe that there is any single entity which may be described as raw, undifferentiated intelligence.

INHERITED OR CREATED?

Many pedigree studies of families noted for high intelligence, and of those noted for low, have suggested that intelligence is largely inherited. Critics of this view have pointed out that intelligence is largely judged by assessing verbal facility and that, since this is environmentally available to one group and not the other, intelligence, whatever it is, may be wholly the result of environmental influences. But studies have shown that identical twins (who have identical genetics) brought up in different families are more alike than non-identical twins (with different genetics) reared in the same family.

There is no denying the importance of environmental influences, but it seems likely that genes matter more. Various estimates of the relative importance of inheritance over postnatal programming have been made, and some are as high as four to one in favour of inheritance.

THE MATURATION OF INTELLIGENCE

Jean Piaget (1896–1980) postulated that intelligence matures in observable, age-related stages, progressing from the earliest perception of sense input and movement, through stages in which a sense of the permanence of objects and of how they fit into groups is established, to the levels of conceptualization and then, finally, abstract thought. Although these stages are not universally agreed, Piaget has been very influential. In particular, most psychologists now agree with his view that the development of intelligence is the result of a dynamic and never-ceasing interaction between the child's very general and unrefined information-processing capacity, and its environment.

PHYSIOLOGICAL CONCERNS

There is no discrete part of the brain which can be said to be the site of intelligence and it is clear from the study of neurological disease that intelligence is a function of the brain as a whole. Local damage to brain matter in certain areas results in loss of specific functions, such as speech or speech comprehension, but does not, in itself, diminish intelligence. But if the general loss of brain substance exceeds about 50 ml, there is a reduction in the speed of mental functions and impairment of reasoning power. Abstract reasoning power is affected adversely if the nerve connections between the frontal lobes and other parts of the brain are damaged. In **Alzheimer's disease** and alcoholic brain damage, the general loss of brain substance is associated with progressive loss of mental function (dementia).

intelligence quotient

The term 'intelligence quotient' (IQ) was introduced by the little-known German psychologist Wilhelm Stern and popularized by Louis Terman (1877–1956), at Stanford University, in 1916. The IQ is obtained by dividing the mental age, as derived from various tests, by the chronological age, and multiplying the result by one hundred. Terman adapted the test formulated by the French psychologist Alfred Binet (1857–1911), which, ever since has been known as the Stanford-Binet test. Current versions of this test include sections for every age level, from two to twenty. There are six items for each test at each age, selected to be appropriate to the age. The examiner starts by determining the level at which all are answered correctly and then presents tests of increasing difficulty until none can be solved.

HOW THEY'RE DONE

Tests for young children involve making copies of simple pictures, putting shapes in appropriate holes, stringing beads and answering questions about everyday objects or activities. Older subjects may be required to identify absurdities in pictures; indicate which pairs of words from a list have some-

thing in common; pair off abstract shapes; predict a symbol complex by identifying sequential patterns of arrangement, and so on. The Wechsler tests include two separate scales for assessment of verbal and non-verbal tasks. This range of tests has now largely replaced the earlier Stanford-Binet series but there are many different kinds of tests designed to assess different aspects of intelligence.

THE DISTRIBUTION OF INTELLIGENCE

The IQ increases with age up to about eighteen, remains fairly static during most of adult life and then, in some people, declines with age. Intelligence, as measured by IQ tests, is distributed, in the population, in accordance with the standard Gaussian distribution curve. This means that there are as many low-scoring people as there are high-scoring people. About 68 per cent of the population have an IQ of between 85 and 110, and 95 per cent have an IQ between 70 and 130.

intensive care

Patients in a critical or unstable condition are liable to die suddenly unless certain danger signs are detected early and appropriate action taken. The dangers include:

- a border-line oxygen supply to the tissues;
- a tendency for the heart to stop beating or to pass into a rapidly fatal state of disorganized twitching;
- a tendency to pass into severe, sustained spasm of the breathing tubes (status asthmaticus);
- a tendency towards changes in the biochemical constitution of the blood;
- severe toxic conditions.

Many such people, if left in a general ward or in their own homes, might well die before appropriate action could be taken to deal with these changes. For this reason, hospitals set up special intensive care departments. These are equipped with all the necessary **monitoring** devices, so that continual surveillance may be maintained, and with all the necessary means of treatment immediately to hand, so that remedial measures may be taken with minimum delay. The ratio of staff to patient is much higher than in any other ward, and the concentration of equipment is also higher.

Highly trained nurses maintain a constant watch on electrocardiogram monitors, automatic blood pressure monitors and pulse and respiration monitors. They check the functioning of positive pressure respirators which are inflating the lungs through tracheostomy tubes; maintain real-time surveillance on blood levels of various substances; and obtain, at intervals, test results from the laboratory. They check physical signs, such as temperature, respiratory rate, pupil reactions and response to stimuli.

Intensive care staff are trained not only to recognize the signals of danger, but to respond to them immediately. They are experienced in diagnosing types of heart stoppage (cardiac arrest) and of applying shock treatment (defibrillation) when appropriate. They are skilled in artificial ventilation and in the emergency use of certain drugs.

Numerous lives have been saved by keeping patients in intensive care units until their condition has improved and stabilized. Intensive care facilities are often given to surgical patients in the immediate post-operative period.

inter-

Prefix meaning 'between' as in intercostal (between the ribs).

intercostal

Between the ribs.

intercourse, painful

See **dyspareunia**.

interferon alfa

An interferon class containing at least 15 functional proteins some of which are used as drugs to treat secondary (metastatic) kidney cancers, chronic myeloid leukaemia, hairy-cell leukaemia, hepatitis B and C, genital warts and AIDS-related Kaposi's sarcoma. Trade names are Intron A, Roferon-A, Viraferon and Wellferon.

interferon beta

An interferon used as a drug to reduce the severity and frequency of relapses of multiple sclerosis. Unfortunately, there is little clear evidence that this interferon can affect the long-term outcome. In addition, it may cause an influenza-like effect for several months after starting treatment. Trade names are Avonex, Betaferon and Rebif.

interferons

These are natural products of the body, produced by cells which have been invaded, and destroyed, by viruses. The reproduction of viruses inside a cell commonly leads to its rupture and this is accompanied by the release of tiny quantities of these powerful chemical substances. Interferons pass to other cells, causing them to arm themselves against invasion, not only by the original virus, but also by any other infecting organism. They also modify various cell-regulating mechanisms and slow down the growth of cancers.

FUNCTION

Interferons have proved successful in the treatment of various conditions including Kaposi's sarcoma, the common cold, Herpes simplex infections, genital warts and an uncommon form of leukaemia, hairy-cell leukaemia.

SIDE-EFFECTS

When injected, interferons cause influenza-like symptoms, possibly because the symptoms of natural flu are caused by interferon release.

TREATMENT POTENTIAL

Genetic engineering techniques are used to produce interferons and, as they become more widely available at lower cost, their full treatment potential may become apparent.

interferon gamma

An **interferon** used as an antiviral drug. A brand name is Immukin.

interleukins

A range of messengers between cells (**cytokines**) secreted by white cells of the immune system. Recipient effector cells have surface receptors for the various interleukins. Interleukins perform many functions. These include:

- action on lymphocytes to increase their ability to respond to antigens;
- resetting the temperature-regulating mechanism at a higher level and thus causing fever;
- promoting the absorption of bone;
- stimulating clonal T cell and B cell division and proliferation;
- activation of natural killer T cells;
- promoting the growth and differentiation of blood-forming cells and the growth of mast cells;
- assisting in the proliferation of activated B cells and eosinophil cells and in the production of IgM and IgA (See **Ig**);
- causing chemotaxis of T cells and polymorph phagocytes;
- promoting the growth and proliferation of T cells;
- inhibiting gamma-interferon secretion and mononuclear cell inflammation.

intermittent claudication

A sudden pain in the leg muscles, often in the calf, associated with temporary loss of the normal power of contraction and a consequent inability to walk.

POSSIBLE CAUSES

Intermittent claudication is caused by an inadequacy in the blood supply to the muscles from narrowing disease of the arteries, usually **atherosclerosis**, and occurs after the affected person walks for a certain, often constant, distance. There is a build-up of waste products in the muscles and these pain-causing substances cannot be dispersed quickly enough. The process is almost identical to that causing **angina pectoris** and there is the same relationship to the amount of exertion. As the arterial disease process worsens, the symptoms come on after walking shorter distances.

> Intermittent claudication is a clear indication that medical attention is required and that the state of the entire cardiovascular system should be investigated.

TREATMENT

Recent evidence suggests that the performance can be improved by deliberately 'walking through claudication'. This does not mean that one should continue to try to walk in spite of the pain, but that one should resume walking as soon as the pain has gone. People with intermittent claudication are advised to walk for an hour every day, and it has been found that those who do so are usually able to walk a progressively greater distance before the pain comes on. The term is derived from the Latin verb *claudicare*, 'to be lame or limping' and immortalized in the name of Claudius, Emperor of Rome, whose limping gait and tendency to stop walking and grimace, as if in pain, must have closely resembled a man with leg artery occlusive disease.

Internet addiction

Compulsive overuse of the personal computer to play Internet games, use chat forums, or to surf the World Wide Web on the Internet. The disorder features loss of control, increased tolerance and typical addictive withdrawal symptoms on deprivation. The full syndrome is said to affect about one Internet user in 400 and features social withdrawal and sometimes low self-esteem, social phobia, depression and attention deficit disorder. Many psychiatrists have questioned the existence of this form of addiction, but the evidence for it appears to be growing.

intersex

A person with bodily characteristics of both man and woman. See **hermaphroditism**.

interstitial pulmonary fibrosis

A serious lung disease in which the normal fine structure is gradually replaced by a homogeneous deposition of fine scar tissue (fibrosis). This severely interferes with the normal passage of oxygen from the air to the blood and with the outflow of carbon dioxide.

POSSIBLE CAUSES

The condition may be caused by chronic irritation from chemical fumes or industrial dusts, but is more usually the result of an unknown process, probably of an auto-immune nature.

RECOGNITION AND SYMPTOMS

There is progressive breathlessness, pain in the chest, cough and clubbing of the fingers, and X-ray shows the typical appearance of widespread fibrosis.

TREATMENT

Treatment may be of little avail if the condition is well advanced, but, in the early stages, treatment directed at the immunological disorder, with immunosuppressive drugs such as azathioprine, can be effective.

intertrigo

An **eczema** occurring in areas where skin surfaces come into contact with each other. This is especially common in obese people and may occur under the breasts, between the buttocks, between the thighs, or even where abdominal fat folds hang down. The resulting moistness from sweat, and the irritation to the skin from rubbing, encourage infection with bacteria and, especially, yeasts (thrush) and these areas may become severely inflamed and damaged.

Intertrigo is difficult to treat, but responds to loss of weight and scrupulous attention to washing and to the care of the skin in the intertriginous areas.

intestinal function deficit

See **gut failure**.

intestinal nerves

See **enteric nervous system**.

intestine

See **oesophagus**, **stomach**, **small intestine**, **large intestine**.

intestine, obstruction of

This may occur in a number of ways. The bowel may become:

- twisted (volvulus);
- strangulated by its own swelling if stuck in a hernia;
- 'telescoped' into itself (intussusception);
- blocked by impacted faeces, especially in the elderly;
- blocked by an internal tumour;
- blocked by a tumour encircling the bowel wall;
- obstructed by a failure of the normal mechanism (peristalsis) which carries the contents along (ileus, adynamic).

Intestinal obstruction may even be present at birth (congenital) as a result of a narrowing at the outlet of the stomach, or of a failure of part of the bowel to form a tube.

RECOGNITION AND SYMPTOMS

Obstruction causes pain in the abdomen which repeatedly rises to a peak and then subsides (colic) as the bowel stretches in trying to overcome the obstruction. Gas forms in the intestine and may cause distention. There may be a visible 'ladder' pattern on the wall of the abdomen caused by prominent loops of small bowel. If the obstruction is near the upper end of the intestine, vomiting occurs early and is bile-stained. Lower obstruction may not cause vomiting. Once the rectum is emptied there is total constipation.

> There must be no delay in seeking medical advice, so that prompt diagnosis and surgical treatment may be given before serious complications occur.

TREATMENT

An operation will be designed to remove the cause of the obstruction and restore normal bowel function. This may involve removing a loop of bowel, and a colostomy or ileostomy.

intestine, tumours of

Benign tumours of the intestine, such as polyps and smooth muscle tumours, cause little trouble. Occasionally, a polyp is pushed along by peristalsis to cause a 'telescoping' of the bowel (an intussusception). Malignant tumours are important and are usually confined to the stomach, colon and rectum. Cancers of the colon are among the commonest of all cancers and, with lung cancer, are the commonest to affect both sexes.

A rare malignant tumour of the small intestine or appendix is the carcinoid tumour, which arises from cells which secrete a powerful neuro-transmitter called serotonin. These tumours secrete large quantities of this substance and cause

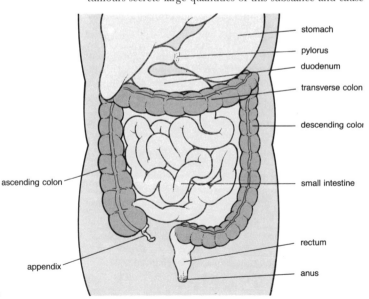

The intestines.

Ways in which the intestine can become obstructed. It would be an unfortunate patient who suffered more than one of these conditons.

alarming flushing, diarrhoea, tightness of the breathing tubes and sometimes heart disorder. Unfortunately, carcinoid tumours spread early to other parts of the body, and about one-third have done so by the time symptoms start.

intoxication

The action of a poison of any kind on an organism. From the Latin *intoxicare*, meaning to smear with poison.

intra-

Prefix meaning 'within' as in intravenous (in a vein).

intracerebral haemorrhage

Bleeding inside the brain, usually from a small artery damaged by atherosclerosis, but sometimes from injury or the rupture of a pre-existing aneurysm. Such bleeding is always serious and usually causes loss of function as a result of damage to brain tissue. Intracerebral haemorrhage is a common cause of stroke.

intractable

Resistant to cure.

intracytoplasmic sperm injection

A method of *in vitro* fertilization (IVF), introduced in 1993, in which a single spermatozoon is injected directly into an ovum, which is then implanted into the womb. The method allows women to become pregnant by partners who may be totally sterile as a result of low sperm counts, poor sperm mobility or even absence of sperms (azoospermia). Anxieties that the method may result in an unacceptably high number of defective babies seem to have been exaggerated. There are indications, however, that there is an increased risk of mild delays in development at one year in babies produced by this method of fertilization. There is also some concern that solitary sperms obtained from an infertile man may carry genes for infertility.

intramuscular

Within a muscle. An intramuscular injection is one in which the needle passes deeply into the substance of a muscle – often in the buttock – before the fluid is injected. Intramuscular injections of a drug usually take effect more rapidly than when the drug is taken by mouth, but less rapidly than when it is given by intravenous injection.

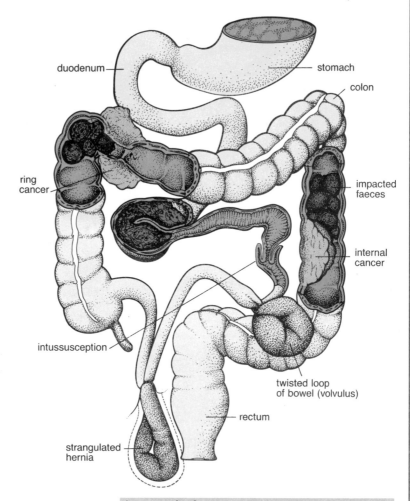

duodenum — stomach — colon — ring cancer — impacted faeces — internal cancer — intussusception — twisted loop of bowel (volvulus) — rectum — strangulated hernia

intra-ocular lenses

Implantable, rigid, or flexible and folding, plastic optical lenses that are placed in the empty lens capsular bag after the opaque natural lens material (the cataract) has been removed either by emulsification or extrusion, and washout. Loss of the natural lens defocuses the eye markedly and additional optical power averaging 15 dioptres is required. This can readily be provided by an intra-ocular lens. Foldable lenses allow the whole cataract operation to be performed through a very short incision that requires no stitching.

intra-ocular pressure

The fluid pressure within the eye necessary to maintain its shape and allow proper optical functioning. Aqueous humour, which is almost pure water, is secreted continuously within the eyeball, and escapes through a filter meshwork just in front of the root of the iris. This filter offers resistance to outflow so that pressure is maintained within the eye. In health, an accurate balance between the rate of aqueous production and the rate of outflow maintains the pressure within narrow limits. Any increase in outflow resistance will cause a rise in the intraocular pressure and this is always dangerous, as the pressure may exceed the blood pressure in some of the small internal blood vessels, so that they collapse and shut off

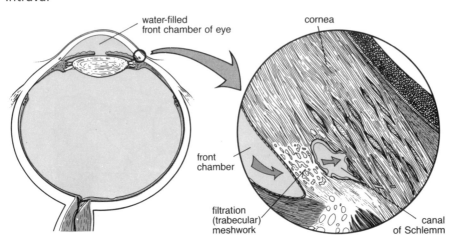

water-filled
front chamber of eye

cornea

*The pressure within the
eye (intra-ocular pressure)
is maintained by constant
secretion of water
(aqueous humour) that
can get out only with
difficulty through the
trabecular meshwork.*

front
chamber

filtration
(trabecular)
meshwork

canal
of Schlemm

the blood supply. The condition in which raised intra-ocular pressure causes damage in this way is called **glaucoma**.

Intraval

A brand name for sodium thiopentone.

intravascular oxygenation

An experimental method of compensating for inadequacies in the lungs or other disorders that cause a dangerous drop in the oxygen levels of the blood and a rise in the levels of carbon dioxide. The method uses a device, the intravenous oxygenator (IVOX), which consists of a bundle of about 1000 very fine siloxane-coated polypropylene hollow fibres through which oxygen is passed. This material is permeable to oxygen so that a proportion of it passes into the blood. And because the concentration of carbon dioxide within the fibres is very low, this gas can pass out of the blood into the fibres. The bundle is about 50 cm long and is inserted into the largest vein in the body, the inferior vena cava, where the gas exchange occurs.

intravascular ultrasonography

The use of ultrasound imaging by means of a miniaturized transducer within a blood vessel. This has become possible by the development of ultrasound probe catheters small enough to be inserted into a coronary artery and other peripheral arteries. The method produces detailed images of the interior walls of arteries and is especially useful in assessing **atherosclerosis**.

intravenous

Into a vein. Intravenous injection of a drug achieves rapid action. It also permits the giving of irritating substances because these are rapidly diluted and dispersed in the blood.

intravenous tube feeding

See **parenteral nutrition**.

introitus

The entrance into a hollow organ or cavity. The term is often used to refer to the entrance to the vagina.

Intron A

A brand name for interferon alfa.

introvert

A person whose tendency is to look inwards, to contemplate the state of his or her own mind and body rather than to seek social intercourse with others. The introvert is often obsessive, anxious, fearful, hypochondriacal, solitary and is always more concerned with thought than with action. Introverts have a small circle of friends and are more interested in how the world affects them than in how they could change the world.

Like most of such broad characterizations, the definition tends to describe a comparatively rare extreme example. None of us is wholly introvert or **extrovert** and most of us are balanced between the two.

intubation

A very common procedure in surgery and in diagnosis and treatment. Intubation is the passage of any tube, such as a catheter, into any organ, passage or tubular structure in the body. This may be done to keep a passage-way open, to withdraw a specimen for analysis, or to administer a drug. Intubation of the airway is common in general anaesthesia and in intensive care situations and is often life-saving. Intubation of blood vessels, even those of the heart itself, is now a common routine, both for diagnostic and treatment purposes.

intussusception

The method by which the intestine passes its contents along (peristalsis) sometimes leads to an internal infolding of the bowel wall so that it slides into itself somewhat in the manner of a pocket telescope. Intussusception in commonest in young children, but may occur as a result of polyps in the adult. Once started, intussusception rapidly progresses until

Intussusception causes colicky pain, vomiting and the passage of blood and mucus. It is a surgical emergency calling for prompt surgical intervention.

the associated blood vessels are also dragged in and become obstructed. Bowel obstruction occurs, but, even more serious, interference with the blood supply may lead to gangrene of the bowel.

invasive

Involving entry to the body through a natural surface. This word is used more often in the negative. Non-invasive methods of diagnosis are those using scanning and other techniques which do not require that the body be entered.

inversion mutation

A mutation resulting from the removal of a length of DNA, which is then reinserted facing in the opposite direction.

in vitro

Literally, 'in glass'. *In vitro* processes or reactions are those, normally occurring in the body, which, for various reasons, are deliberately conducted in a test tube or other laboratory receptacle. The same process in the body is said to occur '*in vivo*'. An example is *in vitro* **fertilization**.

in vitro fertilization

A procedure in which living eggs are taken from a woman's ovary, fertilized by sperm in a sterile glass dish, and replaced in the womb.

SUCCESS RATE
The procedure is fraught with difficulty and, at present, is successful in only about 10 per cent of attempts. *In vitro* fertilization is currently the least successful way of managing **infertility** and is generally regarded as a last resort.

HOW IT'S DONE
Egg production is stimulated with drugs or hormones and the growth of the ovarian follicles checked by ultrasound. When a follicle reaches a size of about 1.5 mm, a dose of hormone is given to prompt the release of eggs. These are collected using a fine needle guided by the ultrasound image.

The eggs are incubated at body temperature in a culture medium for 4 to 6 hours and then the sperm are added. The fertilized egg is kept in the culture medium for about two days, and is then placed in the woman's womb through a fine tube.

in vivo

See *in vitro*.

-ion

Suffix meaning 'action of' as in digestion (digesting).

ion channels

A range of four kinds of protein ports in cell membranes specific to the passage of sodium, potassium, calcium and chloride ions in solution. Protein molecules are chemically large and can take various shapes (conformations). These ports are opened or closed as required, by changes in the conformation of these proteins. Conformational changes result from the attachment of various hormone molecules, from changes in chemical concentration within the cell, or from alterations in local electrical potential. Many diseases result from disordered function of ion channels, and a range of new drugs has been developed by exploiting the ability to bring about conformational changes in the ion channels.

ionizer

An ion is an atom which has become charged by the loss of an orbital electron (positive ion), or gaining an electron (negative ion). Many solutions in water become ionized and gases can be temporarily ionized by means of electrical discharges. The state of ionization of the atmosphere is claimed by some to affect the health, or at least the sense of well-being, and this rather dubious proposition has become the basis for a minor industry producing small machines called ionizers which purport to affect the ionization of the domestic atmosphere in a significant way.

Local ionization does occur and these machines are quite efficient in making dense deposits of fine dust particles on nearby walls. There is little reason to believe, however, that they have any beneficial effect on the health of the body.

Iopidine

A brand name for **apraclonidine**.

ipratropium bromide

An **anticholinergic** drug used to treat asthma. Brand names are Atrovent, Ipratropium Steri-Neb, Respontin, Rinatec.

Ipratropium Steri-Neb

A brand name for **ipratropium bromide**.

iproniazid

An antidepressant drug. A brand name is Marsilid.

IQ

See **intelligence quotient**.

irbesartan

An **angiotensin II antagonist** drug used to treat high blood pressure. A brand name is Aprovel.

iridectomy

The surgical production of a hole in the iris of the eye so that a communication is made between the water-filled chambers in front of and behind the iris. This may be done through a small incision at the edge of the cornea, using forceps and tiny scissors, or more commonly nowadays, by means of a laser. This small peripheral iridectomy is valuable in the treatment of a form of glaucoma in which the iris is pushed forward by the accumulation of water behind it, and obstructs the normal channels through which this water leaves the eye. Once a hole has been made, the fluid can pass easily forward and no longer balloons out the iris.

In some cases the portion of iris removed is larger. This may be for optical purposes – to expose a segment of lens clearer than that behind the pupil, or for the removal of an iris tumour. Broad iridectomies of this kind require the eye to be opened.

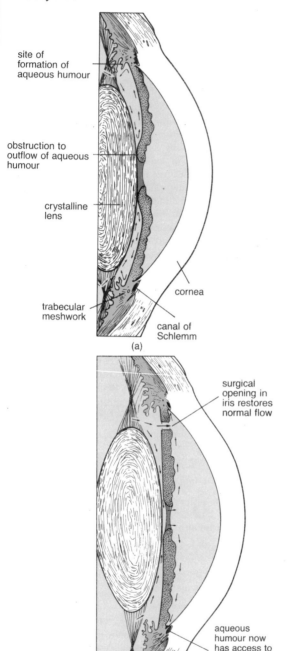

site of formation of aqueous humour

obstruction to outflow of aqueous humour

crystalline lens

trabecular meshwork

cornea

canal of Schlemm

(a)

surgical opening in iris restores normal flow

aqueous humour now has access to canal of Schlemm via trabecular meshwork

(b)

Iridectomy is a minor eye operation done to relieve a form of glaucoma. If pressure of water builds up behind the iris (a) the latter balloons forward to obstruct the outflow angle and a dangerous rise in the pressure within the eye may result. An opening in the iris (b) relieves the situation.

iridocyclitis

See **uveitis.**

irinotecan

An anticancer drug used to treat widespread secondary cancer of the colon or rectum. A brand name is Campto.

iris inflammation

See **uveitis.**

iritis

See **uveitis.**

iron-deficiency anaemia

See **anaemia.**

iron polysaccharide complex

A form of iron used to treat iron-deficiency **anaemia** in premature babies. A brand name is Niferex.

irradiation

Deliberate exposure to radiation either for purposes of treatment, as in radiotherapy, or to sterilize material. Surgical instruments, dressings and other medical equipment which have been sealed up in plastic bags can safely be sterilized by exposure to intense radiation. Gamma rays pass though the outer cover and destroy all living organisms within. Sealed foodstuffs can be sterilized in the same way, and this is now legal in Britain.

irritable bowel syndrome

A persistent disorder associated with recurrent pain in the abdomen and intermittent diarrhoea, often alternating with constipation, for which no organic cause can be found. The condition is also known as *spastic colon*, 'nervous diarrhoea' or 'idiopathic diarrhoea'. The irritable bowel syndrome is a very common disorder responsible for about half the medical attendances for bowel upset.

The condition often begins during a period of emotional stress, as after marital discord, divorce, bereavement or business worry.

INCIDENCE

This distressing disorder most commonly affects women between twenty and forty. Women suffer three times as often as men.

RECOGNITION AND SYMPTOMS

It features rapid transit of food with frequent bowel motions, a sense of fullness, an awareness of the bowel action and often headache and anxiety. The processes of **peristalsis** are stronger and more frequent than normal and there is often intolerance to known kinds of food.

Pain is usually felt in one of the four corners of the abdomen, is sometimes brought on by eating, and is often relieved by going to the toilet. The stools are usually ribbon-like or pellet-like and may contain mucus.

Often, soon after a meal, there is extreme and embarrassing urgency to empty the bowels. There may be loud abdominal rumblings and squeaking (borborygmi), excessive gas production (flatus), headache, tiredness and nausea. Sometimes there is a sense of incomplete emptying after defecation.

Full investigation, including barium meal X-ray, shows no objective abnormality, but, on examination, the colon is seen to be in a state of unusual activity, contracting and relaxing in an abnormally rapid manner.

TREATMENT

A diet high in roughage is helpful in regulating the bowel action, and there are several drugs effective in quieting down the excessive bowel activity and relieving the pain. Drugs can be carried and taken in anticipation of events which might provoke an acute attack. After careful investigation to exclude organic causes, strong reassurance is often, in itself, therapeutic.

ischaemia

An inadequate flow of blood to any part of the body, usually because of narrowing, from disease, of the supplying arteries. Ischaemia is the cause of an immense amount of disease, disability and death and accounts for a high proportion of the morbidity of mankind in the Western world.

Angina pectoris is caused by ischaemia and, when this reaches a sufficiently severe degree, a **heart attack** (coronary thrombosis) may follow. Stroke is caused by ischaemia, as is intermittent claudication. Ischaemia commonly causes infarction.

ischion

Greek root meaning 'hip' as in ischial bone (hip bone of the pelvis).

-ise

Suffix meaning 'make' as in tenderize (make tender).

Isib 60XL

A brand name for **isosorbide mononitrate**.

-isk

Suffix meaning 'diminutive' as in asterisk (little star).

-ism

Suffix meaning 'devotion to' as in alcoholism (devotion to alcohol).

Ismelin

A brand name for **guanethidine sulphate**.

Ismo

A brand name for **isosorbide mononitrate**.

Isocard

A brand name for **isosorbide dinitrate**.

isoconazole

An antifungal drug formulated as a vaginal tablet and used to treat thrush and other vaginal infections. A brand name is Travogyn.

Isogel

A brand name for **isphagula**.

Isoket

A brand name for **isosorbide dinitrate**.

isolation

The deliberate separation of a person suffering from an infectious disease, or carrying potentially dangerous organisms, from those uninfected and possibly susceptible. Isolation is now less commonly used than formerly, as the resources for dealing with infections are now much improved. It is still important, however, used in the reverse direction (reverse barrier nursing), for people who are immunocompromised and who are very susceptible to infection by organisms present on, but unlikely to affect, healthy individuals.

isometheptene

A **sympathomimetic** drug used to treat migraine. A brand name of a preparation with paracetamol is Midrid.

isoniazid

A drug used in the treatment of **tuberculosis**. The drug occasionally produces side-effects such as skin rash and fever, and rarely nerve involvement. Brand names of preparations in combination with other drugs are Rifater, Rifinah and Rimactazid.

isophane insulin

A form of insulin modified by adsorption on to a protein molecule protamine so as to act for up to about 12 hours with delayed onset of action. Brand names are Humulin I, Hypurin Bovine Isophane, Hypurin Porcine Isophane and Hypurin Porcine Biphasic Isophane.

Isophane Hypurin

A brand name for **insulin**.

isoprenaline

An adrenaline-like drug given by injection to treat surgical **shock** and **heart block**. A brand name is Saventrine.

Isopto Carpine

A brand name for **pilocarpine** eye drops in hypromellose.

Isordil

A brand name for **isosorbide dinitrate**.

isosorbide dinitrate

A drug used to prevent or relieve **angina pectoris** and to treat **heart failure**. Brand names are Cedocard Retard, Isocard, Isoket, Isordil, Sorbichew, Sorbid SA and Sorbitrate.

isosorbide mononitrate

A drug used to treat **angina pectoris** and **heart failure**. Brand names are Elantan, Imdur, Isib 60XL, Ismo, MCR-50, Monit, Mono-Cedocard and Monomax.

isotretinoin

A **retinoid** drug used to treat severe acne which has failed to respond to conventional antibiotic treatment. It is not without dangers. Side-effects include skin rashes, muscle pains,dry mouth, conjunctivitis, blurred vision, migraine, convulsions, psychiatric reactions. The oral preparation is used under strictly controlled conditions to exclude pregnancy because of the known risks to the fetus. Brand names are Roaccutane and, for external use, Isotrex and Isotrexin.

Isotrex

A brand name for **isotretinoin** formulated for external use.

Isotrexin

A brand name for **isotretinoin** and **erythromycin** formulated for external use.

ispaghula

A mucilaginous plant that swells in water to provide bulk in the intestine and promote movement of the contents. Ispaghula is used to treat constipation. Brand names are Fybogel, Fybozest, Konsyl and Regulan.

isradipine

A calcium channel blocking drug used to treat high blood pressure. A brand name is Prescal.

-ist

Suffix meaning 'skilled in' as in chiropodist (foot-skilled).

Istin

A brand name for **amlopidine**.

itching

An awareness of a tickling irritation in the skin which prompts one, almost irresistibly, to rub or scratch, although one may be well aware that the relief so obtained is only temporary. Itching is caused by the stimulation of certain nerve-endings in the skin, but the reason for this is unclear. The substances responsible may include various enzymes called *endopeptidases*, which occur naturally in the skin and in the bloodstream, and which may be released by some local skin disturbance.

Severe itching is called *pruritus* and this often occurs in and around the anus or the female genitalia and is commonly associated with thrush (**candidiasis**). Other fungus infections, such as the various forms of tinea, also feature severe itching, and many fungi contain endopeptidases.

Itching is usually remediable if the cause can be established and treated. Scratching often makes things worse and may even set up a vicious cycle which perpetuates the symptom. The use of simple lotions, such as calamine and phenol, are often to be preferred to scratching.

See also **formication**.

-itis

Suffix meaning 'inflammation of' as in bursitis (bursa inflammation).

itraconazole

A triazole antifungal drug use to treat thrush and other fungal infections. A brand name is Sporanox.

-itude

Suffix meaning 'quality' as in amplitude (quality of amount).

-ity

Suffix meaning 'character of' as in acerbity (sharp character).

-ium

Suffix meaning 'diminutive' as in epithelium (little skin).

ivermectin

A drug used to kill microfilaria in the treatment of **onchocerciasis** and other microfilarial diseases. Ivermectin has also been used to treat severe **scabies** in elderly institutionalized people, but an unusually high death rate in this group cast doubt on the safety of the application.

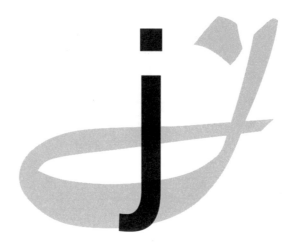

jaundice

A yellowing of the skin and of the whites of the eyes from deposition of a natural colouring substance, bilirubin. This pigment is released from the **haemoglobin** in red blood cells at the end of their working lives, when they are broken down by scavenging phagocyte white cells. In health, the normal continual breakdown of red blood cells does not cause jaundice because the bilirubin is taken up by the liver and passed into the intestine in the bile. It is the bilirubin in the bile which produces the characteristic colour of the faeces.

But if the liver is diseased, so that it cannot secrete the bilirubin, or if the bile ducts are blocked so that the bilirubin cannot get out, it gradually accumulates in the blood and stains the tissues. Jaundice can also be caused by a disease in which red blood cells are broken down more rapidly than normal (haemolytic anaemia) so that more bilirubin is produced than the liver can cope with.

> Jaundice is not, in itself, a disease, but is rather a sign of some other condition. It is, however, always an indication that something significant is happening, and should never be ignored.

POSSIBLE CAUSES

As well as that noted above, a common cause of jaundice is hepatitis – a virus infection of the liver in which the cells are temporarily unable to work properly or to pass the bilirubin through into the bile. As a result, bilirubin accumulates in the blood. The degree of jaundice varies with the severity of the liver disorder, from just visible to obvious yellowing of the skin. Hepatitis seldom causes severe or prolonged jaundice unless it seriously and permanently damages the liver.

Obstructive jaundice, on the other hand, in which the bile outlet is completely blocked by a gallstone or by a tumour near the opening into the bowel, causes severe jaundice. Because none of the bilirubin can get into the bowel, the stools are pale and clay-coloured. The kidneys attempt to get rid of the excess in the blood, and the urine is usually very dark from excess bilirubin.

Dislocation of the hinge joint of the jaw-bone (temporo-mandibular joint) occurs if the head of the mandible is levered out of its socket. This can sometimes occur during an especially wide yawn. The head moves forward and cannot spontaneously return to its proper place.

RECOGNITION AND SYMPTOMS

The cause of jaundice should be found without delay and, if possible, treated. In many cases, as in hepatitis, there will be other symptoms to indicate the cause, but jaundice may be the first sign of some serious disorder such as cirrhosis of the liver or cancer.

jaundice, persistent in baby

See **rhesus factor disease**.

jaw, disorders of dislocation

Sometimes, if the mouth is opened too widely, or if the jaw (mandible) is struck while the mouth is open, this joint may dislocate, the heads of the mandible usually being displaced forward, out of their shallow sockets, just in front of the ears. When this happens the mouth cannot be closed. Dislocation is corrected (reduced) by pressing the lower back teeth downwards with *padded* thumbs.

FRACTURES

Fractures of the jaw are common and are most often caused by road traffic accidents or fighting. There is pain, severe swelling and tenderness and often the mouth cannot close. The strong muscles moving the jaw often pull the fragments apart. Such fractures are usually secured in alignment by wiring the teeth together for about six weeks. The punches to the jaw sustained with seeming impunity on television could never occur in real life.

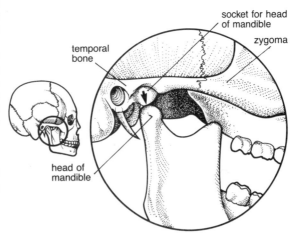

jaw joint replacement

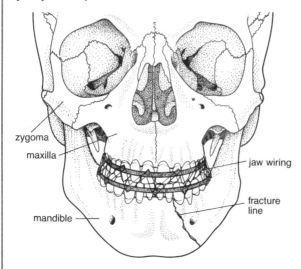

zygoma
maxilla
jaw wiring
fracture line
mandible

Jaw fractures are often best immobilized by wiring the teeth together, thus securing excellent alignment in the proper position. There is usually a gap for tube nutrition but it may be necessary to remove a tooth for this purpose.

jaw joint replacement

See **temporomandibular joint replacement**.

jaw winking

A strange, inherited condition, sometimes called the Marcus Gunn phenomenon, in which a drooping eyelid (ptosis) retracts momentarily when the mouth is opened wide or the jaw is moved firmly to one side. In other cases, a normal eye closes tightly under the same stimulus.

Jaw winking is caused by an abnormal distribution of some twigs of the nerves to the jaw muscles, which are wrongly connected to the muscle which elevates the upper lid.

jealousy in childhood

This is a common result of competition, often between brother and sister, or prompted by the arrival of a new baby. The usual signs are bed-wetting (**enuresis**), a regression to a simpler and more childish mode of behaviour, temper tantrums, or sometimes evident anxiety.

Children should be warned, well in advance, of an expected addition to the family and should be clearly told that time and attention will have to be given to the new baby. Parents must understand and tolerate the signs of jealousy and should give as much attention as possible to the older children. So far as possible, the baby should not be allowed to intrude into the older child's possessions and living area, as this will make the jealousy worse.

jejunal biopsy

This is an important form of investigation in cases in which food is not properly absorbed from the intestine (malabsorption). In many such cases the inner layer of the bowel, through which the digested food is absorbed, has become abnormal and a biopsy can show this.

The biopsy is taken by means of a small device called a Crosby capsule. This is a hollow device, attached to the end of a narrow tube, which is swallowed after an overnight fast. The capsule is allowed to move down, through the stomach and duodenum, into the small intestine. Suction is applied through the tube and this draws a small piece of the wall into the capsule and also activates a spring-loaded knife which painlessly cuts off the specimen. The capsule is then withdrawn and the sample retrieved for microscopic examination. Sometimes the method causes some internal bleeding and, rarely, perforation of the bowel wall.

In some forms of malabsorption the lining of the bowel is atrophied and the small finger-like processes (villi) through which absorption occurs are stunted or absent. This important finding is revealed by a jejunal biopsy.

Jekyll and Hyde disorder

An uncommon schizophrenic-like illness featuring alternating periods of social conformity and strongly antisocial behaviour.

jellyfish stings

Jellyfish carry stinging capsules called *nematocysts* which discharge an irritating substance into the skin when touched. Usually, this causes no more than an itchy rash, which may persist for a day or two. Some species, notably the box jellyfish, *Chironex fleckeri*, of the Pacific and Indian oceans, can cause a severe sting which may lead to vomiting and diarrhoea, a drop in blood pressure, and even paralysis of the muscles of respiration. In such cases, the 'kiss of life' (mouth to mouth respiration) may be literally vital. (See *First Aid.*)

Jellyfish tentacles with their stings should be removed without delay. Vinegar inactivates the sting capsules. An antivenom is available for box jellyfish stings.

jerky eyes

See **nystagmus**.

jet lag

Biological clocks are normally synchronized with local time. Rapid transit, by air, across time zones means that, for a time, the individual's body rhythms, and the biochemical and physiological processes associated with them, are 'out of sync' with local time.

> The problem is worse on an eastward journey, when the need is to shorten the day, and less troublesome when going west. This is partly because the innate circadian rhythm has a period of somewhat more than twenty-four hours.

RECOGNITION AND SYMPTOMS

The most obvious effect is on sleeping, which is commonly disturbed for several days, but other activities, such as digestion, bowel habit and mental functioning are also affected. There is wakefulness during the night, the desire to sleep during the day, a sense of fatigue, inefficiency, lapses of memory and poor physical and mental efficiency.

TREATMENT

The pineal gland in the brain secretes a hormone called melatonin during darkness and suppresses it in the light. This hormone is believed to control some of the biorhythms and has been used experimentally in attempts to prevent jet lag. Although some subjects claim benefit from treatment with this hormone, the evidence is dubious. Not enough is known of the other effects of melatonin to justify its use for purposes such as this.

Jet lag remains a problem. Recovery takes about one day for each time zone crossed, and, if important business is afoot, the journey should, if possible, be advanced appropriately. Avoidance of excessive alcohol and heavy meals during the flight, and the use of a mild hypnotic drug to aid sleep on the aircraft, may help.

jigger flea

See **chigoe**.

joint and spine examination

Joint examination includes a close inspection, with special attention to swelling, deformity, discoloration and wasting, of the surrounding muscles. Movements are checked, both voluntary (active) and those caused by the doctor (passive). If there is any real limitation of joint movement, the doctor may wish to measure the angle through which the affected joint can be moved, using an instrument called a goniometer. Restriction of joint movement may be due to inflammation in the joint, sprain of an external joint ligament or the joint capsule; internal damage, such as wear on the bearing surfaces from **osteoarthritis**, a tear of an internal ligament or of a joint cartilage, loose pieces of cartilage or severe deformity from a condition such as **rheumatoid arthritis**. The doctor tests strength by deliberately resisting various movements.

Spinal movements are tested by asking the subject to bend as far as possible forward, backward and to either side. The range of movement in the upper part of the spine is also checked by systematically noting how far the head can be turned in all directions. Osteopathic practitioners usually carry out a much more detailed examination of the spine than do orthopaedic surgeons, and some of them claim to examine each one of the scores of articular joints between the vertebrae. Spinal movement may be limited by osteoarthritis and, in particular, by **ankylosing spondylitis**, in which the vertebrae tend to fuse together until the flexible spine is replaced by a rigid rod.

The lower back is the site of many medical problems and the source of more aching pain than almost any other part of the body. The lower (lumbar) spine is affected by a number of conditions including inflammation and a healing together of the vertebrae (ankylosing spondylitis), loss of bone density (osteoporosis) and osteoarthritis. Commonest of all is the tendency for the discs between the vertebrae to degenerate so that the pulpy interior is squeezed out to press on the spinal nerve roots and cause pain and disability. This condition is commonly miscalled 'slipped disc' but is more correctly known as prolapsed intervertebral disc. Firm pressure over the area of such protrusion causes an increase in the pain, and there will often be radiation of pain down the leg. The French call this the 'doorbell' sign.

Most of the spinal nerves run down in a large bundle – the sciatic nerve – which passes through the buttock and down the back of the thigh to supply the muscles of the leg. Stretching of this nerve causes severe pain in the back and down the leg, and the doctor tests for this by having the subject lie on his or her back, straighten the knee and raise the leg. If this causes pain, the test is positive and this straight leg-raising test is positive in disc prolapse. The pain is made worse by flexing the ankle backwards – which stretches the nerve more – and is eased by bending the knee, which relieves the tension on the nerve.

joint pain, fleeting

See **rheumatic fever**.

joints

Joints are junctions between bones, and the term is applied whether or not obvious movement is possible. There are three types of joints – fibrous, cartilaginous and synovial. In fibrous joints, such as those between the spines of the vertebral column, the bones of the pelvis or the bones making up the skull, little or no movement is possible because the bones are held firmly together by ligaments. Cartilaginous joints, such as those between the ribs and the breast bone (sternum), have flexible cartilage fusing the bones together, allowing some limited movement. Synovial joints, such as the shoulder, elbow, hip and knee joints, are freely movable. Although the bearing surfaces of synovial joints are covered with cartilage, there is a space between these surfaces which is well lubricated with a fluid known as synovial fluid. The whole joint is enclosed in a capsule of tough fibrous tissue lined with the synovial membrane, which secretes synovial fluid. Synovial joints may be:

- 'ball-and-socket' joints, as in the shoulder and hip, allowing some movement in any direction;
- hinge joints, as in the fingers and knees, allowing movement in one plane only;
- rotating joints, as in the head of the radius at the elbow, and between the upper two vertebrae of the spine;
- sliding joints, as at the wrists and in the feet. Some sliding also occurs at the knee joints.

In all cases, the range of possible movement is restricted by ligaments, which may be external to the joint, internal, or both.

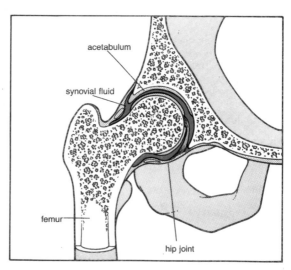

The hip joint. This is an efficient ball-and-socket synovial joint.

joints, disorders of

Diseases of joints, generally, are called arthropathies, the commonest of these being caused by inflammation. Inflammation of joints is called **arthritis** and this is a very common medical problem, the two main classes being **osteoarthritis** and **rheumatoid arthritis**. Other forms of arthritis occur in conjunction with various general diseases such as **Reiter's syndrome**, **psoriasis**, inflammatory bowel disease, **Lyme disease**, meningococcal infections, gonorrhoea, syphilis (see **sexually transmitted diseases**) and **tuberculosis**.

Joints are also susceptible to injury, which may cause dislocation or fracture. The late effect of such injury is commonly some degree of osteoarthritis. The management of severe arthritic and other forms of damage to joints is being revolutionized by the application of engineering skills in the design and production of artificial joint prostheses. The most successful and widely used joint replacement is for injury or arthritic damage to the hip joint.

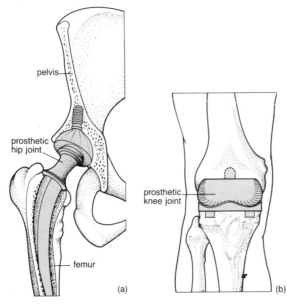

When joints are damaged by arthritis, symptoms and disability may be severe. In many cases the best treatment is to replace the damaged joint by a prosthesis. This illustration shows (a) a prosthetic hip joint and (b) a prosthetic knee joint.

joints, lining of

See **synovial membrane**.

jumping genes,

See **transposons**.

Jungian theory

The Swiss psychologist Carl Gustav Jung (1875–1961) was, at first, a close associate of Freud, but dispute, largely over the significance of sexuality in life and psychological develop-ment, led to a breakaway. Jung was not convinced by Freud's emphasis on erotic factors and believed that this was a reductionist view. He came to recognize Freud's tendency to turn psychoanalysis into a religion, complete with dogmatic articles of faith and immunity from all attack or criticism, and found this incompatible with Freud's claim to be scientific.

As an alternative to Freud's emphasis on sex, Jung proposed a wider definition of *libido* – as a kind of general creative life force, or energy, which could find outlet in various directions. Jung proposed the concepts of extroversion and introversion and suggested a division of mankind into four categories – those most concerned with the intellect, the emotions, intuition and the sensations.

Jung was concerned with symbols which he considered central to the understanding of human nature, recognizing their recurrence in many religions, mythologies and magical systems in many parts of the world and in human history. To account for some of these observations, he found it necessary to postulate the existence of a layered unconscious psyche – the personal and the collective, universal mind. The personal was, he suggested, that acquired during life; the collective unconscious was inherited and was common to all mankind. It was composed of *archetypes* – inherent tendencies to experience and symbolize universal human situations in distinctively human ways. Later in life, Jung suggested that the deepest layers of the unconscious operated independently of space, time and causality and could account for apparently paranormal phenomena such as precognition and telepathy.

Jung was also deeply preoccupied with dreams and fantasies and applied his ideas to his methods of therapy. He believed that patients could, and should, be made aware of both the personal and collective archetypal significance of their symptoms and psychological problems and that, in this way, opposing tendencies could be resolved and personal wholeness could be achieved.

Junifen

A brand name for **ibuprofen**.

Junior Disprol

A brand name for **paracetamol** for children.

junk food

A popular term for highly refined, processed and ready-prepared food, usually containing a fairly high level of sweeteners and a low level of roughage. Junk food has the same calorific value as any other comparative food and is, in itself, likely to be no more harmful than any other kind of food. A diet exclusively of this kind of food may, however, be much too high in saturated fats and relatively deficient in vitamins and minerals and especially in the high cellulose content (roughage) of fresh fruit and vegetables. On such a diet, weight gain occurs readily and the tendency to the deadly arterial disease **atherosclerosis** is enhanced. It should certainly be regarded as less satisfactory than a well-balanced intake.

juxta-

Prefix meaning 'near' as in juxtapose (put near).

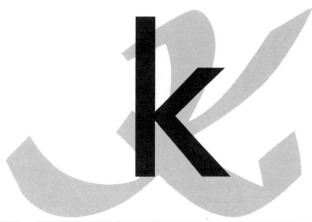

Kabikinase

A brand name for **streptokinase**.

kala azar

A type of **leishmaniasis**, caused by parasites of the genus *Leishmania* and spread by biting sandflies. It occurs in the Mediterranean area, north and east Africa and India, but is now beginning to spread westward into Europe. In endemic areas, stray dogs form a reservoir for the disease. The parasite is present in the human blood and multiplies in scavenging white cells (macrophages), causing fever, malnutrition, loss of immune capacity (immunosuppression), anaemia, enlargement of the lymph nodes, spleen and liver, and damage to the bone marrow.

Kala azar can be diagnosed by the **ELISA test** and is treated with drugs containing antimony.

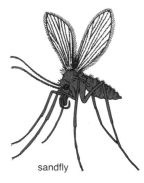

This is a greatly enlarged illustration of the sandfly (Phlebotomus species) that transmits the causal organism of kala azar, the protozoal parasite Leishmania donovani.

sandfly

Kalspare

A brand name for **triamterene** in combination with another diuretic drug.

Kalten

A brand name for **hydrochlorothiazide** formulated with a **beta-blocker** drug.

Kaltogel

A brand name for calcium alginate.

Kaltostat

A brand name for calcium alginate.

Kamillosan

A brand name for **chamomile**.

kanamycin

A broad spectrum aminoglycoside antibiotic derived from the soil actinomycete. Kanamycin is active against Gram negative organisms but is now largely replaced by gentamicin. The aminoglycosides can cause deafness, **tinnitus** and kidney damage. A brand name is Kannasyn.

kangaroo mother method

A method of care for small babies in the first few months of life involving frequent breastfeeding, maximal skin-to-skin contact of mother and baby, and early discharge from the maternity unit. The method requires careful selection after detailed assessment of both mother and baby.

Kannasyn

A brand name for **kanamycin**.

Kaposi's sarcoma

Kaposi's sarcoma has been known for a long time as a rare disease in the Western world (one case per million of the population), usually affecting men over the age of about sixty. The cause is unknown, but it is in some way intimately related to the immune system and probably to cytomegalovirus. In non-AIDS immune deficiency in which Kaposi's is present and in which it has been possible to reverse the immune problem, the disease has disappeared. It is a multiple tumour of blood vessels, primarily affecting the skin, usually on the lower limbs and growing very slowly. Old men, not suffering from AIDS, who get Kaposi's sarcoma usually live for at least ten years and often die from some other disease. Strangely enough, Kaposi's is quite common in parts of tropical Africa where it seems almost like a different disease – amounting to almost 10 per cent of all tumours, affecting young people, and causing death within two or three years. In these cases, the tumour regularly affects the internal organs as well as the skin. Only black people are affected. Whites and Indians living in the same areas do not contract the disease.

This African form of Kaposi's sarcoma bears a striking resemblance to what happens in people with immune deficiency. In **AIDS**, Kaposi's affects about a quarter of the men with the disease, so the average age is about thirty-five. The visible signs are small, circular, pinkish or reddish-brown spots, usually situated on the legs and buttocks. Sometimes the spots are more raised and appear as nodules or plaques of a bluish-purple to dark brown colour. They vary in size from a few millimetres to one centimetre across and vary in number from one to hundreds.

But, in AIDS, Kaposi's is often found, at an early stage, to have involved the insides of the bowels, the mouth, the lungs, the lymph nodes or, indeed, almost any organ of the body. Some of these affected areas seem quiescent, but some may become locally destructive, ulcerating through the skin into the deeper tissues and even sometimes involving the underlying bone.

The clinical evidence on Kaposi's sarcoma is confusing and a fair proportion of people with AIDS have shown no other signs of immune deficiency. In those who do not show opportunistic infections along with the Kaposi's, the outlook is proportionately better and survival is longer. But the discovery of Kaposi's sarcoma in a young man with opportunistic infections is an alarming indication of the severity of the immune deficiency and, until recently, few such patients lasted longer than two years, once the diagnosis was confirmed. Ironically, treatment of the disease in those who do not have AIDS is remarkably effective, and measures such as electron beam radiotherapy and chemotherapy have achieved high cure rates. But in AIDS, the picture is tragically different and the indications are that those who get Kaposi's sarcoma are especially prone, also, to opportunistic infections, for it is from these that, without the best and most energetic treatment, three-quarters of the AIDS patients with Kaposi's sarcoma die.

Kawasaki disease

This disease was first recognized in 1967 by Tokyo paediatrician Dr Tomisaku, in Kawasaki, but is now known to occur world-wide.

RECOGNITION AND SYMPTOMS
It chiefly affects infants and young children and causes fever, a measles-like rash, red eyes, dry cracking lips, swollen lymph nodes and, in about 40 per cent of cases, changes in the coronary arteries. These are local enlargements (aneurysms) and are transient in most cases; only about 10 per cent have long-term involvement of the coronaries.

There is no known laboratory test for Kawasaki's disease but the clinical features are now clear and diagnosis is not difficult.

POSSIBLE CAUSES
The cause remains obscure and, although the features of the disease suggest an infection, no organism has been isolated and there is no response to antibiotics.

Recently, it has been found that children with the disease have an enzyme, reverse transcriptase, which is a feature of a particular class of viruses, the retroviruses. It is also known that viruses can affect the smooth muscle of artery walls. There is some evidence that the disease may be spread by house-dust mites, or cat fleas.

TREATMENT
Aspirin has been found useful in the treatment and appears to reduce the incidence of heart complications. The death rate is less than one per cent and most children make a complete recovery.

Kay-Cee-L

A brand name for potassium (KCl).

Kefadim

A brand name for ceftazidime.

Kefadol

A brand name for **cefamandole**.

Keflex

A brand name for cephalexin.

Keftid

A brand name for cefaclor.

Kefzol

A brand name for cephazolin.

Kelfizine W

A brand name for **sulfametopyrazine**.

keloid

An abnormal response to healing so that scars become markedly overgrown, thickened and disfiguring. Keloids are more common in black people than in white. They are commonest in the upper part of the trunk and may follow any injury or surgical incision, especially for surgery on the thyroid gland.

Unfortunately, surgical removal of keloids is liable to be followed by further keloid formation, so little is gained. They can, however, be helped by injection of steroids and this also relieves the irritation which is a common feature. Keloids left alone tend, very gradually, to flatten.

Kemadrin

A brand name for **procyclidine**.

Kemicetin

A brand name for chloromycetin.

Kenalog

A brand name for **triamcinolone**.

keratitis

Inflammation of the outer lens of the eye (the cornea). Since inflammation is essentially a response in the blood vessels, and since the cornea has none, it is difficult, at first sight, to understand how keratitis can occur. Indeed, many of the conditions previously described as *keratitis* were not, in fact, inflammations of the cornea, although some of them excited an inflammation in the surrounding tissues. Nowadays, these disorders are described as *keratopathies*.

In some cases of corneal disorder, new blood vessels grow into the cornea from the edge and, following this, a true keratitis can occur. New vessel growth is called *vascularization* and is always serious as it usually leads to opacification of the cornea and a major reduction in the clarity of vision. Such *neo-vascularization* occurs in **trachoma** and in the now rare condition of *interstitial keratitis*, which is a feature of congenital syphilis. Keratitis may also follow ulceration of the cornea, especially from the cold sore virus, **Herpes** simplex, as this, if not properly treated, often leads to a persistent and disabling growth of new vessels into the cornea.

See also **keratoconjunctivitis**, **keratopathy**.

> Keratitis tends to be painful and to cause watering and undue sensitivity to light. Vision is not necessarily affected at once, as the condition often starts near the margin of the cornea, but any such symptoms should be reported without delay.

keratoacanthoma

A rapidly growing, alarming-looking skin nodule that affects elderly people, causing much anxiety because of its appearance and size. The keratoacanthoma usually occurs on the face and resembles many people's idea of a cancer. Starting as a small wart-like growth, possibly originating in a hair follicle, it grows rapidly for about two months, until it is over a centimetre in diameter and has developed a bulging convexity with a white, central, horny plug. If left alone, it remains stationary for a month or so and then gradually gets smaller until it disappears altogether, leaving a depressed scar.

The recommended treatment is to scoop out the whole growth with a sharp-edged spoon (curette) and this also allows for pathological examination to confirm that there is no danger. Recurrence is uncommon.

keratoconjunctivitis

Inflammation of the transparent membrane covering the white of the eye (the conjunctiva) associated with a disorder of the outer lens (the cornea).

CAUSE

The commonest cause of keratoconjunctivitis is a virus infection called *epidemic keratoconjunctivitis* or 'shipyard eye', caused by an adenovirus (*adeno* means 'gland') which has an affinity for glandular tissue. This virus is acquired by direct or indirect contact, via mediums such as towels, fingers or eye drops.

RECOGNITION AND SYMPTOMS

Keratoconjunctivitis usually causes a severe inflammation of the conjunctiva with swelling, redness and tearing and often a tender enlargement of the small lymph nodes in front of the ear. A week or two after onset, the cornea may be affected, not with inflammation but with a number of small, whitish opacities which, if central, may disturb the vision. These often last for months, but will, eventually, disappear. Sometimes the inflammation of the conjunctiva is so severe that a false membrane of dead cells and clotted serum forms.

TREATMENT

The virus is not currently susceptible to any treatment, but the inflammation can be controlled by the use of eye drops.

keratoconjunctivitis sicca

Keratoconjunctivitis sicca, or 'dry eye', is a state of persistent inadequacy of the wetting and lubrication of the cornea as a result of defective tear production.

POSSIBLE CAUSES

The glands which produce the tears are affected by the same damaging self-rejecting process (**auto-immune disease**) which causes rheumatoid arthritis, **Sjögren's syndrome**, systemic lupus erythematosus and other related conditions.

Keratoconjunctivitis sicca tends to be a feature of all these disorders.

RECOGNITION AND SYMPTOMS

When the surface tear-film is defective, the outer layer of the cornea becomes rough and irregular and the loss of the optical perfection of the perfectly smooth film of water leads to severe disturbance of vision. There is constant discomfort, foreign-body sensation and sometimes pain. The condition readily progresses to infection and ulceration of the cornea.

TREATMENT

Artificial tears, frequently applied as drops, may be necessary to preserve vision and maintain the health of the corneas.

keratoconus

A corneal growth disorder (dystrophy) leading to a peaking or conicity of the centre of the corneas so that their optical perfection is lost and vision may be severely distorted. A conical lens cannot form a clear image on the retina. Moreover, because the corneas are protruding forward, the effective distance between them and the retinas is increased and the images of distant objects tend to focus in front of the retinas. Near objects can be seen better. This form of 'short sight' (**myopia**) may progress steadily as the keratoconus develops, but the main disability is from image distortion.

Keratoconus is a familial condition and usually starts in adolescence or early adult life. Girls are affected more than boys. Although glasses may help at first, the progressive distortion usually calls for correction with hard contact lenses. These replace the conical refracting surfaces of the corneas with a perfectly spherical surface, and the corneal surface is optically 'lost' within the tear film.

Contact lenses are highly effective for so long as they can be tolerated, but severe keratoconus tends to cause central touch, discomfort, and even opacification of the apices of the cones. When this happens, the best resource is corneal grafting and this can give excellent, and permanent, results.

keratomalacia

Literally, 'softening of the cornea', is a common cause of blindness in severely malnourished children whose body stocks of vitamin A have become exhausted. Vitamin A deficiency causes dryness of the eyes with typical foamy patches (Bitot's spots) in the corners of the whites. So long as some vitamin A remains in the serum, the condition progresses no further, but when none of the vitamin is left, there is 'corneal melt', perforation, a gushing out of the internal fluid and loss of vision. Internal infection follows and the eyes are soon full of pus and irremediably blinded.

This is the fate of millions of children every year. There is a bitter irony in the situation, in that many of these children go blind within easy reach of green leaves containing enough vitamin A to keep their corneas healthy.

keratopathy

Any disorder of the outer lens of the eye (the cornea).

See **corneal abrasion**, **corneal injury**, **corneal ulcer**, **dendritic ulcer**.

keratoplasty

See **corneal graft**.

keratosis

A skin growth caused by excessive local reproduction of the horny outer cells, so that more than the normal amount of keratin is produced. An example is the pre-cancerous condition of solar keratosis, caused by overexposure to the sun.

keratotomy, radial

An operation purporting to reduce shortsightedness (myopia) by making radial cuts in the front lens of the eye (cornea) with the intention of flattening the curvature. The procedure was first performed many years ago in Japan, but the results were so bad that it was soon condemned by all responsible ophthalmologists, and abandoned.

The early lessons were apparently forgotten and, in the 1950s, a second upsurge of interest arose in the USSR. This, too, led to Western disapproval.

Refinements of technique and the use of operating microscopes, diamond knives and precision lasers led some ophthalmic surgeons to participate in a third wave of enthusiasm for this procedure in the 1970s and 1980s and to claim that the operation was, at last, safe and effective. Unfortunately, these claims have been heard before, and many surgeons, although regularly requested by patients to perform these technically simple operations, remained sceptical and unwilling to inflict potentially dangerous damage on healthy tissue for such reasons.

COMPLICATIONS

All ophthalmologists are familiar with the unhappy effects, even serious long-term complications, which can result from such procedures.

Some patients who had radial keratotomy suffered permanent visual flare in dim conditions, as a result of corneal scarring. Some suffered permanent loss of structural strength in the corneas. Many found that their myopia had been reduced but not abolished, while others enjoyed only a temporary improvement.

> The operation is not recommended.

CURRENT THINKING

The current vogue is for the use of the excimer laser to sculpt the corneal curvatures by vaporizing thin layers of tissue so as to modify the optical strength. This ten-minute procedure has now largely displaced radial keratotomy and the claims for the former procedure now sound hollow. It remains to be seen whether the present enthusiasm for the excimer laser is entirely justified.

keraunophobia

Abnormal fear of thunder and lightning.

kerion

A local reaction to fungus infection of the scalp (**tinea** capitis). Kerion is commonest in agricultural areas and is often contracted from farm animals. There is a localized boggy swelling on the scalp with oozing of pus and serum from the hair follicles. This causes the infected hairs to fall out and the condition to cure itself. The suppuration is not caused by infection but by a body reaction to the fungus. Sometimes kerion leads to a permanent small bald patch where the hair follicles have been destroyed.

kernicterus

Jaundice of the brain resulting from **rhesus factor disease** in babies. Rhesus antibodies destroy fetal red blood cells (haemolysis), releasing from them a substance called bilirubin which causes jaundice but which is also highly toxic to nerve cells, if sufficient is able to pass from the blood into the brain. This happens in severe, untreated cases, especially those in which there has previously been a rhesus problem and the mother has built up a high level of antibodies.

RECOGNITION AND SYMPTOMS

Kernicterus causes irritability, an increase in muscle responsiveness to stretch (spasticity) leading to a severe backwards arching of the back and neck, uncontrollable writhing movements (athetosis), reluctance to feed and often death within a week or two of birth. Surviving infants show varying degrees of paralysis, a tendency to **epilepsy**, spasticity of the muscles, athetosis, mental retardation, deafness and blindness.

The diagnosis is suggested by high levels of antibodies in the mother and subsequent amniocentesis.

TREATMENT

Treatment is by exchange transfusion, if necessary while the baby is still in the womb (uterus).

> Kernicterus is always preventable by early diagnosis and treatment of the underlying cause.

Kernig's sign

This is an important sign of irritation of the membranes surrounding the brain and spinal cord (the meninges) and occurs in meningitis. The knee-bending (hamstring) muscles normally bend the knee and straighten the hip joint. Because of irritative spasm in these muscles, attempts to bend the hip with the knee straight are strongly opposed. The sign is best demonstrated with the subject flat on his or her back, one leg straight, and the other bent (flexed) to ninety degrees at the hip and the knee. If there is any meningeal irritation, attempts to straighten the knee of the raised leg will be strongly opposed by muscle spasm.

Ketalar

A brand name for ketamine.

Ketocid

A brand name for **ketoprofen**.

ketoconazole

An imidazole antifungal drug. Ketoconazole is absorbed into the blood from the intestine and can be used to treat internal (systemic) fungal infections as well as skin fungal infections. It can, however, damage the liver. A brand name is Nizoral.

ketoprofen

A drug in the non-steroidal anti-inflammatory (**NSAID**) and pain-killing (analgesic) group. Brand names are Ketocid,

Orudis, Oruvail and, for external use, Oruvail gel and Powergel.

ketorolac

A non-steroidal anti-inflammatory (**NSAID**) drug. Brand names are Acular and Toradol.

ketosis

The presence of abnormally high levels of ketones in the blood. Ketones are produced when there is insufficient available glucose fuel, and fats have to be used. Fats are *triglycerides* and consist of molecules of glycerol to each of which three fatty acids are attached. When fats are used excessively as fuels, these fatty acids are released into the blood where they are converted to the ketones acetoacetic acid, hydroxybutyric acid and acetone.

POSSIBLE CAUSES

Normally the blood ketone levels are low but in starvation, untreated **diabetes**, and when the diet is very high in fats and low in carbohydrates, the levels rise. Ironically, in diabetes, the blood contains large quantities of sugar, but it is in the nature of the condition that this cannot be utilized as fuel. Ketones are volatile substances and confer on the breath the sickly, fruity odour of nail-varnish remover.

RECOGNITION AND SYMPTOMS

The danger, however, is that ketones are acidic and high levels make the blood abnormally acid. This leads to loss of water, sodium and potassium and a major biochemical upset in the body. There is nausea, vomiting, abdominal pain, confusion, and, if the condition is not rapidly treated, coma and death. Mild ketosis may be a feature of excessive morning sickness in pregnancy.

Ketosis can be diagnosed by a simple urine test.

ketotifen

A drug that prevents the release of histamine and other irritating substances from mast cells in allergic conditions. Its action is similar to that of **cromoglycate** but has the disadvantage of causing drowsiness. A brand name is Zaditen.

keyhole surgery

A lay term for **laparoscopic surgery**.

kidney cancer

This may take three main forms, the commonest being the renal carcinoma **hypernephroma**. The second type, the nephroblastoma, or Wilm's tumour, affects young children and is one of the commonest cancers in childhood. The third, the transitional cell carcinoma of the pelvis of the kidney, is a cancer which may be caused by the products of tobacco smoke in the urine or by exposure to aniline dyes.

Kidney cancer often causes blood to appear in the urine and this is a sign which must never be neglected. Blood clots in the urine tubes (ureters) may cause severe loin pain (renal colic). There may be pain, and occasionally swelling and tenderness in the flanks (loins), but kidney cancers may be silent

'Horse-shoe' kidney is a congenital abnormality or variant that may be present throughout life without being suspected or causing any trouble.

until the signs of secondary spread to the lungs, liver or bones appear. In children, the first sign may be a mass in the abdomen.

Kidney cancers are diagnosed by X-ray examination, including intravenous and retrograde pyelography; CT scan; MRI scan; ultrasound imaging; and biopsy. Treatment is by total or partial surgical removal (nephrectomy) and sometimes also radiotherapy and chemotherapy.

kidney cyst

Benign (non-malignant) cysts of the kidney are common. They are filled with fluid and usually cause neither symptoms nor danger.

See **kidney, polycystic**.

kidney disorders

Congenital abnormalities are fairly common. One kidney may be absent or the two kidneys may be joined ('horse-shoe kidney'). Neither need affect life or health. Polycystic kidneys (see **kidney, polycystic**) in which the kidneys become filled with large cysts, usually becomes apparent in the forties or fifties, but may be present in childhood. Hereditary forms of inflammation of the kidneys (nephritis) occur, the commonest being Alport's syndrome. Hereditary kidney tubule defects lead to abnormalities in urinary excretion. Tumours of the kidney include renal cell cancer (see **hypernephroma**) and Wilm's tumour. Inflammation of the kidneys is called nephritis, the commonest forms being acute **glomerulonephritis** and **pyelonephritis**. Kidney tubule damage may be caused by circulating poisons (toxins), surgical shock, infectious disease, hypersensitivity (allergic) reactions, drugs and auto-immune processes.

Obstruction to the outflow of urine will readily lead to back-pressure which can rapidly damage the kidneys. Obstruction can occur in many ways, including severe narrowing (stricture) of the final outlet tube (the urethra),

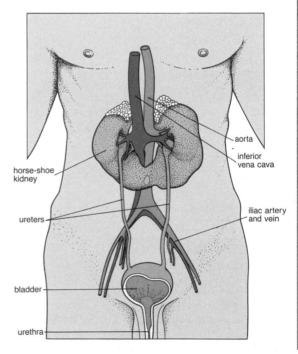

horse-shoe kidney

ureters

bladder

urethra

aorta

inferior vena cava

iliac artery and vein

A marked reduction in the blood flow through the kidneys is a serious matter, giving rise to reduced kidney function and the production of a hormone, angiotensin, which can cause a severe rise in the blood pressure. Such a reduction may be due to narrowing of the kidney arteries from disease, lowered blood pumping rate in heart failure, a reduction in blood volume from haemorrhage or dehydration, an acute drop in blood pressure from shock or severe infection or obstruction of the kidney veins from thrombosis.

enlargement of the prostate gland, stones in the bladder or in the tubes from the kidneys to the bladder (the ureters), and tumours. Sudden obstruction can cause kidney failure in a matter of hours, while partial or progressive obstruction may take months.

Kidney failure leads to an accumulation of toxic products in the blood and eventually to coma and death. Dialysis can, however, often keep patients alive indefinitely. The preferred method of treatment, however, is a kidney transplant.

See also **kidney cancer**, **kidney stones**.

kidney graft

See **kidney transplant**.

kidney inflammation

See **glomerulonephritis**.

kidney, polycystic

A genetic disease in which both kidneys are several times the normal size because of masses of cysts which progressively increase in size. In addition to the cysts, such kidneys often have abnormalities in their blood vessels and extensive scarring (fibrosis).

There are two types – a rare recessive infantile type which is usually fatal within the first year of life, and a commoner dominant adult type in which symptoms often do not develop until much later in life. Polycystic kidney leads to gradual loss of kidney function and to some secondary effects, such as raised blood pressure. Unless maintained by **dialysis**, or given a **kidney transplant**, people with the disorder usually die in middle age from the accumulation of waste products (**uraemia**) or the effects of high blood pressure – stroke or heart failure.

kidneys

The two kidneys are reddish brown, bean-shaped structures, each about 11 cm long, which lie in pads of fat high up on the inside of the back wall of the abdomen, one on each side of the spine. Large arteries run into them directly

from the largest artery in the body (aorta) and large veins run from them, back to the main collecting vein of the body (the inferior vena cava).

The kidneys filter waste material from the blood and adjust the levels of various essential chemical substances, so as to keep them within necessary limits. In so doing, they produce urine – a sterile solution of varying concentration, which passes down from the kidneys to the bladder where it is stored until it can conveniently be disposed of. Urine contains water, urea, uric acids and various inorganic salts in varying concentrations. The kidneys are also largely responsible for ensuring that the body contains the right amount of water and that the blood is of the correct degree of acidity. Most drugs or their breakdown products are eliminated through the kidneys. The kidneys produce a substance, erythropoietin, which stimulates the rate of formation of blood cells in the bone marrow.

Each kidney contains at least a million microscopic structures called nephrons. The nephron is the basic filtering unit of the kidney. Each one consists of a filtering capsule and a long, looped tubule which ends in a urine-collecting tubule. All the collecting tubules run into the pelvis of the kidney. Each nephron capsule contains a roughly spherical tuft of tiny blood vessels and through the walls of these all the components of the blood, except the cells and the larger molecules, pass into the capsules. Proteins, fats and all the cells of the blood remain in the circulation. About 170 litres of filtrate are produced each day.

If this were all that happened, we would very quickly die from fluid and mineral loss, but the kidney tubules have a remarkable power of selectively passing back into the blood vessels surrounding them all the constituents which are required by the body, including much of the water. This selective reabsorption is a highly complicated process which is under the control of various hormones such as aldosterone from the adrenal gland, antidiuretic hormone from the pituitary gland and parathyroid hormone from the parathyroid

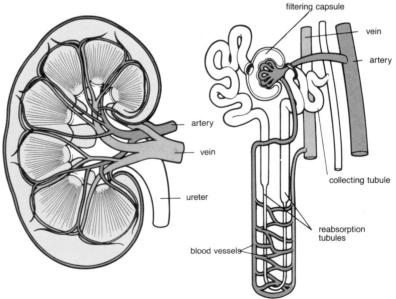

Structure of the kidney. The nephron, the microscopic filtering unit of the kidney, is shown on the right. Each kidney contains about 1,000,000 nephrons.

glands. In the course of reabsorption, sodium, potassium, calcium, chloride, bicarbonate, phosphate, glucose, amino acids, vitamins, many other substances and an appropriate amount of water, are returned to the blood and conserved. Urea, uric acid and many drugs are actively excreted by the tubules.

When the blood pressure falls below normal, or there is excessive loss of fluid from the body, the kidneys release the enzyme renin into the blood. This results in the formation of a further hormone, angiotensin, which, when converted by an enzyme to an active form, rapidly causes blood vessels throughout the body to narrow (constrict). This at once raises the blood pressure. Angiotensin also stimulates the secretion of the hormone aldosterone from the adrenal glands. This hormone acts on the tubules of the kidneys to increase the active reabsorption of sodium into the blood and, as a result, increase water retention in the body.

TREATMENT

Treatment is that of the cause. Diabetics need insulin; starving patients need a normal diet with plenty of carbohydrate; and people on all-fat diets need to take a more common-sense approach to their intake.

kidney stones

Urine is a solution of various substances, often present in such high concentration that crystallization can occur. This is especially likely during periods when the body is short of water and the urine is correspondingly concentrated. Once a small crystal has formed, it may act as a seed for further crystallization and, in this way, stones (calculi) may grow to a large size, sometimes even almost filling the upper part of the urine-collecting system of the kidney (the pelvis). Because of the shape of the collecting system, such stones are called 'staghorn' calculi.

Stones may occur anywhere in the urinary system – in the substance of the kidneys, in the collecting system, in the ureters which carry urine down to the bladder, or in the bladder itself. Small stones may be passed out into the tube from the bladder to the exterior (the urethra). Collections of small stones are known as 'gravel'.

POSSIBLE CAUSES

Dehydration, alone, will not cause stones to form and there is always some other factor such as kidney disease, local infection, a bodily disturbance which alters the amount or character of substances dissolved in the urine, or the taking of a drug which is excreted in high concentration in the urine.

Most kidney stones contain various combinations of calcium, magnesium, phosphorus, and oxalate. Uric acid stones tend to develop when the blood levels of this substance are abnormally high, as in gout. Less commonly, stones may occur in inherited disorders in which abnormal amounts of substances such as cystine and xanthine are excreted.

RECOGNITION AND SYMPTOMS

Stones may cause no symptoms, but if a stone becomes stuck in a ureter, the resulting local muscular contractions cause pain in the loin – ureteric colic – which may be agonizing. The pain may spread to the lower abdomen and the groin. Blood in the urine is a common sign of kidney stones. Stones may cause blockage of the urinary tract and this may have serious secondary effects on the continuing function of the kidney on the affected side. Total obstruction can permanently destroy kidney function.

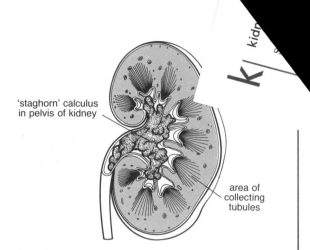

'staghorn' calculus in pelvis of kidney

area of collecting tubules

A large kidney stone, or calculus, formed from substances that have crystallized out from the urine. When the calculus conforms to the shape of the pelvis of the kidney it is called a 'staghorn' calculus.

TREATMENT

Stones which are too large to be passed spontaneously were formerly removed by open operation, but it is now usually possible to break them up into small particles by less invasive means. Fibre optic endoscopes can be passed through the skin to retrieve the stones in a loop or basket, or to break them up by ultrasonic energy. Extracorporeal **lithotripsy**, in which narrowly focused acoustic shock waves are used to break up the stones, is now the preferred method.

> Removal of stones without removal of the cause is bad medicine and stones should always be analysed and the cause ascertained and, if possible, eliminated.

kidney tests

The simplest tests of kidney function involve examination of a sample of urine. The normal composition of urine, and the range of concentrations of dissolved substances in it, are well-known. The presence of substances not normally found – such as blood or protein – or abnormal quantities of substances normally found, can give clear indication of kidney disorders. Abnormalities in the urine can, however, occur for reasons unconnected with the kidneys.

Microscopic examination of the urine may show casts of the kidney tubules, bacteria, pus cells and red cells, all of which may indicate kidney disease. The urine can be cultured for bacteria. The volume of urine produced in 24 hours and the specific gravity of the urine are also important.

The excreting and concentrating power of the kidneys can be tested by measuring the amounts, in the blood, of substances normally disposed of by the kidneys. Urea and creatinine are normally eliminated by the kidneys but rise in quantity if the kidneys are defective. A high blood urea level is a sign of kidney failure.

Plain X-rays of the kidneys can demonstrate enlargement or shrinkage, but a more useful form of X-ray examination is pyelography or urography. In this procedure, an X-ray is taken after injection of a substance which is rapidly excreted by the kidney and which is also opaque to X-rays. This is called an intravenous urogram (IVU) and indicates whether the kidneys are excreting the dye and shows up the internal structure.

435

...ones in, or disorders of, the kidney drainage tubes (the ureters) are also shown. An alternative is to pass fine tubes through the bladder into the ureters and inject the radio-opaque dye directly. This is called retrograde urography.

Ultrasound scanning can show changes in the size of a kidney, and can demonstrate cysts or tumours. CT and MRI scanning provide even more detailed cross-sectional views of the kidney and can reveal disease processes in fine detail.

kidney transplant

Kidney grafting is by far the commonest and most successful of the major organ transplantation operations. It is the final resource for people with total failure of *both* kidneys. The body can function perfectly well with one kidney, so transplantation from a living donor is possible. This, together with the fact that people with kidney failure can be kept alive by the use of the 'artificial kidney' (dialysis machine), allows time for better selection of a donor. For the same reason, the failure of a kidney transplant is less serious than that of a heart or lung transplant.

HOW IT'S DONE

Donor organs can be obtained from both the living and from the recently dead. The requirement for tissue and blood group matching involves so many permutations that efficient use of limited supplies dictates a nationwide, computerized system of coordinating supply and demand. The ideal donor, however, is a close relative.

In most cases, both of the diseased kidneys are removed some weeks before transplantation. The donated kidney is not, however, placed in the normal kidney site, but is accommodated in the lower part of the abdomen, usually on the right side, where there is convenient access to the major

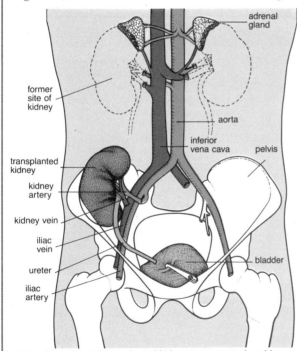

Kidney transplant. Transplanted kidneys are never placed in the normal kidney position. More suitable blood vessels and ready access to the bladder can be obtained if the transplanted kidney is placed in the pelvis, as shown.

artery and vein running down to the leg (iliac artery and vein). The kidney has a very large through-put of blood and the kidney vessels are attached end-to-side to the leg vessels so as to avoid any risk to the leg circulation.

When this has been done and the vessel clamps removed, the donor kidney swells and flushes and soon there is a spurt of urine from the donor ureter. This is pushed obliquely through a stab incision in the wall of the adjacent bladder and stitched in place.

RISKS

The results of kidney transplantation are excellent, with success in more than 80 per cent of cases. Rejection, which is most likely during the first two months, is becoming less common as understanding of immunology improves and new and better anti-rejection drugs are developed. Immunosuppressive regimens have been worked out to provide the maximum security against rejection compatible with the minimum disturbance to the patient's resistance to infection, but these must be continued for life.

killer cells

See **natural killer cells**.

kilocalorie

The amount of heat needed to raise the temperature of a kilogram of water by 1°C. This has been the standard nutritional unit of energy for years, but is now being replaced by the kilojoule. 1 Kcal = 4.187 KJ.

King's evil

The historic term for tuberculosis of the neck lymph nodes (scrofula) which was common at a time when most milk was infected with bovine tuberculosis. The name derives from the belief that scrofula could be cured if the king would only lay hands on the sufferer. This belief persisted until at least the time of Doctor Samuel Johnson (1709–94), who was touched for the scrofula.

Neither the great doctor nor any of the other hundreds of thousands of subjects who were touched by a succession of accommodating kings, enjoyed any direct benefit from the process, but the placebo effect was, undoubtedly, enormous.

Kinidin Durules

A brand name for **quinidine**.

Kinsey reports

The Kinsey reports, the first large-scale studies of sexual behaviour, burst upon a shocked and sometimes disbelieving world in 1948 and 1953. *Sexual Behavior in the Human Male* (1948) by the American zoologist Alfred Charles Kinsey (1894–1956) and his colleagues Wardell B. Pomeroy and Clyde E. Martin, and *Sexual Behavior in the Human Female* (1953) by the same authors and Paul H. Gebhard, were the collated findings of researchers who questioned over 10,000 men and women on matters previously considered too private for general mention – frequency of marital and extra-marital sexual intercourse, methods of intercourse, sexual orientation, masturbation, female orgasm, and so on.

Among their findings were that nearly all males and about 75 per cent of women masturbate at some time; that 4 per

Labels on figure:
adrenal gland
former site of kidney
transplanted kidney
kidney artery
kidney vein
iliac vein
ureter
iliac artery
aorta
inferior vena cava
pelvis
bladder

cent of adult men were exclusively homosexual and another 13 per cent were predominantly homosexual; that more than one man in three had had a sexual interaction leading to orgasm with another male; and that the reported rates of female homosexuality were about half of those for men.

The furore has long subsided and Kinsey and his colleagues are perceived as having made a notable contribution to knowledge of an important aspect of human behaviour. In general, their findings came to be accepted as being a realistic, if not precisely accurate, reflection of the truth, and their pioneering work prompted much further valuable research. Perhaps above all, the Kinsey reports helped people to overcome repressive taboos about open discussion on sex.

kissing disease

See **glandular fever**.

kiss of life

Mouth-to-mouth or mouth-to-nose artificial respiration.
See *First Aid*.

Klean-prep

A brand name for **polyethylene glycol**.

kleptomania

A rare condition characterized by a recurrent failure to resist the impulse to steal, usually from a shop, things not needed or even particularly wanted. The object is often given or thrown away or is carefully hidden. Most kleptomaniacs have the means to pay for the things they steal and the motive is not the same as that of the thief. The disorder, although rare, occurs in all strata of society.

The act is not usually pre-planned and the object of the activity is the theft itself. The stealing is not usually reckless, and reasonable precautions are taken to avoid discovery, but sometimes kleptomaniacs seem to give no thought to the probable consequences of their actions and some of them appear outraged when arrested. In the course of the act there is a rising sense of tension focused on the theft; afterwards, if the act is successfully accomplished, there is relief of tension and a sense of elation. This may, however, be followed by strong guilt feelings and intense fear of discovery.

Kleptomania is often put forward as a defence against an indictment for theft, but it is in fact very uncommon. Less than 5 per cent of people arrested for shoplifting are found, on questioning, to respond in a manner consistent with the diagnosis. The condition is associated with stress, such as bereavement or separation, and kleptomaniacs also tend to suffer from persistent depression and anorexia nervosa. It has also been associated with starting fires (pyromania).

POSSIBLE CAUSES

The cause remains obscure, but many kleptomaniacs feel that they have been wronged, and are unwanted or neglected and are thus entitled to steal. Many explanatory hypotheses have been advanced, especially by psychoanalysts, to explain the phenomenon. It has been suggested that in women it represents a search for a penis; that the disorder is a means of seeking punishment; and that the excitement engendered is enjoyed as a substitute for sexual intercourse.

TREATMENT

Kleptomania tends to be persistent and may, indeed, be a lifelong disorder. In many cases it is compatible with an otherwise apparently normal life and few affected people receive treatment unless this has been ordered by judicial authorities after arrest. Treatment involves a course of psychotherapy designed to provide the affected person with a clear **insight** into the nature of the condition. **Behaviour therapy** has also been successful.

Klinefelter's syndrome

A disorder of male body configuration caused by an abnormality of the sex chromosomes. Instead of the normal X and Y sex chromosomes, men with Klinefelter's syndrome have one or more extra chromosomes, usually an extra X, so that the complement is XXY. This happens in about one male birth in 500. The normal female configuration is XX, and the additional X in the male genome has a feminizing effect. This may not be noticed before puberty, but, thereafter, the testes are seen to be small, and found to be infertile, and the penis is also small. Female breast development and other female sexual characteristics may occur and there is usually diminished sexual interest. Affected men are often tall and slim. The diagnosis can easily be confirmed by chromosomal analysis.

Men with Klinefelter's syndrome often suffer problems of gender identity and some have strong trans-sexual inclinations. Homosexuality and transvestism are common and there is a higher than average incidence of mental retardation. Those who wish to retain a male identity can be helped by surgical removal of the breasts and male sex hormone treatment to promote male secondary sexual characteristics.

knee, disorders of

The knee, although very strong, is readily susceptible to injury. A twisting force can rupture a semi-lunar cartilage and this may 'lock' the knee. Joint surfaces readily become worn and damaged, especially in the overweight, leading to **osteoarthritis**.

Inflammation of the joint lining (synovitis) may result from repeated small injuries and causes an increase in production of synovial fluid, with swelling of the joint. Swelling after injury may also be caused by actual bleeding into the joint (*haemarthrosis*). Sometimes some of the cells of the synovial membrane change their character and become capable of forming lumps of cartilage. These may break off to form 'loose bodies' in the joint.

Inflammation of one or more of the bursas surrounding the knee joint may result from excessive local pressure, especially on the front of the knee. This causes **clergyman's knee**. Fluid may escape from one of the bursas behind the knee to cause a **Baker's cyst**. Adolescent boys often suffer a softening of the kneecap called **chondromalacia patellae**.

knee-locking

When one of the half-moon (semi-lunar or meniscus) cartilages of the knee is torn, as may occur when the foot is caught in the ground and the body twisted, one of the cartilages may remain secured only at one end. In this event, a fragment of cartilage may, at the time or later, slip between the bearing

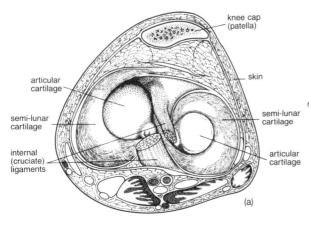

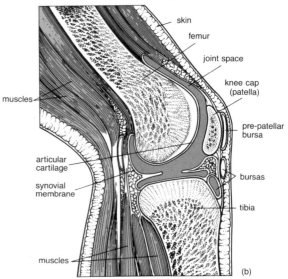

(a) A cross-section, and (b) a longitudinal section, of the knee.
Note the semi-lunar cartilages, the joint space filled with
synovial fluid, the internal crossing (cruciate) ligaments and
the synovial membrane that secretes the fluid.

surfaces of the joint and prevent either full straightening or
full bending. This knee-locking, in a partially bent position, is
very disabling and painful, and is often recurrent. It is a common sign of torn cartilage. In the end, the cartilage may have
to be removed surgically (meniscectomy).

knock-knee

See **genu valgum**.

koilonychia

The Greek word *koilos* means 'concave' or 'hollow' and the
word *onyx* means a finger or toenail. Koilonychia is a condition
which may result from iron-deficiency anaemia or from injury
to a nail bed. The nails are thin, brittle and hollowed out.

Koilonychia may, rarely, be a feature of the inherited
condition dystrophic epidermolysis bullosa and of the
intensely itchy skin disease lichen planus.

Kolanticon

A brand name for a preparation containing **magnesium
oxide** and dimethicone.

Konakion

A brand name for vitamin K (**phytomenadione**).

Konsyl

A brand name for **ispaghula**.

Koplik's spots

Tiny white spots, surrounded by a red base, occurring on the
inside of the cheeks and the inner surface of the lower lip
during the incubation period of **measles**.

koro

A delusional disorder prevalent in South-East Asia, affecting
males and sometimes occurring in epidemics. The sufferer
becomes obsessed with the belief that his penis is shrinking
and that it will disappear into his body, so causing his death.

To prevent this, he will tie his penis to a heavy stone or persuade friends to keep hold of it, in relays. Sometimes he will
even pass a safety-pin through the foreskin.

The delusion is widespread in the areas where koro occurs
and is related to the belief that ghosts have no genitals. Koro,
as distinct from the unrelated condition **kuru**, is a purely cultural and conceptual disorder.

Korotkoff sounds

Blood pressure is measured by listening to the sounds heard
through a stethoscope held over a compressed artery, usually
in the upper arm, as the compression is gradually released.
Compression is achieved with an expandable cuff that is
inflated with air, and the pressure in the cuff is shown on a
column of mercury or a dial. When the cuff pressure exceeds
the peak of blood pressure (systolic pressure) no sounds are
heard, but as the pressure is gradually reduced, blood can get
though the narrowed artery and this causes a sound.

The first pulse sound heard as blood is able to pass
through the narrowed artery is Korotkoff phase I. The sounds
get louder as the cuff pressure continues to fall, but then
there is a sudden muffling. This is Korotkoff phase IV; the
cuff pressure at this point has, in the past, been taken as the
between-beat (diastolic) pressure. Soon after that the sounds
disappear altogether. This is Korotkoff phase V, the cuff
pressure at which there is no compression of the artery. The
pressure shown by the mercury column or the dial at this
point is now generally taken as the diastolic pressure. The
mercury column equipment is called a sphygmomanometer.

Korsakoff's psychosis

See **Wernicke-Korsakoff syndrome**.

Kraurosis vulvae

See **vulvovaginitis**.

Kuntchner nail

A large, strong stainless steel nail used to maintain alignment
in fractures of the shaft of the thigh bone. The nail is inserted
into the hollow canal of the bone.

kuru

One of a group of slow, fatal brain infections, which also includes **Creutzfeldt-Jakob disease**, scrapie in sheep and bovine spongiform encephalopathy in cattle. These are all thought to be caused by a tiny virus-like particle, called a *prion*, which has none of the usual properties of a virus except the ability to produce a characteristic disease process. The prion is resistant to most of the normal methods of sterilization.

Kuru appears to be limited to natives of the highlands of New Guinea among whom it was spread by the practice of eating the brains of dead relatives. This form of cannibalism was confined to women and the virus was transmitted through skin abrasions during the preparation of the meal. This involved removing the brain, squeezing it into a pulp by hand and filling bamboo cylinders in which it was cooked. When first investigated in 1957, the annual mortality from Kuru was about 200. Almost all who died were adult women or children. Only 2 per cent were males. Kuru begins about thirty years after the agent is acquired and kills within a year. It causes progressive inability to walk and, later, even to sit up, headache, aching joints and limbs, inability to speak and to swallow and, in some cases, dementia. Death occurs after months of inexorably progressive disability.

> Some interesting parallels have been drawn between kuru and AIDS. Both are caused by viruses or virus-like agents which were unknown prior to the discovery of the diseases; both are caused by agents with very long incubation periods; both are known to affect the brain in a serious and ultimately fatal manner; in both cases there is good circumstantial evidence that the agents originated in other animals; both seem to have been spread by unusual social behaviour and to have had a devastating effect on the minority groups involved.

kwashiorkor

A serious nutritional deficiency disease of young children which results from a diet with grossly inadequate quantities of protein, but a high content of carbohydrate of low nutritional value. The term derives from a Ghanaian word meaning 'the disease of the child no longer at the breast'. To try to meet the energy needs, the intake has to be of large volume.

Kwashiorkor occurs in underdeveloped areas and is probably the commonest of all dietary diseases. It occurs when children are weaned and thus deprived of the high nutritional value of breast milk, or when the appetite is affected by infections.

RECOGNITION AND SYMPTOMS

The disease causes delayed growth and development, fluid retention (oedema), pigmentary changes in the skin and hair, irritability or apathy, enlargement of the liver and wasting of the muscles. Characteristically the abdomen is markedly protuberant, and the child with kwashiorkor may, superficially, appear to be well nourished. This is an illusion, however, and these children are highly susceptible to severe infectious diseases, which often prove fatal. Loss of protein can reduce the osmotic power of the blood to withdraw fluid from the tissues and these become water-logged. Antibodies are protein molecules and these, too, may be deficient, so that resistance to infection is lowered.

TREATMENT

Kwashiorkor is treated initially with feeds of milk containing vitamin and mineral supplements and then, if possible, a normal balanced diet with adequate protein content.

> Children under two years of age who develop kwashiorkor are likely to suffer lifelong effects.

Kwells

A brand name for **hyoscine**.

kyphoscoliosis

A spinal deformity in which an abnormal degree of backward curvature (**kyphosis**) is combined with curvature to one side (scoliosis).

kyphosis

An abnormal degree of backward curvature of part of the spine. Backward curvature is normal in the upper back (dorsal) region of the spine and in the lowest part (the sacrum). The term 'kyphosis', which comes from the Greek *kyphos* meaning 'bowed or bent', is applied to a degree of backward curvature of the spine sufficient to cause deformity.

Kyphosis is due to downward loading on the spine so that the normal curves are exaggerated. This will not happen unless there is inadequate support, either from poor muscles, faulty posture or softening of the bones. It therefore tends to affect two groups – adolescents, as a result of slouching or slumping, and post-menopausal women as a result of **osteoporosis**. In the case of the latter it is sometimes referred to as a 'dowager's hump'.

Kyphosis usually affects the upper part of the spine causing a disfiguring rounded hump or sometimes a more sharply defined protuberance. The latter is most commonly due to a crush fracture of adjacent spinal bones (vertebrae) or to collapse of the bones from diseases such as tuberculosis or cancer.

TREATMENT

Adolescent kyphosis responds readily to a disciplined and determined attempt to assume an upright posture, together with regular exercises to strengthen the abdominal muscles and those which extend the spine. Later in life kyphosis becomes increasingly difficult to correct, but, at any age, the same approach can help.

Progressive kyphosis from osteoporosis calls for energetic management with hormone replacement therapy, high calcium intake and postural and muscle-maintaining exercises.

> If the condition is neglected, the outcome may be one of serious height loss, gross deformity and sometimes grave disability.

Kytril

A brand name for granisetron.

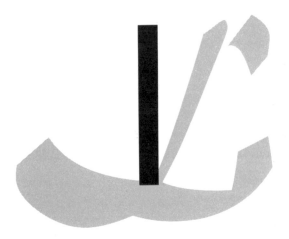

labetalol

A combined alpha- and beta-blocking drug, sometimes found to be more effective in the treatment of high blood pressure than beta-blockers. It is also used to treat **angina pectoris**. A brand name is Trandate.

labia

The labia (singular labium) are the four elongated lips that surround the entrance to the vagina and the external opening of the urine tube (urethra). The inner of the two pairs, the labia minora, are narrow, wrinkled, moist and red and of varying depth. Each one forks, at the front, to form a hood over the front of the head of the clitoris. The outer pair, the labia majora, are long, well padded folds, containing muscle and fibro-fatty tissue, and covered with hair. At the front, they join in the lower part of the pubic mound (mons veneris). As they run back between the thighs, they become more prominent. Behind, they join together a few centimetres in front of the anus. They are normally closed and conceal the rest of the genitalia.

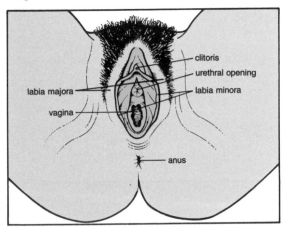

The external genitalia in the female.

labile

Unstable, liable to change. A healthy body and mind has a considerable degree of stability in those features able to vary.

A tendency to sudden, unexpected changes, whether in the biochemical elements of the blood, the action of the heart, the blood pressure or the state of the emotions, is described as lability and indicates an unhealthy state.

labium

Latin root meaning 'lip' as in labial (of the lips).

labour

See **childbirth**.

Labosept

A brand name for **dequalinium**.

labyrinthitis

Inflammation of the part of the inner ear responsible for balance. This is usually caused by a virus infection and may occur in the course of **influenza** or **mumps**. More seriously, the condition may result from the spread of infection through the bone from middle ear infection (**otitis media**).

Labyrinthitis causes a spinning sensation (vertigo) and sometimes unsteadiness or even falling. Vomiting may occur and there may also be deafness and a sense of ringing or hissing in the ears (**tinnitus**). Mild cases caused by viruses usually clear up within a few days. Other infections require specialist treatment.

laceration

A wound which is torn or irregular, rather than one that is cleanly cut (incised).

lacidipine

A **calcium channel blocker** drug. A brand name is Motens.

lacrima

Latin root meaning 'tear' as in lacrimal (of tears).

lacrimal system

The lacrimal system is the tear-production and drainage system of the eyes. Tears are essential for the health of the eyes and without a normal tear film over the cornea normal vision

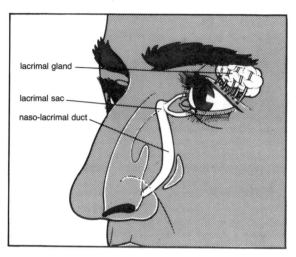

The tear drainage system.

is impossible. Tears are produced by the lacrimal glands which lie in the upper and outer parts of the bony eye socket, behind the upper lids. Tears are also produced by large numbers of microscopic 'accessory' lacrimal glands in the membrane covering the whites of the eyes (conjunctiva).

Excessive tears are disposed of into the nose by way of tiny ducts with openings at the inner corners of the four eyelids. These run into the lacrimal sacs, just inwards of the corners of the eyes, and from there down into the nose. Blockage of this drainage system is a common cause of watering eye.

lactation

The production and secretion of milk after childbirth.
See **breastfeeding**.

lactose intolerance

The effect of a deficiency of the enzyme that breaks down milk sugar (lactose) in the intestine. Because lactose from milk remains unsplit and unabsorbed it accumulates in the gut and is acted on by intestinal bacteria that digest it with the production of much gas. This causes abdominal discomfort, colicky pain and diarrhoea.

Asian and African people who have undergone a change of diet to one with a higher lactose content are often affected in this way.

Lactugal

A brand name for **lactulose**.

lactulose

A disaccharide sugar that acts as a gentle but effective laxative. It is not absorbed or broken down but remains intact until it reaches the colon where it is split by bacteria and helps to retain water, thereby softening the stools. Brand names are Duphalac and Lactugal.

Lamarckism

A now-discredited doctrine, put forward by the French naturalist Jean Baptiste, Chevalier de Lamarck (1744–1829), that species can change into new species as a result of

characteristics acquired as a result of striving to overcome environmental disadvantages. Lamarck claimed, without evidence, that such acquired characteristics became hereditary. The growth of biological and genetic knowledge confirmed his mistake. Lamarck, however, deserved the credit for insisting, long before Charles Darwin, that species were produced by a process of evolution.

Lamictal

A brand name for **lamotrigine**.

laminectomy

An operation to treat the effects of prolapsed intervertebral disk – commonly known as '**slipped disc**'. Through an incision in the back, a small part of one or more of the vertebrae of the spine is removed so as to gain access to the spinal canal. The surgeon can then remove the pulpy material, squeezed out from the centre of the disk, which is pressing on the nerve roots or the spinal cord.

Lamisil

A brand name for **terbinafine**.

lamivudine

A reverse transcriptase inhibitor drug used to treat infections with retroviruses, such as HIV. The drug has also been used to treat hepatitis. Brand names are Epivir and Zeffix.

lamotrigine

A drug used to control the type of epilepsy known as 'petit mal' or absence attacks. It is taken by mouth. Possible side-effects include skin rash, a serious inflammatory condition of the mucous membranes (Stevens-Johnson syndrome), headache, indigestion, double vision, blurred vision, vertigo, drowsiness, reduced white cell count and liver failure. A brand name is Lamictal.

lana

Latin root meaning 'wool' as in lanoline (wool fat).

lance

An old-fashioned term referring to the use of a surgical knife (lancet) to open an abscess or a boil.

lancet

Once a prominent piece of equipment, the lancet has now been replaced almost entirely by the disposable surgical knife or the disposable blade fitted to a reusable handle. A bewildering variety of pre-sterilized disposable blades is available. Such blades are used for one operation only and are then discarded.

Langerhans cell histiocytosis

See **Letterer-Siwe disease**.

Lanoxin

A brand name for **digoxin**.

lansoprazole

A **proton pump inhibitor** drug. A brand name is Zoton.

Lanvis

A brand name for **thioguanine**.

laparoscopic sterilization

Closure of the Fallopian tubes in women by **laparoscopic surgery** so that eggs (ova) cannot be contacted by sperms. This is an established and safe procedure. The tubes may be clipped, cut and sealed with electric cautery or occluded by small circular plastic bands. The latter method allows the possibility of reversal of the sterilization.

laparoscopic surgery

A range of surgical techniques performed through small metal or plastic ports inserted through very short incisions in the skin and often through the navel. The instruments are externally controlled and the operation site is internally illuminated and is commonly viewed on a large computer-type colour monitor. A special range of operating instruments has been designed for this purpose and these are constantly being improved.

Current methods mainly allow two-dimensional viewing, but three-dimensional laparoscopic surgery is under development. This provides the operator with a three-dimensional display of the internal structures, by using an endoscope with two vision channels and two miniaturized video cameras. Active liquid-crystal shutter spectacles are worn to provide a three-dimensional view which improves accuracy, dexterity, speed, and safety.

Most of the pain and discomfort, and the slow convalescence, following earlier surgery was caused by the large incisions through skin and muscle that were considered necessary. These effects are virtually eliminated by laparoscopic surgery, which substantially shortens recovery time. For instance, it is common for a patient to return to work a day or two after a gall-bladder removal by laparoscopic surgery, a procedure formerly requiring long convalescence. This method is, in consequence, deservedly popular with patients. For an increasing range of operations the method has replaced, as the optimum method, earlier and cruder techniques.

Surgery is still in a transitional phase and older surgeons have had to master some entirely new techniques and adapt to the change in the relationship of hand and eye. Some have found this unexpectedly difficult. Pressures on surgeons to adopt the newer methods have, in some cases, led to a higher than acceptable incidence of complications.

laparoscopy

Direct visual examination of the interior of the abdomen, using fibre optic illumination and viewing channels contained in a narrow viewing tube (endoscope), which can be passed through a small incision in the abdominal wall.

Laparoscopy can be used by any specialist concerned with disease of the abdominal organs, but has been especially adopted by gynaecologists for the investigation of disorders of the female reproductive organs in the pelvis. Conditions such as ectopic pregnancy, and sterility from possible obstruction of the Fallopian tubes, which are difficult to diagnose with certainty in any other way short of an exploratory abdominal operation, can be diagnosed in this way. Laparoscopy also allows a range of operations to be performed and is widely used as a means of deliberately closing off the Fallopian tubes to achieve sterilization. Laparoscopy can be valuable in the diagnosis of doubtful cases of appendicitis, or diseases of the gall-bladder or liver.

Laparoscopy is usually done under general anaesthesia. Harmless carbon dioxide gas is passed into the abdomen through a small needle to inflate the abdominal cavity and move the intestines out of the way. The endoscope can then be safely inserted through a small incision. Various instruments, including laser channels, can be passed through the laparoscope, for various purposes. In particular, tissues can be vaporized and cut, without bleeding; local disease, such as

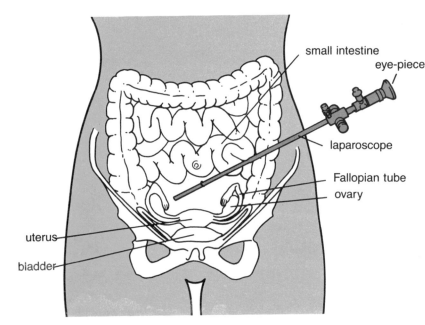

Laparoscopy. This is a valuable method of examination and treatment, especially for gynaecological complaints. The laparoscope is passed through the wall of the abdomen under anaesthesia and gas is used to move the bowels out of the way. The method is commonly used for sterilization, but has much wider applications.

patches of endometriosis, destroyed; and biopsies taken from any organ, including the liver. Eggs (ova) can be taken from the ovaries for *in vitro* fertilization. The pressure of the gas in the abdomen may cause some discomfort for a day or two, until it absorbs.

A development of laparoscopy is videolaseroscopy, in which a video camera is attached to the laparoscope so that the interior of the abdomen can be viewed on a TV monitor and the procedure carried out while watching the screen. This is very convenient for the surgeon who, in the past, has had to spend long periods bending over the patient's abdomen and looking through a single small eyepiece. Zoom magnification of small areas is possible and videotape recordings can be made for record, research and teaching purposes.

LAPAROTOMY

This word 'laparotomy' is really an abbreviation of a phrase, which has come to stand for the phrase. Literally, laparotomy is a cutting through the flank, and properly means a surgical opening into the abdomen. Originally, the phrase was *exploratory laparotomy* but, worn by usage, the phrase is now reduced to the single word, which means any abdominal operation done to discover the cause of an illness which cannot otherwise be determined.

Laparotomy is often necessary in obviously ill people with signs indicating some acute abdominal problem and in whom it is recognized that, once the cause is found, immediate, surgical remedial measures will probably be possible. Thus, laparotomy is usually performed in those cases in which the abdomen would probably have to be opened in any case. In the course of a laparotomy, a wide internal inspection is done to detect other, or associated, disorders.

Often, laparotomy is done because of signs of inflammation of the membrane lining the abdomen (peritonitis) but without indication of the source of the leakage of bowel contents which is causing the trouble. It is also often done to determine whether or not abdominal cancer is present, and, if it is, to determine its extent and operability. The detection of the origin of bleeding within the abdomen, following injury, is another important indication for laparotomy.

In many cases a patient can be spared a laparotomy by having a laparoscopic examination instead.

Largactil

A brand name for **chlorpromazine**.

large intestine

The colon, or large intestine, is called 'large' not because of its length – it is about 1.7 m (5 feet) long compared with the 6 to 7 m (20 feet) of the 'small' intestine – but because of its diameter. The colon forms a kind of festoon in the abdomen, starting on the lower right side at the caecum, rising on the right side (ascending colon), crossing, with a droop, to a point opposite on the left side (transverse colon), descending on the left (descending colon), and curving back and down towards the midline (sigmoid colon) to run into the rectum.

The main function of the colon is to conserve water by extracting it from the bowel contents so that these are turned from a wet mud at the entry, to the familiar firm consistency at the exit. In simple terms, diarrhoea may be considered the result of 'intestinal hurry' with the contents passing through so quickly that there is insufficient time for absorption of water. And constipation may be considered the effect of slow passage with excessive absorption. The process of water withdrawal is very efficient and, if given long enough to act, will turn the faeces into dried pellets. Water conservation is important because although one may drink only a litre or so per day, about another 7 litres are emptied into the bowel from the salivary glands, the liver, the glands of the stomach and intestine and from the pancreas. If all this fluid were lost from the body, severe drying up (dehydration) would result.

The colon contains millions of bacteria and these are useful, producing, among other materials, B vitamins which are readily absorbed. These bacteria also have the ability to ferment some forms of carbohydrate – as found in peas and beans, for instance – that are not digested by the enzymes of the small intestine. This fermentation and other bacterial action produces large quantities of a gas which is a mixture of odourless nitrogen, carbon dioxide, hydrogen and methane, and the far from odourless hydrogen sulphide.

The daily output of faeces varies considerably with the diet, being high if much fibre is present. The average is around 150 g and the weight is mainly made up of bacteria. The faeces also contain cellular debris from the bowel lining, undigested cellulose and some bile pigments and salt. The rectum is the short, but distensible, length of bowel immediately above the anal canal. The latter is about 5 cm long, so the rectum is readily accessible to an examining gloved finger, and rectal examination is an important way of detecting certain disorders, such as internal piles, ano-rectal abscesses, polyps and especially cancers of the rectum. By feeling through the front wall of the rectum, the doctor can easily detect enlargement of the prostate gland. The anal canal is the short terminal portion of the intestinal canal. The anus has two muscle rings (sphincters) by means of which the contents of the rectum are retained until they can conveniently be discharged as faeces.

large intestine ballooning

See **toxic megacolon**.

Lariam

A brand name for **mefloquine**.

larva migrans

See **toxocariasis**.

laryngectomy

Surgical removal of the Adam's apple (larynx). This is hardly ever done except in the extremity of widespread cancer of the larynx, when the operation offers the only hope of saving life. The cut upper end of the windpipe (trachea) is brought out through an opening in the front of the neck to allow breathing.

After the larynx – which includes the vocal cords – has been removed, normal speech is impossible and the person concerned must either learn to produce the necessary vibrations by releasing deliberately swallowed air (oesophageal speech) or use an electromechanical buzzer held against the upper part of the neck. In both cases, the sounds produced are modulated by tongue and mouth movements as in speech, so as to produce intelligible noises.

laryngitis

Inflammation of the voice box (larynx). This is most commonly associated with the sore throat of the common cold or other upper respiratory infection, or may result from overuse of the voice. There is hoarseness, discomfort or pain, cough and difficulty in speaking. In some cases the voice is reduced to a painful whisper.

In the case of acute laryngitis, full recovery may be expected within a few days, especially if the voice is rested. Menthol inhalations or the use of medicated lozenges may be comforting.

More persistent laryngitis from overuse of the voice or long-term irritation from smoking is treated by removal of the cause, if possible. The symptoms may, however, persist and examination by an ear, nose and throat specialist may show the presence of nodules on the vocal cords, which may require treatment.

See also **clergyman's throat, cold, common, singers' nodes**.

laryngoscopy

The voice box (larynx), which causes the protuberance in the front of the neck, known as the Adam's apple, is, fortunately, within reach of visual inspection. Laryngoscopy is the term for examination of the larynx and this can be done using an angled mirror held at the back of the throat (indirect laryngoscopy), or directly by extending the recumbent subject's neck and using a rigid metal instrument which compresses the tongue so that the larynx may be seen from above. This is done under a general anaesthetic. Alternatively, a narrow, flexible, fibre optic viewing tube can be passed down the throat.

Laryngoscopy is important and may be life-saving when it allows the doctor to diagnose and relieve obstruction to breathing or to make an early diagnosis of cancer of the larynx. It is indicated if there is any persistent difficulty in breathing, any unusual inability to produce normal voice sounds, persistent hoarseness or changes in the voice, or unusually noisy breathing (stridor). It can be helpful in finding the cause of persistent pain in the throat or of difficulty in swallowing.

Direct laryngoscopy allows biopsies to be taken from the vocal cords, and polyps, nodules or foreign bodies to be removed.

laryngotracheobronchitis

A widespread inflammation of the upper respiratory tract, involving the voice box (larynx), the windpipe (trachea) and the main air passages of the lungs (the bronchi). In children this is the usual cause of croup.

larynx

Greek root meaning 'throat' as in laryngitis (inflamation of the larynx). The larynx is the structure causing the protrusion on the front of the neck knows as the 'Adam's apple' or voice box. It is situated at the upper end of the wind pipe (trachea), just in front of the start of the **gullet** (oesophagus). At its inlet is a leaf-shaped flap of cartilage, the epiglottis, that closes off the entry to the larynx during swallowing and normally precludes access to food. The larynx has walls of cartilage and is lined with a moist mucous membrane. It contains the vocal cords, two folds of the mucous membrane that can be tensed

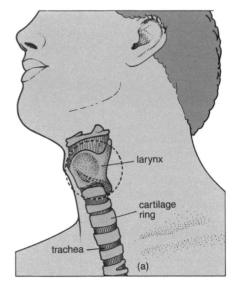

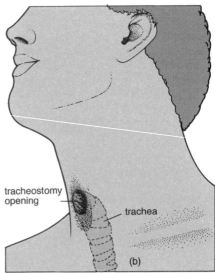

The mutilating operation of laryngectomy is sometimes essential to try to save life when the larynx (a) is affected by cancer. After the operation (b) the patient may have to breathe through an opening in the neck.

by tiny muscles to control their rate of vibration as air passes through them, and hence the pitch of the voice. The gap between the folds is called the glottis.

larynx, cancer of

Cancer of the larynx is comparatively rare and occurs most often in smokers and heavy drinkers. If it affects the vocal cords it causes obvious voice changes and is likely to be diagnosed early. In this case the outlook is favourable. Cancer elsewhere in the larynx is likely to be well advanced before symptoms of breathing or swallowing difficulty arise and the prospects of cure are correspondingly worse.

Small cancers of the vocal cords can often be cured by local treatment, including radiotherapy. Larger cancers usually require **laryngectomy**.

laser

Acronym for Light Amplification by Stimulated Emission of Radiation – a device that produces light of a single, precisely defined wavelength, in which all the waves are in phase with each other (coherent light). This allows the beam to be intensely concentrated, with little tendency to spread out, and permits focusing with a simple lens into a spot of microscopic size and hence of intense heat. Various solids, liquids and gases can be induced to lase light, and the properties of some of the wide range of lasers make them invaluable for a variety of medical and surgical purposes. Medical lasers are all relatively low-power devices and include argon lasers, various YAG lasers, carbon dioxide lasers, various pumped dye lasers and high-precision excimer lasers.

Laser applications in surgery and medicine include:

- simple bloodless tissue cutting;
- destroying or sealing unwanted blood vessels;
- tumour destruction;
- unblocking obstructed Fallopian tubes to restore fertility;
- removal of tattoos and birthmarks;
- removal of atherosclerotic plaque and thrombosis inside arteries so as to restore patency;
- removal of prostate gland tissue causing outflow obstruction;
- precision corneal curvature adjustment to correct refractive errors such as short and long sight;
- treatment of glaucoma by opening eye aqueous drainage channels (see **laser trabeculoplasty**);
- destroying peripheral parts of the retina so as to allow regression of dangerously fragile new blood vessels in diabetic retinopathy;
- attempts to prevent the progression of age-related macular degeneration by destroying leaking retinal vessels;
- attempts to promote healing in sprains, inflamed tendons and painful joints.

Contrary to popular belief, lasers are not used to treat cataract or to correct retinal detachment. They are, however, widely used to seal off areas of retinal degeneration or small retinal holes that might, if neglected, lead to retinal detachment.

laser trabeculoplasty

A treatment for **glaucoma**, using an argon laser to cut multiple tiny holes in the outflow filter of the eye, the trabecular meshwork. This causes scars that, on contraction, widen the channels of the meshwork and increase the facility of outflow of aqueous humour and reduce the pressure in the eye. The method has proved effective in many cases of chronic simple glaucoma that have proved resistant to treatment with beta-blocker and other eye drops.

laser weapon eye injuries

Severe dazzling, after-image formation, visual distortion and permanent blinding caused by military laser rangefinders, target designators, anti-optical sensor systems and anti-personnel laser weapons. Many of the military lasers in current use are capable of immediate and irremediable loss of vision in both eyes. They achieve this by destructive coagulation of the central and most sensitive foveal and macular regions of the retinas. This effect is made more probable because the image of anything that is looked at is focused on the foveas. Protective goggles have been produced but these are effective only if they also eliminate useful vision.

Lasix

A brand name for **frusemide**.

Lasma

A brand name for **theophylline**.

Lassa fever

An infectious disease endemic in many parts of rural west Africa and maintained in the rat population. It is caused by a virus and acquired by contact with infected rat secretions, especially urine. It may also be acquired by contact with the blood, or with the blood-stained secretions, of infected people, and accidental transmission has occurred, in African hospitals, following needle-stick injuries or contamination of broken or abraded skin with the blood of sufferers.

INCIDENCE

Although the mortality in the local population is as high as 20 per cent, the disease may be mild, especially in children and, in endemic areas, about 6 per cent of children have antibodies. Only a few cases have been imported into Britain and there have been no secondary infections from these.

RECOGNITION AND SYMPTOMS

Lassa fever starts, three to sixteen days after infection, with feverishness, aches and pains and sore throat. Between the third and sixth day, thereafter, there is a dramatic worsening with severe pain in the chest and abdomen, high fever, prostration, redness of the eyes, difficulty in swallowing and vomiting. Yellow spots and ulcers appear on the tonsils. The blood pressure drops and there is lethargy, deafness, blurring of vision, and, in severe cases, a faint skin rash.

The high fever lasts for one or two weeks and the most acutely ill patients suddenly deteriorate at some time during the second week, pass into coma and die of inadequate circulation (shock), respiratory insufficiency, or cardiac arrest. Those who survive have a long period of extreme fatigue and some suffer loss of hair and deafness.

TREATMENT

The disease may be treated with plasma taken from former sufferers, but this sometimes aggravates the condition. The drug ribavirin has been much more successful.

lassitude

A disinclination to exert oneself or to make an effort to achieve anything. Lassitude may be a feature of organic disease or depression, but is often due to boredom or the failure to appreciate the importance of interests and enthusiasm.

lateral

Of, at or towards the side. The term comes from the Latin military word *latus* meaning a 'flank' or 'wing'. Unilateral means occurring only on one side; bilateral means relating to two sides. Bilateral pulmonary tuberculosis means TB in both lungs.

latere

Latin root meaning 'side' as in lateral (to the side).

laudanum

A solution of opium in alcohol.

laughing gas

A popular term for the anaesthetic drug nitrous oxide. This gas has useful pain-relieving properties but is a poor anaesthetic and causes loss of consciousness largely by excluding oxygen. On recovery, the subject may experience a sense of omniscience or amusement.

Laurence-Moon-Biedl syndrome

A rare genetic disorder featuring mental retardation, extra toes or fingers, and a retinal degeneration, *retinitis pigmentosa*, that may progress to blindness. There is no treatment for the syndrome and attempts should be made to prevent further transmission of the gene.

laxatives

The subject of constipation is of enduring interest to mankind as well as of enormous commercial importance to the pharmaceutical industry. Like many subjects of wide popular interest, however, it is fraught with fallacy. There is a general belief that some calamity will befall anyone who fails to empty his or her bowels at least once a day. This belief is without foundation. Some people have a satisfying bowel motion three times a day, others three times a week. Some feel the need to go even less often. So long as the passage is easy, without undue straining, and with a satisfying sense of completeness, all these patterns are normal.

Constipation can certainly cause symptoms but these are not, as is alleged by many alternative medicine practitioners, the result of the absorption of 'toxins' from the bowel. These symptoms can be produced by packing the rectum with sterile cotton wool. Constipation does not cause halitosis, distention, abdominal discomfort, belching or headache.

Constipation is as often imaginary as real, and many people, who believe that a daily bowel action is essential to health, severely abuse their lower intestines with laxatives, suppositories and enemas. This response to an imaginary disorder can produce a real one. Anxious, fastidious people, especially those whose food intake is small, often feel that it is essential to get rid of 'unclean' excreta every day. Some become very anxious if there is no bowel motion. The constant use of laxatives in these circumstances can lead to an irritable bowel disorder. Depressed people often excrete less than average and the awareness may, in turn, make the depression worse.

Constipation is, of course, a symptom and not a disease. It has many causes. These include:

- deliberate suppression of evacuation;
- chronic obstruction from tumours or bowel strictures;
- painful piles;
- various neurological disorders such as Parkinson's disease and spinal cord injuries;
- **anticholinergic drugs** such as atropine;
- **analgesic drugs** such as Codeine;
- bismuth salts;
- **anticonvulsant drugs**;
- **antidepressant drugs**.

Constipation is essentially a disorder of civilized societies and is almost unknown among peoples whose diet is largely vegetable with a high fibre content. Such people produce frequent bulky stools and are free from many of the colonic disorders suffered by those who enjoy more expensive diets.

The first step in tackling the constipation syndrome is to ensure adequate bulk in the stools. This is easily done by adjusting the diet so as to replace refined carbohydrate with foods containing much vegetable fibre. Plenty of fruit, vegetables and bran-containing cereals should be taken. The best drug for constipation is bran. This is what is left when flour is extracted from cereals. It contains up to half its weight in cellulose vegetable fibre, which has the property of taking up large quantities of water. So bran should always be accompanied by a good fluid intake. It is hard to eat too much bran. This kind of regime will produce bulky, soft stools and regular motions.

When a laxative is required for long-term use, the only form that should be considered is one of the bulking agents. These are safe, act slowly and gently and are not habit-forming. Bran is the best choice, but most people feel that something more expensive is bound to be better and go in for nicely packaged preparations of methyl cellulose, which is much the same, apart from the price. Isogel is made from psyllium seeds and contains mucilage which, like bran cellulose and methyl cellulose, also swells and bulks up with water.

Other forms of laxative, safe for occasional use, include wetting agents such as Dioctyl and Poloxamer 188, lubricants such as liquid paraffin, and osmotic agents like Lactulose or Epsom, Glauber or Rochelle salts. These agents are not absorbed, but remain in the bowel, retaining and attracting water and thereby increasing the bulk of the stools. Plenty of water should be drunk with all of these. Avoid irritant laxatives, like castor oil, senna, cascara, and so on. These should never be used on a regular basis. Enemas may be needed if you are ill or debilitated, but should be used under medical supervision. Colonic irrigation should probably be regarded as a rather dubious recreational activity.

Laxoberal

A brand name for **sodium picosulphate**.

lazy eye

A lay term, sometimes used to refer to an inturning of the eye (convergent squint or **esotropia**) and sometimes to the defect of vision which often results from untreated squint in young children (**amblyopia**).

-le

Suffix meaning 'diminutive' as in vesicle (little bladder).

lead poisoning

Lead and lead compounds are highly toxic when eaten or inhaled. The symptoms of lead poisoning depend on the dose. Acute poisoning, from a large dose, causes severe intestinal symptoms with abdominal pain, vomiting and diarrhoea, then signs of damage to the nervous system, including convulsions, muscle weakness, coma and death.

Poisoning is, however, usually unsuspected, and most commonly results from small amounts of lead being taken in over long periods. The effects are cumulative and can be disastrous. Although lead is absorbed very slowly, it is excreted even more slowly. So, if there is continued exposure to the fumes of leaded petrol, lead paints, pottery glazes, solder, water from lead pipes, alcohol from illicit stills using lead pipes or other sources, lead accumulates gradually in the body. It is taken up by the red blood cells and circulated through the body to concentrate in the soft tissues, especially the liver, kidneys and brain.

There has been special concern over the risks from tetra-ethyl-lead used as an anti-knocking agent in petrol. Children exposed to the exhaust fumes from such petrol may suffer chronic lead poisoning and this is known to be capable of causing damage to brain function with headache, loss of physical coordination, loss of intellectual ability and memory, and abnormal behaviour. There is now little doubt that large numbers of children have, in the past, suffered varying degrees of loss of intellectual function – even measurable loss of IQ – as a result of prolonged exposure to atmospheric lead. Public awareness of the problem has, however, led to reduced levels of environmental lead and leaded petrol is no longer sold in Britain.

leaky mutant gene

One of a pair of genes (**alleles**) that is less active than its normal partner. A leaky mutation produces only partial loss of a characteristic.

lecithos

Greek root meaning 'egg yolk' as in lecithin (a yolk-like fatty substance).

Ledclair

A brand name for **sodium calcium edetate**.

Lederfen

A brand name for **fenbufen**.

Lederspan

A brand name for **triamcinolone**.

leg, broken

See **femur, fracture of**.

leg fracture traction

See **Steinmann pin**.

Legionnaires' disease

A form of **pneumonia** caused by *Legionella* bacteria, which tend to propagate in large, warm, moist areas such as air-conditioning towers and are spread into the air in water droplets. The first recognized outbreak occurred at an American Legion convention in Philadelphia in 1976 when 221 people were affected, with thirty-four deaths. It is now recognized to be widespread and it is thought to be the cause of as many as 2 per cent of hospital cases of pneumonia.

RECOGNITION AND SYMPTOMS
The disease causes headache, aches and pains, diarrhoea, worsening cough, high fever, pneumonia, mental confusion, and kidney and liver damage. The most serious effects are on the lungs, which may suffer irremediable damage, and this is the common cause of death. The mortality rate is about 4 per cent.
RISK FACTORS
Those especially at risk include the elderly and the infirm, and heavy smokers and drinkers.
TREATMENT
Treatment includes such antibiotics as erythromycin and rifampicin.

leg lengthening

An orthopaedic surgical technique used to equalize leg length in children in cases of severe leg length discrepancy or to correct short stature. An **external fixator** is applied to the leg and the bone is cut through with preservation of the outer bone membrane (periosteum). This membrane is the source of new bone formation. Traction by way of the fixator allows gradual lengthening at a rate of about 1 mm per day. Once the desired length is achieved no further extension is applied but the fixator must be left in place until bone consolidation has occurred. The slow rate of extension is also necessary to allow soft tissue structures, such as muscles, blood vessels and nerves, to adapt. The treatment may take months.

leishmaniasis

A group of infections, caused by single-celled microscopic parasites of the genus *Leishmania*, and spread by sandflies. Leishmaniasis is becoming increasingly important because of the volume of holiday traffic to areas in which it is endemic, especially the Mediterranean. It can affect either the skin (cutaneous leishmaniasis) causing **Delhi boil** or **Oriental sore**, or it may affect the internal organs (**kala azar**).

Espundia, or American leishmaniasis, is caused by *Leishmania braziliensis*. It occurs in south Mexico, Brazil, Paraguay and Peru, causing disfiguring skin ulcers of the face and tissue destruction that extends into the cavities of the nose and mouth. It often persists for years and, if neglected, may lead to death from overwhelming secondary infection.

Lenium

A brand name for a shampoo containing selenium.

lenograstim

Human **granulocyte stimulating factor** produced by genetic engineering and used to treat severe deficiencies of some of the white cells of the blood and the immune system. A brand name is Granocyte.

lenses, contact

Contact lenses are made of plastic – never glass. Hard lenses are made of the acrylic PMMA (poly-methyl-methacrylate or 'Perspex') or the 'gas permeable' material CAB (cellulose acetate butyrate) or co-polymers of various plastics. Soft lenses are also usually acrylic, but the molecule contains a lot of water in a kind of plastic sponge. Most are made of HEMA (hydroxy-ethyl-methacrylate). Hard lenses are always of smaller diameter than the cornea, soft lenses are almost always of greater diameter. 'Permanent wear' lenses are dangerous and should not be worn.

Contact lenses are unlikely to replace spectacles as the definitive correction for the common refractive errors – short sight (**myopia**), long sight (**hypermetropia**) and corneal curvature anomalies (**astigmatism**) – but an increasing proportion of people are using them. Unfortunately, although much more efficient than glasses, contact lenses are liable to cause many more problems for the wearer. And, regrettably, many people acquire contact lenses without a sufficient trial period and without sufficient guidance in the rules of safe wear. Vision with contact lenses is usually better than with glasses – especially in the higher degrees of focusing error.

lenses, folding

See **intra-ocular lenses**.

lens implant

See **cataract surgery**.

Lentard MC

A brand name for **insulin**.

lentigo

A skin blemish similar to a freckle, caused by a local concentration of pigment-containing cells (melanocytes). Lentigos differ from freckles by occurring as commonly on covered as on uncovered parts and they do not become less conspicuous in winter time.

Lentizol

A brand name for **amitriptylene**.

leprosy

See **Hansen's disease**.

leptin

A hormone produced by fat cells, which provides the brain with information about the state of repletion. Leptin receptors are in the hypothalamus on the underside of the brain in an area known to be concerned with satiety and hunger. It is a protein coded for by the ob gene (for 'obesity') and was at first thought to be the complete answer to appetite control, but its action in human beings has been found to be more complex than in rats. Only about one-fifth of people respond to a high concentration of leptin by reducing food intake. Leptin was discovered at the end of 1994 and so much medical and pharmacological interest was aroused that more than 600 papers appeared on the topic within three years.

leptospirosis

Often called Weil's disease, this is an infection caused by a spiral-shaped organism (spirochaete) and transmitted in the urine of rats. The organism can penetrate the intact skin. The disease occurs most often in farm workers, veterinary workers and vagrants. It was formerly a major hazard to fish-market workers, sewer workers and miners, but better working conditions have reduced the incidence in these employments.

RECOGNITION AND SYMPTOMS

Leptospirosis starts about ten days after infection, and may be so mild as to be unsuspected. In more severe cases the onset is sudden with headache, severe muscle aches and tenderness, redness of the eyes, loss of appetite, vomiting and sometimes a skin rash. Many cases settle after a week or two, but in some the liver, kidneys, heart muscle and brain linings (meninges) are affected. **Jaundice**, **heart failure** and **meningitis** are signs of danger. In these cases, the mortality is as high as 20 per cent. Those who recover do so completely.

TREATMENT

The organisms are sensitive to penicillin and treatment with this drug is effective, if given early. It is of little value once organ damage has occurred.

lercanidipine

A calcium channel blocker drug used to treat high blood pressure. A brand name is Zanidip.

lesbianism

Female **homosexuality**. The term comes from the Greek female poet Sappho, who lived on the island of Lesbos with her followers during the seventh century BC. Female homosexuality is sometimes called *sapphism.*

Lesch-Nyhan syndrome

A rare recessive disease of young children in which a deficiency of a particular enzyme causes a severe over-production of uric acid. The high concentration of this substance in the blood causes gout and brain damage with cerebral palsy, mental retardation, bodily writhing and twitching (chorea), and compulsive self-mutilating by biting. The mutated gene is on the X chromosome and, being recessive, is virtually confined to males. This is because males have only one X chromosome so the mutation must have its effect. Females are most unlikely to have the disease as this means that the mutation would have to be present on corresponding genes on both of their X chromosomes.

Lescol

A brand name for **fluvastatin**.

lesion

A word derived from the Latin *laesio* meaning 'an attack or injury'. 'Lesion' is a most useful word to doctors as it covers all forms of disease process, any injury, wound, infection, or any structural or other form of abnormality anywhere in the body.

lethal injection

An increasingly widely used alternative to hanging, gassing or electrocution as a method of execution of condemned criminals. The method involves intravenous skills rarely available to non-medical people, so doctors are commonly asked to advise.

lethal mutation

A mutation whose effect is so serious that the cell is killed. Lethal mutations will often result in the death of the organism concerned.

lethargy

A state of overpowering apathy, drowsiness or lack of energy. In Greek mythology the river Lethe flowed through Hades and the dead were required to drink its water so as to forget their past lives.

letrozole

An **aromatase inhibitor** drug used to treat breast cancer in menopausal women that has resisted anti-oestrogen drugs. A brand name is Femara.

Letterer-Siwe disease

An often fatal disease of infants in which there is fever, generalized lymph node, liver and spleen enlargement, an eczematous skin rash and anaemia. The condition is brought about by an enormous increase in the number of antigen-presenting cells of the immune system known as Langerhans cells. These produce a grossly excessive quantity of **cytokines** resulting in great proliferation. Experts argue as to whether or not the condition is a form of cancer. The preferred name for the condition is now Langerhans cell histiocytosis. The mortality varies but may be as high as 50 per cent.

Leucomax

A brand name for **malgramostin**.

leukaemias

The leukaemias are a group of blood cancers in which certain groups of white blood cells reproduce in an entirely disorganized and uncontrolled way so that they progressively replace, and interfere with, the normal constituents of the blood. The leukaemias are progressive conditions which, unless effectively treated, will usually end fatally either from a shortage of red blood cells (**anaemia**), or from severe bleeding or infection.

POSSIBLE CAUSES
Their cause is unknown but there are definite associations with radiation, with some drugs used in the treatment of other cancers, with certain industrial chemicals such as benzene, and with certain viruses. The different types of leukaemia arise from different white cell types and have different outlooks.

ACUTE AND CHRONIC LEUKAEMIAS
There are two main groups – the acute leukaemias, with a very short life expectancy, and the chronic leukaemias in which the affected person may live for years.

Acute leukaemias often start with influenza-like symptoms, a feeling of great tiredness, sore throat, bleeding from the gums and into the skin, and loss of appetite and weight. There may be enlargement of the lymph nodes in the neck, armpits and groins. A blood check shows severe anaemia and usually large numbers of primitive white cells. It is important for a precise diagnosis to be made of the type of cell involved, as the treatment differs in different types.

Chronic leukaemias are of slow, insidious onset with gradual onset of **lassitude** and fatigue, and a slow increase in the size of the spleen until it becomes massive, causing a dragging weight and pain in the upper left side of the abdomen. There is slow loss of weight, aching in the bones, nose bleeds and sometimes unwanted and prolonged erections (**priapism**) in men. There may be intolerance to heat and undue sweating.

TREATMENT
The treatment of all types of leukaemia is, at present, primarily by chemotherapy. This is especially effective in chronic leukaemias and often maintains life for years. Removal of the spleen is often advised in chronic leukaemias and may be a valuable measure. In the acute leukaemias, 50 to 60 per cent of patients enjoy a remission on chemotherapy. Energetic supportive therapy to treat anaemia and infection is essential and this will usually involve blood transfusions and antibiotics. Other treatments include radiotherapy and white cell transfusions.

New forms of treatment for the leukaemias are being developed, one of the most promising being the removal of the patient's bone marrow, the complete eradication, in the laboratory, of malignant cells, and the replacement of the marrow. Efficient killing of leukaemic cells in patients' marrow has been achieved using **monoclonal antibodies** linked to toxic agents such as ricin-A. Another approach is to treat the removed marrow with powerful chemotherapeutic drugs which leave only normal cells. It has even been found possible in some cases to treat leukaemia by destroying the patient's marrow, by total body radiation, and replacing it with donor marrow. All these methods are still experimental, but workers are optimistic that, eventually, this terrible disease may be conquered.

Leukeran

A brand name for **chlorambucil**.

leukoplakia

A precancerous condition, affecting mainly the mouth, but also the vagina or vulva, in which a small area becomes thickened and whitened as a result of longstanding irritation. In the mouth the disorder involves the tongue, lip or cheek and is usually caused by pipe-smoking, poorly fitting dentures, roughened teeth, overindulgence in spicy and hot food, the use of chewing tobacco or the taking of snuff in the mouth.

> Leukoplakia starts with an inflamed patch which becomes hardened and develops an overgrowth of white surface cells. About 50 per cent of all mouth cancers start in this way. Such areas should always be regarded as danger signs and immediate steps taken to remove the cause. If this is done, the tissues will usually gradually return to normal, but persistent patches must be reviewed regularly and biopsies taken.

leukorrhoea

See **vaginal discharge**.

leukotriene receptor antagonists

Drugs that block the receptors for **leukotrienes** on cell membranes. These drugs have a useful dual effect in relaxing the smooth muscle of the air passages (bronchi) and in combatting inflammation in the bronchial linings – both features of **asthma**. They have also been found useful in hay fever. Examples are montelukast (Singulair) and zafirlukast (Accolate).

leukotrienes

Powerful chemical agents released by **mast cells**, basophil cells and **macrophages** and involved in many allergic and other immunological reactions. Leukotrienes are derived from **arachidonic acid** and cause **chemotaxis** and increase the leakiness of small blood vessels. In asthma they cause the narrowing of the air passages and the secretion of mucus. They can be inhibited by corticosteroid drugs.

leuprorelin

A gonadotrophin-releasing hormone drug used to treat **endometriosis** in women and prostate cancer in men. A brand name is Prostap.

levobunolol

A beta-blocker drug used in the form of eyedrops to treat chronic simple **glaucoma**. A brand name is Betagan.

levocabastine

An **antihistamine** drug formulated as eye and nasal drops for the treatment of allergic **conjunctivitis** and hay fever. A brand name is Livostin.

levocarnitine

A nitrogenous muscle constituent necessary for the transport of long-chain fatty acids across the inner mitochondrial membrane. It is used as a drug to correct a deficiency of carnitine in people on dialysis. A brand name is Carnitor.

levodopa

L-dopa. A drug used in the treatment of **Parkinson's disease**. Levodopa relieves symptoms in the majority of cases and often effects a remarkable reduction in disability. Brand names of the drug, in combination, respectively, with benserazide and carbidopa, are Madopar and Sinemet.

Levonelle-2

A brand name for an emergency contraceptive drug containing 750 micrograms of **levonorgestrel** per tablet. At the time of writing (March, 2000) this drug is licensed as a prescription-only medication, but the company that produces it has hopes that by the end of the year 2000 this preparation will have been granted a licence to be sold in pharmacies without prescription.

levonorgestrel

A **progestogen** drug used in oral contraceptives. Brand names of the progestogen-only product are Microval, Mirena, Norgeston and Norplant. It is also formulated with **ethinyloestradiol** as an oral contraceptive under such brand names as Eugynon 30, Eugynon 30, Microgynon 30, Microgynon 30 ED, Ovran, Ovranette, Schering PC4 and Trinordiol.

Levophed

A brand name for **noradrenaline**.

libido

Sexual desire.

Librium

A brand name for **chlordiazepoxide**.

lice

Common parasites of human and other animals. Lice are small wingless insects which have inhabited man since time immemorial, and it is only recently that the human condition has ceased to be not only nasty, brutish and short, but also, necessarily, lousy.

Even the richest were, until well into the eighteenth century, uncomplainingly infested. When Thomas à Becket (1155–62) was undressed for burial, his shirt was found to be 'silver with lice'. Today, the louse population of the world probably still greatly outnumbers the human population.

There are three kinds of human lice – head lice, body lice and pubic lice – and these differ in their habits.

HEAD LICE

The head louse, *Pediculus humanus capitis*, lives on the scalp and feeds by sucking blood. This causes intense itching and scratching with secondary *dermatitis* and infection of the skin. The females lay eggs (nits) which they glue to the shaft of hairs near the scalp. These hatch in about a week. Spread is by direct contact.

BODY LICE

The body louse, *Pediculus humanus corporis*, lives in the seams of clothing close to the skin, and move on to the body only to feed. The eggs are laid in the clothing. Body lice are easily disposed of by proper cleaning of the clothes. They are, in general, only a problem for those who do not regularly change their clothes. Body lice have been responsible for the maintenance of great epidemics of typhus in times of war and other civil disturbance. They also transmit relapsing fever.

PUBIC LICE

The crab louse, *Phthirius pubis*, so called because of its squat, crab-like appearance, infests the pubic hair and, occasionally, when the infestation is very heavy, the chest hair, armpit hair or even the eyebrows. *Phthirius pubis* is usually transmitted by sexual contact, and once established, likes to stick in one place, causing constant irritation. Heavy infestation is called *pediculosis*. Because of their sedentary habits, crab lice soon

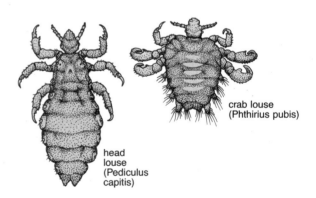

crab louse
(Phthirius pubis)

head louse
(Pediculus capitis)

The pubic, or crab, louse Phthirius pubis *is a squat creature, easily distinguished from the more elongated head louse. The head louse* (Pediculus humanus capitis) *is almost identical in appearance to the body louse* (Pediculus humanus corporis).

become surrounded by louse faeces. The scratching of the infested person inoculates both these and the lice bodies into the skin, leading to a severe dermatitis.

Unlike body lice, crab lice do not transmit any important disease. Lice can be eliminated by the use of suitable lotions or powders and by shaving off the hair or removing eggs with fine-tooth nit combs.

lichen planus

An uncommon skin disease in which intensely itchy, slightly raised patches, of up to 3 mm across and of a shiny reddish-purple hue occur on the skin. These enlarge and run together to form flat-topped plaques of up to 2 cm in diameter. They are commonest on the fronts of the wrists and forearms, the sides of the calves and ankles and the lower back. The cause is unknown.

The itching is easily relieved by hydrocortisone ointment and the disease usually clears up spontaneously within two years.

lichen sclerosus

A form of skin atrophy affecting the vulva in women, genital areas in men (less commonly) and occasionally other skin areas. The skin becomes white, glazed and sometimes severely shrunken and even ulcerated. Although usually painless, the condition may cause itching and sometimes pain. In about 5 per cent of severe cases occurring after puberty the condition progresses to cancer of the vulva, sometimes after it has been present for twenty years or more. Treatment is by local steroid ointment for a limited time, and in some cases, surgery.

lichen simplex

Thickened skin caused by persistent scratching. Lichenification does not occur unless the scratching is abnormally sustained and this may result from any particularly itchy long-term (chronic) skin condition. Scratching, in itself, can cause itching, so that a scratch-itch-scratch-itch cycle can occur. Scratching is often a partly unconscious response to mental agitation.

Lichenification will clear up if itching is controlled by suitable ointments and the area covered.

lid lag

Lid lag is the failure of the normal downward movement of the upper lids to cover the eye on downward gaze. The result is a rather striking staring appearance. Lid lag is often associated with exophthalmos and both are features of thyrotoxicosis – overactivity of the thyroid gland.

lids, puffy

See **blepharochalasis**.

lie detector

The polygraph, as it is properly called, is a collection of devices which simultaneously monitor, and record in graphic form, several changeable features of the human body, such as the pulse rate, the blood pressure, the evenness and rate of breathing and the moistness – and hence the electrical resistance – of the skin.

While this monitoring is in progress, the subject is posed a series of questions to some of which an emotional response is likely. Such a response cannot be concealed by any action on the part of the subject and will be apparent on the tracings.

Emotional responses to certain questions do not, however, necessarily indicate that the subject is lying or concealing the truth, and such results must be interpreted with great care. There is a real danger that wrong inferences may be drawn. The most that can be said for the technique is that it indicates those matters that have an emotional significance for the subject.

life-span

In the absence of disease or injury, the absolute maximum time a human being may expect to live is about 110 years. To some extent this is determined by genetic factors and people with long-lived parents may, in general, expect to live longer than those whose parents died younger. There is no evidence to suggest that life-span is increasing, although the time people *do* live (expectation of life) certainly is. What is happening is that, as a result of a higher standard of nutrition and hygiene, and because of medical advances, more and more people are tending to reach the natural life-span.

There is reason to believe that the natural life-span may be determined by the number of times body cells are capable of dividing. If cells from a young person are artificially cultured, they undergo a certain number of population doublings by division and then cease to divide further and die. Cells from an older person divide less often before dying, and cells from a very old person may not divide at all. The number of population doublings may be relatively fixed and is certainly finite – perhaps around fifty times for some cells. Ironically, certain cancer cell cultures appear to be immortal.

See also **ageing**.

ligaments, disorders of

Ligaments are bundles of a tough, elastic protein material called collagen. They are flexible but extremely strong and, if subjected to excessive strain, will often pull off a fragment of bone at their attachment rather than tear. Major injury to ligaments may require treatment similar to that of fractures – surgical operation and immobilization by plaster cast. Modern materials technology has provided woven artificial ligaments of great strength and flexibility, and these are being increasingly used, in difficult cases, to restore normal function.

ligation

The surgical process of tying off a blood vessel to prevent bleeding, or a duct to close it, with a length of thread or other material (**ligature**). The term is used in the phrase *tubal ligation*, a form of female sterilization in which the Fallopian tubes are tied off.

ligature

Any thread-like surgical material tied tightly round any structure. Ligatures are commonly used to tie off blood vessels in the course of an operation, so as to avoid dangerous or surgically incommoding blood loss. They are also commonly used to tie off other ducts in the body. Ligatures are commonly made of absorbable material, such as catgut, but may be non-absorbable. See also **ligation**.

limbic system

A centrally situated, ring-shaped structure in the brain (hence the name) consisting of a number of interconnected nerve cell nuclei. The limbic system represents much of what constitutes the brain in the lower mammals and is concerned with unconscious and automatic (autonomic) functions such as respiration, body temperature, hunger, thirst, wakefulness, sexual activity and their associated emotional reactions. It is also centrally concerned with emotional responses to incoming stimuli or thoughts. Structural changes in the limbic system from diseases or injury can cause undue and easily induced emotional display, forced or spasmodic laughing and crying, aggression, anger, violence, placidity, apathy, anxiety, fear, depression and diminished sexual interest.

limb injury sequel

See **reflex sympathetic dystrophy**.

Limclair

A brand name for **trisodium edetate**.

Lingraine

A brand name for **ergotamine tartrate**.

Lioresal

A brand name for **baclofen**.

liothyronine sodium

A thyroid hormone preparation used to treat severe thyroid hormone deficiency. A brand name is Tertroxin.

Lipantil Micro

A brand name for **fenofibrate**.

lip cancer

COMMON CAUSES
This is commonest among fair-skinned people who freckle, rather than burn, in sunlight and who are exposed to long periods in the sun. Pipe-smoking and, to a lesser extent, cigarette smoking, are also known causal factors. The danger appears to be in the prolonged application of hot tobacco tars to the lip surface. Formerly, clay pipe smokers commonly developed lip cancer. **Leukoplakia** precedes the cancer in one-third of cases.

RECOGNITION AND SYMPTOMS
Lip cancers appear as persistent ulcers, are cracking and scaly and often preceded by, or associated with, a white patch (leukoplakia). They spread rapidly to the lymph nodes in the neck and under the jaw and, if neglected, may extend to the lymph nodes around the jugular veins in the neck.

TREATMENT
Small local cancers can easily be cured by removal, with little disfigurement, and carry a five-year survival rate of 90 per cent.

> Persistent ulcers on the lip should never be neglected and are an indication for urgent medical attention including biopsy.

If neglected, major surgery and radiotherapy will be required and the chances of survival drop to about 50 per cent.

lip disorders

These include **skin, chapped**, **cheilitis**, **cold sores**, **chancre**, **hard** and **lip cancer**.

lipectomy, suction

A form of body contouring cosmetic **plastic surgery** in which small incisions are made in the skin and a blunt-ended metal sucker is passed through and moved around under the skin to suck out fat cells. The procedure is not without risks, and human frailty being what it is, the effect is usually temporary. A better alternative is the establishment of new and more moderate eating habits.

lipid profile

A laboratory assessment of the levels of fats in a patient's blood. The measurements include total cholesterol, total triglycerides (fats) and high- and low-density lipoproteins. The latter are the tiny spherical vehicles by which lipids are transported in the blood.

lipids

Body fats. The most prevalent of these are the triglycerides, each molecule consisting of a 'backbone' of glycerine (glycerol) to which three fatty acids are attached. Other lipids include phospholipids and the range of sterols, including **cholesterol**.

Lipitor

A brand name for atorvastatin.

Lipobay

A brand name for **cerivastin**.

lipodystrophy

A disorder of fat metabolism in which there may be an abnormal rate of fat breakdown with loss of weight, unduly high levels of fats in the blood, raised blood sugar levels, enlarged liver and abnormal thyroid gland function. Some cases feature breakdown of fat from the upper part of the body and abnormal deposition around the buttocks and thighs.

lipoma

A non-malignant tumour of fatty tissue. Lipomas grow slowly to form soft, smooth swellings and may occur in fat anywhere in the body. They seldom, if ever, cause any problems but can be removed if causing disfigurement.

lipoproteins

Microscopic bodies in which fats and proteins are chemically closely associated (conjugated). The blood lipoproteins are important because they are the cholesterol carriers of the body, and are classified by density in accordance with the proportions of protein. Protein molecules are more dense than fat molecules, so low density lipoproteins (LDLs) contain relatively high amounts of cholesterol and little protein; and high density lipoproteins (HDLs) contain 50 per cent of protein and only 20 per cent of cholesterol. LDLs are viewed as the 'bad' cholesterol carriers and HDLs as the 'good' carriers.

LDLs transport fats to muscles and to fat stores and are associated with the arterial disease atherosclerosis and thus heart disease and stroke. HDLs are protective against these diseases because their main role is to transport cholesterol from the periphery back to the liver. They also carry paraoxanase enzymes that limit oxidative modification of LDLs necessary before cholesterol can be laid down in arterial walls. Blood concentration of HDL cholesterol shows a strong inverse correlation with the risk of coronary heart disease.

liposarcoma

This is the malignant form of the **lipoma** and is very rare.

Lipostat

A brand name for **pravastatin**.

lipping

The formation of a curled edge at the bearing joint surface of a bone in **osteoarthritis** and other degenerative bone disease.

lipreading

An important means of communication with the deaf, who often become highly skilled in obtaining verbal information directly from another person through the medium of vision rather than hearing. Lipreading, or 'speechreading' is not confined to the deaf; in direct conversation we all use vision to supplement what we hear and derive much information from visual clues. But to the deaf, skilled lipreading can be invaluable, and, after training, as many as 60 per cent of spoken words can be discerned. With many subjects, the advantages of lipreading are about equal to those of using a hearing aid, and, with some, great benefit can be obtained from combining both.

HOW IT WORKS

Speech involves placing the jaw, lips and tongue in a rapidly changing sequence of positions. In addition, the changing mental patterns associated with speech are reflected, often quite subtly, in changes of facial expression. English speech involves more than forty distinct sounds but only half a dozen visibly distinguishable mouth patterns can be reliably identified, even if the speaker cooperates by looking directly at the deaf person and talking clearly and slowly.

LEARNING TO LIPREAD

Lipreading is best taught in a class. Instruction involves a detailed analysis of the mouth patterns seen on different faces and as they occur in colloquial speech. It also includes training in the technique of inferring information from an incomplete context.

Liquifilm Tears

A brand name for artificial tears containing polyvinyl alcohol.

lisinopril

An **angiotensin converting enzyme inhibitor** drug used to treat heart failure and high blood pressure. Brand names are Carace and Zestril and, in conjunction with a thiazide diuretic, Carace Plus and Zestoretic.

Liskonum

A brand name for **lithium**.

lisp

A common and easily remedied speech defect. 'Ssss' sounds (sibilants) are produced by placing the tongue high and close to the hard palate, with the tip behind the roots of the upper front teeth. If the tip of the tongue is protruded between the teeth, the hissing 'sss' sound is replaced by a 'th' sound. Thus, the lisp is largely under voluntary control and, should it persist after infancy, speech therapy can be considered.

listeriosis

This is a rare disease which is becoming commoner. It is caused by an organism, *Listeria monocytogenes*, which is remarkable for its ability to survive in adverse conditions. Access to human beings is probably by way of the nose and throat in air-borne droplets and food and there is some evidence, also, of sexual transmission. The organism will survive for long periods in the genital react.

SOURCES OF THE DISEASE

It can resist low temperatures and has been recovered from lamb kept at 0°C for twenty-four days. The organism has been isolated from 50 species of domestic and wild animals and from many birds, fish and crustaceans and from soft cheeses and various precooked foods. It is found in sewage and earth, and in the stools of up to 30 per cent of healthy people. Over half the chickens in Britain carry the organism, either internally or externally, but proper cooking will kill it. The important point, however, is that the organism varies considerably in its ability to cause disease (virulence).

Babies can be infected before birth but this is rare – only about one baby in 18,000 is affected. Many of those who are, however, suffer widespread damage to most of the systems of the body, and about a quarter of those infected in this way, by virulent organisms, are born dead.

RECOGNITION AND SYMPTOMS

Human listeriosis is commonest in babies and old people, affecting the throat, the eyes, the skin and the nervous system. The great majority of cases are mild and probably pass unremarked. Some have an upset similar to **glandular fever**. There is fever, **conjunctivitis**, inflammation of the salivary glands as in **mumps**, and sometimes – especially in veterinary workers – pustules on the skin, and, rarely, arthritis, bone inflammation and abscesses in the brain and spinal cord. A venereal form, with persistent discharge in the urine, may occur.

TREATMENT

Listeriosis responds well to penicillin, erythromycin and tetracycline. These drugs greatly reduce the mortality from listeriosis in infants and the outlook for the disease in adults is good.

Litarex

A brand name for **lithium**.

lithium

An element, the lightest known solid, used as the citrate or carbonate for the control of **manic-depressive** states. Lithium is also used as the succinate in ointments for the treatment of seborrhoeic dermatitis and in shampoos for the control of dandruff. Brand names are Camcolit, Li-liquid, Liskonum, Litarex and Priadel. A preparation for external use is Efalith.

lithotomy

A now largely abandoned surgical operation. Lithotomy, or 'cutting for the stone' means making a cut into the urinary bladder so as to remove a bladder stone. Such a procedure, although common, was once clearly thought to be beneath the dignity of the proper physician. The original Hippocratic oath contains an undertaking not to engage in this barbarous practice, but to leave it to those normally concerned with shaving and cutting hair.

Lithotomy was originally performed through the floor of the pelvis via an incision along the crease at the inside of the top of the thigh. A successful cut was rewarded by a gush of urine and blood and, it was hoped, the appearance of the stone. The position adopted by the patient – lying on the back with the knees up and the thighs spread wide – is still described as the *lithotomy position* and is now much used by gynaecologists. Lithotomy operations have now largely been replaced by **lithotripsy**.

lithotripsy

A method of fragmenting stones in the urinary system and in the gall-bladder, by focused and concentrated ultrasonic shock waves, without the necessity for a surgical incision.

HOW IT'S DONE

If a person's body is immersed in water and an ultrasound wave is generated under water, the continuity between the water and the soft tissues of the body allows the waves to pass, relatively unimpeded, into the body without being significantly reflected from the body surface. Such ultrasound waves can be focused to a point by parabolic reflectors and aimed so that the point of focus, and maximum energy, coincides with the stone. Recent advances in the design of lithotripsy machines mean that it is no longer necessary for the patient to be immersed in water.

The patient is anaesthetized and the position of the stone is accurately determined by an X-ray image intensifier. Shock waves are generated by a high voltage spark discharge and focused on the stone. When the shock is fired, a great deal of energy is liberated and the stone shatters and is reduced to particles small enough to be passed naturally in the urine or into the bile duct and bowel.

Up to 90 per cent of stones which, previously, could have been removed only by open surgery, can now be dealt with by this method.

livedo reticularis

A mottling of the legs in an irregular, wide-mesh, fish-net pattern which occurs in Cushing's syndrome and various collagen diseases. A similar brownish mottling used to be common in women who sat too close to the fire-place. This was called **erythema ab igne**.

liver

This important organ occupies the upper right corner of the abdomen and extends across the midline to the left side. It is a spongy, reddish-brown organ, moulded to fit high under the domed diaphragm so that most of it lies behind the ribs. It is wedge-shaped, with the thin edge pointing across to the left. On the right side, the liver extends down to the level of the lower ribs. The lower edge slopes upwards at an angle, across the front of the stomach, and the wedge-shaped smaller left lobe of the liver lies mainly under the lower part of the breastbone (sternum) and the cartilages for the ribs on the left side. The liver is the largest organ in the abdomen.

Blood from the intestine, the spleen and the stomach passes to the liver by way of a short, wide vein called the portal vein which enters on the underside. At about the same point, a large and important artery from the general circulation, the hepatic artery, also enters the liver. Within the liver, these two vessels divide into tree-like structures, the smallest branches of which end in millions of tiny liver lobules where the blood from them comes into intimate contact with the liver cells. These lobules are the functional units of the liver and in them many complex biochemical processes go on. In parallel with the blood system of the liver is a network of fine, branching drainage tubules – the biliary system. These end up in the bile duct which runs into the small intestine at the duodenum and which has a short side branch to the gall-bladder, under the liver, where the bile is stored and concentrated.

The liver is a kind of processing factory for the body and has an amazing range of chemical skills. The raw materials – glucose, amino acids, fats, minerals, vitamins – enter in the nutrient-rich blood from the intestine. From this blood, the liver takes up glucose and synthesizes from it a highly concentrated storage form of carbohydrate called glycogen. On demand, glucose can immediately be released from this material. The liver also deals with fats and proteins, converting them into forms required by the body, and, when necessary, converting one into the other. Amino acids are built up into the complex proteins required by the blood and the immune system, or broken down and converted to carbohydrate or fat, as the need dictates. The liver takes up the products of old red blood cells, largely from the spleen, and converts these into a pigment, bilirubin, which, together with other substances, forms the bile.

The liver has remarkable powers of breaking down toxic substances into safer forms. Ammonia produced from protein breakdown is converted into urea, which is excreted in the urine. Alcohol and other drugs are altered to safer forms. To a remarkable degree, the liver is able to regenerate itself after disease, toxic damage or injury. But if this capacity is exceeded, the whole function of the body is severely affected.

liver abscess

A localized, walled-off collection of pus in the liver. The commonest cause is the spread of **amoebiasis** from an infection in the large intestine, but abscesses can also be caused by spread of infection from **appendicitis**, **diverticulitis**, pelvic inflammation or from gall-bladder disease. There is high fever, tenderness over the liver, pain in the upper right corner of the abdomen and prostration. Sometimes an amoebic

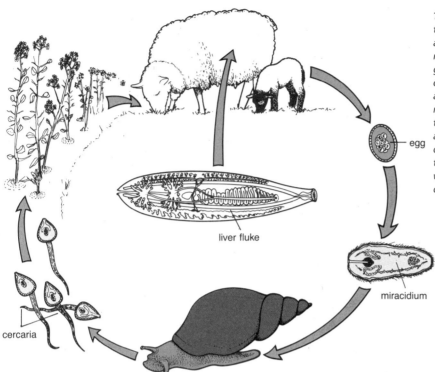

The liver fluke is a trematode parasite of animals and man. A single miracidium in a snail may give rise to thousands of cercariae. If some of these are eaten on plants they migrate up the bile duct to the liver and mature to the adult fluke in about twelve days. Eggs are then passed in the stools. Eggs must reach water before the cycle can continue.

egg

liver fluke

miracidium

cercaria

abscess bursts through the diaphragm into the lung above. The patient may then cough up anchovy-sauce-like pus.

Liver abscesses must be drained, either through a needle or by open operation. In amoebiasis, various drugs are also useful, but are no substitute for removal of the contents of the abscess. Untreated liver abscesses are fatal.

liver biopsy

With the increasing awareness of the importance of precise diagnosis in liver disease and increasing skill in making such diagnosis by microscopic examination and by various tests, liver biopsy has become commonplace. It is now regarded as a straightforward bedside procedure.

Liver biopsy is done by passing a special needle through the lower chest wall, between the ribs, under local anaesthesia. The needle has a sharp-edged, beveled, cutting tip and a solid inner metal core which protrudes beyond the tip. This core is sharply pointed and, just behind the tip, has a long notch into which the soft liver passes. The inner core is drawn back into the needle before removal, so that a short cylinder of liver tissue is cut off and withdrawn with the needle. The procedure can cause internal bleeding.

Liver biopsy is especially valuable in establishing a diagnosis of cirrhosis, in distinguishing between different kinds of hepatitis, in investigating causes of jaundice and of abnormal **liver function test** results, in studying the damage caused by drugs, and in the diagnosis of various forms of cancer, primary and secondary, including lymphomas.

liver cancer

Cancer originating in the liver is rare in Britain, but comparatively common in the tropics where it is believed to be due to two factors – chronic hepatitis B infections and ingestion of food, such as nuts and grains, contaminated with the fungus *Aspergillus flavus*, which produces the poison **aflatoxin**. The great majority of people who develop primary liver cancer have liver cirrhosis and most are males, many of them alcoholics.

PRIMARY CANCER

Primary liver cancer causes loss of appetite and weight, weakness, fever, pain in the abdomen, a swelling of the abdomen both from liver enlargement and from the accumulation of fluid, and secondary effects from liver failure. The concentration of alphafetoprotein in the blood is markedly raised and this is almost diagnostic. Unless the cancer is confined to one lobe and can be surgically removed in its entirety, only palliative treatment is usually feasible.

SECONDARY CANCER

Secondary liver cancer is very common. Usually the tumour has spread from the lung, the breast, the prostate gland, the large intestine (colon) or the womb (uterus). Sadly, in about half the cases, there has been no indication that a primary cancer has been present. The liver usually enlarges rapidly and there is loss of weight, fever and jaundice. Fluid often accumulates in the abdomen and this is frequently found to contain tumour cells.

Secondary liver cancer is an indication of widespread disease for which there is usually little hope of remedy. Chemotherapy can, however, often prolong life.

liver fluke

One of several types of flat worm which can gain access to the liver and cause a feverish illness with liver tenderness and enlargement. The flukes can make their way from the liver into the bile duct system and cause inflammation and obstruction, which may lead to **jaundice**.

The common form of liver fluke, *Fasciola hepatica*, is a parasite of sheep which produces eggs that are passed in the sheep faeces. If these enter water, the eggs hatch after a month or so and a swimming larval stage emerges which bores into the soft underparts of aquatic snails. Two to four weeks later, many individuals of a further larval stage are released from the snails and congregate, in a cystic form, on the leaves of water plants such as cress or water-chestnut. If these are eaten by man, the infestation may be acquired.

Diagnosis is made by finding the characteristic fluke eggs in the stools. Drugs to kill the worms (anthelmintics) are used in the treatment.

liver function tests

A rather inaccurate term for a group of investigations used to determine whether the liver is diseased. Some of the investigations included in this group do not measure liver function and it is impracticable to measure most of the many liver functions. Those tests done are, however, useful, in showing that liver function is defective, although they do not indicate the precise nature of the liver disorder. They are useful in distinguishing between short-term (acute) and long-term (chronic) disorders and between inflammation of the liver (hepatitis) and obstruction to the flow of bile (cholestasis).

The tests most commonly done are those which:

- measure the blood levels of the pigment bilirubin, which is normally removed from the blood by the liver and excreted in the bile;
- assess the levels, in the blood, of certain enzymes, such as aminotransferases, gamma-glutamyl transferase and alkaline phosphatase, which are released into the blood by damaged liver cells;
- measure the levels of the serum proteins, albumin and prothrombin, which are synthesized in the liver;
- check the rate of clearance from the blood of the substance bromsulphthalein, much of which is normally removed within two hours;
- estimate the amount of alphafetoprotein, in the blood, which occurs in high concentrations in liver cancer.

The liver has so many functions that many other tests are possible.

liver transplant

The first liver transplant in Britain was performed in 1968 by the English surgeon Professor Roy Calne (b. 1930) and many hundreds have since been done.

WHY IT'S DONE

Liver transplantation is the only resource for those whose livers are so diseased that they are no longer able to maintain normal living. In most cases, these are people with chronic end-stage liver disease, especially cirrhosis. Acute liver failure and *primary* **liver cancer** are lesser indications.

RISKS

The decision to perform a liver transplant is seldom easy as the risks are great and these must be weighed against the patient's chances with the disease. The risks include a failure of the donated liver to function, acute rejection of the donated liver, the development of hepatitis in the new liver, mainly from one of a variety of infections, and the development of a form of bile obstruction. Strenuous measures are necessary to try to prevent or to treat these complications.

SURVIVAL RATE

The results of liver transplantation are improving steadily. At present, a one-year survival rate of about 75 per cent is achieved, and a five-year survival rate of about 60 per cent is anticipated. Most of the deaths occur early – usually within a month of operation. During that period the death rate is currently about 30 per cent. Patients who survive are able to lead a normal life and, in almost all people, the quality of life is greatly improved.

Livial

A brand name for **tibolone**.

living will

A document in which a competent person requests and directs what should be done in the event of later inability to express his or her wishes on medical management. The purpose of the document is usually to try to ensure that exceptional measures are not taken to maintain his or her life.

Most states in the USA have already enacted legislation to allow this, but, in Britain, such legislation is yet to be considered.

See also **ethics, medical**.

Livostin

A brand name for **levocabastine**.

lobe

A well-defined subdivision of an organ. The brain, the lung, the liver, the pituitary and thyroid glands, and the prostate gland are divided into lobes.

lobectomy

The surgical removal of a lobe.

lobotomy, prefrontal

Sometimes known as pre-frontal leukotomy, this is an operation to separate some of the areas at the extreme front of the brain from those further back. A small opening is made through the bone of the temple and an instrument passed in under careful X-ray control and used to sever nerve tracts. The operation was introduced in 1936 and was much used in the 1940s and 1950s. It was successful in some cases of otherwise intractable mental disorder, but is now used only in a few specially selected, very severe cases in which no other therapy is appropriate. The results are unpredictable and, although the more florid symptoms are usually removed, serious personality changes may be caused.

Locabiotal

A brand name for **fusafungine**.

Loceryl

A brand name for **amorolfine**.

locked-in syndrome

A condition in which the patient is mute and totally paralysed, except for eye movements, but remains conscious and is able to communicate by eye movement codes. This nightmarish state is quite different from coma or the vegetative state.

The locked-in syndrome usually results from a massive haemorrhage, thrombosis, or other damage, affecting the upper part of the brain-stem, which destroys almost all motor function, but leaves the higher mental functions intact. Most patients in this terrible situation survive for only a few weeks or months, but some go on indefinitely. There have been a few cases of recovery from the locked-in syndrome.

lockjaw

A lay term for tight spasm of the powerful chewing muscles which is a feature of the serious infection **tetanus**. The muscle spasm clamps the teeth together so that they can barely be separated. The medical term is *trismus*.

Locoid

A brand name for **hydrocortisone**.

locomotion

Locomotion is a complex mechanical process, calling for remarkable timing in the contraction of a great many different muscle groups. Many muscles must act to brace or balance one part of the skeleton so as to allow another part to move relative to the first. Almost all the voluntary muscles of

severance of connections to pre-frontal region of brain

pre-frontal region

Prefrontal lobotomy, in which fibres from the most forward part of the brain are cut, is now seldom performed. The operation was once commonly used in cases of severe psychotic illness.

the body are involved in the act of walking, although many of them may, at any one moment, be engaged simply in holding some part of the body steady. Such a complex function requires a computer for its control and this is provided by the subsidiary brain, the cerebellum, which hangs down underneath the back of the main brain (cerebrum).

The cerebellum gets input from the cerebrum to tell it what movements are intended. But it also gets input from the eyes, from the position sensors in the inner ears (the semicircular canals) and from all the voluntary muscles of the body.

These various inputs inform the cerebellum about the position of the head relative to the body, and about the position of all the limbs. Having put all that information together, the cerebellum then works out which muscles must be contracted in order to achieve the desired movement. This is a very rough account of what happens, but indicates the complexity of brain function needed to carry out what may, at first sight, seem quite a simple function.

locomotor

Relating to the function of voluntary movement.

Locorten-Vioform

A brand name for **flumethasone** combined with an antibacterial drug.

locus

The position on each of a pair of corresponding chromosomes at which the gene for a particular characteristic resides. The plural is loci. A locus can contain any of the alleles of the gene.

Lodine SR

A brand name for **etodolac**.

lodoxamine

A mast cell-stabilizing drug that prevents the release of **histamine** in allergic conditions, formulated as eyedrops for the treatment of allergic **conjunctivitis**. A brand name is Aldomide.

Loestrin 20

A brand name for an oral contraceptive containing **ethinyloestradiol** and **norethisterone**. See also **contraceptive drugs**.

Loestrin 30

A brand name for an oral contraceptive containing **ethinyloestradiol** and **norethisterone**. See also **contraception**.

lofepramine

A **tricyclic antidepressant drug**. A brand name is Gamanil.

lofexidine

A drug used to control withdrawal symptoms during opiate detoxification. A brand name is BritLofex.

Logynon, Logynon ED

Brand names for oral contraceptives containing **ethinyloestradiol** and **levonorgestrel**.

457

loins

The soft tissue of the back, on either side of the spine, between the lowest ribs and the pelvis.

Lomexin

A brand name for **fenticonazole**.

Lomotil

A brand name for a mixture of **diphenoxylate** and atropine.

longsightedness

See **hypermetropia**.

Loniten

A brand name for **minoxidil**.

loop diuretics

Drugs that lead to a large output of water in the urine by interfering with the reabsorption of sodium and chloride in the loop of Henle tubules in the kidneys. They include **frusemide** and bumetanide.

loose bodies

See **knee, disorders of**.

Loperagen

A brand name for **loperamide**.

loperamide

A synthetic narcotic analogue drug used to control mild diarrhoea. Brand names are Imodium, Loperagen and Norimode.

Lopid

A brand name for **gemfibrozil**.

Lopidine

A brand name for **apraclonidine**.

Lopresor

A brand name for **metoprolol**.

loratadine

An **antihistamine** drug used to treat hay fever and other allergic disorders. A brand name is Clarityn.

lorazepam

A benzodiazepine tranquillizer drug similar to Valium (diazepam). A brand name is Ativan.

lordosis

An abnormal degree of forward curvature of the lower part of the spine, often associated with abnormal backward curvature of the upper part (**kyphosis**). Lordosis and kyphosis exaggerate the normal 'S' shape of the spine and commonly lead to backache or even '**slipped disc**'.

Loron

A brand name for **sodium clodronate**.

losartan

An angiotensin II antagonist drug used to treat high blood pressure. A brand name is Cozaar. The drug is available combined with the diuretic drug **hydrochlorothiazide** under the brand name Cozaar-Comp.

Losec

A brand name for **omeprazole**.

lower leg pain

See **shin splints**.

low molecular weight heparin

Heparin is the natural anticlotting (anticoagulant) agent of the body. Low molecular weight heparin is one of a number of heparins that can be isolated from standard heparin. These differ in their mode of action and pharmacological and immunological properties from normal heparin and are useful in cases in which side-effects of standard heparin have occurred. They have advantages over heparin in the treatment of venous thrombosis. They bind much less avidly to heparin-binding proteins than does standard heparin. This increases their bioavailability at low doses and makes their anticoagulant response more predictable.

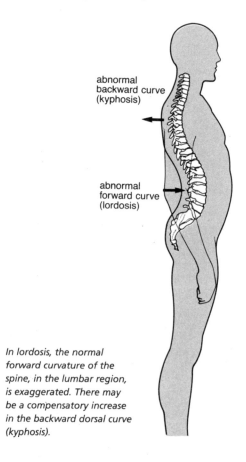

abnormal backward curve (kyphosis)

abnormal forward curve (lordosis)

In lordosis, the normal forward curvature of the spine, in the lumbar region, is exaggerated. There may be a compensatory increase in the backward dorsal curve (kyphosis).

Loxapac

A brand name for **loxapine**.

loxapine

A tricyclic drug used to treat psychotic disorders. A brand name is Loxapac.

LSD

Lysergic acid diethylamide, a hallucinogenic drug derived from lysergic acid, once used in psychiatric research and treatment but now largely confined to illicit use. The drug is a powerful **serotonin antagonist** and can induce a psychotic state with **paranoid** delusions that can last for months.

See **hallucinogenic drugs**.

Ludiomil

A brand name for **maprotiline hydrochloride**.

Ludwig's angina

A spreading bacterial infection of the floor of the mouth which often causes considerable swelling and tenderness of the soft

> The gravest danger in Ludwig's angina is that the swelling might extend to the respiratory passage and cause asphyxia. This can happen within a matter of hours of onset and tracheostomy may be necessary to save life. Early medical attention is thus always required. Large doses of antibiotics will be given and a careful check on the airway maintained.

tissues. It usually starts from an infected tooth, especially a wisdom tooth, or from gum infection, and is uncommon except in people with grossly neglected teeth. There is fever, pain and difficulty in opening the mouth and in swallowing.

lues

An obsolete term for syphilis (see **sexually transmitted diseases**), sometimes used by doctors as a euphemism.

lumbar

Relating to the **loins** and lower back.

lumbar pain

Lumbago, or low back pain, is one of the commonest and most persistent of symptoms, and may vary from mild to excruciating. Severe attacks are often disabling, and the symptom is responsible for the loss of millions of working hours.

POSSIBLE CAUSES

The symptom becomes more frequent with age, and about half of all those over sixty years suffer frequently from it. In most cases it is due to a defective, slouching posture associated with poor development in the large group of muscles surrounding the spine (the paravertebral muscles). In these cases, it can usually be relieved by exercises to strengthen the muscles and by the adoption of a proper, upright posture, both in standing and in sitting. Often, this type of backache is brought on, or made worse, by obesity or by unaccustomed or injudicious work or weight-bearing. It is common in pregnancy.

The fibrous connective tissue of the back muscles, ligaments and tendons is often the site of pain and this may

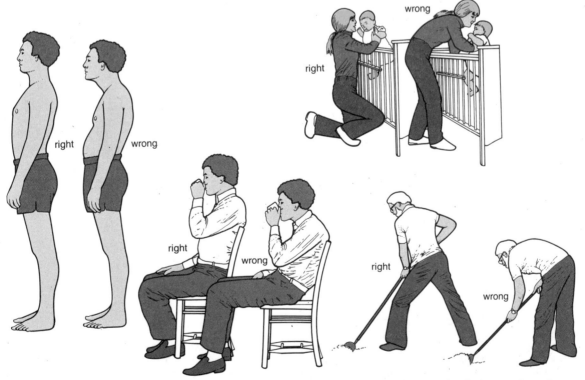

An important cause of lumbar pain is faulty posture, which discourages healthy exercise of the spinal and other muscles and applies abnormal strains to the back. Here are some typical examples of right and wrong postures.

follow unusual or strenuous exercise, especially in sport in the untrained. Lumbar pain can also be related to mental stress, virus infections, sleep disorders and anxiety.

The most common serious form of back pain is caused by what is popularly described as a '**slipped disc**'. This is an inaccurate term as the discs between the bodies of the vertebrae of the spine are very securely attached to the bone and cannot slip. Even the official medical term – prolapsed intervertebral disc – is not quite right. It is not the disc that is displaced, but a variable quantity of the soft, pulpy central material (the nucleus pulposus) which is forced by longitudinal pressure through a localized defect in the outer fibrous ring of the disc and squashed backwards to press on the spinal nerves. Pressure on these nerves causes not only severe backache but also pain which radiates down the course of the nerve – through the buttock, back of the thigh and down as far as the foot. These nerves are bundled together to form the main nerve trunk supplying the leg (the sciatic nerve) and pressure on them causes not only severe backache but **sciatica**. Severe backache and stiffness associated with involvement of the sciatic nerve – pain, numbness or loss of function – indicates a prolapsed disc and calls for proper medical or surgical treatment.

There are many other causes of backache, but these are much less common. They include:

- a tear of a muscle or ligament;
- an actual fracture of one of the facets or processes of a vertebra;
- wearing away of the joint surfaces (chronic **osteoarthritis**);
- inflammation of the spine (**ankylosing spondylitis**);
- minor abnormalities of the lower part of the spine present from birth (congenital bone defects);
- a slipping forward of the lowest lumbar vertebra on the top of the sacrum (spondylolisthesis);
- bone **tuberculosis**;
- bone marrow cancer;
- secondary cancer which has spread to the bone.

TREATMENT

Most attacks of acute low back pain settle in a few days, but it is important to try to determine and avoid the cause as, otherwise, recurrence is likely. This may lead to a permanent (**chronic**) situation.

> In severe and persistent cases it is essential to seek medical advice so that a correct diagnosis can be reached and the appropriate treatment given. Backache is a symptom – an indication of something else, not a disease in its own right.

Osteopaths believe that many backaches are caused by actual displacement of one vertebra relative to another and that they can be relieved by identifying the site of the dislocation and applying pressure to reduce it. Certainly, many people have been relieved of their backache by osteopathic treatment, but most doctors are sceptical of the claimed cause.

> A good osteopath will probably know more about backache than most doctors, but there is always the worry that treatment will be undertaken without an accurate diagnosis. This can be dangerous, if only by delaying access to proper management.

lumbar puncture

This procedure is usually done to obtain a sample of cerebrospinal fluid for laboratory examination in the investigation of disorders of the nervous system. Lumbar puncture also allows the injection of drugs, such as antibiotics, into the cerebrospinal fluid; it allows the doctor to inject fluids opaque to X-rays for radiological examination of the *spinal* canal; and it may be used to achieve widespread local anaesthesia without loss of consciousness, by injecting anaesthetic drugs into the spinal canal. This is known as a spinal anaesthetic.

The patient is placed on his or her side near the edge of an operating table or firm bed, with the head and shoulders bent forward and the knees drawn up. In this way the spine is bent as sharply as possible so that the back parts of the bones of the spine (vertebrae) are pulled as far apart from each other as possible. The area of the lower back is swabbed with an antiseptic solution and the skin is anaesthetized by a small injection of local anaesthetic.

The doctor now feels for the depression between two of the lowest bones and carefully inserts a long needle, containing a wire stylet, exactly in the midline, and perpendicular to the skin. This level is well below the lower end of the spinal cord so there is no risk of damage to that important structure. The needle passes painlessly through the ligaments and between the bones, encountering a slight resistance when the outer covering of the spinal canal (the dura mater) is reached.

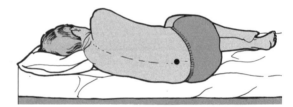

This shows the position of the patient for lumbar puncture and the site of insertion of the needle.

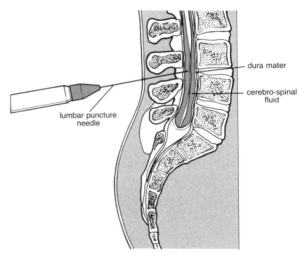

dura mater

cerebro-spinal fluid

lumbar puncture needle

Note how the needle passes between the back processes of the bones of the spine (vertebrae) and through the outer layers of the meninges (the dura mater and arachnoid mater) to enter the sub-arachnoid space which contains the cerebrospinal fluid.

When the needle has entered the canal, the stylet is removed and the cerebrospinal fluid runs out of the needle to be collected in a tube. The pressure of the cerebrospinal fluid can be measured by connecting a pressure gauge (manometer). No more fluid is taken than is strictly needed and when the needle is removed the puncture is sealed with sterile tape. The patient remains lying flat for 24 hours to prevent leakage of cerebrospinal fluid and 'lumbar puncture headache'.

lumbrical muscles

The four small intrinsic muscles of the hand lying between the bones of the palm (metacarpal bones) and acting on tendons of another muscle, the flexor digitorum profundus, to straighten the fingers and bend the joints between the fingers and the palms. Similar muscles, with comparable but more limited actions, occur in the feet and assist in walking.

lumen

The inside of any tube, such as a blood vessel, an air passage (bronchus) or the intestine.

lumpectomy

An operation for breast cancer in which no attempt is made to remove more than the obvious lump. Supplementary treatment with radiation or chemotherapy is then given.

See **mastectomy**, **breast cancer**.

lump in the throat

See **dysphagia**, **globus hystericus**.

lunacy

Psychotic disorder. The term is no longer used by doctors, but remains popular among lawyers. The origins of the word derive from the old belief that madness was caused by the full moon. The Latin word for the moon is *luna*. See also **insanity**.

lung allergy

See **allergic alveolitis**.

lung cancer

Although this is the name commonly used, primary cancer in the lung is not usually a cancer of the lung substance itself, but of the lining of one of the air tubes (bronchi). The medical term is *bronchial carcinoma*.

INCIDENCE AND CAUSE

This is by far the commonest malignant tumour in the lung and accounts for more than half of all male deaths from cancer. The enormous increase in the frequency of this kind of cancer is entirely attributable to the increase in cigarette smoking since the middle of the twentieth century. For many years lung cancer has been commoner in men than in women, but the relative incidence in women has risen and is now coming close to that in men. Most cases occur in people over fifty, so a smoking history going back some thirty to forty years is relevant. During that period the number of women smoking cigarettes has progressively increased. The risk of inducing lung cancer is proportional to the amount smoked and the death rate in heavy cigarette smokers is about forty times that in non-smokers.

RECOGNITION AND SYMPTOMS

The cancer may take various forms and these offer different degrees of danger. The tumour may grow within the bronchus until it causes obstruction and collapse of the part of the lung beyond it, or it may eat its way through the wall to invade the surrounding lung tissue and even the chest wall. When this happens, the involvement of the nerves between the ribs, or of the ribs themselves, causes great pain. The tumour may spread into the partition between the lungs (the mediastinum) to involve the heart, the gullet (oesophagus), the trachea, the great veins returning blood to the heart, or the nerves to the voice box (larynx). The latter complication causes severe loss of the voice, and this may be the first sign of lung cancer. Spread also occurs to local lymph nodes and, by way of the bloodstream, to the bones, brain, skin, liver and other organs.

The presenting sign of lung cancer is usually a productive cough and there is often a little blood in the sputum. When a segment of a lung (**lobe**) or a lung collapses there is breathlessness. Pain in the chest is common, especially if the cancer has spread to the lung lining (pleura) or the chest wall. Often the tumour is initially silent and the first indications are due to remote spread to other parts of the body. Spread to the brain can cause fits, paralysis, personality changes and **dysphasia**. Spread to the liver may cause jaundice and loss of weight. Tumour spread to bone (secondaries) may cause a deep boring pain in the bones, sometimes even a spontaneous fracture. Nodules of secondary cancer may occur in the skin.

X-ray examination usually shows a dense shadow corresponding to the solid tumour or an opaque segment corresponding to a collapsed lobe of the lung. Sometimes the diagnosis can only be made by examining the inside of the bronchi with a bronchoscope. If a tumour is seen, a sample (biopsy) is usually taken for examination. Cancer cells can sometimes be found in the sputum.

TREATMENT

If the tumour is localized to one lobe or one lung, surgical removal of the lobe or lung offers the best chance of survival. Unfortunately, this is so only in about one case in five. Even in these cases, the five-year survival rate is only about 30 per cent. If there has been further spread, the outlook is poor and most patients can expect only a few months of life. Chemotherapy and radiotherapy may sometimes prolong life a little, but cannot cure the condition.

> It is to be hoped that these facts go some way to explaining the difficulty doctors have in maintaining patience with successive governments which allow the apparently conscienceless tobacco lobby to go on advertising its pernicious wares.

lung cancer and smoking

See **health maintenance**.

lung, collapse of

See **atelectasis**.

lung disease, chronic obstructive

Chronic **bronchitis** and **emphysema** commonly occur together. Both cause interference with the normal flow of air into and out of the lungs and, in consequence, with the efficient transfer of oxygen to the blood. In any particular case, the relative importance of each is hard to assess, so they now tend to be classed together as *chronic obstructive airway disease*.

These diseases cause an immense amount of distress, suffering and disability to millions and take a heavy economic toll on the community. The plight of the end-stage respiratory cripple is indeed pitiable. Struggling for breath even when lying down, his shoulders heaving and neck muscles straining to maintain the respiratory effort and his skin blue with **cyanosis**, he knows that his condition can only worsen and that, eventually, even the relief of the oxygen mask will fail.

Chronic obstructive lung disease is largely caused by cigarette smoking.

See also **asthma**.

lung, disorders of

These are common and important and include **actinomycosis**, **anthracosis**, bronchial **asthma**, **bronchitis**, **bronchopneumonia**, **emphysema**, **haemothorax**, **laryngotracheobronchitis**, **Legionnaires' disease**, **lung cancer**, **obstructive airways disease**, pulmonary **embolism**, **respiratory distress syndrome**, **tracheitis** and **tuberculosis**. In immunocompromised people, the lungs may suffer fungus infections such as aspergillosis, histoplasmosis, and **candidiasis**.

Allergic alveolitis is a group of diseases caused by various organic dusts including mouldy hay (farmers' lung), mouldy cane sugar fibre (bagassosis), pigeon droppings (bird fancier's lung) and compost (mushroom worker's lung).

lupus erythematosus

A general disease caused by a severe disturbance of the immune system so that some parts of the body cease to be recognized as 'self' and are attacked by the immune system. In addition, *immune complexes* consisting of clumps of DNA and anti-DNA antibodies are circulating in the blood and causing severe tissue damage, especially to the linings of the blood vessels and to the kidneys. Women are affected much more often than men.

Lupus erythematosus is essentially an inflammatory disease of the body's connective tissue. The skin disorder *discoid lupus erythematosus* (DLE) is one form. In this, red, raised bumps develop in the skin, usually on the face and scalp. In the more serious, and sometimes life-threatening, form, systemic lupus erythematosus, or SLE, there is involvement of the joints and tendons, causing arthritis and sometimes deformities. About two-thirds of patients have a 'butterfly' rash across the bridge of the nose and about half suffer hair loss (alopecia). The heart, lungs, kidneys, liver and nervous system may also be involved.

Severe and life-threatening manifestations of lupus erythematosus call for large doses of steroids. These are highly effective and often life-saving. Patients may, thereafter, be maintained on low doses. Sometimes, immunosuppressive drugs are needed. In general, the outlook in this disease has greatly improved.

lupus pernio

A form of sarcoidosis affecting the skin and causing purple swellings on the nose, ears and cheeks.

lupus vulgaris

Now that milk is reliably free from the tubercle bacillus, this disease is rare. It is a form of skin tuberculosis that was formerly the cause of much facial deformity, especially around the nose and the inside of the mouth. It causes painless ulceration and, unless treated, loss of tissue. In extreme cases, the nose may be lost. Lupus – the name comes from the Latin word for 'wolf' – was once commonly confused with leprosy or syphilis.

Lustral

A brand name for **sertraline**.

Lyclear

A brand name for **permethrin**.

lymecycline

A tetracycline **antibiotic** used to treat acne and general infections. A brand name is Tetralysal.

Lyme disease

This is a more important disease than the scant public attention it has received would suggest.

CAUSE

It appeared first among the inhabitants of Old Lyme, Connecticut, in 1975, and is caused by the spiral organism (spirochaete) *Borrelia burgdorferi*, which is transmitted by the bite of the tick *Ixodes dammini*. The spirochaete is similar in shape to the organism causing syphilis and there are many features of Lyme disease similar to those of syphilis. The Borrelia occurs throughout the temperate regions of the world and has been reported in Europe, Australia, the USSR and China. The natural host seems to be deer, but dogs can also be infected. In the first ten years, about 8000 cases of Lyme disease occurred in America. It is now being increasingly diagnosed in Britain.

RECOGNITION AND SYMPTOMS

Like the causal organism of syphilis, the *Borrelia* organism can affect almost every organ of the body, but most commonly involves the skin, the joints, the heart and the nervous system. The first sign is a slightly itchy red spot at the site of the mite bite. This appears three to thirty days after biting. The red spot expands steadily and then clears centrally so that an expanding ring is formed. In about half the cases other similar spots soon appear and there may be as many as 100 rings, scattered all over the skin, but most frequently in the armpits, groins and thighs. These are not thought to be due to multiple bites, but to be a feature of the disease. The organism can be found in any of the spots or rings. This stage is accompanied by fatigue, a feeling of illness, headaches, fever, stiff neck, aches in the muscles and joints and enlarged lymph nodes. In some cases there is sore throat, cough, **conjunctivitis**, other more severe eye complications and pain in the abdomen with enlargement and tenderness of the liver. Liver tests may show a **hepatitis**.

Several weeks or even months after onset up to 15 per cent of affected people develop nervous system disorders such as **meningitis**, **encephalitis**, paralysis of various nerves, muscle weakness and **shingles**-like pain in the skin. Some develop mental illness and others have a profound sense of fatigue and weakness which may last for months or years. A pattern similar to **multiple sclerosis** may develop, but studies have shown that *Borrelia* is not the cause of that disease. Some authorities believe that the *Borrelia* can cause **dementia**.

The joints are affected in at least half the cases, usually intermittently and mildly, but sometimes severely with joint damage similar to mild rheumatoid arthritis.

Heart involvement occurs in about 8 per cent of cases, usually within a few weeks of onset. The most common effect is **heart block** but heart enlargement and inflammation of the heart capsule (**pericarditis**) also occur.

> There is evidence that Lyme disease can be passed from a mother to her unborn baby, and *Borrelia* have been found in children with severe congenital defects.

TREATMENT

It is a great pity that Lyme disease is not better known. Those familiar with the significance of the characteristic early skin ring pattern can seek immediate confirmation by blood tests and treatment and thus avoid all the complications. Fortunately, the organism is sensitive to many antibiotics, such as penicillin, erythromycin, tetracycline and cefotaxime. These are given for up to three weeks and are usually highly effective.

lymph

The watery or milky fluid that drains from the tissue spaces, along the lymph channels, and is returned to the circulation by way of one of the main veins in the chest. Lymph channels are clear, vein-like vessels that form a network throughout most of the body. Drained lymph passes through **lymph nodes** where most infective organisms in it are dealt with.

lymphadenitis

Infection of lymph nodes. This is usually secondary to infection in the area draining to the affected nodes. Thus an infection in the leg may cause lymphadenitis in the groin.

lymphadenopathy

Any disease process affecting a **lymph node**.

lymphangitis

Inflammation of the lymphatic vessels. This is usually caused by virulent organisms of a type capable of spreading rapidly – often streptococci. The inflamed lymph channels cause conspicuous red streaks under the skin – a sign once dreaded as heralding probable death from **septicaemia**. There is general upset with fever.

> Lymphangitis indicates a severe and potentially dangerous infection and calls for energetic antibiotic treatment.

lymphatic system

The lymphatic system (see illustration on following page) is a subsidiary tissue drainage system of fine tubular channels (lymph vessels) and nodes (the lymph nodes), and is con-

cerned with defence against infection. Lymph is the fluid in the lymph vessels, which drains from the tissue spaces and from the intestine. It varies in constitution in different parts of the body. Lymph from the tissues is largely fluid which has leaked out of the smallest blood vessels (capillaries). It contains large numbers of white cells called lymphocytes (see below), and is usually clear. Lymph from the intestines is milky, especially after a meal, because of the large number of tiny fat globules which it contains. Fat-laden lymph is called chyle.

Lymph nodes are often wrongly called 'glands'. Lymph nodes are small oval bodies, up to 2 cm in length, situated in groups along the course of the lymph drainage vessels. Each node has a fibrous capsule and contains large masses of lymphocytes. The main groups of lymph nodes are situated in the groins, in the armpits, in the neck, deep in the abdomen around the main blood vessels, in the suspensory curtain of the bowels (mesentery) and in the central partition of the chest (the mediastinum).

The lymph nodes are an important defence against the spread of infection from the surface tissues to the deeper parts of the body, and from the internal organs to the bloodstream. Their lymphocytes produce large quantities of antibodies (immunoglobulins) to combat infection and the nodes are often the site of a major conflict with invading organisms. In this event the nodes often become swollen and tender.

Because lymph nodes drain the tissues, cancer cells are often caught up in them and reproduce there, causing enlargement. The lymphocytes themselves may become disordered and may form tumours (lymphomas).

See also **lymphoma in AIDS**.

lymph gland

The incorrect term for a **lymph node**. These are not glands.

lymph nodes

Small bodies, about the shape and size of butter beans, that can be felt when inflamed. They lie mainly in groups in the neck, armpits, groins and around the major blood vessels of the abdomen and chest and are connected by thin-walled lymph vessels. Lymph nodes act as 'filters' to remove infection from the draining body fluids and are packed with **lymphocytes**.

lymphocyte over-production

See **Canale-Smith syndrome**.

lymphocytes

Specialized white cells concerned in the body's immune system. Two main classes, B cells and T cells, and several different subtypes can be distinguished. B lymphocytes (B cells) produce antibodies and are divided into the plasma cells that secrete them, and memory cells. The latter act when the event that originally stimulated antibody selection recurs, and allow faster antibody production than occurred on the first occasion. T lymphocytes (T cells) help to protect against virus infections and cancer and are divided into helper cells, suppressor cells, cytotoxic cells, memory cells and mediators of delayed hypersensitivity. There are also large granular lymphocytes. These are the killer cells (K cells) and the natural killer cells (NK cells).

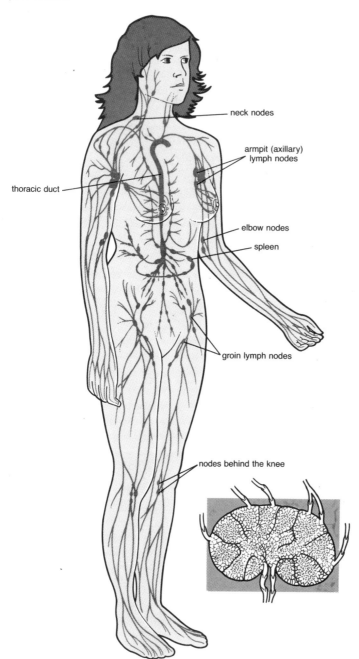

The lymphatic system of the body. Note that the main groups of lymph nodes occur in the armpits, groin and around the main blood vessels of the abdomen. Other groups are found at the elbows and behind the knees. The thoracic duct carries lymph and absorbed fats up from the intestine and discharges it into the main upper vein of the chest. Lymph nodes are commonly, and inaccurately, called 'glands'.

neck nodes

armpit (axillary) lymph nodes

thoracic duct

elbow nodes

spleen

groin lymph nodes

nodes behind the knee

lymphoedema

A persistent swelling of the tissues resulting from blockage or absence of the lymph drainage channels which carry tissue fluid (lymph) from the tissues back into the bloodstream. This may be caused by congenital deficiency of the lymph channels, in which case it usually affects the legs; operative removal, as in the surgical treatment of cancer; obstruction by cancer cells; or obstruction by filarial parasitic worms. The latter causes **elephantiasis**.

Lymphoedema of the arm sometimes follows surgical treatment or radiotherapy for cancer of the breast. It is difficult to treat, but success has been achieved by tight compression of the part with an elastic arm stocking and regular firm massage from the wrist to the armpit. It may be necessary to sleep with the arm raised in a sling above the level of the heart.

lymphogranuloma venereum

See **sexually transmitted diseases**.

lymphokines

Cytokines produced by lymphocytes. Lymphokines attract **macrophages** to the site of foreign material and activate them to kill organisms, cause other T cells to clone, and provide other cells with protection against virus invasion. They include interferons, chemotactic factor, transfer factor and interleukin-2.

lymphoma

One of a group of cancers of the lymph tissue, especially the lymph nodes and the spleen. If the lymphoma contains certain large, irregular cells with multiple nuclei, known as Reed-Sternberg cells, the disease is called Hodgkin's disease (Hodgkin's lymphoma). If not, it is called a non-Hodgkin's lymphoma; in nine out of ten such cases the tumours consist of **clones** of B cells. The remainder are tumours of T cell origin. They vary considerably in their degree of malignancy and have many features in common with certain leukaemias.

Lymphoma features tiredness, loss of weight and sometimes fever. Tumours may enlarge to the point at which they cause pressure on various structures of the body. This may cause paralysis by compression of the spinal cord, difficulty in swallowing from pressure on the oesophagus, difficulty in breathing, obstruction of the bowel causing vomiting, and obstruction of the lymph vessels causing lymphoedema. Treatment depends on the cell type and on the extent of spread. In some cases, no treatment is needed and often patients are watched for years without intervention. But when treatment is required, radiotherapy is often best and may be curative.

lymphoma, Burkitt's

A tumour of B lymphocytes thought to be caused by the Epstein-Barr herpes virus which also causes **glandular fever** (infectious mononucleosis). Burkitt's lymphoma occurs in Central Africa and affects children and young adults. Its discovery, by Dennis Burkitt, aroused great interest as he was able to show that it was almost certainly caused by a virus and spread by insects. This was one of the first human tumours to be shown to be caused in this way.

RECOGNITION AND SYMPTOMS
The tumour commonly and painfully affects the jaw and spreads to the abdomen, where large secondary masses may form, affecting the bowel and collecting behind the membrane covering the bowel (peritoneum). Progress is rapid and anaemia is common from involvement of the bone marrow.

TREATMENT
Immunosuppressive chemotherapy with cyclophosphamide or methotrexate is apparently curative in 80 per cent of early cases and about 40 per cent of those with advanced, widespread disease.

lymphoma in AIDS

Malignant lymphomas are tumours of lymph tissue and consist of masses of monoclonal B lymphocytes and other cells. They may occur anywhere in the body and frequently involve the brain. In AIDS, lymphomas closely resemble a type of tumour previously well-known and described as Burkitt's lymphoma, after Dennis Burkitt who first described the tumour in the middle 1960s and showed that it was related to the Epstein-Barr (EB) herpes virus.

This type of tumour, relatively common in certain parts of Africa, has been extremely rare in the West until it began to appear as a feature of AIDS. Cases have been reported in which the tumour has affected the jaw, the mouth, an eye socket, the lungs, the central part of the chest, the bones, the bowels, the liver and the brain. Cases of AIDS in which lymphomas have occurred frequently show heavy infection with EB virus, but as this is very common in AIDS, the significance, in relation to the tumour, is uncertain. Treatment is difficult but, although most patients who have developed lymphomas have died, some can be saved by energetic chemotherapy based upon existing knowledge of the sensitivity of the different types of lymphomas.

lymphoma, non-Hodgkin's

Any type of cancer of lymphoid tissue other than **Hodgkin's lymphoma**. Non-Hodgkin's lymphomas usually consist of clonal masses of B lymphocytes. They vary considerably in their degree of malignancy and have many features in common with certain leukaemias. Some progress very slowly, but even the more malignant will often respond well to treatment.

RECOGNITION AND SYMPTOMS
Lymphoid tissue anywhere in the body can be involved. The commonest presenting sign is widespread, painless, firm lymph node enlargement. There is tiredness, loss of weight, and sometimes fever. When the disease process reaches a certain stage, there may be pressure on various structures of the body. This may cause paralysis by compression of the spinal cord, difficulty in swallowing from pressure on the oesophagus, difficulty in breathing, obstruction of the bowel causing vomiting, and obstruction of the lymph vessels causing **lymphoedema**.

TREATMENT
In many cases, no treatment is needed and often patients are watched for years without intervention. But when treatment is required, radiotherapy is often best and may be curative.

lymphosarcoma

The term formerly used for **non-Hodgkin's lymphoma**.

Lyon hypothesis

See **X-inactivation**.

lysis

The destruction of a living cell by disruption of its limiting cell membrane. Haemolysis is lysis of red blood cells.

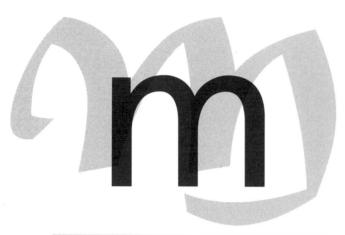

Maalox

A brand name for a preparation containing **aluminium hydroxide** and **magnesium hydroxide**.

Mabthera

A brand name for the monoclonal antibody drug **rituximab**.

machines, intelligent, in surgery

See **robot surgery**.

macro-

Prefix meaning 'large' as in macrophage (large eater).

Macrobid

A brand name for **nitrofurantoin**.

macrobiotics

A system of diet based on the aesthetically pleasing yin-yang (opposing, light-dark, male-female) principle. Scientists do not believe that this is a logical basis for **nutrition**, the principles of which are well established. Over-enthusiastic adherence to a macrobiotic dietary could lead to a unbalanced diet.

Macrodantin

A brand name for **nitrofurantoin**.

macroglossia

An enlarged tongue.

macrophage

Large scavenging cells (phagocytes) of the immune system found all over the body, especially in the liver, lymph nodes, spleen and bone marrow. Some remain stationary within the tissues and are called fixed macrophages or histiocytes; others are free and move about and are attracted to sites of infection. Macrophages in the liver are called Kupffer cells and those in the nervous system are called microglial cells. They readily change shape and flow round bacteria to ingest and destroy them. They take up organic debris in the same way. Macrophages are amoebas. In order to bring about an immune response, most **antigens** must first be processed by macrophages so that their antigenic elements can be presented to **lymphocytes** on the macrophage surfaces.

macrophagic myofasciitis

A recently described apparently new disease featuring fever, muscle and joint pain, muscle and general weakness and infiltration of the tissues around the muscles by sheets of large, finely-granular **macrophages**. The muscle fibres themselves are minimally affected. The microscopic appearances are unlike those of any previous muscle or fibrous tissue plane (fascial) disorder. The condition appears to respond to treatment with various combinations of antibiotics and steroids.

macular degeneration

A disorder of the retina usually affecting elderly people and causing progressive loss of the central part of the field of vision. It is caused by defects in the insulating layer between the retina and the underlying choroid so that leakage of fluid occurs into the retina with progressive destruction of the rods and cones and connecting nerves.

Macular degeneration can affect both eyes simultaneously, but usually one eye is affected weeks or months before the other. In some cases the process can be arrested by laser treatment. Anyone noticing a central gap in the field of vision in one eye should report this at once. The vision should be checked by covering one eye at a time.

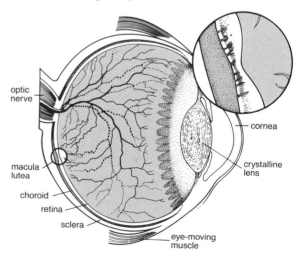

The macula lutea is the tiny, highly sensitive, central area of the retina we use for straight-ahead vision. This means that if the macular function is lost by degeneration only poor-resolution vision surrounding the area of regard remains.

mad as a hatter

This phrase illuminates a point in industrial toxicology now, happily, of historical interest only. Hatters worked with felts made from skins, and an important part of the process involved the use of mercuric chloride. The resulting **mercury poisoning** caused widespread brain damage and symptoms such as staggering gait, speech and emotional disturbances, and fits.

Madopar

A brand name for **levodopa** in combination with **benserazide**.

maggots

See **myiasis**.

Magnapen

A brand name for a mixture of the penicillin antibiotics **ampicillin** and **flucloxacillin**.

magnesium alginate

A drug used to treat **dyspepsia** and heartburn. Trade names of preparations containing it are Algicon and Gaviscon Infant.

magnesium carbonate

A mild antacid drug used to treat **dyspepsia**. Trade names of preparations containing it are Algicon and Topal.

magnesium hydroxide

An antacid and laxative drug. Trade names of preparations containing it are Diovol, Maalox, Mucaine and Mucogel.

magnesium oxide

An antacid drug. Brand name of preparations containing magnesium oxide and dimethicone are Asilone and Kolanticon.

magnesium trisilicate

A drug used as an antacid in the treatment of **dyspepsia**. Trade names of preparations containing it are Gastrocote, Gaviscon and Pyrogastrone.

magnetic resonance imaging

A diagnostic scanning system based on the principle of nuclear magnetic resonance. When certain atoms are placed in a strong magnetic field, the nuclei (core) of the atoms emit a radio signals, the characteristics of which depend on the environment of the nuclei. Hydrogen atoms behave in this way.

This principle is applied to a valuable method of body scanning originally called nuclear magnetic resonance scanning (NMR), but now, to avoid confusion with nuclear radiation, called magnetic resonance imaging (MRI). The method is capable of a degree of resolution of detail greater than that possible with CT scanning and it has the additional advantage over CT scanning that no nuclear radiation is involved.

Every molecule of water contains an atom of hydrogen so the presence of water causes a strong signal to be emitted. Less strong signals are sent out by other materials with proportionately less hydrogen in them. In this way the MRI scanner is capable of resolving subtle differences in the density of soft tissue such as brain and nerves and can detect subtle abnormalities. Differences in tissue composition are easily seen. Thus, for instance, the characteristic plaques of **multiple sclerosis** are clearly revealed. An area of brain deprived of its blood supply, as in a stroke, is easily visible, and in some cases it is even possible not only to show the presence of a tumour,

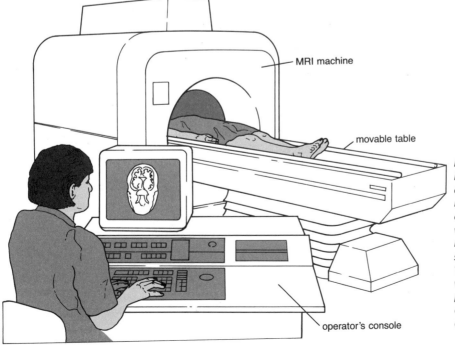

MRI machine

movable table

Magnetic resonance imaging (MRI) is a method of scanning in which X-rays are not used. The equipment is massive and very expensive. Powerful magnetic fields and radio signals are used.
The resolution in imaging with MRI is, for certain purposes, higher than can be obtained in any other way.

operator's console

but to differentiate between benign and malignant types. Details of the heart and of blood vessels, and even the internal structures of the eye, can be made out clearly. Many of the pictures now obtained by MRI closely resemble photographs of sections of the real body as seen in anatomical museums.

So far as is known, MRI is completely safe. The radio waves used are of the same wavelengths as normal short-wave broadcasts and these have been passing through our bodies since birth. The main magnetic field, within which the patient lies, is, however, very strong indeed and all metal objects must be kept well away. Magnetic tapes, credit cards and phone cards are all wiped clean. To produce such a field requires superconducting electromagnets and these are, at present, very bulky and expensive, requiring liquid helium to reach the necessary low temperature. New and more efficient superconducting materials are, however, being developed, which operate at much higher temperatures, so MRI scanners may be expected to become smaller and cheaper.

This is as well, for the principle will certainly be of the utmost importance for the future of diagnostic medicine, offering such striking advantages in the detection of all kinds of tissue abnormality in any part of the body that the CT scanner may become obsolete.

major histocompatibility complex (MHC)

Protein markers on the surface of cells that control the activities of cells of the immune system. These markers, sometime called 'flags', are basic to immune system function, and are coded for by a large cluster of genes on chromosome 6. They indicate tissue type and are important in organ donation, but have wider functions in the immune system.

Infected cells use their MHC sites to signal the fact to helper T cells and cytotoxic T cells that they can be attacked. There are two classes of MHC. Class I MHC molecules are present on virtually all body cells other than red blood cells; class II MHC molecules occur on antigen-presenting cells such as **macrophages** and B cells. Cytotoxic T cell binding sites (CD8) bind to MHC class I, while helper T cells (CD4 sites) bind to MHC class II. MHC variations have been used extensively in human population studies.

malabsorption

A failure of the normal movement of some of the elements of the diet from the small intestine into the bloodstream.
POSSIBLE CAUSES
This may be because of the absence of the chemical substances, enzymes, necessary for the break-up of the food into absorbable form, or to some structural change in the lining of the intestine.

> Malabsorption may lead to malnutrition, even if an adequate diet is taken.

Normal absorption of food ingredients requires that the carbohydrates should be broken down to simple sugars, the proteins to amino acids and the fats to a milk-like emulsion of tiny oily globules. Carbohydrate and protein breakdown requires enzymes and the emulsification of fats requires bile. If any of the digestive enzymes are absent, as in various genetic disorders, such as lactase deficiency (lactose intolerance) or cystic fibrosis affecting the enzyme secretion of the pancreas or the enzyme-secreting glands in the wall of the bowel, failure of absorption will occur. Any failure of the passage of bile to the intestine, as from liver disease or obstruction to the bile ducts from gallstones or other causes, will result in unemulsified fat and this will not be absorbed but will simply be passed in the stools.

Various conditions damage the absorptive power of the inner lining of the bowel. In health this is covered with millions of tiny finger-like processes – the villi – which have the effect of enormously increasing the surface area of the bowel available for absorption. In some malabsorption conditions a sample (biopsy) of the bowel lining, taken with a special spring-loaded capsule on a string, which has to be swallowed, show that the villi are atrophied and reduced in height or even absent altogether. This occurs in coeliac disease, which is caused by an immunological disorder featuring sensitivity to gluten in flour, and in tropical sprue.
RECOGNITION AND SYMPTOMS
People with malabsorption may be generally malnourished, thin and lacking in energy. Children may fail to thrive. The stools are unusually voluminous and often contain fat (steatorrhoea). There may be anaemia, vitamin deficiencies, and mineral deficiencies such as calcium shortage, causing bone distortion (**rickets**) or bone softening (osteomalacia).
TREATMENT
The treatment of malabsorption involves a precise diagnosis of the cause and, if possible, its reversal. High-dosage replacement therapy, with vitamins and minerals, is often necessary.

malaise

In medical textbooks, accounts of the great majority of diseases include, for completeness, a reference to 'malaise'. The authors would not like to be thought to have forgotten that in most diseases the patient feels rotten. That is all the word means. It has no diagnostic value.

malar

Relating to the cheekbone. The Latin word *mala* means the 'cheek or cheekbone', and the term may also relate to the Latin *malum* meaning 'an apple'.

malar flush

High rosy colour, with a bluish tinge, seen on the cheek bones in many patients with narrowing of the mitral valve of the heart (mitral stenosis). This is sometimes called the mitral facies. The sign is by no means diagnostic and, nowadays, is considered of little importance compared with more positive signs of the disease.

malaria

The term 'malaria' comes from the Italian words *mala* meaning 'bad' and *aria* meaning 'air' and reflects the earlier supposition that this widespread disease, which was noted to be commoner in the vicinity of swamps and other areas of stagnant water, was caused by some 'emanation' that polluted the air. Malaria is certainly caused by something in the air and we now know this to be the malarial parasite, carried by certain species of mosquito which breed in stagnant water.
INCIDENCE
The disease occurs anywhere in the world where the *Anopheles* mosquito exists – and that is almost everywhere,

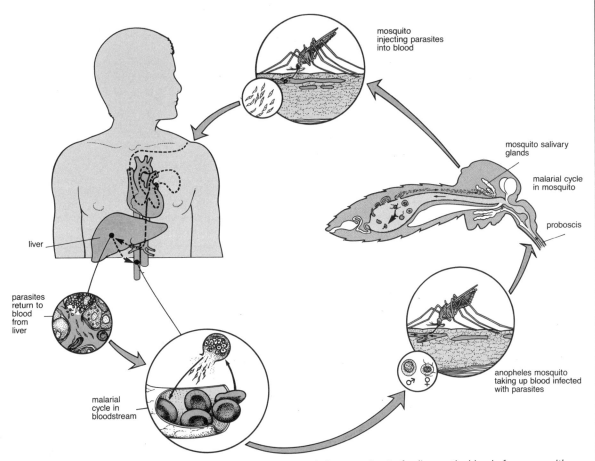

The life-cycle of the malarial parasite in man and in the female Anopheles mosquito. By feeding on the blood of a person with malaria the mosquito takes up red blood cells infected with the parasite. Later, when feeding on another victim, it injects the parasites with its salivary secretions.

including Britain – and where active cases are occurring in people. Malaria is one of the most efficient of all killer diseases and is responsible for at least a million deaths a year, worldwide. It is also responsible for an immense amount of human suffering, debility and ill-health. Some 100 million cases occur every year.

TRANSMISSION

Malarial parasites are single-celled organisms called protozoa. When a female Anopheles mosquito sucks blood from a person with malaria, some of the red blood cells taken up may contain the parasite. If so, these continue their life-cycle in the mosquito, producing large numbers of infective offspring which accumulate in great masses in the mosquito's salivary glands.

The mosquito then flies to settle on its next victim and inserts its proboscis through the skin into a small blood vessel. To clear its proboscis, which is often blocked by malarial parasites, it first injects this material into the blood, then proceeds to feed. The parasites, now in the bloodstream, travel to the liver, settle there and begin to reproduce in some of the liver cells. These, when filled to capacity with newly developed parasites, burst and release them into the blood. The parasites now enter red blood cells, where they also reproduce until the red cells, too, are burst, releasing further parasites to maintain the cycle.

RECOGNITION AND SYMPTOMS

Malaria has something in common with the laser, in that the cycles of invasion and bursting of the red cells, like the light waves in the laser, quickly fall into phase with each other so that the effects, including the symptoms, become regularly periodic. There are several different types of malaria caused by different species of the genus Plasmodium. *Plasmodium falciparum* causes a 24-hour cycle, with bouts of fever, shaking, headache and general aches and pains occurring every day. The common *Plasmodium vivax*, and the *Plasmodium ovale* have a 48-hour cycle and *Plasmodium malariae* a 72-hour cycle.

> Heavy infection can be very dangerous, especially with *Plasmodium falciparum* which can block the small blood vessels of the brain and cause grave illness.

This parasite also often causes so much red blood cell destruction that the released haemoglobin colours the urine dark red or black, giving the name 'blackwater fever'. This is a sign of dangerous disease and is often associated with serious kidney damage. The spleen has to cope with the products of so many destroyed red blood cells that it often becomes greatly enlarged. The 'malarial spleen' is liable to fatal rupture on injury and a blow to the spleen has been a popular method of murder in malarial areas.

TREATMENT

Because of the liver cycle, people who have had malaria and have been inadequately treated may appear to have fully recovered, but may develop severe attacks months or years later, as a result of breeding of parasites in the liver. So good treatment has to be directed not only at control of the current attack, but also at destruction of the parasites in the liver. Malaria can almost always be prevented by taking a small daily dose of an antimalarial drug.

The real solution to malaria is mosquito control and many areas of the tropical world have been rendered entirely free from the disease by the use of insecticides, by the destruction or oiling of areas of mosquito breeding water and by the isolation and effective treatment of residual cases.

Malarone

A brand name for **proguanil** in conjunction with **atovaquone**.

malathion

A poisonous organophosphate insecticide drug used in very low concentration in preparations for external use to destroy lice. Trade names are Derbac-M, Prioderm and Suleo-M.

male sex hormone

See **testosterone**.

malformation

Any bodily deformity, or any structural abnormality, resulting from a defect in development or growth.

malgramostin

A granulocyte and **macrophage** colony stimulating factor used to treat white cell deficiency. It is prepared by recombinant DNA techniques (**genetic engineering**). A brand name is Leucomax.

malic acid

A drug used to clean external wounds and ulcers and remove dead tissue. A brand name is Aserbine.

malignant

A term derived from the Latin *malignus* meaning 'evil' and usually applied to cancerous tumours which spread remotely in the body. The term 'malignant' is opposite in meaning to the term **benign**. It is also used to qualify unusually serious forms of various diseases such as **hypertension**. In general, a malignant disorder is one tending to cause death in the absence of effective medical intervention.

malignant melanoma

About one cancer in 100 is a malignant melanoma. These may occur on the skin or in the eye.

INCIDENCE

Skin melanomas are very rare in childhood and commonest in the middle-aged and elderly. About half develop from pre-existing moles and this is made more likely, in white people, by prolonged exposure to sunlight. Nearly everyone has pigmented moles but only one in a million becomes malignant. Hairy moles hardly ever turn into malignant melanomas.

RECOGNITION AND SYMPTOMS

Malignant change in a mole can be detected by various signs. These include:

- change in shape, especially increasing irregularity of outline; change in size;
- increased protuberance beyond the surface;
- change in colour, especially sudden darkening and the development of coloured irregularities appearing as different shades of brown, grey, pink, red and bluish;
- itching or pain;
- softening;
- crumbling;
- and the development of new 'satellite' moles around the original one.

Those which become nodular are the most malignant as they tend to penetrate deeply.

> Melanomas are commonest on areas exposed to the sun, but may occur anywhere on the skin. Once suspicion has been aroused, there should be no delay in reporting the condition for an expert opinion.

TREATMENT

Melanomas are removed with a wide area of normal-seeming tissue around them and skin grafting may be necessary to cover the defect.

EYE TUMOURS

Malignant melanoma can also affect the choroid of the eye, the layer just under the retina. This is the commonest type of eye tumour. It causes no pain but leads to detachment of the retina and an obvious visual defect. Usually it is necessary to remove the eye, but sometimes a small melanoma can be destroyed by photocoagulation or laser treatment. Untreated choroidal melanomas are often very late in spreading. All medical students are familiar with the association of the glass eye and the enlarged liver from secondary spread of the tumour.

Surprisingly, a substantial proportion of eyes removed for pain and blindness following long-term inflammation from disease or injury are found to contain malignant melanomas. This well-known fact has never been fully explained.

malingering

The conscious pretence to be suffering from a disease, or the simulation of the signs of disease, in order to gain some supposed personal advantage. The motives for malingering include avoidance of work or of unwanted activities, or of real or presumed danger, or to obtain financial advantage by fraudulent claims for compensation.

In most cases, malingering is easily detected by proper medical investigation. Medical attitudes to malingering vary from aggressive determination to unmask the culprit at all costs, to an interested and sympathetic enquiry into the reasons why any human being should behave in such a way.

See also **Munchausen's syndrome**.

Mallory-Weiss syndrome

A tear at the lower end of the gullet (oesophagus) caused by violent movements of the **diaphragm** during retching or vomiting. There is vomiting of blood. In most cases the tear heals well, often without treatment.

malnutrition

The effect of an inadequate diet or of failure to absorb a normal diet or to assimilate absorbed food elements. The term is now sometimes used to describe the taking of a diet damaging in its excess.

Malnutrition from insufficient food intake is a worldwide problem for which there is no medical solution.

POSSIBLE CAUSES

Malnutrition also occurs secondary to a variety of diseased states of the body and mind. Conditions local to the gastrointestinal tract such as sprue, **malabsorption** syndromes, coeliac disease, Crohn's disease and chronic diarrhoea can lead to failure of absorption of food. General conditions such as **diabetes**, thyroid overactivity, cancer and tuberculosis can result in failure of assimilation or an excessive rate of consumption of food elements.

Mental disorders such as **anorexia nervosa** lead to a deliberate reduction of intake; and many prolonged illnesses are associated with a serious lack of interest in eating. Alcoholism is an important cause of malnutrition. The alcohol provides enough calories to remove hunger and alcoholic stomach irritation (gastritis) further discourages eating. But alcoholic drinks provide none of the essential proteins, fats, vitamins and minerals.

RECOGNITION AND SYMPTOMS

In babies, infants and young children, malnutrition causes failure to thrive and to grow to the height otherwise genetically determined. It can interfere with the production of immunoglobulins and hence reduce the efficiency of the body's defence against infection. Vitamin deficiencies, which are a common feature of malnutrition, cause a wide spectrum of specific disorders including **beri-beri**, **pellagra**, **anaemia**, **pernicious anaemia**, **scurvy**, **rickets** and haemorrhagic tendencies. Protein deficiency causes **marasmus** and **kwashiorkor**.

malnutrition in children

See **kwashiorkor**.

malocclusion

Failure of the upper and lower teeth to come together in an acceptable manner. Orthodontic treatment can do much to correct moderate degrees of malocclusion.

malpractice

Professional misconduct including professional negligence. The term may be applied to any professional person, but is most commonly used in connection with the medical profession. In Britain, malpractice has a wide meaning. The term includes:

- the failure to provide proper standards of medical care for patients;
- engaging in reckless or dangerous treatments;
- abuse of professional privileges in prescribing drugs, giving certificates and terminating pregnancy;
- using medical status to exert undue influence on, or to establish sexual or other improper relationships with, patients;
- betraying professional confidences;
- engaging in advertising or other
- disparagement of colleagues.

A doctor suspected of any of these things victed in a criminal court for an offence, before the Professional Conduct Committee of Medical Council (*not* the British Medical Associ asked to answer the allegations. Proceedings are con much as in a civil court, but the PCC has only one senten that the doctor's name be erased from the Medical Regist so that he may no longer legally practise.

Some forms of malpractice are also criminal offences for which a doctor may also have to answer in law.

mamma

Latin root meaning 'breast' as in mammary (of the breast).

mammary artery grafting

A coronary artery bypass procedure used as an alternative to vein bypass surgery. Unfortunately, there is a strong tendency for vein grafts to become arterialized and eventually blocked by atherosclerosis and thrombosis. It has been found that grafts using one or both of the internal mammary arteries instead of a length of leg vein will usually remain open longer and are more resistant than veins to these dangerous disease changes.

mammography

Breast cancer is the commonest cancer in women and takes a terrible toll. Any measure that can reduce the incidence, if even to a minor degree, is of enormous value. Such a measure is mammography, which is a form of X-ray examination used as a screening procedure on groups of women and in cases of suspected breast cancer in individuals. The value of mammography is still questioned by some, but with progressive improvements in instrumentation and methods, these doubts have lessened, and most doctors now acknowledge its value. The results of five trials involving 282,777 women in Sweden, followed for five to 13 years, was published in the *Lancet* in

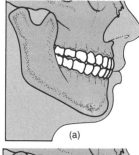
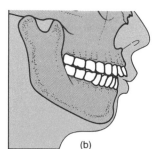
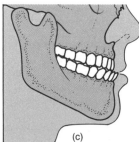

The relationship between the upper and lower teeth is called the occlusion. (a) Shows perfect occlusion; (b) Shows malocclusion from upper teeth overhang; (c) Shows malocclusion from lower jaw prognathism.

(a)

(b)

(c)

overall reduction of
who had mammog-

exclude cancer and
malignant tumours.
s in which sampling
ay, can lead to early
per cent of lumps
ut may be detected
ese contain cancer.
visualized.
nen under 35, but
ended for women
eduction in breast
cancer mortality is greatest – about 30 per cent. The radiation
dosage is very low and offers no significant risk.

The procedure, and position of the patient, varies with the
type of machine, but is painless, although often quite uncomfortable. A variety of methods is used to allow the soft tissue
to be X-rayed without interference from other structures. The
breasts may be laid on top of a flat surface or allowed to hang
down; they may be sucked into a cavity, or may be gently
squeezed between plates.

Mammography is by no means the complete answer to
the breast cancer menace, but it has benefits beyond the
obvious one of early detection and cure. It may allow breast-
conserving surgery in proven cases of small cancers; it may
reduce the need for drug treatment; and it can reduce the
fear of cancer in women with consistently negative results.

Technological advances in recent years, in the design and
construction of mammography equipment, have significantly
improved the value of this procedure as a screening tool
against breast cancer and many of the earlier critics of the
method have revised their opinions.

mammography X-rays without film

See **xeroradiography**.

mammoplasty

See **plastic surgery**.

mandelic acid

An antiseptic drug used in sterile solutions for washing out
the bladder, especially if a permanent catheter is in use. A
brand name is Uro-Tainer.

mandible

The lower jaw.

mandibula

Latin root meaning 'mandible' as in mandible (the jaw bone).

manganese poisoning

An industrial disease of manganese miners who inhale dust
from the ore, and of others exposed to manganese compounds. The condition is essentially one of brain damage
which leads to both psychiatric and neurological effects.
These include delusions, hallucinations and compulsions,
loss of expression, slowness of movement, rigidity of the muscles and impairment of speech.

mania

Greek root meaning 'madness' as in maniacal (raving mad).
It also refers to the manic phase of a **manic-depressive illness**.

manic-depressive illness

A serious disturbance of the emotions (affect) – an affective
psychosis. In some cases the affected person may show only
mania or only depression. Such people are said to have unipolar disorders. If both phases occur the disorder is said to be a
bipolar disorder. The cause is unknown, but studies of identical twins suggest that hereditary factors may be involved.

This illness features an association of diametrically opposite kinds of mood disorder – on the one hand an abnormal
elation (mania), and on the other, one of pathological
depression. The depressive phase usually comes first and
about 10 per cent of people thought to be suffering from
unipolar depression have a manic episode six to ten years
later, usually in the early 30s. No real distinction is now drawn
between the depressive phase of the manic-depressive illness
and psychotic depression generally.

RECOGNITION AND SYMPTOMS

In the depressive phase there is mental and physical slowing;
loss of interest and energy; loss of concentration; sadness; pessimism; self-doubt; self-blame; and thoughts of suicide.
Depressive episodes, if untreated, last for about six months to
one year. The average patient suffers five or six episodes over
a twenty-year period. Most treated episodes clear in about
three months, but if treatment is stopped before about three
months, relapse is very likely. The manic phase, if it occurs,
usually comes after two to four depressive episodes.

During the manic phase the features are:

- speeding-up of thought and speech;
- severely disordered judgement and mental reliability;
- ever-changing flights of ideas;
- constant elation or euphoria;
- inappropriate optimism;
- grandiose notions;
- a gross over-estimation of personal ability.

The latter may be reflected in unrealistic plans and expressed
intentions or even in socially and financially ruinous
behaviour.

The affected person sleeps poorly and may engage in an
unusually high level of sexual activity. About three-quarters
of those with this disorder engage in personal assault or
threatening behaviour, often against people in prominent
positions. They are notoriously unreliable and characteristically engage in deceit and lying.

Both phases may feature the characteristic psychotic elements of hallucinations and delusions.

TREATMENT

The spontaneous recovery rate in manic-depressive illness is
very high – about 90 per cent recover. The relapse rate, however, is also high.

Depression is treated with antidepressant drugs and careful and sympathetic counselling. The doctor is aware of the
ever-present threat of suicide, and advises accordingly. The
mainstay of the treatment of mania is lithium.

manipulation

See **osteopathy**.

manus

Latin root meaning 'hand' as in manual (of the hand).

Manusept

A brand name for triclosan.

mapping

The process of determining the order of genes, and their functions, on the chromosomes. The human **genome** project, currently almost complete, is designed to map the entire collection of human chromosomes, with incalculable potential benefit to humankind, and a huge increase in responsibility for the application of the knowledge.

mapping the human genome

See **genome, human, mapping**.

mapping the X chromosome

See **X chromosome**.

maprotiline hydrochloride

A tetracyclic antidepressant drug. A brand name is Ludiomil.

marasmus

A state of wasting or emaciation, usually in infants.

Marburg disease

See **Ebola virus disease**.

march fracture

A hair-line break in one of the long bones of the foot caused by repeated stress as in marching. The condition was once common in soldiers engaged on long route marches but now occurs more often in joggers. There is pain, tenderness on pressure on the sole of the foot and swelling.

X-ray may not show up the fracture, in the early stages, but during the healing process the X-ray appearance becomes obvious. In most cases there is no displacement and often recovery is possible without the use of a plaster cast.

Marevan

A brand name for the anticoagulant drug **warfarin**.

Marfan's syndrome

A rare genetic disease in which all the collagen connective tissue of the body is abnormally weak. Affected people grow tall and thin and characteristically have very long spidery fingers (**arachnodactyly**). The joints dislocate easily, the suspensory ligaments of the lenses of the eyes break easily so that the lenses become displaced and the main artery of the body, the aorta, is unusually elastic and floppy. There is a strong tendency to develop heart disease.

marijuana

A drug obtained from various species of the hemp grass cannabis, especially *Cannabis sativa*, *Cannabis indica* and *Cannabis americana*. The drug is widely used and has a variety of names in different parts of the world. These include, pot, weed, grass, reefer, hashish, hash, bhang, ganja, kif and dagga. Interestingly, the word 'assassin' derives from the Arabic *hashshashin* – 'a hashish eater', the story being that murderers used hash to give them courage.

Cannabis resin contains many active substances, but the one which causes the desired effects is tetrahydrocannabinol – one of the cannabinoids. Tetrahydrocannabinol causes widening (dilatation) of blood vessels, seen most obviously in the reddened eyes of the cannabis taker, and a fall in blood pressure. There is mild engorgement of the genitals and the heart rate increases.

In most cases, these severe effects arise in people with personalities predisposed to them – people who may have developed the disorders, in due course, without cannabis. But sometimes they occur in people with no apparent psychiatric problem. Young teenagers, especially those under social or other stresses and those suffering emotional disturbances, are especially at risk. Psychiatric patients controlled on drug treatment often suffer severe recurrences on using cannabis.

Other effects include a depression of fertility in both sexes and an immunosuppressive effect. T cell function is depressed (see **AIDS**). Reefer smoke has been shown to be as capable of causing lung cancer as tobacco smoke. Some studies have suggested that it may be more so, but total exposure to marijuana smoke is less than with tobacco. It also causes chronic bronchitis. Oddly enough, the cannabinoids reduce the appetite and can control severe nausea and the drug has some effect on preventing epileptic fits.

The properties of tetrahydrocannabinol have long been exploited for recreational purposes, and they are widely known to recent generations in the West. They are also known for their variability, this being the result of the variety and range of different properties of the many substances present. The main effect is euphoria – the easy promotion of laughter or giggling, often for reasons that seem silly or childish to the observer. Under the influence of the tetrahydrocannabinol there is an apparent heightening of all the senses, especially vision. Colour intensity and contrast are increased, and there is distortion of the dimensions of objects and of the perception of distance. The perception of time, too, is distorted, or sometimes seemingly eliminated. Usually, passage of time is experienced as being slower than reality, so that estimates of periods past are greater than clock time and of future periods less.

One of the much-valued properties among some devotees is the sense of deep philosophical insight conveyed by the cannabinoids. There is a conviction of omniscience, of knowing all the answers to the riddles of the universe, and this is often accompanied by a feeling of calm superiority, so that one hardly bothers to bring the great accessible truths to mind. For those of genuine philosophical bent, however, the inability to retain these insights, as the effects of the drug wear off, is a bitter disappointment. This particular effect is not specific to this group of drugs and is often experienced, for instance, during recovery from a short anaesthetic. The effect is, of course, an illusion. In fact, intellectual performance is impaired during the period of the drug action. Mental arithmetic is less accurate than normal and short-term memory defective. The affected person often forgets the beginning of a sentence before reaching the end.

The effects on performance should be known. Slowing of reflexes, distortion of distance and alteration in the sense of responsibility all have a serious effect on skilled activities such as driving, patient monitoring, air traffic controlling, military surveillance, etc., and it is right that the public should be protected against the use of cannabis by people engaged in these activities. There is little evidence that cannabis promotes criminal activity.

Controversy continues in medical circles as to whether the cannabinoids cause organic brain damage. This has been positively demonstrated in rats and monkeys, but not objectively in humans. Neither CT scanning nor electroencephalography have shown changes. There is, however, plenty of indirect evidence of brain dysfunction in persistent heavy users. Such people can develop the amotivational syndrome and show apathy and loss of interest and concern. Students stop working, suffer a drop in academic performance and give up courses. This effect is to be expected because the cannabinoids are concentrated in the limbic system, which is the motivational centre of the brain and because of the effects on memory and reasoning.

Cannabis withdrawal produces quite severe symptoms, including anxiety, irritability, headaches, sleeplessness, muscle twitching, sweating and diarrhoea, but these will pass and, in most cases, the amotivational syndrome will eventually resolve.

Concern has been expressed about the probability of progress from cannabis use to that of harder drugs. Only a small proportion of casual users do progress, but it is clear that heavy users commonly do progress. Nearly all **heroin** addicts have had previous experience of cannabis. It is unnecessary to propose any pharmacological reason for this, but undoubtedly the cannabis experience in certain predisposed individuals does, for psychological reasons, cause progression to drugs such as heroin. This was accepted by the Canadian Commission of Inquiry into the Non-medical use of drugs, in their 1972 report on cannabis.

At the time of writing there is official consideration of the legalizing the medicinal use of cannabinoids for the relief of symptoms in multiple sclerosis.

marriage guidance counselling

See **partners, counselling of**.

marriage, non-consummation

The failure to achieve penetration of the vagina with the penis. This is commoner than is generally supposed and is believed to be the fate of about one marriage in 100.

Non-consummation occasionally results from ignorance on the part of both partners, remarkable in these outspoken days, as to what should go where. More commonly, it results from physical or psychological problems. The man may suffer **impotence**, of whatever sort, failure to maintain the erection, premature ejaculation or penile abnormality. The woman may have an anatomical abnormality of the vagina or a thick, rigid hymen, or, most commonly, the condition of **vaginismus**. This is an inability to relax the muscles of the floor of the pelvis or even, in extreme cases, the muscles which pull the thighs tightly together. It can usually be overcome by sympathetic advice and careful gynaecological management, including the use of sets of well-lubricated smooth metal rods of gradually increasing diameter (vaginal dilators).

marrow transplant

See **bone marrow transplant**.

masculinization

See **virilism**.

masochism

The achievement of sexual gratification by the experience of physical or mental pain. Many masochists look for personal humiliation and a sense of failure. Masochistic behaviour is often symbolic – grown men may behave as naughty children deserving of punishment – and may involve the wearing of appropriate clothing or suffering tight bondage, verbal abuse and whipping. Such activities are not without danger, especially when, as is often the case, an element of **sadism** is also involved. Deaths, whether accidental or intended, are not uncommon.

Masochism probably derives from a strong consciousness of guilt, partly repressed, which inhibits orgasm, but which can be assuaged by punishment so that orgasm becomes possible. Investigation and explanation can sometimes help, but masochists seldom seek treatment.

massage

Rubbing, stroking, pressing, pummelling, kneading and hand-hammering of skin and muscles. Apart from some increase in the local blood supply, and an easing of tension in muscles, this has very little physical effect, and massage is not a particularly valuable element in physical therapy. But the psychological and symbolic effects of close human touch and contact, with all its powerful associations of childhood comforting and sexuality, are considerable.

Massage is often deeply soothing and can relieve both the physical and mental symptoms of undue muscle tension – symptoms such as headache, backache and a sense of stress or oppression. Such treatment is purely symptomatic and is not associated with any significant organic change.

Massage should be distinguished from orthopaedic and physiotherapeutic manipulation specifically designed to break down actual adhesions.

mast cell

The cell central to the allergic reaction and to many immune system processes. Mast cells are found in large numbers in the skin and mucous membranes and in the lymphatic system. They contain numerous large granules of strongly irritating chemical substances such as histamine and serotonin, and other materials that act as messengers in the immune system.

In people with allergies, the antibody known as immunoglobulin type E (IgE), remains attached to specific receptors on the surface of the mast cells. When the substance causing the allergy (the **allergen**) contacts the IgE, the mast cell is triggered to release the aforementioned chemical irritants and the result is the range of allergic symptoms and signs.

mastectomy

Surgical removal of the breast. Mastectomy is performed almost exclusively for the treatment of cancer. There has been a considerable change in the surgical practice for the treatment of **breast cancer** since the mid-1970s. Today, between 20 and 40 per cent of mastectomy operations are described as 'conservative'.

RADICAL MASTECTOMY

In radical mastectomy, formerly the standard procedure, the whole of the breast tissue and skin, all the underlying pectoral muscles and the lymph nodes in the armpit were removed. This mutilating operation involved a large, elliptical incision sloping diagonally down from the armpit to the lower part of the centre of the chest. Because so much skin cover was lost, it was often necessary to do a major skin graft to cover the bare chest wall, and it was very difficult to achieve even a reasonable cosmetic appearance.

The results of this operation depended on whether, and to what extent, the cancer had spread to the lymph nodes in the armpit. If no nodes were found to be involved the cure rate was about 60 per cent. If one affected node was found, the cure rate was about 48 per cent; if four nodes were affected the cure rate dropped to 38 per cent; and if 20 nodes were affected the cure rate was only about 13 per cent.

MODIFIED RADICAL MASTECTOMY

In the modified radical operation, the breast and lymph nodes are removed but the muscles are left. The results of this operation were no worse than with the radical procedure and in some series were actually better. Some surgeons achieve an 82 per cent cure rate in cases in which none of the lymph nodes are cancerous.

SIMPLE MASTECTOMY

In simple mastectomy, only the breast tissue is removed. An elliptical incision around the nipple is used, and it is sometimes possible to restore a reasonably realistic appearance with an implant.

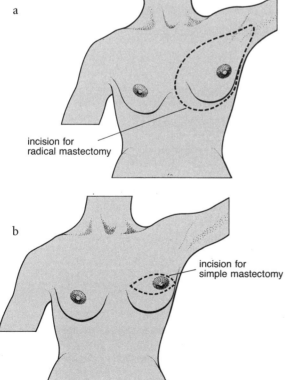

a

incision for radical mastectomy

b

incision for simple mastectomy

The general trend in many cases, today, is to an even less radical procedure called **lumpectomy** in which only the obvious mass is removed through a short radial incision. Ancillary treatment to reduce the chances of regrowth or recurrence of the cancer is essential.

In all cases, the outcome depends, more than on any other factor, on the stage which the cancer has reached when it is detected. This highlights the critical importance of screening by mammography and regular self-examination.

See **tamoxifen**, **anticancer drugs**, **anti-oestrogen drugs**.

Masters and Johnson sex therapy

The American gynaecologist William Howell Masters (b. 1915) and the psychologist Virginia Eshelman Johnson (b. 1925), workers in the field of human sexuality, first came to public notice for their interest in the nature of the physiological changes occurring during sexual arousal. These they were able to record, using a 'lie detector' (polygraph) on volunteer subjects, and much important new information was obtained.

The work has been criticized on the grounds that observation alters behaviour and Masters and Johnson accept this criticism. It has, however, led to some effective methods of sex therapy and to a more realistic public awareness of the nature of human sexuality. In particular, the role of anxiety in male sexual failure has been helpfully demonstrated. Masters and Johnson, who were married in 1971, have trained many thousands of sex therapists.

mastication

Chewing.

mastitis

Inflammation of the breast. This may be an acute condition or it may be persistent (chronic).

POSSIBLE CAUSES

Breast inflammation sometimes occurs as a result of infection elsewhere in the body, with spread by way of the blood, but a woman affected in this way will be obviously very ill. Acute mastitis can also occur as part of a mumps infection, from spread of mumps virus to the breast. This is uncommon.

Chronic mastitis is quite rare and can result from infection with **tuberculosis**, syphilis and **actinomycosis**. The term 'chronic mastitis' is sometimes wrongly applied to a condition in which the breasts are of an irregular rubbery consistency and contain painful or tender nodules or cysts. This is not an inflammation and the condition, which is common, is not a mastitis. It is caused by an upset of the balance of the hormones that control the menstrual cycle and does not normally require treatment.

The common form of acute mastitis occurs during breast-feeding and is caused by infection that gains access through a crack or an abrasion in a nipple. The organisms most commonly involved are *Staphylococcus aureus* – the germs that cause boils and impetigo. These organisms may already be present on the baby's skin, and mastitis is especially likely if the baby has a skin infection.

The mutilating operation of radical mastectomy (a) is now seldom performed. Simple mastectomy through a much smaller incision (b) is commoner.

RECOGNITION AND SYMPTOMS

The symptoms of acute mastitis may be quite severe, with high fever and, in the affected breast, localized redness, hardening and severe pain on pressure (tenderness).

TREATMENT

Unless the infection is quickly controlled by effective antibiotic treatment, a **breast abscess** may form which will have to be opened and drained surgically.

masturbation

Masturbation means self-stimulation of the genitals in order to reach orgasm. In males it is usually accompanied by fantasizing sexually about a woman. There is good evidence that over 90 per cent of males and 75 per cent of females masturbate at one time or another.

Repetitive movement of the skin of the penis or gentle massage of the clitoris is the usual method. Kinsey found that the frequency varied from three or four times a week in adolescence to once or twice a week in adult life.

Attitudes to masturbation have changed somewhat in the past 100 years. Here is an unedited quotation from a family medical encyclopedia, published in the 1880s:

'ONANISM – The crime of Onan – self-pollution – requires no further notice here, than to put parents on their guard respecting their children, in connection with this ruinous vice, acquired at school, and indulged in, in ignorance either of its sin or evil consequences. Some of the most lamentable instances of youthful decrepitude, nervous affections, amaurotic blindness, and mental debility and fatuity in early life, which come before medical men, are traceable to this wretched practice. Whenever young people, about the age of puberty, exhibit unaccountable symptoms of debility, particularly about the lower limbs, with listlessness and love of solitude, look dark under the eyes, &c., the possibility of vicious practices being at the root of the symptoms, should not entirely be lost sight of.'

Masturbation is, of course, a substitute for sexual intercourse with another person and is usually found unnecessary when such intercourse is readily accessible. Even after many years of regular masturbation, the practice will give way to the more satisfying and significant alternative. It is, however, common for people with considerable experience of sexual intercourse to resort to masturbation when a sexual partner is not available. In homosexual intercourse between both men and women, and in those prevented, for any reason, from engaging in heterosexual intercourse, mutual masturbation is important. Masturbation is common in many other animal species.

RISKS

There is no reason to suppose that masturbation is harmful. But some people have suffered mentally as a result of the influence of pious and unfounded statements such as those quoted. It may be that the Victorians were influenced in their opinions on the matter by the observation that mentally deficient people and sometimes schizophrenics occasionally masturbate in public. But, of course, this is simply an indication of mental disturbance and not the cause.

materia medica

An out-dated term for **pharmacology** especially in relation to the treatment of disease by drugs (therapeutics).

maternal mortality

The number of women who die each year, from causes associated with pregnancy or childbirth, for every thousand total births. Deaths during pregnancy from causes unrelated to pregnancy are not included but deaths from associated causes are included, even if they occur months or years later. Maternal deaths occur from such conditions as **ectopic pregnancy**, **abortion**, eclampsia, pulmonary embolism, postpartum haemorrhage and infection of the placental site (puerperal sepsis).

The maternal mortality is a useful index of the standards of medical care in a community. There has been a striking drop in this statistic in the last 50 years, largely because of the developments of antibiotics and because of a better understanding of the management of the various complications of pregnancy and of the management of childbirth.

maternal-only inheritance

See **mitochondria**.

Maxalt

A brand name for the anti-migraine selective serotonin agonist **rizatripan**.

Maxepa

A brand name for **eicosapentaenoic acid**.

Maxidex

A brand name for the steroid drug dexamethasone in the form of eyedrops.

maxilla

Latin root meaning 'jaw' as in maxilla (upper jaw).

Maxitrol

A brand name for **neomycin** with a corticosteroid, for external use.

Maxolon

A brand name for the anti-emetic and anti-nausea drug **metoclopramide**.

Maxtrex

A brand name for **methotrexate**.

McBurney's sign

McBurney's point is the point on the right side of the abdomen two-thirds of the way from the navel to the bony prominence on the front of the hip. Tenderness on gentle pressure at this point is an often reliable sign of appendicitis.

MCR-50

A brand name for **isosorbide mononitrate**.

measles

This is a highly infectious, often epidemic, disease caused by a virus usually acquired by inhalation of infected droplet material. Every two or three years sufficient susceptible children accumulate and an epidemic occurs.

The incubation period is about 14 days and shortly before the rash appears, Koplik's spots may be seen in the mouth. These are small white specks, about the size of grains of salt, surrounded by a red base, and appearing on the inside of the cheeks and the inner surface of the lower lip. If they are seen in a child who has been exposed to a case of measles, the disease can be confidently expected. Koplik's spots occur during the incubation period of the disease.

The established condition features fever, cough, sneezing, general misery, often conjunctivitis, and an irregular, red, mottled, slightly raised rash which lasts for about a week and then fades.

Complications include otitis media, bronchitis and pneumonia, all of which will usually respond to antibiotic treatment, and, much less commonly, inflammation of the brain and spinal cord (encephalomyelitis). There is no foundation in the widely held belief that measles can cause squint (strabismus). Commonly, however, if the underlying cause – such as **hypermetropia** – is present, an attack of measles may precipitate **strabismus**. Most adults have had measles during childhood and a second attack is rare. The disease can be prevented by a vaccine which should be given to all children, aged one to two years, for whom there is no medical objection. Very rarely, measles can result in complications requiring hospitalization.

measles, mumps, rubella vaccination

See **MMR vaccination**.

measles, sign of

See **Koplik's spots**.

meat substitutes

Non-animal protein food products usually designed, flavoured and textured to resemble the natural protein. Vegetable proteins, derived from soya beans, wheat gluten, yeast or other sources, are dissolved in alkaline solutions and then extruded through spinning nozzles so as to form bundles of protein fibres. Fats, emulsifiers, flavouring and colouring substances are then added and a binder, such as egg albumin or vegetable gum is used to hold the fibres together. The resulting mass can then be pressed into various shapes and textures. Sometimes the extra ingredients are added before extrusion and high pressure used to form meat-like strips.

These products are, in general, an adequate substitute for animal protein but may not contain all of the nine amino acids which the body cannot produce for itself (the essential amino acids). Once meat substitutes are digested, their products (amino acids) are indistinguishable from those from animal sources.

meatus

Any passage or opening in the body.

mebendazole

An **anthelmintic** drug used to get rid of roundworms, hookworms, threadworms and whipworms. A brand name is Vermox.

mebeverine

An antispasmodic drug used to treat bowel colic. Trade names are Colofac and Fybogel Meberverine.

mebhydrolin

An antihistamine drug used to treat allergic conditions such as allergic **rhinitis** and **urticaria**. A brand name is Fabahistin.

Meckel's diverticulum

A pouch-like sac, about 5 cm long, protruding outwards from the interior of the lower part of the small intestine (ileum), and present in about one person in 50. As a rule, the diverticulum is harmless, but sometimes it becomes infected and causes a condition indistinguishable from **appendicitis**. Meckel's diverticulum may also lead to telescoping of the bowel (**intussusception**) or twisting (volvulus). Occasionally the diverticulum is lined with the same kind of acid-secreting mucous membrane as is normal in the stomach. In this case, an ulcer may develop.

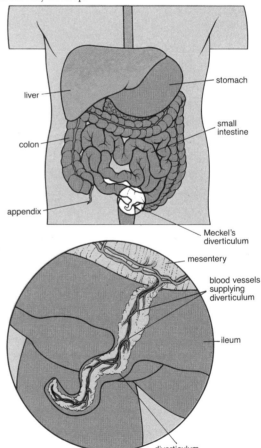

Meckel's diverticulum is rather like an extra appendix, although usually rather wider. It can, however, cause more complications than an appendix.

meconium

The name given to the stools passed by a baby during the first day or two of life, or before birth if there is fetal distress.

Meconium is thick, greenish-black and of a sticky consistency and consists of cells cast off by the lining of the bowel during uterine life, mixed with bowel mucous and stained with bile from the liver. Once feeding is established the meconium is replaced by normal stools.

medial

Situated toward the midline of the body. The antonym is lateral.

mediastinoscopy

This is a method of examining the internal structures of the central compartment of the chest under direct vision, by means of a viewing tube (endoscope) passed through an opening in the base of the neck under general anaesthesia. The mediastinum is the part of the chest containing the heart, the windpipe (trachea) the gullet (oesophagus), some very large blood vessels and many lymph nodes.

The endoscope used provides its own illumination and viewing channels and also allows biopsy (samples) of lymph nodes and other tissues to be taken. This is extremely important in view of the frequency with which mediastinal lymph nodes are involved in disease processes such as cancer, tuberculosis and sarcoidosis.

Mediastinoscopy allows relatively easy access on the right side, but an approach to the left side is more difficult and dangerous and other methods are often preferred.

mediastinum

The central compartment of the chest, flanked on either side by the lungs, and containing the heart, the origins of the great blood vessels, the windpipe (trachea) and the main bronchi, the oesophagus and many lymph nodes.

medical computing

The application of computers to clinical and administrative medicine. Expert system interactive programs have been written that enable a personal computer to take a more detailed and accurate medical history than is possible with the time available to the average doctor. Surprisingly, it has been found that patients will often communicate more freely with a computer than with a doctor.

Most electrocardiogram machines are now equipped with computer programs that can interpret the ECG tracing more accurately than most doctors. Artificial intelligence techniques have been applied to expert diagnostic systems that learn by experience, and these are beginning to rival the best doctors in accuracy. They also provide considerable help in selecting appropriate drugs and dosage. Computers have a major role to play in a wide range of medical administrative tasks.

See also **telemedicine**.

medical database

See **Medline**.

medical diagnosis

Medical diagnosis is the process of identifying a patient's disease so that the best treatment can be given. Diagnosis should always precede treatment and is the most difficult, and the most important, of a doctor's functions. Doctors are never happy about treating patients without knowing exactly what is wrong. Such treatment without diagnosis is called **empirical treatment** and is often necessary, especially in emergency. One form of empirical treatment is known, disparagingly as 'treating symptoms'. This is not considered good medicine. Although it may be effective, it may make matters worse by concealing important clues to diagnosis.

Medical high technology has had a major impact on methods of diagnosis, but it has not changed fundamental principles. The first, and most important, step in diagnosis is the taking of a good history of the complaint and of all related or relevant background particulars, including the family history and the personal circumstances. Technology has, to a limited extent, invaded even this area and there are computer programs, using expert systems, which can take a reasonable history. Comparative trials show that the best of these programs can do better than a less than average doctor but cannot yet compete with a good doctor.

The quality of a doctor may often be judged by the care, persistence and skill with which the history is taken, and by the simultaneous keenness of his or her observation. Good history-taking requires experience and wide knowledge, and the direction the questioning takes will be determined by the doctor's awareness of the significance of certain responses.

HISTORY-TAKING

A doctor uses the word *history* in a special way. A person's medical history is the record of everything that is relevant to his or her health. It includes the details of the present complaint, the previous general medical history, the social history and the family history. An experienced doctor knows the importance of a good history and will often spend at least as much time on the history as on the examination. In taking a history, doctors hope for, but do not always get, clear, simple answers to their questions. Often they are offered a ready-made diagnosis. The patient who informs the doctor that he or she has 'a hepatic liver' tells the doctor nothing; but the patient who says 'When I go for a pee the stream is really feeble and dribbly...' is giving a clear indication of the probable nature of the problem (prostate gland enlargement).

The answer to one question usually brings up a range of possibilities in the mind of the doctor and he or she has to work on the balance of probabilities, knowing which conditions are most common, and thus most likely. A few carefully selected questions will indicate the most promising avenue, and the doctor will follow this route so long as the responses are consistent with this provisional idea. He or she will, if wise, try to avoid leading questions – questions which suggest an answer – but will, at the same time, tactfully keep the patient from straying into irrelevance. If the doctor has not reached a probable diagnosis by the time the history has been taken, the problem is likely to require lengthy investigation.

Good doctors are very particular in their questioning and skilled in the direction their questions take. Effective history-taking is, of course, based on detailed knowledge of the subject and is impossible without it. Taking a good history is a fine art.

FAMILY AND SOCIAL HISTORY

After some brief questioning about the present complaint, the doctor may enquire into the family history. The state of health or cause of death of close relatives is often important because many diseases run in families, even if there is no obvious genetic basis. A family history of conditions such as heart or arterial disease, high blood pressure, diabetes, tuberculosis, cancer or schizophrenia may increase the probability of such a condition and will alert the doctor. If the problem seems psychological, the doctor may ask about the parents and the relationships within the family – questions which may have an important bearing on the personality and medical condition.

Social history, especially occupation and life-style, may be of central importance. Many occupations involve hazards to health, not all of which are obvious. Previous occupations, perhaps followed many years before, may be the cause of current disease. Attitude to, and contentment with, the current occupation may be significant. Work satisfaction, interest in work, a sense of being valued, relations with colleagues, may all be relevant. There may be concealed stress factors, either psychological or ergonomic, which may affect health.

Life-style almost always has a major bearing on health and the history can often bring this out and suggest some of the most important questions the patient may ever have been asked. Matters of concern include:

- kind and quantity of the diet;
- smoking history;
- alcohol intake;
- amount of exercise taken, the exercise tolerance and the response to exercise;
- sleep patterns;
- use of recreational drugs;
- attitudes to sex and the nature of the sex life;
- whether sexual tendencies are monogamous or promiscuous, opportunistic or selective;
- whether sexual preferences are hetero-, homo- or bi-sexual.

Overseas travel may also be highly relevant, as many conditions, rare in Britain, may be acquired abroad and may be developing during the journey back.

THE PREVIOUS HISTORY AND PRESENT COMPLAINT

Of obvious relevance are the details of previous illnesses, injuries, hospital admissions and other medical events, from childhood onwards, as are any previous medical investigations and whether X-rays or scan pictures exist. Previous insurance medical examinations can be helpful for purposes of comparison. Medical treatment given in the past may also have a bearing.

The doctor now returns to the present complaint and will enquire into it in detail, ending up with specific questions based on his or her experience and knowledge of the probable disorder. By now the doctor will probably have a shrewd idea of what is wrong. But this idea must be confirmed by physical examination and, if necessary, by special tests.

A good diagnostician will, in most cases, come to an accurate diagnosis on the basis of the history alone. But this diagnosis is only tentative and will be confirmed or denied as a result of the examination and tests which follow. The experienced doctor is familiar with a great range of characteristic physical signs of disease and will not fail to note their presence.

Doctors distinguish between symptoms, which are what the patient experiences and complains of, and signs, which are bodily changes observable by the doctor, characteristic of, or sometimes positively indicative of (diagnostic of), certain diseases. Symptoms are subjective; signs are objective. There are innumerable well-recognized physical signs, and it would be impossible to list them all.

THE EXAMINATION

The doctor's initial examination involves inspection, feeling (palpation), tapping to determine hollowness or solidity (**percussion**), listening with a stethoscope to heart, lung and blood-vessel sounds (**auscultation**), clinical tests of muscular strength, range of movement, touch and pain sensation, balance, gait, tendon reflexes, and so on. The main constraint is time and, regrettably, many important diagnoses are missed because not enough time can be devoted to detailed history-taking and examination. Specialist examination goes much further than the type of general examination described here.

The history and examination will suggest to the doctor which tests are relevant, and these will then be done or arranged. The tests may include:

- various forms of imaging, such as X-ray, CT scanning, or MRI;
- tests involving detection of changing electrical patterns produced by the body, such as the electrocardiogram (ECG) or the electroencephalogram (EEG);
- various forms of endoscopy, in which the interior of the body is inspected through a variety of types of viewing tubes, inserted through the mouth or anus or through a small surgical incision in the skin;
- removal of a sample of tissue for pathological examination (biopsy);
- taking of specimens or swabs for bacterial culture or growth of viruses;
- any of a wide variety of qualitative and quantitative laboratory tests on the blood or on any of the body secretions;
- skin tests to detect allergic sensitivity or evidence of previous infection;
- tests of the function of various organs, such as thyroid function tests, liver function tests and lung function tests;
- psychological testing or psychiatric investigation.

The final decision on the diagnosis may be made before all investigations are complete and these may then be devoted to determining the degree or extent of the disorder. But sometimes the decision is deferred until all available evidence is to hand, and in such difficult cases it is common, especially in hospital, for doctors to present all the evidence to a small group of colleagues so that the benefit of wider experience and knowledge may be obtained in arriving at a consensus diagnosis and a decision on the best treatment.

General practitioners will, in most cases, be satisfied with their own diagnoses and will proceed to treatment, usually by medicines. In some cases, however, GPs will rightly feel that the advice of a person more knowledgeable in a particular branch of the subject is required and will refer to a specialist. The choice, which is, of course, dictated by the presumptive diagnosis, is wide. All the medical and surgical specialists you are likely to encounter are detailed in this book.

medical ethics

See **ethics, medical**.

medical fear of litigation

See **defensive medicine**.

medical information highway

There is an enormous amount of medical information on the Internet, much of it of dubious accuracy or value. However, the medical information highway is a linked network of thousands of readily accessible medical web pages that can be used to obtain medical information updates.

Caution is still required, but reliability can be assessed in much the same way as in paper publications. Nothing should be regarded as authoritative unless it is published by a recognized and formally licensed medical institution and produced by properly qualified authors of professional status, whose work is subjected to careful and critical review. One approach is to limit browsing to the medical faculties of the better known universities. The full text of nearly all major general medical journals is accessible on the Internet and most now publish regular lists of addresses of reliable medical web sites.

See also **medical computing** and **telemedicine**.

medical misbehaviour

See **malpractice**.

medical rationing

The allocation of scarce or inadequate medical resources to an ever-expanding, and increasingly-demanding, population of patients. The problem is also exacerbated by the increasing proportion of elderly people in populations. The avoidance of rationing, in the sense of denying essential treatment to a proportion of patients, is currently a major preoccupation of the medical profession and has led to a healthy expansion in the use of specialist nurses, nurse practitioners, nurse prescribing, and an increase in the clinical scope of paramedical personnel of all kinds. This is a healthy development that is welcomed by the people concerned as well as by most registered medical practitioners.

medical resources, allocating

See **medical rationing**.

medical thought influenced by awareness of evolution

See **evolutionary medicine**.

medical updates

See **medical information highway**.

medicamento

Latin root meaning 'medicament' as in medication (drugs taken for treatment).

medicina

Latin root meaning 'medicine' as in medicine (subject of this book).

medicine

The combination of science, technology and humanity devoted to the restoration of the sick to normality. Although medicine is a scientific discipline, the effective practice of medicine involves the cultivation of skills and knowledge, and the possession, and exercise, of qualities of human sympathy, understanding and identification, not normally demanded of a scientist.

Medicine is arbitrarily divided into two large classes – the medical specialties and the surgical specialties. In general terms, the former are concerned with the disorders treated by advice or drugs, while the latter constitute those activities likely to climax in a surgical or obstetrical operation or some other form of physical intervention.

The medical specialties include those concerned with the heart (cardiology), with chest diseases, with the skin (dermatology), the endocrine glands (endocrinology), the digestive system (gastroenterology), the blood (haematology), infectious diseases, the nervous system (neurology), cancer (oncology), the diagnosis of disease processes (pathology), mental disorder (psychiatry), the bones and joints (rheumatology) and sexually transmitted diseases.

The surgical specialties include anaesthetics, general surgery, neurosurgery, vascular surgery, childbirth (obstetrics) and the diseases of women (gynaecology), the eyes (ophthalmology), the locomotor and skeletal system (orthopaedics), ear, nose and throat (otolaryngology) and the urinary system (urology).

medicine, Chinese

Traditional Chinese medicine, *chung-i*, is rapidly being overtaken by Western medical practice and pharmacology, especially in the cities, but there is still a wide belief in, and reliance on, the ancient remedies. Every town in the world with any major Chinese population has its traditional medicine shops stocked with an amazing variety of herbs, animal parts and minerals purporting to have medicinal value.

In Hong Kong there are over 8000 practitioners of traditional medicine and they are not subject to any form of legal control. Most of the Chinese population relies on these old remedies and the shops are often crowded.

HOW IT WORKS

Ancient Chinese medicine, the principles of which are followed to this day, classifies drugs according to the tastes and smells appropriate to the 'four energies' and the 'five flavours'. The energies manifest excess (yang) or deficiency (yin) and the flavours – sour, bitter, pungent, salt and sweet – correspond to the five 'elements' – wood, fire, earth, metal and water. Drugs are used, in balanced formulations, to counter effects which are apparent to the patient. 'Cool' drugs, such as extracts of mint and chrysanthemum, are used for 'hot' disorders such as fevers. Sweet herbs deal with 'sour' symptoms, such as dyspepsia, while sour preparations are given for their astringent or 'solidifying' effect.

Balanced formulations rely on the principle that four functions are served – the 'imperial' is the principal active ingredient; the 'ministerial' promotes its circulation and enhances its effect; the 'assistant' neutralizes any toxins; and the servant coordinates and harmonizes the whole prescription. Disease is regarded as an imbalance between the forces of yin and yang and recovery, practitioners believe, is to be obtained by correcting the balance. Diagnosis is made by a subtle and elaborate analysis of the 'pulses' (see **acupuncture**). Other means of treatment used include **moxibustion**, breathing and gymnastic exercises and acupuncture.

DOES IT WORK?

This elegant basis for therapy is far from scientific. Symptoms are not disorders, and metaphors are not facts. No disorder, other than possibly a cardiac one, can be diagnosed simply by feeling pulses. All scientific medical experts know that treating symptoms, without finding and tackling the cause of the disorder, is bad medicine and is likely to delay necessary treatment.

But in rejecting the obviously unscientific basis of traditional Chinese medicine, there is some loss. The Chinese system contains much that is philosophically valuable and some that is empirically useful. Balance, moderation and poise, however defined, are health-giving, and any system that encourages these is to be commended.

medicine, Hindu, ancient

See **ayurvedism**.

medicine, Indian

Early Indian medicine seems to have had a basis in direct observation and practice rather than magic or religion. As a result, the Indians were, at an early stage, well in advance of the rest of the world. The most influential early figure was Susruta who lived some 2000 years ago and who published a treatise on medicine and surgery in which he described more than 100 different surgical instruments including various kinds of scalpel, bone nippers, saws, forceps, scissors, needles, catheters and syringes.

Susruta understood the importance of cleanliness in surgery and directed that cutting instruments should be well polished and kept sharp enough to divide a hair. Surgeons should wash carefully before operating and should keep their clothes clean. He described a design of bamboo splint for fractures of the limb bones, which is useful to this day.

As a result of the efforts of men like Susruta, the early Indian medical tradition was remarkably scientific. A knowledge of anatomy was held to be important and many medical conditions were well understood. Fractures were diagnosed and correctly treated. Inflammation was recognized and treated by poulticing and other means. A wide range of surgery was practised, including operations for cataract, kidney stone, hernia, external tumours, and for restoration of the nose by transposing a flap of tissue, much in the modern manner. The sewing up of wounds was a common practice. **Amputation** and Caesarean section were practised as well as other obstetric operations. Hydroceles and fluid in the abdominal cavity were drained through hollow needles.

The early Indian doctors found it necessary to cloak much of their knowledge in terms of theology and superstition, for social reasons, giving out that medical knowledge and skills were revelations from the gods. Inevitably, an arbitrary fabric of theological belief came to surround the real principles and these suffered in consequence. Modern Indian medicine follows Western scientific practice.

medicus

Latin root meaning 'doctor' as in medical (of medicine).

Medihaler-ergotamine

A brand name for **ergotamine tartrate**.

Medizip

A surgical dressing and wound-closing device in the form of two multi-layered, microporous adhesive supportive strips which are applied one to each side of an incised wound or surgical incision and are then drawn together by closing a slide zip fastener attached to the two inner free edges. Medizip is a trademark of Atrax Medical Group Ltd.

Medline

A large computer database containing a substantial proportion of the professional papers produced in indexed medical journals over a period of years. Medline, which is only one of a number of such databases, contains millions of entries and is accessible, on-line, free of charge to almost any qualified doctor interested enough to wish to consult it. A search, however, requires special skills if one is not to be inundated with references.

Medrone

A brand name for the steroid drug **methylprednisolone**.

medroxyprogesterone

A **progestogen** drug that can be taken by mouth or injection and is used to treat excessive menstrual bleeding (**menorrhagia**), the premenstrual syndrome, **endometriosis**, infertility and oestrogen-dependent cancers. Trade names are Provera, Depo-Provera and Farlutal. It is also available formulated as an adjunct to oestrogen for menopausal hormone replacement therapy under the trade names Premique, Premique Cycle and Tridesta.

mefenamic acid

A non-steroidal anti-inflammatory drug (**NSAID**) and painkilling (analgesic) drug used to treat arthritis, and menstrual disorders. A brand name is Ponstan.

mefloquine

A drug used to prevent and treat **malaria**. The drug is effective but has been criticized for its neuropsychological side- effects which include fatigue, depression, headache, insomnia and distressing dreams. A brand name is Lariam.

mefruside

A diuretic drug similar to the thiazide group, used to relieve the body of excess fluid and to treat high blood pressure. A brand name is Baycaron.

mega-

Prefix meaning 'enlarged' as in megacolon (enlarged colon).

Megace

A brand name for **megestrol**.

megalo-

Prefix meaning 'enlarged' as in megalomania (enlarging madness).

megestrol

A **progestogen** drug used to assist in the treatment of breast or endometrial cancer. A brand name is Megace.

481

meibomian cyst

A hard, pea-like, swelling in an eyelid, caused by a cyst in one of the 30 or so lubricating (meibomian) glands which open on to the lid margin, just behind the line of the lashes. If the outlet of one of these glands becomes blocked, the oily, gelatinous secretions continue to be produced, but cannot escape and accumulate in the form of a tight cyst within the substance of the lid. The resulting meibomian cyst, or chalazion, is harmless but sometimes enlarges to a conspicuous size and may press on the eyeball to produce a temporary blurring of vision.

Meibomian cysts often become infected, causing rapidly increasing swelling, redness and pain. An abscess forms in the lid and the pus usually discharges spontaneously, commonly on the inner surface. This causes no harm to the eye.

Treatment is by a minor operation under local anaesthesia. The cyst is held in a special ring clamp and a tiny incision is make on the inside of the lid, perpendicular to the lid margin. The contents of the cyst are then scooped out with a miniature surgical spoon (curette). No stitching is necessary and healing is rapid.

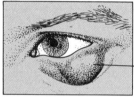

large, lower lid, meibomian cyst

A large meibomian cyst produces an unmistakable swelling in the upper or lower eyelid and is prone to become infected and cause an abscess.

melaena

A blackening of the stools by blood which has been released into the bowel from bleeding points in the oesophagus, stomach, or duodenum. Such blood becomes chemically altered by the action of the hydrochloric acid from the stomach and this produces a characteristic and striking tarry black appearance. About 60 ml of blood is needed to produce a single black stool and a larger single bleed will colour the stools for up to three days.

> Melaena is an important sign which should never be ignored. It is usually an indication of ulceration of the stomach or duodenum but may be caused by cancer.

Stools may also be blackened by iron, bismuth or licorice taken by mouth.

melanoma, malignant

See **malignant melanoma**.

melatonin

A hormone secreted by the pineal gland with a strong circadian rhythm, being produced mainly in the period between about 2100 hours and 0800 hours when the person concerned is not exposed to bright light. Melatonin secretion is suppressed by bright light, and if it is given as a drug it can alter the timing of the body clock for the day/night rhythm. For these reasons melatonin has been proposed as a means of combating jet lag. The results have been disappointing and other methods have been found more generally useful.

Melleril

A brand name for the **phenothiazine** antipsychotic drug thioridazine.

melphalan

A drug used in the treatment of **polycythaemia** vera, chronic **leukaemia** and myeloma. A brand name is Alkeran.

memory loss, brief

See **transient global amnesia**.

memory pill

An informal term for a drug purporting to improve memory. Currently the main interest in the 'ampakines' – drugs that are said to amplify the signal of the neuro-transmitter **glutamate**, which is used in neurons in the memory circuits.

menarche

The start of menstruation in a woman's life, which heralds her ability to become pregnant. The first few menstrual periods may or may not be associated with ovulation.

Ménière's syndrome

An episodic disorder consisting of a combination of dizziness (vertigo), nausea, variable hearing loss, a sense of fullness in the head and singing in the ears (tinnitus). During the episodes of vertigo the deafness and tinnitus temporarily increase. These improve after the episodes are over, but there is a tendency for hearing to decline progressively. Episodes occur with great variability and some people have long periods of freedom. The disorder often starts on one side, but tends later to affect both ears. It is a disease of middle age and affects both sexes equally. One-third of Ménière's sufferers also have migraine.

POSSIBLE CAUSES

Ménière's syndrome is caused by an increase in the amount and pressure of the fluid within the inner ear. This causes distention with damage to the delicate balancing and hearing structures and these may eventually be destroyed. Each episode may cause further damage. The reason for the increase in fluid is often inapparent but, in some cases, it is caused by **otosclerosis**, **Paget's disease** of bone or syphilis.

TREATMENT

Most cases are managed by medical treatment to control the vertigo and nausea. In some cases surgery is advised. Removal of the balancing mechanism on one side (labyrinthectomy) will reliably relieve vertigo, but will produce total deafness on that side.

meningitis

Inflammation of the membranes that cover the brain (the meninges).

POSSIBLE CAUSES

This can be caused by a variety of organisms and may be a feature of **Lyme disease**, **leptospirosis**, **typhus**, **tuberculosis** and other infective conditions. Formerly, meningococcal meningitis (see **meningitis, meningococcal**) was by far the commonest type. Today the commonest cause of meningitis is infection with viruses such as the Herpes simplex virus, the varicella-zoster virus of chickenpox and shingles, the polio virus, echo viruses, Coxsackie viruses and mumps virus. In these cases, the disease often suggests a degree of immune deficiency.

RECOGNITION AND SYMPTOMS

Viral meningitis is often a minor disorder but may be acute, with headache, fever and drowsiness which may progress rapidly to deep coma. In severe cases there may be weakness of the muscles, paralysis, speech disturbances, double vision or partial loss of the field of vision, and epileptic fits.

TREATMENT

Most patients survive, often with complete recovery, but some may have residual effects. There is no specific treatment for most virus infections, but in the case of Herpes meningitis, the drug acyclovir can be valuable.

meningitis, meningococcal

An epidemic form of **meningitis** which may occur in institutions and overcrowded dwellings such as orphanages, barrack-rooms or boarding schools. It is sometimes called cerebrospinal fever and is commoner in children than in adults. The organisms responsible, most commonly *Neisseria meningitidis*, but sometimes *Streptococcus pneumonia* or other bacteria, are present in the nose and throat of many people, but these carriers seldom acquire the disease. The organisms are spread by the aerosol of droplets produced in coughing and sneezing and cause the disease after an incubation period of three to five days.

RECOGNITION AND SYMPTOMS

There is a sore throat, rising temperature, severe headache, marked stiffness of the neck and vomiting. A rash of red spots appears on the trunk, hence cerebrospinal fever is sometimes called 'spotted fever'. The affected person may become gravely ill within a day of onset and pass quickly into a state of confusion, drowsiness and coma.

Babies and infants show fever, vomiting, convulsions and have a characteristic high-pitched cry. In babies, the soft areas on the head between the skull bones (the fontanelles) often bulge outwards and feel much tenser than normal.

> Without treatment, death may occur within days or even hours. In some cases, the acute illness subsides into a persistent (chronic) state which may lead to serious brain damage and mental defect, blindness or deafness. So treatment is always urgent and should never be delayed.

TREATMENT

Fortunately, bacterial meningitis, from *Neisseria meningitidis*, nearly always responds well to antibiotics and treatment is usually successful, with full recovery. Vaccines are available against meningococcal infections but are not in general use. Contacts may have protective antibiotics.

Menogon

A brand name for **menotrophin**.

menopause

The climacteric, 'change of life' or natural end of the sequence of menstrual periods and the end of the fertile years of life in a woman. The menopause occurs at an average age of about 50 but the usual range is from 47 to 52. Occurrences outside this range are quite common. Sometimes the menopause is delayed to 55 or later; quite often it occurs at 40 or earlier. If the periods started earlier than usual, the menopause is usually later than average; and if the periods started late, the menopause is usually early. A premature menopause occurs if the ovaries are removed surgically (oophorectomy).

The menopause involves a cessation of egg production (ovulation) by the ovaries and the resultant hormonal changes which alter the inner lining of the womb (uterus). Ovulation usually becomes irregular, with non-ovulating cycles occurring frequently as the menopause approaches. For this reason, pregnancy is very rare after 50. The periods do not usually stop suddenly, although this sometimes happens. As a general rule, the periods first become more scanty, then the odd period is missed; then they stop.

EFFECTS

The main effect of the menopause is a reduced production of the hormone oestrogen by the ovaries. After the menopause the ovaries cease altogether to produce this hormone and most women have no oestrogen production. A few women continue to produce some oestrogens from the adrenal glands or other sources.

Most of the physical effects associated with the menopause are due to oestrogen deficiency, but some women also suffer psychologically from the awareness that they have come to the end of reproductive life, and have reached what may seem to be a significant stage in ageing. Other women regard the menopause as a stage of liberation from the nuisance of menstruation and the responsibilities of parenthood.

OESTROGEN DEFICIENCY

Oestrogen deficiency has many effects. It leads to a gradual shrinkage (atrophy) of the genitalia. Pubic hair becomes more sparse, the labia flatten, the wall of the vagina becomes thinner and smoother and the secretions more acidic, the womb becomes smaller and its lining thin. Even the ligaments that support the womb become weaker and, as a result, the tendency for the womb to 'come down' (prolapse) increases, especially if the pelvic floor has been weakened in childbirth. The changes in the vagina and the reduction in lubricating secretions can cause difficulty and discomfort in sexual intercourse. The reduction in acidity from lactic acid deficiency often leads to changes in the bacterial population of the vagina, and this can result in bladder infection (cystitis). Much of the bladder trouble in post-menopausal women is now recognized as originating in this way.

During the reproductive period, women are strongly protected by oestrogens against the major arterial disease **atherosclerosis**. As a result heart attacks and strokes are rare, in non-smoking women, during this span of life. Unfortunately, this protection is lost after the menopause, and the incidence of these diseases soon rises to equal that in men. Loss of bone bulk and **osteoporosis** is a natural feature of ageing, but loss of oestrogen accelerates the process in post-menopausal women. Men, on the other hand, continue to enjoy the anabolic effect of their sex hormones.

HORMONE REPLACEMENT THERAPY

For these and other reasons, there is a strong case to be made for **hormone replacement therapy**. Some women object to this on the grounds that it is unnatural. But it is worth remembering that almost the whole of human evolution occurred during a period of millions of years in which few if any women lived long enough to reach the menopause. There were thus no evolutionary pressures to alter the existing system. In evolutionary terms, the number of Graafian follicles in the ovaries was quite sufficient to last a lifetime. Looked at in this way, it may be considered *more* natural to ensure that oestrogens persist in the body.

Most women pass easily, and relatively unaffected, through the menopause, relieved of the risk of pregnancy and anxious to get on with their lives. Perhaps a quarter suffer in some way, mainly from hot flushes affecting the face and neck. These vary greatly in frequency and duration. For some women they are very brief and infrequent; others may have many episodes in a day that last for as long as 15 minutes. Flushes do not indicate a rise in blood pressure, but merely a rise in the flow of blood through the affected parts. The cause of flushes remains uncertain but many doctors are convinced that they have something to do with oestrogen deficiency (see below).

Other presumed menopausal symptoms include night sweats, insomnia, headaches and general irritability. Often these symptoms are severe enough, in themselves, to justify treatment. It is by no means certain that these symptoms are due to oestrogen deficiency – this has never been proved. But the **placebo** effect of oestrogen treatment is so strong that most people believe it responsible for the resulting improvement.

Weight gain after the menopause is not hormone-related, but it is fairly common and is probably the result of having less physical work to do without changing established eating habits. There is no evidence that the menopause is associated with a marked increase in psychiatric disturbance.

Menorest

A brand name for **oestradiol**.

menorrhagia

This means excessive bleeding during a menstrual period. Heaviness of periods is, of course, relative. For some women, bleeding for seven or eight days with frequent passage of clots is normal. But for a woman whose normal period is three to four days of light bleeding, a period like this would represent menorrhagia. There are, of course, limits to what can be considered normal.

> A period that, at its most severe, required a change of tampon or pad every hour, for a continuous period of more than a few hours, would, in any woman, be regarded as abnormal and would require medical attention.

POSSIBLE CAUSES

There are several possible causes for menorrhagia. These include:

- early abortion;
- **fibroids** of the womb;
- **endometriosis**;
- infection of the fallopian tubes and ovaries (salpingo-oophoritis);
- the presence of an IUD;
- polyps;

- cancer of the womb lining;
- hormonal problems;
- thyroid gland underactivity (myxoedema);
- **leukaemia**;
- **purpura**.

Spontaneous abortion often occurs without pregnancy being suspected. Up to 10 per cent of pregnancies end in this way, and the retained products may cause heavy bleeding. In this case, the menorrhagia can be cured by a **D and C**. Fibroids commonly cause excessive bleeding, but polyps and cancer of the endometrium are more likely to cause irregular bleeding, rather than menorrhagia. Blood diseases such as leukaemia and purpura are very rare causes of menorrhagia.

A much commoner cause of menorrhagia is an excessive build-up of the inner lining of the womb – the endometrium. This is controlled by oestrogen. Progesterone, from the follicle in the ovary after the ovum is released, controls the bleeding. At the menarche and near the menopause, periods often occur without ovulation, so, on these occasions, no progesterone is secreted and the periods may be very heavy. Hormonal imbalance can also occur at other times. Progesterone can be used to control this type of menorrhagia in young women.

See also **menstruation, irregular**.

menotrophin

A gonadotrophin drug used to treat both female and male infertility and inadequate development of the sex organs. Trade names are Menogon and Pergonal.

menstrual disorders

The control of menstruation involves complex and easily upset hormonal changes and balances which operate on the lining of the womb. Since the womb, itself, is liable to various diseases, the possibilities for menstrual disorders are considerable.

AMENORRHOEA

Amenorrhoea is the absence of menstruation and this may, of course, be due to the fact that the periods have not yet started. But if the absence continues after the time at which the periods ought to have started, this is called primary amenorrhoea. Secondary amenorrhoea occurs in women who have already had periods. Primary amenorrhoea may be due to hormonal causes, stress, excessive athletic activity or, rarely, a complete (imperforate) hymen that closes off the vaginal outlet. The commonest cause of secondary amenorrhoea is, of course, pregnancy. In the Third World secondary amenorrhoea is commonly caused by severe nutritional inadequacy, but in the West **anorexia nervosa** is a common cause. Secondary amenorrhoea also occurs in athletes engaged in sustained, very vigorous training. Infrequent or very scanty menstruation is called oligomenorrhoea.

DYSMENORRHOEA

Dysmenorrhoea is the term for painful menstruation. Pain occurring at the time of ovulation – that is, in the middle of the menstrual cycle – is known as *mittelschmerz*, from the German term meaning 'middle pain'.

MENORRHAGIA

Menorrhagia means excessive bleeding during periods occurring at normal intervals. Polymenorrhoea means having periods more often than every three weeks. Metrorrhagia is bleeding between periods.

See also **premenstrual syndrome**.

menstruation

Menstruation is the periodic casting off of the inner lining of the womb (uterus) in women of reproductive age. Between the start of the bleeding in one cycle and the start of the next, the time, on average, is 28 days. The range, however is wide and the periods may be as short as 21 days, or, in extreme cases, as long as 60.

The pituitary gland of the brain secretes a follicle-stimulating hormone (FSH) which acts on one of the ovaries to cause an egg-containing collection of cells (a Graafian follicle) to develop. This follicle secretes increasing amounts of oestrogen hormone during the first half of the menstrual cycle and this hormone causes a thickening and increased glandularity of the lining of the womb.

In the middle of the cycle the egg (ovum) is released from the follicle in the ovary, but the follicle has not yet fully served its purpose. The cells of the empty follicle develop into a mass, the corpus luteum, which begins to secrete progesterone, a hormone necessary to maintain the lining of the uterus so that it is suitable to support a pregnancy. If the ovum is not fertilized, the corpus luteum degenerates and progesterone production drops off. This causes the lining of the uterus to be discarded, as menstruation, about 14 days after the time of ovulation.

The vaginal blood loss that occurs when the body's level of progesterone or oestrogen hormones drops suddenly is called withdrawal bleeding. Normal menstruation is preceded by withdrawal of both oestrogen and progesterone. The withdrawal bleeding that occurs at the end of each cycle of combined oral contraceptive pill mimics menstruation, but is usually shorter and lighter. It is the withdrawal of progesterone that produces this blood loss. Discontinuation of an oestrogen-only preparation also produces bleeding, which may differ from normal menstruation in amount and duration.

Menstruation normally starts between the ages of about nine and 16, usually between 12 and 14 years. This is called the menarche. The early menstrual cycles periods are often of irregular duration and period of bleeding, but within a few months will usually settle down to a 28-day cycle with bleeding for three to seven days. The menstrual periods are suspended during pregnancy and, usually, while breastfeeding is continuing.

menstruation, irregular

This is especially common at the beginning of the menstrual life and at the time of the menopause, but is also commonly due to an occasional missed period from unsuspected pregnancy followed by miscarriage (spontaneous abortion) at a very early stage.

Irregular bleeding, which is not actually menstrual irregularity, may also be due to:

- womb infection;
- **fibroids**;
- malignant tumours;
- polyps;
- **endometriosis**;

- bleeding after intercourse from trauma to the cervix;
- the presence of an IUD.

Periods missed as a result of anorexia, excessive dieting or strenuous athletics may also cause irregularity. Another common cause of seeming irregularity is midcycle bleeding, when, at the time of ovulation, oestrogen levels may briefly drop sufficiently to allow the endometrium to break down.

mental retardation

Human beings vary greatly in intellectual ability and it is impossible to draw a definite line between normality and deficiency. There are, however, many people whose mental ability is so much below average that they are unable consistently to perform even simple work or other social functions and require constant supervision and guidance if they are not to fall into distress or danger. Such people are said to suffer from mental deficiency.

POSSIBLE CAUSES

The deficiency is the result of brain defect or malfunction and is often present from birth. It may result from genetic factors directly or indirectly affecting the brain, from injury to the brain before, at, or soon after birth – often from oxygen deprivation – or from subsequent injury or disease of the brain. Infection and poisoning, severe nutritional deficiency, radiation or other environmental hazards and severe sensory or emotional deprivation early in life may all affect the structure or function of the brain in such a way as to produce mental deficiency.

CLASSIFICATION

There are degrees of mental deficiency and the mentally retarded are usually classified by intelligence quotient (IQ). Mildly defective people have IQs from 70 down to about 55; moderately defective people have IQs from 54 to 40; and severely defective people have IQs below 40. These figures are somewhat arbitrary as it is very difficult to measure intelligence reliably in these groups.

People of low mental capacity should be strongly encouraged to try to master some form of useful or other work under supervision. Work can be a source of pride and satisfaction to the retarded, and training in work activities often reveals a higher capacity than had been expected.

menthol

A volatile oil used as a local application to relieve itching or as an embrocation. Menthol can also be used as an inhalant to relieve nasal congestion. Excessive inhalation can be dangerous and menthol can cause skin allergy. Trade names of preparations for external use containing menthol are Balmosa, Fradol, Radian B and Salonpas.

meprobamate

A mildly tranquillizing carbamate drug with muscle-relaxant properties used in combination with pain-killing drugs to treat muscle and joint pain. A brand name is Equagesic.

Meptid

A brand name for the mild narcotic-like painkiller meptazinol.

mequitazine

An **antihistamine** drug used to treat hay fever and other allergic conditions. A brand name is Primalan.

Merbentyl

A brand name for **dicyclomine hydrochloride**.

mercaptopurine

A **cytotoxic** drug used in combination with others in the treatment of acute **leukaemia**. A brand name is Puri-Nethol.

Mercilon

A brand name for **ethinyloestradiol** formulated with the **progestogen** drug desogestrel as an oral contraceptive.

mercury poisoning

Acute poisoning, as from the accidental swallowing of a mercury compound – but not metallic mercury – causes nausea and vomiting, bleeding from the intestine, pain in the abdomen, diarrhoea, kidney failure and collapse.

Long-term (chronic) poisoning with small doses, as from the inhalation of mercury vapour in industrial processes, causes damage to the nervous system, leading to loss of sensation, staggering, tunnel vision, deafness, garbled speech and severe tremor. It may also cause irritability, excitability and other emotional disturbances.

Concern has been raised, from time to time, as to the possible risks of chronic mercury poisoning from amalgam in teeth. This is an alloy of liquid mercury with another metal such as powdered silver and has been widely used for over a century. Repeated suggestions that amalgam might be dangerous have been repudiated by the British Dental Association, but the authorities in other countries have suggested that its use should be discontinued or minimized. The American Food and Drug Administration (FDA) considered the matter in 1990, and other public bodies did so in succeeding years. None made any particular recommendations. In 1993 the American Public Health Service published a major review on dental amalgam and made various suggestions as to research, education and regulations but without concluding that the material was unsafe.

> It has been suggested, but without convincing clinical evidence, that mercury in dental amalgam might be responsible for causing Alzheimer's disease and some experts have suggested that it may do so by interfering with the synthesis of a substance necessary for the normal functioning of brain cells. According to an editorial in the *British Medical Journal*, no firm evidence of any association between dental amalgam and Alzheimer's disease has been published.

Merocets

A brand name for **cetylpiridinium chloride**.

Meronem

A brand name for **meropenem**.

meropenem

A carbapenem antibiotic drug. A brand name is Meronem.

mesalazine

A salicylate drug used to treat, and prevent recurrences of, **ulcerative colitis**. Trade names are Asacol, Pentasa and Salofalk.

mesna

A drug used to prevent damage to the urinary tract of people being treated with the anticancer drugs cyclophosphamide or ifosfamide. A brand name is Uromitexan.

messenger RNA

The molecule, usually referred to as mRNA, that reads the genetic code from DNA and carries it to the next stage in the process of protein synthesis. Before mRNA can function the DNA double helix must separate into two single strands. One of these carries the same sequence of bases as the mRNA and is not used. This strand is called the coding strand. The other is called the template, or antisense, strand and it is this strand that directs the synthesis of the mRNA by complementary base pairing (see **base pair**).

The messenger RNA molecule then leaves the cell nucleus and passes out through one of the many pores in the nuclear membrane to the site of protein synthesis, the ribosomes. There the appropriate **amino acids** are selected from the cell fluid and linked together in the right order by **transfer RNA** which, using its anticodons, reads the code on the messenger RNA. Ribosomes, with their own ribosomal RNA move along the messenger RNA linking the selected amino acids together into a polypeptide chain, the sub-unit of a protein.

messengers between cells

See **interleukins**.

mesterolone

A male sex hormone (androgen) drug used to treat male infertility from androgen deficiency. A brand name is Pro-Viron.

mestranol

An oestrogen drug, used in combination with a **progestogen** as an oral contraceptive or as a hormone replacement therapy for post-menopausal women. A brand name is Norinyl-1.

meta-

Prefix meaning 'changing' as in metamorphosis (changing shape).

meta-analysis

An impressive name for a simple matter. Many similar medical trials of drugs, treatments, etc., are done and these may give a wide scatter of broadly similar results. It is thus often thought useful to combine the results of a range of trials in a manner that hopefully, complies with the rules of statistics. Such a combination is called a meta-analysis. Care must be taken to ensure that the method does not give misleading results. This may occur if the trials are not strictly comparable. A meta-analysis of many badly conducted trials is not likely to provide more reliable information than the trials considered individually.

metaraminol

A **sympathomimetic** drug used as a heart stimulant in states of abnormally low blood pressure (hypotension) or to relieve paroxysmal **tachycardia** caused by hypotension. A brand name is Aramine.

metastasis

The spread of any disease, but especially cancer, from its original site to a remote point in the body where the disease process starts up anew. The word is also used to describe the new focus of disease. It is a feature of **malignant** tumours that they have a strong tendency to metastasize. This they do by 'seeding off' small clumps of tumour cells from the primary tumour. These are then carried elsewhere to start up a new, secondary, tumour. Cancers commonly metastasize to the lungs, the liver, the brain and the bones, but secondaries can occur literally anywhere in the body. Metastasis may occur by way of the bloodstream, by spread along the lymphatic vessels, or, in the case of lung cancer, by coughing and re-inhalation of affected particles to other parts of the lung.

Metenix

A brand name for **metolazone**.

-meter

Suffix meaning 'measurer' as in manometer (pressure measurer).

metformin

A biguanide oral **hypoglycaemic** drug used in the treatment of maturity onset diabetes. The drug may be dangerous to those with liver or kidney disease or a high alcohol intake. A brand name is Glucophage.

methadone

A synthetic narcotic pain-killing (analgesic) drug with properties similar to those of morphine. It is also used as a substitute for **heroin** in attempts to manage addiction, but is widely abused. A brand name is Physeptone.

methionine

A drug used in combination with paracetamol to protect the liver against the serious damage that is caused by deliberate overdosage. A brand name of the combination is Paradote.

methocarbamol

A centrally acting muscle relaxant drug used to treat conditions of severe muscle spasm. A brand name is Robaxin.

methotrexate

An **antimetabolite** and **immunosuppressant** drug used to treat cancer and help in the treatment of **rheumatoid arthritis**. It acts by interfering with the metabolism of **folic acid**. A brand name is Maxtrex.

methotrimeprazine

A phenothiazine derivative anti-psychotic drug. A brand name is Nozinan.

methoxamine

An alpha-adrenergic agonist drug that constricts arteries and is sometimes used in emergency to raise falling or dangerously low blood pressure. A brand name is Vasoxine.

methyl cellulose

An inert and non-absorbable substance that has been used to bulk out meals in the hope of achieving weight loss. It is also used as a laxative and in artificial tears. A brand name is Celevac.

methyldopa

An alpha adrenergic agonist drug that, paradoxically, is effective in the treatment of high blood pressure. The drug is said to act centrally on the brainstem by stimulating adrenergic receptors in such a way as to reduce the normal action of the sympathetic nervous system on arteries. This explanation is not universally accepted. A brand name is Aldomet.

methylphenidate

A nervous system stimulant drug that, paradoxically, has been found effective in the management of **attention deficit hyperactivity disorder** in children. A brand name is Ritalin.

methylphenobarbitone

A long-acting sedative drug useful in controlling all forms of **epilepsy** apart from absence seizures (petit mal). A brand name is Prominal.

methylprednisolone

A corticosteroid drug used in a wide range of conditions to control severe inflammation, treat allergies and replace steroid deficiencies. It is commonly used in depot form for long-term action. Trade names are Medrone, Depo-Medrone and Solu-Medrone.

methyl salicylate

An aromatic compound used externally as an embrocation, often in combination with other ingredients. Also known as Oil of Wintergreen. Trade names of formulations containing methyl salicylate are Balmosa, Monphytol, Phytex, Radian B and Salonpas.

methysergide

A **serotonin antagonist** ergot derivative drug used to treat resistant cases of migraine and some cases of persistent diarrhoea. A brand name is Deseril.

metipranol

A beta-blocker drug formulated as eye drops to treat **glaucoma**. A brand name is Minims metipranol.

metoclopramide

An **anti-emetic** drug also useful in the control of severe **heartburn** (reflux oesophagitis) in **hiatus hernia**. Trade names are Gastrobid Continus, Gastromax and Maxolon. The drug is also formulated with paracetamol as a migraine treatment under the brand name Paramax.

metolazone

A diuretic drug similar to the thiazide group used to treat high blood pressure. A brand name is Metenix.

Metopirone

A brand name for **metyrapone**.

metoprolol

A cardioselective beta-blocker drug used to treat **angina pectoris**, heart irregularities, high blood pressure and migraine. Trade names are Betaloc and Lopressor. The drug is also formulated with the diuretic **hydrochlorothiazide** under the brand name Co-Betaloc.

Metosyn

A brand name for **fluocinonide**.

Metrogel

A brand name for **metronidazole** formulated for external use only.

metronidazole

An antibiotic drug effective against *Trichomonas vaginalis* and *Entamoeba histolytica* as well as many other organisms. It is especially useful in the treatment of amoebic dysentery and amoebic liver abscesses as well as anaerobic infections. Trade names are Elyzol, Flagyl and Zidoval. The drug is also formulated with the antifungal drug nystatin under the brand name Flagyl Compak and, for external use only, under the trade names Anabact, Metrogel, Metrotop and Rozex.

Metrotop

A brand name for **metronidazole** formulated for external use.

metyrapone

An **aldosterone** inhibitor drug used to treat aldosterone-induced oedema and **Cushing's syndrome**. A brand name is Metopirone.

mewing baby cry

See **cri du chat syndrome**.

mexiletine

An anti-arrhythmic drug used in the treatment or prevention of severe heart irregularity arising in the ventricles. A brand name is Mexitil.

Mexitil

A brand name for **mexiletine**.

mibefradil

A calcium channel blocking drug used to treat **angina pectoris** and high blood pressure. A brand name was Posicor. In mid-1998 this drug was voluntarily withdrawn by the manufacturers Roche because of concern over possible interactions with other drugs.

miconazole

An imidazole antifungal drug. It can be taken by mouth or given by intravenous injection in severe **systemic** fungus infections and is used as an oral preparation for mouth infections. A brand name is Daktarin. The drug is also formulated for external use with benzoyl peroxide for the treatment of **acne** under the brand name Acnidazil; with hydrocortisone as Daktacort; and as a lacquer for dentures under the brand name Dumicoat. A vaginal preparation for the treatment of thrush is available under the brand name Gyno-Daktarin.

microbiologist

An ancillary health professional or doctor concerned with the study of micro-organisms that can affect health. The medical microbiologist may be concerned with the identification of certain classes of viruses, bacteria, fungi and protozoa and with providing advice to assist in the treatment of the diseases caused by these organisms.

microcephaly

Abnormal smallness of the skull. This often reflects poor brain growth and is usually associated with some degree of **mental retardation**.

Microgynon 30, Microgynon 30 ED

Trade names for low-dose oral contraceptive pills containing **ethinyoestradiol** and **levonorgestrel**.

Micronor

A brand name for **levonorgestrel** as an oral contraceptive.

Micronor-HRT

A brand name for the progestogen drug norethisterone intended for use as an adjunct to oestrogen **hormone replacement therapy**.

microscope as clinical tool

See **biomicroscopy**.

microsurgery

Operative surgery carried out at magnifications of two to about 20 times, using an operating microscope and appropriately miniaturized operating instruments.

WHY IT'S DONE

Microsurgery allows a degree of precision in the cutting, manipulation and approximation of small parts which is unobtainable by other means. It makes possible procedures which would almost certainly fail if attempted using conventional techniques and has, in certain fields, allowed major advances.

Microsurgery is now universally used in almost all eye (ophthalmic) operations and has revolutionized the results in **cataract surgery**, **glaucoma** surgery, and the management of severe eye injuries. Delicate operations on the middle and inner ears, often to cure conductive deafness, are now commonplace, and the joining up of small arteries (vascular microsurgery) has reached the stage at which it is now often possible successfully to re-attach severed arms or legs. Microsurgery is also being employed in gynaecology and urology.

HOW IT'S DONE

The operating microscope is either ceiling-mounted or is supported on a heavy portable stand to eliminate vibration. It is a binocular instrument and may provide binocular facilities for both surgeon and assistant. The microscope cannot be sterilized but the surgeon is able to control focus, movement and zoom magnification by means of a panel of controls operated by his or her feet. The operating field is brightly illuminated by a beam of light from the microscope itself, often following the same path as the viewing optics.

Microval

A brand name for **levonorgestrel** as an oral contraceptive.

Mictral

A brand name for **nalidixic acid** formulated with alkalizing drugs.

micturating cystogram

An X-ray taken while the subject is actually urinating. Prior to the examination an injection is given into the bloodstream of a dye that is opaque to X-rays and that is rapidly excreted in the urine. The method can provide important information about abnormalities of the bladder and of the urine tubes entering it (ureters) and leaving it (urethra). It is especially useful in investigating reflux flow of urine back up the ureters from the bladder in children.

midazolam

A **benzodiazepine** drug given by intravenous injection as a sedative for minor surgery or to induce general anaesthesia. A brand name is Hypnovel.

middle ear disease

See **otitis media**.

middle ear effusion, persistent

See **otitis media**.

Midrid

A brand name for **isometheptene**.

midwife

A nurse trained and qualified in the conduct of antenatal care, labour and childbirth. The function of the midwife differs from that of the medically qualified obstetrician to the extent that it is concerned primarily with the normal. Complications and undue difficulties are managed or supervised by doctors specializing in obstetrics.

mifepristone

A progesterone antagonist drug also known as RU-486, or the 'abortion pill'. When given in early pregnancy mifepristone causes the detachment of the early pre-embryo (blastocyst), and the production of prostaglandins that prompt contraction of the womb and softening of the cervix. The result is loss of the conceptus and termination of the pregnancy. A trade name is Mifegyne.

migraine

See **headache**.

Migraleve

A brand name for the antihistamine buclizine formulated with paracetamol and codeine.

Migranal

A brand name for a mixture of **paracetamol**, atropine, **papaverine** and nicotinic acid.

Migril

A trade name for a mixture of the anti-migraine drugs ergotamine, **caffeine** and **cyclizine**.

milk

The secretion from the mammary gland (breast) of any mammal. Because of its similarity to human milk, cow's milk is a unique food, providing an excellent balance of carbohydrate, fat, protein, minerals and vitamins. As a result, it has been commercially exploited on an enormous scale.

Although close in composition, cow's milk is not identical to human milk, the chief difference being in the composition of the milk fats. The human milk fats contain a higher proportion of long chain and unsaturated fatty acids, and these provide greater resistance to organisms commonly affecting the bowel, such as those causing dysentery, than do fatty acids from cow's milk. Even more important, human milk contains protective **immunoglobulins** (antibodies) produced by the mother's immune system, which provide the baby with protection against many organisms, until such time as the baby can produce its own.

The main carbohydrate in milk is lactose. Some people do not have the enzyme which breaks this down to simpler sugars and, since the unaltered lactose cannot be absorbed, it remains in the bowel and ferments, causing bloating, distention, pain and diarrhoea. This is called lactose intolerance.

Milk protein allergy occurs in some infants and can cause **eczema** or vomiting and diarrhoea.

milk-alkali syndrome

A rare condition caused by excessive intake of alkali and calcium by people being treated for stomach or duodenal ulcer with antacids and milk. There is excessive calcium in the blood and a partial breakdown of the mechanism controlling the acidity of the blood, so that it becomes more alkaline. Calcium is deposited in various tissues including the kidneys, and this may lead to kidney failure.

milk from baby's breasts

See **milk, witches'**.

milk intolerance

See **lactose intolerance**.

milk, witches'

Surprisingly, the breasts of newborn babies sometimes produce milk. The reason is interesting. Throughout the pregnancy, the output of the milk-promoting hormone, prolactin, by the mother's pituitary gland has been rising steadily. At the time of birth, peak concentrations of this hormone are circulating freely in the mother's blood. Some of this hormone gets through the placenta into the baby's blood and acts on the baby's breasts in exactly the same way as it acts on the mother's. The baby, however, produces no prolactin of its own and the effect soon wears off.

milrinone

A **phosphodiesterase inhibitor** drug. A brand name is Primacor.

minerals

Chemical elements necessary in the diet in adequate amounts to maintain health. The amounts needed are small, and deficiency is comparatively rare. As in the case of vitamins, to take much more than the required amounts serves no useful purpose and can be dangerous. The essential minerals are calcium, iron, magnesium, phosphorus, potassium, sodium, and zinc. Shown on the table below are daily requirements and rich sources.

Mineral	Recommended daily allowance	Rich source
CALCIUM	800 MG	MILK
CHLORIDE	2000 MG	SALT
COPPER	2 MG	MEAT
FLUORIDE	2 MG	WATER
IODINE	0.15 MG	VEGETABLES
IRON	18 MG IN WOMEN, 10 MG IN MEN	MEAT
MAGNESIUM	350 MG	MILK
PHOSPHORUS	800 MG	MILK
POTASSIUM	1800 TO 5700 MG	MILK
SODIUM	1000 TO 3500 MG	SALT
ZINC	15 MG	HAZELNUTS, CASHEWS, PISTACHIOS

minimal access surgery

See **laparoscopic surgery**.

minimally invasive coronary bypass surgery

The performing of a coronary artery bypass operation by **laparoscopic surgery** without stopping the heart or using a cardiopulmonary bypass machine. The left internal mammary artery is connected (anastomosed) to the left anterior descending coronary artery. The operation is appropriate only for a blockage of this artery near the upper part of the heart.

Minims

A brand name for a range of eyedrop preparations dispensed in single-dose plastic vials. The range, which is very large, includes atropine, castor oil, chloramphenicol, **fluorescein**, **neomycin**, **pilocarpine**, **prednisolone** and **sulphacetamide**.

Minims Benoxinate

A brand name for **oxybuprocaine**.

Minims Chloramphenicol

A brand name for **chloramphenicol**.

Minims Fluorescein

A brand name for **fluorescein**.

Minims Homatropine

A brand name for **homatropine**.

Minims Lignocaine fluorescein

A brand name for **fluorescein** eyedrops compounded with a local anaesthetic.

Minims Metipranol

A brand name for **metipranol**.

Minims Neomycin

A brand name for **neomycin**.

Minims Phenylephrine

A brand name for **phenylephrine**.

Minims Pilocarpine

A brand name for **pilocarpine**.

Minims Prednisolone

A brand name for **prednisolone**.

Minims Proxymetacaine

A brand name for **proxymetacaine**.

Minims Proxymetacaine Fluorescein

A brand name for **fluorescein** compounded with a local anaesthetic.

Minims Rose Bengal

A brand name for **rose Bengal**.

Minims Tropicamide

A brand name for **tropicamide**.

Minocin

A brand name for **minocycline**.

minocycline

A **tetracycline** antibiotic used to treat **acne** and general infections. Trade names are Aknemin, Dentomycin and Minocin.

Minodiab

A brand name for **glipizide**.

minoxidil

A **vasodilator** drug used in the treatment of high blood pressure. Used externally on the scalp, the drug has a somewhat exaggerated reputation as a hair-restorer and must be used continuously if any advantage gained is to be retained. A brand name is Loniten and, for external use to restore hair, Regaine or Rogaine.

Mintezol

A brand name for **thiabendazole**.

Minulet

A brand name for **ethinyloestradiol** formulated with a progestogen drug as an oral contraceptive.

Mirena

A brand name for **levonorgestrel** as an intrauterine, three-year contraceptive.

mirtazapine

An antidepressant drug that acts by increasing the release of serotonin and noradrenaline. A brand name is Zispin.

misbehaviour, child

Around 10 per cent of children consistently behave in a manner unacceptable to their parents, but many of these children are merely 'difficult' and will turn out well in the end. Less than 2 per cent of children regularly behave in such a way as to interfere with normal educational progress or to damage social relationships. Most commonly, these children show aggressive non-cooperation, a pattern of automatic opposition to suggestion, unwillingness to adapt to changing circumstances, outbursts of anger and periods of sulkiness.

POSSIBLE CAUSES
Sometimes the problem lies with the parent rather than the child. Many parents have an unrealistic idea of normal behaviour and of what may be expected of a child at various stages. Many are overprotective to the point of interfering with the child's need to explore and seek information and stimulation. This induces boredom and frustration in the child. At the same time, parents of problem children often feel guilty and helpless. Most are unaware that tensions of this kind are, to a greater or lesser degree, almost universal.

DISCIPLINE
Problems of this kind should not be tolerated for long. The longer they persist, the more difficult they are to deal with. Professional advice from a child psychologist or psychiatrist, at an early stage, can completely alter the outlook. Parents will be advised to make reasonable but firm rules and stick to them, to avoid obvious expression of annoyance or anger and to spend more time actively engaged in play and other activities with the child. Children are always happier if there is no doubt in anyone's mind about the rules. They will, of course, always try to break or bend the rules and to extend the limits of what they can get away with. Such attempts must be blocked with firmness, but, if possible, with good humour.

PUNISHMENT
Physical punishment may be useful as an ultimate sanction but should be a rare and noteworthy event. When applied, it should be unequivocally clear to the child that the punishment actually does hurt the inflictor more than the victim. Positive reinforcement is useful, for general disciplinary purposes. The object of punishments, such as brief, timed periods of banishment to a boring place, must be carefully and unemotionally explained to the child prior to the sentence, and at the end of the punishment, the child should be asked to state the reason for it. Soon after, if possible, the child should be praised for some action. Positive reinforcement of this kind can be highly effective.

> To be avoided at all cost is the common emotional outburst – shouting, scolding, striking – in response to the child's stubborn aggressiveness and indiscipline. This induces a vicious cycle in which the child will seek for, and find, all sorts of ways to hit back – sullenness, refusal to eat, tantrums, the eating of soil or dirt, deliberate defaecation into the clothes, refusal to go to bed, bedwetting, night waking, and so on. This cycle must be broken, but to do so may call for unusual control on the part of the parents.

Tantrums and refusal of food must be ignored. Food should be cleared away at the normal time and should not be available until the next meal. There need be no concern about the effect on the child's health. Appetite will assert itself.

> However difficult, the parent must at all times bear in mind the critical importance of maintaining the child's sense of security and of being loved.

See also **temper tantrum**.

miscarriage, spontaneous

See **cervical incompetence**.

mismatched organ transplant

See **CTLA4-Ig**.

miso-

Prefix meaning 'hatred' as in misogamist (hater of marriage).

misoprostol

A **prostaglandin** drug used to treat peptic ulcers especially those caused by non-steroidal anti-inflammatory drugs (**NSAIDs**). A brand name is Cytotec. The drug is also formulated with **diclofenac** under the brand name Arthrotec, and with **naproxen** under the brand name Napratec, for the treatment of **rheumatoid arthritis**.

missense mutation

A mutation caused by a change in a DNA sequence in any group of three bases (any **codon**) specifying a particular **amino acid** into one that specifies a different amino acid. The change of even a single amino acid out of hundreds may render an enzyme inactive or malfunctioning.

mitochondria

One of the microscopic cell organs (organelles) found in large numbers in the cytoplasm of all nucleated cells.

Mitochondria may be rod-shaped, spherical, branched or ring-shaped and have double-layered walls, the inner layer being deeply infolded to form compartments. They contain genes and some protein-forming bodies, the mitoribosomes and are the site of cell respiration. **Mitochondrial DNA** is transmitted only from the mother and, apart from mutations, remains unchanged through the generations.

mitochondrial DNA

A small circular DNA molecule of which all the **mitochondria** in cells have several copies. It contains 16,569 base pairs and, being present in the cytoplasm of the cell, is transmitted exclusively by the mother. A mature ovum contains about 100,000 copies of mitochondrial DNA but sperms contain none. Its main function is to code for enzymes needed by the mitochondrion. Its **genome** has been completely sequenced, and the sites of common mutations, especially deletions, are known, as are a number of diseases caused by these genetic defects. See also **mitochondrial DNA diseases**.

mitochondrial DNA diseases

Diseases caused by mutations in **mitochondrial DNA** (mtDNA) or by nuclear DNA mutations that affect the function of mitochondrial processes. Because both mitochondrial and nuclear genes may be involved, inheritance may be maternal or Mendelian. They are all rare.

Pure mitochondrial diseases caused by point mutations include a form of blindness from optic nerve atrophy; various muscle disorders; a brain disorder featuring lactic acid excess and stroke-like episodes; a neurological disorder causing weakness with staggering (ataxia) and retinitis pigmentosa; paralysis of eye movements; and excessive ageing.

Mitoxana

A brand name for **ifosfamide**.

mitoxantrone

A **cytotoxic** anticancer drug. A brand name is Novantrone.

mitral valve, disorders of

The mitral valve is the valve on the left side of the heart, between the upper chamber which receives blood from the lungs (left atrium) and the lower, powerful pumping chamber (left ventricle) which sends blood to all parts of the body.

The mitral valve may, rarely, be defective from birth, or may develop various disorders as a result of damage, especially from rheumatic fever. This disease can cause it to be either narrowed (mitral stenosis) or distorted and leaky (mitral incompetence). Both conditions have marked secondary effects on the heart muscle, which has to work harder to maintain the circulation, and which often thickens as a result. So long as this compensatory enlargement and increased power permits full recirculation of all the blood returning from the lungs, reasonable health is maintained. When the heart is no longer able to do this, it is said to be in failure.

The floppy valve syndrome (mitral valve prolapse) is a condition of the mitral valve present in about one person

The mitral valve, with its two cusps, is said to resemble an inverted bishop's mitre. It lies on the left side of the heart between the upper and lower chambers.

in 20. Although it causes a characteristic heart murmur, it is usually of no consequence. In a small proportion of cases it may lead to valve leakage, chest pain, pulse irregularity, bacterial **endocarditis** and, rarely, **heart failure**.

Mivacron

A brand name for **mivacurium**.

mivacurium

A non-depolarizing muscle-relaxant drug used by anaesthetists. The drug acts within three to four minutes and its effect lasts for about 15 minutes. Mivacurium is rapidly broken down by cholinesterase in the blood. A brand name is Mivacron.

Mixtard

A brand name for a preparation of **insulin** with a prolonged action.

MMR vaccination

A protective active immunization against measles, mumps and rubella that should be routine for all children unless contraindicated by a strong medical reason. Concern was raised in 1998 that MMR vaccination could lead to an intestinal disorder that allows the absorption of otherwise non-permeable peptides capable of causing autism and other developmental problems. The evidence was reviewed by the Joint Committee on Vaccination and Immunization and no case was found for abandoning a vaccine of proved effectiveness and safety.

Mobiflex

A brand name for **tenoxicam**.

Mobilan

A brand name for the non-steroidal anti-inflammatory drug (**NSAID**) **indomethacin**.

mobilization

After illness or injury it is always important to ensure that, whenever possible, the full range of mobility and activity, either of the whole body or of a part, is restored. Movement

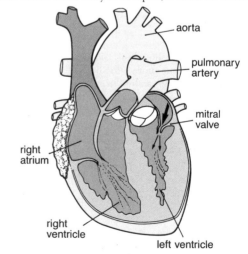

is life and the longer movement is prevented, the harder it is to recover it. On enforced rest, muscles waste and weaken, joints stiffen and lose range of movement, and mental motivation may be lost. After a period in bed, it will take, at the very least, an equal period to get back to the prior state of mobility, so bed rest should always be minimized. Stroke victims often become permanently bed-ridden as much because of failure to mobilize early as because of the damage to the nervous system.

Local mobilization after fractures, joint or joint capsule disorders, or other injuries may involve active help from physiotherapists or sometimes even manipulation under anaesthesia.

moclobemide

A reversible mono-amine oxidase inhibitor drug used to treat severe depression and social phobia. A brand name is Manerix.

modafinil

A non-amphetamine nervous system stimulant used to treat narcolepsy. A brand name is Provigil.

Modalim

A brand name for **ciprofibrate**.

Modecate

A brand name for the tricyclic antipsychotic drug **fluphenazine**.

Moditen

A brand name for **fluphenazine**.

Modrasone

A brand name for **alclometasone**.

Modrenal

A brand name for **trilostane**.

Moducren

A brand name for **hydrochlorothiazide** formulated with a beta-blocker drug.

Moduret 25

A brand name for **hydrochlorothiazide** formulated with another diuretic.

Moduretic

A brand name for a mixture of the potassium-sparing **diuretic** drug **amiloride** and the thiazide diuretic **hydrochlorothiazide**.

Mogadon

A brand name for the benzodiazepine hypnotic drug **nitrazepam**.

molar pregnancy

See **hydatidiform mole**.

Molcer

A brand name for **docusate sodium**.

mole

A birthmark (naevus) containing pigment. Moles may be large, disfiguring and sometimes hair-bearing, and if cosmetically undesirable can easily be removed under local anaesthesia. Hairy moles never become malignant.

molecular biology

The study of cellular phenomena, and especially genetics, at a molecular or chemical level. As knowledge has progressed the term has become more and more synonymous with 'biology', for biology today aims at nothing less than a full understanding of the functioning of living things in terms of the nature and interactions of their molecules.

molecule binding agent

See **annexin**, **annexinopathies**.

Molipaxin

A brand name for **trazodone**.

molluscum contagiosum

An infectious skin condition featuring groups of small, white, painless encapsulated, hemispherical, pearl-like lumps, 2–3 mm in diameter, each with a central dimple. If squeezed, a white, cheesy material is expressed. The condition is caused by a type of pox virus and is acquired by direct or indirect contact with another infected person, often in a public swimming pool. The infection can also be transmitted by sexual contact.

Treatment consists in squeezing out the contents of the lumps and touching the centre with a sharpened orange-stick dipped in phenol. In untreated cases the infection tends to spread to other parts of the body, on fingers, clothes or towels. The condition has no effect on the general health.

mometasone

A corticosteroid drug used as a nasal spray to treat hay fever. A brand name is Nasonex. The drug is also formulated for external use under the brand name Elocon for the treatment of **psoriasis** and atopic **eczema**.

mongolian spot

A kind of pigmented birth-mark (naevus) found on the buttocks or lower part of the back. Mongolian spots have a bluish-black appearance and are caused by a local accumulation of the normal skin pigment. They are commonest in coloured children and have usually disappeared by the age of about four.

mongolism

The outdated name for **Down's syndrome**.

moniliasis

See **candidiasis**.

Monistat

A brand name for a cream containing **miconazole**.

Monit

A brand name for **isosorbide mononitrate**.

monitoring

Since it is often possible to reverse or correct dangerous trends in people who are seriously ill or injured, it is essential that such trends should be detected as quickly as possible. Continuous monitoring, whether by direct observation, or by the use of instruments, enables changes to be noted and appropriate action quickly taken. Such monitoring is usually done in an intensive care unit, often on people in danger of developing potentially lethal alteration of heart action. The display of the **electrocardiogram** of several patients may be shown on screens, placed close together at a nurses' station, so that a constant check can be kept. Other bodily functions or physical signs can also be monitored. These include pulse rate, temperature, respiration rate, the condition of the pupils, various blood gas concentrations such as oxygen and carbon dioxide, the level of consciousness and the degree of appreciation of pain.

In some cases monitoring is done for diagnostic, rather than for life-saving, purposes and in these cases a 24-hour record of some parameter, such as the electrocardiogram, may be recorded on tape even while the person concerned goes about his or her business. Analysis can then be done by computer.

monkey HIV

See **SIV**.

mono-

Prefix meaning 'one' as in monocular (one eye).

monoamine oxidase inhibitors

Drugs that interfere with the action of the enzyme monoamine oxidase. This enzyme plays an important part in the breakdown of the neurotransmitters **noradrenaline** and 5-hydroxytryptamine (serotonin), both substances that can elevate mood. The MAO inhibitor drugs are used in the treatment of **depression** and anxiety.

See also **antidepressant drugs**.

Mono-Cedocard

A brand name for **isosorbide mononitrate**.

Monoclate-P

A brand name for **Factor XIII**.

monoclonal antibody

Antibodies (**immunoglobulins**) are produced by B cells (B lymphocytes). From the natural population of B cells in the body, one which best fits the invading organism (antigen) is selected and from this cell is formed a large population of identical cells (a clone) of antibody-producing cells. In this way a large quantity of the correct antibody (immunoglobulin) is formed.

This collection of identical immunoglobulin molecules is called a monoclonal antibody.

There is a type of cancer, called myelomatosis, in which a single B cell develops into a tumour (a myeloma) of antibody-secreting cells. This results in enormous quantities of a single immunoglobulin – a monoclonal antibody. Mice readily develop myelomas and these have provided workers with unprecedented quantities of monoclonal antibodies. Their usefulness was at first limited because these antibodies were specific to a particular, unknown, antigen and could not be used for other antigens.

In 1975, however, the German-born Cambridge immunologist Georges Kohler (b. 1946) and the Argentinian-born Cambridge molecular biologist Cesar Milstein (b. 1927) found a way of taking normal mouse B cells and fusing them with cultured myeloma cells so as to form immortal lines of cells that continue indefinitely to generate the particular antibody produced by the B cell concerned. In this way it became possible to produce hybrid cell tumours, called hybridomas, that grow like myelomas but produce large quantities of a chosen and identifiable monoclonal antibody. This is one of the most important biotechnological advances of the century. It is now possible to obtain monoclonal antibodies that can recognize individual antigenic sites on any organism, indeed on almost any molecule, and the research implications of this advance have been enormous.

SIGNIFICANCE

In practical terms, monoclonal antibody production has made possible tests for the presence of an almost unlimited range of organisms and for different types of cells, including cancer cells. Unfortunately, human myeloma cells do not grow well in culture. Human B cells infected with the virus of glandular fever do, however, grow in culture and continue to produce antibodies. This is a major growth zone in research.

Since monoclonal antibodies can be made to seek out and recognize cancers, wherever they might be in the body, much research has been done into the possibility of using this method to carry a toxic agent to the tumour cells and destroy them. Reports of progress appear regularly in the medical press.

See also **ELISA test**.

Monomax

A brand name for **isosorbide mononitrate**.

Mononine

A brand name for **Factor IX**.

mononucleosis, infectious

See **glandular fever**.

monorchism

Having only one testicle in the scrotum. This is most commonly due to a failure of one testicle to descend into the scrotum before birth. This affects about one boy in 50.

See **testicle, disorders of**.

Monophane

A brand name for an **insulin** preparation used in the control of **diabetes**.

monosodium glutamate

This is the sodium salt of glutamic acid and is produced by the action of acids or enzymes on vegetable protein such as wheat gluten or soya bean.

It is also known as 'Ajinomoto', 'Vetsin', 'Chinese seasoning', 'Accent' and 'Zest'. It is a white crystalline powder with a meat-like taste which imparts a meat flavour to blander foods if used with a little salt. It has also been used to improve the flavour of tobacco.

Monosodium glutamate has been suspected of being the cause of the **Chinese restaurant syndrome**.

Monotard

A brand name for **insulin**.

Monotrim

A brand name for **trimethoprim**.

Monozide 10

A brand name for **hydrochlorothiazide** formulated with a **beta-blocker** drug.

montelukast

A drug that binds to the receptors for certain leukotrienes thus blocking both phases of the **asthma** response. It is used in the treatment of asthma that shows an inadequate response to inhaled steroids. A brand name is Singulair.

mood disorders

See **depression, mania, manic-depressive illness**.

mood swings

See **bipolar disorder**.

moon face

A chubby, hamster-like appearance of the face caused by excessive doses of cortico-steroids or by excessive production of the natural adrenal cortical hormone in **Cushing's syndrome**. When the effect is caused by steroid drugs, doctors often refer to it by the inelegant term 'Cushingoid'.

morbid anatomy

The branch of pathology concerned with the gross changes which are caused in body tissues and organs by disease and injury and which are, in general, discernible at post-mortem examination.

morbidity

The state of being diseased. The morbidity rate is the number of cases of a disease occurring in a given number (usually 100,000) of the population. The annual morbidity figures for a disease, in a particular population, are the **incidence** figures – the number of new cases reported – in the year.

morbilli

Another name for measles.

morbo

Latin root meaning 'disease' as in morbid (diseased).

Morcap SR

A brand name for **morphine**.

morning-after pill

See **postcoital contraception**.

moron

A person of a mild degree of **mental retardation**. A person with an IQ between 50 and 70. The term is no longer used in medicine but has been widely adopted in popular speech.

-morphic

Suffix meaning 'shaped' as in anthropomorphic (man-shaped).

morphine

A powerful pain-killing and narcotic drug used to control persistent pain that cannot be relieved by lesser drugs. It can be taken by mouth or given by injection. Morphine has a valuable effect on the emotional response to pain and in relieving the anxiety associated with the contemplation of the implications of severe pain. It is a respiratory depressant and is never given in cases of head injury or in other conditions in which respiration may be prejudiced. When appropriately prescribed addiction is unlikely. Trade names are Morcap SR, MST Continus, MXL, Oramorph, Rapiject, Sevredol and Zomorph. The drug is also formulated with the anti-emetic cyclizine under the brand name Cyclimorph.

morphine antidote

See **naloxone**.

morpho-

Prefix meaning 'shape' as in morphogenesis (shape development).

morphoea

A localized form of scleroderma in which areas of skin and underlying tissue are replaced by hardened patches (plaques) of fibrous tissue, with loss of the normal skin constituents, such as sweat glands and hair follicles.

Morphoea is commoner in women than in men and, although sometimes disfiguring, does not offer any danger to life.

RECOGNITION AND SYMPTOMS
The affected areas are usually round or oval, but may take the form of bands or stripes, sometimes running the whole length of a limb. They are smooth, white and hard and the surrounding skin may be pinkish or violet. Sometimes the plaques become adherent to the underlying bone. In severe cases they may involve the whole of one side of the face. After a long time they tend to become softer and may acquire a brownish colour.

TREATMENT
There is no effective treatment for morphoea but ointments can be helpful.

mortality rate

In any particular population, the mortality rate is the ratio of the total number of deaths from one or any cause, in a year, to the number of people in the population. 'Crude mortality' is the number of deaths in a year per 1000 total population. The age-specified mortality rate is the number of deaths occurring in a year in people of a particular age or in a particular age-group.

Mortality rates are invaluable as a means of determining the comparative state of health of a population and of assessing any changes in disease trends. Rates for the whole population may be compared with rates within certain socio-economic groups or in certain occupations, thus highlighting possible causes of disease or death.

See also **infant mortality**.

mosquito bites

See **flies**.

Motens

A brand name for **lacidipine**.

Motifene

A brand name for **diclofenac**.

Motillium

A brand name for the **anti-emetic** drug **domperidone**.

motion sickness

A general term applied to nausea or vomiting induced by any form of passive motion of the body, whether by boat, car, aircraft, swing, space-rocket or simulator. Interestingly, the word 'nausea' derives from the Greek word *naus*, meaning a 'ship'.

RECOGNITION AND SYMPTOMS

After a variable period of exposure to unaccustomed motion there is abdominal discomfort, progressive nausea, pallor, sweating of the face and hands, increased salivation, a sense of depression and vomiting. If the motion continues, the symptoms persist for several days, with variable severity. There is apathy, depression, total loss of appetite and sometimes a loss of the will to live, so that action to maintain personal safety may be abandoned.

POSSIBLE CAUSES

The cause of motion sickness is unknown, but it is not experienced by people whose inner-ear balancing mechanisms are destroyed. The condition seems to be related to a sustained loss of any fixed base by which to judge bodily position and head orientation, and it is relieved if the eyes can be focused on some unmoving point or line, such as the horizon.

TREATMENT

Motion sickness is best treated with small doses of one of the drugs found, by experience, to be effective. Useful drugs include atropine (Belladonna) and its derivative hyoscine (Kwells), and atropine-like antihistamine drugs such as cyclizine (Marzine), promethazine (Phenergan or Avomine), or dimenhydrinate (Dramamine).

Sometimes the phenothiazine tranquillizers and the barbiturates may be used. Any drugs must be taken at least an hour before the motion starts and great care should be taken to avoid overdosage, especially in children, by repeating the dose too frequently.

Motipress

A brand name for **fluphenazine** formulated with **nortriptyline**.

Motival

A brand name for **fluphenazine** formulated with **nortriptyline**.

motor

The medical term for anything that causes movement. A motor nerve is one which stimulates muscles into contraction. The motor pathways in the nervous system are the large pyramidal tracts of nerve fibres sweeping down from the part of the surface of the brain subserving movement (the motor cortex) to the spinal cord to link with the nerves running out of the cord to the muscles.

motor neuron disease

A rare disorder of unknown cause in which the nerve cells concerned with causing the muscles to contract suffer a gradual and progressive loss of function and structure. This may affect **motor** neurons in the brain and in the spinal cord.

INCIDENCE

The condition is rare before 40 and affects men twice as often as women.

RECOGNITION AND SYMPTOMS

When motor neurone disease affects the brainstem fibres it causes difficulty in swallowing and in speaking. There is hoarseness, reduction in the strength of the voice and wasting of the tongue. Involvement of the long motor tracts and nerve cells in the spinal cord causes wasting and weakness of the small muscles of the hands, spreading to the forearms, and increased muscle tension (spasticity) in the legs.

In all forms of the condition, progressive worsening occurs until there is widespread paralysis affecting all four limbs and eventually the muscles of respiration. However severe, there is never any effect on intellectual function or awareness.

TREATMENT

There is, unfortunately, no treatment for motor neuron disease and, depending on the area first affected, the survival time varies from two to ten years.

The shortest course is in those in whom the condition starts in the brainstem.

Motrin

A brand name for the non-steroidal anti-inflammatory drug (**NSAID**) **ibuprofen**.

mountain sickness

See **altitude sickness**.

mould

Any one of a large group of fungi that form multi-cellular, filamentous colonies.

Moulds will grow readily on organic matter, especially if moist, and most of them are harmless. Some of them, such as the common mould *Penicillium notatum*, secrete useful antibiotics. Others can cause allergic disease, such as **farmer's lung**, cork worker's lung and malt worker's lung.

mousy-smelling baby

See **phenylketonuria**.

mouth cancer

This most commonly involves the lip and the tongue, less often the floor of the mouth, the inside of the cheeks or the palate. It may start in one of the salivary glands.

> Mouth cancer must be diagnosed early if extensive surgery is to be avoided. If major surgery is needed it may be impossible to restore a normal appearance or full mouth function. Tongue cancer spreads rapidly to the local lymph nodes and from there to other parts of the body. Prolonged delay in diagnosis may be fatal.

POSSIBLE CAUSES
Mouth cancer is usually tobacco-induced, and switching from cigarettes to a pipe or cigars, or using snuff or oral tobacco, does not reduce the risk. Keeping a quantity of tobacco in one place in the mouth for long periods is dangerous and often causes **leukoplakia**, a well-recognized pre-cancerous condition. The consumption of alcohol, ill-fitting dentures and poor state of the teeth, especially if teeth are rough or jagged, also increase the likelihood of developing mouth cancer.

RECOGNITION AND SYMPTOMS
Any persistent local spot, whether whitish or inflamed, hard or soft, or any persistent crack, fissure, ulcer or other abnormal area on the lip or in the mouth must be considered a potential cancer and reported for expert advice. Developing tumours may be painless, but will extend and form ulcers which may bleed. Cancers of the tongue tend to be painful and there is constant consciousness of the tongue which may feel unnaturally inflexible. There may be difficulty in speaking properly or in swallowing.

TREATMENT
Early treatment, by surgery and sometimes radiotherapy, gives good results but with delay the outlook rapidly worsens.

mouth, dry

Dryness of the mouth is a normal response to fear and may be caused by taking belladonna (atropine) or any one of the many atropine-like drugs which temporarily cut down the rate of secretion of the salivary glands. It may also be caused by salivary gland disorders or by general disorders affecting glandular tissue, such as **Sjögren's syndrome**.

Permanent dryness makes swallowing difficult and may affect speech. It tends to promote tooth decay (dental caries) and to make dentures ill-fitting. Relief can be obtained by the use of frequent sips of fluid which is held in the mouth.

mouth-to-mouth resuscitation

See *First Aid*.

mouth signs

Much is to be learned by a look inside a person's mouth. Red, peeling areas, at the line of contact of the lips, suggest a vita-

min B deficiency. Inflamed cracks at the corners may indicate thrush infection, especially if there is corner dribbling. A crack in the lip persisting for more than three or four weeks, especially in an elderly person, might be caused by cancer and should be investigated.

The state of the teeth speaks volumes about the standards of personal hygiene and gives away the smoking history. Obvious decay indicates dental neglect. Brownish mottling can be caused by excess fluorine and by the antibiotic drug tetracycline given in infancy while the teeth are developing. Swollen, inflamed gums, with discharge of pus (pyorrhoea), usually indicates gross neglect of the teeth, as pyorrhoea is usually secondary to dental calculus. Swollen gums which bleed easily may indicate vitamin C deficiency (scurvy). A blue line appears along the gum margin in lead poisoning.

In dehydration the tongue is dry and furred. Furring, by itself, is of no significance. Certain kinds of anaemia cause the tongue to be smooth, shiny, and sometimes sore. Blueness of the tongue suggests insufficient oxygenation of the blood. Enlargement of the tongue occurs when there is excessive hormone production (acromegaly) and is a feature of **Down's syndrome**. Firm, white, thickened patches on the tongue, which cannot be removed, could be leukoplakia – a pre-cancerous condition.

mouth ulcers

These are very common and appear as painful white, grey or yellow open sores that may develop anywhere on the mouth lining (mucous membrane) – on the inside of the lip or cheek or on the floor of the mouth.

RECOGNITION AND SYMPTOMS
The ulcers are shallow, round or oval, with an inflamed red border. They may occur singly or in clusters.

POSSIBLE CAUSES
Known causes include Herpes simplex virus infection, **Behçet's syndrome** and Vincent's infection of the mouth. Severe ulceration may accompany **regional ileitis** (Crohn's disease), **ulcerative colitis** and coeliac disease. Most mouth ulcers occur for no known reason, often in perfectly healthy people. Sometimes they are precipitated by emotional stress and in women they sometimes occur regularly before the menstrual period.

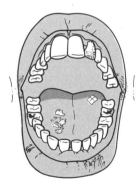

No medical examination is complete without a thorough inspection of the inside of the mouth. This can reveal not only a variety of local mouth and dental disorders, but can often give valuable information about more general conditions such as dehydration, anaemia, lead poisoning, scurvy, Down's syndrome and acromegaly.

> It is important to distinguish temporary ulceration of the mouth from a possible early cancer. People over 40 should be especially wary of any apparent ulcer which persists for more than a month.

TREATMENT

These usually respond well to hydrocortisone ointment.

See also **mouth cancer**.

mouthwash

Mouthwashes are popular and are widely advertised but, like eye-washes, are unlikely to achieve more than nature is already doing – providing a flow of cleansing and washing fluid to the area. Nature, moreover, has the advantage of constancy. Mouthwashes are, however, mainly harmless and often leave the mouth feeling pleasantly refreshed for a few minutes.

Mouthwashes are often used for the treatment of real or imagined bad breath (**halitosis**), but this has many causes, and persistent halitosis is unlikely to be eradicated by a mouthwash. Real medical indications for a mouthwash are few and are a matter for the dentist.

Movelat

A brand name for **mucopolysaccharide polysulphate**.

Movicol

A brand name for **polyethylene glycol**.

Moxacin

A brand name for **amoxacillin**.

moxibustion

A primitive form of treatment involving the burning of a cone of dried leaves close to the skin. Any local irritant of this kind has a minor effect in promoting an increased blood supply to the area and so helping to relieve inflammation. Although widely practised in many parts of the world, moxibustion is of little medical value and has no place in scientific medical practice.

moxonidine

A drug that causes arteries to relax by influencing the action of the sympathetic nervous system. It is used to treat high blood pressure. A brand name is Physiotens.

MRI

See **magnetic resonance imaging**.

MRSA

A term originally referring to strains of the common disease-producing organism *Staphylococcus aureus* that were not killed by the antibiotic methicillin (methicillin-resistant *S. aureus*). The term is now generally taken to mean multiple-resistant *S. aureus*. MRSA is a strain of the germ that is capable of resisting treatment with almost all antibiotics. Over 90 per cent of hospital strains of *S. aureus* have long been penicillin-resistant and some strains are also resistant to other antibiotics. This is a matter for great concern as MRSA, which is commoner in hospital than anywhere else, is responsible for many deaths.

MST Continus

A brand name for **morphine**.

Mucaine

A brand name for a preparation containing **aluminium hydroxide** and **magnesium hydroxide**.

mucin

A glycoprotein that is the main constituent of **mucus**. The term is also used as a generic name for the substance used as a drug formulated with xylitol as artificial saliva under the brand name Saliva Orthana.

muco-

Prefix meaning '**mucus**' as in mucopurulent (mucus and pus).

mucocoele

A benign and usually harmless cyst-like body filled with **mucus** which is produced by mucus-secreting cells in its lining. Mucocoeles occur in various parts of the body when normally secreted mucus is unable to escape though its normal channels. They are likely to do harm only if unable to expand without compressing or displacing other structures.

Mucogel

A brand name for a preparation containing **aluminium hydroxide** and **magnesium hydroxide**.

mucolytic drugs

Drugs which make mucus more liquid and less sticky. They are used most to assist in the coughing up of sputum, but are occasionally used for other purposes where excess mucus is a problem. The most commonly used mucolytic drug is **acetylcysteine** (Parvolex, Airbron).

Mucomyst

A brand name for **acetylcysteine**.

mucopolysaccharide polysulphate

A drug formulated with salicylic acid as a cream or gel for external application in minor muscle and joint disorders. A brand name is Movelat.

mucous membrane

The inner lining of many of the cavities and hollow internal organs of the body. Mucous membrane lines the mouth, the nose, the eyelids, the intestine, the gall-bladder, the urinary bladder, the urethra, the vagina, the uterus and many other structures. It contains large numbers of goblet-shaped cells. These secrete **mucus** which keeps the surface moist and lubricated.

mucus

A slimy, jelly-like material, chemically a mucopolysaccharide or glycoprotein, which is produced by the goblet cells of mucous membranes. It has essential lubricating and protective properties and life would be unpleasant, and perhaps impossible, without it. Mucus prevents acid from destroying the stomach wall and prevents enzymes from digesting the intestine. It assists in the conditioning of inhaled air and in the clearance of smoke and other foreign particles from the lungs. It eases swallowing and the movement of the bowel contents by peristalsis and makes possible comfortable sexual intercourse.

mucus

Latin root meaning 'phlegm' as in mucus (secretion of mucus glands).

multi-

Prefix meaning 'many' as in multipara (many births).

multiple sclerosis

This chronic disease of the central nervous system affects about one person in 2000 in Britain. Multiple sclerosis (MS) may occur at any age, but it is rare before puberty and after 60. In most cases it starts between the ages of 20 and 40.

Multiple small scattered 'plaques' – areas of degeneration and loss of the insulating myelin sheath of nerve fibres – occur in a random manner anywhere in the brain or spinal cord. These can be seen on MRI scanning. Where these plaques occur the conduction of the nerve fibres is blocked and the function served by them is lost. As a result, affected people develop any of the wide range of disabilities resulting from loss of nervous system function – weakness, paralysis, loss of sensation, visual loss, incoordination and mental disturbances. Attacks do not destroy the whole of the function concerned, because only a proportion of the nerves is affected, but if repeated attacks occur, the disability is usually progressive.

In spite of intensive research and many advances in understanding, the cause remains unknown.

RECOGNITION AND SYMPTOMS

Limb weakness is a common initial feature, as is a central area of visual loss caused by involvement of an optic nerve (retrobulbar neuritis). There may be patches of skin without sensation, double vision, vertigo, staggering, disorders of speech, facial paralysis or epilepsy.

The disease is characterized by long periods of freedom followed, in many cases, by recurrences. The course is very variable. Some people have an attack and then are free from trouble for up to ten years or longer. The condition can even be found on post-mortem examination in a person who had never suspected that anything was wrong.

> Research into the cause takes account of a number of known facts. The incidence of MS varies widely in different parts of the world, being very low in the tropics. People who, before adolescence, move from high incidence to low incidence areas enjoy a reduced risk; and young people who move from areas of low incidence to those of high incidence acquire the greater risk. After the age of 15, a move of location does not affect one's chances of developing MS. There is a higher incidence of the disease in people of certain tissue type groups (HLA groups) than in the general population, and there is also a higher incidence in relatives of MS sufferers. It seems probable, from this and other evidence, that the disease may occur in people with a genetic susceptibility who become infected, early in life, with an unknown slow virus.

Usually, the early symptoms clear up spontaneously in about six weeks and this is followed by a period of freedom. Relapses may occur at any time and in some cases each of these seems to be followed by complete recovery. In other cases relapses lead to increasing disability. Eventually, about half of all those with MS become permanently and increasingly affected. The disease is often associated with unexpectedly high morale, even euphoria, but appropriate depression is also common. Late in the disease there may be intellectual impairment.

TREATMENT

Unfortunately, there is no effective treatment for MS but much may be done to support and encourage those affected and to relieve or ameliorate many of the symptoms and effects. Undue bed rest should be avoided and mobility maximized. Walking frames, wheelchairs and adapted motor vehicles should be used, together with all required physical aids. Association with other sufferers and the promotion of the highest attainable degree of intellectual activity are important in the attempt to promote the best possible quality of life.

multivitamin preparations

Combinations of vitamins, most of which are purchased and consumed by people who have no need for them and derive no benefit from them.

People on normal diets do not suffer from vitamin deficiency unless they are suffering from a rare malabsorption disorder. Vitamins A and D are dangerous if taken in excess. Hypervitaminosis A and D are well recognized clinical syndromes. All the B vitamins are co-enzymes and are needed for many of the chemical reactions of the body. But the amounts required are very small and are adequately provided by all but extremely inadequate or grossly unbalanced diets. Any taken in excess of the requirements are wasted. The B vitamin folic acid, however, will prevent neural tube defects (**spina bifida** and other serious congenital defects) if taken immediately before and in the first few weeks of pregnancy. The amounts of vitamin C in multivitamin preparations are quite inadequate if they are being taken as **anti-oxidant** drugs; at least 1000 mg a day are required for this purpose. Vitamin E, taken as an antioxidant, should be taken separately in a dose of about 400 mg for an adult. Large doses of vitamin E are dangerous for babies.

mumps

A virus infection, most commonly affecting children, which causes fever and swelling of the main pair of salivary glands (the parotids) so that the face assumes a hamster-like appearance. In adult males, mumps is also often associated with a painful inflammation of the testicles (orchitis). An attack of mumps confers permanent immunity.

The disease is spread by aerosol droplet transfer during coughing and sneezing and the first symptoms appear after an incubation period of about three weeks. The period of fever is brief – two or three days – and the illness is often very mild, perhaps no more than a slight discomfort in front of the ears and on chewing. If more severe, there may be headache. The swelling of the parotid glands resolves in about ten days. Occasionally a mild form of meningitis (inflammation of the menges) may occur, but this is seldom serious.

Munchausen's syndrome

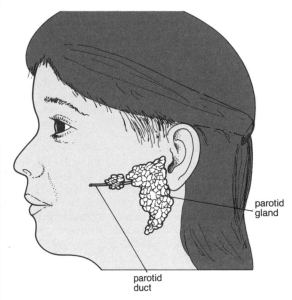

*Mumps is an inflammation of the main salivary gland –
the parotid – on each side as a result of a virus infection. The
swelling of the glands produces a striking broad-faced,
hamster-like appearance.*

The complication most commonly causing concern is
orchitis. This does not affect young boys but occurs in about
a quarter of the adolescent or adult males who contract
mumps and it may cause much distress. As a rule, only one
testicle is affected, but this may become considerably swollen,
exquisitely tender and painful and may remain so for several
days, before returning to its normal state. Padding with much
loose cotton wool may be needed. Occasionally mumps orchitis leads to sterility of the affected testicle, but this seldom
affects fertility. Total sterility from this cause is very rare.

Munchausen's syndrome

A sustained course of deliberate and calculated deception of
the medical profession for the purposes of obtaining attention, personal status and free accommodation and food.
People with this condition make a career of simulating disease. They read books like this one with admirably close attention and then report to a doctor complaining of the symptoms
of a specific disease, preferably a serious one. Such people are
usually very plausible and sometimes subtle, and if previously
unknown to the doctor or hospital
concerned, are likely to carry conviction and succeed in their desire to
be admitted for investigation and
treatment.

Participators in the Munchausen's
syndrome have a preference for surgical conditions and often carry an
unusual number of surgical scars
upon their persons – a circumstance
viewed with suspicion by most doctors,
if the patient is new to them. On being
detected, as they invariably eventually
are, these people immediately discharge themselves from hospital.

Baron Karl Friedrich Hieronymus von Munchausen
(1720–97) was a German soldier, liar and retailer of outrageous pseudo-autobiographical tales. These were popularized
in 1785 by the German novelist Rudolf Eric Raspe (1737–94)
and have remained in print ever since.

Munchausen's syndrome by proxy

Illness or injury in a child caused by a parent or other person
in charge for the purpose of obtaining attention and possibly
sympathy, or for other unimaginable reasons. The most common effects seen in such unfortunate children are bleeding,
diarrhoea and vomiting, rashes, seizures, apparent respiratory failure, and near-coma. These are brought about by such
means as the application of blood or the use of anticoagulants such as warfarin rat poison, the administration of drugs,
poisoning, pressure on the neck or partial suffocation. The
child is brought, often repeatedly, for medical attention and
if suspicion is raised any responsibility for the child's medical
condition is strongly denied. Separation from the parent or
person in charge, however, quickly leads to the child's recovery
unless he or she is too seriously affected. Covert closed-
circuit TV monitoring has been used to detect the crime.

mupirocin

A broad-spectrum antibiotic used externally on the skin and
as a nasal ointment to treat carriers of staphylococci. Trade
names are Bactroban and Bactroban nasal.

muscarinic antagonists

A group of drugs that oppose the action of acetyl choline (see
anticholinergic drugs) and are used to treat certain cases of
urinary frequency and incontinence.

muscle

Between 40 and 50 per cent of the body weight consists of
muscle – a tissue made from cells with the power of rapidly
changing shape. Muscle fibres are elongated cells which,
under a suitable stimulus, either from a nerve or as a result
of being stretched, shorten and thicken without change of
volume. Muscles fibres cannot contract to a variable degree.
Either they contract fully or not at all. Body muscles are
made up of considerable bundles of fibres and the force
exerted varies with the number contracting at any time.
Under maximum effort, almost all the fibres in the muscle
will contract.

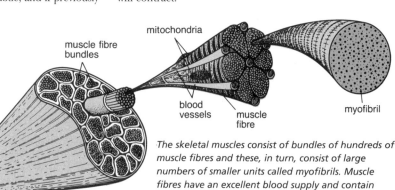

*The skeletal muscles consist of bundles of hundreds of
muscle fibres and these, in turn, consist of large
numbers of smaller units called myofibrils. Muscle
fibres have an excellent blood supply and contain
many mitochondria that are essential for the
production of energy from fuel.*

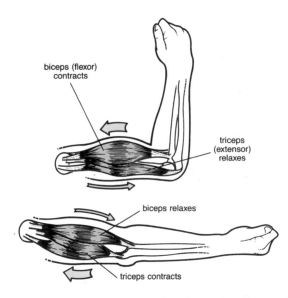

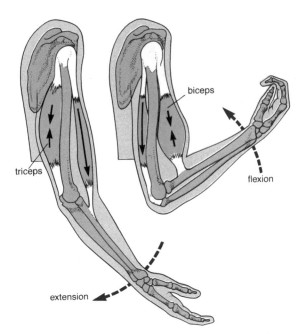

Above: Muscle action. On contraction, the muscle thickens and shortens but does not change in volume. When a muscle contracts, its opponent relaxes.

Above: Most muscles operate across joints in such a way that shortening of the muscle causes the joint to bend (flex) or straighten (extend). The illustration shows how the biceps is a flexor, and the triceps is an extensor, of the elbow.

Left: The muscles of the shoulder and arm. Those above the elbow move the shoulder and elbow or rotate the forearm; those below act mainly to open and close the hand by way of tendons passing over the wrist.

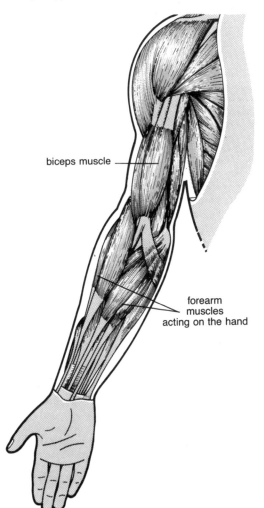

Muscle fibres convert chemical energy into mechanical energy and their main function is to produce movement in the body. For this reason, most muscles are connected to bones and lie across a joint with one end attached on either side.

Contraction of the muscle thus causes the joint to bend (flex). Muscle action of this kind is never unopposed and there is always another muscle, or group of muscles, on the other side of the joint, exerting an opposite and balancing effect on the joint. Muscles which bend a joint are called flexors and those which straighten it are called extensors. There are three kinds of muscle:

- striated, or voluntary, muscle which is attached to bone;
- smooth, or involuntary muscle, which occurs in such places as the walls of blood vessels, the intestine and the urinary tract;
- heart muscle (myocardium), which is a kind of network of muscle fibres with special power of automatic regular contraction without external stimulus.

The body contains hundreds of muscles. Here are some examples.

The biceps is the prominent and powerful muscle on the front of the upper arm which bends the elbow and rotates the forearm outwards, as in using a screwdriver. The triceps is a three-headed muscle, which extends the elbow and opposes the action of the biceps.

501

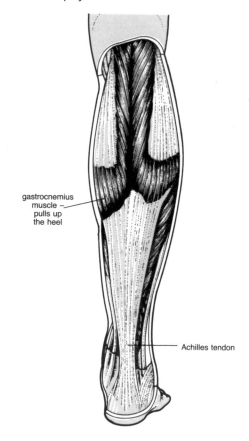

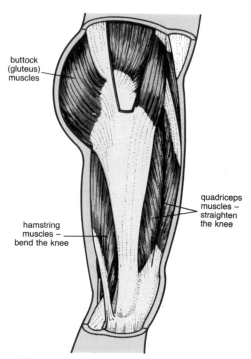

Above: The muscles of the buttocks and thighs. The buttocks are built up of three layers of muscles.

Left: The muscles of the lower leg. Those on the back of the leg extend the ankle and pull down the toes. They act on the foot by way of tendons passing over the ankle or inserted into the heel bone.

The buttocks are the twinned masses of powerful muscle at the base of the trunk, behind, each consisting of three gluteal muscles – gluteus maximus, gluteus medius and gluteus minimus. These muscles arise from the back of the bony pelvis and run into the upper end of the back of the thigh bone (femur). Their action, therefore, is to straighten the flexed hip joint during walking, running or climbing stairs and to raise the trunk from the stooping, bowing or sitting position. They are often well developed, and correspondingly prominent, in dancers and athletes.

The quadriceps muscle is the massive muscle group forming the front of the thigh. It consists of four muscles, which take origin from the thigh bone (femur), and from the front of the pelvis. All four muscles end, below, in a stout tendon – the quadriceps tendon – which is large enough to accommodate the kneecap (patella) and which is firmly attached to a bump on the upper end of the front of the main bone of the lower leg (tibia). In contracting, the quadriceps muscles therefore exert a powerful straightening action on the knee, lifting almost the whole weight of the body and allowing walking. The 'quads' need to be used to maintain their bulk and strength and are very well developed in runners and other athletes.

The hamstring muscles are the three long, cylindrical muscles at the back of the thigh, whose prominent tendons can be felt at the back of the knee on either side. These muscles are the 'hams' and the name 'hamstrings' refers to the tendons rather than to the muscles. All three muscles arise from bony bumps on the underside of the pelvis and their tendons are inserted into the back of the upper end of the

bone of the lower leg – the tibia. The hamstring muscles, on contracting, bend the knee and straighten the hip joint.

Because the tendons are prominent and superficial, they can easily be cut by deliberate intention, a barbaric practice common in earlier warfare and often inflicted on horses. When the hamstrings are cut, the knee collapses.

The calf muscles, consisting of the gastrocnemius and the soleus muscles, arise from the back of the lower leg bones and run down to be inserted into the back of the heel bone. The common tendon, by which both these muscles are joined to the heel bone, is called the Achilles tendon. This is the prominent tendon just above the heel.

The Achilles tendon is essential in walking and running and is easily strained or torn.

In mythology, the baby Achilles was dipped in the river Styx by his mother, to make him invulnerable. Unfortunately, she held him by the heel, the immersion was incomplete, and he later perished by a wound in the unprotected area. The eponymous tendon often proves to be the 'Achilles heel' of over-enthusiastic athletes and ball-game players.

The size of the individual muscles is determined in youth and early adult life almost entirely by the amount of physical work that the muscles are called upon to do. Sustained, hard muscular work will ensure that, within the limits of the size and strength of the skeleton, large, healthy muscles are produced.

muscle atrophy

See **amyotrophic lateral sclerosis**.

muscle-attacking cells

See **macrophagic myofasciitis**.

muscle biopsy

This valuable method of investigation involves removal of a small sample of muscle for examination. The muscle sample may be taken under local anaesthesia with little discomfort and, in certain conditions, provides information obtainable in no other way. A wide range of investigations may be performed on the sample and this can throw light on conditions such as muscular dystrophies, rheumatoid arthritis, malnutrition, alcoholism, kidney failure and various endocrine disorders.

Electron microscopy is now revealing subtleties in the ultrastructure of muscle cells, especially in the **mitochondria**, which are throwing new light on the nature of many previously obscure conditions.

muscle cell death

See **Zenker's degeneration**.

muscle, disorders of

See **cardiomyopathy**, **intermittent claudication**, **compartment syndrome**, **cramp**, **dermatomyositis**, **fibroids**, **gangrene**, **muscle spasm**, **muscular dystrophy**, **myasthenia gravis**, **myocarditis**, **myoma**, **tetany**, **tics** and **trichinosis**.

muscle disorders, rare

See **mitochondrial DNA diseases**.

muscle relaxant

A drug capable of reducing tension in muscle or even of causing temporary paralysis. Muscle relaxants have an important place in modern anaesthesia and allow smaller and safer doses of general anaesthetics to be used.

muscle-relaxant drugs

Anaesthetists commonly use drugs, such as tubocurarine (Curare), pancuronium, gallamine and suxamethonium (Scoline) to paralyse muscles and allow safer anaesthesia (see also **depolarizing drugs**). In more general use are some drugs which reduce spasm of voluntary muscles without affecting voluntary movements. These may be useful in nervous system diseases, such as stroke and cerebral palsy, which cause the muscles to go into spasm, and in rheumatic and other diseases featuring painful sustained contraction of muscles. These drugs include baclofen (Lioresal), which is a derivative of one of the body's nerve activators (neuro-transmitters) (GABA), and dantrolene (Dantrium) which acts directly on the muscles.

Other muscle-relaxing drugs are diazepam (Valium), chlormezanone (Trancopal), carisoprodol (Carisoma) and methocarbamol (Robaxin).

muscle spasm

An abnormal state of sustained contraction of a **muscle**. In health, nerve connections from the brain normally exert a dampening or controlling influence on the natural tendency of voluntary muscles to go into spasm. When these connections are damaged, as in **stroke**, cerebral palsy or severe head injury, the controlling influence is removed and a spastic condition of the muscles results. Spastic paralysis is a common feature of stroke.

Muscle spasm can also result from local irritation to the spinal nerves supplying them, as may occur in nerve root pressure from a **slipped disc** (prolapsed intervertebral disc).

muscle spasm, widespread

See **stiff man syndrome**.

muscle wasting

See **motor neuron disease**.

muscle weakness

See **ragged red fibres**, **muscular dystrophy**.

muscular dystrophy

A group of hereditary muscle disorders in which slow, progressive degeneration occurs, leading to increasing weakness and disability. There are three main types of muscular dystrophy.

DUCHENNE

The Duchenne type of dystrophy is caused by a gene on one X (sex) chromosome. Because females have two sex chromosomes and the gene is recessive, this condition is almost confined to males – who have only one X chromosome. The first signs usually appear before the age of three and in most cases the muscles appear bulkier than normal (pseudohypertrophy). The bulk of actual muscle tissue is not, however, increased and there is progressive weakening. This initially affects the buttocks and leg muscles, causing a characteristic waddle in walking. The weakness causes the child to get up from lying in a typical way – by rolling on his or her face and using the arms to push himself or herself up by 'hand-walking' up the legs. Unfortunately, nothing can arrest the progress of the disease, which is usually fatal by the mid teens.

The healthy female carriers of this gene (in one of the X chromosomes) can be detected and counselled. Half the sons of such carriers will develop the disease.

LIMB GIRDLE

Another main form of muscular dystrophy, the limb girdle type, affects the shoulders, pelvic and uppermost limb muscles, has a recessive inheritance and affects both sexes, usually causing severe disablement within 20 years.

FACIO-SCAPULO-HUMERAL

The facio-scapulo-humeral type of muscular dystrophy affects the muscles of the face, upper back and upper arm, and is caused by a dominant gene. It progresses very slowly and does not necessarily shorten life.

musculo

Latin root meaning 'muscle' (meat, contractile tissue).

Muse

A brand name for **alprostadil**.

musicians' overuse syndrome

This common disorder causes pain and loss of function in the upper limb muscles in pianists and string players, or, in the case of wind players, in the muscles of the lips, cheeks, soft palate or throat. It is usually caused by an increase in the workload of playing or practising. The pain may be severe and disabling and may wake the musician at night, hours after a musical session. The pain may spread to muscles not primarily involved in the musical activity. There is often swelling over the affected muscles and sometimes some loss of sensation. Loss of accuracy, agility and speed are common and the loss of function leads to depression.

> Competition in music is so fierce that many young players drive themselves into overuse. But muscles cannot continue to be used indefinitely without harm and continuous sessions of longer than about half an hour are undesirable. A five-minute break every half hour will allow recovery.

TREATMENT

Once the overuse syndrome has developed, much more stringent restrictions have to be applied. Any activity causing pain must be stopped immediately, even if this means, initially, that periods of playing must be limited to about five minutes. Players should, if possible, avoid other activities using the affected muscles. In some cases a radical rest programme, lasting for weeks or months, may be required, and resumption must be very gradual and progressive.

Overuse syndrome is sometimes related to the lack of proper support for the instrument. Supporting posts for clarinets and body-mounted supports for violins and violas may allow musicians to continue to play comfortably.

mutation

Any change in the genetic material (DNA) of a cell is called a mutation. The word comes from the Latin verb *mutare*, meaning 'to change'. A mutation most commonly involves a single gene on a chromosome, but may affect the whole, or a major part of, a chromosome, even causing reduplication so that the number of chromosomes is increased. An extra chromosome 21 (trisomy-21), for instance, causes **Down's syndrome**. Mutations occurring in the chromosomes of the reproductive tissues are inherited if the affected cell happens to take part in fertilization. This is more likely to happen if the mutation occurs in a precursor cell of sperms or ova so that more are affected. Mutations in the DNA of cells other than sex cells cannot be inherited, but can cause cancer.

Agents that raise the probability of mutation above the spontaneous rate are called mutagens. These are present in the environment. Mutagens include X-rays, gamma radiation, ultraviolet light and many chemical substances including some of the 3000 or so compounds in tobacco smoke, and a large number of industrial chemicals. Mutations are rare and most are unfavourable, often leading to the death of the cell or interfering with its power to reproduce. Mutation, however, provides the basis for the variations necessary for evolution by natural selection.

Mutation in a cell in the testes that gives rise to a spermatozoon or an egg (ovum), will be passed on to a clone of sperms or eggs and one of these may take part in fertilization so that the mutation is passed on to every cell in the body of the future individual, including the sex cells. New mutations occurring in the sex cells (germ line mutations) may thus lead to hereditary abnormalities. Mutations in body cells

(somatic mutations) cannot do this but can cause cloned abnormalities including cancers.

See also **frameshift mutation**, **insertion mutation**, **inversion mutation**, **leaky mutant gene**, **lethal mutation**, **missense mutation**, **nonsense mutation**, **point mutation**.

mutism

Dumbness. The inability, or refusal, to speak. Mutism can occur in congenital deafness, an elective refusal to speak, **mental retardation**, severe **manic-depressive illness**, **schizophrenia**, certain forms of brain tumour, water on the brain (**hydrocephalus**) and as a type of **hysteria**.

MXL

A brand name for **morphine**.

Myadec

A brand name for a multivitamin and mineral preparation.

myambutol

Myambutol was formerly a brand name for ethambutol but is now a generic name.

myalgia

Pain in muscle. The term is usually applied to long-term (chronic) conditions, in which there is persistent muscle inflammation (**myositis**) rather than to the muscle pains which commonly follow unaccustomed use or minor injury. Myalgia is a feature of polymyositis and **dermatomyositis**.

See also **polymyalgia rheumatica**.

myalgic encephalitis

Encephalitis means 'inflammation of the brain' and *myalgic* means 'relating to muscle pain'. The concept of myalgic encephalitis (ME) has deeply divided the medical profession for years and has provoked sometimes acrimonious and dismissive argument between those who believe the condition entirely imaginary and those who think it has an organic basis.

There is no questioning the existence of a common entity, affecting predominantly women, although some men – and interesting, both male and female members of the medical profession have been affected – featuring severe **fatigue** and emotional disturbance and made worse by exercise, a single act of which may cause fatigue for weeks. Unfortunately, these effects have been variously associated with a great number of other symptoms and signs, and a range of names has been applied to what may or may not be the same condition. These names include the Royal Free disease, epidemic neuromyasthenia, Otago mystery disease, Icelandic disease, institutional mass hysteria, benign myalgic encephalomyelitis and the post-viral fatigue syndrome.

POSSIBLE CAUSES

Virus infection has been widely proposed as a cause of the syndrome and a wide range of viruses including Coxsackie, herpes, polio, varicella-zoster (chickenpox and shingles) and Epstein-Barr (glandular fever) have been cited. Unfortunately, the finding of antibodies to these or other viruses in people with ME proves nothing – the world is full of people with such antibodies who do not have ME.

Moreover, it is well known that psychological stress increases susceptibility to infection, so even a higher than normal prevalence of these antibodies in ME sufferers would not prove that this was the cause. Extensive immunological studies into people with ME have been inconclusive.

Although the condition is called an encephalitis, none of the normal neurological tests, such as electroencephalography, show that this is present. Some tests on muscle fibres have shown abnormalities in some cases but these have not been universally accepted.

RECOGNITION AND SYMPTOMS

It is clear that the fatigue experienced by ME sufferers is not a matter of the muscles alone and is quite different from the weakness experienced in muscular disorders such as **myasthenia gravis**. The fatigue of ME has a strong cognitive element and is commonly associated with mild to severe depression. A comparison of the bodily (somatic) effects of depression – fatigue, headache, breathlessness, chest pain, dizziness and often bowel upset – with those of ME shows a striking similarity. The prevalences of ME and of depression are also very similar. In some cases the syndrome has responded well to treatment with antidepressant drugs.

THE MEDICAL DEBATE

The basic difficulty, so far as medical attitudes are concerned, stems from two points – medical awareness that complaint of persistent fatigue is often a feature of 'non-organic', 'neurotic' illness in which the sufferer is seeking a resolution of some major personal or social problem; and the failure of medical investigation to find a cause.

Pejorative attitudes on the part of doctors and others have not been helpful and have caused great distress to sufferers who have often been forced to turn to alternative therapists. Whether the condition is of external organic origin or otherwise is, currently, the central point at issue. But it is surely equally important to acknowledge that people whose lives are as severely affected as those of ME sufferers, deserve as much help as any similarly affected people, whatever the cause. Such a gross and persistent disruption of normal living indicates a major disorder of the whole person and can, in no sense, be considered to be 'all in the mind'.

myasthenia gravis

A disease in which muscles weaken abnormally rapidly on use. The symptom becomes worse towards the end of the day and after exercise.

Myasthenia gravis is an **auto-immune disease** caused by an abnormal antibody which blocks or damages the sites at which nerves act on muscle fibres to make them contract. These are called receptor sites and they are stimulated by the **neuro-transmitter** acetylcholine released by the nerve endings. In some cases, the abnormal antibody production is known to be due to an abnormality in the thymus gland, which processes T lymphocytes. In about 15 per cent of cases there is a **benign** tumour of the thymus gland.

INCIDENCE

Myasthenia usually appears after the age of 15 and may start at any age up to about 50. Women are affected about three times as often as men.

RECOGNITION AND SYMPTOMS

In the early years, the disorder tends to be intermittent. Often the first sign is drooping of the eyelids or double vision. Other early signs are difficulty in swallowing, rapid fatigue of

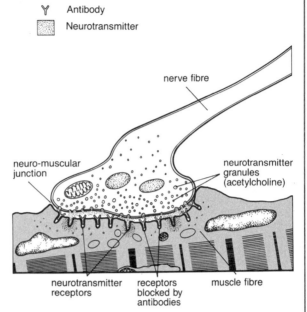

Y Antibody

▨ Neurotransmitter

The problem in myasthenia gravis is that the acetylcholine receptor sites are blocked by abnormal antibodies. The acetylcholine released by the nerve cell ending is thus prevented from starting a muscle fibre contraction.

the chewing muscles, difficulty in speaking and general weakness of the limbs. If weakness of the muscles of respiration occurs, life may be threatened. The ability to cough may be so reduced that there is a risk of asphyxia from accumulated secretions.

The diagnosis of myasthenia is often confirmed by observing the effect of a small injection of the drug Tensilon (edrophonium hydrochloride) which has a brief but specific effect at the nerve-endings, causing an improvement in muscle power within half a minute.

TREATMENT

Acetylcholine is broken down by an enzyme, cholinesterase, and this can be antagonized by drugs such as neostigmine and pyridostigmine. These are called anticholinesterase drugs and are useful in the treatment of myasthenia. Removal of the thymus gland can be helpful and in some cases a procedure to remove the antibodies from the blood (**plasmapheresis**) may be justified.

myc-

Prefix meaning 'fungus' as in mycology (fungus study).

Mycardol

A brand name for pentaerythitol tetranitrate.

-myces

Suffix meaning 'fungus' as in dermatomycosis (skin fungus).

mycetoma

An uncommon tropical disorder in which a tumour-like mass of fungus, or of bacteria that form fungus-like colonies, forms in a limb. The mycetoma is a hard swelling, often involving bone, and with multiple discharging channels from which pus emerges. Amputation may be necessary if surgical drainage and antibiotic or antifungal treatment fail.

Mycifradin

A brand name for **neomycin**.

Myciguent

A brand name for an ointment containing the antibiotic **neomycin**.

mycobacterium avium-intracellulare infection in AIDS

The mycobacteria cause tuberculosis and this member of the family normally causes TB in birds. In the past it has been a rare disease in humans, although not unknown, but in immunocompromised people this infection comes high on the list of probabilities. Post-mortem examinations on people who have died of **AIDS** show that up to 50 per cent have widespread infection with mycobacterium avium-intracellulare (MAI). The lungs, the lymph nodes, the bones, the liver, the blood – all contain the organism – and all parts of the body may show areas of tissue breakdown to form the typical, cheesy masses of dead cells characteristic of TB. Large cavities are likely to be found in the lungs, and abscesses in the muscles or skin. The neck lymph nodes may be severely involved and these may fester and cause a drainage channel (sinus) running to the outside of the skin – a condition called scrofula.

AIDS patients with MAI infection are likely to be very ill, with a number of different conditions, and this particular aspect of opportunistic infection may be concealed by other, more acute, infections. MAI is slow in developing and may be overtaken by pneumocystis pneumonia before it has had time to progress far. Unfortunately, the MAI organism is more resistant to treatment than human TB and a variety of the known anti-tuberculous drugs, used in arbitrary combination, have to be tried in the hope that some effect can be obtained. If the patient survives, treatment will usually have to be continued for at least two years.

Mycobutin

A brand name for **rifabutin**.

mycology

The study of fungi.

mycoplasma

A genus of micro-organisms with the distinction of being the smallest known organism capable of independent existence. Although about the size of some viruses, they can be cultured outside cells. They differ from bacteria, however, in having no cell wall.

One species, *Mycoplasma pneumoniae* often causes outbreaks of pneumonia in institutions and barracks, affecting especially children and young adults. Another, *Mycoplasma hominis*, is thought to be a possible cause of urethritis (see **sexually transmitted diseases**). These organisms are susceptible to tetracycline and erythromycin.

mycophenolate mofetil

An **immunosuppressant drug** used to help to prevent rejection of the donated organ after kidney grafting. A brand name is Cellcept.

mycosis

A disease caused by a fungus.

mycosis fungoides

A **lymphoma**, of T lymphocyte origin, affecting the skin with multiple flat tumours. It usually affects middle-aged men and remains confined to the skin for many years, spreading inwards to the glands and other structures only at a late stage. It may affect any part of the skin, but is commonest on the buttocks, back, or shoulders.

The condition may simulate **eczema** or **psoriasis**, appearing as patches of inflamed, scaly skin. The affected areas may be of odd and variable contour. Only in the late stages do frank tumours appear, with ulceration and sometimes severe itching. Progress to internal malignancy is so slow that affected people often die of other conditions before the disorder can do much harm. Anticancer treatment may be needed.

Mycostatin

A brand name for **nystatin**.

Mydriacyl

A brand name for eye drops containing **tropicamide**.

mydriasis

Widening (dilatation) of the pupil of the eye, whether occurring naturally in dim light or as a result of disease, injury or drugs. See also **Adie's pupil**.

myelin

The fatty, whitish, insulating material surrounding most nerve fibres. Accumulations of nerve cell bodies have a grey appearance but bundles of myelinated fibres look white. Demyelination is the loss of the myelin sheath and is a feature of nerve degeneration and certain nerve diseases. The most important of the demyelinating diseases is **multiple sclerosis** in which plaques of demyelination occur, affecting many adjacent nerve fibres.

myelitis

Inflammation of the spinal cord. This is usually the result of virus infection and the inflammation most commonly involves either the cells at the front of the cord, which are the cell bodies of nerves to the muscles (**motor** nerves), or the cells at the back of the cord – the sensory nerve cells. Myelitis affecting the motor cells at the front is usually called 'polio' (anterior **poliomyelitis**). Posterior poliomyelitis is more usually referred to as **shingles**. Transverse myelitis, affecting a complete cross-section of the cord, often follows a viral infection but may occur for no obvious reason. It causes paralysis of the body below the level involved. Recovery is variable, but may be complete.

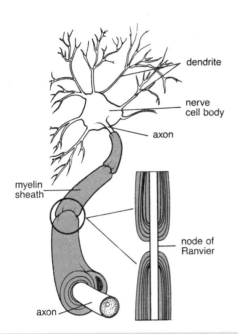

Myelin is a fatty material that acts as a kind of insulator for long nerve fibres (axons) so that nerve impulses can pass normally. Damage to myelin blocks the passage of nerve impulses with serious results.

been used extensively in the investigation of 'slipped disc', tumours of the spinal cord, and various disorders of the nerve roots. Since the development of the CT and MRI scanners myelography is less often done as the newer and less invasive imaging methods are safer and more comfortable.

myeloma, multiple

See **lymphoma**.

myelomeningocele

See **myelocele**.

Mygdalon

A brand name for the **anti-emetic** drug **metoclopramide**.

myiasis

Infestation of any of the tissues of the body by the larvae of **flies**. Human myiasis is rare in temperate climates, but in the tropics it is common for wounds to become fly-blown and maggoty. Although unpleasant to observe, surface maggots seem to have

myelo-

Prefix meaning 'spinal cord' as in myelitis (cord inflammation).

myelocele

The spinal cord and its coverings, the meninges, lie within a bony canal running down inside the spine (vertebral column). If, as a result of a failure of normal development of the spine, some of the bone forming arches around the back of the spinal cord is missing, the cord and the meninges can protrude backwards to form a swelling under the skin. This is called a myelocele. The bony defect is called **spina bifida**. More correctly, the term should be meningomyelocele or myelomeningocele.

myelodysplasic syndrome

A group of uncommon bone marrow disorders featuring reduced blood cell production with abnormal granular white cells, especially the neutrophil polymorphonuclear leukocytes, and resulting in **anaemia** which is very difficult to treat. The neutrophils have reduced activity against organisms, so there is increased risk of infection. The syndrome affects elderly people and tends to progress to acute myeloid **leukaemia**. Bone marrow transplantation can produce long-term remission in younger patients.

myelography

Plain X-rays show little if any detail of the spinal cord, the spinal nerves or other soft tissues within the spinal canal. These tissues are surrounded by bone, which is much more opaque to X-rays than the soft tissue. By injecting a liquid opaque to X-rays (a contrast medium) into the cerebrospinal fluid, however, the outline of this fluid can readily be shown and protrusions into it demonstrated.

The radio-opaque liquid contains iodine and is introduced by lumbar puncture. By tilting the patient, the fluid can be moved to different parts of the spinal canal surrounding the cord, and X-ray pictures taken. The method has

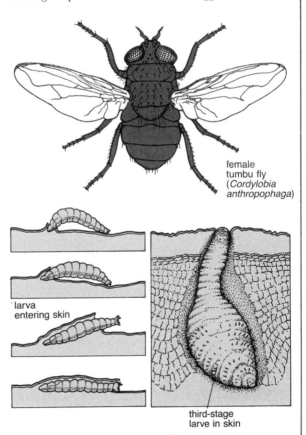

female tumbu fly (*Cordylobia anthropophaga*)

larva entering skin

third-stage larve in skin

Myiasis is body infestation with fly larvae. This illustration shows the African tumbu fly whose first-stage larva can penetrate the skin and grow to form a boil-like swelling.

a cleansing effect and remove dead and devitalized tissue. Maggoty wounds usually heal well after the maggots are removed.

The larvae of the African tumbu fly penetrate the skin to produce boil-like swellings, each with an opening through which the larva breathes. On maturity, the adult fly emerges. The botfly lays its eggs on a mosquito, which leaves them on human skin while feeding. The larvae then penetrate, producing a painful, itchy spot like a severe mosquito bite. Close inspection may show the end of the larva protruding through the skin.

Some fly larvae have the power to penetrate deeply into areas such as the sinuses around the nose, causing great destruction to the face. Others may be swallowed and cause abdominal pain, cramps, vomiting and diarrhoea.

Mylanta

A brand name for a mixture of aluminium hydroxide, magnesium hydroxide and simethicone.

Myleran

A brand name for **busulphan**.

Mynah

A brand name for the anti-**tuberculosis** drug ethambutol.

myo-

Prefix meaning 'muscle' as in **myalgia** (muscle pain).

myocardial infarction

See **heart attack**.

myocarditis

See **heart, inflammation of**.

myoclonus

An involuntary sudden muscle contraction causing a limb or other part to make a rapid, uncontrollable jerk or movement. Myoclonus is common in normal healthy people, usually occurring just before falling asleep. It is also a feature of epilepsy and of certain other nerve diseases.

Myocrisin

A brand name for **sodium aurothiomalate**.

myoma

A noncancerous (benign) tumour of muscle. The commonest sites for this type of tumour are in the womb (uterus) and in the intestine. The operation for removal of a myoma is called 'myomectomy'.

myopathy

Any disease of muscle, such as **muscular dystrophy**.

myopia

Short-sightedness. The origins of the term *myopia* have been disputed, but it probably comes from the Greek word *myo-*

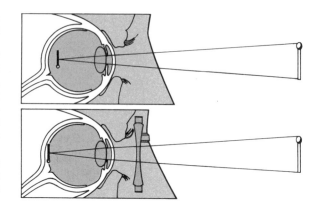

In myopia, or short sight, the converging power of the eye is too strong relative to its length. Vision in myopia is corrected with weakening lenses that allow less strongly converging rays to enter the eye so that they can focus on the retina.

meaning 'muscle' and *opia* means vision. Prior to the introduction of spectacles, myopes had no resource except to peer through narrowed lids and so producing the 'muscular eye'.

Myopia is a condition in which the focusing power of the eye is too strong so that the images of distant objects come to a focus in front of the proper focal plane (the retina). Rays from near objects, however, are diverging more when they enter the eye, and these focus further back, often on the retina. The result is that a myopic person cannot see distant objects clearly, but sees near objects well.

POSSIBLE CAUSES

The condition is not, as is usually stated, invariably due to the eyeball being too long, but is the result of a failure of the proper relationship between the curvature of the cornea, the axial length of the eye, and the power and position of the internal crystalline lens. The corneal power in normally myopic people varies over a wide range, having a radius of curvature anywhere from about 6 mm to over 8 mm. So myopia may occur in an eye with a very steeply curved cornea, even if the length is less than average. In the less common higher degrees of myopia, the eyeball is always too long and may be from 2 – 14 mm longer than normal. To compensate for myopia, weakening (minus or concave) lenses are needed.

COURSE

Myopia usually appears around puberty, but may present at any age up to about 25. It is rare for myopia to appear after body growth is complete. The earlier it starts, the higher the final degree is likely to be. People with high degree myopia have almost always started in early childhood or infancy. Those whose myopia appears late in adolescence never develop high myopia. Since the condition is of dimensional origin, it is not surprising to find that it runs in families.

COMPLICATIONS

Myopia is, in most cases, no more than a nuisance, calling for contact lenses or spectacles. But in the higher degrees there is a significantly raised probability of eye trouble such as **retinal detachment**, retinal degeneration and bleeding (haemorrhages).

TREATMENT

Myopia is increasingly being treated by corneal 'sculpturing' with an excimer laser that vaporizes the surface layers in a controlled manner so as to flatten the curvature and reduce the optical power of the eye, thereby making it less short-sighted. The results appear to be good and the incidence of side-effects low.

It is worth noting, however, that the opinions of people lucratively engaged in performing this ten-minute operation might possibly be biased in its favour. The same degree of enthusiasm was formerly shown by some ophthalmologists engaged in the operation of radial keratotomy for myopia, and this procedure has now been generally abandoned.

myopia cure

See **excimer laser refractive surgery**.

Myoquine

A brand name for quinine.

myos

Greek root meaning 'muscle' as in myalgia (muscle pain).

myositis

Inflammation of muscle. This may occur as a result of virus infection, as in **Bornholm's disease**, or it may be a response to cancer elsewhere in the body.

myotonia congenita

A dominantly inherited genetic disease in which the only symptom is the inability to relax muscles normally after they have been contracted. If something is grasped, it can be released only slowly and with great difficulty. If the eyes are tightly shut, it may be many seconds before they can be opened again. In early life, the muscles are sometimes unusually powerful.

myringoplasty

The surgical repair of a hole (perforation) in an eardrum, usually by **microsurgery**. This is done to improve hearing. Various materials may be used to repair the defect, including a small piece of the tendinous sheath (fascia) of the temporal muscle. The term is sometimes also used to refer to a more extensive and elaborate repair involving not only the drum but also the tiny, delicate chain of middle ear bones (the ossicles) which link the drum to the inner ear.

myringotomy

A surgical incision made in the eardrum. This may be done to allow the insertion of a grommet in cases of 'glue ear'

(secretory **otitis media**) so as to drain the middle ear and relieve deafness. Rarely, the operation may be needed to release pus and relieve pressure in the middle ear in cases of acute otitis media, so as to prevent dangerous internal spread of infection. This is seldom required, nowadays, but was a common operation in the pre-antibiotic era.

Myringotomy is usually performed under general anaesthesia, using an operating microscope and a fine scalpel, with a very small blade, which is introduced through a conical **speculum** pushed into the ear canal.

Mysoline

A brand name for the **anticonvulsant** drug primidone, used in the control of **epilepsy**.

Mysteclin

A brand name for a mixture of the **antifungal** drug **nystatin** and the antibiotic **tetracycline**.

myxa

Greek root meaning 'phlegm' as in myxomatosis (disease featuring mucus).

myxoedema

A term used to describe the general effects of severe underactivity of the thyroid gland. This occurs in women five times as often as in men. The skin is dry and scaly, cold, thickened and coarse. The hair is scanty, coarse and brittle. Often the eyebrows are greatly thinned or even partly absent. The lips are thickened and mauve-coloured and there is **halitosis**. The affected person does not complain, but is lethargic, readily fatigued, slowed in body and mind and suffers muscle aches, loss of menstruation, deafness, **angina pectoris**, **heart failure**, **anaemia** and **constipation**.

All these effects can be reversed by the administration of thyroid hormones.

myxoma

An uncommon, jelly-like benign tumour consisting of soft mucoid material. Myxomas are most commonly found under the skin but are of special interest as they may, rarely, occur within one of the chambers of the heart. In this situation a myxoma may give rise to blood clots which can be released as emboli to cause trouble by obstructing small blood vessels in various parts of the body. A myxoma in the heart may also interfere with the flow of blood through the heart, but may be removed by a surgical operation.

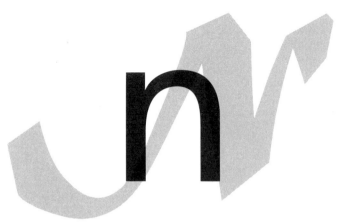

nabumetone

A non-steroidal anti-inflammatory drug (**NSAID**) used to treat **arthritis** and other painful conditions. A brand name is Relifex.

nadolol

A non-selective beta-blocker drug that acts on all beta-adrenergic receptor sites. A brand name is Corgard.

nafarelin

A gonadotrophin releasing hormone analogue drug used to treat **endometriosis** and infertility. A brand name is Synarel.

naftidrofuryl

An artery-widening drug used to improve the blood supply to the brain and to the limbs. A brand name is Praxilene.

nail-biting

A common habit-pattern, symbolic of anxiety, but no more than a mild habit disorder, or an indication of boredom. Nail-biting may start as early as one year of age and becomes increasingly common up to about the age of 12. There is no reason to suppose that nail-biting is an indication of any emotional disorder.

Some nail-biters, however, carry the habit to the extremity of causing actual damage to the fingertips by nibbling at the cuticles and causing secondary infection of the fingers and nail beds. The effect is markedly unsightly and, with growing consciousness of the importance of personal appearance, the adolescent nail-biter will often find the discipline to desist. Bitter-tasting applications may help to remind the biter of the resolution.

Nail-biting is a feature of severe mental retardation and of some cases of paranoid **schizophrenia**.

nails

The nails are protective covers for the vulnerable finger and toe ends and provide useful tools for many manipulative purposes: When we feel with the fingertips, the nails exert counter-pressure.

The nail consists of a curved plate of a tough protein called keratin, resting on the nail bed and growing outwards from the growth zone (nail matrix). The base of each nail shows a variable-sized 'half moon'. The inturned skin edge

around the nail is called the nail fold. The cuticle is the free skin edge over the half moon.

Fingernails take four to five months to grow from matrix to fingertip, growing at a rate of about 1 cm in three months. Toenails take about three times as long.

nails, disorders of

Because of their position, and the constant use of the hands, fingernails are vulnerable to injury. Commonly, as a result of injury, a collection of blood (a **haematoma**) forms under the nail, and this may affect nail adhesion. Detachment of the nail from its bed is called onycholysis. Apart from injury, this may be caused by **psoriasis**, fungus infection and **thyrotoxicosis**. The separation usually starts at the tip and extends backwards. Air under the nail gives it a greyish-white colour. A complete, spontaneous shedding of one or more nails can occur in any severe illness as this can lead to a sudden cessation of nail growth and lack of adhesion of the plate to the bed.

Toenails are also susceptible to injury, often repeated, and this may lead to a condition of very marked thickening and claw-like curving, known as **onychogryphosis**.

Paronychia, the infection of the soft tissue around the nail, is probably the commonest of all nail disorders. There is pain, swelling and inflammation, and sometimes pus appears at the nail edge. The condition usually results from repeated minor injury and working conditions which make hand care difficult. Fungus infection of the nails (onychomycosis) is common and causes thickening, distortion and separation. It is hard to treat but will respond to the drug griseofulvin which must be taken for at least a year. Unfortunately there may be side-effects.

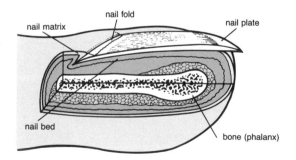

Section of a fingernail.

Small point-like depressions (pits) occur in **psoriasis** and in **alopecia** areata. Single horizontal ridges that move along, with growth, towards the tip may indicate a previous illness. Multiple horizontal ridges suggest infection in the skin around the nail bed. Longitudinal ridges occur in alopecia areata, psoriasis and **lichen planus**. Nail thickening is common in psoriasis and fungus infection.

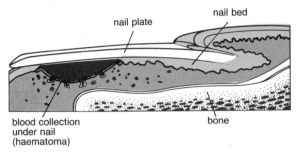

Trauma to the tip of a finger or toe commonly results in a local collection of blood under the nail plate. Such a haematoma may result in sufficient separation of the plate from the bed that the nail becomes loose.

nails, pseudo-splinters under

Often called splinter haemorrhages, these are actually streaks of blood, but closely resemble splinters. They may occur in healthy people as a result of injury but can be a sign of a serious heart disorder, infective endocarditis. If these occur, it would be as well to seek medical advice.

nalbufine

An opiate drug used to control moderate to severe pain. A brand name is Nubain.

Nalcrom

A brand name for **sodium cromoglycate**.

nalidixic acid

A quinolone antibiotic drug, effective against gram negative bacilli, including Proteus species, and much used for urinary infections. Trade names are Negram, Uriben and, formulated with alkalizing drugs, Mictral.

Nalorex

A brand name for **naltrexone**.

naloxone

A narcotic antagonist drug that can be life-saving in cases of **morphine** or other opioid poisoning. The drug is similar to morphine in chemical structure and occupies morphine receptor sites on cell membranes, so preventing morphine from acting. A small dose of the drug, given to a morphine addict, can induce withdrawal symptoms within a matter of minutes. A trade name is Narcan.

naltrexone

A narcotic antagonist used as a maintenance therapy in former narcotic addicts. A brand name is Nalorex.

nandrolone decanoate

A male sex hormone with **anabolic** properties. The drug is sometimes used also to stimulate blood cell production in **aplastic anaemia**. A brand name is Deca-Durabolin.

nanobacteria

Exceptionally small micro-organisms that resemble bacteria but are less than 0.1 micrometre long and are surrounded by a mineralized shell. It is claimed by some experts that cells infected with these bacteria develop mineral deposits, and may be the cause of kidney stones and other diseases that feature calcification. Others have suggested that these are simply normal bacteria that have shrunk and become calcified.

naphazoline

An **adrenergic** drug that causes small blood vessels to constrict and thus reduces congestion in mucous membranes. It may be taken as a nasal spray. A brand name is Antistin Privine.

nappy rash

Simple nappy rash may affect the whole nappy area or may be localized to the area around the anus. There will be obvious discomfort and much crying. An extensive rash is usually caused by prolonged contact with a wet nappy in which bacterial decomposition of the urine has resulted in the formation of ammonia. One can readily smell the ammonia in these cases, and it is highly irritating to tender baby skin.

The remedy is to change the nappies frequently and to try to keep the nappy area as clean and free from contamination as possible. Disposable nappies are preferable to towelling, but are more expensive. Disposable liners are helpful. Since the problem is primarily due to breakdown of urea by bacteria, a mild antiseptic in conjunction with good standards of hygiene will help. Terry cotton nappies must be very carefully washed and sterilized. Biological washing powder will sometimes act as an irritant, so thorough rinsing is important.

A rash confined to the area around the anus may be due to irritants in the baby's faeces and this is likely to be associated with **diarrhoea**. There may be obvious pain on bowel movement. The diarrhoea must be attended to without delay, and the area kept as clean as possible. A bland protective barrier cream (e.g., zinc and castor oil) can be valuable. Waterproof pants should be used only when strictly necessary.

Persistent rashes in the nappy area encourage secondary infection with thrush (candidiasis). *Candida albicans* infection is common in babies and the fungus may be present in the bowel. Rashes lasting for over two weeks should arouse suspicion and professional advice should be obtained.

Naprogesic

A brand name for **naproxen**.

Naprosyn

A brand name for **naproxen**.

naproxen

A non-steroidal anti-inflammatory drug (**NSAID**). Trade names are Naprosyn, Nycopren, Synflex and, formulated with the prostaglandin drug **misoprostol**, Napratec.

naratriptan

A serotonin agonist drug used to treat migraine. It is believed to act by narrowing the brain arteries that are widened during a migraine attack. A brand name is Naramig.

Narcan

A brand name for **naloxone**.

narce

Greek root meaning 'numb' as in narcotic (drug that numbs pain).

Nardil

A brand name for the antidepressant drug **phenelzine**.

narcissism

Exaggerated self-regard. A narcissistic person is so much in love with himself or herself that normal relationships with others, and especially love relationships, are impossible. Freud used the concept to account for the inability of the subject of psychoanalysis to fall in love with the analyst (transference). As in other cases, Freud derived this term from his knowledge of mythology. Narcissus was a handsome youth who fell in love with his own image reflected in a pond, and died of frustration at its lack of response.

The narcissistic personality disorder features an overwhelming sense of one's own importance, a constant and exhibitionistic need for attention, admiration and praise, high sensitivity to criticism, a tendency to over-value one's accomplishments and often a habit of fantasizing about one's own amazing success in the world of wealth and power. The narcissistic approach to life is fostered and reflected by much of the glossy advertising to which we are now all exposed.

narcolepsy

See **cataplexy**.

narcosis

This term is derived from the Greek word *narke* meaning 'numbness'. It means a sleep-like or stuporous state, caused by a drug, from which the affected person cannot immediately be fully aroused.

narcotic

A drug which, in appropriate dosage, produces sleep and relieves pain. Overdosage of narcotics may cause coma and death. Most narcotics are derived from opium or are synthetic substances chemically related to **morphine**.

narcotic drugs

See **analgesic drugs**.

Naropin

A brand name for **ropivacaine**.

Narphen

A brand name for the narcotic **analgesic** drug **phenazocine**.

Nasacort

A brand name for **triamcinolone**.

nasal congestion

'Stuffiness' of the nose caused by a variable degree of obstruction to the air flow from swelling of the lining mucous membrane. This is most commonly caused by a common cold virus infection, but may be due to **hay fever** (allergic **rhinitis**) or **sinusitis**.

Nasal congestion can be temporarily relieved by decongestant drugs taken as drops or sprays, but these are liable to cause 'rebound' congestion, which may be worse than before. Once the cause has resolved the congestion should settle. If it does not, medical advice should be sought.

nasal discharge

Watery discharge, becoming thick and yellow from pus formation as secondary infection develops, is a feature of the common cold. The discharge in **hay fever** (allergic **rhinitis**) is usually watery and clear.

nasal obstruction

The commonest cause of obstruction to the nasal airway is **nasal congestion**, but this may also result from greatly enlarged **adenoids**, nasal polyps, or, rarely, a tumour in the nose. One-sided blockage is very common and this is usually due to deflection to one side of the central partition of the nose (the nasal septum). This may be natural or the result of injury.

> A constant, clear, watery drip from the nose following an injury may indicate a fracture of the base of the skull with leakage of cerebrospinal fluid from between the membranes surrounding the brain. In such a case, there is a danger of meningitis and treatment is essential.

nasal septum, disorders of

The nasal septum is the thin, central partition that divides the airway of the nose into two passages. At the front, the skeleton of the septum is made of a thin plate of cartilage; behind it is made of bone. The whole septum is covered with **mucous membrane**.

A degree of deflection of the septum to one side (deviated septum) is very common and usually causes no trouble. If breathing is obstructed, the septum can be straightened surgically. Sometimes a blow to the nose may cause blood to collect between the cartilage and the mucous membrane and form a **haematoma**. This may obstruct breathing and may become infected to cause an abscess, which might have to be opened surgically. Sometimes a hole develops in the septum as a result of damage from persistent infection or from sniffing cocaine.

Bleeding often occurs from small blood vessels on the septum, near the front, especially if there is persistent nose-picking. Severe bleeding from this site may require cauterization of the small artery concerned.

NASOGASTRIC TUBE

Sometimes called a 'Ryle's tube', this is a soft rubber or plastic tube about half a millimetre in diameter. When one end is lubricated, it can easily be passed through the nose and down the gullet (oesophagus) into the stomach.

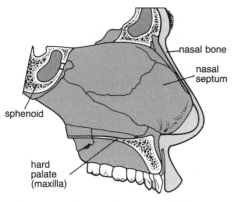

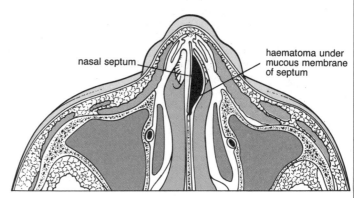

The partition between the two nasal air passages, the nasal septum, is part bone, part cartilage and is covered with a mucous membrane. A blow to the nose can cause bleeding between the septum and the mucous membrane and a haematoma may develop.

A nasogastric tube may be used to supply nutrition to a person too ill to swallow easily, or to take samples of the stomach contents by suction with a syringe. In obstruction to the bowel, it is essential to keep the stomach empty, and this is one of the most important uses of the nasogastric tube.

The nasogastric tube is too narrow in bore to be suitable for stomach washout in cases of poisoning and a wider tube, inserted through the mouth, is used in these cases.

naso

Latin root meaning 'nose' as in nasal (of the nose).

Nasobec

A brand name for **beclomethasone**.

Natrilix

A brand name for the thiazide **diuretic** drug **indapamide**.

natriuretic factor

People with persistent **heart failure** have higher than normal levels of a protein-like substance, known as atrial natriuretic factor, in their blood. This substance, which was discovered in 1981 and has been intensively studied ever since, causes blood vessels to widen and increases the output of urine. It appears to have a selective action on the kidneys which, by relieving oedema, is beneficial to those with heart failure and shows promise of being useful in treatment.

Natulan

A brand name for the anticancer drug procarbazine.

natural childbirth

This term was used by pioneers of prepared, or educated childbirth, such as the English gynaecologist Grantly Dick-Read (1890–1959) and others, including Margaret Gamper and Elizabeth Bing, to try to attract women to the concept that giving birth is, or should be, a normal and natural process rather than a kind of medical or surgical disorder. The work of these pioneers has proved invaluable to countless millions of women who have found that a clear and full understanding of what to expect, and instruction in relax-

ation and cooperation, can make labour much less difficult and painful, and more rewarding.

The preparation is primarily psychological and is based, in part, on an understanding of the nature of pain and of how this is influenced by the state of mind and the condition of tension in the muscles. Women are shown how fear and ignorance breed muscle tension and a state of mind in which the perception of, and sensitivity to, pain are much higher than necessary.

The movement is now part of the routine of childbirth and is available to almost all women who want it. Those approaching a first labour are strongly advised to attend classes.

natural killer cells

A class of large granular lymphocytes that bind directly to cells bearing foreign **antigens** and kill them. Natural killer cells do not require prior exposure of the immune system to the antigen and kill their victims by programmed cell death (**apoptosis**). They are components of innate immunity rather than of acquired immunity.

natural remedies

HISTORY

Natural remedies go back a long way. Many must have been known to man since the dawn of civilization. First came the accidental finding that many plants or minerals were dangerous, causing alarming symptoms and sometimes death, but did occasionally seem to help in various disorders. The berries of the deadly nightshade, *Atropa belladonna*, caused blurred vision, dry mouth, red skin, convulsions and death. *Cascara sagrada* beans caused violent purgation. Ergot of rye caused gangrene and, in pregnant women, abortion. Chewing the leaves of the coca plant numbed the mouth, but relieved hunger and fatigue and induced a pleasant state of mind. Eating the bark of the Chinchona tree caused excitement, confusion, singing in the ears and deafness.

Later, word of mouth knowledge of this kind was systematized in medical and other herbals and much empirical but valuable knowledge was preserved. There were many of these herbals – they date back at least to early Roman times – and the later versions, such as those of Konrad von Megenberg (1475), John Gerard (1597) and John Parkinson (1640), drew heavily on earlier books. Extensive borrowing can be traced from works as early as those of Pliny the Elder or

Dioscorides. Unfortunately, the tendency to allow imagination and wishful thinking to fill the gaps in real knowledge was as common in authors then as it is today. So, much dross was mixed with the gold and, as always, the items most reliably perpetuated from century to century were those prompting the greatest wonder and amazement.

But some of the empirical fact was remarkable. The foxglove, *Digitalis purpurea*, was widely recommended and used for the dropsy (oedema), long before Dr William Withering published an account in 1785 of the action of the dried seeds on the heart. Today it is a medical commonplace that the oedema of heart failure can be cleared by the action of digitalis in improving the heart's efficiency. Nicholas Culpeper (1649), perhaps the most celebrated of all the herbalists, knew of the drug but warned readers about the side-effects: 'The operation of this herb is often violent even in small doses: it is best not to meddle with it, lest the cure should end in the churchyard.'

In the 19th century, those natural remedies with obvious action, and no immediate tendency to kill off patients, were enthusiastically embraced and were extensively recommended – not always for appropriate purposes. Laudanum (tincture of opium), a powerful analgesic and tranquillizer, was, until 100 years ago, wildly popular for the treatment of everything from cancer to tuberculosis. Hashish, too, had a wide and uncritical following. But some applications were sensible. *Claviceps purpurea* (ergot) was used in obstetrics and in the symptomatic treatment of migraine. *Datura stramonium* (jimson weed) and *Hyoscyamus niger* (henbane) were used to relax muscle spasm, relieve travel sickness and treat Parkinsonism. *Veratrum album* (white hellebore) was used for high blood pressure.

PHARMACEUTICALS OF TODAY

The entire pharmaceutical industry was, of course, initially founded on natural remedies. Until the 1930s the pharmacist's shop was a child's delight of hundreds of mysterious drawers and rows of beautiful bottles labelled with strange names such as Fol. Rosmarini (rosemary leaves), Ext. Rhubarb., Ext. Glycyrrh. (liquorice), Cinnamon bark, Tinct, Capsic.(Cayenne Pepper), Tinct. Benz, Co., Senna Pod, Balsamum Peru., Gentian Violet, Tinct. Nux. Vom. (strychnine) and so on. These and hundreds of other plant derivatives were all natural remedies, and were compounded by the pharmacist, on the spot, into pills, powders, draughts, infusions, tinctures and mixtures in accordance with an elaborate prescription.

But by the 1950s, the active ingredients – mostly alkaloids – of the valuable plant drugs had all been isolated and their pharmacology worked out. By then, most of the old and much-tried natural 'remedies' had long since been abandoned as largely useless. Pharmaceuticals were becoming big business and there was a large and ready market for any drug of real value. Nothing of clinical or commercial use was wasted. The search was on, and every useful natural preparation was incorporated into the Pharmacopoeia.

Rightly, the remainder – things like *Sambucus nigra* (elder), *Matricaria chamomilla* (camomile), *Allium sativum* (garlic), *Anisum vulgare* (anise), *Anethum graveolens* (dill), *Thymus vulgaris* (thyme) – were either junked or relegated to the back shelves as of minor medical importance.

TWENTIETH-CENTURY RESURGENCE

People with a revulsion against scientific medicine are inclined to turn back to the 'natural remedies'. There is little harm in this so long as the selected 'remedies' are not biochemically active. It should be remembered that those natural plant and animal products with pharmacological action are all liable to be dangerous. They should on no account be selected from nature. Packaged 'remedies' are, on the whole, safe, but there have been many reports of undesirable side-effects.

naturopathy

A philosophy featuring the justifiable suspicion that the body can be damaged by artificial additives to the diet, insecticides, hormones, fertilizers and other environmental contaminants. To that extent naturopathy is acceptable. But some proponents go further and claim that all disease can be cured by restricting oneself to a 'natural' diet, largely vegetarian, and free from all possible contaminants. This, regrettably, is manifest nonsense and adherence to such a view can be dangerous.

nausea

The feeling of sickness which often precedes vomiting.
See **anti-emetic drugs**.

nausia

Greek root meaning 'sea sickness' as in nausea (feeling of sickness). The root *naus* means 'a ship'.

Navelbine

A brand name for **vinorelbine**.

Navoban

A brand name for **tropisetron**.

Navridex

A brand name for thiazide **diuretic** drug cyclopenthiazide.

Nazen

A brand name for **naproxen**.

nebulizer

A form of inhaler used mainly in the control and treatment of **asthma**. Nebulizers deliver an aerosol of the active drug in water or other vehicle. Some are electrically operated.

neck, broken

Fracture, with dislocation, of any of the vertebrae of the neck. This commonly results from car accidents, diving into shallow water, crushing industrial injuries or gunshot wounds. The significance of a broken neck is not in the bony injury but in the almost inevitable associated injury to the spinal cord. The head is much heavier than is generally appreciated, so a powerful shearing force may be applied to the soft nerve tissue in the event of a fracture. For the same reason, 'whiplash' injuries are dangerous and sometimes cause severe injury to the spinal cord.

When the spinal cord is completely severed, in the course of a neck fracture, there is paralysis of the whole body below the neck (quadriplegia). All voluntary movement and sensa-

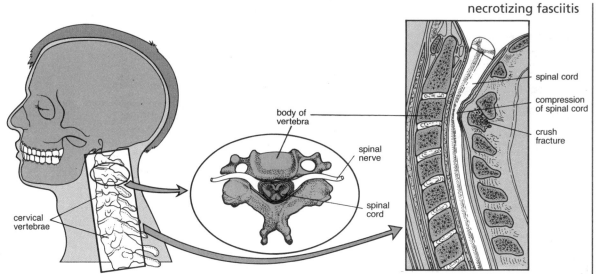

The major danger of a broken neck is injury to the spinal cord by compression or even severance. This causes paralysis of the body below the level of the cord injury. High cord injuries are often fatal.

tion subserved by nerves joining or leaving the cord below the level of the injury are immediately and permanently lost.

neck instability

See **atlanto-axial instability**.

neck, rigid

See **meningitis**.

neck rigidity

Stiffness and pain on movement caused by spasm of the neck and spinal muscles. This is a cardinal sign of **meningitis**.

neck swelling

Because the structures within the neck are packed so closely together, swelling of any of them may be dangerous. Swelling may arise from inflammation, allergy, bleeding, or tumours and may cause interference with breathing. Swelling (oedema) of the mucous membrane lining of larynx from a bee sting or allergy may close off the air passage altogether and **tracheostomy** may be necessary to save life. Tumours or other swellings in the neck may also interfere with swallowing.

neck vertebra, second

See **axis bone**.

neck vertebra, upper

See **atlas bone**.

necrophilia

A form of sexual deviation in which sexual intercourse is performed with a dead body. On the face of it, this would seem a somewhat limiting propensity and the likelihood is that necrophilia is more often a product of gothic romance than of actuality.

necropsy

An alternative term for an **autopsy**, or postmortem examination, of a body. The term is little used.

necrosis

Death of a body tissue. Gangrene. The commonest cause of necrosis is inadequacy or loss of blood supply (ischaemia), but tissue death can result from overwhelming local infection; physical injury from heat, cold or trauma; chemical injury, as from corrosive substances; or radiational injury from X-rays, gamma rays or other forms of radiation.

necrotizing enterocolitis

A serious disorder featuring patches or diffuse area of tissue death (necrosis) in the small or large intestine, especially in premature infants but also sometimes in full-term babies. It is most likely to affect babies that are poorly, especially those with congenital heart disease or respiratory distress syndrome. A severe infection with the organism is almost always present. The condition has been ascribed to overdosage with the antioxidant vitamin E, which may interfere with the oxygen free radicals needed by **phagocytes** to perform their immunological function.

necrotizing fasciitis

An uncommon but severe form of tissue damage caused by a streptococcus of Group A. The superficial **fascia** is the layer of fatty tissue under the skin. Fasciitis is inflammation of this layer and, in this form of the condition, the effect is so intense that the tissue appears, in places, almost to be 'eaten away'.

RECOGNITION AND SYMPTOMS

There is severe pain, marked general upset and intense redness of the overlying skin. Surgical exploration shows grey, swollen fat that can be stripped out easily with the finger.

> Surgical shock and failure of various organs, such as the kidneys, may occur and the outcome, in inadequately managed or late treated cases, is often fatal.

TREATMENT

Treatment is by massive doses of antibiotics such as 2500 mg of benzyl penicillin four hourly and Clindamycin

515

600–1200 mg six-hourly, by early radical surgery to remove infected tissue and by exposure to high oxygen concentrations in a special chamber (**hyperbaric oxygen treatment**). The latter is the most important part of the treatment; inadequate surgery results in a mortality of 30 to 60 per cent.

nedocromil

An anti-inflammatory drug used to treat hay fever, seasonal allergic **conjunctivitis** and bronchial **asthma**. Trade names are Rapitil and Tilade.

needle exchange programmes

AIDS and **hepatitis B** are commonly spread among intravenous drug abusers by cross-infection as a result of sharing needles for drug abuse. An effective public health measure to reduce the prevalence of these conditions is the free provision of sterile needles and syringes in exchange for used equipment. It is now estimated that about half of new HIV infections are caused by needle sharing, and many research studies have shown that this is a valuable measure that does not encourage illegal drug usage. Almost alone among developed countries, the USA continues, presumably for political reasons, to refuse to adopt these programmes.

nefazodone

A **selective serotonin re-uptake inhibitor** drug used to treat depression. A brand name is Dutonin.

nefopam hydrochloride

A pain-killing drug. A brand name is Acupan.

Negram

A brand name for **nalidixic acid**.

Nembudeine

A brand name for a mixture of the painkillers **paracetamol** and codeine and the sedative **pentobarbitone**.

Nembutal

A brand name for the barbiturate sedative **pentobarbitone**.

Neo-Cortef

A brand name for a preparation, for external use, containing the anti-inflammatory **hydrocortisone** and the antibiotic **neomycin**.

Neo-Cytamen

A brand name for **hydroxocobalamin**.

Neo-Hycor

A brand name for eye preparations containing the anti-inflammatory drug **hydrocortisone** and the antibiotic **neomycin**.

Neo-Medrol

A brand name for a skin preparation containing the steroid drug **methylprednisolone** and the antibiotic **neomycin**.

Neo-Mercazole

A brand name for **carbimazole**.

neomycin

An aminoglycoside antibiotic drug derived from a strain of *Streptomyces fradiae*. Neomycin can be given by mouth to destroy organisms in the bowel or can be used in solution to irrigate the bladder. It is poorly absorbed into the bloodstream. It is much too toxic to be given by injection and can have seriously damaging effects on hearing and on the kidneys. The drug is widely used as a surface application in ointments, usually with other ingredients such as steroids. Trade names are Nivemycin and Minims neomycin. Preparations of neomycin with a corticosteroid, for external use, include Betnesol-N, Dermovate-NN, Maxitrol, Neo-Cortef, Predsol-N and Synalar-N.

neonatologist

An American term, beginning to be used in Britain, for a doctor specializing in the care of newborn babies. This important branch of paediatrics handles the special problems of premature or low-weight babies and those born with congenital abnormalities. The neonatologist takes charge during the first four weeks of life, after which the child comes under the care of a general paediatrician.

Neophryn

A brand name for **phenylephrine**.

neoplasm

Literally, a 'new growth'. This is the result of an abnormal local increase in the numbers of body cells so that a mass of cells develops called a tumour or neoplasm. A neoplasm may be malignant (cancerous) and spread both locally and distantly; or it may be benign and form a local, usually encapsulated mass. See also **cancer**.

Neoplatin

A brand name for cisplatin.

neostigmine

A drug used to treat **myasthenia gravis**. Neostigmine interferes with the enzyme that breaks down the neuro-transmitter acetylcholine and so prolongs its action. A brand name is Robinul neostigmine.

Neotigason

A brand name for **acitretin**.

Nepenthe

A brand name for **morphine**.

nephrectomy

Surgical removal of a kidney. *Nephros* is Greek for kidney.
WHY IT'S DONE
Nephrectomy may be necessary because of cancer of the kidney or of the urine-collecting system (the pelvis of the kidney

and the ureter), severe infection of the kidney with malfunctioning, especially if this is causing raised blood pressure, multiple large kidney stones interfering with kidney function, or severe injury and uncontrollable bleeding.

HOW IT'S DONE

The operation is performed under general anaesthesia and the incision is made in the loin just under the lower ribs. The kidney is freed from its capsule of fat and brought up into the wound. The ureter and the major blood vessels of the kidney are identified and clamped, the artery being clamped before the vein. **Ligatures** are then applied round each clamped part and each is tightly tied and cut. The kidney can then be removed. A drainage tube is left in place and the incision is closed in layers.

One healthy kidney provides more than enough kidney function to maintain health and allow full activity.

Nephril

A brand name for the thiazide **diuretic** drug **polythiazide**.

nephritis

See **glomerulonephritis**.

nephroblastoma

See **kidney cancer**.

nephrolithiasis

See **kidney stones**.

nephropathy

Any disease or damage to the kidneys.
See **kidney disorders**.

nephros

Greek root meaning 'kidney' as in nephritis (kidney inflammation).

nephrosis

See **nephrotic syndrome**.

nephrotic syndrome

A kidney disorder characterized by heavy loss of protein (albumin and globulin) in the urine with lowered protein levels in the blood and resultant accumulation of fluid in the body tissues (**oedema**). In health, no protein is lost in the urine.

RECOGNITION AND SYMPTOMS

If the kidneys become permeable to protein and the rate of loss exceeds the rate at which the liver can synthesize protein, blood levels of protein will drop. The protein dissolved in the blood is one of the main elements in maintaining the tendency for blood to draw water from the tissues and retain it (osmotic pressure). If the osmotic pressure drops, fluid remains in the tissue spaces which become waterlogged and prone to infection. The skin becomes swollen and puffy and

In nerve block local anaesthesia, the drug is injected around the sensory nerve at a point remote from the operation site. Pain impulses arising in the course of the operation cannot pass to the brain and nothing is felt.

pits on pressure. Fluid accumulates in the abdomen and chest and produces secondary effects. The protein loss may be so severe as to cause malnutrition.

POSSIBLE CAUSES

The kidney damage in the nephrotic syndrome may be a feature of **glomerulonephritis** or may be caused by various other conditions including **diabetes**, severe high blood pressure (hypertension), metallic and other forms of poisoning and adverse drug reactions.

TREATMENT

The mainstay of treatment of the nephrotic syndrome is the use of diuretic drugs to increase the urinary output of water and reduce the oedema. The outlook depends on the cause and severity of the kidney damage.

nephrotoxicity

The liability of a substance, such as a drug, to cause damage to the kidneys. A nephrotoxic effect is more likely if existing kidney damage reduces the rate of excretion of the toxic agent so that it acts for longer periods on the kidneys.

The most important of the nephrotoxic drugs are the aminoglycoside antibiotics, such as neomycin, gentamycin and amikacin. These are unlikely to do harm, however, unless used in very large dosage or in the presence of kidney disease.

Nerisone

A brand name for **diflucortolone valerate**.

nerve block

A method of producing local anaesthesia without having to inject directly into the area to be operated upon. This is done by injecting local anaesthetic around the main nerve carrying pain and touch sensation from the area concerned back to the brain. The effect is to cause a temporary obstruction to the passage of nerve impulses so that, whatever is done to the area from which the nerve is running, nothing is felt.

Nerve blocks are commonly employed in dentistry. The mandibular nerve block, given high up on the back of the jaw bone, internally, on one side, will anaesthetize one complete half of the lower jaw (mandible) so that operative dentistry can be done painlessly. Other examples of nerve block anaesthesia are **epidural anaesthesia**, commonly used in childbirth, and **spinal anaesthesia**.

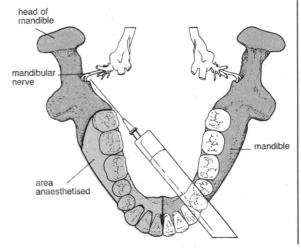

head of mandible

mandibular nerve

mandible

area anaesthetised

nerve cell

See **neuron**.

nerve cells, junctions between

See **synapse**.

nerve gases

Powerful pharmacological agents, chemically related to the organophosphorus insecticides, that cause extreme salivation, nausea, vomiting and diarrhoea, sweating, giddiness and tightness in the chest. The pupils of the eyes constrict and the vision blurs. Breathing fails and there are convulsions, coma and death. Very small doses can be fatal. Nerve gases are usually produced as volatile liquids that operate after inhalation or after absorption through the skin. A single drop on the skin can be fatal.

These agents are inhibitors of the enzyme cholinesterase. This prevents the breakdown of the ubiquitous nerve synapse transmitting agent acetylcholine, which thus continues to act strongly, with the effects described.

nervo

Latin root meaning 'nerve' as in nerve (conducting tissue).

nervous breakdown

This is not a recognized medical condition but rather a popular term of uncertain definition. It is used to describe a range of emotional crises varying from a brief attack of 'hysterical' behaviour to a major psychoneurotic illness with severe, long-term effects on the life of the victim. The term is also sometimes used as a euphemism for a frank psychiatric illness such as **schizophrenia**.

nervous system

The central nervous system (CNS) consists of the **brain** and its downward continuation, the spinal cord, which lies in the spinal canal within the **spine** (vertebral column). Together, and in conjunction with the **endocrine system**, these form the major controlling and coordinating elements of the body.

The CNS is entirely encased in bone and is continuous with the peripheral nervous system, which consists of the 12 pairs of **cranial nerves** arising directly from the brain and the 31 pairs of spinal nerves running out of the spinal cord. The peripheral nervous system also includes all the multitudinous branches of these peripheral nerves, and the autonomic nervous system which supplies the heart, the glands and all involuntary muscle in the body.

The functioning of the nervous system predicates the constant arrival of a great deal of information. Indeed, the surface of the human body is one large information-gathering entity. The whole skin, the eyes, the ears, the nasal lining and the mouth are all concerned, continuously, in receiving stimuli and prompting nerve impulses which convey these stimuli to the brain. The stimulus-response phenomenon is a basic attribute of the brain and nervous system without which normal life would be impossible. The nervous system is essentially a responsive mechanism which, in the absence of input stimuli, sinks into an abnormal state of torpor and, probably, coma. Total sensory deprivation cannot, in practice, be

achieved, so the latter point is not established, but all the evidence suggests that consciousness and normal living depend on a constant input of information. Much of the functioning of the nervous system occurs, fortunately, without our conscious awareness.

A reflex is an automatic and predictable response to a stimulus impinging on the body or arising within it. The jerking away of the hand from unexpected contact with a very hot surface is a reflex and, unless warning is given, it cannot be inhibited. Standing would be impossible without the spinal reflexes which automatically tense muscles when their opponent muscle groups contract. Without these tensing reflexes, joints would collapse and we would fall down. This kind of spinal reflex is easily demonstrated by putting a sudden stretching pull on the quadriceps muscle group by firmly tapping the tendon of this group below the knee. The stretch causes a sudden reflex contraction of the quadriceps muscles and the lower leg is jerked upwards. Spinal reflex arcs involve the spinal cord only and the integrity of the input and output channels of these arcs, to and from the cord, can be tested by tapping muscle tendons anywhere in the body.

But reflex action goes much further than this. Sneezing and coughing are reflexes. Sudden movements to preserve balance are reflexes. The response of the pupils to light and dark are reflexes, as are the blink or the screwing up of the eyelids in response to immediate threat to the eyes. Complex activities, such as walking, while partly under voluntary control, do involve much necessary automatic reflex activity and would be impossible without it.

Proprioception is the name given to the process of continuous monitoring of the position and movement of the limbs and the state of muscle tension, so that information is constantly supplied to the brain about the relative orientation of the parts of the body and their position in space.

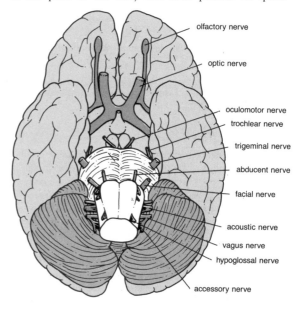

olfactory nerve

optic nerve

oculomotor nerve

trochlear nerve

trigeminal nerve

abducent nerve

facial nerve

acoustic nerve

vagus nerve

hypoglossal nerve

accessory nerve

The origins of the cranial nerves from the base of the brain. Testing of the functions of these nerves provides vital information about diseases of the brain and nervous system.

Proprioceptive information comes from sensory nerve endings and special receptors in the joints, tendons and muscles, and this information is integrated with other data coming from the balancing, gravitational and acceleration receptors in the inner ears and visual information from the eyes.

Fortunately, proprioception, too, is largely unconscious and the corrective action taken, in response to it, automatic and reflex. Functions such as walking, or even standing, would be impossible without an efficient proprioceptive system providing feedback and controlling information. Many of the disabling effects of disease or damage to the nervous system are due to interference with normal proprioceptive function.

Much of the internal control of biochemical stability (homeostasis) is reflex in nature, making use of crude and automatic responses to change, which are then refined by negative feedback loops. Conditioned reflexes are those that are built up, over a period, as a result of experience. Many conditioned reflexes are associational in nature and operate without reference to reason or logic. If one has been repeatedly burgled by teenage boys, one is likely to come to regard all teenage boys with suspicion. It is probable that conditioned reflexes are the basis of human prejudices and social responses. Observation of human behaviour suggests that much of this, too, is reflex and predictable, even up to the highest levels. Many of us live 'on autopilot' for quite long periods, even making verbal responses which are predictable. Some thinkers believe that all human functioning is reflex, but it is more comforting to think that a large measure of reflex activity is necessary to free the mind for engagement with 'higher things'.

nervous system examination

This includes tests of brain function, examination of motor ability and tests of sensory nerve function. Tests of brain function include a check of memory, orientation, comprehension, speech production and cranial nerve function.

MEMORY AND ORIENTATION

Memory is tested by questions of which the answers are highly likely to be known by a normal person. Once obvious questions are correctly answered, more difficult, or specialized questions may be asked. The doctor wishes to establish whether the person being examined retains an appropriate fund of knowledge and the power of forming general concepts from particular examples. The powers of concentration and attention are also assessed. Tests of orientation are enquiries into whether the person knows where he or she is, knows his or her name and address, knows the month and date, major current affairs, and so on.

COMPREHENSION AND SPEECH PRODUCTION

The examiner is interested in the quality of the speech and, if there appears to be a problem, whether it is a defect of language or of speech production. In language defect, the subject may be unable to recollect the names of common objects, or may use words inappropriately. He or she may readily understand what is said but may find it difficult to produce the right words in replying. This is called **dysphasia** and is due to damage to the speech area in the dominant half of the brain – nearly always the left hemisphere. In truly left-handed people, the right side of the brain may be dominant. Dysphasia may be receptive or expressive or both. In receptive dysphasia, comprehension of the speech of others is impaired, but this always leads to a defect in the patient's own use of language, since verbal symbolism and syntax usage are impaired. In expressive dysphasia, the patient knows what he or she wants to say, but is unable to say it. Dysphasia is a common feature of stroke.

Another form of speech difficulty is called **dysarthria**. In this, there is difficulty in coordinating the lips and tongue so that speech production is defective. This, too, may be caused by nervous system disease.

THE CRANIAL NERVES

Twelve pairs of nerves arise directly from the brain and are called the cranial nerves. These are concerned with smell, vision, movements of the eyes, sensation in the face, facial expression, hearing, taste, movement of the palate and tongue and movement of the upper neck muscles. All these are tested systematically and in turn.

Smell is tested, one nostril at a time, by asking the subject to identify characteristic, strong-smelling liquids. Vision tests are done with standard vision-testing charts. Visual field tests are often of prime importance in neurological examination and are almost always done unless the diagnosis is obvious. The three pairs of nerves that cause eye movements can be checked by asking the subject to follow an object with the eyes while keeping the head still. Facial sensation is tested to light touch and pin-prick, the sensitivity on the two sides being compared. The doctor tests facial movement by asking the subject to wrinkle up the forehead, screw up the eyes, raise the upper lip in a snarl, and turn down the corners of the mouth. Again, the two sides are compared and should show equal strength. Hearing is tested by tuning fork tests or by audiometry. Taste is rarely affected and complaints of loss of taste are usually due to loss of smell. Palate movement is checked by asking the subject to open the mouth and say 'Ah'. If one of the cranial nerves responsible for palate movement is affected, the hanging process at the back of the palate (the uvula) will deviate to the normal side. Movements of the upper neck muscles are tested by asking the subject to move his or her head forwards, backwards and from side to side.

MOTOR ABILITY

The power of movement (motor ability) is now checked, and the doctor will particularly note any differences in muscle power on the two sides of the body, asking the subject to grip both hands, to push the arms and legs in various directions against resistance and to demonstrate the ability to walk normally.

Normal walking is possible only if several different, but integrated, parts of the nervous system are intact. These are the voluntary motor centres in the brain; the nerve pathways which connect these centres directly, and indirectly via the cerebellum, to the spinal nerves supplying the muscles; the feedback nerve pathways for position information from the muscles and joints and from the eyes and the balancing apparatus in the inner ears; and the cerebellar computer which coordinates all this information. Any defect anywhere in this complex system is likely to be reflected in changes in the gait. An unsteady, reeling gait, with the feet wide apart, suggests a disorder of the cerebellum, and the affected person may veer consistently to the affected side if the problem affects one half of the cerebellum. **Parkinsonism** causes a slow, shuffling gait, with small steps, sometimes becoming increasingly rapid as if the person is about to fall forwards. The arms do not swing.

An unstable knee from weakness of the surrounding muscles, as may follow poliomyelitis, causes the person to fling the leg forward, like a flail. High-stepping, with both feet, results from loss of position sense, as may occur in late syphilis. Foot drop, due to conditions such as slipped disc (see disc, intervertebral, prolapse) or neuritis, causes the affected person to lift the foot higher than normal, so as to clear the ground in walking.

Weakness on one side of the body (hemiparesis) such as is commonly caused by a stroke, produces a characteristic gait with the arm on the affected side held bent across the chest and the affected leg stiff and being swung outwards and forwards, rather than being bent at the knee.

SENSORY NERVES

These are the nerves which carry sensory information from the body to the brain. They are concerned with touch, pain, temperature, vibration and position sense, and their integrity must also be checked. Again, the doctor will compare one side with the other, as marked differences between the two sides are more meaningful than an apparently equal loss on both. Testing is done with light touch and pin-prick, with small hot and cold objects and with a tuning-fork. Position sense is checked by asking the subject to close the eyes and then passively moving fingers and toes into different positions. The subject is then asked to indicate the position.

The doctor will also test the tendon jerk reflexes, at the wrists, fronts and backs of the elbows, the knees and the ankles and will perform the **Babinski's test**.

nervous system stimulants

See **analeptic drugs**.

Netilin

A brand name for **netilmicin**.

netilmicin

An **aminoglycoside antibiotic drug** derived from gentamicin. It is slightly less likely to damage the kidneys than gentamicin and is often effective against organisms resistant to that drug. A brand name is Netillin.

Neulactil

A brand name for **pericyazine**.

Neupogen

A brand name for **filgrastim**.

neuralgia

Pain originating in a sensory nerve, as distinct from the more common type of pain which originates outside the nerve but is conveyed by it. Neuralgia is a result of an abnormality of the nerve so that a stimulus is set up within it. This may be caused by injury to the nerve; by some unknown nerve abnormality; or by infection, especially by viruses, or other agency causing nerve inflammation (**neuritis**).

Neuralgia tends to be episodic and in some cases is triggered by a minor external stimulus such as a light touch to the area supplied by the nerve. Neuralgic pain is referred to the area from which the affected nerve would normally con-

vey pain impulses. Thus, in the post-herpetic pain, which commonly follows an untreated attack of **shingles**, although the nerve damage occurs near the entry of the nerve to the spinal cord, the pain is felt in the skin. **Trigeminal neuralgia** is a severe, one-sided facial pain originating in the nerve which conveys sensation from one half of the face.

Certain drugs, such as Tegretol (carbamazepine) are capable of interfering with the passage of nerve impulses along sensory nerves, and these can be useful in the management of neuralgia. In extreme cases, nerves may be cut surgically.

neural networks

Artificial electronic or software systems, capable of self-modification as a result of being used, that can simulate some of the more complex neurological functions, including a crude form of vision. In conjunction with expert software systems, involving artificial intelligence, neural networks will inevitably prove important in medicine in the future. Humanoid robots worthy of the name, which are now beginning to appear, require neural networks.

neural tube defect prevention

See **folic acid**.

neurasthenia

An old-fashioned term based on an early and unsophisticated notion that psychological fatigue, loss of motivation and energy and other associated symptoms were, in some unspecified way, caused by a disorder of the nerves. 'Nervous exhaustion', the literal meaning, seemed to imply that a person had run out of 'nervous energy'.

Such notions are currently considered naive, but, as knowledge of brain function increases, it seems increasingly likely that psychological symptoms are mediated by some disorder of the nerves, most probably of a biochemical nature and concerned with changes in **neuro-transmitters**. Already, a number of psychiatric conditions are known to be caused in this way.

neuritis

Inflammation of a nerve. This may be due to infection, injury, **auto-immune** attack, vitamin deficiency, poisoning, or to other poorly understood processes, such as the cause of the demyelination occurring in **multiple sclerosis** and other conditions.

neurodermatitis

Another name for **lichen simplex**.

neurofibromatosis

This disease, which is also called von Recklinghausen's disease, has a prevalence of about one case in 3000 people. It is a genetic disorder with dominant inheritance but about half the cases occurring result from a new mutation. The disease varies in severity from a few minor skin features to severely disfiguring and dangerous involvement of other parts of the body, including the nervous system.

RECOGNITION AND SYMPTOMS

Diagnosis is usually made by observing six or more *café au lait* patches, more than 15 mm in diameter, on the skin, and freckles in areas, such as the armpits, not normally exposed to the sun. In the fully established condition, the fibrous sheaths of numerous nerves in the skin and elsewhere develop soft tumours called neurofibromas. In most cases these are confined to the skin and have cosmetic significance only. But in about 20 per cent of cases serious complications arise from massive skin involvement or involvement of the central nervous system. The celebrated Elephant Man, made famous by the English surgeon Sir Frederick Treves (1853–1923) probably had neurofibromatosis.

The tumours can involve the brain and spinal cord; the eye sockets, leading to increasing protrusion of the eyes; the bones, leading to spontaneous fractures; and the spine, causing severe deformity and sometimes paralysis. Mental retardation, usually mild, occurs in a proportion of cases.

TREATMENT

Regrettably there is no practical treatment for a condition that features hundreds or thousands of benign tumours of nerve sheaths. Surgery is theoretically possible, but it would be difficult to remove tumours without affecting the function of the nerves concerned.

COPING

People with neurofibromatosis need support and help and, in Britain, this is supplied by such organizations as the Neurofibromatosis Association.

neurologist

A doctor trained in neurology, who has a detailed knowledge of the structure and function of the nervous system and is skilled in the diagnosis and treatment of its disorders. Neurologists are physicians and do not engage in operative treatment, but often work in close association with a neurosurgeon.

neurology

The medical discipline concerned with the nervous system and its disorders. Neurology is based on a detailed knowledge of the complex structure of the brain, the spinal cord and the peripheral nerves and their plexuses and distribution. An understanding of what may go wrong with these structures requires, in addition to an extensive knowledge of the many neurological diseases, a good knowledge of the basic medical sciences of body function (physiology), of disease processes (pathology), of the body's defensive response to infection (immunology) and of the inheritance of disease (genetics).

Neurology has made great strides in recent years and has changed from a rather academic discipline of presumptive diagnosis, but little curative ability, to a precise science capable of doing much for its patients. Modern methods of imaging and wider understanding of the nature of neurological disorder make possible an increasing range of effective treatments.

neuroma

A non-malignant (benign) tumour of nerve tissue.

neuron

A nerve cell, and the functional unit of the nervous system. A neuron is a single cell with a very long, fibre-like extension of its body, called an axon, and one or many short body extensions called dendrites. The axon, or nerve fibre, may be 100,000 times as long as the diameter of the cell body. Some axons are as long as 1 metre, making the nerve cell by far the longest cell in the body.

Nerve impulses are electrical in nature but are not electric currents. They are zones in which the normal negative charge on the outside of the fibre has become less negative because of movement of charged ions across the membrane. These are called zones of depolarization. These zones travel outwards along the axon from the cell body. Incoming impulses travel to the cell body along the dendrites.

Neurons interconnect with each other at specialized junctions called **synapses**, situated mainly between the end of an axon of one neuron and the cell body or the dendrites of another. Many neurons have as many as 15,000 synaptic junctions, some more, and it is this richness of interconnection that allows the brain to exhibit properties that may seem preternatural. Most synapses are interneurons connecting with other nerve cells, rather than with muscles or glands.

Neurontin

A brand name for **gabapentin**.

neuropharmacology

The study of drugs that act on the nervous system.

neuropsychiatry

The branch of medicine concerned with the psychiatric effects of disorders of neurological functional or structure. Increasingly, the correlation is being drawn between demonstrable brain changes and the resulting effects on the mind. It is the function of the growing speciality of neuropsychiatry to investigate this relationship.

Neuroremed

A brand name for **tryptophan**.

neurosis

An overall term for any persisting mental disorder which causes distress to the person concerned, which is recognized by the sufferer as being abnormal, but in which contact with reality is retained. There is no obvious causal factor and the behaviour of the sufferer does not grossly violate social norms. The breadth of this definition is necessary because of a progressive appreciation of the inadequacy of older, mainly Freudian, ideas about neurosis.

Freud's classification included anxiety neurosis, phobic neurosis, obsessive-compulsive neurosis, hysteria, depressive neurosis, narcissistic neurosis, depersonalisation and others, but experience showed that, in practice, it was often impossible accurately to apply these labels, and the tendency, today, is to recognize that most neurotic people suffer from anxiety which is either experienced directly or expressed through **defence mechanisms**, and appears as one or more of a variety of symptoms, such as a phobia, an obsession, a compulsion or as sexual dysfunction.

The modern classification of mental disorders does not include an overall class of neuroses. The disorders formerly included in this group are now described as anxiety disorders;

somatoform or conversion disorders (formerly **hysteria**); **dissociative disorders** (**amnesia**, **fugue**, multiple personality, depersonalization); sexual disorders; and dysthymic disorder (neurotic depression). Psychoanalysis has conspicuously failed to have any real value in the treatment of these conditions and orthodox medicine gives little credence to Freud's speculations as to their origins. These various conditions are probably best regarded as being the result of a form of conditioning or programming inappropriate to the mores of society. The most hopeful form of treatment would seem to be some form of **behaviour therapy**.

neurosurgeon

A surgeon specializing in brain surgery and surgery on the spinal cord and peripheral nerves.

neurosurgery

This is the specialty popularly thought of as 'brain surgery', but the reality is rather different from the popular image. Neurosurgery is concerned with the surgical treatment of those conditions of the nervous system which can be relieved or cured by operative intervention.

WHY IT'S DONE

Conditions which can be cured or relieved by neurosurgery include head injury with bleeding inside the skull, tumours of the brain or spinal cord, abnormalities of the arteries of the nervous system, such as **aneurysms** around the base of the brain, congenital disorders such as **hydrocephalus** or **spina bifida**, and infections of the nervous system which have led to the formation of abscesses.

HOW IT'S DONE

Neurosurgery usually involves long operations, often of many hours duration, and the physical labour undertaken by the surgeons is often considerable. Bone has to be cut through and removed, many bleeding points have to be tied off and secured, pulped and destroyed brain tissue sometimes has to be sucked out and work has to be done often in what are sometimes the most awkward and inaccessible parts of the body.

neuro-transmitter

A neuro-transmitter is a chemical substance selectively released from a nerve ending by the arrival of a nerve impulse. The neuro-transmitter then interacts with a receptor on an adjacent structure to trigger off some kind of response. The adjacent structure may be another nerve, a muscle fibre or a gland. Nerve action, mediated by neuro-transmitters, is a sensitive process that can be increased or decreased as needed. And because the chemical structure of many of the neuro-transmitters is known, they can be used as drugs to modulate some of the most important actions of the nervous system. In addition, many highly effective drugs act by simulating the action of neuro-transmitters, by modifying their action or by blocking the receptor sites at which they normally act. Some neuro-transmitters are broken down by enzymes so that their action ceases. Others are taken up again into the region from which they were released. The drug fluoxetine (Prozac), for instance, blocks the re-uptake of serotonin so that its stimulatory action is greatly prolonged.

The main neuro-transmitters are acetylcholine, dopamine, noradrenaline, serotonin, GABA (gamma-amino-butyric

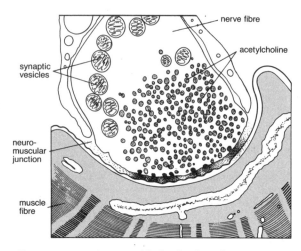

The neuro-transmitter acetylcholine is released from the nerve ending and diffuses across the narrow gap between the nerve and the muscle fibre, to stimulate the fibre into contraction.

acid), the endorphins, the enkephalins, glycine, glutamate, aspartine, adrenaline, histamine, vasopressin and bradykinin.

Knowledge of neuro-transmitters and their action is growing apace and is throwing light on many aspects of brain function and neurological disorders. An increasing number of diseases of the nervous system are being shown to be due to disorders of neuro-transmitters' production or action.

Neutrexin

A brand name for **trimetrexate**.

nicardipine

A **calcium channel blocker** drug used to treat **angina pectoris** and high blood pressure. A brand name is Cardene.

nickel dermatitis

A severe skin allergy, causing **eczema**, from direct contact with the metallic element nickel. This was once common at a time when nickel was widely used as a plating for metallic articles worn on the body, such as watch-straps, underwear fastenings and spectacle frames. The condition is now rare.

nickel poisoning

Foods can be contaminated with nickel during processing and cooking, but this is rare. Nickel carbonyl is highly toxic and is the only nickel compound readily absorbed. It is a hazard to workers in the nickel industry. Nickel absorbed into the body is stored mainly in the brain and spinal cord, the lungs and the heart. Acute poisoning causes headache, dizziness, vomiting, chest pain, cough, short rapid breathing, blueness of the skin (cyanosis) and severe weakness.

> Nickel has been shown to be capable of causing cancer of the nasal passages and sinuses, and nickel platers have about 150 times the normal incidence of these cancers.

niclosamide

A drug used to remove tapeworms. Unlike earlier treatments, it is free from major side-effects. A brand name is Yomesan.

nicorandil

A **potassium channel activator** drug used to treat **angina pectoris**. A brand name is Ikorel.

Nicorette

A brand name for chewing gum containing **nicotine**. This is intended to make the abandonment of cigarette smoking a less painful procedure for those deficient in resolution.

nicotine

A powerful alkaloid drug derived from the leaves of the tobacco plants *Nicotiana tabacum* and *Nicotiana rustica*. It is a colourless to amber oil with a strong smell of tobacco and an intensely bitter taste. Nicotine is highly toxic and is sometimes used as an insecticide. Nicotine poisoning causes severe nausea and vomiting, spontaneous emptying of the bladder and bowels, mental confusion and convulsions. It is not responsible for causing cancer.

Like many other poisons, nicotine, taken in very small dosage, is valued for its stimulant properties. In smoking, the drug passes rapidly into the bloodstream and gives a quick 'lift' by its **neuro-transmitter**-like action on the brain until broken down in the liver and excreted in the urine. In those who are habituated, it increases the heart rate and raises the blood pressure by narrowing small arteries. This effect can be dangerous in certain arterial diseases.

Nicotine is not a powerfully addictive drug and enforced deprivation produces only minor withdrawal effects, which soon pass. Its use, nevertheless, is so important to many that they continue to smoke cigarettes although well aware of the major risk to health.

nicotinyl alcohol tartrate

A **vasodilator** drug used to treat disorders caused by peripheral arterial spasm. A brand name is Ronicol.

nicoumalone

An **anticoagulant** drug of the coumarin group. A brand name is Sinthrome.

Nidazol

A brand name for **metronidazole**.

nifedipine

A **calcium channel blocker** drug used to control the symptoms of **angina pectoris** and to treat high blood pressure. It has a powerful effect in widening (dilating) arteries, including the coronary arteries, and this improves the blood supply to the heart muscle. The drug, however, causes flushing, headache, skin itching and dizziness. It is often used in combination with a **beta-blocker**. Nifedipine has been used effectively to prevent high altitude lung oedema, a feature of mountain sickness. Trade names are Adalat, Adipine MR, Angiopine MR, Cardilate MR, Coracten, Fortipine LA, Tensipine MR and Unipine XL.

Niferex

A brand name for **iron polysaccharide complex**.

nifurtimox

A drug used in the treatment of South American trypanosomiasis (Chagas' disease). The drug is effective against the causal agent *Trypanosoma cruzi* but its use is associated with side-effects such as nausea, vomiting, loss of appetite, abdominal pain, muscle and joint aches, headache and vertigo.

night blindness

Poor vision in dim light. The medical term is nyctalopia and the condition is quite common in people with no discernible eye disorder. It is also common in short-sighted people, and is a feature of vitamin A deficiency. More serious forms of nyctalopia may be caused by a range of degenerative retinal diseases including **retinitis pigmentosa**.

nightmare

The Anglo-Saxon word *maere* means an evil male spirit or demon, intent on sexual intercourse with a sleeping woman, i.e., an incubus. This idea of the incubus seems to be central to the historical concept of the nightmare which is an intensely vivid and unpleasant dream, suffered more by children than by adults.

Nightmares, in fact, seldom have a sexual content but, in adults, are often connected with some prior event of a highly traumatic nature such as an assault, a car accident, imprisonment or torture. They may be caused by the withdrawal of sleeping tablets.

Nightmares are anxiety dreams and occur during the periods of rapid eye movement (REM) sleep. They are distinguished from **night terrors** which occur in the early part of the night during the period of deep, non-REM sleep.

night sweat

Drenching perspiration occurring at night or during sleep. Night sweats may be a feature of any feverish illness but have no specific significance in suggesting any particular diagnosis.

night terrors

Night terrors produces much more powerful physiological effects than the **nightmare** – the heart rate accelerations have been among the highest recorded, the respiratory rate is very high and there is marked sweating. There is often loud screaming. The deeper the non-REM sleep, the more severe the night terror tends to be. The content of the night terror is usually a conviction of suffocation, choking, entrapment in a small space or impending death. Night terrors are commonest around the age of five or six and tend to stop in adolescence.

night waking

About a quarter of all British children, of one to two years of age, regularly disturb their parents' sleep during the night. In some other countries, the age range is greater.

Management is difficult, but recommendations have included changing the domestic routine so as to reduce daytime naps; sedatives for the child or the mother or father, or all; leaving the child to cry; and behaviour modification methods such as rewarding the child for not disturbing the mother or introducing a fixed bedtime ritual.

Rituals are effective with children and should, preferably, involve both parents. They might include an agreement not to cry during the night.

Sedatives are widely used for this problem but they work only while they are being given. They do not induce 'habits' of all-night sleep and if they are replaced by a placebo, the former behaviour returns. The antihistamine drug Vallergan (trimeprazine) is widely used in children.

Nilstat

A brand name for the antifungal drug nystatin.

nimodipine

A **calcium channel blocker** drug used to minimise brain damage after subarachnoid haemorrhage. A brand name is Nimotop.

Nipent

A brand name for **pentostatin**.

nipple, disorders of

The nipple is the central prominence of each breast, larger in women than in men. The word derives from the Anglo-Saxon *nib*, meaning 'a little beak'. In women, 15 to 20 milk ducts pass from the milk-producing lobes of the breast out through each nipple. The area surrounding the nipple is called the areola and this is a pinkish colour in those who have not been pregnant, but darker in those who have. Erection of the nipple occurs in the cold, on light touch, on sexual excitement and on the stimulus of breast feeding.

Nipples are sometimes naturally turned inwards (inverted) and this can cause feeding problems. Inverted nipples should be regularly pulled out.

> A naturally inverted nipple should be distinguished from a previously normal nipple which becomes indrawn or distorted. This may be a sign of cancer and should be reported to a doctor at once.

Cracked and sore nipples are common features of breastfeeding. Cracked nipples can allow access to infective organisms and may lead to breast inflammation (**mastitis**) or a **breast abscess**. They should be allowed to heal even if breastfeeding must be stopped for a day or two and the milk expressed and given from a bottle. Sore nipples sometimes occur when the nipple is pulled from the baby's mouth instead of breaking the suction with a finger. Teething babies should be firmly stopped from biting. Sore nipples should be exposed as much as possible and allowed to dry after feeds.

nisoldipine

A **calcium channel blocker** drug used to treat **angina pectoris** and high blood pressure. A brand name is Syscor MR.

The nipple is penetrated by 15 to 20 fine ducts that carry the milk to the exterior. During feeding, the ducts just behind the nipple become swollen with milk.

nit

A louse egg. See **lice**.

Nitradisc

A brand name for a preparation of the angina-relieving drug **glyceryl trinitrate**.

Nitrados

A brand name for **nitrazepam**.

nitrate and nitrite drugs

The action of these drugs is to relax the circular layers of smooth muscle in the walls of arteries. The effect of this is that the arteries widen so more blood can flow though. This is called 'vasodilatation'. The nitrates are short-term vasodilators but are valuable in treating **angina pectoris**, in which the blood flow to the heart muscle is reduced by coronary arteries narrowed by the artery disease atherosclerosis. The nitrates are also of value when the pumping efficiency of the heart is reduced (heart failure).

One of the most commonly used nitrates is nitroglycerine, the explosive, which, for medical purposes, is mixed with inert (inactive) material and made safe. This is best taken in a tablet placed under the tongue from which absorption into the blood is rapid. Amyl nitrite is a volatile liquid supplied in thin-walled glass capsules which must be broken before the liquid can be inhaled. Isosorbide dinitrate (Cedocard), and

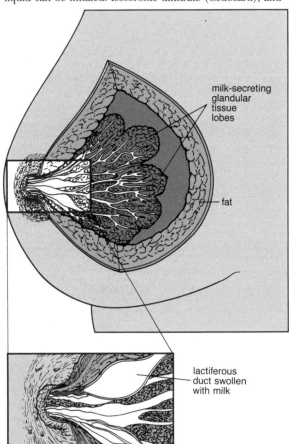

milk-secreting glandular tissue lobes

fat

lactiferous duct swollen with milk

isosorbide mononitrate (Elatan) are used to try to prevent anginal attacks.

Because they widen many of the arteries in the body, nitrates can cause fainting and collapse by reducing the blood pressure too suddenly and too much. This is likely only if they are taken in excessive dosage or if you have become hypersensitive to them. Nitrates may cause severe headaches by stretching the pain-sensitive tissues around the brain arteries – a kind of drug-induced migraine.

nitrazepam

A long-acting **benzodiazepine** hypnotic drug, widely used to promote sleep in insomnia. A brand name is Mogadon.

nitric oxide

An important physiological mediator found, in 1987, to be a relaxant of smooth muscle in the walls of blood vessels andto be derived from the inner lining (endothelium) of blood vessels. Further research showed that nitric oxide was synthesized from endothelium, from nerves and from large phagocyte cells called macrophages by three different enzymes and that it had actions all over the body. Nitric oxide is involved in:

- controlling blood pressure;
- the phagocytic action of macrophages;
- inhibiting clumping of blood **platelets** and hence blood clotting;
- limiting the development of **atherosclerosis**;
- controlling the heart action;
- relaxing the smooth muscle in the air tubes of the lungs and the walls of the intestine;
- a range of brain functions;
- promoting erection of the penis (see **sildenafil citrate**).

Nitro-bid

A brand name for a preparation of the angina-relieving drug **glyceryl trinitrate**.

Nitrocine

A brand name for nitroglycerine (**glyceryl trinitrate**).

Nitro-Dur

A brand name for **glyceryl trinitrate**.

nitrofurantoin

A drug that damages bacterial **DNA** and is used to treat urinary tract infections. Trade names are Furadantin, Macrobid and Macrodantin.

nitrogen

A chemically inert, colourless and odourless gas making up about 80 per cent of the Earth's atmosphere. Nitrogen is a constituent of various important body elements, especially proteins, and it appears in the urine in the form of urea, the main nitrogenous waste product of the body.

See **decompression sickness**.

nitrogen narcosis

The toxic effects on the brain of the high concentrations of nitrogen occurring in the blood in divers breathing air at depths of 30 metres or more. This effect is different from **decompression sickness**. There is a sense of detachment from reality, loss of concentration and slowing of mental processes. The condition is relieved by ascending to about 10 metres.

Nitrolate

A brand name for a preparation of the angina-relieving drug **glyceryl trinitrate**.

Nitrolingual

A brand name for **glyceryl trinitrate**.

Nitromin

A brand name for **glyceryl trinitrate**.

Nitronal

A brand name for **glyceryl trinitrate**.

nitrous oxide

See **laughing gas**.

Nivaquine

A brand name for chloroquine.

Nivemycin

A brand name for **neomycin**.

nizatidine

An **H2 receptor antagonist** drug used to prevent and treat peptic ulcers. Trade names are Axid and Zinga.

Nizoral

A brand name for **ketoconazole**.

Nobrium

A brand name for medazepam.

nocardiosis

An infection by the bacterium *Nocardia asteroides* and other members of the same genus, which are commonly found in soil. It causes discharging abscesses under the skin (Madura foot) and abscesses in the lungs in people with reduced resistance to infection (immunodeficiency). Lung nocardiosis may spread to other parts of the body, including the bowels and the brain. The bacterial colonies have a fungus-like appearance but are susceptible to antibiotics and sulphonamides.

nociceptors

Nerve endings in or under the skin that selectively respond to **pain**.

nocturia

Getting up during the night to pass urine. This has several causes including:

- excess fluid intake;
- **cystitis** with heightened awareness of bladder filling;
- enlargement of the **prostate** gland with obstruction to the outflow of urine so that the bladder is only partly emptied at each urination;
- excess evening alcohol intake (alcohol is a diuretic, increasing the urinary output);
- inadequately treated **diabetes**;
- kidney failure;
- insomnia leading to a normal awareness of a full bladder.

> Nocturia can be symptomatic of a dangerous condition and medical advice should be sought.

nocturnal emission

The 'wet dream'. The spontaneous orgasm and ejaculation occurring during sleep, often at the climax of an erotic dream.

Nocturnal emission is experienced by almost all adolescent males except those so sexually active that they have nothing much to ejaculate. It is also common in older men of restricted sexual opportunity.

No Doz

A brand name for a preparation of caffeine.

nodule

A small, hard or soft lump of tissue in, or under, the skin or occurring in other tissues of the body. The term is purely descriptive and says nothing about the nature of the lump.

no-fault compensation system

Indemnification of the victims of medical accidents and mishaps in which no legal claim can exist against doctors or medical institutions. Such a system has been introduced in France and is a topic of regular discussion among doctors and lawyers interested in this field of jurisprudence.

noise, effects of

> The risks of noise-induced damage to hearing should be known to all. After exposure to noise loud enough to cause temporary deafness, most of the hearing loss is restored, usually in a matter of hours; but some permanent loss occurs and there is no evidence that any form of medical treatment can reverse this. This damage is the result of structural injury to the delicate hair cells in the inner ear which may, in some cases, be literally shaken to pieces.

The degree of permanent damage depends on the noise intensity and on the length of exposure. Thus, a very high sound intensity lasting only for milliseconds (as in an explosion) could equal, in its effects, lower levels of sound intensity applied for hours, weeks or months. All loud noise is potentially damaging and the danger can rise critically as one comes closer to the source of the sound.

The range of possible sound intensity is so great (the loudest being about a thousand million million times greater than the quietest) that a logarithmic scale of comparison (a scale rising by equal multiples rather than by equal additions) is necessary. This is known as the decibel scale. Note that a decibel is not a unit of sound intensity but a unit of comparison with a fixed standard. Prolonged exposure to levels over 90 decibels above the standard is liable to cause permanent **tinnitus** and deafness. Lower levels may possibly be harmful.

Gun-fire is a major concern. Ear defenders are now mandatory in the Armed Forces, where bitter experience has shown how readily damage can be caused t o the organ of hearing in the inner ear (the cochlea). But many civilians are still apparently unaware of the dangers and fire off shotguns and rifles with little concern that each shot chips another fraction of a decibel off their hearing acuity. Explosive fireworks, too, are highly dangerous to hearing and children should never be allowed to handle them. Indeed, there is a strong case for banning them altogether.

> Measurements have shown that many people exposed to rock band and disco music have suffered inner ear damage. These people will suffer from noises in the head (tinnitus) and hearing loss in the future. Effective legislation to control noise of this kind is badly needed.

The evidence for the danger of personal earphones which, because of the close proximity to the eardrums, can produce high effective intensities is conflicting, but there are good reasons to suspect danger.

The typical early sign of noise-induced inner ear damage is a moderate loss of hearing acuity, as shown by audiometry, in the middle to upper frequency range. This is commonly associated with tinnitus, but the hearing loss is often not noticed at this stage. As exposure continues, the zone of damage extends in both directions, with the greater emphasis on the higher frequencies, and this process goes on until all high frequency hearing is lost.

Nolvadex

A brand name for **tamoxifen**.

noma

See **cancrum oris**.

nonaccidental injury

See **child abuse**.

non-nuclear DNA

See **mitochondrial DNA**.

nonoxynol-9

A **surfactant** spermicidal drug intended for use in conjunction with barrier contraceptives. It is available as a foam, pessary, gel, or cream. Trade names are Delfen, Double Check, Ortho-Forms, Duragel, Gynol II and Ortho-Creme.

nonsense mutation

A **point mutation** which changes a **codon** that specifies an amino acid into one that marks the position where translation of a messenger RNA sequence should stop (a termination codon). The result is a gene with a segment lopped off. Such a gene will code for a protein that may have missing amino acids and may thus be functionally defective.

nonspecific urethritis

See **sexually transmitted diseases**.

Nootropil

A brand name for **piracetam**.

noradrenaline

An important adrenergic **neuro-transmitter** released by post-ganglionic adrenergic nerve endings and secreted by the medulla of the adrenal gland. Noradrenaline acts chiefly on alpha-adrenergic receptors and causes constriction of arteries and a rise in the blood pressure. This is a **sympathomimetic** action. One of the catecholamines. A brand name is Levophed.

noradrenaline re-uptake inhibitors

A class of drugs that function by increasing the available amount of the neuro-transmitter **noradrenaline** at synapses. This is achieved by interfering with the normal physiological reuptake mechanism that brings about the removal of noradrenaline from the synaptic gap. Selective noradrenaline re-uptake inhibitors can have a useful antidepressive effect. They include **amitriptyline**, **clomipramine**, **doxepin**, **imipramine**, **amoxapine**, desipramine, maprotiline and **nortriptyline**.

Norcuron

A brand name for **vecuronium**.

Norditropin

A brand name for **somatotropin**.

norethandrolone

A synthetic **anabolic steroid** similar in chemical structure to **testosterone**.

norethisterone

A **progestogen** drug used to treat premenstrual tension (PMT), excessive menstrual bleeding, endometriosis, painful menstruation, metastatic breast cancer, and as an adjunct to oestrogen hormone replacement therapy. Trade names are Micronor-HRT, Primolut N, Micronor and Utovlan. The drug is also used in combination with an oestrogen as an oral contraceptive. It is formulated with ethinyloestradiol under such trade names as Binovum, Brevinor, Loestrin 20, Norinyl-1, Otho-Novin 1/50, Ovysmen, Synphase and Trinovum; and with oestradiol valerate under the trade names Climagest and Climesse.

norfloxacin

A quinolone antibacterial drug used to treat urinary tract infections. A brand name is Utinor.

Norgalax

A brand name for **docusate sodium**.

Norgesic

A brand name for **orphenadrine**.

norgestrel

A **progestogen** drug used as an oral contraceptive. A brand name is Neogest.

Norimin

A brand name for **ethinyloestradiol** formulated with a **progestogen** drug as an oral contraceptive.

Norimode

A brand name for **loperamide**.

Norinyl-1

A brand name for **mestranol** in combination with **norethisterone** as an oral contraceptive.

Normacol Plus

A brand name for **frangula** formulated with the bulking agent sterculia.

Normison

A brand name for **temazepam**.

Norplant

A brand name for **levonorgestrel** in an implantable form as a long-term, reversible contraceptive. This product has been withdrawn.

Norprolac

A brand name for **quinagolide**.

Nortap

A brand name for **nortriptyline**.

nortriptyline

A tricyclic antidepressant drug. A brand name is Allegron. The drug is also formulated with the phenothiazine drug fluphenazine under the trade names Motipress and Motival.

Norval

A brand name for the antidepressant drug myaserin.

Norvir

A brand name for **ritonavir**.

nose bleed

See *First Aid*.

nose, broken

Fracture of the nose is a common consequence of external violence and requires treatment only if there is visible deformity or if the nasal septum is deviated so much to one side as to obstruct breathing. Broken noses are fairly easily moulded back into shape by manipulation under anaesthesia, if this is done soon after the injury. After about two weeks, bone healing makes this more difficult. In some cases it is necessary to apply a plaster cast for two or three weeks.

nose reshaping

See **rhinoplasty**.

nosology

The science of the classification of diseases. The word comes from the Greek *nosos* meaning 'disease'. Nosocomial infection is one acquired in hospital.

notexin

An enzyme from snake venom that attacks muscle cells and motor nerve terminals. It has been proposed for the treatment of upper lid droop (blepharoptosis) in mitochondrial muscle weakness, to encourage the proliferation of satellite muscle cells, which contain mostly normal mitochondria.

notifiable disease

Any condition required by law to be reported to a central medical authority by the doctor who diagnoses it.

The notification of certain potentially harmful infectious diseases, such as **typhoid fever** or **poliomyelitis**, is important, as it enables public health officers to take immediate steps to control the spread of infection by isolating infected individuals and by offering protection to their contacts.

Notification also provides important statistical information about the incidence and prevalence of a disease. This may provide the information on which health policies are based, for example, immunization programmes or improvements in sanitation.

Some categories of disease other than infections are also notifiable. These include all cancers and certain occupational diseases.

Novantrone

A brand name for **mitoxantrone**.

Novocain

A brand name for the local anaesthetic drug procaine hydrochloride.

Novoseven

A brand name for **eptacog alfa**.

Noxyflex S

A brand name for **noxythiolin**.

noxythiolin

An antifungal and antibacterial drug used to treat **peritonitis**. A brand name is Noxyflex S.

Nozinan

A brand name for the antipsychotic drug ethotrimeprazine.

NSAIDs

Non-steroidal anti-inflammatory drugs. The range of NSAIDs includes aspirin, benorylate, diflunisal, fenbufen, fenoprofen, ibuprofen, naproxen, diclofenac, indomethacin, phenlybutazone and piroxicam.

See **analgesic drugs**, **anti-inflammatory drugs**.

Nubain

A brand name for the narcotic analgesic **nalbufine**.

nuchal translucency test

A method of ultrasound screening for the detection of fetuses with a chromosomal abnormality, especially **Down's syndrome**. The examination consists of the assessment of small collections of fluid at the back of the neck and spine of the fetus that increase translucency to ultrasound. About three-quarters of cases of Down's syndrome can be detected in this way.

nuclear magnetic resonance (NMR)

See **magnetic resonance imaging**.

nuclear medicine

A medical specialty in which radioactive substances are used in diagnosis and treatment. Radioactive materials have the advantage that their presence in the body can easily be traced and their concentration, at any particular point, determined by the intensity of radiation emitted from that point.

In the diagnostic technique called radionuclide scanning, the materials used consist of compounds incorporating small, and safe, quantities of artificially made radioactive isotopes of common elements. These are given, by mouth or by injection, and their distribution in the body is detected and measured by an instrument called a gamma or scintillation camera. This is a radiation detection device, of which the sensitive element is a large crystal of sodium iodide, nearly a metre in diameter in some cases. The crystal produces tiny sparks of light whenever it is struck by a gamma ray emitted by the isotope. Associated apparatus detects the light flashes, noting the location and strength, and converts them into electrical impulses. These data are used to produce a picture or image of the origins of the gamma rays within the body.

Specific radioactive elements or compounds containing them are selectively concentrated in different organs. For instance, iodine is concentrated in the thyroid gland. So it is possible to obtain images that represent the functional activity of the organ.

Making use of the same principle, nuclear medicine is able to provide methods of local treatment, using more strongly radioactive substances, which rely on the way the body concentrates these substances in the organ which requires to be irradiated. This is a common and highly selective form of radiotherapy.

nuclear medicine physicist

An ancillary health professional scientist or doctor concerned with the use of radioactive substances for the diagnosis and treatment of disease. Radioactive isotopes can be incorporated into compounds that selectively concentrate in different organs, or in particular disease tissues where they can be detected or can produce useful effects.

nuclear radiation

The radiations and particles emitted from the cores (nuclei) of radioactive atoms during radioactive decay and nuclear reactions. They are the nuclei of helium atoms (alpha particles), electrons (beta particles), and electromagnetic radiation of wavelength shorter than visible light or X-rays (gamma rays). These three types of radiation have different powers of penetration, the beta particles being least penetrative and the gamma rays most.

Ionizing radiations such as these are capable of dislodging atomic particles, such as linking electrons, from molecules and thus breaking them into smaller molecules. The effect of this on the body is to produce biological changes in structures such as the chromosomes, in which mutations may occur, or to form active or toxic products in the cells. In general, radiations are most destructive to those cells most rapidly dividing. They thus tend to have their greatest effect on the reproductive organs, on the lining of the digestive tract and on the skin.

See also **radiotherapy**.

nucleoside

A molecule compounded of a purine or pyrimidine base (see **base pair**) attached to a sugar (ribose or deoxyribose). A **nucleotide** without the phosphate group.

nucleoside analogue

A drug that resembles a **nucleoside** (see **nucleotide**) and that can be taken up in place of the natural nucleosides in viruses so as to alter their DNA, making it fragile and susceptible to breakage. Drugs of this class, which include famciclovir, didanosine, idoxuridine and penciclovir, require the action of an enzyme carried by the target virus, before they become functional.

nucleotide

A molecule, that is a part of DNA, formed from the bonding of a purine or a pyrimidine base (see **base pair**) with a sugar and a phosphate group. The bases link in pairs to form the 'rungs' of the double helix 'ladder', while the alternating sugar and phosphate groups form the longitudinal helices. There are four nucleotides. They differ from each other by virtue of the four different bases. The full names for the four nucleotides refer to their full chemical constitution and are clumsy (e.g., 2'-deoxyadenosine 5'-triphosphate). For convenience, their names are commonly abbreviated to A, G, C and T (respectively for the variable parts adenine, gua-

nine, cytosine and thymine). The order of the bases along the DNA strand, taken three at a time, form the genetic code.

A nucleotide without the phosphate group is called a nucleoside.

nucleus

Nucleus is the Latin word for a little 'nut' or 'kernel' – something right at the centre of something else.

The nucleus of a body cell is the central structure consisting of the tightly bundled chromosomes surrounded by a nuclear membrane.

Nuelin

A brand name for **theophylline**.

Nulacin

A brand name for a mixture of calcium carbonate and magnesium trisilicate. An antacid preparation.

nullipara

A woman who has never given birth to a viable child.

Nupercaine

A brand name for the local anaesthetic drug cinchocaine.

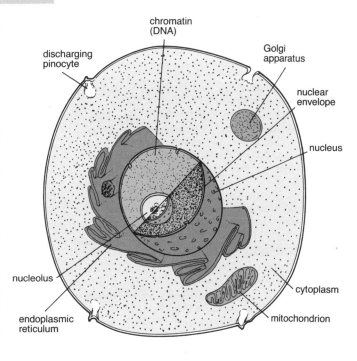

Most cells have a single nucleus consisting of a mass of fine-stranded chromatin that coils into chromosomes at the time of cell division. The nucleus has an envelope and contains a small body called a nucleolus. Some cells have more than one nucleus.

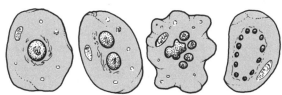

Nurofen

A brand name for **ibuprofen**.

nurse

A health care professional who has undergone a specified period of training in a hospital approved by the General Nursing Council and has passed an examination before qualifying for registration as a Registered General Nurse (RGN) with the United Kingdom Central Council for Nursing, Midwifery and Health Visiting. Nurses are the most immediate ancillaries to the medically qualified members of the profession. Their responsibilities extend far beyond that of providing assistance to doctors, and include:

- continuing personal medical education;
- ensuring the well-being and safety of patients;
- assisting in their recovery from illness;
- the promotion of positive health;
- care of the unconscious patient;
- care of the elderly and the dying;
- respect for patients' rights, privacy and confidentiality;
- the formation and maintenance of an ethical basis of behaviour.

The administrative and clinical levels in the nursing profession have been changing over the years. Domestic ward work is done by Health Care Assistants who do not have a nursing qualification. A nurse working for her or his Registered General Nurse (RGN) qualification is called a student nurse. After qualifying the nurse may become a staff nurse and may then advance to become a Team Leader or Ward Manager (informally, Sister). Above the Team Leaders is the Hospital Manager (formerly Matron) or the Director of Nursing Services.

The nursing process is a formal description of the actions involved in nursing, and provides the basis of most nursing in the UK and the USA. The stages in the process consist of obtaining information about the patient; using this information to identify problems and determine objectives; writing a nursing care plan; providing the planned care; and assessing the effectiveness of the care provided.

The scope of nursing is rapidly expanding as many qualified nurses are now university graduates. Many nurses are becoming specialists in particular fields that now extend far beyond midwifery and district nursing.

nurse-anaesthetist

A nurse trained to administer general anaesthetics. Historically, nurse-anaesthetists were once common in the USA but were never adopted in the UK. In the USA, the nurse-anaesthetist, who worked under the supervision of a specialist, has been largely replaced by medically qualified specialist anaesthetists. Increasing demands for medical services, however, are now prompting a re-appraisal of the concept of the nurse-anaesthetist.

nurse-practitioner

A fully qualified and experienced nurse graduate who carries out most or all of the functions of a medically qualified general practitioner, referring patients who need emergency or specialist care to appropriate doctors or facilities. Experience in the USA suggests that the idea is feasible. The nursing profession in both the UK and USA has responded warmly to the idea but there has been some medical opposition. Many group practices, however, have found that a capable nursing sister, allowed an appropriate degree of autonomy, can provide invaluable assistance to busy practitioners and can safely relieve them of much routine work.

nurse-prescribing

A change in medical practice in 1994, authorized by The Medicinal Products: Prescribing by Nurses Act (1992) that allows registered nurses, health visitors and midwives to prescribe drugs from within an agreed formulary.

nursing, barrier

Local isolation of a patient with an infectious disease so as to avoid spread to society in general, and the local hospital environment in particular. The 'barrier' takes the form of coverings (gowns, caps, overshoes, gloves, masks) which are donned before approaching the patient and discarded, for safe disposal or sterilization, before returning to the normal environment. For medical and economic reasons, direct access to such patients is strictly limited.

Barrier nursing is also used when it is essential to protect patients especially susceptible to infection. In this case, although the barrier takes a similar form, its purpose is to prevent organisms carried on the visitors' clothes or persons from gaining access to the patient. All those working in or visiting hospital carry potentially dangerous organisms. This form of isolation is necessary for patients with extensive burns and for those with a severe deficiency in the normal immunological protective mechanisms.

nutrition

The nutritional requirements are for appropriate amounts of water, carbohydrates, fats, proteins, vitamins, minerals and fibre. In the poorer parts of the world, malnutrition implies deficiencies, in the richer, excess. Both forms are equally harmful. Most people in the Western world eat far too much and suffer in consequence. Pregnant women should, however, remember that they are also supplying a growing passenger.

CARBOHYDRATES

Complex carbohydrate foods such as bread, potatoes, cereals and starches should form the largest part of the diet, and are important sources of energy. Glucose, the simplest of all carbohydrates, and the one to which most carbohydrates are eventually broken down, is the principal fuel of the body.

Carbohydrates vary in chemical complexity: the simpler the form, the more easily digested and absorbed. Glucose is ideal for quick refuelling, but, for normal purposes, slowly absorbed fibrous polymer carbohydrates, such as those found in fruits and vegetables, are more desirable. Some long-chain complex carbohydrates (polysaccharides) like cellulose and pectins are not digested and form roughage.

PROTEINS

Proteins are the chief structural material of the body, but the amount needed to effect repair is small. Growing children need protein to form muscles, bones, skin and other structures. Proteins are complex molecules built from smaller molecules called amino acids, of which the body uses 20 different types. Eleven of these amino acids can be synthesized in the body but the other nine must be provided in the diet.

FATS

Fats are a concentrated fuel, and should form less than one-third of the calorie intake. Fats from fish and vegetable sources (polyunsaturated fats) are less harmful, quantity for quantity, than saturated fats from dairy products and meat. **Cholesterol** is an essential ingredient for health. It is synthesized in the liver and only a small dietary intake is needed.

Saturated fats encourage a rise in the levels of low-density lipoproteins (LDLs) in the blood. LDLs encourage the deposition of cholesterol in the walls of arteries – a feature of arterial disease (**atherosclerosis**). Unsaturated fats encourage a rise in the levels of high-density lipoproteins (HDLs) and these are protective against cholesterol deposition.

VITAMINS AND MINERALS

Except when used as treatments or as antioxidants, taking more **vitamins** than the quantities required to maintain health is pointless and can be dangerous. Vitamins do not generally enhance health unless there is a deficiency. A reasonably varied diet will contain enough vitamins and minerals for normal purposes and to prevent deficiency. The mineral requirements are small – in most cases a few thousandths of a gram.

CALORIES

Calorie requirements vary with sex, body size and weight, and with the degree of activity. **Calories** are used up in maintaining body heat, in keeping all the bodily processes going, and in performing muscular work. A sedentary woman may require as little as 1600 calories a day, while a lumberjack working in snow might need 5000 calories a day. We consume about 100 calories an hour, just sitting; 250 walking; and 600 running.

nutrition, early, and later health

See **Barker hypothesis**.

Nutrizym GR

A brand name for **pancreatin**.

nymphomania

Excessive or pathological desire for copulation, affecting a woman. There is usually an implication that the woman is indifferent as to the partner. There is some reason to believe that the concept of nymphomania is a male-fantasy-engendered fiction. Certainly, there are women who engage in a great deal of sexual activity, but who is to say what is excessive? Those women, claimed to be nymphomaniacs, whose cases have been studied, were usually unable to achieve orgasm or were suffering an intense fear of losing love. It seems probable that women who behave promiscuously are often attempting to satisfy a need for dependency, rather than seeking sexual gratification.

Nyspes

A brand name for **nystatin**.

nystagmus

Persistent jerky or wobbling movement of the eyes, usually together. The movement is most commonly horizontal, but may be vertical, or even circular. The commonest type of nystagmus, 'sawtooth' nystagmus, involves a repetitive slow movement in one direction followed by a sudden recovery jerk in the other. This kind can be observed daily, as a normal phenomenon, in underground railway passengers trying to read the station name from a moving train. Permanent sawtooth nystagmus is almost always present from birth and seldom implies anything serious. Although the eyes are normal, it is, however, usually associated with a slight reduction in visual acuity.

Nystagmus, of a searching type, as if the affected person is constantly looking for something, is a feature of very severe visual defect, such as might occur from dense congenital **cataract** or other serious eye defects present from birth.

> Nystagmus appearing for the first time later in life indicates a probably serious disorder of the nervous system and should prompt immediate medical attention.

Nystan

A brand name for **nystatin**.

nystatin

A drug used in the treatment of fungus infections, such as thrush (**candidiasis**). Nystatin is useful for external infections only as it is not absorbed when given by mouth and is too toxic to be given by injection. A brand name is Nystan. Nystatin is produced in various formulations with other drugs such as **neomycin** (Gregoderm), **metronidazole** (Flagyl Compak), **triamcinolone** (Nystadermal), **oxytetracycline** (Terra-Cortril Nystatin) and the steroid clobetasol propionate (Dermovate-NN).

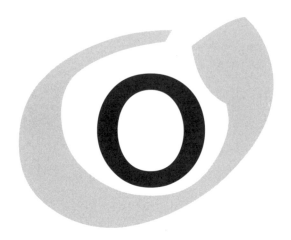

oat-cell carcinoma

A kind of lung cancer feared for its extreme malignancy. About a quarter of lung cancers are of this type and, usually, by the time the diagnosis has been made, the cancer has already spread widely to other parts of the body. In such a case, surgery usually offers no advantage and the only hope is to use anticancer chemotherapy, sometimes with radiotherapy.

Oat-cell carcinoma is also known as 'small-cell' carcinoma because it consists of a mass of small, undifferentiated cells, which multiply rapidly and in an uncontrolled manner. Most cases are caused by cigarette smoking.

obesity

See **health maintenance**.

obesity gene

See **ob gene**.

obesity measurement

See **skinfold thickness measurement**.

ob gene

A gene on chromosome 7 that codes for the hormone **leptin**, which is produced in adipose tissue and which exercises control over food intake and energy expenditure. Ob is an abbreviation of 'obesity'.

obsessive-compulsive disorder

An obsession is an intrusive thought or feeling, recurring constantly with little relevance to present events. One may, for instance, be obsessed with the idea that one is constantly being observed. A compulsion is an intrusive and recurrent prompting to perform some act, such as hand-washing or repeatedly checking that the front door has been locked. Many of us have obsessions; most of us have compulsions, and these are normal and often invaluable aids to success.

The obsessive-compulsive disorder is the state in which these recur with sufficient frequency and irrelevance to cause distress or disability. The sufferer, who is usually of above average intelligence and educational level, may have an obsession, a compulsion, or both, and is perfectly aware that the situation is irrational, but is unable to control it. Complying with the compulsion does not relieve the associated anxiety.

RECOGNITION AND SYMPTOMS

People with the obsessive-compulsive disorder are often deeply preoccupied with cleanliness and fear of contamination, especially with faeces. Some are driven by repeated washing to produce a severe dermatitis of their hands. The checking compulsion is also common and can severely interfere with the normal conduct of life. The obsession that actions must be performed meticulously and slowly can also be very disabling. Affected people are also often preoccupied with aggression and are prone to the phenomenon of 'magical thinking' – the feeling that events can be brought about by thinking about them. This results in much concern over aggressive thoughts.

The obsessive-compulsive disorder usually starts in early adult life often after a stressful event such as a bereavement or a sexual problem of some kind. Usually the sufferer keeps quiet about the matter and often does not seek help for as long as ten years. One-third develop depression and suicide is not uncommon.

POSSIBLE CAUSES

The condition has long been classified as a neurosis, but the tendency, these days, is to avoid this term and simply refer to the problem as a behaviour disorder. There is some evidence that this condition is associated with subtle brain damage, possible, in some cases, from birth injury.

TREATMENT

Treatment with tricyclic antidepressant drugs, especially clomipramine, can be valuable, but the best results have been achieved by behaviour therapy and family therapy. There is no evidence that psychoanalysis can cure the condition.

See also **cognitive behaviour therapy**.

obstetrics

The branch of medicine concerned with childbirth and with the care of the woman until her reproductive organs have returned to normal, about six weeks after the birth.

obstructive airways disease

See **lung disease, chronic obstructive**.

Occam's razor

A principle in science and philosophy, first propounded by the English philosopher William of Occam (c. 1290–1349), and much applied in medicine. The principle states that one should try to account for an observed phenomenon, or a number of simultaneous phenomena, in the simplest possible way and should not look for multiple explanations. For instance, a range of symptoms and signs occurring together should always, if possible, be attributed to a single disease rather than to several different diseases occurring at the same time.

Occlusal

A brand name for **salicylic acid**.

occlusion

A closing off or covering of an opening, or the obstruction of a hollow tube or part of the body. The term is also used by dentists to describe the way the biting and grinding surfaces of the teeth of the two jaws come together. Malocclusion is when the teeth do not fit together correctly. Occlusion, in the sense of deliberately covering one eye for long periods, is an important method of treatment of **amblyopia** in **orthoptics**.

occult

Concealed or obscure. The term is often applied to concealed traces of blood in the faeces or sputum whose presence can only be detected if special tests are used, but which may be of high significance.

occupational diseases

Diseases resulting from exposure to occupational hazards such as toxic, irritating or cancer-producing substances – whether dusts, liquids, solids or gases, bacterial and other infecting organisms, heat, cold, noise, vibration, high or low atmospheric or gas pressure or radiation of any kind. Certain of these diseases are notifiable, by law, to the Chief Employment Medical Adviser. These are aniline poisoning, **anthrax**, arsenic poisoning, **berylliosis**, bitumen ulceration, cadmium poisoning, carbon bisulphide poisoning, chrome ulceration, chronic benzene poisoning, compressed air illness, **lead poisoning**, **manganese poisoning**, **mercury poisoning**, mineral oil ulceration, paraffin ulceration, phosphorus poisoning, pitch ulceration, tar ulceration, toxic anaemia and toxic jaundice.

The range of occupational diseases is wide. Occupational lung diseases, for instance, are an important group and are known to be caused by many industrial substances, including acid anhydride, amine hardening agents, ammonia, animal excreta, asbestos, beryllium, cadmium, chlorine, coal dust, cotton dust, flax dust, fungal spores, grain mites, hemp dust, iron oxide, isocyanates, mouldy straw, mouldy hay, mushroom compost, nitrogen dioxide, phosgene, platinum salts, proteolytic agents, rosin, silica, sulphur fumes and tin dioxide.

Some thousands of substances are thought to be capable of causing **cancer**, often at long intervals after exposure, so that the causal link may not be very apparent.

Industrial conditions due to biological agents include anthrax, **brucellosis**, **farmer's lung**, **glanders**, viral **hepatitis**, **hookworm infestation** (ankylostomiasis), **hydatid disease**, **leptospirosis** and **tuberculosis**.

occupational medicine specialist

A doctor engaged in the branch of medicine concerned with people at work, with the effects of work on health, and of health on the ability to work. This is essentially a branch of preventive or environmental medicine based on a knowledge of working conditions and a concern to detect and remedy work hazards.

occupational therapist

An ancillary health professional engaged in the teaching and supervision of selected occupations to exercise mind and body of the sick and injured, to arouse and sustain interest, to promote confidence and to overcome disability. The aim of the occupational therapist is to inculcate new work interests leading to complete rehabilitation.

octreotide

A hormone inhibitor analogue of the natural substance somatostatin. Octreotide has a much longer effective time of action than somatostatin and is selective in its action on secretion of growth hormone, gastrin, secretin and motilin. It is also effective against various tumours of the **endocrine system**. A brand name is Sandostatin.

Ocufen

A brand name for **flurbiprofen**.

ocular

Relating to the eye. Ocular pathology is any disease process affecting the eye. The term is also used to refer to the eyepiece of an optical device such as a microscope. A binocular telescope is a double telescope for use with both eyes.

ocular equipment advance

See **ophthalmic digital imaging system**.

oculo

Latin root meaning 'eye' as in ocular (of the eye).

Ocusert

A brand name for a device that leaches **pilocarpine** into the conjunctival sac, for the treatment of glaucoma.

-ode

Suffix meaning 'like' as in nematode (thread-like, worm).

odontos

Greek root meaning 'tooth' as in dental (of the teeth).

Odrik

A brand name for **trandolapril**.

oedema

Excessive accumulation of fluid, mainly water, in the body. The accumulation may be general, or in a particular location. In generalized oedema, fluid accumulates in any of the tissues, but especially in the air spaces of the lungs and in the spaces in the abdomen surrounding the bowels and other organs (peritoneal cavity). This cannot occur in a healthy person, however much fluid is drunk, because the kidneys simply dispose of the surplus fluid in the urine.

POSSIBLE CAUSES

Generalized oedema occurs if loss of dissolved substances from the blood, such as protein and salt, reduces the power of the blood to withdraw fluid from the surrounding tissues by the process known as osmosis. This may result from kidney disease such as the **nephrotic syndrome** or acute **glomerulonephritis**; from liver disease, such as cirrhosis, in which the synthesis of protein is reduced; or from starvation, in which the intake of protein is inadequate. Oedema also occurs in **heart failure**, in which the heart is unable to pump blood round fast enough to clear fluid from the tissues. There is a rise in back pressure in the veins and fluid accumulation. Stagnating blood always results in a net outflow of water to the tissues. Oedema of the legs occurs in varicose veins for this reason.

> Any unexplained oedema should be investigated, whether local or general.

RECOGNITION AND SYMPTOMS

Generalized oedema, historically known as *dropsy*, causes weight increase. In mild cases there may be no more effect than this, but more severe oedema can cause difficulty with breathing.

> If the lung oedema becomes severe the situation may become life-threatening and the affected person may literally drown in his or her own body fluid.

TREATMENT

Oedema is treated by correcting the cause, if possible, and by the use of drugs which increase the urinary water output. These are called diuretics.

> Local oedema is the result of injury to a part of the body and results from an increase in the water permeability of the injured blood vessels, which is a normal feature of inflammation. In most cases local oedema settles as the inflammation resolves.

Oedipus complex

The Freudian notion that all sorts of evils, including all the *psychoneuroses*, spring from the young boy's unconscious wish to kill his father and have sexual intercourse with his mother. Freud got the idea from his own experience, and the name from the mythical hero of Sophocles' tragedies. Much of the edifice of Freudian psychoanalysis was built up on this concept, but it is now rarely invoked.

oesophagal cancer

Cancer of the oesophagus occurs most often in people between the ages of sixty and seventy and usually affects the lower part of the gullet. Unfortunately, it has often spread to other local structures by the time a diagnosis has been made. The first sign is obstruction to the passage of solid food with discomfort in the lower chest. Later, there is obstruction to liquids. Usually, this is not reported for several months, by which time there has been considerable weight loss.

A barium swallow X-ray will readily suggest the diagnosis and this can be confirmed by direct examination through an endoscope (oesophagoscopy). Treatment is by surgery and radiotherapy, but often only palliative measures are possible.

oesophagitis

Oesophagitis is inflammation of the lining of the oesophagus, usually from regurgitation of the highly irritating acid from the stomach (reflux oesophagitis). This is a common feature of **hiatus hernia**. The main symptoms are heartburn, acid in the mouth (waterbrash) and difficulty in swallowing, and the condition may be complicated by ulceration, scarring and narrowing of the oesophagus.

A severe form of oesophagitis is caused by the swallowing, accidental or deliberate, of corrosive poisons.

VARICES

Most of the blood from the intestine returns to the heart by way of the liver so that nutrients can be taken up and processed. When the liver develops extensive fibrosis (**cirrhosis**), this flow is dammed back and the blood has to find other pathways back to the great vein of the abdomen (the inferior vena cava). One such pathway is via the veins at the lower end of the oesophagus and these become greatly widened and distorted (varicose) to form oesophageal **varices**. Should these varices be injured there is a danger of severe bleeding and vomiting of large quantities of blood. This occurs in about 40 per cent of all cases of cirrhosis of the liver.

Bleeding oesophageal varices are treated by direct pressure from special internal balloons, blood transfusion, lowering of the blood pressure by drugs and then surgical measures to prevent further bleeding. These include closure of the varices and shunt operations to bypass the area.

oesophagos

Greek root meaning 'gullet' as in oesophagus.

oesophagus

The gullet, or swallowing tube, which extends downwards from the throat (pharynx) to pass through the diaphragm and enter the stomach, is called the oesophagus. It is about 24 cm long and is a muscular tube lying just in front of the spine and behind the wind pipe (trachea). After food has been swallowed, it is carried down by controlled contraction of the muscular walls of the oesophagus. The circular muscles of the tube wall relax in front of the lump of food and contract behind it (peristalsis). This action forces the food to slide along the tube and is, of course, essential, if the tube is not to get totally blocked. When peristalsis becomes disordered and acts against itself severe colic develops.

At the bottom of the oesophagus, immediately above the **stomach**, is an important muscle ring, the cardiac sphincter, which normally closes after swallowing, to prevent the stomach contents from returning.

oesophagus, disorders of

The oesophagus is the gullet, or swallowing tube. It may suffer spasm, which causes pain like a heart attack and which may interfere with swallowing. A diverticulum of the oesophagus is a local out-pouching of the lining, usually as a result of infection in adjacent lymph nodes spreading to damage and weaken the outside of the tube.

oestradiol

A natural oestrogen drug that can be taken by mouth as a hormone replacement therapy and to control menopausal symptoms. Trade names are Climaval, Ellest Solo, Menorest, Progynova, Sandrena, Vagifem and Zumenon. Preparations of oestradiol for external use as a transdermal patch include Estelle Solo MX 40, Estraderm MX, Evorel, Fematrix 40 and Femseven. The drug is also used externally in a vaginal ring for post-menopausal vaginitis, under the brand name Estring.

oestriol

An **oestrogen** used to treat infertility due to inadequate penetration of the cervical mucus by spermatozoa. A brand name is Ovestin.

oestrogen

One of a group of steroid sex hormones secreted mainly by the ovaries, but also by the testicles. Oestrogens bring about the development of the female secondary sexual characteristics and act on the lining of the uterus, in conjunction with progesterone, to prepare it for implantation of the fertilized **ovum**. They have some **anabolic** properties. Oestrogens are used to treat ovarian insufficiency and menopausal symptoms, to limit postmenopausal **osteoporosis**, to stop milk production (lactation) and to treat widespread cancers of the **prostate gland**. They are extensively used as oral contraceptives. Trade names are Premarin and Prempac-C.

oestrogen drugs

A group of female steroid sex hormones secreted mainly by the ovaries, but also by the testicles. Oestrogens bring about the development of the female secondary sexual characteristics. In conjunction with progesterone, they act, each month in the non-pregnant, to prepare the lining of the womb for implantation of the fertilized egg (ovum). They have some anabolic properties (see **anabolic steroids**).

Oestrogen drugs are substances chemically related to the natural hormones. They include oestradiol, ethinyloestradiol, mestranol and diethylstilboestrol. They can be given by mouth, by implants under the skin, by vaginal pessaries and by skin patches. They are used to treat inadequate ovary function. They are the basis of hormone replacement therapy (HRT) for menopausal symptoms and to limit postmenopausal osteoporosis. They are used to stop milk production (lactation) and to treat widespread cancers of the prostate gland. Most of all, they are used as oral contraceptives (see **contraceptive drugs**).

Oestrogen therapy rarely produces serious complications, but there may be side-effects. These include:

● nausea and vomiting;
● weight gain;
● bloating due to water retention;
● painful breasts;
● increased blood clotting with a higher risk of thrombosis;
● gallstones;
● high blood pressure.

Oestrogens given as hormone replacement therapy may increase the risk of cancer of the womb and may encourage the growth of any existing breast cancer. Some experts believe that the addition of progesterone eliminates the risk of womb cancer. You should be sure that no breast tumour is present before starting HRT.

oestrogens from plants

See **phyto-oestrogens**.

oestrogens, non-biological

See **xeno-oestrogens**.

ofloxacin

An antibacterial drug. Trade names are Exocin for an eye drop preparation and Tarivid to be taken by mouth for general infections.

-oid

Suffix meaning 'like' as in sarcoid (flesh-like).

olanzapine

A thienobenzodiazepine drug used to treat **schizophrenia**. it is similar to **clozapine**. A brand name is Zyprexa.

Olbetam

A brand name for **acipimox**.

old age, good quality of

See **eugeria**.

Olestra

A non-digestible fat substitute that was given approval by the US Food and Drug Administation (FDA) in 1996 but which does not appear to be the final solution to the obesity problem. About 20 per cent of those eating it are said to have abdominal symptoms such as cramping or diarrhoea. There is also concern that Olestra might inhibit the absorption of fat-soluble antioxidant carotenoids.

oligospermia

An abnormally low concentration of sperms (spermatozoa) in the seminal fluid. The average ejaculate, in a young man, is about 3 ml and contains about 300 million sperms. Men with fewer than about 20 million sperms per ml are likely to be infertile. See also **sperm count**.

oliguria

A reduction in the normal output of urine. The daily urine output, in a healthy person, varies between about 700 ml and 2 litres. Oliguria is most commonly the result of increased fluid loss through the skin due to sweating, or inadequate fluid intake. In such a case the urine is concentrated. Similarly, severe fluid loss in diarrhoea or vomiting or severe blood loss can also cause oliguria, with concentrated urine resulting.

Apart from these cases, oliguria is usually due to sudden failure of kidney function (acute renal failure), or to the end stage of long-term kidney disease.

olsalazine

A salicylate drug used to treat ulcerative colitis. A brand name is Dipentum.

-oma

Suffix meaning 'lump, growth' as in carcinoma (hard lump).

omeprazole

The first of the class of proton pump inhibitor drugs used to control the production of stomach acid and treat stomach and duodenal ulcers and especially the **Zollinger-Ellison syndrome**. Omeprazole can be effective in cases that have failed to respond to H-2 receptor blocker drugs such as **ranitidine**. The drug is long-acting and need only be taken once a day. A brand name is Losec.

Omnopon

A brand name for **papaveretum**.

Omnopon-scopolomine

A brand name for **hyoscine** and **papaveretum**.

onchocerciasis

Commonly called 'river blindness', this is a tropical parasitic disease caused by the microfilarial worm *Onchocerca volvulus*. The disease occurs only within about 500 metres of turbulent rivers because it is spread by the biting black fly *Simulium damnosum*, which breeds only in well-oxygenated rivers and which has a limited flying range.

Onchocerciasis is so called because it causes lumps or nodules under the skin. *Oncho* is Greek for 'a lump'. Each *oncho* contains at least one male and one female adult worm.

INCIDENCE
The disease occurs mainly in certain areas of West Africa, notably Nigeria and Ghana, but is also found in East Africa, South Mexico, Guatemala, Venezuela, and Columbia. At least 20 million people have onchocerciasis and hundreds of thousands are blinded by it. In many villages almost all the adults are blind and are led about by children who have not yet been blinded.

RECOGNITION AND SYMPTOMS
The male adult worm is 2 to 4 cm long and the mature female is 30 to 50 cm long. After impregnation, the female worm releases millions of microscopic microfilaria which wander about under the skin. Those on the head enter the eyes and swim about in the ocular fluids, causing little upset. On dying, however, they set up a severe and destructive inflammation which opacifies the corneas, causes adhesions between the irises and the internal lenses, and destroys the function of the retinas, leading to irremediable blindness. The microfilaria also often block lymph vessels and cause **elephantiasis**.

TREATMENT
The worms can be killed by drugs such as diethylcarbamazine and suramin but such treatment is dangerous and must be used with caution. If communities can be persuaded to move away from rivers, the disease dies out, but an alternative water source must be provided and such a move is often strongly resisted on cultural grounds.

oncogene

One of a number of genes that contribute to cancerous changes in cells. Oncogenes are mutations of normal cell genes and must work together to cause cancer. Similar or identical genes are found in viruses known to be able to cause cancer. If one of the three virus genes, gag, pol or env, is replaced by an oncogene, such as ras, the virus becomes capable of causing cancer. The normal allele of an oncogene is called a proto-oncogene.

oncological surgeon

A surgeon who specializes in cancer treatment.

oncologist

A doctor who specializes in the study of the causes, features and treatment of cancer. An oncologist is a cancer specialist, knowledgeable in the latest advances in cancer management and skilled in applying this knowledge.

oncology

The study of the causes, characteristics and treatment of **cancer**. The Greek root *onco* means 'a lump'.

Oncovin

A brand name for the anticancer drug **vincristine**.

ondansetron

A serotonin antagonist drug used to relieve nausea and vomiting caused by anticancer chemotherapy and radiotherapy and to prevent sickness after surgery. A brand name is Zofran.

One-alpha

A brand name for **alfacalcidol**.

onychogryphosis

Claw-like finger- or toenails resembling the talons of the mythological griffon. This may occur for no obvious reason, but is often associated with **candidiasis** of the nails or with repeated injury.

onycholysis

Loosening or separating of the nail, or part of it, from its bed. See also **nails, disorders of**.

onychos

Greek root meaning 'fingernail' as in onychogryphosis (griffon fingernails).

oon

Greek root meaning 'egg' as in oophoritis (ovary inflammation).

oophorectomy

Surgical removal of an ovary or of both ovaries. This is done if the ovaries are affected by cancer, cysts or other disease. Removal of one ovary has little effect, either on fertility or on

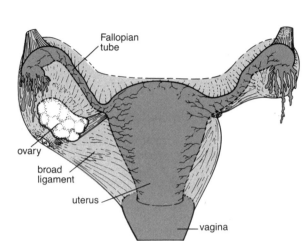

Surgical removal of an ovary is called griffon. This involves tying off the blood supply to the ovary and cutting the broad ligament.

the hormonal situation. Removal of both ovaries causes sterility and has secondary effects from the loss of sex hormones, especially **oestrogen**.

operating theatre

A room, or suite of rooms, set aside for the performance of surgical operations. The first consideration, in the design of an operating theatre, is the safety of the patient, especially by avoiding infection of the open surgical wound. For practical reasons it is impossible to achieve sterilization of floors, walls, tables and other major equipment, but these are all designed to be easily washed down each day, so as to keep the bacterial count low. Walls are tiled and floors are covered with washable material of a kind not liable to build up charges of static electricity. X-ray and scan viewing boxes are often built into the walls.

An operating lamp, designed to produce shadowless illumination, is suspended from the ceiling in such a way as to be freely adjustable, and in some operating rooms an operating microscope may also be ceiling mounted. Supplementary lamps, on mobile floor stands, are used, when necessary.

The operating table, although of heavy construction, and immobile while in use, is so designed that it can be moved freely to clear the theatre for cleaning. It is generally made of stainless steel and has a wide range of adjustments so that the whole table may be raised or lowered, tilted about its long or central axis, or tilted independently up or down at either end. The table is covered with a thick slab of conductive rubber for the comfort and protection of the patient.

Near the operating table is the anaesthetic machine, a wheeled trolley fitted with cylinders of oxygen and anaesthetic gases and with valves and gauges for controlling the rate of delivery of the anaesthetic agents. The machine also contains a mechanical ventilator by means of which the respiration of the anaesthetized and paralysed patient may be maintained, and an electrocardiogram monitor, often with an audible bleep. The anaesthetic machine is so designed that it can be connected to the patient in the adjacent anaesthetic room and wheeled into the theatre alongside the patient's trolley. Many operating theatres are equipped with

outlets for anaesthetic gases directly piped from a central depot in the hospital.

Several stainless steel, wheeled tables are necessary for the layout of instruments. These are covered with sterile towels before use. A diathermy machine, used by the surgeon to control bleeding or to make bloodless incisions, is commonly present, and there may also be a laser cutter. Various other items of equipment are brought in, depending on the kind of operation to be performed. These may include special frames for the support of the patient, various imaging devices, fibre optic endoscopes, powerful electromagnets for the removal of metallic foreign bodies and heart-lung machines.

Adjoining the central operating room are various ancillary rooms – scrub-up annexes with foot- or elbow-operated water taps where the surgeons, the assistants and nurses meticulously clean their hands and arms before donning sterile gowns and rubber gloves; the sterilizing room, where the autoclaves are installed; the changing rooms where staff leave normal clothing and put on clean operating garments; the anaesthetic room, where patients are anaesthetized; store rooms for instruments, sutures, drugs and equipment; and rest and coffee rooms for the theatre staff.

Traditionally, a senior and experienced nursing sister is in charge of the theatre and junior surgeons in training quickly learn to accord her the high respect which is usually her due.

operation

The act or process of performing anything. A surgical operation is a procedure, performed on the body of a patient, usually by means of instruments, but sometimes with the hands only, to effect some beneficial change. Most surgical operations would involve pain and so are performed under anaesthesia which may be local or general.

operon

A row of consecutive genes on a chromosome that operates as a single functional unit. The structural genes in the operon, that code for the protein, are preceded by two regulatory sites occupied by regulatory genes, the promoter and the operator. These are essential for the expression of the operon. The genes in an operon have related functions that occur sequentially. All the genes in the operon are turned on and off together. All are transcribed into one large segment of **messenger RNA**.

Ophthalin

A brand name for **sodium hyaluronate**.

ophthalmia

An old-fashioned term for an inflammatory eye disorder. The term has been abandoned now that the precise nature of all the different eye disorders is known, and specific and meaningful terms have been applied to them.

ophthalmic digital imaging system

A piece of equipment whereby a camera capable of imaging the retina or cornea of the eye or an ophthalmic diagnostic microscope (slit lamp ophthalmic microscope) is coupled to a personal computer. This system allows an immediate, high-resolution, colour, digital bit-mapped image of all visibly accessible parts of the eye to be displayed on the computer monitor for convenient study, and the file of the image may be saved for clinical record-keeping and training purposes.

The system, which runs under Windows 98 or Windows 2000 software, has been described as the most important advance in ophthalmic imaging since the invention of the retinal camera.

ophthalmic optician

An ancillary health professional qualified to test vision, to establish the type and degree of refractive error, to examine the eyes for disease and to prescribe glasses and contact lenses. Also known, especially in the USA, as an optometrist.

ophthalmic surgeon

An ophthalmologist who regularly treats eye disorders such as corneal opacities, cataracts, glaucoma, retinal detachment and vitreous opacities by surgery.

ophthalmologist

A doctor practising the combined medical and surgical specialty concerned with the eye and its disorders. The ophthalmologist has a detailed knowledge of the structure, function and diseases of the eyes, of the associated neurological systems concerned with vision and of the range of non-ocular diseases that affect the eyes. He or she is skilled in ophthalmic optics and in the medical and microsurgical skills and techniques used in the treatment of the many ophthalmic conditions.

ophthalmology

The specialty concerned with the eye and its disorders. Ophthalmology is a combined medical and surgical discipline practised by doctors who, after basic qualification, have undertaken training in ophthalmic optics, in the structure, function and diseases of the eyes and in the associated neurological systems concerned with vision. They are also versed in the wide range of different general conditions which affect the eyes and in their detection within the eye.

Ophthalmologists must also acquire the delicate skills of microsurgery so as to be able to perform the range of operations to treat conditions such as **cataract**, **glaucoma**, opacity of the cornea, squint (**strabismus**), retinal detachment, major eye injuries and disorders of the **lacrimal system**.

ophthalmoplegia

Paralysis of the muscles which move the eye. This is sometimes referred to as external ophthalmoplegia, to distinguish it from internal ophthalmoplegia, in which the internal focusing muscles and the muscles of the iris are paralysed.

ophthalmos

Greek root meaning 'eye' as in ophthalmology (study of eyes).

ophthalmoscopic 'cattle-trucking'

The ophthalmoscope is an optical instrument which allows inspection of the inside of the eye, especially the retina. With this instrument, the blood in the small arteries and veins of the retina, at the back of the eye, can easily be seen. At, or shortly before, death, the blood ceases to flow in these vessels

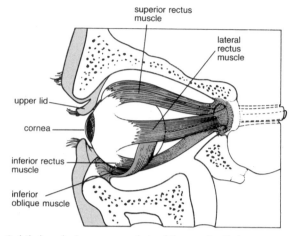

Ophthalmoplegia means paralysis of the muscles that move the eye. There are six of these tiny, but precisely acting, muscles to each eye.

and the blood column breaks up into short segments like railway trucks. This is a sign that the circulation of the blood has ceased.

Opilon

A brand name for **thymoxamine**.

opium derivatives

Crude opium as a solution in alcohol, known, expressively, as laudanum was once the only major narcotic **analgesic drug** and was widely used for all sorts of appropriate, and inappropriate, purposes. Purified preparations containing a mixture of the many opium alkaloids are still used. These include Nepenthe, Papaveretum and Omnopon.

The main alkaloid narcotic derived from opium is morphine, and this is still extensively used. It is a valuable drug both for its powerful painkilling property and for the calm euphoria, and relief from shock and anxiety, it gives to those who are the victims of severe accidents or other dangerous and painful misfortunes. Heroin (diamorphine) is even more powerful, but has long been banned for medical use in most countries in the world as offering no advantage over morphine except increased solubility. Heroin, still used medically in the UK, is converted into morphine in the body.

In addition to relieving pain and distress of mind, morphine adversely affects breathing, sometimes fatally, stops coughing, promotes sleep, causes vomiting and constipation, and makes the pupils small.

Codeine, a mild narcotic analgesic drug, is another opium derivative. It is used mainly for relief of moderate pain and to check diarrhoea and irritable, nonproductive coughing.

opportunistic infection

Infections by organisms that are normally effectively repelled by the body's defence mechanisms, but which are able to establish themselves because these mechanisms are temporarily or permanently defective.

Opportunistic infections occur in conditions of immunodeficiency such as AIDS and hypogammaglobulinaemia, but are also common in people who, for good reason, are given immunosuppressive drugs. They occur in people suffering from prolonged debilitating diseases, in alcoholics, in people with cancer, diabetes, cirrhosis of the liver, kidney and heart failure and severe burns; and they are common in people who have to have long courses of antibiotics and in those who have prolonged intravenous therapy.

Most of the organisms concerned are normally fairly harmless and many are regular inhabitants of the body. They include *Pneumocystis carinii*, histoplasma, cytomegalovirus, *Candida albicans*, *Herpes simplex* and the tubercle bacillus. In most cases, effective treatment is available for opportunistic infections, but recurrence is, of course, common.

ops

Greek root meaning 'eye' as in myopia ('muscular eye').

opsis

Greek root meaning 'appearance' as in autopsy (appearance after death).

optic atrophy

Degeneration of the optic nerve. This may be due to injury, hereditary or acquired disease, poisoning or local pressure. Common causes are **multiple sclerosis**, **glaucoma**, **retinitis pigmentosa** and poisoning with quinine or methylated spirits (wood alcohol or methanol). On examination with an ophthalmoscope the readily visible head of the optic nerve is white instead of its usual pink colour.

optic disc oedema

The optic disc is the head of the optic nerve, conspicuously visible at the back of the inside of the eye when examined with an ophthalmoscope. In disc oedema, the disc swells and protrudes forward so that it ceases to be in the same plane of focus as the retina.

> This is an important clinical sign of a rise in the pressure within the skull from any cause – such as a brain tumour – and many lives have been saved by the observation of this early sign.

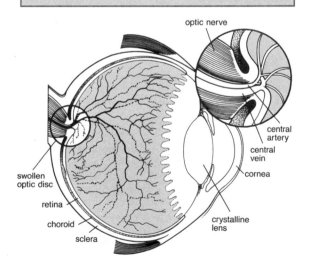

optician

In Britain there are two kinds of optician, the ophthalmic optician and the dispensing optician. The former is able to test vision, determine any defects of focusing and prescribe appropriate glasses or contact lenses. Ophthalmic opticians also carry out brief medical examinations of the eyes and refer to a doctor any cases in which eye disorder is suspected.

Dispensing opticians are skilled in the correct fitting of spectacle frames and in making the measurements necessary if lenses are to be properly centred in the frames. They also fit and supply contact lenses, but do not determine the lens power of these.

optic neuritis

Inflammation of the optic nerve. This may be due to spread of infection from the adjacent sinus, but is most commonly due to **multiple sclerosis**. There is often little or no pain, but usually some tenderness on pressing on the closed lids or on extremes of movement of the eye. Inflammation interferes with the passage of nerve impulses and because most of the optic nerve fibres come from the central part of the retina, neuritis causes loss of the centre of the field of vision in the affected eye, resulting in a 'hole' in the image. Recovery is usual but this may take six weeks or longer.

Treatment with corticosteroid drugs may hasten the return of vision, but is unlikely to affect the long-term outcome.

Opticrom

A brand name for **sodium cromoglycate**.

Optilast

A brand name for **azelastine**.

Optimine

A brand name for **azatadine**.

optometrist

See **ophthalmic optician**.

Orabet

A brand name for the antidiabetic drug metformin.

Oradexon

A brand name for dexamethazone.

oral

Relating to the mouth.

oral contraceptives

See **contraceptive drugs**.

Swelling (oedema) of the head of the optic nerve (optic disc) is an important sign of raised pressure within the skull. Disc oedema is readily visible with the ophthalmoscope.

Oraldene

A brand name for **hexetidine**.

oral hypoglycaemic drug

See **antidiabetic drugs**.

Oramorph

A brand name for **morphine**.

Orap

A brand name for the antipsychotic and movement disorder drug **pimozide**.

Orbenin

A brand name for cloxacillin.

orbital cellulitis

The orbit is the bony cavern which encloses and protects the eyeball. This cavern contains much fat and the eye-moving muscles, and when these become involved in a spreading inflammation, the condition is called orbital cellulitis. The orbit is separated from the skin and the eyelids by a tissue plane, called the orbital septum, and this offers some barrier to the spread of infection backwards. The veins of the face, however, pass through the orbits and provide one route of infection to the orbital tissues and, through them, to the cavernous sinus behind.

POSSIBLE CAUSES

The commonest source of infection of the orbital tissue, however, is the collection of bony sinuses which surround the orbits. In particular, on the inner side, separating the two orbits, are the ethmoidal sinuses or air cells. These are separated from the orbits by paper-thin bony walls (the *lamina papyracea*) and infection in these sinuses spreads readily to the orbits. Infection may also spread from the frontal sinuses, which form the roofs of the orbits, and from the maxillary sinuses (antrums) which form the floors.

RECOGNITION AND SYMPTOMS

Orbital cellulitis causes the eyeball to be pushed obviously forwards, but the lids are often so swollen that the eye remains tightly shut. On gently separating the lids, the conjunctiva, which normally lies flat and inconspicuous on the white of the eye, will be seen to be full of fluid and bulging forward between the lids so that the cornea appears to be at the bottom of a circular pit. Eye movement may be paralysed and the vision severely reduced. There is often general upset with fever, headache and nausea.

> Orbital cellulitis is a serious emergency calling for urgent intensive antibiotic and occasionally surgical treatment. If an abscess forms within the orbit, this must be opened and the pus drained out. Nowadays, this is rarely necessary. The major risk to life is of the development of cavernous sinus thrombosis.

orchidectomy

The surgical removal of a testicle. Sometimes called *orchiectomy*. This may be done for tumour of the testicle itself or, more commonly, both testicles may be removed to reduce secretion of the male sex hormone testosterone. Cancers of the prostate gland, and secondary spreads from these cancers, are sex-hormone dependent, and orchidectomy is often effective in assisting in the treatment of such cancer.

When only one testicle is removed, potency and fertility are retained.

orchidopexy

The testicles are formed inside the abdomen and normally descend into the scrotum before birth, by passing down a tube called the inguinal canal. Sometimes one or both testicles fail to descend, remaining in the abdomen or in the inguinal canal. Orchidopexy is an operation to bring an undescended testicle down into the scrotum and to fix it in place. A testicle which remains in the abdomen will become sterile because the lower temperature of the scrotum is necessary if normal sperms are to be produced.

Ten per cent of undescended testicles remain in the abdomen and in such cases, orchidopexy is difficult and has to be done in stages, but most lie in the canal and can usually be brought down in a single-stage operation. This should ideally be done before the age of three.

orchis

Greek root meaning 'testicle' as in orchidectomy (testicle removal).

orchitis

Inflammation of the testicle. The commonest cause is the **mumps** virus and at least 20 per cent of men who contract mumps after puberty suffer orchitis. The testicle becomes swollen, sometimes greatly so, and acutely painful and there is usually high fever. These effects last for three to seven days and then gradually subside. In some cases, orchitis is followed by atrophy of the testicle, but sterility is uncommon unless both testicles are severely affected in this way. Orchitis may also be caused by other viruses including the lymphocytic choriomeningitis virus.

There is no specific treatment for orchitis, but great relief can be obtained by the use of pain-relieving drugs (analgesics) and by careful padding of the testicle in wool.

orciprenaline

A non-selective beta-adrenoceptor agonist that can be used as a heart stimulant. A brand name is Alupent.

Orelox

A brand name for **cefpodixime**.

Orexin

One of a pair of centrally acting neuropeptides produced by the lateral hypothalamus where the sensation of hunger is mediated. Rats given orexin will eat about ten times the normal amount of food and rats starved for 48 hours have more than twice the normal concentrations of orexin. There are also specific receptors for the two orexins. These facts are being exploited in the design of drugs that can both stimulate and reduce appetite.

organelle

Any one of the bodies forming the internal functional components of cells. The term means 'little organs'.

The organelles include:

- **mitochondria**;
- the golgi apparatus, which packages and moves proteins;
- the endoplasmic reticulum, which pervades the cell interior and carries ribosomes;
- ribosomes, which construct proteins on the instruction of the genetic code;
- lysosomes, which package digestive enzymes and break down dead cells;
- centrioles, which assist in cell division.

The physiology and biochemistry of the organelles is a major science, by comparison with which pre-electron microscope physiology of the whole body was simple. The study of organelle function and of the interaction of cells now constitutes the greater part of human physiology.

organic brain syndrome

See **brain damage**.

organism

Any living animal or plant. The most elaborate known example is man. Micro-organisms include the single-celled protozoa, the fungi, the bacteria and the viruses. Most of these are harmless to man, but medicine is much concerned with those which are capable of causing disease. Other organisms of medical importance are the parasitic worms, the bugs, the lice, the fleas, the flies, the spiders, the mites, the ticks and the snakes.

orgasm

A sequence of bodily processes, occurring at the climax of sexual intercourse, and involving the pleasurable release of heightened muscle tension. In men, the orgasm features a succession of spasmodic muscle contractions which cause the **ejaculation** of seminal fluid.

In female orgasm, the cervix contracts rhythmically, which can help to draw the sperm into the uterus. It is not, however, necessary for conception and plays no essential role in ensuring fertilization. Up to 50 per cent of women do not experience orgasm.

It is rare for men, even those who are impotent, to fail to achieve orgasm. Orgasmic problems in men are more often connected with failure to control the onset of orgasm so that this occurs prematurely.

Women may fail to experience orgasm through failure of sexual arousal, but absence of orgasm is common even if arousal is high. The female orgasm is promoted by clitoral stimulation which may be direct or indirect. Vaginal stimuli are less effective, but movement of the vagina causes indirect massage of the clitoris via the hood which joins the two **labia** minora. Many women can achieve orgasm only by masturbation or by the use of a mechanical aid (vibrator). In most cases, the female orgasm consists of a relatively low peak of sexual excitement centred in the clitoris. This may be single or multiple with one peak running into another. Rarely, the male-type experience occurs – an intense peak which precludes the desire for further stimulation.

Oriental sore

Cutaneous **leishmaniasis**, or Oriental sore, is caused by the single-celled microscopic parasite *Leishmania tropica* and is transmitted by the bite of the sandfly. It occurs in the Mediterranean area, China, and parts of India, but is gradually spreading westward and cases are beginning to occur in the west Mediterranean holiday resorts. Unlike *visceral* leishmaniasis, the infection normally remains localized to the region of the sandfly bite – usually on the face, arms or legs.

RECOGNITION AND SYMPTOMS

The condition starts as a small, raised, red area (papule) that gradually increases in size until it is up to 10 cm in diameter. This develops into an ulcer with an overlying crust. In many cases a number of small surrounding papules also occur.

TREATMENT

Healing takes from three months to three years, and leaves a depressed and often disfiguring scar. Some forms of the disease never heal spontaneously. Treatment is by the application of local heat and the use of organic antimonial drugs.

-orium

Suffix meaning 'place for' as in vomitorium (vomiting place).

orlistat

An anti-obesity pill that acts in the intestine by inhibiting the action of intestinal pacreatic fat-splitting enzymes (lipases) so that up to one-third of dietary fat is not absorbed but is excreted in the faeces. People who are taking the drug and continue to eat fats may regret may suffer oily stools, anal leakage and problems flushing the toilet. Another disadvantage is that the absorption of fat-soluble vitamins (A, D, E and K) and beta carotene may be interfered with. Almost 6 per cent of people on orlistat for two years had abnormally low levels of vitamin D, beta carotene or vitamin E. The latter two may be important as antioxidants. The drug is certainly effective, however, and if it encourages people to eat less fat it will serve a very useful purpose. A brand name is Xenical.

Ormetan

A brand name for **aminoglutethamide**.

Oroxine

A brand name for the thyroid hormone **thyroxine**.

orphenadrine

A drug used to relieve muscle spasm, especially in **Parkinson's disease**. Trade names are Biorphen and Disipal.

-orrhagia

Suffix meaning 'flooding' as in menorrhagia (flooding periods).

Ortho Dienoestrol

A brand name for **dienoestrol**.

orthodontics

The dental specialty concerned with the cosmetic and functional state of the position of the teeth, and the relationship of the upper teeth to the lower (**occlusion**). Orthodontics takes advantage of the remarkable degree to which tooth positioning can be influenced by sustained pressure, and several different kinds of appliances are used to apply such pressure. These include various types of braces, springs, wires and harnesses. Sometimes small metal attachments are cemented to the teeth so that force may be applied, and sometimes teeth are deliberately extracted to make room.

Pressure applied to a tooth causes absorption of socket bone on the side opposite to the pressure, and new bone production on the same side. The process is slow, but the effect on the position of the tooth is permanent.

orthodontist

A dentist specializing in the correction of irregularities of tooth placement and in the relationship of the upper teeth to the lower (**occlusion**). The orthodontist organizes the movement of teeth by sustained pressure from braces, springs, wires and harnesses. The process, which produces permanent results, sometimes involves removal of crowded teeth.

orthopaedic collar

A collar is commonly prescribed for the treatment of inflammation or arthritis of the neck bones (**cervical spondylosis**), but is of value only if firm and severely restrictive. Soft collars which allow much movement do no good at all.

> Collars are of benefit if they relieve pain. If a collar makes pain worse, the doctor who prescribed it should be informed, for it may need alteration or re-appraisal.

Collars should have washable coverings. A silk scarf worn over the collar may improve comfort and appearance. Collars are seldom worn for more than about two months.

orthopaedics

This word derives from the Greek for a 'straight child', not 'straight foot', as is commonly thought. Orthopaedics is the branch of surgery concerned with the correction of deformity caused by injury, disease or congenital abnormality of the bones, joints and associated ligaments, muscles and tendons.

Orthopaedic surgeons treat fractures, dislocations, joint disorders of all kinds, including those of the spine and intervertebral discs, back problems generally, foot problems, degenerative diseases of bones and joints, tumours of bone, congenital defects of the skeleton, and many other conditions. Orthopaedics is increasingly concerned with the replacement of damaged and degenerate joints with prosthetic devices, and hip, knee and even finger-joint replacements are now commonplace. Increasingly, too, joint instability from tendon defects are being treated by the use of very strong synthetic, woven, carbon-fibre materials.

orthopaedic surgeon

A surgeon specializing in the treatment of fractures, dislocations, joint disorders of all kinds, back problems generally, foot bone disorders, congenital defects of the skeleton and many other conditions. The orthopaedic surgeon is greatly concerned with the replacement of damaged and degenerate

joints with prosthetic devices, especially artificial hip and knee joints.

orthoptics

A specialty, ancillary to **ophthalmology**, concerned mainly with the management of squint (**strabismus**) in childhood and the avoidance of the visual loss (**amblyopia**) which readily results from squint. Orthoptists are experts in the diagnosis of inapparent squint and in obtaining information about the state of the visual acuity, in both eyes, in children. They are also able to determine the degree to which the child is able to perceive simultaneously with the two eyes (binocular vision).

The avoidance of amblyopia is achieved largely by the judicious covering, for variable periods, of the better-seeing eye (occlusion). Orthoptists use a variety of ingenious instruments in their work.

orthoptist

An ancillary health professional who works with an ophthalmologist to diagnose squint, to measure the angle of squint, to assess visual acuity in young children and to determine the degree to which children are able to perceive simultaneously with the two eyes (binocular vision). The orthoptist works to avoid or overcome the defects of vision that arise from squint and other early disorders of the eyes.

Orudis

A brand name for **ketoprofen**.

Oruvail

A brand name for **ketoprofen**.

Oruvail gel

A brand name for **ketoprofen** formulated for external use.

os (bone)

Latin root meaning 'bone' as in osteomyelitis (bone inflammation).

os (mouth)

Latin root (pl. ora) meaning 'mouth' as in oral (of the mouth).

-ose

Suffix meaning 'condition of' as in varicose (like varix).

Osgood-Schlatter disease

A knee disorder affecting mostly boys, usually around puberty. The bulky group of muscles on the front of the thigh run down together into a heavy tendon which contains the kneecap and which is inserted into a bony lump on the front of the main bone of the lower leg (the tibia). Repetitive strong pulls on this tendon, as the knee is straightened against resistance (an inevitable occurrence in normal boyhood activity) sometimes cause damage at the point of insertion of the tendon. Some authorities believe this to be due to interference with the blood supply of the region. There is swelling of the upper end of the tibia and sometimes acute tenderness on pressure.

Fortunately the problem resolves rapidly with no more treatment than a period of avoidance of activities such as climbing, cycling and rugby-playing. If these are persisted in, an unsightly protuberance may develop below the knee. In severe cases a plaster cast to prevent bending may be required.

-osis

Suffix meaning 'disease of' as in sclerosis (hardness disease).

osmosis

An important principle in physiology. The movement of fluid in various directions, under the influence of osmosis, underlies a considerable part of the functioning of the body. Unless osmosis is understood, many aspects of body function, both at a cellular and at an organic level, will be mysterious.

A semi-permeable membrane is one which allows liquid, such as water, to pass through but does not allow certain substances dissolved in the liquid to pass. Most of the membranes in the body are semi-permeable, and osmosis is occurring constantly everywhere in the body. If such a membrane, placed vertically, separates a pure liquid from one in which substances are dissolved, the pure liquid will pass through the membrane to dilute the solution on the other side. This will cause the level to rise on the side of the solution, and the level will continue to rise until the extra weight of liquid on that side just balances the tendency of the liquid to pass through. The pressure exerted by the extra liquid is said to be equal to the 'osmotic pressure' of the solution. Osmotic pressure is determined by the number of molecules dissolved in a particular quantity of the solution.

Since the interior of the body is a fluid medium, and since every cell in the body is surrounded by a semipermeable membrane, the effect of osmosis is universal. Biological membranes, in general, do not allow passage of substances of high molecular weight. Thus, in general, inorganic molecules pass easily but organic molecules do not. Membranes can, however, by consuming energy, transmit various substances actively, against the direction of osmotic pressure.

Osmosis is readily shown by placing living cells in solutions of various osmotic pressures. If cells are placed in solutions of low pressure, such as distilled water, water flows into them and they swell up and may burst. If placed in solutions of high pressure, they shrink and collapse. For most cells, a 0.9 per cent solution of salt will cause no net movement of fluid either way, and this is called an *isotonic* solution. Such a solution, used for infusion, is called 'normal' saline.

ossification

The process of the formation of bone. This is a dynamic process, continuously occurring throughout life, but is more active during the period of body growth and following a fracture. Ossification sometimes occurs in tissues not normally associated with bone, and may follow long-term inflammation.

Ossopan

A brand name for **hydroxyapatite**.

osteitis

Inflammation of bone. Infection of bone, with involvement of the bone marrow, is called **osteomyelitis**.

osteoarthritis

A degenerative joint disorder involving damage to the cartilaginous bearing surfaces and sometimes widening or re-modelling of the ends of the bones involved in the joint.

Osteoarthritis is closely age-related and many people of thirty show early osteoarthritic changes. By age sixty-five, about 80 per cent of people have objective evidence of the disorder, but only a quarter of these have symptoms. In the elderly, women tend to be more severely affected than men.

POSSIBLE CAUSES

Osteoarthritis is the commonest form of **arthritis** and the cause is unknown. It is, however, commonly associated with injury or deformities of the skeleton which disturb the normal mechanics of the joints and the relationships of the joint surfaces. Obesity is an important aggravating factor. In spite of the name, there is little inflammation. Bony spurs often develop at the margins of the affected joints.

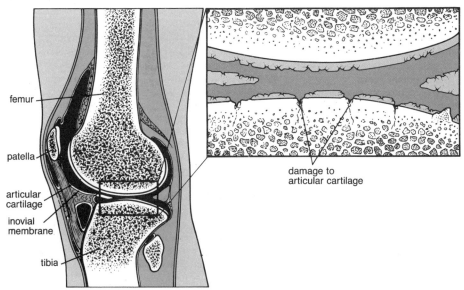

femur

patella

articular cartilage

inovial membrane

tibia

damage to articular cartilage

In osteoarthritis the cartilaginous bearing surfaces of the bones becomes roughened and worn so that the raw bone is exposed. This causes pain and disability.

RECOGNITION AND SYMPTOMS

Osteoarthritis most commonly involves the spine, the knee joints and the hip joints. Symptoms come on gradually, with pain which at first is intermittent and then becomes more frequent. Joint movement becomes progressively more limited, initially because of pain and muscle spasm, but later because the joint capsule becomes thickened and less flexible. Movement may cause audible creaking, and swelling results from quite minor injury.

TREATMENT

Short of joint replacement, there is no specific remedy for osteoarthritis, but much can be done to relieve the symptoms. It is important to avoid undue stress or injury to the joints. Loss of excess weight is very helpful. Rubber heels can reduce jarring and a walking stick can be valuable. A change of occupation may be necessary. In some cases, injection of corticosteroids into the affected joint can markedly reduce pain and disability.

osteochondritis dissecans

The release of small fragments of cartilage or bone (loose bodies) into the interior of a joint, causing swelling, pain and restriction of movement. If troublesome, the loose bodies may have to be removed surgically.

osteoclast inhibition

See **osteoprotegerin (OPG)**.

osteogenic sarcoma

See **bone cancer**.

osteomyelitis

An infection of bone and bone marrow, usually with staphylococci spread from a boil or other skin infection, but sometimes with other organisms including Salmonella species. It can also result from an open (compound) fracture. The disease is commonest in children and starts abruptly with fever and severe pain at the affected bone site. An adjacent joint may swell and stiffen and confuse the diagnosis. X-ray changes do not occur for several days or weeks, but isotope scanning can establish the cause of the trouble.

> Intensive antibiotic treatment is necessary if osteomyelitis is not to become long-term (chronic), with abscess formation and death of an isolated piece of bone (sequestrum formation). In pre-antibiotic days osteomyelitis was almost always permanent and was curable only by amputation.

osteon

Greek root meaning 'bone' as in osteosarcoma (bone cancer).

osteopathy

A system of medical management founded in the United States in 1874 by Andrew Taylor Still (1828–1917) and based on the idea that health will result if the structures of the body, especially those of the spine, bear a proper relationship to each other. Still believed that displaced vertebrae obstruct 'the flow of the life-forces through the nerves'. Most osteopaths put much emphasis on the importance of the function of the spinal column as a whole and on its relationship to the pelvis and the limb bones. Osteopathic treatment is manipulative and is aimed at freeing and loosening joints and re-establishing proper relationships.

Although these basic premises are not generally accepted, and the objective value of manipulation is widely questioned, osteopathy is not fundamentally at variance with orthodox medicine and such opposition as exists within the medical profession arises mainly from concern that danger may arise if treatment is undertaken without proper diagnosis.

Qualified osteopaths have had years of training in the basic medical disciplines of anatomy, physiology and pathology and, because of their narrow concentration on skeletal and muscular disorders, many become highly skilled in the effective treatment of these conditions, so far as they are amenable to manipulative treatment. It must, however, be said that the psychological and placebo effect of the 'laying on of hands' can hardly be overestimated, and that many disinterested critics believe that this is the main reason for such success as is obtained. Nevertheless, most doctors now have no objection to referring patients to osteopathic practitioners once a firm diagnosis has been made.

osteoporosis

A reduction in the density of the protein (collagen) scaffolding of the bones and of the calcium salts deposited on the protein. Like other tissues of the body, the bones are in a state of constant physical and chemical change, losing and gaining calcium and protein, to and from the bloodstream.

POSSIBLE CAUSES

These changes are controlled by various growth and sex hormones, and alteration in the amounts of these in the body affects the strength of the bones. As a result, diseases of the hormone-producing glands may cause osteoporosis and this is a feature of overactivity of the thyroid and parathyroid glands; of disorders of the adrenal glands; of reduced output of sex hormones; and of disorders of the pituitary gland. Osteoporosis occurs in **Cushing's syndrome**, **acromegaly**, prolonged **thyrotoxicosis**, and **diabetes**.

The bones are thickest and strongest in early adult life. Thereafter, they become gradually thinner with age, as a result of progressive loss of the protein structure and of calcium. Bones stay strong by being used so that physical forces are applied to them. Under-use, such as occurs in the bed-ridden or in astronauts living in zero gravity, leads to osteoporosis. Even a change from an active to a sedentary life can cause osteoporosis, as do the ordinary processes of aging, with associated loss of activity and reduced hormone levels.

Women are worse off then men in this respect because while men continue to secrete sex hormones into old age, women have an oestrogen shut-down at the menopause and begin to lose calcium in the urine, with progressive weakening of the bones. Adequate dietary calcium in youth is important in minimizing the risk, especially in women.

RECOGNITION AND SYMPTOMS

In most cases of osteoporosis there are no symptoms until some effect of the weakening in the bones occurs. This may be a loss of height from shrinkage of the bones of the spinal column, severe curvature of the spine, sudden collapse of one of the bones of the spine with severe pain and disfigurement, a wrist or forearm fracture or, perhaps commonest of all, an unexpected fracture of the neck of the hip bone as a result of a quite minor stumble or fall. About one woman in four over the age of seventy-five suffers this misfortune and the consequences are often very serious, often shortening life.

TREATMENT

There is still controversy about oestrogen hormone replacement therapy to reduce the risk of osteoporosis in women after the menopause. Oestrogens certainly retard the process of bone loss, but do not increase bone bulk. They have some disadvantages, however, especially in causing a slight increase in the risk of thrombosis and cancer of the uterus. Most doctors, however, are strongly in favour of oestrogens and often prescribe them in combination with progesterone. Such combined therapy minimizes the risk of uterine cancer but restores periodic bleeding and may slightly increase the risk of breast cancer.

Male sex hormone treatment, in men, is useful only in those relatively rare cases in which osteoporosis is due to inadequate production of natural sex hormone. In both sexes, calcium supplements are valuable and help to prevent further loss of bone.

See also **hormone replacement therapy**.

osteoprotegerin (OPG)

A secreted protein that inhibits the development of the cells that break down old bone (osteoclasts) prior to the growth of new bone. The **cytokine TRANCE** binds to osteoprotegerin.

-ostomy

Suffix meaning 'making mouth' as in colostomy (mouth in the colon).

otalgia

Pain in the ear from any cause.

otitis externa

Inflammation of the skin of the ear canal. The skin of the external ear (pinna) may or may not be involved.

POSSIBLE CAUSES

Otitis externa may be a local disorder or part of any general inflammatory disorder of the skin. These include a wide variety of infections.

Staphylococci may cause a painful boil in the canal, herpes viruses, both simplex and zoster, may cause the characteristic blisters (vesicles) and crusting, and fungi of various kinds, including thrush (*Candida albicans*), may cause persistent and sometimes intractable inflammation. This is called otomycosis. **Eczema** and seborrhoeic **dermatitis** are common causes of otitis externa.

RECOGNITION AND SYMPTOMS

Most forms of the disorder cause pain, sometimes severe, and there is usually a discharge from the ear (otorrhoea). Unless the canal becomes blocked, hearing is not usually affected.

TREATMENT

Otitis externa may be persistent (chronic) and difficult to treat, and the management varies with the cause. Thorough cleaning of the canal and specific antibiotic or anti fungal treatment are often necessary, and solutions of such drugs may be applied locally on gauze 'wicks'.

otitis media

Inflammation in the middle ear cavity, usually as a result of spread of infection from the nose or throat by way of the Eustachian tube. Although this is the route of access, outward drainage through the Eustachian tube is also important in maintaining the health of the middle ear, and blockage commonly leads to infection.

POSSIBLE CAUSES

Eustachian tube obstruction may be caused by the adenoids or by inflammation in the tube itself as a result of repeated infection.

> Acute suppurative otitis media is a form in which the onset is sudden with a rapid production of pus in the middle ear so that the pressure rises and the eardrum bulges outwards. There is severe pain and fever with general upset and a risk of perforation of the drum. Urgent treatment with antibiotics is necessary.

In chronic suppurative otitis media, there is a perforation in the drum, usually with a persistent discharge (otorrhoea). Deafness and **otitis externa** are common complications.

GLUE EAR

'Glue ear' is a persistent and insidious condition of the middle ear, mainly affecting children. The term is a popular but useful one, describing the condition of secretory otitis media, and indicates that the structures of the middle ear – the drum and the three small linking bones (the auditory ossicles) – which transmit sound vibrations from the air to the cochlea in the inner ear, are impeded from free movement by a 'glue' of sticky mucus produced by the inflammation.

The condition arises mainly because the middle ear is unable to drain its secretions into the nose by way of the Eustachian tube. Glue ear is not primarily caused by infection, as are the other common forms of otitis media.

Glue ear can be treated fairly easily, and normal function restored, by a simple operation in which a tiny cut is made in the eardrum (myringotomy) and a small plastic drainage tube – a *grommet* – is inserted. This allows immediate equalization of pressure on the two sides of the drum and free drainage of middle ear secretions.

The condition is usually symptomless, the only effect being deafness, and this, too, may be unsuspected as the affected child is often unaware that anything is wrong and may not complain. Such children are often accused of inattentiveness. A high proportion of young children who fail to meet their parents' educational expectations suffer from glue ear and are found, on audiometric testing, to be incapacitated by deafness.

> Undetected severe glue ear is particularly disastrous if it occurs in the first two years of life, for normal hearing is essential for the development of speech and learning. Sensory deprivation during this period may have a lifelong effect, not only on comprehension and speech, but on actual intellectual development. Language problems starting in this way persist and cause irremediable later difficulties in acquiring a vocabulary. Severe childhood inattention may be due to deafness.

Audiometry under the age of five is very difficult, but simpler tests can demonstrate hearing defect and draw attention to the condition of the ears and the state of the throat.

-otomy

Suffix meaning 'cutting into' as in tracheotomy (cut into the trachea).

otoplasty

A plastic surgical operation to correct prominent, bat-like ears, usually performed on children. Ugly ears may be a serious matter for a young child, who may suffer taunting and isolation from his or her peer group. Children's ears are always relatively large – the ear is three-quarters grown at the age of three and almost fully grown by eight – so any unusual prominence is more obvious than in an adult.

HOW IT'S DONE

The skeleton of the ear is a single piece of gristle (cartilage) of complicated shape, and this is covered with skin which is firmly stuck to the front surface but more loosely attached behind. This is convenient, because, to conceal the scars, the surgeon will do the operation on the back of the ear. Great care will be taken to ensure that any incisions made on the back do not come right through to the front where the skin would be marked.

If the prominence is due to a folding outwards of the cartilage, the principle is to thin, or weaken, it along an almost vertical line so that it can easily be bent backwards towards the head. The surgeon makes a vertical cut through the skin on the back of the ear and exposes the cartilage. The weakening can be done in various ways. Some surgeons actually cut a thin vertical strip out of the cartilage, but this is apt to cause rather sharp bending, when the cartilage is folded back, with a very prominent ridge. Others prefer to weaken the cartilage by making a large number of fine cuts with the point of a sharp scalpel. Alternatively, the line of bending can be thinned by the use of a tiny rasp, or file, or the line can be carefully pared thin.

Once the cartilage is thinned in the right place, it will bend back easily and, to keep it back, the surgeon will remove a vertical ellipse of skin from the back of the ear and then sew the edges together. Because there is now less skin on the back of the ear, the edges of the incision can only be brought together if the cartilage folds back. The degree to which it will bend back does, of course, depend on the width of the ellipse of removed skin, and this must be skilfully judged to get the amount of bending just right. Quite often there is a difference in the prominence of the two ears and, in such a case, the width of the ellipse will have to be varied accordingly.

If the ear prominence is due solely to a large angle between the ear and the head, a different operation is necessary. In this case, the skin removal behind the ear is more extensive, and it is necessary to take away some skin covering not only the back of the concha but also some skin over the adjacent mastoid bone of the head. When this is done, the bared area includes the angle between the ear and the head. When the free edges of this area are sewn together, vertically, the ear will be brought close against the head and will be less prominent. In very severe cases, where both angles are large, both procedures may have to be combined.

otorhinolaryngology

The full title for the surgical specialty concerned with the diseases of the ear, nose and throat. Also known as otolaryngology.

otorrhoea

A discharge, or running, from the ear.
See **otitis externa**, **otitis media**.

otos

Greek root meaning 'ear' as in otitis media (middle ear inflammation).

otosclerosis

A hereditary ear disease leading to progressive deafness of the 'mechanical' or 'conductive' type. The vibration of the eardrum, under the influence of sound waves, is conveyed to the inner ear by a chain of three small bones, known as the auditory ossicles. The innermost of these, the stapes, is shaped like a stirrup and the 'footplate' of this bone fits into an oval window, in the outer wall of the inner ear, in such a way that it is free to vibrate in the window. In otosclerosis, the fibrous seal surrounding the footplate becomes replaced by bone so that the stapes becomes progressively immobilized. People with otosclerosis can hear best in noisy surroundings, but eventually become severely deafened.

TREATMENT

The condition can be treated only by a microsurgical operation. In one procedure, the loop of the stapes is detached and a small hole is drilled in the footplate to take an artificial metal or plastic piston. This is then linked to the middle ossicle so that when the eardrum vibrates, the piston moves in its hole. The results of this delicate operation can be excellent.

ototoxicity

Damage to ear function by drugs or other toxic agents. These act on the inner ear, causing injury to both hearing and balancing mechanisms. The main ototoxic agents are the aminoglycoside antibiotics (streptomycin, gentamycin, neomycin, etc.); some diuretic drugs (frusemide and ethacrynic acid); salicylates, including aspirin; and quinine. All of these have to be taken in larger than usual dosage to cause ear damage. They may, however, have this effect if the kidneys are unable to excrete them normally, as may occur in certain kidney diseases.

Otrivine-Antistin

A brand name for **antazoline**.

outer ear disease

See **otitis externa**.

ovarian cysts

These may occur at any age, but are commonest between the ages of thirty-five and fifty-five. Most of them produce no symptoms and the only sign is a gradual increase in the size of the abdomen which may be attributed to simple obesity. In some cases, however, they may lead to varicose veins or piles (**haemorrhoids**) or may cause breathlessness and abdominal discomfort. Women sometimes mistake this enlargement for a pregnancy.

Cysts may be caused by slight disorders of **ovulation** or by distention of the delicate outer lining of the ovary from fluid collection. Such swellings are usually harmless. Cysts caused in this way usually pass unnoticed, but occasionally they grow big enough to cause pain. Treatment is seldom required.

The commonest true ovarian cysts are serous cysts containing watery fluid. These occur late in the reproductive life or after the menopause and may be of almost any size up to an enormous bulk, filling and distending the abdomen. The similar pseudomucinous cysts contain a viscous mucoid fluid and may also grow very large. These cysts cause trouble mainly by their bulk, but may cause severe complications if they become twisted and their blood supply is cut off or if they rupture or become infected. Care must be taken during the removal of pseudomucinous cysts to avoid damaging the capsule, as the contents are very irritating to the peritoneum and cells can be released which can set up new cysts elsewhere in the abdomen.

Ovarian cysts may result from **endometriosis** of the ovary. These contain altered blood and almost always cause pain. Surgical treatment is usually necessary.

ovarian cysts, multiple

See **Stein-Leventhal syndrome**.

ovaries

The ovaries are the female gonads – paired organs situated in the pelvis, one on each side of the womb, just under, and inward of, the open ends of the Fallopian tubes. They are almond-shaped and about 3 cm long, with prominent blood vessels. Once a month, one (or sometimes more than one) ovum site (Graafian follicle) matures and releases an egg (ovum). This is called ovulation. Each ruptured follicle is replaced by a yellow body known as a corpus luteum. In addition to the production of ova, the ovary synthesises three types of steroid hormone – oestrogens, progesterones (female sex hormones) and androgens (male sex

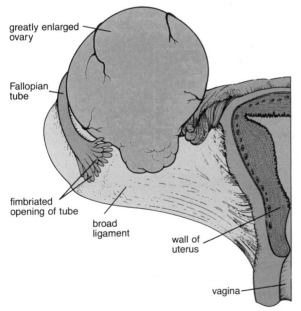

greatly enlarged ovary

Fallopian tube

fimbriated opening of tube

broad ligament

wall of uterus

vagina

The ovaries are particularly prone to cyst formation. Most of these are innocent (benign) but they can grow to a very large size and may cause problems simply on account of their bulk. Some are inherently dangerous.

hormones). Ovulation may be associated with pain ('middle pain' or *mittelschmerz*).

ovary, cancer of

Cancer of the ovary is commoner in women who have never had children than in those who have. It may occur at any age but is most usual between fifty and sixty. Unfortunately, ovarian cancer tends to be 'silent' until it has grown and spread, displacing and invading the womb (uterus) and spreading widely within the pelvis and abdomen. Diagnosis is usually made by direct endoscopic visualization (laparoscopy). Treatment is surgical and the uterus and both ovaries must be removed (see **hysterectomy** and **oophorectomy**), as the second ovary often also contains a tumour. Ovarian cancer is often very susceptible to anti-cancer chemotherapy. Radiotherapy is seldom useful.

overactivity, child

See **attention deficit hyperactivity disorder**.

overdose

A quantity of a drug well in excess of the recommended dose.

overeating

See **health maintenance**.

over-the-counter (OTC) drugs

These are drugs that can be bought without prescription. This is not to imply that such drugs are harmless; many of these OTC preparations contain powerful drugs, and they should all be used responsibly and in the exact dosage recommended. Government decisions to save money in this way have not been uniformly approved by doctors. To quote from a leading Lancet article in June, 1994: 'The unthinkable is happening at the pharmacy counter. Drugs that no one would have dreamed would take the route can be bought over-the-counter (OTC), and more will follow...'

In Britain, the following are some of the potent drugs that can now be bought over-the-counter:

- various non-sedating **antihistamine drugs**;
- some steroid drugs for **hay fever**;
- nicotine patches;
- acyclovir cream for **herpes** simplex;
- imidazole **antifungal drugs**;
- **hydrocortisone** cream;
- sodium cromoglycate eyedrops;
- **H2 receptor antagonists**;
- chloroquine phosphate for **malaria** prevention;
- various non-steroidal anti-inflammatory drugs (**NSAIDs**).

These recently released drugs are obtainable only from a registered pharmacy where advice can be obtained from the pharmacist. Doctors anticipate that pharmacists will spend more time talking to customers than before. In pharmacological trade circles drugs are classified as POM (prescription-only medication), or OTC, or P (pharmacy-only). So there are really three categories.

The range of drugs available over the counter also includes many preparations in such categories as painkillers; indigestion remedies; symptomatic treatments for coughs and colds; drugs for hay fever, ear, eye and mouth care remedies; skin, hair and scalp medications; sun protection drugs; sedatives; travel sickness remedies; vitamin and mineral preparations; and aids to smoking avoidance.

Doubts have been expressed about the safety of some of these changes, mainly on the grounds that patients may be denied the advice normally given by a doctor when such drugs are prescribed. Concern has also been voiced over the risk of adverse interactions of these drugs with prescribed drugs. Some doctors are worried that symptoms of a more serious disorder may be concealed by the use of such drugs. Others, however, view the change favourably.

overweight

See **health maintenance**.

Ovestin

A brand name for the oestrogen drug **oestriol**.

Ovran

A brand name for **levonorgestrel**, a **progestogen** drug formulated with **ethinyloestradiol** as an oral contraceptive.

Ovranette

A brand name for **levonorgestrel**, a **progestogen** drug formulated with **ethinyloestradiol** as an oral contraceptive.

ovulation

The development of an ovum (egg) in the ovary is called oogenesis, and its release is called ovulation. Ovulation usually occurs about 14 days before the start of the next period. A released ovum is swept into the fallopian tube and carried along towards the womb. While in the tube, it may be met by sperms (spermatozoa). If not, the ovum is simply discarded during the next menstruation.

If pregnancy does occur, the placenta, almost as soon as it is established, begins to secrete a hormone called chorionic gonadotrophin. This is similar to the luteinizing hormone of the pituitary gland and its function is to keep the corpus luteum going so that the right hormones are secreted to prevent further ovulation and menstruation during the remainder of the pregnancy. At the end of pregnancy, the placenta is lost, and, with it, the supply of chorionic gonadotrophin.

Absence of ovulation means that the woman concerned is sterile. Ovulation can, however, often be induced artificially. Tests for ovulation include the measurement of blood progesterone levels, which rise in the second half of the cycle, and examination of the mucus in the cervix, which changes at ovulation. Home testing kits, based on detecting a hormone in the urine, are now very accurate. A check of follicle breaking by ultrasound scanning is also useful. Sometimes the pain on ovulation (*mittelschmerz*) is severe and positive enough to be indicative. In general, regular menstruation suggests that ovulation is occurring.

See also **menstruation**.

ovum

Latin root meaning 'egg' as in ovulation (egg production).

The egg, or ovum, is the female reproductive cell (gamete), produced by the ovary about halfway between two menstrual periods. Human ovaries usually produce one egg per month, but often produce more than one. The egg contains half the chromosomes required by the new individual, and the other half are supplied by the sperm at the moment of fertilization. The egg is a very large cell, much larger than a sperm, and is about 0.1 mm in diameter. Its size is determined by the need to contain nutritive material (yolk) to supply the embryo in its earliest stages before it can establish a supply from the mother via the placenta.

At birth the ovaries contain about a million immature ova. New ova are not produced during life and all those fertilized are the same age as the mother. This is why the incidence of

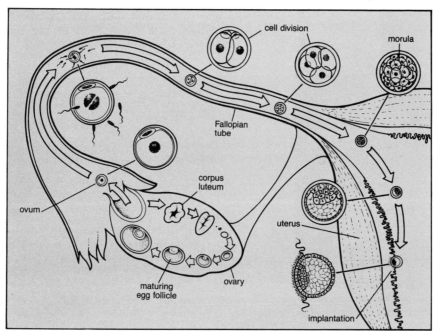

The sequence of ovulation, fertilization, ovum division and implantation in the lining of the womb (uterus).

genetic abnormalities rises in babies born to older women – the ova have had a longer period in which mutation can occur. Only about 400 of these immature ova become mature and are released.

The process by which egg cells are produced in the ovaries and are prepared for release and fertilization is called oogenesis. Oogenesis includes the process by which the number of chromosomes is reduced to half the normal, so that, on fertilization the full complement will be restored by a half-number contribution from the sperm.

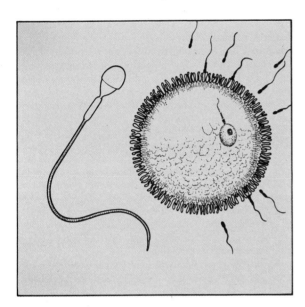

Ovum and sperm (spermatozoon) under huge magnification and not to scale. The ovum is many hundreds of times the size of the sperm.

ovum donation

The provision of human eggs (ova) by harvesting them from living donors, or by obtaining them from the ovaries of women who have recently died or from aborted fetuses. Donated ova could be used to relieve infertility or for important research purposes. The topic is highly controversial and has aroused strong reactions on both sides of the argument.

ovum production, multiple

See **superovulation**.

Ovysmen

A brand name for **ethinyloestradiol** formulated with a **progestogen** drug as an oral contraceptive.

oxazepam

A **benzodiazepine** tranquillizing drug. A brand name is Serenid.

oxerutin

A bioflavonoid drug used to treat oedema from poor venous drainage. A brand name is Paroven.

oxidative stress

The widespread and damaging effects of oxygen **free radicals** on any part of the body. Oxidative stress is limited by natural body antioxidants and may be reduced by dietary supplements of antioxidant vitamins (C and E) and flavonoids.

Oxis Turbohaler

A brand name for **eformoterol**.

oxitropium

An **anticholinergic** drug used from an inhaler to treat asthma and chronic obstructive lung disease. A brand name is Oxivent.

Oxivent

A brand name for **oxitropium**.

oxpentifylline

A xanthine drug that relaxes smooth muscle and is used to improve blood flow in peripheral blood vessel disorders. A brand name is Trental.

oxprenolol

A beta-blocker drug used to treat **angina pectoris**, high blood pressure and disorders of heart rhythm. Trade names are Slow-Trasicor and Trasicor.

oxybuprocaine

A local anaesthetic drug used as eyedrops to effect rapid anaesthetization of the cornea for pressure measurement in glaucoma (tonometry), foreign body removal and other purposes. A brand name is Minims benoxinate.

oxybutynin

An anticholinergic antispasmodic drug used to treat urinary urgency, frequency and incontinence and bed-wetting in children. Trade names are Cystrin and Ditropan.

oxygen

An invisible, odourless gas constituting about one-fifth of the earth's atmosphere. Oxygen is the most vital necessity for life, and deprivation for more than a few minutes is fatal. It is taken into the body in inspiration and conveyed to all parts by the blood, in the form of oxyhaemoglobin – a loose combination with the haemoglobin in the red blood cells.

Much of medicine is concerned with circumstances and factors which, actually or potentially, prejudice the supply of oxygen to the tissues. These include lung disorders, blood diseases, disorders of the heart and the blood vessels, many poisons, and injuries involving loss of blood and interference with air access to the lungs.

Oxygen is needed for the fundamental process of oxidation of fuel to release energy. This is a highly complex biochemical process known as oxidative phosphorylation and involving the synthesis of the universal energy carrier ATP (adenosine triphosphate) in the inner membranes of the mitochondria of the cells. In energetic terms, however, it is similar to the release of energy, as heat, which occurs when hydrogen is burned in oxygen to form hydrogen oxide, more commonly known as water (H_2O).

oxygen concentrators

The development of molecular sieves of silica and alumina, which selectively adsorb the components of air, have made possible reasonably efficient oxygen concentrators, producing medically acceptable oxygen at a cost competitive with that of current methods of fractionation of liquid air.

These concentrators work by virtue of the fact that if air under pressure is passed through a column of molecular sieves, oxygen passes through at a faster rate than nitrogen. The output consists of 95 per cent oxygen and 5 per cent of the inert gas argon. Concentrators were developed, initially, for use in military aircraft, and small concentrators, of the type used in aircraft, have been available for some time now for patients in their own homes who need supplementary oxygen. These deliver oxygen at a small fraction of the cost of oxygen in cylinders.

oxygen supply, emergency

See **transtracheal oxygen catheterization**.

oxygen supply, improving

See **intravascular oxygenation**.

oxygen therapy

This is used to treat conditions in which the oxygen concentration in the blood is reduced, and also to help to improve the oxygen supply to tissues, even when the haemoglobin is fully saturated, by increasing the amount carried in solution in the blood plasma. This may be valuable in very ill patients with **anaemia**.

Oxygen is given by light plastic masks or by double tubes fitting comfortably into the nostrils. Oxygen tents are now rarely used.

Oxymycin

A brand name for **oxytetracycline**.

oxyphenbutazone

A non-steroidal anti-inflammatory drug (**NSAID**) limited to external use in ointment form. A brand name is Tanderil.

oxytetracycline

A broad-spectrum tetracycline antibiotic derived from the mould-like bacterium *Streptomyces rimosus*. The drug is effective against a range of gram positive and gram negative organisms including Rickettsiae and is widely used to treat acne. A brand name is Terramycin.

oxytocin

An oxytocic hormone produced by the pituitary gland. The hormone promotes contraction of the womb and is used as a drug in obstetrics to bring on labour at term and to augment slow labour. It is given by intravenous infusion. A brand name is Syntocinon.

ozaena

An uncommon form of inflammation and atrophy of the mucous membrane lining of the nose, featuring a thick discharge, crusting of the lining and a foul smell, of which the sufferer is, by habituation, usually unaware. This is one of the causes of **halitosis**. Ozaena requires skilled management by an ENT specialist.

ozone

A powerful and unstable gas produced by the action of ultraviolet radiation or electrical discharge on oxygen in air. The molecule consists of three oxygen atoms (O_3), and only a small quantity is normally present in atmospheric air. This is fortunate, as ozone is a highly poisonous, irritating gas, sometimes used as a disinfectant. The idea of health-giving ozone, at the seaside, is a myth.

There is a layer of ozone in the stratosphere produced continuously by the action of ultraviolet radiation from the sun. This layer forms a protective barrier, cutting down the intensity of the ultraviolet component in sunlight. The ozone shield lies in the region between 10 and 50 km above the earth's surface, and is most concentrated at an altitude of 20 to 25 km. This shield maximally absorbs ultraviolet light of wavelength about 250 nanometres, which is biologically very damaging. Without the ozone layer human beings would suffer serious biological effects from solar radiation, including a large increase in the incidence of skin cancer and irritating eye disorders, such as **pterygium**.

Ultraviolet light is known to cause **rodent ulcer** of the skin (basal cell carcinoma), squamous cell skin cancer and **malignant melanoma**.

Under normal circumstances, the rate of production of ozone is balanced by the rate of its natural breakdown, so the layer remains unchanged. Chlorofluorocarbons (CFCs), such as Freon, released from aerosol sprays, plastic foam blowers and refrigerators, drift slowly upwards and release chlorine free radicals – chemical groups with an unpaired electron. These radicals act as catalysts, breaking down ozone to oxygen and then being released unchanged to go on acting. Although the million tonnes or so of CFCs released annually represent a mere drop in the ocean in the context of the volume of the atmosphere, catalysts can have powerful effects even in very low concentration. These free radicals survive for more than 100 years. Released CFCs take decades to reach the ozone layer.

The concern is that the ozone shield may be significantly reduced, and recent observations of 'holes' in the stratospheric layer over the Antarctic have aroused widespread concern. Calculations suggest that an 85 per cent reduction in CFC production would be necessary to stabilize atmospheric concentrations at their *present* level. Under the auspices of the United Nations, the major industrial countries of the world have now signed the Vienna Convention on the Ozone Layer, but there is little agreement on action. European ministers have committed themselves to a freeze on increase in CFC production and a 20 per cent reduction after five years. The Americans insist on a 50 per cent reduction. Both proposals may yet prove to be too little and too late.

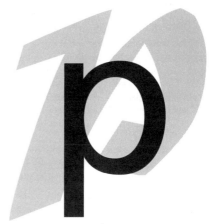

pacemakers

Permanent, implanted, artificial heart pacemakers are small, battery-driven electronic oscillators which deliver short pulses of electricity, at 3 to 4 volts, to cause the heart muscle to contract. They are used in people with a defect of the conducting system of the heart (**heart block**). The pulse generator is buried under the skin of the chest and often forms one contact. The electrode, which is well insulated except for the tip, runs into a large vein and from there into the heart, usually the upper right chamber.

Pacemakers may run at a fixed rate, but these limit physical activity, 'and most, nowadays, are triggered by the demands of the heart or are programmable from the outside by means of radio signals. The battery, in the generator, lasts for about ten years.

External pacemakers are widely used in the emergency treatment of heart block to maintain heart action until the block recovers spontaneously or more permanent arrangements can be made. External pacemakers are connected to the heart by an insulated electrode which is inserted into a vein and moved, under X-ray control, into the heart.

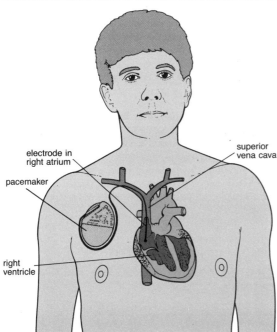

A pacemaker is an electronic pulse generator, complete with battery, that is implanted under the skin of the chest wall. An insulated electrode with a bare tip carries the pulse current into the heart by way of a vein.

Pacitron

A brand name for the antidepressant drug tryptophan.

paclitaxel

A taxane anticancer drug used mainly to treat ovarian cancer and widespread breast cancer. A brand name is Taxol.

paediatrician

A doctor who specializes in all aspects of childhood diseases and disorders and with the health and development of the child in the context of the family and the environment.

paediatrics

The medical specialty concerned with the care of children. Paediatrics is concerned with more than simply the diseases that affect children. It covers all aspects of child health and development in the context of the family and the whole environment. The specialty calls for a knowledge of:

- genetics and the whole range of genetic disorders;
- normal and abnormal physical and mental development;
- the special aspects of bodily function (physiology) of the child;
- child psychiatry;
- behaviour and learning problems;
- the special nutritional requirements and problems of childhood;
- immunization;
- the infectious fevers and other disorders common to childhood;
- the whole range of diseases that affect people of all ages, but have special features or dangers in childhood.

With the growth of medical knowledge, paediatrics, like other medical and surgical disciplines, has become too large to be mastered by single individuals and is rapidly becoming fragmented into subspecialties.

paedophilia

Recurrent sexual urges towards a child under thirteen by a person over the age of sixteen and at least five years older than the child. Most child sexual molestation involves fondling of the genitals and oral intercourse. Vaginal or anal intercourse is relatively infrequent except in cases of incest. Most children physically molested are thought to be male, but most reported cases involve female children.

Almost all paedophiles are heterosexual and in at least half of the incidents reported there has been some degree of alcohol intoxication. Paedophiles are often also involved in voyeurism, exhibitionism or rape.

Paedophilia is not a medical or psychiatric condition. It is, and should remain, as much a matter for criminal prosecution as any other act performed, for selfish advantage, against the interests of others.

Paget's disease

A bone disease, sometimes called osteitis deformans because of its tendency to cause softening and distortion of any of the bones of the body.

INCIDENCE

It affects men more often than women and often runs in families. It is rare before the age of forty, but increasingly common thereafter, affecting up to three per cent of the elderly population.

POSSIBLE CAUSES

Recent evidence suggests that the disease may be due to a virus infection of one of the two types of cells which organize bone (osteoclasts).

RECOGNITION AND SYMPTOMS

The bones most often involved are the skull, the collar bones (clavicles) the spine (vertebral column), the pelvis and the leg bones. Sometimes the bones of the face become distorted to produce the lion-like appearance known as leontiasis ossea. There is an increased blood flow though the affected bones and the area involved may feel unusually warm. Affected bones are enlarged and distort under pressure. The legs may become bowed; spinal distortion may affect the spinal cord, causing paralysis; spontaneous fractures may occur; and skull enlargement and thickening may cause headache and deafness from compression of the acoustic nerves.

TREATMENT

Paget's disease is treated with pain-relieving drugs and with the hormone calcitonin, which decreases the rate of bone turnover and allows more calcium and phosphorus to be lost in the urine. People with Paget's disease who are confined to bed often develop very high levels of calcium in the blood and are at risk from kidney stones and other complications. A high fluid intake, and measures to reduce blood calcium, are important.

Paget's disease of the nipple

It is quite common for an itchy skin rash to affect both breasts. This is often a form of **eczema**, calling for treatment with ointments. But if a patch of reddened skin, resembling eczema, appears on only one nipple, it is possible that, under it, is a small cancer. This may be so even if no mass can be felt. This is called Paget's disease of the nipple.

Such a patch should always be reported. Usually a **biopsy**, to exclude or confirm cancer, is required. Paget's does not readily spread beyond the breast tissue, but should always be removed.

pain

An unpleasant sensation, often localized, caused by strong stimulation of sensory nerve endings by an event or process damaging to, or liable to damage, tissue. The term comes from the Latin *poena* meaning 'punishment'. Pain, unless very persistent (chronic), commonly serves as a warning of danger and leads to action tending to end it. Such action may be reflex, involuntary and very rapid, or conscious, deliberate and purposeful.

EFFECTS

Pain causes distress and anxiety and sometimes fear, and the psychological and physiological changes associated with it may be similar to those experienced during anger and aggression. The significance of the pain is often more closely related to the quality of these secondary effects than to the actual intensity of the pain itself. The psychological reaction to pain is often considerably modified by past experience. If pain is separated from its mental reaction, as is possible by the use of drugs such as morphine, it may still be felt but may no longer be unpleasant. The distress caused by pain depends also, to a large extent, on the sufferer's awareness of the cause. Thus, the effect of even minor pain inflicted by a torturer may be much more severe than if the same pain were the result of an innocent cause such as an accident.

THE PROCESS OF PAIN

The nerve endings for pain are called nociceptors and these are stimulated into sending pain messages to the brain by the chemical action on them of substances, such as prostaglandins, released from local tissues damaged by the injury causing the pain. Different nociceptors show different sensitivities, some being stimulated by low-grade 'warning' events, such as firm pressure or temperatures not high enough to burn. These cause a sensation of threat rather than pain. Other pain nerve endings respond only when strongly stimulated, as by skin cutting, pricking, or

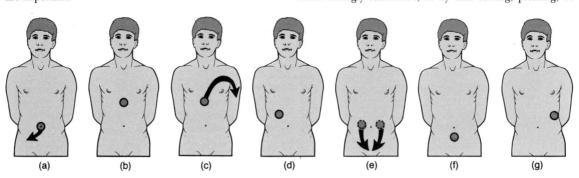

The location of pain in the abdomen can be an aid to diagnosis. This illustration shown typical pain sites for (a) appendicitis; (b) duodenal ulcer; (c) coronary thrombosis; (d) cholecystitis or gallstones; (e) kidney stone; (f) cystitis; and (g) shingles.

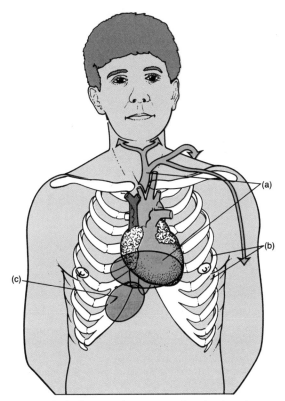

Chest pain due to angina pectoris (a) typically radiates up into the neck, through to the back and down the arms. Pleurisy (b) causes a sharp, stabbing pain on deep breathing. Chest pain is often due to abdominal disorders such as duodenal ulcer (c).

burning. In both cases, the stronger the stimulus, the more powerful the nerve impulses sent to the brain.

Pain impulses can also arise from stimuli affecting the nerve fibres at a point nearer the nervous system than the remote nerve ending. Stimuli of this kind occur in diseases such as shingles and are also responsible for one form of referred pain.

Although the nerves carrying pain impulses terminate in the brain, and give rise to neurological activity there, the pain is usually felt in the region in which the nerve endings are situated.

PAIN CONTROL

Nerve impulses passing to the brain may be blocked by local anaesthetics, by electrical stimulation applied through the skin, by acupuncture, and by the inhibitory action of other nerve fibres coming down from the brain.

The latter are believed to release blocking substances called *endorphins* and *enkephalins*. Morphine and other similar drugs are believed to relieve pain by acting on nerve receptor sites in a manner similar to that of endorphins. Pain control can also be effected by hormones, since removal of the pituitary or adrenal glands increases sensitivity to pain. The hormones involved have not been positively identified, but are believed to be endorphins.

> Experts on pain control emphasize that it should be treated by the simplest and safest available means, but that attempts should always be made to relieve it once the cause is known. Prolonged pain is demoralizing and debilitating and should be controlled as early as possible.

Neglected pain becomes more difficult to control. Pain-controlling drugs work best if they are used as soon as the pain reappears, and they should not be withheld until pain becomes unbearable. Different forms of pain control, used in combination, are more effective than methods used in isolation. Authoritative reassurance by a doctor, when appropriate, increases the effectiveness of pain control measures.

Local anaesthetic injections can control pain, but the effect is brief and this is not a practicable method. They may, however, be useful as a preliminary trial before resorting, in extreme cases, to permanent nerve destruction by alcohol injection or by surgical severance. In general, surgical methods of pain control are to be avoided. They inevitably involve unpleasant permanent loss of sensation and, even when the pain fibres are cut in the spinal chord, do not necessarily succeed in controlling the pain.

THE GATE THEORY

Many electronic devices, such as computers, operate by an elaboration of logical *gates* through which the passage of a stream of electrical impulses is permitted, or blocked, by a secondary controlling electrical signal. Most physiologists believe that the nervous system contains analogous arrangements of nerve cells and fibres (neurones), operating as gates, and that pain impulses travelling up the spinal chord pass through such gates and can be blocked by signals coming from elsewhere. This theory provides an explanation for some of the physical methods of pain control.

Many physical methods of pain control are effective, probably by blocking neurological gates in the spinal cord. These include skin rubbing with a soft cloth, electrical stimulation of the skin using a variety of machines, acupuncture or acupressure, massage, or cold sprays to the skin.

pain below knee

See **Osgood-Schlatter disease**.

pain control therapist

A doctor, often an anaesthetist but sometimes a general physician, who specializes in the management of long-term severe pain or of pain in terminally ill people.

painkillers

See **analgesic drugs**.

pain, long-term

See **chronic pain syndromes**.

pain relief, non-drug

See **TENS**.

Painstop

A brand name for a mixture of the painkiller drugs **paracetamol** and codeine.

Paladac

A brand name for a preparation of **vitamins**.

Paldesic

A brand name for **paracetamol**.

Palfium

A brand name for the narcotic **analgesic** drug **dextromoramide**.

Palladone

A brand name for **hydromorphone**.

palma

Latin root meaning 'palm' as in palmar (of the palm of the hand).

palpebra

Latin root meaning 'eyebrow' as in palpebral (of the eyelid).

palpitation

Consciousness of the heart beat, either because it is faster than normal or because it is irregular. A rapid heart rate is normal during exercise or emotion. Brief periods of irregularity are common and are usually due to premature beats followed by unusually prolonged pauses (extrasystoles). These are felt as a fluttering or thumping in the chest, sometimes with a brief but alarming sense that the heart has stopped beating. Extrasystoles do not normally indicate disease of the heart.

Another cause of palpitation is atrial tachycardia, a condition in which, for periods of seconds to days, the heart beats very rapidly – sometimes over 200 beats per minute. The onset is sudden and causes faintness and breathlessness and the affected person becomes very anxious. The rate can be controlled by medical treatment.

Atrial fibrillation is a condition in which the upper chambers of the heart (the atria) beat in a wholly disorganized manner and only the strongest impulses are passed down to the main lower pumping chambers (the ventricles). The result is a grossly irregular heartbeat. In the early stages, affected people have palpitation with unpleasant awareness of the irregularity of the heart's action, but, with time, usually become accustomed to the symptom and fail to notice it.

palsy

An old term for **paralysis**, a condition of absent or defective muscular action, commonly due to a failure of the normal motor nerve supply from the brain, or to a peripheral nerve disorder. The term persists in the conditions of **Bell's palsy** and cerebral palsy (congenital **spastic paralysis**).

Paludrine

A brand name for the antimalarial drug proguanil.

Pamergan P100

A brand name for **pethidine** formulated with **promethazine**.

Pameton

A brand name for a mixture of **paracetamol** and its antidote methionine.

pamidronate

A **bisphosphonate** drug that prevents bone reabsorption by interfering with the action of osteoclasts. The drug has been used to treat cancer bone metastases and multiple myeloma. A brand name is Aredia.

Pamine

A brand name for **hyoscine**.

Panadeine

A brand name for a mixture of **paracetamol** and codeine.

Panadol

A brand name for **paracetamol**.

Panamax

A brand name for the pain-killing drug **paracetamol**.

Panasorb

A brand name for a readily absorbable form of **paracetamol**.

Pancoast's tumour

A tumour in the lower part of the neck, near the apex of a lung which, because of its situation, involves a number of important structures and causes a characteristic group of physical signs.

RECOGNITION AND SYMPTOMS

Physical signs include pain in the shoulder, the upper chest, the lower neck, the armpit and the arm, caused by spread of the tumour to the lung covering (pleura), ribs and spine. There may be hoarseness, when the tumour spreads to involve the nerves to the larynx. A common feature is Horner's syndrome (drooping of the lid and smallness of the pupil of one eye with absence of sweating on the same side of the face), caused when the tumour interferes with the sympathetic chain of nerves in the neck. Spread to the network of nerves deep in the armpit (the brachial plexus) causes weakness and atrophy of the muscles of the arm and hand.

> Pancoast's tumour is most commonly a lung cancer (bronchial carcinoma) and is an indication that the disease has reached an advanced and probably incurable stage.

pancreas

The pancreas produces digestive enzymes which pass into the first part of the small intestine (duodenum). But it is also an endocrine gland, containing groups of specialized cells, in areas known as the Islets of Langerhans, which monitor the concentration of glucose in the blood and secrete appropriate amounts of the hormones insulin and glucagon to lower or raise the amounts of sugar, as necessary.

Glucagon is a protein hormone produced by the islet cells of the gland, which has an effect opposite to that of insulin. By causing glycogen, stored in the liver, to break down to glucose, a process known as gluconeogenesis, it increases the amount of sugar in the bloodstream. Glucagon is also involved in the mobilization of fatty acids for energy purposes. It is used as an emergency measure when the blood sugar levels are dangerously low (hypoglycaemia) and must be rapidly raised. A glucagon injection can prevent brain damage or even save life.

Insulin acts by forming 'ports' on cell membranes which allow glucose to pass in. In its absence, glucose, which is the main fuel of the body, cannot get into the cells and accumulates in the blood. The body responds to its need for glucose by releasing more from the muscles, which waste away. This wasting disorder caused by insufficient insulin is called diabetes and is corrected by injections of insulin.

Pancrease

A brand name for **pancreatin**.

pancreas transplant

A method of treating **diabetes** by grafting healthy pancreatic tissue from a donor. Currently, this procedure is feasible only in people who require immunosuppression for other purposes, usually kidney transplants, because unfortunately, the immunosuppressive treatment needed to prevent graft rejection is more dangerous than the diabetes. Several thousand successful transplants have, however, been achieved in diabetics who had to have immunosuppression.

pancreatic duct X-rays

See **endoscopic retrograde cholangiopancreatography (ERCP)**.

pancreatin

A preparation of pancreatic digestive enzymes that can be taken by mouth. This may be required by people who have had a pancreatectomy or whose pancreatic enzyme production is inadequate. Trade names are Creon, Nutrizym GR, Pancrease and Pancrex V.

pancreatitis

Inflammation of the **pancreas**. This may be a sharp, short illness (acute pancreatitis) or a persistent disorder (chronic pancreatitis).
POSSIBLE CAUSES
Half the cases of acute pancreatitis are caused by interference with the outflow of pancreatic secretion by **gallstones**. The retained enzymes in the pancreas begin to digest the gland itself and this process may spread to adjacent organs. The enzymes also get into the blood and can cause remote damage. As may be expected, severity varies considerably. One-fifth of cases are due to alcoholism, but, in these cases, there is usually a history of pancreatic trouble.
RECOGNITION AND SYMPTOMS
The onset is sudden with severe pain high in the centre of the abdomen. This often occurs within twelve hours of a heavy meal with alcohol. The pain spreads through to the back and may extend to the shoulder and then to the whole abdomen. There is nausea and vomiting and sometimes severe surgical **shock**. Bleeding may occur into the bowel or this may become obstructed. Bile duct obstruction may cause **jaundice**. The condition so closely resembles a perforated **peptic ulcer** or acute **appendicitis** that the true diagnosis is frequently discovered only in the operating theatre. Acute pancreatitis is sometimes mistaken for a coronary thrombosis (see **heart attack**).

> Pancreatitis occurs most commonly in men of thirty to forty-five who drink fifteen to twenty units of alcohol a day and who enjoy a rich diet, high in fats and protein.

The condition starts with episodes of pain, high in the abdomen, and spreading through to the back, usually lasting for at least a day. A short period of jaundice usually occurs and an X-ray or CT scan shows that the pancreas is full of cysts, many of them filled with chalky stones. The attacks tend to recur and the pain may be very severe. Because the pancreas is the only source of insulin in the body, severe damage of this sort is liable to cause **diabetes**. Other disasters may occur, such as damage to the nearby bowel, which may become narrowed or completely blocked. The mortality, in those people who go on drinking after developing chronic calcifying pancreatitis, is very high.

Pancrex V

A brand name for **pancreatin**.

Pancuronium bromide

A muscle-relaxing drug of the non-**depolarizing** class, used during general anaesthesia. A brand name is Pavulon.

pandemic

An epidemic of world wide proportions.

panic disorder

A condition featuring spontaneous, intense, episodes of **anxiety**, usually lasting for less than an hour and occurring about twice a week or more often. About two-thirds of people with **agoraphobia** also have panic attacks.
RECOGNITION AND SYMPTOMS
The attacks consist of an acute sense of fear, with a conviction of impending death, and mental confusion. The heart beats rapidly, breathing is fast and deep, and there is sweating and great distress. Overbreathing (**hyperventilation**) often makes the attack worse.
POSSIBLE CAUSES
The condition has a genetic basis, and brain imaging has shown that there is an increased blood flow in a particular part of the brain, on the non-dominant side, during a panic attack. An injection of sodium lactate brings on a panic attack in 70 per cent of those who are subject to the disorder but in only 5 per cent of others. This substance is thought to lead to a marked increase in adrenaline production in the susceptible individuals. About half of those who suffer from panic attacks have a minor abnormality of the mitral valve of the heart (mitral valve prolapse) which occurs in only 5 per cent of the general population, usually harmlessly. Overactivity of the thyroid gland is also associated with panic attacks.
TREATMENT
Panic attacks are treated with antidepressant drugs, especially tricyclics and monoamine oxidase inhibitors. Properly used, these are effective and may completely remove the attacks. Anxiety from anticipation of further attacks can be controlled by behaviour therapy.

panic, treatment of

See **cognitive behaviour therapy**.

Panoxyl

A brand name for benzoyl peroxide.

Pantheline

A brand name for **propantheline**.

pantoprazol

A **proton pump inhibitor** drug used to treat peptic ulceration and other disorders due to excess stomach acid. A brand name is Protium.

papaveretum

A mixture of purified opium alkaloids. Papaveretum has the same pain-killing and narcotic properties as **morphine** and is mainly used for surgical premedication. Also known as Omnopon. A brand name of the drug combined with aspirin (see **analgesic drugs**) and **papaverine** is Aspav.

papaverine

An opium derivative used as a smooth muscle relaxant and to treat heart irregularities following a heart attack. Papaverine has been used to treat organic impotence by direct injection into the corpora cavernosa of the penis. A brand name of the drug combined with aspirin (see **analgesic drugs**) and **papaveretum** is Aspav.

papilloedema

Swelling and forward protrusion of the front end of the optic nerve, visible within the eye by means of the ophthalmoscope. Papilloedema is an important sign of increased pressure within the skull. This raised pressure is transmitted along the sheaths of the two optic nerves, interfering with the normal internal flow of material along the nerve fibres and causing swelling.

> Raised pressure within the head is always serious, often being caused by a tumour. Early observation of papilloedema may be life-saving.

papillomavirus and cancer of the cervix

The human wart-causing papillomavirus is widespread and causes various forms of **warts** (verrucae) anywhere on the skin, including the hands, the face and the soles of the feet. It is also sexually transmitted and infects the genitalia of many people who are sexually promiscuous. In these it may cause venereal warts and changes in the cells lining the neck of the womb (cervix) which can be detected by a cervical smear test.

Women with such changes are more than fifteen times as likely to develop cancer of the cervix, within six years of the test, as other women. The normal incidence of cervical cancer is about two women in a thousand. In those with papillomavirus changes, the incidence is over 30 per 1000.

PAPNET

An automated cervical smear test involving an electronic neural net. The system is a supplement to smear examination by human pathologists but saves a great deal of time and expertise. PAPNET checks every cell on the microscope slide, comparing it with a normal standard. It then selects the 128 that are most abnormal and displays them on a monitor where they are checked by an expert. The system has been able to identify abnormal cells previously reported as normal up to twelve years before a positive diagnosis was reached.

papule

This term comes from the Latin *papula*, meaning 'a pimple' and is used for any small, well-defined, solid, slightly raised area of skin. Papules are normally less than 1 cm in diameter and may be domed or flat, smooth or warty. Many skin diseases feature papules.

para-

Prefix meaning 'beside, beyond' as in paramedic (beside the doctor).

paracentesis

The surgical puncture of a body cavity, with a needle or cannula, so that fluid may be removed. This may be required for the relief of symptoms, to release unwanted or infected material, or to obtain a sample for examination. In heart failure and other conditions, fluid commonly accumulates in excessive quantity in the peritoneal cavity. This is called ascites, and paracentesis may afford great relief.

Fluid may collect in the pleural space and may cause collapse of the lung, or in the pericardial space where it may interfere with heart action. In both cases, paracentesis may be an essential part of the treatment.

Paracentesis of other cavities is also common. In bladder outlet obstruction it may be used to remove urine and relieve acute symptoms; in acute otitis media paracentesis of the eardrum can allow pus to escape from the middle ear.

paracetamol

A drug widely used to relieve pain and reduce fever. The drug does not irritate the stomach, as aspirin (see **analgesic drugs**) does, but overdose causes liver and kidney damage and may cause death from liver failure (15 g or more is potentially serious). The victim remains well for a day or two and liver failure develops between the third and fifth day. Trade names are Alvedon, Calpol Disprol Paediatric, Infadrops, Medinol and Salzone. Preparations that include paracetamol include Cosalgesic, Distalgesic, Domperamol, Fortagesic, Kapake, Midrid, Migraleve, Paradote, Paramax, Remedeine and Solpadol.

Paradex

A brand name for a mixture of **dextropropoxyphene** and **paracetamol**.

Paradote

A brand name for **methionine** in combination with **paracetamol** as an antidote.

Paralgin

A brand name for the painkiller **paracetamol**.

paralysis

Temporary or permanent loss of the power of movement of a part of the body. This is usually due to damage to the nerves or nerve tracts which carry impulses to the muscles to cause them to contract, but may be due to disorders of the muscles themselves. Nerve damage may occur in the brain or spinal cord (central nervous system) or in the nerves running from the central nervous system to the muscles (peripheral nerves).

POSSIBLE CAUSES

Paralysis of the right or left half of the body (hemiplegia) is very common and is almost always the result of a **stroke**. Severe injury to the spinal cord may cause paralysis of both sides of the body below the level of the injury. This is called paraplegia. If the level of the injury is high in the neck and all four limbs are paralysed, the condition is known as quadriplegia. In very rare cases, the whole of the body is paralysed, as in the **locked-in syndrome**.

Paralysis caused by nerve damage outside the central nervous system is called flaccid paralysis and the muscles are floppy and soon atrophy. Paralysis due to damage within the brain and damage to the long tracts in the spinal cord does not deprive the muscles of the primitive reflex arc via the cord. The result is called spastic paralysis and the muscles tighten up and the limbs tend to become fixed in bent positions due to contractures.

Paralysis is also caused by brain injury at birth, by brain tumours and injuries, by **multiple sclerosis** and by various infections such as **poliomyelitis**, **diphtheria**, untreated syphilis and **encephalitis**.

Paramax

A brand name for **metoclopramide** formulated with **paracetamol**.

paranoid disorders

Paranoia is a delusional disorder without identifiable organic cause. The main feature is a conviction of persecution. The delusion lies in the basic idea – that one is being spied upon, followed, drugged, maligned, prevented from succeeding, and so on – and the consequent beliefs follow logically from this basic premise. There are no other mental disturbances and no **hallucinations**. Other types of paranoid disorder include:

- the grandiose type, in which there is a conviction of personal grandeur, often unrecognized by society;
- jealous type, featuring a conviction of sexual infidelity in a partner;
- somatic type, with a conviction of some bodily defect, body smell or body parasitization;
- erotic type, which features a conviction that someone, usually a notable personality, is in love with one.

POSSIBLE CAUSES

Factors that might promote delusional disorder include:

- social isolation;
- distrust and suspicion of others;
- envy and jealousy;
- lowered self-esteem;
- perceiving one's own defects in others;
- undue rumination over meanings and motivation.

To people too greatly oppressed by such factors, a delusional system offers a comfortable relief.

People with paranoid disorders are often highly intelligent and may be effective professional workers. They are usually well dressed and show no sign of other personality disintegration. They are often hostile, suspicious and appear eccentric. They frequently resort to the law in pursuit of redress of believed wrongs.

TREATMENT

Treatment is very difficult, probably because the basic delusion is so important to the sufferer. Psychotherapy seems to offer the best chance of cure, but this calls for a degree of wisdom, sensitivity, patience and experience in the therapist, which cannot be widely available.

paraphilia

Any deviation from what is currently deemed to be normal sexual behaviour or preference. Thus, paraphilia may include bestiality, exhibitionism, fetishism, homosexuality, masochism, paedophilia, sadism, transvestism and voyeurism.

paraphimosis

Tight constriction of the neck of the glans of the penis by the narrowed outlet of a very tight foreskin (prepuce) which has been drawn back. The blood in the arteries of the penis, which is under pressure, is able to enter the glans, but because of the constricting ring, the veins, which are softer and contain blood under lower pressure, are compressed and the blood cannot escape. As a result, the glans swells progressively and the situation rapidly becomes worse. The condition is painful and there is some danger of gangrene of the glans unless the paraphimosis is rapidly reduced.

The treatment is to return the foreskin to its normal position by squeezing fluid back out of the swollen glans until it is small enough to allow the narrowed opening of the foreskin to pass over it. Usually, squeezing with the fingers, supplemented, if necessary, by an injection of an enzyme that aids the dispersion of fluid by breaking down the cement substance in tissues (hyalase), will succeed, but surgery under general anaesthesia may be necessary.

After the paraphimosis is reduced, it is wise to agree to **circumcision**.

paraplegia

See **paralysis**.

paraplegic walking

A method of movement for people paralysed in both legs (see **paralysis**), in which the legs are braced in splints and lifted and moved forward by the strength of the arms, which are also bearing crutches. Great strength is needed and the process is exhausting. In some experimental systems power assistance is provided but this raises the problem of heavy batteries.

Attempts have been made to cause paralysed leg muscles to contract effectively, so as to permit paraplegic walking, by electrical stimulation. This method has had some success, especially in the hands of some workers in the former Yugoslavia, and various devices are being developed and evaluated in Britain.

parapsychology

A term which appears to give scientific status to various obscure 'phenomena' such as extrasensory perception, telepathy, clairvoyance, spoon-bending and the movement of objects without physical force (telekinesis). The danger is that the uncritical may infer that these phenomena are accepted by scientific people – which, in general, is not the case.

parasites

Organisms living on or in the body of another living organism. Ectoparasites live on the surface, endoparasites live inside. Parasites derive their nourishment from the host but do not contribute anything to the host's welfare. They are often harmful. Hundreds of human diseases are caused by parasites, which include many different viruses, a wide variety of bacteria, some fungi, various protozoa, a range of different kinds of worms, a few types of flukes, some ticks, four types of lice, some bugs, a few burrowing flies and a variety of leeches.

Protozoal parasites include amoebae which cause dysentery, flagellata which cause vaginal discharge and irritation, ciliata which are often harmless, and sporozoa which cause malaria. Worms include tapeworms, roundworms, hookworms and threadworms. See also **parasitology**.

parasitology

The study of organisms which use other organisms as their living environment. Although bacteria and viruses are **parasites**, they are so important as to deserve a separate discipline and are not normally included in medical parasitology. This is concerned with the larger, and often visible, parasites of man such as the various worms, and the microscopic protozoal and microfilarial parasites.

Parasitic diseases, include the worm conditions ascariasis, clonorchiasis, fascioliasis, **Guinea worm** infestation, **hookworm** disease, paragonimiasis, **schistosomiasis, strongyloidiasis, taeniasis** and **trichinosis**; and the protozoal conditions **trypanosomiasis, trypanosomiasis, South American amoebiasis, leishmaniasis, malaria and trichomoniasis**.

Paraspen

A brand name for the painkiller **paracetamol**.

parathyroid glands

These are four small, bean-shaped organs, each about half a centimetre long, which lie in the substance of the thyroid gland. They secrete a hormone called parathormone which regulates the fate of calcium and phosphorous in the body. This hormone is automatically produced if the level of calcium in the blood drops, and its presence causes the blood calcium levels to rise again by the release of calcium from the bones, a reduction in calcium loss by the kidneys and increased absorption from the bowel. Excess phosphorous is excreted in urine so that the correct balance between the two is maintained.

Sometimes the parathyroids enlarge or develop tumours and secrete too much parathormone. The result is excessive loss of calcium from bones resulting in softening. Surgery is usually necessary to remove some of the glands. Insufficient parathormone results in low blood calcium – a potentially dangerous condition featuring abnormal muscle excitability and spasm (tetany).

parenteral

Referring to drugs or nutrients, taken or given by any route other than by the normal alimentary canal. Parenteral routes include the intramuscular and the intravenous.

parenteral nutrition

Feeding by the infusion of sterile nutritional solutions directly into a vein. Also known as intravenous feeding. Parenteral nutrition is necessary when the normal intestinal (enteral) route cannot be used. The earliest attempts at intravenous feeding by way of the limb veins were all frustrated by the fact that the strong sugar solutions used invariably led to vein inflammation with clotting of the blood and closure of the veins (thrombophlebitis) within a matter of hours. This was overcome by the use of a vein cannula that passed inwards to enter the large central vein. More recent developments in the design of cannulas and new feeding solutions, with calorie-rich emulsified fats (lipids), amino acids and weaker carbohydrates may, it is hoped, allow safe peripheral vein feeding.

Parfenac

A brand name for bufexamac, a drug used to relieve skin irritation.

Parkinsonism and Parkinson's disease

A syndrome, sometimes called paralysis agitans, characterized by involuntary tremor of the hands at rest, with finger movements resembling 'pill-rolling', rigidity of the muscles and slowness of body movements.

RECOGNITION AND SYMPTOMS

The rigidity causes the face to become mask-like but the intellect is not affected. The speech becomes slow and the voice quiet and monotonous. The handwriting becomes minute. On standing, there is a strong tendency for the body to incline forwards and there may be great difficulty in starting to walk. The steps are short and tottering, sometimes as if the affected person were falling forwards.

INCIDENCE

Parkinsonism usually starts between the ages of forty and seventy, and progresses steadily over the years, eventually causing severe physical disability. It affects one person in 1000 and, in those over sixty, one in 100.

POSSIBLE CAUSES

It is due to changes in the connections between the areas of the brain called the substantia nigra and the corpus striatum, with loss of pigment and dopamine-producing cells. It may be caused by:

- certain drugs used in psychiatric treatment;
- synthetic heroin **designer drugs** containing MPTP;
- possibly by arterial disease affecting the brain;
- carbon monoxide, manganese or other substances;
- tumours;
- head injuries;
- the 'punch-drunk' syndrome;
- **encephalitis**.

In most cases, the cause of Parkinsonism is unknown and these cases are called Parkinson's disease.

TREATMENT

The condition is treated by dopamine replacement. The drug levodopa can produce striking improvement in two-thirds of affected people. Other drugs, which stimulate dopamine receptors in the brain, can be used. Experimental treatment with transplantation of a sample of the patient's own adrenal tissue, or implantation of fetal cells, to try to restart dopamine production in the substantia nigra, have been tried, but the results are, at the time of writing, uncertain. Mexican workers claimed remarkable improvement, but the reports have been criticized.

Parlodel

A brand name for **bromocriptine**.

Parlovex

A brand name for **acetylcysteine**.

Parmid

A brand name for **metoclopramide**.

Parmol

A brand name for the painkiller **paracetamol**.

Parnate

A brand name for the monamine oxidase inhibitor antidepressant drug **tranylcypromine**.

parotid glands, disorders of

The parotid produces less than the normal amount of saliva when the body is short of water (dehydration) and in **Sjögren's syndrome**. Severe lack of secretion causes abnormal dryness of the mouth (xerostomia). Inflammation of the gland is called parotitis and this is most commonly due to infection with the mumps virus, but may also result from bacterial infection.

Sometimes an abscess forms, which may have to be opened and drained surgically. The glands may enlarge in sarcoidosis.

The most common tumour of the parotid gland contains elements both of a tumour of surface lining (carcinoma) and of a tumour of connective tissue (sarcoma). It is thus called a *mixed salivary tumour* and presents as a slow, painless enlargement of one of the parotids. The degree of malignancy varies and the tumour should always be removed as early as possible.

-parous

Suffix meaning 'giving birth to' as in multiparous (many deliveries).

paroxetine

A serotonin re-uptake inhibitor drug. A brand name is Seroxat.

parthenogenesis

The development of an unfertilized egg into an adult organism. A normal ovum, having half the usual number of chromosomes (haploid), cannot produce an organism, so some change is necessary in the early cell divisions (meiosis) to produce the full number. If such a cell continues to divide as does a fertilized cell, the result will be parthenogenesis. The resultant organism will be a clone of the mother and will be identical to her in all respects. Only females can be produced by parthenogenesis, as no Y chromosome is present.

Parthenogenesis is common in bees and ants and sometimes chickens and turkeys and has been produced experimentally in frogs, mice and rabbits. Ova can sometimes be induced to begin to divide by pricking them with a fine glass fibre. Human parthenogenesis is a theoretical possibility and, if achieved, would make men biologically redundant.

partners, counselling of

Much discord between partners arises from difficulty, or refusal, to see matters from the other's point of view, and differences can sometimes be resolved if an agreed third person, who is able to take a detached and unbiased view, is brought into the situation. Communication blockage between partners can be re-established and damaging behaviour patterns, obvious to an outside observer but inapparent to the participants, can be pointed out and examined.

Effective counselling calls for experienced, wise and unprejudiced counsellors – people who can gain the respect of, and whose advice can be accepted by, even the most apparently unreasonable. No special school of psychology need be involved, but the ideas of the behaviourists, which are largely based on common sense, seem to be more fruitful, in application, than most. Sexual problems can also often be resolved by counselling.

To a large extent, success in counselling is dependent on a genuine desire for reconciliation and on the importance each partner places on the relationship. Often, unfortunately, it is much more important to one than to the other.

Partobulin

A brand name for **anti-D immunoglobulin**.

passive smoking

The rate of lung cancer in non-smokers rises significantly if they are regularly exposed to other people's cigarette smoke, as, for instance, by living with a smoker or by working in an office where others smoke. It has the advantage over smoking cigarettes that a fairly high proportion of the tars and other dangerous ingredients will have been retained in the body of the smoker, but enough remain in the exhaled air to pose a threat to the health of others. An increasing number of people, aware of this fact and of the dangers inherent in cigarette smoke, are expressing their objections to anyone smoking in their immediate environment.

There is no safe threshold for the effects of carcinogens, and non-smokers who breathe environmental cigarette smoke are exposed to known carcinogenic substances. Such non-smokers are found to have nicotine and other tobacco products in their urine. Although nicotine is not a carcinogen, some of the other 3000 or so chemical substances in cigarette smoke are, and these are being inhaled also. Ten separate studies have shown an increase of up to 30 per cent in the risk of lung cancer among non-smokers living with smokers, compared with non-smokers living with non-smokers.

pasteurization

A method of destroying bacteria and other micro-organisms in milk and other liquid foods. The method most commonly used today is the high-temperature, short-time process. Milk is passed, in one direction, between thin, stainless steel plates separated by gaskets, while hot water is pumped in the other direction, on the other side of the plates. In this way, the milk is rapidly heated to about 78°C (176°F) and maintained at that temperature for fifteen seconds. It is then rapidly cooled to below 10°C (50°F).

Standards of pasteurization in milk are tested by checking for the presence of a milk enzyme which is destroyed at the correct temperature and for the presence of the bacterium *Coxiella burnetti*. Pasteurized liquid eggs are tested for the presence of two species of Salmonella bacteria.

Other food products can be pasteurized by blowing in high-temperature steam.

patella, disorders of

The patella (kneecap) may be fractured by direct violence and may be the seat of the common conditions of **chondromalacia patellae** and **Osgood-Schlatter disease**, which occur in adolescence and early adult life.

paternity tests

When a man alleged to be the father of a child has been wrongly named, normal blood-grouping tests can provide proof of nonpaternity in 97 per cent of cases. They cannot, of course, prove that a particular man *is* the father, but they can offer evidence to help to establish paternity.

The paternity index is the ratio of the chance the putative father has of producing, in a sperm, the genes required to father the child to the chance of his doing so if he is not related to the child. Ratios vary from less then one in ten to up to many thousands to one. High values are virtual proof of paternity.

In only a small number of cases is the technique of DNA fingerprinting necessary to prove paternity, but since technology is often employed simply because it exists, genetic fingerprinting is likely to be increasingly used in the future.

pathological gambling

See **gambling, pathological**.

pathologist

A doctor specializing in the branch of medical science dealing with bodily disease processes, their causes, and their effects on body structure and function. The pathologist may subspecialize in post-mortem work (morbid anatomy), histopathology (see **histopathologist**), haematology (see **haematologist**), clinical chemistry or forensic pathology (see **forensic pathologist**).

pathology

The branch of medicine dealing with disease processes in the body, their causes, and their effects on bodily structure and function. Pathology includes three main branches – morbid anatomy (including histopathology), haematology and clinical chemistry. Morbid anatomy is the process of diagnosing disease from examination of diseased organs or tissue removed at operation, from biopsies, or from specimens obtained at post-mortem examination. Histopathology is the examination of such tissue under the microscope so as to diagnose the disease present.

Haematology and clinical chemistry are laboratory disciplines, now largely automated, in which blood, body fluids, discharges and secretions are examined to determine the concentration and state of various normal and abnormal cells and of the wide range of biochemical substances in them.

Forensic pathology is concerned with applying all three subdivisions in the interests of criminal investigation or in the assessment of suspicious deaths.

patient's charter

A document produced by the Department of Health in 1992, and revised in 1995, that affirms the Government's acknowledgement of certain rights for patients (see **patients' rights**) and its expectations for the achievement of certain standards in patient care. The charter deals with such matters as:

- waiting list times for surgery;
- waiting times for outpatient appointments after referral;
- waiting times in routine clinics and in Accident and Emergency Departments;
- waiting times for provision of a bed after a decision to admit to hospital.

Regrettably, although these rights are acknowledged they are not by any means always fulfilled.

patients' rights

People in contact with doctors, especially in hospital, often feel they have little control over what happens to them, but are reluctant to make demands or to object to proposed treatment or investigation. But patients do have rights, and these include the right to considerate and respectful care and to full information about what is going on. Adult patients are entitled to know the diagnosis and the outlook (*prognosis*), explained in terms they can reasonably be expected to understand. In some cases doctors may consider it inadvisable to give the full facts, but these ought to be made available to a suitable person, such as a close relative or spouse.

Patients are entitled to all information necessary to give informed consent to any operation, procedure or treatment. They are entitled to know the nature and probability of all significant risks and the probability of success, as well as the likely duration of incapacity afterwards. They should also be made aware of possible alternatives to the proposed procedure.

Patients have the right to refuse treatment and to be informed of the probable consequences of such refusal. They are entitled to privacy and confidentiality over their medical details and are entitled to protest if these rights are not respected by medical and nursing staff. Patients have a right to be told if the medical staff propose to engage in any form of medical trial or experiment in which they are involved, and have a complete right to refuse to participate in such research.

Patients also have the right to discharge themselves from hospital at any time, but may properly be required to sign a document stating that they do so in full knowledge of the possible consequences.

-pause

Suffix meaning 'end' as in menopause (end of menses).

Pavacol-D

A brand name for **pholcodine**.

Pavulon

A brand name for **Pancuronium bromide**.

Paxadon

A brand name for pyridoxine (vitamin B6).

Paxane

A brand name for **flurazepam**.

Paxofen

A brand name for **ibuprofen**.

peak expiratory flow measurement

This test is widely used to assess the degree of any kind of obstruction to the air passages, especially of the kind caused by asthma and chronic bronchitis. The test gives a valuable indication of the severity of the disease and of response to treatment.

In a normal person, asked to breathe out as forcibly as possible through the mouth, the rate of flow of the air rises rapidly to a peak and then declines steadily to zero. A normal person can breathe out at a peak rate of up to 8 litres a second, but in certain lung diseases, because of narrowing or partial obstruction of the bronchial tubes or other causes of respiratory weakness, the figure is much lower. Peak flow meters, which measure the maximum flow rate of air on expiration, are simple devices that measure the speed of air movement through them and record the highest figure.

The person being tested is asked to take a very full breath, put the wide nozzle of the device in the mouth, and blow through it as rapidly and forcefully as possible. Providing there is no gross weakness in the respiratory muscles, which prevents the taking of a full breath or making a full expiratory effort, a reduction in the peak flow rate indicates probable disease of the air passages, such as asthma, bronchitis or bronchiectasis, or a lung disorder, such as emphysema or fibrosis, that affects the natural recoil of the lungs.

peanut allergy

An often severe form of allergy in which up to one-third of sufferers experience potentially dangerous **anaphylaxis**. Peanut allergy is no more common than other food allergies, all of which are rare, affecting about 1 person in 100,000 per year. It is, however, liable to be more severe than most, and is especially dangerous in asthmatic children. Peanut proteins may be found in a wide variety of foodstuffs, from chocolate spread to Scotch eggs.

peau d'orange

A characteristic orange-skin-like change in an area of the skin of the breast found in certain kinds of cancer. Such an appearance should be reported at once.

pectore

Latin root meaning 'breast' as in angina pectoris (chest pain).

pede

Latin root meaning 'foot' as in pedal (of the foot).

pellagra

A vitamin deficiency disease common in underdeveloped countries, but sometimes occurring in the West in chronic alcoholics who derive all their calorie requirements from alcohol. It is due to a deficiency of the B group vitamin niacin (nicotinamide) for periods of as short as six weeks. The medical student mnemonic for pellagra is the 'three Ds' – diarrhoea, dermatitis and dementia.

RECOGNITION AND SYMPTOMS

The skin appearances usually first suggest the diagnosis. There is generalized redness, like severe sunburn, in areas exposed to light, and this may progress to blistering, cracking and crusting with oozing of serum. There is loss of appetite, nausea and swallowing difficulty, soreness of the mouth, and a generalized inflammation of the bowel which causes diarrhoea. In the most severe cases, brain involvement causes delirium. In prolonged, but less severe cases, brain damage progresses to the stage of dementia.

TREATMENT

Pellagra responds rapidly to nicotinamide by mouth or injection and there is often a striking improvement within a day. Unfortunately the economic conditions or the alcoholism which led to the disease are less easily dealt with. In the southern United States where, fifty years ago, pellagra was widespread among the rural poor, the disease has been almost eradicated, partly by economic improvement and partly by fortification of bread and maize with nicotinic acid.

pelle

Latin root meaning 'skin' as in pellicle (any, thin skin or film).

-pellent

Suffix meaning 'drive off' as in repellent (again, drive off).

pelvic girdle and leg structure

The pelvis is the bony girdle formed by the junction of the two hip bones (innominate bones), on either side, with the triangular curved sacrum, behind, at the sacroiliac joints. The innominate bones are held together in front by a midline joint called the symphysis pubis. Each innominate bone contains a deep, spherical cup, called the acetabulum, into which the head of the thigh bone (femur) fits.

The sacroiliac joints are the semi-rigid ligamentous junctions, at the back, holding the two outer bones of the pelvis to the side surfaces of the sacrum. The coccyx, or tail bone, consists of four small vertebrae fused together and joined to the curved sacrum. Normally, little movement occurs at the sacroiliac joints, but late in pregnancy the strong ligaments holding the joints together become a little lax, to allow easier childbirth. The width of the hips is determined by the width of the pelvis and by the angle at which the heads of the two femurs join it. The thigh bones (femurs) are the longest and stoutest bones in the body. Each has an almost spherical head

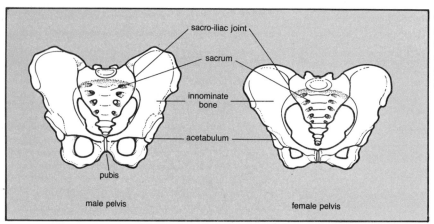

Comparison of the male and female pelvis. The latter is shallower and with a wider canal and so is better adapted for the downward passage of a baby's head in childbirth.

which fits into a cup (the acetabulum) on the side of the pelvis. To the bottom end of each femur, at the knee, is attached the two lower leg bones, the stout tibia and the slender fibula – corresponding to the two bones of the forearm. The bottom ends of these bones join the eight tarsal bones – corresponding roughly to the eight wrist bones, then the five metatarsal bones and the fourteen phalanges of the foot and toes. The big toe has two phalanges; the others three. In front of the knee joint, between the femur and the tibia, lies the flat kneecap (patella) within the tendon of the thigh muscles.

Anatomists can readily distinguish the female pelvis from the male, by its proportions. The female pelvis is relatively wider and shallower than the male and the cross-section of the opening is better shaped to allow the passage of a baby's head. The lower part of the sacrum is also more flexible in the female.

pelvic internal viewing

See **culdoscope**.

pelvimetry

The assessment of the area of the outlet of the female pelvis so as to anticipate difficulty in delivery of the baby. A rough assessment can be made by checking the distance between the prominent bones behind the buttocks (the ischial tuberosities) on vaginal examination. More precise measurements can be made by various X-ray techniques, but the use of X-rays in this region is avoided, if possible, during pregnancy, and the method is seldom used nowadays.

Even so, radiological pelvimetry may occasionally be justified in women with a history of difficult or prolonged labour, when safer methods of imaging are not available. It may even be needed for women already in labour if the fetal head has failed to engage, or in breech presentation with a large baby. The later in pregnancy, the lower the radiation risk to the fetus.

Penbritin

A brand name for **ampicillin**.

penciclovir

A **nucleoside analogue** drug used to treat cold sores (herpes simplex infection) of the lips. A brand name is Vectavir.

Pendramine

A brand name for **penicillamine**.

penetrance

The frequency with which an abnormal gene manifests its effect. A completely penetrant dominant gene will always produce its effect. The failure of a mutation to produce its usual effect may result from the modifying effect of other genes or from environmental influences. Penetrance is measured as the proportion of individuals in a population with a particular mutated gene who show the corresponding effect. The eye cancer retinoblastoma, for instance, is a genetic disease with incomplete penetrance. Of 100 children with the gene for the disease, only 90 will develop retinoblastoma. The penetrance in this case is 90 per cent. This indicates that the gene does not cause the disease directly, but causes a strong susceptibility to it, and that other factors are necessary.

-penia

Suffix meaning 'shortage of' as in leukopenia (low on white cells).

penicillamine

A chelating agent used to treat poisoning with metallic salts or disorders such as **Wilson's disease**. Trade names are Distamine and Pendramine.

penicillin antibiotic drugs

An important group of antibiotic drugs. The original natural penicillin was derived from the mould *Penicillium notatum* but the extensive range of penicillins in use nowadays is produced synthetically. The original penicillin was penicillin G (Crystapen), which had to be given by injection. This was followed by the phenoxymethyl derivative, penicillin V, which could be taken by mouth. The semisynthetic penicillins followed from the discovery that 6-aminopenicillanic acid could be obtained from cultures of *Penicillium chrysogenum*. The penicillin molecule contains a beta-lactam ring and many organisms produce an enzyme, beta-lactamase, that can inactivate the drug by breaking this ring. Side chains are added to the basic molecule to try to frustrate the action of this enzyme. Penicillins act by interfering with the synthesis of the walls of bacteria. See also **antibiotic drugs**.

penicillium

One of a range of common blue-green moulds of the genus *Penicillium* that grow on decaying fruits and ripening cheese. *Penicillium* species such as *P. notatum* and *P. rubrum* were originally studied by the Scottish bacteriologist Alexander Fleming (1881–1955) in investigating the properties of the antibiotic penicillin.

penile outlet, narrow

See **phimosis**.

penis

The penis is the erectile male organ of copulation and urination. It is a triple structure, consisting of two main longitudinal cylindrical bodies of sponge-like tissue, the corpora cavernosa, lying side by side, and, beneath them, a single, central, smaller column, the corpus spongiosum, through which runs the tube for urine and semen (urethra). The corpora cavernosa are connected by a wall of fibrous tissue, which is incomplete in places, to allow blood to pass from one to the other and thus equalize the pressure. In other mammals this wall contains a bone, the os penis. The corpus spongiosum, also of spongy tissue, expands near the tip of the penis into a conical cap-shaped swelling called the glans (glans penis).

The urethra runs along the centre and opens at the tip of the glans as a vertical slit. At the root of the penis, the two corpora cavernosa separate and the corpus spongiosum expands to form the bulb of the penis, where the urethra enters it from above. Into each of these three bodies runs an artery capable of supplying blood under pressure. The penis is firmly attached to the pelvis by fibrous tissue continuous with the sheaths surrounding the three corpora. It is covered with thin, dark-coloured, freely mobile skin, under which are some large veins and branches of the arteries supplying the corpora.

penis, disorders of

In **hypospadias** the urethra opens anywhere on the undersurface of the penis. In **epispadias** the urethra opens on the upper surface. **Phimosis** is an abnormal narrowing of the opening of the foreskin (prepuce) and may require **circumcision**.

Balanitis is an inflammation of the glans penis. Penile warts may occur anywhere on the organ but are commonest on the glans or the foreskin (prepuce). They are caused by the human papovavirus, which is sexually transmitted. In syphilis, the initial sore, the hard **chancre**, may also occur anywhere on the penis, but is commonest on the glans.

Cancer of the penis is rare and is almost unknown in circumcised men. It presents as a single painless warty lump or persistent ulcer on the glans or the foreskin and progressively enlarges. Sometimes, the first sign is a blood-stained discharge.

Injury to the penis may occur in various ways. Strangulation by a tight string or rubber band may cause gangrene. Rupture of the fibrous sheaths of the corpora occasionally occurs in impetuous coitus or from direct injury. Most injuries cause severe bruising and the formation of a free blood pool (a haematoma) is common. Amputation is rare, but is sometimes performed as an act of self-mutilation.

Priapism is an abnormally sustained erection, which will not subside – a state calling for urgent medical attention.

Commoner is the inability to achieve or sustain a[n] (**impotence**). **Peyronie's disease** is a condition of un[known] cause in which the erect penis becomes deformed with [a] bend to one side.

Pentacarinat

A brand name for **pentamidine**.

Pentalgin

A brand name for a mixture of **paracetamol**, codeine and **pentobarbitone**.

pentamidine

A drug used in the treatment of *Pneumocystis carinii* pneumonia and **trypanosomiasis**. A brand name is Pentacarinat.

Pentasa

A brand name for **mesalazine**.

pentazocine

A synthetic pain-killing drug with actions similar to those of **morphine**. A brand name is Fortral.

pentobarbitone

A now little-used barbiturate sedative and **hypnotic** drug of medium duration of action. It is occasionally given as a premedication before surgery. A brand name is Nembutal.

pentostatin

An **adenosine deaminase inhibitor** anticancer drug. A brand name is Nipent.

Pentothal

The former brand name for the rapid-acting barbiturate drug thiopentone sodium commonly used to induce general anaesthesia. The drug is now known as Intraval.

Pepsid

A brand name for **famotidine**.

pepsis

Greek root meaning 'digestion' as in dyspepsia (indigestion).

Peptard

A brand name for hyoscyamine.

peptic ulcer

An ulcer in the lining of the stomach, duodenum or at the lower end of the gullet (oesophagus). Peptic ulcers involve local loss of the **mucous membrane** lining, with some penetration into the underlying muscular layer.

INCIDENCE

The condition is common, affecting about 10 per cent of all adult males and 2 to 5 per cent of women.

POSSIBLE CAUSES

Ulcers result when the stomach juices, which are highly acid and contain a powerful digestive enzyme called pepsin,

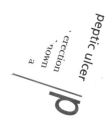

of the bowel wall. Normally, they are ... because they are present in insuffi- ... se the lining is protected by mucus ...onate secreted by the lining cells. A ...rfere with the ability of the lining to ... include the taking of certain drugs, ... alcohol, and the reflux of bile and secre- ...intestine into the stomach. The organism ... ...losely associated with peptic ulceration (see below). Sev... ...d injury, burns, major operations and severe infections are all known to promote peptic ulcers. Cigarette smoking interferes with the healing of ulcers and may contribute to their causation. Ulceration of the lower oesophagus occurs only when there is reflux of acid from the stomach.

The duodenum is the C-shaped tube which constitutes the first part of the small intestine. The stomach contents empty directly into the duodenum, and the first 3 cm take the brunt of this highly irritating mixture. Soon, however, the acid is neutralized by the alkaline secretions from the pancreas, which enter the duodenum about its mid point. Duodenal ulcers are usually found within 3 cm of the stomach outlet and are local areas in which the bowel wall is being digested by the acid and the pepsin. Ulcers do not occur in people who do not secrete stomach acid.

Duodenal ulcers are usually single, but two or more may occur simultaneously. They are usually about 1 cm in diameter and penetrate the wall at least as far as the muscular coat immediately under the lining. In severe cases they may pass right through (perforating ulcer), leaving a hole through which the contents of the bowel can escape into the sterile peritoneal cavity of the abdomen. This causes the serious condition of **peritonitis**.

As in gastric ulceration, causal factors include the amount of acid secreted, the efficiency of the mucus, secreted by the lining, in protecting its own surface from digestion and the presence of *Helicobacter pylori*. To what extent, and by what means, these and other factors are influenced by the psychological or emotional state of the affected person, or by life stress, is not entirely clear, but it is common experience that some forms of stress make symptoms worse.

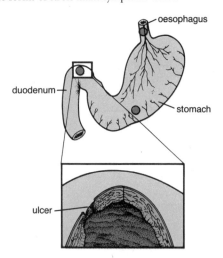

Peptic ulcer. This illustration shows the three sites at which ulceration may occur – at the lower end of the gullet (oesophagus), in the stomach and in the duodenum.

RECOGNITION AND SYMPTOMS

Peptic ulceration causes a burning, boring, gnawing pain high in the abdomen, in the angle between the ribs. The pain usually comes on about two hours after a meal. Duodenal ulcer pain is characteristically relieved by taking a small amount of food. This causes the stomach outlet to close, temporarily, so that the new food can be retained for digestion. The pain is not present on waking in the morning but tends to come on around the middle of the morning. It is also common for duodenal ulcer pain to wake the sufferer two or three hours after falling asleep. The diagnosis is often apparent from the history but may be confirmed by **barium X-ray examination** and by **endoscopy**.

TREATMENT

The great majority of gastric and duodenal ulcers heal in four to six weeks. A range of treatments is used, including the eradication of *Helicobacter pylori* organisms with antibiotics and bismuth, antacid drugs to neutralize stomach acid, histamine H-2 blockers to reduce acid secretion, proton pump inhibitor drugs such as omeprazole (Losec), drugs which form a protective coating on the base of the ulcer and promote healing, drugs which reduce painful spasm, and certain prostaglandin drugs which reduce acid. In some cases, surgical treatment, such as bypassing the duodenum (**gastroenterostomy**), reshaping the stomach outlet (pyloroplasty), removing an affected part of the stomach (partial **gastrectomy**) or cutting some of the nerves to the stomach which promote acid secretion (selective or truncal **vagotomy**) may be very helpful. In addition, treatment with tranquillizing drugs may help by relieving anxiety or depression.

The nature of the diet seems to be of little relevance. Strict diets are not required, only common-sense avoidance of items known to cause symptoms.

> Unfortunately, in spite of treatment, chronic peptic ulceration often persists for life, with relapses every two years or so. Relapses are said to be less common if *Helicobacter pylori* organisms are eliminated. In all cases, the outlook will be greatly improved if smoking is abandoned, aspirin tablets thrown away, alcohol taken only in moderation and in reasonable dilution and dietary intake reduced.

per-

Prefix meaning 'through' as in percutaneous (through the skin).

percussion

A method of clinical examination used by doctors since 1761 when Leopold Auenbrugger of Vienna, adapting the trick the wine merchants used to check the amount of wine in their barrels, published his *Inventum Novum* and achieved immortality.

In percussion, the fingers of the left hand are spread out on the skin with the middle finger pressing firmly down on the area of interest. The middle finger of the right hand is now slightly bent and used as a hammer to tap briskly on the back of the left middle finger. If firm pressure is used, a percussion note, which varies in resonance with the hollowness or solidity of the underlying structure, is heard.

Percussion is especially valuable in the examination of the chest and can easily detect areas of the lung which have become solidified by pneumonia, or demonstrate fluid accumulation in the space between the two layers of the lung coverings (pleural effusion). It can be used to elicit several other signs of disease including air in the pleural cavity (pneumothorax) and fluid in the abdomen.

Percutol

A brand name for **glyceryl trinitrate** in a formulation for absorption through the skin.

Perfan

A brand name for **enoximone**.

perforation

A hole through an organ or tissue, made by a disease process or by accidental or deliberate injury. The term is also used for the act of making a hole through a part. Perforation may occur as a result of ulceration, inflammation or cancer of the wall of structures such as the stomach, duodenum, gallbladder or appendix, and is a serious complication.

It may also occur as a result of inflammation or other processes causing a rise in the pressure of fluid or pus within a structure. Perforation of the eardrum (tympanic membrane) occurs in this way.

Perforating wounds are penetrating wounds which extend into a body cavity or an organ, and are always serious. Surgical exploration is usually necessary.

pergolide

A drug that simulates the action of dopamine and is used to treat **Parkinsonism**. A brand name is Celance.

Pergonal

A brand name for **menotrophin**.

peri-

Prefix meaning 'around' as in perioral (around the mouth).

Periactin

A brand name for the **antihistamine** and appetite-stimulating drug cyproheptadine.

pericarditis

Inflammation of the membranous sac which encloses the heart (the pericardium). The pericardium has an outer, tough, inelastic, fibrous layer and an inner smooth layer separated into two sheets. Of these, the innermost is firmly attached to the heart and the outer is attached to the fibrous layer. Between the two inner layers is the pericardial space containing a small quantity of pericardial fluid to lubricate the movements of the heart in contracting.

POSSIBLE CAUSES

Pericarditis may be the result of:

- damage to the underlying muscle during a **heart attack** (coronary thrombosis);
- infection by Coxsackie B viruses, bacteria or fungi;

- indirect injury, as from a swallowed foreign body or a stab wound;
- a condition spread from the lung or breast or by lymphomas;
- immunological disorder.

> Pericarditis may complicate rheumatoid arthritis or systemic lupus erythematosus. Sometimes, pericarditis is followed by a progressive thickening and fibrosis of the pericardium so that there is severe mechanical interference with normal heart action. This is called constrictive pericarditis and may require surgical correction.

RECOGNITION AND SYMPTOMS

Pericarditis always affects the inner smooth layers of the pericardium and it may do this in several ways. There may be a local roughness causing a scratching sound with heart movement, which can be heard with a stethoscope. There may be an excess production of fluid between the layers so that the heart is compressed and unable to fill properly from the veins. The fluid may be fibrinous (containing the ingredients for the formation of scar tissue) so that the two layers become locally stuck together, causing restriction in the heart's movement. In pericarditis caused by tumour there may be release of blood into the pericardial space, and when certain infections are the cause, pus may collect there.

There is fever and a characteristic pain behind the breastbone (sternum) which may spread to the neck and shoulders. The pain may be worse on deep breathing or on changing the position of the body, or even on swallowing. It may be relieved by sitting up and leaning forward. If the heart action is impeded, heart output will fall and with it the blood pressure. **Shock** may develop. If there is much fluid in the pericardial sac, X-ray shows enlargement of the heart shadow. The echocardiogram is helpful in diagnosis, and there are typical changes on the electrocardiogram.

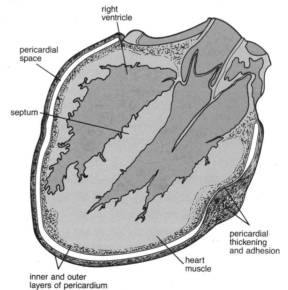

The pericardium is a double-layered bag enclosing the heart. Note how the inner layer is fixed to the heart but is separated by a layer of lubricating fluid from the outer layer. These layers may adhere if the membrane is inflamed (pericarditis).

TREATMENT

The treatment of pericarditis varies with the cause, as does the outlook. Pain can be relieved by analgesics or by anti-inflammatory drugs. If the heart action is being seriously affected by excess fluid in the pericardial sac, this may have to be drawn off through a needle.

pericyazine

A **phenothiazine derivative** drug used to treat psychotic disorders. A brand name is Neulactil.

perindopril

An **angiotensin converting enzyme inhibitor** drug used to treat **heart failure** and high blood pressure. A brand name is Coversyl.

periodontal disease

The disorders of the tissues surrounding and supporting the teeth – the gums (gingiva), the structure that holds the teeth firmly in their sockets (the periodontal membrane) and the tooth sockets (the alveoli). Periodontal disease includes inflammation of the gums (**gingivitis**) and the more serious inflammation of periodontitis, which causes a discharge of pus (pyorrhoea).

Periodontal disease is a consequence of poor oral hygiene with neglect of brushing so that dental plaque forms, leading to **dental calculus**, enamel damage, infection and loss of teeth. **Malocclusion** may lead to dental stresses which weaken the periodontal membrane and promote disease.

period pain

Pain caused by cramping contractions of the womb which interfere with the blood supply to the muscles and other cells and cause them to be slightly damaged. Whenever any cell in the body is damaged, substances called **prostaglandins** are released from the cells. Prostaglandins have a variety of actions, but the one we are interested in, here, is the pain-stimulating effect. Injected prostaglandins cause severe headache and pain in the blood vessels.

The common pain relievers – **aspirin** and **ibuprofen** – are similar in their action. These drugs block the production of prostaglandins by damaged cells, and this is how they relieve pain. Drugs like **morphine** act on the brain; others act on nerve conduction. But the aspirin-like drugs act directly on damaged cells and work solely by preventing the production of the substances which cause the pain.

The aspirin-like drugs are powerful and should be treated with respect. Never use ordinary aspirin, only the soluble variety, and never use aspirin if you have indigestion or a previous history of ulcer trouble. Sensitivity to aspirin, especially in people with other allergies, is rare, but can cause alarming and often dangerous reactions, including severe asthma and dangerous swelling inside the Adam's apple. This can obstruct your breathing. So if you have genuine allergies, beware of aspirin and the aspirin-like drugs. Polyps in your nose are a special warning of this danger. Remember that such side-effects are common to the whole group of aspirin-like drugs.

The popular painkiller **Panadol** or **paracetamol** also has its dangers. The drug is broken down in the liver and an overdose can cause liver failure and death, after a few days. There is an antidote, called **methionine**, but this must be taken early. The safest form is called **Pameton**, in which paracetamol is combined with the liver-protecting methionine.

Brufen, or **ibuprofen** has, in the past, been taken primarily for relief of joint pain, but it has other uses and seems to be better than aspirin for menstrual period pain. It is certainly safer than aspirin, although it causes tummy upset in about one person in ten. Like aspirin, it can prolong bleeding time and people sensitive to aspirin such as asthmatics, can react to it in exactly the same way. It should be taken very cautiously by people with liver disease.

These drugs are most effective if taken one or two days before menstruation starts and continued for one or two days after the onset of the period. Should they give insufficient relief, try a little codeine as well. If all else fails, you may need to have your ovulation temporarily suppressed by a low-dose, oestrogen-progesterone contraceptive pill. This, of course, is a matter for your doctor.

peripheral nerves

Nerves are bundles of **neurons**, outside the central nervous system, bound together and enclosed in fibrous sheaths. The individual neurons are usually insulated by a layer of white material called myelin, which gives the nerve a white, shiny appearance.

Most nerves contain neurons running outward from the central nervous system to all parts of the body and others running from the body inwards to the central nervous system. The outgoing neurons mostly go to **muscles** to stimulate them to contract. These neuron bundles are called the motor part of the nerve. Most of the ingoing neuron bundles are carrying information to the **brain** and form the sensory part of the nerve. So most major nerves are mixed motor and sensory nerves, but near their endings the motor and sensory part separate. Within the central nervous system neuron bundles form neural tracts. The white matter of the spinal cord and brain consists of many neural tracts.

Coming directly from the brain are twelve pairs of cranial nerves, and coming directly from the spinal cord are thirty-one pairs of spinal nerves. These eighty-six nerves connect to all the muscles in the body and receive information from the whole area of the skin and from all internal organs. A ganglion is a large collection of nerve cell bodies, from which emerges bundles of nerve fibres. Ganglia are present in many parts of the body, some of the most conspicuous being located near the spinal cord and containing the cell bodies of the large spinal nerves entering the cord. Another chain of ganglia, the sympathetic ganglia, lie on either side of the vertebral column, and are linked together by nerve fibres.

peristalsis

A coordinated succession of contractions and relaxations of the muscular wall of the gullet (oesophagus), small intestine or urine outlet tube (ureter), producing a wave-like pattern whose effect is to move the contents along. When gut peristalsis fails, a serious condition of intestinal blockage soon develops.

peritonitis

An acute inflammation of the membrane which lines the abdominal cavity and forms the outer coating of the abdomi-

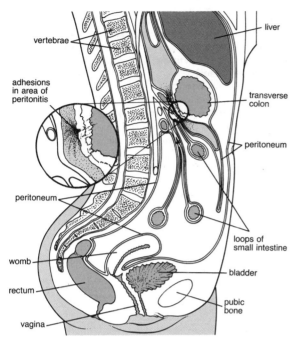

The peritoneum is a complex membrane surrounding, investing and, in some cases, suspending the abdominal organs. Local inflammation (peritonitis) causes adhesions between the layers.

nal organs (the peritoneum). By contrast with the contents of the bowel, this membrane is sterile and is very susceptible to infection.

POSSIBLE CAUSES

Peritonitis usually results from perforation of some part of the intestine so that the contents are able to gain access to, and infect, the peritoneum. Perforation of an inflamed appendix, or of a gastric or duodenal ulcer, are the commonest causes of peritonitis, but it can also result from perforating injury as may occur in a stabbing assault or a criminal abortion

RECOGNITION AND SYMPTOMS

Peritonitis causes paralysis of **peristalsis** (paralytic ileus) and this effectively blocks the bowel. Fluid from the blood accumulates in the abdominal cavity and the loss of fluid from the circulation may cause shock. There is severe abdominal pain, board-like rigidity of the abdominal muscles and high fever.

> Unless effectively treated, peritonitis is rapidly fatal. Treatment involves fluid infusion to control shock, surgery to drain the peritoneal cavity and repair the cause, and antibiotics to deal with the infection.

permethrin

A drug used externally in a hair rinse to get rid of head lice. A brand name is Lyclear.

pernicious anaemia

Also known as megaloblastic anaemia, this type is due to the failure of absorption of vitamin B_{12}, which is necessary for the correct synthesis of DNA in the maturation of red blood cells in the bone marrow. The result is the production of a smaller number of abnormally large cells which do not last as long as normal. The absorption failure results from the absence of an internal factor (intrinsic factor) produced in the normal stomach. This is a glycoprotein synthesized by the stomach lining cells. In people with pernicious anaemia, the stomach lining is defective and produces neither acid nor intrinsic factor.

RECOGNITION AND SYMPTOMS

There is soreness of the tongue, loss of weight, skin pallor, often with a lemon tint, and intermittent diarrhoea. The nervous system may be affected, causing tingling of the fingers and toes, muscle weakness, staggering, calf tenderness, confusion and, eventually, sometimes **dementia**.

TREATMENT

Treatment is highly effective. The form of vitamin B_{12} known as hydroxocobalamin is given twice a week for the first week and then weekly until the blood is normal. In very severe cases, blood transfusion may be necessary and extra iron may also be needed. Maintenance dosage of vitamin B_{12}, every three months for life, is necessary.

Pernivit

A brand name for a mixture of nicotinic acid and acetomenaphthone, used to treat chilblains.

perphenazine

A phenothiazine derivative drug used in the treatment of **schizophrenia** and other psychotic conditions. It is also used to relieve severe vomiting and control persistent hiccups. A brand name is Fentazin.

Persantin

A brand name for the antiplatelet drug **dipyramidole**, used to prevent **thrombosis**.

persistent aches and pains

See **fibromyalgia syndrome**.

persistent vegetative state

The state of a patient who, because of severe damage to those parts of the brain concerned with volition, awareness, wakefulness and what is generally regarded as consciousness, is unable to experience any of these things and can have no appreciation of his or her situation.

This may be hard for relatives and friends to accept because patients in a persistent vegetative state can breathe without mechanical assistance. The heart, kidney and intestinal functions may be normal and the bladder and bowels will empty automatically. At times such patients appear to be awake. They will respond to painful stimuli by opening their eyes, moving their limbs, breathing more quickly, and occasionally grimacing.

The type and degree of brain damage, and the length of time for which these patients remain totally inaccessible to any human interaction, indicate, however, that they cannot perform any of the higher neurological or mental functions known to be essential for any mental activity.

personal computer, medicine and

See **telemedicine**.

personality changes

See **Jekyll and Hyde disorder**.

personality, over-reacting

See **cluster B personality**.

Pertofran

A brand name for the tricyclic antidepressant drug desipramine.

pertussis

The medical term for **whooping cough**.

pessary

A vehicle for medication that is placed in the vagina. Medicated pessaries are often made of cocoa butter which melts under body heat. They contain drugs to treat vaginal disorders, such as thrush (**candidiasis**) or **trichomoniasis**, or spermicides for contraceptive purposes.

pesticide

A poison used in the attempt to eradicate pests of any kind, including unwanted birds, rodents, insects, plants, fungi, and micro-organisms. Modern agriculture is dependent on pesticides for its efficiency, as are public health authorities for the control of the many insect-borne diseases, but much concern has arisen because of the scale of usage, especially of insecticides, herbicides, and fungicides, and because of the potential or actual dangers of residual poisons to human beings and wildlife. Pesticide residues in food, dangers to agricultural workers, ecological damage and many other concerns relating to pesticides are an increasing preoccupation of governments throughout the world.

petechiae

Tiny, round, purplish or red points in the skin or in a mucous membrane, less than 2 mm across, caused by bleeding from the smallest blood vessels (the capillaries). Petechiae may result from multiple small points of damage from infective emboli, as occur in bacterial **endocarditis**, but are more commonly an indication of a bleeding disorder such as **purpura**.

pethidine

A synthetic narcotic pain-killing drug somewhat less powerful than morphine. Pethidine is widely used during childbirth and as a premedication. Overuse may lead to addiction. A brand name of pethidine in a formulation with promethazine is Pamergan P100.

petit mal

Minor **epilepsy**, or 'absence' attacks, fairly common in children and adolescents but rare in adults. The attacks are brief, usually two to ten seconds in duration, and are often unobserved by the suffered and may be taken, by the observer, to be moments of inattention or absentmindedness.

As many as 100 attacks may occur in a day and the total loss of time and educational input may be serious. By causing gaps in consciousness, these attacks also derange thinking and this, too, can affect educational performance, especially if the diagnosis is unsuspected. Attacks tend to diminish in frequency towards adolescence and may disappear.

Unfortunately, petit mal often progresses to major epilepsy (grand mal).

RECOGNITION AND SYMPTOMS

There is a complete interruption of consciousness. The child remains motionless, stares, stops talking, ceases to respond, and is, for the duration of the attack, inaccessible.

Sometimes the attacks feature small, jerky contractions of the muscles of the eyelids, face or fingers at a rate of about three per second. The associated abnormality of brain electrical activity shows up prominently on the electroencephalogram. There may be lip-smacking or chewing movements, especially if the attack is brought on by voluntary over-breathing (**hyperventilation**) – a process which some children learn to use purposefully.

In a petit mal attack, the affected child does not usually fall and may even continue to walk or ride a bicycle.

TREATMENT

Petit mal can be managed by attempting to eliminate any known precipitating factors; by ensuring regular sleep, a good balanced diet and a physically active life; by the promotion of healthy family attitudes and the avoidance of over-solicitude and over-protection. The drugs Zarontin (ethosuximide) and Diamox (acetazolamide) are useful and can greatly reduce the tendency to attacks.

Peutz-Jeghers syndrome

A genetic disorder featuring multiple polyps in the small intestine. The condition is often symptom-free, but sometimes the polyps bleed or cause abdominal pain. Rarely, a polyp may turn cancerous.

Pevaril, Pevaril TC

Trade names for the antifungal drug **econazole**.

peyote

A Mexican cactus of the species *Lophophora williamsii* from the flowering heads of which the hallucinogenic drug mescaline is prepared.

Peyronie's disease

Angulation of the penis, on erection, caused by a nodular contraction in part of the fibrous sheath surrounding the erectile tissue. The penis is unable to enlarge uniformly as it fills with blood, and bends upwards or to one side. Sexual intercourse may be impeded or painful. The local fibrous thickening may extend into the columns of erectile tissue so that the normal passage of blood is obstructed and the erection compromised. The cause is unknown.

Some cases settle without treatment after several months. Surgical removal of the scar tissue has been tried, but the results have not been uniformly good. Local injections of corticosteroids are sometimes successful.

phaeochromocytoma

A tumour of the cells which produce **adrenaline**. Phaeochromocytomas usually occur in the adrenal glands, but may arise elsewhere, and are usually nonmalignant.

Tumours are often multiple and may develop from adrenaline-producing cells in the sympathetic nerves, in the brain, around the main arteries of the body and elsewhere.

RECOGNITION AND SYMPTOMS

Phaeochromocytomas do not usually secrete the hormone continuously, but when they do, the affected person has a sharp rise in blood pressure, a fast pulse with palpitation, severe headache, nausea and vomiting, a cold clammy skin, and sometimes **angina pectoris**. There may be a feeling of impending death. These effects can often be brought on by pressing on the area of the tumour but they may also be induced by emotional upset, change of posture and sometimes even by urinating. Beta-blocking drugs can bring on an attack.

TREATMENT

The treatment of choice is the surgical removal of the tumours. Unfortunately, even giving an anaesthetic can induce an outflow of adrenaline and the blood pressure must be continuously monitored so that, if necessary, drugs can be given to control the heart action.

-phage

Suffix meaning 'eater' as in macrophage (big eater).

phagocyte

An amoeba-like cell of the immune system that responds to contact with a foreign object, such as a bacterium, by surrounding, engulfing and digesting it. Phagocytes occur widely throughout the body wherever they are likely to be required. Some wander freely throughout the tissues. They include macrophages and neutrophil polymorphonuclear leukocytes ('polymorphs').

phagocyte, giant

See **macrophage**.

phakoemulsification

A method of minimally invasive cataract surgery, which allows the procedure to be performed via a very short incision near the edge of the cornea and that may not require stitching. A fine probe capable of ultrasonic vibration is inserted into the eye and this breaks up the opaque lens (the cataract) within its capsule, converting it into a fine emulsion that can be removed by suction and washing. A replacement plastic lens is then slipped into the capsule. A rolled-up or folded soft plastic lens may be used, allowing the shortest possible incision. Phakoemulsification, which is performed under the operating microscope, is progressively displacing cruder, although still highly effective, methods.

phalanx

Greek root meaning 'aligned' as in phalanges (finger or toe bones).

phallos

Greek root meaning 'penis' as in phallic (of a penis).

phantom limb

An illusion that a limb which has been amputated is still present. The illusion is dispelled by looking or feeling with the hands, but may, otherwise, be powerful. It occurs because the nerves which formerly carried information from the limb are still able to convey impulses from the lower limits of the stump. If such nerves are stimulated by pressure or irritated by scar tissue, the impulses reaching the brain are interpreted in the only way possible to the brain – as if they were coming from the original limb. An amputee may thus experience touch, pressure or pain referred to the position in the limb formerly occupied by the endings of these nerves and will have the impression that the limb is still present.

pharmacist

An ancillary health professional or doctor concerned with drugs – with their origins, isolation, purification, chemical structure and synthesis, effects, uses, side-effects and relative effectiveness. In hospital the pharmacist orders stock and supplies drugs, and provides an advisory service on drug treatment to doctors and others.

pharmaco-economics

The application of health economics to the selection and supply of medical drugs, with special reference to cost-effectiveness in prescribing. The topic, which includes such matters as measures to promote the prescription of generic drugs rather than the higher-priced branded equivalent trade, has become increasingly important as medical costs escalate.

pharmacogenomics

The interaction of genetics and pharmacology and, in particular, the recognition of the fact that the effect of therapeutic drugs on people may be considerably affected by their genetic variability. A person's genes may affect a drug's absorption into the body, its distribution in the body, and the rate of its breakdown (metabolism) and excretion. As a result, many drugs that work very well in some people work poorly in others. At present, the best that doctors can do is to prescribe a drug and then wait and see how well the patient responds. Fuller knowledge of pharmacogenomics will, in future, allow more reliable treatment and avoid expensive waste.

pharmacokinetics

The study of how a **drug** is absorbed into, distributed and broken down in, and excreted from, the body.

pharmacology

The science of **drugs**. Pharmacology is concerned with the origins, isolation, purification, chemical structure and synthesis, assay, effects, uses, side-effects, relative effectiveness of drugs and the influence of genetic factors on drug action. It thus includes, among other disciplines, genetics, organic chemistry, pharmacokinetics, therapeutics and toxicology.

pharmacon

Greek root meaning 'drug' as in pharmacology (study of drugs).

pharmacopoeia

A book, known as a formulary, that lists and describes the characteristics of drugs used in medicine. The major pharmacopoeias, such as the *British Pharmacopoeia* (BP), the *Pharmaceutical Codex* and the *Extra Pharmacopoeia*, are large volumes dealing with all important drugs and offering a semi-official guide to pharmacists, doctors and others as to their uses and disadvantages.

pharmacy

The process of preparing, compounding and dispensing drugs, usually to the prescription of a doctor. Also, a place where these activities are performed.

Pharmorubicin

A brand name for **epirubicin**.

pharyngeal pouch

A disorder in which a blind-ended sac of mucous membrane bulges backwards and downwards from the back of the throat, at the junction of the pharynx and the oesophagus, to lie between the oesophagus and the spine. The pouch seldom occurs before middle age and when fully formed pushes the oesophagus forward and causes difficulty in swallowing. A person with a pharyngeal pouch has a constant sense of something stuck in the throat and on swallowing the neck swells and a gurgling sound may be heard. Food accumulates in the pouch and becomes offensive so that there is often severe **halitosis**. Because of the proximity of the larynx, the pouch may also cause interference with breathing, and inhalation of the contents of the sac may lead to pneumonia.

The treatment is surgical and aims to remove the pouch and to close off the opening completely. This must be done with great care, as subsequent leakage into the central partition of the chest (the mediastinum) is dangerous.

A pharyngeal pouch is a sac-like protrusion from the lower part of the throat into which food can pass and be trapped, causing an unpleasant sense of incomplete swallowing and of something stuck in the throat.

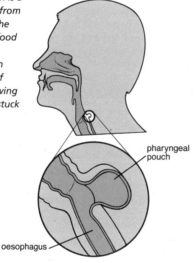

pharyngeal pouch

oesophagus

pharyngitis

Sore throat. This is a common condition, usually caused by viruses or bacteria, which normally responds well to simple treatment. There is discomfort on swallowing, occasional earache, redness and swelling of the throat, enlarged and tender lymph nodes in the neck, and slight fever. Pharyngitis is often the starting sign in **glandular fever**, **influenza** and scarlet fever but may also be caused by scalding from hot fluids or contact with corrosives or abrasive foreign material in the food.

Although commonly of minor importance, pharyngitis is sometimes serious, with high fever, general upset, swelling (oedema) of the soft palate or larynx – a potentially life-threatening emergency which may require tracheostomy – and the formation of an adherent, dirty-white membrane over the throat. Diphtheria is an uncommon but serious form of pharyngitis, which is becoming more prevalent in some countries because of a decline in immunization. It may also lead to a hard swelling of the soft tissues in the floor of the mouth (Ludwig's angina).

pharynx

Greek root meaning 'throat' as in pharyngeal (of the throat).

Phasal

A brand name for **lithium**.

Phazyme

A brand name for the silicone preparation dimethicone, used to treat indigestion from intestinal gas.

phenazocine

An opiate pain-killing drug used to relieve severe pain. A brand name is Narphen.

phenelzine

An **antidepressant** drug of the **monoamine oxidase inhibitor** group. A brand name is Nardil.

Phenergan

A brand name for **promethazine**.

phenindione

An **anticoagulant** drug that can be taken by mouth. Now little used due to allergic side-effects. A brand name is Dindevan.

phenobarbitone

A **barbiturate** drug now used mainly as an **anticonvulsant**. Phenobarbitone is no longer used as a sedative or **hypnotic**. A brand name is Luminal.

phenothiazine derivative drugs

An important group of drugs widely used to treat serious mental (psychotic) illness and to relieve severe nausea and vomiting. Examples are chlorpromazine (Largactil), thioridazine (Melleril) and perphenazine (Fentanyl).

phenoxybenzamine

An alpha-**adrenergic blocking drug** with a powerful and persistent action, used to treat bladder neck obstruction and the effects of the adrenaline-producing tumour, the **phaeochromocytoma**. A brand name is Dibenyline.

phenoxymethylpenicillin

A synthetic **penicillin**. A brand name is Crystapen V.

Phensedyl

A brand name for a mixture of codeine, **ephedrine** and **promethazine**.

phentermine

A drug with an **amphetamine**-like action used for appetite control in obesity. A brand name is Duromine. There is evidence that phentermine may be associated with heart valve disease and pulmonary hypertension.

phentolamine

An alpha-**adrenergic blocking drug** used in the treatment of **phaeochromocytoma**. A brand name is Rogitine.

phenylbutazone

A non-steroidal anti-inflammatory drug (**NSAID**) once widely used but that is now available for use in hospitals only because of its tendency to cause **heart failure** from fluid retention and severe blood disorders. It is used, under specialist supervision, in cases of **ankylosing spondylitis**. A brand name is Butacote.

phenylephrine

A **sympathomimetic** drug used as eye drops to dilate the pupils for ophthalmic examination of the interior of the eyes. A brand name is Minims phenylephrine.

phenylketonuria

A genetic disease in which a normal component of protein, the amino acid phenylalanine, is present in abnormal amounts in the blood. The excess phenylalanine is converted to phenylpyruvic acid and other substances which are very toxic and cause mental retardation. Phenylketonuria results from the absence of a body enzyme which normally converts this amino acid to a simpler and safe compound. The absence of this enzyme is the result of a defective gene with a recessive transmission.

> About one baby in 16,000 has phenylketonuria and because some of the phenylalanine, and several of its breakdown products, are excreted in the urine, a simple urine test with a special paper test strip on a wet nappy will detect the abnormality. This test becomes positive at the age of four to six weeks, but a more sensitive test is available for babies at birth. This is called the Guthrie test.

RECOGNITION AND SYMPTOMS

Newborn babies with phenylketonuria show little sign of disorder and are often strikingly blond with blue eyes. A rash resembling eczema is common. But early in infancy there are indications of mental retardation and neurological disturbance including the two main forms of **epilepsy**, grand mal and absence attacks (**petit mal**). Because of the secretion of phenylpyruvic and phenylacetic acid in the sweat and urine, affected children often have an unpleasant 'mousy' odour.

TREATMENT

Phenylalanine is a natural constituent of food, being present in all proteins, and any affected baby taking milk will receive enough to cause damage to the brain. It is thus essential to ensure that the diet is free from phenylalanine. Complete foodstuffs, with protein free from this amino acid, are available and the affected child may supplement these with natural foods, including fruit and selected vegetables and cereals low in protein.

To prevent any damage to the nervous system, however, such a diet must be substituted for milk in the first few days of life. There is dispute as to how long it must be continued, some authorities claiming that once the brain nerve fibres are fully sheathed with myelin – by about eight years of age – a normal diet can safely be taken. The current recommendation is that the special diet should be continued until the age of ten and for as long afterwards as the child will tolerate.

phenytoin

An **anticonvulsant** drug widely used as a long-term suppressant of major epilepsy. A brand name is Epanutin.

Philadelphia chromosome

An acquired chromosomal defect in which the long arm of chromosome 22 is deleted and attached (translocated) to another chromosome, usually number 9. Clones of cells with this defect apparently cause chronic myeloid **leukaemia**.

phimosis

A very narrow outlet in the foreskin (prepuce) so that the skin cannot be pulled back over the glans of the penis. This is commonly congenital, but may result from swelling (oedema), infection or scarring. Phimosis is normal in infancy but later is liable to cause trouble. If full retraction is eventually achieved, the tight prepuce may become fixed around the neck of the glans (**paraphimosis**) and this may have serious consequences.

Phimosis also interferes with the important hygienic necessity to wash away accumulated smegma and this becomes offensive, irritating and possibly carcinogenic. Phimosis persisting after the age of four or five is an indication for **circumcision**.

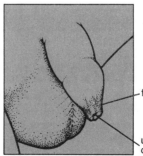

An abnormal narrowing of the outer opening in the foreskin (prepuce) is called phimosis. If such a foreskin is pulled right back, a paraphimosis may result.

foreskin

urethral orifice

phlebitis

Inflammation of a vein wall, commonly with resulting clotting of the blood in the vein (thrombophlebitis). This is usually secondary to infection in the surrounding tissues. Blood clot formation (thrombosis) results in partial or total occlusion of the vein, the latter being preferable. The main danger from thrombosis is that part of the blood clot may break free and be carried to the heart and from there to the lungs. Sometimes a long, soft, snake-like clot forms in an inflamed vein, and this is particularly dangerous and a common cause of death by pulmonary embolism.

phlebos

Greek root meaning 'vein' as in phlebitis (vein inflammation).

phobias

Intense, irrational fears which cannot be ignored or overcome even when the sufferer is fully aware, as is usually the case, that there is no reason for the fear.

Phobias take many different forms and include fear of humiliation or embarrassment (social phobias), fear of high places (acrophobia), fear of open places (**agoraphobia**), fear of spiders (arachnophobia), fear of enclosed places (**claustrophobia**), fear of cats (gatophobia), fear of water (hydrophobia), fear of dead bodies (necrophobia), fear of darkness (nyctophobia), fear of crowds (ochlophobia) and fear of animals (zoophobia).

> Phobias may relate to almost any situation, idea or object and most people have at least one mild phobia. Severe phobias are, however, very disabling and can seriously disrupt normal living.

POSSIBLE CAUSES
Freud interpreted phobias by suggesting that they are the effect of a hidden and forbidden unconscious drive striving for expression, but being strenuously repressed. They are, he thought, the result of conflict arising from an infant oedipal situation with castration anxiety.

It seems more likely that a phobia is a simple, forgotten conditioned reflex which is kept active (reinforced) by the repeated drive to avoid the unpleasant experience. This view is supported by the success of behaviour therapy in removing phobias.
TREATMENT
The physiological responses to phobias – fast pulse, sweating, high blood pressure, and so on, can be controlled by the use of beta-blocking drugs.

phocomelia

A major congenital abnormality in which the limbs are replaced by short, flipper-like stumps. This is a very rare disorder, but was a common feature of children born to mothers who took the drug thalidomide in early pregnancy.

pholcodine

An opioid drug used mainly for cough suppression. Trade names are Galenphol and Pavacol-D.

Pholcomed

A brand name for a mixture of **papaverine** and the cough suppressant pholcodine.

phosphodiesterase inhibitor

A drug used to prevent inactivation of the cell messenger cyclic amp and thereby increase its stimulating effect on the heart. It is useful to strengthen the heart's action in certain cases of heart failure. Trade names are Perfan and Primacor.

photosensitivity

A state in which an abnormal reaction occurs on exposure to sunlight. The commonest reaction is a skin rash occurring as a combined effect of light and some substance that has been eaten or applied to the skin. Such substances are called photo sensitizers and include various drugs, plant derivatives, dyes or other chemicals.

phototherapy

Treatment with light, especially in conjunction with a sensitizing drug such as the psoralen methoxalen. This is known as PUVA (psoralen ultraviolet-A) therapy and is useful in the management of **psoriasis**. Ultraviolet therapy is sometimes used in the treatment of acne.

-phyll

Suffix meaning 'leaf' as in chlorophyll (green leaf).

Phyllocontin

A brand name for **aminophylline**.

Physeptone

A brand name for **methadone**.

physical medicine specialist

A doctor specializing in the branch of medicine concerned with the treatment and rehabilitation of people disabled by injury or illness. The physical medicine specialist is assisted by **physiotherapists**, **occupational therapists** and **speech therapists**.

physician

A doctor, in Britain usually a Member or a Fellow of the Royal College of Physicians (MRCP or FRCP), who is practising hospital medicine and who may specialize in any one of the non-surgical disciplines. Outside Britain, and especially in the USA, the term is used to refer to any qualified doctor.

physician-assisted suicide

See **doctor-assisted suicide**.

physiology

The study of every aspect of the functioning of the body. Physiology has become so large a subject that it has had to be subdivided into separate disciplines such as molecular biology, cell biology, biological control systems, biochemistry, biophysics, neurophysiology, immunology and physiological psychology.

Physiotens

A brand name for **moxonidine**.

physiotherapist

An ancillary health professional who uses physical methods such as active or passive exercises, gymnastics, weight-lifting, heat treatment, massage, ultrasound, short-wave diathermy and hydrotherapy to promote recovery from disease and injury. The physiotherapist aims to restore the maximum possible degree of function to any disabled part of the body and is much concerned with patient motivation. (See also **physical medicine specialist**.)

Phytex

A brand name for **tannic acid** formulated with other drugs.

phytomenadione

A vitamin K derivative used to treat haemorrhagic disease in newborn babies. A brand name is Konakion.

phyto-oestrogens

A range of naturally occurring oestrogen-like substances derived from plants and present in the diet. Phyto-oestrogens have anticancer properties. Research has shown, for instance, that the risk of breast cancer is substantially lower in women with high levels of phyto-oestrogens, as measured by urinary secretion of these substances, than in those with a low intake.

The main phyto-oestrogens are isoflavonoids, which are high in soya products, and lignans, which are high in whole grains, fruit, vegetables and berries. It has been found that the phyto-oestrogen genistein, found in soya, binds preferentially to the oestrogen receptors occurring mainly in the heart and the blood vessels (cardiovascular system) rather than in those in the breast and womb. This has encouraged the hope that phyto-oestrogens might be valuable in controlling **atherosclerosis** and **osteoporosis** without increasing the risk of cancer.

phytopharmaceuticals

Drugs derived from plants.

phytotherapy

Those who are sensitive to the concept of **evolutionary medicine** will recognize the importance of the fact that during almost the whole of human evolution the typical diet must have consisted of a high intake of plant products punctuated by occasional gorging on animal protein and fats. Modern epidemiological medicine has shown that a diet based on a high intake of vegetables and fruit is to be recommended. There is strong scientific evidence that such a diet will reduce the risk of cancer, intestinal disorders, heart attacks and strokes.

Phytotherapy is medical treatment based on plant extracts and products. Unfortunately, as an alternative therapy, it is often based on inadequate knowledge and on the unjustified premise that because plants are 'natural' they must be 'good' for us and are unlikely to be harmful. Many important drugs used in orthodox medicine are derived from plants, but in scientific medicine these are purified and analysed and their effect is known and can be predicted. Treatment using crude plant extracts can be dangerous because of the wide and uncontrolled range of potency involved in seemingly identical samples of the same plant. There is a growing literature on these dangers and many cases of serious illness and even death have been reported.

pica

A persistent tendency to eat non-nutritional substances such as earth, ice, match-heads, coal, chalk or wood. Pica is common in children under eighteen months of age and, in these, is not considered abnormal. Pica in pregnancy has been known throughout the ages and the bizarre catalogue of substances eaten include mothballs, soap, insects, clay, baking soda and excrement. Pica is a feature of nutritional deficiency and iron-deficiency anaemia and sometimes succeeds in providing a needed supply of minerals.

Pica will often stop if anaemia is effectively treated. It is a feature of mental deficiency and may also occur in severe psychiatric disorders.

> In most cases, pica does little harm, but there have been many medical reports of obstruction or perforation of the bowel, lead poisoning, parasite infestation and other misfortunes from this cause. No satisfactory explanation of many types of pica has been produced.

piles

See **haemorrhoids**.

pill-rolling

The coarse tremor of Parkinson's disease often affects the forearm muscles in such a way that the thumb and forefinger rub against each other as if the affected person were trying to make a small ball from plasticine or dough. This was how pills of medication were once made.

pilocarpine

A drug used in the form of eye-drops to treat **glaucoma**. Pilocarpine causes extreme constriction of the pupils so that traction is exerted on the root of the iris so as to open up the drainage channels for aqueous humour. Trade names are Minims pilocarpine, Pilogel, Salagen, and, in the form of a sustained-release insert placed behind an eyelid and left for a week at a time, Ocusert Pilo.

Pilogel

A brand name for **pilocarpine**.

pilonidal sinus

A small, midline skin opening in the upper part of the cleft between the buttocks (natal cleft) leading in to a small cavity full of hairs. The term literally means 'nest of hairs'. Pilonidal sinuses are probably caused by the ingrowth of body hair, or to a mechanical process by which hair is forced in through the skin. They are prone to become infected and form abscesses. They may have to be removed surgically.

Pilopt

A brand name for eye drops containing **pilocarpine**.

pilos

Greek root meaning ' hair' as in pilosebaceous (of fatty hair lubrication).

pilus

Latin root meaning 'fur' as in pilomotor (causing hair to rise).

pimozide

A long-acting phenothiazide antipsychotic drug of the diphenylbutylpiperidine group that is also used in the treatment of the **Gilles de la Tourette's syndrome**. A brand name is Orap.

pimple

A small area of localized inflammation in the skin often caused by accumulation of sebaceous material in the dermis, in a person suffering from **acne** vulgaris. The irritation causes a red papule and this may progress to an accumulation of sterile pus, when it is known as a 'yellow head' (pustule). A pimple may also result from infection of a hair follicle in the skin to produce a **pustule**, or furuncle.

Sebaceous material (sebum) contains fatty acids and it is important that it should not be released into the tissue surrounding the hair follicle and the sebaceous gland. This is the real reason why squeezing blackheads can make the effects of acne worse. Pimples that form in the region of a squeezed blackhead are more likely to be due to fatty acid irritation than to infection.

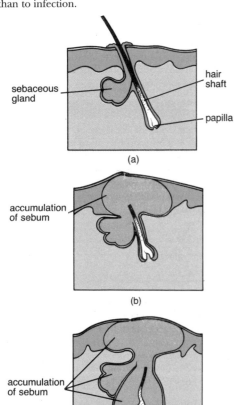

Each hair follicle is associated with a small sebaceous gland (a). Over-secretion of sebaceous material and blockage of the outlet (b) leads to the large accumulation of sebum under the skin (c) that constitutes a pimple.

pindolol

A **beta-blocker** drug used in the treatment of **angina pectoris**, high blood pressure and heart irregularity. A brand name is Visken.

pinguecula

A harmless, raised, yellowish patch in the conjunctiva on the exposed areas of the white of the eye, usually on the inner side. Pingueculas are common in and after middle age, especially in people living in tropical areas. They are due to damage to the cell nuclei by ultraviolet radiation in sunlight. Occasionally a pinguecula enlarges enough to prevent the upper eyelid from sweeping evenly over the cornea. In this case, the cornea adjacent to the pinguecula tends to dry and to lose its surface cells and become raw. The pinguecula can then extend on to the cornea to cause a **pterygium**, and the process can progress towards the centre of the cornea, sometimes affecting vision. For this reason, surgical removal of enlarged pingueculas, which is easy and safe, may be justified.

pinkeye

A common name for **conjunctivitis**.

pinna

The auricle or visible part of the external ear.

pinworms

See **threadworm infestation**.

piperacillin

A broad-spectrum **penicillin**. A brand name is Pipril.

piperazine

An **anthelmintic** drug used to get rid of **roundworms** and **threadworms**. The drug paralyses the worms which are then passed with the faeces. A brand name for the drug formulated with the laxative senna is Pripsen.

Pipril

A brand name for **piperacillin**.

piracetam

A drug that simulates the action of the **neuro-transmitter GABA** and is used to treat **myoclonus**. A brand name is Nootropil.

pirenzepine

A drug used to cut secretion of acid by the stomach in the treatment of **peptic ulcer**.

Piriton

A brand name for the **antihistamine** drug **chlorpheniramine**.

piroxicam

A non-steroidal anti-inflammatory drug (**NSAID**) used mainly to control symptoms in the various forms of **arthritis**. A brand name is Feldene.

Pitressin

A brand name for vasopressin.

pituitary gland

The pituitary is a small, pea-sized organ connected to the middle of the underside of the brain by a short stalk and lying in a hollow in the central bone of the base of the skull (sphenoid bone), just behind the nose cavity. It is connected to the hypothalamus area of the brain, immediately above it, and is the central hormone-producing gland and the controller of all the other glands which secrete hormones into the bloodstream (endocrine glands, or glands of internal secretion). The pituitary is the nodal point of the whole endocrine system and, in conjunction with the hypothalamus, forms the link between the nervous system (movement, sensation, mental activity) and the chemical control system (all metabolic, growth and regulatory processes) of the body.

The pituitary gland secretes a variety of different hormones. They are:

- growth hormone, which controls growth;
- prolactin, which promotes milk production at the end of pregnancy;
- thyroid-stimulating hormone, which controls the output of thyroid hormone;
- follicle-stimulating hormone, and luteinizing hormone, which control the production of eggs (ova) from the ovary and the maintenance of pregnancy after fertilization;
- adrenocorticotrophic hormone (ACTH), which controls the output of cortisol from the adrenal glands;
- oxytocin, which releases milk from the breast and causes the womb (uterus) to contract;
- vasopressin, also called the antidiuretic hormone, which increases the reabsorption of water in the kidneys and controls water loss;
- melanocyte-stimulating hormone which stimulates the growth of pigment cells in the skin.

If growth hormone is absent during early life, pituitary dwarfism results. Excess during this period causes gigantism. After the end of the growth period, excess growth hormone causes the disease acromegaly. Pituitary failure has widespread effects, including failure of normal sexual development at puberty, loss of steroid (cortisol) production and consequent weakness, a low metabolic rate from thyroid underaction, an excessive urinary output (diuresis) and bleaching of the skin. Cushing's syndrome is the result of excessive output of some of the pituitary hormones, usually from a tumour. Simmond's disease is the result of extreme underfunction of the gland, usually from loss of blood supply or destruction by tumour. The effect is severe weight loss, great weakness, and underactivity of the thyroid and adrenal glands. Diabetes insipidus is the result of lack of production of the hormone vasopressin. There is an abnormally large output of urine, resulting in extreme thirst. Deficiency of this hormone causes the tubules of the kidneys to lose their power to concentrate urine.

Prompted by the pituitary, the other endocrine glands, in turn, produce their own hormones, such as:

- adrenaline from the inner part of the **adrenal glands**;
- cortisol (corticosteroid) from the outer part of the adrenals;
- thyroxine, tri-iodothyronine from the thyroid gland;

- calcitonin from the **thyroid gland**;
- insulin and glucagon from the **pancreas**;
- parathyroid hormone from the **parathyroid glands**;
- oestrogen and progesterone from the **ovaries**;
- testosterone from the **testes**.

All have specific functions. The levels of these hormones in the blood are monitored by the hypothalamus so that the normal balance (homeostasis) is achieved.

pituitary gland failure

See **Sheehan's syndrome**.

pituitary gland removal

See **hypophysectomy**.

pizotifen

An antihistamine drug used in the treatment of severe migraine. A brand name is Sanomigran.

placebo effect

As awareness of the power of the placebo effect has grown, the definition of the term has been extended. Formerly, the word was used only in two senses. A placebo was defined as a substance with no pharmacological effect made to appear indistinguishable from a real drug and used in clinical trials, in comparison with the real thing, to determine how far the effects of the new drug under trial were genuinely due to its pharmacological action. The term was also used for a prescription given to please the patient when there was no organic disorder but it was thought that a prescription was expected. It derives from the Latin verb *placere* meaning 'to appease or placate'.

> It is now recognized that the placebo effect is much more widespread and is present in almost all interactions between a therapist of any kind and a person in the role of patient. It even operates between lay people when one claims medical knowledge, and comments, encouragingly or optimistically, on another's condition. The placebo effect operates on the brain and can modify the symptoms of many conditions, sometimes more profoundly than can active drugs.

This is especially true of **pain**, in which the psychological component is often as important as the sensory in determining the significance of the pain to the individual.

Opiate drugs, including the natural opiates, the endorphins, do not necessarily remove the pain, but they may so modify the attitude to it that the affected person ceases to be concerned about it. It is highly significant that people receiving 'pain-killing' tablets of milk sugar, which they believe to be strong analgesics, show raised opioid (endorphin) levels in their blood.

The implications of all this are profound, especially in relation to the great range of unorthodox 'therapies' and the placebo effect of 'the laying on of hands' may be very great and the sufferer may derive remarkable, although usually transient, relief. It may be well, however, to appreciate that subjective effects of this kind ought not necessarily to be taken as scientific validation of the method.

placental-blood transplantation

The use of umbilical cord blood as a source of blood cell-producing stem cells and progenitor cells. These can be used to restore bone marrow function in patients whose bone marrow has ceased to form blood cells as a result of disease, especially leukaemia. The procedure has the unique advantage that the immunological immaturity of the source makes rejection less likely. The method has been found useful and effective even if the donor is unrelated to the recipient.

plague, bubonic

One of the great scourges of mankind, bubonic plague has occurred in **pandemics** throughout recorded history, sometimes killing a third of whole populations. Known as the 'Black Death', the 'Great Mortality' or the 'Pestis', bubonic plague struck London in 1665 and China in 1860. This pandemic spread to Hong Kong and India and then sprang up in Brazil and California. In all, over ten million people died. In Vietnam, between 1970 and 1980, 14,000 cases occurred, and during the same period, nearly 3000 cases occurred in Burma, 1400 in Brazil, 300 in Peru, 220 in Bolivia and just over 100 cases in the United States.

CAUSES

Plague is caused by an organism, *Yersinia pestis*, which naturally infects rats, squirrels, mice and wild dogs causing, in them, a mild but persistent disease. The disease is harboured in rats all over the world and there are still regular small outbreaks, especially in Africa, Asia and South America.

RECOGNITION AND SYMPTOMS

The danger sign, in urban areas, is when the rats begin to die off. Rat fleas leave the dead rats and turn to man for their nutrition.

Two to five days after infection there is sudden fever, shivering and severe headache. Soon the buboes appear, mainly in the groin, as a result of flea bites on the legs, less often in the armpits, neck, behind the knees or at the elbows. They are smooth, oval, acutely painful swellings, from 1 to 10 cm long, stretching and reddening the overlying skin. They are exquisitely tender to the touch and the sufferer avoids any movement which might cause pressure on them.

The buboes are lymph nodes, massively infected with yersinia organisms, and with their appearance comes the release of a powerful bacterial poison (toxin) which causes first restlessness, then delirium, fits, coma and death. The toxin is so virulent that many die within a day or two of the first appearance of the buboes. The mortality, in untreated cases, is about 60 per cent.

TREATMENT

Happily, the yersinia is highly sensitive to antibiotics such as chloramphenicol, tetracycline or streptomycin, and these can reduce mortality to less than 5 per cent.

PREVENTION

Plague prevention involves rodent control by:

- secure storage of food and poisoning;
- treatment of rat holes and floors with residual insecticides against fleas;
- use of insect repellents;
- reporting of patients to public health authorities so that control measures can be adopted;
- segregation of people with yersinia lung infection (pneumonic plague);

- use of a plague vaccine for those travelling in areas of high endemicity.

> Pneumonic plague is highly infectious and can spread directly from person to person. All contacts of cases of this form of the disease must be kept under close watch and the temperature checked four times a day for a week. Antibiotics are given on the first suspicion of illness. Some authorities believe that all contacts of cases of pneumonic plague should be given antibiotics.

-plakia

Suffix meaning 'flat, broad' as in leukoplakia (white, flat area).

Planequil

A brand name for the antimalarial drug **hydroxychloroquine**.

planta

Latin root meaning 'sole' as in plantar (of the sole of the foot).

plantar wart

A wart (verruca) on the sole of the foot. Like other common warts, the plantar wart is caused by a papillomavirus of the papovavirus family. The infection is commonly acquired from contaminated wet floors, changing room showers or duckboards in swimming pools.

RECOGNITION AND SYMPTOMS

Were it not for their situation, plantar warts would appear identical to other warts. But because of pressure from the weight of the body, plantar warts are flattened and forced into the thickened skin of the sole. They may occur as single warts or as a 'mosaic' of many tiny warts closely packed together.

Plantar warts are always a nuisance and may be disabling from extreme tenderness, so that a plastic foam or felt ring or pad may have to be used to avoid pressure and allow comfortable walking. Sometimes they are confused with corns, but the distinction becomes clear on attempts at paring, when the wart will bleed.

TREATMENT

Various methods of treatment may be tried include freezing with liquid nitrogen, the use of salicylic acid plasters or trichloroacetic acid applications, electrodesiccation or cutting out with a sharp-edged spoon (curettage). Unfortunately, none is entirely satisfactory and recurrence is common because it is almost impossible to eliminate the virus. It is important that the treatment should not cause permanently sensitive scars.

plasmapheresis

A method of treatment used in certain diseases in which improvement can be achieved by removing unwanted substances from the blood. It is also known as plasma exchange, because the process essentially involves separation of the blood cells from the fluid part of the blood (the plasma), rejecting the latter and re-transfusing the cells in fresh plasma or a plasma substitute, such as an albumin solution.

HOW IT'S DONE

Clearly, the whole of the blood cannot be removed at once, so the process has to be done a little at a time. Blood is withdrawn from a vein and the plasma removed in a machine called a cell separator. The cells are then suspended in the new medium and re-transfused.

WHY IT'S DONE

The method is expensive and involves some risk, but is useful in some diseases which cannot be treated in other ways. These include the muscle-weakening disease **myasthenia gravis**, the serious kidney condition Goodpasture's syndrome, and other diseases caused by antibodies to the body's own tissues (**auto-immune diseases**), the B cell tumour multiple myelomatosis and certain genetic diseases featuring dangerously high blood cholesterol levels (familial **hyperlipidaemia**).

plastic (including cosmetic) surgeon

A surgeon concerned with the repair and reconstruction of injured, diseased or malformed tissue so as to restore normal appearance and function. Many plastic surgeons also perform cosmetic surgery, which is surgery devoted to the improvement or alteration of the human appearance.

plastic surgery

The branch of surgery concerned with repair and restoration of defects of the skin and the underlying tissue, whether present from birth (congenital) or from disease or injury. The primary aim of plastic surgery is not, as is commonly believed, to modify the healthy human face or body for aesthetic reasons – this is the province of cosmetic surgery, which is a branch of plastic surgery – but rather to restore to those with obvious organic defects, the maximum possible functional capacity and the best possible appearance.

WHY IT'S DONE

Plastic surgical treatment is most commonly indicated for tissue damage from burning, mechanical injury, cancer, or mutilating surgery, and is often, in the first instance, concerned with providing cover for areas denuded of skin. To achieve this, a wide variety of techniques of skin transfer is used, including split skin or full-thickness skin grafting, Z-plasty to lengthen an area of skin at the expense of width, skin flap transfer of many different types, and pedicle grafts (skin tubes fashioned for transfer as a two-stage procedure). Various methods of skin expansion may also be used. Breast reconstruction after mastectomy (see below) is one of the more difficult techniques.

COSMETIC SURGERY

The cosmetic branch of plastic surgery is concerned with the removal, or the improvement of the appearance of, birthmarks, moles, scars, tattoos, warts (papillomas), cholesterol skin deposition (xanthelasmas) and other blemishes; with the correction of disfiguring congenital defects; and with the **elective** correction of real or fancied defects of appearance. In pursuance of the latter, surgeons may perform **face lift** (rhytidectomy), nose reshaping (**rhinoplasty**), correction of ear defects (**otoplasty**), removal of redundant eyelid skin (**blepharoplasty**), skin sandpapering to remove superficial defects and foreign bodies (**dermabrasion**), chemical peel of the face, hair implants, scalp bald spot removal, silicone breast implant or surgical removal of excess breast skin and fat (augmentation or reduction mammoplasty) and various kinds of body contour surgery.

BODY SHAPING

The body shape is determined by the skeleton, the muscle bulk and the amount and distribution of the layer of fat immediately under the skin (subcutaneous fat or superficial fascia). Only the latter is readily capable of alteration, and for those distressed by the results of their own overindulgence, but unable to apply the obvious remedy, body contour surgery now offers a new, if expensive, alternative.

Intervention may be radical, with a major surgical assault on sagging aprons of abdominal skin and subcutaneous fat and on buttocks and flabby limbs. Inevitably, such operations involve long incisions with correspondingly extensive scars.

Body contour surgery does not necessarily involve such massive intervention. Instead, fat may be sucked out through small incisions. (See **suction lipectomy**.)

> These are radical procedures not to be undertaken lightly, for they carry a small but by no means negligible risk of complications. There is even, as with all major surgery, some risk to life, and this equates very largely to the experience and responsibility of the surgeon.

BREAST CONTOUR AND RECONSTRUCTIVE SURGERY

WHY IT'S DONE

Because female breasts vary so much in size and shape, they cause a good deal of dissatisfaction to women and, sometimes, to their partners. They may be considered to be too small, too pendulous, too large, too heavy or lacking in symmetry. There may also be dissatisfaction with other features such as fullness, roundness and nipple positioning.

HOW IT'S DONE

Enlargement is easy; reduction is sometimes difficult and usually involves fairly major surgery. Cosmetic breast operations must achieve more than simply an alteration in the outline; it must also preserve the normal consistency and 'feel' of the breast and it must not interfere with the way in which the shape and position of the breasts are affected by gravity and by changes in the position of the body and the arms. Surgery must also preserve the position of the nipple and the surrounding darker circle (the areola). If possible, it should also preserve the special sensitivity, to touch, of this part. The nipple should be of adequate size and projection and milk production should not be affected. In general, it is easy to meet most or all these criteria when the operation is to enlarge the breast; it may be difficult or impossible to do so when major breast reduction is required.

AUGMENTATION MAMMOPLASTY

This is the impressive term used for breast enlargement. The breakthrough in augmentation mammoplasty came in 1963 with the development of an implant consisting of a silicone rubber capsule loosely filled with a soft silicone gel. Silicone rubber is very strong and leakage of the gel is unlikely. Until recently, no one doubted that this method was safe and more satisfactory than any other, and it has been widely used. Over a million women, mostly in the United States, have had the operation.

HOW IT'S DONE

Implants are buried as deeply as possible, behind the fat and breast tissue and even sometimes behind the flat pectoral muscles which lie deep to the breast. The operation may be done either under local or general anaesthesia and the implant is pushed in through a short incision made near the crease on the underside of the breast. just a little in front of the crease. The incision can be very short because the implant moulds easily and can be squeezed through a cut only 3 cm long.

The surgeon is careful to check that there is no bleeding. If there is, blood will collect in the cavity around the implant and may cause all kinds of trouble including infection and abscess formation. Once the implant is nicely in position the incision can be closed with a few small stitches.

RISKS

The main long-term complication of augmentation mammoplasty is the development of a hard fibrous capsule around the implant, leading to an unnatural and undesirable feel in the breast and even some distortion of its shape. This is usually noticed within about six months of the operation, but may occur even years afterwards. The complication is common – about one woman in four experiences it – and an injection of steroids into the breasts at the time of the implant may be given in an attempt to prevent it. Daily breast massage may also help. Sometimes it is necessary to have the hard capsule forcibly broken up by external pressure.

> Reports of severe adverse reactions to leakage of silicone gel or even to the silicone of the capsule have excited much media attention. The conditions concerned – auto-immune diseases such as rheumatoid arthritis, systemic lupus erythematosus and scleroderma – are all serious and have aroused great alarm among women who have had silicone implants. They have also aroused alarm in the manufacturers of these products. The risk seems to have been exaggerated. By the end of 1992, of the more than a million women who had had implants, only about eighty-eight cases had, according to a report in the *Lancet*, been reported. By February 1994, however, more than 25,000 lawsuits had been brought against the firms making the implants, especially the largest US manufacturer, Dow Corning. These firms were forced to put up billions of dollars into compensation funds. The American Food and Drugs Administration (FDA) prohibited silicone gel implants in January 1992. Saline implants are still allowed. Many women have had implants removed, probably unnecessarily.

REDUCTION MAMMOPLASTY

Although breast reduction may be a daunting prospect, there are many women for whom it can offer great relief. Unduly large, heavy and pendulous breasts cause embarrassment, discomfort, a stooping tendency, awkwardness when hurrying or running and skin rashes from constant skin to skin contact (**intertrigo**). They force the wearing of tight bras with heavy pull on the straps and even arthritis in the neck vertebrae from the constant need to brace back the spine.

HOW IT'S DONE

In women seeking reduction mammoplasty the nipples always sit very low and have to be re-implanted at a higher level. As much breast tissue and skin have to be removed, there is also the problem of leaving conspicuous scars. This is ingeniously solved by cutting right round the areola so that the nipple and underlying breast tissue are freed, and can be moved up to occupy a circular hole cut at a suitable level in the skin above. From this hole, a vertical cut must then be made downwards and the bottom of this is extended to either side to make an anchor-shaped incision. The required amounts of breast tissue and skin are then cut away and the incision closed with fine stitches. If the breasts are very large, the areola and nipple may have to be completely separated

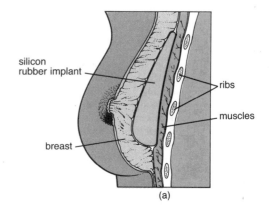

(a)

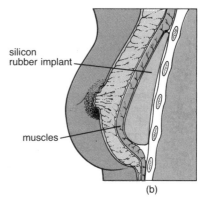

(b)

The apparent size of the breast can be increased by inserting a silicone rubber (silastic) bag filled with silicone oil, either between the breast tissue and the muscles (a) or under the muscle layer (b).

and replaced as a free graft. In this case, all nipple sensation and the possibility of later breastfeeding are lost.

BREAST RECONSTRUCTION AFTER SURGICAL REMOVAL

The most difficult breast operation of all is that done to provide a cosmetically acceptable breast appearance after radical or modified radical **mastectomy**. Women who have had to have a breast removed because of cancer require the more complex process of breast reconstruction. Today, breast cancer surgery is often less extensive than it used to be, and reconstruction operations are correspondingly easier. But radical mastectomy, in which all breast tissue and often the underlying muscles, too, are removed, leaves a woman sadly mutilated. The reconstitution of a symmetrical breast, in such a case, is difficult and may involve both tissue transplantation and plastic augmentation. Much work of this sort is undertaken by NHS consultant plastic surgeons.

In reconstruction operations, because so much tissue has already been lost, the main difficulty is to achieve reasonable symmetry. A perfect result is impossible and the limitations of breast reconstruction must be understood or disappointment is inevitable. If the other breast is large, there may be much to be said for reducing its size. This, of course, means more scars. Breast reconstruction is usually deferred until at least three months to a year after the breast removal operation, especially if radiotherapy, which interferes with healing, has been given.

After a simple mastectomy without removal of the muscles, a straightforward implant may be sufficient. But if more radical surgery has been done, it will be necessary to find real tissue to bulk out the breast.

This may be taken from the back where, on either side, is a thick, broad muscle called the *latissimus dorsi*. If the incision is made in the direction in which the muscle fibres run, it is possible safely to take a fairly large ellipse of skin from the back wall of the armpit with its underlying muscle. This can be moved round to the front without detaching itself from its blood supply. The free edges of the skin and muscle are brought together with stitches without too much tension. The donated skin allows the necessary increase in skin area for the new breast and the muscle, together with an implant, provides the necessary bulk.

As an alternative, skin, fat and muscle can be taken from the front of the abdomen. There is usually plenty of tissue here and an implant is often unnecessary, but because the blood supply cannot be preserved there is a greater risk that the graft will fail to take. The loss of muscle from the abdominal wall can weaken it and a later hernia is possible.

There is, of course, no nipple to transplant and it is not easy to fashion a viable and convincing substitute, but this can be done. Women who feel they have had enough surgery will sometimes settle for a **prosthesis** that can be stuck on, if required.

Platamine

A brand name for cisplatin.

Platelet GPIIb-IIIa blockers

Drugs that interfere with an early stage in the formation of a blood clot within a blood vessel – the clumping together of small cell fragments called platelets. The drugs are used to prevent, or reduce the risk of, clot formation in the coronary arteries of people at risk of heart attacks and in people who have had recent heart attacks. They are also useful in reducing the likelihood or severity of strokes in susceptible people.

platelet production stimulant

See **thrombopoietin**.

platelets

Important constituents of the blood derived from the break-up of large cells called megakaryocytes. Each cubic millimetre of the blood should contain between 150,000 and 300,000 platelets. Platelets are not cells but have an essential function in bringing about blood clotting. They have an average life of about 10 days, so failure of continuous production soon leads to deficiency, a state known as thrombocytopenia.

Platelet deficiency is one of the causes of spontaneous bleeding into the tissues. This is usually visible on the skin as tiny red spots (petechiae) or more extensive areas bleeding (ecchymosis). Platelet disorders also include intrinsic platelet abnormalities, both congenital and acquired, and the disorders caused by an excess (thrombocytosis). Several syndromes include thrombocytopenia, platelet membrane disorders or giant platelets. Platelet disorders may be of genetic origin or may be acquired and may involve reduced platelet production or increased platelet consumption.

See also **purpura**.

Platosin

A brand name for the anticancer drug cisplatin.

Plavix

A brand name for the anti-stroke and anti-heart attack drug **clopidogrel**.

Plendil

A brand name for **felopidine**.

Plesmet

A brand name for **ferrous glycine sulphate**.

pleura

Greek root meaning 'side or rib' as in pleurisy (inflammation of lung covering).

pleura, disorders of

Inflammation of the pleura is called pleurisy, or pleuritis, and this usually occurs if there is some disease process in the

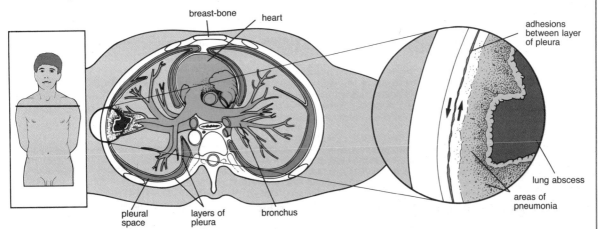

The pleura, or lung covering, has two layers. One is firmly attached to the lung and the other to the inside of the chest wall. These two layers move smoothly over one another lubricated by a thin layer of fluid.

underlying lung, such as pneumonia, cancer or tuberculosis. Pleurisy causes roughening of the surfaces in contact and as these rub against one another there is a sharp pain. This usually occurs at a particular point on breathing in. Inflamed patches of pleura can become permanently stuck together (pleural adhesion). Pleurisy is treated by treating the underlying cause.

A pleural effusion is a collection of excessive pleural fluid between the layers, forcing them apart and collecting in the lower parts so that the lung on the affected side may be compressed and partially collapsed. Fluid can also collect in the pleural space as part of a generalized body **oedema** in heart failure. Blood can also collect between the layers.

A spontaneous pneumothorax occurs when a bleb on the layer of pleura over the lung bursts and releases air into the pleural space. This can cause a severe collapse of the lung on that side. The same serious outcome can result from a penetrating wound of the chest wall.

pleurisy

See **pleura, disorders of**.

pneuma

Greek root meaning 'air' as in pneumatic (of air).

Pneumocystis carinii pneumonia

Pneumocystis is a protozoon – a single-celled parasite – which hardly ever causes trouble in people with normal immune systems. But in those who are immunocompromised, the organism frequently produces a dangerous infection. In AIDS patients the trouble starts with a persistent, annoying, dry cough and breathlessness on quite minor effort. Characteristically, a formerly fit person becomes breathless even when at rest and the doctor is puzzled as to how to account for this effect, for careful examination of the chest seems to reveal none of the usual signs of bronchitis or pneumonia. Even the X-ray of the chest may be entirely clear, but sometimes this will show some shadowing. In spite of the absence of signs, the disease process is actually having a serious effect in that it is preventing the normal amount of oxygen from getting through from the atmosphere to the blood. Tests of the amount of oxygen in the blood will show that this is unusually low and this is why people with this condition are often breathless, even at rest, and sometimes show a bluish colour in the skin.

In the lungs, a thick frothy liquid forms in the vital air sacs and prevents the air from reaching the thin-walled blood vessels through which it should pass to get into the blood. The condition is dangerous because very rapid deterioration can occur if it is not diagnosed quickly and treated, and the outcome can be fatal. The difficulty in diagnosis adds to this danger. But doctors are now becoming more familiar with the possibility of pneumocystis infection and, if there is the least suspicion that this might be the cause of the illness, will not hesitate to pass a tube down into the lungs (a bronchoscope) in order to get a sample of the material causing the problem. When the infection is present the material brought up is found to be teeming with the pneumocystis organisms.

Pneumocystis pneumonia

The *Pneumocystis carinii* is a single-celled microscopic parasite which has been known to biologists for many years, but which was considered of little or no importance until 1981 when cases of pneumonia caused by this organism began to occur with great frequency in promiscuous homosexual men in Los Angeles and New York.

The organism is an opportunistic invader, harmless to people with normal immune systems, but very dangerous to the immunocompromised. Pneumocystis pneumonia is a lung inflammation common in people with AIDS, in whom it is a frequent cause of death. The condition causes fever, rapid breathing, cough and debility and may progress rapidly to death in about half the cases. The condition is treated with a combination of the drugs trimethoprim and sulphamethoxazole.

pneumon

Greek root meaning 'lung' as in pneumonia (lung inflammation).

pneumonectomy

Surgical removal of a lung, usually for cancer. This is possible because the remaining lung, if healthy, is capable of transferring enough oxygen to the blood to sustain life. The person concerned will not, however, be able to undertake more than mild exertion.

HOW IT'S DONE

The operation is performed under general anaesthesia through a long incision from below the shoulder blade around under the arm to below the nipple. The muscles are cut and the chest is entered usually between the fifth and sixth ribs, the ribs being spread with retractors after the bone lining (periosteum) is stripped off. The layer of pleura lining the chest wall is cut through.

Once access has been achieved, the main air tube of the lung (bronchus) is cut close to its origin so as to avoid a residual stump in which secretions would accumulate, and is closed with stitches or staples. The arteries and veins are tied off and cut through and the lung removed. Often a drain is left, temporarily, in the pleural cavity so that accumulating fluid can escape.

pneumonia

See **bronchopneumonia**.

podophyllotoxins

A range of powerful substances derived from the mandrake root (*Podophyllum peltatum*). Podophyllotoxins act as **topoisomerase** inhibitors causing breaks in **DNA** strands. Ironically in view of John Donne's famous reference to mandrake, podophillotoxins are also used locally to treat genital **warts** in both sexes. Trade names of preparations for the latter purpose are Condyline and Warticon.

podophyllum resin

A drug used externally to destoy **warts**. A brand name is Posalfilin.

podos

Greek root meaning 'foot' as in podopompholyx (small blisters on the foot).

point mutation

The replacement of one **nucleotide** with another. This need not necessarily cause any change in the protein produced by the affected gene because 18 of the 20 amino acids have more than one coding triplet of base pairs (codon). Glycine, for instance, is coded for by GGA, GGU, GGG and GGC. This redundancy feature of the genetic code arises because the four bases, taken three at a time, allow for 64 triplets that could code for the twenty amino acids and the three stop codons. It is called degeneracy.

poisoning with nitrogen

See **nitrogen narcosis**.

poisons

See *First Aid*.

poisons from germs

See **toxin**.

poliomyelitis

An infectious disease caused by one of a group of viruses known as the *enteroviruses* because they inhabit the intestine and are passed in the stools in large numbers for up to six weeks after the start of the illness. At one time, poliomyelitis was by far the commonest cause of paralysis in young people and, for this reason, was known as 'infantile paralysis'. The proper name is usually abbreviated to 'polio', but the full term is *anterior poliomyelitis*. The anterior pole cells of the spinal cord are concerned with the nerves to the muscles (motor nerves) and it is these cells which are affected, causing paralysis, which may be extensive.

> Polio was also once a common cause of death, but the widespread use of oral vaccine has greatly reduced its incidence. Just as the dangerous viruses were once spread by direct faecal contamination of food by fingers and by coughing, so the modified viruses in the oral vaccine are also spread. In this way, many more people acquire protection than simply those who have the two drops of vaccine on a sugar lump.

RECOGNITION AND SYMPTOMS

Even in the unprotected, most cases of polio are mild, causing a brief, unidentified illness with headache, fever and sometimes vomiting, which comes on one or two weeks after infection, lasts for a few days, and passes with no ill effects. But in some cases, this stage is followed by a more major illness, the effects of which can be devastating. If the body's immunity is insufficient, the viruses multiply in the throat and the bowel and invade the bloodstream to be carried to the nervous system. Serious illness is more likely if the tonsils have recently been removed or some other inoculation has been given, or if there is much physical exertion at the time the viruses reach the nervous system. A strenuous game of squash to 'sweat out the fever' may lead to death or permanent total paralysis.

There is severe headache, neck stiffness, high fever and progressive muscle weakness. The paralysis is worst at the end of the first week of the severe symptoms and, thereafter, there may be gradual recovery. Any muscle which has shown no sign of movement by the end of a month is, unfortunately, permanently paralysed. If the upper part of the spinal cord or the brain stem are involved, death may occur from paralysis of respiration during the acute stage, unless some form of artificial respiration is used.

TREATMENT

The 'iron lung' was once the only way of saving the lives of those in this situation, but has now been superseded by better methods.

Oral polio vaccine is completely successful in preventing such a catastrophe and should be given to everyone.

pollex

Latin root meaning 'thumb' as in pollux (thumb or thumb bone).

pollutants

Environmental pollutants are substances, produced by human activity, which are in any way dangerous or damaging to people, animals or plants. The most serious are those which are difficult or impossible to remove.

Many thousands of substances can pollute the environment, but the major pollutants fall into a comparatively small number of groups. These include metal poisons such as lead, cadmium and mercury; organic solvents like carbon tetrachloride, trichloroethylene, toluene, benzene and xylene; and, especially, the halogenated organic compounds. These are chemicals in which chlorine, bromine, iodine or fluorine are incorporated in organic molecules.

They are used as pesticides, herbicides, solvents and fire retardants and in the manufacture of plastics. Many of those most widely used are very toxic to the nervous system. Widespread pollution of water has occurred, for instance, from the dumping of polychlorinated biphenyls (PCBs), used in electrical appliance manufacture. The fire retardant polybrominated biphenyl (PBB) has contaminated animal feed, leading to the necessity to destroy thousands of affected farm animals. Residents in the affected areas still retain this substance in their bodies.

The most dangerous of the organo-halogen compounds is probably dioxin. This substance was present in the herbicide Agent Orange, which was used by the United States' Army to defoliate large areas in South Vietnam. Much suffering was caused to the local population from the dioxin, which killed many animals and is believed to have been responsible for a high abortion rate and an increase in the incidence of congenital defects in Vietnamese babies. Another dioxin disaster resulted from a factory explosion in Italy.

Aromatic hydrocarbons, such as benzene, are known to cause cancer, leukaemia and brain damage. These compounds are released when petrol and various waste materials are burned. Other pollutants include radioactive fallout from nuclear accidents, asbestos, arsenic and sulphites.

polyacrylic acid

A substance used to formulate artificial tears and supplied as eye drops for the relief of dry eye syndromes. A brand name is Viscotears.

polyarteritis nodosa

An inflammatory disease of the walls of medium-sized arteries usually affecting middle-aged men. The arteries suffer numerous areas of weakening that become locally expanded causing nodular swellings (aneurysms) along the length of the affected vessels. The condition is due to a disturbance of the immune system sometimes triggered by the hepatitis B virus. There is marked general upset with loss of appetite and weight, obstruction to the blood flow causing raised blood pressure, muscle pain and weakness and sometimes gangrene. Involvement of the coronary arteries may cause a heart attack. Treatment is with large doses of corticosteroid drugs.

Polybactrin

A brand name for a mixture of the antibiotics bacitracin, **neomycin** and polymyxin. For external use.

Polycrol

A brand name for a mixture of the antacid drugs aluminium hydroxide and magnesium hydroxide and the antifoaming agent dimethicone.

polycystic disease of the ovaries

This rare condition features numerous small cysts under the surface of the ovaries, which cause the organs to be smoothly enlarged. The cysts are seldom more than about 5 mm in diameter. More important than the presence of the cysts is the fact that the condition is associated with failure of production of the oestrogen hormone. As a result, affected women have infrequent or absent periods, may be infertile and tend to grow hair excessively in a male distribution. Obesity also occurs.

polycythaemia

An abnormal thickening of the blood due to an increase in the concentration of red cells. Some degree of polycythaemia is a normal compensatory process in people living at high altitudes, but the condition may occur, as a disease, if the regulation of the rate of red cell production by the bone marrow becomes defective.

The effect of excessive red cells is to cause a plethoric appearance due to excessive redness of the skin, headache, high blood pressure and a tendency to stroke and to other complications arising from blockage of the arteries.

The treatment is to bleed the affected person at intervals or to reduce the rate of red blood cell production by chemotherapy or radiotherapy.

polydactyly

Having more than the normal number of fingers or toes. This is not uncommon and affects about one person in 200. It may be a harmless familial trait or it may occur as part of a more serious genetic disorder, such as the **Laurence-Moon-Biedl syndrome**.

polyethylene glycol

A substance used with other ingredients as a laxative. Trade names are Klean-prep and Movicol.

Polyfax

A brand name for a mixture of the antibiotics bacitracin and polymyxin B, used externally.

polygraph

See **lie detector**.

polymerase chain reaction

A method for the rapid production of very large numbers of copies of any required sequence of DNA, and one of the most powerful techniques currently in use in biological science. DNA is separated by heat into its two strands. The required sequence is isolated on one of the strands by the attachment of small molecules called primers to each of its ends. An enzyme, DNA polymerase, is then used to build a new copy of the strand of the section between the primers. Each copy becomes a template for the production of further strands, so that the number produced increases logarithmically. In twenty cycles a million copies are made. The polymerase chain reaction was invented one evening by the American biochemist Karry B. Mullis while he was driving a car. It earned him the Nobel Prize for Chemistry in 1993.

polymyalgia rheumatica

A persistent condition, featuring pain and stiffness in the shoulders, neck, back and arms, which is associated with another, more dangerous condition, giant cell arteritis.

RECOGNITION AND SYMPTOMS

The stiffness is often present on waking or after prolonged sitting, and may be so severe that the affected person can hardly get out of bed. The morning stiffness and disability are severe. Patients describe how they get their husbands (women are affected almost three times as often as men) to pull them out of bed, or, if they are alone, how they gradually make their way to the edge of the bed by a snake-like wriggling manoeuvre and then get out by a controlled fall.

There is low-grade fever, anaemia, **malaise**, loss of appetite (anorexia) and weight loss. The condition is remarkable for the absence of organic signs. There is no real muscle weakness and wasting is from disuse only. Muscle **biopsies** are normal as are serum tests for the presence of muscle enzymes which occur in cases of muscle damage. Electrical tests on muscles (electromyograms) are also normal. Tests for rheumatoid arthritis and antibodies to DNA are negative. The one constant and significant feature is that the sedimentation rate of the blood (the ESR) is very high – often over 100 mm in the hour. The normal ESR is less than 10 mm in the hour. When a short segment of an artery is removed, as a biopsy, in people with polymyalgia, about 40 per cent are found to have the obstructive changes in the artery known as giant cell arteritis.

TREATMENT

The response to the timely administration of steroids is so striking as almost to confirm the diagnosis. On a maintenance dose of steroids there is dramatic relief of stiffness and

People with the condition, however, are at risk of suffering sudden blindness, especially if the arteries on the temples are inflamed and tender. In such cases, urgent high steroid dosage can be sight-saving.

disability and this is sustained for periods of up to two years. Sudden blindness from giant cell arteritis is due to blockage of the end-branches of the main arteries to the eyes (ophthalmic arteries), but this does not usually occur until after some weeks or months of local symptoms such as transient visual loss (amaurosis fugax), double vision and headache. The headache is increasingly severe, is often worst in the areas of the affected arteries, persists through the day and is worse at night. When a facial artery is involved, there is pain on chewing – 'jaw claudication'. This is a very suggestive symptom which, in any patient over fifty, warrants an urgent sedimentation rate test.

polynoxylin

An antibacterial and antifungal drug used externally to treat skin infections. A brand name is Anaflex.

polyp

A normally benign and often harmless tumour, usually occurring on a mucous membrane and attached to the underlying tissue by a narrow stalk. Polyps occur in the nose, nasal sinuses, voice box (larynx), stomach, bladder, large intestine and womb (uterus) and may sometimes cause obstruction or may bleed. Nasal polyps are associated with long-term hay fever (allergic **rhinitis**) and may result in infection and discharge. Rarely, a polyp may become malignant. If necessary, polyps may be removed surgically, often with cauterization of the base.

polypharmacy

A mildly facetious term for the generally disapproved practice of prescribing several different drugs to one person at the same time. Polypharmacy increases the risk of unwanted side-effects and of dangerous interactions between different drugs.

Polytar

A brand name for coal tar.

polythiazide

A thiazide diuretic used to relieve oedema and treat high blood pressure. A brand name is Nephril.

Ponderax

A brand name for the weight-control drug fenfluramine.

Ponstan

A brand name for **mefenamic acid**.

population explosion

By general consent, this is the greatest menace facing mankind today. If the world population continues to grow at the present rate, all other medical, social and political problems will fade into insignificance beside this one. It is not generally appreciated that populations do not grow by addition but by multiplication. Each additional individual means the potentiality for several others. This means that it is not only populations that get larger; the rate of growth of populations also increases.

In the 1960s, world population was increasing by about a million every eight days. Today, the rate of increase has dou-

bled and a million more babies are born every four days. Every year there are far more women to have babies. At the beginning of the nineteenth century the world's population was less than one billion. In 1975 the world's population was about 4 billion. In 1995 the population was 5.5 billion, and each year the number of babies born increases by 93.5 million. Within a decade the total will be 6 billion. This is what is meant by exponential population rise.

EFFECTS

The effects of such a population explosion are devastating. It means starvation for increasing millions of people. Half of these billions of people will live in towns, many of them in poverty. Already there are 100 million homeless children desperately trying, by any means, to scrape a living. The population growth will exacerbate environmental damage, with accelerating deforestation, depletion of fresh water and degradation of the oceans.

Damage to ecosystems will inevitably mean serious damage to health, let alone damage to the quality of life. The growth in the prevalence of AIDS means that millions of these additional children will be left as orphans, abandoned to poverty, malnutrition and emotional deprivation.

THE CONTRACEPTION DEBATE

In the face of this appalling prospect of human suffering, it is hard to contemplate with equanimity the attitude of fundamentalist groups that oppose any attempt to limit population growth by contraceptive methods. The United Nations Cairo Conference on population in September 1994 was the occasion for a new offensive by the Vatican against contraception. The organizers were accused of promoting abortion, contraception and sexual immorality. The condom, now widely acknowledged as one of the principal weapons in the fight against AIDS, is viewed by the Vatican as an instrument of the devil.

UNICEF predicts that by 1997 AIDS will kill more children than malaria. Forty million people could be infected by the year 2000, 90 per cent of them in the Third World. Meantime, one-third of African women are desperate to limit their families but are denied the means. So millions of them are condemned to pregnancy that is often ruinous to their health, or to dangerous abortions and soaring maternal mortality.

The Catholic Church supplies enormous funding for medical relief in the Third World but this is often conditional on its anti-contraception policies being respected by governments. It was able successfully to block discussion on population control at the Rio Earth Summit in 1992.

The Catholic position on contraception springs from various sources, including the Old Testament story of Onan, who incurred God's wrath by practising coitus interruptus, and the writings of St Augustine (AD 354–430), especially his book *Marriage and Concupiscence* (AD 418). More recently, Catholic doctrine on the subject was moulded by the theologian Arthur Vermeersch who drafted much of Pope Pius XI's encyclical *Casti Connubi* (1930). This condemned all contraception except periodic abstinence as 'grave sin', and much of the content of this encyclical was restated by Pope Paul in his encyclical *Humanae Vitae* of 1968.

The author of the Onan story and St Augustine did not have reason to anticipate the recent appalling consequences of their teachings. But latter-day repressive Catholic theologians must be driven to consider very closely whether the grounds for their views and actions can be justified in the light of the terrible, and increasing, burden of human suffering that is their inevitable consequence.

Porcine Biphasic

A brand name for **insulin**.

Porcine Neutral

A brand name for **insulin**.

pore

Any small opening. The word is commonly used to refer to the small openings in the skin through which the sweat passes from tiny glands situated in the deepest layers of the skin or just under it. Other pores in the skin are the hair follicles into which open the sebaceous glands producing the oily secretion sebum. In the skin of the nose, the hairs in these follicles are usually small in comparison with the sebaceous glands, so that the pore appears to be concerned solely with sebum production.

In the margin of each eyelid is a row of pores, just behind the line of the lashes. These are the openings of the meibomian glands. Sebaceous glands in the areola of the breast, in the labia minora, and in the foreskin (prepuce) discharge through pores which are also independent of the hair follicles.

Pork Insulatard

A brand name for pig **insulin**.

Pork Mixtard

A brand name for pig **insulin**.

pornography

Pornography, or obscenity, is defined legally as any material, textual, graphic, cinematographic, or in any other medium, which tends to deprave or corrupt. Obscenity is not necessarily concerned with the representation of sexual activity, and a representation of violence, for instance, may be deemed obscene.

The difficulty is to determine whether or not any item has a corrupting tendency, so the definition tends to beg the question. An attempt was made, in the United States, to introduce the idea that pornography was material essentially lacking in redeeming social or artistic values, but this proved unworkable. In Britain the first antipornography legislation, the Obscene Publications Act, was passed in 1857. Under the current Obscene Publications Act 1959 and 1964, it is an offence to publish an obscene article.

The medical interest in pornography lies in the questions as to whether erotic imagery, of whatever kind, can corrupt and whether it may legitimately, and properly, be used in the treatment of sexual disorders. There is no ready answer to these questions, but the view is widely held that pornography teaches defective attitudes to sexuality which should, ideally, be based on mutual human respect and love, rather than primarily on the impulse to personal gratification. It can hardly be questioned that pornography, at a 'popular' level, which depicts the active association of sexuality with any form of violence, is to be deprecated.

A new impetus has been given to the study of the subject by the realization that a great deal of pornographic material is now being circulated among children and others in the form of personal computer software passed on in floppy disks and by way of Internet communication.

porphyria

Any one of several rare hereditary diseases featuring excessive production of porphyrins. These are important to the body, as haemoglobin and other biochemicals are made from them. Excess porphyrins occur because the enzymes which convert them to haemoglobin are missing. Some porphyrias are of dominant transmission, some are recessive.

RECOGNITION AND SYMPTOMS
The effect is to cause various combinations of digestive upset, severe skin disorders, with sensitivity to light, and brain damage. In some cases the symptoms are brought on by various drugs. Porphyrins in the urine cause it to turn dark red on standing.

TREATMENT
Treatment is difficult, but much may be done by avoiding known precipitating factors. Some types can be relieved by deliberate bleeding (venesection) and some are improved by administration of the drug panhaematin.

> King George III, King George IV and other members of the royal family are believed to have suffered from porphyria, which is sometimes called the royal malady.

portal hypertension

The portal vein is the main channel for blood returning from the intestine and it carries all absorbed nutrition to the liver. In the liver, the portal vein breaks up into many small branches so that the blood can be distributed throughout the organ. In cirrhosis of the liver, these small branches become narrowed by surrounding and constricting fibrous tissue and this greatly restricts the flow of blood though the veins. As a result there is a rise in back pressure, called portal hypertension, and the blood has to find an alternative route back to the heart. In so doing it causes veins in the lower end of the gullet (oesophagus) and elsewhere to widen and become varicose (oesophageal varices), and leads to the accumulation of fluid in the abdominal cavity (ascites).

> Oesophageal varices are dangerous, as they may rupture and bleed profusely. The treatment of this emergency involves the use of a special inflatable balloon to compress the bleeding veins, followed by surgery. Sometimes, threatening veins can be closed by injecting clotting fluid (sclerosant).

Portal hypertension can also be treated by means of a liver bypass or shunt, which allows some of the blood to return by way of the main abdominal drainage vein (the inferior vena cava).

port-wine stain

An extensive, flat, reddish-purple birthmark (naevus) caused by a patch of widening (dilatation) of the smallest of the skin vessels, the capillaries. The medical term is a capillary haemangioma. The port-wine stain can often be treated by laser destruction of the dilated vessels or, if the skin is lax, by surgical removal of all or part. Sometimes a port-wine stain is an outer sign of a more extensive and serious type of blood vessel tumour affecting the brain (the **Sturge-Weber syndrome**).

Posalfilin

A brand name for **podophyllum resin**.

Posicor

A brand name for **mibefradil**. This drug was withdrawn in mid-1998 after reports of interactions with other drugs.

post-

Prefix meaning 'after' as in postpartum (after delivery).

postcoital contraception

Prevention of pregnancy after sexual intercourse has occurred. If conception has occurred, the measure is not, strictly, contraceptive. Methods include:

* taking two high-dose contraceptive pills as soon as possible and then, 12 hours later, taking a single dose of mifepristone;
* the insertion by a doctor of a copper-releasing intrauterine contraceptive device.

Mifepristone is used for legal termination of pregnancy in the UK but is currently not licensed anywhere outside China for postcoital contraception.

Postcoital contraception is also known as emergency contraception or the 'morning-after pill'.

postconcussional syndrome

A range of symptoms occurring after what appears to be a minor head injury with brief loss of consciousness and little or no immediate memory loss (retrograde or post-traumatic amnesia). The syndrome, which may last for a year or longer, includes headache, depression, loss of concentration and the power of attention, memory loss, anxiety, dizziness and low tolerance to noise.

postnasal drip

Popularly known as 'nasal catarrh', this is a trickle of watery or mucinous fluid produced in the nasopharynx in chronic infective, and other forms, of **rhinitis**. The fluid passes down the back wall of the **pharynx**, sometimes with difficulty because of its viscidity, causing an uncomfortable awareness of its presence. When infection is active, the post-nasal drip fluid contains pus as well as mucus.

POSSIBLE CAUSES

Post-nasal drip is also a feature of vasomotor rhinitis in which the mucous membrane of the nasopharynx becomes overactive and secretes excessively. This may be due to allergy, stress, infection, sexual excitement ('honeymoon rhinitis'), drugs for high blood pressure (**hypertension**), and the overuse of decongestant nasal sprays and drops, which produce a *rebound* congestion of the mucous membrane.

post-traumatic stress disorder

This is the current terminology for what used to be called 'shell-shock', 'psychiatric battle casualty' or 'battle fatigue'. It may affect any person who has suffered a major psychological

trauma, such as long exposure to gun-fire, severe assault, rape, fire danger, earthquake, shipwreck. The onset may be weeks or months after the event.

RECOGNITION AND SYMPTOMS

The condition features initial numbness followed by the inability to respond emotionally to other experiences and to other people, a sense of guilt at surviving, irritability, depression, and recurrent nightmares which feature the traumatic event or circumstances. There may be outbreaks of violence and the reactivation of earlier emotional problems. Affected people often have an exaggerated startle response and are abnormally vigilant. They may have recurrent, intrusive memories of the event and a recurrent sense of reliving it. They suffer severe emotional distress at being reminded of it and are much aware of anniversaries. They will try to avoid activities or situations that bring back such memories.

TREATMENT

About 30 per cent of affected people recover completely, 40 per cent have mild persistent effects and 30 per cent remain unchanged or get worse. Treatment with antidepressant drugs and with beta-blockers can be helpful, as can psychotherapy, especially behaviour therapy and group therapy. Psychotherapy can help the sufferer to come to terms with, and accept, the past.

Potaba

A brand name for **aminobenzoic acid**.

potassium channel activators

A new class of drugs that greatly enhance the movement of potassium ions through channels in cell membranes. The action on the membranes of smooth muscle cells in arterial walls is to cause hyperpolarization so that the cells' sensitivity to the normal stimuli to contraction is reduced. The muscle fibres are thus relaxed and the arteries widened. Drugs in this class are useful in improving the blood supply to the heart muscle in **angina pectoris**. A typical drug in this group is nicorandil (Icorel).

potassium channel blockers

These drugs close the channels in cell membranes through which potassium ions pass out of cells. The effect of this is to increase the excitability and probability of action of the cells. Potassium channel blockers include the sulphonylurea group of drugs used to treat maturity-onset diabetes. These increase the output of insulin from the beta cells of the Islets of Langerhans in the pancreas.

potency

The strength of a drug based on its effectiveness to cause change. Also, the claimed increase in the power of homoeopathic remedies with increasing dilution and shaking.

Pott's disease

A tuberculous infection of the bones of the spine which used commonly to lead to collapse of one or more of the bodies of the vertebrae, causing acute angulation of the back. This was once a common cause of the disfigurement known popularly as 'hunchback', but is now, happily, rare. The infection was usually acquired from bovine tuberculosis in milk, now largely eliminated by **pasteurization**.

Pott's fracture

A now obsolete term for a fracture, or fracture-dislocation, of the lower leg, involving the ankle, with injury to the main bone (the tibia) and sometimes also the slender fibula.

povidone-iodine

An antiseptic drug suitable for application to the skin or, in the form of pessaries, to the vagina. It is also used as a mouthwash or gargle to treat mouth infections. Trade names are Betadine and Inadine.

Powergel

A brand name for **ketoprofen** formulated for external use.

Prader-Willi syndrome

A rare genetic disorder caused by the abnormal removal (deletion) early in development of a small segment from the long arm of chromosome 15. At birth the baby is very floppy and initial physical development is very slow. Later in childhood, however, there is a rapid increase in weight progressing to obesity. The face is narrow with a thin upper lip and down-turned mouth. The genitalia are underdeveloped, especially in males, and puberty is delayed. Older children may show severe obsessive-compulsive behaviour problems, temper tantrums and stubborn resistance to discipline.

Pragmatar

A brand name for a mixture of coal tar, the skin-softening agent salicylic acid and sulphur.

Pramin

A brand name for **metoclopramide**.

Praminil

A brand name for **imipramine**.

pravastatin

One of the class of statin cholesterol-lowering drugs. A brand name is Lipostat.

Praxilene

A brand name for the **vasodilator** drug **naftidrofuryl**.

prazosin

A drug that widens the arteries (vasodilator) and is used in the treatment of high blood pressure, **heart failure** and **Raynaud's phenomenon**. A brand name is Hypovase.

pre-

Prefix meaning 'before' as in precordial (in front of the heart).

precancerous

Having a tendency to progress to cancer. Many conditions are known to be precancerous. These include:

- **leukoplakia** of the mouth which sometimes progresses to carcinoma of the mouth or tongue;

- persistent damage to the linings of the air tubes (bronchi) of the lungs from smoking, with loss of the normal character in the lining cells, which often progresses to lung cancer;
- certain changes in the lining cells of the neck of the womb (the cervix) associated with venereal warts which may progress to cancer of the cervix;
- **ulcerative colitis** and polyposis of the colon, which are associated with an increased incidence of multiple cancers of the large intestine (colon) and the rectum;
- **Down's syndrome** which predisposes to **leukaemia**;
- **xeroderma pigmentosum** which nearly always proceeds to multiple basal cell carcinomas (**rodent ulcers**), squamous carcinomas, and sometimes melanomas and **angiomas**;
- von Recklinghausen's disease (**neurofibromatosis**) and tuberous sclerosis which have an increased incidence of gliomas, meningiomas, and various endocrine tumours;
- papillomas of the bladder which may proceed to bladder cancer.

Knowledge of precancerous conditions provides an opportunity either to avoid the causes or to be especially aware of the possibility of cancer and to seek treatment before this happens.

Precortisyl Forte

A brand name for **prednisolone**.

Predenema

A brand name for **prednisolone**.

Predfoam

A brand name for **prednisolone**.

Pred Forte

A brand name for **prednisolone**.

Prednefrin Forte

A brand name for eye drops containing **prednisolone** and **phenylephrine**.

Prednesol

A brand name for **prednisolone**.

prednisolone

A semisynthetic corticosteroid drug derived from the natural steroid hormone cortisol and used in the treatment of a wide range of inflammatory disorders. Prednisolone may be given by mouth or injection, but many preparations are formulated for application to the skin or the eyes or ears and the drug may also be given as an enema. Trade names are Deltacortril, Deltastab, Minims prednisolone, Precortisyl Forte, Pred Forte, Predenema, Predfoam, Prednesol, and Predsol.

prednisone

A synthetic corticosteroid drug used to reduce inflammation and relieve symptoms in rheumatoid arthritis, ulcerative colitis and many other conditions. A brand name is Decortisyl.

Predsol

A brand name for **prednisolone**.

Predsol-N

A brand name for **neomycin** with **prednisolone**, for external application.

Prefil

A brand name for the bulk-forming antidiarrhoeal agent sterculia.

Pregaday

A brand name for **ferrous fumarate** in conjunction with **folic acid**.

pregnancy

Pregnancy is the period from conception to the birth of the baby. It begins when a single sperm (spermatozoon) penetrates the outer layer of an egg, and usually ends 266 to 270 days (about forty weeks) later when the baby is delivered. After fertilization, the combined egg and sperm cell begins to split repeatedly into two and is called an embryo. Some development of the embryo is necessary before it can implant into the lining of the womb. So if fertilization has occurred too near the point where the Fallopian tube enters the womb, there may be insufficient time for the ovum to develop to the stage at which it can implant. In this case, the pregnancy ends at that point.

About a week after entry of the sperm, the fertilized ovum becomes implanted in the endometrium, usually in the upper part, which has been prepared by the hormone stimulation from the corpus luteum of the ovary.

HEALTHY LIVING DURING PREGNANCY

Ideally, it should be unnecessary to make any substantial changes in your lifestyle during pregnancy, except, perhaps to eat more than usual (see below). The latter is unlikely to be a problem, but it is important to pay particular attention to the rules for healthy living. These are all detailed in this book. As your pregnancy advances you will naturally modify your exercise programmes on common-sense grounds. Your antenatal clinic staff will advise you on special exercises to strengthen the pelvic floor. Now is the time, also, to learn all you can about the care of your breasts and about the advantages of **breastfeeding**.

PREGNANCY TESTS

As soon as the embryo begins to implant it sends out tiny fingerlike processes called chorionic villi which help to anchor it into the womb lining and which later become the placenta. Within about a week of conception, these villi are producing a hormone called human chorionic gonadotrophin. This is necessary to maintain the corpus luteum in the ovary (see above) so as to prevent menstruation and termination of the pregnancy.

Nearly all the early tests for pregnancy depend on the presence of chorionic gonadotrophin. This hormone is first present in the blood, but soon afterwards appears in the urine. A simple dipstick test into fresh morning urine can detect pregnancy with about a 98 per cent certainty. Kits for performing these tests are available over-the-counter from pharmacies. Even more delicate immunological tests to

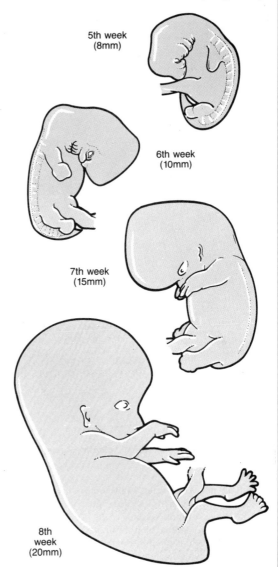

5th week
(8mm)

6th week
(10mm)

7th week
(15mm)

8th
week
(20mm)

Growth of embryo showing approximate head to rump length at different ages.

detect the hormone by its combination with pre-prepared specific antibodies to it, can confirm pregnancy within a week of conception. These include the **ELISA test** and a radioimmunoassay test. These are normally done in a hospital laboratory.

If these tests are positive the accuracy is nearly 100 per cent certain; if the test is negative, about 80 per cent certain.

SIGNS OF PREGNANCY

In addition to using hormone tests, doctors can confirm pregnancy by noting certain physical changes (signs) and by taking a history of a few symptoms. The woman concerned will usually be aware that she has missed one or more menstrual period. This is the most obvious early sign of pregnancy. Most women suffer some nausea and vomiting in early pregnancy, but this does not necessarily occur in the mornings. 'Morning sickness' varies greatly in severity and may be seriously disabling, but it usually settles by about twelve weeks. Severe

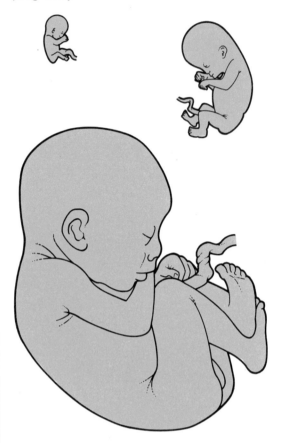

The relative sizes of the fetus at 3 months, 5 months and 9 months.

vomiting may necessitate admission to hospital and this, alone, is usually effective (see excessive vomiting below).

Because the womb lies close to the bladder, an increase in its size often causes bladder irritability with increased frequency of emptying of the bladder. Other signs and symptoms of pregnancy include:

- engorgement and enlargement of the breasts;
- breast soreness;
- tiredness, sometimes severe;
- progressive enlargement of the womb;
- visualization of the fetal outline by ultrasound scanning at about six weeks;
- detection of the fetal heartbeat with a stethoscope, usually at about the twentieth week;
- browning of the pink zones round the nipples (areolas);
- perception by the mother of fetal movements (quickening).

Quickening is usually perceived at about the eighteenth week in a first pregnancy, and about two weeks earlier in later pregnancies. By this time the womb has enlarged enough to be in contact with the inside of the wall of the abdomen so that impulses are transmitted to the touch receptors near the surface. The sensations are, at first, feeble and barely perceptible, and are often confused with 'wind', but as the fetus matures and its jerky movements increase in strength, the source of the sensation ceases to be in doubt.

Quickening is, however, one of the least reliable sign of pregnancy and one that often misleads. It should never be accepted as a proof in the absence of other indications. A woman anxious to conceive may easily become convinced that she is feeling fetal movements, when, in fact, she is not pregnant.

ANTENATAL CARE

All pregnant women should have proper antenatal care, the functions of which are to:

- ensure, as far as possible, the health of the mother and fetus;
- detect and deal with problems as early as possible;
- prepare the mother for birth;
- help the mother with subsequent baby care.

At the first visit, a full history will be taken of previous medical problems; of family disorders; of previous pregnancies; and of whether there have been any problems with the present pregnancy. A full general examination is then carried out, including an examination of the abdomen. A vaginal examination and a Pap smear test are sometimes done. An assessment of the pelvis is sometimes made at this stage and any possible difficulties from disproportion between the baby's head and the pelvis anticipated. This, however, is often left until later. A check is made as to whether the dates given by the mother correspond to the physical state.

All or most of the following tests may be performed:

- blood pressure check;
- check for oedema;
- urine examination for sugar, protein and organisms;
- blood test for blood grouping and rhesus factor status;
- blood test for anaemia and other blood disorders;

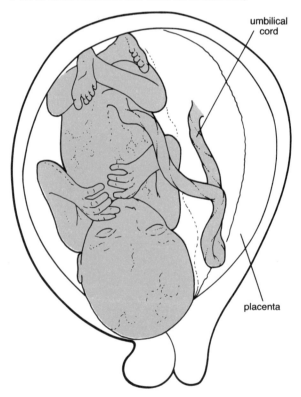

The pregnant uterus near term.

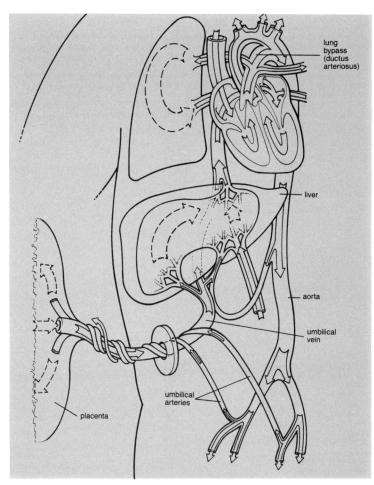

The connections between the umbilicus and the fetus. Note that blood passes to the placenta by two arteries coming from the main arteries to the legs of the fetus and returns by the large umbilical vein into and through the liver of the fetus. At this stage the lungs are mainly bypassed and the oxygenated blood from the placenta is shunted to all parts of the body of the fetus.

lung bypass (ductus arteriosus)

liver

aorta

umbilical vein

umbilical arteries

placenta

- rubella antibody test;
- blood test for syphilis;
- alphafetoprotein blood test;
- hepatitis B test;
- HIV test in women at special risk.

Ultrasound screening is generally offered between the sixteenth and the twentieth weeks to confirm the dates and to detect any gross fetal abnormality. Follow-up attendances are shorter and the examination is much less extensive. Blood pressure, urine tests, ankle oedema and the height of the top of the womb are all checked. Excessive weight gain would be monitored. A blood test for anaemia is repeated towards the end of pregnancy. Failure of normal growth of the fetus is fully investigated, and any abnormal findings are dealt with. If necessary, the mother is admitted to hospital for further investigation and treatment.

THE STAGES OF PREGNANCY

Although pregnancy is a continuous, slow process of embryonic and then fetal growth, doctors and nurses find it convenient to divide the whole gestation period arbitrarily into three periods, each of three months, called trimesters.

From the point of view of the future health and normality of the baby, the first trimester is by far the most important. This is because all the major structures of the body form during this period and any agency that can interfere with this formation – such as a rubella virus infection, a toxic drug, high maternal blood alcohol or maternal smoking – may have

serious and permanent effects on the body and brain of the future child. Such damage is, in general, less serious later in the pregnancy. By the end of the first trimester the fingers, toes, external genitalia, facial features and ears are visible.

During the second trimester, the fetal heart action is strong enough for its sounds to become audible through a stethoscope and an experienced examiner can feel the fetus carefully through the abdominal wall. Because of the rapid growth of the womb and the extra space it takes up in the abdomen, there is unusual pressure on the internal organs and this may cause discomfort and various symptoms. Pressure on the stomach, for instance, may force some stomach acid up into the gullet causing severe heartburn to the mother. Pressure on the bladder may increase the desire to pass urine.

Irregular, painless contractions of the womb, readily felt by the mother, may occur from this time on. These are called **Braxton-Hicks contractions** and they are perfectly normal. They do not imply that labour is starting. During the second trimester the developed fetal organs begin to function. The skin is still quite transparent and, on laparoscopy, blood vessels can easily be seen through the skin. Scalp hair begins to grow. During this stage the bones become more solid and become conspicuous on ultrasound scanning.

The Braxton-Hicks contractions become more frequent in the third trimester and all the symptoms worsen due to a growing increase in pressure within the abdomen. Upward pressure on the diaphragm prevents it from moving downwards fully during respiration and this limits full expansion of the lungs. For this reason a heavily pregnant woman will often suffer breathlessness. During this trimester, the growth rate of the fetus is at a maximum and all the normal external features of a baby – fingernail and toenails, testicles in boys, labia in girls and ear lobes – can be seen on laparoscopy.

During the last month of the pregnancy many women in their first pregnancy experience a sense of relief from the symptoms caused by abdominal fullness. This occurs because the baby is normally lying head-down and it may move downwards as its head sinks naturally into the pelvis. This sense of relief from abdominal pressure is called lightening. Now the mother's diaphragm is able to descend more fully and the lungs to expand so that breathing is easier. The cost of this, however, is that the pressure on the bladder and rectum may be worse. Lightening may not occur with second or subse-

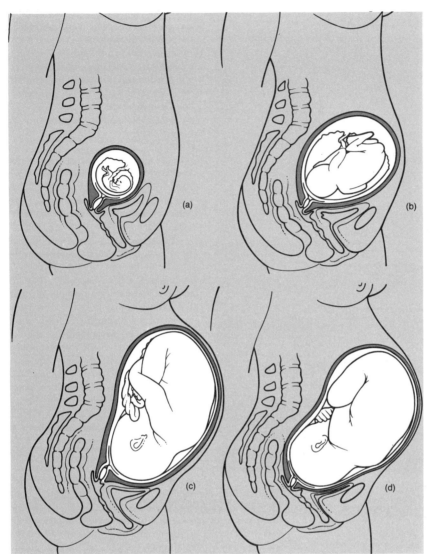

Relative sizes of the womb (uterus) at the end of the third (a), sixth (b), and ninth (c) month. In (a), (b) and (c) the head of the fetus is above the brim of the pelvis, but near the end of pregnancy the head usually sinks down into the pelvis (d), relieving pressure in the abdomen and making breathing easier. This is called 'lightening'.

quent pregnancies. In these, it is quite common for the baby's head to fail to 'engage' until labour has actually started.

WEIGHT GAIN IN PREGNANCY

Most women gain 20–30 lb (9–14 kg) by the end of pregnancy. Weight gain depends on many different factors, including body size and eating habits. Weight gain during pregnancy is by no means all due to increased fat deposition

Weight gain in pregnancy		
FETUS	6–8 lb	(3–4 kg)
WOMB	2 lb	(1 kg)
PLACENTA	1.5 lb	(0.5 kg)
AMNIOTIC FLUID	2 lb	(1 kg)
BREASTS	1–2 lb	(0.5–1 kg)
BLOOD AND BODY FLUID		
VOLUME INCREASE	5–7 lb	(2–3 kg)
FAT AND OTHER		
BODY STORES	4–6 lb	(2–2.5 kg)

and much of it is lost after the baby is born. The approximate distribution of the additional weight can be seen in the table. Most pregnant women require an additional intake of about 300 calories per day to provide for the growth of the fetus, placenta, womb and breasts.

MULTIPLE PREGNANCY

Twins can occur in two ways. If two eggs are released at the same time and both are fertilized and survive, non-identical twins are produced. Because such twins arise from different eggs and different sperms they are genetically no more similar than any two children of the same parents. They may be of the same or of different sexes and can have very different characteristics. Each has its own placenta and each occupies a different membrane sac (see below). Such twins are known as dizygotic twins because they come from two zygotes. A zygote is the cell that results from the union of a sperm with an ovum.

If, however, only one egg is released and this is fertilized in the usual way by a single sperm, and if, after the first cell division, the two resulting cells separate so that each forms a new individual, the resulting twins will be genetically identical

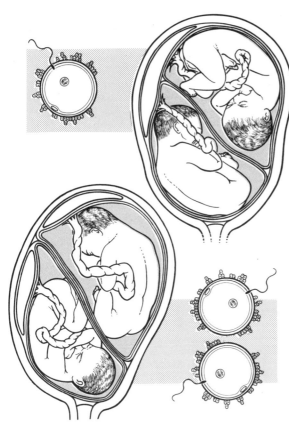

The difference between uniovular and binovular twins. The former come from a single ovum and sperm and share a placenta. They have identical genes. Binovular twins come from separate ova, are separately, but simultaneously, fertilized and have separate placentas. Binovular twins have different genetic material.

and will, in all respects, resemble each other. They are clones. They have exactly the same chromosomes with the same genes and they share a placenta with two umbilical cords. Usually, however, each is surrounded by a separate bag of membranes. Identical twins are known as monozygotic twins.

Triplets usually occur from a combination of these possibilities so may be identical or contain both identical and non-identical siblings. Quads and quins are very rare unless multiple ovulation has been caused by drugs used to treat infertility. The more recent drugs used, however, are less likely to have this dramatic effect. The various complications of pregnancy, especially prematurity, are commoner in multiple than in single pregnancies.

COMPLICATIONS OF PREGNANCY

The great majority of pregnancies go from start to finish without any real problems. Although many things can go wrong, it is remarkable that such a complicated process usually proceeds without a hitch.

Stretchmarks, known as striae, are broad lines on the abdomen, thighs and breasts that affect about three-quarters of all pregnant women. At first red and slightly raised, they later become purplish and flattened. During pregnancy striae are known as striae gravidarum. After delivery they become silvery white and are then known as striae albicans.

Striae are said to be due to stretching of the skin and the resulting damage to the elastic protein collagen in the skin. It is notable, however, that striae do not occur when the skin of the abdomen is stretched in most other ways, even if this stretching occurs rapidly. Large ovarian cysts, for instance, can grow as quickly as a pregnancy but do not cause striae. It seems clear, therefore, that there are other causes and it is believed that these are probably hormonal. The condition of Cushing's syndrome, in which there are long-term high levels of steroids, similar to the hormones of pregnancy, in the blood, features striae. Unfortunately, striae are permanent.

Pregnancy outside the womb is known medically as ectopic pregnancy. Ectopic simply means 'in the wrong place'. It comes from the Greek *ek*, 'out of' and *topos*, 'a place'.

In about 1 pregnancy in 200 the fertilized ovum burrows into a body tissue other than the lining of the womb (the endometrium), and an ectopic pregnancy results. The commonest place for this to occur is in a Fallopian tube which has been narrowed or otherwise affected by inflammation. Much less commonly, ectopic pregnancies can occur in an ovary or even within the abdominal cavity (see **abdominal gestation**).

Ectopic pregnancy is a very dangerous condition. The early embryo is a most energetic burrower and is seeking blood vessels so that it can form a placenta and link up with the mother's blood circulation. To do this, the embryo produces substances called enzymes that actually partially digest the tissues to promote burrowing. The womb has evolved to cope with this but the other tissues of the body have not, and the result of this process occurring in the wrong place is often massive internal bleeding. Early diagnosis and surgical treatment of ectopic pregnancy are essential. Untreated ectopic pregnancies can end fatally from uncontrollable haemorrhage and surgical shock.

Ectopic pregnancy usually starts with cramping period-like pains and slight vaginal bleeding occurring soon after the first missed period. These are much more likely to be indications of threatened abortion than ectopic pregnancy, but if they are followed by a more severe pain in the lower

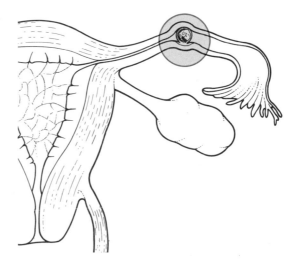

Sometimes a fertilized ovum sticks in the Fallopian tube (or elsewhere other than in the womb) and begins to develop. This is called an ectopic pregnancy and is very dangerous as severe bleeding is inevitable.

abdomen, localized to one side, and a deterioration in the woman's general condition, the diagnosis of ectopic pregnancy must be seriously considered. Urgent hospital management is needed.

Gynaecological examination, blood and urine tests and ultrasound scanning and laparoscopy, can establish what is happening. If the diagnosis is confirmed, surgical removal of the mass can be done immediately. Unfortunately, this may mean removing a length of Fallopian tube. If this is so, every effort is usually made to join up the cut ends to preserve continuity and function, so that subsequent pregnancy is possible.

Maternal rubella in early pregnancy is one of the most distressing things that can happen. Rubella is an infection of the mother with the German measles (rubella) virus, and this mild and usually harmless condition can have devastating effects on the early fetus if the viruses get to it. These viruses enter the cells of the developing embryo and early fetus and can cause a wide range of damage that may result in such conditions as:

● congenital heart disease;
● congenital cataracts;
● congenital deafness;
● visual defects;
● neurological defects;
● mental retardation;
● defects in the skeleton.

The term 'congenital' means 'present at birth'. These things are likely only if the infection is acquired during the first few weeks. Lesser degrees of damage can occur from rubella later in pregnancy, but the more fully the organs are developed the less the likelihood of damage. Even so, studies have shown that 23 per cent of children exposed to early rubella but apparently normal at birth, were found to have various defects by the age of two.

Because of these risks it is essential that pregnant women should, at the first antenatal check, have a special immunological test to see whether they have previously had the infection or have been successfully immunized. Those who are found to be susceptible should be particularly careful to avoid contact with any possible case and should be immunized as soon as the pregnancy is over. Any susceptible women who develop a rash and swollen glands in the back of the neck early in pregnancy should be checked to discover whether the condition is rubella. If this is confirmed by immunological testing the question of termination of the pregnancy will have to be considered.

All young girls should have rubella immunization as a matter of course. Boys should also be immunized. If they became infected they could pass the virus to pregnant women.

Excessive vomiting is another distressing complication of pregnancy. Most pregnant women suffer 'morning sickness' to a greater or lesser degree and this is considered normal. Vomiting of a degree and frequency that precludes normal life is a rare complication of pregnancy and is known as hyperemesis gravidarum. No one really knows what causes this kind of uncontrolled vomiting in pregnancy and many experts believe it has a psychological basis. Pregnant women who suffer much sickness, or anyone who has experienced severe seasickness, will appreciate that a condition like this is quite enough to produce an extremely disturbed state of mind.

Hyperemesis can be very serious and may even threaten survival. The constant loss of stomach acid and bowel con-

tents in the vomit causes fundamental biochemical changes, and these are made worse by the accompanying starvation and dehydration. An acidic condition of the blood (ketosis) similar to that occurring in severe untreated diabetes may result. This can also endanger the fetus.

Hyperemesis may require hospital treatment and it is sometimes necessary to replace lost fluids by intravenous infusion. In many cases, however, the mere fact of admission to hospital will cure the condition. Less severe cases can be managed at home. Interestingly, hyperemesis is now very much less common than it was twenty-five years ago and it is almost unknown in developing countries.

An excess of the normal fluid in the womb (hydramnios) occurs in about one pregnancy in 150. The fetus normally floats in, and is cushioned by, a liquid called amniotic fluid produced by one of the membranes (the amnion) that surround it. This fluid is regularly swallowed and the fetus regularly urinates into it. In this way, the volume of the fluid is partly regulated by the fetus itself. Usually, there is just enough of this to serve its protective purpose, but occasionally an abnormal excess volume of amniotic fluid occurs in the womb.

The normal volume of fluid towards the end of pregnancy is about 800 to 1000 ml. In hydramnios this may rise to well over 2 litres. In most cases the excess occurs gradually and is not noted until about the thirtieth week. Often the cause is unknown, but hydramnios may occur if, for any reason, the fetus cannot swallow amniotic fluid. This may be because its gullet is abnormally narrowed or closed. Hydramnios is also common in the severe congenital abnormality in which the brain is largely absent (anencephaly). Anencephaly can, of course, be detected quite early in the pregnancy by scanning or fetoscopy through an endoscope. In the case of such a disaster the pregnancy is usually terminated.

In hydramnios, the fetus is free to move more freely than normal and, as a result, will often present for birth in a position other than the normal head-down and back-of-the-head-to-the-front orientation. The greater freedom of movement also increases the probability that the placenta will separate from the wall before delivery. As may be expected, hydramnios also leads to a tendency to premature rupture of the membranes, and this may be associated with the dangerous condition in which the umbilical cord partly comes out before delivery of the baby.

Ultrasound examination is mandatory in hydramnios. This will show up any gross abnormalities in the fetus. If there is severe discomfort near term, labour may be deliberately induced a little early. Some obstetricians remove the excess fluid, by way of a needle passed through the abdominal wall. This, they believe, makes delivery safer. Occasionally, a Caesarean section operation (see **childbirth**) is necessary.

Cervical incompetence is the condition in which the upper part of the narrow canal that runs through the neck of the womb – the cervical canal – remains a little open, perhaps sufficiently to admit an object, such as a surgical dilator, about 1 cm in diameter. This abnormal widening is present at all times and remains so during pregnancy. As the pregnancy progresses, the internal pressure from the increasing volume of fluid and fetus tends to open the outlet further. As a result, women with this problem may, repeatedly, suffer the disappointment of having painless, spontaneous miscarriages usually around the fourth or fifth month. These miscarriages are painless because the cervix is abnormally lax and open and does not need to be stretched.

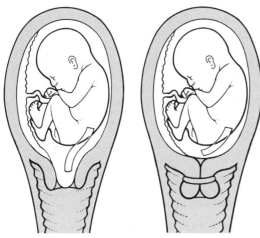

A common cause of miscarriage is an incompetent cervix which opens too easily. If diagnosed, the pregnancy can often be saved by means of a temporary encircling stitch.

Cervical incompetence may also lead to premature rupture of the membranes. Usually, but not always, cervical incompetence is due to previous damage during delivery or to previous surgery such as repeated dilatations and curettage (D & C); a cone biopsy for suspected cancer; or an amputation of the cervix. Fortunately, once recognized, this condition is easily treated. Before the sixteenth week of pregnancy, but after the twelfth week (when most spontaneous abortions have already occurred) a single, strong stitch of non-absorbable material is sewn around the cervix in an in-and-out 'purse-string' manner. This procedure is known as the Shirodkar operation. The suture keeps the cervix firmly closed until such time as the baby can safely be delivered. The stitch is then simply cut and pulled out – a procedure that takes only a few minutes.

The term pre-eclampsia has, for many years, been given to a set of physical signs that gives warning of one of the most dangerous conditions that can affect a pregnant woman. The established condition – eclampsia – is the major cause of maternal death in Britain, America and other advanced countries. Fortunately it is very rare.

Eclampsia is a disorder originating in the placenta that, once under way, causes widespread upset of the functioning of the circulatory system of both mother and fetus. The effects are devastating. The possible features of eclampsia include:

- major epileptic fits;
- cerebral haemorrhage;
- serious kidney damage;
- possible blindness from retinal damage;
- rupture of the liver;
- widespread clotting within the blood vessels;
- separation of the placenta;
- death of the mother and fetus.

The maternal mortality rate in established eclampsia is about 3 per cent and the baby death rate about 15 per cent. Eclampsia must be avoided at all costs and an important reason for antenatal examination is that it provides the opportunity for the detection of the signs that are known to herald it.

The most important sign of pre-eclampsia is a significant rise in the blood pressure. The other signs are the presence of the protein albumin in the urine – this is always abnormal – and the occurrence of excessive fluid retention in the tissues (oedema). These signs do not necessarily imply that eclampsia may occur, but if they are detected, a particularly close watch is maintained, often in hospital.

Other more subtle signs can be helpful in the diagnosis. These include a rise in the uric acid in the blood, a drop in the number of the tiny platelet cell fragments in the blood necessary to promote blood coagulation and various abnormalities in the enzymes produced when the liver is damaged.

The one pressing necessity is to get rid of the placenta. This means, in effect, inducing labour or performing a Caesarean section so that the baby and the placenta can be delivered. The aim, of course, is to produce a live baby, as mature as possible, while preventing injury to the mother. If at all possible, the pregnancy is maintained until the thirty-sixth week. Rest in bed is an important measure. Drugs to reduce blood pressure are avoided, if possible, as they may interfere with the supply to the fetus through the placenta. Imminent eclampsia is a signal for energetic measures to sedate the mother, get the blood pressure down and deliver the baby as soon as possible.

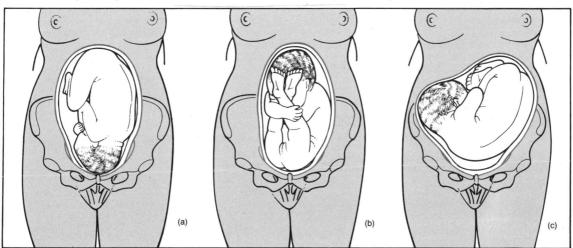

At full term, the fetus should lie head down with the neck bent and the back of the head to the front (a). Malpresentations such as breech presentation (b) or transverse lie (c) can cause complications.

Unfortunately, in spite of intense research, the exact cause of pre-eclampsia and eclampsia remains one of the mysteries of medicine. We know that the condition is three times as common in the first pregnancy as in later pregnancies, and a great deal is also known about the effects of various forms of treatment. But until the cause is known no completely effective way of avoiding this distressing condition can be devised.

Unusual positioning of the baby before birth is known as malpresentation. This simply means that the baby is in such a position in the womb that a part of it other than the usual back of the head threatens to be born first. At the time of the great majority of births, the baby lies head down with the chin tucked in and the back of the head to the front. Alternatives to this are the breech presentation in which the buttocks appear first; a face-front presentation; a shoulder presentation; a transverse lie; or a presentation with the neck extended instead of flexed and the back of the head to the rear. Sometimes the baby's arm presents first.

Breech presentations are usually allowed to proceed and in most cases there is no real trouble. Other presentations may, however, cause difficulty in labour, or even a complete hold-up. In these cases it may be necessary to try to turn the baby in the womb – a procedure not without danger – or, more commonly, to deliver by Caesarean section. Turning the baby, whether by internal or external manipulation, can lead to separation of the placenta and requires great skill and experience.

Any vaginal bleeding during pregnancy is always worrying. In the early stages, bleeding is called threatened abortion (see **abortion and miscarriage**) and may or may not imply that the pregnancy will terminate. Bleeding from the womb after about the twenty-fourth week of pregnancy is called antepartum haemorrhage.

Antepartum haemorrhage implies that the attachment of the placenta to the inner wall of the womb is not as secure as it should be. This may be due to an abnormality in the placement, or in the security of attachment of the placenta and occurs in about 3 per cent of pregnancies. The risk to the fetus from inadequate blood supply depends on the degree of separation and this can usually be judged by the amount of bleeding. If severe bleeding occurs, the risk to the fetus is considerable and there may also be a risk to the mother.

Antepartum haemorrhage calls for close monitoring of the state of the fetus and a careful watch on the condition of the mother. If things go badly, an emergency Caesarean section may be necessary to save the baby.

pregnancy outside the womb

See **abdominal gestation**, **ectopic pregnancy**.

pregnancy tests

See **pregnancy**.

Pregnyl

A brand name for chorionic gonadotrophin.

Premarin

A brand name for a preparation of conjugated oestrogens. The name is said to derive from the source – pregnant mare's urine.

premature babies, lung disorder

See **bronchopulmonary dysplasia**.

premature ejaculation

See **ejaculation, disorders of**.

prematurity

Babies whose birth weight is less than 2.5 kg (6 lb) are usually referred to as 'low birthweight babies'. Those weighing less than 1.5 kg (3 lb) are often called 'very low birthweight babies'. Babies born with a weight which is significantly low for the dates, are known as 'small-for-dates babies'.

About 10 per cent of babies born are premature. The average weight of a baby at birth is about 3.3 kg (7 lb). There is, however, much natural variation and many babies are heavier than average because their mothers are naturally heavy or diabetic. The cause of prematurity is by no means always apparent. In about half of all cases, however, prematurity can be attributed to such factors as:

- poor maternal health;
- maternal smoking;
- excessive maternal alcohol intake;
- maternal drug addiction;
- maternal toxaemia (pre-eclampsia);
- maternal high blood pressure;
- placental inadequacy;
- twin or triple pregnancy;
- abnormal attachment of the placenta;
- infection in the uterus;
- genetic defects.

Premature babies are more likely to have problems than full weight babies. In particular, they are apt to lose temperature very readily, are unusually prone to infection and have difficulty in swallowing or coughing. They are also especially prone to respiratory distress syndrome, to retrolental fibroplasia and to sudden infant death syndrome (cot death).

Premature baby care units are special care facilities staffed by medical and nursing personnel with specialized training and experience in the management of babies with special needs. Because of their ready tendency to hypothermia, premature babies are kept in temperature-controlled environments in incubators. These are designed to allow careful and continuous monitoring of all the important bodily functions.

The staff in premature baby care units are particularly careful about personal hygiene and wash their hands scrupulously before approaching their charges. Any of the staff who develop upper respiratory tract infections are automatically excluded from the unit. Masks are no longer considered essential, however.

Staff are also skilled in the feeding of premature infants and are very much aware of the dangerous tendency for such tiny babies to inhale liquid food. Many premature babies are fed exclusively by means of a fine, soft PVC tube that is passed through the nose and down into the stomach. Breast milk expressed from the mother may be used. Continuous feeding by this method may be used until the baby is mature enough to develop a suckling reflex. Vitamin supplements, folic acid and iron are usually given. Injections of vitamin K are given routinely to prevent a bleeding tendency.

Since the middle 1980s many babies born with a birth-weight of less than than 750 grams have survived, and it is now possible to assess the effects of such low birthweights on development. Regrettably, it has been found that, as they develop, such children, on average, suffer a serious disadvantage compared to those of normal birthweight. They have a substantially higher incidence of mental retardation, spastic paralysis, visual defect and reduced physical skills. They do less well academically, have inferior social skills and suffer from attention and behavioural problems. About 20 per cent of such children have below-normal mental abilities and almost half of them require special educational attention.

Doctors are now beginning to appreciate that it is not enough to be concerned only with saving the life of a fetus; the avoidance of extreme prematurity at birth is also of critical importance for the future well-being of the individual.

See also **immunization**, **immunodeficiency disorders**, **incubator**, **neonatologist**, **retina**, **disorders of**.

premenstrual syndrome

This is a constellation of variable symptoms which include:

- irritability;
- headaches;
- depression;
- general emotional upset;
- loss of concentration;
- inefficiency at work;
- sleeplessness;
- a sense of fullness in the abdomen (bloating);
- backache;
- breast tenderness;
- weight gain of up to 1 kg (2 lb).

Premenstrual syndrome (PMS) is also said sometimes to be associated with antisocial reactions and even with violence. This has been accepted in some courts of law as grounds for the defence of diminished responsibility in criminal cases.

PMS affects up to three-quarters of women, especially those over thirty, during the late phase of the menstrual cycle when the corpus luteum is formed. When severe, these symptoms, and the associated psychological effects, can sometimes be disabling. The symptoms improve as soon as the period has started and usually pass altogether until about ten days before the next period.

Medical opinion is still divided on the reality of PMS but many women will testify that they suffer badly at this time. Some doctors believe that PMS is due to a relative overproduction of oestrogen, compared with progesterone, in the second half of the cycle. Treatment with progesterone and with diuretic drugs to remove fluid can be helpful.

Premique, Premique Cycle

Brand names for **medroxyprogesterone** formulated in conjunction with conjugated oestrogens for post-menopausal hormone replacement therapy.

Prepidil

A brand name for **dinoprostone**.

Prepulsid

A brand name for **cisapride**.

presbyacusis

Progressive loss of hearing associated with advancing age. The upper frequency limit of hearing, in childhood, is at least 16,000 cycles per second (Hertz), but this drops progressively with age so that few people over seventy can hear much above 5000 Hertz.

Superimposed on this natural loss of sensitivity to high tones is the effect of several other possible factors which may exaggerate the loss. These include prolonged exposure to high noise levels, brief exposure to very high noise levels such as explosions, the effect of diminished blood supply to the inner ear from arterial disease, toxic damage to the inner ear from drugs, and hereditary influences.

As a result of these factors, many people in the middle fifties have already suffered so much high tone loss that normal conversation may be difficult or impossible for them. Background noise increases the difficulty, and loud sounds often produce an unpleasant, almost painful blasting effect, called recruitment. This is one reason why people with presbyacusis often resent being shouted at. Another reason is the tendency, because of the very gradual progression of the condition, not to recognize that deafness exists and to blame external factors, such as the failure of others to speak clearly enough.

Presbyacusis is associated with progressive loss of function of the microscopic hair cells and nerve fibres in the *organ of Corti*, which is part of the cochlea in the inner ear. Unfortunately, nothing can be done to restore such loss. Modern hearing aids are often, but not always, helpful.

presbyopia

The effect, usually noticed around the age of forty-five, of the progressive loss of the ability to focus the eyes for near vision (accommodation). The power of accommodation is greatest in childhood and gradually weakens with age until, around the age of sixty-five, very little focusing power remains.

The effect of this is that the nearest point at which clear vision is possible gradually moves away. Print which is large enough will still be able to be read, but the diminishing effect of perspective may make small print impossible to make out.

Simple lenses of low magnification, prescribed as reading glasses, are used to compensate for presbyopia. Assuming the distance vision is normal, the first prescription, at about age forty-five, will be lenses of the power of one dioptre (a lens of focal length 1 m). These will need to be progressively increased in strength, at intervals of a few years, over the course of about twenty years, until, eventually, all the focusing is being done by the glasses.

It should seldom be necessary to change the reading glasses more often than about once every four or five years, the power rising by about half a dioptre each time. The usual reading correction, at age sixty, for a person with normal distance vision, is about two and a half dioptres. Lenses of this power focus at 40 cm – a convenient reading distance – with no accommodation. The power needed in the reading glasses is affected by the basic refraction at distance. A hypermetropic person (see **hypermetropia**) will need stronger lenses and a short-sighted person (see **myopia**), weaker lenses. A person with two or three dioptres of myopia will never need reading glasses.

Prescal

A brand name for **isradipine**.

prescription

An instruction to a pharmacist, written by a doctor, to dispense a stated quantity of a particular drug in a specified dose. A prescription also contains instructions to the patient indicating how the drug is to be taken, how often, and for how long. These are usually computer-printed on the label by the pharmacist.

prescription-free medication

See **over-the-counter (OTC) drugs**.

Preservex

A brand name for **aceclofenac**.

pressure sores

See **bed sores**.

Prestim

A brand name for a mixture of the thiazide diuretic drug bendrofluazide and the beta-blocking drug timolol.

Priadel

A brand name for **lithium**.

priapism

Prolonged and painful penile erection in the absence of sexual interest. Priapism results from the failure of the normal return of blood from the corpora cavernosa of the penis to the circulation at the termination of a period of sexual excitement (*detumescence*).

POSSIBLE CAUSES
This may happen for a variety of reasons. In some cases there is a disturbance of the nervous control of blood flow, to and from the penis, due to disease of the spinal cord or brain. In others, blood disorders, such as **leukaemia** or **sickle-cell disease** may be causing partial clotting (coagulation) of the stagnant blood in the penis, or there may be other disease processes, such as inflammation of the **prostate gland** (prostatitis), stone (calculus) in the bladder, or urethritis, which interfere with the normal outflow of blood from the penis.

> Long-sustained erection is dangerous because of the risk of clotting in the corpora cavernosa of the penis. Such thrombosis produces serious and permanent loss of erectile function, so treatment must be prompt and effective. Considerations of embarrassment must not occasion delay.

TREATMENT
Unfortunately, treatment is not always easy, often because the cause of the problem remains obscure, or cannot be quickly established. The first priority is to achieve normal detumescence and the longer this is delayed the more difficult it becomes, for the blood soon acquires the consistency of thick oil. Spinal anaesthesia may help but surgical decompression, by letting out blood through a wide-bore needle, may be necessary. The bulb (glans) of the penis is never affected and it is sometimes possible to drain the corpora internally into the glans.

prickly heat

Heat rash, medically known as *miliaria rubra*. This is the result of sweat duct blockage in conditions of high humidity and high temperature, usually in the tropics. It may, however, affect people in less extreme conditions, if they are unsuitably dressed. The blockage is thought to be due to excessive sogginess (over-hydration) of the skin. In the most severe forms, salt crystals may form in the sweat gland ducts, producing small blisters.

RECOGNITION AND SYMPTOMS
The condition features multiple small red bumps and a constant prickling or itching sensation from over-stimulation of the nerve endings.

TREATMENT
As acclimatization to the adverse conditions occurs, prickly heat usually resolves. Air conditioning, the choice of suitable clothing to encourage evaporation of sweat, and plenty of open-air swimming are all helpful.

prilocaine

A local anaesthetic drug normally given by injection. A brand name is Citanest. The drug can also be applied in a cream for surface anaesthesia under the brand name **Emla cream**.

prim-

Prefix meaning 'first' as in primigravida (first pregnancy).

Primacor

A brand name for the **phosphodiesterase inhibitor** drug **milrinone**.

Primalan

A brand name for **mequitazine**.

Primaxin

A brand name for **cilastatin**.

primidone

An **anticonvulsant** drug used in the treatment of **epilepsy**. A brand name is Mysoline.

Primodian

A brand name for the male sex hormone **testosterone**.

Primogyn

A brand name for the female sex hormone **oestradiol**.

Primolut N

A brand name for **norethisterone**.

Primoteston

A brand name for **testosterone**.

Primperan

A brand name for the **anti-emetic** drug metoclopramide.

Prioderm

A brand name for a preparation containing **malathion** for external use.

prion protein disease

A disease, such as **Creutzfeldt-Jakob disease** (CJD), Gerstmann-Straussler syndrome, **kuru**, **bovine spongiform encephalopathy** (BSE) and **fatal familial insomnia**, generally believed to be caused by an abnormal form of a protein that is a normal constituent of the brain. Prion protein is resistant to digestion by protease enzymes. It was isolated by Stanley Prusiner in 1982, the term 'prion' (an abbreviation of 'proteinaceous infectious particle') being proposed by him to make the point that the agent he was describing was not a virus.

An abnormal form of the normal prion protein (PrP) is found in high concentration in brains affected with spongiform encephalopathy, and forms **amyloid** deposits in these brains. This structurally simple, seemingly infectious agent of simpler constitution than any virus, is apparently capable of changing the shape of the normal, and essential, prion protein into the abnormal, insoluble form, which leads to the formation of the amyloid masses and causes these severe and invariably fatal diseases of the nervous system. Prions resist sterilization by normal methods and have been spread on surgical instruments and in donated human growth hormone. It has been discovered that normal methods of high temperature sterilization of surgical instruments can actually fix prion proteins, making them more stable and harder to destroy.

A new variant of CJD with a shorter incubation period appeared in the late 1980s and by February 1998, 24 cases had been reported, 23 of them in Britain. There is clear evidence that this form is either caused by, or in some way involves, the same strain of prion as bovine spongiform encephalopathy. Recent research suggests that normal prion protein may be essential in preventing nerve cells from undergoing programmed suicide (see **apoptosis**). The abnormal PrP cannot do this so there is widespread destruction of brain cells leading to the spongy appearance.

Prusiner was awarded the Nobel Prize in 1998 for his work on prions.

Pripsen

A brand name for a mixture of the **anthelmintic** drug **piperazine** and the laxative senna.

pro-

Prefix meaning 'in front of' as in progeria (premature aging).

Pro-Actidil

A brand name for the **antihistamine** drug triprolidine.

probenecid

A drug used in the treatment of gout. Probenecid acts by increasing the rate of excretion of uric acid in the urine and thus lowering its levels in the body. A brand name is Benemid.

probucol

A cholesterol-lowering drug. A brand name is Lurselle.

procainamide

A local anaesthetic-like drug used intravenously to control heart irregularities by its action to diminish the excitability of the conducting bundles in the heart muscle. A brand name is Pronestyl.

procarbazine

An anticancer drug used especially in the treatment of **lymphomas**. A brand name is Natulan.

prochlorperazine

A **phenothiazine derivative** antipsychotic drug used to treat **schizophrenia** and **mania** and to relieve nausea and vomiting. Trade names are Buccastem and Stemetil.

proctos

Greek root meaning 'anus' as in proctology (surgery of anal region).

procyclidine

An **anticholinergic** drug used to treat **Parkinson's disease**. Trade names are Arpicolin and Kemadrin.

Profasi

A brand name for chorionic gonadotrophin.

Proflex

A brand name for **ibuprofen** in a preparation for external use.

progeria

An extraordinary condition of accelerated ageing in which the usual processes of bodily decline and deterioration take place over the course of only a few years. Progeria is very rare and occurs in two forms. In the Hutchinson-Gilford syndrome, the condition appears before the age of four and by ten or twelve the affected individual has all the physical characteristics of old age – lax, wrinkled skin, loss of hair, and all the other common degenerative changes including widespread **atherosclerosis**. Death usually occurs about the age of thirteen, from coronary thrombosis or **stroke**.

Adult progeria, or Werner's syndrome, starts in early adult life and follows, over the course of about a decade, the same rapid progression to senility, with balding or grey hair, deafness, arthritis, **cataract**, loss of teeth, and atherosclerosis. In both forms there is severe resistance to administered insulin. Werner's syndrome also features increased levels in the tissues of hyaluronic acid – a substance that interferes with the development of small blood vessels, especially during development.

POSSIBLE CAUSES

Little is known of the cause of progeria. Both the Hutchinson-Gilford syndrome and Werner's syndrome can be transmitted by autosomal (non-sex-linked) recessive inheritance but many occur as a fresh dominant mutation.

Cultures of cells, such as the normally rapidly reproducing skin fibroblasts, taken from people with progeria, undergo only a few cell divisions and then cease. Cell cultures from normal children produce fifty or more generations before reproduction stops.

Progesic

A brand name for the non-steroidal anti-inflammatory drug (**NSAID**) fenoprofen.

progesterone

The hormone secreted by the corpus luteum of the ovary and by the placenta. Progesterone acts during the menstrual cycle to predispose the lining of the womb (endometrium) to receive and retain the fertilized ovum. During pregnancy, progesterone from the placenta ensures the continued health and growth of the womb and promotes the growth of the milk-secreting cells of the breasts. Progesterone-like substances (progestogens) are widely used in medicine and are common constituents of oral contraceptives. The hormone is used to treat menstrual symptoms and infertility and as an adjunct to oestrogen in post-menopausal hormone replacement therapy (HRT). Trade names are Crinone, Cyclogest and Gestone.

progestogen drugs

A group of drugs chemically similar to the natural hormone progesterone. They are used in oral contraceptives (see **contraceptive drugs**, **oestrogen drugs**) to help to prevent ovulation and to make the mucus in the cervix less easily penetrable by sperms. They are also used to treat menstrual disorders.

prognathism

Fixed forward protrusion of the lower jaw (mandible) or of both the lower and upper jaws. This is most commonly due to an abnormal increase in the length of the mandible but may be caused by an under-developed upper jaw in conjunction with a normal mandible. Prognathism often results in the inability to bring the upper and lower teeth into proper relationship (**malocclusion**). Mandibular prognathism can be corrected by removing sections from both sides of the jaw (osteotomy).

prognosis

An opinion, forecast, or known fact as to the course and outcome of a disease. The prognosis is always based on a knowledge of the natural history of the disease present and on the clinical state and attitude of the patient. Expression of a prognosis is usually qualified, and may vary from 'excellent', through 'uncertain' or 'gloomy', to 'hopeless'. In every case, however, the prognosis is no more than an informed assessment and the doctor is not always right.

Progout

A brand name for **allopurinol**.

proguanil

An antimalarial drug mainly used for prevention (as a prophylactic). A brand name is Paludrine. Formulated in conjunction with **atovaquone**, it is produced under the brand name Malarone.

Progynova

A brand name for **oestradiol**.

prolactinoma

A benign tumour (**adenoma**) of the **pituitary gland**. A prolactinoma secretes excessive quantities of the hormone prolactin, and this may cause milk secretion (**galactorrhoea**), absence of menstrual periods (**amenorrhoea**) and **infertility**, in women.

A prolactinoma may also occur in men, causing **impotence** and breast enlargement (**gynaecomastia**). In both cases, the tumour may cause headache and may be associated with **diabetes insipidus** by interfering with the production of the associated antidiuretic hormone of the pituitary. It may also press on the optic nerve crossing, causing loss of the fields of vision on both sides.

Prolactinomas may be detected by measurement of the prolactin levels in the blood and by X-ray, CT or MRI scan examination of the bony hollow in the middle of the skull (sella turcica) in which the pituitary gland lies.

prolapse

The displacement, often downwards, of the whole or part of an organ, from its normal position. Prolapse occurs because of weakness or laxity of some supporting structures, such as muscles or tendons. The commonest examples of prolapse are of the rectum and womb (uterus), but the bladder may prolapse into the vagina; the pulpy nucleus of an interverte-

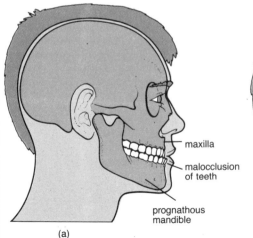

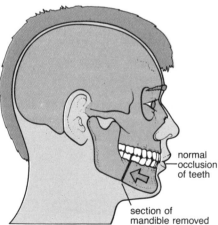

maxilla

malocclusion of teeth

prognathous mandible

(a)

normal occlusion of teeth

section of mandible removed

(b)

Prognathism is the condition in which one jaw protrudes abnormally forward. A prognathous mandible (a) can be corrected by removing a section of bone from either side (b).

bral disc may prolapse through the outer fibrous ring (see **slipped disc**); a haemorrhoid may prolapse through the anus; the umbilical cord may prolapse from the uterus during birth; and the iris may prolapse through a corneal wound.

Proleukin

A brand name for **aldesleukin**.

Proluton

A brand name for **hydroxyprogesterone hexanoate**.

promethazine

An **antihistamine** drug used to relieve itching, to control motion sickness and as a sedative. A brand name is Phenergan.

Prominal

A brand name for the barbiturate **methylphenobarbitone**.

pronation

Turning into the face down (prone) position. Applied to the hand and arm, the term means rotating the forearm so that the palm of the hand faces downward. The opposite of pronation is *supination*.

Prondol

A brand name for the antidepressant drug iprindol.

Pronestyl

A brand name for the **anti-arrhythmia** drug **procainamide**.

propafenone

A drug used to treat heart irregularities (arrhythmias). A brand name is Arythmol.

propamidine

An antibacterial drug used externally in the form of eye drops to treat eye infections. A brand name is Golden Eye.

Propanix

A brand name for **propranolol**.

propantheline

An antispasmodic drug used to relieve bowel spasm and to treat the irritable bowel syndrome and urinary incontinence caused by an irritable bladder. A brand name is Pro-Banthine.

Propess-RS

A brand name for **dinoprostone**.

Propine

A brand name for **dipivefrin**.

propiverine hydrochloride

A smooth muscle relaxant drug that allows bladder capacity to increase so that urination can occur less frequently. It is used to treat urinary incontinence and excessive urinary urgency. A brand name is Detrunorm.

propofol

A general anaesthetic drug given by injection. A brand name is Diprivan.

propranolol

A beta-blocker drug used to treat anxiety, migraine, high blood pressure, **angina pectoris** and heart irregularities (cardiac arrhythmias). Trade names are Beta-Prograne, Inderal and Propanix.

proprioception

The process of continuous monitoring of the position and movement of the limbs and the state of muscle tension, so that information is constantly supplied to the brain about the relative orientation of the parts of the body and their position in space. Proprioceptive information comes from sensory nerve endings and special receptors in the joints, tendons and muscles, and this information is integrated with other data coming from the balancing, gravitational and acceleration receptors in the inner ears and visual information from the eyes.

Fortunately, proprioception is largely unconscious and the corrective action taken, in response to it, automatic. Functions such as walking, or even standing, would be impossible without an efficient proprioceptive system providing feedback and controlling information. Many of the disabling effects of disease or damage to the nervous system are due to interference with normal proprioceptive function.

proptosis

Protrusion of an eyeball. An alternative term is **exophthalmos**.

Proscar

A brand name for **finasteride**.

prostaglandins

A group of unsaturated fatty acid hormones occurring throughout the tissues and body fluids. They are produced by the action of the enzyme phospholipase A2 on a fatty acid in cell membranes. Prostaglandins have many different actions. These include:

- constriction or widening of arteries;
- stimulation of pain nerve endings;
- promotion or inhibition of the aggregation of blood **platelets**, hence influencing blood clotting;
- induction of abortion;
- reduction of stomach acid secretion;
- relief of asthma;
- stimulation and inhibition of immune system responses.

Some pain-killing drugs, such as aspirin, act by preventing the release of prostaglandins from injured tissue. Prostaglandins have such a wide range of actions that they have, inevitably, been exploited as drugs. Synthetic prostaglandins are used to induce labour or procure abortion, to treat persistent ductus arteriosus and to relieve stomach and duodenal ulcer.

prostate enlargement and cancer test

See **prostate-specific antigen (PSA)**.

prostate enlargement surgery

See **TURP**.

prostate gland

The prostate is a gland, comparable in size, shape, colour and consistency to a chestnut, which surrounds the first few centimetres of the urine tube (urethra) in males. The prostate thus lies immediately under the bladder and close in front of the wall of the rectum, through which it can easily be felt and its size estimated. The prostate secretes a thin, milky, slightly alkaline fluid which helps to keep the spermatozoa active while they are waiting.

prostate gland, disorders of

The prostate is very liable to enlarge, especially after the age of about sixty, probably because of a falling off in the secretion of male sex hormone. About a quarter of men over sixty-five have moderate to severe symptoms from this cause.

ENLARGEMENT

Enlargement is liable to interfere with the outflow of urine from the bladder by narrowing the urethra, or even by expanding upwards into the bladder so as to form a kind of ball-valve. There is reduction in the force of the urine stream and incomplete emptying of the bladder, leading to much increased frequency of urination, with repeated necessity to get up at night. Sudden acute stoppage may occur, requiring an emergency passage of a **catheter** or, if this is impossible, drainage of the bladder through a wide needle passed through the abdominal wall. Back pressure can damage bladder function and the kidneys.

Enlargement of the prostate often has to be treated by removal of part or all of the gland. This is most commonly done through the urethra, using a special viewing and cutting instrument called a *resectoscope*. If the enlargement is considerable, a direct surgical approach through the lower part of the wall of the abdomen and the wall of the bladder may be necessary. The results are usually excellent.

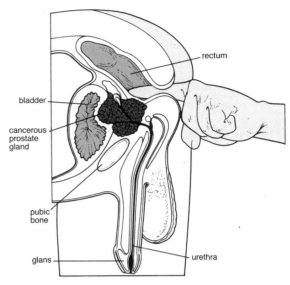

A hard, irregular enlargement of the prostate from cancer can readily be felt by rectal examination with a gloved finger.

CANCER

Cancer of the prostate is the second most common cancer in men. It presents in the same way as simple enlargement, but on rectal examination the gland is felt to be very hard and there may even be indications that the tumour has already spread to other parts of the body, often to the bones. Treatment of prostatic cancer may involve removal of the prostate and elimination of the male sex hormones, on which prostate cancer is dependent. This is done by **castration** – removal of both testicles (bilateral orchidectomy) – or by giving female sex hormones (oestrogens). Enlargement of the breasts (**gynaecomastia**) may complicate this treatment but the effect on the tumour is usually valuable.

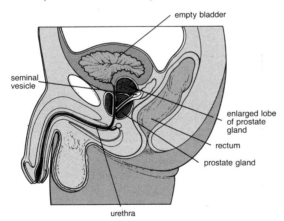

The prostate gland surrounds the urine tube (urethra) immediately under the bladder. Enlargement, as shown, can seriously obstruct the outflow of urine, and can even act as a valve preventing emptying of the bladder.

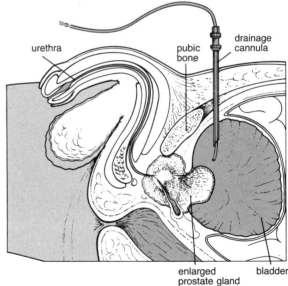

Enlargement of the prostate gland may so obstruct the outflow of urine that the bladder may have to be emptied through a cannula passed in through the wall of the abdomen just above the pubic bone.

prostate-specific antigen (PSA)

An enzyme produced by the lining (epithelial) cells of the prostate gland to liquefy the seminal fluid. The amounts produced are proportional to the size of the gland, whether this is increased benignly, as in simple age-related prostatic enlargement, or by prostate cancer. Small quantities of PSA enter the bloodstream and the levels can be accurately measured. Raised levels imply an increase in the bulk of prostate tissue and can thus be used as a marker for simple enlargement (prostatic hyperplasia) or prostate cancer. High levels do not necessarily imply cancer but indicate the need for full urological investigation.

See also **prostate gland, disorders of**.

prosthesis

An artificial part used to replace a missing or diseased organ, tissue or other structure of the body either for cosmetic or for functional purposes. Many prostheses are used, from artificial eyes, which are of cosmetic value only, to artificial limbs, which are often highly functional. Other prostheses include artificial joints, especially hip joints, artificial heart valves, breast implants, woven Teflon artificial blood vessels, silicone rubber sheets to maintain body tissue boundaries, breast implants, artificial nipples and dental appliances.

Prostigmin

A brand name for **neostigmine**.

Prostin

A brand name for **alprostadil**.

Prostin E2

A brand name for **dinoprostone**.

prostitution and sexually transmitted disease

A great deal of attention has been given to the role of prostitution in the heterosexual spread of AIDS and this is now known to be a major factor in developing countries. The role of prostitutes and the noncommercially sexually promiscuous in the West is gradually assuming greater importance as the HIV load in Western countries increases. Prostitutes continue to transmit other sexually transmitted diseases.

One study of fifty London prostitutes, who agreed to attend a clinic fortnightly for up to a year, showed that, during the period, 28 per cent had at least one episode of gonorrhoea. Forty-six per cent of the women had a genital chlamydial infection; 6 per cent had genital warts; 10 per cent had PAP smear evidence of early cancerous change in the lining of the cervix; 12 per cent had pubic lice; 2 per cent had active syphilis and 2 per cent had evidence of treated syphilis; 4 per cent had evidence of previous hepatitis B infection.

Female prostitutes are, of course, at considerable risk of contracting HIV infection and the percentage infected is steadily rising. In 1988 a study showed that the percentage of prostitutes who were HIV positive was reported as zero in Paris, 5 per cent in Seattle, 6 per cent in Athens, 40 per cent in Florida and 88 per cent in Rwanda. Today, the European percentages are much higher. Ironically, the greatest risk of HIV infection to European prostitutes is still from shared needles and syringes.

Many prostitutes have now recognized the value of condoms for protection against infection and these are increasingly being insisted upon.

Prosulf

A brand name for **protamine**.

protamine

A drug that acts as an antidote to the anticoagulant **heparin**. A brand name is Prosulf.

protamine zinc insulin

A slow-release form of insulin with an action lasting for up to 24 hours. A brand name is Humulin Zn.

Protaphane

A brand name for a form of **insulin**.

protease inhibitors

A range of drugs that interfere with the action of the enzyme protease, used by HIV to activate the synthesis of its polymer protein coat. These drugs slow the progression of the infection and lengthen life. An undesirable direct or indirect effect is the abnormal laying-down of body fat and high levels of lipids in the blood, which may lead to coronary artery disease and strokes. Brand names are indinavir, nelfinavir, ritonavir and saquinavir.

See also **HIV-protease inhibitor drugs**.

protein, abnormal, in Alzheimer's disease

See **tau protein**.

protein building block

See **amino acid**.

proteins

Proteins are large organic molecules essential to the structure and function of the body. The term comes from the Greek word *protos* meaning 'first' or 'earliest'. They are the most important constituent of cells, and thus of the whole body. Proteins are found everywhere in the body, but in the largest quantity in muscle cells.

The structure of bone is founded on a scaffolding of a protein, called collagen, impregnated with calcium and phosphorus. Collagen is also the main ingredient of tendons and ligaments and forms a major part of the skin. The hair and the nails are made of keratin, which is a protein. There is protein in haemoglobin, hormones are often made of protein, and all the **antibodies** and **enzymes** in the body are made of protein. The basic monomers of protein are the **amino acids**. Body proteins can be broken down into twenty different amino acids. Some of these can be synthesized by the body but some cannot and, in a nutritional context, the latter are known as essential amino acids and must be obtained from protein in the diet. A protein is a long chain or polymer of amino acids linked together. A few amino acids linked together form peptides. Dipeptides have two amino acids, polypeptides have many. Polypeptides join to form proteins.

p | proteins

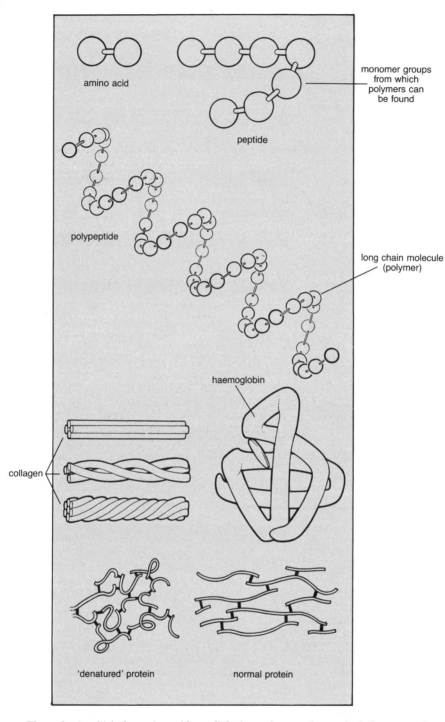

Protein molecules form the most important structural elements in the body. Amino acids link together to form peptides and these link as polymers to form complex, often strand-like molecules, such as collagen. Other protein molecules take different forms.

amino acid

monomer groups from which polymers can be found

peptide

polypeptide

long chain molecule (polymer)

haemoglobin

collagen

'denatured' protein

normal protein

The order in which the amino acids are linked together varies from protein to protein and determines the type and properties of the protein. It is this sequence that is laid down in the genetic code of the DNA molecule in the nucleus of the cell. Proteins are formed on a kind of mould, or template, produced by the **DNA**. The transcription of protein from DNA is not direct, but involves, first, the production of strands of nucleic acid called **RNA** (ribonucleic acid). RNA is processed, and edited, to form messenger RNA (mRNA), and is moved out of the nucleus to one of cell organs in the cyto-

plasm called ribosomes, where the translation into chains of amino acids – the synthesis of new protein – occurs. The amino acids needed to form the proteins are picked up from the cell fluid where they are present in enormous numbers.

The amino acids, linked firmly together, are also arranged in such a way as to form other, weaker, attractions between occasional pairs. This leads to a particular three-dimensional structure such as a complex folded shape, as in the haemoglobin molecule, or gives rise to more regular secondary structures, such as a single helix or triple helices. The keratin of hair and the myosin of muscles are regularly repeating single helices. The strong collagen of bones and tendons is a triple helix.

Protein, in the form of collagen, is the major structural element of the body. Collagen fibres make up much of the connective tissue of the body. When formed into bundles, as in tendons, they provide remarkable tensile strength. The collagen fibres, themselves, are composed of bundles of fibrils which, in turn, are assembled from collagen molecules. Each of these consists of a triple helix of three polypeptide chains coiled together, and the polypeptides are linked series of amino acids. The stability and strength of the helix depends on cross-linkages between certain of the amino acids and the linkages depend on vitamin C. Scurvy is a disorder of weakened collagen caused by a deficiency of vitamin C.

When proteins are heated or affected by strong chemicals they become denatured and can never recover their original shape or properties. This is why, for instance, the transparency of egg white can never be restored once boiled, or the crystalline lens of the eye healed once it has developed a cataract.

Prothezine

A brand name for **promethazine**.

Prothiaden

A brand name for the tricyclic antidepressant drug **dothiepin**.

Protium

A brand name for **pantoprazol**.

proton pump inhibitor drugs

A class of drugs that controls the production of stomach acid. The proton pump is the chemical activator (enzyme) hydrogen-potassium ATP-ase. This is involved in the final stage of acid production by the specialized cells of the stomach lining (the parietal cells). A proton pump inhibitor is a drug that blocks the action of this enzyme. The first, and still most widely used, drug with this action is omeprazole (Losec). This drug can be used in cases in which H2 receptor blocker drugs have failed to reduce acid sufficiently (see **antacid drugs**).

proto-oncogene

Any gene capable of becoming a cancer-producing gene (an oncogene). Proto-oncogenes have important functions in the normal cell, but, if they suffer mutation or acquire genetic control elements from cancer-causing viruses (oncoviruses) that have invaded the cell, they can lose their normal regulatory functions, which can lead to the uncontrolled multiplication of the cell – cancer.

Protostat

A brand name for **metronidazole**.

protozoa

A group of microscopic, single-celled organisms widely distributed in nature, some of which are parasitic and may cause disease. Some protozoa, such as the parasite causing **malaria**, live inside human cells for part of their life cycle; some,

such as the organism causing amoebic dysentery, *Entamoeba histolytica*, invade tissues but do not enter cells. Other protozoa of medical importance include *Trichomonas vaginalis*, which causes vaginal and penile inflammation; *Giardia lamblia*, which infects the intestine causing diarrhoea and loss of appetite and weight; *Toxoplasma gondii*, which infects the nervous system and the eyes, causing **toxoplasmosis**; *Pneumocystis carinii*, which causes pneumonia in immunocompromised people; and *Leishmania donovani* which causes **leishmaniasis**.

Protran

A brand name for **chlorpromazine**.

protriptyline

An antidepressant drug used especially to treat narcolepsy or depression associated with pathological lethargy. A brand name is Concordin.

Pro-Vent

A brand name for the asthma-control drug theophylline.

Provera

A brand name for the **progestogen** drug methylprogesterone.

Provigil

A brand name for **modafinil**.

Pro-Viron

A brand name for the male sex hormone drug **mesterolone**.

proxymetacaine

A local anaesthetic drug used as eye drops for ophthalmic procedures. A brand name is Minims proxymetacaine.

Prozac

A brand name for **fluoxetine**. This widely used mood-controlling drug can interact dangerously with drugs of the MAO inhibitor group and some other antidepressants.

Prozac neuro-transmitter

See **serotonin**.

prurigo

A description of the changes in the skin which result from scratching following prolonged itching from any cause. Prurigo is not, in itself, a disease, but may follow allergic conditions such as atopic **eczema**; parasites such as **scabies**; cancer; and endocrine disorders. The skin shows many small, firm papules capped by small blisters (vesicles) which then crust over.

pseudoephedrine

A decongestant drug used to relieve nasal stuffiness (congestion) and contained in many cold remedies. A brand name is Galpseud. It is also formulated with antihistamine drugs under the trade names Dimotane and Sudafed.

pseudogout

True gout is caused by the deposition of sodium urate crystals in joints. In pseudogout there is deposition of calcium pyrophosphate. The symptoms and signs are often indistinguishable from those of true gout, and can be correctly diagnosed only by obtaining a sample of the joint fluid and showing that the crystals differ from those of gout.

Pseudogout may occur as a complication of overactivity of the parathyroid glands (hyperparathyroidism), in cases of iron deposition in the tissues (haemochromatosis) and in other metabolic diseases, including **diabetes**.

pseudohermaphroditism

In true **hermaphroditism**, the affected person has both male and female external genitalia, but in pseudohermaphroditism only those of one sex are present, but there is a congenital abnormality of the genitalia so that they resemble those of the opposite sex. Thus a woman may appear to be a hermaphrodite because of an enlarged **clitoris**, which looks like a **penis**, and enlarged **labia** which resemble a scrotum. A man with a very small penis and a divided scrotum, simulating labia majora, may also appear, wrongly, to be a hermaphrodite.

Psilocybin

A powerfully hallucinogenic phosphorylated tryptamine present in the fungi contaminating some types of mushrooms, especially in *Psilocybe mexicana*. It is a powerful hallucinogenic drug with properties similar to those of LSD.

psittacosis

A form of pneumonia which can be fatal to human beings. This is primarily a bird infection caused by *Chlamydia psittaci*. It is usually acquired directly from infected parrots, budgerigars or pigeons but can be passed on to people handling birds for the food industry.

An outbreak in a Texas turkey processing plant, in 1948, caused twenty-two cases with three deaths. In 1980, nineteen cases occurred among duck industry workers in Norwich and in the same year fifteen veterinary surgeons, on a course on poultry processing plant inspection, came down with the infection. A recently discovered new strain of the organisms, found initially in Taiwan, causes miscarriage in women who are in contact with the aborted products of sheep infected with it. These products are teeming with the organisms and are highly infectious. This strain is called TWAR agent (*Taiwan acute respiratory disease agent*).

Psittacosis is treated with tetracycline antibiotics.

Psoradrate

A brand name for a mixture of the antipsoriasis drug dithranol and urea.

psoralen treatment

Use of a plant derivative (coumarin) which, when applied to the skin or taken internally, increases the tendency of the skin to pigment under the action of ultraviolet light. This effect is exploited in the treatment of **psoriasis** and other skin conditions.

psoriasis

A common, non-infectious skin disease featuring non-itching, bright red or pink, sharply outlined, dry plaques with silvery scaling surfaces.

RECOGNITION AND SYMPTOMS

These plaques affect mainly the elbows, knees, shins, scalp and lower back. The nails can also be affected, causing severe distortion. The plaques are caused by increased thickness, from rapid growth, of the skin outer layers (the epidermis and the keratin surface). This is associated with the abnormal presence of nucleated cells in the skin above the basal cell layer. There are also widened (dilated) blood vessels and sometimes migration into the plaques of white blood cells (polymorphs) to produce sterile pus. The patches vary in size from a few millimetres to many centimetres.

POSSIBLE CAUSES

The cause of psoriasis is unknown. It may start at any age, but usually shows itself in early adult life, often after a period of severe stress, including illness or childbirth. There is sometimes a family history. Plaques often appear at the site of a minor injury and usually clear on exposure to sun. Psoriasis is sometimes associated with arthritis of the fingers and toes, or of a single large joint.

TREATMENT

Psoriasis is usually very persistent (chronic) and difficult to treat. Severe cases require management by a dermatologist. Coal tar is a long-established remedy for simple psoriasis and the tar may be supplemented by salicylic acid which helps to reduce scaling. Dithranol is widely used and is highly effective, but is damaging to normal skin and must be applied with great care. Some doctors advise a 'short-contact' application for no more than half an hour, followed by a bath. Other treatments include ultraviolet light in association with psoralens (PUVA), derivatives of vitamin A called retinoids, hydrocortisone and, in very stubborn cases, the powerful cytotoxic drug methotrexate. Recurrence is common.

Psorin

A brand name for a mixture of the antipsoriasis drug **dithranol**, coal tar and the skin-softening agent **salicylic acid**.

psychiatric detention

See **sectioning**.

psychiatric disorder, poison-induced

See **toxic psychosis**.

psychiatrist

A doctor specializing in the branch of medicine concerned with the diagnosis and treatment of mental illness, including psychotic and psychoneurotic disorders, and with the management of emotional and behavioural problems.

psychiatrists' bible

See **DSM IV**.

psychiatry

The branch of medicine concerned with behavioural and emotional disorders whether attributable to known disease of the brain or not. Psychiatry is concerned with a range of conditions including:

- **schizophrenia**;
- delusional disorders, with paranoia;
- mood disorders, especially **depression** and **manic-depressive illness**;
- **anxiety** and **phobias**;
- psychosomatic (somatoform) disorders;
- **sexual deviation**;
- **dissociative disorders**;
- personality disorders;
- **mental retardation**;
- eating and sleep disorders;
- **tics**;
- mental disturbance caused by organic brain damage (organic mental syndromes).

THE NATURE OF PSYCHIATRIC DISORDERS

Psychiatrists are medically qualified and, on the whole, wish to view their specialty as closely analogous to other medical disciplines which deal with clearly recognizable diseases, mostly of known cause and with accepted remedies. Most psychiatrists prefer to think of, and deal with, psychiatric patients as being mentally ill, and of psychiatric disorders as being formal diseases. This is easily done in the case of the organic mental syndromes and disorders in which there is either a known neurological cause or the pattern of symptoms and signs strongly suggests that such a cause is operating.

But there are difficulties in pursuing such a course for all mental and emotional disorders, and there is a wide school of thought which holds that 'pure' psychiatric conditions – excluding the organic syndromes – cannot legitimately be considered as diseases. Many believe that at least some of these disorders are patterns of behaviour adopted, by the sufferer, to deal with a hostile or unacceptable social environment, or with the emotional responses to such an environment. There are those who say that people described as schizophrenic are perfectly entitled, if they wish, to enter, and remain in, an alternative and more comfortable world of their own making. This view tends to ignore the immense suffering of the mentally ill, especially of those with pathological depression.

The uncertainty as to the true nature of psychiatric disorder is reflected in the wide divergences of opinion among psychiatrists about the causes of some psychotic illnesses, especially schizophrenia, about the best methods of treatment and even, in particular cases, on the diagnosis. Some schools of psychiatry emphasize the biological and genetic factors in behavioural disorders while others concentrate on psychological or social factors.

TREATMENT OF PSYCHIATRIC DISORDERS

Drugs are widely and effectively used in the treatment of depression and other major psychiatric disorders. Electroconvulsive treatment and enforced incarceration in an institution are now much less widely employed. **Psychoanalysis**, in the Freudian sense, is gradually being seen to be of little therapeutic value. **Psychotherapy**, under the aegis of a spectrum of philosophies, while useless in the management of florid psychotic disorder, is widely regarded as being helpful to those with less fundamental problems. Interestingly, apart from behavioural therapy, the formal basis on which psychotherapy is conducted seems to have

little or no bearing on its success. The quality of the therapist, on the other hand, does. We may infer that it is usually the human interaction, rather than the application of any scientific principle, that does the good.

psychoactive drugs

Drugs whose action modifies in some way the state of the mind. They include mental stimulants such as amphetamine, cocaine, caffeine, and nicotine; depressants such as the **benzodiazepine drugs**, the **barbiturates**, alcohol, and **tranquillizer drugs**; the narcotic **analgesic drugs**, such as morphine, pethidine and methadone; and the **hallucinogenic drugs**, such as LSD, mescaline and psilocybin.

psychoanalysis

Since Sigmund Freud invented and first described this procedure early this century, it seems only fair to limit the definition of this word to Freudian analysis.

Psychoanalysis is based on a number of assertions which, in the minds of adherents, have become axioms. These are that:

- many important events in the mental life of the individual take place in the unconscious mind;
- most of what goes on in the unconscious is concerned with sex and aggression;
- 'unconscious thoughts', 'wishes' and 'impulses' are a constant potential source of neurosis;
- these are constantly being revealed by symbolism in dreams and by significant errors and puns ('Freudian slips'), which are often subtle expressions of sexual and aggressive impulses;
- most of the troubles of mankind can, ultimately, be traced to little boys' repressed jealousy of their fathers' sexual access to their mothers (the Oedipus complex).

Freud claimed that the unconscious mind was accessible by a process of free association and that when repressed painful material was 'brought to the surface' and contemplated, the harm that it had been causing would be resolved. The analyst's function was a passive, detached, non-commenting and non-participatory guidance.

Whatever the merits of Freud's theories – and his contribution to thought was certainly important – the value of the application of them to the practical management of psychological disorder is now seen to be negligible. Significantly, Freud recognized, and taught, that unless a *transference* was achieved – that is unless the patient fell in love with, or otherwise became emotionally involved with, the analyst – psychoanalysis would fail. Experience, in other areas of human interaction, has shown that it is precisely the quality of the interpersonal relationship between the participants that is therapeutically effective.

psychologist

An ancillary health professional concerned with the scientific study of behaviour and its related mental processes, including memory, rational and irrational thought, intelligence, learning, personality, perceptions and emotions and their relationship to behaviour. A clinical psychologist applies this knowledge to help in the assessment of the mental state and capabilities of patients and in their treatment.

psychoneuro-immunology

The discipline concerned with the effect of the emotions on the immune system and hence on the development of disease. Psychoneuro-immunology is based on the growing recognition that mental and physical events are so inextricably inter-related that nothing of importance can happen to one without affecting the other.

psychopath

The term 'psychopath' has become unfashionable, but there is still a need for a succinct word for the person whose behaviour is wholly self-centred and antisocial and who appears incapable of any form of emotional identification with others. Descriptions such as 'sociopath', 'moral defective' or 'patient with a personality disorder' tend to diffuse the clarity of the concept and discourage study of what has, through the ages, been a source of enormous harm to society and distress to its members. History is full of examples of the ill perpetrated by psychopaths.

RECOGNITION AND SYMPTOMS

The psychopath has no defect of intellectual function and may be highly intelligent. There are no abnormalities of perception, memory or imagination, no delusions, hallucinations nor any signs of organic brain disorder. The electroencephalogram is normal. The psychopath is found in every level of society and in every walk of life. Although often identified as a common criminal, the more intelligent and successful psychopath is to be found in the armed forces, in the police, in the worlds of finance and politics, in the medical and legal professions – everywhere. Many psychopaths have had appallingly deprived childhood circumstances – not necessarily deprived in the material sense, but deprived of love, affection, discipline, rules, emotional security, and a clear and unequivocal program of ethical principles.

> The psychopath commonly reveals himself (or, more rarely, herself) by outbursts of explosive rage and violence or by reckless disregard for the safety or well-being of others. But this is not an invariable sign. Equally often, the psychopath manifests ruthless, cold, manoeuvring and heartless dealings by which he gains a social or commercial advantage over others. It has been claimed that modern social pressures and the emphasis on material factors in contemporary society have brought about a sharp increase in the incidence of psychopathy.

TREATMENT

There is also ample evidence that, even well into adult life, psychopaths can be helped by therapy. In the therapeutic community at Henderson Hospital, Sutton, Surrey, for instance, success has been achieved in the rehabilitation of young adult psychopaths by a process of analysis followed by sociotherapy in a stable, supportive and disciplined environment.

psychotherapist

An ancillary health professional or doctor engaged in any purely psychological method of treatment of mental or emotional disorders. There are many schools of psychotherapy but results appear to depend on the personal qualities, experience and worldly wisdom of the therapist rather than on the theoretical basis of the method.

psychotherapy

The application of any nonphysical or nonpharmacological technique or method that purports to cure or relieve any mental, emotional or behavioural disorder. There are many different schools of psychotherapy, much sought after by the unhappy, the anxious, the depressed, the alienated and the lonely. These include Freudian **psychoanalysis**, Jungian analysis, the Adlerian school, Gestalt psychotherapy, psychodynamic therapy, behavioural therapy, client-oriented therapy and existential therapy.

As the dominance of Freud and the other major schools has declined, an eclectic and pragmatic tendency has emerged – one in which what appear to be the best features of various systems, however fundamentally at variance, are adopted and employed.

There is growing evidence that effectiveness in therapy is primarily dependent on the quality of the relationship between therapist and patient and that this, in turn, depends on the quality of the therapist. The results of psychotherapy are, however, difficult to assess, especially since many or most of the conditions treated naturally improve with time. There can be little doubt that many people can benefit greatly from wise and considered counselling by an educated and experienced life-guide. Whether there is any school of psychotherapeutic training which can induce such qualities is another matter entirely.

psychotherapy-induced fictions

See **false memory syndrome**.

psychotropic analgesic nitrous oxide

The use of the anaesthetic gas nitrous oxide to assist in the management of drug and alcohol withdrawal, in amounts below those necessary to induce general anaesthesia. Nitrous oxide acts on opioid receptor systems in the brain to regulate local accumulation of the neuro-transmitter dopamine. This is said to be directly related to the withdrawal state.

Also known as PAN.

psychotropic drugs

Drugs which effect the state of the mind, including sedatives, **tranquillizers**, antipsychotic drugs and **hallucinogenic** drugs.

pteron

Greek root meaning 'wing' as in pterygium (wing-shaped eye membrane).

pterygium

A disorder of the cornea in which a wing-shaped fold of conjunctiva is attracted across the margin of the cornea and extends progressively towards the centre. Pterygium is caused by radiational damage from the ultraviolet component of sunlight and is common in equatorial areas. Vision is seldom markedly affected, if the pterygium is left alone, but surgical removal of a pterygium is usually followed by a recurrence which is larger than the original and which may encroach upon the central optical zone of the cornea. This complication can be avoided by applying beta rays from a strontium 90 source, but this, too, has its dangers.

The persistent discomfort associated with pterygium is not caused by the pterygium but by the underlying tissue damage from solar radiation. It is not relieved by removal of the pterygium. Pterygia are best left alone, but the eyes should be protected from direct or reflected sunlight.

ptosis

An abbreviation for *blepharoptosis*, which means a drooping of the upper eyelid. Ptosis may be present at birth (congenital) or may occur later in life, either spontaneously or as a result of disease or injury. It is due to a weakness of the levator muscle of the upper lid, or to interference with the nerve supply to this muscle.

Congenital ptosis of such degree as to cover the pupil calls for immediate surgical elevation of the lid or there will be severe and irremediable failure of visual development (**amblyopia**).

Acquired ptosis, without obvious cause, may be a sign of **myasthenia gravis**, diabetic nerve damage (neuropathy), brain tumour, or an **aneurysm** on an artery at the base of the brain.

pudendal block

A form of local anaesthesia used during childbirth, especially to allow painless forceps delivery. Injections of a local anaesthetic drug are given either through the side walls of the vagina or through the skin on either side of the **labia** majora into the area on either side of the vagina.

Pulmadil

A brand name for the bronchodilator drug rimiterol.

Pulmicort

A brand name for the corticosteroid drug bursonide.

pulmonary

Relating to the lungs.

pulmonary fibrosis

Scarring and thickening of lung tissue usually as a result of previous disease, such as silicosis, **asbestosis**, **pneumonia** or **tuberculosis**. The effect is a reduction in the ease with which oxygen can be transferred from the atmosphere to the blood and, depending on the severity of the fibrosis, a proportional reduction in physical capacity.

Fibrosis causes breathlessness, at first on effort, but later even at rest, and may be severely disabling. Oxygen therapy may be necessary.

pulmonary hypertension

Raised blood pressure in the arteries carrying blood to the lungs as a result of narrowing or damage from disease. A gradual onset of pulmonary hypertension often follows **pulmonary fibrosis** or **emphysema**, and the condition can arise suddenly as a result of pulmonary **embolism**. The increased resistance to blood flow in the arteries means that the right side of the heart has to work harder – contract more strongly than normal – and the wall of the pumping chamber (the right ventricle) becomes thickened and stronger (right heart enlargement).

It should be remembered that all the blood passes through the lungs and that it does so at the same rate as it is pumped by the left side of the heart to the rest of the body. While the enlargement and strengthening of the right side of the heart is able to keep the blood circulating, the situation is said to be compensated and no further symptoms arise. But, as the condition progresses, the point is likely to be reached at which the right heart is unable to do this. This is known as right heart failure and the result is that blood returning to the right side of the heart from the rest of the body cannot be moved on fast enough and dams back.

RECOGNITION AND SYMPTOMS

This damming back, seen best in the jugular veins of the neck, also causes enlargement of the liver and a generalized collection of fluid in the tissues (**oedema**).

The ankles and the small of the back will pit when pressure is applied by a finger and the fluid will collect in the bases of the lungs, increasing the problem of oxygen transfer to the blood.

There will also be symptoms of the underlying cause – coughing, wheezing, breathlessness and sometimes blueness of the skin (cyanosis).

TREATMENT

Pulmonary hypertension is treated by measures to remove oedema fluid, to strengthen the right side of the heart, and to deal with the underlying cause, so far as that is possible. Diuretic drugs, which increase the urinary fluid output, are helpful.

pulmone

Latin root meaning 'lung' as in pulmonary (of the lung).

Pulmozyme

A brand name for **dornase alfa**.

pulseless disease

See **Takayasu disease**.

pulse oximeter

A safety device used during general anaesthesia for the continuous monitoring of the blood oxygen levels. This is done by means of a small transducer device clipped to, or pushed over, a finger of the patient and connected to the main equipment by a light cable. A very small drop in blood oxygenation is immediately apparent, both by visible and audible signal, so alerting the anaesthetist. This is a major aid to the elimination of the main danger to a patient during surgery under general anaesthesia – a drop in the supply of oxygen to the brain.

pulso

Latin root meaning 'pulse' as in pulse (repetitive pressure wave in blood).

pumactant

A lung surfactant drug. A brand name is Alec.

pupil, disorders of

Many conditions affect the size and shape of the pupil. It may be congenitally displaced to one side, or may be 'keyhole' shaped (coloboma) due to a missing radial segment, usually below. Penetrating corneal injuries usually distort the pupil as do adhesions of the iris to the lens in **uveitis**. In Adie's pupil, a harmless condition, there is dilatation with poor constriction to light and slow dilatation in the dark. The now rare Argyll Robertson pupil, once commonly caused by syphilis, is small, irregular, and non-reactive to light, but contracts when an effort at close viewing is made.

Many drugs affect the size of the pupil. It is widely dilated by belladonna (atropine), hyoscine, cyclopentolate and tropicamide and constricted by pilocarpine, acetylcholine, carbachol, eserine and physostigmine.

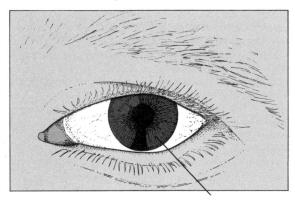

iris with missing segment

A congenital coloboma of the iris causing a 'keyhole' pupil. This is usually present on both sides and may be associated with absence of a strip of retina. Vision is not necessarily seriously affected.

pupil, white in baby

See **galactosaemia**.

purgative

A strong **laxative** drug.

Puri-Nethol

A brand name for the anticancer drug **mercaptopurine**.

purpura

A group of bleeding disorders which cause haemorrhages into the tissues from small blood vessels. These may often be seen under or in the skin either as the tiny pin-head *petechiae* or as larger 'black and blue' bruises (ecchymoses).

Purpura arises in two ways – from damage to small blood vessels or from a shortage of blood platelets (thrombocytes), which are necessary for normal clotting.

SIMPLE PURPURA

'Simple' or 'senile' purpura is the commonest of all bleeding disorders and is seen most often in post-menopausal women. Unsightly, and sometimes extensive, bruising is readily seen through the thinned skin, often on the thighs or arms. Bleeding may also occur under the lining mucous membrane of the mouth. This form of purpura is due to increased fragility of small blood vessels and is sometimes related to oestrogen deficiency.

ALLERGIC PURPURA

Allergic purpura, or Henoch-Schonlein purpura, often follows a streptococcal infection in children and is due to damage to the lining of small blood vessels by the resulting immune complexes (antibody linked to the material causing the reaction). In addition to the signs of bleeding, the skin may show redness and **urticaria**. This form of purpura causes local inflammation and itching and may affect a wide range of organs, especially the kidneys, the joints and the bowels. Kidney disease occurs in about 10 per cent of cases. There may be swollen and painful joints, abdominal pain and sometimes blackening of the stools from altered blood (**melaena**). Sometimes there is bleeding into the brain, causing headaches, dizziness and confusion.

PLATELET DEFICIENCY

Platelet deficiency (**thrombocytopenia**) is a common cause of purpura and can occur in many ways. These include inadequate production by the bone marrow, as a result of tumour, infection, drug reaction or radiation; increased platelet destruction by drugs, alcohol or other causes; and increased usage, as in burns, septicaemia and severe injuries. Thrombocytopenia from increased platelet destruction often occurs for no determinable reason, but the condition commonly follows a virus infection, especially in children and young adults, and is probably the result of an antibody-antigen reaction. This is called acute idiopathic thrombocytopenia.

Platelet deficiency interferes with normal clotting and the result is an abnormal tendency to bleed anywhere in the body. The skin shows petechiae and bruising, there may be nose bleeding, bleeding into the bowel, urinary system, vagina, brain, spinal cord and joints. Such haemorrhages cause effects varying with the site, but, in addition, the persistent blood loss tends to lead to anaemia with fatigue, weakness and even heart failure.

The condition is very variable in severity, showing, at the one extreme, only a few petechiae, and at the other, severe and barely controllable bleeding.

OTHER CAUSES

Purpura has other causes. It may result from vitamin C deficiency, when it is called **scurvy**; it may be caused by hereditary blood vessel weakness; by excessive antibodies in the blood (hypergammaglobulinaemia); and by an auto-immune reaction to the person's own red blood cells.

TREATMENT

The treatment of purpura depends on the type. Common purpura in menopausal women may be helped by hormone replacement therapy or by corticosteroids. Immunosuppressive therapy has been found helpful in severe cases, as has **plasmapheresis**. Thrombocytopenic purpura is treated according to the cause. In many cases it is necessary to transfuse platelet concentrates. Scurvy is cured by vitamin C.

purulent

Relating to **pus**.

pus

A yellowish or greenish creamy liquid formed most commonly at the site of bacterial infection, and usually heavily infected, but occasionally occurring in sterile locations, without infection. Pus consists of millions of scavenging white blood cells, mostly *polymorphs*, which have died in the defence of the area; particles of dead tissue partly digested by enzymes released by the white cells; white cells digested by their own enzymes; nucleic acid; bacteria, both alive and dead; and bacterial toxins. A localized, encapsulated collection of pus, in solid tissue, is called an **abscess**.

The main pus-forming organisms are staphylococci, some streptococci, pneumococci, meningococci, gonococci, and *Escherichia coli. Pseudomonas aeruginosa (pyocyaneus)* produces pus with a bluish tinge. Many other related bacteria also produce pus. All these organisms produce substances that strongly attract white blood cells and then kill them, giving rise to pus.

It is a general surgical principle that collections of pus should be released. Often, an infection will not settle until this is done. Antibiotics are not, in themselves, effective in dealing with abscesses.

pustule

A small, pus-filled skin blister, commonly resulting from staphylococcal infection of a hair follicle, but sometimes, as in **acne**, prompted by chemical irritation rather than infection, and containing sterile pus. A **stye** is a pustule forming at the root of an eyelash.

pyelography

Often called urography. People who repeatedly have infections of the urinary system, who pass blood in their urine or who have other symptoms, such as pain in the loin, suggestive of kidney trouble or kidney stones, are usually investigated by X-ray pyelography. In addition, this may be necessary in young people with high blood pressure to check whether this might be caused by kidney disease.

The kidneys, ureters and bladder are not easily seen on plain X-rays, so an iodine-based contrast medium is commonly used. This may be introduced into the urinary system in two ways – by way of the bloodstream (intravenous pyelography or IVP), or backwards up the urinary tract by means of a fine tube or catheter inserted through a viewing instrument called a cystoscope.

In IVP a radio-opaque dye is injected into a vein in the arm. The dye travels in the bloodstream to the kidneys where it is rapidly excreted. An X-ray picture is taken immediately, and further pictures are taken five, ten, and thirty minutes later. The dye passes down the ureters from the kidneys and accumulates in the bladder where it shows up conspicuously on the X-ray. When the bladder has filled with dye, another X-ray picture is taken while urine is being passed, and a final one after the bladder has apparently emptied.

IVP shows whether the kidneys are of normal size and shape, and whether they are in the right position. It shows the exact course of the ureters, and indicates any narrowing or obstruction. Any major abnormality of the bladder may be shown up, and the X-ray taken after urination shows whether the bladder has emptied completely.

Retrograde pyelography requires an anaesthetic so that a cystoscope can be passed into the bladder. A fine tube is then threaded through the cystoscope into the bladder and, under direct vision, is pushed carefully up the ureter to the kidney. A small quantity of radio-opaque dye is now injected through the tube so that it is released in high concentration, and X-rays are taken. Retrograde pyelography is

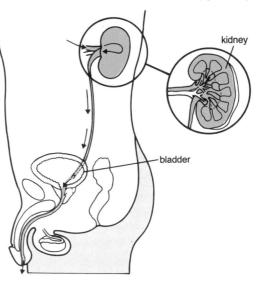

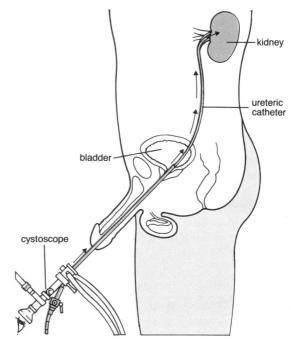

There are two kinds of pyelography – intravenous and retrograde. In the former, the radio-opaque dye is injected into the blood and is excreted and concentrated in the kidney and urine-collecting tubes. In the latter, the dye is passed back up the ureter to the kidney.

especially useful for showing up obstructions of the upper part of the urinary tract and the urine-collecting systems of the kidney, and for demonstrating stones in any part of the drainage system.

pyelonephritis

Infection and inflammation of the urine-collecting system (the pelvis) of the kidney, usually with small abscesses in the substance of the kidney. The condition causes sudden pain in the back, under the ribs (the loin), radiating to the lower quadrant of the abdomen on the same side, difficulty in passing urine, with burning or scalding, high fever, shivering, vomiting and, in children, sometimes convulsions.

Pyelonephritis may progress to **pyonephrosis** or to a kidney abscess. This causes bulging of the back wall under the ribs and an acute worsening of the condition, and the abscess may burst through the wall of the back to the exterior.

Pyelonephritis is treated with antibiotics and any possible underlying cause is investigated and, if possible, removed.

pyloric stenosis

Narrowing of the muscular outlet from the stomach (the pylorus) so that the passage of food into the first part of the small intestine – the duodenum – is obstructed. The condition may be present at birth, calling for an urgent operation to relieve the obstruction, or may be acquired as a result of repeated attacks of ulceration in the area. In this case, an operation known as pyloroplasty may be needed. Pyloric stenosis is occasionally caused by cancer of the stomach.

Congenital pyloric stenosis is commonest in children of mothers who also had the disease, and occurs most often in first-born male babies. It usually shows itself by projectile vomiting at about six weeks of age. The vomiting occurs immediately after a feed and the baby remains very hungry. A firm swelling below the ribs on the right side, about the size and consistency of an olive, can usually be felt. Abnormal movement of the intestine (reverse peristalsis) can also be seen through the abdominal wall.

Treatment is by Ramstead's operation, a surgical procedure in which the tight ring of thickened muscle is cut. The results are excellent.

Pylorid

A brand name for **rantitidine bismuth citrate**.

pyoderma gangrenosum

A rare condition occurring as a complication in 5 per cent of patients with **ulcerative colitis**. Boils appear on the skin and, as the condition progresses, hard, painful areas form surrounded by discoloured skin. These areas are undermined by the destructive process.

pyonephrosis

A condition in which a kidney becomes filled with pus, as a complication either of kidney stones, **hydronephrosis** or acute **pyelonephritis**. The enlarged kidney causes a swelling in the side and great pain. The affected person is severely ill, with high fever, signs of urinary infection and anaemia. There is likely to be pus in the urine. The condition is unlikely to respond to antibiotics and it is usually necessary to operate in order to drain the pus from the kidney or even, if the damage to the organ is sufficiently severe, to remove it altogether.

pyos

Greek root meaning 'pus' as in pyodermatitis (skin inflammation with pus).

Pyralvex

A brand name for a preparation of **anthraquinone glycosides** and **salicylic acid**.

pyrantel

An anthelmintic drug used to treat intestinal worm infestations, especially **roundworms** and **threadworms**. A brand name is Combantrin.

pyrazinamide

An antituberculosis drug that diffuses well into the cerebrospinal fluid and is used to treat tuberculous **meningitis**. Trade names are Zinamide and, with other antituberculosis drugs, Rifater.

pyrazolone drugs

A group of non-steroidal anti-inflammatory drugs (**NSAIDs**) that includes phenylbutazone and azapropazone.

pyretos

Greek root meaning 'fire' as in pyrexia (fever).

pyrexia

See **fever**.

pyridostigmine

A cholinergic drug used in the treatment of **myasthenia gravis**. A brand name is Mestinon.

pyrimethamine

A drug used in the treatment of **malaria** and **toxoplasmosis**. Trade names are Daraprim and, with other antimalarial drugs, Fansidar and Maloprim.

Pyrogastrone

A brand name for a mixture of the antacid drugs aluminium hydroxide, sodium bicarbonate and magnesium trisilicate, the antifoaming agent alginic acid and the ulcer-protective drug carbenoxolone.

pyrogen

Any substance causing fever. The immediately acting pyrogen is now known to be the substance interleukin-1 which is released by macrophage cells following infection with bacteria, viruses, yeasts, or spirochaetes, or in the presence of progesterone, certain drugs and other substances. All these substances are also called pyrogens (exogenous pyrogens).

Interleukin-1 acts on the temperature-regulating centres in the hypothalamus of the brain, resetting the thermostat at a higher level, so that the blood temperature is interpreted as being too low. Heat production action, by shivering, then rapidly raises the body temperature.

pyuria

Pus cells in the urine. This is a feature of any urinary infection, whether it involves the urethra, the bladder or the kidneys.

PZI Hypurin

A brand name for protamine zinc **insulin**.

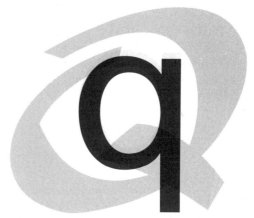

Q fever

The name of the disease arose before the cause was known. 'Q' stands for 'query'. It is an illness of sudden onset, characterized by high fever lasting up to three weeks. The mortality is below 1 per cent, even in untreated patients, and with antibiotics, it is much less.

CAUSE

Q fever is caused by a small organism called *Coxiella burnetii* which is harboured by farm animals such as sheep, cattle and goats and passed in the faeces, urine and milk. It is also found in the meat of these animals. The organism occurs in great numbers in the placentas of infected animals. In dry areas, the disease may be contracted by inhaling dusts contaminated with dried faeces, urine or products of conception. Untreated milk is another source. The disease may also be acquired by the bite of various insects, such as ticks, which are also commonly infected.

RECOGNITION AND SYMPTOMS

There is high fever lasting for up to three weeks, severe headache, muscle and chest pain and cough. In the second week of the illness a form of pneumonia develops, but recovery is usual. In some cases the disease is very prolonged and, in these, one-third of the people affected develop **hepatitis** and some suffer **endocarditis**.

Diagnosis is made on the symptoms and by finding specific antibodies to *C. burnetii* in the blood.

> It is important for people working with farm animals to be aware of the risks of drinking untreated milk or of exposure to dusts from animal excreta and placentas. Workers in slaughter houses, rending plants, dairies, and wool processing plants are also at risk.

TREATMENT

The antibiotics tetracycline and chloramphenicol are effective against the infection. There is an effective vaccine.

quack

A person who fraudulently claims to have medical knowledge, skills or remedies. The history of medicine abounds in quackery and many of the most notable quacks became rich and famous.

quadrantopia

Loss of a pie-shaped quarter segment of the field of vision, usually an upper quadrant. Corresponding quadrants are usually lost in *both* eyes (homonymous quadrantopia). This effect is due to damage, by disease, to a portion of the nerve tracts (the optic radiations) carrying neurological information from the eyes to the visual area at the extreme back of the brain (the visual cortex). The lower halves of these nerve fibres make a detour into the temporal lobe of the brain and it is these which are affected.

Quadrantopia is less common than loss of half the field of vision of each eye (**hemianopia**), but both are usually the result of interference with a full blood supply to this part of the brain. In hemianopia, however, it is usually the visual cortex that is affected.

quadriplegia

Paralysis of the muscles of both arms, both legs and of the trunk. This results from severe damage to the spinal cord above the level at which the nerves to the arms come off, so that no nerve impulses are able to pass down from the brain to the levels below the region of damage.

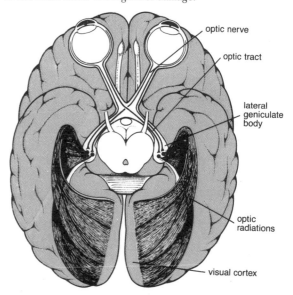

Quadrantopia: the visual nerve pathways from the eyes to the visual cortex, right at the back of the brain. The optic radiations are well spread out and contain fibres from both eyes. As a result, visual field loss resulting from damage to the radiations involves corresponding sectors of the fields of both eyes.

Quadriplegia is most commonly caused by a fracture-dislocation of the neck, often from accidental injury, but may also result from disease, such as **poliomyelitis**.

See also **paralysis**.

quarantine

The period for which people who have been in contact with an infectious disease are required to be isolated before being allowed to move freely among the population. The term comes from the French word for 'forty', this being the number of days for which ships' crews were isolated if they arrived flying a yellow flag indicating disease on board (the 'yellow jack'). Quarantine must last for a time equal to the longest known **incubation period** of the disease. If the isolated person does not develop the disease during this period, he or she may safely be released, as offering no threat of infection to others.

In a context of an ever-increasing volume of international travel, quarantine, even if it were useful, would be impracticable. In some instances, such as a risk of spreading yellow fever, the problem is solved by compulsory immunization. Fortunately, with the decline in bacterial infectious disease and the ease with which most can now be treated, the large-scale quarantining of people has become almost a historic procedure – almost, but not quite. With the appearance of new and virulent human diseases, such as **Lassa fever** and **Ebola virus disease**, it is still, from time to time, necessary.

Animals are still subject to quarantine, mainly because of the **rabies** risk, and, unfortunately, the incubation period of this disease is very much longer than most.

quartan

Recurring on the fourth day. Quartan **malaria** produces bouts of fever every seventy-two hours. If the day of the fever is counted as day one, the next bout will be on day four.

Queensland tick typhus

A mild to moderately severe infectious disease occurring in rural north-eastern Australia, caused by *Rickettsia australis* and transmitted by the tick *Ixodes holocyclus*. The condition is very similar to **Rocky Mountain spotted fever** and features a conspicuous spot at the site of the bite that heals slowly. The symptoms include fever, enlarged lymph nodes and a generalized rash involving the palms and the soles. Most cases recover completely.

quetiapine

A dibenzothiazepine antipsychotic drug used to treat **schizophrenia**. A brand name is Seroquel.

quinagolide

A drug with properties similar to those of dopamine used to treat infertility in women with excess levels of the hormone prolactin. A brand name is Norprolac.

quinalbarbitone

A barbiturate drug used for brief periods of treatment of insomnia in people addicted to barbiturates. A brand name is Seconal Sodium.

quinapril

An **angiotensin converting enzyme inhibitor** (ACE inhibitor) drug used to treat heart failure and high blood pressure. A brand name is Accupro.

Quinate

A brand name for quinine.

Quinbisul

A brand name for quinine.

quinghaosu

A Chinese herbal drug used for 2000 years to treat **malaria**. The active ingredient is a sesquiterpene lactone that, in a manner not yet understood, appears to reduce greatly the number of malarial parasites in the blood. The pharmacology is being investigated and trials of the drug have recently started in the West.

Quinidex SA

A brand name for **quinidine**.

quinidine

A drug derived from quinine and used to control irregularity or excessive rapidity of the heart beat by depressing the excitability of the muscle. A brand name is Kinidin Durules.

Quinidoxin

A brand name for **quinidine**.

Quinoctal

A brand name for quinine.

quinolone drugs

A group of synthetic antibiotic drugs that includes nalidixic acid, ofloxacin and enoxacin. These drugs act by inactivating an enzyme, **DNA** gyrase, necessary for replication of the organisms. They are often useful for treating infections with organisms that have become resistant to other antibiotics. They are administered by mouth. Possible side-effects include nausea, vomiting, diarrhoea and abdominal pain, headache, restlessness and tiredness. Psychiatric disturbances occasionally occur.

Quinsul

A brand name for quinine.

quinsy

An abscess between the capsule of the tonsil and the adjacent wall of the throat (**pharynx**). Quinsy usually follows a severe attack of **tonsillitis**.

RECOGNITION AND SYMPTOMS

The abscess is almost always on one side only, and the swelling appears above the tonsil, near the soft palate, so that the small floppy tongue of the soft palate (the uvula) is pushed across to the unaffected side. The throat is extremely painful and there is high fever, headache and

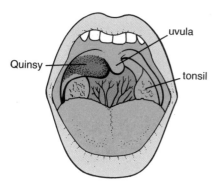

A quinsy is an abscess in the back wall of the throat. In this case the swelling lies above the tonsil and pushes the uvula of the soft palate to the opposite side.

other signs of general upset. The speech is impaired and there is much salivation and dribbling. The neck lymph nodes are enlarged and tender.

TREATMENT

Antibiotics, given at an early stage before the abscess has fully developed, may bring the infection under control, but once the quinsy is established they are of little value and surgical drainage is necessary. This is followed by rapid relief. When the condition has fully settled it is advisable to have the tonsils removed, to avoid recurrence.

quintuplets

Five babies born in a single gestation. Quins are rare. Prior to the introduction of 'fertility' drugs, to promote ovulation, triplets occurred once in 10,000 pregnancies and quadru-
plets once in 500,000. The incidence of quintuplets was too small to be assessed. Since the size of the baby is, in general, inversely proportional to the number in the gestation, the chances of survival drop sharply with increasing numbers.

The survival of the Dionne quins, born in Canada in 1934, was a unique phenomenon, never before reported. The Dionne quins arose from a single fertilized egg (ovum) which divided and separated three times, giving rise to six genetically identical individuals. The sixth fetus aborted spontaneously during the third month of the pregnancy. The five babies were, necessarily, all of the same sex and physical constitution and this added greatly to their commercial value – a value successfully exploited for years.

Fertility drugs cause multiple pregnancies, not in this way, but by stimulating the ovaries to produce multiple ova, which may be fertilized separately. In this case, the siblings are genetically dissimilar. The risk of high multiple pregnancies is slight with the commonly used drug clomiphene, but is much greater when gonadotrophins are used to stimulate the ovaries. Quintuplet, sextuplet, septuplet and octuplet pregnancies are not uncommon when the latter drugs are used, but these fetuses are often too small at birth to survive.

quotidian fever

A fever occurring every day. None of the types of malaria can, by itself, cause quotidian fever, but a mixed malarial infection can do so.

Qvar

A brand name for **beclomethasone**.

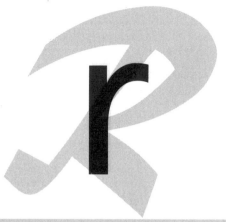

rabies

Hydrophobia. A disease of the nervous system affecting a wide range of animals. Rabies is an inflammation of the brain (**encephalitis**) caused by a virus which enters the nervous system at the site of a bite by a rabid animal and travels slowly to the brain. Once the disease is established, it is almost always fatal.

The rabies virus is a bullet-shaped organism of the family of rhabdoviruses, and commonly infects foxes, wolves, jackals, skunks, mongooses, raccoons and vampire bats. Almost any animal can, however, be infected and domestic dogs and cats readily acquire the infection if exposed to wild animals with the disease. The saliva of an infected animal is teeming with the virus and contact with an abrasion or cut is sufficient for infection.

The virus remains for a variable period at the site of the bite, but because it then travels slowly along the interior of nerves to reach the brain, the time between biting and the start of the symptoms (the **incubation period**) varies with the distance of the bite from the head. Severe bites on the head or neck may result in rabies in as short a period as nine days; bites remote from the head are followed by a much longer incubation period, perhaps as long as several months. The incubation period also varies with different strains of the virus, but the average time between bite and onset is four to eight weeks. Only a proportion of infected people suffer the disease.

INCIDENCE

The incidence of human cases closely parallels the incidence in animals in the area. Some thirty countries are now classified as rabies-free, largely because of strict animal control.

RECOGNITION AND SYMPTOMS

The disease begins with a low fever, loss of appetite, headache, and often a recurrence of pain or tingling at the site of the bite. During the next few days there is a growing sense of anxiety, jumpiness, disorientation, neck stiffness, and sometimes epileptic seizures. Within a week many cases show the characteristic fear of swallowing. The patient may be consumed with thirst, but any attempt to drink at once induces violent spasms of the diaphragm, pharynx and larynx, with gagging, choking and a growing sense of panic – hence the term *hydrophobia*. As the condition worsens, even the sight or sound of water prompts these effects and there are intervals of maniacal behaviour with thrashing, spitting, biting and raving. Delusions and hallucinations develop.

These attacks alternate with periods of lucidity in which the patient suffers acute anxiety and mental distress. The nerves controlling eye movement and facial expression become paralysed and coma and death occur, usually within a week of the onset of the severe symptoms.

TREATMENT

Once the symptoms start, the mortality is almost 100 per cent, but a very small number of patients with established rabies have been successfully treated, using heavy sedation and intensive care facilities to maintain the action of the heart and the respiratory system. Full recovery has been reported in a small number of cases. No antiviral agent is directly effective against the virus.

> In an attempt to minimize the risk after biting, experts recommend that animal bites should be thoroughly cleaned with soap, detergent, cetrimide, benzalkonium solutions or hydrogen peroxide, and that they should then be surgically opened up and left unstitched. The biting animal should be secured, locked up and not killed.

Rabies can usually be prevented from developing if proper treatment is started within a day or two of the biting. Both hyperimmune serum (human anti-rabies globulin) and rabies vaccine are used, so as to provide both passive and active protection. The serum is injected around the bite and also into muscles (intramuscularly) elsewhere. The safest vaccine is human diploid cell strain vaccine and this is given three, seven, fourteen, thirty and ninety days after biting.

The animal is watched. If still healthy after five days, it does not have rabies and the treatment is stopped. If it has been killed or dies, the brain is examined for the typical inclusion bodies seen in the brain cells in rabies. If the animal escapes before the five days are up, the treatment is continued.

PREVENTION

The most important preventive measure is stringent public health control of stray animals and the movement of possibly infected animals across frontiers into uninfected regions. The mortality is so high and the mode of death so distressing that sentimental considerations have no place in deciding control measures. The importation of animals into safe countries should be allowed only after six months of quarantine and heavy penalties should be imposed on those contravening the regulations. In endemic areas, domestic dogs should be vaccinated annually and stray dogs shot.

All who handle potentially infected animals, and those at particular risk in endemic areas, should have anti-rabies vaccination. Initial protection is provided by two injections given four weeks apart and, thereafter, annual booster injections are needed.

rachitic

Affected by **rickets**.

rad

A unit of dosage of absorbed ionizing radiation. The rad is the energy absorption of 0.01 joule per kilogram of the material being irradiated.

radial keratotomy

See **keratotomy, radial**. See also **myopia**.

radiation

The emission and propagation of electromagnetic waves or particles. Radiation covers a wide spectrum of wavelengths, from those of radio waves, which may be thousands of metres long, to those of X-rays and gamma rays with wavelengths of the order of millionths of millionths of millimetres. Radiation is a form of physical energy and it interacts with any matter it encounters. Radiation of relatively long wavelength, such as that from radio transmitters, microwave ovens, ultrasound machines, electric light bulbs, the sun and ultraviolet light sources, is described as non-ionizing radiation.

This means that such radiation, although it may cause atoms and molecules of the body to vibrate strongly, does not actually break up molecules.

IONIZING RADIATION

Short wavelength radiation, such as X-rays, gamma rays, neutrons or charged particles (alpha and beta particles), can displace linking electrons from molecules and cause them to break up into smaller charged bodies or chemical groups called ions or free radicals. For this reason it is called ionizing radiation.

The sources of ionizing radiation include:

- outer space and the sun (cosmic rays);
- medical X-ray machines;
- radioactive elements such as uranium and radium;
- radioactive isotopes, many of which are man-made;
- radioactive fall-out from atomic explosions and industrial accidents;
- leakage from atomic power stations.

Ionizing radiation can damage any molecules in the body, including the large **DNA** molecules which make up the chromosomes of our body cells. Radiation which kills cells causes dozens of breaks in, and other damage to, the DNA. Lesser damage can, up to a point, be repaired by the cells, but the risk of a permanent and inheritable change (a genetic mutation) is always there. Cells which are dividing rapidly, such as those in the blood-forming tissue of the bone marrow, the testicles, intestine and skin, are more susceptible to radiation damage than cells which are dividing infrequently, or not at all. On the other hand, when cells are killed by radiation, those which divide most rapidly can more easily make up the losses and resume normal function. Others may be replaced by scar tissue or sustain permanent damage, as in the greying of hair, the formation

of cataracts, or the production of cancers under the influence of high radiation dosage.

The higher the radiation, the higher the percentage of cells killed, and if the dose is high enough, death of the individual occurs. A burst of high-level radiation, lasting for a few minutes and covering the whole body, might be fatal. But if the same whole-body dose were spread over a month, death would not result, although life might be shortened. The size of the area of the body exposed to radiation is also very important. An intensity of radiation which, if applied to the whole body, would certainly cause death, can be safely applied, for purposes of treatment, to a small area.

radiation therapy

See **radiotherapy**.

radical surgery

Surgery designed to root out the whole of the disease process, usually a cancer. The term derives from the Latin word *radix*, meaning a root. Radical surgery will often involve widespread removal of tissue. In radical mastectomy, for instance, the whole of the breast, together with the underlying muscle and the lymph vessels and lymph nodes in the armpit, are removed. This is seldom done nowadays. In radical dissection of the neck, the surgeon exposes the great vessels and strips away all the possibly affected lymph nodes, often removing, in the process, sections of the jugular veins, parts of the salivary glands on the floor of the mouth, and some of the muscles.

Gangrene, or the presence of a highly malignant tumour, often makes the radical procedure of a major amputation necessary. In the past, this has involved removal of an entire hindquarter or even, in a few cases, the whole of the lower part of the body (hemicorporectomy). With advances in management, such procedures are now almost unknown.

radiographer

An ancillary health professional who takes X-rays for medical diagnosis. The radiographer is skilled in the positioning of patients and in making correct exposures. He or she also performs imaging using ultrasound, CT, MRI and PET scanners, as well as radionuclide scanning methods using a gamma camera.

radiologist

A doctor who specializes in medical imaging and is skilled in the interpretation of X-ray, CT scan, MRI, PET scan, ultrasound and radionuclide scanning films. He or she is a specialist in nuclear medicine, familiar with the use of radioactive isotopes and with electronic imaging and intensifying methods, and an expert in the insertion of arterial and cardiac catheters. Some radiologists also practise radiotherapy (see **radiotherapist**).

radionuclide scanning

See **nuclear medicine**.

radiotherapist

A doctor who specializes in the treatment of cancer, and some other conditions, by ionizing radiation. He or she is skilled in the direction, collimation and shielding of radiation and the size and timing of the dosage to cause maximal damage to the tumour and the minimal damage to the patient. The radiotherapist uses high voltage X-ray machines, linear accelerators and powerful radioactive isotopes such as cobalt-60.

radiotherapy

A medical specialty concerned with the treatment of cancer, and, to a much lesser extent, other conditions by the use of ionizing **radiation**. Radiation affects both normal and cancerous tissues, but almost all cancers are more sensitive to radiation than are normal cells. It is this difference in sensitivity that makes radiotherapy possible. In addition, radiation can be directed accurately at a tumour with minimal exposure of non-malignant tissues, and a total dose of radiation can, with relative safety, be applied to one localized area, although the same dose, applied body-wide, might be fatal. The doses selected, their timing and directions of application are calculated to produce the maximum damage to the tumour and the minimum to the host.

HOW IT WORKS

The radiation sources used are high energy (high voltage) X-ray machines, linear accelerators and radioactive isotopes, such as cobalt-60 and iodine-131, which emit gamma rays. The patient is carefully shielded with lead so that only the area of the tumour is irradiated and the dosage is usually spread over a period of some weeks. The effect on the patient, generally, is monitored in various ways, especially by checking on the rate of blood cell production by the bone marrow, which is sensitively affected by radiation.

Small and well-localized tumours can be effectively treated by direct application of radioactive sources in or around them. This radioactive material can be inserted, in a tube, into the neck of the womb (cervix) or can sometimes be placed, in the form of 'needles' of iridium-192 or caesium-137, within the tumour itself. Skin tumours can be treated by direct application of radioactive materials.

RISKS

In many cases, modern radiotherapy is curative. Unfortunately, about half the patients presenting for radiotherapy have little prospect of cure because the disease is already so advanced or widespread. Radiotherapy can however, even in these cases, bring about a considerable improvement in the condition, palliate symptoms and prolong life.

radius, fracture of

The radius, one of the two long forearm bones, is one of the most commonly broken bones in the body, mainly because of the frequency with which people fall on their outstretched hands. In such a fall, the radius takes most of the strain and commonly breaks just above the wrist causing a backward displacement of the wrist and the hand – the 'dinner-fork' deformity of the Colles' fracture. In young people, the disc-shaped head of the bone, at the elbow joint, is often fractured. If this part of the bone is shattered, it may be necessary to remove some or all of the fragments.

Fracture of the shaft of the radius, with separation and over-riding of the bone ends, is also common. Re-alignment, by manipulation under anaesthesia, or even by open operation and wiring, is necessary if full function is to be restored.

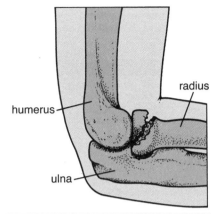

One of the less common types of fracture of the radius – a fracture of the rotating head. Removal of a bone fragment may be necessary.

Rafen

A brand name for **ibuprofen**.

ragged red fibres

A feature of several **mitochondrial DNA** disorders in which a high proportion of the muscle fibres contain **mitochondria** that are both structurally and functionally abnormal. When stained and examined under the microscope these fibres appear ragged and readily take up a red stain.

Ragged red muscle fibres are commonly associated with slowly progressive weakness of the muscles of the limbs, defects of ocular movements, abnormally rapid tiredness on exertion, and a marked rise in the levels of lactic acid in the blood on exertion or even at rest.

raltitrexed

A folate analogue drug used in the palliative treatment of advanced cancer of the colon or rectum. A brand name is Tomudex.

ramipril

An **angiotensin converting enzyme inhibitor** drug that has been shown to be capable of greatly extending life after heart attack. A brand name is Tritace.

ranitidine

An H-2 (histamine-2) receptor antagonist drug used to reduce acid secretion in cases of peptic ulceration. A brand name is Zantac.

ranitidine bismuth citrate

A drug that combines the properties of **ranitidine** with the protectant action of bismuth. A brand name is Pylorid.

ranula

A cyst-like swelling under the tongue caused by the obstruction of the duct of one of the salivary glands and its ballooning out with secretion. Salivary gland duct obstruction is usually caused by a salivary stone (**calculus**).

rape

Definitions vary in different countries. In Britain, rape is defined as sexual intercourse with a woman who does not, at the time, consent to it, by a man who knows she does not, or who is reckless as to whether or not she does. The offence requires that there should have been some penetration of the vagina with the penis, however slight, but does not require that there should have been ejaculation of semen. Rape need not be forcible and can be effected by a trick, such as by impersonating a husband. It is no longer a defence to rape to submit that one is married to the victim.

In some American states, the definition has been broadened to include other forms of sexual contact and to include acts against wives and acts by women against males. In the USA, statutory rape is sexual intercourse with a person below a specified age, which may vary, in different states, from twelve to eighteen. Intercourse with a mentally deficient or unconscious person may also be statutory rape. In Britain, such offences as these are described as sexual offences.

THE RAPIST

The motives for rape are more complex and varied than is generally supposed. It is not engaged in exclusively for erotic reasons or as a result of uncontrollable sexual appetite or the desire to demonstrate virility. Rape is nearly always a violent act, often motivated by anger and aggression against a person, a sex or a class. In many cases the victim is regarded as a symbol or scapegoat. Some rapists act to gratify sadistic impulses and it is common for the rape to be associated with the infliction of cruel physical and mental pain.

THE VICTIM

For centuries, rape has been concealed by women as shameful. It has also been concealed because male rationalizations have suggested that raped women have invited the act. Although rape is still under-reported, there is now a strong movement towards better understanding of the plight of the rape victim and sympathy for her, both on the part of society generally and by the police. As a result, women are encouraged to bring about prosecutions. The psychological effects of rape are now better understood and effective counselling is more readily available. Most of the sexually transmitted diseases that can be acquired in the course of rape can be effectively treated. Unfortunately, this does not apply to **AIDS** and to genital **herpes**. In many societies pregnancies resulting from rape can usually be terminated. Even with the highest standard of care, however, the mental distress associated with rape may be severe and prolonged.

Rapidard

A brand name for **insulin**.

Rapifen

A brand name for **alfentanil**.

Rapiject

A brand name for **morphine**.

Rapilysin

A brand name for **reteplase**.

Rapitil

A brand name for **nedocromil**.

Raynaud's disease

A disorder of the small arteries supplying fingers and toes, in which exposure to cold causes them to go into spasm so that blood flow is restricted. The cause is unknown. Raynaud's disease is commonest in young women and usually affects both hands. The toes are less often affected.

RECOGNITION AND SYMPTOMS

In cold conditions, there is tingling, burning and numbness in the affected parts and the fingers are very pale from lack of blood. As slow blood flow is resumed and the oxygen is withdrawn from the blood, the characteristic purplish colour of deoxygenated blood (cyanosis) is seen. When the parts are warmed and the spasm of the blood vessels passes off, the vessels open widely, allowing a flush of fresh blood to pass. In this stage, the fingers or toes become red.

In the early months or years, no organic change occurs in the affected blood vessels, but eventually the vessel walls may become thickened and the flow of blood permanently reduced. Arteries may block off altogether, from blood clotting (**thrombosis**), and this can lead to tissue death (**gangrene**) at the tips of the affected fingers or toes.

> People suffering from Raynaud's disease must avoid cold and keep the extremities well insulated. Cigarette smoking is especially dangerous as nicotine increases the constriction of the small arteries.

TREATMENT

Various drugs to relax the smooth muscle in the walls of the arteries are useful in Raynaud's disease. These include calcium antagonists, reserpine, tolazoline, and the vasodilator nitroglycerine in ointment form. The thyroid hormone tri-iodothyronine has been found effective and this has been usefully combined with reserpine. Cutting of the sympathetic nerves which supply the vessel wall muscles (sympathectomy) can be helpful, especially when the disease affects the lower limb.

RAYNAUD'S PHENOMENON

When the symptoms are an effect of known causes, they are called Raynaud's phenomenon. This occurs in any form of occlusive disease of the arteries, such as **atherosclerosis** or Buerger's disease (**thromboangiitis obliterans**) or any cause of obstruction, such as **embolism**, **thrombosis** or diabetic large vessel disease. Small artery occlusion also occurs in **rheumatoid arthritis**, systemic **lupus erythematosus** and **scleroderma** and it may result from repeated vibration or physical trauma to the fingers. Raynaud's phenomenon sometimes affects musicians, typists or those using vibrating power tools or pneumatic drills. It may also be caused by drugs such as ergotamine, methysergide or beta-blockers, which narrow arteries, and it can be caused by toxic industrial agents such as polyvinyl chloride.

Raynaud's phenomenon is treated by correcting the cause, if this is possible, but treatment of the symptoms, as described for Raynaud's disease, may also be necessary.

Raynaud's sign

The red, white and blue sign of arterial spasm. A temporary closure, on exposure to moderate cold or vibration, of the arteries of the extremities, such as those in the fingers, causes whiteness, coldness and insensitivity. This is followed by blueness (cyanosis) as the blood in the tissues loses its oxygen, and redness, on recovery, as the flow of blood is restored. This sequence is a feature of the circulation disorder **Raynaud's disease**.

re-

Prefix meaning 'back' as in reversed (turned back).

rebound tenderness

In bowel inflammation, such as appendicitis, it is often possible to apply gentle but increasing pressure on the front of the abdomen with the flat of the hand, without causing too much pain. If this is done carefully and the hand is then suddenly and sharply removed, a definite pain may be felt in the position of the inflammation, even if this is at some distance from the point at which the pressure is applied. Thus, in appendicitis, pressure may be applied to the left side of the abdomen and the rebound tenderness felt in the lower right quadrant – the site of the appendix.

reboxetine

A selective **noradrenaline re-uptake inhibitor** antidepressant drug. A brand name is Edronax.

receding chin

A congenital condition caused by disproportion between the size of the lower jaw bone (mandible) and the rest of the skeleton of the face. The condition is of cosmetic concern only. The appearance can be improved by various plastic operations, either to lengthen the side pieces of the mandible, to increase the bulk of the bone at the front by bone grafting, or to implant a plastic prosthesis between the soft tissue of the chin and the bone.

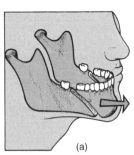

(a)

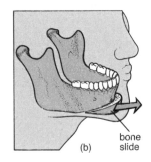

(b) bone slide

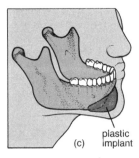

(c) plastic implant

Cosmetic treatment of a receding chin may involve (a) an angled cut with forward slide of the front part of the mandible; (b) cutting off the tip of the bone with forward slide; or (c) the use of a plastic implant.

recombinant DNA

See **genetic engineering**.

recommended daily amounts (RDAs)

The daily intake of a particular nutrient, whether carbohydrate, protein, fat, vitamin, mineral or trace element, that is, at the time of publication, considered adequate to maintain health. RDAs are decided upon by various official nutritional committees and commonly shown by later research to have erred in either direction. This uncertainty is reflected in the fact that RDA tables are regularly revised. Even the name cannot be agreed upon and has recently changed to reference nutrient intake (RNI), which does not, on the whole, appear to be an improvement, unless the members of the committees concerned are anxious to avoid responsibility for making recommendations.

The matter is more complicated than might at first appear. Nutritional requirements differ at different stages in life and differ between the sexes. They differ for different people of different weight and body build. Pregnancy also imposes its own special requirements. Different people, even those of identical sex, weight and age, may also have different requirements. And when the effects of various illnesses are also considered, the matter becomes even more complicated. It is necessary to decide on a figure that will always be adequate, not for everyone, but for an agreed percentage of the population, commonly 97 per cent. Most people's requirements are less than this, so to avoid the risk of recommending too much, tables of estimated average requirement (EAR) are produced.

Her Majesty's Stationery Office (HMSO) publishes a book called *Dietary Reference for Food Energy and Nutrients for the United Kingdom.*

recreational drugs

A dubious term that trivialises the dangers and serious social implications of the use of drugs such as **cocaine**, **amphetamine**, various **hallucinogenic drugs** and **marijuana**.

rectal bleeding

> This is one of the health danger signs which should never be ignored unless the cause is known.

Fortunately, the commonest cause of blood on the stools is the minor condition of piles (**haemorrhoids**) which need occasion no alarm. But there are other causes of rectal bleeding, the most important being cancer of the rectum (see **rectal cancer**) or large intestine (see **colon, cancer of**). This occurs most often in people over sixty and can be effectively treated if caught early.

Other causes of rectal bleeding include the painful condition of cracking at the edge of the anus (fissure in ano), **rectal prolapse**, **diverticulitis**, rectal polyps, **ulcerative colitis**, and amoebic and bacillary dysentery (**shigellosis**).

rectal cancer

Cancer of the rectum is uncommon before the age of forty, but in later years, together with cancer of the colon (see **colon, cancer of**), becomes second only to cancer of the lung as a cause of death in Britain and the USA. Over 70 per cent of large intestine cancers occur in the rectum and lower colon (sigmoid colon).

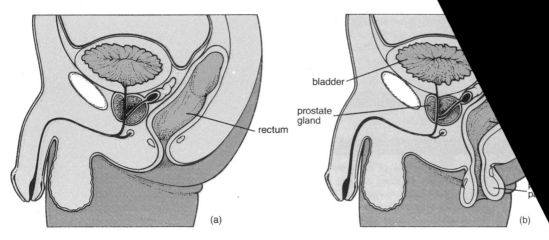

(a) The normal position of the rectum. (b) The lower part of the rectum can be everted and forced out of the anal canal, so that the mucous membrane lining is exposed.

Cancers may be of three types – ring growths, which narrow the bowel; polyp-like growths which protrude into the bowel; and ulcerative tumours which eat into the wall. Rectal cancers may spread through the bowel wall to the lining membrane of the abdomen (peritoneum); they may spread to the local lymph nodes and from there up the chain of lymph vessels and nodes surrounding the large arteries and veins of the pelvis; or they may spread remotely, by way of the bloodstream, to other parts of the body.

RECOGNITION AND SYMPTOMS

The important signs of rectal cancer are any change in the bowel habit and **rectal bleeding**. Commonly, there is early morning urgency with a repeated strong desire to empty the bowel, which has little effect except for the passage of some mucus and blood. This may occur several times before more normal stools are passed. There is often a sense of incomplete evacuation and the stools may sometimes be ribbon-like.

Complete obstruction of the bowel may occur.

TREATMENT

Rectal cancer is treated by surgery with removal of the affected segment of the bowel and an end-to-end joining up, if this is possible. When the cancer is very low in the rectum, the anal canal must also be removed, to prevent recurrence, and in that case an artificial opening, bringing the bowel out through the front wall of the abdomen (a **colostomy**) is necessary.

rectal examination

If the medical history suggests a disorder in the pelvis, anal or lower rectal region, a doctor will almost certainly perform a rectal examination. This is also important if there is any suggestion of enlargement of the prostate gland, which is usually a benign condition, but is sometimes due to cancer. Rectal examination is only mildly uncomfortable and need not occasion distress. The doctor uses disposable plastic gloves and a lubricant such as K-Y jelly. There is a slight sensation as if the bowels are moving.

Rectal examination can reveal disorders, such as cancer, in the rectum itself, but also provides information about disorders in adjacent structures, such as the neck of the womb (cervix) and the prostate gland. The wall of the rectum is thin, and other parts can be felt through it. Enlarged ovaries can sometimes be felt, and tenderness, from inflammation or other disorders in the pelvis, can be localised. An inflamed appendix, or an appendix abscess, can often be felt on rectal examination. Sometimes a simultaneous vaginal examination is done. Rectal examination is an important part of any general examination.

rectal prolapse

A condition in which the mucous membrane lining of the anus, or the lower part of the rectum turns inside-out and passes out of the anus. In incomplete prolapse, only the lining of the anus appears, but in complete prolapse the whole thickness of the bowel protrudes as a thick cylindrical mass with the mucous membrane lining on the outside.

Incomplete prolapse is common in young children and usually requires no treatment, or, at the most, strapping together of the buttocks or a small injection to encourage internal adhesion of the lining.

Complete prolapse occurs in adults, mostly in women, because of weakness of the muscle ring around the anus (anal sphincter), or of the supporting floor of the pelvis, following childbirth. Anal surgery or **haemorrhoids** may also predispose to the condition in adults.

Prolapses are easily pushed back in but tend to recur, and complete prolapses usually require a surgical operation to tighten the anal sphincter or to carry out internal fixation of the rectum.

red eye

See **conjunctivitis**.

Redoxon

A brand name for vitamin C (ascorbic acid).

reduction

The restoration of a displaced part of the body to its proper position by manipulation or other surgical procedure. Closed reduction of a bone fracture, usually under anaesthesia, involves only external pulling (traction) to overcome muscle spasm, and local pressure to re-align the broken ends. Open

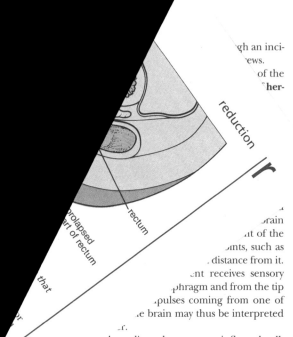

gh an inci-
...ews.
of the
...her-

reduction

prolapsed
part of rectum

rectum

that

...rain
...t of the
...ints, such as
...distance from it.
...nt receives sensory
...phragm and from the tip
...pulses coming from one of
...e brain may thus be interpreted
...r.

that a liver abscess or an inflamed gall-
...se pain in the right shoulder. The pain of
...ris is often felt in the left arm and pain from a
...r the urine tube from the kidney to the bladder (the
...er) is often felt in the lower abdomen on the same side or
...ven, in men, in the testicle.

Referred pain may also occur if a nerve coming from a remote part of the body is stimulated at a point nearer the brain. In this case the pain will seem to be coming from the remote point.

In the phantom limb syndrome after an amputation, stimulation of the cut ends of the nerves by scar tissue can cause a powerful impression that the limb is still there. Pressure on the nerve roots in the spinal canal, by pulp squeezed out of an intervertebral disc can cause pain in the lower leg or foot.

See also **pain**.

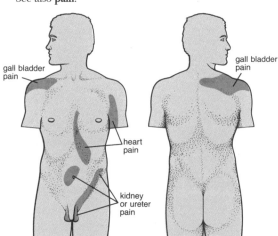

Areas to which pain is commonly referred from other sites of origin. Right shoulder pain is often referred from the gall-bladder, heart pain may be experienced in the left arm or upper abdomen, and kidney or ureter pain may be referred to the lower abdomen or testicle.

reflexes, primitive

Automatic movements made by newborn infants, in response to various stimuli applied to the body as a whole. These reflexes disappear during the first months of life, but provide useful guidance to the state of health of the immature and developing nervous system.

They include:

the automatic closure of the hand around an object such as ...finger (grasp reflex);
...udden bending up of the legs and embracing movement of the arms in response to a noise or to momentary lack of support to the head (Moro reflex);
● the walking or stepping reflex, when the baby is held upright with its feet on the ground;
● and the turning of the head and sucking actions when the cheek is stroked (rooting reflex).

The periods during which these responses are present are well-known to paediatricians and the absence or undue prolongation of these primitive reflexes provides valuable clinical information.

reflex sympathetic dystrophy

A condition that may follow severe injury to a limb. It features pain, tenderness, swelling, abnormal blood flow, disorders of sweating, involuntary movements and tissue atrophy of a kind known as trophic change.

The disorder is also known as Sudeck's atrophy, complex regional pain syndrome and algodystrophy.

reflux

Abnormal, and usually undesirable, reverse movement of fluid within the body. Reflux of urine from the bladder up the ureters to the kidneys can cause kidney damage. Sustained pressure on the abdomen may cause reflux of blood into the jugular veins, suggesting right heart failure (hepatojugular reflux). The most commonly experienced example of reflux is the movement of the acid stomach fluid (gastric juice) back up into the gullet (oesophagus) to cause the inflammatory pain of **heartburn** (reflux oesophagitis).

Refolinon

A brand name for **folinic acid**.

refraction tests

See **vision tests**.

Refrane

A brand name for lobeline.

Regaine

A brand name for **minoxidil** in a preparation for external use as a hair restorer.

regenerative cell therapy

Treatment claiming to rejuvenate the skin. Various methods are used, including injections of extracts of the endocrine glands of animals (monkey gland therapy) or of chick embryos. There is no proof that these treatments have any beneficial effect and every reason to believe that they are futile. Similar claims have been made for equally worthless skin creams containing extracts of embryo or placenta, which are alleged to make the skin firmer and more supple.

regional block anaesthesia

A form of local anaesthesia in which loss of sensation is achieved in a part or region of the body by injecting an anaesthetic drug at a remote point around the nerves carrying sensory impulses from the area.

regional ileitis

A bowel disease in which segments become inflamed and ulcerated and then greatly thickened. Between these affected segments the intestine remains normal. The condition commonly affects the lower part of the small intestine (the ileum), and is sometimes called **Crohn's disease**. All probable causes of regional ileitis have been investigated, but neither infection, immunological disorder nor diet can be conclusively implicated.

RECOGNITION AND SYMPTOMS

Regional ileitis causes fever, persistent diarrhoea, loss of appetite and weight and a feeling of fullness and pain in the lower part of the abdomen. In the early stages it is often mistaken for **appendicitis**. Unfortunately, the effects of the disease are not confined to the bowel. Complications include **arthritis**, red swellings in the skin (**erythema nodosum**), mouth ulcers, eye inflammation, a persistent inflammation of the spinal column leading to fusion of the bones (**ankylosing spondylitis**), gallstones, kidney stones and a strong tendency to urinary infection.

TREATMENT

The condition lasts for a lifetime and no treatment is known which will eradicate it. There may be long periods of quiescence, but flare-ups are always liable to occur. These may be greatly helped by appropriate treatment. Methyl cellulose or psyllium preparations help to firm up the stools, antibiotics may be given to combat infective complications, and steroid drugs to control inflammation. In some trials, drugs which interfere with the immune system (immunosuppressive drugs) have been found valuable.

Surgical treatment is avoided unless major complications such as obstruction or abscess formation make it essential. Surgery usually prompts a flare-up of the disorder and repeated operations, usually at the same site, are almost always required.

regression

A term used by psychoanalysts to describe what they take to be a return to childish or to a more primitive form of behaviour or thought. Freud believed that many people, although ostensibly mature, may be unconsciously stuck (fixated) at one of the earlier (Freudian) levels, such as the anal or oral stage. Under adverse conditions such people are liable to return to this stage. Some psychoanalysts suggest that regression is a fleeing from reality to a more infantile and less responsible state.

The cognitive school of psychology use the term to refer to a temporary falling back to an earlier and less mature form of thinking in the process of learning how to deal with some new complexity. Cognitive psychologists view regression, in this sense, as a normal part of the process of mental development.

Regulan

A brand name for **ispaghula**.

regurgitation

A reverse movement, or reflux, of material or fluid within the body. The bringing up of partly digested food from the stomach into the mouth is an example of regurgitation, as is the abnormal movement of blood back through a leaking (incompetent) valve in the heart.

rehabilitation

The process by which the physically, mentally or socially disabled are, so far as is possible, restored to a normally functional life. Rehabilitation, as a 'physical medicine' speciality, deals with the treatment of disorders of the musculoskeletal and nervous systems and attempts to restore the physically disabled to the highest possible level of function.

Much can be done to improve the function of those suffering from severe disabilities resulting from brain and spinal cord injuries, multiple sclerosis, strokes, spina bifida, cerebral palsy, muscular dystrophy, arthritis, amputations and many other conditions. Other forms of rehabilitation are concerned with the restoration to normal social activity of those suffering from drug or alcohol dependence or psychiatric disorder.

Rehabilitative treatment is most successful if provided by a multidisciplinary team, often working in a rehabilitation centre, which includes, as necessary, physiotherapists, occupational therapists, speech therapists, clinical psychologists, psychiatrists, social workers, vocational advisers and teachers. The emphasis is always on the achievement of the maximal mobility and the greatest degree of usage of body and mind, assisted, when appropriate, by all available technological aids.

Bioengineering is being widely applied to improve the quality of life of the disabled. Bioengineers have designed new and improved artificial limbs and braces, better engineered wheelchairs, modifications to motor vehicles and electronic systems for communication, environment control and education. The computer has become a major tool for the disabled and has allowed many to lead a fuller and more satisfying, and sometimes creative, life.

reimplantation, dental

The immediate replacement of a dislodged tooth in its socket in the hope that it may be retained. The tooth must have a root. A broken tooth cannot be reimplanted. The tooth should be thoroughly washed, pushed back into the cavity and held in place until a dentist can apply splinting. Success depends on various factors, but the sooner the tooth is replaced the better. Dental splinting, for several weeks, may be necessary.

Reiter's syndrome

A condition affecting people of the tissue type HLA B-27, mainly men, and featuring joint inflammation (**arthritis**) and a discharge from the penis or, in women, from the urethra or the neck of the womb (**cervicitis**). Formerly, **conjunctivitis** was also thought to be an essential part of the syndrome, but it is now accepted that the condition can occur without this feature. The arthritis in Reiter's disease is of the sero-negative type: the test for the rheumatoid factor is negative.

The condition occurs one to three weeks after a venereal infection or an attack of bacillary dysentery (**shigellosis**) or a Salmonella infection, but Reiter's syndrome is not an infection in the ordinary sense. It is a local inflammation induced in a genetically predisposed person by an infecting agent. In the venereal type, this agent is thought to be an organism of either the chlamydia or mycoplasma groups, and in the dysenteric type is either *Shigella dysenteriae*, *Shigella flexner* or one of the other dysentery-producing bacilli.

RECOGNITION AND SYMPTOMS

Reiter's disease is the commonest cause of arthritis in young men and occurs in about 2 per cent of men with inflammation of the urethra not caused by gonorrhoea. The arthritis most commonly affects only a knee or an ankle, and there is often fever and general upset. The affected joints are warm, red and painful, and the trouble persists for days, weeks or months. In addition to the joints, tendons and ligaments may become inflamed, and even the tendinous sheets (fascia) of the soles of the feet may be involved. The Achilles tendon behind the ankle is commonly affected and the heel bone (calcaneum), to which it is attached, sometimes develops a bony spur which may cause great discomfort in walking. Skin rashes also occur.

The conjunctivitis is usually quite mild, affects both eyes and settles spontaneously after about a month. In about 10 per cent of cases, a more serious eye inflammation, **uveitis**, may occur. This can be severely damaging to the eyes and calls for urgent specialist attention. Uveitis causes deep eye pain and blurring of vision. Conjunctivitis never affects vision.

TREATMENT

Reiter's syndrome is treated symptomatically – there is currently no specific remedy. Pain-killing drugs (analgesics) and non-steroidal anti-inflammatory drugs are helpful, but may have to be used over a long period. After apparent recovery, recurrences are common, especially in those who acquire further venereal infection. A tenth of the affected men still have evidence of active disease twenty years after the onset. In about 20 per cent of cases there is some permanent disability, usually from heel problems or distortion of the feet.

relapse

The re-appearance or worsening of a disease after apparent recovery or improvement.

relapsing fever

An infection with a spirochaete of the *Borrelia* genus, transmitted from person to person by the bite of a louse or a tick, and causing acute attacks, occurring in cycles, with normal intervals in between. Louse transmission occurs when the insect, having taken blood, passes to another host and is crushed into the skin during scratching. Tick transmission is by the *Ornithodoros species* of soft ticks. These acquire the spirochaetes by feeding on infected people, or rodents, and harbour them for years, passing them on to subsequent generations of ticks. Infection occurs when the tick bites another human, at night. The bite is painless.

INCIDENCE

The condition is very rare in civilized communities but is liable to flare up and occur in epidemics in times of civil disorder, war or famine, when refugees are crowded together. Tick-borne relapsing fever occurs sporadically in the western USA and the disease is endemic in Ethiopia.

RECOGNITION AND SYMPTOMS

There is a sharp rise of fever, up to 40°C, with shivering, headache, aches and pains, vomiting and sensitivity to light. The fever and symptoms continue for three to six days and then, after a brief worsening of the illness, during which collapse and death may occur, everything settles back to normal. Seven to ten days later, the whole cycle is repeated. In louse-borne relapsing fever there is usually only one relapse, but in the tick-borne disease there may be several recurrences, each being shorter and milder than the previous.

The end of each episode is associated with the clearance of the spirochaetes from the blood by antibodies, and each recurrence indicates that a new strain has appeared on which the previously produced antibodies have no effect. The spirochaetes can be demonstrated on a stained blood film, on a microscope slide.

TREATMENT

The *Borrelia* spirochaetes are highly sensitive to a range of antibiotics, but treatment with these may be dangerous because the clearance of the organisms is often associated with a severe reaction similar to, but more acute than, that occurring at the end of each period of fever. This occurs particularly in louse-borne relapsing fever and is thought to be due to a release of toxins from the killed spirochaetes. The reaction may be fatal. Because of this, antibiotic treatment must be cautious, and a slow-release penicillin, giving a gradual reduction in the spirochaetes, is safest. Ticks can be killed by lindane applied to floors and across the thresholds of houses.

relaxant

Anything, but especially a drug, that induces muscle relaxation or relieves tension. Relaxant drugs are widely used in general anaesthesia so as to avoid the necessity for deep levels of unconsciousness. They include tubocurarine, **suxamethonium chloride** and **dantroline**. See **muscle-relaxant drugs**.

relaxation

Anxiety causes tensing of muscles, almost anywhere in the body and sustained tension causes symptoms. The process is not, however, one way only and ample experience shows that the release of tension in muscles can relieve anxiety.

Because of the intimate interrelationship between the state of the mind and the state of the muscles, the achievement of adequate relaxation is not easy, and practice, and even training, may be necessary. It is likely that voluntary relaxation of the muscles can only be achieved if there is a simultaneous relaxation of the mental processes. This may be why techniques such as Hatha Yoga or various forms of meditation have been more successful than methods based on attempts at purely muscular control. **Biofeedback** from the muscles is helpful and, again, the mental component is involved.

Relaxation is always safe, though not to be regarded as a universal or very powerful method of treatment. It may certainly be an aid to other forms of therapy, and is probably of value even to the healthiest of us.

Relifex

A brand name for **nabumetone**.

remedio

Latin root meaning 'remedy' as in remedial (causing recovery).

remifentanil

A narcotic painkiller used during the induction or maintenance of general anaesthesia. The use of painkillers during general anaesthesia is not, as it may seem, pointless. Painful stimuli act on the autonomic nervous system causing effects that can interfere with the smooth conduct of the anaesthetic and the post-operative period. A brand name is Ultiva.

remission

A reduction in the severity, or even a temporary disappearance, of the symptoms or signs of a disease.

REM sleep

Rapid eye movement **sleep**. REM sleep periods are those in which the eyeballs can be seen to be moving constantly behind the closed lids, the muscles twitch, dreaming occurs and, in men, the penis becomes erect. REM sleep occurs in periods totalling about 20 per cent of the sleeping time, and is necessary for health. Sleepers are hardest to wake during these periods, and if awakened will admit that they have been dreaming.

renal

Pertaining to the **kidneys**.

renal calculus

See **kidney stones**.

renal cell carcinoma

See **kidney cancer**.

renal colic

A severe, rhythmical pain in the loin usually caused by the spasmodic muscular efforts of the tube from the kidney to the bladder (the ureter) to force an obstructing body, such as a kidney stone (calculus), downwards. Renal colic may also be caused by blood clots in the ureter.

renal disorders

See **kidney disorders**.

renal failure

See **kidney disorders**.

renal transplant

See **kidney transplant**.

rene

Latin root meaning 'kidney' as in renal (of the kidney).

Renitec

A brand name for **enalapril**.

Reopro

A brand name for the drug **abciximab**.

reperfusion injury

The damage and loss of function that commonly occurs in the heart muscle when, after a heart attack, the flow of blood to the muscle is restored (reperfusion). This damage, which may severely add to the degree of muscle function loss, is generally agreed to be due mainly to the action of oxygen free radicals. These have been demonstrated to be present in large quantity during this phase of the heart attack. There is some evidence that antioxidant therapy with vitamins C and E can reduce the degree of damage.

The condition is also known as myocardial stunning.

repetitive strain injury

Initially, the condition explicitly, and by definition, excluded all disorders of known cause, but this led to many legal and other difficulties, and accounts now list numerous causes. RSI is, however, often stress-related and in many cases no muscular, tendon or neurological abnormality can be found, except that affected people often have raised thresholds for the appreciation of vibration. Changes in the proportions of the different types of muscle fibres and an increase in the number of muscle cell **mitochondria** have been described. The condition is usually managed by rest and rationed periods of work.

Replenine

A brand name for blood clotting **factor IX**.

reproductive system

The term genitalia usually refers to the external genitalia – the **labia** majora and minora and the **clitoris** of the female and the **penis** and scrotum of the male. Strictly speaking, however, the genitalia include all the organs of reproduction – the **ovaries**, **Fallopian tubes**, **womb** (uterus), **vagina** and external parts in the female; and the testicles (**testes**),

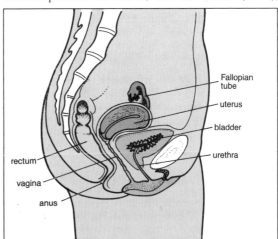

The organs of the female pelvis in section.

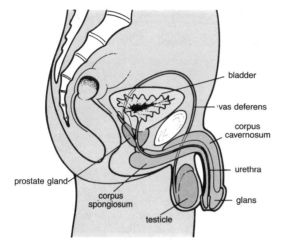

The male pelvic organs in section.

spermatic cord (including the vasa deferentes), the seminal vesicles, the **prostate gland** and the **penis**, in the male.

In the male the reproductive organs are closely associated with the urinary system and the same tube, the urethra, serves as a channel for both semen and urine.

reproterol

A **beta-adrenoceptor** stimulating drug used to treat **asthma**. A brand name is Bronchodil.

Requip

A brand name for **ropinirole**.

resection

Surgical removal of any part of the body or of diseased tissue.

resectoscope

A surgical instrument which is passed along the urine tube (urethra) in the penis and which allows both a view of the enlarged **prostate gland** and the means of removing the excess tissue. The resectoscope is essentially a cystoscope through which an electrically heated wire loop can be used, under direct supervision, to cut away redundant tissue and allow the free outflow of urine. The results are excellent and potency is seldom affected.

resorcinol

A drug used externally that softens and helps to remove the horny outer layer of the skin. A keratolytic drug. A brand name for a preparation containing resorcinol is Eskamel.

Resperidal

A brand name for **risperidone**.

respiration, Cheyne-Stokes

A type of periodic breathing which occurs in people with severe heart failure or brain damage or who are under the influence of narcotics. Cheyne-Stokes respiration often occurs in dying people. Breathing becomes shallower and then ceases for a period. After a few seconds, breathing is resumed and, with each breath, becomes deeper until it reaches a maximum then quickly decreases in depth until it stops. The cycle is then repeated indefinitely.

The phenomenon is due to a reduced sensitivity of the respiratory centre in the brain stem to the stimulus of carbon dioxide in the blood. This has to rise to a higher than normal level before breathing is stimulated, but when it is, the response is excessive.

respirator

A mechanical device used to maintain the breathing movements or the regular supply of oxygen to the lungs, in those incapable of breathing spontaneously, by reason of temporary or permanent paralysis.

HOW IT WORKS

Nowadays, almost all respirators are of the intermittent positive pressure type. In these, air or oxygen is blown into the lungs through a tube fitted tightly into the windpipe (trachea) through the nose, mouth or through a **tracheostomy** opening in the neck. The pressure is applied, intermittently, at the normal rate of breathing and, during release periods, the air is expelled from the lungs by the collapse caused by their normal elasticity.

Respirators of the iron lung or cuirass type are obsolete nowadays.

respiratory arrest

Cessation of breathing.

See *First Aid*.

respiratory distress syndrome

A condition of increased fluid in the lungs, so that the normal passage of oxygen into the blood is impeded, and the lungs become stiffer. The fluid in the lungs comes from the blood and may contain the clotting protein fibrinogen which encourages collapse of the air sacs, thereby further reducing the passage of oxygen to the blood.

POSSIBLE CAUSES

In newborn babies the respiratory distress syndrome may occur in those born before term whose lungs are immature and do not inflate fully after birth. This is the result of the deficiency of a substance known as a surfactant which acts as a kind of detergent, or wetting agent, to lower the surface tension of the fluid in the lungs.

In adults, the syndrome may be caused by any form of lung infection; by inhalation of irritant fluids such as vomit, or irritant gases such as chlorine, phosgene, ozone or smoke; by breathing high oxygen concentrations; by partial drowning; by narcotic overdose; by certain other drugs, such as nitrofurantoin; and by certain auto-immune disorders (see **auto-immune disease**).

RECOGNITION AND SYMPTOMS

Reduced oxygen in the blood prompts a reflex increase in the rate of breathing, but the increased stiffness of the lungs makes breathing much more difficult and the affected person is forced to make much stronger efforts to breathe than normal. The result is increasing distress. Fatigue of the muscles used for breathing leads to a worsening of the situation. Breathing becomes increasingly heavy and laboured, and the accessory respiratory muscles in the shoulders and neck have to be used. As the condition progresses, the skin becomes blue-tinged from deoxygenated blood (**cyanosis**) and when the muscular efforts fail, the level of carbon dioxide in the blood rises and, in the absence of effective treatment, death occurs.

TREATMENT

In the early stages, the administration of oxygen by mask can raise the blood oxygen levels and if the condition does not progress, this is all that is required. If the condition worsens, a tube must be passed into the windpipe (trachea), and sealed in place, and mechanical ventilation (see **ventilator**) used to force oxygen into the lungs and inflate the air sacs, so that the volume of the lungs actually increases. In some cases, sedation, or even deliberate paralysis by drugs, may be necessary so that spontaneous attempts at breathing do not interfere with the mechanical ventilation.

RISKS

The outcome depends on the severity of the condition and the effectiveness of treatment. In newborn babies, complications are common and the respiratory distress syndrome is still a common cause of death in premature babies.

respiratory system

Every cell in the body needs a constant supply of oxygen and it is important to understand how this is accomplished. The greater part of the chest cavity is occupied by the two lungs – paired, air-filled and expansile organs situated on each side of the heart, in which the blood takes up oxygen and gives off carbon dioxide and other unwanted gases. The respiratory system consists of the nose, the larynx, windpipe (trachea) and the lungs.

Air drawn in though the nose is warmed, moistened and cleaned. The inside of the nose is divided into two passages by a central plate (nasal septum) and is complicated by three pairs of internal plates, the turbinates, attached to the insides of the outer walls. These plates are covered with a moist and mucus-secreting membrane, and this conditions the air. The inspired air then passes down the throat (pharynx) and forward into the larynx. This is the 'Adam's apple' or voice box, situated at the upper end of the windpipe (trachea), and has, at its inlet, a sensitive and rapidly acting flap mechanism, the

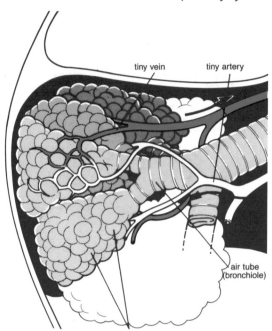

The air sacs (alveoli) through which oxygen passes into the blood and waste gases pass out.

epiglottis, which directs swallowed food into the gullet (oesophagus) and prevents it from entering the air passages.

The larynx extends from the throat to the top of the trachea. It has walls of cartilage and is lined with a moist mucous membrane. The vocal cords, situated in its upper region, are two folds of the mucous membrane, extending from the wall. Tiny muscles, in the cords and in the adjoining larynx, control the tension and rate of vibration of the cords as air passes through them. In normal breathing the vocal muscles remain loose, so that air can pass easily in and out. The tighter the vocal cords, the higher the pitch of the sound produced when we speak or sing. The gap between the folds is called the glottis.

The trachea and all the larger air tubes (bronchi) are supported and kept open by rings, or partial rings, of cartilage. As the size becomes less, these reinforcements are lost. The smaller, self-supporting air tubes are called bronchioles. The lining of the air tubes is covered with a specialized layer of cells bearing cilia (fine, motile hairs) and mucus-secreting goblet cells. The combination of mucus production and hair movement is essential to keep the air tubes clear. Fine particles of foreign material in the inspired air are trapped by the mucus and carried upwards, by the action of the cilia, into the larger passages from which they may be removed by coughing.

At each bronchial division, the area of the two branches is greater than that of the parent, and the branching is so profuse that when the air sacs (alveoli) are reached, the area available for gas exchange is very large. The terminal small bronchi (bronchioles) end in alveolar ducts and alveolar sacs, the latter bearing the many tiny alveoli. It is in these that the air comes into intimate contact with the blood and it is here that the interchange of gases occurs.

The lungs are rather like a pair of bellows, containing hundreds of thousands of alveoli all communicating, by means of this branching tree of tubes, with the nose and mouth and, through them, with the outside air. Between the chest and the

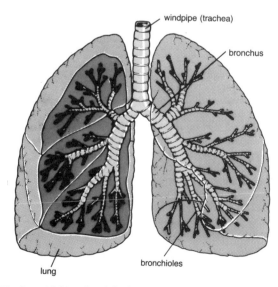

The bronchial 'tree' and the lungs.

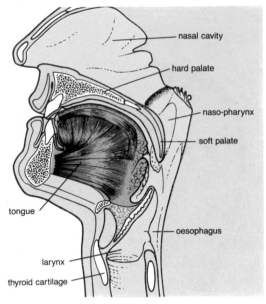

The mouth and nasal cavities, back of nose (naso-pharynx), throat (pharynx) and voice box (larynx).

Labels on diagram: nasal cavity, hard palate, naso-pharynx, soft palate, tongue, oesophagus, larynx, thyroid cartilage

abdomen is an upwardly domed sheet of muscle and tendon called the diaphragm. The chest cavity is air-tight and, by virtue of the way in which the ribs can spread outwards and upwards and the diaphragm can flatten downwards, the inside volume of this cavity is, during breathing, capable of great expansion. Because the lungs are elastic this increase in volume means that, during the expansion phase, new air will be sucked in to fill the tiny air sacs, only to be expelled again when the volume of the chest returns to normal.

Blood enters the lungs for two purposes – to supply the lung tissues with oxygen and nutrition in the normal way, and to recharge the haemoglobin with oxygen. Because of this, the lung receives a dual blood supply, the minor portion being by way of the bronchial arteries from the left side of the heart, and the major being the massive pulmonary circulation to which the right side of the heart is dedicated. The pulmonary arteries also form a tree-like structure, mirroring that of the bronchi, and end in capillaries which form a network around each alveolus.

The surfaces of the alveoli consist of little more than the walls of the blood capillaries so there is little hindrance to the passage of oxygen from the alveolar air spaces to the red blood cells and of waste gases from the blood to the air. The transfer of oxygen to the blood is an automatic process resulting from the higher concentration of oxygen in the air than in the blood.

The chemical properties of the haemoglobin in the red cells are also important. Haemoglobin will combine with oxygen or discard it, depending on whether it is in an environment of high or low oxygen level. Haemoglobin in red cells carried to the lungs, having been supplying the tissues of the body, is low in oxygen. In passing through the capillaries of the alveolar walls, it enters an environment of high oxygen tension and at once takes up the gas.

By a similar process, carbon dioxide and other gases, which are present in higher concentration in the lung blood than in the alveolar air, pass from the former to the latter.

Each lung is enclosed in a firmly adherent membrane called the visceral pleura. On each side, a separate layer of pleura, the parietal pleura, lines the inside of the chest wall, the sides of the central, solid zone of the chest (the mediastinum which contains the heart), and the upper surface of the diaphragm. The two layers of pleura are in close contact but the interface is lubricated with pleural fluid so that the lungs may slide freely during respiratory movement. The trachea and the bronchi are studded with lymph nodes which drain the tissues of the lungs.

respiratory tract infections

All of us are susceptible to infections of the respiratory tract, especially the upper part of the respiratory tract.

UPPER RESPIRATORY TRACT INFECTIONS

Doctors have to refer to these so often that they call them URTIs – upper respiratory tract infections. URTIs are usually caused by viruses and are seldom dangerous. They include the common cold (see **cold, common**), **tonsillitis**, sore throat (**pharyngitis**), **sinusitis**, **laryngitis** and **croup**.

Most URTIs lead to nasal congestion – oedema of the mucous membranes lining the nose and covering the internal nasal cartilages and bones (turbinates) – and this causes distress, mouth breathing and, in babies, difficulty in both breast- and bottle-feeding. Nasal catarrh, with mucus accumulation, will cause similar problems and these can be relieved by the judicious and sparing use of decongestants containing volatile oils.

> Decongestants containing drugs like ephedrine (sympathomimetic amines) should not be used in young children. They may be dangerous and the rebound effect leads to increased congestion.

TREATMENT OF UPPER RESPIRATORY TRACT INFECTIONS

Cough, which is a constant feature of URTIs, should not automatically be treated, as the cough is part of the defensive mechanism of the respiratory system. But tiring and distressing coughing may helpfully be relieved in children over one year, who are not otherwise unwell, by a mild antihistamine and soothing (demulcent) mixture. Antihistamine and sympathomimetic mixtures are helpful for older infants and may help to avoid middle ear infection (**otitis media**) which often follows Eustachian tube blockage from mucosal inflammation.

The widespread practice of treating URTIs with antibiotics is generally deplored by microbiologists who are justifiably alarmed that this will lead to a more rapid increase in antibiotic resistance than new antibiotics can be developed to deal with. On the other hand, streptococcal infections of the throat can lead to serious conditions such as **rheumatic fever** and **glomerulonephritis** and antibiotics, in such cases, are strongly indicated.

LOWER RESPIRATORY TRACT INFECTION

Lower respiratory tract infections are, in general, more serious. They affect the breathing tubes (trachea and bronchi) and the lungs, and include acute **bronchitis**, acute bronchiolitis and various kinds of **pneumonia**.

Respolin

A brand name for **salbutamol**.

Resprim

A brand name for cotrimoxazole.

rest

Ideas have changed, in recent decades, about the importance of bed rest for the sick. Clearly it is a comfort for the acutely ill, the fevered or the weak to be rested in a well-made bed, but it is now seen to be a mistake to infer from this that all those suffering from any disease, whatsoever, should automatically be so confined.

> It is now known that bed rest often does more harm than good. Prolonged rest is, in itself, harmful and it will take at least as long to recover from it as the period spent in bed.

Elderly people confined to bed may never recover their former state of vitality. Muscles weaken and lose bulk; bones decalcify and lose bulk (**osteoporosis**) and become more liable to fracture; pressure sores (**bedsores**) may develop; the efficiency of the heart declines; and there is a markedly increased tendency for clotting to occur in the large veins of the legs (deep vein thrombosis). The latter is especially common after surgical operations in the elderly. Vein thrombosis commonly leads to the formation, within the veins, of a loose, gelatinous and ever-lengthening snake-like blood clot which, initially attached at one end, may break loose and be carried up to the heart whence it is pumped to the lungs to cause a highly dangerous obstruction to one of the main arteries (pulmonary embolism). This is often fatal.

The body, at any age, is responsive to the physical demands made upon it, and its capacity for work will, within limits, adapt to these demands. Thus enforced bed rest, unless clinically necessary, is usually damaging and often leads to a notable decline in fitness.

Restandol

A brand name for **testosterone**.

restless legs

A condition associated with insomnia in which the legs ache and are constantly moved about in the attempt to achieve comfort. The cause is obscure but the condition is not dangerous and relief can be obtained by the use of the alpha adrenergic blocker drug tolazoline.

restriction fragment length polymorphism (RFLP)

Variations within a species in the lengths of fragments of **DNA** produced when a length of DNA is broken down into pieces by enzymes that cut it at recognized points (restriction enzymes). The variations from the normal are caused by mutations that either abolish the normal sites of breakage or create new ones, characteristic of the mutations. Analysis of RFLP is a valuable genetic tool and may allow genetic abnormalities to be detected, often before birth, even if the location of the mutated gene or genes is unknown.

resuscitation

See *First Aid*.

reteplase

A drug that dissolves blood clots. A fibrinolytic drug used in the early stages of a heart attack to try to restore patency to a coronary artery branch that has been blocked by a blood clot. A brand name is Rapilysin.

Retin-A

A brand name for **tretinoin**.

retina, disorders of

Many different disease processes may affect the retina and because of its essential role in vision, these are often serious. Modern methods of examination, by ophthalmoscopy, retinal photography and fluorescein angiography, have made precise diagnosis of many of these conditions possible, and many can now be successfully treated.

Any intrinsic disorder of retina is called a retinopathy. Retinal disorders include:

- diabetic retinopathy (see **retinopathy, diabetic**); retinopathy resulting from high blood pressure;
- **retinal detachment**, which is often associated with degeneration, thinning and hole formation and high degrees of short-sightedness (**myopia**);
- **macular degeneration** – a progressive spontaneous destruction of the central and most important part of the retina, which is regrettably common, and, in most cases of which, little can be done to halt the inexorable loss of central vision;
- colour perception, popularly called **colour blindness**, which is usually congenital and affects men far more often than women, but which may be acquired as a result of macular disease;
- pigmentosa;
- of prematurity, which results from exposure of the premature baby to excessive oxygen concentration and which causes abnormalities in the retinal vessels, the formation of blinding masses of fibrous tissue (**retrolental fibroplasia**), and retinal detachment;
- a highly malignant tumour affecting young babies;
- the worm infestation **toxocariasis**;
- actinic retinopathy, sometimes called eclipse blindness, which is a permanent burn of the macula occurring when the image of the sun is focused on the retina in the course of staring directly at it;
- retinopathy from drugs, such as the antituberculous drug ethambutol, the antimalarial and antirheumatoid drug chloroquine, or methyl alcohol;
- serous retinopathy, which usually affects young adults, causing depression or distortion of a small area of central vision in one or both eyes for a period of a few weeks.

retinal detachment

An accumulation of fluid under the retina with forward movement, separating it from the underlying nutritional layer (the choroid). The fluid accumulation is almost always the result of the development of a hole, break or tear in the retina, and this may be due to natural degeneration or to local traction on the retina by contracting strands in the vitreous gel.

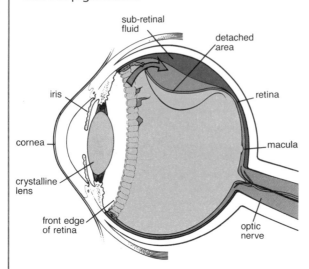

Retinal detachment most commonly follows the development of a hole in the retina through which fluid passes to accumulate under the retina and balloon it off. A retina separated from the choroid cannot function and must be re-flattened.

POSSIBLE CAUSES

Occasionally, retinal detachment occurs in the course of major injury to the eye, but the condition is usually spontaneous. It is commonest in very short-sighted people who often have thinned retinas with areas of degeneration. It is also common following cataract surgery, but improved methods of surgery have reduced this risk.

RECOGNITION AND SYMPTOMS

Retinal detachment is entirely painless and the only symptoms are disturbance of vision. Detachment is usually heralded by bright flashes of light as the sensitive membrane is stretched. These are seen usually at the periphery of the field .of vision, and are often accompanied by a shower of dark floating spots. These symptoms may be absent, and the affected person may be unaware that anything is amiss until the classic indication of retinal detachment occurs – the appearance as of a black curtain coming up, down or in from one sidè, to obscure vision. The curtain descends if the lower part of the retina is detaching, ascends with an upper retinal detachment, comes in from the right if the left part is detaching detachment, and from the left if the right side is detaching.

> Retinal detachment calls for urgent specialist attention before the central macula becomes detached, for once this has happened, normal central vision cannot be restored.

RISKS

When the field defect is above (lower detachment) the upright posture is safe, but if the field loss is below (upper detachment) or to the sides, there is a risk that the accumulating fluid will strip off the macula, and it is better to lie flat.

TREATMENT

Retinal holes and tears which threaten to cause detachment can be sealed and made safe with the ophthalmic laser, but established detachment almost always involves a surgical operation. The sclera overlying the detachment is indented with a tiny, soft silicone rubber sponge sewn in place on the outside. This causes the absorption of the sub-retinal fluid

and the retina settles back into place. Applications of extreme cold to the area (cryopexy) result in an inflammatory adhesiveness of the underlying tissues, so that the retina is fixed in place. If the macula has not been detached, the results are usually excellent.

retinitis pigmentosa

A slow degeneration of the rods and cones of the retinas of both eyes, starting at any time from adolescence to late middle age, and progressing to a variable degree. In some cases there is little disability, but in many the eventual loss of vision is profound. The condition usually has a genetic basis but spontaneous cases occur.

The first sign of the disease is defective night vision due to loss of function of the rods, which are necessary for vision in dim light. This observation usually leads to ophthalmic examination and the visual field test shows a ring-shaped area of loss, well out from, but surrounding, the point of regard. At first, this is narrow, but, over the years, it gradually extends, both outwards and inwards, to destroy an increasing area of the field. This ring *scotoma* corresponds to an area on each retina in which the retinal pigment, normally evenly distributed, has become clumped into scattered masses. Fortunately, central vision is retained, often for many years.

There is, as yet, no treatment for retinitis pigmentosa.

retinoblastoma

A tumour arising from the primitive cells which form the retina, some of which fail to develop normally and become malignant. It appears in the early years of life, usually before three years, affecting about one baby in 20,000, and often first shows itself as a visible whiteness in the pupil – the 'cat's eye' reflex. An eye affected in this way is usually blind and often develops a squint (**strabismus**). In about one-third of cases, both eyes contain the tumour.

Retinoblastoma may appear in more than one child in the same family and siblings should always be examined. It is a highly malignant tumour which can spread from the eye to the orbit and along the optic nerve to the brain. It may also spread to remote parts of the body. Because of its high malignancy, early removal of the affected eye is often advised. If the tumour is present in both eyes, radiotherapy is usually applied to the less severely affected eye.

> The occurrence, however uncommon, of retinoblastoma makes it imperative that every baby with squint should be carefully examined by an ophthalmologist.

retinoid drugs

A class of drugs related to vitamin A that act on the skin to cause drying and peeling and a reduction in oil (sebum) production. These effects can be useful in the treatment of acne, psoriasis, ichthyosis and other skin disorders. They are administered by mouth or applied as a cream. Possible side-effects are many and some are serious. They include severe fetal abnormalities (if taken by pregnant women), toxic effects on babies (if taken by breast-feeding mothers), liver and kidney damage, excessive drying, redness and itching of the skin, and muscle pain and stiffness. A brand name is Retin-A, Roaccutane.

retinopathy, diabetic

Diabetic retinopathy, which is now one of the commonest causes of blindness in the world, is a disease of small retinal blood vessels. Damage to these vessels causes blood leakage (haemorrhages) which may be small and confined to the retina, or which may extend forward into the jelly which fills the main cavity of the eye (the vitreous gel) with grave effects on vision.

The growth of fronds of new and fragile blood vessels on the surface of the retina, especially around the head of the optic nerve (the optic disc) is also a feature of this kind of retinopathy and these bleed readily. Haemorrhage into the vitreous gel may allow new blood vessels and fibrous tissue to grow forward into the gel, causing serious and permanent damage, including retinal detachment.

One of the important reasons for routine eye examinations is that if new vessel formation is detected early, it may be treated effectively, and the dangerous vessels dispersed, by applying multiple laser burns to the periphery of the retina.

Retinova

A brand name for **tretinoin**.

RET oncogene

A **proto-oncogene** on chromosome 10. Several mutations are known and all of them are associated with thyroid tumours. A number of children living in the Chernobyl region at the time of the power station disaster have been found to have rearrangements of the RET oncogene. Thyroid cancers, formerly very rare in children, are now occurring much more frequently than usual.

retractor

An instrument used to hold surgical incisions open or to keep tissue out of the way of the operator. A wide range of retractors, in a variety of sizes and designs, is needed in modern surgery, and few operations could proceed satisfactorily without them. Some retractors are double-bladed and have catches which hold them open. One of the chief duties of the surgical assistant is to maintain vigilant retraction so that the surgeon has continuous good access to the tissues being operated upon.

retro-

Prefix meaning 'backward, behind' as in retrosternal (behind the breastbone).

retrobulbar neuritis

Inflammation of the optic nerve, usually caused by the demyelinization process of **multiple sclerosis**. This is the local loss of the insulating fatty outer sheath of nerve fibres. Retrobulbar neuritis causes loss of the centre of the field of vision of the eye, usually for a period of about six weeks, but in most cases vision is restored. The condition may also be caused by infection in the adjacent sinuses.

retrolental fibroplasia

The most important feature of the retinopathy that may affect premature babies who have been treated with high oxygen concentrations after birth. It appears within a few weeks of birth. When such babies are incubated or treated for the **respiratory distress syndrome**, it is often necessary, as a life-saving measure, to provide them with oxygen at a concentration higher than atmospheric. The immature retinal tissues respond to this by closing off their blood vessels. When normal oxygen concentrations are resumed, these tissues now have an inadequate blood supply and bud out fronds of new vessels and strands of fibrous tissue. Fully mature tissues do not respond in this way to high oxygen concentrations.

The fibrous tissue may extend into the vitreous gel behind the lens, seriously interfering with vision and leading, later, to retinal detachment and other serious consequences. Research, mainly done in Japan, has suggested that early freezing treatment can prevent **retinal detachment** in this condition.

retrovirus

A virus with a **genome** consisting of one or two single strands of RNA from which duplex **DNA** is synthesized under the catalytic influence of an enzyme called **reverse transcriptase**. This is the reverse of the much more common DNA to **RNA** process. The **AIDS** virus HIV is a retrovirus. Special interest was aroused in the genetic community by the discovery of retroviruses and reverse transcriptase because Francis Crick, who, with James Watson, elucidated the structure of DNA in 1953, had propounded the rule, often described as the central dogma of genetics, that the direction of transcription was always from DNA to RNA and never in the opposite direction.

Rett syndrome

A serious brain disorder affecting only girls between the ages of nine months and three years. It causes a gradual loss of acquired skills, such as speech and walking; epileptic seizures; repetitive writhing (athetoid) movements; autism; and progressive disablement. These defects are caused by a significant reduction in the profusion of the interconnection between the brain cells in two layers of two regions of the brain near the surface (the cortex) concerned with the motor and some of the higher functions. The cause of Rett syndrome remains obscure, but it is thought to be the result of a fresh mutation rather than an inherited genetic defect.

Revanil

A brand name for lysuride.

reverse transcriptase

An enzyme that allows certain viruses, notable HIV, to synthesize double strand **DNA** from the virus's own single strand of RNA so that it can be incorporated into the genome of the host cell. It is called reverse transcriptase because its action operates in the reverse of the usual transcription direction, which is from DNA to **RNA**. Viruses of this kind are called retroviruses for the same reason. Some of the drugs used to treat AIDS are inhibitors of reverse transcriptase. These drugs, known as **reverse transcriptase inhibitors**, include lamivudine, stavudine, zalcitabine and zidovudine.

reverse transcriptase inhibitor

One of a range of drugs that interfere with the process by which retroviruses, such as **HIV**, convert their **RNA** genomes into duplex **DNA** which can then be incorporated into the DNA of the attacked cell. By delaying this process the progress of a retroviral infection can be slowed. Trade names are lamivudine, stavudine, zalcitabine and zidovudine.

reward deficiency syndrome

A name for a partial failure of the brain-reward, or satisfaction, mechanism. This is believed to be a feature of various conditions, such as **drug** and alcohol abuse, smoking, obesity, pathological gambling and **attention deficit hyperactivity disorder**, in which the subject seems to be unusually concerned to achieve reward. The syndrome results from a defect in the dopamine receptor gene which causes dysfunction of dopamine receptors. The gene is on chromosome 11 and has several known abnormal **alleles**. Variants (**mutations**) of the gene have been correlated with these and other reward-seeking behaviours.

Reye's syndrome

The serious condition that has resulted in the prohibition of **aspirin** to children suffering from viruses infections. Reye's syndrome is a disease of childhood in which swelling of the brain and a form of liver inflammation (**hepatitis**) occur following infection with one of several viruses including **chickenpox**, **influenza**, **rubella**, **herpes** simplex, and echovirus.

Because the skull prevents the brain from expanding, swelling rapidly interferes with brain function. The liver disorder is also severe and there is some reason to believe that the effect on the brain may be secondary to the liver damage. The rise in the level of liver enzymes in the blood, which is a characteristic of liver damage, may be extreme.

POSSIBLE CAUSES

The condition comes on just as the child is recovering from the virus infection and it is clearly related to viruses. But there is clear evidence that Reye's syndrome is also connected with aspirin-taking and this evidence is now so strong that the medical authorities in Britain and the United States have advised that children suspected of having chickenpox or influenza should not be given aspirin. Some have gone further and have recommended that aspirin should never be given to children. The British pharmaceutical industry appears to have accepted this advice, and paracetamol has replaced aspirin in paediatric painkillers.

RECOGNITION AND SYMPTOMS

Brain swelling causes uncontrollable vomiting, delirium and disorientation and rapid onset of stupor and coma. There are signs of increasing brain damage with local or general seizures, and the disorder may progress to deepening coma. In fatal cases, the average time between admission to hospital and death is four days.

TREATMENT

Treatment is directed at the control of brain swelling by steroids and withdrawal of fluid from the brain by the transfusion of strong sugar solutions into the blood. Artificial ventilation may be needed.

With increasing understanding of the condition and its management the death rate from Reye's syndrome has dropped from about 50 per cent to about 10 per cent. Some children, unfortunately, suffer residual brain damage.

rhesus factor disease

After the A, B, AB and O blood groups, the rhesus factor is the most important. The gene that makes a person rhesus positive is called D. This is present is 85 per cent of the population. The gene is dominant, so a person is rhesus positive even if only one of the gene pair is D. All the offspring of a rhesus-positive father with two D genes (homozygous) will be rhesus positive. If the father has only one D allele (heterozygous), each pregnancy will have a 50 per cent chance of producing a rhesus-positive baby.

HOW IT OCCURS

When a rhesus-positive father produces a rhesus-positive baby in a rhesus-negative mother, the baby's red blood cells will act as antigens capable of causing the mother to produce antibodies against them. These antigens do not normally reach the mother's blood until labour so they are unlikely to cause serious harm in the first pregnancy. But in subsequent pregnancies, the levels of these antibodies in the mother's blood rise rapidly and soon reach a point at which they are able to destroy the red cells of the fetus.

EFFECT ON THE FETUS

In the most severe cases, the fetus dies in the uterus, usually after the twenty-eighth week. If born alive, the child is deeply jaundiced with an enlarged liver and spleen and a low haemoglobin level in the blood. Excess haemoglobin in the blood leads to excess bile pigment (bilirubin) production and this has a much more serious effect than merely to stain the skin and cause jaundice. Bilirubin is very toxic to the brain, which becomes bile-stained (**kernicterus**) and leads to paralysis, spasticity, mental retardation and defects of sight and hearing.

A badly affected baby can have an exchange transfusion, via the umbilical cord, as soon as it is born, or even while still in the uterus. This corrects the anaemia and gets rid of the bilirubin. Exposure to intense blue light soon after birth assists in converting the bilirubin in the skin to a form which is harmless to the brain.

ANTI-D

Rhesus-negative women can be prevented from developing antibodies by being given an injection of anti-D gamma globulin within sixty hours of the birth of a rhesus-positive baby. In order to protect future babies, this is done in all such cases. Gamma globulin is also given when there has been an abortion or if there is any other reason to believe that rhesus-positive fetal blood may have gained access to the woman's circulation, as in obstetrical procedures like turning the baby (external version). The injection is given if an amniocentesis shows blood-stained amniotic fluid.

Rheumacin

A brand name for **indomethacin**.

rheumatic fever

In spite of the name, rheumatic fever does not seriously affect the joints, and, although **arthritis** does occur, this does not produce any permanent disability.

Rheumatic fever is important because of the frequency with which the heart is affected and because of the severity and permanence of the resulting damage. The nervous system may also be involved, causing 'Saint Vitus' dance' (Sydenham's chorea) which is a gradually progressive nervous system disorder, resulting from rheumatic inflammation, and featuring uncontrollable, jerky movements of the limbs and body and usually emotional upset.

INCIDENCE

Rheumatic fever is becoming steadily less common in developed countries where housing conditions have been improved and overcrowding reduced.

POSSIBLE CAUSES

The cause of the disease is unknown, but rheumatic fever always follows a throat infection with a particular strain of streptococcus – the Group A haemolytic strep. It is not caused by the normal processes of infection and is generally believed to be some form of **auto-immune disease** induced by streptococci. No positive proof of this has yet appeared. It can always be prevented by prompt treatment of the streptococcal throat infection with antibiotics. The avoidance of overcrowding and of other conditions promoting the spread of respiratory infection is also important in prevention.

RECOGNITION AND SYMPTOMS

According to an old medical students' maxim, rheumatic fever 'licks the joints and bites the heart'. There is fever and inflammation of one or more of the larger joints, with pain and swelling. As the symptoms settle in one joint they tend to start up in another. Sometimes several joints are affected at the same time. The heart involvement is often insidious and there may be no symptoms until a much later stage, when the heart is found to be damaged. The commonest and most serious effect on the heart is a fibrous thickening and scarring of the valves, with narrowing (stenosis) or leakage (incompetence). This may seriously interfere with the heart's action and cause severe secondary effects on the health of the affected person. Heart valve replacement may be necessary.

TREATMENT

Acute rheumatic fever is treated with bed rest, aspirin, sodium salicylate and corticosteroids, after antibiotics have been used to destroy any streptococci present. Children who have had rheumatic fever should be protected from further damage by long-term preventive penicillin, taken until they are about twenty years of age. Sydenham's chorea is helped by tranquillizer drugs and sedatives.

rheumatoid arthritis

A general disease of unknown cause that affects 1 to 3 per cent of the population. The usual age of onset is between thirty and forty, but the disease may start at any age and may even involve children (juvenile rheumatoid arthritis or Still's disease). Women are affected three times as often as men and about 16 per cent of the female population over sixty-five have the disease.

POSSIBLE CAUSES

The cause remains unclear, but there appears to be a genetic predisposition and an immunological disorder, probably triggered by an infection. No causal organisms have been identified, but all sufferers have antiglobulin antibodies circulating in their blood. These are called rheumatoid factors and are important in making the diagnosis. The great majority of people with swollen and painful joints do not have rheumatoid arthritis.

RECOGNITION AND SYMPTOMS

Rheumatoid arthritis causes joint deformities and disability as a result of a long-term destructive process affecting typically the small joints of the fingers and hands, but progressing to involve the wrists, elbows, shoulders and other joints. The finger joints near the palms of the hands are affected rather than those near the tips, and this causes a characteristic 'spindle-like' appearance. There is constant pain and spasm of the muscles and the latter contributes to the deformity. The fingers become deviated to the side of the little finger with tight bending of the joints near the tips and extension of those nearest the hand. Clawing of the toes and other foot distortion also occurs.

Rheumatoid arthritis does not only affect the joints. There is loss of appetite (anorexia) and weight, lethargy, muscle pain, the development of nodules under the skin, tendon inflammation, **bursitis**, and often eye inflammation, which may be severe and damaging. The condition may also be complicated by **pericarditis**, **vasculitis**, **anaemia** and Raynaud's phenomenon. **Sjogren's syndrome** with dryness of the mouth, eyes and genitalia is often associated with rheumatoid arthritis.

TREATMENT

As the cause is unknown, treatment is limited to control of inflammation and complications and the relief of pain. This may involve the use of drugs, rest, splinting, physiotherapy and even surgery. Corticosteroids can have dramatic effect, lasting for weeks or months, but can lead to further joint destruction and other important side-effects. Non-steroidal anti-inflammatory drugs are widely used, as is aspirin in large dosage for those who can tolerate it. The anti-malarial drug chloroquine can be valuable, but, in the dosage needed, may damage the retina unless monitored carefully. Penicillamine and gold are also widely used, but both have side-effects.

> The immunosuppressive drugs azathioprine, cyclophosphamide and methotrexate are used in severe cases. These are powerful drugs with potential dangers and must be carefully monitored.

The outcome in rheumatoid arthritis is very variable. About one-quarter of affected people enjoy full remission within ten years and 40 per cent suffer only moderate disability. About 10 per cent become severely disabled.

rheumatologist

A doctor engaged in the medical specialty concerned with the causes, pathology, diagnosis and treatment of diseases affecting the joints, muscles and connective tissue.

Rheumox

A brand name for **azapropazone**.

rhinitis

Inflammation of the mucous membrane lining of the nose. This causes swelling, so that the air flow is obstructed, and over-activity of the glands in the mucous membrane causing excessive mucus production and a watery discharge.

Rhinitis is a feature of the common cold and of **hay fever** (allergic rhinitis), which is not caused by hay, and is not a fever. It is an allergy to grass, weed and tree pollens, moulds, hair, feathers, skin scales (dander), house mites, house dust or other airborne substances. It causes sneezing, stuffiness and a watery nasal discharge.

Vasomotor rhinitis is an intermittent condition due to disturbance of the function of nerves controlling blood vessels that supply the mucous membrane. The membrane becomes over-responsive to stimuli, which may be psychological, hormonal or climatic, and there is sneezing and a watery discharge. It is common in immigrants from the tropics and in those taking oestrogens, including the oestrogen-progestogen contraceptive pill. It may be brought on by sexual arousal or eating highly spiced foods.

Hypertrophic rhinitis is the result of long-term inflammation or repeated infection. There is thickening and congestion of the lining and persistent symptoms. Atrophic rhinitis, in which there is shrinkage and loss of the mucous membrane, can result from sarcoidosis, **tuberculosis** or excessive surgery to the nose. There is dryness, crusting, loss of the sense of smell, and an unpleasant odour (ozaena) of which the affected person is often unaware.

Rhinolast

A brand name for **azelastine**.

rhinophyma

A form of **rosacea**, occurring almost exclusively in elderly men, in which the sebaceous and connective tissues in the skin of the nose become greatly overgrown so as to produce a bulbous deformity in which the enlarged openings of the skin pores are readily visible ('potato-nose'). Over-secretion of the sebaceous glands causes the skin to become oily, and wide dilation of small blood vessels produces permanent redness.

In spite of the grotesque appearance, rhinophyma is easily treated. Under anaesthesia, the redundant tissue is boldly pared away until the nose is reduced to an acceptable size and shape. Skin grafting is unnecessary as regeneration readily occurs from residual skin tissue and healing is rapid.

rhinoplasty

An operation to alter the structure of the nose for cosmetic reasons, either to correct a deformity caused by injury or disease or to improve the appearance of a healthy nose.

HOW IT'S DONE

The surgery is performed within the nose to avoid visible scarring. Under a general anaesthetic, incisions are made in the mucous membrane to uncover the wall of cartilage and bone that divides the nose into two cavities (the nasal septum). The cartilage is reshaped and surplus bone removed with a chisel or, if necessary, built up with bone grafts from elsewhere in the body. The new shape of the nose is retained with a plaster mould for about ten days.

rhinorrhea

Runny nose. This is usually due to the **rhinitis** of the common cold or to allergic or vasomotor rhinitis.

> Following a head injury, a persistent drip from the nose may be due to leakage of cerebrospinal fluid from the brain cavity, through a fracture in the thin plate of bone forming the roof of the nose. In such cases, measures to avoid **meningitis** are necessary.

rhinos

Greek root meaning 'horn or nose' as in **rhinitis** (nose inflammation).

rib fracture

Rib fractures are common, especially from direct violence, or in crushing injuries. They cause pain with a sharp catch on deep breathing, and overlying swelling and tenderness on light pressure. Fractured ribs show up readily on X-ray and the ends are seldom displaced, so immobilization is not required. Rarely, the sharp end of a fractured rib may penetrate a lung, causing it to collapse.

ribozyme

One of a unique class of **RNA** molecules that have the extraordinary property of being able to act as cleaving enzymes in addition to storing genetic information. This is a notable exception to the general rule that all enzymes are proteins. Ribozymes form complementary base pairs in the normal manner but can cleave segments of nascent RNA during the splicing process of the formation of mature RNA transcripts of **DNA**. They can be used in various ways as treatment modalities.

Because enzymes play such a large and fundamental part in all living systems, the discovery that simple non-protein molecules could act as enzymes excited great interest, especially among scientists concerned to elucidate the processes by which life originated on earth.

ribs

In the chest area, the vertebrae of the spinal column provide attachment for the twelve pairs of ribs, and most of these connect to the breast bone (sternum) in front, thus forming the chest bony wall (thoracic, or rib, cage). The articulation of the ribs with the spine (vertebral column) behind, and the breast bone in front, their shape, and the way each is suspended by a muscle from the one above, results in a considerable increase in the internal volume of the rib cage when the muscles between the ribs (intercostal muscles) contract.

The upper seven pairs of ribs are attached by flexible cartilages to the sternum. The next three pairs, known as false ribs, are each connected by cartilage to the pair of ribs above. And the last two pairs, known as the floating ribs, are shorter and are not attached at the front. Occasionally, there is an

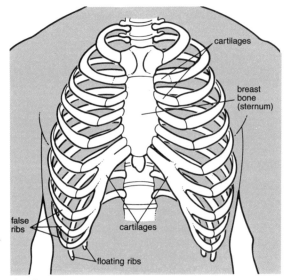

cartilages

breast bone (sternum)

false ribs

cartilages

floating ribs

The rib cage.

extra pair of ribs, lying above the normal top pair. These cervical ribs may cause problems by compressing nerves or arteries running into the arm.

rickets

A disorder affecting body calcium and phosphorus, mainly involving the bones, and caused by a deficiency of vitamin D. This vitamin is necessary for the absorption of calcium from the intestine. Vitamin D (calciferol) is a fat-soluble vitamin found in dairy products and fish oils. Vitamin precursors in the diet are also converted to vitamin D by the action of sunlight on the skin, and poorly nourished children, such as vegans, who are also deprived of sunlight are more likely to be affected.

RECOGNITION AND SYMPTOMS

Rickets involves diminished deposition of calcium in the bones and a consequent weakening and softening. The result may be bowing of the legs, a pigeon breast deformity, curvature of the spine, an increased tendency to bone fracture and softening, and squaring off and flattening of the skull. There is delay in the eruption of teeth and softening of the enamel after eruption.

TREATMENT

Rickets is treated by adequate, but not excessive, doses of vitamin D and plenty of calcium-containing food, such as milk.

rickettsia

A type of micro-organism, spread by ticks and small insects, and causing **typhus**, **Q fever**, and **Rocky Mountain spotted fever**.

Ridaura

A brand name for **auranofin**.

rifabutin

A drug used to treat tuberculosis of the lungs and to prevent the development of lung TB in **AIDS** patients. A brand name is Mycobutin.

Rifadin

A brand name for **rifampicin**.

rifampicin

An antibiotic drug used mainly to treat **tuberculosis** and leprosy (**Hansen's Disease**), but also **Legionnaires' disease**, prostatitis, **endocarditis** and **osteomyelitis**. Rifampicin acts by inhibiting transcription of bacterial nucleic acid. It interferes with the action of oral contraceptives. Trade names are Rifadin and Rimactane.

Rifater

A brand name for a formulation of **rifampicin** and **isoniazid**.

Rifinah

A brand name for a formulation of **rifampicin** and **isoniazid**.

rigor

A powerful attack of shivering caused by a rapid rise of fever.

rigor mortis

The stiffening of muscles which occurs after death. When the supply of blood stops, the glucose in the muscles is reduced to lactic acid and this causes the muscle plasma to coagulate and the muscles to lose their elasticity. Strenuous exercise before death causes an increase in muscle lactic acid and hastens the onset of rigor mortis.

On average, rigor starts three to four hours after death and reaches a maximum within twenty-four hours, usually after about twelve hours. But during this time, enzymes are starting to work to break down and soften the muscles and the stiffness gradually lessens over the next two to three days.

A number of factors, especially the effect of environmental temperature on the temperature of the body, affects the timing of these biochemical changes and these factors must be taken into account if the state of rigor mortis is being used to help in establishing the time of death for medicolegal purposes.

riluzole

An antiglutamate drug used to slow the rate of progress and prolong life in **amyotrophic lateral sclerosis**. A brand name is Rilutek.

Rimactane

A brand name for **rifampicin**.

Rimactazid

A brand name for a formulation of **rifampicin** and **isoniazid**.

rimexolone

A steroidal anti-inflammatory drug formulated in eyedrops for the relief of post-operative eye inflammation and other inflammatory eye disorders. Rimexolone is claimed to be less likely to raise the intraocular pressure than other steroid eyedrops. As in the case of other steroids, it should not be used in virus infections. A brand name is Vexol.

rimiterol

A **bronchodilator** drug used in the treatment of **asthma** and **bronchitis**. A brand name is Pulmadil.

Rimso-50

A brand name for a solution of **dimethylsulfoxide** (DMSO).

Rinatec

A brand name for **ipratropium bromide**.

ringing in the ears

See **tinnitus**.

ringworm

See **dermatophytosis**.

Rinstead

A brand name for **chloroxylenol**.

risperidone

A benzisoxazole antipsychotic drug used to treat **schizophrenia** and other psychotic disorders. The drug acts by interfering with serotonin and dopamine receptors. A brand name is Resperidal.

Ritalin

A brand name for **methylphenidate**.

ritodrine

A drug that relaxes the muscles of the womb and is used to prevent onset of premature labour. A brand name is Yutopar.

ritonavir

A **protease inhibitor** drug used in combination with other drugs to treat **AIDS**. A brand name is Norvir.

rituximab

A genetically-engineered monoclonal antibody used to treat non-Hodgkin's lymphomas. A brand name is **Mabthera**.

rivastigmine

An acetylcholinesterase inhibitor drug used to treat early **Alzheimer's** dementia.

river blindness

The popular term for the disease **onchocerciasis**, so called because the disease is spread by a species of biting black fly found only in fast-flowing water.

Rivotril

A brand name for **clonazepam**.

rizatripan

A selective serotonin agonist that narrows intracranial arteries widened in migraine. A brand name is Maxalt.

RNA

Ribonucleic acid. RNA may be a double chain like deoxyribonucleic acid (DNA), but in the cell RNA usually exists as a single chain of **nucleotides**, like one strand of the double helix of DNA. RNA carries coded instructions, derived from the genetic code in DNA, for the synthesis of specific proteins from **amino acids**. Whereas in most cells DNA carries the permanent, inheritable code for cell reproduction, RNA most commonly acts as a transcriber or as **messenger RNA** (mRNA), carrying the code within the cell to the ribosomes where proteins are actually formed. In some viruses, however, the inherited code for replication occurs in the form of RNA.

Transfer RNA (tRNA) picks up and carries amino acids to the ribosomes to be inserted in the correct sequence of the protein. Ribosomes contain ribosomal RNA (rRNA) and proteins. RNA polymerase is an enzyme that catalyses the joining of appropriate nucleotides to form a molecule of RNA, using DNA as a template. RNA replicase is another enzyme that catalyses the synthesis of RNA, using RNA as a template. This enzyme is used by RNA viruses for the replication of their **genome** within a cell.

Roaccutane

A brand name for **isotretinoin**.

Robaxin

A brand name for **methocarbamol**.

Robertson's sign of malingering

The pupils will normally widen if a sudden pain is experienced. The absence of this normal reaction when pressure is exerted over an area alleged to be tender or painful is known as Robertson's sign of malingering. This sign, on its own, would not be considered final proof.

Robinul

A brand name for **glycopyrronium bromide**.

Robinul neostigmine

A brand name for **glycopyrronium bromide** compounded with **neostigmine**.

robot surgery

A technology, currently in its infancy, to use robotic devices in surgery, based on those currently in wide use in automobile manufacture. Some devices have been used to perform some of the simpler functions in surgery, and they promise to improve the precision and ease of surgery. Robotic arms have been used to replace surgical assistants holding retractors, and m ore advanced devices are in the experimental stage.

Rocatrol

A brand name for calcitriol.

Rocephin

A brand name for **ceftriaxone**.

Rocky Mountain spotted fever

An acute infectious disease, sometimes called 'tick typhus', which is caused by the organism *Rickettsia rickettsii*, and transmitted to man by the bite of certain species of hard ticks (*Ixodid* ticks) from a reservoir of infection in small rodents and dogs. The disease occurs in southeastern USA and South America and is becoming progressively more common.

RECOGNITION AND SYMPTOMS

Symptoms start about a week after the tick bite. There is fever, loss of appetite, irritability and headache, and the attack may be so mild that the affected person remains up and about. In some cases, however, symptoms come on suddenly and with great severity and there may be prostration, severe headache, severe aching and tenderness in the muscles, nausea and vomiting. Widespread haemorrhages and **gangrene** of the fingers, ears or genitalia may occur. In severe cases, especially if the fever is very high, death may occur within a week of onset. More often, however, the fever remains high for about two weeks and then subsides.

Two to six days after onset, a rash appears, first on the wrists and ankles and then spreading all over the body. Initially, the rash consists of small, round, pink, slightly raised spots, but these soon become darker, purplish and then haemorrhagic. The rash begins to fade when the fever settles, but may take some weeks to disappear altogether.

TREATMENT

A suspicion of the correct diagnosis may be critically important, because, although many of the commonly used antibiotics, such as penicillin, streptomycin, garamycin, and cephalosporin, have no effect on the disease, early treatment with chloramphenicol or a tetracycline antibiotic may be life-saving. Prompt use is essential and usually cures the disease within a few days with few complications.

> Delayed diagnosis in severe cases is dangerous, as major life-threatening complications may arise very quickly.

rocuronium bromide

A non-**depolarizing** muscle relaxant drug used in general anaesthesia. A brand name is Esmeron.

rodent ulcer

Referred to, medically, as a basal cell carcinoma, this is one of the commonest of all cancers and one of the least dangerous. It affects the skin, mainly in areas exposed to the sun, and especially on the nose and around the eyes. It is a slowly growing, raised-edged swelling, with a dimple in the centre and often with small blood vessels visible below the surface. Although the tumour can, if neglected, spread widely, causing extensive tissue damage, it hardly ever shows the feature, common to almost all other cancers, of seeding off tumour cells and thus spreading to remote parts of the body.

The diagnosis of rodent ulcer is confirmed by **biopsy**. The tumour can be treated by direct surgical removal, by radiation, or by freezing. The method advised is likely to depend on whether the patient has been seen by a surgeon or by a dermatologist, but, in good hands, all are equally effective.

Roferon-A

A brand name for **interferon alfa**.

Rogitine

A brand name for **phentolamine**.

Rohypnol

A brand name for **flunitrazepam**.

Romberg's sign

A normal person, asked to stand upright with the feet together, the arms outstretched and the eyes closed, will not show any strong tendency to sway or fall over when given a gentle push. If the person sways, tends to fall, or opens the eyes and spreads the feet, this suggests a defect of the position sense resulting from disease of the nervous system or the inner ear balancing mechanism. Such a reaction is known as Romberg's sign.

Ronicol

A brand name for **nicotinyl alcohol tartrate**.

ropinirole

A drug with dopamine-like action used to treat **Parkinson's disease**. A brand name is Requip.

ropivacaine

An aminoamide local anaesthetic drug similar to **bupivacaine** but with a less toxic effect on the heart and a reduced tendency to block the function of motor nerves. A brand name is Naropin.

Rorschach test

See **ink blot test**.

rosacea

A blushing skin disorder of unknown cause, featuring redness, myriads of tiny dilated blood vessels and acne-like pustules on the central areas of the face and forehead. It affects especially the nose, which may become thickened, red, pitted and oily. Rosacea affects both sexes in middle age and later life and may be complicated by inflammation of the conjunctivas of the eyes and by the growth of blood vessels into the corneas. In men, the condition of **rhinophyma** may develop.

RECOGNITION AND SYMPTOMS

The disorder involves both the facial blood vessels and the sebaceous glands of the skin. There is a ready tendency to blush and the affected area becomes gradually redder with progressive widening (dilatation) and irregularity of the blood vessels of the skin.

TREATMENT

Rosacea persists for years, but may be kept under control, as may the eye complications, by a small daily dose of the antibiotic tetracycline. It should not be inferred from this that rosacea is an infection. The action of the drug is not well understood, but its effectiveness is unquestioned. Steroids, however, make the condition worse and should be avoided, as should unnecessary exposure to sunlight and wind. Circumstances which cause blushing should, if possible, be avoided. Rosacea is not associated with any general disease and is not made worse by alcohol. It is not hereditary.

rose Bengal

A biological stain that can be applied to the cornea as eye drops to reveal subtle damage to the outer layer (epithelium). A brand name is Minims Rose Bengal.

roseola infantum

A common but transient disorder of unknown cause, which affects toddlers. No virus has been isolated, but the disease has been transmitted by filtered blood. It is sometimes called 'sixth disease' or *exanthem subitum*. There is high fever for three days, sometimes starting with a convulsion, lymph-node enlargement, general upset and, after two or three days as the fever settles, a pink rash resembling that of **rubella**. This is present only for a short time and may easily be missed. Roseola is almost always harmless and complete recovery is the rule.

rotator cuff injury

The rotator cuff is the tendinous structure around the shoulder joint comprising the tendons of four nearby muscles. These tendons blend with the fibrous capsule of the joint and provide additional support during movement of the shoulder.

Injury to the rotator cuff of tendons may result from a fall. It is more common in the elderly when these tendons have worn a little. A partial tear may cause pain when the arm is moved away from the body (abduction) at a particular angle. A complete tear may prevent abduction altogether, although other shoulder muscles usually compensate by tilting the shoulder blade (scapula) and allowing some outward movement. If a complete tear causes severe disability, surgical repair by stitching (suturing) may be required.

roundworms

Roundworms, a form of *nematode*, are common human intestinal parasites. The common roundworm, *Ascaris lumbricoides*, has a life span of about a year and inhabits the small intestine. The females pass eggs in the faeces and, under suitable conditions, as in moist soil, these can survive for three years or more. Crops or hands are commonly contaminated by eggs, and eggs may occasionally be transmitted by dust or paper money.

Ingested eggs hatch in the small intestine and the larvae penetrate the bowel lining and are carried in the blood to the lungs where, after two moults, on the sixth and tenth days, they migrate up the air passages to the pharynx and are swallowed. During this migration the larvae are growing rapidly. On return to the small intestine, they mature into adult worms and start copulating.

INCIDENCE
So many people are infested that the human parasitic roundworm population of the world must greatly exceed the human population. It is estimated that 98 per cent of people either have a nematode infestation or have had one at some time.

RECOGNITION AND SYMPTOMS
The commonest symptoms are abdominal discomfort and pain, nausea, vomiting, irritability, loss of appetite and disturbed sleep. These symptoms occur only if more than a few worms are present. In heavy infestations, of 500 to 1500 worms, pneumonia or obstruction of the bowel may result.

TREATMENT
Roundworms are easily disposed of by means of the drugs piperazine, levamisole or mebendazole, but unless social conditions are improved, re-infestation is inevitable.

See also **ascariasis**.

Rowatinex

A brand name for a mixture of the essential oils camphene, pinenes, borneol, fenchone, anethol and cineole used to treat urinary stones.

Royal Society of Medicine

A unique British medical society, founded in 1805, of which full Fellowship is available to all registered medical, dental and veterinary practitioners. The RSM is independent of government or of any university. It does not train medical students or award degrees but it is deeply concerned with post-graduate medical education. It contains 40 specialty sections covering all disciplines, each with a distinguished consultant as President, and holds 400 meetings each year. Fellows have the right to attend any meeting in any discipline.

The Society, through the RSM Press, publishes a wide range of medical books, journals, distance-learning materials and CD-ROMs. The premises are at 1 Wimpole Street, London where, among other facilities, the largest medical library in Britain – and one of the largest postgraduate medical libraries in Europe – is to be found.

Rozex

A brand name for **metronidazole** formulated for external use only.

-rrhoea

Suffix meaning 'flowing' as in diarrhoea (flowing through).

rubella

German measles. This infectious disease is caused by a virus which infects the respiratory tract and, during a long incubation period of up to three weeks, multiplies and spreads to local lymph nodes, especially those in the back of the neck.

RECOGNITION AND SYMPTOMS
There is a mild illness, swollen nodes and a scattered rash of slightly raised red patches where the virus has settled in the skin. The disease is so mild that it often passes unnoticed. In adults, the virus sometimes attacks the joints causing an arthritis which may occasionally become persistent (chronic). The natural infection produces lifelong immunity.

PREVENTION
Immunization against rubella could eliminate this disease. All seronegative people of childbearing age should be vaccinated, but vaccination should never be done during pregnancy as it is thought possible that the vaccine can affect the fetus. If there is a risk of pregnancy, effective contraception should be used for three months after vaccination.

> The chief importance of rubella is that, in pregnant women, viruses circulating in the blood can localize in the placenta and infect the fetus. Until this fact was known, rubella was a major cause of congenital heart disease and other malformations, blindness, deafness and mental retardation. The fetus is especially susceptible to the toxic effects of the virus during the first three months of pregnancy and if the virus is circulating at the time that the brain, the eyes, the ears and the heart are undergoing their early development, serious effects are likely. In the combined results of five separate studies, the incidence of congenital defects, when rubella occurred during the first month, was 50 per cent; during the second month, 25 per cent; during the third, 17 per cent; during the fourth, 6 per cent; and after the fourth month, less than 2 per cent.

ruga

Latin root meaning 'wrinkle' as in rugose (wrinkled).

rupture

A popular term for **hernia**.

Rynacrom

A brand name for **sodium cromoglycate**.

Rythmodan

A brand name for **disopyramide**.

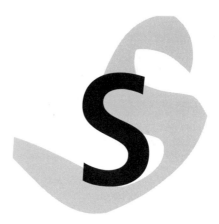

Sabril

A brand name for **vigabatrin**.

sadism

An aggressive sexual abnormality in which pleasure and sexual excitement are derived from the infliction, or contemplation, of physical or mental pain. The term is derived from the name of the French soldier and writer, the Marquis de Sade (1740–1814), who wrote pornographic accounts of sexual tortures coupled with pseudo-philosophic justifications, and who died in a madhouse.

POSSIBLE CAUSES

The causes of sadism vary and include an inability to cope with feelings of disgust or shame associated with sex, normally repressed hostility towards parents or others in authority, a strong feeling of inferiority, and a distorted macho image of the male-female relationship.

In sadomasochism, sexual arousal is also caused by submitting to physical or mental abuse. The term masochism derives from the name of the Austrian lawyer Chevalier Leopold von Sacher-Masoch (1836–95) who wrote at great length about the pleasure he gained from being subjugated and physically abused. In this deviation, the pain suffered may be minor – perhaps only a ritual humiliation – or may be severe, but usually the masochist retains control and can end the act before suffering serious injury. Sometimes one or both participants are carried away, with fatal results.

INCIDENCE

The sadomasochist is usually male and often has other sexual deviations, such as fetishism. Research suggests that up to about 5 per cent of men and 2 per cent of women have sadistic or sadomasochistic inclinations. The popularity of sadomasochistic video tape recordings, of which millions are watched every day, suggests that these leanings may be more widespread than this. Prior to the video revolution, sadomasochistic literature was extensively read.

SADS

Seasonal Affective Disorder Syndrome (SADS) is a postulated disorder in which the mood of the affected person changes according to the season of the year. Typically, with the onset of winter, there is depression, general slowing of mind and body, excessive sleeping and overeating. These symptoms resolve with the coming of spring. The phenomenon may partly account for the known seasonal variation in suicide rates.

SADS is not yet generally accepted and the prevalence is unknown. There is, however, evidence that mood is related to light, which suppresses the release of the hormone melatonin from the pineal gland. Exposure to additional lights during the day is said sometimes to relieve symptoms.

saeta

Latin root meaning 'bristle' as in setal (bristly).

safe sex

Measures taken to try to minimize the risk of sexually transmitted disease, especially **AIDS**. These include the avoidance of promiscuity, fidelity to the partner, the use of condoms, non-penetrative sexual activity and avoidance of contact with body fluids such as blood, genital secretions and saliva. It is worth bearing in mind that, since late 1999, the majority of HIV infections in Britain have resulted from heterosexual, rather than homosexual, intercourse. It is also notable that the incidence of gonorrhoea in London rose by 30 per cent in the last three years of the 20th century.

Saizen

A brand name for **somatotropin**.

Salagen

A brand name for **pilocarpine**.

Salamol Steri-Neb

A brand name for **salbutamol**.

Salazopyrin

A brand name for the drug **sulphasalazine** used to treat **rheumatoid arthritis**, **ulcerative colitis** and **Crohn's disease**.

Salbulin

A brand name for **salbutamol**.

salbutamol

A **bronchodilator** drug used to treat **asthma**, chronic **bronchitis** and **emphysema**. It is also sometimes used to relax the muscle of the womb and prevent premature labour. Trade names are Aerolin Autohaler, Airomir, Asmasal, Salamol Steri-Neb, Ventmax SR, Ventodisks, Ventolin and Volumax.

salicylates

A group of anti-inflammatory, mildly **analgesic** and fever-reducing (antipyretic) drugs that includes aspirin, sodium salicylate and **benorylate**.

salicylic acid

A drug that softens and loosens the horny outer layer of the skin (the epidermis) and is used in the treatment of various skin disorders such as **acne**, **psoriasis**, **ichthyosis**, **warts** and **callosities**. Trade names are Acnisal, Occlusal, Pyravlex and Verugon. Numerous skin preparations contain salicyclic acid in conjunction with other ingredients.

Saliva Orthana

A brand name for a **mucin** preparation.

salivary glands

The processing of food starts with the cutting and grinding action of the teeth, the lubrication of food with saliva and the beginning of its biochemical breakdown with the action of the first enzyme. Food meets a variety of digestive enzymes on its way down the intestinal tract, and although these act on different types of food, they all act in much the same way, to break the food down, chemically, to simpler materials.

There are three pairs of salivary glands. These open into the mouth, and provide a fluid to clean the mouth, lubricate chewing, and moisten the mucous membranes. Saliva contains the digestive enzyme amylase, which starts the process of breaking down the carbohydrate starch in the food. The paired salivary glands are the parotids, the sublinguals and the submandibular glands. The parotid glands lie in the cheeks, just in front of, and below, the ears and their ducts open on the inside of the cheeks opposite the molar teeth. The sublingual glands are in the floor of the mouth, and discharge though openings near the lower front teeth. The submandibular glands are situated in the neck and discharge into the mouth at the base of the tongue. Salivation is under the control of the autonomic nervous system.

salivation

The production of saliva by the six **salivary glands** that open into the mouth.

salmeterol

An adrenaline-like drug used to treat **asthma**. A brand name is Serevent.

Salmonella

A genus of rod-shaped bacteria, of which over 1500 species have been identified. There are over 700 different species known to cause food poisoning and these may infect the intestines of poultry – especially chickens and turkeys – pigs, cattle, dogs, tortoises, terrapins and other animals. The organism may be present in processed domestic pet food.

Salmonella organisms are responsible for a variety of human diseases, including typhoid and paratyphoid fevers, gastroenteritis and food poisoning. Common contaminants of food include *Salmonella typhimurium*, *S. hadar*, *S. enteritidis*, and *S. virchow*. *Salmonella dublin* is especially associated with cattle.

Salmonella agona was imported into Britain from Peru in the late 1970s in fishmeal chicken feed and rapidly became a major cause of Salmonella gastroenteritis in Britain.

> After an attack of Salmonella gastroenteritis, the person concerned usually excretes the organisms in the faeces for six weeks or longer and, if careless of personal hygiene, will transmit the infection to others. Food handlers are especially dangerous.

Salmonella gastroenteritis has become very common in modern industrial societies largely because of developments in the food industries, especially in relation to mass production and poultry feeding methods. Salmonella are frequently present in poultry, meat, sausages and eggs.

> Inadequate kitchen hygiene, inadequate thawing of frozen food before cooking and inadequate cooking all contribute to outbreaks of gastroenteritis.

Salofalk

A brand name for **mesalazine**.

salt

Common salt, sodium chloride (NaCl), is important in the body in maintaining the tendency of the blood to take up water. The electrically charged sodium and chloride ions, into which the compound dissociates when dissolved in water, also play a major role in initiating and transmitting impulses along nerves. Excessive dietary salt intake can cause fluid retention (oedema) and may contribute to high blood pressure (hypertension). Loss of salt from excess sweating and inadequate intake can cause heat exhaustion.

See *First Aid*.

salve

A popular, and old-fashioned, term for an ointment or lotion intended to soothe and heal. Modern skin medications are, or should be, prescribed with more specific intent once an accurate diagnosis has been made.

Sabril

A brand name for **vigabatrin**.

Sandimmun

A brand name for cyclosporin.

Sandocal

A brand name for a calcium preparation.

Sandostatin

A brand name for **octreotide**.

Sandrena

A brand name for **oestradiol**.

sanguine

Latin root meaning 'blood' as in sanguinary (bloody).

sanitary protection

Sanitary protection is the use of anything that will contain the menstrual flow and prevent bloodstaining of clothing. Historically, women have had to use rags or other absorbent material which could be washed and re-used. The need is so great that major commercial pressures are now involved in what is a multi-million pound industry. Present methods are to employ various designs of disposable sanitary pad for external use or compressed tampons that are inserted into the **vagina**. Due attention is paid to the varying requirements needed to cope with heavy, moderate or light bleeding. On average, ten to fifteen tampons or pads are required for each period, but the range is wide. There have been considerable improvement in the design of pads and tampons in recent years, driven largely by competitive market forces.

PADS

The trend in external pads today is for a slim-line design of layered structure using various materials of suitable absorptive power in a layered structure and with a waterproof cover. Artificial cotton wool and absorptive paper are commonly used, enclosed in a surrounding layer of fabric. A major advance in design and function was achieved with the idea of using a fine polyacrylate powder to absorb and retain fluid. These self-adhesive or winged pads are intended to fit securely into close-fitting underpants. Thick pads are still used in many maternity units and are preferred by some women. Thick pads can chafe the inner thighs, and are conspicuous under tight-fitting clothing. Pads, of whatever type, must be changed every four to six hours or bacterial action on the blood causes them to become offensive.

TAMPONS

Tampons are also made from absorbent fibrous material and are of a generally cylindrical shape. Some of them are compressed into a tubular container so designed that after insertion of the container into the vagina, the tampon can be released. Others are moulded so as to have a rounded point at one end to facilitate insertion. Because a forgotten tampon can cause infection it is important that they should be easy to remove (see below). In most, a string tail is attached to act as a reminder and facilitate removal. Tampons have the advantage of being entirely inconspicuous.

Tampons can be used by women who have not had sexual intercourse, but some virgins may find insertion difficult because of a tight or rigid hymen. Tampons are probably the preferred method of sanitary protection in women prone to thrush, because this infection thrives in the moist environment encouraged by a pad. Not infrequently, a tampon is accidentally left in the vagina at the end of a period. This may be a cause of **vaginal discharge**.

> Heavy staphylococcal infection of tampons is one of the causes of the dangerous toxic shock syndrome. For this reason manufacturers have been discouraged from making very highly absorbent tampons.

sanitate

Latin root meaning 'health' as in sanitation (study of health preservation).

Sanomigran

A brand name for **pizotifen**.

saquinavir

A **protease inhibitor** drug used in conjunction with other anti-HIV drugs to treat **AIDS**. Saquinavir acts by blocking the enzyme aspartic protease, so preventing the cleavage of gag and gag-pol polyproteins into functional proteins. The result is the production of immature and non-infectious viral particles. A brand name is Invirase.

sarcos

Greek root meaning 'flesh' as in sarcoma (hard cancer).

Saroten

A brand name for **amitriptyline**.

satyriasis

This is the male equivalent of **nymphomania** and is said to be manifested by an uncontrollable craving for sexual intercourse, without discrimination as to the sex, age, or even species, of the partner. As in the case of nymphomania, the condition is more likely to be a product of a disordered imagination than a disordered psyche, but both conditions are sometimes solemnly 'treated' by psychoanalysts.

Saventrine

A brand name for **isoprenaline**.

Saw-scaled viper venom

A snake venom with a powerful effect in inactivating the action of blood platelets in forming clots within the circulation. A synthetic drug tirofiban (Aggrastat) has been developed from this venom which has been shown to have a substantial advantage over the anticoagulant **heparin** in preventing heart attacks and deaths in cases of **unstable angina**.

scab

A crust formed on skin or mucous membrane when serum leaks from a damaged or infected area, becomes mixed with skin scales, pus, and other debris, and dries.

scabies

Infestation of the skin with the human mite parasite *Sarcoptes scabei*. This burrows in the skin, often on the hands or wrists, to lay eggs and feed on dead epidermal scales. Transmission is by direct close contact and scabies is often acquired by sexually promiscuous people. Scabies in one member of a family is likely to pass quickly to all the others.

The infestation causes intense itching and promotes constant

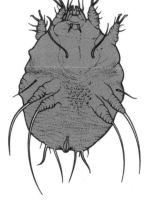

This illustration shows, greatly magnified, the Sarcoptes scabei mite that causes human scabies and mange in domestic animals. The short, strong forelegs end in digging claws by which the mite burrows into the skin.

scratching, with resultant damage to the skin and inoculation of the mite bodies, promoting severe local reaction. Treatment, with insecticide lotions, is highly effective, but all close contacts and all members of the family must be done at the same time.

scalpel

A surgical knife. Scalpels are used to cut any of the soft tissues of the body and are available in a wide variety of sizes and shapes appropriate to work of varying degrees of delicacy. At one extreme, they are used in the microsurgery of the middle ear and the eye and, at the other, in the amputation of a limb. Modern scalpels often consist of a handle to which can be fixed pre-sterilized, disposable blades supplied in sealed packs. These blades are intended to be used once only. In other cases, the scalpel has a cheap plastic handle and the whole knife is disposable. Most scalpel blades are made of high-quality, non-corrosive steel, but for certain purposes the superior sharpness possible with diamond or ruby blades makes the high cost of these justified. Diamond knives are commonly used in ophthalmic surgery.

In the pre-disposable era, scalpel blades were integral with the handle and had to be regularly sharpened by skilled cutlers.

scanner advance

See **spiral computed tomography**.

scaphoid fracture

The scaphoid, or navicular, bone, so called because of its resemblance to a boat, is one of the eight bones of the wrist – the outermost, on the thumb side, in the row nearest the body. It is a curved bone, narrower in proportion to its length than the other wrist bones and is readily fractured across its waist by a fall on the outstretched hand. This causes tenderness on the back of the wrist between the two tendons which extend the thumb.

Early scaphoid fractures often show up poorly on X-ray, and delay in treatment may result, sometimes with serious consequences, such as osteoarthritis and limitation of movement. Repeat X-rays are ordered by wary doctors, especially if wrist tenderness persists.

scapula

Latin root meaning 'shoulder blade' as in scapular (of the shoulder blade).

Schering PC4

A brand name for **ethinyloestradiol** formulated with **levonorgestrel** as an oral contraceptive.

schistosomiasis

A parasitic worm disease, formerly called bilharziasis, common in most tropical countries of the world. The schistosome trematode worms, or flukes, are so called because the body of the male worm splits longitudinally to form the gynaecophoric canal in which the female worm lies during copulation (Greek *schizo-* means 'split' and *soma* means 'body'). There are three species of schistosome worms, each with its own individual species of intermediate host water snail in which the larval forms develop. Each species also predominantly affects a particular part of the body. The worm eggs are excreted in the urine and faeces and, if water is contaminated, these pass to the snails.

RECOGNITION AND SYMPTOMS

The disease is acquired during immersion in water contaminated with the larval forms of the worms, released by the snails, which are able to penetrate the skin, causing a dermatitis in the process. The larvae travel to the bowel, the bladder, the liver and other organs, where they inhabit the veins and grow to adult size – 1–2.5 cm long – depositing eggs and causing bleeding into the urine or the faeces.

Late complications include fibrosis and loss of normal function of the bladder, persistent **cystitis**, bladder stones, cancer of the bladder, kidney failure and cirrhosis of the liver. The Far East species of schistosome, *Schistosoma japonicum*, can cause bowel and liver upset and, in some cases, involves the nervous system, producing epilepsy, blindness, spinal cord damage with paralysis, coma and death.

PREVENTION AND TREATMENT

Schistosomiasis is prevented by avoiding immersion in water which might possible be contaminated with human excreta. The drug praziquantel is highly effective in killing the adult worms.

schizoid personality type

This is the term used to describe people who show a life-long pattern of withdrawal, social isolation, solitariness and sometimes eccentricity. They often seem aloof and cold and avoid involvement in the affairs of others. Men of this type seldom marry and may pursue only a fantasy sexual life. Schizoid women sometimes marry dominating aggressive men. People of schizoid personality are unable to express anger directly and tend to fantasize revenge.

It is believed that about 10 per cent of people of this personality type develop florid **schizophrenia**.

schizophrenia

This is the commonest major psychiatric disorder and affects about 1 per cent of the population of the western world. It usually shows itself before the age of twenty-five and lasts for life. About half the patients in mental hospitals are schizophrenics, as are many of the homeless who inhabit city streets. Schizophrenia is not a disease in the normal medical sense and has no fixed characteristics. Definitions vary widely and the condition is constantly being officially redefined. At one time it was called 'premature dementia' (*dementia praecox*), but it is in no sense a dementia and the intellectual powers are not affected. There is no laboratory test for schizophrenia and no observable change in the nervous system. The diagnosis is based entirely on the behaviour of the person under consideration.

RECOGNITION AND 'SYMPTOMS'

It is not easy to discuss schizophrenia in the same terms as an organic disorder as it is impossible to be as certain of the reality of 'symptoms' as with organic disease, and much must be inferred from the affected person's behaviour and statements. Schizophrenics are said to suffer from false beliefs (**delusions**), false sensations (**hallucinations**), disordered thinking and loss of awareness of reality. They have a tendency to ramble in speech, with non-logical free associations, loss of the distinction between literal and metaphorical meaning, the use of invented words (neologisms) and unusual applications of common words.

POSSIBLE CAUSES

Current thinking favours the idea of social environmental stress or life experience of a kind rendering the individual incapable of relating 'normally' to society or the world in general. The finding of biochemical changes in the nervous system of schizophrenic people – excess of the **neuro-transmitter** dopamine, for instance – by no means necessarily indicates that this is the cause of the disease. Alteration in neuro-transmitter may be no more than a correlate of 'abnormal' behaviour as may be the lack of increased blood flow in the frontal lobes of the brain, shown by positron emission tomography (PET scanning), in schizophrenics.

On the other hand, since brain abnormalities can certainly cause most, if not all, of the manifestations of schizophrenia and, since brain abnormalities can result from unsatisfactory programming, or information input, during the developmental period of the nervous system, the causation may involve both external and internal factors.

The evidence of genetic studies suggests that genes exist which confer a susceptibility to the disorder. The closer the genetic relationship to a person with schizophrenia, the more likely one is to suffer the disorder oneself. Identical twins show the highest concordance rate. It should, of course, be remembered that the closer the genetic relationship, the more similar the environmental influences. There have been a few studies of identical twins one of which was reared separately from the parents. These suggest that the adopted twin is as likely to develop schizophrenia as the twin remaining with the natural parents.

INCIDENCE

Schizophrenia certainly runs in families. In the children of one schizophrenic parent the incidence is about 10 per cent. When both parents are affected, the incidence is about 50 per cent. About 10 per cent of the brothers or sisters of a schizophrenic develop the condition. In the case of identical twins, the figure is about 50 per cent. But heredity cannot explain the causes of schizophrenia.

CLASSIFICATION

Classically, three varieties of schizophrenia are described:

- paranoid schizophrenia, with delusions usually of persecution or grandeur;
- hebephrenic schizophrenia, with extreme mental disorganization, silliness of emotion and behaviour and ideas of bodily deterioration;
- catatonic schizophrenia.

This kind of classification is no longer relevant and the condition cannot be so neatly divided. Paranoid schizophrenia is still very common, hebephrenic, much less so.

Catatonic schizophrenia characterized the conventional notion of 'madness'. It occurred after a long period of gradual loss of interest in life with growing apathy and indifference which drifted into stupor and a tendency to remain unmoving in one position in a state of trance-like immobility and unresponsiveness. There was parrot-like repetition of words spoken (echolalia) or imitation of actions performed (echopraxia). The affected person was said to remain unmoving, allegedly for hours, in any position in which he or she had been placed, even if the position was bizarre and awkward. The limbs displayed an odd, stiff flexibility, and the joints bent slowly but unresistingly, under pressure, into new positions. Food was refused and faeces retained indefinitely.

There was often urinary incontinence. Every command was resisted. Such people were, however, fully aware of everything said to them and could recall the details later when, weeks or months later, there was sudden recovery.

Today, catatonic schizophrenia is very rare, and recent studies have shown that depression is a far commoner cause of catatonia than schizophrenia. That organic brain disease can cause catatonia has been viewed by some as evidence that schizophrenia is a neurological disease. Others have found that the nature of catatonia strongly suggests that, on the contrary, it is a reactive response to intolerable circumstances.

TREATMENT

Schizophrenia is treated mainly with anti-psychotic drugs which, although not bringing about a cure, can, while they are being taken, usually restore the affected person to a state generally acceptable to society. They are often given by injection as depot preparations. Electroconvulsive therapy was widely used until the late 1950s, but was displaced by the development of the drug largactil and is now rarely employed. Largactil was the fore-runner of a wide range of anti-psychotic drugs. Psychoanalysis has no value in the treatment of schizophrenia.

sciatica

This is not a disease, as is often thought, but a symptom. The sciatic nerve is the largest nerve in the body and runs down through the buttock and the back of each leg from the spinal cord, to supply all the muscles of the lower limb. It also carries sensory information back from the leg to the cord, and, via the cord to the brain.

Each sciatic nerve is made up from six or seven large nerve roots emerging from the bottom of the spinal cord (in the lumbar and sacral region) and sciatica is usually caused by

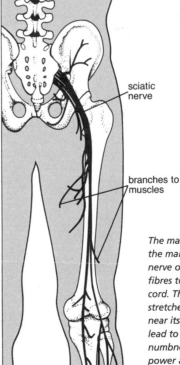

sciatic nerve

branches to muscles

The massive sciatic nerve is the main motor and sensory nerve of the leg carrying fibres to and from the spinal cord. The nerve is often stretched or compressed near its origin and this may lead to local pain, and numbness or loss of muscle power anywhere in the leg.

pressure on these nerve roots due to squashed-out pulp from the centre of one of the discs lying between the vertebrae of the spine (**slipped disc**). Depending on the degree of pressure, this may cause symptoms ranging from minor backache to the most severe pain, extending right down to the foot, associated with considerable loss of muscle power.

POSSIBLE CAUSES

Sciatica can also be caused by nerve pressure from other sources such as a tumour.

TREATMENT

Since sciatica is a symptom, the correct treatment is to remove the cause, if possible. Nerve root pressure is often relieved by lying down as the weight of the body is no longer acting to press out the pulp from the disc. Surgical removal of the prolapsed material may be necessary.

scissors gait

See **spastic paralysis**.

sclera, disorders of

The sclera is the white of the eye, the strong outer coating, made of densely packed and interwoven collagen fibrils, and remarkably resistant to injury. Under great violence, however, the sclera may rupture, usually along a circular line concentric with, and behind, the margin of the cornea. It is fairly easily penetrated by sharp objects.

The sclera is also remarkably free from disease. It may be unusually thin and show a bluish tinge from the pigment in the underlying choroid layer, an effect which is obvious and striking. This is so in the condition of *fragilitas ossium*, a hereditary collagen disorder in which bone fractures occur from minor force. In certain collagen diseases such as **rheumatoid arthritis**, lupus erythematosus, **herpes** zoster ophthalmicus and polyarteritis nodosa, the sclera may become intensely inflamed. This is called scleritis. Rarely, it may weaken and become so thinned that the choroid bulges through and the integrity of the eye is threatened. This sometimes happens in Wegener's granulomatosis.

Scleritis is usually persistent but often responds well to corticosteroid eye drops, although, in severe cases, these may sometimes increase the danger of perforation.

sclerosis

Hardening of a normally soft tissue. Sclerosis is usually due to the deposition of fibrous tissue, following inflammation. Examples are **atherosclerosis**, in which arteries become hardened, and **multiple sclerosis**, in which plaques of nerve tissue are replaced by fibrous tissue.

Scop

A brand name for **hyoscine**.

scotoma

A blind spot in the field of vision. A negative scotoma is an area of absent vision of which the affected person is unaware, and most scotomas, including the normal 'blind spot', are of this kind. A positive scotoma causes a grey or black spot which is fixed in relation to the point of gaze, but moves with eye movement. A central scotoma results from disease of the optic nerve – most of the fibres of which arise from the cen-

tre of the retina (the macula) – or from disease of the macula itself, such as **macular degeneration**. Peripheral scotomas result from disease of the peripheral retina or optic nerve and these occur in such conditions as chronic simple **glaucoma**, **retinitis pigmentosa**, or pituitary tumour. A scintillating scotoma is an expanding area of visual field loss, with a sparkling edge, persisting for about twenty minutes. This is a common feature of migraine and is usually harmless.

scrofula

Tuberculous infection of the lymph glands of the neck. The condition, now uncommon, was formerly usually caused by bovine tuberculosis and acquired by drinking infected milk. As a result, the term scrofula has become quite uncommon.

Any of the neck nodes may be involved but most commonly affected are those high up, just under the angle of the jaw, which drain the tonsils. Lymph nodes infected with tuberculosis usually feel rubbery or hard to the touch but are not tender. It is rare, nowadays, for infected nodes to cause breakdown of the overlying skin, but in former times, when repeated infection from contaminated milk was the rule, scrofula commonly involved the skin, causing scarring and multiple openings which discharged tuberculous pus. Scrofula used to be known as 'the King's evil' and the monarch was supposed to have the power to cure the condition by mere touch. Today, anti-tuberculous chemotherapy is more generally effective.

scrotum, swellings in

Swellings in the scrotum may be hard or soft. Apart from the tender and painful swelling of mumps **orchitis**, hard swellings are liable to be dangerous and must be urgently investigated. Cancer of the testicle is always a possibility. Soft swellings may be due to **varicocele** or to **hydrocele**.

scrotum-wrinkling muscle

See **dartos muscle**.

scurvy

A deficiency disease caused by inadequate vitamin C (ascorbic acid) in the diet. Prior to the discovery of the importance of the vitamin, scurvy was most strikingly evident in seamen, subsisting on long voyages on a diet of salt pork and sea biscuits. Today, it is comparatively rare but still occurs in people in poor circumstances, especially the elderly and toothless, living alone on a poor and unvaried diet of tea and toast.

Most animals are able to synthesize ascorbic acid from sugar, but primates, including man, cannot do this and a certain minimum is required in the diet if disease is to be avoided. Signs of scurvy will appear one to three months after intake of a source of vitamin C stops, the period depending on the previous body stores.

RECOGNITION AND SYMPTOMS

Vitamin C is necessary for the production of stable collagen, an important structural protein in the body, and in its absence there is weakness of small blood vessels and poor healing of wounds. As a result, bleeding into any of the tissues of the body may occur, and this is most obvious in the skin in which widespread bruising may be seen. Gums bleed, teeth loosen and recently healed wounds may break down. Bleeding into muscles and joints causes much pain.

The condition is even more serious in children who tend also to bleed into the membranes surrounding the long bones. This may cause separation of the growing ends of the bones and interference with body growth. Major, and possibly fatal, haemorrhages into and around the brain sometimes occur in children. Scurvy is often associated with other vitamin deficiencies and anaemia is common.

TREATMENT

Vitamin C occurs so widely in fruit and vegetables that a modest intake of these will provide more than the amount needed to prevent scurvy. It is also found in milk, liver, kidney and fish. At least half of the vitamin C content of these foods survives cooking and preserving. The response to treatment with large doses of ascorbic acid is rapid. Bleeding stops within a day, wound healing occurs, and muscle and bone pain quickly settle.

sea sickness

See **motion sickness**.

sebaceous cyst

A harmless soft swelling, of variable size, within the skin, caused by the gradual accumulation of a cheesy, fatty material called sebum which is secreted by the sebaceous glands of the skin. Sebaceous cysts occur if the opening of a sebaceous gland into a hair follicle becomes blocked. The cyst commonly occurs on hair-bearing areas, such as the scalp, face, ears, back of neck and scrotum, and may become secondarily infected to form a discharging abscess.

Sebaceous cysts are often apparently cherished by their owners and allowed to grow to an impressive size. They are easily removed through a small incision made painlessly under local anaesthesia.

Seconal sodium

A brand name for the barbiturate drug **quinalbarbitone**.

sectioning

Certification of insanity was abolished in Britain in 1959 and replaced by a Mental Health Act, which makes provision for compulsory admission to hospital for periods of observation of up to 28 days (Section 25), or for longer periods, if necessary (Section 26). This is done on application by the nearest relative or by the Mental Welfare Officer supported by the recommendation of two doctors.

Sectral

A brand name for **acebutolol**.

security objects

These are particular items which bring comfort and a sense of security to young children, often for a number of years. They are especially important when children are ill. Security objects are usually associated in some way with bed and are often made of soft material which is good to feel and cuddle. Typical security objects include: scrap of an old blanket; scrap of a former night garment; a teddy bear; a soft toy; or an old nappy.

Security objects are often pressed to the face as the child settles down to sleep. Some children claim that they like the smell of the comforter. Most who use security objects are clearly emotionally attached to them and resent attempts to deprive them of the object.

Later a kind of ambivalence develops as the child comes to see that the security object is 'rather silly' and 'babyish'. Around the age of six or seven, the security object is usually repudiated and there may even be a ritual destruction. In some cases the use of the security object may even persist into adolescence or even adult life.

There is no reason to suppose that security objects are in any way undesirable, at any age, and enforced removal may be cruel. A sick child who is already weaned of a security object may well revert to it during the illness. This should be respected and accepted as a matter of course.

Securon

A brand name for the drug **verapamil**.

Securon SR

A brand name for **verapamil** in a sustained release form.

Securopen

A brand name for **azlocillin**.

sedation

The use of a mild drug to calm, alleviate anxiety and promote sleep.

sedative drugs

A group of drugs that includes antianxiety drugs, sleeping drugs, antipsychotic drugs and some antidepressant drugs.

See **anti-anxiety drugs**, **anti-emetic drugs**, **barbiturates**, **benzodiazepine drugs**, **beta-blocker drugs**, **hypnotic drugs**.

seizures

See **epilepsy**.

seizures, hereditary

See **benign familial neonatal convulsions**.

seizures, monitor-induced

See **video game epilepsy**.

selective serotonin re-uptake inhibitors (SSRIs)

A range of drugs that act at the clefts of synapses in the brain preventing released serotonin from being removed and thus increasing its action as a **neuro-transmitter**. Serotonin, or 5-hydroxytryptamine (5-HT), is a neuro-transmitter and hormone found in many tissues, especially the brain, the intestinal lining and the blood platelets. It is concerned in controlling mood and levels of consciousness. Its action is disturbed by some hallucinogenic drugs and imitated by others. It constricts small blood vessels, cuts down acid secretion by the stomach and contracts the muscles in the wall of the intestine. The best known drug in this group is Prozac. Generic names are **citalopram**, **fluoxetine**, **fluvoxamine**, **nefazodone**, **paroxetine**, **sertraline** and **venlafaxine**.

selegiline

A selective **monoamine oxidase inhibitor** drug used in the treatment of **Parkinsonism and Parkinson's disease**. Selegiline is thought to retard the breakdown of dopamine. Trade names are Eldepryl and Vivapril.

selenium sulphide

An anti-**dandruff** agent formulated as a shampoo. Trade names are Lenium and Selsun.

self-deception, protective

See **defence mechanisms**.

self-gratification failure

See **reward deficiency syndrome**.

Selsun

A brand name for a selenium-containing shampoo used to treat dandruff.

Semi-daonil

A brand name for **glibenclamide**.

Semilente MC

A brand name for **insulin**.

seminal fluid

Semen, or seminal fluid, is the creamy, greyish or yellowish, sticky, gel-like material ejaculated from the penis during the sexual orgasm. It is secreted by the prostate gland, the storage seminal vesicles, the lining of the sperm tubes (epididymis and vas deferens) and some small associated glands.

The volume of the ejaculate varies considerably, especially with age, and ranges from 2–6 ml in youth to almost nothing in elderly men. The volume rises after ten days or so of continence and drops if ejaculation occurs more than twice a day. Each millilitre contains from 50 million to 150 million sperms (spermatozoa).

After ejaculation semen remains gel-like for about twenty minutes, but then liquefies. Until it does the sperms hardly move. Ejaculate contains the sugar fructose which provide the spermatozoa with energy. Seminal fluid spilt on soft material has a hardening effect when it dries.

Semitard MC

A brand name for a form of **insulin** having medium duration of action.

Semprex

A brand name for **acrivastine**.

Sengstaken tube

A tube with two inflatable balloons near one end that is passed down the gullet until the lower balloon is in the stomach and the higher one at the lower end of the gullet. The balloons are then inflated to exert pressure on the lower end of the gullet (oesophagus) and the upper part of the stomach, so as to control bleeding from the varicose veins that may result from obstruction to the flow of blood from the intestine to the liver. These abnormal veins are called oesophageal varices and commonly occur when there is cirrhosis of the liver.

senility

The word 'senile' comes from the Latin *senilis* meaning old and should carry no negative connotation. The Romans respected their aged and appointed many of them to the 'Senate' – a revered council of elderly men. But senility has come to imply the deterioration in intellectual power and the rigid, restricted and repetitive pattern of thought often, but not inevitably, associated with old age. See also **dementia**.

senna

A stimulant laxative drug used to treat constipation. A brand name is Senokot.

Senokot

A brand name for **senna**.

sensate focus technique

The concentration of the attention on a particular sensory experience, especially a pleasurable sensual one. Sensate focus has been widely applied by sex therapists in the treatment of sexual dysfunction such as impotence in men and lack of sexual desire or satisfaction in women.

The method, which is often highly successful, involves a preliminary prohibition of coitus, or even of attention to the genitalia, and a concentration on the art and experience of sensual mutual massage. The removal of the need to demonstrate performance ability relieves the anxiety which is at the root of much sexual dysfunction, and introduces a new pleasurable element, which is often highly erotic in its effect.

See also **Masters and Johnson sex therapy**.

sensory deprivation

The state in which there is a major reduction in incoming sensory information. Prolonged sensory deprivation is very damaging as the body, being an essentially reactive entity, depends for its health and normal function on constant stimulation. The main input sensory channels are the eyes, the ears, the skin and the nose. If input from all of these is blocked, there is loss of the sense of reality, distortion of time and imagined space, hallucinations, bizarre thought patterns and other indications of neurological dysfunction.

Even minimal sensory deprivation in early childhood can have a devastating effect on the future personality. An eye covered for a few months in infancy remains effectively blind for life. Early deprivation of normal hearing can produce severe intellectual and educational damage. Deprivation of the normal contact and stimulation provided to the baby by the mother can cause personality disturbance in later life.

sentinel node

An important new concept in the management of breast cancer. The sentinel node is a lymph node presumed to be the first to which a breast or other cancer will extend by lymphatic spread. In the case of breast cancers, sentinel nodes in the armpit can be identified prior to surgery by injecting near the site of a breast tumour a small quantity of harmless serum albumin tagged with a low-intensity radioactive marker. The normal lymph drainage carries the tracer substance to a particular node, which can then be located and identified by a hand-held gamma-ray detector probe. Alternatively, a blue dye can be injected, and this, too, will be carried to the sentinel node.

Sentinel node biopsy is the identification and removal for examination of the sentinel node. It is claimed that examination of this single lymph node can accurately predict in 97.5 per cent of cases whether or not a breast cancer has spread to the lymph nodes. The false negative rate is 4.6 per cent. It also been used in the management of malignant melanoma.

separation anxiety

A childhood disorder in which excessive and inappropriate anxiety is shown whenever there is separation, or the threat of separation, from one or both parents, or from someone *in loco parentis*. The child suffers unrealistic fears of abandonment, and of danger to the parent. In addition to dramatic demonstration of concern at the time of separation, a demonstration suggesting terror or panic, the child may complain of symptoms such as headaches, abdominal pain and nausea, and may often vomit. Such children make greater than normal demands to be held and cuddled and can obtrude unduly into adult affairs. They will persistently refuse to go to school or to sleep away from home and may refuse even to go to bed unless accompanied by the attachment person.

Separation anxiety is treated by constant reassurance of love and support, fairness, especially in relation to siblings, explanation, firmness and natural responses. Occasionally, tranquilliser drugs and night sedatives may have to be used.

septicaemia

'Blood poisoning'. The circulation of large numbers of disease-producing micro-organisms in the blood. There is high fever, shivering, headache, rapid breathing and sometimes delirium. It is treated with intensive antibiotic therapy but may progress to the very dangerous condition of **septic shock**.

septic shock

When infective organisms enter the bloodstream, it is called bacteraemia, and if these organisms multiply in the blood the affected person has **septicaemia**, a condition popularly described as 'blood poisoning'. Organisms can get into the blood from infection in many different parts, especially the middle ear, the sinuses, the skin, the lungs, the urinary system, the bowel when **diverticulitis** is present, and the gallbladder. It is especially common in people who have partly lost their defence against infection (immunocompromised people) from immunological disorders or treatment involving immunosuppressive drugs; in people with widespread cancer, leukaemia, diabetes, cirrhosis of the liver or major burns; or in women who have had inept illegal abortions.

Septicaemia tends to cause secondary areas of infection as organisms are deposited in the bones, the liver, the brain and the heart valves, but there is another serious effect. Many organisms which cause septicaemia contain powerful poisons (toxins) which can severely damage any of the cells of the body.

In this case, the effect of the toxins is mainly on the walls of the small blood vessels, causing them to become leaky so that much fluid is lost into the tissue spaces. The loss of fluid from the blood may be so great that the normal circulation cannot be maintained (acute circulatory failure) and the blood pressure drops. This is called shock. Surgical shock is commonly caused by loss of blood from injury, or loss of fluids from burns. In this case, because it is caused by bacterial toxins, it is called septic shock. Another dangerous effect of bacterial toxins is widespread clotting of the blood within the small blood vessels. This is called disseminated intravascular coagulation.

RECOGNITION AND SYMPTOMS

Shock features collapse, a rapid, very weak pulse, pallor and a cold clammy skin. The failure in the supply of blood to all parts of the body leads to organ failure, especially of the kidneys, liver, lungs and brain and the mortality in septic shock may be over 60 per cent.

> Septic shock calls for urgent treatment with antibiotics, given in large dosage. Transfusion of fluids to maintain the circulatory volume is also essential. To help to reduce the damaging effect of the bacterial toxins on cells, steroids are also used and these, too, can be life-saving.

See also **toxic shock syndrome**.

septoplasty

An operation to correct deflection to one side of the normally central bone and cartilage partition of the nose (the nasal septum). The mere presence of a deflection is not, in itself, a reason for operating, but if symptoms, such as one-sided blockage of the airway, are troublesome, the operation may be performed.

HOW IT'S DONE

The mucous membrane covering of the septum is cut through and all abnormal attachments to the cartilage are freed so that the partition can be repositioned centrally. The surgeon removes as little bone or cartilage as possible, so as to minimise risk of collapse of the nose.

Septrin

A brand name for the antibacterial drug cotrimoxazole.

Serc

A brand name for the drug betahistidine used in the treatment of **Ménière's syndrome**.

Serenace

A brand name for the tranquillizing drug **haloperidol**.

Serepax

A brand name for **oxazepam**.

serious illness in a child

Serious illness in children is uncommon and is usually obvious, even to people without medical knowledge. The seriously ill child remains quiet. Loud crying or screaming is seldom, if ever, a feature of serious illness. When seriously ill, the child must harbour all his or her resources to combat the problem and this means lying still, and not wasting energy in crying.

Parents are often worried that symptoms such as fastidiousness in diet, loss of appetite, colic and pallor of the skin imply serious illness. Such concern is nearly always unjustified.

The following points are especially important:

- unrousable coma;
- uncharacteristic and inappropriate drowsiness;
- any alteration in the state of consciousness;
- any interference with easy breathing;
- weak or inadequate breathing efforts;
- any obstruction to breathing;
- the onset of blueness of the skin;
- convulsions (but see **fever fits**);
- irregularity of the pulse;
- weak, thready and rapid pulse after bleeding, severe vomiting or diarrhoea;
- sudden projectile vomiting for no apparent reason, especially if associated with headache.

If any of these occur in your child, urgent medical attention in hospital is probably needed.

sermorelin

A growth hormone releasing factor used to treat growth failure. A brand name is Geref.

Serophene

A brand name for the drug clomiphene, used in the treatment of infertility.

Seroquel

A brand name for **quetiapine**.

serotonin

The neuro-transmitter and hormone 5-hydroxytryptamine (5-HT) found in many tissues, especially the brain, the intestinal lining and the blood **platelets**. Serotonin is concerned in controlling mood and levels of consciousness. Its action is disturbed by some hallucinogenic drugs and imitated by others. It also constricts small blood vessels, cuts down acid secretion by the stomach and contracts the muscles in the wall of the intestine. It is the only neuro-transmitter whose name is widely familiar outside medical circles. This is because of the public interest in the claims of those promoting the drug Prozac and the popular explanations that have been published about its mode of action. Prozac, generic name fluoxetine, is a **selective serotonin re-uptake inhibitor** and results in more persistent action in the brain of this neuro-transmitter.

serotonin antagonist drugs

Serotonin, or 5-hydroxytryptamine (5-HT) is an adrenaline-like nerve stimulator (neuro-transmitter) that has a marked effect on mood and excitability. Serotonin-antagonist drugs oppose the action of this substance and produce a variety of effects, including reduction of depression and the control of migraine. The action is not clearly understood.

sertraline

A **selective serotonin re-uptake inhibitor** drug used to treat depression and severe premenstrual syndrome. A brand name is Lustral.

setting sun sign

A characteristic downward deviation of the eyes so that the irises appear to descend behind the 'horizon' of the lower lids, with the whites of the eyes showing above the corneas, is a sign of raised pressure within the skull or irritation of the brain stem. The sign is commonly found in infants with hydrocephalus.

severe combined immunodeficiency disorder (SCID)

A congenital immunodeficiency that has nothing to do with **AIDS**. It is the result of a genetic defect that causes a failure of the enzymes essential for the production of the receptors for the vital immune system cells, the T cells and the B cells. As a result neither of these classes of lymphocytes can become immunologically functional and the affected child is gravely susceptible to infections of all kinds.

severe throat abscess

See **quinsy**.

Sevredol

A brand name for **morphine**.

sex, attitudes to

Men and women, in common with all the other higher animals, experience recurrent inclination to copulate. In the past, these inclinations were, to some extent, held in check by social taboos and by the fear of pregnancy. The virtual abolition of these two factors and the universal access to alcohol have made it easy to yield to this inclination, even when it is not particularly strong.

There is no denying that the earlier sexual taboos were a cause of much unhappiness and psychological ill-health. But the casual indulgence in sex does, unfortunately, cause psychological problems. Sex can never be entirely divorced from normal human feelings of loyalty, fidelity, trust and so on, and the use of sex for purely erotic purposes will invariably offend against these values.

The hedonistic 'philosophy' propagated by people who see the commercial advantage of pandering to men's wish for sexual variety without responsibility, is a cynical travesty of the truth. It has had a damaging effect on human happiness, especially that of women. The explosive spread of **sexually transmitted disease** in the last fifty years, and of **AIDS** in the last twenty, has been one of the consequences of a radically altered attitude to sexual relationships, fostered by such ideas. Indeed the word 'relationship' has become inappropriate, with the growing emphasis on sex as a source of erotic or purely sensual pleasure rather than as a principal component in a love association. Today, it is often a matter of taking rather than of giving and of using others for one's own gratification.

sex chromosomes

There are 23 pairs of chromosomes in humans. Twenty-two of the pairs are known as autosomes. The other pair are the sex chromosomes and they determine gender. Women have two sex chromosomes of similar appearance called X chromosomes (XX). Men have one X chromosome and another, much smaller chromosome, called a Y (XY). Sperms have 23 chromosomes, rather than 23 pairs, and thus have half the normal complement. One of these is either an X or a Y chromosome. If an X chromosome enters the egg (ovum) during fertilization the result will be a female, if a Y, a male. Eggs also have 23 chromosomes, but the sex chromosome is always an X. At fertilization, the full complement of 46 chromosomes is restored. See also **X chromosome, X-inactivation**.

sex glands

Puberty is the period, occurring usually between the ages of ten and fourteen, when the sexual organs mature, the secondary sexual characteristics begin to develop, the significance of sexuality begins to become apparent to the young person, and reproduction becomes possible. The time scale varies considerably, especially in boys, so that at the age of fourteen one boy may appear sexually mature while another may still have infantile genitalia.

In both female and male, puberty is initiated by the production, by the pituitary gland, of hormones, called gonadotrophins, which cause the ovaries and the testicles to increase production of their own hormones, respectively oestrogen and testosterone.

In girls, the first sign of puberty is breast budding or the appearance of pubic hair. One breast may develop more rapidly than the other, but inequalities normally disappear as growth continues. It is usually about a year before the ovaries are mature enough for ovulation to occur so that the first menstrual period is induced. By this time the breasts are usually well advanced and pubic and underarm hair are fully grown. During this period, there is an acceleration of growth with a widening of the pelvis and characteristic deposition of fat under the skin. When the menstrual periods are fully established at regular intervals, puberty is complete. The first sign of puberty in boys is an increase in the rate of growth of the testicles and scrotum. This is followed by the beginnings of a beard and the appearance of pubic hair extending upwards in a diamond pattern toward the navel. The penis then begins to grow, reaching its adult size in about two years. Sperm production gets under way, under the influence of testosterone, and this also prompts the maturation of the prostate gland and the seminal vesicles, and the enlargement of the voice box (larynx) so that the voice deepens.

About 80 per cent of the adult height is reached before sexual maturation starts, but a considerable spurt in growth, and even more in weight gain, occurs during the period around puberty. The body weight may be almost doubled during this period. In boys, this is mainly due to the increase in the weight of muscle. In girls, muscle weight increases by about 50 per cent but there is also a large increase in fat deposition. By around eighteen years of age this amounts to over 20 per cent of the body weight, compared to 10 per cent in young men.

sex hormones

Hormones that bring about the development of bodily sexual characteristics and regulate sperm and egg production and the menstrual cycle. They are steroids of three main types, androgens (male), oestrogens (female) and progestogens that prepare women for, and maintain, pregnancy. Sex hormones or chemically similar substances are widely used in medicine for a variety of purposes such as contraception, treatment of menstrual disorders, discouragement of cancers, improving muscle bulk and so on. Male sex hormones are anabolic steroids.

sex hormones, male

See **androgens**.

sex hormone, male, receptor

See **androgen receptor gene**.

sex-linkage

Inheritance in which the gene for the condition is carried on one of the X or, very rarely, Y sex chromosomes. For this reason, sex-linkage is virtually the same as X-linkage. Recessive sex-linked conditions almost always affect males, are carried on the male X chromosome and thus cannot be transmitted directly from father to son because only Y-bearing sperms result in boys. The male X chromosome comes, only in the egg, from the mother. The best-known sex-linked recessive condition is **haemophilia**. Recessive sex-linked conditions become manifest in males because the the gene concerned is on its own. There is no corresponding **allele** on the Y chromosome. Y-linked conditions are rare because the Y chromosome is very small and carries few genes.

sex reassignment surgery

Surgical treatment sometimes given to transsexuals, usually males, to people with ambiguous genitalia and to those convinced that they are of the wrong anatomical sex. Such people have a profound wish to be rid of their genitalia and to live as a member of the opposite sex.

Before any question of surgery arises, the transsexual person is given a detailed psychiatric and psychological evaluation to ensure that the desire is genuine and permanent and has been present for at least two years.

HOW IT'S DONE

Male-to-female sex change surgery involves removal of the structures within the penis, but not the skin, reimplantation of the urine tube (urethra), removal of the testicles and most of the skin of the scrotum, and the fashioning of an artificial vagina from the inverted skin of the penis, and labia minora from the scrotal skin. Female sex hormones are given. This causes changes in the skin and hair and a re-distribution of fat on the hips, buttocks and breasts. Breast implantation (augmentation **mammoplasty**) is also often done.

The 'female genitalia', so provided, are far from perfect. Artificial lubrication is likely to be needed in the vagina and there will be a tendency to shrinkage. Orgasm may not be possible and there will, of course, be no menstruation or the possibility of conception.

Female-to-male surgery involves mastectomy to remove the breasts, followed by removal of the uterus and ovaries. Construction of a penis may then be attempted by grafting abdominal skin over a catheter. Operations for ambiguous genitalia are usually done as soon as possible after birth.

sex selection

The determination of the sex of a future individual before conception by the separation of sperms bearing Y chromosomes (male) from those bearing X chromosomes (female). Such techniques are still experimental and uncertain and raise major ethical issues. A more sinister form of sex selection has been widely practised in some areas since medical technology made it possible to determine the gender of the embryo or fetus at a very early stage in the pregnancy. If the sex is what is wanted, well and good. If not, the pregnancy is aborted.

sex selection before birth

If an ovum is fertilized by a sperm carrying an X chromosome, the result will be a girl; if by a sperm carrying a Y, the baby will be a boy. 'Female' sperms contain about 3 per cent more DNA than 'males' and are heavier and slower moving, but can travel further.

Attempts to make use of these facts to select the sex of the future child – by depositing semen further away from the site of fertilization in the Fallopian tube if a girl was desired – have not been universally successful.

The separation of sperms into X-bearing and Y-bearing types can be done in the laboratory by various methods and this can increase the percentage of Y-bearing sperms from fifty to about eighty. Artificial insemination, with the Y-enriched semen, can then be used. X-enrichment is also possible. Women can be 'immunized' against proteins present only in the Y-bearing sperms, but this is not thought to have been a successful method of sex-determination. The overall success rate in sex determination, by the most effective current methods, is less than 80 per cent.

A more reliable method of sex selection that is being practised in many countries in which males are preferred is to check the sex by intrauterine scanning and abort the females. This practice was prevalent in India where, in mid-1994, Government reports suggested that 50,000 female fetuses were aborted every year. As a result, a bill was passed in Parliament under which doctors who participated in this practice would be struck off the medical register, fined £200 (10,000 rupees) and imprisoned for three years. Pregnant women who had tests to detect the sex of their fetus would be liable to the same fine and sentence. Doubts have been expressed as to whether such a law can be enforced. In Delhi alone there are 2000 private clinics, many offering such tests. These facts raise major ethical problems. Should sex selection be widely practised, an undesirable change in the balance between males and females might possibly occur.

sex therapy

See **sensate focus technique**, **Masters and Johnson sex therapy**, **impotence**, **ejaculation, disorders of**.

sexual abuse

The subjection of an individual to sexual activity that is likely to cause physical or psychological harm.

See also **child abuse**, **rape**.

sexual deviation

A term of somewhat uncertain meaning, sometimes taken to apply to any form of physical sexual activity outside the convention of heterosexual, penile/vaginal intercourse. Thus, some people still regard as sexually deviant any form of homosexual activity and any heterosexual act involving an alternative orifice to the vagina. Widely regarded as deviant are sexual activity with children (**paedophilia**) or animals (bestiality), **exhibitionism**, **sadism**, **masochism**, sexual **fetishism** and **transvestism**.

Other deviations include watching the sexual activity of others (**voyeurism**), making obscene telephone calls (telephone scatologia), rubbing the penis against women in crowded places (**frottage**), the use of enemas for sexual stimulation ('high colonic lavage'), and taking sexual pleasure in defecating on a partner or in being defecated upon (coprophilia).

The term usually has a pejorative content and its application varies with the sexual tastes and orientation of the user.

See **paraphilia**.

sexual intercourse

The totality of the physical and mental interplay between human beings in which the explicit or implicit goal is bodily union and, by this means, the mutual expression of love and affection. Regrettably, the term is more often used to refer to nothing more than the act of copulation. 'Intercourse' implies mutuality.

sexuality

A term having varying meanings in different contexts. In biology it is often limited to an indication of the structural (anatomical) differences between male and female or the capacity to transmit genetic material from one organism to another. In everyday speech it is commonly used to describe an individual's sexual attitudes, drive, interest or activity.

In general psychology the term is used to cover all those behaviour patterns, drives, emotions and sensations connected with reproduction and with the use of the sex organs. Freudian psychology gives the term a still wider meaning, based on the idea that all drives connected with bodily satisfaction are essentially sexual.

Heterosexuality prompts a sexual interest in people of anatomically opposite sex, while homosexuality directs attention to those of the same bodily sex. The term bisexuality refers to those capable of responding physically to members of either sex.

sexually transmitted diseases (STDs)

PREVALENCE
The steady overall rise in the number of people contracting these diseases is a reflection of changed social attitudes to sex. It is also a reflection of the not always healthy commercial pressures imposed on young people, by the entertainment and advertising media, to believe that 'instant sex', dissociated from affection or responsibility, is an acceptable, even desirable, norm. As a result of these and other influences, the age at which sexual activity starts continues to drop. Another factor is increased personal mobility. People travel more, both at home and abroad, and this separation from the normal environment encourages sexual promiscuity, as does the increasing alcohol consumption among the now affluent young of the Western world.

Contraception is available to all, and, in spite of official advice on protection against AIDS and increasing evidence of the protective value of condoms, many men continue to expect women to use oral contraceptives, intrauterine devices and diaphragms, rather than agree to use condoms.

Finally, there is a strong link between the prevalence of sexually transmitted diseases and the use of recreational drugs. One trend is the exchange of sex for drugs by young women who have become addicted and who engage in many sexual encounters to support their habit. Gonorrhoea, syphilis, AIDS and chancroid are especially linked with the use of **crack** cocaine. AIDS, also, is strongly associated with **heroin** needle-sharing.

There has been a notable change in the pattern of occurrence of sexually transmitted disease over the last half century. Syphilis has been declining in prevalence for much longer than that. Indeed the decline has been steady for over 100 years. Since 1940, the incidence of **general paralysis of the insane** (GPI) and other forms of the particularly nasty tertiary stage of syphilis has dropped by 99 per cent in the Western world. In the same period the incidence of syphilis, generally, has dropped by about 90 per cent. This is mainly due to the use of antibiotics. The figures for early syphilis have not fallen so dramatically but continue to drop, and this unpleasant disease is much less common than it used to be. A low point was reached in 1957, after which the incidence rose to a new peak in 1982. This rise was largely due to increases among homosexual men.

Genital herpes is booming. Antibodies to HSV-2 – the genital strain – occur in 20 per cent of people thirty to forty-four years of age in the USA. Consultations for genital herpes amounted to 3.4 per 100,000 of the population in 1966; in 1979, this figure was 29.2. In Britain, 9000 new cases were reported in 1980, 16,000 in 1983. Today the figure must be many times that number. The prevalence of herpes is increasing faster than that of any other sexually transmitted disease. Chlamydial infections – most cases of **nonspecific urethritis** are chlamydial – are also flourishing. They are well up at the top of the list with a record of about 150,000 victims a year in Britain. In the USA chlamydial infections are even commoner than gonorrhoea and there, also, it is by far the most prevalent sexually transmitted disease. It is a major cause of pelvic inflammatory disease and sterility in women. Up to 70 per cent of infected women and 25 per cent of infected men may have the disease without being aware of the fact. Sexually promiscuous people should be checked for this infection.

Gonorrhoea, popularly known as 'the clap', once the scourge of the promiscuous, seems to be falling back a little, but is still in second place with about 60,000 transmissions a year in Britain. In the USA the disease has reached pandemic proportions. Ninety per cent of cases occur in teenagers and young adults. Forty per cent of men who have sexual intercourse with infected women, acquire the infection. Gonorrhoea, however, has, for years, been developing resistance to penicillin, a drug which was once a 100 per cent sure cure. Resistance to ampicillin, tetracycline, cefoxitin and spectinomycin is also commonplace. These organisms have mutated and evolved to produce an enzyme that interferes with antibiotic action. Over 20 per cent of gonococci are now resistant to penicillin and tetracycline. Doctors continue to be seriously worried about the emergence of strains of the organism which are totally resistant to ordinary penicillin. These strains were first noted in 1976 and the number of cases caused by the totally resistant strains has doubled each year since then.

Candidiasis (thrush), although, of course, not necessarily a sexually transmitted disease, is very commonly spread by sexual intercourse, and the figures, at well over 50,000, are only a little lower than those for gonorrhoea. Genital warts are also flourishing, at about 35,000 cases a year. **Trichomoniasis** is also running strongly at just over 20,000, but, again, trichomoniasis is not necessarily sexually spread.

That leaves a miscellaneous group of infestations: crab **lice** – 10,000 cases; **scabies** – 2500 cases; and infections such as **gardnerella vaginalis infection**, **molluscum contagiosum**, lymphogranuloma venereum, chancroid and **yaws**.

Sexually transferred **hepatitis** is steadily becoming more common. There are an estimated 200 million carriers of hepatitis B in the world and in the USA it is believed that 300,000 new cases occur every year. The incidence of this disease has not declined since 1982, in spite of a sharp drop in homosexual contacts. The reason for this is the increase in heterosexual transmission and transmission by infected needles.

Worst of all is the acquired immune deficiency syndrome (**AIDS**) whose incidence has been doubling yearly. Concern about AIDS resulted in a decrease from 1982 to 1986. There was then a sharp rise, which, in the USA, amounted to about fifteen cases per 100,000 of the population.

This catalogue suggests that sexually transmitted diseases are difficult to avoid. This is true for people engaging in regular promiscuous sexual activity who will certainly, sooner or later, and probably sooner rather than later, acquire a sexually transmitted disease. The question is whether the disease is just a minor annoyance, easily cured, or whether it is one which seriously, and perhaps permanently, affects health.

PSYCHOLOGICAL EFFECTS

There is much more to the matter than this. Sexually transmitted disease is never simply a matter of physical health. By definition, such an infection involves at least one other person, and raises major ethical problems. When an STD is acquired or passed on there will inevitably be blame and recrimination. Third parties – often an unsuspecting spouse – may be involved. The normal reaction is one of guilt or deep resentment and even if the latter is not openly expressed, it is almost certain to damage relationships.

Many people react to the discovery that they have a sexually transmitted disease by developing a distaste for sexual intercourse, especially with the person from whom the disease was acquired. Some men become impotent – not from the sexually transmitted disease but from the psychological reaction to it or to the other person's infidelity. Often the impotence is 'relative', that is, occurs only with the partner who was the source of the disease. Some people become very angry when they find that they have acquired a sexually transmitted disease and some men become violent. Assault on women partners is not uncommon. All these are major problems having an important bearing on health in the wider sense. Relationships are of basic importance to health and happiness and anything that damages them is disastrous to well-being.

SYPHILIS

This disease is six times as common in men as in women because, nowadays, most new cases occur in homosexual males. Syphilis is caused by the spirochaete *Treponema pallidum*, and the first signs usually appear about three weeks after exposure. The incubation period may, however, be as long as three months. The first sign is the chancre. This is a single, small, red area, slightly raised and entirely painless, occurring on any part of the penis or the vulva or even on the cervix. The chancre may be inconspicuous and can be missed entirely. After a few days the raised area breaks down, still painlessly, to leave a clean, round wet crater with a hardened edge and base that looks like wet chamois leather. This base is teeming with spirochaetes. The chancre heals within three to ten weeks and during this time the lymph nodes in the groin often enlarge and feel rubbery. They are, however, never painful or tender.

The secondary stage starts four to eight weeks after the appearance of the chancre, and, if the chancre has been missed, provides another chance of appreciating that something serious has happened. The commonest feature of secondary syphilis is a skin rash of circular spots, up to 1 cm in diameter and either rosy pink or coppery red, scattered over the chest, back, abdomen and arms. They occur even on the palms of the hands and soles of the feet. This rash occurs in 75 per cent of affected people. Its extent is an indication of how widely the spirochaetes have spread throughout the body. The spots are painless and not even itchy so they have to be looked for. In areas where two layers of skin are in contact these spots may expand and become large and fleshy (condylomata lata), and on the lips or in the mouth or on the genitalia shallow, painless ulcers, resembling snail tracks, may form. Even if nothing is done, these signs will eventually disappear and the uninformed or unwary may think that that is the end of the matter.

Fortunately, the third and fourth, or tertiary and quaternary, stages of syphilis have now become rare. They are, however, much too dangerous to risk. The tertiary stage occurs some ten years later and involves the skin, soft tissues and bones, in which masses of rubbery, tumour-like tissue form. These are known as gummas. In those unfortunate people who proceed to the quaternary stage, several very unpleasant things may occur. The late effects of syphilis may be delayed for many years, but if they occur they do so with a vengeance. They include:

- ballooning and fatal bursting of the major artery of the body (**aneurysm** of the aorta);
- **tabes dorsalis**;
- blindness;
- incontinence;
- impotence;
- inability to maintain balance;
- personality changes;
- delusions of grandeur;
- severe defect of judgement;
- paralysis.

These effects are due to long-term damage to the arteries and the brain. Although late syphilis is no longer the common disease it was a century ago, it is a fate to be avoided at all costs. Anyone who suspects that he or she might have contracted syphilis, however long before, should report to a doctor and ask for a test. The usual test is the VDRL (Venereal Disease Reference Laboratory) test. If this is positive, antibiotic treatment will be arranged. Even in the comparatively late stages this can be effective.

HERPES
There are two strains of the Herpes simplex virus – HSV-1 and HSV-2. The former cause cold sores and the latter genital herpes. Nowadays, the two strains are not so well-separated as they used to be. Both are capable of causing either disorder.

Genital herpes appears, so far, to be an incurable disease and every effort should be made to avoid infection.

The first sign, which appears within a week of exposure, is a red, painful rash anywhere on the genitals or the surrounding skin. This may be confined to the genital area or may extend also to the thighs or buttocks. The pain may be severe and is in proportion to the extent of the rash.

Soon a succession of crops of blisters develops. The fluid in these blisters contains millions of herpes viruses. When the blisters break they leave raw ulcers which may join up to form quite large areas of shallow cratering. At this stage the sores are very sensitive, especially if urine comes in contact with the raw areas. Local neurological upset may also occur temporarily and this may even lead to retention of urine. There are often enlarged and tender lymph nodes ('glands') in the groin, showing that the infection has spread deeply into the body. Some people have slight fever and general illness. Finally, about three weeks after the beginning of the attack, the ulcers crust over and begin to heal. The pain usually goes away about two weeks after the rash first appears.

The first recurrence usually appears about four months after the initial infection and is often heralded by a local tingling sensation with great sensitivity of the skin in the areas about to be affected. After two or three days the sequence described above is repeated. Fortunately, recurrences are hardly ever as severe as the first attack and do not last as long. The new blisters usually heal in just under two weeks. Whenever blisters or rash are present, the affected person is highly infectious to others. Recurrences may be brought on by various factors including menstruation, stress or even sexual intercourse.

Once the virus is established in the body, indefinite recurrences are likely.

The drug acyclovir, taken by mouth, can greatly reduce the severity of attacks and shorten their duration, but it cannot cure the condition. It is the most effective treatment developed to date and is apparently quite safe.

CHLAMYDIAL INFECTION AND GONORRHOEA
Chlamydial infections are caused by *Chlamydia trachomatis* and gonorrhoea by *Neisseria gonorrhoea*. Both can cause acute or chronic pelvic inflammatory disease in women and lead to serious and persistent illness. The consequences of this may be permanent sterility.

The early signs are usually vaginal and urethral discharges and severe irritation, occurring two to five days after intercourse in the case of gonorrhoea, and seven to twenty-one days in the case of chlamydia. In men, the discharge may be yellow (pus) or clear, but should not be confused with the clear mucoid discharge noted after sexual excitement.

Many women have a vaginal discharge unconnected with an STD, but if there is a change in the character of the discharge, especially a few days after a new sexual contact, one of these conditions should be suspected. Unfortunately, in women especially, these diseases may occur without the affected person being aware of it.

In women, gonorrhoea and chlamydial disease start as an infection of the cervix and produce a **cervicitis** with discharge. In about 10 per cent of cases, the infection spreads up into the womb and along the fallopian tubes to cause inflammation (salpingitis). This can damage the linings and promote narrowing of the already narrow canals so that fertilized eggs may not be able to move along normally. This increases the risk of a pregnancy occurring in the tube (**ectopic pregnancy**). Repeated attacks of gonorrhoea or chlamydial infection are likely to cause sterility. After three or more attacks, about three-quarters of women have totally blocked tubes.

In women, the organisms causing these conditions often spread further to cause persistent inflammation of the inside of the pelvis. This is called chronic pelvic inflammatory disease (PID). It features a distressingly constant, dragging abdominal pain, tenderness on pressure and bouts of fever. In addition, there is likely to be discomfort, or even pain, on sexual intercourse. Another effect of these organisms is to cause abscesses in the lips at the entrance to the vagina.

Men usually get off more lightly. The discharge, which at first may be profuse with severe discomfort on urination, will gradually become less, and complications are not very common. A proportion of men, however, do suffer spread of infection to the testicles or prostate and these infections may last for months or years. Some men, after repeated attacks of gonorrhoea, develop a local narrowing (stricture) of the urine tube (urethra). This can obstruct the flow of urine and may have serious long-term consequences. In addition, about one man in 100 with chlamydial infection develops a severe form of arthritis affecting mainly the ankles, knees and feet and possibly involving also the eyes and even the heart. This condition is called **Reiter's syndrome**.

If caught early, both gonorrhoea and chlamydial infections will respond well to treatment with suitable antibiotics, and cure is to be expected. But once the secondary complications have developed, treatment is difficult. Surgery may be required and even this may be unsuccessful.

LYMPHOGRANULOMA VENEREUM

This disease is comparatively rare in Western countries but occurs in many parts of the tropics, especially in Africa, India, South-East Asia, South America and the Caribbean. Like non-gonococcal sexually transmitted disease it is caused by the organism *Chlamydia trachomatis*. Cases occasionally occur in Britain.

The first sign appears one to five weeks after contact, as a small and usually inconspicuous ulcer on the genitalia, which soon heals. The chlamydial organisms have, however, moved to the regional lymph nodes in the groin and these soon become inflamed, enlarged and matted together. The skin overlying the infected nodes becomes discoloured and dusky pink. In neglected cases the nodes may become so severely infected that pus accumulates in them and abscesses form. These are liable to break through to the surface leaving multiple discharging openings on the skin known as sinuses. These are very persistent and may take months to heal. Some affected people develop a rash, fever, headache, aches and pains, loss of weight and an enlarged spleen.

The condition is treated with tetracycline for about two weeks and usually clears up. This is best given before the groin nodes become too severely affected.

CHANCROID

Caused by the bacterium *Haemophilus ducrei*, chancroid is uncommon in Britain, but is a major health problem in many parts of the tropical developing world, where it is often commoner than syphilis.

The word chancroid means 'chancre-like' and the early sore often closely resembles the hard **chancre** of syphilis (see above). Three to five days after exposure an inflamed pustule develops on the genitalia which rapidly develops into a painful spreading ulcer. The floor of the ulcer is covered with a greyish membrane and the edges are ragged and undermined. Soon afterwards, the lymph nodes in the groin become enlarged and tender and form abscesses called buboes. These often burst externally so that, without effective treatment, permanent drainage channels (sinuses) are formed.

Chancroid can be treated with sulphonamides or antibiotics.

sexual problems

The proportion of sexual problems attributable to organic or structural disorder is small: the majority are of psychological or inter-relational origin. They include **impotence**, **ejaculation disorders**, especially premature ejaculation, lack of orgasm in females, inability to relax the muscles of the genitalia (**vaginismus**), and various forms of sexual deviation.

Organic disease such as neurologically or diabetically induced impotence, **Peyronie's disease** in males, or drying or shrinkage of the vagina in the elderly woman from oestrogen deficiency (*kraurosis vulvae*), can cause serious sexual difficulties.

Sezary syndrome

A rare condition featuring a malignant spread of excessive numbers of abnormal T cells (T lymphocytes) in the blood, with enlarged lymph nodes and lymphoid deposits in the skin, liver and spleen. There are red, scaly patches on the skin extending to form a widespread, itchy and flaking rash, hair loss and distortion of the nails. The condition is thought to be caused by a retrovirus, HTLV-I. Treatment is with anticancer drugs and radiotherapy.

shaken infant syndrome

The presence in a small baby of unexplained fractures of the long bones and blood clots under the main membrane surrounding the brain (subdural haematoma). These injuries are caused by whiplash and excessive rotational movement of the head, caused by violent shaking. A baby's head is very heavy relative to the strength of the neck muscles and the latter can offer little or no resistance to brutal treatment of this kind. Such trauma may lead to bleeding within the cranial cavity and an expanding blood clot which, unless treated by surgery, will produce progressive signs of brain compression with irritability, convulsions, coma and death.

shaking, drug-induced

See **tardive dyskinesia**.

shave, dirty

See **sycosis barbae**.

Sheehan's syndrome

The effects of destruction of the front part of the pituitary gland by loss of its blood supply (infarction) following severe bleeding from the womb after delivery of a baby (postpartum haemorrhage). There is failure of milk production, loss of body hair, absence of menstruation, lethargy and other effects of the underaction of the endocrine glands. Treatment is by comprehensive hormone replacement therapy.

shigellosis

Dysentery caused by bacteria of the Shigella genus. Shigellosis is often called bacillary dysentery and should be distinguished from amoebic dysentery (see **amoebiasis**). It occurs all over the world especially in areas where standards of hygiene and sanitation are poor. It is a highly infectious disease, especially prevalent in closed communities such as children's play-schools, institutions for old people and mental hospitals. Male homosexuals are frequently infected. Many outbreaks have been caused by food contamination.

RECOGNITION AND SYMPTOMS

Shigellosis may vary from mild watery diarrhoea to a severe illness with high fever. It usually begins suddenly, one to seven days after infection, with pain in the abdomen, nausea, vomiting, generalized aching and fever. Initially, the diarrhoea is watery, but after a few days, frequent small stools containing mucus and blood are passed and there are repeated spasms of the rectum with the desire to empty the bowel (**tenesmus**). The diarrhoea reaches a maximum in about a week, and then subsides. Untreated patients usually continue to pass Shigella organisms for one to four weeks, but a small proportion remain carriers for much longer. The death rate is very low and a fatal outcome is rare except in babies and old people not properly treated.

TREATMENT

If fluid loss is severe, the first concern is to correct dehydration. Fluids are best given by mouth, but those unable to drink may require transfusion. This is particularly important in children and the elderly. In many cases, shigellosis settles without treatment, but antibiotics will shorten the illness and reduce the risk of spread. Many antibiotics are effective but bacterial resistance to the most commonly used drugs is common. Tetracycline is one of the most useful.

shingles

A painful and sometimes debilitating disease caused by the same virus that causes chickenpox (the *varicella-zoster* virus). In a progressively ageing population, shingles is an increasing problem, for most sufferers are over fifty and the frequency rises with age. Half of those who reach eighty-five will have had at least one attack, and an attack does not necessarily confer permanent immunity. Every year some 200,000 people in this country suffer an attack of shingles and about half of them will suffer severe and persistent pain.

The name *shingles* comes from the Latin *cingulum* meaning 'a girdle', in reference to the common distribution of shingles along one or more strips of skin supplied by a single nerve root (dermatome) on the chest wall. The Greek word *zoster* means the 'belt' of a soldier and the medical term for shingles is *Herpes zoster*. The Greek verb *herpein* means 'to creep', a reference to the tendency of both forms of herpes – **herpes** simplex and herpes zoster – to spread in a creeping manner.

Shingles is not, in the ordinary sense, an infection. The virus is acquired, as a general rule, during childhood when it causes an attack of chickenpox – usually a very mild and transient illness and one which may even go unnoticed. In the course of the attack of chickenpox, varicella-zoster virus is believed to enter the sensory nerve endings in the skin and travel up the nerves to the collections of nerve bodies (the ganglia) near the spinal cord. The virus has been isolated from these ganglia at postmortem examination of patients who died while suffering from shingles. Later, often many years later, the viruses become reactivated and produce an acute ganglionitis (inflammation in the ganglion). This is the cause of the pain experienced in the area supplied by the nerve, prior to the onset of the rash. Reactivation occurs because of a drop in the efficiency of the immune system which had been keeping the virus in check.

Replication of the viruses now produces a large number of new individuals and these travel down the nerve to the skin where further reproduction occurs and the characteristic rash, from cell damage, appears.

RECOGNITION AND SYMPTOMS

The first indication of shingles is usually a tingling sensation (hypersensitivity) in the area to be affected and this is followed by pain, often severe, in the same area. The area involved is the skin distribution of one or more sensory nerve roots supplying a strip of the skin of the chest or abdominal wall on one side, or on the face, above the eyebrow, also on one side. There is often fever and sickness and on the fourth or fifth day after the onset, the skin becomes red, and typical crops of small blisters (vesicles) appear in the area affected.

These vesicles are initially full of clear fluid, which is teeming with herpes viruses, but about three days after appearing, they turn yellowish and within a few days flatten, dry out and crust over. In the following two weeks or so, the crusts gradually dry up and drop off, leaving small, pitted scars. Occasionally, the rash is more widespread and the vesicles may join up to form large confluent areas of damaged skin. In these cases healing may take many weeks and residual scarring may be severe. Widespread rash should arouse the suspicion of an underlying malignancy or a compromised immune system.

Herpes zoster of the face, which occurs in 10 to 15 per cent of cases, is especially distressing, for the eye may be involved, and the vision affected.

COMPLICATIONS

The complications of shingles include:

- rash infection, by secondary organisms, causing deep tissue damage and scarring;
- skin contractures around the chest and eye;
- local loss of skin pigment, leaving white areas;
- involvement of the external ear with occasional damage to the middle and inner ears, with deafness and vertigo;
- the Ramsay-Hunt syndrome, in which there is ear involvement together with paralysis of the facial nerve (**Bell's palsy**) on the same side;
- ulceration and permanent scarring of the cornea;
- loss of sensation in the cornea;
- inflammation of the iris and ciliary body (**uveitis**);
- persistent pain in the site of the rash.

The latter misfortune, which is known as post-herpetic pain, is the real reason why shingles is so important. As a rule, the pain and discomfort of shingles settles in two or three weeks from the onset. But in a proportion of cases this is not so and the pain continues for months or sometimes even for years. This affects about 30 per cent of shingles patients over the age of forty, and the older the person, and the more severe the pre-rash pain, the more likely this is to happen.

Persistent pain of this kind can have a devastating effect on the life of the unfortunate sufferer. Many are old and frail and ill-equipped to tolerate the resulting debility and the deeply depressing effects of unremitting pain. For many, the will to live may, all too easily, be lost.

TREATMENT

Shingles can hardly be avoided, but an important recent advance has made it possible to ensure that the effects are mild and the post-herpetic pain minor. This is the development of the anti-herpes drug acyclovir, which should be given in large dosage as soon as the diagnosis becomes clear. The earlier the drug is given, the more effective the results will be.

shin splints

A lay term for pain in the lower leg muscles and bones occurring in runners and football players and made worse by exertion. Causes include expanding muscle bulk within constricting fibrous sheaths (compartment syndrome), muscle tear, muscle inflammation (myositis), inflammation of the bone covering membrane (periostitis) or tendon inflammation. The condition will settle with rest. Occasionally it may be necessary to cut open the sheaths of muscle compartments to allow muscle expansion.

shivering

An important means of heat production in the body. Shivering is a rapid succession of contractions and relaxations of muscles. This occurs automatically when extra heat is required to maintain body temperature and is thus a feature of exposure to cold. The power of the contraction depends on the rate of heat production needed and may be considerable, leading to a rigor (violent shivering). The correct response to shivering from cold is to improve the body's insulation by suitable clothing and so reduce heat loss.

The body contains a thermostat, in the form of certain temperature-sensitive nerve cells in the hypothalamus of the brain and a drop in the temperature of the blood is sensed by these nerves, and the shivering reflex initiated. In fever, the bacteria, toxins etc., release from some of the white cells of the blood a substance called interleukin-1, and this resets the thermostat at a higher point. The nervous system then responds as if the blood were too cold and shivering results. In this case, the extra heat production may or may not be beneficial, depending on the cause, but, in general, heat loss from the body should be encouraged.

shock, surgical

This is a condition poorly understood outside medical circles, mainly because the word has a separate, but associated, lay usage – emotional shock (see **post-traumatic stress disorder**). Shock is a dangerous and often critical medical condition caused by a reduction in the volume of the circulating blood. This may be due to:

- severe blood loss after an injury;
- loss of fluid as a result of major burns or damage to the blood vessels from severe infection (**septic shock**);
- the presence of bacterial poisons (toxins) in the blood (**toxic shock syndrome**);
- failure of the heart to function properly, as after a **heart attack** (coronary thrombosis);
- abnormal loss of tension in the blood vessels;
- obstruction in major arteries, as in blockage of a pulmonary artery by a blood clot in the lungs (pulmonary embolism).

In shock there is a drop in blood pressure, the heart beats rapidly, to try to maintain the circulation, but the pulse is weak. The skin is pale but moist and the production of urine drops. Unless rapidly reversed, shock is likely to be fatal.

When shock is due to fluid loss, or burns, prompt transfusion, not necessarily of blood, but sometimes simply of salty water (saline), can be life-saving. Septic shock calls for urgent, intensive antibiotic treatment. Pulmonary embolism is treated with anti-clotting drugs or enzymes that dissolve the clot. In acute emergency it may be necessary to remove the clot surgically, but patients seldom survive long enough to allow this.

shock therapy

See **electroconvulsive therapy**.

short bowel syndrome

A disorder caused by the surgical removal of a segment of intestine. It features weight loss, diarrhoea, fatty stools (steatorrhoea), and deficiencies of sodium, potassium and trace elements. Affected people must eat several small meals a day, of readily-absorbed, finely chopped or ground foods supplemented by vitamins and minerals. Bowel-lengthening surgery or bowel transplant may be feasible.

short-sightedness

See **myopia**.

shoulder girdle and arm structure

Lying over the upper ribs of the back are the two flat shoulder blades (scapulas), and these are also supported, from the front, by the two collar bones (clavicles) which link the top of the sternum, on each side, to a bony process on each scapula. Without the scapulas and clavicles we would have no shoulders. This incomplete ring of bones is called the shoulder girdle.

Each scapula bears on its upper and outer angle a shallow cavity in which the head of the upper arm bone (the humerus) sits. Because the cavity is so shallow, movement of the arm at the shoulder can occur in an arc of 360 degrees. The bottom end of the humerus joins with the forearm bones, the radius and ulna and the bottom ends of these with the eight carpal bones of the wrist. Beyond these are the five metacarpals

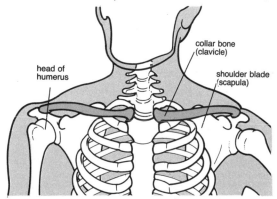

The shoulder girdle. This provides suspension for the arm bones and attachment for several muscles.

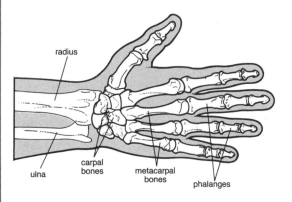

The bones of the wrist and hand.

(meta means 'beyond') of the palm of the hand and the fourteen phalanges (singular phalanx) of the fingers and thumb. Each finger has three phalanges; the thumb has two.

shunt

A bypass allowing blood or other fluid to be diverted from its normal direction of flow. An arterio-venous shunt allows blood to go directly from an artery to a vein without passing through the capillaries, in the normal way. Such a shunt may be made artificially in the arm in those who have to be repeatedly connected to a dialysis machine, or may occur as a result of penetrating injury, such as a gunshot wound, involving both vessels.

A shunt commonly occurs in congenital heart disorders when an abnormal opening, such as a defect in the wall between the two sides – a 'hole in the heart' – allows blood to pass from the left side of the heart to the right. Sometime shunting occurs in the opposite direction so that the lungs are bypassed.

Shunts are successfully used in treating 'water on the brain' (**hydrocephalus**) to allow free drainage of cerebrospinal fluid, by way of a plastic tube containing a pressure-operated valve, from the brain spaces to the heart or the abdominal cavity. A shunt may also be used between the por-

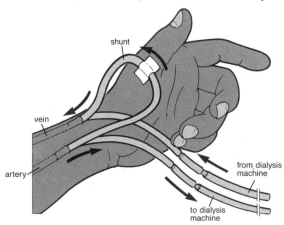

One form of arterio-venous shunt – that used in patients who need regular dialysis because of kidney failure. Between treatments the blood from the artery is allowed to run directly back into a vein through the artificial shunt.

tal vein of the liver and the main vein of the body (portacaval shunt) in order to prevent the development, in cirrhosis of the liver, of dangerous varicose veins at the lower end of the gullet (oesophagus).

Siamese twins

Twins joined together at birth. The junction is usually along the trunk or between the two heads, at the front, back or sides. In some cases, organs are shared and this makes separation difficult or impossible. Sometimes, one twin is normal and the other is a severely underdeveloped parasite, relying on its host for nutrition. In such a case it may be decided to remove the smaller twin in the interests of the other.

The name derives from the male twins Chang and Eng, born in Siam in 1811 and surviving until they were sixty-three. Chang and Eng were joined face to face from breastbone to navel but both married and each contrived to father several children.

Siamese twins are derived from a single fertilized ovum and are uniovular, identical twins. In the normal case, at the time of the first division of the ovum, the two resulting daughter cells either remain joined to produce one individual, or separate completely to produce two identical individuals, which then develop separately. In the case of Siamese twins, this separation is incomplete. The surprise is not that the phenomenon occurs, but that it should be so rare.

sick building syndrome

A rather vague concept, probably related psychologically to awareness of Legionnaire's disease, that has never been realistically formalized. It refers to a varied group of symptoms sometimes experienced by people working in modern office buildings and attributed to some property of the building. These include fatigue, headache, dryness and itching of the eyes, sore throat and dryness of the nose.

No convincing explanation has been offered and it may be that this is an attempt to rationalize employees' dissatisfaction with boredom and unacceptable working conditions. Some workers have experienced symptoms from ozone produced by photocopiers, inadequate air conditioning, poor lighting, un-ergonomic seating at desks, lack of privacy due to open-plan office design, hatred of personal computers, secondary smoking, excessive coffee intake, or dislike of their colleagues. The truth may be that the problem lies in the relationship of the workers to the building rather than in the building itself.

sickle-cell disease

This is an autosomal recessive genetic disorder mainly affecting Africans and their descendants. Its essential feature is an abnormal form of haemoglobin (haemoglobin S) in the red blood cells. When the red cells are low in oxygen, this form of haemoglobin goes into a crystal-like structure that causes the red cell membrane to distort. As a result, the blood becomes thicker, blocking small arteries (thrombosis) and causing severe pain and swelling in the tissues thus deprived of blood.

Normal haemoglobin is designated haemoglobin A and, in this context, a normal person is said to have the genotype AA. A person with sickle-cell disease has the defective gene for haemoglobin S in both of the relevant paired chromosomes (is homozygous). Such a person has the genotype SS. A person heterozygous is SA. The latter is said to have the sickle-cell trait D a much less serious condition.

SYMPTOMS

These usually start in early infancy and include pallor, jaundice, breathlessness, enlarged spleen, fatigue and headaches. Crises may be precipitated by infections, dehydration or cold weather, and feature bone pain, blood in the urine, and sometimes stroke or epileptic seizures. Anaemia may be severe and even life-threatening. Children with sickle cell anaemia are prone to pneumonia.

TREATMENT

Anaemia is treated with folic acid and iron and infection may be prevented with routine antibiotics. Crises may call for fluid transfusions, oxygen therapy and pain-killers. An exchange blood transfusion may be necessary in severe cases.

MALARIA AND SICKLE CELL DISEASE

People with the sickle-cell trait show considerable resistance to the normally lethal effects of falciparum **malaria** in early childhood. This is because the malarial parasite cannot thrive normally in the abnormal red cells. This surprising fact accounts for the frequency with which the sickle-cell gene is found in areas, especially in equatorial Africa, where falciparum malaria is endemic. People with the sickle-cell trait (SA) have been naturally selected relative to normal people and there is a close correlation between the distribution of the haemoglobin S gene and the past prevalence of falciparum malaria.

This is a striking example of the way in which genetics, the environment and evolution can interact.

Siddha medicine

A system of medicine practised in Tamil areas of South-east India and by Tamil-speaking people elsewhere. The system has something in common with the early medical notion of the four humours, but is based on wind, bile and phlegm. Diagnosis is made by the analysis of the pulse and the appearance of the urine: the darker the urine, the more severe the disease. Siddha medicine includes yogic practices, faith in the miraculous alchemical properties of mercury and sulphur and the ability to prolong life through rejuvenating treatments especially the regulation of the breathing. It is believed that eternal youth is to be achieved by 21,600 respirations a day.

sight, partial

Permanent loss of vision, not amounting to total blindness, but of such degree as to cause substantial handicap. The loss may involve either visual acuity or **visual field**, or both. A person may be registered partially sighted although able to read the bottom line on the eye testing chart, if the peripheral vision is severely restricted.

Sigmacort

A brand name for **hydrocortisone**.

sildenafil citrate

An oral therapy for impotence in men. During sexual stimulation nitric oxide is released in the corpora cavernosa of the **penis**. Nitric oxide activates the enzyme guanylate cyclase, which leads indirectly to higher levels of cyclic guanosine monophosphate. This substance relaxes smooth muscle in the corpora cavernosa so that blood can flow in easily under arterial pressure. The monophosphate is, however, broken down by a phosphodiesterase enzyme (type 5) which limits its action. Sildenafil is a selective inhibitor of this type of enzyme, resulting in prolonged action of cyclic guanosine monophosphate and a more substantial and better-sustained erection. The drug has its maximum effect about an hour after ingestion. It is said to have no effect in the absence of sexual stimulation. The drug increases the blood pressure-lowering effect of nitrates and should not be taken by patients using organic nitrates in any form. Other side-effects include headache and transient blue-green colour perception defect. A trade name is Viagra.

silent mutation

A change in **DNA** that has no effect.

silent site

In a gene, one of the positions at which a mutation does not change the product.

silicone and breast implants

The silicones are polymeric (long-chain), organic compounds of silicon and oxygen in which each silicon atom is linked to an alkyl group (one of the paraffin series from which a hydrogen atom has been removed). Silicones may be produced as oils, greases or rubbers. Silicone rubbers, such as Silastic, are valuable prosthetic surgical structural materials as they are inert, permeable to oxygen and well tolerated by the tissues. They are widely used in surgery and cause little or no adverse effects.

In spite of enormous public and legal interest, and the massive awards that have been made to women claiming that silicone breast implants have caused serious disorders, the current expert view is that there is no causal connection between these implants and the disorders.

silver sulphadiazine

An antibacterial drug used externally to treat skin infections, burns, pressure sores and ulcers. A brand name is Flamazine.

Simeco

A brand name for a mixture of aluminium hydroxide, magnesium hydroxide and simethicone.

Simulect

A brand name for **basiliximab**.

simvastatin

A statin drug used to treat raised blood cholesterol levels. A brand name is Zocor.

Sinemet

A brand name for **levodopa** in combination with carbidopa.

Sinequan

A brand name for the tranquillizing drug **doxepin**.

singer's nodes

Small whitish swellings or nodules on the vocal chords resulting from prolonged use of the voice in a strained or unnatural manner. High-pitched voice sounds, as used by some pop singers, can be obtained by vibrating the front part of the vocal cords, while the rear parts remain pressed together. This practice, however, leads to trauma to the cords which respond by a protective production of fibrous tissue in the form of singer's or screamer's nodes.

The resultant increase in the mass of the vocal cords causes hoarseness and loss of voice and this can be restored only by microsurgical removal of the nodules. Training in the proper use of the voice is necessary if recurrence is to be avoided. The removed tissue is sent for examination as a **biopsy**, because nodes on the vocal cords are sometimes cancerous.

See also **clergyman's throat**, **laryngitis**.

single sperm injection

See **sperm injection IVF**.

single strand binding proteins

Proteins that keep single strands of DNA apart during replication, in spite of the tendency for complementary **base pairs** to stick together. These proteins work by attaching to the separated strands at the point of separation (the replication fork) so as to seal them off from each other and prevent immediate re-linking.

Singulair

A brand name for **montelukast**.

Sinthrome

A brand name for nicoumalone.

Sintisone

A brand name for **prednisolone**.

sinusitis

Inflammation, almost always from infection, of the linings of the bone cavities of the face (sinuses).

Sinusitis is often a complication, due to secondary bacterial infection, of the common cold. The inflammation of the mucous membrane lining causes swelling and this may lead to obstruction of the narrow outlet so that discharge – mucus and pus – cannot easily escape. The result is a feeling of fullness or even pain, which is felt in the forehead, cheeks or between the eyes, depending on which sinuses are affected. Severe sinusitis causes fever and general upset. The symptoms are usually compounded with those of the associated common cold.

Complications of sinusitis are rare and any tendency for spread of infection to adjacent bone can usually be easily controlled by antibiotics.

Sinutab Antihistamine

A brand name for a mixture of **paracetamol**, **pseudoephedrine** and **chlorpheniramine**.

Sinuzets

A brand name for capsules containing **paracetamol**, **pseudoephedrine** and **phenylephrine**.

-site

Suffix meaning 'eating, food' as in parasite (eating along with).

SI units

Scientific units of the Système Internationale. SI units have long replaced earlier systems of units and are now almost universally used in British, European and American medicine. They include the metre for length, the kilogram for weight, the mole for the amount of a substance in a solution, the joule for energy and the pascal for pressure. These units are qualified by decimal multipliers or divisors such as mega- (a million), kilo- (a thousand), deci- (a tenth), centi- (a hundredth), milli- (a thousandth), micro- (a millionth), nano- (a thousand millionth), pico- (a million millionth), and femto- (a thousand million millionth).

SIV

Simian immunodeficiency virus. This is an organism, similar to HIV, that affects monkeys.

Sjögren's syndrome

Dryness of the eyes, mouth and vagina, associated with immune system disorders, such as **rheumatoid arthritis**,

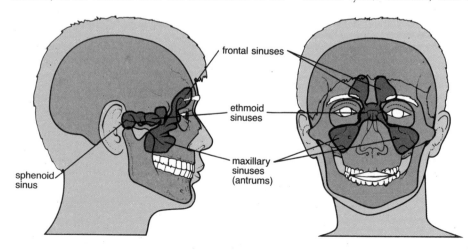

frontal sinuses
ethmoid sinuses
maxillary sinuses (antrums)
sphenoid sinus

The position of the various bone sinuses surrounding the nose. The sinuses are very variable in size. Sinusitis most commonly affects the frontal and maxillary sinuses.

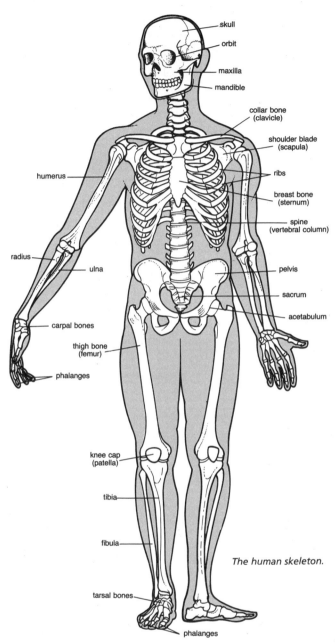

The human skeleton.

the mouth, difficulty in mastication, soreness of the tongue and swelling of the **salivary glands**. There is commonly loss of the senses of taste and smell. Dryness of the nose can be painful and is often associated with a hoarse voice and persistent chest infection. Dryness of the vagina causes difficulty and discomfort in sexual intercourse.

TREATMENT

Sjögren's is an immunological disorder, and the dryness results from reduced secretion of various kinds of glands following invasion and damage by immune system white cells (lymphocytes). There is no specific treatment to restore the glands to normal function, but much may be done by the use of artificial tears, frequent sips of fluid or polyvinyl alcohol sprays in the mouth, careful dental hygiene, and the use of K-Y jelly for vaginal lubrication.

skeleton

The skeleton is the framework of connected bones that gives the body its general shape, and provides support and protection for the internal organs and attachments for the muscles. There are 206 bones in the skeleton, which is organized on the axis of the spine (vertebral column) to which the **ribs** are attached. The **skull** rests on the upper end of the spine and the pelvis is firmly attached to the lower end. The shoulder girdle (see **shoulder girdle and arm structure**) consists of the shoulder blades (scapulas) and collar bones (clavicles) and provides attachment for the arm bones. The leg bones are attached to the pelvis. There is a close structural similarity between the arms and the legs.

See also **pelvic girdle and leg structure**.

Skelid

A brand name for tiludronic acid.

skills, loss of, in baby girls

See **Rett syndrome**.

skin

The skin is much more than just a waterproof cover for the body. It is a major organ, 1.5 – 2 square metres in area, self-renewing and self-repairing, providing heat regulation for the body and protection from the outside world. It is exquisitely sensitive to touch, pressure, pain, irritation, heat and cold and is an important sensory interface between the body and the outer world, endlessly sending environmental information to the brain. In addition to preventing undue loss of water – the interior of the body is largely watery – it controls loss of some small soluble molecules (electrolytes) and proteins.

The skin screens against light damage by absorbing light energy into the pigment melanin, and is a complete barrier against the alpha particles of radioactivity. Bacterial attack is resisted by the healthy skin, and the constant shedding of the outer horny layer of the outer layer of the skin (epidermis) also actively dislodges micro-organisms. The skin synthesizes vitamin D.

systemic **lupus erythematosus**, **myasthenia gravis**, dermatitis herpetiformis or auto-immune liver or thyroid disease.

INCIDENCE

Twenty-five to 50 per cent of people with rheumatoid arthritis have Sjögren's syndrome and 90 per cent of those affected are women, usually middle-aged and often post-menopausal. The peak incidence is between forty and sixty and the cause is unknown. About two per cent of the population is affected, but the condition is often missed.

RECOGNITION AND SYMPTOMS

The most obvious feature of Sjögren's syndrome is the dry eye condition keratoconjunctivitis sicca. There is a sense of grittiness in the eyes, a burning and itching sensation, redness, dimness of vision and sensitivity to light. The mouth involvement features a lack of saliva, and causes a sense of dryness in

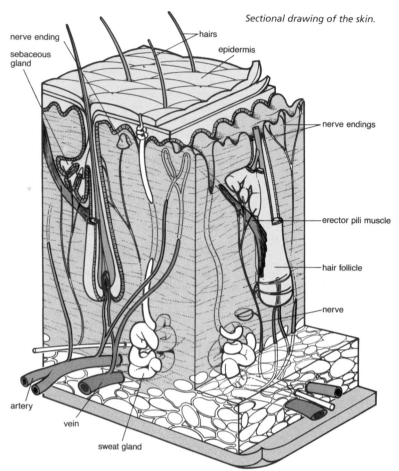

Sectional drawing of the skin.

nerve ending
sebaceous gland
hairs
epidermis
nerve endings
erector pili muscle
hair follicle
nerve
artery
vein
sweat gland

Apocrine glands are the type of sweat glands found in the hairy parts of the body, especially in the armpits and the groin. They develop after puberty and produce sweat which is broken down by skin bacteria to substances responsible for unpleasant body odour. Apocrine sweat should be washed off daily and may be inhibited by antiperspirant deodorants.

skin ache syndrome

A persistent and debilitating disorder of unknown cause in which pain is brought on by pressing on, or pinching certain small areas of the skin. The most common 'trigger' sites appear to be on the knee, over the shoulder blade and on the skin of the abdominal wall. The pain is abolished by the injection of a local anaesthetic under the relevant point and this often effects a permanent cure.

skin, air under

See **surgical emphysema**.

skin blisters, sticky

See **impetigo**.

skin, chapped

In healthy skin, the water content of the outer horny layer is 10 to 15 per cent and this is normally maintained by the action of cells which contain water-attracting (hydroscopic) substances. If the water content of the skin drops below about 10 per cent, there is a loss of elasticity and softness and the skin tends to crack. This is called chapping. Once cracks have formed, they tend to be maintained by the entry of soap and other irritating material.

The water content of the skin can drop as a result of excessive dryness in the atmosphere, especially in very cold weather, or of the overuse of household detergents, which dissolve an essential fatty acid component essential for the plasticity of the outer layers of the skin. Chapping is much less likely in warm conditions. The higher the atmospheric temperature, the more water it can contain.

Chapping can be reduced or avoided by bearing these facts in mind and acting accordingly. Rubber or plastic gloves will protect the skin from detergent damage and will help to maintain a local micro-climate of higher humidity. Excessive hand washing should be avoided.

skin, disorders of

Disorders of the skin the province of **dermatology**. This is a major discipline dealing with a wide range of disorders, covering much of the spectrum of tissue disease including inflammations, allergies, benign and malignant tumours, degenerative disorders, ageing effects, blood-supply deficiencies, and so on. The largest group are the inflammations and these are all grouped under the term **dermatitis**. This is not, as is commonly thought, a particular disease. The term sim-

Skin pores are the small openings in the skin through which the sweat passes from tiny glands situated in the deepest layers of the skin or just under it. Other pores in the skin are the hair follicles into which open the sebaceous glands producing the oily secretion sebum. In the skin of the nose, the hairs in these follicles are usually small in comparison with the sebaceous glands, so that the pore appears to be concerned solely with sebum production.

In the margin of each eyelid is a row of pores, just behind the line of the lashes. These are the openings of the oil-secreting meibomian glands. Sebaceous glands in the areola of the breast, in the labia minora, and in the prepuce discharge through pores which are also independent of the hair follicles.

The epidermis is the outermost layer of the skin. As the name implies, it lies beyond or outside the true skin, or dermis. The epidermis is structurally simple with no nerves, blood vessels, or hair follicles, and acts as a rapidly replaceable surface capable of tolerating much abrasion and trauma. The deepest layer of the epidermis is called the basal cell layer and it is this layer which grows abnormally in the common skin cancer basal cell carcinoma or rodent ulcer. This layer contains the pigment melanin in concentration which varies from person to person, thereby occasioning the characteristic skin colour. Above the basal layer is the prickle cell layer, and it is the prickle cells which grow abnormally in common warts. The outermost cells of the epidermis are dead and are continuously shed.

ply means 'inflammation of the skin'. It relates to a multitude of causes and includes all skin disorders in which the skin is inflamed. Although the causes are legion, the effects may be quite similar. Dermatitis may be caused by:

- infection by almost any kind of organism – viruses, bacteria, fungi and protozoa;
- allergy to a wide range of contact materials;
- physical or chemical injury;
- heat;
- intense ultraviolet light;
- other forms of radiation.

Eczema is also a form of dermatitis but has specific features. It is often allergic in origin and may start in infancy. **Urticaria** (hives or nettle-rash) is the common skin reaction to allergy, whether from contact, insect sting or ingestion.

Bacterial skin infection is very common. Different organisms produce recognizably different effects. *Staphylococci* cause pimples, boils and carbuncles. *Streptococci* produce an enzyme that breaks down tissue planes allowing the organisms to invade widely and cause spreading skin inflammation (**cellulitis**). Some can cause **necrotizing fasciitis**. Both staphylococci and streptococci can cause **impetigo**. Human papilloma viruses cause most forms of skin **warts**. Although these may take various quite distinct forms, they are all essentially the same. The herpes zoster **chickenpox** virus causes **shingles**. **Herpes** simplex viruses cause **cold sores** and venereal herpes.

Fungus infection, or epidermophytosis, causes the various forms of **tinea**. Fungus also commonly infects the nails.

Infestation with various mite and insect parasites, such as the **scabies** mite, *Sarcoptes scabiei*, fleas, bed bugs and lice, cause damage to the skin and this is often compounded by damage and secondary infection from scratching.

See also **acne**, **malignant melanoma**, **mole**, **nappy rash**, **port-wine stain**, **prickly heat**, **psoriasis**, **purpura**, **rodent ulcer**, **rosacea**, **sebaceous cyst**, **squamous cell carcinoma**, **ultraviolet light**, **vitiligo**, **xanthelasma**.

skin flap

When more than a small area of skin is lost through disease, injury or surgical removal, the first priority is to obtain skin cover of the bare area left. In some cases this may be done by a free graft of skin taken from another part of the body, but often this cannot provide either the bulk filling needed, or good matching of skin colour and texture. The bare area, too, may be inadequately supplied with blood vessels so that a free graft would not take. This might be so, if tendons, or even bone, are exposed.

The solution often rests in the repositioning, over the bare area, of a skin flap, left connected at one end so that an adequate blood supply is preserved, but rotated into position, or bridged over or tunnelled under normal skin. Sometimes this has to be done in stages, using an intermediate position which is maintained until new blood vessels have grown into the flap. More commonly, nowadays, microsurgical techniques are used to allow free thick tissue grafts to be employed, the blood supply being provided by joining up small arteries and veins. Many ingenious procedures have been designed to solve these difficult problems and the results are often cosmetically superior to the results of free skin grafting.

skinfold thickness measurement

A method of assessing the amount of fat under the skin by means of special calipers, sprung to exert a standard amount of pressure and fitted with a scale. If the primary interest is in the actual amount of subcutaneous fat, skinfold thickness measurements will more accurately assess obesity than weighing.

skin loosening and shedding

See **toxic epidermal necrolysis**.

skin malignancy

See **malignant melanoma**, **squamous cell carcinoma**.

Skinoren

A brand name for **azelaic acid**.

skin pallor

Skin colour depends on several factors including its thickness, the amount of pigment present in the form of cells containing the substance melanin, and, especially, the profusion and state of openness of the underlying small blood vessels. While it is true that extreme pallor may be caused by intense constriction of these blood vessels in the dangerous condition of surgical shock, this condition never occurs in otherwise healthy children but only follows serious injury or grave illness. It follows that skin pallor, by itself, has no medical significance. Much the same applies to 'dark rings under the eyes' which is due to the thinness of the skin of the lids and the profusion of the blood flow though the underlying vessels.

skin peel

A cosmetic procedure to improve the appearance of the facial skin by removing small wrinkles, scars, freckles and other blemishes. A paste containing carbolic acid is used to remove the surface layer of the epidermis and thin the skin. Protection against the ultraviolet in sunlight is necessary for some weeks after the procedure.

skin, scaly in children

See **eczema**.

skin, slate-blue coloured

See **Mongolian spot**.

skin spot, spidery

See **spider naevus**.

skin, undue sensitivity of

See **skin ache syndrome**.

skin, yellow

See **jaundice**.

Skitz

A brand name for benzoyl peroxide.

skull

Because the brain is the most important organ in the body it is correspondingly well protected and entirely enclosed in, and supported by, the hollow skull. The interior of the skull fits precisely to the shape of the brain and contains three descending shelves to support the frontal lobes, the middle part of the brain, the rear lobes and the hind brain (cerebellum).

In the centre of the middle shelf is a hollow to accommodate the pituitary gland, and in the centre of the deep rear shelf is a large opening, the foramen magnum, through which the downward continuation of the brain, the spinal cord, passes into the canal of the spine. In the centre of the upper shelf, on either side of the midline, are two thin perforated bony plates through which the many fibres of the nerves of smell (olfactory nerves) pass down into the nose.

Lying immediately under the outer parts of the front shelf are the two bony sockets (the orbits) which accommodate and protect the eyes. At the back of the orbits are holes in the bone to allow the optic nerves to pass back to the brain and to allow the nerves which move the eye muscles to run forward from the brain. To the inner side of each orbit, and separated from them by paper-thin sheets of bone, are two sets of sinuses, or air cells, the ethmoidal sinuses.

The back wall of the nose is formed by the front of the bone (the sphenoid) forming the central shelf of the skull. This bone is hollow and contains one or two sinuses. The pituitary gland is accessible, surgically, from the nose, through this wall. The floor of the nose is formed by the bony palate and this forms the roof of the mouth. The hard palate is a plate of bone which forms part of the upper jaw (maxilla). It is transversely ridged in young people but smooth in the old. The back edge of the hard palate is easily felt, in the mouth, and has a small protruding bump at each side.

Under the orbits are the paired maxillary bones of the upper jaw. Like the sphenoid, these are hollow. They contain the maxillary sinuses, or antrums, and bear the upper teeth. The hinged lower jaw (mandible) carries a corresponding set of lower teeth. The jaw bone joins with the base of the skull at hinge joints high up in front of each ear. The heads of the mandible can be seen bulging the skin, just in front of the ears, when the mouth is opened widely. The mandible is pulled upwards by wide powerful muscles running down to it from the base of the skull and the outside of the temple bones. The latter can be felt to contract, on either side of the forehead, when the teeth are clenched.

The vault of the skull consists of the wide forehead bone (frontal bone) containing the frontal sinuses – air spaces between the two layers of hard bone of which the vault of the skull is made; the paired, upper and rear side bones (parietal bones); the paired lower front temporal bones; and the single lower rear occipital bone. Infants have a gap, called a fontanelle, between the upper parts of these bones.

The prominence of the cheeks and part of the outer walls and floors of the orbits are formed by the zygomatic bones. The prominent bony process, which may be felt behind the lower part of the ear, is called the mastoid process. This is honeycombed with air cells and these communicate with the middle ear.

skull, pressure rise in

See **benign intracranial hypertension**.

sleep

The regular, daily period of unconsciousness, which occupies one-quarter to one-third of the duration of each person's life. Sleep requirements vary considerably, the limits, in health, being about four to ten hours in each 24-hour period.

On falling asleep, the level of consciousness declines gradually, through a half-awake stage to a loss of awareness of external events and then a stage in which brain electrical activity is markedly diminished. This level is interrupted several times each night by periods in which much neurological activity occurs, showing itself by an increase in blood flow though the brain, rapid changes in heart and respiration rates, quick, roving eye movements and erection of the penis in males. These periods are called rapid eye movement (REM) sleep and it is here that dreaming occurs. The state of the brain during REM sleep is similar to that during emotional arousal.

The purpose of sleep is unknown but prolonged deprivation of non-REM sleep is harmful, causing lethargy, depression, seizures and severe mental disturbances, including hallucinations. Less severe deprivation causes fatigue, irritability, loss of concentration and skills and deterioration of work performance. Repeated short periods of 'dropping off' occur.

Sleep apnoea is a rare disorder in which the breathing of the sleeping person stops spontaneously many times during the night, causing sudden waking. The stoppage may be due to obstruction to the airway in snorers or to a more serious

The skull, showing sutures between the bones of the vault and internal shelving to accommodate the brain.

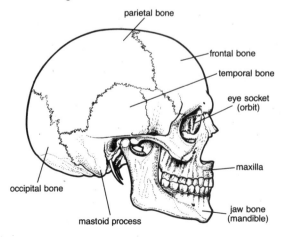

parietal bone
frontal bone
temporal bone
eye socket (orbit)
maxilla
jaw bone (mandible)
mastoid process
occipital bone

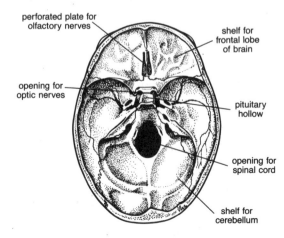

perforated plate for olfactory nerves
shelf for frontal lobe of brain
opening for optic nerves
pituitary hollow
opening for spinal cord
shelf for cerebellum

failure of the rhythmical nerve impulse drive from the brain to the muscles of respiration.

Narcolepsy features an irresistible desire to sleep; the affected person tends to fall asleep several times a day, but is readily awakened. In the associated condition of sleep paralysis, the affected person is unable, for a time, to move on waking from sleep, although fully conscious.

Sleepwalking, or somnambulism, is quite rare in adults, but common in children, especially boys, most of whom have an occasional episode. Some children sleepwalk regularly. The episode usually lasts for only a few minutes and is not purposeful. Sleepwalking is of little significance so long as precautions are taken to avoid danger from potential falls, and sleepwalking children need not be wakened, but should be guided gently back to bed.

sleeping drugs

Drugs used to promote sleep. The group includes many **benzodiazepines**, some **antihistamines**, antidepressants and chloral hydrate. The **barbiturates**, once widely used for this purpose, have mainly fallen into disrepute. See also **hypnotic drugs**.

sleeping sickness

A disease caused by a spindle-shaped, single-celled, parasite, the *Trypanosoma brucei*, which is transmitted by the bite of the tsetse fly. Sleeping sickness is endemic in a very large area of Central and West Africa. In some areas, the organism is passed from person to person, but in others the reservoir is the bushbuck antelope. The disease also affects cattle and renders millions of square miles of Africa uninhabitable.

When the infected fly bites, it deposits the parasites under the skin where they reproduce and cause local damage and ulceration. As the organisms multiply, they escape, in waves, into the circulation, causing fever. They settle in the small blood vessels of the heart and brain causing myocarditis, which is often fatal, and extensive brain inflammation (**encephalitis**), with loss of the outer sheath of the nerve fibres (demyelinization).

RECOGNITION AND SYMPTOMS

There is severe headache, loss of concentration, and insomnia and, after a long interval, the gradual development of serious brain damage with lassitude, a vacant expression, drooping eyelids and progressive loss of attention. Eventually, no spontaneous action is taken, and the patient will starve to death unless fed. Speech becomes slurred and indistinct and then ceases, paralysis and seizures occur, and coma and death inevitably supervene.

TREATMENT

Without treatment, the disease is generally fatal. If the nervous system has not been affected, suramin or pentamidine are the drugs of choice, but these do not penetrate to the brain and in brain involvement another, more toxic drug, melarsoprol, must be used. This may cause dangerous reactions.

sleep, twilight

A state of light anaesthesia and mental calm produced by a mixture of morphine and scopolamine, formerly used during childbirth.

sleepwalking

See **sleep**.

sling

A support to rest and immobilize the arm, either as a first aid measure following injury or as a definitive form of treatment, to place the arm in an appropriate position for the healing of a fractured collar bone (clavicle).

Slings are also used to rest an arm which has sustained muscle or other soft tissue injury, or which is severely infected.

slipped disc

This commonly used term is misleading, for there is no question of the disc slipping. Between the bodies of each of the bones of the spine (the vertebrae) is a cushioning pad called the intervertebral disc. Each disc consists of an outer ring of tough fibrous tissue firmly fixed to the bone, above and below, and an inner, pulpy core made of squashy, rubbery material called the nucleus pulposus. Normally, the outer fibrous ring is strong enough to keep the pulpy nucleus in place, and together, they form an efficient and elastic shock-absorber which allows movement between the two bones, while preventing them from grinding together.

Immediately behind the main front part of each vertebra is a hole running vertically downward through the bone. The column of vertebrae, with their intervertebral discs, thus contains a flexible tube called the spinal canal. Within this tube lies the all-important spinal cord with its thirty-one pairs of spinal nerves, emerging from it, running downward and then coming out through holes between the bones.

In intervertebral disc prolapse, partial degeneration of the back part of the fibrous ring allows some of the pulpy centre (the nucleus pulposus) to bulge through under pressure. This seldom occurs directly backwards, because there are strong retaining ligaments running up and down the fronts and backs of the bodies of the vertebrae. But often the pulp will squeeze through to one side and bulge into the spinal canal just where the spinal nerves are bunched together. This happens most often in the small of the back and it is the pressure of the disc pulp on these nerves that causes the main symptoms and dangers of 'slipped disc'. Protrusion of pulp may also occur from a disc or discs in the neck, but this is less common.

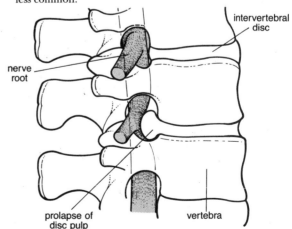

Slipped disc. The disc between the vertebral bodies does not, in fact, slip. Degeneration of the outer fibrous ring allows some of the pulpy inner matter of the disc to protrude backwards and press against the nerve roots, as shown.

RECOGNITION AND SYMPTOMS

In lower back disc pulp protrusion there is severe pain in the back and usually down the back of the leg, on the affected side, along the line of the sciatic nerve, which is made up from the lower spinal nerves. This pain is made worse by moving, coughing and straining. Even laughing can cause a shoot of pain. Raising the leg while lying flat will stretch the sciatic nerve and will cause pain in the back and down the leg. In addition to the pain, tingling and numbness occurs in the region supplied by the nerves – and this may be as far down as the foot.

> The muscles moved by the affected nerve eventually can become weak and wasted and there may even be interference with proper bladder control. This is a serious sign calling for urgent treatment.

TREATMENT

Continued activity at this stage can be dangerous. Strict bed rest, lying on the back on a firm surface for at least two weeks, is the first step. If the trouble persists, traction in hospital may be necessary and possibly an operation to remove the offending pulp. In neck protrusion, traction, a collar and head halter may be needed.

slipped vertebra

See **spondylolisthesis**.

Slo-Bid

A brand name for **theophylline**.

Slo-Fe

A brand name for the iron preparation **ferrous sulphate**.

slough

Dead tissue which is being, or has been, cast off or separated from its original site. The term is also used as a verb. Thus, sloughing of dead tissue commonly occurs following gangrene of an extremity or when a segment of bone, deprived of its blood supply in the course of a fracture, or as a result of infection, is cast off. A slough may remain sequestrated within the tissue from which it came. This is common in bone.

Slow-Fe Folic

A brand name for **ferrous sulphate** in conjunction with **folic acid**.

Slow-K

A brand name for a potassium preparation.

Slow-Trasicor

A brand name for **oxprenolol**.

Slozem

A brand name for **diltiazem**.

small head

See **microcephaly**.

small intestine

The beginning of the small intestine, the duodenum, is so called because it is said to be twelve finger-breadths' long. It is the widest, shortest and most immobile part of the small bowel and forms an almost circular curve from the outlet of the stomach to the beginning of the jejunum. It ends just below and to the left side of its starting point. About the middle of the descending curve, the duodenum is entered by the ducts from the pancreas and the gall-bladder (see **liver**), thereby receiving a plentiful supply of digestive juices (pancreatic enzymes) and a quantity of a detergent-like emulsifying agent (bile salts) which break up ingested fats into a milky emulsion which is easily absorbed.

The small intestine is elaborately folded up and suspended by a remarkable membrane, the mesentery, which is only a few centimetres long at its point of attachment to the back wall of the abdomen, but is more than 6 m long at the border attached to the bowel. In consequence, the much folded tube resembles a mass of sausages, and that was the origin of the name bowel – from the Latin *botulus*, meaning 'sausage', by way of the French *boel*.

The jejunum is the part of the small intestine that lies between the duodenum and the ileum. The name jejunum means 'empty' and in this part of the bowel the contents are very fluid and pass quickly along under the influence of peristalsis. The jejunum is wider and thicker-walled than the ileum and occupies the middle part of the abdomen. Like the rest of the small intestine, it consists of four layers – an inner, deeply folded layer of mucous membrane, covered with millions of tiny finger-like processes called villi; a sub-mucous coat containing blood vessels, glands and nerves; a double muscular layer of circular and longitudinal fibres; and a thin outer coat of transparent peritoneum.

Much of the digestion of food, and most of the absorption, has taken place before the end of the jejunum. Absorption occurs through the thin walls of the villi. Because the villi are so numerous, the total area available for absorption is very large. The whole surface area of the small intestine approximates to that of a tennis court.

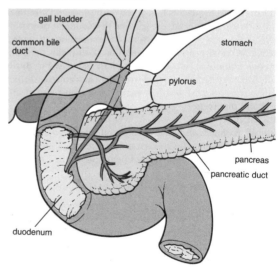

The duodenum. This is the start of the small intestine. The ducts from the pancreas and from the liver and gall-bladder enter the duodenum together, bringing digestive juices and bile.

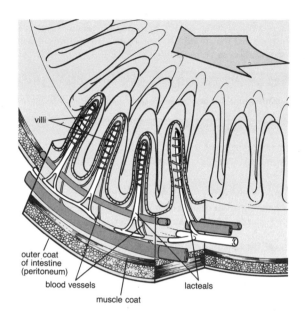

villi

outer coat
of intestine
(peritoneum)

blood vessels

muscle coat

lacteals

A microscopic section of the wall of the small intestine. The finger-like processes are called villi and it is through these that nutrients are absorbed from the digested food. Fats are absorbed into the lacteals and the other nutrients directly into the blood vessels.

The third, and lowest, part of the small intestine is the ileum and this part joins the large intestine (colon) at the wide, sac-like caecum, from which the appendix protrudes.

smallpox

A disease with the unique distinction of having been totally eradicated. Once a major scourge of mankind, causing enormous mortality and widespread distress from disfigurement and blindness, smallpox ceased to exist in 1978 as a result of an intensive international campaign coordinated by the World Health Organization. With the exception of six smallpox cultures in various parts of the world, laboratory stocks of the virus have now been destroyed.

Smallpox was a severe, highly infectious, virus disease, spread mainly by droplet infection, and causing fever, headache, generalized muscle aches, and then an apparent recovery followed by the appearance of a severe rash. This rash started as small macules scattered on the face and arms which progressed to **papules**, enlarging and spreading widely to the extremities and then to the trunk, then crusting, scabbing and ulcerating the skin and leaving the patient with deep pitted scars. The rash frequently became secondarily infected and this increased the tendency to scarring.

Smallpox had a very variable mortality. In some epidemics hardly any patients died, while in others the mortality was as high as 20 per cent. Its eradication was a triumph of enlightened international cooperation and it is hoped that other diseases occurring in man only may similarly be conquered.

small round viruses

A term used to refer to a varied group of poorly characterized small viruses of about 25–35 mn in diameter, because little is known about them. They are divided into small round structured viruses (SRSV) in which some internal details can be discerned on electron microscopy, and small round nonstructured viruses. They include the Norwalk agent and are known to be responsible for many cases of food poisoning and gastroenteritis.

smegma

A cheesy-white, sebaceous gland secretion that accumulates under the foreskin of an uncircumcised male with poor standards of personal hygiene. Smegma that is not washed away, preferably daily, becomes infected, foul-smelling and irritating and can cause local inflammation.

For a time smegma was believed by some researchers to be capable of causing cancer of the penis and of the cervix in sexual contacts. This belief was based partly on the observation that horse smegma could cause skin cancer in shaven mice. Later studies suggest that a far more likely explanation is that papillomaviruses present in smegma may be the cause. These viruses cause various kinds of warts, including venereal warts. Papillomavirus infections are thought to be the probable reason for the higher incidence of cancer of the cervix in women with many sexual partners.

smell, sense of

The nose is the normal entry route for inspired air, which carries the tiny chemical particles conveying smell. In the highest part of the roof of the nose lie many hair-like nerve fibres. These are the sensitive receptors of the paired olfactory nerves – the nerves of smell. Particles are trapped by the mucus and fluid covering these nerve endings and act chemically on them in a very specific way, producing many different frequencies, amplitudes and combinations of nerve impulse which pass to the brain. See illustration on following page.

smoking cigarettes

See **health maintenance**.

smoking, objection to

See **tobacco-free social norm**.

snake bite

See **antivenin**.

snake venom drug

See **notexin**.

sneezing

A barely controllable reflex caused by irritation, from any cause, within the nose. The effect of sneezing is to tend to remove the cause of the irritation. Sneezing is important in young children, who have not yet learned to blow their noses, as it is the means of removing excess mucous, dried secretions, or other irritating material.

The reflex response begins with a deep indrawing of breath followed by tight closure of the vocal cords. The air in the chest is then compressed by elevation of the diaphragm and lowering of the ribs, the tongue is pressed against the roof of the mouth, and the vocal cords are suddenly separated. The resulting blast of air through the nose is the sneeze.

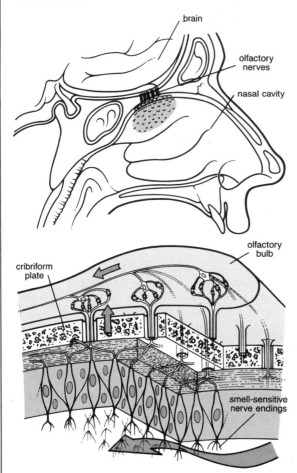

The olfactory system. The olfactory nerves are the first pair of cranial nerves. Chemical stimulation of the sensitive nerve endings in the lining of the upper part of the nose sets up nerve impulses which pass along numerous fine nerve fibrils. These pass through holes in the cribriform plate of bone, separating the nose from the brain, and into the olfactory bulbs which then run back to enter the underside of the brain.

Sno Phenicol

A brand name for chloramphenicol antibiotic eye drops.

snoring

A noise caused by vibration of the soft palate during sleep when a current of air passes over it during breathing through the open mouth. Anything which prevents normal breathing through the nose may thus contribute to snoring and may have to be corrected if the snoring is to be cured. Acoustically, snoring can vary from a soft, barely audible sound, to a nerve-shattering reverberation which echoes round the bedroom, changing its character at intervals. Snoring is never heard by the person causing the sound.

POSSIBLE CAUSES

Nasal obstruction may be caused by swelling of the mucous membrane lining, due to polyps, fracture of the nasal bone or allergic **rhinitis**, or it may be caused by enlarged **adenoids** or nasopharyngeal carcinoma. Snoring is more likely to occur if the sleeper is lying on his or her back, when there is a tendency for the mouth to drop open. Any measure which prevents this can be helpful.

Sodium Amytal

A brand name for **amylobarbitone**.

sodium aurothiomalate

A gold preparation given by injection for the treatment of **rheumatoid arthritis**. A brand name is Myocrisin.

sodium calcium edetate

A chelating agent used to treat poisoning with lead and other heavy metals. A brand name is Ledclair.

sodium cellulose phosphate

A drug that removes excess calcium from the body by an ion-exchange process. A brand name is Calcisorb.

sodium clodronate

A drug that prevents bone loss by interfering with the cells (osteoclasts) that break down bone. Trade names are Bonefos and Loron.

sodium cromoglycate

A drug used to treat **hay fever** (allergic rhinitis), allergic **conjunctivitis**, food **allergy** and allergic asthma. Cromoglycate stabilizes the **mast cell** membrane and prevents the release of **histamine**. Trade names are Cromogen, Hay-Crom, Intal, Intal Syncroner, Nalcrom, Opticrom and Rynacrom.

sodium fusidate

An antibacterial drug used both generally and for local application. Trade names are Fucidin and Fucithalmic.

sodium hyaluronate

A viscous, gel-like material used in ophthalmic surgery to protect the important inner lining of the cornea and maintain the front chamber of the opened eye. A brand name is Ophthalin.

sodium perborate

An antiseptic drug used as a mouthwash. A brand name is Bocasan.

sodium picosulphate

A stimulant laxative drug used to treat constipation. A brand name is Laxoberal.

sodium tetradecyl sulphate

A sclerosing substance that can be injected into segments of emptied varicose veins so as to close them off and relieve symptoms. A brand name is Fibro-vein.

sodium valproate

An anticonvulsant drug used to treat **epilepsy**. A brand name is Epilim.

Sofradex

A brand name for eye or ear drops or ointment containing dexamethasone, **framycetin** and **gramicidin**.

Soframycin

A brand name for the antibiotic drug **framycetin**.

Solcode

A brand name for a mixture of aspirin (see **analgesic drugs**) and codeine.

Solian

A brand name for **amisulpride**.

Solone

A brand name for **prednisolone**.

Solprin

A brand name for aspirin (see **analgesic drugs**).

Solu-Cortef

A brand name for **hydrocortisone**.

Solu-Medrone

A brand name for **methylprednisolone**.

Solvazinc

A brand name for **zinc sulphate**.

solvent abuse

The deliberate inhalation of the vapour from various solvents for the sake of their narcotic effect. Substances used in this way include any of the solvent-based commercial adhesives, volatile cleaning fluids, lighter fuel, petrol, paint thinner solvents, marking ink, anti-freeze, nail varnish remover, butane gas and toluene. Usually, a small quantity of the solvent is poured into a polythene bag which is held tightly against the nose and mouth, so as to exclude additional air and avoid reducing the vapour concentration.

The effects vary, but are generally intoxicant, with loss of full awareness of the surroundings, incoordination and loss of muscle control and, sometimes, hallucinations. Unconsciousness may occur and episodes can end fatally, usually by asphyxiation, inhalation of vomit, or accident. Many reports have been published of brain, liver and kidney damage from solvent abuse. Addiction can occur and habituation is rapid so that ever larger doses are required to produce the desired effect. These large doses are liable to cause organ damage.

soma

Greek root meaning 'body' as in somatic (of the body).

somatic gene therapy

Genetic treatment that affects only the general body (somatic) cells but not the sex cells, and thus is limited in its effect to the individual treated. The alternative form – genetic treatment affecting the germ cells in the ovaries or testes – may be perpetuated through succeeding generations. For this reason it is currently prohibited.

somatization disorder

This is the current term for **hysteria**.

somatotropin

A growth hormone produced by recombinant **DNA** techniques (genetic engineering) and used to treat growth defects. Trade names are Genotropin, Humatrope, Norditropin, Saizen and Zomacton.

somatotype

A body type. The description of somatotypes was an interesting attempt to correlate personality types and the tendency to develop certain patterns of mental illness, rather than others, with the bodily configuration. In the 1920s, the German psychiatrist Ernst Kretschmer (1888–1964) described the tall, thin (asthenic), round-bodied (pyknic) and burly (athletic) types and W. H. Sheldon, in the 1940s, selected the roughly corresponding ectomorph, endomorph and mesomorph.

Although there seems to be some correlation between an asthenic build and a tendency to schizophrenia, and a pyknic build and a tendency to **cyclothymia**, the somatotypes do not offer any useful guidance in diagnosis and interest in the matter has dropped off.

Sominex

A brand name for the antihistamine drug **promethazine** used as a sedative.

somnambulism

See **sleep**.

somno

Latin root meaning 'sleep' as in somnolent (sleepy).

Somophyllin

A brand name for **aminophylline**.

Sone

A brand name for **prednisone**.

Soneryl

A brand name for the barbiturate drug butobarbitone.

Sorbichew

A brand name for **isosorbide dinitrate**.

Sorbid SA

A brand name for **isosorbide dinitrate**.

Sorbitrate

A brand name for **isosorbide dinitrate**.

[]0

Sorbosan

A brand name for calcium alginate.

sore

Any ulcer, diseased spot, septic wound or other infected breach of the surface of the skin or a mucous membrane. **Bedsores** are skin ulcers caused by pressure over bony points. A **cold sore** is a flare-up or outbreak of infection with **herpes** simplex and a 'desert sore' is a form of tropical ulcer. A 'running sore' is any discharging ulcer. The term 'soft sore' is applied to the sexually transmitted infection chancroid.

See **sexually transmitted diseases**.

sore throat

See **pharyngitis**, **tonsillitis**.

Sotacor

A brand name for **sotalol**.

sotalol

A long-acting beta-blocker drug used to treat irregularity of the heart action. Trade names are Beta-Cardone and Sotacor.

Span K

A brand name for a potassium preparation.

spasm

From the Greek root *spasmos*. Involuntary contraction of a muscle or a group of muscles. This may result from disease of the nervous system, as in **spastic paralysis**, **myoclonus** and **chorea**, but may be caused in other ways. The word is also used metaphorically, as in the phrase 'a spasm of pain'.

Habit spasms, or **tics**, are repetitive, purposeless contractions. A reduction in the level of calcium in the blood causes **tetany**, a condition characterized by powerful muscle spasms. In **tetanus**, the infecting organisms release a powerful toxin which enhances nerve impulses and also acts directly on muscle cells to cause contraction. Severe and widespread spasms result. Similar effects on the nervous system occur in **rabies** and in strychnine poisoning.

Vasospasm is the tightening of the circularly arranged muscle fibres in the wall of an artery, so that passage of blood is impeded. This commonly causes symptoms, as in migraine, or even death, as in coronary artery spasm. Spasm of the circular muscles of the lung air tubes (bronchi) is the central feature of **asthma**.

Spasmonal

A brand name for **alverine citrate**.

spastic paralysis

Also known medically as cerebral palsy. This is a form of non-progressive loss of function of the motor part of the brain affecting about one child in 500. Spastic paralysis appears early in life and is not associated with any readily visible brain abnormality. It is extremely variable in effect. Some children suffer only the slightest of disability, others are almost totally disabled.

RECOGNITION AND SYMPTOMS

The principle feature is a lack of proper movement control usually with stiff spasticity of the muscles, less commonly with lack of coordination and sometimes involuntary jerks and movements. There is almost always difficulty in walking, varying from trivial to total. Commonly the legs press tightly together, causing the characteristic 'scissors gait'. Often the articulation of speech is affected. Speech may also be affected by sub-normal intelligence, which affects about half of all children with cerebral palsy. About a quarter also suffer seizures.

Babies with spastic paralysis are often 'floppy' (see **floppy infant syndrome**) and show feeding problems. When the paralysis (palsy) becomes apparent it may be a diplegia, affecting mainly the legs, a paraplegia, affecting all four limbs, or a hemiplegia, affecting one side of the body only. In general, the more widespread the paralysis, the more likely, and the more severe, the mental retardation. Muscle spasms (spasticity) appears at about six months, and the limbs take up characteristic abnormal positions which result from certain muscle groups being stronger than others. The ankles tend to be extended, as if the child were trying to walk on tip-toe and the affected arms are bent at the elbow and flexed at the wrist.

POSSIBLE CAUSES

The cause of spastic paralysis has, for many years, been accepted as birth brain injury, especially from oxygen lack during delivery. This view is being increasingly challenged by obstetricians, neurologists and paediatricians. Major improvements in obstetrical techniques and in the care of newborn infants, in the last twenty years, have resulted in no consistent reduction in the incidence of spastic paralysis. Research studies have shown that physical malformations, unconnected with the brain, and present before labour began, are significantly more frequent in children with cerebral palsy than in the general population. In one large study, only one child in five with spastic paralysis had a clear history of signs of asphyxia, such as slow heartbeat and delay in crying for five minutes after birth. Many babies who develop spastic paralysis are small – less than 2 kg.

So it seems likely that birth injury is a less important cause than has been thought, and that events occurring during pregnancy may be more relevant. Rhesus incompatibility, leading to haemolytic disease of the newborn, with severe jaundice and brain damage from blood breakdown product (bilirubin) deposition, is a well-recognized cause, as are infections such as **encephalitis** and **meningitis**, and head injury early in life.

COPING

Cerebral palsy, if severe, can impose a terrible burden on parents but attitudes should always be as positive as possible. Much can be done to help children to control muscular action and to prevent deformity from muscle contractures. Special equipment, and in some cases even surgery, may be needed. Mildly spastic children should attend normal schools, but those with severe defects will only benefit from attendance at institutions dedicated to their management.

speaking in tongues

See **glossolalia**.

specialists

In Britain, a physician is a doctor who practises medicine (that is, who deals with those diseases that are treated by other than surgical means and mainly by drugs). Thus, in

British hospitals the clinical specialists are mainly divided into physicians and surgeons. In the USA, the term 'physician' simply means any doctor. In Britain, clinical doctors are also divided into two large groups, the general practitioners, who are concerned mainly with family doctoring and who work usually in group practises, and the specialists, who work mainly in hospitals and special clinics.

Specialists are not necessarily consultants; there is a well-marked hierarchy in hospital medicine, each specialty being staffed by doctors at various stages in their training. The consultant is the head of any 'firm' and is clinically autonomous. Below him or her are senior registrars, well advanced in their training, and registrars who have already had considerable experience. Below the registrars are young doctors who are beginning their training in the particular specialty. Registrars and senior registrars commonly see referred patients. If they are in doubt, they will discuss the case with the consultant. Some of the specialties are also staffed by senior and experienced specialists who have not achieved consultant status but who function very much as consultants.

spectacles

Frames fitted with simple thin lenses used for the correction of short sight (**myopia**), long sight (**hypermetropia**), **astigmatism** and **presbyopia**. Myopic eyes focus too strongly and need concave, weakening lenses (minus lenses); hypermetropic eyes may not be able to focus strongly enough either for reading or even for distance viewing, and require convex, strengthening lenses (plus lenses). In astigmatism, the eye has a maximal focus for lines oriented at a particular angle and a minimal focus for lines at right angles to this orientation. Correction is required for one, and sometimes both, orientations. So astigmatism needs lenses more steeply curved in one direction than in the other (cylindrical, or toric, lenses).

In presbyopia the eye is unable to make sufficient adjustment to increase its power for near viewing, so lenses of the same type as are used in hypermetropia are needed. Superimposed on the distance correction – which may be zero – presbyopes aged forty-five, need, on average, an addition of one **dioptre**; those of fifty, one and a half dioptres; those of fifty-five, two dioptres; and those of sixty, two and a half dioptres. A lens of two and a half dioptres focuses at 40 cm, which is a convenient reading distance, so the near addition should seldom exceed this power.

Bifocal glasses are capable of focusing at two distances and are prescribed for presbyopes who also need a distant correction. They are essentially glasses for distance but with a small reading segment, placed below, of stronger power, which brings near objects into focus. It is natural to look down, and a little inwards, when reading, so the lower segment is set on the inner side of each lens and should, ideally, be as small as possible. A lower segment extending right across the lens is optically pointless and can cause annoyance when the wearer is going downstairs or stepping off curbs.

Bifocal glasses are very convenient and are worn appreciatively by millions, but many people are illogically discouraged by the 'granny' stereotype and prefer to burden themselves with separate pairs of spectacles.

SPECTACLES IN CHILDHOOD

Many children hate wearing glasses and it is common for behavioural problems to arise when parents, on the advice of opticians, insist that they do. Reasonable parents dislike imposition without explanation, but often feel hopelessly uninformed and are concerned that damage to their children's vision may result if glasses are not worn.

After the age of about eight years, glasses are needed only by those who cannot see clearly without them. However poor the vision, no harm is done to the eyes if glasses are not worn or if the prescription is incorrect. The worst that can happen, physically, is a feeling of discomfort, strain or dissatisfaction. Education may, of course, suffer if vision is defective.

During the period from birth to eight, glasses may be critically important, not primarily for purposes of seeing clearly, but to allow the full visual function to develop normally. The full link-up between the eye and the brain is not present at birth and is not complete until about the age of eight, and this link-up will not occur unless young children form sharp images on their retinas. This is why glasses may be important in childhood for the long-term quality of vision. Any focusing errors, or differences in focus between the two eyes, present in young children, may result in the failure of full neurological link-up with the brain and the production of a form of defective vision known as amblyopia.

Ophthalmologists and skilled opticians can determine the refraction objectively in a small child, without any more cooperation than that the eyes are kept open. In cases of extreme difficulty, it may be justified to give a child a general anaesthetic, but this is rarely necessary. Children accommodate so strongly that it is often necessary to use drops which temporarily paralyse the accommodation before doing the test. This will always be done in children found to have squints. Atropine is generally used, other drugs seldom being strong enough to prevent this powerful focusing.

speech, nasal

See **adenoids**.

speech therapist

An ancillary health professional who is concerned with treatment designed to help people with a communication difficulty that arises from a disturbance of language, a disorder of articulation, difficulty in voice production or a defective fluency of speech.

spermatic cord

A cord-like structure consisting of the **vas deferens** surrounded by a dense plexus of veins and other blood vessels, lymphatic vessels and nerves. The spermatic cord runs upwards from the back of the testicle through a canal in the groin (the inguinal canal) into the abdominal cavity where the vas leaves it to run into the prostate gland.

spermatozoa

A spermatozoon is a male reproductive cell (gamete), carrying all the genetic contribution from the father and bearing either an X chromosome to produce a daughter, or a Y chromosome to produce a son. Only one sperm in hundreds of millions succeeds in fertilizing an ovum. All the others are wasted. Sperms contain half the number of chromosomes present in a normal

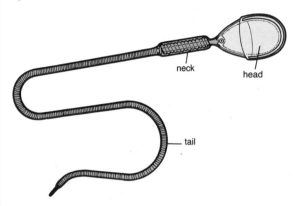

A spermatozoon, greatly magnified.

cell, but so do ova, and on fertilization, when the sperm and the ovum combine, the normal number is made up.

Sperms are microscopic, about 0.05 mm long, and are present in millions in the seminal fluid. They have thrashing tails by which they achieve mobility and move actively towards the ovum in the Fallopian tube, taking anything from a few minutes to about three hours to do so. Only the most active and healthy of sperms reach the ovum. Even so, thousands surround a single ovum, trying to break in, but only one enters. A protective barrier then forms in the ovum membrane, preventing any other sperm from entering.

sperm count

Sperm counting is an important part of infertility investigation. A semen sample is obtained by masturbation. A known dilution of the sample is made and a drop is allowed to flow on to a counting slide, microscopically engraved with squares of a known size. The number of sperms on several of these squares is counted, under a microscope, and averaged. From this figure, the total sperm count can easily be calculated. Fertility is unlikely if the count is below 20,000,000 per ml.

sperm donation

Seminal fluid provided by a donor, usually anonymous, for the purposes of fertilization of women whose husbands or partners are sterile. Seminal fluid is obtained by masturbation and can be preserved indefinitely frozen in a glycerol cryoprotectant in phials, or plastic straws and kept in liquid nitrogen sperm banks. After thawing, the semen is injected, using a sterile syringe, on to the surface of the cervix or into the cervical canal. This is done when ovulation is most likely to occur. The success rate of this procedure is exactly the same as for ordinary sexual intercourse.

sperm injection IVF

A method of *in vitro* fertilization in which an ovum is held steady by a microscopic suction device while a single sperm is injected directly into it through a very fine needle. The method, which was adopted to ensure fertilization in cases in which the father's sperm count is too low, has been criticized on the grounds that it may increase the likelihood of birth defects. It is suggested that it interferes with the natural selection process in which only the fittest sperms are able to penetrate the egg. Concerns were raised in 1999 that sperms

taken from men with very low sperm counts may carry a gene mutation that could convey male infertility to future generations. There may also be the potential for the transmission of other genetic diseases.

See also **androgen receptor gene**.

sperms, absence of

See **aspermia**.

sperm, single, injection

See **intracytoplasmic sperm injection**.

sperm tube

See **vas deferens**.

sphygmomanometry

The procedure for measuring the blood pressure.

sphygmos

Greek root meaning 'pulse', as in sphygmomanometer (device for measuring blood pressure).

spider fingers

Abnormally long thin fingers and hands, known as arachnodactyly – literally 'spider fingers', may be a sign of Marfan's syndrome. This is a genetic disease featuring weakness of collagen connective tissue in the body so that the joints are unusually lax and the large arteries abnormally elastic. Often the internal lenses of the eyes become dislocated.

See **arachnodactyly**, **Marfan's syndrome**.

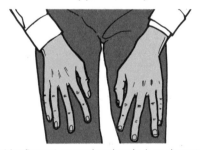

'Spider fingers', or arachnodactyly, is so characteristic of Marfan's syndrome as to be almost diagnostic.

spider naevus

A common, tiny skin blemish consisting of a small, central, slightly raised, bright red area from which fine red lines, like spider legs, radiate. Numerous spider naevi occur in serious liver disease, such as cirrhosis, and sometimes in pregnant women or those receiving hormone replacement therapy.

spina

Latin root meaning 'spine' as in spinal of the spine (vertebral column).

spina bifida

A developmental defect in which the rear part of one or more of the vertebrae of the spine remain incomplete. The term

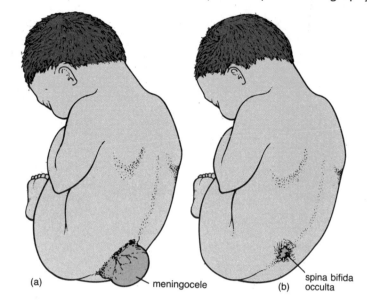

In the most severe form of spina bifida a large protrusion is seen in the lower back containing part of the spinal cord and its membranes. This is called a meningomyelocele. If only the linings protrude, as in (a), the condition is called a meningocele. In the most minor degree, spina bifida occulta (b), little external evidence is seen and the bony defect can be revealed only by X-ray or ultrasound scanning.

(a) meningocele (b) spina bifida occulta

was first used by Professor Nicolai Tulp, now best known as the central figure in Rembrandt's famous picture *The Anatomy Lesson*, of 1632.

RECOGNITION AND EFFECTS

As a result of the bony defect, the spinal cord, which runs down through a series of holes in the vertebrae, is relatively unprotected in the affected area. In spina bifida occulta, the condition is hidden and usually discoverable only on X-ray. In more serious cases, the coverings of the cord (the meninges) pass back through the opening to form a cyst-like swelling (a meningocele). In the worst cases, the spinal cord itself is exposed. This is called a myelocele.

The effects vary with the type and severity. When there is a myelocele there is usually paralysis of the legs and loss of sensation. In the worst cases there may be total paralysis of the lower part of the body and incontinence. Repeated urinary tract infections lead to kidney damage. An associated failure of normal circulation of the cerebrospinal fluid leads, in many cases, to 'water on the brain' (**hydrocephalus**) and subsequent brain damage with **epilepsy**, **spastic paralysis** and retardation.

> Several studies have shown conclusively that a small daily intake of folic acid, taken before pregnancy and during early pregnancy, will substantially reduce the risk of spina bifida. The dose usually found in over-the-counter multivitamin preparations is probably enough to achieve this advantage. It appears to be sufficient to take the vitamin for twenty-eight days before and after conception. No more than 0.4 mg is required.

TREATMENT

Spina bifida, especially if severe, is easily diagnosed before birth by amniocentesis, alphafetoprotein estimation and ultrasound examination. Surgery to correct the defect may be performed as soon as possible after birth. In severe cases, detected early on in the pregnancy, the option of termination of the pregnancy may be considered.

spina bifida prevention

See **folic acid**.

spinal anaesthesia

A major form of local anaesthesia, performed by injecting an anaesthetic drug between two of the vertebrae of the lower back into the cerebrospinal fluid. This blocks nerve transmission in the adjacent spinal nerves.

spine

The spine, or vertebral column, is a curved column of individual bones, called vertebrae, all of the same general shape but varying progressively in size and proportion from the top of the column to the bottom. Each vertebra consists of a stout, roughly circular body in front, and an arch behind, enclosing an opening to accommodate the spinal cord. The bones fit neatly together, the bodies being separated by the intervertebral disc and the arches making contact by four smooth surfaces, two above and two below.

The vertebrae in the neck are the smallest but have the largest cord opening. Those at the bottom of the column are massive. There are seven vertebrae for the neck, twelve for the back and five for the lumbar region. The fifth lumbar vertebra sits on top of the sacrum, which is formed from the fusion of five vertebrae into one bone and which forms the centre of the back of the pelvis. The coccyx, hanging from the lower tip of the sacrum, is the fused remnant of the tail.

See illustrations on following page.

spine inflammation

See **spondylitis**.

spiral computed tomography

A development of CT scanning that is so rapid that it allows scanning of a large body volume on a single breath-hold. The resolution is such as to provide high-quality two- and three-dimensional images. The X-ray tube rotates around the patient in a spiral, taking less than a second to complete one rotation. Up to 60 rotations are possible. A special surface-shading display technique reveals astonishing detail of the internal structures of the body, especially of bones.

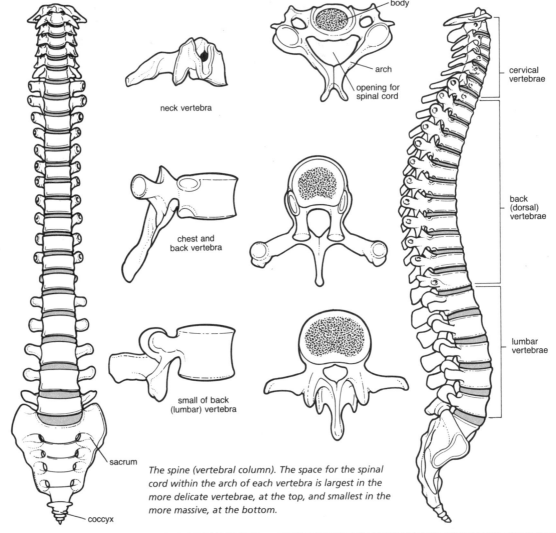

The spine (vertebral column). The space for the spinal cord within the arch of each vertebra is largest in the more delicate vertebrae, at the top, and smallest in the more massive, at the bottom.

Spiretic

A brand name for the diuretic **spironalactone**.

spirochaete

A class of bacteria notable for their spiral form. Spirochaetes are highly motile by means of a lashing tail. The three most important groups are the Treponema genus which includes the causal agent of syphilis *Treponema pallidum*; the Leptospira, which include *Leptospira icterohaemorrhagiae*, the cause of **leptospirosis**; and the Borrelia, which include the cause of relapsing fever, *B. recurrentis*, and of **Lyme disease**, *B. burgdorferi*.

Spiroctan

A brand name for **spironolactone**.

spironolactone

A diuretic drug that does not lead to loss of potassium from the body. It is an antagonist of the hormone aldosterone. A brand name is Aldactone.

splanchna

Greek root meaning 'bowels' as in splanchnic (of the bowels).

spleen

The spleen is a solid, dark purplish organ, situated high up on the left side of the abdomen, close to the outer wall and immediately under the diaphragm. It lies immediately under the lower ribs between the stomach and the left kidney. A large artery, arising from a branch of the aorta, runs along behind the stomach, to supply it with blood.

The spleen has an elastic fibrous capsule with many fibrous bands running inwards to form a kind of sponge. In the spaces between these bands is the largest collection of lymph tissue in the body – a mass of pulpy material consisting mostly of lymphocytes, phagocytes and red blood cells. The spleen is the main filter of the blood, clearing from it the products of the constant breakdown of red blood cells, and other foreign and unwanted semi-solid material. It is also a source of new lymphocytes and a major site of antibody formation.

The spleen thus serves a double purpose – as a blood filter and as an important part of the immune system. In its filtering role, the spleen acts on the blood in much the same way as the lymph nodes act on the tissue fluid (lymph) returning from the tissue spaces. The muscle fibres in the outer parts of the spleen can cause it to contract so that blood cells within it can be forced into the circulation. It thus acts as a minor reservoir of blood.

The spleen varies in size in different people and, in health, weighs an average of 170 g. In a person who has had repeated attacks of malaria the spleen is enlarged, sometimes greatly, and may weigh as much as 9 kilos.

Formerly, it was supposed that no particular harm resulted from the loss of the spleen or from the loss of its function. This was considered fortunate, because removal of the spleen (splenectomy) is necessary if it, or its supplying blood vessels, are severely injured. There are also certain medical conditions for the treatment of which splenectomy is valuable. A common cause of spleen malfunction is sickle cell disease in which the rate of breakdown of red blood cells may be much greater than normal. The situation is not quite so simple as was thought. It is now known that up to 5 per cent of people who have had their spleens removed, or whose spleens are, for any reason, non-functioning, may suffer a severe and possibly fatal infection. This is called overwhelming post-splenectomy infection (OPSI). This condition may come on with dramatic suddenness and urgent life-saving treatment may be necessary.

Because of the risk of OPSI it is recommended that people without spleens, or with non-functioning spleens, should be offered preventive treatment against infection in the form of daily doses of an antibiotic such as penicillin V. This is especially important in people with any degree of immune deficiency, for such people are, of course, particularly prone to infections. As an alternative, people at risk of OPSI should be clearly aware that on the early signs of an infection – such as fever, sore throat or cough – they should take antibiotics at once. In addition it is recommended that such people should be immunized with polyvalent pneumococcal serum against the organism causing pneumonia. This should ideally be done before the spleen is removed.

spleen, disorders of

Because of its position and consistency, a normal spleen cannot easily be felt, but many conditions cause it to enlarge so that it becomes firmer and can be felt under the ribs on the left side. The spleen becomes enlarged in **malaria**, **typhoid fever**, **typhus**, **tuberculosis**, infectious mononucleosis (**glandular fever**), **septicaemia**, syphilis, **schistosomiasis**, trypanosomiasis and **kala azar**. Excessive white cell production, as in **leukemia** or increased red cell destruction, as in haemolytic anemia or **thalassaemia**, will also lead to enlargement, as will tumours of any of the normal constituents of the spleen. The commonest of these tumours are **Hodgkin's disease**, lymphosarcoma and other malignant **lymphomas**. Some of these conditions are benefited by removal of the spleen.

Rupture of the spleen occurs most commonly in the course of serious road or industrial accidents, and in falls from a height and contact sports. If the spleen is enlarged for any reason, rupture is much more likely. Because of the size of the artery supplying the spleen, the major danger from rupture is severe haemorrhage. This may be fatal unless urgent surgical treatment, to tie off the artery and remove the spleen, can be provided.

In malarial areas, where enlargement of the spleen was once almost universal, murders were commonly committed by striking a blow under the ribs, on the left side, with a heavy blunt iron instrument called a larang, so as to rupture the spleen.

splen

Greek root meaning 'spleen' as in splenomegaly (spleen enlargement).

splint

A temporary support or reinforcement for an injured part, designed to prevent movement at the site of the injury. In the case of a fracture of a bone, a splint, whatever its form, will be effective only if it immobilizes the joint above, and the joint below, the fracture. Immobilization is necessary because movement at an injury site can cause not only great pain but may lead to increased bleeding, **shock** and further soft tissue damage.

Splints take a variety of forms and, in an emergency, may be improvised from any suitable material to hand. Ready-made splints may be of inflatable material, wire frame lattice, wood strips, malleable metal, polystyrene foam, etc. Plaster of Paris is often fashioned into splints. Splints are secured by firm wrapping with bandages, scarves, cloth strips or other available material. Bony points, over which the splint passes, should be well padded.

See *First Aid*.

split personality

A phrase which acquired credence mainly on account of the interest of the concept. In fact, 'multiple personality' is very rare indeed. The term was once much used, in a descriptive way, in relation to cases of **schizophrenia** (literally, 'split mind') in which there was a dissociation of thought and emotion, but has now fallen into disuse.

spondylitis

Inflammation of any of the joints between the vertebrae of the spine. This may occur in **osteoarthritis**, **rheumatoid arthritis** or, more specifically, in **ankylosing spondylitis**.

spondylolisthesis

The abnormal forward displacement of a vertebra relative to the one under it, most commonly of the lowest, the fifth lumbar vertebra, over the top of the sacrum. This is due to a symptomless congenital weakness, knows as spondylolysis, of the bony arch that bears the facets by which the vertebrae articulate together. Spondylolisthesis causes severe backache on standing and leads to nerve pressure effects. The condition may also, less commonly, affect vertebrae in the neck.

spondylos

Greek root meaning 'vertebrae' as in spondylitis (spine inflammation).

Sporanox

A brand name for **itraconazole**.

sports medicine

The branch of medicine concerned with the physiology of exercise and its application to the improvement of athletic performance and fitness, and with the prevention, diagnosis and treatment of medical conditions caused by, or related to, sporting activities of all kinds. Regrettably, sports medicine has recently had to concern itself disproportionately with the problem of the illegal use of performance-enhancing drugs by athletes.

sprue

A disorder in which nutrients are not absorbed properly from the intestine. There are two types: coeliac sprue (see **malabsorption**) and **tropical sprue**.

squalamine

A drug extracted from the dogfish that has been claimed to be capable of killing a range of sexually transmitted bacteria including the gonococcus and chlamydia and of killing cells invaded by viruses.

squama

Latin root meaning 'scale' as in squamous (scaly).

squamous cell carcinoma

A form of skin cancer which, like **rodent ulcer** (basal cell carcinoma) and malignant melanoma, is related to sunlight exposure. A squamous cell cancer starts as small, firm, painless lumps occurring most commonly on the lip, ear, or back of the hand and slowly enlarging. Surgical removal and examination is important as, unlike the rodent ulcer, this tumour may spread to other parts of the body, with fatal consequences. Malignant melanoma is, of course, even more likely to spread.

squint

See **strabismus**.

squint treatment

See **orthoptics**.

staging

The process of determining the stage to which a disease, especially a cancer, has progressed. Staging is important as an indication of the likely outcome (prognosis) and because it may have an important bearing on the most effective form of treatment. This may differ markedly at different stages.

stammering

See **stuttering**.

standard deviation

A measure of the amount by which a set of observed values differs from the average of them, that is widely used in medical statistics. Standard deviation is the square root of the arithmetic average of the squares of the deviations of the members of a sample from the mean.

Stanford-Binet test

A type of **intelligence quotient** test.

stanozolol

An anabolic steroid drug used to treat the effects of deep vein thrombosis and systemic sclerosis. A brand name is Stromba.

stapedectomy

An operation for the treatment of **otosclerosis**, a condition in which deafness is caused by growth of bone into the elastic ligament surrounding the footplate of the innermost of the three small bones in the middle ear (the auditory ossicles), the stirrup-shaped stapes.

HOW IT'S DONE

In the operation most of the outer part of the stapes bone is removed and a fine hole is drilled through the thickened footplate left fused by disease into the temporal bone. A tiny cylindrical plastic or stainless steel piston, bearing a fine wire hook, is now pushed into the hole and the hook is attached to the incus (the middle ossicle). Vibration of the eardrum is now transmitted, by way of the piston, to the inner ear, and the hearing is restored.

RISKS

The operation has a high success rate, but about 5 per cent of patients suffer permanent hearing loss as a result. Because of this, it is often recommended that the operation should be done only on the less severely affected ear.

Staphlipen

A brand name for the antibiotic **flucloxacillin**.

Staphylex

A brand name for **flucloxacillin**.

staphylococcal infections

A very common group of infections, predominantly affecting the skin, but sometimes causing serious internal disorders. Staphylococci clump together in bunches – the name comes from the Greek word *staphyle*, meaning 'a bunch of grapes' – and contaminate the skin of all humans, from time to time. Usually the concentration of staphylococcal bacteria is insufficient to do any harm, but sometimes they invade the deeper tissues to cause boils, abscesses, styes and carbuncles.

Staphylococcal organisms in the bloodstream (bacteraemia) may lead to **septic shock**, infective **arthritis**, **osteomyelitis**, **pneumonia**, widespread abscesses, and **endocarditis**.

Staphylococcal **food poisoning** is caused by the toxin produced by the organism, and the usual source of contamination is a pustule or boil on the skin of a food-handler. The organisms continue to reproduce on the food, even at normal room temperatures, and to secrete the toxin. Severe vomiting, and often diarrhoea, occurs within two to six hours of eating the food, but the symptoms seldom persist for more than about twelve hours.

Staphylococcal infection of the vagina may cause the toxic shock syndrome.

Staril

A brand name for **fosinopril**.

statins

See **hydroxymethyl glutaryl co-enzyme A reductase inhibitors**.

statin drugs

See **hydroxymethyl glutaryl co-enzyme A reductase inhibitors**.

status asthmaticus

If the normal treatment to control **asthma** fails, or if obvious worsening of symptoms occurs in spite of normal treatment, there is a real danger that the asthma may progress to the life-threatening condition of *status asthmaticus*. This involves severe, prolonged and sometimes uncontrollable spasm of the circular muscles of the air tubes of the lungs (bronchi), and requires urgent hospital treatment.

In this condition, the level of oxygen in the blood rapidly drops to a dangerous degree and there is extreme respiratory distress. Oxygen is administered, and large doses of steroids and bronchodilators are given directly into a vein. Mechanical ventilation may be necessary.

status epilepticus

A repeated sequence of major epileptic seizures without recovery of consciousness between attacks. Status epilepticus is commonest in children and in people with organic brain disease, but it also tends to occur in epileptics who suddenly stop taking their tablets or who take them irregularly.

> The condition is very dangerous and may prove fatal unless urgent measures are taken to control the seizures and ensure a clear airway. The fits are stopped by the use of Valium (diazepam), given by intravenous injection, or by means of more powerful drugs, if necessary.

stavudine

A **reverse transcriptase inhibitor** drug used to treat **HIV** infections. A brand name is Zerit.

Stein-Leventhal syndrome

A condition associated with multiple cysts in the ovaries, which features menstrual disturbances or absence of menstruation, sterility, obesity and a male distribution of body hair from hormonal disturbances. Insulin resistance appears to be an important causal factor. Possible late manifestations include **diabetes**, high blood pressure, heart disease and cancer of the womb lining (endometrial carcinoma). Treatment is by the removal of large wedges from both ovaries. This is usually effective. Also known as polycystic ovarian syndrome.

Steinmann pin

A fine surgical nail passed through the lower end of the thigh bone (femur) or the upper end of the main lower leg bone (tibia) and held under tension in a steel stirrup so that traction can be applied in the treatment of fractures of the femur. The presence of the pin is painless.

Stelazine

A brand name for the phenothiazine antipsychotic and **anti-emetic** drug **trifluoperazine**.

stem cell

A progenitor or parent cell from which a whole class of different cells develop by a process of differentiation. A single type of stem cell in the bone marrow, for instance, gives rise to the entire range of immune system blood cells (neutrophils, eosinophils, basophils, monocytes, macrophages, **platelets**, T cells and B cells) and the red blood cells (erythrocytes). Stem cell transplantation can be used to correct deficiencies.

Stemetil

A brand name for the phenothiazine antipsychotic drug and **anti-emetic** prochlorperazine.

stenting

The use of a physical device, such as a tubular stainless steel or plastic mesh or coil of wire, to keep a body tube fully open. Stents are most commonly used in arteries such as the coronary arteries, the aorta, the renal arteries and the femoral arteries, but there has been a considerable expansion of their use for other purposes in recent years.

Self-expanding metallic stents have been successfully used to keep the intestine open, especially the gullet, in cases of swallowing difficulty, but also to overcome narrowing in the colon or rectum. They are used to prevent the urine tube (urethra) from healing closed, to maintain patency in narrowing of the bile ducts, and to keep the tear-drainage duct (naso-lacrimal duct) open in cases of persistently watering eyes. Silicone rubber stents have been used in narrowing of the trachea and bronchi. Stents in arteries are liable to blockage by blood clotting, and anticoagulant treatment is required.

stercore

Latin root meaning 'excrement' as in stercolith (stony-hard stool).

stereotaxic surgery

Operations, especially on the brain, in which fine instruments are guided with precision to the required point by three-dimensional scanning methods. An elaborate harness may be attached to the head to support the directional guides for the instruments which determine the exact orientation of the axes along which the instruments will pass.

sterilization

The process of rendering an object or area free from living micro-organisms. The term is also used for any process, such as **hysterectomy**, ligation of the Fallopian tubes, **vasectomy** or **castration** by which a person is incapable of having children.

Bacterial, viral and fungal sterilization may be achieved by dry heat, boiling, autoclaving in a steam pressure vessel, immersion in one of many different antiseptic chemical solutions, exposure to toxic vapours or gases, irradiation with gamma rays or short-wavelength ultraviolet light, or exposure to intense ultrasound waves. Liquids can be sterilized by forcing them through filters of such small pore size that even viruses cannot pass. Some organisms form resistant spores which are able to survive some of the methods of sterilization. Some are also capable of surviving temperatures many degrees below freezing.

See also **operating theatre**.

673

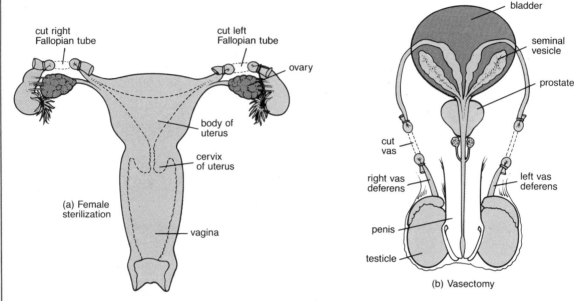

cut right
Fallopian tube

cut left
Fallopian tube

ovary

body of
uterus

cervix
of uterus

(a) Female
sterilization

vagina

bladder

seminal
vesicle

prostate

cut
vas

right vas
deferens

left vas
deferens

penis

testicle

(b) Vasectomy

(a) The commonest form of female sterilization in which the Fallopian tubes are cut.
(b) The corresponding operation, vasectomy, in the male, in which both vasa deferentes are cut.

sternon

Greek root meaning 'sternum' as in sternum (breastbone).

sternum

Latin root meaning 'breastbone' as in sternum.

sternum, fracture of

The sternum is the breastbone. Fracture of the sternum may be caused by direct violence and the broken bone may be driven inwards, reducing the volume of the chest. Urgent realignment (reduction), by hooking the fragments outwards, may be necessary. More commonly, the sternum is fractured in the course of an acute forward bending injury, with fracture of the spine and vertical compression of the rib cage.

steroids

A popular term for the group of steroid drugs known as the corticosteroids. These were first isolated from the outer layer (cortex) of the adrenal gland, where the natural hormone cortisol is produced – hence the name. A steroid is a member of the large chemical group, related to fats, which includes sterols such as cholesterol, bile acids, sex hormones, many drugs and the adrenal cortex hormones. Corticosteroid drugs are chemically similar to the natural steroid hormones.

These drugs have many uses and can be given by injection, by mouth, in the form of ointments or creams or as eye or ear drops. They are highly effective against inflammation, and are prescribed for many conditions in which inflammation may cause damage to the body. These include:

- inflammatory diseases of the bowel, such as regional ileitis (**Crohn's disease**) and **ulcerative colitis**;
- joint inflammation, such as **rheumatoid arthritis**;
- inflammation of arteries, as in **temporal arteritis;**
- inflammation in the eye (**uveitis**);

- **asthma**;
- **hay fever** (allergic rhinitis);
- **eczema**.

The steroids are used to help to suppress the immune responses which lead to the rejection of a donated organ transplant and are often life-saving in conditions of severe stress in which the production of natural hormones is inadequate. And they are given as hormone replacement therapy to people with disease of the adrenal glands (**Addison's disease**).

It seems to be a law of nature that anything capable of a powerful effect can also do a lot of harm. Powerful drugs nearly always have major side-effects and the corticosteroids, given in large dosage, are no exception. But you need to view this with a sense of proportion. Steroid skin ointments and creams, used occasionally, are unlikely to do any harm and, indeed, some steroids for local application are considered so safe that you can buy them over the counter without a doctor's prescription. Powerful steroids used on the skin, however, are liable to cause skin atrophy and thinning. Steroids used in an inhaler are also unlikely to have any significant general side-effects, as the dose is very small and, properly used, the drug goes only where it is needed. But steroids in high doses for long periods will inevitably cause some side-effects and these vary with the dose and how the drug is given.

The more important of these include:

- suppression of the body's production of natural steroids;
- reactivation of latent infections;
- increased susceptibility to new infections;
- breakdown of partly-healed stomach or duodenal ulcers;
- **osteoporosis**;
- **diabetes**;
- high blood pressure;
- excessive **hairiness** (hirsutism);
- **glaucoma**;
- **cataract**.

Suppression of natural steroid production doesn't matter too much so long as steroid is being taken, but suddenly stopping the treatment is very dangerous. All patients on long-term steroid treatment should carry a card indicating, in detail, the treatment they are having. In the event of a severe accident or other major stress, this knowledge can be life-saving. The risks of side-effects of steroids vary considerable from person to person and may be minimal. Doctors, however, will always balance the risks against the risks and disadvantages of not using high-dose, long-term steroids.

The decision to give long-term steroids to young children must be balanced against the fact that these drugs cause severe stunting of growth. It must be remembered that the same effect may be caused by serious childhood illnesses, for which steroids may be needed.

sterculia

A bulking agent used to treat constipation. A brand name is Normacol.

Sterofrin

A brand name for eye drops containing **prednisolone**.

Ster-Zac Bath Concentrate

A brand name for **triclosan**.

Ster-Zac D.C.

A brand name for **hexachlorophane** in a hand cream formulation for pre-operative hand cleansing.

Ster-Zac Powder

A brand name for **hexachlorophane** dusting powder.

Stesolid

A brand name for diazepam.

stethos

Greek root meaning 'chest' as in stethoscope (instrument for chest listening).

Stiedex lotion

A brand name for desoxymethasone.

Stiedex LP

A brand name for desoxymethasone.

stiff man syndrome

A rare nervous system disorder characterized by muscle spasm, rigidity, pain and severe bodily stiffness. The condition is related to stress and is often precipitated by being startled. The spasm usually starts in one muscle group and then spreads progressively to other parts of the body. Often the whole of the trunk becomes involved and the spasms may become almost continuous so that the disability is severe. Sixty per cent of patients have antibodies to an enzyme that operates on one of the 20 **amino acid** 'building blocks' of protein (of which muscle is largely constructed). The condition

is as common in women as in men, so it might be better to rename it 'the stiff person syndrome'.

stilboestrol

A synthetic oestrogen drug similar in action to the natural hormone oestradiol. Stilboestrol is used to treat cancer of the **prostate**, some types of breast cancer and postmenopausal atrophic **vaginitis**. A brand name of a preparation used in pessary form is Tampovagan.

stillbirth

Birth of a dead baby. The distinction between stillbirth and miscarriage (see **abortion**) is arbitrary and in Britain is set at twenty-eight weeks of pregnancy. Stillbirths must be registered, the cause of death established, if possible, sometimes by autopsy, and a certificate of stillbirth provided before burial may take place.

In many cases, the cause of death of the fetus is not established. **Diabetes** or high blood pressure in the mother, **rhesus factor disease**, eclampsia, severe fetal malformations, inadequacy of the placenta, or infections such as **toxoplasmosis**, **rubella**, syphilis or **herpes** simplex are all well-recognized causes.

Stilnoct

A brand name for **zolpidem**.

stimulation

See **analeptic drugs**.

stings, bee

Bee venom contains highly irritating protein amines, including histamine and 5-hydroxytryptamine. These, together with other proteins, cause a local area of blanching surrounded by a red swelling.

> The black sting may be seen in the centre of the swelling and, to avoid possible injection of further venom, this should be removed by a careful scraping action with a fingernail or credit card rather than by pulling. The use of eyebrow tweezers is liable to compress the sac and inject any remaining venom, and is best avoided.

Antihistamine or cortisone skin cream, or even an ice cube, will reduce pain.

> Over 100 simultaneous stings would be needed to provide a potentially lethal dose, but it should be remembered that people who have been stung before may have become hypersensitive. In such cases, a single sting may be fatal. Also dangerous are stings on the inside of the throat. These may occur from bees floating on the surface of drinks. Stings in this area are liable to cause such severe swelling of the tissues around the vocal cords that the breathing is cut off. If this happens, life can be saved only by cutting into the wind pipe (trachea) centrally, just above the notch of the breastbone. This procedure is called tracheostomy.

Stokes-Adams attacks

Repeated, brief episodes of loss of consciousness from transient failure of an adequate blood supply to the brain, due to cessation or extreme slowness of the heart beat. Stokes-Adams attacks occur in cases of severe heart beat irregularity or complete **heart block**. Most cases are treated by the fitting of an artificial **pacemaker**.

stoma

Greek root meaning 'mouth' as in stomatitis (mouth inflammation).

stomach

From the **oesophagus**, food enters the stomach, the bag-like organ which lies immediately under the diaphragm in the left upper part of the abdomen. The stomach acid, hydrochloric acid, and its digestive juices (enzymes) work together to process food. These chemicals also protect against infection, many organisms being destroyed by the acid. This strong acid is secreted by cells in the lining of the stomach to assist in the break-up of food and the formation of a solution called chyme. The action is largely on the connective tissue and cell membranes of the food, so as to cause mechanical rather than biochemical breakdown. Acid has little action on the breakdown of proteins, polysaccharides and fats. The stomach enzyme pepsin, acting in the acid medium, begins to break down proteins.

The onward passage of partially digested food is controlled by the pyloric sphincter at the lower outlet of the stomach. Unduly large lumps of food tend to cause the pyloric sphincter to close so that they are retained longer in the stomach for further chemical action. The average stomach can hold about 1.5 litres, but heavy eaters and drinkers often have stomachs of much greater capacity. The stomach empties into the duodenum, which is the first part of the small intestine.

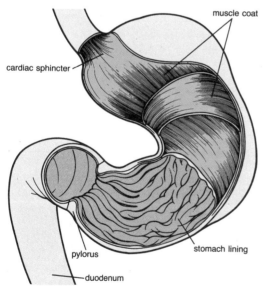

The stomach. Note the longitudinal and circular muscle coats and the greatly corrugated mucous membrane lining which secretes acid and digestive juice.

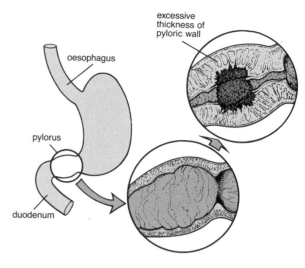

Pyloric stenosis may be a congenital severe narrowing of the outlet of the stomach with undue thickening of the muscle layer, or it may be an acquired condition resulting from scarring and narrowing as a result of ulceration. Congenital pyloric stenosis is readily treated by a fairly simple operation.

stomach, disorders of

The stomach secretes a strong acid, hydrochloric acid, and digestive juices (enzymes) to process food. Because of these and its efficient, self-protective, mucus layer, the stomach has remarkable built-in protection against infection and other causes of damage. Many viruses, bacteria and fungi are destroyed by the acid. The price paid for this protective power, however, is the common tendency for the stomach to attempt to digest itself, causing **peptic ulcer**. Ulceration around the outlet of the stomach can cause scarring and narrowing. This is called *pyloric stenosis* – a condition that may also occur at birth (congenital pyloric stenosis) This can be cured by a simple operation.

Cancer of the stomach is fairly common in the elderly and because the effects are seldom striking in the early stages, the diagnosis is often not apparent until a fatally late stage. Warning signs include any new symptoms of pain, discomfort or indigestion, especially in a person previously free of such symptoms, unexplained vomiting, and blackening of the stools. Non-malignant polyps also occur in the stomach.

Enlargement (dilatation) of the stomach is commonly caused by persistently excessive intake of food or liquid, but may occur in a more serious form as a complication of several diseases and as a result of severe injury or the wearing of a body plaster cast. Very large volumes of fluid collect in the stomach and so much may be lost from the circulation that shock develops. Removal of fluid from the stomach, by suction through a tube, is an urgent requirement in this condition.

Atrophy of the stomach lining, so that the cells which normally produce acid and the enzyme pepsin have disappeared, is a constant feature of **pernicious anaemia**. One of the tests for pernicious anaemia is to demonstrate the complete absence of acid in the stomach.

stomachos

Greek root meaning 'stomach'.

stomach pump

A popular misconception. See **stomach washout**.

stomach washout

Also known as gastric lavage. Washing out the stomach with water is usually done to remove poisons taken by mouth. It is an emergency procedure, usually carried out in the home or the casualty department of a hospital.

The person to be treated lies face down, preferably with the head below the level of the stomach. A wide-bore rubber or plastic tube is lubricated and pushed steadily down over the back of the tongue to pass into the gullet (oesophagus) and then down into the stomach. A small funnel is attached to the top of the tube.

A half to one litre of water is then poured into the stomach. The top of the tube is then lowered so that the water may drain from the stomach into a bucket. This procedure is repeated until the water returns clear. A sample of fluid from the stomach is kept for analysis. Stomach washout is avoided if a corrosive poison has been swallowed, because the passage of a tube may cause additional damage to the oesophagus or stomach.

stoma nurse

A qualified nurse specially trained to assist people who have had a colostomy operation and whose bowel excretions must be evacuated into a bag. The nurse is concerned with giving dietary advice to minimize bowel problems; with the day-to-day care of the colostomy opening (stoma) on the abdominal wall; with the health of the surrounding skin, to which the colostomy bag must be attached; and with the supply of necessary appliances and materials.

stomatitis

The word *stoma* is new Latin from the Greek word for 'mouth'. Stomatitis is inflammation or ulceration of the mouth. The commonest cause is **herpes** simplex virus infection, which usually causes the typical crusting and blistering cold sores on the lips only, but which may also affect the gums and the tongue. Thrush infection (**candidiasis**) is another form of stomatitis. It is common in debilitated babies and is likely to occur in immunocompromised people or in those being treated with broad-spectrum antibiotics. Both herpes and candida mouth infections are features of **AIDS**.

The term angular stomatitis is applied to the infected, moist cracks at the corners of the mouth, caused by constant drooling of saliva. Aphthous stomatitis is a fairly common condition in which round or oval shallow ulcers, up to half a centimetre across, appear on the lips, insides of the cheeks, floor of the mouth, or soft palate. These ulcers occur either singly or in groups, cause considerable discomfort or pain, and then heal within ten to fourteen days. Aphthous stomatitis also occurs in **Behçet's syndrome** and **Reiter's syndrome**.

stools, black

See **black stools**.

stop codon

One of three **nucleotide** triplets that marks the end of every gene and indicates that protein synthesis ends at that point.

strabismus

The condition, commonly known as 'squint', in which only one eye is aligned on the object of interest. If the other eye is directed too far inward, the condition is called convergent strabismus, and if too far outward, divergent squint. Occasionally, one eye will be directed upward or downward, relative to the fixing eye. This is called vertical strabismus.

RECOGNITION AND SYMPTOMS

Squint most commonly starts in early childhood, usually because the brain mechanisms underlying binocular vision (fusion of the two images into one) have not yet developed fully at a time when new stress factors begin to operate. The most important of these is hypermetropia, a focusing error in which the relaxed lens system of the eye is not strong enough to bring the image to a focus on the retina. Hypermetropia forces the child to exert strong accommodation to see clearly and the result is a convergent squint. The strong accommodation actually prompts the brain to turn the eyes in. But the child is trying to look at an object further away, so one eye remains straight while the other turns in.

> Such a squint causes double vision and, to overcome this, the brain immediately rejects the signals from the deviating eye. From that moment on, visual development stops in the squinting eye, and the result, unless effective treatment is given, is a severe and permanent defect of vision in that eye, known as amblyopia. By the age of eight the whole system has firmed up and nothing can be done to correct amblyopia after this age. The earlier amblyopia is treated the easier it is to correct.

TREATMENT

The treatment involves stopping the child from making this excessive accommodative effort by prescribing a full spectacle correction for the hypermetropia. This is one of the cases in which spectacles are sight-saving (see **spectacles**).

After glasses have been prescribed, the 'lazy' (amblyopic) eye has to be forced to make a seeing effort. This is done by covering up the good eye (patching or occlusion) for varying periods, until vision is restored to its former level in the squinting eye. At this stage, the squint will often alternate from one eye to the other. This is an encouraging sign and a muscle balancing operation at this stage will often complete the cure. But glasses must still be worn at least until the neurological control system is fully mature and stable.

> Squint acquired later in life almost always causes double vision and requires urgent investigation for it implies organic disorder, either of the brain, such as cerebrovascular disease or diabetic neuropathy, or of the eye-moving muscles or their nerves.

strapping

The use of adhesive tape to maintain the desired relationship of parts of the body or to rest an injured or inflamed part. Strapping may be helpful in avoiding undue pull on a muscle, tendon or ligament or to restrict the movement of joints.

Strapping is also sometimes used to prevent the pooling and stagnation of blood in the legs in the treatment of **varicose veins** or varicose ulcers.

Streptase

A brand name for the blood clot dissolving enzyme drug **streptokinase**.

streptococcal infections

Infections caused by bacteria of the genus Streptococcus. These are among the commonest bacteria causing disease in humans and are responsible for **tooth decay**, **cellulitis**, **tonsillitis**, **pharyngitis**, scarlet fever, **impetigo**, **erysipelas**, **endocarditis**, **necrotizing fasciitis** and urinary tract infections. In addition to causing infections, streptococci give rise, by an auto-immune process, to the serious conditions of **rheumatic fever** and **glomerulonephritis**. Unlike **staphylococci**, which tend to cause localized infections, such as abscesses, streptococci are essentially *spreading* organisms. They achieve this by means of **enzymes** such as streptokinase, which digests fibrin, and hyaluronidase (hyalase), which increases the permeability of tissues.

streptodornase

A protein-splitting **enzyme** used externally to clean wounds. A brand name is Varidase.

streptokinase

A protein-splitting **enzyme** used as a drug to dissolve blood clot in a coronary artery so as to minimize the degree of myocardial infarction during a heart attack. It is also used to treat pulmonary embolism. Trade names are Kabikinase and Streptase.

stress

There is wide debate as to what constitutes a stress and to what extent some claimed stresses may be purely internal – in the mind of the individual, created by fears and imagination.

EFFECTS

There is no debate about the stressful nature of many life events and about the temporary effects these have on the body – increased cortisol and adrenaline production, with raised heart rate and blood pressure, muscle tension and raised blood sugar. The difficulty is to decide to what extent these responses are harmful. Many people are obviously able to sustain high levels of stress for long periods with apparent impunity. Others seem to succumb, and it is claimed that stress states, if prolonged, can lead to organic disease such as **peptic ulcers**, **hypertension**, **asthma**, **rheumatoid arthritis**, **thyrotoxicosis**, **ulcerative colitis** and neurodermatitis. Very little convincing evidence has, however, ever been produced to show that these disorders are actually caused by external stress factors.

WHO DOES IT AFFECT?

Some people, of certain personality types, seem to attract stress – most notably, the driving, time-urgent, hostile, aggressive personalities, especially those who repress aggression – these people suffer a higher than average incidence of heart attacks. In addition, people who habitually achieve stress situations by their behaviour or by abusing their bodies with alcohol, drugs and overeating are, of course, more likely than average to develop organic disorders. This, however, may be to broaden the definition of stress so widely as to lose any specific meaning. There may also be some confusion between cause and effect.

CAN STRESS CAUSE ILLNESS?

The intimate inter-relationship of body and mind is undeniable and there is no question that people burdened by an overwhelming sea of troubles do break down and develop severe symptoms and disabilities. The **post-traumatic stress disorder** is a case in point, but this occurs in people who have suffered emotional or physical stress that would be very traumatic to anyone. Notwithstanding all the claims of the stress industry, this remains the only condition unequivocally known to be actually caused by a stressful event.

stress genes

A general term for genes that are caused to turn on and to transcribe following exposure to the action of DNA-damaging agents such as radiation or oxygen free radicals.

stress ulcers

Acute, rapidly developing stomach ulcers that develop as a consequence of surgical **shock**, burns or severe illness or injury.

striae

Broad lines on the skin, most commonly affecting pregnant women, and occurring on the abdomen, breasts or thighs. They are often called stretchmarks. Striae are initially red and slightly raised, but later become purplish, eventually flattening to form shiny streaks, usually between 6 and 12 mm wide. The appearance is the result of local alteration in the fibrous protein, collagen, which give the skin its natural elasticity. Striae can also be caused by corticosteroid medication or by the excess steroids present in **Cushing's syndrome**. Striae become less conspicuous with the passage of time.

stroke

This is the result of acute deprivation of blood in a part of the brain, by narrowing or **thrombosis** in an artery, or of physical damage to part of the brain by internal or external bleeding.

POSSIBLE CAUSES

Cerebral haemorrhage – bleeding into or around the brain – is the cause of the most serious kinds of stroke and is often fatal. Bleeding into the brain is usually the result of the rupture of a small artery, damaged and weakened by **atherosclerosis**, which gives way under the influence of raised blood pressure. High blood pressure contributes to atherosclerosis and is the main risk factor for stroke. The bleeding can occur almost anywhere in the brain and the effect varies with the location.

The pumping action of the burst vessel forces blood into the brain tissue which is disrupted and compressed. The effect is most obvious in those parts in which the nerve tracts concerned with movement, sensation, speech and vision are situated close together and so are involved in common. Haemorrhage into the brain-stem, where the centres for the control of the vital functions of breathing and heartbeat are situated, is the most immediately dangerous to life.

The first sign of a cerebral haemorrhage is usually a sudden severe headache. This is quickly followed by obvious functional loss such as paralysis down one side of the body, loss of vision to one side, fixed turning of the eyes to one side and perhaps a major epileptic-type fit. Often consciousness is lost early and when the haemorrhage is large, this may never be regained – more than half of the people affected in this way die within a few hours or days. Those who recover consciousness always have an initial defect of function which is often severe. Smaller haemorrhages produce less damage and there may be no loss of consciousness, but simply the signs of functional injury to the nervous system.

This is almost always worst at the beginning and much of it is caused by recoverable and temporary loss of function in brain tissue surrounding the area of damage. Brain swelling (oedema) occurs and this temporarily interferes with nerve conduction. Recovery also occurs, to some extent, as a result of reabsorption of the released blood. As these recovery processes proceed there is a slow, but usually substantial improvement and, unless further haemorrhages supervene, the end result may be good. Some degree of permanent disability is, however, usual. Strokes may be caused by bleeding from a ruptured **aneurysm** on one of the arteries supplying the brain (see **subarachnoid haemorrhage**).

Cerebral **thrombosis**, or a minor **embolism**, produces effects similar to, but generally less severe than, those of cerebral haemorrhage and recovery is common. Strokes due to thrombosis or repeated embolism may occur in people with atherosclerosis of the carotid arteries or their branches, or in people with diseased heart valves on which small blood clots form, and then break loose to be carried up to the brain.

RECOVERY

After a stroke, the emphasis should always be on the restoration of maximum function by sustained efforts to achieve as much activity as possible. A person who consistently attempts to walk after a minor stroke is much more likely to recover mobility than one who stays in bed.

stroke in progression

Brain damage caused by an obstruction to its blood supply that increases progressively over the course of hours, days or weeks. Stroke in progress has also been defined as 'a stroke in which the neurological deficit is still increasing in severity or distribution after the patient is admitted to observation'.

strongyloidiasis

A very persistent intestinal infection with the tiny parasitic worm *Strongyloides stercoralis*. The parasite is common in many parts of the Far East and thousands of Second World War former prisoners of war of the Japanese still harbour the infestation, fifty years later.

The worms are acquired by walking barefoot over ground contaminated by human faeces carrying the worm larvae. These larvae can penetrate the skin, causing an itchy rash ('ground itch'), and gain access to small blood vessels, from whence they are washed along in the veins carrying blood back to the heart. They are then taken to the lungs where they first encounter the obstruction of small capillaries and are trapped. The active worms are, however, easily able to pass through the walls of the capillaries into the lung air sacs (alveoli) and they then have free passage upwards to the pharynx to be swallowed.

In the small intestine the larvae mature and copulate and the pregnant females burrow into the wall of the intestine to lay their eggs in crevices. When the eggs hatch, most of the larvae are released in the faeces, but some convert to the infective form and pass directly through the bowel lining into blood vessels, to initiate a new cycle. When T cell immunity is reduced, this autoinfection can result in a very heavy worm load with the whole of the small and large intestine harbouring a lining of actively reproducing worms. It is believed that the females can also reproduce by virgin birth (**parthenogenesis**).

RECOGNITION AND SYMPTOMS

Moderate numbers of worms in the bowel may cause no symptoms, but heavy infestation causes discomfort and distention. Very heavy infection may cause diarrhoea, but in some cases more serious effects, such as **septicaemia**, **meningitis**, or severe bleeding from the lungs, may occur. Because they can reproduce within the host, strongyloides worms are much more dangerous than other parasitic worms, and a person may die from one of these complications many years after acquiring the infection, having, in the meantime, been unaware that anything was wrong.

Strongyloidiasis is diagnosed by microscopic examination of stool samples for larvae, adult worms and eggs. Populations at risk may be screened using the **ELISA test**.

TREATMENT

Treatment with thiabendazole is effective against adult worms but not larvae, so repeated courses must be given and the stools examined several times, at monthly intervals, to confirm that the infection has been eradicated.

Stugeron

A brand name for **cinnarizine**.

Sturge-Weber syndrome

The association of a large purple birthmark (haemangioma) on one side of the face with a similar malformation of blood vessels in the brain. There may be weakness on the opposite side of the body, epileptic seizures, **glaucoma** and sometimes mental retardation.

stuttering

A condition featuring intermittent inability to produce smooth and normal speech. There may be repetition or prolongation of syllables and sometimes complete blocking, so that no sound is uttered. Stuttering almost always starts before the age of eight and tends to be worse in conditions of social stress, or when the affected person is in a conspicuous situation. It does not occur during singing and is usually absent when the affected person speaks to an animal.

Stuttering is not caused by any organic disorder and appears to be the result of unsatisfactory early conditioning during speech learning. The great majority of stutterers achieve normal speech by the end of adolescence, but about 20 per cent remain severely disabled.

Speech therapy is highly effective in treating stuttering and this should be started as soon as the condition is established, no matter how young the child.

stye

An infection around the root of an eyelash. A stye is a small abscess, usually caused by staphylococcal bacteria, the follicle being stretched painfully by the collection of pus. This often causes a small 'yellow head' at the base of the eyelash. In such cases relief may sometimes be obtained by pulling out the lash and so discharging the pus.

Styes tend to recur because of spread of infection to adjacent lash follicles. Antibiotic eye ointment, applied to the lid margins two or three times a day for two or three weeks, will help to prevent this. If styes prove very persistent, attention should be paid to the general health and the urine should be tested for sugar to eliminate diabetes.

subarachnoid haemorrhage

The arachnoid matter is the middle of the three layers of the meninges – the membranes which form an enclosure for the brain and the spinal cord. The main branches of the arteries which supply the brain with blood lie in the space under the arachnoid and this space also contains the cerebrospinal fluid in which the brain and cord are bathed. A subarachnoid haemorrhage is bleeding from one of these arteries into the fluid. The condition is rare before early adult life and reaches its peak incidence between the ages of thirty-five and sixty-five.

POSSIBLE CAUSES
The commonest cause of subarachnoid haemorrhage is the rupture of a pre-existing berry-like swelling (**aneurysm**) on one of the arteries or of a tumour-like malformation on an artery, and this usually occurs spontaneously without injury.

RECOGNITION AND SYMPTOMS
Blood from the artery floods under pressure over the surface of the brain, causing sudden very severe headache usually followed rapidly by loss of consciousness or other signs of neurological damage. There may be paralysis of eye movement, a dilated pupil on one side, a drooping eyelid, neck stiffness, vomiting or any of the signs and symptoms of **stroke**.

The condition can often be recognized by its effects, but confirmation of the diagnosis is best made by CT scanning.

TREATMENT
The outlook is always serious and the death rate high. The affected person is nursed under strict bed rest in a darkened room. Measures are taken to avoid any strain or exertion, and drugs are given to keep the blood pressure reasonably low, to control any tendency to seizures, to relieve the headache, to prevent blood vessels from going into spasm – which is a most dangerous complication – and to prevent the clot forming in the aneurysm from dissolving. Antifibrinolytic drugs, such as aminocaproic acid, will often prevent re-bleeding from a dissolving clot. Rarely, bleeding can be controlled surgically.

subclavian steal syndrome

The main arteries that supply the head arise from large arterial trunks which go on to supply the arms. If one of these trunks is partially blocked by **atherosclerosis**, the blood flow both to the head and to the arm may be restricted. In such a case, use of the arm may divert ('steal') so much blood from the limited common supply that it leaves an insufficient flow to the brain. This may cause various symptoms, such as vertigo, headache, skew deviation of the eyes, double vision, and nausea and vomiting.

The narrowing can be detected by X-ray examination after a radio-opaque dye has been injected into the bloodstream (angiography). The pulse at the wrist on the affected side will be weak. The subclavian steal syndrome is a clear indication of serious risk of stroke and active treatment of the obstruction, perhaps by **endarterectomy**, may be indicated.

subconjunctival haemorrhage

Release of blood under the membrane covering the white of the eye (the conjunctiva) so that a local area, or even the whole of the white, becomes bright red. The conjunctiva contains many small blood vessels which are relatively poorly supported and it is common for a vessel to rupture spontaneously and for a variable quantity of blood to be released and retained between the conjunctiva and the eyeball. Because the conjunctiva is transparent, this blood is readily visible and conspicuous. Usually, the area of blood is sharply delineated and, round about it, the normal white coat (sclera) shows through the normal transparent conjunctiva. If bleeding is brisk, the whole of the subconjunctival space may fill up, giving a dramatic appearance. Subconjunctival haemorrhage sometimes occurs on sneezing or straining at the toilet, but usually there is no obvious explanation. It does not indicate high blood pressure.

The condition is painless and there is no effect on vision. The blood begins to absorb at once and will usually have disappeared within two weeks. Recurrence is common and it is occasionally necessary to have a bleeding vessel treated by an ophthalmologist.

subconscious

The very large database of information, of which only a small part is in consciousness at any one time, but which may be drawn upon, with varying degrees of success, at will. The term is also used as an adjective applied to data which can be made conscious.

Freud is popularly attributed as being the 'discoverer' of the subconscious, but the existence of a large memory store has, of course, been apparent to the thoughtful throughout the ages. Freud's writings on the subject were preceded by hundreds of publications, spanning about 2000 years, postulating the existence of a subconscious mind.

In psychoanalytic theory, the subconscious is considered to be a 'level' of the mind through which information passes on its journey 'up' to full consciousness from the unconscious mind.

subdural haemorrhage

One of the most dangerous complications of **head injury**. Sudden accelerative forces to the head, such as may occur in boxing, car accidents, etc., even without fracture of the skull, may cause tearing of the large veins under the dura mater, which is the outermost of the three meninges covering the brain and spinal cord. The blood gradually accumulates and, over the course of days or weeks, may form an expanding clot which slowly compresses the brain.

The classic sign of subdural haemorrhage is recovery of consciousness from the original injury, followed by a relapse into coma some time later. Such a sequence indicates the urgent requirement for investigation and possible surgery to open the skull, remove the clot and stop the bleeding.

sublimation

Any socially acceptable re-direction of normally unacceptable impulses or energy. Sublimation is an important concept in psychoanalysis in which it is considered to be the process by which primitive sexual urges are redirected into new, learned channels such as artistic and creative activities. Effective sublimation is considered to be a healthy feature of maturity of personality.

Sublimaze

A brand name for **fentanyl**.

submucous resection

An operation for the removal of displaced cartilage and bone from underneath the mucous membrane covering the central partition (septum) of the nose. This is done if the septum is deviated so much to one side as to cause nasal obstruction. Care must, however, be taken to ensure that sufficient supporting structure is left to prevent collapse of the tip of the nose. Submucous resection is therefore avoided in young children. Even in adults, the surgeon may prefer a less radical procedure if resection would involve weakening the profile of the nose.

substance

A well-understood general term which has, in recent years, acquired a new sense. The term, in this restricted sense, is applied to any chemical, solid, liquid or gas capable of affecting the state of the mind. A psychoactive material. The term is used most often in the phrases 'substance use' or 'substance abuse', the latter referring to the non-medical and 'recreational' use of drugs such as **amphetamine**, **cannabis**, **cocaine**, methylenedioxymethamphetamine (**Ecstasy**), **heroin**, lysergic acid diethylamide (**LSD**), organic solvents by inhalation, and so on.

The term 'substance abuse' is also applied to an intake of alcohol that is likely to prove harmful. Oddly enough it is not currently applied to a commonly-used substance which is more dangerous than most of these – tobacco. Another phrase containing this new usage, and originating in the USA, is 'substance use disorder' This refers to addiction to drugs or alcohol, or both.

sucking wound of chest

An open wound in the chest wall through which air is drawn in and expelled as a result of respiratory movements. When the muscles of respiration – the diaphragm and the intercostal muscles – contract, they increase the internal volume of the chest cavity and air is sucked in, or, more accurately, forced in by atmospheric pressure. If the chest wall is intact, the only route for air entry is into the lungs and these expand passively.

An opening in the chest wall provides an alternative route for air entry into the chest cavity, but, in this case, the air does not have access to the system of bronchial tubes and does not enter the lungs. Because the lungs are separated from the inside of the chest wall by the two layers of the pleura, air passing through an open wound of the chest wall enters the pleural cavity and the lung on that side collapses. The central partition of the chest (the mediastinum) may also shift to the other side, resulting in a partial collapse of the other lung.

> The effect of an open wound of the chest wall may be very serious, causing grave embarrassment to respiration. The urgent first-aid measure is to close the opening, so as to allow the lungs to resume normal action and this should be done immediately using the hand. The opening should not be uncovered until some form of air-tight seal can be applied or medical attention obtained.

sucralfate

A drug that forms a protective coating over the stomach or duodenal lining. Sucralfate is used in the treatment of peptic ulceration. A brand name is Antepsin.

suction

A means of removing unwanted or excess fluid, or semi-fluid material, from a cavity or organ. Suction may be by syringe or mechanical pump and is often applied by way of a container which acts both as a trap and as a receptacle. After most surgical operations under general anaesthesia, the anaesthetist will use suction to clear accumulated secretions from the throat (pharynx). A similar procedure is often necessary for newborn babies. Suction is used to clear the windpipe in people who have had a **tracheostomy** and continuous suction is commonly necessary to maintain adequate drainage from the abdominal or chest cavity.

suction lipectomy

A cosmetic operation performed to remove excess fat from under the skin. Human fat is a liquid oil at body temperature, the oil being contained in thin-walled fat cells. In suction lipectomy, small incisions are made through the skin at strategic points and through these are passed a blunt-ended metal tube (cannula) connected to a powerful vacuum pump. The cannula is moved around under the skin so as to break down the fat cell walls and vacuum out unwanted fat. This is a fairly traumatic procedure that will inevitably damage other structures, especially blood vessels. Bruising may be considerable and occasionally a **haematoma** may form.

> Infection and haemorrhage can occur; there can be haematoma formation and skin laxity. There is a small possibility of abscesses forming, and oedema.

Sudafed

A brand name for **pseudoephedrine** with **triprolidine**.

sudden infant death syndrome

Cot death. The sudden death of an apparently well baby. The child, not more than a few months old, is found dead in the cot and no apparent cause can be found, even by a detailed post-mortem examination.

INCIDENCE
The sudden infant death syndrome is now, after major congenital abnormalities and severe prematurity, the commonest mode of death for infants between one month and one year of age. Each year, about 1500 babies die in Britain in this way and the distress to parents and relatives is incalculable.

The unexpected death of a baby affects boys more often than girls and is commoner in winter than in summer. Premature babies are at greater risk. This disaster strikes families in the lower socio-economic groups more often than the better off, black families more often than white. Maternal smoking during pregnancy and narcotic addiction or alcoholism leads to greater risk. Breastfed babies are less often affected than bottle-fed babies.

POSSIBLE CAUSES
In spite of agonized public concern and intensive study, the causes remain unknown. From ancient times, cot deaths have been attributed to suffocation from 'overlying' by the mother, and countless women have been unjustly accused of causing, either accidentally or intentionally, the deaths of their infants in this way. But in more recent years it has become apparent that sudden death commonly occurs in a baby sleeping alone.

Many theories have been put forward to account for the deaths of these babies. These include:

- over-soft bedding, in which the baby's face becomes buried;
- high environment temperatures causing heat stroke;
- the fear paralysis reflex, brought on by separation from the mother, especially in the dark;
- sensitivity to cow's milk;
- botulinum poisoning;
- unnoticed chest or bowel infection.

None of these has been accepted as a major cause, although all have been implicated in some cases. Some experts believe that some cot deaths result from a transient disorder of the nerve control of breathing and heartbeat.

Investigation of babies found dead shows that many of the deaths can be explained by well-known processes. Cases have been reported of overlying by mothers affected by extreme tiredness, epilepsy, drug abuse or obesity. In some there has been a reasonable assumption of accidental death from asphyxiation by toys or plastic bags or by wedging between unsuitable foam pillows. Some resulted from excessive environmental temperature leading to excessive body temperature (hyperthermia), and some from possible child abuse. By definition, none of these can be classed as the sudden infant death syndrome, but the conclusion may be that much more attention needs to be given to the recognition and avoidance of the many avoidable dangers which put at risk the lives of helpless infants.

> Research done in the Netherlands, in New Zealand and in Bristol in the early 1990s showed that there was a correlation between the sleeping position and the risk of cot death. Infants sleeping face-down (prone) were more liable. The official recommendation is now that babies should not be put down to sleep in the prone position.

COPING

In most cases of the sudden infant death syndrome, death occurs during sleep and without any suffering on the part of the child. But the effect on the family is devastating and close support is needed. Inevitably, the sense of loss is compounded by feelings of guilt and remorse for real or imagined failure to anticipate danger. This is seldom justified. Counselling and supportive visits from others who have suffered the same kind of bereavement is helpful in making the necessary adjustment to the prospect of having further children.

sudore

Latin root meaning 'sweat' as in sweat (secretion of sweat glands).

suffocation

Deprivation of oxygen as a result of mechanical obstruction to the passage of air into the lungs. This may occur by occlusion of the nose and mouth, as by a pillow or plastic bag, by blockage of the throat (pharynx) or voice box (larynx), by a foreign body or swelling (oedema), or by blockage of the windpipe (trachea). See also **asphyxia**.

sugar cane dust lung disease

See **bagassosis**.

sugars

Sugars are carbohydrates and make up about 1 per cent of the weight of body cells. They are more important as fuels than as structural materials. Nearly all the carbohydrate in the diet is broken down to the basic fuel, glucose and, for storage purposes, glucose molecules are linked together into a polymer called glycogen which is stored in the liver and can release glucose on demand. Surplus glucose – and there is usually plenty of this – is converted into fat, for long-term storage in fat cells under the skin and in the abdomen.

Carbohydrates are often combined with protein to form the important ground substance in which fibrous proteins are embedded. Combined carbohydrates and proteins are called mucopolysaccharides. A polysaccharide is a long-chain molecule, a polymer made up of many molecules of a simple sugar such as glucose, linked together. The 'muco' part is the protein.

suicide

Intentional self-killing. This may be done directly, or by neglect of action necessary for self-preservation, or by persuading another person to perform the killing. Suicide is on the increase and seems to be a feature of modern civilization. It is rare in more primitive cultures, although in some it is considered honourable. Hara-kiri was valued in Japan as a highly proper and atoning response to shame and disgrace.

INCIDENCE

In the West, suicide was formerly commoner among the elderly, but in the past thirty years the rates have risen steeply among adolescents and young adults. The published rates are not reliable because of a natural tendency to try to conceal the fact of suicide, and the real rates are certainly higher than those reported. Roman Catholic countries publish apparently low suicide rates because suicides are excluded from Christian burial.

> Apparent suicides are often accidents and were not intended to succeed. The use of hypnotic drugs, such as barbiturates, may lead to a drowsy state of mind in which tablets continue to be taken in an almost unconscious manner. Suicides by hanging or asphyxiation, too, may be gestures which went wrong. On the other hand, throat-cutting or wrist-cutting gestures seldom cause death, as the motivation to make the necessary depths of cut have to be very strong.

POSSIBLE CAUSES

Depression is one of the commonest causes of suicide and the severely depressed should always be considered at risk from this. Suicide is also common among alcoholics, people with **schizophrenia**, and people with severe personality disorders.

TREATMENT

Attempted suicide should never be considered as merely a manipulative act, but ought to be regarded as a non-verbal cry for help. People who go to this extreme are people who need skilled help and guidance and this should be acknowledged and help provided. When the attempt seems to have been genuinely directed to self-destruction, every effort must be made to secure the affected person in safety and to remove any means of repetition of the act. Psychiatric help is always urgently needed in such cases.

Suleo-M

A brand name for a preparation containing **malathion** for external use.

sulfadoxine

A **sulphonamide drug** used as an adjunct to chloroquine in the treatment of Falciparum **malaria**. A brand name is Fansidar.

sulfametopyrazine

A **sulphonamide drug** taken weekly to control infection in chronic bronchitis. A brand name is Kelfizine W.

sulindac

A non-steroidal anti-inflammatory drug (**NSAID**). A brand name is Clinoril.

Sulparex

A brand name for **sulpiride**.

sulphacetamide

A **sulphonamide drug** limited to external use. A brand name for a vaginal cream preparation also containing sulphathiazole and sulphabenzamide is Sultrin.

sulphamethoxazole

A **sulphonamide drug** used in combination with the folic acid inhibitor drug trimethoprim in the treatment of various infections, especially urinary infections. Trade names are Chemotrim and Septrin.

sulphasalazine

A compound of a **sulphonamide drug** and 5-aminosalicylic acid used to treat **rheumatoid arthritis**, **ulcerative colitis** and **Crohn's disease**. A brand name is Salazopyrin.

sulphinpyrazone

A uricosuric drug used to reduce the frequency of attacks of **gout**. A brand name is Anturan.

sulphonamide drugs (sulpha drugs)

The sulphonamides, which initially appeared in the 1930s, were the first effective antibacterial drugs that could safely be taken by mouth. They saved millions of lives by their action against streptococci and staphylococci and other organisms, until they were largely supplanted by the **antibiotic drugs**.

Sulphonamides are now used to a limited extent, but are still valuable for urinary infections where their high concentration, as they are excreted from the body, makes them efficient.

Certain sulphonamides are very poorly absorbed from the intestine and so are useful and safe in treating some intestinal infections. The group includes **sulfadoxine**, **sulphacetamide**, sulphadiazine, sulphadimethoxine, sulphadimidine, sulphamerazine, sulphamethazine, sulphamethizole, **sulphamethoxazole** and sulfathiazole.

sulphonylurea drugs

A class of drugs used in the treatment of maturity onset (Type II), non-insulin dependent diabetes. They are taken by mouth. Also known as oral hypoglycaemic drugs.

sulpiride

An antipsychotic drug used to treat **schizophrenia**. Trade names are Dolmatil, Sulparex and Sulpitil.

Sulpitil

A brand name for the antipsychotic drug **sulpiride**.

Sultrin

A brand name for **sulphacetamide** in combination with sulphathiazole and sulphabenzamide.

sumatripan

A **serotonin antagonist** drug, effective in the symptomatic treatment of acute migraine. A brand name is Imigran.

sunburn

The damaging or destructive effect of solar ultraviolet light on the skin. Sunburn is more likely in those unaccustomed to bright sunlight and in those with minimal melanin skin pigmentation. Carefully graduated exposure, for periods starting with no longer than fifteen minutes a day and increasing progressively as the skin pigmentation builds up, can prevent it.

> It should be remembered, however, that even if sunburning does not occur, all intense sunlight is damaging to the skin and may have permanent undesirable effects. The elastic collagen of the skin is changed, causing permanent loss of elasticity and wrinkling. The DNA of deep epidermal cells may be altered so that tumours such as rodent ulcers (basal cell carcinomas), squamous carcinomas and malignant melanomas are more likely to occur.

Sunscreens and protective clothing can effectively minimize skin damage, but people in tropical and sub-tropical areas are well aware of the advantages of remaining indoors.

superantigen

One of a class of molecules that react with a substantial proportion of the whole population of T cells in the body. Among the most striking superantigens are the toxins (enterotoxins) produced by the germ Staphylococcus aureus. Staphylococcal enterotoxin A (SEA) is a powerful T-cell promotor (mitogen) and can give rise to the release of large quantities of **cytokines**. This is believed to be one of the bases of the **toxic shock syndrome**.

superbug

An informal term for an infective micro-organism that has become resistant to antibiotics and is capable of causing serious infection. Rapid evolutionary natural selection forces have ensured that some organisms, such as *Staphylococcus aureus* (see **MRSA**) and various Enterobacteriaceae, are now resistant to virtually all the earlier antibiotics. Resistance to a range of antibiotics has arisen in numerous other organisms, including those causing bacillary dysentery, food poisoning, gonorrhoea and tuberculosis.

superego

The psychoanalytic term for the conscience.

superfecundation

The fertilization of more than one ovum within a single menstrual cycle by separate but closely associated acts of coitus. This would normally produce fraternal twins with the same father, but the possibility arises of twins born with different fathers.

superfetation

The very rare occurrence of two or more fetuses of different ages in a womb. This can happen as a result of fertilizations occurring in different menstrual cycles. The phenomenon is extremely rare because the establishment of the first pregnancy almost always leads to the suppression of ovulation.

Superglue

See **cyanoacrylate**.

Superglue sterilization

The use of methylcyanoacrylate adhesive ('Superglue') to achieve closure of the Fallopian tubes as a method of female sterilization. A small balloon pump device is used to apply the material by way of the cervix. The method was developed as an alternative to the much-criticized but widespread practice of inserting pellets of the now discredited antimalarial drug quinacrine to achieve closure by inflammatory healing. Tests of toxicity have been passed.

superinfection

A second infection, often with a fungus or virus, complicating an existing infection. The superinfecting organism is usually one which is resistant to, or not susceptible to, the drugs being used to treat the original infection.

superiority complex

An exaggerated and unrealistic belief that one is better than others. The Austrian psychologist Alfred Adler (1870–1937) suggested that a superiority complex develops in some people in response to the natural feelings of inferiority present in us all.

superovulation

The production of more than one or two ova at one time. Superovulation is a common effect of the use of drugs to stimulate ovulation in the treatment of infertility.

superoxide dismutase

A natural body antioxidant enzyme that converts the superoxide free radical to hydrogen peroxide, which is then catalyzed to water. The gene for superoxide dismutase is on the long arm of chromosome 21 near the Alzheimer's locus. Brain tissue is highly susceptible to free radical damage. People with Alzheimer's disease have reduced levels of superoxide dismutase.

suppository

A vehicle for a drug in the form of a block of cocoa butter or gelatin of a variety of shapes and sizes that is solid at room temperature but melts at body temperature. Suppositories are placed in the vagina or rectum and release drugs either for local action or to be absorbed. They may contain antibiotics and antifungal agents, local anaesthetics, corticosteroids, non-steroidal anti-inflammatory drugs (**NSAIDs**) and **anti-emetic drugs**.

Supradyn

A brand name for a multivitamin and mineral preparation.

suprapubic catheterization

Prostate enlargement may give rise to such extreme closure of the urine outlet tube (the urethra) that urinary outflow is completely blocked. Suprapubic catheterization is an emergency procedure offering immediate relief to a patient with an agonizingly full bladder. Such a person is also at risk of kidney damage from back pressure.

Under local anaesthesia a sharp-pointed metal rod surrounded by a snugly-fitting tube (trocar and cannula) is pushed firmly through the abdominal wall in the mid line at a point about one third of the distance up from the upper edge of the pubic bone to the navel. When the end of the instrument is in the bladder the trocar is removed so that urine can flow out through the cannula. In children a much smaller cannula normally used for intravenous infusion can be used.

supraventricular tachycardia

Episodes of abnormally fast heart-rate lasting for hours or days. The rate may be as high as 300 beats per minute, but is usually between 140 and 180. It is caused by fast spontaneous impulses, arising in the upper chambers of the heart, that over-ride the natural pacemaker. The condition may cause chest pain, breathlessness, alarming consciousness of the heart action (palpitations) and faintness. Attacks may be stopped by holding the breath and compressing strongly (**valsalva manoeuvre**) or by the use of antiarrhythmic drugs. Sometimes electrical **cardioversion** is necessary. Attacks of this kind call for urgent medical attention.

Suprax

A brand name for **cefixime**.

Surem

A brand name for the benzodiazepine drug **nitrazepam**.

surfactant

Any substance that reduces surface tension and promotes wetting of surfaces. The lungs contain a surfactant to prevent collapse and sticking together of the walls of the tiny air spaces (alveoli). The natural surfactant may be deficient in premature babies and the deficiency may lead to the **respiratory distress syndrome**. Surfactants can also be used to interfere with the motility of spermatozoa and so act as supplementary contraceptives with a spermicidal action.

Surgam

A brand name for **tiaprofenic acid**.

surgery, non-cutting

See **blunt dissection**.

surgery, precise location

See **stereotaxic surgery**.

surgical cutting and coagulation

See **laser**.

surgical emphysema

Localized volumes of air or gas in the tissues giving rise to a characteristic crackling effect when the affected area is pressed with the fingers. Surgical emphysema occurs most commonly in the neck as a result of leakage from a lung, or from injury to the gullet (oesophagus) or from fracture of the wall of one of the air sinuses surrounding the nose. Surgical emphysema is not, in itself, harmful and the air soon absorbs if further leakage from the source is prevented, but the cause must be established and, if necessary, treated.

surgical shock

See **shock, surgical**.

surgical stabber

See **trocar**.

Surmontil

A brand name for the tricyclic antidepressant drug **trimipramine**.

surrogacy

The deliberate undergoing of pregnancy so as to produce a child that will be surrendered to others. Fertilization may be by seminal fluid provided by the future adoptive father, or an ovum fertilized *in vitro* may be implanted in the surrogate mother. Surrogacy for gain is illegal in Britain and in some other countries. Surrogacy may be an act of great philanthropy or may be a way of raising money. In the latter case it commonly occurs that the surrogacy agreement is not kept because of the natural desire of the biological mother to retain the baby as her own. Surrogacy, which is an inherently unnatural process, has given rise to much unseemly legal wrangling.

Suscard

A brand name for the artery-dilating drug **glyceryl trinitrate** (nitroglycerine).

Sustac

A brand name for the artery-dilating drug **glyceryl trinitrate** (nitroglycerine).

Sustamycin

A brand name for the antibiotic **tetracycline**.

Sustanon

A brand name for the male sex hormone drug **testosterone**.

suture

A length of thread or thread-like material used for surgical sewing. The term also refers to the process of stitching. In spite of advances in technology, suturing still remains the preferred method of closing surgical incisions and other clean wounds, in most cases.

Sutures may be made of catgut, collagen, strips of human fascia, linen, silk, nylon, polypropylene, polyester and stainless steel, and most of these are available in a wide range of thicknesses. Sutures vary in diameter from almost a millimetre, when great strength is required, down to a barely visible one hundredth of a millimetre for delicate ocular and fine blood vessel surgery. Many sutures are produced swaged into the hollow end of an eyeless needle of appropriate size and shape. These are called atraumatic sutures, and the needle and remaining suture are discarded after use.

Needles may be straight, but the majority of surgical needles are curved and many have points with cutting edges so as to pass more easily through the tissues. Remarkable advances in needle technology, especially in the smaller sizes, have made possible many important surgical advances. Large needles may be held in the fingers, but most surgical sutures are inserted with the needle held in specially designed needle-holders which come in a wide range of sizes, for different purposes. The edges of the tissue being sutured are almost always held in forceps.

The term suture is also applied to the complex interlocking junctions between the various bones of the skull.

suxamethonium chloride

A **depolarizing** muscle relaxant drug used in general anaesthesia. A brand name is Anectine.

swab

A quantity of cotton, or other absorbent material, used in surgical operations to apply cleaning and antiseptic solutions to the skin before making the incision, and to mop up free blood, and other fluids, in the course of the operation so as to improve visibility. The term is also applied to small sterile twists of cotton wool on orange sticks used to obtain bacterial samples for culture and examination.

The surgical swab, or sponge, is commonly of very loosely woven cotton gauze, folded several times, and is held either in the fingers or in a long-nosed clamp. It is often necessary to leave swabs temporarily inside the body during an operation, and to prevent such swabs being overlooked, a careful count is made before the start of the operation and before the incision is closed. Surgical swabs often contain a thin strip of material opaque to X-rays.

swallowing, difficulty in

See **dysphagia**.

Swan-Ganz catheter

A soft, flexible, double-bore tube with a small balloon at one end. The catheter is passed along a vein to the upper right chamber of the heart (right atrium) and the balloon is inflated. The force of the blood flow then carries the balloon down into the lower chamber (right ventricle) and then up into the pulmonary artery, allowing important pressure measurements to be made.

sweating, excessive.

See **hyperhidrosis**.

swelling on baby's head

See **caput**.

swellings around eyes

See **dermoid cysts**.

swinging eyes

See **nystagmus**.

swollen glands

A term based on the mistaken notion that lymph nodes are glands. They are not. Lymph nodes are small bean-like bodies packed with immune system cells (**lymphocytes**) and have no glandular function. 'Swollen glands' are lymph nodes that are enlarged by inflammation or by infiltration with parasites or cancer. Inflammation of lymph nodes is called lymphadenitis, but even this term perpetuates the mistake. The root 'aden' means 'a gland' and the suffix '-adenitis' means 'inflammation of glands'. Purists use the term 'lymphadenopathy', which causes ultrapurists to smile. A new term is needed but no one seems to have come up with it.

-sy

Suffix meaning 'name of' as in epilepsy (seize-upon sickness).

sycosis barbae

An old-fashioned term, still in use, for the condition popularly known as barber's itch. This is an infection of hair follicles in the beard area, usually with *Staphylococcus aureus*, acquired from infected razors or towels. Treatment is with antibiotic drugs and temporary avoidance of shaving. The increase in the prevalence of MRSA infections in hospital calls for extra care with patients' shaving equipment.

Symmetrel

A brand name for **amantadine**.

sympathectomy

Sympathectomy is an operation to destroy the sympathetic nerve supply to an area in order to prevent sympathetic constriction of the blood vessels and thus improve the blood supply to the part. This may be done by actual cutting of the nerves or by chemical injections to destroy them. Sympathectomy can be valuable in the treatment of conditions in which the supply of blood to the skin is dangerously reduced. It does not increase blood flow to the muscles. Sympathectomy is also valuable in the management of intractable pain in the abdomen.

sympathomimetic drugs

Drugs which act on the body to cause effects similar to those of adrenaline or of the sympathetic part of the autonomic nervous system (see **anticholinergic drugs**). These effects are generally stimulating and include:

- increase in the heart rate;
- increase in the blood supply to the voluntary muscles;
- slowing of digestion;
- widening (dilatation) of the pupils of the eyes;
- widening of the lung air tubes (bronchial tubes);
- tightening of the muscle rings (sphincters) around the outlet of the bladder and the bowels.

These effects are produced by the natural hormones adrenaline and noradrenaline and by drugs such as amphetamine, ephedrine, isoprenaline, methoxamine, salbutamol, phenylephrine, metaproterenol, terbutaline and salmeterol. All these are called sympathomimetic drugs. The effects are complicated by the fact that there are several different receptors for adrenaline-like substances. Some drugs stimulate some of these receptors, but not others. Some stimulate all adrenoreceptors. In general, drugs which block the adrenoreceptors (see **beta-blocker drugs**) are antagonistic to the sympathomimetic drugs.

symptoma

Greek root meaning 'symptom' as in symptom (sensation associated with a disease).

Synacthen

A brand name for **tetracosactrin**.

Synadrin

A brand name for the **calcium channel blocker** drug prenylamine.

Synalar

A brand name for the steroid drug **fluocinolone**, used for local applications.

Synalar C

A brand name for **fluocinolone** with the antifungal drug **clioquinol**.

Synalar N

A brand name for **fluocinolone** with **neomycin**.

Synandone

A brand name for the steroid drug **fluocinolone**, used for local applications.

synapse

The very narrow gap between two connected nerves, or between a nerve and a muscle fibre or a gland. The synaptic gap contains fluid across which nerve impulses are transmitted by means of a chemical **neuro-transmitter** such as acetylcholine or noradrenaline. Synapses allow impulses to pass in one direction only and a single brain cell may have more than 15,000 synapses with other cells. This complexity, allowing logical 'gate' operation, partly or wholly underlies the computational and storage abilities of the brain.

Synarel

A brand name for **nafarelin**.

syncope

The medical term for fainting.

syndactyly

An abnormal fusion of two or more adjacent fingers or toes, present at birth. In mild cases the fusion involves skin only and surgical separation is easy, but in more severe cases the bones may also be fused.

syndrome

A unique combination of sometimes apparently unrelated symptoms or signs, forming a distinct clinical entity. In most cases the elements of a syndrome arise from a common cause and are merely distinct effects of that cause. Sometimes the relationship is purely one of observed association and the causal link obscure and not yet understood.

syndrome, premenstrual

See **premenstrual syndrome**.

Synflex

A brand name for the non-steroidal anti-inflammatory drug (**NSAID**) **naproxen**.

Synopessin

A brand name for the drug lypressin used in the treatment of **diabetes insipidus**.

synovial membrane

The secretory membrane that lies within the capsule of a joint and produces the clear, sticky, lubricating synovial fluid without which smooth joint movement would be impossible. The synovial membrane covers all the internal structures of the joint except the bearing surfaces (the articular cartilages). Also known as the synovium.

synovitis

Inflammation of the synovial membrane, which lines the capsule of joints. Synovial membranes produce a lubricating fluid for the joint, and inflammation, as well as causing pain, warmth and redness, leads to a considerably increased secretion of synovial fluid and swelling of the joint. Synovitis may be caused by infection, by any form of arthritis, by overuse or by injury. The treatment depends on the cause, but will in all cases involve rest and support for the joint. In very persistent cases, resistant to drug treatment, it may be necessary to resort to surgical removal of the synovial membrane (synovectomy) or radiotherapy.

Synphase

A brand name for **ethinyloestradiol** formulated with a **progestogen** drug as an oral contraceptive.

Syntaris

A brand name for the corticosteroid drug **flunisolide**.

Syntocinon

A brand name for the womb muscle stimulating drug **oxytocin**.

Syntometrine

A brand name for **ergometrine**.

syphilis

See **sexually transmitted diseases**.

Syraprim

A brand name for the antibacterial drug trimethoprim.

Syrette

A brand name for a squeezable tube with a hypodermic needle attached, containing a single dose of a drug, such as **morphine**, for use in emergency or wartime situations by unskilled persons, or for self-medication.

Syscor MR

A brand name for **nisoldipine**.

systemic

Pertaining to something that affects the whole body rather than one part of it. Of a drug taken by mouth or given by injection, as distinct from a drug applied externally.

Sytron

A brand name for the iron preparation, sodium iron edetate, used in the treatment of **anaemia**.

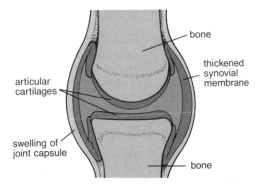

In synovitis, the synovial membrane becomes inflamed and thickened and secretes excess fluid into the joint. This causes joint swelling (effusion).

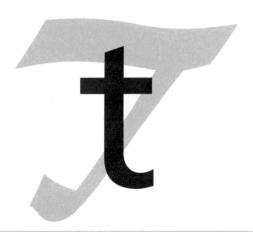

tabes dorsalis

A degenerative disorder of the nerve pathways in the spinal cord that carry sensory information up to the brain. Tabes, which is also called *locomotor ataxia*, is caused by untreated syphilis and, if it occurs, it does so five to twenty years after acquiring the infection.

RECOGNITION AND SYMPTOMS

The first indication is a series of episodes of severe, stabbing *lightning* pains in the legs or around the lower trunk. Loss of sensory information leads to unsteadiness and walking defects and the affected person lifts the feet high, stamps forcibly and proceeds with the feet well apart, so as to avoid falling. Loss of bladder control is common. The joints become damaged and unstable and there may be painless ulcers on the feet. Eye coordination is affected, leading to double vision, and the eyesight may fail from damage to the optic nerves.

TREATMENT

Treatment with penicillin can arrest the progress of the disease and may bring about some improvement, but recovery of function in destroyed nerve tissue is not to be expected.

See **sexually transmitted diseases**.

tacalcitol

A vitamin D analogue drug used to treat **psoriasis**. A brand name is Curatoderm.

tachycardia

A rapid heart rate, whether as a normal reaction to exertion or caused by heart disease.

tacrolimus

A potent immunosuppressant macrolide compound isolated from a bacterium. Tacrolimus is effective in reducing the risk of rejection of solid-organ transplants, especially liver transplants. It has also been used in ointment form for atopic dermatitis. A brand name if Prograf.

tactu

Latin root meaning 'touch' as in tactile (of touch).

taeniasis

Tapeworm infestation. The common human tapeworms are *Taenia solium*, the pig tapeworm, and *T. saginata*, the beef tapeworm. The fish tapeworm *Dibothriocephalus latus* occurs in some parts of Europe, Africa and South America.

A tapeworm is a ribbon-like population of joined flatworms, of the class Cestoda, all derived from a common head (scolex) equipped with hooks or suckers by which it is attached to the lining of the bowel. The body of the worm is composed of segments of increasing size, known as proglottids, each of which is a separate individual containing both male and female reproductive organs. *T. solium* extends to about 4 m in length and has 800 to 1000 segments.

The younger, smaller proglottids release sperm which fertilize the eggs contained in the older proglottids. Segments with developing embryos break off and are passed in the faeces. If these are eaten by an animal (the intermediate host), the larvae develop, travel to the animal's muscles and form cysts. Pork meat containing taenia cysts is called 'measly pork' and if this is eaten when it is undercooked the worm is released in the intestine, attaches itself, and the life cycle is continued.

TREATMENT

Tapeworms can be eliminated fairly easily with anthelmintic drugs. A more serious situation occurs, however, if a person ingests the fertilized proglottids. In this case, the affected person becomes the intermediate host and the larvae will form cysts, which may be up to 4 cm in diameter, in the brain, muscles, lungs, liver or other organs. Serious complications, including **epilepsy**, can result.

Tagamet

A brand name for cimetidine.

Takayasu disease

A disease of young women, rare except in Japan, that causes inflammation and narrowing of the major arteries of the upper part of the body. The result is diminished blood supply to the head, brain and arms, causing headache, faintness, muscle wasting and defective vision. The arteries are so narrowed that pulses in the upper limb can hardly be felt. Corticosteroids may help but the outlook is poor. Also known as pulseless disease or the aortic arch syndrome.

talipes

Clubfoot. A congenital deformity affecting the shape or position of one or both feet. The commonest type is called *talipes equinovarus* and in this the entire foot, including the heel, is twisted inward, so that the inner border lies horizontally.

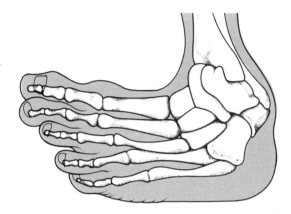

Talipes is a congenital foot deformity in which the whole skeleton of the foot is twisted.

The arch of the foot is greatly exaggerated. *Talipes* is the Latin word for 'clubfoot' and *equinovarus* combines the word for a horse with the word for an inward deviation.

POSSIBLE CAUSES

Talipes is thought to be caused by a lack of balance in the muscles which stabilize the foot, and the condition has a definite familial tendency.

TREATMENT

Treatment must begin at, or as soon as possible after, birth, and consists of repetitive deliberate manipulations in which the inturn and the high arching are gently but positively corrected, followed sometimes by the application of a splint. If started during the first week of life, splintage may not be necessary and the mother, after careful instruction, may be able to continue the manipulation herself. If the start of treatment is delayed for three weeks, splintage will probably be required. Longer delay means greater difficulty in correction. Failure to achieve full correction at six months of age means that surgical correction will be needed.

Talpen

A brand name for the penicillin antibiotic talampicillin.

talus

Latin root meaning 'heel or ankle' as in talus (bone of foot above heel bone).

Tambocor

A brand name for **flecainide acetate**.

Tamofen

A brand name for **tamoxifen**.

tamoxifen

A drug that blocks oestrogen receptors and is useful in the treatment of certain cancers, especially breast cancer. Research involving 37,000 women has shown that tamoxifen substantially improves the survival figures after breast cancer and substantially reduces the probability of cancer in the other breast. The drug also stimulates egg production from the ovaries and can be used to treat infertility. Brand names are Nolvadex, Soltamox and Tamofen.

tampon

See **sanitary protection**, **toxic shock syndrome**.

tamponade

The heart is enclosed in a firm, fibrous sac called the pericardial sac. If this becomes inflamed (**pericarditis**) it produces an excess of its normal lubricating fluid and this leads to compression of the heart, a condition known as tamponade. The same effect can result from injury with bleeding into the sac. Tamponade prevents normal heart filling and seriously prejudices its function, leading to breathlessness and sometimes collapse from reduced heart output. Pericardial fluid or blood can, in an emergency, be withdrawn through a needle.

Tampovagan

A brand name for **stilboestrol**.

tamsulosin

A selective alpha-adrenergic smooth muscle relaxing drug that is used to relieve the symptoms of enlargement of the **prostate gland**. A brand name is Flomax MR.

tannic acid

An antifungal drug, used externally to treat fungus infections of the skin. A brand name of a preparation containing tannic acid and other drugs is Phytex.

tantrum

See **temper tantrum**.

tapeworm infestation

See **taeniasis**.

tardive dyskinesia

A side-effect of some antipsychotic drugs such as the phenothiazine derivatives. Tardive dyskinesia is involuntary repetitive shaking movements that persist or become worse after the drug is withdrawn. The condition usually affects elderly people after years of treatment with the drug.

Targocid

A brand name for **teicoplanin**.

tarsal tunnel syndrome

Entrapment of the nerves to the foot by pressure from the fibrous band that restrains the tendons, at the ankle, of the leg muscles that are inserted into the foot. This band is called the flexor retinaculum and its pressure on the nerves causes weakness of the muscles of the foot and numbness. The effect is similar to the **carpal tunnel syndrome**.

tarsorrhaphy

Surgical sewing together of the eyelids after removing strips of marginal surface skin (epidermis), so that the raw areas heal together and remain closed after the stitches are removed. Tarsorrhaphy is sometimes done to conceal an unsightly and blind eye, but is also used as a temporary measure to aid in the healing of a severe ulcer on the cornea or to protect the cornea from drying and damage in conditions of protrusion of the eye (**exophthalmos**).

taste, sense of

Taste is seldom experienced in the absence of the sense of smell, but when it is, it will be found to be an unrefined and crude sensation, in which only four different modalities can be distinguished – sweet, sour, salt and bitter. Combinations of these extend the range, but it is still very limited. When, however, these four are associated with the enormous range and subtlety of the sense of smell (olfactory sense) the full aesthetic possibilities of the 'palate' become apparent.

Taste results from the stimulation of specialized nerve endings, mainly on the tongue but also on the back of the throat and palate, called taste buds. The sensation of sweetness is experienced around the tip of the tongue, sour and salt on the edges and bitter at the back.

Actual loss of the sense of taste happens very rarely and complaints of loss of taste almost always originate from the loss of the sense of smell, either as a result of temporary causes, such as a cold, or from permanent damage to the olfactory nerve filaments in the roof of the nose, as a result of injury.

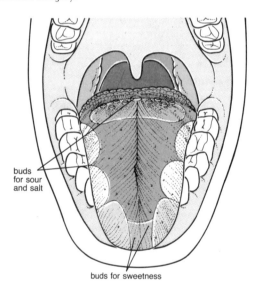

buds for sour and salt

buds for sweetness

Location of the taste buds.

tattooing

The deliberate or accidental insertion of coloured material into the deeper layers of the skin, so producing a permanently visible effect.

Tattooing may be done deliberately for decorative or other purposes, such as tribal identification. Most decorative tattooing is acquired by young people and is sometimes regretted, but removal of the tattoo is not always easy. Tattooing may also be incidental to injuries of various kinds, especially those involving deep abrasions or where particles are driven in by explosions. Proximity to exploding fireworks or blank cartridges, and gun shot injuries often cause tattoo-

ing. Brown or black particles buried deep in the skin cause a blue colouring.

RISKS

Professional tattooing is not without potential danger and concern has been expressed over the possible transmission of **hepatitis B** and **AIDS**. Other possible, if unlikely, complications include skin sepsis, **septicaemia**, and the transmission of syphilis and warts. **Psoriasis** and **lichen planus** and discoid **lupus erythematosus** often appear at tattoo sites.

Skin reactions have occurred to the metallic pigments sometimes used in tattooing, including salts of mercury (red), chromium (green), cobalt (blue), manganese (purple) and cadmium (yellow). Cadmium salts often react badly to sunlight.

REMOVAL

Small tattoos can be removed along with the whole of the involved skin, and the defect closed by stitching. Larger areas may sometimes be managed by the process of **dermabrasion**, by cutting off the surface layers of the skin, by vigorously rubbing in salt on a swab until the surface of the skin is removed and then covering with a sterile dressing, or by vaporizing the particles with a laser. The results are not always satisfactory.

tau protein

An important protein associated with the microtubules that form the skeletal structure of nerve cells (the cytoskeleton). In **Alzheimer's disease** an abnormal form of the protein, with a shorter molecule, is found in the filaments of the abnormal neural plaques and fibrillary tangles that are features of the disease. Tau protein is also found in the cerebrospinal fluid of people with dementia, but it is present in higher concentration in Alzheimer's disease than in other forms of dementia.

Abnormal tau protein binds strongly to the normal protein and the latter then becomes shortened by nerve cell protein-splitting enzymes into the abnormal form, which cannot be split by these enzymes.

Tavegil

A brand name for **clemastine**.

taxane and taxoid drugs

One of a group of diterpene substances derived from the Pacific yew tree *Taxus brevifolia* that have been found useful in cancer treatment. Taxanes have a unique action in permanently stabilizing the microtubule assembly in cells. This prevents the movement of chromosomes and halts the process of cell division. One of the taxanes, **paclitaxel** (Taxol), has been licensed for use and has been found to be helpful in the treatment of cases of cancer of the ovary that have proved to be resistant to other treatment.

Taxoid drugs, such as paclitaxel and docetaxel, are extracted from the needles of the yew *Taxus baccata*. These drugs enhance cellular microtubule assembly and interfere with the breaking up (depolymerization) of the tubular protein tubulin. The result of this is that cells are unable to form the normal mitotic spindle (see **mitosis**) that organizes the movements of the chromosomes into an arrangement necessary for cell division. Cells affected in this way are unable to divide. As with most other anticancer drugs, the effect is greatest on the most rapidly dividing cells.

Taxol

A brand name for **paclitaxel**.

Tay-Sachs disease

A recessive genetic disorder, common among Ashkenazi Jews, which appears in the early months of life and leads to blindness, deafness, progressive dementia, seizures, paralysis and death, usually before the age of three years. The condition is due to the absence of an enzyme which breaks down a substance called ganglioside present mainly in the nervous system. It is the accumulation of this material that is so damaging.

Unfortunately, there is no treatment for Tay-Sachs disease so it is very important for carriers or possible carriers to have genetic counselling. Antenatal diagnosis by **chorionic villus sampling** can be done and, if the diagnosis is confirmed, termination of pregnancy can be offered. Some Jewish communities have successfully organized premarital counselling services and testing in the hope of preventing the occurrence of this autosomal recessive disorder.

tazarotene

A **retinoid** drug used externally to treat **psoriasis**. A brand name is Zorac.

tazobactam

A beta-lactamase inhibitor penicillin antibiotic. A brand name is Tazocin.

Tazocin

A brand name for **tazobactam**.

TB

See **tuberculosis**.

T cell activator, universal

See **superantigen**.

T cell development

See **thymus**.

tears, artificial

Solutions of various substances such as methyl cellulose, hypromellose, dextran or polyvinyl alcohol, which are more viscous and persistent than plain salt solutions, and are used to maintain the moistness of the exposed surfaces of the cornea and conjunctiva in conditions in which the tear secretion is inadequate.

teeth

From the centre outwards, a full set of permanent teeth consist, in each jaw, of four biting teeth (incisors), six tearing teeth (two canines and four premolars) and six grinding teeth (molars). So the full complement is thirty-two, but it is

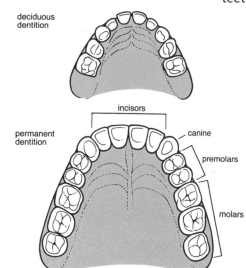

There are three kinds of teeth – cutters (incisors), tearers (canines) and grinders (premolars and molars).

common for one or more of the third molars, at the back ('wisdom teeth'), to remain within the gum (unerupted) until well into adult life.

The 'milk' teeth (primary, or deciduous, teeth) which begin to appear about halfway through the first year of life and are all present before the age of three number only twenty and consist of four incisors, two canines and four molars. In most cases, the first teeth – the central incisors – appear around six to nine months, followed, in a month or two, by the other incisors. Around ten to sixteen months, the first molars appear and at sixteen to twenty months, the canines appear. The second molars usually erupt some time between the second and third years of life. Around the age of six, these begin to be replaced by the permanent teeth, being pushed out as the permanent teeth erupt.

The greater part of a fully developed tooth consists of a hard material called dentine. The part of the dentine above the level of the gums (the crown of the tooth) is covered with

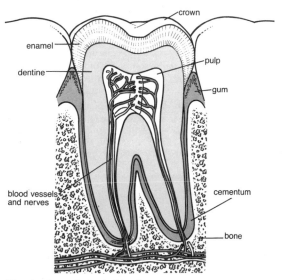

The structure of a typical tooth.

the extremely hard, visible enamel, and that part which lies in the socket in the jawbone is covered with a sensitive, bone-like material called the cementum. The cementum is secured to the bone of the socket by a series of fine strands called the periodontal membrane.

The dentine is hollow, leaving a central pulp space in the tooth, and this contains blood vessels, and nerves, which run in and out of the tooth at the tips of the root or roots.

In spite of its hardness and resistance to abrasion, enamel can be damaged by the acids produced when food particles, especially carbohydrates, left in the crevices between the teeth after eating, are broken down by mouth bacteria. This leads to tooth decay (caries).

teeth, artificial

See **dentures**.

teeth deformities

See **malocclusion**, **orthodontics**.

Tegretol

A brand name for **carbamazepine**.

teicoplanin

A glycopeptide antibiotic used to treat serious infections in people with penicillin allergy or in those who are not responding to a penicillin or a cephalosporin. A brand name is Targocid.

telangiectasia

A localized increase in the size and number of small blood vessels in the skin. Often incorrectly called 'broken veins', the condition most commonly affects the skin of the nose and the cheeks, causing permanent redness. In many cases a tendency to telangiectasia is present from birth but it also results from loss of support to the blood vessels from collagen damage due to undue exposure to sunlight and adverse environmental conditions. Persistent flushing from the effects of alcohol is also said to be a cause.

Telangiectasia is the main feature of the blushing disorder **rosacea**, but occurs in a number of other disorders, including **psoriasis**, **lupus erythematosus** and **dermatomyositis**. When the condition is restricted to a number of very small patches it produces the characteristic spots known as spider naevi. Large numbers of these suggest liver disease. In the rare condition of *hereditary haemorrhagic telangiectasia*, frequent bleeding occurs from small rounded patches of dilated vessels situated around the mouth and nose.

Teldane

A brand name for terfenadine.

telemedicine

Long-range multimedia medical communication, between doctor and patient, or between medical personnel, via a communication network such as the Internet or an intranet. Such communication may be by printed text, or by audible and visual means, and allows a previously unprecedented freedom of long-range interchange between medical personnel.

This communication can include teleconferencing, teleconsultation, teleradiology, distance learning and even the performing of surgical operations at a remote distance from the patient. Telemedicine broadens the scope of consultation and makes access to experts easier. It can effect considerable savings in medical costs. See also **medical computing**.

Telfast

A brand name for **fexofenadine**.

telomeres

The short sections of **DNA** that form the natural end of a chromosome so that they resist union with fragments of other chromosomes. Telomeres consist of repeated groups of the base sequence TTAGGG, where T, A and G represent the bases thymine, adenine and guanine, respectively (see **base pairs**). Whenever telomeres are formed some junk DNA is shaved off the end of the chromosome. There is, however, a limit to the number of times that this can occur before essential DNA is lost. This is believed to be the reason for the upper limit in the number of times cells can divide and reproduce. Fibroblasts from a young person, grown in culture, will divide no more than about 80 times.

Telomerase is an enzyme that can reform the telomeres at the ends of chromosomes. This enzyme is found in cancers and is able to prevent the shortening that would otherwise occur with repeated replication, thus allowing cancerous cells in culture to achieve immortality.

Temaze

A brand name for **temazepam**.

temazepam

A benzodiazepine drug used to treat insomnia. A brand name is Normison.

Temgesic

A brand name for **buprenorphine**.

temperature

See **fever**.

temperature measurement

Clinical thermometers have, in the past, consisted of a thick glass tube with a very fine bore (capillary tube), expanded at one end to form a reservoir and sealed at the other. The tube contains mercury or coloured alcohol and a rise in temperature causes the fluid to expand so that the free end moves along the tube. Because the bore is narrow, a small temperature rise causes a comparatively large movement of the indicating fluid. The thermometer is calibrated against a standard and a scale is engraved on the glass. The thick glass wall forms a cylindrical lens which acts as a magnifier, making the thread-like fluid column easier to see. Clinical thermometers are calibrated either in Celsius or Fahrenheit units and may be used in the mouth or rectum.

There has been a trend, in recent years, towards the use of cheap disposable skin thermometers employing heat-sensitive compounds which become visible at known temperatures.

These are generally less useful than mercury thermometers and are more likely to be affected by external factors. More satisfactory is the modern electronic thermometer using a heat-sensitive transducer and a digital readout.

temperature regulation

The process by which body temperature is kept within narrow limits. Blood temperature is monitored by a kind of thermostat situated in the hypothalamus, a part of the brain on its under surface just above the **pituitary gland**. If the blood temperature tends to drop, the hypothalamus immediately arranges for skin blood vessels to close and for the muscles to undergo rapid alternation of contraction and relaxation (shivering). This produces a rapid rise in heat production and the closure of the skin vessels ensures that the heat is retained. If the blood temperature rises the skin vessels open up and there is skin flushing and sweating so that heat is lost by radiation and evaporation.

In fevers, the normal control is affected by the fact that the hypothalamic thermostat is set high. The result of this is that normal temperatures are interpreted as if they were low temperatures and the heat production and retention mechanisms come into play.

temper tantrum

The expression of frustration in a toddler who has reached the stage of wishing to demonstrate independent action but is prevented from doing so. Tantrums may be very noisy and, especially in public, embarrassing, as they seem to imply lack of parental discipline or effectiveness. The toddler soon learns to exploit the power of screaming, floor-rolling, head-banging and **breath-holding** and, if injudiciously handled, may come to dominate a household.

Occasional tantrums are normal and acceptable, but a pattern should not be allowed to develop. Tantrums must be handled calmly, firmly and consistently with minimal necessary restraint, and the child's demands, unless reasonable, should never be met. If necessary, a short period of banishment to a safe cot or playpen in a separate room until the tantrum has passed may be tried. Once adequate communication has been achieved, temper tantrums should settle, as the child can express his or her wishes and can be reasoned with.

temples, tender streaks on

Elderly people who develop tenderness to touch on the temples should waste no time in seeking medical advice. Inflammation of the arteries of the temples may be a sign of a more generalized disease of the arteries, called *giant cell arteritis*, which can cause serious effects, including blindness. These can be prevented by early treatment with steroids, but delay is dangerous. Tender temples is an urgent indication for checking the blood sedimentation rate. If this is very high, the diagnosis is clinched.

temple, tender red streaks on

See **temporal arteritis**.

temporal arteritis

A potentially serious disease, also known as *giant cell arteritis*, mainly of elderly people, in which the walls of certain arteries in the head become severely inflamed and thickened so that blood flow is reduced or stopped. The arteries of the temple become prominent, red and exquisitely tender, so that the wearing of a hat becomes intolerable. The importance of recognizing this condition is that there is a serious danger that the nearby arteries to the eyes may become affected and cause blindness. The diagnosis is assisted by a raised blood sedimentation rate. Urgent treatment with steroids is necessary to save the sight.

temporal lobe epilepsy

See **epilepsy**.

tempore

Latin root meaning 'temple' as in temple (side of forehead).

temporomandibular joint replacement

A surgical procedure to replace the hinge joint of the jaw bone with a prosthesis in cases of severe limitation of mouth opening from disease or derangement of this joint.

temporomandibular joint syndrome

The temporomandibular joint is the joint just in front of the ear at which the jaw bone (mandible) articulates with the temporal bone on the base of the skull. The temporomandibular joint syndrome is thought to be due to spasm of the chewing muscles as a result of emotional tension and is one of the more obscure causes of headache, facial pain and pain in the ear.

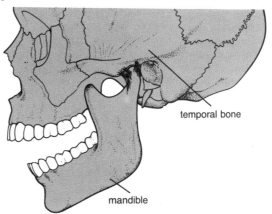

temporal bone

mandible

The lower jaw articulates high in front of the ear in a hollow in the temporal bone. Undue tension on the muscles that pull up the jaw can cause pain in this area.

Tempra

A brand name for **paracetamol**.

ten day rule

The regulation, observed in all X-ray departments, that radiological examination of the lower abdomen in women of childbearing age should be performed only during the ten days immediately following the first day of the last menstrual period. This is to avoid the risk of exposing a young embryo to radiation.

pressure on the affected area, or abnormal
touch or pressure.

...jerks

So long as the nerves from the spinal cord to the muscles, and
those from the muscles to the cord, are intact, the sudden
stretching of a muscle tendon, by striking it with a rubber hammer, will cause the muscle to tighten, because these nerves are
linked, by other short nerves, within the substance of the cord.
This nerve circuit is called the reflex arc and it is normally
damped down by controlling impulses coming down the cord
from the brain and acting on the linking nerves. If these controlling influences are removed, as in brain damage from a
cerebral thrombosis or haemorrhage, the reflexes become
much brisker and more prominent than normal. If, on the
other hand, there is damage to, or pressure on, the nerves running to or from the spinal cord, the reflex jerk will be absent.

tendons, disorders of

Tendinitis is inflammation of a tendon and the lining of
its sheath, causing pain and limitation of movement. It
is most commonly caused by injury or overuse, and is
often associated with inflammation of an adjacent fluid-filled
sac (**bursitis**). Treatment includes non-steroidal anti-
inflammatory drugs (**NSAIDs**), other pain-killing drugs
(analgesics), local heat and sometimes injections of a depot
corticosteroid preparation around the affected tendon.

The Achilles tendon may be ruptured during strenuous
athletic activity, especially jumping. Other tendons may be
torn, or pulled off their
attachment, by unaccustomed
sudden exertion. Tendons
are often cut in the course of
injuries involving sharp-edged
instruments. Such injuries
cause severe disability and
require careful surgical repair
and prolonged immobiliza-
tion. Tendon grafting is
sometimes necessary.

*The main calf muscles are
inserted into the heel bone
by way of the strong Achilles
tendon, but this tendon
undergoes severe strain in
extending the ankle and
may rupture, as shown here.*

gastrocnemius
muscle

Achilles
tendon

tendon transfer

An operation to disconnect a tendon from its normal insertion and connect it to a new site, so that, after retraining, its
muscle can be made to perform a different function, such as
restoring movement to a paralysed part.

Tenesmus

A continuing, or frequently recurrent, sensation of wishing to
empty the bowels. Tenesmus causes ineffective straining with

the occasional passage of small amounts of faeces. It is a
feature of **shigellosis**, **haemorrhoids,** the **irritable bowel syndrome**, rectal polyps, prolapse of the rectum, inflammation
of the anal region, **ulcerative colitis** and sometimes tumour of
the rectum.

tennis elbow

Inflammation in the region of the bony prominence on the
outer side of the elbow from which several forearm muscle tendons arise. Excessive use of the muscles which extend the wrist
causes trauma at this point. There is pain and tenderness in the
elbow, on the thumb side, and in the back of the forearm, made
worse by use of the elbow and hand.

The treatment involves temporary avoidance of the activity
which caused the problem, rest, support, painkillers and anti-
inflammatory drugs. If the inflammation resulted from playing sport, professional advice on technique may be necessary.

tenon

Greek root meaning 'tendon' as in tenosynovitis (tendon
sheath inflammation).

Tenopt

A brand name for eye drops containing **timolol**.

Tenoretic

A brand name for **atenolol**.

Tenormin

A brand name for **atenolol**.

tenosynovitis

Inflammation of a tendon sheath, usually due to overuse.
Tenosynovitis causes pain, swelling and a grating or creaking
sensation, or even sound, on movement of the tendon in its
sheath. The condition is commonest in the tendons of the
hand and wrist. There is often some limitation of movement,
and sometimes adhesions form between the tendon and its
sheath, leading to persistent restriction.

Tenosynovitis calls for rest, immobilization, the use of
anti-inflammatory drugs, including corticosteroids injected
around the affected tendon. Occasionally, surgical freeing of
an adherent tendon is required. Rarely, tenosynovitis is
caused by infection following an injury. This is liable to cause
serious disability unless effectively treated by surgical
drainage and antibiotics. Many cases of alleged **repetitive
strain injury** (RSI) are, in fact, tenosynovitis.

tenoxicam

A non-steroidal anti-inflammatory (**NSAID**) used to treat
arthritis and other painful conditions. A brand name is
Mobiflex.

TENS

An abbreviation for Transcutaneous Electrical Nerve
Stimulation. This is a method of treating long-persistent pain
by passing small electric currents into the spinal cord or sensory nerves by means of electrodes applied to the skin. The

necessary equipment is miniaturized and is readily portable.

See also **barbotage**.

tension

A sense of strain, usually associated with anxiety and reflected in a general or local tightening of muscles. Tension is a response to **stress**, difficulty, frustration, unhappiness and unrelieved anger and is a potent cause of symptoms, which result from the sustained muscular contraction. Most cases of persistent **headache** are caused in this way. Often the cause cannot be remedied, but a clear awareness of what is happening, an analysis of the circumstances, and deliberate attempts to relax the tension can be helpful. In some cases severe tension may be an indication of an **anxiety** disorder.

Tensipine MR

A brand name for **nifedipine**.

Tensium

A brand name for diazepam.

Tenuate dospan

A brand name for the appetite-reducing drug diethylpropion.

terazosin

A selective alpha-adrenergic blocker drug used to treat high blood pressure and to relieve the symptoms of simple enlargement of the **prostate gland** (benign prostatic hyperplasia). Trade names are Hytrin and Hyrin BPH.

terbinafine

An antifungal drug that acts by causing leakage of the fungal cell contents through the fungal cell wall. It is especially useful against **tinea** of the skin and nails for which it is said to be more effective than clotrimazole. A brand name is Lamisil.

terbutaline

A bronchodilator drug used in the treatment of **asthma**, **bronchitis** and **emphysema**. It is also used to relax the womb muscle and prevent premature labour. A brand name is Bricanyl.

Terence Higgins Trust

A charitable community-based aid organization that provides current information to HIV-infected and at-risk individuals. It was named after one of the earliest victims of **AIDS** in the UK.

terlipressin

A drug that releases vasopressin over a period of hours. This is used to help to control bleeding from oesophageal varices (see **oesophagitis**) by constricting the small arteries in the intestinal tract. A brand name is Glypressin.

terminal care

See **dying, care of the**.

termination of pregnancy

See **abortion and miscarriage**.

Terramycin

A brand name for the tetracycline antibiotic **oxytetracycline**.

Tertroxin

A brand name for **liothyronine sodium**.

testes

Behind and below the penis is the scrotum, the hanging skin and muscle receptacle for the testicles and the beginning of the tubes (vasa deferentes – singular, vas deferens) which carry the sperm produced in the testicles up to the seminal vesicles for storage. Each testicle is divided into about 250 wedge-shaped lobes and each of these contains one to three narrow, coiled-up tubes called the seminiferous tubules, each about 60 cm long. Sperms develop in the walls of these, the more mature passing to the centre of the tubule. In each testicle these tubules join to form the epididymis. This, too, is a long, elaborately coiled-up tube and lies along the outer rear border of the testicle, connecting it to the vas deferens. By its length, the epididymis allows time for maturation of the sperms produced in the testicle, as they proceed on their long, slow upward passage, forced by the pressure of more sperms from below, by way of the vas.

The thin layer of muscle under the skin of the scrotum is called the dartos muscle and when this contracts, the scrotum tightens and becomes smaller.

testicle, disorders of

The testicles develop in the abdomen and descend into the scrotum soon before birth. It is not uncommon for one, sometimes both, to fail to descend. Testicles remaining in the abdomen become sterile and should be brought down surgically during infancy. Sometimes the testicle has partly descended, but remains in the canal in the groin through which it normally descends. Again correction is necessary if fertility is to develop.

Inflammation of the testicle (**orchitis**) is fairly common as a complication of **mumps**. Torsion of the testis is the acutely painful condition in which the spermatic cord becomes twisted within, or just above, the scrotum. The veins in the spermatic cord are soon occluded and the return of blood

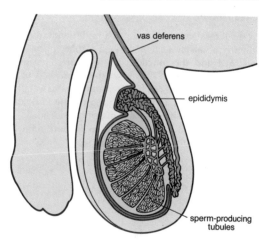

The testicle in section.

obstructed. There is great swelling, tenderness and bruising. Early surgical correction is necessary if fertility, in the affected testicle, is to be preserved. The other testicle may be secured, as a precaution.

Cancer of the testicle is uncommon, but occurs more often in testicles that have not descended. It affects young and middle-aged men and appears as a hard swelling on one side which is often entirely painless, but may be associated with inflammation, pain and tenderness. Unless routine self-examination is being performed regularly, a testicular cancer is likely to be missed until well advanced. The outlook, in early cases, is excellent, but worsens with delay in diagnosis. Any new lumps should be reported at once. Treatment involves removal of the affected testicle (**orchidectomy**) and often radiotherapy or chemotherapy.

See also **cryptorchidism**, **epididymitis**.

testicle-lowering operation

See **orchidopexy**.

testicular feminization syndrome

A rare condition, causing male **pseudohermaphroditism**, in which a man with the normal male chromosomes physically resembles a woman. The testicles are present, but have not descended into their normal position. They may lie in the abdomen or in what appear to be labia majora. They do, however, secrete male sex hormones (androgens). There is no uterus, but a short, blind-ended vagina and the penis is rudimentary. The breasts may be well developed.

Body cells carry, on their surfaces, specific receptors for androgens. The testicular feminization syndrome results from an X-linked, genetically induced defect of these receptors so that the male hormones are unable to act and normal male characteristics cannot develop. Because there is a tendency for cancer to develop in the testicles of these men, it is usual to remove the testicles and to give female sex hormones (oestrogens). These promote full development of the characteristics of the assumed, and accepted, sex.

testicular pain, severe, sudden

See **torsion of testis**.

test meal

A small meal, left in the stomach for a standard period and then removed by suction through a tube so that it can be analysed and the function of the stomach assessed. The presence or absence of acid in the stomach is of medical importance and this can be determined in this way. If no acid is found following an injection of histamine, then the stomach is deemed to be incapable of acid production.

The test meal had been replaced by more refined methods of examination.

Testomet

A brand name for methyltestosterone.

testosterone

The principal male sex hormone (androgen) produced in the interstitial cells of the testis and, to a lesser extent, in the **ovary**. Testosterone is **anabolic** and stimulates bone and mus-

cle growth and the growth of the sexual characteristics. It is also used as a drug to treat delayed puberty or some cases of infertility or to help to treat breast cancer in post-menopausal women. It may be given by mouth, depot injection or skin patch. Trade names are Andropatch, Restandol, Sustanon and Virormone.

tests for baby development

See **reflexes**, **primitive**.

test tube baby

A popular term for a baby derived from an ovum fertilized outside the body (*in vitro* **fertilization**).

tetanus

A serious infection of the nervous system caused by the organism *Clostridium tetani* which is found in cultivated soil and manure. This organism forms tough spores which are resistant to environmental influences, and germinates in deep wounds where the oxygen supply is poor. It gains access to the body by way of penetrating wounds, which may be small and seemingly trivial, and causes the disease two days to several weeks later.

INCIDENCE

The disease is rare in Britain but is still a common cause of death in developing countries where the mortality from the disease is around 50 per cent. Babies are commonly infected through the stump of the umbilical cord, and in these the mortality is nearly 100 per cent.

RECOGNITION AND SYMPTOMS

The tetanus organism produces a powerful **toxin** which triggers off the nerves supplying voluntary muscles, or the nerve endings on the muscles, causing them to go into violent spasms of contraction. The chief early sign is a spasm of the chewing muscles (trismus), causing great difficulty in opening the mouth – hence the name of 'lockjaw'. This spasm spreads to the muscles of the face and neck, producing a snarling, mirthless smile known as the *risus sardonicus*. The back muscles then become rigid and, in severe cases, the back becomes strongly arched backwards so that the abdominal wall becomes tight, rigid and board-like. Spasms of contraction occur every few minutes and increase in severity and frequency over the course of a week. There is also fever, difficulty in swallowing, severe stiffness of the limbs, sore throat and headache. Death from exhaustion or from **asphyxia** in the course of convulsions is common.

TREATMENT

Tetanus is treated by giving tetanus antitoxin, preferably human antitetanus globulin (antibodies), and large doses of antibiotics or metronidazole as soon as the diagnosis is suspected. Spasms are controlled by diazepam (Valium), given into a vein, and every effort is made to handle the affected person gently so as to avoid promoting spasms by unexpected stimuli. In severe cases it may be necessary deliberately to paralyse the patient with curare and to maintain respiration artificially. General measures to maintain the airway and the nutrition are also important. Tetanus is a terrifying ordeal and much reassurance is necessary.

Tetanus is easily prevented by safe immunization with tetanus toxoid and all should be protected.

tetany

A characteristic form of muscle spasm most commonly caused by abnormally strong nerve conduction resulting from low levels of blood calcium. It can also result from a reduction in blood acidity, which in turn affects calcium levels, from deliberate or hysterical over-breathing (**hyperventilation**). Tetany usually affects the hands and the feet, producing a claw-like effect with extension of the nearer joints and bending of the others (*carpopedal spasm*). If severe, it may, however, extend to involve the facial muscles, the larynx, or even the spinal muscles. The initial minor spasms are painless, but, if they persist, they become painful and may even lead to muscle damage.

Tetany is a feature of underaction of the parathyroid glands and was once common following surgical operations on the thyroid gland. Underaction of the gland may occur for other reasons.

tetracosactrin

An analogue of ACTH used as a test of adrenal function. An injection of the drug is given and the resulting rise in serum cortisol is monitored. A brand name is Synacthen.

tetracycline

One of a group of antibiotic drugs originally derived from *Streptomyces species*. They are used to treat a wide range of infections including **rickettsia** diseases, **cholera**, **brucellosis**, **Lyme disease** and most of the **sexually transmitted diseases**. They have the disadvantage that they are deposited in bones and teeth and will cause permanent yellow staining of the latter if given to young children. They will similarly affect fetuses if given to women in late pregnancy. The tetracyclines have a useful effect on **acne** and **rosacea**. This does not imply that acne is an infection. Tetracyclines are effective in acne because nonpathogenic bacteria present in the sebum in acne produce enzymes that separate fatty acids from the fats and these acids cause inflammation. Tetracyclines are concentrated in sebum, while penicillins are not. Trade names are Achromycin, Deteclo and, for external use, Topicycline.

See also **antibiotic drugs**.

tetrahydrofuryl salicylate

A formulation of drugs for external use that cause reddening of the skin and increase the blood flow in the underlying tissue (a rubefacient). A brand name is Transvasin.

tetralogy of Fallot

See **Fallot's tetralogy**.

Tetralysal

A brand name for **lymecycline**.

Tetrex

A brand name for **tetracycline**.

thalassaemia

A condition of abnormal haemoglobin in the red blood cells, leading to unduly rapid breakdown of the cells and severe anaemia. The disorder is common in the area surrounding the Mediterranean sea, hence the name (*thalassa* is Greek for 'the sea', *haima* is Greek for 'blood').

Haemoglobin is the pigment in red blood cells which transports oxygen. It contains two kinds of protein (globin), alpha chain globin and beta chain globin. Abnormal alpha globin is very rare and often fatal. Most cases of thalassaemia involve defective beta chains. The haemoglobin abnormality can take various forms, but all are due to the inheritance of an abnormal gene. Inheritance is recessive.

RECOGNITION AND SYMPTOMS

The presence of one defective gene (heterozygous state) causes a minor disturbance (thalassaemia minor), inheritance of both genes (homozygous state) causes a much more serious type (thalassaemia major), with breathlessness, ready fatiguability, jaundice and enlargement of the spleen. Red cells are broken down in the spleen and the enlargement is due to accumulation of red cell products. These symptoms and signs are caused by the anaemia and the reduced oxygen-carrying capacity of the blood. The body responds by attempting to produce more red cells in the bone marrow and this may cause characteristic enlargement of bones, such as *bossing* of the skull in children.

TREATMENT

Thalassaemia in children may require a blood transfusion so as to allow normal development. Accumulation of iron in the body, from red cell breakdown, must also be treated, or this will cause complications including cirrhosis of the liver.

thalidomide

A drug (Distaval and many other trade names) that was widely advertised as the first really safe sedative, particularly suitable for pregnant women. In 1961, however, it was found that when given during early pregnancy it caused severe bodily malformation of the fetus with stunting of the limbs, which were often replaced by short flippers (phocomelia). This medical disaster was instrumental in drawing much closer attention to the unwanted side-effects of powerful drugs and to the necessity for much closer investigation into such possible effects before releasing new drugs for general use.

Thalidomide has since been found of real value in the treatment of certain forms of leprosy and of Behçet's syndrome. In 1997 it was approved by the US Food and Drug Administration (FDA) for the treatment of leprosy.

Theo-Dur

A brand name for **theophylline**.

Theograd

A brand name for **theophylline**.

theophylline

A bronchodilator drug used to treat asthma and to assist in the treatment of **heart failure** by increasing the heart rate and reducing **oedema** by promoting excretion of urine. Trade names are Lasma, Nuelin, Slo-Phyllin, Theo-Dur and Uniphyllin Continus. Franol and Franol Plus are theophylline preparations with **ephedrine**.

Thephorin

A brand name for the antihistamine drug phenindamine.

Theraderm

A brand name for the anti-**acne** drug benzoyl peroxide.

therapeutic community

An imaginative way of trying to improve the situation of people with personality disorders that produce antisocial behaviour. The therapeutic community is a small local population of such people, set up in a nonclinical environment under the supervision of medical staff. The object is to make plain to those concerned the effects that such behaviour has on one other and on themselves, and to try to instil constructive patterns of conduct and improve social and interpersonal skills. Results have been promising.

therapy

The attempted treatment of disease or of conditions supposed to be diseases. Within medicine, forms of therapy include **chemotherapy**, hydrotherapy, physiotherapy, radiotherapy, psychotherapy and occasionally hypnotherapy.

thiabendazole

An **anthelmintic** drug used to get rid of worms such as *Toxocara canis*, *Strongyloides stercoralis* and *Trichinella spiralis*. A brand name is Mintezol.

thiazide diuretic drugs

See **diuretic drugs**.

thinking simply

See **Occam's razor**.

thioguanine

A drug used in the treatment of acute myeloblastic leukaemia. A brand name is Lanvis.

thiopentone sodium

A barbiturate drug widely used as a pleasant and rapid induction agent for general **anaesthesia**. The drug is given by slow intravenous injection. A brand name is Intraval.

Thioprine

A brand name for **azathioprine**.

thioridazine

An antipsychotic drug used to treat **schizophrenia** and **mania**. A brand name is Melleril.

thioxanthene drugs

A group of antipsychotic drugs related to the **phenothiazine derivative drugs**. The group includes flupenthixol and clopenthixol.

thirst

A strong desire to drink water or other liquid, arising from a degree of dehydration (water shortage) in the body, or from an increase in the concentration of substances dissolved in the blood, or a drop in blood volume. Thirst may thus result from inadequate intake or excessive loss of water, as in profuse sweating or severe and prolonged diarrhoea. It may also result from excessive intake of salt or other materials readily absorbed into the bloodstream. Any medical condition which causes dehydration or an increased concentration of the blood will cause thirst. Such conditions include **diabetes mellitus** and **diabetes insipidus**.

When concentrated blood passes through certain areas in each side of the hypothalamus in the brain, certain nerve receptors, sensitive to changes in the osmotic pressure of the blood, are stimulated and thirst is induced by a nerve reflex. From the same area of the brain, and prompted by the same stimulus, the antidiuretic hormone vasopressin is released and is carried to the kidneys where it controls water loss. In addition to raised blood concentration, a drop in the actual volume of the blood, as occurs in severe haemorrhage, will also stimulate the hypothalamus to produce thirst.

When the sensation of thirst is abolished by damage to the hypothalamus, the affected person will make no attempt to drink adequate amounts of water and will soon become seriously dehydrated.

Although thirst normally causes dryness of the mouth, dryness will cause thirst, even in the absence of dehydration, and may be relieved merely by moistening the mouth.

thoracic outlet syndromes

A group of conditions in which nerves and arteries emerging from the upper outlet of the rib cage are compressed or angulated so that their function is impaired. Compression may be caused by an extra upper rib (cervical rib), an abnormal first rib, the borders of muscles in the region or by a band of tissue running from the side of the lowest neck vertebra to the first rib. The effects include pain, tingling and numbness in the arm and hand, on the little finger border and weakness or even atrophy of the small muscles of the hand. Surgical treatment may be needed to relieve the pressure.

thoracic surgeon

A surgeon who specializes in operations performed within the chest cavity, especially on the wind pipe, the lungs, the heart and the gullet.

thoracotomy

Surgical opening of the chest, usually for the purpose of performing an operation on one of the structures within. Most thoracotomies are made from the side, with access between spread ribs, after the muscles over and between them are cut. Sometimes it is necessary to cut through, and open, the covering membrane of a rib (periosteum) and remove a short length of bone. If access is required to the heart, thoracotomy is done from the front. This involves splitting the breastbone (sternum) from top to bottom and prising the halves apart. Afterwards the two halves of the sternum are wired together.

thorax

The part of the trunk between the neck and the top of the abdomen. The thorax contains a central compartment, the mediastinum, which houses the heart and separates the two lungs. It also contains the wind pipe (trachea), the gullet (oesophagus) and a number of large arteries and veins connected to the heart. Its walls consist of the dorsal vertebrae of the spine, the breastbone (sternum) and the rib cage.

thought disorders

These are characteristic of **schizophrenia** and various forms of **dementia**. Some kinds of thought disorder also occur in **mania**. They may be divided into disorders of content, form and process.

Disorders of content include false beliefs and ideas (**delusions**), and a loss of the sense of the limits of one's power and influence. Disorders of form are manifested by the use of meaningless or invented words (neologisms), incoherent language, abnormal verbal associations, word repetition, and by mutism. Disorders of process include loss of memory, poverty of thought content, thought blocking, sudden flight of ideas from one to another, loss of attention, loss of abstracting ability and the relating of words by their phonetic resemblance rather than by logical association (clang associations).

threadworm infestation

Threadworms, or pinworms, are intestinal parasites which commonly infest children in all parts of the world. The threadworm, *Enterobius vermicularis*, is the commonest worm parasite of children in temperate areas.

INCIDENCE
At least 20 per cent of all children are affected at any one time. The mature female worm is about a centimetre long, white, and with a blunt head and a fine, hair-like, pointed tail. The male is shorter and is rarely seen, as he remains in the intestine.

RECOGNITION
The pregnant female worms moving on the skin around the anus to deposit their eggs cause a strong tickling sensation. The child scratches and the eggs adhere to the fingers and nails. These are then transferred, either directly to the mouth to cause re-infestation, or, by way of toys, blankets, etc., to other children. The eggs can survive for three weeks and will sometimes hatch on the skin and re-enter the bowel. Swallowed eggs hatch in the intestine and the worms reach adult size, and begin to reproduce, after two to six weeks.

Diagnosis is easy, as the worms are readily seen and may appear on the faeces. In cases of doubt, sticky tape can be applied to the skin around the anus to pick up eggs, which can then be identified microscopically.

TREATMENT
It is unlikely that threadworms ever do any real harm except to disturb the sleep of children and the sensibilities of fastidious parents and, if re-infestation is avoided, the problem will disappear spontaneously within a month. Ointments may be used to allay the anal itching and there are various effective de-worming drugs, such as mebendazole, piperazine or pyrantel. Treatment of all the members of the family is, however, necessary.

throat

See **pharynx**, **pharyngitis**, **tonsillitis**.

throat inflammation, dangerous

See **diphtheria**, **epiglottitis**.

throat, lump in the

See **globus hystericus**.

thrombectomy

Surgical removal of a clot from an artery following **thrombosis**.

thromboangiitis obliterans

Sometimes called Buerger's disease, this uncommon condition, in which the arteries become progressively obstructed by blood clots, is almost entirely confined to men who are heavy cigarette smokers. The disease usually starts before the age of forty and causes a progressive reduction in the blood supply to the limbs, especially the legs, with pain, coldness and blueness of the skin. At first, the pain is on exercise only (claudication), but as the condition worsens, pain occurs on rest. Later, the diminution of the blood supply is often so great that **gangrene** develops and amputation may be necessary.

The exact nature of the disease process in thromboangiitis obliterans remains obscure, but the clotting in the arteries is preceded by a concentration of white blood cells of the polymorph variety in the wall of the vessel. The adjacent vein is also often involved in the inflammatory process. The role of cigarette smoking is unequivocal, but the mechanism is not understood.

Aggrieved victims of the disease, feeling that they have not been sufficiently warned of the dangers of smoking, have brought actions for damages against cigarette manufacturers.

thrombocytopenia

A diminution in the number of platelets in the blood. The blood platelets are tint cell fragments necessary for normal clotting of the blood. Thrombocytopenia, if sufficiently severe, leads to spontaneous bleeding from the smallest blood vessels (the capillaries).

See also **purpura**.

thrombolytic drugs

Drugs that dissolve blood clots and can be useful in the treatment of **thrombosis** or **embolism** affecting any part of the body. Also known as fibrinolytic drugs.

thrombophlebitis

Localized inflammation of a vein (phlebitis) with resulting clotting of the blood within the affected part (**thrombosis**). When this affects a vein near the surface (superficial vein), there is obvious redness and swelling and often acute tenderness to touch. There may be fever and general upset but serious complications are uncommon.

Thrombophlebitis of the deep veins – usually those of the lower limb – may affect sick people on prolonged bed rest, paralysed people, mothers after delivery, people with cancer, and those taking oestrogens, including oral contraceptives. Deep vein thrombophlebitis is more worrying because of the risk of formation of a long, eel-like blood clot which may separate and be carried to the heart, to be pumped to the lungs where it may block the arteries (pulmonary **embolism**). Anticoagulant treatment with heparin is important in the management of deep vein thrombosis, to minimize the risk of clot enlargement and separation.

thrombopoietin

A hormone responsible for the growth of colonies of the large cells, the megakaryocytes, which break down into fragments to form the blood platelets. The existence of thrombopoietin had been suspected for 30 years, but it was only discovered in 1994. In 1997 the results of a trial of genetically engineered (recombinant) thrombopoietin were published. It had been found to have a powerful stimulatory effect on platelet production.

thrombos

Greek root meaning 'clot' as in thrombosis (blood clot within a vessel).

thrombosis

Clotting of blood within an artery or vein. This is always abnormal and often very dangerous as it may restrict, or even totally cut off, the flow of blood. Thrombosis, when it affects vital arteries, such as the coronary arteries (coronary thrombosis – **heart attack**) or the arteries supplying the brain with blood (see **thrombosis, cerebral**), is a major cause of death and serious illness, such as **stroke**. Thrombosis of arteries supplying the limbs leads to pain, disability and, if severe, even loss of the limb by **gangrene**. The arteries to the intestines sometimes suffer thrombosis, leading to gangrene of a segment of bowel, calling for emergency surgical treatment.

POSSIBLE CAUSES

In general, thrombosis seldom occurs in a healthy artery, because the smooth inner lining prevents the sequence of events leading to blood coagulation from starting. Injury to a vessel, or any disease process affecting the smoothness of the inner lining, or allowing the local release of blood, may initiate thrombosis. By far the commonest cause of thrombosis is the common artery disease **atherosclerosis**. Even when arteries are normal, a clotting tendency may occur as a result of hormonal or biochemical changes in the blood. The tendency to thrombosis in arteries may be greater during pregnancy, in women using oral contraceptives, in people with cancer which has affected vessels, and in people whose blood is more viscous than normal (**polycythaemia**). Thrombosis in veins is encouraged by local pressure, inflammation (**thrombophlebitis**) and stagnation of blood flow, as occurs in **varicose veins**.

TREATMENT

The thrombus which forms in arteries is called a white thrombus. It is secure and tends to progress to occlude the artery. Thrombi in deep veins are red, soft, loose and easily detached, and may cause **embolism**. Thrombosis may be helped by the use of anticoagulant drugs, such as heparin and warfarin, and may, to some extent, be prevented by regular small doses of aspirin. The use of enzymes to break down the thrombus (fibrinolytic therapy), as soon as possible after its formation, is a growth zone in treatment. There is good evidence that the combination of fibrinolytic drugs, such as streptokinase, with aspirin can significantly reduce the death rate from coronary thrombosis.

thrombosis, cavernous sinus

The two cavernous sinuses lie within the cranial cavity, immediately behind each eye socket (orbit) and on either side of the pituitary gland. They are actually large veins and connect with the veins of the face and those of the brain. As well as containing blood, the cavernous sinuses contain the nerves running forward to control the eye-moving muscles and to provide sensation to part of the face and a major artery, the internal carotid.

RECOGNITION AND SYMPTOMS

The network of veins which runs back to join the cavernous sinuses drains mainly from a triangular area centred around the nose. Any infection in this area, as from a pimple or boil in the nostril or on the upper lip or nose, may cause a local tissue inflammation, known as cellulitis, from which infection may spread backwards by way of the veins to reach, and involve, one of the cavernous sinuses. If this happens, the blood in the sinus may turn to an infected clot, with grave consequences. There is high fever, severe pain behind and around the eye, paralysis of eye movement, forward protrusion of the eyeball (proptosis), severe blurring or loss of vision, and gross swelling of the lids and of the membrane covering the white of the eye (the conjunctiva).

RISKS

In the days before antibiotics, the development of cavernous sinus thrombosis was almost invariably a death warrant. The infection would soon spread to the other sinus and then into the brain veins, causing **meningitis** and extension into the brain substance itself. In those days, doctors used to speak of the central triangle of the face as the 'danger triangle' and would warn seriously of the dangers of interfering with infected spots in this area. These dangers remain, but happily, in the event of any backward spread it is almost always possible, by the use of antibiotics, to control the infection and restore normality.

See also **orbital cellulitis**.

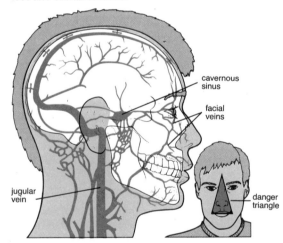

The cavernous sinus is an important part of the vein system of the head. It contains several nerves and part of the internal carotid artery. Thrombosis, as a result of the spread of infection from the central part of the face, is very serious.

thrombosis, cerebral

The brain is critically dependent on a good blood supply for normal function and is easily damaged by any diminution in that supply. Four arteries, running up the neck – the two carotids and the two vertebrals – provide that supply, and any obstruction, or even severe narrowing, of these arteries or of any of their many branches within the skull can be disastrous.

The most common cause of obstruction is the formation of a blood clot, or thrombosis, on top of a patch of **atheroma**, in an artery affected by **atherosclerosis**.

Since this disease, when present, affects all the arteries in the body in a patchy manner, it is a matter of chance whether it causes cerebral thrombosis, by blocking an artery supplying the brain, or whether it closes off one of the branches of the coronary blood supply to the heart muscle and causes a coronary thrombosis (**heart attack**). The coronary arteries are narrower than the carotids or vertebrals and coronary thrombosis is a commoner cause of death than cerebral thrombosis, even in people who have clear signs, in the form of **transient ischaemic attacks**, that they are in danger of the latter.

Blockage of the cerebral arteries by cerebral thrombosis, or by clots or other material carried in the blood from elsewhere (emboli), is the major cause of **stroke**. This is a commoner cause of stroke than cerebral haemorrhage (see **haemorrhage, cerebral**). When a brain artery is blocked, the area of brain supplied by it may or may not be able to be maintained by other nearby arteries. If these, too, are narrowed by disease, they are unlikely to be able to provide the necessary additional blood. The result is death of the nerve tissue and loss of its former function. This loss of function is worst at the beginning. If the affected person survives, there is usually slow, progressive improvement, at least up to a point.

thrombosis, coronary

See **heart attack**.

thrombosis, deep vein

See **thrombophlebitis**.

thrombus

See **thrombosis**.

thrush

See **candidiasis**.

thumbsucking

A harmless habit, common and normal in young children, which may safely be ignored unless persisted in after the age of six or seven, when it may lead to some displacement of the central teeth (incisors). In this case, the child may require orthodontic treatment and possibly the use of a dental appliance at night.

thunderclap headache

A very severe headache that occurs suddenly and without warning. Such headaches, especially if never previously experienced, may signal one of a number of dangerous possibilities including bleeding into the fluid space around the brain (subarachnoid haemorrhage), splitting of the wall of a vertebral or carotid artery (dissection) or clotting of the blood in one of the large veins around the brain (cerebral venous sinus thrombosis). Fortunately, in most cases the thunderclap headache implies nothing more grave than a severe migraine.

thunder, fear of

See **keraunophobia**.

thymoxamine

A drug that widens blood vessels (vasodilator) and may be useful in the management of **Raynaud's disease**. A brand name is Opilon.

thymus

A small flat organ of the lymphatic system situated immediately behind the breastbone. It is apparent in children but shrinks to inconspicuous dimensions after puberty. The thymus processes primitive **lymphocytes** so that they differentiate into the T cells of the immune system.

thyroid cancer gene mutation

See **RET oncogene**.

thyroidectomy

Surgical removal of a part, or of the whole of, the thyroid gland. Thyroidectomy is done to reduce the output of thyroid hormones in some cases of **thyrotoxicosis**, in the treatment of some cases of goitre, and in the treatment of thyroid cancer. If the whole gland is removed, replacement thyroid hormone (thyroxine) must be given, or hypothyroidism will result.

thyroid function tests

The function of the thyroid gland is to synthesize the thyroid hormones – the iodine-containing amino acid, thyroxine (T4), which has four iodine atoms in each molecule, and tri-iodothyronine (T3), with three iodines per molecule. The most direct way to test thyroid function is to measure the rate at which iodine is accumulated by the gland. This is conveniently done using a radioactive isotope of iodine which, although chemically identical to the normal element, can easily be assessed by measuring the level of radioactivity at the gland, with a radiation counter held in front of the neck. This is called thyroid scanning and the measurement is usually taken half an hour after administering a dose of the isotope by mouth. The amounts of the two hormones, T4 and T3, in the blood can be measured in the laboratory using samples of serum taken from the patient.

Because the thyroid gland has such a marked influence on the metabolic rate, its function may be assessed by taking measurements of the rate of oxygen consumption in the resting state. This is called the basal metabolic rate (BMR), and its estimation was once widely used as a test of thyroid function. Other tests have now replaced BMR measurements.

The pituitary gland not only controls thyroid gland activity, but is also influenced by the levels of thyroid hormones in the blood. Thus, a measurement of the amount of thyroid stimulating hormone (TSH) produced by the pituitary gland can be a valuable indirect test of thyroid function.

thyroid gland

This lies in the neck just under the 'Adam's apple' (larynx). The thyroid produces two iodine-containing hormones, thyroxine and tri-iodothyronine, which act directly on almost all the cells in the body to control the rate at which they break down and build up chemical substances (metabolism). Excess thyroid hormone causes an abnormal rate of breakdown (anabolism) and increased heat production. Fuel stores become depleted and muscles waste. There is a rapid pulse, hyperactivity, jumpiness, anxiety and loss of weight. This is called hyperthyroidism. Insufficient thyroid hormone in adults (hypothyroidism) causes both physical and mental slowing, sensitivity to cold, weight gain and puffiness of the tissues (myxoedema). In babies, lack of thyroid hormone causes cretinism and, in older children, failure of growth and development.

The production of thyroid gland hormone is controlled by thyroid-stimulating hormone (TSH) from the pituitary gland. There is a feedback mechanism by which the levels of thyroid hormone in the blood also control the pituitary, reducing its output of TSH.

A third hormone, calcitonin, is secreted by cells in the thyroid gland and is released into the blood, but has nothing to do with the thyroid hormones. Its action is on bone, where it interferes with the release of calcium. The specialized cells in the thyroid gland which produce calcitonin also monitor the blood calcium level continuously. If the level falls, less calcitonin is produced and there is less interference with calcium release by the bones. If the blood calcium rises, more calcitonin is secreted and calcium release inhibited. This kind of negative feedback control mechanism is very common in the body.

Calcitonin control of calcium blood level acts in opposition to the parathyroid hormone system. It is less important in calcium balance than the parathyroids.

thyroid gland, disorders of

IODINE DEFICIENCY
Iodine is an essential element in the thyroid hormone and a deficiency of this, although rare, can cause serious trouble. Iodine deficiency from birth causes *cretinism*, a condition of physical and mental retardation featuring poor feeding, constipation, a characteristic cry, a large tongue and eventual signs of brain damage. Cretinism also occurs as a result of a genetically induced failure of thyroid gland development.

Treatment with thyroid hormones, if begun early, can reverse many of the changes.

HYPOTHYROIDISM
Underaction of the thyroid gland, in the adult, usually the result of **auto-immune disease**, is known as hypothyroidism. This features an overall slowing of the physical and mental processes, sensitivity to cold, obesity, absence of sweating with scaly dry skin, loss of hair, puffiness of the face (**myxoedema**), premature ageing, coronary artery disease, and an eventual descent, unless treatment is given, into immobility and coma. Thyroid hormone, given early enough, will restore normality. Overproduction of thyroid hormones is called hyperthyroidism or **thyrotoxicosis**.

GOITRE
Enlargement of the thyroid gland, from any cause, is called **goitre**. Some small degree of goitre often occurs, as a normal event, around puberty or during pregnancy, but this usually settles without treatment. Relative deficiency of iodine, as may occur in areas remote from the sea, was once a common cause of goitre, but table salt is now iodized and goitres from this cause are now rare. Goitre is now more often caused by inflammation of the thyroid gland (thyroiditis) from virus infection or auto-immune disease. It may also be caused by a hereditary defect in an enzyme necessary for the synthesis of thyroid hormones (dyshormonogenesis). The commonest form of thyroiditis is **Hashimoto's thyroiditis**.

CANCER
Thyroid cancer is comparatively rare and presents as a single firm lump in the neck around the Adam's apple (larynx). If more than one lump is felt, the condition is unlikely to be cancer, but all lumps in this area must be properly investigated. Cancers grow gradually to form an increasing, irregular mass which is adherent to the adjacent structures and which spreads quickly to the lymph nodes in the neck. The nerves supplying the muscles of the vocal cords in the larynx may be involved, causing severe hoarseness or loss of the voice. Spread to the gullet (oesophagus) may cause difficulty in swallowing.

Thyroid cancer is treated by surgical removal, by giving thyroid hormone, which restricts tumour growth, and by the use of radioactive iodine, which concentrates in the thyroid gland and in any secondary deposits of thyroid cancer elsewhere in the body.

thyrotoxicosis

The thyroid hormones, thyroxine and tri-iodothyronine, act on all the cells in the body which are consuming energy, to speed up the processes of fuel consumption. Normally, the amount of thyroid hormone in the blood is carefully controlled so that these metabolic processes occur at a correct rate. Thyrotoxicosis, or hyperthyroidism, is a thyroid disorder in which there is excessive production of thyroid hormones, so that all these cellular processes are accelerated. In most cases the gland is either generally enlarged or contains many nodules of overactive thyroid tissue.

POSSIBLE CAUSES
The causes of thyrotoxicosis have not been fully explained, but it is believed that an **auto-immune disease** process is involved.

RECOGNITION AND SYMPTOMS
Thyrotoxicosis is very much commoner in women than in men. The symptom picture is typical and is usually easy to recognize as the affected person appears jumpy, anxious and overactive. Typically, there is constant body movement, as of severe anxiety, a fast and sometimes irregular pulse, sweating, shakiness, loss of weight in spite of good appetite and large intake and **palpitations**. There is great dislike of hot weather. A common feature is a staring appearance of the eyes, caused by retraction of the upper lids. Sometimes, the eyes may protrude markedly (**exophthalmos**) as a result of swelling of the tissues behind them, but this may occur long after the acute illness has subsided.

Thyroid function tests show abnormal levels of the thyroid hormones in the blood.

TREATMENT
Thyrotoxicosis is treated with drugs, such as carbimazole, methimazole and thiouracil, which cut down the activity of the gland, and sometimes by surgical removal of part of the gland (partial **thyroidectomy**). Gland activity can also be reduced by the use of a radioactive isotope of iodine. While treatment is having effect, many of the symptoms can be relieved by the use of beta-blocker drugs (beta-adrenergic blocking agents).

thyroxine

The principal thyroid hormone. Thyroxine has four iodine atoms in the molecule and is often known as T4. The sodium salt of thyroxide is sold as a drug used to treat thyroid deficiency disorders (hypothyroidism) under the brand name Eltroxin.

tiagabine

A drug that interferes with the uptake by nerves of the neurotransmitter GABA. The result is reduced excitability of nerves, which is helpful in the management of epilepsy. A brand name is Gabitril.

tiaprofenic acid

A non-steroidal anti-inflammatory drug (**NSAID**) of the propionic acid group, used to treat a wide range of arthritic and muscular inflammatory disorders. A brand name is Surgam.

tibia, fracture of

The tibia, the main bone of the lower leg, has a surface just under the skin, so it is common for fractures of the shaft of the tibia to be in communication with the outside world, and hence infected (compound fractures). This increases the probability of complications and of delayed healing.

POSSIBLE CAUSES
Fractures may be caused by direct violence or, commonly, by a twisting injury which causes an oblique or spiral break in the bone, often with dislocation of the ankle and a fracture at the lower end of the fibula – the slender bone on the outer side of the tibia. Crack fractures may occur during long periods of running or even walking.

TREATMENT
Fractures of the tibia are often unstable, mainly because the powerful calf muscles tend to pull the foot upwards so that the fragments over-ride. To get the fragments into alignment, it is necessary to exert a strong pull on the foot, under anaesthesia. If this fails it is necessary to exert a sustained pull (traction) by the application of a steel pin through the heel bone, using weights. This is usually successful, but sometimes open operation and the use of steel plates and screws may be necessary.

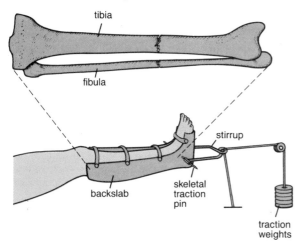

Fracture of the tibia is almost always accompanied by fracture of the delicate fibula. Skeletal traction to prevent over-riding of the broken ends is a common method of treatment.

tibolone

A synthetic sex hormone drug used to treat menopausal and postmenopausal symptoms and disorders and to reduce the tendency to osteoporosis. A brand name is Livial.

ticarcillin

A penicillin antibiotic useful for its action against the organism *Pseudomonas aeruginosa*. The drug is formulated with the clavulanic acid under the brand name Timentin.

tic douloureux

See **trigeminal neuralgia**.

tick bite ulcer

See **tularaemia**.

tics

Repetitive, twitching movements occurring at irregular intervals and always at the same site. Simple tics occur in about a quarter of all children and usually disappear within a year. They are three times as common in boys as in girls and are absent during sleep and when the child is deeply absorbed. They are worse during stress and when the child is aware of being observed. A small proportion persist into adult life and most of these are minor. Some, however, become so severe and widespread as to call for medical assistance. Such major tics occasionally affect the diaphragm causing a grunting sound.

RECOGNITION AND SYMPTOMS
Tics do not indicate any organic disorder, but reflect a psychological disturbance. They can be controlled by an effort of will, but since they appear to release emotional tension, such control is unpleasant. A tic commonly affecting adults is a spasmodic closure of one or both eyes, known as blepharospasm.

Neurotic blepharospasm can be very disabling, the affected person sometimes being unable to open the eyes at all, even in very dim conditions. Any attention given to the phenomenon makes it worse and the condition is a trial for the examining doctor trying to establish whether there is any ocular cause. It is not the result of fear of light (photophobia) and is not abolished by drops which anaesthetize the cornea. It is often associated with other tics such as hitching up a shoulder, jerking up the chin, or turning or tilting the head to one side. Frank psychiatric signs are absent and, although the cause seems to be buried deep in the unconscious, psychotherapy, hypnotism and even **aversion therapy** usually fail. In desperation, some victims have submitted to having the muscle concerned deliberately paralysed by injections of **botulinum toxin**.

The most severe form of tic is called the **Gilles de la Tourette's syndrome**. This usually starts in childhood and involves multiple twitchings, especially of the face, neck, and shoulders, with involuntary grunting, yelping or other utterances. An extraordinary feature is that, in most cases, these noises are eventually altered to brief, common swear-words, and sometimes the movements turn to obscene gestures.

Once fully established, the Gilles de la Tourette's syndrome is usually permanent and may cause extreme embarrassment to the sufferer. Treatment is difficult but some major tranquillizing drugs are helpful, although not without risk. Behaviour therapy is claimed to be effective in the management of severe tics.

Tiempe

A brand name for **trimethoprim**.

Tietze's syndrome

Persistent inflammation of rib cartilages causing pain and tenderness in the front of the chest wall, made worse by movement. The condition is treated with pain-killing drugs and non-steroidal anti-inflammatory drugs (**NSAIDs**) and passes off after a few months.

Tigason

A brand name for the retinol anti-**psoriasis** drug etretinate.

Tilade

A brand name for **nedocromil**.

Tildiem

A brand name for the calcium channel blocker anti-**angina** drug **diltiazem**.

Tiloryth

A brand name for **erythromycin**.

tiludronic acid

A bisphosphonate drug used to treat **Paget's disease** of bone. A brand name is Skelid.

time interval, infection to onset

See **incubation period**.

timolol

A beta-blocker drug used to treat high blood pressure, angina pectoris, migraine and, as eye drops, to treat **glaucoma**. Trade names are Timoptol, Betim, Blocadren and Glaucol.

Timopotol

A brand name for eye drops containing **timolol**, used to control **glaucoma**.

Tinacidin

A brand name for **tolnaftate**.

Tinaderm-M

A brand name for a mixture of the antifungal drugs **nystatin** and **tolnaftate**, used to treat skin fungus infections.

tincture

An alcoholic solution of a drug. Little used nowadays, tinctures were once popular. Laudanum was a tincture of opium.

tinea

This condition is often called 'ringworm', but is not a worm and does not necessarily form rings. It is an infection of the skin by fungi, especially *Microsporum*, *Trichophyton* and *Epidermophyton species*, collectively known as dermatophytes. These fungi attack the dead outer layer of the skin, or the skin appendages – the hair and the nails – causing persistent and often progressively extending areas of scaling and inflammation.

RECOGNITION AND SYMPTOMS

The common sites of infection are the feet ('**athlete's foot**' or *tinea pedis*), the groin (*tinea cruris*), the trunk (*tinea corporis*), the scalp (*tinea capitis*) and the nails (*tinea unguium*). Kerion of the scalp is an inflamed circular area caused by a immunological reaction to the fungus, which soon brings about healing.

Tinea pedis affects the areas between the toes, usually starting between the third and fourth toe and spreading to the other spaces. Tinea cruris is a dermatophyte or yeast infection, encouraged by tight clothing, obesity and insufficient washing. The edge of the area of inflammation often extends gradually outwards from the groin, but the scrotum is not usually involved. It is intensely itchy. Tinea of the nails is usually a *Trichophyton* infection and causes loss of lustre, thickening and an accumulation of debris under the free edge. The nail often becomes separated from its bed and may be cast off. The condition is very persistent and identification of the fungus type is essential if treatment is to be effective. Fungus infections of the trunk tend to form rings because affected areas heal centrally leaving normal skin relatively resistant to the infection, which must thus spread outwards.

TREATMENT

Tinea is usually treated with the drug griseofulvin, which is taken by mouth. Some infections, especially those of the nails, may require more than a year of treatment for eradication. As this drug is of no value in the treatment of **candidiasis** of the nails, a correct species diagnosis is essential. Tinea corporis may respond to imidazole cream or other local applications.

Tineaderm

A brand name for **tolnaftate**.

Tineafax

A brand name for **tolnaftate**.

tinea versicolor

An infection with the yeast fungus *Pityrosporon orbiculare* which causes multiple, slightly scaly skin patches, varying in colour from white to brown, on the trunk, neck and sometimes the face. The infection is commonest in young adults and often becomes apparent only when it is noted that the affected areas do not tan in summer time. The areas fluoresce in ultraviolet light and skin scrapings show yeast fungus.

The condition is treated with selenium, most conveniently in the form of a selenium shampoo applied directly to the skin at bedtime and washed off in the morning. Three or four days' treatment will usually suffice. This remedy may prove too irritating and milder measures are available.

tinidazole

An antibacterial and antiprotozoal drug similar to **metronidazole** but with a longer duration of action. It is used to treat **amoebiasis**, **trichomoniasis** and **gingivitis**. A brand name is Fastigyn.

tinnitus

A hissing, whistling or ringing sound heard in one or both ears, or in the centre of the head. In most cases, the sound is continuous, but awareness of it is usually intermittent and the degree of distress caused is largely determined by the personality. Tinnitus is almost always associated with some degree of deafness and is related to damage to the hair cells of the cochlea of the inner ear. Often it starts spontaneously, but it may be caused by any of the factors known to cause deafness, such as nearby explosions, prolonged loud noise, aminoglycoside antibiotics and various ear disorders, such as **Meniere's syndrome**, **otosclerosis** and **presbyacusis**.

Tests have shown that the impression of the loudness of tinnitus, as experienced by sufferers, is misleading, and that the actual levels, as judged by comparison with external sounds, are, in fact, very low. Nevertheless, tinnitus can be very trying, especially in quiet conditions, and sufferers often resort to external sounds to cover it. Personal headphones may be useful and *white noise* generators, known as tinnitus maskers, have been found useful by some.

Certain drugs, such as local anaesthetics and others which interfere with nerve conduction, have been found to have an effect on tinnitus and some patients have been greatly relieved by the use of the drug carbamazepine (Tegretol). Such measures do not, however, have a major part to play in the management of the disorder. The great majority of tinnitus sufferers learn to live with it without distress.

Tinset

A brand name for the antihistamine drug oxatomide.

tinzaparin

A **low molecular weight heparin** drug that interferes with the action of Factor X in the blood coagulation cascade and can be used to prevent blood clotting within the blood vessels in people undergoing surgery. A brand name is Innohep.

tioconazole

An **imidazole** antifungal drug used externally to treat nail infections with **tinea** and *Candida albicans* fungi. A brand name is Trosyl.

tirofiban

An experimental anticoagulant drug with the brand name Aggrastat. See **saw-scaled viper venom**.

tissue culture

The artificial growth of sheets of human tissue in the laboratory. This is done on the surface of a carefully formulated bacteriologically sterile growth medium that contains all necessary ingredients in solution. Living cells are seeded on to the surface and the whole is kept at normal internal body temperature in an incubator.

Tumour cells are readily cultured; some appear to be immortal and can be grown indefinitely. These are widely used for laboratory purposes. For surgical purposes, normal skin cells (keratinocytes) can be cultured and used for grafting. Three-layered arteries have been grown, as have sheets of urethral endothelium for purposes of urethral reconstitution in **hypospadias**. It has even been possible to grow a new ear around a mould of polymer mesh.

Cultured tissue retains the immunological typing of the person from whom the seeding sample was taken. This means that if the cultured tissue is used to treat the same person there will be no rejection problems.

tissue damage by free radicals

See **oxidative stress**.

tissue death in intestine

See **necrotizing enterocolitis**.

tissue plasminogen activator

A naturally occurring chemical activator (enzyme) that can dissolve blood clots. Since so many serious conditions are caused by clotting (thrombosis) within arteries, or the breaking free of clots in veins (see **anticoagulant drugs**), obviously a substance that can break down clots and restore the blood flow is of major medical importance. Other clot-dissolving enzymes, such as streptokinase and urokinase, have been in use for many years. These have achieved some success if given within an hour or two of the thrombosis. TPA appears to have several major advantages over these earlier drugs. It is believed to be responsible for opening up (recanalizing) blood vessels blocked by thrombosis, and it is much more effective in dealing with mature blood clot – a mass of the protein fibrin – than either streptokinase or urokinase. TPA can be produced by genetic engineering methods and is marketed under the name alteplase (Actilyse).

Many important studies have now been done on patients with recent coronary thromboses, people with unstable angina and people in whom blood clots have travelled to the lungs causing the dangerous condition of pulmonary embolism. TPA can open up blocked coronary arteries within 19–50 minutes of being injected, restoring the blood supply to the heart muscle. If the affected area of muscle has not been killed, function is restored. TPA can dissolve large clots carried to the lungs from the veins, and it can stop these clots from forming (deep vein thrombosis). The drug does not produce antibodies. The results are uniformly excellent and there is no doubt that TPA is an important advance in treatment.

All this sounds wonderful, but nothing is ever perfect in this world. TPA has one major side-effect – a tendency to cause bleeding. Because of this the drug is dangerous in people who have recently had a stroke, in those with any bleeding tendency and in people with a history of stomach or duodenal ulcer. TPA drugs do not, of course, distinguish between an unwanted thrombosis and a naturally occurring sealing plug of clot. So bleeding readily occurs at any point of blood vessel injury such as a recent injection site or at the points of insertion of blood vessel catheters.

tissue type

See **major histocompatibility complex (MHC)**.

tissue typing

The first known example of the existence of tissue types was the A, B, AB and O blood groups, discovered in 1901 by the Austrian-born American pathologist Karl Landsteiner (1868–1943). It was not until much later in the century that it was realized that every cell in the body carries on its surface chemical markers called antigens which are specific to the individual. The human leukocyte antigens (HLAs) are the antigens, first found on white blood cells, such as the lymphocytes, but now known to occur on virtually all nucleated cells of the body. These antigens fall into one of a number of distinct categories, similar to the blood groups.

Just as blood groups are of critical importance when blood from one person is donated and introduced into another, so the HLA group is important if tissue, or whole organs, are donated. The immunological response to these antigens is the cause of most graft rejection. Tissue typing is a test for tissue groups and is used to check a person's suitability to receive an organ transplant from a particular donor, if the tissue type of the donor is known. The HLA is also of value in cases of disputed parentage and can be helpful to doctors who are aware that certain diseases are much commoner in some HLA groups than in others. For instance, the diseases ankylosing spondylitis and Reiter's syndrome hardly ever occur except in people who are HLA-B27. People with the arthritis that occurs in psoriasis are often HLA-B13 or HLA-B17 and there is an association between systemic lupus erythematosus and dermatitis herpetiformis and HLA-B8.

The HLA test merely involves the collection of a small sample of blood, either from a vein, by needle and syringe, or by pricking a finger or ear-lobe and drawing a drop or two into a fine tube. A range of antibodies, each of which attaches itself only to an antigen of its own type, is held in the laboratory. If lymphocytes from the blood to be tested are added to a solution containing the right antibody, they will react by clumping together or by taking up a protein substance called complement. Both the clumping and the absence of complement can easily be detected and thus the tissue type discovered.

tizanidine

A muscle relaxant drug used to treat muscle spasm in multiple sclerosis or spinal injury. This drug is said to reduce spasm without reducing strength. A brand name is Zanaflex.

tobacco

See **health maintenance**.

tobacco advertising

The medical profession, aware that cigarette smoking is the cause of about one-sixth of all deaths from all causes, is rightly incensed that there should legally exist a sustained campaign to persuade people, especially young people, to smoke. The attitude of the Government is anomalous. Revenues from tobacco are so large (£4000 million a year in Britain) that to take the only respectable step – making smoking illegal – would have major economic consequences. On the other hand, the Government accepts the medical advice and pays a kind of token respect to it by legislation requiring public warnings of the danger. As a result we have the ludicrous spectacle of advertising which explicitly implores people to kill themselves.

The tobacco and advertising industries appear to have succeeded in rationalizing and concealing the truth from themselves, so that they are able to claim that the medical evidence is wrong. Many maintain, disingenuously, that the only purpose, and effect, of advertising is to encourage loyalty to a particular brand of cigarette, or to persuade existing smokers to change to the brand advertised. This view cynically disregards the whole ethos and obvious effectiveness of advertising in persuading impressionable people. The plain truth is that the industry must recruit several hundred new smokers every day to make up for those it kills. There can be no doubt that cigarette advertising recruits new smokers, provides stimuli for increased consumption, makes it more difficult for smokers to give up and encourages former smokers to resume the habit.

Cigarette sponsorship of sport on television is popular with the manufacturers because it neatly circumvents the ban on TV advertising and allows the names of brands to be shown. There is clear evidence that this form of covert advertising is about as effective as any other and conveys, especially to the young, a spurious kind of respectability for the products.

The tobacco lobby is rich and proportionately powerful in its effect on governmental decisions. Some members of parliament have links with advertising or have constituency interests in tobacco, and some have used their influence to block positive legislation against smoking, brushing aside as irrelevant the unequivocal recommendations of the medical Royal Colleges, the British Medical Association and the World Health Organization that cigarette advertising should be banned.

tobacco-free social norm

A concept, gaining ever-wider general acceptance, that the avoidance of smoking should be generally regarded as natural and normal, and smoking as harmful and undesirable. The establishment of such a norm is especially important as a means of discouraging young people from smoking.

Tobralex

A brand name for eye drops containing **tobramycin**.

tobramycin

An antibiotic drug similar in use to Gentamicin, but useful in the treatment of gentamicin-resistant infections. A brand name is Nebcin.

tocainide

An antiarrhythmic drug used to treat or prevent heart beat irregularities. A brand name is Tonocard.

toe, disorders of

See **bunion**, **hallux valgus**, **hammer toe**, **ingrown toenail**.

toenail, ingrowing

See **ingrown toenail**.

Tofranil

A brand name for **imipramine**.

Tolanase

A brand name for **tolazamide**.

tolazamide

A sulphonylurea drug used to treat maturity-onset, non-insulin-dependent **diabetes**. A brand name is Tolanase.

tolfenamic acid

A non-steroidal anti-inflammatory drug (**NSAID**) used to treat migraine. A brand name is Clotam.

tolnaftate

An antifungal drug used to treat **tinea**. A brand name is Tinaderm-M.

Tomudex

A brand name for **raltitrexed**.

tongue, disorders of

Inflammation of the tongue is called **glossitis**. Soreness, redness and smoothness of the tongue is a feature of various anaemias. Enlargement occurs in cretinism and **Down's syndrome**. 'Black hairy tongue' is caused by enlargement and discoloration of the papillae on the surface. The condition, although unsightly, is harmless and can be improved by regular brushing with a toothbrush.

Mouth ulcers may sometimes affect the tongue and are usually harmless, but any persistent ulcer or hardness or any persistent white patch (**leukoplakia**) lasting for more than a month, should be reported for full investigation as there is always the possibility that these may be an early sign of cancer. Tongue cancer is always serious because of its tendency to spread rapidly. It most commonly occurs in people over forty who smoke heavily, neglect their teeth and who have a long history of soreness of the tongue. The cancer may present as a small ulcer with raised edges, as leukoplakia, or as a thickened, raised mass. The cancer itself is rarely painful. Spread is rapid and the tumour quickly extends to adjacent structures in the mouth, including the lower jaw, and to the lymph nodes in the floor of the mouth and in the neck. By the time this has happened, only radical and mutilating surgery is likely to save life.

Tongue-tie is a rare defect in which the soft partition under the tongue (the frenulum) extends too far forward and is too tight, thereby limiting tongue movement. This may affect speech, but is easily corrected by snipping the frenulum.

tonic

There is a widespread belief that there exists a class of medicines, called tonics, which, in some unspecified way, can improve the general state of the health or safely and permanently increase the feeling of well-being.

Tonocard

A brand name for the antiarrhythmic heart drug **tocainide**.

tonsillectomy

The surgical operation for the removal of the tonsils.

WHY IT'S DONE

In childhood, the tonsils serve a useful purpose in defending a common portal of entry to the body against infection. In so doing, they become inflamed and enlarged, but this is not now considered justification for removing them unless the attacks are frequent and severe or prolonged or are causing complications such as obstruction to breathing or swallowing. The condition of **quinsy** is also a reason for removing the tonsils.

HOW IT'S DONE

Tonsillectomy is done under general anaesthesia. The mouth is held open by a ratchet *gag* and each tonsil is grasped, in turn, by forceps and separated from its bed by blunt dissection and minimal cutting.

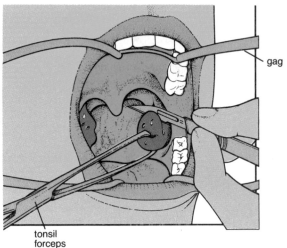
gag

tonsil forceps

Tonsillectomy can be done using a tightening wire loop (snare) or, as shown here, by dissection with a scalpel.

RISKS

Bleeding from the raw areas left is sometimes a problem, and it is occasionally necessary to tie off a small bleeding artery. Rarely, severe bleeding occurs some hours after the operation. Tonsillectomy is followed by a period of severe discomfort, especially on swallowing, but this settles in two or three weeks.

tonsillitis

Inflammation of the tonsils. Acute tonsillitis is often caused by streptococcal bacteria but may be caused by other organisms.

RECOGNITION AND SYMPTOMS

The tonsil become swollen and red and the surfaces may show spots of pus exuding from the clefts (tonsillar crypts). Sometimes material from the crypts forms a whitish membrane over the surface. The lymph nodes in the neck, just behind or under the angle of the jaw, are swollen and tender to the touch.

There is sore throat, pain on swallowing, headache, fever, which may be very high in young children, and a feeling of unwellness (**malaise**). Constipation and earache are common. The tongue is often furred and the breath unpleasant. There may be slight difficulty in opening the mouth and thickened speech.

COMPLICATIONS

Complications of tonsillitis are uncommon, but may include abscess behind the tonsil (**quinsy**), abscess in the back of the throat, **otitis media**, **rheumatic fever**, **glomerulonephritis** and **septicaemia**.

TREATMENT

Tonsillitis responds well to antibiotic treatment and this should always be given if the infection is streptococcal. Recurrent, severe or complicated tonsillitis may justify **tonsillectomy**.

tonsil removal

See **tonsillectomy**.

tooth abscess

A late complication of neglected **tooth decay** (dental caries). Infection, which has gained access to the root canal of the tooth, causes an inflammation in the tissues surrounding the tip of the root (periapical periodontitis) leading to local tissue destruction and a collection of pus. The abscess may involve the bone of the socket. There is pain, especially on biting and chewing, and the surrounding gum is usually inflamed, tender and swollen. There may be swelling of the face and fever.

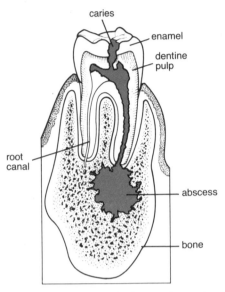

Tooth abscess. This is a late stage of infection of the pulp of the tooth which communicates with the tooth socket, by way of the canal for the blood vessels and nerves, causing a pus-filled sac around the root.

Often a tooth abscess will spread sideways under the gum to cause a 'gumboil' and if this opens and discharges into the mouth there will be much relief of the pain. Sometimes treatment of the abscess requires removal of the tooth so that the abscess can drain, but it is often possible to save a tooth by drilling down through it into the abscess to release the pus and then to treat with antibiotics and root filling. Antibiotics alone are of no value in the treatment of established abscesses.

toothache

Pain in a tooth usually from **tooth decay** (caries) in which the hard enamel or the underlying dentine has been breached so that infecting organisms have reached the central pulp and caused inflammation. The pulp contains sensory nerves and it is the stimulation of these that causes the pain.

Caries reduces the thickness of the hard material between the exterior and the tooth nerve and leads to undue sensitivity to cold, heat, acid materials or even to sweet substances. In the presence of caries, all of these can cause toothache. Toothache can also be caused by a broken tooth or by inflammation of the supporting tissue around a tooth (periodontitis). The roots

> Toothache is a symptom indicating that something is wrong, probably with one or more teeth. Neglect will usually lead to a worsening of the situation and possibly to the loss of an otherwise reclaimable tooth. Toothache is an indication for an immediate visit to a dentist.

of the upper teeth project into the sinuses (maxillary antrums) in the cheeks and inflammation in these sinuses can cause toothache.

tooth decay

Dental caries. Damage to the enamel and underlying dentine of teeth so that cavities form. If neglected, these will allow infection to reach the pulp of the teeth and destroy the internal blood vessels and nerves on which the survival of the teeth depend. Dental caries is always avoidable.

A small proportion of people who do not regularly brush their teeth appear, nevertheless, to be immune to dental caries. But the majority who, by neglecting brushing and flossing, allow **plaque** to develop, will eventually lose all or most of their teeth. Plaque is a mixture of dried saliva, food debris and bacteria which forms around the necks of teeth at the gum margins. The bacteria produce **enzymes** which act on sugary (carbohydrate) food residues to produce acid, and it is this which causes the caries, by eating into enamel and dentine. At this stage, bacteria infect the pulp, causing damage to the fine blood vessels and nerves within, and sometimes leading to abscesses in the bone socket at the tips of the roots. Destruction of the pulp leads to death of the tooth.

Proper brushing after meals and the use of dental floss will prevent the accumulation of plaque and the further stage of **calculus** formation. Regular dental inspection will ensure that plaque is revealed, calculus removed by scaling and early cavities cleaned and filled. Fluoride is protective.

tooth extraction

Modern dentists try to be as conservative as possible and remove teeth only as a last resource, or for purposes of correcting overcrowding, improving appearance or allowing another tooth to erupt. Teeth may be extracted under general or local anaesthesia, the latter being preferred if many teeth have to be removed.
HOW IT'S DONE
Teeth may be removed by means of dental forceps or sometimes using a rotating instrument with a small metal protrusion at one end, called an elevator. Dental forceps are provided in a range to be used on specific teeth. They are designed so that, on being tightened, the blades divide the membrane securing the tooth to the bone (periodontal membrane) and expand the socket. Sometimes a slight twist is given to assist in breaking the membrane. Elevators apply considerable leverage, as the transverse handle is many times longer than the short elevating end which engages the tooth. It is sometimes necessary to cut a flap in the gum and remove a small piece of bone from the edge of the tooth socket, so as to allow access to broken off roots or a very tight tooth.

toothpaste

Sometimes called dentifrice, this material contains a fine abrasive powder, such as chalk, and a little soap or detergent. Together, these assist in the removal of plaque. It also contains some flavouring, often peppermint, and some sweetening agent and, ideally, a fluoride salt. Many toothpastes also contain a chemical to coagulate protein in the dentine tubules and desensitize them to acids and temperature changes.

tooth plaque demonstration

See **disclosing agents**.

tooth replacement

See **reimplantation**, **dental**.

Topal

A brand name for a mixture of **aluminium hydroxide**, **alginic acid** and **magnesium carbonate**, used to treat **dyspepsia**.

Topamax

A brand name for **topiramate**.

tophi

Chalky excrescences that appear on the skin of the ear and elsewhere in **gout**. Tophi are collections of uric acid crystals.

topical

Relating to something, usually some form of medication, applied to the surface of the body rather than taken internally or injected. Skin ointments or creams, eye and ear drops or ointments and vaginal pessaries are topical applications.

Topicycline

A brand name for **tetracycline** for external use.

Topilar

A brand name for the corticosteroid drug fluclorolone, used for local (topical) applications.

topiramate

A drug that reduced the sensitivity to firing of nerve cells and is used to prevent epileptic seizures. A brand name is Topamax.

topoisomerase

A term, pronounced 'topo-isomerase', for the range of enzymes that assist in changing the shape of the double helix **DNA** molecule, necessary during replication. This is called topological manipulation. Before DNA can replicate it must be unwound. This occurs in short segments and is achieved by a Type I topoisomerase that cuts one strand so that the free end can unwind around the unbroken strand. The broken strand then rejoins. Type II topoisomerases cut both strands.

Topoisomerase inhibitor drugs interfere with DNA replication by inhibiting the action of the topoisomerase enzymes. They thus prevent cells from reproducing and are used as anticancer drugs and, by local application, to treat warts.

topotecan

A **topoisomerase** inhibitor drug used to treat cancer (see **cytotoxic drugs**). A brand name is Hycamtin.

toracemide

A **loop diuretic** drug used to treat high blood pressure or oedema from any cause. A brand name is Torem.

Toradol

A brand name for **ketorolac**.

TORCH

An acronym for 'Toxoplasmosis, Rubella, Cytomegalovirus and Herpes simplex' virus infections. This group of infections is often routinely looked for in investigating ill infants, especially if there is a possibility of congenital or neonatal infection. The practice has, however, been criticized as being wasteful and inefficient.

Torecan

A brand name for the **anti-emetic** drug thiethylperazine.

Torem

A brand name for **toracemide**.

toremifene

An anti-oestrogen drug used to treat oestrogen-dependent breast cancers that have spread. Most breast cancers are oestrogen-dependent. A brand name is Fareston.

torsion

Twisting. Parts of the body which hang loosely on a narrow support are liable to suffer torsion. Torsion of a testicle or of a loop of bowel are the commonest examples. The danger in torsion is that the blood vessels supplying the suspended part may become obstructed. Veins are softer and more easily compressed than arteries, but if veins become obstructed in this way, the continuing arterial inflow under pressure leads to great swelling and a rapidly worsening situation.

> Torsion often presents an acute surgical emergency calling for quick action before gangrene supervenes.

torsion of testis

Twisting of the **spermatic cord** within, or just above, the scrotum. This causes occlusion of the veins so that return of blood pumped in by the artery is obstructed and there is great swelling, pain, tenderness and bruising. Early surgical correction is necessary if the affected testicle is not to become permanently sterile.

torticollis

Sometimes called 'wry neck', this condition features a sustained abnormality in the position of the head caused by a persistent or permanent twisting of the neck. Common causes of torticollis include damage, at birth, to one of the main longitudinal muscles of the neck (the sternomastoid muscle) so that it is shortened and the head tilted to one side; whiplash injury to the neck with painful muscle spasm; a vertical imbalance in the eye muscles so that a tilt is needed to avoid double vision; or severe scarring and shortening of the skin of the neck.

The treatment of torticollis depends on the cause. Congenital muscle shortening from injury should be corrected by early stretching and perhaps surgery, otherwise permanent asymmetry of the skull and face may result. Skin contractures call for plastic procedures and eye imbalance requires squint surgery. Traumatic muscle spasm will generally settle with rest and time.

Totamol

A brand name for **atenolol**.

Tourette's syndrome

See **Gilles de la Tourette's syndrome**.

tourniquet

Any encircling band which can be tightened enough to compress blood vessels and control blood flow. A tourniquet can be used in an emergency to control severe bleeding from an artery or a large vein or it may be used to impede flow in veins only, so as to cause them to become engorged and thus make injections, or blood removal, easier.

> Tourniquets are dangerous and if applied tightly enough to impede flow in the arteries and left in place for more than an hour or so, will always cause gangrene and loss of the part of the limb beyond the point of application. If severe bleeding cannot be stopped in any other way, a tourniquet may be applied, but the fact must be known to all concerned. In most cases bleeding can be controlled by direct pressure, and tourniquets are not now recommended in first aid.

toxaemia

The presence of bacterial poisons (**toxins**) in the blood, which can lead to the dangerous condition **toxic shock syndrome**.
See also **septicaemia**.

toxic epidermal necrolysis

A severe skin disorder featuring inflammation, peeling, blistering, loosening and shedding of large sheets of the outer layer (the epidermis). In children it was believed to be due to a circulating staphylococcal toxin and is often called staphylococcal scalded skin syndrome (SSSS). It is now thought that the condition is usually a severe adverse reaction to a drug.

toxicity

The property or degree of poisonousness. Toxicity refers to any poisonous substance whether it be a **toxin** of bacterial origin, a plant poison, or any other poisonous chemical substance. The unit of toxicity is the LD50 (50 per cent lethal dose) – the dose of the poison which kills half of a group of animals exposed to it.

Toxicity is almost always a matter of the dosage. A very large range of substances not normally considered toxic are poisonous if taken in sufficient amount. Highly toxic substances are those which are dangerous if taken in very tiny amounts. The 'pleasure poisons' such as nicotine, alcohol, cocaine, heroin and so on, are taken in doses sufficient to produce their desired effect (intoxication) but not usually in sufficient doses to kill immediately.

toxic megacolon

A dangerous ballooning or dilatation of the large intestine (colon) with gas that may occur as a complication of inflammatory bowel disease such as **ulcerative colitis** or **Crohn's disease**. The danger is of perforation of the intestine, which carries a high mortality. The condition can often be relieved by turning the patient into the prone position.

toxicology

The study of the nature, properties and biological effects of poisons.

toxic psychosis

An organically induced psychotic breakdown caused by the effect on the brain of any poison or drug. Possible causes include alcohol, lead, mercury, cocaine, amphetamine, cannabis and hallucinogenic drugs.

toxic shock syndrome

Bacterial **toxins** are among the most dangerous poisons known and when they enter the bloodstream in more than the most minute quantities the effects are always serious. The toxic shock syndrome is an acute and dangerous condition caused by the absorption into the bloodstream of toxins from bacteria of the *Staphylococcus aureus species*. Fortunately, the condition is very rare.

An epidemic of the toxic shock syndrome occurred among young menstruating women in the early 1980s and investigation showed that it was associated with high-absorbency vaginal tampons and a considerable increase in the number of staphylococcal organisms in the vagina.

RECOGNITION AND SYMPTOMS

S. aureus produces three different kinds of toxins, producing three different syndromes – food poisoning, the *scalded skin syndrome* in newborn babies and small children, and the toxic shock syndrome. Ninety per cent of cases of the toxic shock syndrome occur in menstruating women. Others occur in people with severe staphylococcal infections of the bone or the heart valves, or following operations. Staphylococcal toxin produces widespread damage throughout the body. Among other effects, it causes the involuntary muscles in the walls of arteries to relax so that the vessels widen, and the small blood vessels to become more leaky so that fluid passes out. The net effect of the increase in the capacity of the circulatory system and the reduction in blood volume may be insufficient filling of the vessels, and the heart may be unable to keep the blood circulating. This is what is meant by surgical **shock** and the condition may be rapidly fatal unless the volume of the circulation is maintained by transfusion of fluid such as saline or by a blood transfusion.

There is a fever of 40°C or above, an acute drop in the blood pressure, a rapid but very weak pulse, a blotchy red rash which becomes scaly (desquamated), dizziness, vomiting and diarrhoea, muscle pain, inflammation of the vagina, liver damage and sometimes disorientation and confusion.

PREVENTION AND TREATMENT

Since the cause and nature of the condition, and the appropriate treatment have been understood, the mortality has been greatly reduced and is now no more than about 2 to 3 per cent. But because the trouble is caused by the toxins which have already been released from the organisms, killing the staphylococci with antibiotics has little effect on the course of the illness. It does, however, reduce the likelihood of recurrence and such treatment is always given. The most urgent requirement, however, is the restoration of the full blood volume by transfusion. This is life-saving.

The history of the toxic shock syndrome has taught that high-absorbency tampons should be avoided and that all tampons should be changed frequently. This lesson appears to have been learned. Other cases arose from burns, wounds, abscesses and **bronchopneumonia**.

toxin

Any substance produced by a living organism that is poisonous to other organisms. Bacterial disease is largely the result of poisoning by the toxins they produce. Some bacteria release soluble exotoxins that act remotely. Others produce only endotoxins which solely operate locally. Some bacterial toxins are among the most poisonous substances known.

toxocariasis

Infestation with the juvenile forms of the common puppy worm *Toxocara canis*. The condition is largely confined to children who come into contact with puppy fur and contaminated soil. London parkland has been shown to be extensively and uniformly contaminated with toxocara worm eggs deposited by dogs. Soil samples taken from almost anywhere within the parks are found to contain ova.

When the eggs are ingested they hatch in the intestine and the juveniles penetrate the wall of the bowel to gain access to the bloodstream. They are carried to every part of the body and can remain alive in the tissues for many weeks, where their movement produces tracks of haemorrhage, inflammation and dead cells. Eventually they die, and at the sites of death, small abscesses and collections of fibrous tissue and new blood vessels (granulomas) occur. In some cases, live juveniles may remain walled up for years only to resume their migration at a later date.

INCIDENCE

Human infestation is commoner than has been supposed for many cases are free of symptoms. Surveys have shown that in some groups of children (black youngsters in the southern states of the USA) up to 25 per cent have antibodies to toxocara (white children in the same areas show a prevalence of about 5 per cent). Whether or not symptoms occur is determined by the number of live eggs swallowed and by the resistance of the child.

RECOGNITION AND SYMPTOMS

The migration of the juvenile worms causes a transient illness known as visceral larva migrans. There is fever, pallor, lassitude, loss of appetite and weight and often cough and wheezing. Rarely, epileptic seizures – usually of the **petit mal** type – may occur. *Poliomyelitis* and heart muscle inflammation (myocarditis) have been described.

EYE INVOLVEMENT

The chief interest has been in those comparatively few cases in which the eye has been involved. If a juvenile worm happens to lodge in the layer of blood vessels behind the retina, and dies, the result is a tumour-like mass at the back of the eye which may cause great damage to vision. In addition, the mass may be mistaken for the highly malignant **retinoblastoma**. In the past, many children's eyes were removed because toxocariasis was not recognized for what it was and the clinical appearances could not be distinguished from this form of cancer. This tragedy is now rare, as toxocariasis is now well understood and tests, such as the **ELISA test**, can point to the correct diagnosis. Taken in combination with other clinical and laboratory findings, this test now enables doctors to make the diagnosis with considerably more confidence.

Treatment of eye involvement is a difficult problem, and if severe damage has been done to the eye, little of benefit can be done. Steroids may be used to attempt to minimize the inflammatory damage. Laser treatment or photocoagulation have been used to destroy the juvenile worm and to prevent its migration to the more important central area of the retina.

PREVENTION

Prevention is, of course, better than cure. Many puppies are infested *in utero* and require de-worming, with the anti-worm (anthelmintic) drug piperazine adipate, at two, three, four and eight weeks after birth and then twice more between three and six months. Thereafter, one further dose is desirable. Pregnant bitches should also be repeatedly treated with the same drug. As the eggs can survive for years in soil, all dog faeces should be collected and destroyed.

It has been proposed that special dog exercise areas should be set aside in parks, from which children would be excluded, and both parents and children should be aware of the dangers associated with puppies. Eating earth (**pica**) should be discouraged.

Toxoplasma gondii infection in AIDS

Human infection with this single-celled protozoon parasite is widespread. Most people are probably harbouring some of the organisms, harmlessly. Many, however, have small foci of the infection in the eyes and these occasionally flare up and sometimes cause damage to vision. The case is much more serious in the immunocompromised and, in **AIDS**, the chief danger is to the brain. About 10 per cent of AIDS victims are affected in this way. The lesions may be small and widespread or there may be a large abscess-like mass. If the patient survives, there is usually a slowly progressive dementia that often becomes seriously disabling. *T. gondii* also produces a pneumonia and, like cytomegalovirus, commonly leads to variable degrees of visual loss.

Treatment is difficult, for the organism is very resistant and the best currently available drugs are neither very effective nor very safe. Daraprim (pyrimethamine) is a drug normally used to treat malaria, which is caused by a similar protozoon, but both this and the sulphonamide Sulphadiazine, used along with it, are liable to interfere with bone marrow blood cell production. Daraprim can also cause fetal abnormalities and should not be used in pregnant women. So, although these drugs do have some action against the toxoplasma organism, they can hardly be said to be highly effective.

Prevention of new infection is very important in immunocompromised people. Toxoplasmosis is commonly acquired from undercooked meat – practically every known mammal, bird and fish has been shown to be prone to infection – so all sorts of meat, game and fish should be thoroughly cooked. Another important source of infection is domestic cats, who can be relied upon to consume any wild rodents or birds they can catch and thus acquire the toxoplasma. Infected cats excrete the cystic collections of *T. gondii* in their droppings and these are highly infectious. So immunocompromised people should not keep cats and should keep away from cat boxes or soil used by cats. Although the general danger is minimal, to those with less than the normal degree of immunity, the poor results of treatment make this an organism to be avoided at all costs.

toxoplasmosis

A common infection with the microscopic organism *Toxoplasma gondii*, often acquired before birth, but sometimes passed on by cats or acquired by eating undercooked meat from infected animals. The organism infects all known mammals and most of us have antibodies to it. Toxoplasmosis can affect the nervous system and, especially, the eye and is a common cause of permanent damage to the retina, causing a blind spot of variable size, which may enlarge at intervals throughout life. The condition should not be confused with **toxocariasis**, which is a worm infestation, also capable of affecting the eye.

RECOGNITION AND SYMPTOMS

In most cases, the infection causes no symptoms or observable effects, as the immune system is capable of controlling it and preventing significant damage. Antibodies, however, operate less efficiently in the internal tissues of the eye than elsewhere, and damage to the retina and the underlying layer (the choroid) is fairly common. Recurrences, which tend to cause further permanent damage to the retina, are a feature of the condition. But it is only when the central (macular) part of the retina is involved that loss of vision is apparent.

Apart from eye damage, toxoplasmic infection sometimes causes widespread lymph node enlargement in people with apparently normal immunity. The node enlargement may be accompanied by fever, headache, malaise, muscle and joint aches, and liver enlargement.

> When heavy infection occurs before birth, the fetus often suffers extensive damage to the nervous system and elsewhere, and miscarriage or stillbirth is common. For the same reasons, toxoplasmosis in people with immune deficiency, either from AIDS or other factors, may be a severe disorder, with tissue destruction in the brain, lungs and heart caused by the rapidly spreading organisms. About 10 per cent of patients with AIDS suffer a severe encephalitis (brain inflammation) from toxoplasmosis.

TREATMENT

Ocular toxoplasmosis is treated with pyrimethamine, an antimalarial drug, used in conjunction with Sulphadiazine or another similar sulpha drug. The treatment is not very effective and may suppress bone marrow blood cell production, but this danger may be reduced with folinic acid or baker's yeast.

trabeculectomy

An eye operation to treat cases of **glaucoma** that cannot be controlled by medication. In glaucoma the pressure of the watery fluid (aqueous humour) within the eye is excessive and this can slowly and painlessly destroy vision by its effect on the tiny blood vessels that nourish the nerve fibres from the retina. Trabeculectomy provides a new outlet route for the aqueous humour.

tracheia

Greek root meaning 'wind pipe' as in tracheal (of the wind pipe).

tracheitis

Inflammation of the lining of the wind pipe (trachea), usually as an extension of an infection of the throat or voice box (larynx). It is also commonly associated with **bronchitis**. Tracheitis is usually caused by a virus infection but some cases are due to organisms susceptible to antibiotics. It causes **croup** in young children.

Tracheitis causes pain in the upper part of the chest, hoarseness, sometimes wheezing, and a painful dry cough. In very small children there may be some risk of asphyxia. This was a common cause of death when tracheitis was caused by **diphtheria**.

Treatment involves antibiotics, if appropriate, the use of soothing inhalations and sometimes drugs to control ineffective coughing. Most cases settle without treatment.

tracheo-oesophageal fistula

An abnormal connection between the wind pipe (trachea) and the gullet (oesophagus), occurring as a birth defect due to an abnormality of development. Swallowing is impeded and food may enter the trachea so that the baby is at risk from choking, asphyxia, pneumonia and collapse of the lungs. The condition is often associated with other congenital defects and, unless of a very mild degree, calls for early surgical correction.

tracheostomy

An operation, also called a tracheotomy, in which an artificial opening is made in the front of the wind pipe (trachea), through the skin of the neck, and a tube inserted, through which breathing may continue until the normal airway can be

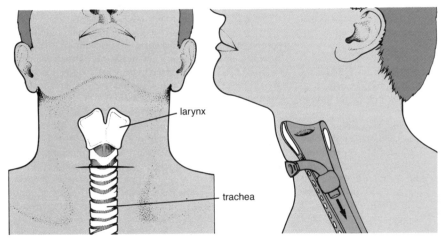

larynx

trachea

Tracheostomy may be a life-saving procedure in an emergency. An opening is made into the trachea just below the larynx, and this is kept open by a curved tube through which the subject breathes.

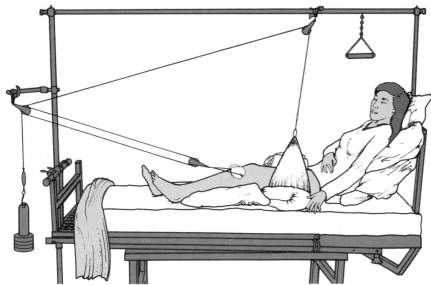

Traction is a common method of treating long bone fractures and is most commonly applied by way of a steel pin passed through the end of a bone and secured firmly in a stirrup. The force of the traction is varied, as needed, by changing the weights.

restored. It is often carried out as an emergency when life is threatened by obstruction to the airway. Tracheostomy is also commonly performed on people unable to breath spontaneously so that the respiration can be maintained artificially by an air pump. A permanent tracheostomy is necessary after the voice box (larynx) has been removed surgically.

Because it readily becomes blocked with dried secretions, the tracheostomy tube is double-lined. The inner lining may be removed regularly for cleaning and then replaced.

trachoma

An eye infection with the organism *Chlamydia trachomatis* which probably causes, or contributes to, more blindness, worldwide, than any other agency.

INCIDENCE

Trachoma is highly infectious, and in some areas of the world the infection rate in children is 100 per cent. Some 400 million people are affected in the less developed areas of Africa and Asia. Transmission is by eye contact with infected fingers, flies and contaminated materials (fomites) and occurs between people living in conditions of squalor. Trachoma presents no problem, even in endemic areas, to those fortunate enough to enjoy a high standard of living, and can be effectively treated.

RECOGNITION AND SYMPTOMS

The primary infection is in the conjunctiva, especially of the upper lids, and the result is a persistent (chronic) inflammation that spreads to the corneas, eventually leading to scarring and blindness. Scarring of the inner lining of the upper lids causes the lids to curl inwards (**entropion**) so that the lashes rub against, irritate and ulcerate the corneas, opening the way to secondary infection with other organisms. The result is often deep, penetrating corneal ulcers, sometimes with spread of infection into the inside of the eye and permanent destruction of the globe. Trachoma entropion is a misery to millions, whose only resource is to try to pull out the offending eyelashes.

TREATMENT

Like many other widespread and devastating diseases, trachoma is essentially a consequence of poverty and ignorance. Although the organism is susceptible to antibiotics, the real remedy lies in raising the standards of living and of elementary conceptions of hygiene.

Tracrium

A brand name for **atacurium besylate**.

traction

The exerting of a sustained pull on a part of the body, usually for purposes of maintaining proper alignment of parts. Traction is mainly used in the management of **fractures** which cannot be effectively immobilized by plaster casts and in which the broken ends of the bone tend to over-ride.

Fractures of the shaft of the thigh bone (femur) are commonly treated by traction, which is often applied to a stirrup connected to a steel pin passed though the upper end of the main lower leg bone (the tibia). Traction is also often necessary in the treatment of fractures of the spine. In this case, the traction may be applied to tongs fitted into holes drilled in the skull. Traction can also be valuable in the management of intervertebral disc disorders (see **slipped disc**).

tramadol

A centrally acting synthetic opiate pain-killing drug. It is less likely to cause respiratory depression, constipation, euphoria and addiction than many of the opioid agonists. It is currently the fourth most commonly prescribed analgesic in the world. Trade names are Tramake, Zamadol and Zydol.

Tramake

A brand name for tramadol.

Tramazoline

A **sympathomimetic** drug used to treat **hay fever**. A brand name of a preparation of tramazoline combined with dexamethasone and **neomycin** is Dexa-Rhinaspray.

TRANCE

An acronym for tumour-necrosis-factor-related activation-induced **cytokine**. This cytokine stimulates the development of

713

the cells concerned in the breakdown of bone as a preliminary to new bone formation (osteoclasts). It offers the possibility of developing new control over bone loss in **osteoporosis**.

Trancopal

A brand name for the benzodiazepine anti-anxiety drug chlormezanone.

Trandate

A brand name for the beta-blocker drug **labetalol**.

trandolapril

An **angiotensin converting enzyme inhibitor** drug used to treat high blood pressure and weak function of the left ventricle following a **heart attack**. Trade names are Gopten and Odrik.

tranexamic acid

A drug that interferes with the dissolution of blood clot (fibrinolysis) and can be used to prevent bleeding during minor operations such as tooth extraction in people with **haemophilia**. A brand name is Cyclokapron.

tranquillizers

The term 'tranquillizer' is not really scientific but is useful as a grouping for a range of drugs having mild muscle-relaxing and anxiety-relieving action. The major **antidepressant drugs** and antipsychotic drugs are excluded from this group. So the tranquillizers include such drugs as the **benzodiazepine drugs**, the **barbiturates**, the **beta-blocker drugs** and some of the mild **hypnotic drugs**. Other drugs such as meprobamate (Equanil) and buspirone (Buspar), are also used.

See also **anti-anxiety drugs**.

transactional analysis

A psychological theory, or interpretation, based on a study of social interactions. The general idea is that, in interactions, individuals tend to assume one of three roles, in relation to each other: that of 'adult', 'parent' or 'child'. These roles correspond roughly to Freud's **ego**, **superego** and **id**. Relationships are said to be balanced and satisfactory if properly complementary roles are adopted, but are disruptive and damaging if the people concerned refuse to play the game and instead take up non-reciprocal roles.

HOW IT WORKS

In their relations with others, people are said to take up four basic positions – 'I'm OK, you're OK'; 'I'm OK, you're not OK'; 'I'm not OK, you're OK'; and 'I'm not OK, you're not OK'. Lives are structured to obtain certain desired 'payoffs' and there is a need for a minimum score in social gratification. The games people play are designed to score these points and achieve satisfaction from them.

Transactional analysis explores the way people play these life games and identifies bad play which may be damaging to the quality of life.

transcriptase

Any enzyme that catalyses the transcription of a molecule, as in the process of producing a copy of **RNA** from **DNA**.

Reverse transcriptase is an enzyme found in viruses, such as HIV, that catalyses DNA from an RNA template. This is the reverse of the usual procedure.

transference

The passing on, or transferring, of an emotion or emotional attitude, experienced in relation to one person, to another person or object. A common example is the transference of attitudes or emotions, originating in childhood in relation to a parent, to a person in adult life. Transference may be positive when the transferee is regarded with approval, or negative when disliked.

Freud came to regard transference in psychoanalysis as central to its success.

transfer RNA

The shortest of the three types of **RNA** (ribonucleic acid), a single-strand molecule folded into a four-armed, clover-leaf-like structure, capable of combining with a specific **amino acid** in cell fluid and positioning it appropriately in a protein chain that is being synthesized in a ribosome (see **organelle**). Transfer RNA (tRNA) occurs in at least 20 different varieties, one for each of the 20 amino acids. At the end of one of the arms is an anticodon, complementary to the **codon** for an amino acid in **messenger RNA**. At the end of the opposite arm is a site to which the appropriate amino acid can be chemically linked. The identity of the passenger on a particular tRNA molecule is determined by its anticodon rather than by its attached amino acid. Ribosomes, with their own ribosomal RNA, move along the messenger RNA linking the right amino acids together.

transfusion

Strictly, this word means the replacement of blood lost by haemorrhage or disease, by donated blood from another person. But the term is often used to refer also to the infusion of other fluids such as plasma, saline, glucose saline, etc. Blood transfusion is often life-saving and in cases of severe, life-threatening blood loss or continuing bleeding, blood may be given very quickly, sometimes under pressure, and often into more than one vein simultaneously.

See also **blood** and **rhesus factor disease**.

transfusion with own blood

See **autologous blood donation**.

Transiderm-Nitro

A brand name for **glyceryl trinitrate**.

transient global amnesia

A state, lasting for less than twenty-four hours, in which there is an inability to form new memories and loss of memory for periods of up to years (retrograde amnesia) prior to the attack. After the attack there is permanent memory loss for the period of the attack but the earlier memory is restored. The condition may be brought on by emotional upset, physical exertion, sexual intercourse or strong compression while holding the breath (**valsalva manoeuvre**) as in defecating when constipated.

transient ischaemic attacks

Brief periods of disturbance of body function, of less than twenty-four hours, resulting from localized nervous system defects.

RECOGNITION

These defects occur because the blood supply to part of the brain is temporarily interrupted or reduced. The disturbances may take many forms – weakness in an arm or leg, local numbness, speech difficulty, loss of the ability to name objects, visual obscuration, loss of part of the field of vision, and so on. The type of disturbance gives a clue to the area of the brain affected and usually indicates which arteries are involved.

An attack lasting for several hours suggests that an actual permanent blockage has occurred but that neighbouring vessels have been able to open up sufficiently to maintain function. Even so, it is likely that some permanent damage to brain function has occurred. In some cases, repeated ischaemic attacks of this kind lead to progressive loss of function. When this deterioration is rapid, the condition is known as *stroke in evolution*.

POSSIBLE CAUSES

Transient ischaemic attacks are caused either by temporary vessel blockage from **embolism**, often by showers of very small emboli, or by intermittent reduction in blood supply to part of the brain. The latter occurs in vessels narrowed by **atherosclerosis**. Emboli may consist of cholesterol crystals or clumped blood platelets and these come from the linings of diseased neck (carotid) or other arteries, or from the heart itself.

Impending closure of any branch of the carotid or vertebral artery systems may cause transient ischaemic attacks.

> Transient ischaemic attacks must always be taken seriously as they are a clear warning that a stroke may occur soon. They should always be investigated and the cause ascertained and, if possible, treated.

translocation

A form of mutation in which a detached part of a whole chromosome becomes attached to another chromosome. Alternatively, parts of two chromosomes may be joined. Translocations may be inherited or acquired. In many cases they cause no effect on the body because all the normal chromosomal material is present. But if a translocation results in a deficiency or excess of chromosomal material the results are serious.

transplantation

The introduction of donated organs or tissues into the body in the hope that they may survive and continue to function or maintain structure. Two main advances have made successful transplantation possible – developments in microsurgical techniques, especially in the joining up of arteries, and developments in the understanding of the immunological processes that lead to the rejection of 'foreign' tissue.

Transplants between identical twins do not lead to rejection problems because the tissues are immunologically identical. The discovery of the **tissue types** based on the histocompatibility antigens soon led to the finding that transplants between tissue-matched siblings do almost as well as those between identical twins.

Immunosuppression is the deliberate and artificial blocking of the reactions which lead to rejection, and drugs exist which effectively achieve this. Such drugs are universally used in transplantation, but are clearly not without disadvantage.

Kidney grafting has been the most successful type of organ transplantation, and the results have been excellent, especially since the introduction of the selective immunosuppressive drug cyclosporin. Failure in kidney grafting is also less serious than in the case of heart transplantation, because patients with kidney failure can be sustained by regular use of the artificial kidney (haemodialysis).

See also **heart transplantation**, **heart-lung transplant**, **kidney transplant**.

transposons

Discrete sequences of **DNA** that can transport themselves directly from one part of the genome to another without the use of any vehicle. They move by making normal **RNA** transcripts and then making DNA copies of these, which are then incorporated into the **genome** at a new site. Sometimes called 'jumping genes'. Transposons can affect gene activity, probably by separating a gene from the adjacent sequences necessary for its function.

transsexualism

A persistent conviction that one's true gender does not correspond to one's anatomical sex. Transsexualism is largely confined to men, who often seek **sex reassignment surgery** so that they can live fully as members of the opposite sex. The condition is often associated with depression, anxiety and various personality disorders.

transtracheal oxygen catheterization

Maintenance of a supplementary oxygen supply to the body by means of a fine tube passed through a tracheostomy opening in the front of the neck into the trachea. The method has substantial advantages over nasal cannulas or facemasks and is preferred by many patients.

transvaginal ultrasound

Ultrasound imaging of the pelvic structures in women by means of a transducer placed in the vagina. Transvaginal imaging of the lining of the womb (endometrium) can provide valuable information about thickness and texture in women with abnormal bleeding. Unduly thick endometrium suggests cancer or hyperplasia.

Transvasin

A brand name for **tetrahydrofuryl salicylate**.

transvestism

The desire, in men, to wear women's clothing. In theory, the desire, on the part of a woman, to wear men's clothing is also transvestism, but this common inclination is not normally referred to as transvestism. Transvestites are not necessarily, or even often, transsexuals. Some limit their indulgence to the wearing of female underwear; others for elaborate couture and exaggeratedly feminine dress. Some feel more relaxed when transvestured; others derive sexual excitement from it. Most are heterosexual and have a sexual relationship with a woman.

Tranxene

A brand name for the benzodiazepine antianxiety drug clorazepate.

tranylcypromine

A **monoamine-oxidase inhibitor** (MAO) antidepressant drug. A brand name is Parnate.

Trasicor

A brand name for the beta-blocker drug oxprenolol.

Trasylol

A brand name for **aprotinin**.

trauma

Greek root meaning 'injury' as in traumatic (of injury).

travellers' diarrhoea

A lay term for gastroenteritis usually caused by faecal contamination of food or water. The organisms most commonly involved are *Escherichia coli*, *Campylobacter jejuni*, *Salmonella species*, and *Shigella species*.

travel sickness

See **motion sickness**.

Travogyn

A brand name for **isoconazole**.

Traxam

A brand name for **felbinac**.

trazodone

An antidepressant drug. A brand name is Molipaxin.

Treacher-Collins syndrome

A dominant genetic disorder also known as incomplete mandibulo-facial dysostosis or the Collins-Franceschetti syndrome. It features a characteristic facial configuration with down-sloping eyes, notches (colobomas) in the eyelids, a small mouth and lower jaw, small mis-shapen external ears and often deafness. The mutated gene and its protein product were identified in 1996. It is on the long arm of chromosome 5. Over 20 different mutations have been found.

treatment, reliable

See **evidence-based medicine**.

Tremonil

A brand name for the anticholinergic drug methixene, used to control the symptoms of **Parkinson's disease**.

tremor

A rhythmical oscillation of any part of the body, lasting for at least a few seconds, and affecting especially the hands, the head, the jaw or the tongue. Tremor is very common, especially in the elderly, and does not necessarily imply disease. A minor degree of tremor, known as physiological tremor, is normal, and everyone, from time to time, experiences exaggeration of this into an obvious, coarse shake, especially when the muscles concerned are being tensed. Tremor during excitement or anxiety, due to raised adrenaline levels, is an exaggerated physiological tremor.

Essential-familial tremor is an embarrassing condition which runs in families and produces an effect of nervousness. It does not progress to more serious disease and is usually temporarily relieved by alcohol. It may be suppressed by beta-blocking drugs such as propranolol.

POSSIBLE CAUSES

Persistent tremor at rest, with a frequency of four or five cycles per second, may indicate **Parkinson's disease**, even if the tremor disappears on complete relaxation. Such tremor may be extreme but has less effect on voluntary movement than would be expected and a person who normally has a violent tremor may be able to drink from a glass without mishap. Severe tremor is also a feature of **multiple sclerosis**, **Wilson's disease**, cerebellar ataxia, **encephalitis**, mercury poisoning, and **thyrotoxicosis**. Tremor caused by brain disorder (encephalopathy) from liver failure or other metabolic disorders is called *asterixis*.

A variety of drugs can cause tremor. These include amphetamines, antidepressant drugs, caffeine, corticosteroids and lithium. A marked tremor is a common feature of patients under drug treatment for certain psychiatric disorders.

Trental

A brand name for **oxpentifylline**.

trephine

A tubular, cylindrical cutting instrument with the edge at one end sharpened or saw-toothed. The cutting end of the trephine is pressed hard against the tissue to be cut and the instrument rotated. Trephines are used to cut a circular hole in bone, cornea or other tissue. In corneal grafting, the same trephine is used to cut the opening in the cornea and the disc from the donated eye so that the graft fits perfectly.

Trephines have been widely used to make holes in the skull which can then be joined with saw cuts so that a flap of bone may be removed. Trephining, or trepanning, of the skull to release evil spirits has been performed throughout the ages and many very old skulls with trephine holes have been found.

tretinoin

A **retinoid** drug used to treat **acne**, scaly skin conditions such as **ichthyosis**, skin ageing and certain forms of **leukaemia**. Trade names are Retin-A, Retinova and Vesanoid.

Triadene

A brand name for **ethinyloestradiol** formulated with a **progestogen** drug as an oral contraceptive.

triage

A selection process, used in war or disaster situations, to divide casualties into three groups so as to maximize resources and avoid wastage of essential surgical skills on hopeless cases. In triage, an experienced surgeon or other person rapidly sorts cases into those needing urgent treatment, those that will survive without immediate treatment, and those beyond hope of benefit from treatment. Triage is also used to assign treatment in the event of the simultaneous appearance of a number of men suffering acute chest pain.

triamcinolone

A corticosteroid drug used to treat inflammatory disorders, asthma, thrombocytopenia and some forms of leukaemia. Trade names are Adcortyl, Adcortyl in Orabase, Kenalog, Lederspan and Nasacort. Triamcinolone is also an ingredient is a range of preparations for external use.

Triam-Co

A brand name for **triamterene** formulated with **hydrochlorothiazide**.

triamterene

A potassium-sparing diuretic drug used to relieve the body of excess water and to treat mildly raised blood pressure. Triamterene is formulated with another diuretic drug under the trade names Diazide, Dytide, Frusene, Kalspare and Triam-Co.

triazolam

A benzodiazepine sedative drug used to relieve insomnia. A brand name is Halcion.

Trib

A brand name for co-trimoxazole.

tribavirin

A drug used to treat severe respiratory syncytial virus infections. A brand name is Virazid.

trichiasis

A condition in which the eyelashes, instead of turning outwards, grow, or are directed in, an inward direction so that they rub against the cornea of the eye (see also **entropion**). This causes severe discomfort and may lead to abrasion, infection and ulceration – a sequence that often occurs in the condition of **trachoma** in which trichiasis is very common.

The usual response to trichiasis is to pull out the offending lashes, but this is not an effective remedy as lashes soon grow again, and short, stubby lashes may be more damaging than more flexible longer lashes. The proper treatment of trichiasis is a plastic procedure on the lid, by which the lid margin is turned outwards, carrying the lashes away from the eye. If only a few lashes are involved, electrolytic destruction of them may be effective.

trichinosis

A parasitic disease caused by the roundworm *Trichinella spiralis*, and usually acquired by eating undercooked infected pork or pork products. These contain tiny oval cysts, about half a millimetre long, containing the dormant forms of the worm.

When pig meat containing Trichinella cysts is eaten, the larva break out of the cysts when the meat is digested in the stomach. This causes fever and nausea. Two days later, sexual maturity is reached and the worms, 2 to 4 mm long, have attached themselves to the lining of the small intestine. After copulation the smaller male dies but the female lives for a month during which one worm can produce 1500 larvae. These pass into the blood circulation and are carried to all parts of the body, settling in the muscles to form cysts in which they can survive for 30 years. The process of migration and cyst formation lasts for about three months during which a range of symptoms may occur.

RECOGNITION AND SYMPTOMS

In most cases, the infestation is light and the symptoms minimal, but in a heavy infestation there may be sustained or intermittent fever; swelling (oedema) of the face, especially the eyelids and the conjunctivas; invasion of the diaphragm causing cough, breathlessness and pain; generalized muscle invasion with pain, stiffness and tenderness in any muscle group; invasion of the brain causing **encephalitis**; and invasion of the heart causing myocarditis. Intense infestations may be fatal, but those who recover do so completely.

trichomoniasis

A genital infection, mainly of the vagina, with the single-celled organism *Trichomonas vaginalis*. This pear-shaped organism with an undulating membrane down one side is able to move about actively by lashing with several long, hair-like flagella. The infection is usually transmitted by a male carrier during sexual intercourse. In contrast to other sexually transmitted conditions, this one can be acquired from contaminated objects such as toilet seats. Although it most commonly affects the vagina, it may also involve the urine tube (urethra) in either sex and the prostate gland in men.

RECOGNITION AND SYMPTOMS

Trichomoniasis causes sudden onset of severe genital irritation, burning and itching and a profuse, frothy, yellowish, offensive discharge. It is one of the common causes of vaginal discharge. If the urethra is affected, there is burning on urination and some urethral discharge. Vaginal trichomoniasis often causes discomfort or pain during sexual intercourse. It may affect women of any age and is common during pregnancy. Positive diagnosis is made by spreading a small quantity of the discharge on a microscope slide and identifying the characteristic moving organism.

TREATMENT

Men with a prostatic infection can act as carriers of the infection and if one of a pair of sexual partners has the infection, both must be treated or no advantage will be gained. The drug metronidazole (Flagyl) is the mainstay of treatment and is highly effective.

See also **sexually transmitted diseases**.

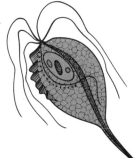

A greatly enlarged drawing of the common microscopic protozoal parasite Trichomonas vaginalis – a common cause of vaginal irritation and discharge.

trichos

Greek root meaning 'hair' as in trichology (study of hair).

Trichozole

A brand name for **metronidazole**.

triclosan

A disinfectant drug used externally in staphylococcal and other skin infections. Trade names are Aquasept, Manusept, Ster-Zac Bath Concentrate.

tricyclic antidepressant drugs

A group of drugs whose structure is based on three six-carbon rings. The tricyclics produce an elevation of mood but this does not occur until the drugs have been taken for two to three weeks (an important point as depressed people may commit suicide during this period). These drugs have an anticholinergic effect and may cause dry mouth, constipation, urinary retention and blurred vision. The tricyclic antidepressants are the most widely used group for depression. They act by blocking the re-uptake of noradrenaline and serotonin at synapses thus allowing these stimulatory neurotransmitters to act for longer. With use, actual changes occur in the synapses that are of benefit. **Fluoxetine** (Prozac) is not a tricyclic. It has only two rings and is a selective re-uptake inhibitor of serotonin only. Other tricyclic antidepressant drugs are **amitriptyline**, **doxepin**, **imipramine**, **nortriptyline**, and **trimipramine**. Up to 50 per cent of patients have genetic variations that prevent them from responding to these drugs.

See also **antidepressant drugs**.

Tridesta

A brand name for **medroxyprogesterone** formulated as an adjunct to oestrogen.

Tridil

A brand name for **glyceryl trinitrate**.

trifluoperazine

An antipsychotic drug used mainly to treat **schizophrenia**. A brand name is Stelazine.

trigeminal neuralgia

A poorly understood disorder in which sudden nerve impulse discharges occur in the sensory nerve of the face – the fifth, or trigeminal, cranial nerve – on one side. These discharges cause episodes of excruciating stabbing pain in the cheek, lips, gums, chin or tongue lasting for only a few seconds or, at the most, a minute or two, but usually so intense that the affected person is arrested. The severity of the pain causes the muscles of the face to wince, hence the earlier name of *tic douloureux*.

RECOGNITION AND SYMPTOMS

The condition affects middle-aged and elderly people, almost exclusively, causing repeated attacks over periods of several weeks. During these periods, the affected person may be constantly 'on edge' in anticipation of the next stab of pain. There is a tendency for the periods of freedom between series of attacks to become shorter with time.

A feature of the condition is that it may be brought on by touching a particular part of the face or any other area supplied by the trigeminal nerve, such as the lips, gums or tongue. It may thus be precipitated by chewing, swallowing, or even speaking.

TREATMENT

The cause of trigeminal neuralgia is uncertain and treatment is difficult. The drug carbamazepine (Tegretol) is effective in most cases, but about 20 per cent of sufferers develop resistance and some are unable to tolerate a high enough dosage to relieve the pain. When drug treatment fails, an injection to destroy the root of the nerve, or operative cutting of the nerve, may be necessary. These procedures cause permanent numbness of one side of the face and complications are common.

trigger finger

An effect caused by localized swelling of the tendon by which the finger is bent (flexor tendon), and of the tendon sheath. The swelling in the tendon occurs near the base of the finger and when the finger is bent, the swollen tendon is able to slip normally out of the end of its sheath, but cannot easily slip back in again. The finger thus remains bent unless straightened passively, which may cause an audible click.

Permanent correction is possible by surgical opening (decompression) of the tendon sheath so that the tendon is no longer obstructed.

Trilafon

A brand name for **perphenazine**.

Trilisate

A brand name for the anti-inflammatory and pain-killing drug choline magnesium trisalicylate.

trilostane

A drug that interferes with the natural synthesis of steroids and is used to treat breast cancer in postmenopausal women. A brand name is Modrenal.

trimeprazine

An antihistamine drug used to relieve itching in allergic conditions and as a sedative for children. A brand name is Vallergan.

trimethoprim

An antibacterial drug used to treat urinary and other infections. Trade names are Monotrim and Trimopan. Combined with sulphamethoxazole it is sold as co-trimoxazole (Septrin) and Chemotrim.

trimetrexate

An inhibitor of the enzyme dihydrofolate reductase. It is used to treat *Pneumocystis carinii* pneumonia in people with **AIDS**. A brand name is Neutrexin.

Tri-Minulet

A brand name for **ethinyloestradiol** formulated with a **progestogen** drug as an oral contraceptive.

trimipramine

A tricyclic antidepressant drug with a strong sedative effect. A brand name is Surmontil.

Trimogal

A brand name for **trimethoprim**.

Trimopan

A brand name for **trimethoprim**.

Trinordiol

A brand name for **ethinyloestradiol** formulated with **levonorgestrel** as an oral contraceptive.

Trinovum

A brand name for **ethinyloestradiol** formulated with a **progestogen** drug as an oral contraceptive.

Triominic

A brand name for a mixture of the nasal decongestant drug phenylpropanolamine and the antihistamine drug pheniramine.

Triperidol

A brand name for the antipsychotic drug trifluperidol.

triple-X genome

See **XXX configuration**.

Triplopen

A brand name for the penicillin antibiotic benethamine penicillin.

tri-potassium di-citrato bismuthate

A drug, used to treat stomach and duodenal ulcers, that reacts with the gastric secretions to provide a protective barrier for the bowel lining (a cytoprotectant drug). Trade names are DeNol and DeNoltab.

Triprim

A brand name for **trimethoprim**.

triprolidine

An antihistamine drug used to treat allergy and to relieve the symptoms of colds. A brand name of a preparation combined with **pseudoephedrine** is Sudafed.

Triptafen

A brand name for the tricyclic antidepressant drug amitryptyline and the antipsychotic and **anti-emetic** drug perphenazine.

triptorelin

A synthetic gonadotrophin-releasing hormone used to treat advanced cancer of the **prostate gland**. A brand name is Decapeptyl SR.

trismus

Lockjaw. Tight closure of the mouth as a result of uncontrollable spasm of the muscles used in chewing. This may be caused by any painful condition around the jaw joint, just in front of the ear, or by any inflammation in the soft tissues surrounding the chewing muscles. Thus, trismus may be a feature of **tonsillitis**, **quinsy**, **mumps**, severe ulcerative **gingivitis**, acute **tooth decay** affecting the molars, or even cancer of the back of the nose (nasopharynx).

Trismus is a classic sign of the serious infection **tetanus**, and is sometimes troublesome in **Parkinson's disease**. Occasionally trismus occurs as a hysterical condition and is sometimes a feature of **anorexia nervosa**. The treatment of trismus is the treatment of the underlying cause.

trisodium edetate

A **chelating agent** used to reduce excess body calcium and treat calcareous deposits in the corneas. A brand name is Limclair.

trisomy

The chromosomes occur in twenty-three matched and identifiable pairs. Trisomy is the condition in which there are three, instead of two, of a particular chromosome. This is always serious and has effects varying from death of the fetus in the womb to a range of structural abnormalities affecting parts of the body such as the heart, the face, the skeleton or the brain. Trisomy can be detected by **chromosome analysis**.

See also **Down's syndrome**.

trisomy 13

The presence of three copies of chromosome 13 in every cell of the body. This causes the Patau syndrome in which there is an abnormally small head (microcephaly), cleft lip or palate, deafness, blindness, extra fingers and finger deformity. Infants with trisomy 13 rarely survive for more than a few weeks.

trisomy 18

The presence of three copies of chromosome 18 in every cell of the body. This causes the Edwards syndrome in which there is failure to thrive, severe mental deficiency, anomalies of the face, hands, breastbone and pelvis, persistent contraction of muscles with clenching of the hands. Survival beyond a few months is uncommon. This trisomy leads to spontaneous abortion in nine cases out of ten.

trisomy 21 syndrome

see **Down's syndrome**.

trocar

A sharp-pointed surgical stilette normally used within a tubular instrument (a cannula) to allow its insertion into a body cavity. After the trocar and cannula have been inserted into the body, the trocar is withdrawn, leaving the cannula in place.

Tropergen

A brand name for **diphenoxylate**.

tropical diseases

A number of tropical diseases depend on the coincidence of a parasite and the specific agent responsible for its spread (vector). These include diseases such as **malaria** – coincidence of the malarial parasite in man and the *Anopheles* mosquito; **onchocerciasis** – the larval worms (microfilaria) in man and the biting black fly *Simulium damnosum*; **yellow fever** – the yellow fever virus in man and the *Aedes egypti* mosquito; and **leishmaniasis** – the leishmania parasites in man and the phlebotomus sandfly. At least some of these vectors can, however, survive in temperate zones – malaria was once common in the south of England – and often the condition can be eliminated by removal of either the parasite or the vector.

A number of conditions are caused by exposure to tropical sunlight. The commonest of these is skin collagen damage from the ultraviolet component of sunlight. This causes an unnatural degree of wrinkling, loss of skin elasticity, and an increased tendency to **rodent ulcer** (basal cell carcinoma), squamous epithelioma, and **malignant melanoma**. Ultraviolet light is also damaging to the eye and may lead to the development of **pinguecula** and **pterygium**. Heavy physical work in the tropics, with inadequate water and salt replacement, may lead to heat exhaustion, and prolonged exposure of the unacclimatized to high temperatures may lead to heat-stroke.

Most of the diseases considered as 'tropical', however, are not primarily the result of tropical geographic factors, but occur mainly because in many tropical areas large sections of the population live at a low socio-economic level, suffering poor nutritional standards in conditions of unsatisfactory hygiene and sanitation. Many of the diseases which currently take an enormous toll in suffering and mortality in tropical areas – diseases such as lung and bone **tuberculosis**, malnutrition, **typhoid fever**, **plague**, **shigellosis**, **cholera**, **amoebiasis**, **diphtheria**, **typhus**, **rabies** – were once common in temperate zones when these were still at a low level of social and economic development, and it is clear that diseases such as these are not specifically related to tropical conditions.

Parasitic diseases, such as **schistosomiasis**, **strongyloidiasis**, **hookworm** and tapeworm infestation, are also largely maintained by social conditions which encourage water and soil contamination with human excreta and the barefoot habit. Parasitic disease is also encouraged by low standards of public health administration, food inspection and food handling. A high proportion of all 'tropical diseases' are caused by infective agents and, given adequate resources of finance and education, almost all of these diseases can be brought under control.

Tropical ulcer is common in malnourished people who are unable to maintain normal standards of hygiene or personal care.

tropical sprue

A disease in which there is a failure to absorb some of the elements in the food, so that nutritional deficiency occurs. It is similar to non-tropical **sprue** (see **malabsorption**) except that it occurs only in those living in or visiting tropical areas. It may, however, begin months or years after residence in the tropics. The cause is unknown.

Tropical sprue causes loss of appetite, weight loss, anaemia, distention of the abdomen and fatty diarrhoea. The unabsorbed carbohydrate in the bowel tends to ferment, causing a sense of fullness, the passage of gas (flatus) and explosive defecation. Deficient absorption of iron and vitamins often leads to inflammation of the tongue (glossitis) and mouth (stomatitis).

Tropical sprue responds well to various forms of treatment, such as antibiotics, vitamin B12 and folate.

tropical ulcer

A general term for a range of conditions in which there is localized loss of skin and underlying tissue. This may be due to untreated or neglected bacterial infection, cutaneous **leishmaniasis**, **diphtheria** of the skin, **yaws**, or other chronic infection.

tropicamide

A drug used in the form of eye drops to dilate the pupil so that the inside of the eye can more easily be examined or operated upon. Trade names are Minims tropicamide and Mydriacyl.

tropisetron

A **serotonin** receptor blocker drug used to treat severe nausea and vomiting, especially that induced by anticancer chemotherapy. A brand name is Navoban.

tropism

An automatic movement made by an organism or a cell towards or away from a source of stimulation.

Tropium

A brand name for the benzodiazepine antianxiety drug chlordiazepoxide.

Trosyl

A brand name for **tioconazole**.

Trusopt

A brand name for **dorzolamide**.

truss

A padded appliance worn on the body to hold a 'rupture' (**hernia**) in place, once the protruding bowel has been pushed back into the abdomen. The truss is an inherently unsatisfactory way of managing a hernia and is used only when, for some reason, surgical correction cannot be provided, or has to be delayed.

trypanosomiasis

See **sleeping sickness**, **trypanosomiasis, South American**.

trypanosomiasis, South American

Often called Chagas' disease after the Brazilian physician and microbiologist Carlos Ribeiro Chagas (1879–1934) who first described it, South American trypanosomiasis occurs only in scattered areas of South and Central America, including Chile, Argentina and Mexico. Fifteen to 20 million people are affected in endemic areas.

The disease is transmitted by the 'kissing' or 'assassin' bug which resides in the thatch and the cracks of dwellings. The kissing bug bites the sleeping person painlessly, usually around the mouth, and the *Trypanosoma cruzi* parasite enters the bite wound from the deposited faeces of the insect.

RECOGNITION AND EFFECTS

As in African trypanosomiasis (sleeping sickness), this species of trypanosome can cause nervous system damage, but in many cases the main effects are on the heart. In children, the disease may be acute, with severe neurological effects, and the involvement of the heart is often fatal. In adults, acute illness, with inflammation of the brain (**encephalitis**), meninges (**meningitis**) and heart muscle (myocarditis), kills 5 to 10 per cent of affected people within a few days. The remainder gradually recover and appear to be well, but are, in fact, harbouring the parasite.

The long-term results may be extremely serious. In the affected geographic areas, Chagas' disease is the main cause of heart disease and is responsible for a quarter of the deaths in people twenty to forty years old. The parasite causes progressive damage to the heart muscle, often very slowly over the course of many years, but in the end, **heart failure** or sudden cardiac arrest are common.

TREATMENT

There is no treatment which can safely eliminate the trypanosomes, but the long-term effects of Chagas' disease can be minimized by the use of various drugs.

Tryptanol

A brand name for **amitriptyline**.

Tryptizol

A brand name for **amitryptyline**.

tryptophan

An antidepressant drug. L-tryptophan, sold in the USA as a nonprescription food additive, was withdrawn by the American Food and Drugs Administration (FDA) because of reports of a severe muscle disorder apparently caused by an unidentified contaminant. A brand name is Optimax.

tubal pregnancy

A form of ectopic pregnancy.

tube, interior of

See **lumen**.

tuberculin test

A skin test used to discover whether or not an individual has already had a tuberculous infection and has thus acquired a degree of immunity. The great majority of people have a minor, low-dose, *primary* tuberculous infection, usually of the lungs or tonsils, which, in most cases, heals completely and does no harm. In addition, the small primary infection provides a useful degree of immunity against a more serious later massive infection from contact with an active case.

The purpose of tuberculin testing is to discover whether or not this primary infection, or a later infection, has occurred. It is important in the investigation of family contacts. People who react negatively to the test can be given normal immunity by **BCG** vaccination.

The test is done with a solution of *old tuberculin* or purified protein derivative tuberculin – substances which have the antigenic properties of the tubercle bacillus without the dangers of causing the disease. In the *Mantoux* test the material is injected into – rather than under – the skin with a fine needle. In the Heaf test, or the multiple puncture test, instruments with a number of sharp tines are used to introduce the tuberculin into the skin. The Heaf gun does this with a spring-loaded device. None of these procedures causes more than a very slight pain.

The test is read after three days. A positive reaction is shown by the development of a hardened swelling around the site. Negative reactors can be retested with a stronger solution of freshly prepared tuberculin. A repeated negative test practically rules out tuberculosis, except in old people, in people with sarcoidosis, or in those taking immunosuppressive drugs. A strongly positive reaction, in a person with other suggestive symptoms, may indicate current tuberculosis infection.

tuberculosis

A once common infection caused by the organism *Mycobacterium tuberculosis*, often called the tubercle bacillus. Until effective antituberculous drugs were introduced some fifty years ago, tuberculosis was one of the main causes of death, and hospitals dedicated to the treatment of the condition (tuberculosis sanatoria) were to be found everywhere. Since the advent of streptomycin and other drugs, these have all been closed or devoted to some other purpose. Tuberculosis is still a scourge in many underdeveloped countries.

Tuberculosis can affect the lungs (pulmonary tuberculosis) or other parts of the body, such as the lymph nodes (tuberculous adenitis or **scrofula**), the skin and the bones. Pulmonary tuberculosis is, in general, derived from other people who cough out tubercle bacilli, while general (systemic) tuberculosis is usually derived from infected milk from cows with bovine tuberculosis. In most cases human lung infection is well localized, controlled by the immune system, and is symptomless. Active lung disease occurs if immunity drops. The great majority of people have had a primary infection with tuberculosis, as is shown by a positive tuberculin skin test. Those who are tuberculin negative are more susceptible and may benefit from **BCG** inoculation. Tubercle bacilli can remain dormant for years before producing active disease.

RECOGNITION AND SYMPTOMS

Symptoms of pulmonary tuberculosis include fever, fatigue, loss of appetite and weight, night sweats and persistent cough. Sputum may be streaked with blood. Tuberculous pleurisy leads to an accumulation of fluid in the pleural cavity and partial collapse of the lung. Occasionally, the destructive process in the lung may involve a large artery, causing massive haemorrhage. Tuberculosis may spread widely throughout the body (miliary tuberculosis). Tuberculous **meningitis** is another dangerous complication.

TREATMENT

Tuberculosis is treated with various regimens of drugs in combination. Isoniazid, para-aminosalicylic acid (PAS), rifampicin, ethambutol, pyrazinamide and streptomycin all have their place in the now highly effective management of this disease. Treatment is needed for nine to twelve months.

tuberous sclerosis

See **epiloia**.

tularaemia

A disease of wild animals, caused by the organism *Francisella tularensis*, and occurring in the USA, Japan and most European countries other than Britain. It may, rarely, be contracted by human beings through contact with infected animals, inhalation of infected material or bites from infected insects. The disease features an ulcer at the site of the bite, enlargement and suppuration of the local lymph nodes and scattered, small, localized areas of tissue death in all parts of the body. Pneumonic and ocular forms occur, depending on the route of entry. Tularaemic septicaemia is highly dangerous. Treatment is with antibiotic drugs such as streptomycin or gentamicin.

tumour lysis syndrome

The release of damaging cell breakdown products that occurs when tumour cells are killed by effective anticancer treatment. There is a rise in blood potassium, uric acid and phosphates and a drop in calcium. The effect may be a severe metabolic disturbance that can cause prolonged illness and may prove fatal. Severe kidney damage may occur from the deposition in the kidneys of urate crystals.

tumour markers

Abnormal levels of substances in the blood or urine that suggest the presence of a malignant tumour in the body. Tumour markers include:

- proteins such as thyroid hormone (thyroglobulin) and antibodies (immunoglobulins);
- glycoproteins such as the **prostate-specific antigen** (PSI) and CA-125;
- hormones such as beta-human chorionic gonadotrophin and adrenocorticotrophic hormone;
- enzymes such as lactate dehydrogenase and prostatic acid phosphatase;
- tumour-associated carbohydrate antigens;
- neuro-transmitters such as noradrenaline;
- oncogenes;
- oncofetal antigens such as **alphafetoprotein** and carcino-embryonic antigen;
- cytogenic markers such as the **Philadelphia chromosome**.

In many of these cases the marker is a normal body constituent but is present in abnormal quantity.

tumour necrosis factor

One of two related **cytokines** capable of killing certain cancer cells and which also have regulatory functions on the immune system. Tumour necrosis factor is implicated in various inflammatory diseases including rheumatoid arthritis. A tumour necrosis factor antagonist is a fusion protein, produced by recombinant DNA technology, consisting of the tumour necrosis factor receptor, p75, linked to the antibody IgG.

tumour-specific antigens

Substances produced by specific kinds of tumours that can be detected in the blood and may act as indicators or markers of the presence of tumours or of recurrences of tumours. The method is not wholly reliable because these substances can sometimes occur in the body apart from tumours.

tunnel vision

When we look straight ahead and avoid moving the eyes, our fields of vision should extend out to about 90 degrees on either side. Perception in the peripheral visual fields is vague and the power of resolving detail (visual acuity) low, but the fields of vision are important in providing us with information and warnings about what is happening round about us. Tunnel vision is the lay term for a severe constriction of the fields of vision. The central vision may be, and often is, entirely normal and the visual acuity high.

POSSIBLE CAUSES

Visual field loss may be caused by any disorder of the peripheral parts of the retinas, or any disorder that restricts the function of the optic nerves or their connections with the brain (visual pathways). The commonest cause of tunnel vision is **glaucoma** in which raised pressure within the eye causes damage to optic nerve fibres. **Retinitis pigmentosa** causes peripheral retinal damage. Brain tumour, **stroke**, severe head injury or **multiple sclerosis** may also result in tunnel vision by affecting the optic nerves or visual nerve pathways.

Severe tunnel vision, even if the central visual acuity is normal, is usually justification for a person to be registered blind.

Turner's syndrome

A genetic disorder affecting females and caused by a sex chromosome abnormality. The normal female has two X (sex) chromosomes and in most females with Turner's syndrome one of the X chromosomes is missing. Sometimes both X chromosomes are present, one being normal and the other defective. Turner's syndrome may also result from an abnormal distribution of sex chromosomes occurring in normal females at the time of one of the early cell divisions. In this case, some cells have the normal number and some not. This is called *mosaicism*. Unlike Down's syndrome, Turner's syndrome has no relationship to maternal age.

RECOGNITION

Girls with Turner's syndrome are short of stature, have webbed neck skin, misshapen ears, increased outward angulation at the elbows, and a failure of development of the sexual characteristics – underdevelopment of the uterus, vagina, and breasts, lack of pubic and axillary hair and absence of the menstrual periods. There is localized narrowing of the largest artery in the body (coarctation of the aorta), abnormalities of the eyes and of the bones, and usually some degree of mental retardation.

TREATMENT

Attempts have been made to increase growth with anabolic steroids or growth hormone, but these are liable to cause the growing bone ends to fuse prematurely and so ensure dwarfism. Coarctation of the aorta should be treated by early surgery.

TURP

An abbreviation for Trans-Urethral Resection of the Prostate. This is the commonest type of operation for enlargement of the prostate gland. See **prostate gland, disorders of**.

Tussinol

A brand name for **pholcodine**.

tussis

Latin root meaning 'cough' as in pertussis (whooping cough).

twilight sleep

A now outdated popular term for a state of relative insensitivity to pain and partial consciousness, induced by drugs such as morphine and scopolamine, to ease the pains of childbirth.

twins

Two offspring from a single pregnancy. The incidence of twins is about one in ninety pregnancies. If a fertilized ovum begins to divide and the two cells produced separate, each will produce a new individual. These will be genetically identical, and necessarily of the same sex. They have to share a single placenta. They may, for purely environmental reasons, be different sizes at birth, but they will, otherwise, closely resemble each other. They will share every characteristic that is inherited. Because such identical twins come from a single **zygote** they are called monozygotic. They may also be called monovular because they both come from the same egg.

Non-identical twins occur when two different eggs are produced at the same time and each is fertilized by a separate sperm. Such twins may be of different or of the same sex but do not resemble each other any more than do any pair of siblings from separate pregnancies. They are called dizygotic or binovular twins. Each dizygotic twin has its own placenta.

Very rarely, the two cells produced by the first division of a single fertilized egg separate partially but not completely. If this happens, the result is **Siamese twins**. Some families have a history of dizygotic twins, but there seems to be no special familial incidence of monozygotic twins.

The incidence of pregnancy and birth complications is a little higher in twin pregnancies than in single pregnancies.

twins, joined

See **Siamese twins**.

twins with different fathers

See **superfecundation**.

twisted neck

See **torticollis**.

twitch

The result of a sudden spontaneous impulse in a nerve supplying a group of muscle fibres, so that they give a single, simultaneous, strong contraction, causing visible movement or rippling of the muscle.

Twitching need not necessarily indicate any important disorder. The common *fasciculation* of the fibres of the flat muscle surrounding the eye, for instance, is seldom of any significance. Diseases of motor nerves, however, often produce a state of hyperexcitability with spontaneous passage of strong nerve impulses, causing twitching, and this may be a feature of **poliomyelitis**, amyotrophic lateral sclerosis, progressive spinal muscular atrophy, polyneuritis and pressure on the spinal nerve roots from prolapsed intervertebral disc. Twitching of the muscles is a feature of kidney failure, and is caused by the effect of the raised level of urea in the blood on the brain.

Tylex

A brand name for a mixture of the pain-killing drugs codeine and **paracetamol**.

tympanoplasty

Middle ear disease, especially severe infection and **cholesteatoma**, may so damage the chain of three tiny bones (ossicles) which bridge across the inner ear that the linkage is broken and the vibrations of the drum are only very poorly conveyed to the fluid in the inner ear. Tympanoplasty is an operation to reconstitute the linkage between the eardrum and the oval window of the inner ear, so that hearing again becomes possible. The procedure adopted in tympanoplasty depends on the extent of the damage. Often, one or two of the bones remain intact and sometimes the gap can be bridged by reshaping one of them. In difficult cases, it may be necessary to use plastic implants or ossicles taken from a cadaver. Such grafts, sometimes complete with eardrum, are being used increasingly.

Loss of the normal middle ear mucous membrane lining seriously reduces the chances of success, as recurrent adhesions are likely. Even in the most favourable cases, restoration of hearing cannot be guaranteed.

typhoid carrier

A 'carrier' is a person who carries the organisms of an infectious disease, and passes these on to infect others, while remaining immune to it. In most cases, carriers will have suffered an attack of the disease concerned and recovered.

Typhoid carriers develop a permanent infection in the gall-bladder where the *Salmonella typhi* organisms breed freely without causing any apparent harm to the host. These bacteria pass down the bile duct with the bile and enter the intestine where they contaminate the bowel contents and are excreted with the faeces.

Thus the stools of typhoid carriers are heavily infected with typhoid organisms and so, in the course of normal activity, are the fingers. Any failure in scrupulous standards of hand washing after visiting the toilet inevitably means that these unwelcome and invisible agents are passed on to others.

Unfortunately, not all food handlers are noted for the high standards of their personal hygiene, and unwanted donations are to be expected.

Many different organisms can be transmitted by short- or long-term carriers. These include hepatitis A and B (respectively in stools and blood); staphylococci (in the noses of hospital staff and others); the diphtheria organism, *Corynebacterium diphtheriae*, (in noses and on the skin); and, of course, the human immunodeficiency virus which causes AIDS (in blood and other body secretions).

typhoid fever

A serious infectious disease occurring only in human beings and acquired by consuming food or water contaminated with the organism *Salmonella typhi*. Other Salmonella organisms commonly affect many of the lower animals, but this species occurs only in man. A disease identical to, but usually milder than, typhoid, and known as paratyphoid is caused by different strains of Salmonella.

Typhoid results from the ingestion of organisms derived from the faeces of people with the active disease or from those of symptomless carriers. During the acute illness, the organisms accumulate and multiply in the gall-bladder, and are released in enormous numbers into the bowel to appear in the faeces. In most cases, this gall-bladder reservoir clears up, but in about 3 per cent of cases, the Salmonella continue to multiply there, without causing any symptoms. For many years, often for the rest of their lives, such people remain the source of the disease to others. Such a person is called a **typhoid carrier**. Women carriers exceed men, three to one.

POSSIBLE SOURCES

The organisms can resist freezing and drying and may be transmitted from faeces to food by flies or other insects, or by direct contamination of food, by food-handlers with low standards of personal hygiene. Epidemics have been caused by faecal contamination of tinned meat products. Water supplies are a common source and even ice can transmit the disease. Shellfish may be contaminated by sewage containing infected faeces. It is estimated that about ten million Salmonella organisms are required to cause infection.

RECOGNITION AND SYMPTOMS

Typhoid varies in severity from a mild upset lasting a week to a major illness persisting for two months. Headache is commonly the first symptom and is often severe. Fever, loss of appetite and malaise follow and there is abdominal discomfort, a bloated feeling and constipation. The fever often rises a little higher each day for the first week. As the fever continues, the patient's mind often becomes dulled and there may even be delirium. The initial constipation soon gives way to diarrhoea.

During the second week of the disease a crop of small, raised red spots appears on the front of the chest and upper abdomen. These are called *rose spots* and last for two or three days. At about the same time, the liver and spleen enlarge and may be felt on either side, just below the ribs. The abdomen is always tender but pain is moderate. Severe pain suggests the possibility that the bowel may have perforated causing **peritonitis**. In most cases, symptoms begin to subside after three weeks and the temperature has usually returned to normal by the end of the fourth week.

The diagnosis may be made by culturing the Salmonella organisms directly from the blood during the first week of the disease or later. Organisms may also be cultured from the stools, and sometimes from the urine, especially in the third or fourth week of the disease. Antibodies to *Salmonella typhi* may be detected about a week after the onset and these rise steadily in concentration for several weeks thereafter.

PREVENTION

Because typhoid is an infection confined to human beings, it could, in theory, be eliminated by the identification and treatment of carriers and by the isolation of those with the active disease. Official notification, followed by repeated stool culture, is important. A knowledge of the mode of spread is helpful in prevention. Immunization offers protection against small numbers of the organism, but is overcome by large numbers. Two doses of vaccine are given, at one- or two-week intervals, and a yearly booster dose is needed.

TREATMENT

Typhoid responds well to antibiotic treatment and can usually be brought under control, within a matter of days, with chloramphenicol. Resistance to this drug may occur, but other antibiotics, such as ampicillin, are also effective. In severely ill patients this treatment may have to be supplemented with a dose of corticosteroids.

The serious complication of bowel perforation may be difficult to manage and surgery is avoided if possible. Under adequate antibiotic control, small perforations may seal off spontaneously, but an operation may be necessary if there is widespread peritonitis or severe bleeding. Given early diagnosis and proper treatment, the outlook, for people with typhoid, is usually excellent. Deaths occur mostly in untreated patients, in the old and debilitated, and in those developing major complications such as peritonitis, severe haemorrhages, and liver and kidney failure.

typhus

An infectious disease causing high fever, a mottled rash, severe headache, delirium and coma, and sometimes death. Epidemic, or louse-borne typhus has been known and feared throughout history, killing thousands, especially during times of war when conditions led to close herding of large numbers of refugees. It is now rare except in times of famine and population migration, but occurs in poor areas of tropical Africa, Asia, and South America, especially in the highlands.

Other forms of typhus, spread in different ways, occur in many parts of the world. The quite different disease **typhoid fever** – the name means 'typhus-like' – was often confused with epidemic typhus. All forms of typhus are caused by micro-organisms of the genus Rickettsia, different species of which are transmitted by different insects. Thus, epidemic typhus and trench fever are spread by lice, **Rocky Mountain spotted fever** is spread by ticks, Scrub typhus is transmitted by mites, and endemic typhus by fleas. **Q fever** may be spread by ticks or by inhalation of infected material.

Epidemic typhus is caused by *Rickettsia prowazeki*, which is taken up by human lice feeding on infected patients. When fever occurs, the lice find the host less tolerable and pass to another person. Louse faeces, heavily contaminated with the Rickettsia, are deposited on the skin and are inoculated by scratching. Sometimes the infected faeces are inhaled. Overcrowding and close personal contact greatly encourage spread. Between epidemics, the disease is maintained by mild or inapparent cases and by small mammals such as rats and flying squirrels.

RECOGNITION AND SYMPTOMS

Twelve to fourteen days after infection there is sudden headache, pain in the back and limbs, shivering, cough and constipation. The temperature rises steadily, the face becomes flushed, the eyes red and the mind confused. On the fourth to the sixth day of the disease a measles-like rash appears, usually on the front folds of the armpits and the backs of the hands, and spreads to the flanks and forearms. In the second week the symptoms become increasingly severe, with prostration, weakness of heart action, and often delirium and stupor. The mouth becomes very dry and the tongue shrunken, and pneumonia often develops. In untreated cases, death, from toxaemia, heart or kidney failure, or pneumonia, is common.

TREATMENT

Antibiotics are effective and life-saving in typhus. One of the tetracyclines is commonly used. General measures to control fever and relieve headache are also required. Severe headache may necessitate lumbar puncture and delirium may require control by drugs. Oxygen may be needed in pneumonia.

tyrothricin

An antibiotic obtained from the soil bacterium *Bacillus brevis* and used by local application to treat gram positive infections and mouth and throat infections. It is too toxic for systemic use. It is formulated with benzocaine under the brand name Tyrozets.

Tyrozets

A brand name for throat lozenges containing tyrothricin and the local anaesthetic drug benzocaine.

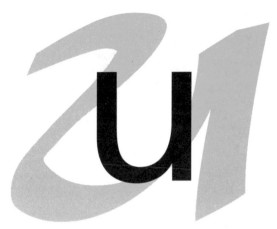

Ubretid

A brand name for **distigmine**.

Ukidan

A brand name for **urokinase**.

ulcer

An area of the skin or of a mucous membrane that has lost its surface covering as a result of local destruction of tissue, an open sore. Once the protection of the surface layers has gone, infection is inevitable and this often makes the ulcer worse. Ulcers may be caused by mechanical, chemical or biochemical damage, by loss of blood supply and by bacterial or other infection. Ulcers of the stomach or intestine (gastrointestinal tract) are called **peptic ulcers**.

Sustained pressure over bony points, as occurs when a debilitated person lies unmoving for long periods, interferes with the local blood supply and causes **bedsores** (decubitus ulcers). Arterial diseases such as **atherosclerosis** can so reduce blood supply to a limb, that the skin readily breaks down to form ulcers. This is also more likely in **diabetes**. Skin ulcers are commonly caused by bacterial toxins, such as those produced by the organisms of **anthrax, tuberculosis, diphtheria** or syphilis (chancre).

Leg ulcers are common in cases of severe **varicose veins**. In this condition, blood stagnates and the nutrition and oxygenation of the skin and underlying tissue suffer. For the same reasons, varicose ulcers are often very persistent and slow to heal.

See also **tropical ulcers**.

ulcerative colitis

A disease of unknown cause, usually occurring between the ages of twenty and forty and featuring recurrent attacks of abdominal discomfort, diarrhoea with blood, mucus and pus in the stools, and a constant desire to empty the bowels (tenesmus). When severe, the attacks may be exhausting and the loss of fluid so great that dehydration results. After many attacks, the bowel becomes permanently damaged by internal scarring and becomes rigid and unable either to reabsorb water from the contents or to store faeces. This scar tissue can sometimes resemble cancer of the large intestine (colon).

RECOGNITION

In ulcerative colitis the lining of the colon becomes inflamed, swollen and extensively ulcerated. The ulcers may be deep and may spread sideways under the surface of the lining.

Sometimes parts of the lining are destroyed and come away and the bowel may be dangerously thinned. Perforation of the bowel may occur.

> Ulcerative colitis predisposes to cancer of the colon: in people with widespread severe disease the risk of cancer may be increased by forty times. Careful follow-up can detect the majority in time for treatment to be effective.

TREATMENT

The condition is treated with corticosteroid drugs, given locally in the form of suppositories or enemas, or given by mouth. These are very effective in controlling attacks. In severe and worrying cases they may be given by intravenous injection. A less effective, but useful, drug is salazopyrin. In some cases it is necessary to remove the affected parts of the bowel surgically.

ulcers, stress-activated

See **stress ulcers**.

Ulcol

A brand name for **sulphasalazine**.

-ule

Suffix meaning 'diminutive' as in papule (little bubble).

-ulous

Suffix meaning 'tending to' as in edentulous (almost without teeth).

Ultralente MC

A brand name for a long-acting **insulin**.

ultrasound in arteries

See **intravascular ultrasonography**.

ultrasound scanning

Unlike electromagnetic radiations such as X-rays and gamma rays which pass easily through a vacuum, sound is a vibration of the molecules of a gas, liquid or solid. Vibrations between about 16 cycles per second (Hz) and 20,000 cycles per second are perceptible as sound, but we are deaf to those of a higher frequency. Audible sound waves have long wavelengths –

often several metres long – and can only be reflected by very large surfaces, such as the side of a mountain, causing echoes. The higher the frequency of the vibration, the shorter the wavelength and the smaller the area needed for reflection.

In ultrasound scanning, a beam of 'sound' – of a frequency of about three to ten million cycles per second – is projected into the body. Whenever it meets a surface between tissues of different density, echoes are created and these return to the source. The time taken to do so depends on the distance. The ultrasound waves are produced by feeding short pulses of alternating current, at the frequency desired, to a piezoelectric crystal in the scanner head. The electrical variations cause the crystal to vibrate at the same frequency. Piezoelectric materials have the property of working in both directions – they change shape when electricity is applied to them, but they also generate electricity if their shape is distorted. So the returning echoes cause the crystal to act as a microphone and this, in turn, generates a tiny electric current. The length of time between the emitted pulse and the returning echo is a measure of the distance to the interface. Any device which converts one mode of energy into another is called a transducer and this is the term used for the scanner head.

The earliest scanners used a simple cathode-ray tube display which merely showed a series of 'blips' on a horizontal line, corresponding to returning echoes ('A' scan). These were capable of highly accurate measurements, but did not produce any pictorial representation. In the next development ('B' scan), the ultrasound was focused into a narrow parallel beam which was scanned from side to side in one plane of the body. The returning echoes were correlated, in a computer, with the corresponding angle of the beam, and this enabled a two-dimensional picture to be built up. Later developments of great sophistication have produced ever higher resolution and great improvement in the standards of the display. Even so, ultrasound scans are still only representations of interfaces and require to be interpreted by experts. The quality of resolution is much poorer than CT scans or MRI and it is mainly their high safety level that recommends them.

So far as is known, ultrasound, of the intensity and frequency used in scanning, is completely harmless. There are no recorded instances of any damage being caused, and millions of pregnant women, and their fetuses, have had scans with no apparent indications of harm. Ultrasound of higher intensity can, however, cause tissue warming and is sometimes used for treatment purposes by physiotherapists, so ultrasound is not entirely free from internal effect.

A report in the *Lancet* in October 1993 suggested that women who had repeated examinations of a type known as continuous-wave Doppler flow studies might produce babies which, on average, were slightly smaller than those of women who had not had repeated ultrasound examinations. The authors did not suggest that this method of examination, which provides valuable information on the flow of blood in the placenta, should not be used, but advised that repeated examinations of this type should be limited to women in whom the information obtained was likely to be of clinical benefit.

Routine ultrasound screening significantly reduces birth mortality, mainly through the early detection of fetal abnormalities.

USES IN OBSTETRICS

This is one of the chief applications of ultrasound scanning and, today, the majority of pregnant women are screened by ultrasound, usually around the 16th to 20th week of pregnancy.

Ultrasound can detect twins, can confirm that the fetus is of a size appropriate to the stage of pregnancy, can detect major fetal abnormalities such as anencephaly and spina bifida. It can even measure the rates of blood flow through the heart valves and the large arteries of the fetus and can sometimes detect certain forms of congenital heart disease. The position of the afterbirth (placenta) can be determined and trouble from malposition, such as placenta praevia, anticipated. Ultrasound is also used to facilitate amniocentesis, fetal blood sampling, chorionic villus sampling and fetoscopy.

Under ultrasound control, fetal blood samples can be obtained through a fine tube, and analysed to detect coagulation disorders, infections, haemoglobin abnormalities and immunodeficiency disorders. Antibody levels, in the blood, can provide indications of infections such as rubella and toxoplasmosis. Biopsies can be taken for pathological examination. Exchange blood transfusion in rhesus disease can be done in the uterus, drug treatment given, and even certain forms of surgery performed – all under ultrasound visualization.

OTHER USES

Ultrasound is useful for examining fluid-filled organs such as the gall-bladder, and soft organs, such as the liver, pancreas and kidneys. Gallstones and kidney stones are easily detected. Cirrhosis of the liver, liver cysts, abscesses and tumours can all be readily displayed. Echocardiography is a sophisticated method of heart examination which reveals the heart's action in detail in scans taken from different directions. Defects of the heart valves and changes in the walls of the main pumping chambers (ventricles) are shown.

Ultrasound waves cannot easily pass through bone or gas, so parts of the body surrounded by bone – such as the brain and spinal cord – cannot be studied by this means. The lungs and the intestines are also unsuitable for ultrasound examination.

ultrasound scanning via vagina

See **transvaginal ultrasound**.

ultrasound treatment

A method of physiotherapy in which high-frequency sound waves are used to achieve a degree of deep heating of inflamed soft tissues such as muscles, tendons and ligaments. Local heat has some limited value in inflammation, by dilating blood vessels and improving the blood supply. This is helpful in inflammation caused by infection, as tissue nutrition is improved and the supply of antibodies and combating white cells is increased. The value of ultrasound treatment in the management of soft-tissue injury, without infection, is less clear.

Ultratard

A brand name for a long-acting form of **insulin**.

ultraviolet light

Electromagnetic radiation of shorter wavelengths than visible light, but longer wavelength than X-rays. Ultraviolet light (UVL) is invisible to the human eye and is sometimes called black light. The spectrum of UVL is arbitrarily divided into three zones. That nearest to visible light (UVA) covers wavelengths from 380 down to 320 nanometres (billionths of a metre); UVB extends from 320 down to 290; and UVC from 290 down to one-tenth of a nanometre. UVC is especially penetrating and harmful to human tissue but is strongly absorbed by the ozone layer in the earth's stratosphere. Most of the UVB content is also filtered out by this layer.

RISKS

Ultraviolet light causes sunburning and, in excessive dosage, can damage the elastic protein, collagen, in the skin, leading to excessive wrinkling and premature ageing. UVL is also a major factor in the development of the skin condition solar keratosis, and the skin cancers **rodent ulcer**, **malignant melanoma** and **squamous cell carcinoma**. The eyes are especially susceptible to UVL because of the transparency of the outer tissues. **Pingueculas** and **pterygium** are the result of excessive exposure to UVL. Although the incidence of **cataract** is much higher in areas of high sunlight than in temperate zones, there is no clear evidence that UVL causes cataract.

Fluorescent and mercury-vapour lamps can produce large amounts of UVL, but there is no biological danger from ordinary domestic fluorescent lighting. Artificially produced UVC can be used to sterilize air and the surface of materials.

uncertain sex

See **pseudohermaphroditism**.

unconscious

A person's total data storage, in memory, is very great and, if present in consciousness at all times, would be overwhelming and disabling. Most of these data must, therefore, be held in a data store which is accessible only when needed. Processing of these data also occurs without conscious awareness and we are regularly able to draw on the new information derived from correlation and association of information. These facts have been self-evident through the ages and it has also been apparent that the information in the unconscious mind has a profound effect on behaviour.

The work of Freud drew general attention to these matters and prompted much thought and speculation as to the real nature of the unconscious mind. By no means all of his assertions, however intriguing and interesting they may be, are generally accepted. Freud's model divided the mind into conscious, preconscious and unconscious regions. The conscious mind contained ideas of which one was immediately aware; the preconscious mind contained ideas, not currently in consciousness, but immediately accessible by directing attention to them; and the unconscious mind had a content that was not accessible because it was unacceptable and thus repressed.

Freud saw the unconscious as a dark world of primitive urges and desires, constantly struggling for expression and fulfilment and able to surface only in dreams, everyday errors and psychoneurotic symptoms.

unconsciousness

A state of unrousability caused by temporary or permanent damage to brain function and associated with reduced activity of the nerve cells and fibres in the part of the brain stem called the *reticular formation*. Levels of unconsciousness vary from a very light state, in which movements or even protesting sounds are made when the unconscious person is disturbed or subjected to pain, to a state of profound **coma** in which even the strongest stimuli evoke no response.

POSSIBLE CAUSES

Causes of unconsciousness include: **head injury**; inadequacy of blood supply to the brain from arterial disease, **thrombo-**sis, **embolism** or fainting; poisoning; asphyxia; near drowning; starvation; lowered blood sugar (**hypoglycaemia**); diabetic **ketosis**.

TREATMENT

See *First Aid*.

undecylenic acid

An antifungal drug used to treat external fungal infections. A brand name is Tineafax.

Unicap T

A brand name for a multivitamin and mineral preparation.

Unihep

A brand name for the anticoagulant **heparin**.

Unimycin

A brand name for antibiotic drug oxytetracycline.

Uniparin

A brand name for **heparin**.

Unipine XL

A brand name for **nifedipine**.

Unisomnia

A brand name for **nitrazepam**.

Univer

A brand name for the calcium channel blocker drug **verapamil**.

unstable angina

A severe and dangerous form of angina pectoris due to breakdown of a plaque of atherosclerosis in the coronary arteries and the formation of blood clot (thrombosis) on the raw surface. There may also be coronary artery spasm from products derived from blood **platelets**. Pain becomes more frequent and prolonged, and may occur at rest. The accurate predictability of pain onset in terms of its relation to a given amount of exertion is lost, and the risk of a heart attack is high.

upper respiratory tract infection

This group includes any infection of the nose, throat, sinuses and larynx. Upper respiratory tract infections are among the commonest of all illnesses, especially in young children, the most familiar being the common **cold**, sore throat (**pharyngitis**), **tonsillitis**, **sinusitis**, **laryngitis** and **croup**.

uraemia

The result of failure of the kidneys to excrete nitrogenous waste so that it accumulates dangerously in the blood causing a range of effects. These include nausea and vomiting, **oedema** of the tissues, an increased tendency to bleeding, anaemia, itching, apathy, mental confusion, twitching of muscles, seizures, drowsiness and coma. If unrelieved, uraemia is fatal. Blood analysis shows high levels of urea, uric acid, phosphorus and creatinine.

Urantoin

Kidney failure will, in most cases, be diagnosed early and an artificial kidney (haemodialysis) used to maintain the normal state of the blood so that uraemia does not occur. If a person is found to have uraemia, dialysis is urgently indicated, together with full investigation into the cause.

Urantoin

A brand name for the antibacterial drug nitrofurantoin.

Uremide

A brand name for **frusemide**.

ureteric colic

See **renal colic**.

ureterolithotomy

The removal of a stone from the tube (the ureter) which carries urine down from the kidney to the bladder. This may be done by open operation or by crushing the stone, under direct vision, through a cystoscope. Such stones are now commonly dealt with by shock wave **lithotripsy**.

urethral discharge

The appearance of yellow pus, mucus and pus (*muco-pus*) or clear mucus at the opening of the urine tube (urethra). Urethral discharge suggests one of the **sexually transmitted diseases** such as gonorrhoea or chlamydial non-specific urethritis, but need not necessarily imply this. Sexual interest or excitement promotes a crystal-clear discharge of lubricating mucus from the urethra in the male. This is normal. A yellow discharge appearing a few days after a new sexual contact is almost certainly a sign of a sexually transmitted disease.

urethral stricture

A local narrowing of the bore of the tube leading from the urinary bladder to the exterior (urethra). Urethral stricture was once the common sequel to untreated or inadequately treated gonorrhoea (see **sexually transmitted diseases**) but is now uncommon. Stricture can seriously interfere with the outflow of urine and can lead to back-pressure effects which can damage the kidneys. It may be treated by repeated dilatations with a solid, round-tipped instrument (a *bougie*), or by an operation to remove scar tissue or reconstruct the urethra.

urethral syndrome

A condition, mainly affecting women, in which symptoms suggesting cystitis or urethritis occur but in which no infecting organisms can be found in the urine. There are several possible causes including local allergies and congestion of the urethra from sexual intercourse.

urethritis

See **sexually transmitted diseases**.

When the bladder has had to be removed provision must be made for disposal of urine. In (a) the ureters have been implanted into the lower end of the large intestine. In (b) an artificial bladder has been fashioned from an isolated length of bowel.

urethroplasty

Plastic surgical repair of the urine outlet tube (urethra).

Urex

A brand name for **frusemide**.

Uriben

A brand name for the antibacterial drug **nalidixic acid**.

urina

Latin root meaning 'urine' as in urinary (of urine or urinary system).

urinal

A container into which urine can conveniently be passed for subsequent disposal. Urinals are used only by men and are useful for the bedridden or the frail. Incontinent men may use an appliance consisting of a thick condom connected by a tube to a plastic drainage bag attached to the leg.

urinary bladder, disorders of

The commonest bladder disorder is **cystitis** – an infection more frequent in women than in men because women have a much shorter urine output tube (urethra) than men and germs can get into the bladder more easily. Cystitis is also promoted after the menopause by oestrogen deficiency causing vaginal changes that encourage infection.

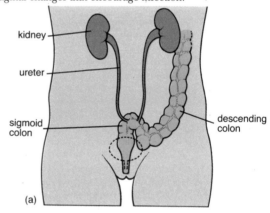

(a)

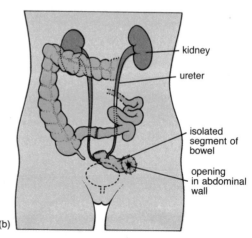

(b)

Another distressing disorder is obstruction to urinary outflow. This is essentially a male problem and is one of the commonest disorders of elderly men (see **prostate gland, disorders of**). Bladder stones, too, can cause obstruction and commonly result in infection, but many remain unrecognized. Most bladder stones consist of aggregated crystals of calcium oxalate or uric acid. The ancient operation of 'cutting for the stone' (lithotomy) has now been largely replaced by internal crushing or the use of focused shock waves of ultrasound (extracorporeal **lithotripsy**).

Rupture of the bladder is rare but may occur in the course of a severe crushing injury, such as a car accident, if the bladder is full. See also **bladder cancer**, **incontinence, urinary**.

urinary catheterization

The passage of a blunt-ended, rubber or plastic tube along the urine outlet tube (urethra) into the bladder so as to release urine in cases of obstruction to outflow or inability to pass urine voluntarily for other reasons (urinary retention). See also **catheterization**, **intermittent** and **suprapubic catheterization**.

urinary diversion

When the normal temporary storage or outflow of urine is interfered with by disease, injury or necessary surgical treatment such as removal of the bladder, it is essential that the urine coming from the kidneys should be redirected. Such redirection is called urinary diversion and may be done, either temporarily or permanently, by bringing the urine tubes (ureters) out on to the surface of the abdomen, or implanting them into the colon or the rectum, or into a substitute bladder formed from a loop of small bowel, with an outlet through the skin or the anus.

Several bowel implant operations have been designed but, because of the probability of infection passing upwards to the kidneys, and the strong tendency for the new connections to become narrowed, none of these is entirely satisfactory. The more elaborate procedures with an isolated loop of bowel can give better results.

urinary drainage system

From each kidney, a tube, called a ureter, descends to the back of the lower part of the urinary bladder. The ureters are distensible and contain circular muscle fibres by which they can milk urine downwards. A kidney stone in the ureter stimulates powerful contraction of these muscles and causes great pain.

The bladder is a muscular bag situated in the midline of the pelvis at the lowest point in the abdomen, immediately behind the pubic bone. It continuously receives urine from the kidneys, by way of the two ureters, relaxing progressively to accommodate the urine, and storing it until it may conveniently be disposed of. A full bladder contains about 350 ml of urine and, in spite of pressure, this is retained by the sustained contraction of the first part of the outlet tube (urethra) which acts as a compression cock (sphincter). Under normal circumstances, the accumulation of urine occurs unconsciously until the pressure in the bladder reaches a level of about 20 cm of water, at which point the desire to urinate obtrudes on consciousness. Voluntary relaxation of the sphincter allows the urine to pass to the outside by way of the urethra. If this signal is ignored, the bladder relaxes a little and the impulse ceases. This sequence then repeats at ever shorter intervals until there

is a continuous and urgent demand for release, accompanied by rhythmical contraction of the bladder muscle, and controlled only by a major effort on the part of the now wholly preoccupied subject. Eventually, whatever the circumstances, at a pressure of about 100 cm of water, the sphincter relaxes and the bladder empties spontaneously by way of the urethra. The urethra occupies the underside of the penis in the male. In the female it runs down just in front of the front wall of the vagina, opening between the vagina and the clitoris.

urinary infection

See **cystitis**, **pyelonephritis**.

urinary system function investigation

See **urodynamics**.

urinary system X-ray

See **urography**.

urination, excessive

Production of excessive quantities of urine, or *polyuria*, may simply be due to the excessive intake of fluid, as in the common case of the over-enthusiastic beer drinker, but it can also be a sign of diseases such as **diabetes mellitus**, **diabetes insipidus** or certain diseases of the kidney, known as 'salt-losing' states. Excessive urine output also occurs when **oedema** from any cause is treated with diuretic drugs to get rid of the excess fluid accumulated in the tissues of the body.

Excessive urination is not necessarily the same as abnormally frequent urination. In the latter, it is common for the affected person to be able to pass only small quantities of urine on each occasion. Frequency of this kind may be stimulated by the irritation of a bladder infection (**cystitis**). In elderly men, the commonest cause is enlargement of the **prostate gland** which so obstructs urine outflow that only a small quantity can be passed each time. As a result, the desire to urinate soon recurs.

urination, painful

This is always abnormal and should be reported. The pain experienced, which is usually described in such terms as 'burning' or 'scalding', is often accompanied by difficulty in getting starting or by a sense of not being quite finished. *Dysuria*, as it is known medically, is most commonly caused by bladder infection (**cystitis**), but has several other possible causes. These include:

- urethritis;
- inflammation of the prostate gland (prostatitis);
- inflammation of the glans of the penis (balanitis);
- **candidiasis** of the vulva;
- bladder polyps;
- bladder cancer;
- stone in the bladder;
- the passage of blood clots or small urinary stones.

Even highly concentrated urine, as may occur in fever or excessive fluid loss in sweat, may cause discomfort.

> Persistent pain on urination should never be neglected.

urine

On average, a little over 1 ml of urine is formed per minute with a daily output of 1200 to 2000 ml. This figure varies greatly with variations in fluid intake and the amount of sweating.

Urine is usually acid and contains creatinine and various products of blood breakdown. The yellow colour comes from the pigment urochrome. The constituents of the urine vary characteristically in various diseases and laboratory examination of it can provide valuable information.

Urine is a solution in water of many organic and inorganic substances, most of which are the waste products of the chemical processes occurring in the course of the buildup and breakdown of body substances (metabolism). By getting rid of these waste products and by adjusting the rate of loss of water from the body, urine production accurately controls the internal state of the body (the milieu) and maintains a remarkable constancy in the composition and amount of the body fluids.

Healthy urine is crystal clear but will vary considerably in density of colour depending on its concentration. This, in turn, depends on the requirement for fluid loss. If the body is relatively short of water, the urine will be concentrated and dark; if water is plentiful, the urine is dilute and light-coloured. Urine normally has a specific gravity in the range 1.017 to 1.020. After heavy sweating and inadequate fluid replacement, the urine can, however, also be affected by certain items in the diet and by certain drugs.

About 60 per cent of the dissolved substances are organic materials including urea, uric acid, creatinine and ammonia. About 40 per cent are inorganic, mainly sodium chloride, potassium, calcium, phosphates and sulphates. Urine is usually slightly acid but this, too, is affected by the diet. Its acidity or alkalinity is adjusted automatically so as to correct any tendency for the internal milieu to move away from neutrality.

One of the most important constituents of urine is urea. The formation of this substance by the liver, and its elimination in the urine, is the method by which the body gets rid of excess nitrogenous material formed from amino acids when protein is broken down. About half of the molecular weight of urea consists of nitrogen and about 30 grams of urea is lost each day by the average meat-eating male. In the condition of kidney failure, the levels of urea in the blood rise to dangerous levels and, unless removed by dialysis, the outcome is a fatal uraemia.

Another important constituent, uric acid, is the main metabolic end-product of the breakdown of the purine bases adenine and guanine – two of the four bases that form the genetic code in DNA. Uric acid is not readily soluble and can crystallize out within the body if, for any reason, the levels in the body become too high. In the condition of gout, the crystallization occurs in the joints.

urine opening on underside of penis

See **hypospadias**.

urine release, emergency

See **suprapubic catheterization**.

urine release, self-help

See **urinary catheterization**.

urine retention

The inability to pass urine voluntarily or to empty a full bladder. This is a problem predominantly affecting males. There is constant discomfort or pain in the lower abdomen and the bladder can often be felt as a swelling above the pubis.

POSSIBLE CAUSES

Retention may be due to an actual mechanical obstruction to the outflow of urine, as in **phimosis**, from a tight prepuce in small boys, urethral stricture from gonorrhea, inflammation of the prostate (prostatitis) in young adult males, or enlarged prostate in elderly men. The latter may be due to simple enlargement (benign hypertrophy) or to cancer of the prostate. Retention is common in bedridden people, especially after surgery, and particularly in elderly men who have been given large quantities of fluids so that excessive distention of the bladder occurs.

Retention of urine may also be due to a disease of the nervous system involving the spinal cord or the nerves supplying the bladder. More commonly it may be due to a temporary nervous system defect resulting from the use of drugs that relax the bladder wall and tighten the urinary sphincters, or to a surgical operation or a general or spinal anaesthetic.

Urinary retention is uncommon in women but may be due to narrowing of the urethra from infection, pressure from uterine fibroids, obstruction from cancer, or neurological or psychological causes.

urine tests

See **kidney tests**.

Urisal

A brand name for sodium citrate, a drug used to make the urine less acid.

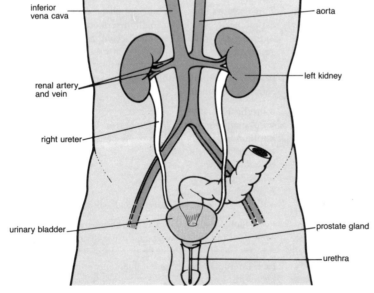

The urinary system.

Urispas

A brand name for the urinary **antispasm** drug flavoxate.

urodynamics

The quality of functioning of the urinary bladder, the output control muscle ring (urethral sphincter) and the pelvic floor muscles. Urodynamic studies, which may be made in various ways, involve measurement, over a period, of such parameters as:

- urine flow rates;
- total bladder capacity;
- bladder urine volume before voiding;
- residual urine volume;
- bladder pressure before and during voiding;
- bladder contractability;
- urethral sphincter pressure;
- patient's perception of bladder fullness;
- ability to inhibit voiding.

urography

X-ray examination of the urinary system using a substance in the urine that is opaque to X-rays (a contrast medium) to show the outline of the interior of the urinary drainage system and the bladder. The contrast medium is usually an iodine-containing solution given either by way of a vein (intravenous urography) or passed back up the tubes from the bladder to the kidneys (ureters) using a fine tube inserted through a cystoscope (see **cystoscopy**). The latter procedure is called retrograde urography.

urokinase

An enzyme found in human urine that is used as a drug to dissolve blood clots occurring within blood vessels. Urokinase is a member of the class of plasminogen activators. The actual enzyme that breaks down the clots is plasmin. Urikinase converts plasminogen to plasmin.

urological surgeon

A surgeon who specializes in the diagnosis and treatment of disorders of the kidneys, the urine drainage system and the prostate gland.

urologist

A doctor trained in the medical and surgical treatment of disorders of the kidney, urinary bladder and urethra, and also concerned with disorders of the male sexual organs, including **sexually transmitted diseases**. In recent years, urologists have become deeply involved in the AIDS epidemic.

The urologist treats many patients with bladder disorders, the emphasis being on cystitis and incontinence in women and prostate problems in men. Urological investigations involve X-rays using dyes that are opaque to X-rays (contrast media) given either by injection (intravenous pyelogram, or IVP) or passed back up the ureters from the bladder (retrograde pyelogram). The urologist frequently examines the interior of the bladder using an illuminating endoscope (cystoscope), under general anaesthesia, and is by this means able to diagnose conditions such as bladder polyps, stones and cancers, and to take biopsy specimens.

A major concern of the urologist is benign prostatic enlargement (hypertrophy) in men. This is treated surgically by prostatectomy, usually through the urethra itself (transurethral prostatectomy), but sometimes through the bladder via an incision in the lower part of the abdomen, or directly by way of an incision through the skin immediately behind the scrotum. The urologist also treats cancer of the prostate, using similar methods, but also by removal of the testicles (**orchidectomy**) to get rid of the male sex hormone-producing cells, and by the use of female sex hormones (oestrogens).

Uromide

A brand name for a mixture of the pain-relieving drug phenazopyridine and the sulphonamide drug sulphaurea, used to treat urinary infections.

Uromitexan

A brand name for **mesna**.

uron

Greek root meaning 'urine' as in urinary (of urine or the urinary system).

Uro-Tainer

A brand name for a fluid containing the antiseptic **mandelic acid**.

Ursofalk

A brand name for ursodeoxycholic acid.

URTI

See **upper respiratory tract infection**.

urticaria

An allergic skin condition commonly called 'nettle rash' or 'hives'. Urticaria features raised, intensely itchy, pinkish areas, surrounded by paler areas of skin, which last for half an hour to several days and then disappear completely.

POSSIBLE CAUSES

It can be caused by heat, cold, sunlight, food allergy, drug allergy, parasitic infestation such as **scabies**, insect bites, jellyfish stings and contact with plants. Apart from the latter, contact urticaria is rare, as is urticaria from inhaled allergens. In many cases, the cause of urticaria is not apparent. Emotional factors are often cited as being a cause, but this is uncertain; urticaria often induces a major emotional reaction.

TREATMENT

Short-term (acute) urticaria is treated with antihistamine drugs or sometimes with steroids. In very severe cases these drugs may have to be given urgently by injection.

Persistent (chronic) urticaria is often more difficult to treat and the sufferer's diet may have to be carefully analysed for possible stimulating factors (allergens). These may include a variety of foods, food dyes such as tartrazine, food preservatives, yeast, nickel, aspirin, penicillin and other drugs. Long-term antihistamine treatment may be needed, but side-effects, such as drowsiness, may be a problem.

uterine dystocia

Inadequately strong and badly coordinated womb contractions during childbirth. Dystocia affects about 4 per cent of all births and is one of the commonest indications for emergency Caesarean section. The cause often remains obscure.

uterine tube

See **Fallopian tube**.

uterus

Latin root meaning 'womb' as in uterus (womb).

uterus, cancer of

CERVICAL CANCER
INCIDENCE

Cancer of the neck of the womb (cervix) is a common female cancer, second only to cancer of the breast. After falling steadily for many years, the incidence and mortality have now started to rise steeply in young women.

> Over 2000 women die each year in Britain from cancer of the cervix and the disease is becoming commoner. In the United States about 13,500 new cases of invasive cervical cancer occur every year and about 40 per cent of these eventually die from the disease. These deaths are particularly tragic when one considers how accessible is the site of the cancer and how easily it can be detected in the early stages if it is looked for.

RECOGNITION AND SYMPTOMS

Cancer of the cervix is preceded, *for many years,* by a recognizable and easily diagnosable pre-invasive condition, known as *carcinoma in situ* (CIN). About 55,000 cases of CIN occur each year in the USA. Half of all cancers of the female reproductive system are in the cervix.

Unfortunately, cancer of the cervix often causes no symptoms until it has spread and may, indeed, cause no symptoms at all before reaching an incurable stage. Sometimes there is bleeding between periods or following sexual intercourse, but there are no dramatic early signs. Pain and general upset are rare until a late stage is reached. The moral is clear: cancer of the cervix has to be looked for. **Cervical smear** screening (Pap test) for the precancerous stage should be done on all women.

Practical considerations dictate some restrictions, but those especially at risk should have the test at least every five years, or more often if abnormalities are found. Pap smear tests should ideally be accompanied by microscopic examination of the cervix (colposcopy). This allows accurate localization of the abnormal surface tissue.

POSSIBLE CAUSES AND RISK FACTORS

Cigarette smoking and exposure to cigarette smoke (passive smoking) is associated with a raised incidence of cervical cancer, but the strongest positive correlation is with a history of **sexually transmitted disease**. Cancer of the cervix is commonest in women with genital warts, those who have had many sexual partners, or whose sexual partner has genital warts, those who smoke heavily, or who became pregnant at an early age and who have had three or more pregnancies. Two viruses are implicated – the human papilloma (wart) virus, and the Herpes simplex (genital herpes) virus. There have also been suggestions that some men have carcinogenic sperm.

TREATMENT

Established cancer is difficult to treat successfully and there is no firm agreement on the relative merits of surgery or radiotherapy. Radiotherapy is widely used and this is usually provided by means of sealed containers of radioactive caesium or radium that are placed in the vault of the vagina and in the cavity of the womb. The curability depends on the extent of spread at the time of diagnosis. Early cancer, confined to the cervix, offers an excellent prognosis, with a cure rate of over 85 per cent. But if there has been spread to the vagina and surrounding tissues, the cure rate drops to about 50 per cent. Extensive spread to the organs of the pelvis, and remote spread to other parts of the body, have a very poor outlook. In only about 10 per cent of such cases is the patient still alive five years later.

ENDOMETRIAL CANCER
INCIDENCE

Cancer of the lining of the womb (endometrial cancer) has quite different features from cervical cancer and is much less common. It is essentially a disease of older women and occurs most often between the ages of fifty and seventy. It is commoner in women who have not had children. The peak incidence is at age sixty-one.

POSSIBLE CAUSES AND RISK FACTORS

It affects mostly those who, in spite of being postmenopausal, have high blood levels of oestrogen. Known risk factors are a late menopause, obesity, certain cysts of the ovary, ovarian tumours that secrete oestrogen, and oestrogen **hormone replacement therapy** (HRT) unopposed by progesterone.

> The first sign is usually irregular bleeding from the vagina or a blood-stained discharge. This is a critically important sign after the menopause and must never be ignored.

RECOGNITION AND SYMPTOMS

Again, early diagnosis is essential. This is done by a **D and C**. If the diagnosis is made reasonably early and **hysterectomy**, with removal of the Fallopian tubes and ovaries, is done, the outlook is usually excellent. Some endometrial cancers, however, are highly malignant and rapidly invasive; in these cases the outlook is much less favourable. Surgery may be supplemented with radiotherapy.

uterus, disorders of

Congenital abnormalities of the womb (uterus) affect about one woman in 100. Most of these are minor and unimportant, but sometimes the uterus is absent, doubled, or divided into two separate halves by a partition. Infections of the lining of the uterus may follow trauma, as in illegal attempts at **abortion**, or may occur in the raw area left when the placenta separates after childbirth. **Cervicitis** may be caused by gonorrhoea, syphilis or a chlamydial or herpes infection. **Cervical erosion** is a popular misconception and, although common, is usually unimportant.

Functional disorders of the lining of the womb (endometrium) are mostly menstrual disorders of endocrine origin. Overgrowth (hyperplasia) and atrophies are common as is the growth of areas of uterine lining elsewhere in the abdomen (**endometriosis**).

Cancer of the womb, especially of the cervix, is a common and important disorder. Cancer of the lining is less common. (See **uterus, cancer of**.) Tumours of the body of the uterus are common and most of them are benign. The commonest tumours are **fibroids** (leiomyomas), which affect 10 per cent of women of reproductive age. They are benign growths of smooth muscle and fibrous tissue, of widely varying size, which may be symptomless or may cause abnormal bleeding. Large fibroids may have local pressure effects on other organs and may interfere with pregnancy, labour or delivery. Endometrial polyps are benign, single or multiple masses which often bleed.

Other disorders include downward displacement (see **uterus, prolapse of**), and backward displacement (see **uterus, retroverted**).

uterus, prolapse of

A prolapse is a sinking down of an organ from its normal position. The womb is normally retained in position by various ligaments by which it is suspended from the walls of the pelvis.

POSSIBLE CAUSES

Prolapse is very rare in women who have not had children, and the more children born, the more likely it becomes. It is almost always due to damage to these supporting structures which can be stretched and permanently lengthened during pregnancy. This is not the sole cause, however, as prolapse often does not occur until after the menopause, and it must be assumed that further weakening, from the usual postmenopausal genital atrophy is necessary.

RECOGNITION AND SYMPTOMS

These changes may allow the womb to descend. As it does so it turns the vagina inside out. A descent into the vagina only is called a first degree prolapse; if the womb protrudes beyond the vaginal opening the prolapse is said to be of the second degree. In a third degree prolapse the whole uterus remains outside and the surface becomes dried, whitened and thickened.

Prolapse of the womb causes a distressing feeling of lack of support down below and there may even be a sense that something is coming down. Because the womb and the bladder are closely adjacent, prolapse causes distortion of the latter and commonly leads to **incontinence** and **cystitis**.

TREATMENT

The treatment of prolapse involves a surgical operation to strengthen the floor of the pelvis and to shorten and tighten the supporting ligaments. In very severe cases, removal of the uterus (**hysterectomy**) may be advised. In women who do not wish surgery or in whom surgery is thought undesirable, the womb may often be kept in place by means of a polythene ring pessary that stretches the back wall of the vagina upwards.

uterus, retroverted

The canal of the womb is usually directed forwards at about a right angle to the canal of the vagina. If the two are in line, or if the womb canal is directed backwards, the uterus is said to be *retroverted*. This is the case in about one woman in five. The discovery of a retroverted uterus used to be taken to be an explanation for all sorts of symptoms, from backache to painful intercourse (dyspareunia), and was even assumed to be a cause of infertility. Gynaecologists now know better and these myths have been dispelled. The condition is now considered entirely normal.

> Retroversion can be caused by some other gynaecological disorder and this condition may be causing symptoms. In such a case, full investigation is called for.

Uticillin

A brand name for the penicillin-type antibiotic carfecillin.

Utinor

A brand name for **norfloxacin**.

Utovian

A brand name for **norethisterone**.

uveitis

Uvea is the Greek word for a peeled black grape and this is the appearance of the layer of the eye under the white outer coat (the sclera). This layer, called the uvea or uveal tract, consists of the choroid, the ciliary body near the front of the eye, and the coloured iris diaphragm. Acute uveitis is a short-term or severe inflammation of the uvea – mainly in the iris and the circular muscle at its root. Uveitis is not an infection, but usually an immunological problem.

RECOGNITION AND SYMPTOMS

The pupil on the affected side is smaller than the other and often of irregular outline. The iris may appear to be of a slightly different colour from the healthy one. There is blurring or mistiness of vision and, almost always, a dull aching pain in the eye itself.

TREATMENT

Treatment is urgent because in uveitis the iris forms adhesions to the front surface of the crystalline lens behind it and if these become firm, permanent damage will result. Such adhesions can cause acute glaucoma and must at all costs be avoided.

Prolapse of the womb (uterus) may occur to varying degrees. In a first degree prolapse (a) the cervix remains well up in the vagina; in a second degree prolapse (b) the cervix reaches the outlet; and in a third degree prolapse (c) the whole of the uterus is external.

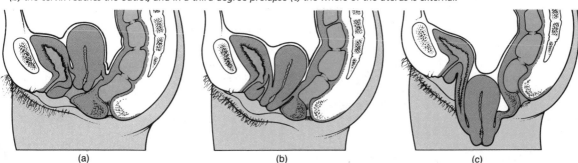

(a)   (b)   (c)

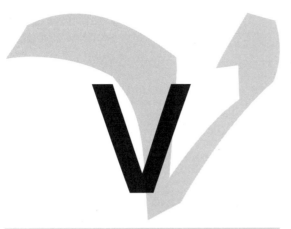

vaccination

See **immunization**.

vaccinia

A mild disease, sometimes called 'cowpox', which affects the udders of cows and the hands of milkmaids. In the 1790s, the British physician Edward Jenner (1749–1823) overheard a milkmaid state that she could never get smallpox because she had had the cowpox, and it was this that led him to conduct his successful experiments with vaccination, using vaccinia virus. This was the beginning of the now major science of immunology.

Vagifem

A brand name for **oestradiol**.

vagina

This is a mucous membrane-lined, muscular passage, 7 to 10 cm along its front wall and 12 to 15 cm along its rear wall. Normally, the front and rear walls are in contact. The vagina slopes upwards and backwards, pointing into the hollow of the sacrum of the pelvis. The neck of the womb (cervix) protrudes well into the upper end of the vagina and there is a deep cul-de-sac (fornix) around it.

The vagina is supported by the muscles of the floor of the pelvis and these can tighten firmly around the entrance. Further up, the vagina stretches easily. The walls of the vagina are normally covered with a creamy material consisting of mucoid secretions from the cervix, cast-off cells from the lining, lactic acid and many bacteria.

During sexual excitement, the vaginal blood vessels become engorged and the lining thickened and hot. The upper vagina dilates and the secretion of mucus from glands near the vaginal entrance increases. During orgasm, the muscles around the vagina contract reflexly and repeatedly.

vagina, disorders of

Congenital defects of the vagina are rare but sometimes the vagina is absent or double. Inflammation of the vagina (vaginitis) is common and causes discharge and itching (see **vaginal discharge**). Most cases are caused by infection, especially with the *Trichomonas vaginalis* (**trichomoniasis**) and with Candida fungi which causes thrush (**candidiasis**) or other yeast fungi such as monilia. Gonorrhoeal vulvovaginitis may affect women who have been exposed to a gonococcal infection, but little girls are more susceptible because of the thinness of the vaginal lining. The usual source of infection in infantile gonococcal vaginitis is the mother, and infection may be acquired during birth.

Vaginitis is also common in elderly women who suffer from oestrogen deficiency and develop thinning and atrophy of the mucous membrane of the vagina. **Vaginismus** is a psychological disorder in which attempts at sexual intercourse lead to painful, and sexually disabling, involuntary spasm of the vaginal muscles. Primary cancer of the vagina is uncommon but cancer of the cervix commonly spreads to the vagina.

vaginal bleeding

This entry is concerned with bleeding other than menstrual bleeding. Occasionally, if sexual intercourse is unusually vigorous or violent, bleeding may occur from the wall of the vagina or from an area of so-called **cervical erosion**, but this is rare. Women using the contraceptive pill may experience occasional unexpected 'spotting' of blood at odd times, possibly because they are not taking a pill with the optimum dosage.

Bleeding in early pregnancy indicates a threatened abortion. Towards the end of pregnancy, bleeding is also a potentially serious sign as it may be caused by separation of the placenta or by the condition of *placenta praevia* in which the placenta lies over the outlet of the womb.

> Non-menstrual bleeding should always be taken seriously because it nearly always implies that something is going wrong. The real concern is that it may indicate cancer of the cervix, cancer of the lining of the uterus (the endometrium) or endometriosis. Bleeding occurring after the menopause, other than that caused by HRT with balanced oestrogens and progesterone, is an especially important sign as it may indicate endometrial cancer.

See also **uterus, cancer of**.

vaginal discharge

It is important to distinguish between normal secretion from the womb and vagina and a discharge due to a local disorder.

Sometimes the normal secretions are profuse enough to persuade the woman concerned that something is wrong. Normal secretions are not offensive and do not cause irritation. Even so, vaginal discharge is one of the commonest of women's complaints.

The wall of the vagina is kept moist, not by producing its own fluids, but by water that passes through from the tissue fluid in the pelvis. This is called a *transudate* and as it passes, it carries away cast-off cells from the vaginal lining and these make it look white or creamy. This transudate becomes mixed with mucus secreted by glands in the lining of the cervix and by glands in the lining of the womb. Cervical mucus is usually fairly viscous but becomes more watery around the time of ovulation.

The normal vaginal secretion varies in amount at different times in the menstrual cycle, being most profuse in the few days before the onset of menstrual bleeding. During sexual excitement the area around the entrance to the vagina is lubricated by further clear mucus from the two Bartholin glands lying in the labia. This source may add to the amount of the discharge. Vaginal secretions are also inclined to be more profuse during pregnancy. The term *leukorrhoea*, which does not imply any disease process but which was once used as synonymous with abnormal vaginal discharge, is now often applied to the normal condition. Vaginal discharge is sometimes caused by a forgotten tampon which has been pushed up into the cul-de-sac (fornix) behind the cervix.

Before the menopause, discharge resulting from bacterial infection of the vagina is uncommon. This is because the vagina is kept at a significantly acid pH by lactic acid formed by normal **commensal** bacteria from sugars in the lining. The loss of these 'healthy' bacteria is undesirable and is one of the reasons for vaginal problems, especially after the menopause. The commonest cause of abnormal vaginal discharge is thrush (**candidiasis**), and another cause, which is becoming increasingly common, is infection with the *Trichomonas vaginalis* organism. This is known as **trichomoniasis**.

vaginal hysterectomy

An operation to remove the womb, performed by way of the vagina so that no external scar is visible. The operation, however, leaves more extensive scars in the wall of the vagina than in the case of a hysterectomy performed through the front wall of the abdomen. Hysterectomy is now commonly performed by keyhole surgery (**laparoscopic surgery**).

vaginismus

A partly or wholly involuntary rejection of attempted sexual intercourse or gynaecological examination in a woman who may express no or feel no emotional disinclination. The response to such an attempt includes straightening the legs, pressing the thighs together, and a tightening up of the muscles in the floor of the pelvis and surrounding the vagina.

Such women often claim that their sexual inclinations are strong and all appears normal until actual penetration is tried.
POSSIBLE CAUSES
Vaginismus tends to affect anxiety-prone women who have never been able to insert a tampon or even a finger into the vagina, because of the anticipation of pain. Sometimes there are guilt feelings about sex induced by unimaginative and ignorant childhood teaching. Rarely, vaginismus stems from an earlier traumatic sexual experience or from a history of rape or sexual abuse during childhood. In a few cases, vaginismus is the result of actual disease of the vulva or vagina which causes pain on contact.
TREATMENT
Vaginismus is treated by full explanation followed by training in the insertion of vaginal dilators of gradually increasing size. So long as this is tactfully done, the results are usually good.

Vaginyl

A brand name for the drug **metronidazole**.

vagotomy

An operation to cut some or all of the branches of the vagus nerve to the stomach. The left vagus nerve stimulates the production of stomach acid and the digestive enzyme pepsin, and a reduction in the secretion of these is valuable in the treatment of **peptic ulcer**.
HOW IT'S DONE
Depending on the requirement, vagotomy may involve complete severance of the nerve (truncal vagotomy) or may be selective or highly selective. Major vagotomies interfere with the stomach's ability to relax its outlet **sphincter** (the pylorus), and are usually done in conjunction with a procedure to widen the outlet (pyloroplasty).
WHY IT'S DONE
Vagotomy can be highly effective in promoting the healing of peptic ulcers of the stomach and duodenum.

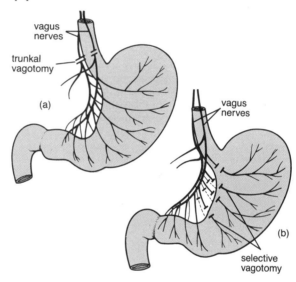

Vagotomy means cutting the vagus nerves to the stomach to reduce acid secretion. This may be truncal, as in (a), or selective, as in (b).

valaciclovir

An antiviral drug used to treat genital herpes and **shingles**. A brand name is Valtrex.

Valclair

A brand name for diazepam.

Valcote

A brand name for **sodium valproate**.

valgus

The term for an abnormal displacement, in an outwards direction, from the midline, of the part beyond a joint. The *hallux* is the big toe. In **hallux valgus** the big toe hinges outwards, at the joint nearest the foot, so as to point towards the little toe. In **genu valgum**, or knock knee, the lower legs are displaced outwards. The opposite term is *varus*. 'Bow legs' are called *genu varum*.

Valium

A brand name for diazepam.

Vallergan

A brand name for the antihistamine drug **trimeprazine**.

Valoid

A brand name for the **anti-emetic antihistamine** drug cyclizine.

valproic acid

An **anticonvulsant** drug used to prevent all kinds of epileptic seizures. A brand name is Convulex.

valsalva manoeuvre

The attempt to breathe out forcibly with the mouth and nose firmly closed or with the vocal cords pressed tightly together. This happens frequently in everyday life, as when we lift heavy weights or strain to empty the bowels, and is normally harmless.

At the beginning of the valsalva manoeuvre the blood pressure rises because the increased pressure in the chest is added to the pressure in the main arteries. But this raised chest pressure also compresses the large veins so that the return of blood to the heart is impeded and the heart output drops. This soon results in a drop in blood pressure and the pressure receptors in the large arteries prompt the heart to beat more rapidly to try to compensate.

> At the end of the manoeuvre, the blood in the great veins rushes back to the heart and this and the increased heart action causes a second sharp rise in blood pressure. Because of these changes, the valsalva manoeuvre may be dangerous in people with heart disease, and should be avoided. Such people are advised to breathe out deliberately instead of compressing the breath.

valsartan

A drug that interferes with the action of angiotensin II and is used to treat high blood pressure. A brand name is Diovan.

Valtrex

A brand name for **valaciclovir**.

valve replacement

See **heart valve replacement**.

Vancocin

A brand name for the antibiotic **vancomycin**.

vancomycin

An antibiotic effective against many Gram positive bacteria. It is toxic and its use is limited to infections that fail to respond to the common antibiotics. A brand name is Vancocin.

variation from the average

See **standard deviation**.

varicella

See **chickenpox**.

varices

Twisted, distorted sections of vessels, most commonly veins. Veins affected by varices are called **varicose veins**. These occur mainly in the legs, but other veins may become varicose. Oesophageal varices are the dangerous varicosities that affect the veins at the lower end of the oesophagus when the vein drainage through the liver is impeded by cirrhosis.

varicocele

A collection of enlarged veins in the scrotum, usually on the left side. This common condition of varicosity in the plexus of veins that surrounds the testicle is usually of no significance but sometimes causes a dragging ache and may contribute to infertility. In these cases surgical correction of the problem is justified.

varicose veins

A varicosity is a local irregular expansion and distortion, most commonly affecting the veins. It occurs most frequently in the legs but can occur elsewhere, most notably at the lower end of the gullet (*oesophageal varices*) or in the scrotum (see **varicocele**).

The pressure of the blood is high in the arteries but is almost zero in the veins. This is because the force of the heart beat is almost entirely expended by the time the blood has passed through the capillary beds and has reached the veins. So blood flow in the veins is largely the passive result of the

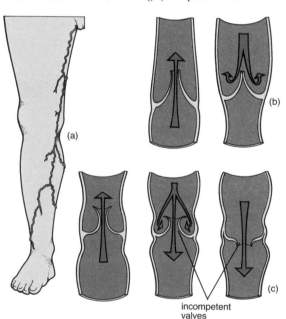

Varicose veins (a) are caused by leaking vein valves. Normal valves (b) support short columns of blood and reduce the pressure on the walls. Incompetent valves (c) lead to greater pressure on the vein walls.

volume moving in the circulation. This low pressure is reflected in the structure of the veins, which are thin-walled and collapse easily. Blood returning to the heart from the lower part of the body must do so against gravity, and the veins of the legs must support a heavy column of blood. The movement of this column is, however, helped by a series of one-way valves that allow the blood to move only in the direction of the heart.

Because of these valves, any compression of the veins causes the blood to move and it can only do so in the direction allowed by the valves. This external compressive force comes from the changing shape of the surrounding muscles as they contract, and most of the vein pumping is done by the contraction of the calf muscles during walking.

So, although increased consumption of oxygen and fuel may cause symptoms, as already described, it is equally true that the symptoms of varicose veins are often relieved by walking. If the blood flow can be normalized by muscle action, varicosity need not lead to pain from the accumulation of metabolites.

If vein valves are leaky, this mechanism is seriously interfered with. Unless the blood column is broken into segments by efficient valves, all the pressure from the weight of the column of blood from the heart to the lower legs is exerted on the thin walls of the veins. It is hardly surprising that this leads to bulging, lengthening and tortuosity of the relatively unsupported veins just under the skin. Fortunately, the most important veins – those deep within the muscles – are well supported and, apart from valve defects, usually remain structurally normal. The deep leg veins can, by themselves, convey all the returning blood, and form an effective pump. The surface veins, however, do not receive the same all-round compressive force and become varicose.

The surface veins are connected to the main deep veins in the groin and at various levels in the legs. These cross-connections are called the *perforating veins* and they, too, contain valves that allow flow from the surface to the deep veins but not vice versa. Normally, there is free movement of blood from the surface to the deep veins by way of the perforators. But if the valves in the perforating veins are defective the muscle pump pressure in the deep veins is transferred to the less well-supported surface veins. The cause of vein incompetence is complex as it, also, is known to be a result of varicosity. In most cases, however, the defect in the veins obviously comes first.

PREVALENCE

Varicose veins of the legs affect millions of people and are especially troublesome to women, to whom much distress is caused by their unsightly appearance and the associated symptoms.

RECOGNITION AND SYMPTOMS

Varicosity does not simply mean the cosmetic problem of ugly, purplish, bulging veins. For many, varicosity means aching and tiredness, persistent swelling of the ankles, brownish-blue discoloration of the skin, a strong tendency to ulceration after minor knocks or abrasions and sometimes, although happily rarely, profuse and even dangerous bleeding from a ruptured vein.

POSSIBLE CAUSES

Varicosity implies stagnation of blood flow, a poor supply of oxygen, glucose and other nutritional requirements to the surrounding tissues, and the accumulation of toxic products of metabolism which, normally, are diluted and washed away by a brisk blood flow. It is this combination of inadequate nutri-tion and local damage that causes both the symptoms and the liability of the skin to break down to form persistent ulcers.

Varicose veins tend to run in families and it is probable that there is a genetic tendency to weakness and incompetent valves. Obesity certainly contributes, as does any factor that impedes the free flow of blood up the veins, such as pregnancy, prolonged standing and local constriction from underwear elastic or garters. Insufficient exercise, with resulting stagnation of blood in the veins, is another known factor.

TREATMENT

Adequate external support of the surface veins – as by well-designed and properly selected compression hosiery – can be a great help in the treatment of varicose veins. This will prevent blood stagnation, relieve local oxygen lack and help to prevent accumulation of pain-causing metabolites. It will divert blood from the surface into the deep veins where the muscle pump works better and prevent the undesirable reflux of blood from the deep veins. Symptoms are relieved, and even established varicose ulcers will often heal. The most effective support hosiery applies the greatest compression at the ankle with a progressively graded reduction in pressure up the leg to the thigh. Many people are dissatisfied with the relief given by external support. A more radical approach is to cause the blood in the affected veins to clot by injecting a special solution. This, if successful, closes them off altogether. The definitive treatment for varicose veins, however, is to remove them by an operation known as *stripping*. So long as tests show that the deep veins are working properly, these can be relied on to carry all the blood back to the heart. An incision is made, high in the groin, to expose the upper end of the vein, which is then tied off. Another incision is made at the lower end of the vein at the ankle. An instrument, called a vein stripper, consisting of a long flexible cable with a metal, half-acorn-like knob at its bottom end, is pushed right up the vein to the groin. The lower end of the vein is securely tied to the cable close to the knob. The surgeon returns to the groin end and pulls the cable slowly but firmly up the leg and out of the incision. As the lower wide end of the stripper passes upwards it carries the concertinaed vein with it, up and out of the wound.

The results of this operation are usually excellent.

Varidase

A brand name for a mixture of **streptokinase** and **streptodornase** used locally to remove blood clots and organic debris from wounds.

variola

See **smallpox**.

Vascace

A brand name for **cilazapril**.

Vascardin

A brand name for the nitrate **vasodilator** drug isosorbide dinitrate, used to treat **angina pectoris**.

vascular endothelial growth factor (VEGF)

A remarkable example of the way feedback operates in the body, in this instance involving lack of oxygen in the tissues, blood vessel production and active genetics. Vascular endothelial growth factor is a naturally occurring protein-like substance (polypeptide) that promotes the production of tiny new blood vessels by stimulating the growth, migration and proliferation of body lining cells (endothelial cells). It opens up existing vessels through the mediation of **nitric oxide**. Local shortage of oxygen to the tissues prompts a local increase in the gene expression of VEGF, which causes new blood vessels to form and increases the available oxygen.

vasculitis

An inflammatory disorder of blood vessels which is the central feature of a range of conditions including **rheumatoid arthritis**, polyarteritis nodosa, **erythema nodosum**, **temporal arteritis**, certain forms of **purpura** and Buerger's disease (**thromboangiitis obliterans**).

Vasculitis damages the lining of vessels, causing narrowing, so that the blood flow is slowed or even stopped. The effects on the tissues supplied by these vessels may be serious. In temporal arteritis, for instance, the blood supply to the eyes may be cut off and permanent blindness result.

Foreign material, such as bacteria, act as *antigens* and stimulate the production of antibodies, which normally adhere to the antigens and destroy them. Sometimes, however, the antigen-antibody combinations (immune complexes) circulate in the blood until they settle on the wall of a small artery and excite a severe inflammatory response. Immune complexes are believed to be important in the production of vasculitis.

Corticosteroid drugs are of great importance in the management of cases of vasculitis.

vas deferens

The fine tube that runs up the **spermatic cord** on each side from the epididymis of the testicle, over the pubic bone and alongside the bladder to end by joining the seminal vesicle near its entry to the prostate gland. The vas deferens conveys spermatozoa from the testicle to the seminal vesicle.

vasectomy

This is the common operation for male sterilization, in which the vas deferens (plural, vasa deferentia) on each side is cut. The vas deferens is the tube which carries sperms from the testicle, where they are formed, up to the seminal vesicle, adjoining the prostate gland, on each side, where some of the seminal fluid is stored. Sperms pass up each vas deferens in a kind of slow-moving sludge that is forced upwards by the pressure of new production below. Both vasa deferentia must be cut if the operation is to succeed and the cut ends must be kept well apart so that there is no possibility of their joining up again.

The lower parts of the vasa deferentia lie almost entirely within the scrotum and just under the skin, so the operation is simple and can be done readily under local anaesthesia. Each vas deferens is exposed through separate small skin incisions or through a small central incision, on the upper part of the scrotum, and brought out to be completely cut through. Often a short segment is removed, or the ends may be turned back and secured with a tie. Sometimes the cut ends are burned with a cautery. The skin incision or incisions are now closed with a few stitches.

The operation is often followed by bruising and aching in the testicles for a day or two, but this soon passes. A small number of men experience chronic testicular pain after the operation. Sperms still active above the level of the incision may allow fertilization for some weeks afterwards and three ejaculation samples should be examined for absence of sperm before sterility can be assured.

The operation has no direct effect on male sexual sensation, and the orgasm and the volume of the ejaculate are unchanged. The male sex hormone production from the testicles is not affected by the operation. Some men feel diminished from the knowledge that they are now sterile, but most are unaffected in this way. Reversal of the operation is possible but cannot be relied upon to be successful.

Vasectomy has made it easy for men to accept the burden of responsibility for contraception. Female sterilization is a more major procedure requiring general anaesthesia, and should not be insisted upon by husbands or partners, for purely contraceptive reasons, when this option is open to them.

vasoconstriction

Active narrowing of small arteries so that the flow of blood through them is diminished. The narrowing is caused by the shortening (contraction) of circularly arranged smooth muscle fibres in the walls of the vessels. Vasoconstriction is the principal way in which the body purposefully reduces the supply of blood to a particular area. In cold weather, for instance, the blood supply to the skin, by which much heat may be lost, is markedly cut down by vasoconstriction.

The opposite of vasoconstriction is called vasodilation.

vasoconstrictor drugs

Drugs which cause the circular smooth muscle coat in the walls of arteries to contract so that the vessel is narrowed and the rate of blood flow though it reduced. The natural hormones adrenaline and noradrenaline act on particular alpha-adrenergic receptors (see **sympathomimetic drugs**) to cause vasoconstriction.

Both nicotine and cocaine are powerful vasoconstrictors and the former has been implicated in the gangrene-producing disease **thromboangiitis obliterans** (Buerger's disease).

See also **decongestant drugs**.

vasodilator drugs

Drugs which cause arteries to widen so that the blood flow through them is improved. Vasodilator drugs are often valuable, but sometimes cause alarming effects by lowering the blood pressure too much. They include **nitrate and nitrite drugs**, drugs such as prazocin and hydralazine, and **calcium channel blocker drugs** such as nifepidine.

vasovagal attack

A common type of fainting. Vasovagal attacks usually occur during strong emotion, personal distress or pain or by witnessing a shocking event. Fainting is promoted by poor health, fasting, **anaemia**, prolonged bed rest and unfitness and is most likely to occur in crowded, close, warm rooms.

RECOGNITION AND SYMPTOMS

The attack occurs while the person concerned is standing or sitting upright. There is yawning, perspiring, nausea, deep and fast breathing, dimness of vision and ringing in the ears, followed by loss of strength, confusion and loss of consciousness. The face is very pale and the affected person falls, usually with sufficient control to avoid injury. The pulse is often very weak and can barely be felt.

POSSIBLE CAUSES

These symptoms are caused by a temporary shortage of blood supply to the brain, which is exquisitely sensitive to lack of oxygen. This occurs because the large network of blood vessels in the limb muscles and the abdomen, normally kept in a state of narrowed tension (**vasoconstriction**) by the action of the autonomic nervous system, become widely dilated so that a large proportion of the total blood is pooled in the lower part of the body. There may also be slowing of the heart rate.

> Fortunately, the attack is of the nature of a 'fail-safe' mechanism in that falling flat will restore the brain supply by gravity. Indeed, a faint can often be aborted by laying the subject down and elevating the legs. For the same reason, it is dangerous to prevent a fainting person from lying down or to raise a person who has fainted before full recovery has occurred.

Vasoxine

A brand name for **methoxamine**.

VD

Short for venereal disease, an outmoded euphemism for **sexually transmitted diseases**.

vecturonium

A non-**depolarizing** muscle relaxant used in general anaesthesia. A brand name is Norcuron.

Veganin

A brand name for a mixture of the pain-killing drugs aspirin (see **analgesic drugs**), codeine and **paracetamol**.

vegetarianism

The deliberate exclusion from the diet of meat (animal muscle protein) and sometimes of other animal products. The diet of vegetarians thus consists of vegetables, cereals, nuts, legumes and fruit, and sometimes eggs and dairy products. Soya bean, in various forms, such as bean curd (tofu) or fermented bean paste (miso) are popular sources of protein and are eaten as meat substitutes.

Degrees of vegetarianism vary. Vegans consume no meat, dairy products or eggs and wear no animal products, such as leather. Lacto-vegetarians take milk and cheese but not eggs. Ovo-vegetarians will eat eggs but will not eat dairy products. Motives also vary. In some cases there are religious prohibitions, in others the conviction that a vegetarian diet promotes better health. Some people are vegetarian for purely humane reasons, being unable to accept, emotionally, the concept of a diet which includes parts of the bodies of other animals. Some are vegetarian for ecological reasons, arguing against the expense and waste of the production of animals for food.

Man evolved as a carnivorous animal and the human digestive system is 'designed' to cope with animal protein. It secretes specific proteolytic enzymes for the purpose of breaking down such protein into absorbable form. At the same time, it must be said that in the Western world we are certainly injuring our health by over-indulgence in food of animal origin. The evolutionarily unnatural element today, presumably, is the great ease with which we can now obtain animal protein and fat and the resulting abnormally high proportion of these elements in our diet. A much higher proportion of cellulose roughage and carbohydrate would be greatly to our benefit, as it undoubtedly was to our forebears, who could get animal sources of food only by first undergoing the physical exertion involved in catching and killing them.

vegetative state

The condition of living like a vegetable, without consciousness or the ability to initiate voluntary action, as a result of brain damage. People in the vegetative state may sometimes give the appearance of being awake and conscious, with open eyes. They may make random movements of the limbs or head and may pick or rub with the fingers, but there is no response to any form of communication and no reason to suppose that there is any awareness of the environment.

Voluntary movement, all forms of sensation, vision and hearing, and the higher functions such as thought and memory, all depend on the normal functioning of the outer layer of the brain (the cortex). The vegetative state results when this part of the brain is extensively damaged while the deeper structures, which maintain the more primitive functions – breathing, heartbeat, maintenance of body temperature, and crude response to stimuli – continue to operate normally.

The vegetative state should be distinguished from apparently similar conditions such as the psychiatric state of catatonia, in which consciousness is retained and from which full recovery is possible, and the **locked-in syndrome** from damage to the brain stem, in which the patient is conscious but unable to speak or move any part of the body, except for blinking and eye movements, which permit signalling.

vein obstruction

See **veno-occlusive disease**.

veins

The veins are thin-walled compared to the arteries and carry blood from the capillaries back to the heart. The main veins run in conjunction with the corresponding arteries supplying an area and are usually larger than the artery. Many of them contain valves which prevent the backflow of blood, especially in the legs.

The veins of the head, neck, arms and upper chest empty into the large draining vein, the superior vena cava. Those from the rest of the body run into the inferior vena cava. Both caval vessels empty into the right atrium of the heart, as do those returning blood from the coronary supply. The veins bringing oxygenated blood back from the lungs run into the left atrium.

veins, disorders of

See **haemorrhoids**, **phlebitis**, **thrombophlebitis**, **varices**, **varicocele**, **varicose veins**.

Velbe

A brand name for the anticancer drug **vinblastin**.

Velosulin

A brand name for **insulin**.

vena

Latin root meaning 'vein' as in vein (low-pressure, thin-walled blood vessel).

vena caval filter

A wire mesh filtering device that is inserted into the lower of the two major veins of the body (the inferior vena cava) to prevent the passage of dangerous blood clots from the leg veins and elsewhere to the lungs, via the heart (pulmonary embolism). Long, snake-like blood clots are liable to form in the leg veins, especially if a patient remains immobile after surgery. If such a clot breaks off to form an embolus, the situation is very dangerous and commonly causes death. Vena caval filters, which can be inserted by way of a vein in the groin, can prevent this disaster.

venepuncture

The common procedure to gain access to the bloodstream for the purpose of obtaining a sample of blood or giving an injection directly into it. Venepuncture is an elementary medical skill, commonly performed by doctors, nurses, pathology laboratory technicians and others.

HOW IT'S DONE

The selected vein may be at the front of the elbow, on the back of the hand or elsewhere. An elbow vein is often selected because, at that site, some large veins lie just under the skin and these can conveniently be engorged by the use of a **tourniquet** around the upper arm. When engorged, these veins are easily felt.

After the skin over the vein has been cleaned with alcohol, the needle, which is attached to a syringe, is passed through it, alongside, or immediately above, the vein, being held at a small angle to the skin so that it does not penetrate deeply. The point of the needle is then passed carefully through the wall of the vein and pushed along, for a short distance, inside the vessel. If the plunger is now pulled back, blood will flood backwards into the syringe and a sample may be taken or the injection given. In another commonly used method a vacuum container, without plunger, is employed.

After a vein at the elbow has been entered and the needle withdrawn, local pressure with a sterile cotton swab will soon stop the bleeding. The common practice of bending the elbow over the swab should be avoided as this encouraged bleeding into the tissues and bruising.

venereal diseases

See **sexually transmitted diseases**.

venereology

The medical speciality concerned with the **sexually transmitted diseases**.

venesection

Bloodletting. The deliberate removal of blood to obtain quantities for **transfusion**, or for purposes of treatment. The latter is seldom called for but is useful in the condition of polycythaemia, a disorder in which there is too much haemoglobin and the blood is too 'thick'. Venesection, for treatment, is also used in the rare conditions of **haemochromatosis** and **porphyria**. In prescientific days, venesection was commonly used as an alleged remedy and was often a contributory cause of the patient's demise.

venlafaxine

A **serotonin** and **noradrenaline** re-uptake inhibitor drug used to treat depression. A brand name is Efexor.

venom

A poison produced by a few snakes, spiders, insects and scorpions. Venoms may affect the nervous system to cause paralysis or may affect the blood, causing either extensive clotting or bleeding (haemorrhage). Venoms are seldom fatal unless the victim is very young or debilitated, or the dose very large, as in multiple bee, wasp or hornet stings.

veno-occlusive disease

A liver disorder in which the small branches of the hepatic vein within the liver become closed off, but not by blood clotting. The condition can be caused by drinking 'bush tea', which contains pyrrolizidine alkaloids, and in other ways. The effects are almost identical to those of the **Budd-Chiari syndrome**.

Ventide

A brand name for a mixture of the steroid drug beclomethazone and the **bronchodilator** drug salbutamol, used to control **asthma**.

ventilator

A mechanical device consisting essentially of an electric motor driving an air pump or bellows, which provides an intermittent flow of air or oxygen under pressure.

WHY IT'S USED

Ventilators are commonly used in operating theatres to maintain the respiration of patients who are paralysed by anaesthetic agents. In such cases, the ventilator will pump anaesthetic gases as well as oxygen. Ventilators are also used to maintain respiration in people who have, through brain damage or other causes, lost the power of spontaneous breathing and who would, without artificial respiration, quickly die.

HOW IT WORKS

The outlet of the ventilator is attached to a tube which has been inserted into a person's wind pipe (trachea), and the pressure is sufficient to expand and fill the person's lungs. The tracheal tube may have been inserted through the mouth or nose or through an artificial opening in the neck (**tracheostomy**). At the end of each input cycle, which can be adjusted in volume and time, the pressure is suddenly released and the elastic collapse of the lungs drives out the air, which can leave easily through a light valve.

Ventmax SR

A brand name for **salbutamol**.

Ventodisks

A brand name for **salbutamol**.

Ventolin

A brand name for the bronchodilator drug **salbutamol**.

ventral

Relating to the front of the body. The term comes from the Latin word *venter* meaning 'the belly'.

ventre

Latin root meaning 'belly' as in ventral (of the belly).

ventricular fibrillation

A heart disorder incompatible with life and usually occurring as a result of a severe **heart attack**. In ventricular fibrillation, the main lower chambers of the heart, the ventricles, instead of contracting forcefully to pump the blood, undergo a rapid fluttering, or twitching, which is ineffective in moving blood. Ventricular fibrillation is a form of cardiac arrest and unless quickly reversed by electric shock defibrillation, is soon fatal.

Vepeside

A brand name for **etoposide**.

Veractil

A brand name for the antipsychotic drug methotrimeprazine.

Veradil

A brand name for **verapamil**.

verapamil

A calcium channel blocker drug used to correct irregularities in the heart beat. There is evidence that verapamil and other calcium channel blockers are anti-atherogenic and can prevent recurrent narrowing of arteries, such as the coronary arteries after these have been widened by **coronary angioplasty**. Trade names are Cordilox, Securon, Securon SR and Univer.

vermicide

A drug that kills worms.

vermifuge

A drug that drives out intestinal worms.

Vermox

A brand name for the anthelmintic drug **mebendazole**.

vernix

Properly called vernix caseosa, this is the layer of greasy material, fine hairs and skin scales with which fetuses and newborn babies are covered. It is easily washed off and does not recur.

verruca

A **wart**, from the Latin root meaning 'wart' as in wart (benign skin excrescence). It is widely believed that veruccas occur only on the soles of the feet. These are, however, only one of the several varieties of verruca affecting any part of the skin.

See **plantar wart**.

vertebra

Latin root meaning 'backbone' as in vertebral (of the spine).

vertebra, slipped

See **spondylolisthesis**.

vertebrobasilar insufficiency

An inadequate blood supply to the brainstem and lower part of the brain resulting from atherosclerosis in the pair of vertebral arteries that run up through holes in the side processes of the bones of the neck. This causes dizziness (**vertigo**) and loss of balance, double vision, weakness or paralysis on one side of the body, speech disturbances and sometimes loss of consciousness. See also **carotid artery disease**.

vertigo

Latin root meaning 'giddiness' as in vertigo. An illusion that the world, or sometimes oneself, is spinning round. The effect may be slight and only just noticeable, or may be so severe that one falls to the ground as if thrown down. Mild vertigo is very common and such cases are seldom due to underlying disease, or require any treatment. Vertigo can be caused by fear of heights, by **motion sickness**, by overbreathing (**hyperventilation**) brought on by anxiety or by alcohol or drugs.

More severe vertigo may indicate disorder of the balancing mechanisms in the inner ears, such as **Ménière's syndrome** or **labyrinthitis**, or a disorder of the neurological mechanism subserving balance in the cerebellum or its connections, resulting from **vertebrobasilar insufficiency** or other cause, such as tumour or **multiple sclerosis**.

Vertigon

A brand name for the phenothiazine antiemetic drug prochlorperazine.

Verugon

A brand name for **salicylic acid**.

Vesanoid

A brand name for **tretinoin**.

vesica

Latin root meaning 'bladder' as in vesical (of a bladder).

vesicle

A small blister filled with clear serum or similar fluid, which may form when cells disintegrate locally as a result of damage. The term comes from the Latin *vesiculum*, the diminutive of *vesica* meaning a 'bladder' or 'bag', and is also applied to a number of small pouches of various organs. Thus, the seminal vesicles are the small bladders which store semen.

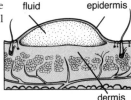

A vesicle is a small fluid-filled blister between the dermis and the epidermis.

vestigio

Latin root meaning 'trace' as in vestigial (of non-functioning parts from earlier evolution).

Vexol

A brand name for ocular anti-inflammatory drug rimexolone.

Viagra

A trade name for the oral drug sildenafil citrate. The drug, which is made by the firm Pfizer, and has been dubbed 'the Pfizer riser', has attracted considerable attention. United States prescription figures, in April, 1998, soon after the drug was issued, were about 100 times the average for most new drugs and outstripped both Prozac and Rogaine. Since then the drug has gone from strength to strength and, although it is intended to be a prescription-only drug, is readily available on the Internet.

Viazem XL

A brand name for **diltiazem**.

Vibramycin

A brand name for the tetracycline antibiotic **doxycycline**.

vibration-induced disorders

A range of disorders that include deafness, vibration-induced nerve damage (neuropathy), 'white finger' (Raynaud's phenomenon) and, in the case of whole body vibration, motion sickness, low-back pain, visual disturbances and insomnia. The hand-arm vibration syndrome (HAVS) features spasm of blood vessels with white fingers, sensory and motor nerve damage and even muscle, bone and joint changes.

vibrator

An electrically operated reciprocating device which can apply low-frequency repetitive force to any part of the body. Vibrators are sometimes used ostensibly to 'tone' muscles, but this word has no scientific meaning. More commonly, vibrators are used to stimulate the clitoris and induce orgasm, as an alternative to sexual intercourse, or as a convenient method of masturbation. They are said to be of value in sex therapy for orgasmic problems, particularly in women, and in the treatment of some cases of ejaculatory incompetence in men. Vibrators are available in varying shapes and sizes, to suit their intended purpose.

video game epilepsy

Epileptic attacks triggered by watching the screen when playing video games on a TV set or PC or in an amusement arcade. The stimulus that prompts the epileptic attack may be regularly changing lights (intermittent photic stimulation) or pattern alone. These activities cannot cause epilepsy but may precipitate attacks in susceptible children and others. The nearer the screen, the more powerful the stimulus, so children should view TV screens from a distance of 2 metres. Such children should be prohibited from playing computer games.

Videx

A brand name for **didanosine**.

vigabatrin

A drug that simulates the action of the **neuro-transmitter** GABA and is used to treat epilepsy resistant to other controlling agents. A brand name is Sabril.

viloxazine

A drug that inhibits the re-uptake of **noradrenaline** and is used to treat depression. A brand name is Vivalan.

vinblastine

An anticancer drug used mainly in the treatment of **Hodgkin's disease** and other. A brand name is Velbe.

vinca alkaloids

A group of drugs that interfere with cell division and are of value in the treatment of certain cancers. They are used especially in acute leukaemias and malignant lymphomas. They include vinblastine and vincristine. Possible side-effects include:

- inflammation and clotting in veins at the site of injection;
- hair loss;
- interference with nerve function;
- interference with bone marrow blood cell production.

Vincent's disease

A painful inflammation of the mouth caused by infection with two organisms, a spindle-shaped bacterium, *Bacillus fusiformis*, and a **spirochaete**, *Borrelia vincenti*. These organisms are commonly present in the mouth and are unlikely to cause the infection unless there is some underlying cause, such as vitamin B deficiency.

RECOGNITION AND CAUSES

Vincent's disease is also called trench mouth, and features painful ulcers and an acute destructive inflammation of the gums (necrotizing gingivitis). It is treated with the antibacterial drug metronidazole, an antiseptic mouthwash and dental scaling to remove **calculus**. See also **stomatitis**.

Vincent's powders

A brand name for aspirin (see **analgesic drugs**).

vincristine

A vinca alkaloid anticancer drug used to treat **leukaemia**. A brand name is Oncovin.

vindesine

A vinca alkaloid anticancer drug (see **cytotoxic drugs**) used to treat leukaemia. A brand name is Eldisine.

vinorelbine

A vinca alkaloid anticancer drug (see **cytotoxic drugs**) used to treat lung and breast cancer. A brand name is Navelbine.

Viokase

A brand name for **pancreatin**.

violence in the home

This is much more common than is generally appreciated. For obvious reasons violence is more often directed at women than at men, but husband-beating is by no means unknown. Such cases are increasingly coming to court. There are some indications of the prevalence of domestic violence and these suggest that about one woman in 100 is regularly exposed to violent assault.

POSSIBLE CAUSES

The causes of domestic violence are numerous, but there are some obvious patterns. There are, of course, people, men far more than women, who have, from early in life, established a pattern of resorting to violence as an automatic response to **frustration**. This is a conditioned reflex that can often be eradicated by **behaviour therapy** or **group therapy**. There are others who require far less annoyance than most to respond with **anger**. Such people with a 'short fuse' are creatures of a habit that is easily acquired, but which can be broken if suitable **insight** is gained by good psychotherapy.

Men who readily resort to domestic violence are often, but not necessarily, inarticulate or are in a situation in which they find communication very difficult. In such cases violence can be regarded as an attempt at communication. Often, however, such men are simply unable to deal with the normal problems of life and fall back on the only resource they have – their physical strength.

RECOGNITION

Domestic violence against women follows a fairly predictable escalating pattern. Quarrelling and increasingly severe verbal abuse is followed by a slap or a vigorous and aggressive push. On the next occasion there may be a slap or a punch. Many recorded case histories show that this is not the end of the downward progression. Less and less provocation is needed to induce an assault and the degree of injury tends to become ever greater. Women who attempt to defend themselves are liable to suffer more as men will often see this as justification for their anger.

Although a severe assault is often followed by a period of remorse and even an attempt to re-establish good relations, the common pattern is one of continuing escalation. Women in this situation are often in real danger of serious injury or even of murder. Official advice is that they should always threaten legal action and, if necessary, take it. But these women are often in a desperate situation, as, for many of them, the violence may seem preferable to the alternatives – poverty, humiliation, ostracism, loneliness, seemingly unsympathetic official prying. Wives who go to the police also face painful alternatives – a partner in prison who is not earning or a partner who is acquitted and who returns to her more resentful than ever.

Vira-A

A brand name for virarabine.

Viraferon

A brand name for **interferon alfa**.

viral enzymes

See **reverse transcriptase inhibitor**.

Virazid

A brand name for **tribavirin**.

virgin

A virgin is a person who has never had sexual intercourse. Since the term derives from the Latin *virgo*, a maiden, it should, strictly, apply only to a female, but popular usage allows extension to males also. The claimed physical sign of virginity in women, an intact hymen, is by no means proof that sexual intercourse has never occurred. The normal hymen is subject to wide anatomical variations. But in most cases the hymen is torn during the first sexual penetration.

See also **hymen reconstruction**.

virginity

The state of a person who has never had sexual intercourse.

The physical sign of virginity in a woman – an intact hymen – can be misleading, as hymens vary considerably in thickness, extent and rigidity and in some cases may stretch, without tearing, during sexual intercourse. In addition, a hymen may be torn in the course of an accident or fall involving trauma to the area. In most cases, however, the hymen is torn during the first sexual penetration.

virginity restoration surgery

See **hymen reconstruction**.

Viridal

A brand name for **alprostadil**.

virilism

The secondary sexual characteristics and the general configuration of the body are determined by whether the sex hormones are male or female. This may be so, regardless of the actual genetic sex. Virilism is the condition of masculinization in the female brought about by an excess of male sex hormones (androsterones).

POSSIBLE CAUSES

If this occurs during fetal life, the result is one form of **pseudohermaphroditism**. After birth, the phenomenon may be caused by a genetic disorder that interferes with the normal production, by the adrenal glands, of cortisol. As a result, the pituitary gland, which monitors hormone levels, tries to drive the adrenal gland to produce more cortisol. The only effect is to produce abnormal amounts of male sex hormone and this leads to masculinization.

Later in life, virilism may be caused by anything that causes a rise in male sex hormones in a woman. It may occur in tumours of the adrenal glands, and, to a lesser extent, of the ovaries. A proportion of male sex hormone is normally present in the female, but in these conditions the amount is grossly excessive. Virilization can also occur from the use of anabolic steroids by female athletes and body-builders. These steroids are chemically related to male sex hormones.

RECOGNITION AND SYMPTOMS

High male hormone levels have several distressing effects on the female. These may include:

● broadening of the shoulders;
● a general increase in muscular development;

- loss of the typically female distribution of fat on the hips and breasts;
- deepening of the voice from enlargement of the larynx;
- increased growth of body hair;
- redistribution of body hair in the male distribution;
- receding of hair at the temples;
- reduction or cessation of the menstrual periods;
- enlargement of the clitoris;
- acne.

> Virilism in a woman implies a potentially dangerous disease process or the abuse of anabolic drugs. It should always be investigated.

virion

A rudimentary virus particle, the smallest known infectious agent. Virions are smaller than the smallest **viruses** and differ from viruses in that they have no protein capsule (capsid). In spite of their small size, virions can replicate and produce disease when they enter cells. Most of those so far identified infect plants.

virology

In a medical context, virology is a sub-division of clinical microbiology and is concerned with the study of the characteristics, and especially the disease-producing ability, of **viruses**.

Viruses can grow and reproduce only in living cells and this makes their culture more difficult than that of bacteria. Because of this, isolation and identification of viruses is a much larger problem than the identification of bacteria. Virus diseases are mainly diagnosed by the identification of the antibodies produced by the body in response to viruses. In this way all the virus diseases, including such common conditions as **warts**, **herpes** simplex infections, **shingles** (herpes zoster), **chickenpox**, **glandular fever**, the common cold (see **cold, common**), **influenza**, viral conjunctivitis, **rubella** and many respiratory infections such as viral **pneumonia**, can be diagnosed.

Virormone

A brand name for the male sex hormone drug **testosterone**.

virulence

The capacity of a particular infective microorganism to injure or kill a susceptible host. Virulence cannot be considered except in the context of the ability of the infected person (the host) to resist. So any particular organism may have a high virulence to one person – who may be immunocompromised – and a low virulence to a person with high immune competence.

Virulence also depends on other factors such as the numbers of the organism present, the site at which the organisms present themselves (portal of entry) and whether local defensive factors are operating well.

Thus, certain organisms may be harmless if confined to the inside of the bowel, but may exert a highly virulent effect if an opening in the wall of the bowel allows them access to the peritoneal cavity of the abdomen. Our skins, at most times, carry highly potentially virulent organisms, but these may remain harmless unless access occurs through a cut or an abrasion.

viruses

Viruses are so small that ordinary units of measurement are far too large to measure them. A red blood cell – of which there are about five million in every cubic millimetre of blood – is about 7500 nanometres in diameter, while small bacteria, like cocci, are 1000 nanometres across. A nanometre is a millionth of a millimetre. The largest viruses of all are around 300 nanometres in length, although they go down in size to about 10 nanometres.

Around 1940, when the electron microscope made it possible to actually see viruses, some were found to be roughly spherical, some bullet-shaped, some loaf-shaped and some polyhedral. Many have a strict geometrical and symmetrical shape. Analysis has shown that each virus has a definite composition, the larger viruses being more complex than the smaller ones, and containing, in addition to a nucleic acid core, outer capsules consisting of variable amounts of protein, fat (lipid) and carbohydrate. While not all viruses contain all these elements, all have nucleic acid. The protein components of viruses are mainly responsible for their ability to stimulate antibody production within the body, and consist of repeating amino acid subunits

Viruses are fundamentally different from bacteria. Each of the cells in our bodies contains all the apparatus necessary for its own functioning and reproduction. Cells are like tiny chemical engineering factories, full of enzymes, power-supply units, digestive elements and so on. The central part of the cell, the nucleus, contains the blueprint for reproduction – **DNA**. Viruses, also, have a blueprint with the plans for future individuals, but very little else.

The essential point about viruses is that they do not have any of the chemical equipment necessary to provide for their nutritional and energy needs. They are not even able to reproduce on their own. Incredibly, they simply take over the internal equipment of a living cell and put it to use for their own purposes.

It is by no means certain that viruses are alive. They occupy a shadowy area between chemical molecules and living organisms, and as knowledge of viruses grew it became apparent that our definition of life was inadequate. Unless a virus particle can get into a cell it can't do any of the things that qualify it to be described as living. Once in a cell, however, a virus can effectively feed (take up necessary materials and assimilate them) and then reproduce itself hundreds of times.

Considering the damage they can do, viruses have a remarkably simple structure – apart, that is, from the central core of nucleic acid that carries the cloning program. This part is called the genome. The Greek word *genos* means 'born of a certain kind'. Some viruses have a DNA core, but others have a slightly simpler genetic core called **RNA** (ribonucleic acid) and this can be thought of as being like one strand of the double helix of DNA. The HIV that causes AIDS has two separate copies of these single strands. The central core of the virus is surrounded by a protective coat of protein arranged in regular lumps – rather similar to corn on a cob. This coating of protein is called the capsid and this, in turn, is usually covered by a smooth fat and protein envelope of varying shape. And that's about all there is to virus structure.

Viruses enter cells by making use of specific proteins of the kind that all cells have in their outer cell membranes. The virus's own protein links up with the cell protein but this has to be of the right kind for the virus. This is why certain viruses can only enter certain cells. Once attached, the virus injects its genome into the cell. By taking over vital cell chemical mechanisms, viruses commonly kill cells. Often the cell manages to survive, although in a sadly altered state, and unable to carry out its proper function within the body. Sometimes, the presence of viruses inside cells causes them to begin to divide in an uncontrolled manner and a number of well-known types of cancer may be caused in this way.

Some viruses can stay inside human cells without doing any harm. Many, like the virus that causes chickenpox and shingles, can lie dormant in cells for years. Viruses that can do this, for a variety of reasons, may cause trouble later.

Since viruses have DNA or RNA cores and little else, their basic purpose is to reproduce themselves. After the genome enters the cell there is a short period during which an infectious virus cannot be recovered from the cell. This is when the various parts of the new virus progeny are being assembled. The enzymes which do this are called polymerases. In some cases the virus brings its own polymerases, but often it uses those already present in the cell it has invaded. In this way, a virus which has entered a cell is able to transcribe its DNA or RNA and replicate itself, manufacturing, for each of the new virions (free virus particles) formed, a new envelope from the materials of the host cell.

Under suitable conditions, viruses can produce so many offspring that the host cell is packed to capacity, then stretched until it bursts, releasing enormous numbers of free viruses into the surrounding tissue fluid or blood. Some viruses produce the first offspring in as short a period as two hours. Most take rather longer. Herpes viruses, for instance, reproduce in about five hours, while the AIDS virus, if it is reproducing, takes about ten hours from the time of entering the cell to the time of the appearance of the first new virus.

The most important virus diseases are cold sores (**herpes simplex** infections of the skin), **shingles** (herpes zoster), **chickenpox**, cytomegalovirus infections, **glandular fever**, the now extinct **smallpox**, **vaccinia**, orf, **molluscum contagiosum**, equine encephalitis, **yellow fever**, **poliomyelitis**, the common **cold**, some forms of **gastroenteritis**, **influenza**, para-influenza, **mumps**, **measles**, **rabies**, arthropod-borne fevers, **Lassa fever**, aseptic **meningitis**, Burkitt's lymphoma (see **lymphoma, Burkitt's**), 'shipyard' conjunctivitis (epidemic **keratoconjunctivitis**), **warts**, and progressive multifocal leukoencephalopathy.

See also **astrovirus**, **Chinese avian influenza**, **Ebola virus disease**, **hantavirus disease**, **HIV**, **oncogene**, **retrovirus**, **reverse transcriptase**, **RNA**, **SIV**, **small round viruses**, **transcriptase**, **virus interference**.

virus interference

Protection of cells against virus infection, resulting from prior virus infection of nearby cells. The original viral infection stimulates the infected cells to produce proteins, called interferons. These become attached to the membranes of other, uninfected cells and prompt them to produce enzymes which interfere with the genetic replication of subsequent viral invaders. Interferons also stimulate killer lymphocytes to attack and destroy cells which have been invaded with viruses and, in this way, to limit further viral production.

viscera

The plural of *viscus* from the Latin root meaning 'bowels' as in visceral (of the bowels). A viscus is an organ within a body cavity, especially an organ of the abdomen concerned with digestion. Thus, the term 'viscera' is often used to refer to the stomach and intestines.

Viscotears

A brand name for **polyacrylic acid**.

Viside

A brand name for **cidofovir**.

vision

Vision provides one of the chief sources of information to the brain. Since the development of reading, printing and the representation of information by other forms of graphic imagery, this channel has also taken over some of the functions of hearing.

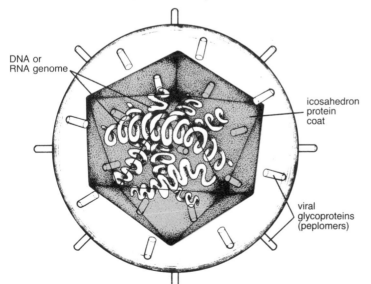

DNA or RNA genome

icosahedron protein coat

viral glycoproteins (peplomers)

A typical virus. Many have a different structure. The genetic blueprint (genome) is surrounded by a 20-sided protein coat and the whole is enclosed in a membrane bearing 'spikes' or peplomers of glycoprotein.

Environmental information, coded in terms of form, size, colour, movement and perspective, is constantly flooding into our brains for analysis and storage. The eyes are sensitive to the narrow band of electromagnetic radiation, lying between 380 and 720 nanometres, which we call visible light.

A close analogy can be made between the eye and a video camera. The eye has a lens system (the cornea and internal crystalline lens) with focal length of about 25 mm and a maximum aperture of about f2.8. The cornea is the more powerful lens. Between these two lenses is an iris diaphragm. Both focusing (accommodation) and light control (pupil reaction) are automatic. Focusing is done by altering the curvature of the elastic internal lens. The iris is the coloured part of the eye, a pigmented diaphragm with a central opening called the pupil. It contains circular muscles, surrounding the pupil margin, which, on contracting, constrict it, and radially placed muscle fibres which, on contracting, enlarge (dilate) it.

Eye colour is not a matter of different pigments, but simply of different amounts, and distribution of a single brown pigment, melanin. In dark-coloured eyes there is a large amount of this pigment scattered throughout the full thickness of the iris, much of it being near the front. In blue eyes, there is very little pigment and it is placed in the deeper layers so that it has to be viewed through a variable thickness of semi-transparent iris tissue. Eye colour is also influenced by the layer of water

and transparent cornea through which light, by which the eye colour is seen, must pass twice. In so doing, it acquires a bluish tinge, by absorption of the longer (red) wavelengths. Every eye surgeon is familiar with the dull, muddy appearance of the iris, viewed directly in the opened eye.

The converter (transducer) in the focal plane, corresponding to the film, or vidicon, in a camera, is called the retina and this, too, is capable of variable sensitivity and a speed of several thousand ISO. It contains millions of photocells, called rods and cones. Cones are colour-sensitive and of three kinds, each producing maximum electrical output on being exposed to light of a particular waveband. This is the basis of colour vision. The output from the retina is a multichannel, frequency-modulated signal which passes along the optic nerve to the brain.

The eyes are coordinated in their movements by the brain, so that both align on the object of interest, changing the degree of convergence with altering distance. In this way the two images overlap accurately. They are, however, viewed from slightly different points and differ slightly. This provides for a sense of the solidity of objects (stereopsis). Optic nerve fibres from the inner half of each retina cross to the opposite side, in a nerve junction behind the eyes. Those from the outer halves do not cross. The effect of this is that the left half of the brain receives information from the right field of

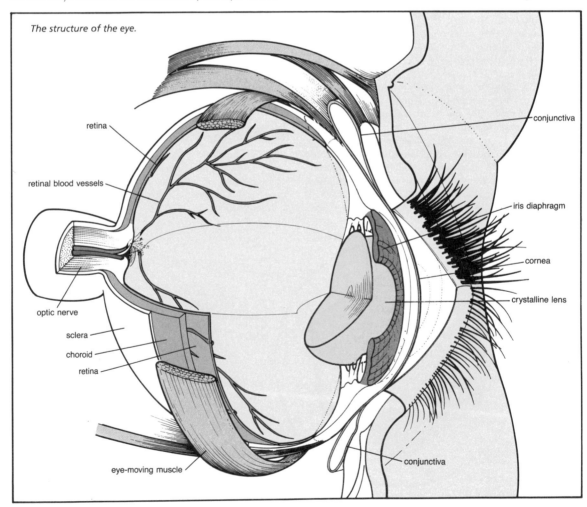

The structure of the eye.

vision, and vice versa. Both halves also receive information from the small central zone of immediate visual interest. The part of the brain concerned with vision is at the back (occipital cortex) and the visual pathways have to pass right through the brain to reach this region. This arrangement has important implications in the diagnosis of many brain disorders. Mapping the visual fields can often localize brain damage.

The natural blind spot is the projection into space of the head of the optic nerve (optic disc) which consists solely of nerve fibres and has no rods or cones. The blind spot occurs, in the field of vision of each eye, about 15 degrees to the outer side of whatever point we are looking at. If an eye is turned outwards to align itself on the point which was previously the projection of the optic disc, the blind spot will simply move 15 degrees farther out. It is mainly because of this that we are unaware of it. The eyeball is sealed off from the environment by the conjunctiva – a transparent membrane which covers the white of the eye and the inner surfaces of the eyelids in one continuous sheet. The conjunctiva is firmly fixed around the cornea and is tightly adhered to the lids, but elsewhere lies loosely on the eyeball, allowing free movement of the globe. The term 'conjuntiva' means 'connecting, or joining, together'.

vision, disorders of

Blurred vision is most commonly caused by a failure of the optical system of the affected eye to form a sharp image on the retina of the object being looked at, as a result of the refractive errors, **myopia**, **hypermetropia** and **astigmatism**. Blurred near vision is also commonly caused by **presbyopia**. These errors can all be compensated for by glasses.

Other causes of blurred vision, which cannot be corrected by appropriate spectacles or contact lenses, are:

- opacification of the outer lens of the eye (corneal opacities) from ulceration, scarring or disease;
- interior **uveitis** with cell deposits on the inside of the cornea and milky aqueous humour;
- bleeding into the aqueous humour;
- internal lens opacities (**cataract**);
- opacities in the inner jelly of the eye (vitreous opacities);
- bleeding into the vitreous;
- active retinal disease;
- disease of the optic nerve, such as **retrobulbar neuritis**.

Slow, progressive loss of vision is common in old age, as a result of loss of transparency of the crystalline lenses of the eyes (cataract). Other common causes of gradual loss of vision are **macular degeneration**, for which there is no remedy, and chronic simple **glaucoma**. The latter is now one of the major causes of blindness in the Western world.

Progressive opacification of the cornea from destructive disease, such as herpes simplex **dendritic ulcer**, also causes gradual visual loss. A hereditary degeneration of the retinas, called **retinitis pigmentosa**, causes a variable degree of visual loss in both eyes. Sudden loss of vision may be caused by both optical and neurological disorders. Bleeding into the water (aqueous humour) in the front chamber of the eye (**hyphaema**) usually results from injury and normally resolves completely, but recurrent bleeding often leads to blindness in the affected eye.

Sudden loss of vision from spontaneous bleeding into the jelly of the eye (vitreous haemorrhage), usually from

fragile newly grown blood vessels in long-term diabetics (diabetic retinopathy) is another common cause of blindness. Retinal disorders may also reduce vision suddenly (see **retina, disorders of**).

Optic nerve inflammation (optic neuritis), from **multiple sclerosis** or other causes can severely reduce central vision in one eye within hours. Any damage to the nerve connections between the eyes and the brain, or to the visual area of the brain itself, causes loss of vision. In this case, the loss usually involves the vision in the right or left halves of the field of each eye, or loss of the two outer halves, rather than centrally. Damage to these nerve tracts may result from inadequate blood supply (ischaemia), primary or secondary cancer of the brain, brain abscess, or the loss of the fatty (myelin) sheath of nerve fibres as in multiple sclerosis. Ischaemia is commonest, and is the most frequent cause of stroke. A warning sign of possible incipient stroke is given by **transient ischaemic attacks** in which brief episodes of visual loss occur.

Much blindness is caused by severe ocular injury, especially from penetrating wounds. Windscreen glass, in car accidents, has blinded many, but the incidence of this kind of injury has dropped markedly since the introduction of seat belts.

A less common, but no less seriously disabling form of visual impairment is visual **agnosia**. This is a strange effect of extensive damage to the brain areas concerned with vision and visual associations in which the person concerned, although totally blind, often appears to be unaware of it. Such a person denies blindness, and behaves as if vision is normal, often bumping into objects. There appears to be no regret at the loss of sight, and difficulties are rationalized away by such explanations as that the light is poor or that the spectacles have been lost.

visione

Latin root meaning 'sight' as in vision (faculty of seeing).

vision in dim light

See **dark adaptation**.

vision, machine

See **neural networks**.

vision, peripheral

See **visual fields**.

vision tests

These include tests of the sharpness of vision (visual acuity) and tests of the extent and completeness of the peripheral vision (visual field tests). The former are commonly done, the latter relatively rarely, although they can be of critical importance in assessing diseases of the eye and of the nervous system.

In the course of vision testing, it is often necessary to discover the nature and degree of any focusing defect (refractive error) which may be present. This may lead to the prescription of spectacles.

VISUAL ACUITY TESTING

Visual acuity is tested using a standard letter chart at a standard distance so that the size of the images of the letters formed on the person's retina is standardized. Under these conditions, correct recognition of a whole line of letters may be taken as a measure either of the degree of sharpness of the retinal image or of the resolving power of the retina, or both.

Acuity is measured, in each eye separately, before and after any focusing error is corrected by spectacle lenses placed in a trial frame. The standard Snellen's chart, well-illuminated, is used at a standard distance of 6 metres. People who correctly read the whole of a line of letters near the bottom of the chart, and known by experience to be readable by those with normal visual acuity, are said to have 6/6 vision. The line above this, with larger letters, could be resolved by a normal person at a distance of 9 metres. If the subject, at 6 metres distance, is only able to resolve this line, the acuity is 6/9. Higher lines have progressively larger letters which could be made out at greater distances. The top letter on the chart is of such a size that a normal person could read it at 60 metres. If only this letter can be resolved at 6 metres, the visual acuity is 6/60 – one tenth of normal.

VISUAL FIELD TESTS

The difficulty in visual field testing is to ensure that the person under test does not look directly at the object or light he or she is being asked to perceive. It is instinctive to do this, and various ingenious arrangements are used to overcome the difficulty. Most field testing machines involve the use of a large, white-painted hemisphere on the inner surface of which small spots of light may be projected so as to appear for brief periods in various places or to be moved inwards from the periphery. The subject's head is secured in a central head-rest, one eye is covered, and the other is directed to a point at the centre of the inside of the bowl. The eye must not move during the test.

The subject is given a press-switch, and signals, by pressing the button, when the peripheral targets are seen. Because the chin is supported, speaking causes the head to move. Most machines allow some form of automatic recording, on a chart, of the points on the field at which the targets are seen.

Visual field tests can demonstrate disorders of the retinas and optic nerves and of the nerve tracts (optical pathways) conveying nerve impulses to the back of the brain (occipital cortex). These nerve tracts pass though the whole of the brain, from front to back, spreading out as they do so, and are, in consequence, commonly involved in a wide range of brain disorders, including tumours, cerebral thromboses and haemorrhages (stroke) and the effects of injuries and infections. Visual field testing may thus provide important, sometimes life-saving, information about the presence of a progressively damaging condition.

REFRACTION TESTS

These are done to discover whether the person has a refractive error, such as 'long sight' (hypermetropia), 'short sight' (myopia), or astigmatism, and whether there is a deficiency in the power of accommodation. The test is often done simply by putting different lenses in front of each eye in turn and finding, by trial and error, which are most effective in sharpening the vision. The definitive method, however, is the technique known as retinoscopy. A narrow beam of light is projected into the eye from an instrument which allows the retina to be illuminated and the light reflected back through the pupil to be observed by the person performing the test. Small deliberate movements of the light are made. If the reflected light moves in the same direction as the incident light, the eye is hypermetropic; if it moves in the opposite direction, the eye is myopic; and if it moves differently in different meridia, the eye is astigmatic. Different lenses are now

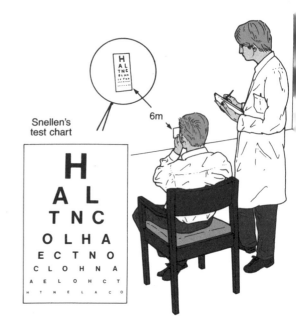

Vision tests. These are performed at a fixed standard using charts with letters of a standard size. The eyes are tested one at a time, with and without glasses.

held in front of the eye and the test repeated, in different meridia, until the movement of the reflected light ceases. The appropriate spectacle correction can be calculated from the power and type of the lenses needed to neutralize the movement of the light.

Accommodation is the faculty of changing the focus of the eyes so that near objects can be seen clearly. Unaccommodated eyes, of normal refraction, are in focus for the distance. Young people have powerful accommodation and can clearly see objects held close to the eyes. The power of accommodation falls off progressively with age so that most people of about 45, unless moderately short-sighted (myopic), need glasses to read comfortably.

Accommodation is tested by asking the person concerned to try to read small print at short range. Once the refraction is known and any distance error corrected, the correction for near sight is largely predictable on the basis of the person's age, and suitable glasses can be prescribed.

Visken

A brand name for the beta-blocker drug pindolol.

Visopt

A brand name for eye drops containing **phenylephrine** and hypromellose.

visual fields

The area over which some form of visual perception is possible while the subject looks straight ahead. The visual fields normally extend outwards to about 90 degrees on either side but are more restricted below and above, depending on how deeply set the eyes are and how large the nose is. Parts of the fields may be lost as a result of **glaucoma**, retinal damage, optic nerve disease and brain disease.

Visual acuity in the peripheral visual fields is low and does not allow the resolution or discrimination necessary for reading or for recognizing faces, reading time on clocks, and so on. Peripheral vision is, however, important for purposes of safe movement and 'navigation'. People whose visual fields are contracted to leave only the small area of direct, straight-ahead vision are severely disabled and may qualify for blind registration, although able to read the whole of an eye-testing chart correctly.

vital signs

Indications of life. Vital signs include indications of breathing, the presence of a palpable pulse and constriction of the pupils in response to bright light. Any response to a strong painful stimulus, such as a vibratory pressure of the knuckles on the breastbone, is also a vital sign, as is the indication of electrical activity in the brain on the electroencephalogram.

vital statistics

Figures of birth, marriage and death rates for a population. Vital statistics are concerned with the rate of natural increase in a population, the number of births per childbearing woman (fertility rate), the marriage and divorce rates, the life expectancy at birth, and the major causes of death.

Accurate birth rates and absolute death rates are comparatively easy to obtain, but figures for the causes of death are always approximate. These have to be obtained from death certificates completed by doctors who, with the best intentions, cannot be expected always to know the precise cause of death, or to be able to represent the various contributory causes in the right order. Nevertheless, for most administrative and planning purposes, the accuracy is sufficient.

Death rates, for the various diseases and causes, are given in numbers per 100,000 of the population. The table gives estimated figures for the United Kingdom for 1987.

CAUSES OF DEATH	RATE PER 100,000
Heart and circulatory diseases (including coronary artery disease)	568
Cancer	282
Stroke	148
Respiratory diseases (including pneumonia)	131
Diseases of the digestive system	131
Accidents	26
Endocrine diseases (including diabetes)	19
Genito-urinary diseases	16

The great preponderance of deaths from diseases of the heart and circulation highlights the importance of attention to factors leading to the arterial disease **atherosclerosis**.

vitamins

Chemical compounds necessary for normal body function. Vitamins take part in many of the enzyme systems of the body, operating within the cells, and are necessary for the synthesis of tissue-building material, hormones and chemical regulators, for energy production and for the breakdown of waste products and toxic substances. The B group of vitamins function as *co-enzymes* – substances without which the vital enzyme-accelerated chemical processes of the body cannot occur or do so abnormally. The result of a co-enzyme deficiency is always serious.

Vitamins are largely derived from the diet and are present in food in small but usually adequate quantities. They have been analysed and can be made synthetically with exactly the same chemical structure, and, consequently, biochemical function, as the natural substances. The quantities needed for health are very small and are almost always present in adequate amounts in normal, well-balanced diets. With the exceptions of vitamins C and E, if vitamins are taken in excess of the minimum requirement, no advantage is gained. In some cases, notably those of vitamins A and D, there may be danger. A major, and almost entirely wasteful, industry has been built up on the fiction that supplementary vitamins are 'good for us'.

Vitamin deficiency is uncommon in well-nourished populations but is very common in underdeveloped areas. It can, however, occur in people who cultivate fad diets or extreme forms of **vegetarianism**; in those with malabsorption disorders; in alcoholics who derive sufficient calories from alcohol to fulfil their energy requirements and who feel no need to eat; in people taking certain drugs, such as hydralazine, penicillamine and oestrogens; and in the urban poor.

Vitamins are conventionally divided into the fat-soluble group A, D, E and K; and the water-soluble group, vitamin C (ascorbic acid) and the B vitamins – B1 (thiamine), B2 (riboflavine), nicotinic acid, B6 (pyridoxine), pantothenic acid, biotin, folic acid and B12. Because of their metabolic function, they are found in highest concentration in the most metabolically active parts of animal and plant tissues – the liver and seed germs.

FAT-SOLUBLE VITAMINS

Vitamin A is a pale-yellow alcohol, readily destroyed by cooking and prolonged storage. It is best derived from fish-liver oils in which it is present in high concentration. Plants contain several carotenoid pigments which are converted to vitamin A in the intestine. Vitamin A deficiency causes defective growth of bones and teeth, eye inflammation, softening and perhaps perforation of the corneas and night blindness.

Vitamin D is one of two chemically similar sterol-like (steroid) compounds, calciferol (D2) and activated 7-dehydrocholesterol (D3). Sunlight activates 7-dehydrocholesterol in the skin, and the vitamin D3 thus formed becomes available for body use. Vitamin D2 is formed by the action of ultraviolet light on ergosterol, a precursor found in many plants. Vitamin D is also found in large quantities in fish liver oil. Deficiency in growing children causes **rickets**, in adults it causes softening of the bones (osteomalacia) and tooth problems. Vitamin E is a group of eight closely related compounds called tocopherols. These function as antioxidants to prevent damage to cell membranes. They are found widely in nature especially in vegetable oils, and are stable to cooking, acids and alkalies. Deficiency is said to cause reproductive failure and damage to the testicles, but there is no real proof of this.

There is some evidence that vitamin deficiency may cause anaemia. The vitamin has been recommended, usually without convincing proof, for the treatment of cataracts, liver damage, anaemia, pancreatitis, nerve and muscle disease, lung disease, retrolental fibroplasia, hyperlipidaemia and protection against air pollution. Recent research into the effects of chemical groups called *free radicals*, which are known to be damaging to the body, suggests that vitamin E – which can 'mop up' free radicals – may indeed be valuable in various conditions (see below).

Vitamin K is one of two naturally occurring yellow oils found in green leafy vegetables, cereals and fruit. It is also synthesized in the large intestine by bacteria. Deficiency causes a decrease in the clotting component prothrombin in the blood and results in prolongation of the time taken for blood to clot. The result is spontaneous bleeding into the skin and the muscles. The vitamin is, however, so ubiquitous in vegetables, and so efficiently produced in the body, that deficiency is rare except in newborn babies or when there is liver disease and the bile necessary for its absorption is unavailable. Antibiotics can affect production.

WATER-SOLUBLE VITAMINS

Vitamin C (ascorbic acid) is plentiful in citrus fruit, tomatoes, green peppers and salad greens. Its function is to maintain the cement substance between the cells of bone, cartilage and other tissues and to take part in the synthesis of the body building protein collagen. Deficiency causes **scurvy**. There is much controversy as to whether 'megadoses' of vitamin C are valuable. Linus Pauling, the chemistry Nobel prize-winner, believes they are and reminds us that primitive man often had an intake of several grams of vitamin C daily. Vitamin C, as a powerful oxidizing agent, deals effectively with dangerous **free radicals**.

Vitamin B1, or thiamine, is found in pork, offal, whole grains, peas and beans. It is involved in chemical reactions concerned with the removal of the waste product carbon dioxide from cells. A deficiency causes **beri-beri** with heart failure, oedema and inflammation of the peripheral nerves.

Vitamin B2 (riboflavine), which is found in most foodstuffs, is a co-enzyme necessary for the production of energy in cells, the breakdown and utilization of carbohydrates, proteins and fats and the synthesis of adrenal hormones. It is found in most foods. Deficiency causes reddening and cracking of the lips, cracks at the corners of the mouth, soreness of the tongue, abnormal sensitivity to light and sometimes visual loss (nutritional amblyopia).

Nicotinic acid is a co-enzyme in the chemical reactions concerned with the metabolism of carbohydrates and fats, the proper functioning of the nerves and the intestines, the synthesis of sex hormones and the maintenance of normal skin. It is plentiful in liver, lean meat, grains and pulses. Deficiency causes **pellagra**, a disease featuring disorders of the bowels and the skin and nerve and mental malfunction.

Vitamin B6 deficiency causes poor growth, dermatitis around the eyes, anaemia, kidney stones, irritability, muscle twitching and epileptic convulsions.

Pantothenic acid has functions similar to those of riboflavine and it, too, is present in most foodstuffs. Both are particularly prevalent in liver, offal – especially heart and kidney, egg yolk, fish, wheat germ and brewer's yeast. Deficiency of pantothenic acid causes fatigue, headache, muscle cramps, impaired coordination, sleep disturbances and nausea. **Peptic ulcers** can occur in severe cases.

Biotin is a co-enzyme necessary for the synthesis of fat and the glucose storage polymer glycogen, and for the excretion of the waste products of protein breakdown. It is found in vegetables, pulses and meat, and a deficiency causes fatigue, depression, nausea, dermatitis and pains in the muscles.

Folic acid is a co-enzyme involved in the production of the genetic material in cells (DNA) and in amino acid metabolism. It is necessary for the healthy functioning of the nervous system and for the production of normal red blood cells. It is found in green leafy vegetables such as spinach and broccoli, and in liver, egg yolk, mushrooms and wheat grains. Deficiency causes poor growth in children. In adults, deficiency causes anaemia, soreness of the mouth and diarrhoea.

Vitamin B12 is a group of dark red, crystalline, cobalt-containing compounds, often called cyanocobalamin. It is necessary, as a co-enzyme, in DNA synthesis, in red blood cell production, in the utilization of folic acid and carbohydrates and in the normal functioning of nerves. It is present in meat, eggs and dairy products, but not in plants. Deficiency causes **pernicious anaemia** and neurological disorders. Pernicious anaemia occurs in people lacking a factor secreted in the normal gastric juice which allows vitamin B12 to be absorbed.

Vitamin C and E are powerful antioxidants and there is increasing evidence that daily doses of the order of 2000 mg of C and 400 mg of E can have a substantial effect in countering the oxygen free radicals that mediate so much of the bodily damage effected by disease and environmental factors. In particular, it is now widely accepted that the process of arterial damage leading to atherosclerosis, with all its dire consequences, involves free radical action and can be countered by anti-oxidant vitamins. Ageing is also thought to be partly mediated by free radicals.

See also **anti-oxidants and vitamins**.

vitiligo

A disfiguring skin condition in which white patches, of variable size and shape, appear on the skin in childhood or adult life. These occur especially on the face, the backs of the hands, the armpits and around the anus. In white people, in winter, vitiligo may be almost invisible, but in black people or tanned whites it is very conspicuous and a source of embarrassment.

POSSIBLE CAUSES

Skin colour is caused by pigment cells called melanocytes and in the areas of vitiligo these are absent. The reason remains obscure but it seems likely that an immunological mechanism is involved. People with vitiligo often have pigment abnormalities in their retinas and inner ears and most have antibodies to pigment cells circulating in their bloodstreams.

TREATMENT

The treatment of vitiligo is difficult and many affected people use cosmetic cream applications. Artificial local tanning with Covermark (dihydroxy acetone in alcohol) can be useful. Local steroids sometimes help. Recently, it has been found that repigmentation can be achieved by giving L-phenylalanine, a precursor of melanin pigment, and then exposing the skin to ultraviolet light (UVA) or sunlight. The effect is not apparent for several months.

vitreous detachment

Separation of the rear part of the vitreous body of the eye from the retina as a result of the natural shrinkage that occurs in elderly people. This is much less serious than retinal detachment and gives rise to trouble in only about one case in twenty. Symptoms of vitreous detachment are the perception of floating specks or moving clouds and sometimes flashing lights. Both of these may be a conspicuous feature of the process but are often temporary.

Vivalan

A brand name for **viloxazine**.

Vivapril

A brand name for **selegiline**.

vivisection

Experimental surgery on animals. The contemplation of any act involving cruelty or damage to, or mutilation of, any animal is abhorrent and there has been much public outcry against any such practices, whatever the motive.

Essentially, the use of animals in medical research involves a balance between the expectation of the relief of the suffering of human beings, on the one hand, and the sacrifice of often anaesthetized animals, on the other. Gratuitous cruelty is as abhorrent to scientists as to anyone else and is certainly less common in laboratories than outside them. Few thinking people question that animal experiments, especially in cancer and drug research, benefit mankind and most recognize the scientist's responsibility to society in the conduct of such work. Scientists, however, are as liable as any other class of people to become blunted in their sensibilities by custom and fascination with their work, and have a strong obligation to avoid the use of animals when there is any feasible alternative.

vocal cords, disorders of

Vocal overuse, as in prolonged shouting or talking, or improper use of the voice, as in certain types of pop singing, commonly results in the development of polyps on the vocal cords (**singer's nodes**).

> Overuse in the presence of laryngitis is especially dangerous and may cause permanent damage to the muscles which tense the cords. Singers or actors with laryngitis should never try to perform.

Excessive smoking sometimes causes persistent (chronic) laryngitis with thickening of the vocal cords and hoarseness of the voice.

Paralysis of the muscles which tense the vocal cords prevents them from being pressed together and the voice becomes breathy, toneless, hoarse, or is lost altogether.

> Such paralysis is usually caused by interference with the nerves supplying the muscles of the larynx (recurrent laryngeal nerves) and this must always be regarded as a possible sign of serious disease, such as cancer, in the region around and below the larynx.

These nerves pass well down into the chest before running up again close to the wind pipe (trachea), the gullet (oesophagus) and the large blood vessels to reach the larynx. Laryngeal paralysis may thus occur in lung cancer, cancer of the oesophagus, cancer at the base of the skull or cancer of the thyroid gland. It may also be caused by enlargement of the heart or by aneurysm of the aorta or other major vessels.

> Hoarseness or loss of voice is, of course, common from innocent causes, but sudden loss of phonation, in the absence of obvious cause, should be urgently reported.

Primary cancer of the vocal cords will cause hoarseness, and examination of the larynx (laryngoscopy) will reveal the tumour. If this is confined to the soft tissue and no cartilage is involved, cure is possible by radiotherapy in 90 per cent of cases. If spread is more extensive, removal of the larynx (**laryngectomy**) may be necessary.

See also **larynx, cancer of**.

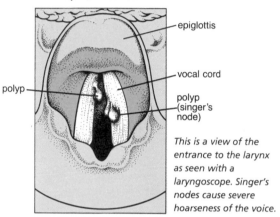

This is a view of the entrance to the larynx as seen with a laryngoscope. Singer's nodes cause severe hoarseness of the voice.

voice box, internal viewing of

See **laryngoscopy**.

voice, loss of

See **vocal cords, disorders of**.

Volkmann's ischaemic contracture

A permanent shortening of some of the muscles on the front of the forearm, leading to a disabling deformity in which the wrist and fingers become fixed in a bent position. Volkmann's contracture is caused by lack of an adequate blood supply (ischaemia) to the muscles of the forearm as a result of damage to the main artery of the arm, just above the elbow (the brachial artery), usually from a fracture of the upper arm bone (the humerus) or a dislocation of the elbow.

Volkmann's contracture is a very serious disability, constantly borne in mind by doctors dealing with such fractures. The state of the circulation in the forearm and hand is always a preoccupation after fractures around the elbow and particular attention is paid to the colour of the skin, the pulses at the wrist and the finger movements. Sometimes, the re-alignment (reduction) of fractures above the elbow becomes an emergency requirement and occasionally the surgeon must open the arm, expose the brachial artery and ensure, by vessel grafting if necessary, that continuity of blood supply is maintained.

In established contracture, major reparative surgery, sometimes involving shortening of the arm, muscle transplants or fusion of the wrist, may be necessary.

Volraman

A brand name for **diclofenac**.

Volsaid Retard

A brand name for **diclofenac**.

Voltarol

A brand name for **diclofenac**.

Volumax

A brand name for **salbutamol**.

volvulus

The rotation or twisting of a loop of intestine, on its suspending membrane (mesentery), so that the passage of its contents is impeded and the blood vessels supplying it are in danger of being obstructed. Blood vessel obstruction is called strangulation and leads to **gangrene**. Volvulus is most likely to occur if the mesentery has been shortened by previous adhesions, or is abnormal from birth.

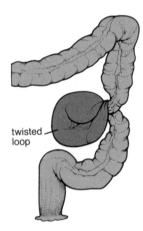

twisted
loop

Volvulus is a dangerous twisting of a loop of bowel, in this case of the descending colon. Twisting causes occlusion of the blood vessels and may lead to gangrene of the loop.

RECOGNITION AND SYMPTOMS
Bowel obstruction leads to severe pain in the abdomen, occurring at intervals of a few minutes, rising to a peak and then settling. Between peaks, the pain is absent. Vomiting follows the pain at an interval which depends on the site of the obstruction. The lower the blockage, the longer the interval, and several hours may elapse between the onset of pain and the start of the vomiting.

TREATMENT
Volvulus is often a surgical emergency and sometimes it may be necessary to remove the affected loop of bowel and join the ends.

vomiting

Involuntary expulsion of the stomach contents via the oesophagus and the mouth. Vomiting is usually, although not always, preceded by severe nausea and indications of overactivity of the parasympathetic nervous system – sweating, excessive salivation, pallor and slowing of the heart rate. The brain mechanism for vomiting consists of a vomiting centre, which receives information from the digestive tract and other parts of the body, and a chemoreceptor trigger zone, which responds to vomit-stimulating substances in the blood and then prompts the vomiting centre to initiate the act.

The stomach plays an almost passive role in vomiting, the ejection of the contents being brought about by sudden pressure on it from the surrounding structures, as a result of forceful simultaneous downward movement of the diaphragm and inward movement of the wall of the abdomen. At the same time, the upper part of the stomach, and the sphincter between the stomach and the oesophagus, relax, while the sphincter at the lower outlet of the stomach closes tightly.

To prevent the dangerous entry of stomach contents into the lungs, the vocal cords are pressed tightly together during vomiting and breathing is temporarily impossible. The process of retching, which often precedes vomiting, is, in part, an attempt to overcome this reflex and to take breath.

POSSIBLE CAUSES
Vomiting may result from undue distention of the stomach from over-eating, and is a common feature of severe indigestion, stomach or duodenal ulcer, acute appendicitis, or **peritonitis**. Infection of the intestine, as in **gastroenteritis**, **shigellosis**, or parasitic worm or other infestation, commonly causes vomiting. Intestinal obstruction, from causes such as congenital narrowing of the outlet of the stomach (pyloric stenosis), **volvulus**, **intussusception**, or tumour, will, unless relieved, inevitably lead to vomiting.

Certain foods, especially fatty foods, often cause people with dyspepsia to vomit, but many ingested substances will do so, either by irritating the stomach lining or by stimulating the vomiting centres in the brain. These include a wide range of drugs and chemicals and the toxins of various bacteria, including those causing food poisoning. Alcohol is one of the commonest causes of vomiting, both by its irritant action on the stomach and by its central action.

Inflammation in structures connected with the digestive tract will also cause vomiting – as in hepatitis, gall-bladder inflammation, gallstones and pancreatitis.

Conditions remote from the digestive system can cause vomiting and the most important of these is a rise in the pressure within the skull from any cause such as brain tumour, **encephalitis** or **hydrocephalus**. A sudden rise in the intracranial pressure will cause unexpected, forcible, 'projectile' vomiting, often without nausea. Disorders of the balancing mechanism in the inner ear, such as **Ménière's syndrome**, or acute labyrinthitis, regularly cause vomiting.

Vomiting is common in endocrine disorders and is a feature of acidosis in **diabetes**, **Addison's disease** and early pregnancy – 'morning sickness'. Hyperemesis gravidarum is the serious, and sometimes life-threatening, excessive vomiting in **pregnancy**. Cyclical vomiting is a condition, tending to run in families, which causes recurrent attacks of vomiting and headache. It often starts in childhood and is associated with migraine.

Psychogenic vomiting may occur as a result of a passing emotional upset, or may be a feature of a more permanent psychiatric disorder. It may occur in anorexia nervosa in spite of the low food intake, and is a constant feature of bulimia.

> Particular attention should be paid to persistent vomiting in babies and young children. This may be a sign of unsuspected disorders of the digestive or nervous systems. Persistent vomiting may also lead to dangerous dehydration and changes in the acidity of the blood.

TREATMENT

Vomiting should not be considered a disorder in its own right, but rather a sign of some particular disorder. There is always a cause and this should, if possible, be found and removed. Because vomiting is sometimes purposive, leading to rejection of toxins, poisons or irritants, deliberate suppression of vomiting, without knowledge of the cause, may worsen the situation.

The most effective drugs for the control of vomiting – drugs such as metoclopramide – act on the chemoreceptor trigger zone by blocking its chemical receptors. Such drugs are highly effective in the control of both nausea and vomiting, but are used only when the cause of the vomiting cannot immediately be relieved.

See also **vomiting blood**.

vomiting blood

> This is a serious physical sign, which should never be disregarded.

Doctors must distinguish between blood actually vomited, and blood in the vomit, but originating from the nose or mouth. Occasionally, there may be confusion with coughed-up blood.

RECOGNITION

Vomited blood is seldom bright red as it has almost always been acted on by the stomach acid and altered so that it resembles dark coffee grounds.

People who vomit blood almost always show the associated sign of tarry-black stools (**melaena**) and this confirms that the bleeding is in the stomach or bowel. Melaena, too, should always be reported.

POSSIBLE CAUSES

Vomiting of blood is called haematemesis and is a sign of stomach ulcer, severe gastritis – often from irritation by alcohol or aspirin – bleeding from varicose veins in the stomach or oesophagus, or from a tear in the oesophagus lining caused by powerful retching or vomiting (the **Mallory-Weiss syndrome**). Cancer of the stomach causes bleeding but is less likely than these conditions to lead to vomiting of blood.

vomiting in pregnancy

See **pregnancy**.

von Recklinghausen's disease

See **neurofibromatosis**.

von Willebrand's disease

A genetically induced bleeding disorder, similar to **haemophilia**, due to insufficiency of a factor in the blood necessary for normal clotting of the blood.

voyeurism

Sometimes called *scoptophilia*. The voyeur obtains sexual stimulation by covertly observing people undressing, naked or engaging in sexual intercourse. The observation is accompanied by masturbation and the practice often starts in childhood. Almost all voyeurs are men and are commonly known as peeping Toms. Voyeurism tends to be a persistent habit which generally occurs in isolated and lonely people.

vulnere

Latin root meaning 'wound' as in vulnerable (susceptible to injury).

vulva, disorders of

The vulva are the external female genitalia – the labia and the clitoris. The opening of the vagina is only a centimetre or two in front of the anus and, however scrupulous the personal hygiene, it is impossible to avoid some contamination of the vulva with faecal organisms. In spite of this, infection and inflammation (vulvitis) is uncommon, usually being controlled by natural local resistance. Other organisms can, however, cause infection. The commonest vulval infections are genital **herpes** and thrush (**candidiasis**). The latter is especially common in diabetics.

Vulval inflammation also occurs from post-menopausal oestrogen deficiency (*kraurosis vulvae*), or contact allergies to soaps, vaginal deodorants, washing powder residues on underwear and sometimes solutions used for douching. Other causes of inflammation include bartholinitis and the various causes of vaginitis, especially **trichomoniasis**.

See also **sexually transmitted diseases**, **vagina, disorders of**.

vulva, skin atrophy in

See **lichen sclerosus**.

vulvovaginitis

Inflammation of the vulva and the vagina. The condition is commonest in childhood as a result of poor hygiene, or a foreign body in the vagina or sexual assault. There is soreness on urination, redness and sometimes a slight discharge. Daily washing is often all that is necessary but medical attention is called for to establish the cause.

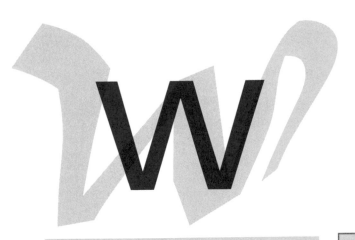

warfare, eye risks in

See **laser weapon eye injuries**.

warfarin

An **anticoagulant** drug used to prevent blood from clotting in the blood vessels. A brand name is Marevan.

Warticon

A brand name for **podophyllotoxin**.

wart on sole of foot

See **plantar wart**.

warts

Warts, or verrucae, are caused by different strains of the human papilloma virus and are all essentially the same, although they have a different appearance in different kinds of skin. The viruses cause an overgrowth of the layer at the base of the epidermis of the skin, called the prickle cell layer, and the result is an excessive local production of the horny material keratin. The form the wart takes depends on the thickness of the skin and on its location.

Warts appear and disappear apparently spontaneously, but in reality under the influence of changes in the resistance to the virus (changing immunological status). They occur in large numbers in people whose immune systems are compromised by disease or medical treatment by immunosuppressive drugs. Genital warts are associated with cancer of the cervix, but there is no positive proof that they actually cause it. Other factors common to the sexually promiscuous may equally be responsible. There is no evidence that warts elsewhere on the body have any connection, whatsoever, with cancer.

TYPES OF WARTS

The common wart, verruca vulgaris, can occur anywhere. Verruca plana is the round, flat-topped, yellowish wart occurring mainly on the back of the hands. Verruca filiformis is the long, slender, fir-tree-like wart common on the thin skin of the eyelids, armpits or neck.

Venereal warts (condylomata acuminata) are pink cauliflower-like growths on the penis or vulva, but, again are essentially the same as other warts. Plantar warts (verruca plantaris) are ordinary warts modified by the pressure of the weight of the body which forces them deeply into the thick skin of the sole of the foot.

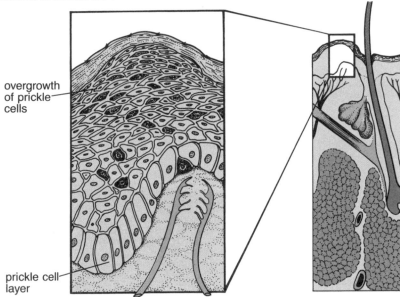

overgrowth of prickle cells

prickle cell layer

Warts are benign growths (papillomas) caused by a local overgrowth of the prickle cell layer of the skin.

TREATMENT

Most warts resolve without treatment, 30 per cent of them within six months. Some persist for five years or more. Several forms of treatment are available. These include salicylic acid in collodion, salicylic acid plasters, formalin soaks, podophyllin, freezing with liquid nitrogen and burning with a cautery under anaesthetic. Plantar warts may require ring pads to relieve pressure and are sometimes removed by cutting them out with a sharp-edged spoon (a curette).

wasp stings

See **insect and mite bites and stings**.

water

Water is one of the commonest chemical compounds in the world and is essential for life. Ninety-nine per cent of the molecules in the body are water, but water represent a smaller proportion of body weight. In the obese, about 50 per cent of body weight consists of water; in the lean, the figure is nearer 70 per cent. The body of an average man (70 kg) contains just over 40 litres of water.

A little over half the total body water is within the cells and the remainder outside, partly in the blood, but mainly in the tissue spaces surrounding the cells. Water molecules are so small that they move freely across all cell membranes and redistribution is constantly occurring. Even when no net movement of water occurs, many molecules are actually moving across cell membranes in both directions.

Water is actually produced within the body, by the oxidation of nutrients and almost as much is acquired by eating so-called solid food as by drinking. Water is lost by four routes, the proportion leaving the body by each of these varying with the circumstances. Most water is lost in the urine, but a considerable volume leaves in the form of vapour in the breath and 'insensible' evaporation from the skin. Loss in sweat varies with the environmental conditions and a small amount is lost in the faeces.

The maintenance of the normal body water volume is largely achieved by automatic alteration in the quantity of urine passed, and by thirst, which prompts additional intake when body water is depleted. A persistent state of excess water in the tissues is called **oedema**. The presence of less than the normal amount is called dehydration.

WATER POLLUTION

Population and industrial growth have greatly increased the risk and actuality of adding undesirable substances to natural water. These substances alter the biological safety of this vital element, both to man and to water life, and may, in consequence, endanger health and even human life. Natural water contains considerable oxygen in solution. This is essential for the respiration of fish and other aquatic life forms, and is depleted by raised temperatures and by the presence of many pollutant substances. Many waste materials deposited in water are broken down by bacteria which, in the presence of such nutrients, multiply enormously, using dissolved oxygen for respiration. If the oxygen is entirely consumed, all larger living forms are destroyed and the water becomes septic and offensive.

Inadequately separated domestic waste contributes faeces and urine, kitchen waste, household cleaning agents and detergents and may promote the risk of water-borne disease, especially **typhoid fever** and **dysentery**. Industrial waste water may contain a very wide range of toxic and water-degrading material. Pollution control is entirely a matter of applied science and financial expenditure. No pollution problem is beyond solution, given motivation, money and realistic legislation to prevent industrial profits being made without regard to public amenity. But we should remember that all of us are contributing to the problem and we should be willing to pay for its solution.

water-borne infection

Diseases commonly spread by water include a number of intestinal infections such as **typhoid fever** and other Salmonella infections, **cholera**, **hepatitis A**, amoebic **dysentery** and worm parasite infestations. Diseases acquired by contact with water include Weill's disease (**leptospirosis**), **schistosomiasis** and **Guinea worm.**

waterbrash

The regurgitation of acid into the mouth from the stomach. Waterbrash is associated with heartburn (reflux **oesophagitis**) and is a feature of **hiatus hernia** and various stomach disorders.

watering eye

A common sign either of excessive tear production (lacrimation) or of an obstruction to the normal tear drainage channel (lacrimal duct). The lacrimal ducts run from the inner corners of each eyelid, down into the nose. Watering from overproduction of tears is treated by removing the cause, if possible.

POSSIBLE CAUSES

Lacrimation is caused by any irritating stimulus, such as strong emotion, a foreign body, a corneal ulcer or **conjunctivitis**. Lacrimal duct obstruction causes tear overflow (epiphora) and may result from swelling of the lining of the narrow tear passage, obstruction by mucus, pus or cellular debris, or, unfortunately, by infective damage to the lining which has led to permanent closure by healing. It can also be caused by obstruction from swelling of the lining of the nose, at the lower end of the duct.

TREATMENT

Lacrimal duct obstruction may respond to a wash-through with salt water. If this fails, the duct can, especially in babies, be opened by the careful passage, along the duct, of a blunt metal probe. This is seldom successful in adults, however, and a more radical procedure, in which a new opening is made through into the nose (dacryo-cysto-rhinostomy) is often necessary.

water on the brain

See **hydrocephalus**.

water on the knee

A lay term for an accumulation of fluid (effusion) within the knee joint as a result of injury or an arthritic problem. Excess fluid in the region of the knee can also occur when, as a result of inflammation, fluid accumulates in one of the fluid-secreting sacs (bursas) situated around the knee joint.

See also **bursitis**, **clergyman's knee**.

Watson-Crick model

The double helix concept of the **DNA** molecule, proposed by two scientists in Cambridge in 1953, which triggered off a revolution in biology and medicine and led to an explosive succession of advances in genetics. The men concerned were the American ornithologist turned molecular biologist James D. Watson, and the English biochemist Francis H. C. Crick, now a neurophysiologist interested in brain function.

wax bath

A form of local heat treatment used by physiotherapists in the treatment of **rheumatoid arthritis** and other joint conditions. It is questionable whether the method differs particularly in its effect from any other form of local heat application, but the build-up of the coating, as the affected part of the body is dipped repeatedly into the container of molten wax, is impressive and interesting to the sufferer and probably distracts somewhat from the pain. Wax baths have sometimes been used in the treatment of burns of the hands.

wax, ear

The secretion of the ceruminous glands in the skin of the wall of the external auditory canal (meatus). The glands are modified sweat glands, producing a sticky fatty secretion which protects the eardrum by trapping dust and small objects. Normal soft wax makes its way out of the ear and is removed by washing. Hard, or dried wax tends to accumulate. The rate of secretion of wax is affected by irritation to the skin, and constant exploration of the ears with physical objects will tend to produce more wax. Some people naturally produce more than the normal amount of wax. Those who do so sometimes suffer deafness from occlusion of the meatus and such wax accumulation tends to recur even after complete removal by a doctor.

Deafness is not caused by wax until the meatus is completely obstructed, but this may occur suddenly if water gets into the ears. Ear wax is hygroscopic, absorbs water and swells up. Removal of wax by syringing can give great relief, but this should be done by an expert aware of the risks. Many ENT specialists prefer to avoid syringing, in case infected material should be carried into the middle ear through an unseen perforation in the drum, and choose instead to remove waxpiece meal by instruments, or by suction.

Waxsol

A brand name for **docusate sodium**.

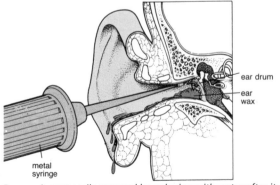

Ear wax is most easily removed by syringing with water after it has been softened with oil. This must be done carefully to avoid rupturing the eardrum, and there is always a risk that infected material may be carried into the middle ear through a perforation in the drum.

waxy brain masses

See **amyloid**.

weakness

The state of debility brought about by serious illness, prolonged bed rest, muscle disease or wasting, anaemia, starvation or a strong disinclination to exert oneself. The latter is a common cause of a sense of weakness or fatigue and is an unhappy state engendered by boredom, dislike of one's work or social situation, or a close personal relationship. The absence of motivation to work is as disabling as any organic cause of weakness and may occur without any obvious physical disorder. In time, however, it is likely to give rise to disuse atrophy of body, or mind, or both.

weaning

The substitution of solid foods for milk in an infant's diet.

webbed neck

See **Turner's syndrome**.

Web browsing, excessive

See **Internet addiction**.

Wegener's granulomatosis

An inflammatory disorder of the small blood vessels (vasculitis) in which nodular masses of cells, buds of blood capillaries and fibrous tissue form in various parts of the body, including the nose, the lungs, the heart and the kidneys. These masses are known as granulation tissue and they may cause local damage and become gangrenous.

RECOGNITION AND SYMPTOMS
The symptoms of the disorder include bleeding from the nose and the kidneys (haematuria) and occasionally pain in the chest. Kidney failure can occur.

POSSIBLE CAUSES
The vasculitis which underlies this condition is thought to be due to an auto-immune process in which parts of the small arteries cease to be regarded by the immune system of the body as 'self' and are attacked by antibodies and white cells.

TREATMENT
Wegener's granulomatosis responds well to the immunosuppressive drug cyclophosphamide, but this may have to be used long term.

weight

Body weight varies with height and with skeletal shape and bulk and should not vary with age. The parameter which causes the largest variation in body weight in Western societies, however, is the amount of fat storage. Excess fat storage is dangerous and significantly increases the risk of developing several serious diseases including **diabetes**, high blood pressure (**hypertension**), **atherosclerosis**, **angina pectoris**, coronary thrombosis (**heart attack**) and **osteoarthritis**. Efforts should therefore be made, at all costs, to avoid obesity.

weight loss

Weight loss arises when dietary calorie intake is smaller than calorie expenditure. This may be the result of a deliberate, weight-losing policy in the interests of health (see **health maintenance**), a pathological reduction in food intake as in **anorexia nervosa** or **depression**, or unavoidable starvation. Weight loss, from excess of tissue breakdown (catabolism) over build up (anabolism), is also a feature of many diseases, particularly **thyrotoxicosis**, cancer, **tuberculosis** and **diabetes**. Reduced calorie intake may also result from **malabsorption** disorders or from intestinal disorders, such as persistent vomiting or diarrhoea.

> Unexplained weight loss is one of the warning signs of possible serious disease and should never be disregarded.

weight problems

See **health maintenance**.

Weil's disease

See **leptospirosis**.

welder's eye

An acute **conjunctivitis** with damage to the outer layer of the cornea (the epithelium) caused by the intense ultraviolet light radiation emitted by an electric welding arc. Welder's eye occurs in those incautious enough to engage in electric arc welding without the normal eye protection. A few hours after exposure, the eyes become intensely red and painful, with tearing, spasm of the lids, and a sensation as if they are full of sand. The radiation damage causes the outer cell layers of the corneas to strip off, exposing the underlying nerve endings.

Recovery is the rule, but it is usually necessary for the affected person to remain quiet with both eyes kept closed under pads for two or three days. Antibiotic eye drops are used to prevent infection.

Welldorm

A brand name for the sleeping drug **chloral betaine**. Also a brand name for elixir **chloral hydrate**.

Wellferon

A brand name for **interferon alfa**.

Wellvone

A brand name for **atovaquone**.

wen

See **sebaceous cyst**.

Werner's syndrome

A rare hereditary, probably autosomal recessive, condition featuring premature ageing, dwarfism, atrophy of the skin, cataracts, severe arterial disease, osteoporosis, atrophy of the testicles and diabetes.

Wernicke-Korsakoff syndrome

A brain disorder affecting long-term alcoholics who rely solely, or mainly, on alcohol for their nutrition. One effect is a deficient intake of **vitamin** B1 (thiamine), necessary for among other things, normal functioning of the nervous system.

The syndrome may present in one, or both, of two forms. The more immediately dangerous of these is called Wernicke's encephalopathy. This starts suddenly, and features areas of congestion and bleeding in the brain resulting in states of confusion, loss of bodily coordination, staggering, and, particularly, paralysis of eye movements. Unless urgently treated the condition soon progresses to stupor and death. An intravenous injection of a large dose of thiamine will reverse most of the effects, sometimes within hours, and is life-saving.

In Korsakoff's psychosis, the other form, the main change is in mental function and this may, at first, be subtle. There is a severe memory defect with almost total loss of the capacity to store new information, but this is concealed by the, initially effective, process of confabulation, in which the affected person makes up stories to fill in the gaps in the memory. People with Korsakoff's psychosis may talk convincingly to strangers, but those who know them soon become familiar with the constantly replayed 'tape recording'. Unfortunately, this form is usually irreversible and proceeds to profound **dementia** and the need for constant supervision.

Wernicke's encephalopathy

See **Wernicke-Korsakoff syndrome**.

Wernicke's sign

The *visual pathways* are the nerve tracts running from the eyes to the back of the brain. These are extensive and are often damaged in brain disorders such as cerebral thrombosis or tumours. So long as the parts concerned with 'straight-ahead' vision are unaffected, people with even major visual pathway loss are often unaware that half the field of vision is missing in each eye. If a narrow beam of light is projected on to the blind halves of the retinas, the pupils will not show the normal narrowing (constriction). Light shone on the normal halves, however, causes the pupils to constrict. This is known as Wernicke's sign.

wetting agent

See **surfactant**.

whiplash injury

Because of the flexibility of the neck and the considerable weight of the head, sudden accelerative or decelerative forces applied to the body will almost always cause violent bending of the neck in a direction opposite to the direction of the force. This is immediately followed by a reflex contraction of the overstretched muscles, so that the head then jerks in the opposite direction. Whiplash injury is usually caused by a frontal car collision, in which the head first swings forward as the body is decelerated, or by a collision from the rear, in which the head first swings back.

Often the degree of neck bending exceeds the normal range of movements imposed by the structure, and the ligaments connecting the bones (vertebrae) may be stretched or even torn. In the worst cases, a fracture of one or more of the neck vertebrae may occur. Whiplash injury causes much persistent pain and disability, often for weeks, and the support of an orthopaedic collar may be needed for a month or two. (See illustration overleaf.)

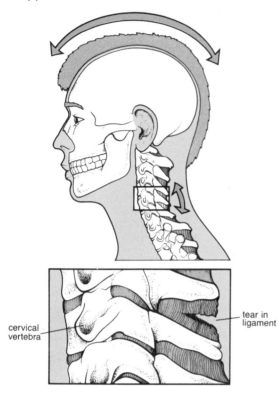

cervical vertebra

tear in ligament

In whiplash injury a tear may occur in the ligaments between the back processes of the neck vertebrae. This may cause weeks of pain and disability.

Whipple's disease

A **malabsorption** disorder, also called intestinal lipodystrophy, which causes fever, loss of weight, abdominal pain, diarrhoea, **arthritis**, enlarged lymph nodes, **anaemia** and abnormal skin colouring (pigmentation). Men are affected more often than women and joint problems often precede the intestinal disorder, sometimes by months or years.

The cause is unknown, but a **biopsy** from the small intestine shows characteristic changes in the immune system cells which ingest foreign material (the macrophages). The condition responds well to prolonged treatment with antibiotics, such as tetracycline.

whipworm infestation

Infestation with *Trichuris trichiura*, an intestinal parasitic worm, universally found in underdeveloped areas. The adult worms are 2.5 to 5 cm long and have a whip-like appearance, the 'tail' being the head. In the male worm, the 'handle' of the whip is also spiralled. Each pregnant female lays about 2000 eggs a day and these survive in moist soil contaminated with faeces. In conditions of poor hygiene and sanitation, the eggs readily find their way into the mouths of children and others.

RECOGNITION AND SYMPTOMS

Whipworms inhabit the lower bowel and usually cause no trouble, but in very large infestations with hundreds of worms, there may be a wasting diarrhoea which, in children suffering from malnutrition, may be serious. The characteristic barrel-shaped eggs are easily identified in the stools, by microscopy.

TREATMENT

Treatment with mebendazole will drive out the worms. The real solution, of course, is to improve, if possible, the social conditions.

white coat hypertension

Abnormally high blood pressure caused by the act of measuring it. People with white coat hypertension show normal pressures when these are recorded on a cassette during 24-hour ambulatory monitoring measurements. But when the blood pressure is measured by a doctor or nurse it is found to be higher than normal. Assuming that ambulatory methods show acceptable levels, white coat hypertension will usually not require treatment. But close follow-up is necessary as it has been found that some of the affected people develop later complications such as kidney impairment or enlargement of the left ventricle of the heart.

white pupil

See **cataract**, **galactosaemia**, **retinoblastoma**, **retrolental fibroplasia**.

white skin and hair

See **albino**.

whitlow

An infection in the pulp of the fingertip usually resulting from a prick or a small cut and often leading to abscess formation.

> The condition, which is also called a felon, is potentially serious and should never be neglected as it may lead to infection of the bone of the fingertip (osteomyelitis).

Pulp space infection causes a dull pain, worse when the hand is hanging, and redness and swelling of the finger. At this stage, the condition may often be controlled by antibiotic treatment. If untreated, the pain quickly becomes more severe and throbbing, and there is great tenderness on pressure. Hardening of the pulp indicates that pus is present and that surgical drainage will be required. A persistently discharging opening suggests that part of the bone has died and must be removed. If this is done, the wound will heal, but the finger will be shortened and the nail curved and disfiguring.

The term 'whitlow' is also used to refer to an infection of the finger skin, in the region of the nail, or of the skin at the edge of the nail, by Herpes simplex viruses.

whooping cough

This is an acute, highly infectious, disease occurring almost exclusively in children under five years of age and spread by droplet infection. It is also known as pertussis and is caused by the organism *Bordetella pertussis*. The early, infectious stage cannot be distinguished from a cold, so epidemics commonly occur in susceptible children. The incubation period is seven to ten days.

The disease, which can be very distressing, lasts for about six weeks. After the first week or two of cold symptoms, the characteristic cough begins and the number of paroxysms of coughing varies from two or three to as many as fifty. These bouts are commoner at night. The child is seized by an uncontrollable succession of short, sharp coughs, so insistent and rapid in sequence that there is no time to draw breath between them. The lungs thus become almost emptied of air and the cough sequence is followed by a long, deep inspiration which often features a whooping sound. The final paroxysm in a series is often followed by vomiting. The process is exhausting to child and parent alike.

Whooping cough may be complicated by pneumonia, collapse of a segment or lobe of a lung, epileptic seizures from lack of oxygen in the brain, ulceration of the central membrane under the tongue and pushing out (prolapse) of the rectum. Antibiotics are of no value once the paroxysmal stage has been reached, unless secondary infection occurs. Vomiting may interfere with nutrition, but feeds are usually retained if given immediately after vomiting.

In very rare cases, whooping cough vaccine has been said to cause epileptic-like seizures or brain damage, and public knowledge of this led to a decline in acceptance of vaccination in Britain. It is important to state that the risks of vaccination are much less than the risks of whooping cough. Prior to the introduction of the vaccine in 1957 over 100,000 cases of whooping cough were officially notified each year, and many more occurred which were not notified. The death rate was about one per 1000, overall, but the rate was much higher in children under one year of age. By 1973, vaccination of 80 per cent of children had led to a reduction to about 2400 cases. But public anxiety thereafter caused a drop to 30 per cent vaccination, and major epidemics occurred from 1977–1979, and from 1981–1983. Since then, acceptance has again risen and in 1986 was 67 per cent.

Most doctors advise that this disease should be prevented by active immunization of all infants, from three months of age, unless the child is suffering from any other acute illness or shows an adverse reaction to the first injection of the vaccine. Decisions may be difficult in the case of children with a history of brain damage or seizures or a family history of epilepsy. In these the risk of vaccination may be higher, but so may be the risks of whooping cough.

Babies under three months should be protected, as far as is possible, from contact with children who may be infected with whooping cough. They do, however, have considerable protection from antibodies acquired from the mother before birth.

wife-battering

See **violence in the home**.

Wilms' tumour

See **kidney cancer**.

Wilson's disease

Sometimes called hepato-lenticular degeneration, this is a rare genetic disorder in which excessive amounts of copper accumulate in the body, especially in the liver and brain. The copper is also deposited in the margins of the corneas, causing a ring of greenish-brown discoloration known as the Kayser-Fleischer ring. This is diagnostic of Wilson's disease.
RECOGNITION AND SYMPTOMS
Episodes of **hepatitis**, culminating in cirrhosis of the liver and liver failure, occur. The brain copper accumulation leads to

behaviour changes, twisting movements of the limbs (athetoid movements), muscle rigidity and contractures, and personality changes progressing to **dementia**.

Untreated, the disease is invariably fatal.

TREATMENT
Wilson's disease, if diagnosed before serious liver and brain changes have occurred, responds well to reduction in intake of copper-containing foods and the use of the drug d-penicillamine, which binds copper into a form which is excreted in the urine. Oral zinc sulphate is also effective.

'wind'

See **colic**.

wind chill

The additional cooling effect produced by wind in conditions of low atmospheric temperatures. Wind chill may cause rapid heat loss from the body and adds to the danger of hypothermia.

Winsprin

A brand name for aspirin (see **analgesic drugs**).

witches' milk

See **milk, witches'**.

withdrawal bleeding

In the menstrual cycle the ovarian secretion first of oestrogen then, after ovulation, of progesterone leads to the build-up of the womb lining to a state suitable for implantation of a fertilized egg. But if fertilization does not occur there is a sudden drop in the levels of both hormones and this leads to the casting off of the womb lining as a menstrual period. The bleeding that results from this drop in the levels of sex hormones is sometimes called *withdrawal bleeding*. The term is applied to any circumstance in which uterine bleeding is brought about in this way, as in cessation of hormonal treatment or at the end of each cycle of the contraceptive pill.

withdrawal syndrome

The complex of symptoms experienced on withdrawal of a drug on which a person is physically dependent. Symptoms of heroin withdrawal include craving for the drug, restlessness, depression, running nose, yawning, pain in the abdomen, vomiting, diarrhoea, loss of appetite, sweating and gooseflesh ('cold turkey'). Those caused by withdrawal of other narcotic drugs are similar but less intense.

See also **detoxification under anaesthesia**.

wives, battered

See **violence in the home**.

Wolff-Parkinson-White syndrome

The heart beat stimulus is conducted down through the heart muscle by a band of specialized muscle cells so that the chambers contract in an organized manner. The Wolff-Parkinson-White syndrome is a heart disorder caused by an abnormal channel of conductive tissue in the muscle that can by-pass the controlling and timing node, the atrio-ventricular node, that lies between the upper and lower chambers. The result can be a kind of feedback oscillator that may produce fatally rapid heart rates. Treatment is by drugs such as amiodarone or disopyramide, to slow the heart.

womb

The womb, or uterus, is a hollow, pear-shaped organ about 8 cm long before childbirth and larger after. It has thick, muscular walls and is suspended by ligaments between the bladder and the rectum. The lower part, the cervix, protrudes into the vagina. The inner lining, the endometrium, is soft and velvety to the touch and contains many blood vessels and mucous glands. This lining undergoes considerable changes in the course of the menstrual cycle and much of it is cast off during menstruation. At the upper (fore) end of the uterus, on either side, the two Fallopian tubes emerge.

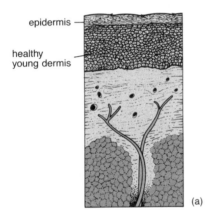

epidermis

healthy young dermis

(a)

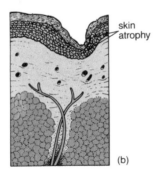

skin atrophy

(b)

womb cancer

See **uterus, cancer of**.

womb contractions, weak

See **uterine dystocia**.

womb lining destruction

See **endometrial ablation**.

womb removal

See **vaginal hysterectomy**.

word blindness

See **dyslexia**.

wrinkle

A small furrow in the skin lying between ridges caused by skin laxity. The line of the wrinkle indicates the attachment to the deeper tissue.

Wrinkles are a natural feature of the ageing skin and arise from the loss of the youthful elasticity conferred by healthy collagen – the body's structural protein. The degree of wrinkling varies considerably from one person to another and this is due at least in part to damage from ultraviolet radiation from sunlight. Wrinkling is particularly common in white-skinned people living in areas of high sun intensity such as the Middle or Far East, the south-west United States, South Africa and Northern Australia.

There is no medical or surgical way to restore elasticity to the skin, but the effect of laxity can be temporarily overcome by undermining, stretching, and removal of the excess skin – a **face lift** (*rhytidectomy*) – or by removal of excess eyelid skin (**blepharoplasty**).

wrist, disorders of

See **Colles' fracture**, **carpal tunnel syndrome**, **tenosynovitis**, **scaphoid fracture**.

wry neck

See **torticollis**.

Healthy young skin (a) compared with elderly skin (b) that has been damaged by undue exposure to ultraviolet light. Local atrophy causes wrinkles.

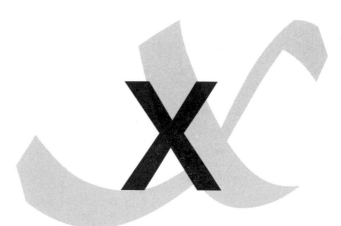

xamoterol

A beta-adrenergic stimulant drug used to treat mild degrees of **heart failure**. The drug has been used as a stimulant by athletes to try to improve performance and is on the International Olympic Committee's list of banned substances. A brand name is Corwin.

Xanax

A brand name for the benzodiazepine anti-anxiety drug.

xanthelasma

A common eyelid blemish due to deposition of cholesterol in the skin. This causes unsightly, thick yellow patches that are often very conspicuous. They occur mostly above and below the inner corner of the eye, and tend to enlarge slowly but inexorably, with time. Many people are worried that these indicate a seriously high level of cholesterol, but this is not usually so.

> There is, however, a comparatively rare genetic condition known as familial hypercholesterolaemia in which xanthelasma is a constant feature and in which cholesterol levels are dangerously high. For this reason, people with xanthelasma should always seek medical advice and have a check of the blood cholesterol.

In people with lax, redundant lid skin the cosmetic treatment of moderately sized plaques of xanthelasma is easy; the affected skin is simply removed. Unfortunately, these plaques commonly recur. There is also a danger, with over-enthusiastic surgery, that the eyelids might be unduly shortened so that eye-closure is impossible. This is a disaster that will lead to corneal drying and possible loss of vision.

xanthomatosis

A metabolic disorder in which collections of cholesterol-containing fatty material, known as xanthomas, are deposited in various parts of the body, including the arteries, the skin, the corneas, the internal organs and the brain. In severe cases xanthomas may develop in areas of skin pressure such as the elbows and knees.

The most serious effect of xanthomatosis is the deposition of cholesterol in the linings of the blood vessels so that the obstructive disease **atherosclerosis** occurs at an unusually early age. In familial hypercholesterolemia, for instance, **heart attack** from coronary thrombosis is common in the thirties in men and in the forties in women. By the age of sixty, about 85 per cent of men with familial hypercholesterolaemia have had a coronary thrombosis.

POSSIBLE CAUSES

Xanthomatosis can result from a range of disorders causing raised levels of fats and cholesterol in the blood (hyperlipidaemia). These include several common genetically induced disorders such as familial hypercholesterolaemia – excess cholesterol in the blood – and familial hypertriglyceridaemia – excess fat in the blood, and various other causes, some of which are of unknown origin.

The condition of **xanthelasma**, in which cholesterol is deposited in the eyelids, is also a feature of xanthomatosis, but commonly occurs in people with normal levels of blood cholesterol.

TREATMENT

People with xanthomatosis should have full investigation to establish the cause. Treatment is, in general, directed to lowering the abnormally high levels of lipoproteins in the blood. The diet should be low in cholesterol and high in polyunsaturated fats. A drug, such as cholestyramine, can help. This binds bile acids, formed by the liver from cholesterol and secreted into the bowel, preventing reabsorption, and so lowering the blood cholesterol. Newer agents which block an enzyme necessary for cholesterol synthesis, show great promise for the future.

Xatral

A brand name for **alfuzosin**.

X chromosome

The chromosome which, with the Y chromosome, determines the sex of the individual. About 50 per cent of sperms carry an X chromosome and 50 per cent a Y. The sex of the future child is determined by whether an X-carrying or a Y-carrying sperm happens to fertilize the ovum. The ovum carries only an X chromosome. Females have two X chromosomes in each body cell, males have one X and one Y. The X chromosome is large and contains about 6 per cent of the whole of the genomic **DNA**. The Y is about half the size. Well over a hundred disorders are known to be determined by mutated genes on the X chromosome. These are called X-linked conditions. See also **X-inactivation**.

Xenical

A brand name for **orlistat**.

xenograft

A tissue or organ graft taken from an animal of a different species from the host. Xenografts include pig heart valves and pig kidneys. Catgut, made from sheep intestine, is not a graft as it is intended to be absorbed. Transplantation sources may include transgenic animals specifically engineered for the purpose. A major setback has been the discovery that potentially dangerous retroviruses related to HIV may be transmitted with the organ. Xenografts are also known as heterografts.

xeno-oestrogens

Substances with oestrogenic properties derived from other than biological sources. A number of organochloride compounds, for instance, have been found to be sufficiently oestrogenic to cause a rise in the incidence of breast cancer in groups of women exposed to them. The insecticide dieldrin is a case in point. **Phyto-oestrogens** are not xeno-oestrogens.

Xepin

A brand name for the antidepressant and antihistamine drug **doxepin** formulated as a cream to relieve eczema.

xeroderma pigmentosum

A rare genetic skin disease featuring excessive sensitivity to sunlight, premature ageing of the skin and the development of skin cancers. The unfortunate victims are almost confined to an indoor existence and have to rely on protective covering and skin sunscreen creams.

xerophthalmia

See **dry eye**.

xeroradiography

A form of X-ray screening for breast cancer in which the image is formed on special photographic paper instead of on transparent film. Xeroradiographs can be viewed directly without special lighting. Also known as xeromammography.

xerostomia

See **mouth, dry**.

X-inactivation

In females, one X chromosome is derived from the mother and one from the father. There is good evidence, however, that early in development of the female one of these is randomly rendered inactive and that it remains so in all subsequent daughter cells. The inactivated chromosome is visible microscopically as the Barr body and the two X chromosomes in each mature cell are derived from one of the original pair. This effect explains a number of observed phenomena in genetics and is now generally accepted as true. Its implications include a degree of polarization in inheritance from the parents.

xipamide

A thiazide diuretic drug. A brand name is Diurexan.

X-linkage

See **sex-linkage**.

X-linked disorders

Genetically caused disorders in which the gene is located on the large X (sex) chromosome. Examples are **agammaglobuli-** naemia, albinism (see **albino**), Alport syndrome, Charcot-Marie-Tooth peroneal muscular atrophy, **colour blindness**, **diabetes insipidus**, ectodermal dysplasia, glucose-6-phosphate dehydrogenase deficiency, Fabry disease, glycogens storage disease VIII, gonadal dysgenesis, **haemophilia** A, one form of **hydrocephalus**, hypophosphataemia, **ichthyosis**, **Turner's syndrome**, various forms of mental retardation, Becker and Duchesse **muscular dystrophy**, one form of **retinitis pigmentosa**, the **testicular feminization syndrome**, familial premature ovarian failure and a type of **thalassaemia**. There is evidence that the X chromosome also carries genes which regulate the function of genes on other chromosomes.

XO configuration

The state of the chromosomes when only one sex chromosome, an X, is present. This is the sex chromosome abnormality most commonly found in **Turner's syndrome**. Also known as monosomy X.

X-ray examination

When a high-speed beam of electrons, accelerated by a high voltage, strikes a metal, such as copper or tungsten, electromagnetic radiation, called X-radiation, is produced. This has the power to penetrate matter to varying degrees, depending on its density, and to act on photographic film in much the same way as does visible light. These properties make X-radiation extremely valuable in medical diagnosis. X-rays have been in use for almost a century, and many millions of X-ray photographs are taken each year.

We are now more concerned than formerly about the health hazards of radiation, and X-rays are avoided if any alternative form of imaging is available and suitable. X-rays are particularly avoided in early pregnancy as they are known to increase the risk to the fetus of later cancer, especially leukaemia. CT scanning is a form of X-ray examination.

See **angiography**, **barium X-ray examination**, **bone imaging**, **bronchography**, **chest X-ray**, **cystogram**, **micturating**, **digital radiography**, **mammography**, **pyelography**.

X-ray fetal safety rule

See **ten day rule**.

X-ray while urinating

See **cystogram, micturating**.

XXX configuration

The state of the body cells when an additional X chromosome is present. Females possessing this chromosome configuration often have learning difficulties, but their children, if any, do not.

Xylocaine, Xylocard

Trade names for the local anaesthetic drug lignocaine.

XYY configuration

A male chromosome abnormality in which an additional male sex chromosome is present in every body cell. This configuration has been found in symptomless men, but is often associated with learning difficulties and behavioural problems.

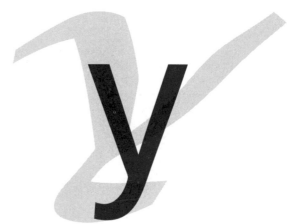

yawning

A normally involuntary act of slow, deep breathing associated with a strong desire to open the mouth widely. Yawning is associated with sleepiness, but its purpose remains a matter of speculation. It has been suggested that it may serve to stretch, open out and ventilate the air sacs of the lungs which, in the somnolent state, are apt to collapse. Yawning helps to improve the return of blood to the heart by way of the large veins. This reduces stagnation and improves the level of oxygen in the blood.

yaws

A persistent (chronic) infectious disease occurring throughout the underdeveloped areas of the world and caused by the spirochaete responsible for syphilis. It is not, however, a venereal disease, but is spread from case to case by finger contamination of areas of skin, the surface of which has been breached by minor injuries, abrasions or insect bites. The infection is almost always acquired in childhood.

RECOGNITION AND SYMPTOMS
After an **incubation period** of three to four weeks, a raised, irregular, reddish, warty patch appears at the site of inoculation. This is teeming with spirochaetes and is highly infectious. Unfortunately, the patch is also very itchy and, inevitably, further patches arise elsewhere on the skin from scratching. The primary patches heal, but are followed by secondary similar patches, which also heal. As in syphilis, there is a dangerous tertiary stage several years later. This features deep skin ulcers with much tissue destruction, bone changes and a leprosy-like deformity.

TREATMENT
In the decade 1950 to 1960, the World Health Organization mounted mass campaigns in which over 60 million people were treated for yaws with penicillin or tetracycline to which the organisms are very sensitive. The disease was eradicated from many areas but, unfortunately, flared up again in the 1980s in West and Central Africa.

yeasts

Single-celled plants classified with the fungi. The chief medical interest in the yeasts arises from the strong tendency for those such as the Candida and Monilia species to cause skin infections commonly known as thrush (**candidiasis**).

Yeasts contain powerful enzymes which, in the process known as fermentation, break down carbohydrates to form alcohol and carbon dioxide – the source of the 'ferment' as well as the fizz. They grow easily and quickly and are also cultivated as a source of food rich in B **vitamins**.

yellow fever

An acute infectious disease occurring in tropical America and Africa, caused by the flavivirus and transmitted by the bite of the mosquito *Aedes aegypti*. The reservoir of infection is believed to be the 'canopy' monkeys who inhabit the tops of trees. Canopy mosquitos occasionally transmit the disease to a forest worker who returns to a town and starts an epidemic.

INCIDENCE
It has been a plague to mankind through the ages, and has caused millions of deaths. In the early 1960s an epidemic in Ethiopia affected over 100,000 people with 30,000 deaths. In Brazil, in 1971, 21,000 people were infected.

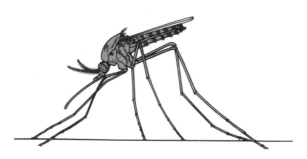

This shows the (greatly enlarged) mosquito Aedes aegypti, *a blood-sucking fly that transmits yellow fever.*

RECOGNITION AND SYMPTOMS
The disease may be mild and over in three days, but yellow fever is often a severe illness with high fever, a slow pulse rate, severe headache, general aches and pains, bleeding from the nose and gums, nausea and vomiting. The liver is commonly severely damaged by fatty degeneration and the pigment normally excreted by the liver accumulates to cause yellowing of the skin (jaundice). The kidneys are also affected and kidney failure (see **kidney disorders**) may result. Usually, the temperature drops to normal about the third day of illness, but then rises again. Intestinal bleeding often causes vomiting of blood from and black stools. Severe bleeding from the bowel and the womb (uterus) may occur and these are grave signs, often followed by agitation, delirium, coma and death.

TREATMENT

The mortality varies from 5 to 10 per cent and those who recover are immune for life. There is no specific treatment, but vaccination confers protection for at least ten years.

> The first attempt to cut the Panama Canal was abandoned after thousands had died from yellow fever. In 1901, the American worker Walter Reed and his colleagues discovered the mode of spread (vector) and control measures became possible. It remains a mystery why yellow fever has never occurred in Asia, in spite of the widespread presence of the main vector mosquito *Aedes aegypti*.

yellow skin

A definite yellow tinge to the skin, especially if the whites of the eyes are also yellow, suggests jaundice and some upset of the liver such as gallstones or hepatitis. In severe jaundice, the yellow tinge becomes very marked and then the colour deepens into a greenish tint.

See **jaundice**.

yew trees, anticancer drugs from

See **taxane and taxoid drugs**.

yin and yang

See **medicine, Chinese**.

yoga

The word comes from the Sanskrit and means 'yoking, as of oxen' or 'union'. Yoga is one of the six orthodox systems of Indian philosophy which aims to free the soul from further migration and unite it with the supreme being. In the West, the term is usually applied to Hatha Yoga in which the emphasis is on physical preparation for spiritual advancement. Hatha yoga is not a series of exercises but of 'poses', known as 'asanas', calculated to maintain youthful flexibility of the body and achieve physical and mental control, relaxation and peace. Many of these poses have names, derived from the appearance of the posture, and each has a specific purpose.

The purpose of the asanas is to train the subject to remain immobile in an unnatural pose so that the mind can be freed from any concentration on the body or its functions. The

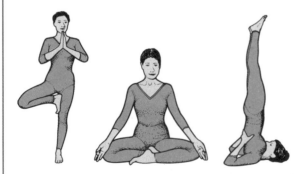

Three of the many Hatha yoga poses (asanas) that, regularly performed, help to maintain bodily flexibility, good posture, physical and mental control and calmness.

achievement of this is the third of the eight stages on the path to a state of *samadhi* – a trance-like condition of perfect concentration and dissociation from bodily awareness.

Of the thirty-two or more asanas, probably the best known and most used is the *padmasana* or 'lotus posture'. This is a cross-legged sitting position, with the arms extended by the sides and the palms facing forward. The 'full lotus', in which the outer edge of each foot rests on the thigh of the other leg may, if forced, lead to damage to the ligaments of the knee joints.

Properly and conscientiously followed, Hatha yoga can confer benefit, but it should be noted that some of the poses may be dangerous for people with certain diseases, or if attempted without adequate preparation and knowledgeable tuition. Back disorders, high blood pressure (see **hypertension**) and **glaucoma** are known hazards. People with glaucoma should not practise head or shoulder stands as these raise the pressure within the eyes.

yoghurt

A slightly acid product fermented from concentrated milk by the action of the *Lactobacillus bulgaricus*. In the late nineteenth century, it was suggested that since many diseases were caused by toxins produced by putrefactive bacteria in the intestine (untrue), health could be enhanced by replacing these with the harmless *Lactobacillus bulgaricus*.

This view was thought to be supported by the longevity of certain Bulgarian peoples whose diet featured a large intake of yoghurt. There is no reason to believe that the Lactobacillus does, in fact, colonize the bowel, and good reason to believe that it is inhibited by bile salts.

Yoghurt has recently found another use and is commonly employed as a vaginal cream in the treatment of thrush.

yohimbine

An **alkaloid** derived from the yohimbe tree, yohimbine has long had a reputation as an effective treatment for erectile impotence. It is now known that this substance blocks a certain type of cell membrane receptor for adrenaline. In technical terms, it is an alpha2 adrenoceptor antagonist, and its effect is to increase the blood pressure and promote arousal and anxiety. Although the corpora cavernosa of the penis are rich in alpha adrenoreceptors, no mechanism by which yohimbine could cause erection has yet been worked out. Research continues.

There is some evidence that yohimbine is of value in the treatment of psychogenic impotence. In one double-blind trial, in which twenty-four patients were given yohimbine three times a day and twenty-four a placebo, 62 per cent of those receiving the drug claimed some improvement in sexual function, while only 16 per cent of those receiving the dummy tablets admitted to an improvement. None of the trial subjects knew whether they were taking the drug or the placebo. This result is somewhat better than is usually achieved by sex therapy.

Yomesan

A brand name for the **anthelmintic** drug niclosamide.

Yutopar

A brand name for the womb-relaxing drug **ritodine**.

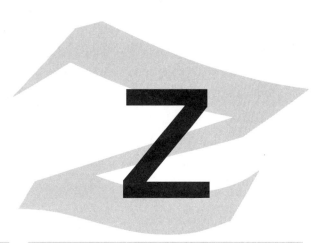

Zaditen

A brand name for **ketotifen**.

zalcitabine

A **reverse transcriptase inhibitor** drug used in combination with other drugs to treat AIDS. A brand name is Hivid.

Zamadol

A brand name for **tramadol**.

Zanaflex

A brand name for the muscle-relaxing drug **tizanidine**.

Zanidip

A brand name for **lercanidipine**.

Zantac

A brand name for the stomach acid-reducing drug **ranitidine**.

Zarontin

A brand name for the antiepilepsy drug **ethosuximide**.

Zavedos

A brand name for **idarubicin**.

Zenker's degeneration

Death of segments of muscle cells that sometimes occurs in prolonged fevers such as **typhoid**, or in **hepatitis**. Also known as hyaline necrosis.

Zestoretic

A brand name for the **angiotensin converting enzyme inhibitor lisinopril** formulated in conjunction with the diuretic drug **hydrochlorothiazide**.

Zestoretic 20

A brand name for lisinopril formulated with **hydro-chlorothiazide**.

Zestril

A brand name for **lisinopril**.

Zidoval

A brand name for **metronidazole**.

zidovudine

An antiviral drug used to try to retard the progress of **AIDS**. Also known as azidothymidine or AZT. A brand name is Retrovir.

Zinamide

A brand name for the antituberculosis drug pyrazinamide.

zinc

In recent years it has become apparent that the metallic element zinc is a nutrient of importance. Although zinc deficiency is comparatively rare, its effects may be serious. Acute deficiency has been reported in people on long-term intravenous feeding and it also occurs in certain **malabsorption** states, alcoholism, **anorexia nervosa**, **diabetes**, severe burns, prolonged feverish illness, and severe malnutrition in childhood.

In such cases, low zinc levels in the blood are associated with atrophy of the thymus gland, poor wound healing, diarrhoea, apathy, eczema and loss of hair. There is an association between zinc deficiency and dwarfism.

The recommended intake in adults is 15 mg a day, and foods high in zinc include meat, whole grain cereals and pulses. Oysters contain exceptionally high amounts. Fats, sugar and white bread are very low in zinc.

Zincaps

A brand name for a **zinc** preparation.

Zincfrin

A brand name for eye drops containing **zinc** sulphate and **phenylephrine**.

zinc sulphate

A drug used as a source of **zinc** in zinc-deficiency states. Trade names are Solvazinc and Z Span Spansule.

Zineryl

A brand name for **erythromycin** formulated with other drugs for external use only.

Zinga

A brand name for **nizatidine**.

Zinnat

A brand name for the cephalosporin antibiotic **cefuroxime**.

zip fastener for wounds

See **Medizip**.

Zirtek

A brand name for cetirizine.

Zispin

A brand name for **mirtazapine**.

Zita

A brand name for cimetidine.

Zithromax

A brand name for **azithromycin**.

Zocor

A brand name for **simvastatin**.

Zofran

A brand name for **ondansetron**.

Zoladex

A brand name for **goserelin**.

Zollinger-Ellison syndrome

A condition caused by a hormone-secreting tumour of the pancreas, known as a gastrinoma. This tumour produces large quantities of the hormone gastrin, which is a powerful stimulator of acid production in the stomach. The result is a massive outpouring of stomach acid, inevitably leading to severe ulceration of the stomach and duodenum (peptic ulceration). In most cases the diagnosis is not made until normally effective treatment for peptic ulceration is followed by severe recurrence.

A test of the gastrin levels in the blood will show these to be high. Gastrinomas are often multiple and most of them are malignant, although usually slow-growing.

The ideal treatment is the complete surgical removal of the tumours, but this is possible only in about a quarter of the cases. Total gastrectomy can be helpful, and much relief is obtained from the use of drugs in the H-2 receptor antagonist group, such as cimetidine.

zolmitriptan

A drug that stimulates **serotonin** receptors and is used to treat migraine. A brand name is Zomig.

zolpidem

An imidazopyridine **hypnotic** drug used for the short-term treatment of **insomnia**. A brand name is Stilnoct.

Zomacton

A brand name for **somatotropin**.

zombification

The induction of a state, purportedly by magical means, in which the awareness of an individual is retained by a sorcerer in a bottle or jar while the body, lacking will or agency, becomes the slave of the sorcerer. In Haiti, where the practice has been common, zombification is deemed to be murder even if the victim is manifestly still alive. The delusional state is induced either by various poisons or by strong suggestion, or both, in a context of powerful superstitious belief. Some zombies have, however, been found to be schizophrenics and it is possible that this psychosis may sometimes be induced by the process of zombificaton.

Zomig

A brand name for **zolmitriptan**.

Zonivent

A brand name for **beclomethasone**.

Zonulysin

A brand name for the protein-splitting enzyme alpha-chymotrypsin that is made up in a solution for the purposes of dissolving the zonule as a preliminary to the intracapsular removal of a cataractous lens. This method is now rarely used in developed countries.

zoon

Greek root meaning 'animal' as in zoology (study of animal life).

zoonoses

Infectious diseases of animals which can, in some conditions, also affect people. The zoonoses do not include those diseases which are primarily human and which are transmitted from person to person by animals.

Examples of zoonoses are **anthrax** from cattle, **brucellosis** and **Q fever** from goats and sheep, **glanders** from horses, **leptospirosis** and **plague** from rats, **psittacosis** from parrots, **rabies** from any mammal, **Rocky mountain spotted fever** from rabbits and other small mammals, **toxocariasis** from dogs, **toxoplasmosis** from cats, **tuberculosis** from cows and **yellow fever** from monkeys.

Zoton

A brand name for **lansoprazole**.

Zovirax

A brand name for the antiviral drug **aciclovir**.

Z-plasty

A valuable technique in surgery for relieving skin tension, changing the direction of a scar, or lengthening a contracture line and so correcting deformity. The principle involves cutting a Z-shaped incision, so as to make two V-shaped flaps, freeing the skin by separating it from the underlying tissue (undermining) and transposing the points of the flaps. The effect of this is to relieve tension in the direction of the central arm of the Z while increasing tension in the direction perpendicular to this.

Various modifications of this method are commonly used. In the case of a long, narrow scar, a series of small, connected Z-plasties may be more effective than a single large one.

Z Span Spansule

A brand name for **zinc sulphate**.

zuclopenthixol

A thioxanthene antipsychotic drug used to treat schizophrenia and other psychotic disorders. A brand name is Clopixol.

Zumenon

A brand name for **oestradiol**.

Zydol

A brand name for **tramadol**.

zygote

An egg (ovum) which has been penetrated by a spermatozoon so that fusion of the nuclear material has occurred. The zygote thus contains all the genetic code for a new individual. In this context, the ovum and sperm are called gametes. The chromosomes in the gametes are unpaired so gametes contain half the normal number of chromosomes of a body cell (haploid). The fusion of the two gametes to form the zygote restores this number to the normal forty-six (diploid). Each chromosome from the male gamete is paired with a chromosome from the female gamete, so the inherited characteristics are a mix of those of both parents.

The term 'zygote' is applied only to the fertilized ovum before it begins on its programme of division to form a new individual. After cell division starts, it is called an embryo.

Zyloprim

A brand name for **allopurinol** that blocks the formation of uric acid and is used in the prevention of **gout**.

Zyloric

A brand name for the drug **allopurinol**.

Zyprexa

A brand name for **olanzapine**.

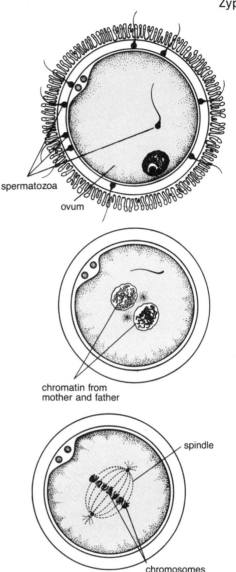

spermatozoa

ovum

chromatin from mother and father

spindle

chromosomes

The beginning of a new individual by the fusion of a single spermatozoon with an ovum. Two sets of 23 chromosomes are, in this way, brought together to make up the full complement. The bottom illustration shows the beginning of cell division.

Useful Addresses

The information listed below was correct when this book went to press.

Additional health support groups may be found in The Health Address Book (ISBN 1-85315-455-5), published by The Royal Society of Medicine in association with the Patients Association.

Adoption

After Adoption
12–14 Chapel Street
Manchester
Greater Manchester M3 7NN
Tel: 0161 839 4932
Helpline: 0161 839 4930

Coram Family (adoption, fostering, children in care)
49 Mecklenburgh Square
London WC1N 2QA
Tel: 020 7520 0300

Age concern

Age Concern
Astral House
1268 London Road
London SW16 4ER
Tel: 020 8765 7200
Helpline:0800 7314931
www.ace.org.uk

Age Concern Cymru
4th Floor, 1 Cathedral Road
Cardiff CF1 9SD
Tel: 029 2037 1566
www.accymru.org.uk

Aid for the Aged in Distress
54 London Road
Morden
Surrey SM4 5BE
Tel: 020 8640 5523
www.agedistress.org.uk

Help the Aged
16–18 St James Walk
Clerkenwell Green
London EC1R 0BE
Tel: 020 7253 0253
www.helptheaged.org.uk

Independent Living (1993)
Fund
PO Box 183
Nottingham NG8 3RD
Tel: 0115 942 819112
funds@ilf.org.uk

Association for Residential Care
(ARC)
ARC House
Marsden Street
Chesterfield S40 1JY
Tel: 01246 555 043

AIDS and immune deficiency

Terence Higgins Trust
52–54 Grays Inn Road
London WC1X 8JU
Tel: 020 7831 0330
Helpline: 020 7242 1010
www.tht.org.uk

Primary Immunodeficiency
Association (PIA)
Alliance House
12 Caxton Street
London SW1H 0QS
Tel: 020 7976 7640
pimmune@dial.pipex.com

Alcohol, drugs and smoking

Action on Smoking and Health
(ASH)
102 Clifton Street
London EC2A 4HW
Tel: 020 7739 5902
www.ash.org.uk

Alcohol Concern
Waterbridge House
32–36 Loman Street
London SE1 0EE
Tel: 020 7928 7377
alccon@popmail.dircon.co.uk
www.alcoholconcern.org.uk

Alcohol Advisory and Counselling
Service
62 Dee Street
Aberdeen AB11 6DS
Tel: 01224 573 887
info@aacs.co.uk
www.aacs.co.uk

Alcoholics Anonymous
PO Box 1
Stonebow House
Stonebow
York Y01 7NJ
Tel: 01904 644 026
www.alcoholics-anonymous.
org.uk

Alcohol Counselling and
Prevention Services
34 Electric Lane
London SW9 8JT
Tel: 020 7737 3579
acaps.uk@virgin.net

Alcohol Problem Advisory Service
(APAS)
309 Grays Inn Road
London WC1X 8QF
Tel: 020 7530 5900

Alcohol Recovery Project
68 Newington Causeway
London SE1 6DF
Tel: 020 7403 3369
www.arp-
charity.demon.co.uk/arp.htm

Drugs Aid
16 Clive Street
Caerphilly
Wales CF83 1GE
Tel: (029) 2088 1000
drugaid@talk21.com

Quit
Victory House
170 Tottenham Court Road
London W1T 7NR
Tel: 020 7388 5775
Helpline: 0800 002 200
www.quit.org.uk

The Advisory Council on Alcohol
and Drug Education (TACADE)
1 Hulme Place
The Crescent
Salford M5 4QA
Tel: 0161 745 8925

Arthritis and rheumatism

Arthritic Association
First Floor Suite
2 Hyde Gardens
Eastbourne
East Sussex BN21 4PN
Tel: 01323 416 550
info@arthriticassociation.org.uk

Arthritis and Rheumatism Council
Copeman House
St Mary's Court
St Mary's Gate
Chesterfield
Derbyshire S41 7TD
Tel: 01246 558 033
info@arc.org.uk
www.arc.org.uk

Arthritis Care
18 Stephenson Way
London NW1 2HD
Tel: 020 7916 1500
Helpline: 0808 800 4050
arthritis.care@virgin.net
www.arthritiscare.org.uk

Children's Chronic Arthritis
Association
47 Battenhall Avenue
Worcester WR5 2HN
Tel: 01905 763 556

Fibromyalgia Association UK
PO Box 206
Stourbridge
West Midlands DY9 8YL
Tel: 01384 820 052
Benefits Helpline 01254 832 463
www.ukfibromyalgia.com

Lady Hoare Trust (for children
with arthritis and limb disabilities)
1st Floor
89 Albert Embankment
London SE1 7TP
Tel: 020 7820 9989
info@lhtchildren.org.uk

L'Arche
10 Briggate
Silsden, Keighley
West Yorkshire BD20 9JT
Tel: 01535 656 186
info@larche.org.uk

National Ankylosing Spondylitis
Society
PO Box 179
Mayfield, East Sussex TN20 6ZL
Tel: 01435 873 527

National Osteoporosis Society
PO Box 10
Radstock, Bath BA3 3YB
Tel: 01761 471 771
Helpline: 01761 472 721
info@nos.org.uk

Perthes Association
15 Recreation Road
Guildford
Surrey GU1 1HE
Tel: 01483 534 431
Helpline: 01483 306 637
Admin@perthes.org.uk
www.perthes.org.uk

Psoriasis Arthropathy Alliance
PO Box 111
St Albans AL2 3JQ
Tel: 01923 672 837
www.paalliance.org

Repetitive Strain Injury
Association
380–384 Harrow Road
London W9 2HU
Tel: 020 7266 2000
Helpline: 0800 018 5012
rsia@dial.pipex.com

Scoliosis Association UK
2 Ivesbury Court
325 Latimer Road
London W10 6RA
Tel: 020 8964 5343

Blindness

Action for Blind People
14–16 Verney Road
London SE16 3DZ
Tel: 020 7732 8771
central@afbp.org
www.afbp.org.uk

Birmingham Focus on Blindness
48–62 Woodville Lane
Harborne
Birmingham B17 9AT
Tel: 0121 428 5000

British Wireless for the Blind
Gabriel House
34 New Road
Chatham
Kent ME4 4QR
Tel: 01634 832 501
info@blind.org.uk
www.blind.org.uk

Catholic Blind Institute
Christopher Grange Centre
for the Adult Blind
Youens Way (off East Prescot Road)
Liverpool L14 2EW
Tel: 0151 220 2525

Deafblind UK
100 Bridge Street
Peterborough PE1 1DY
Tel: 01733 358 100
Textphone: 01733 358 858
Helpline: 0800 132 320
info@deafblind.org.uk
www.deafblind.org.uk

Guide Dogs for the Blind
Association (GDBA)
Hillfields
Burfield Common
Reading RG7 3YG
Tel: 0118 983 5555
guidedogs@gdba.org.uk

Henshaw's Society for the Blind
John Derby House
88–92 Talbot Road
Old Trafford, Manchester M16 0GS
Tel: 0161 872 1234
info@henshaws.org.uk

International Glaucoma Association
108C Warner Road
London SE5 9HQ
Tel: 020 7737 3265
www.iga.org.uk

National Federation for the Blind
of the UK
215 Kirkgate
Wakefield, West Yorkshire WFl 1JG
Tel: 01924 291 313
nfb@globalnet.co.uk
www.users.globalnet.co.uk/~nfbuk

National Library for the Blind
Far Cromwell Road
Bredbury, Stockport SK6 2SG
Tel: 0161 355 2000
enquiries@nlb.org

Royal London Society for the Blind
Dorton House
Seal, nr. Sevenoaks
Kent TN15 OED
Tel: 01732 592 500
www.rlsb.org.uk

Royal National College for the Blind
College Road
Hereford HR1 lEB
Tel: 01432 265 725
Textphone:01432 276 532
md@rncb.ac.uk
www.rncb.ac.uk

Royal National Institute for the
Blind (RNIB)
224 Great Portland Street
London W1N 6AA
Tel: 020 7388 1266
www.rnib.org.uk

RNIB Customer Services
PO Box 173
Peterborough PE2 6WS
Tel: 0345 023 153
Helpline: 0345 669 999
cservices@rnib.org.uk
www.rnib.org.uk

RNIB Cymru
Trident Court
East Moors Road
Cardiff CF24 5TD
Tel: 029 2045 0440

Scottish National Institute
for War Blinded
50 Gillespie Crescent
Edinburgh EH10 4HZ
Tel: 0131 229 1456
enquiries@rbas.org.uk

Scottish National Federation for
the Welfare of the Blind
50 Gillespie Crescent
Edinburgh EH10 4HZ
Tel: 0131 229 1456

SENSE (The National Deafblind
Rubella Asssociation)
11–13 Clifton Terrace
London N4 3SR
Tel: 020 7272 7774
Textphone: 020 7272 9648
enquiries@sense.org.uk
www.sense.org.uk

SENSE Cymru
Shand House
20 Newport Road
Cardiff CF2 1DB
Tel: 029 2045 7641

SENSE Scotland
5th Floor
45 Finnieston Street
Clydeway Centre
Glasgow G3 8GU
Tel: 0141 564 2444
Textphone: 0141 564 2442
admin@sensescotland.org.uk

The Partially Sighted Society
9 Plato Place
72–74 St Dionis Road
London SW6 4TU
Tel: 020 7371 0289
london@partsight.org.uk

West of England School for
Children with Little or No Sight
Countess Wear
Exeter, Devon EX2 6HA
Tel: 01392 454 200

Bone disorders

Brittle Bone Society
30 Guthrie Street
Dundee DD1 5BS
Tel: 01382 204 446
Helpline: 0800 028 2459
bbs@brittlebone.org
www.brittlebone.org

Child Growth Foundation
Affiliated with: Bone Dysplasia
Group
Growth Hormone Deficiency
Group
Premature Sexual Maturation
Group
Russell Silver Society
Sotos Syndrome Society
Turner's Syndrome Society
2 Mayfield Avenue
London W4 1PW
Tel: 020 8994 7625
or 020 8995 0257
cgflondon@aol.com
www.cgf.org.uk

National Association for the Relief
of Paget's Disease
323 Manchester Road
Manchester M28 3HH
Tel: 0161 799 4646
director@pagets.org.uk

Bowel problems

Association for Continence Advice
Winchester House
Kennington Park
Cranmer Road
The Oval, London SW9 6EJ
Tel: 020 7820 8113
info@aca.uk.com
www.aca.uk.com

British Colostomy Association
15 Station Road
Reading, Berks RG1 1LG
Tel: 0118 939 1537
Helpline:0800 328 4257
www.bcass.org.uk

Coeliac Society of UK
PO Box 220
High Wycombe
Bucks HP11 2HY
Tel: 01494 437 278
admin@coeliac.co.uk

Crohn's in Childhood Research
Appeal (CICRA)
Parkgate House
356 West Barnes Lane
Motspur Park
Surrey KT3 6NB
Tel: 020 8949 6209
support@cicra.org

NASCPS (Charity of Incontinent
and Stoma Children)
51 Anderson Drive
Valley View Park
Darvel
Ayrshire KA17 ODE
Tel: 01560 322 024
john@stoma.freeserve.co.uk

National Association for Colitis and
Crohn's Disease
4 Beaumont House
Sutton Road
St Albans
Herts AL1 5HH
Tel: 01727 844 296
nacc@nacc.org.uk
www.nacc.org.uk

The Continence Foundation
307 Hatton Square
16 Baldwins Gardens
London EC1N 7RJ
Helpline: 020 7831 9831
continence.foundation@dial.pipex.
com
www.continence-foundation.
org.uk

The Oesophageal Patient
Association
16 Whitefields Crescent
Solihull
West Midlands B91 3NU
Tel: 0121 704 9860

Cancer

Anthony Nolan Bone Marrow
Trust
2–3 Heathgate Place
London NW3 2NU
Tel: 020 7284 1234
www.anthonynolan.com

Breakthrough Breast Cancer
Level 6
Kingsway House
103 Kingsway
London WC2B 6QX
Tel: 020 7430 2086
info@breakthrough.org.uk
www.breakthrough.org.uk

Breast Cancer Care
Kiln House
210 New Kings Road
London SW6 4NZ
Tel: 020 7384 2984
Helpline: 0808 800 6000

Cancer BACUP
(British Association of Cancer
United Patients)
3 Bath Place
Rivington Street
London EC2A 3JR
Tel: 020 7696 9003
Glasgow Counselling Telephone:
0141 553 1553
Freephone Outside London:
0808 800 1234
Information Line for London:
020 7613 2121
info@cancerbacup.org
www.cancerbacup.org.uk

Cancer Research Campaign
10 Cambridge Terrace
London NW1 4JL
Tel: 020 7224 1333
Cancer Information Nurses:
020 7317 5027
Health Promotion Materials:
020 7317 5076
cancer.info@crc.org.uk
www.crc.org.uk

Cancerlink
11–21 Northdown Street
London Nl 9BN
Tel: 020 7833 2818
Support Link Service:
0808 808 0000
cancerlink@cancerlink.org.uk

Imperial Cancer Research Fund
PO Box 123
Lincoln Inn Fields
London WC2A 3PX
Tel: 020 7242 0200
www.icnet.uk

Leukaemia Care Society
2 Shrubbery Avenue
Worcester WR1 1QH
Tel: 01905 330 003
Careline: 0800 169 6680
leukaemiacare@ukonline.co.uk
www.leukaemiacare.org

Lymphoedema Support Network
St Luke's Crypt
Sydney Street
London SW3 6NH
Tel: 020 7351 4480
adminlsn@lymphoedema.
freeserve.co.uk
www.lymphoedema.org/lsn

Lymphoma Association
PO Box 386
Haddenham
Aylesbury
Bucks HP20 2GA
Tel: 01296 619 400
Helpline: 0808 808 5555
www.lymphoma.org.uk

Macmillan Cancer Relief
89 Albert Embankment
London SE1 7UQ
Tel: 020 7351 7811
postmasters@macmillan.org.uk
www.macmillan.org.uk

Marie Curie Cancer Care
7th Floor
89 Albert Embankment
London SE1 7UQ
Tel: 020 7599 7777
www.mariecurie.org.uk

Sargent Cancer Care for
Children
Griffin House
161 Hammersmith Road
London W6 8SG
Tel: 020 8752 2800
care@sargent.org

Terminal Care Hospice
Information Service
St Christopher's Hospice
51 Lawrie Park Road
Sydenham
London SE26 6DZ
Tel: 020 8778 9252
info@his2.freeserve.co.uk
www.hospiceinformation.
co.uk

769

Useful Addresses

WCT Line for Testicular Cancer
Support (formerly Mind Over
Matter)
14 Blightmont Crescent
Southampton S015 8RH
Tel: (023) 80 77 5611

Women's Nationwide Cancer
Campaign
Suna House
128 Curtain Road
London EC2A 3AQ
Tel: 020 7729 4688
admin@wnccc.org.uk
www.wnccc.org.uk

Carers

Carers National Association
20–25 Glasshouse Yard
London EC1A 4JT
Tel: 020 7490 8818
Freephone Carers Line:
0808 808 7777
(10am–12pm, 2–4pm)
info@ukcarers.org
www.carersnorth.demon.co.uk

Care and Repair – England
3rd Floor, Bridgford House
Pavillion Road
West Bridgford
Nottingham NG2 5GJ
Tel: 0115 982 1527
careandrepair@freenetname.co.uk
www.careandrepair-england.org.uk

Care and Repair – Cymru
Norbury House
Norbury Road
Fairwater, Cardiff CFS 3AS
Tel: 029 2057 6286
enquiries@careandrepair.org.uk
www.careandrepair.org.uk

Care and Repair Cymru
– North Wales
1 Lon Polsky
Bangor
Gwynedd LLS7 1HR
Tel: 01248 371 528

Foundations
(carers co-ordinating body)
Bleaklow House
Howard Town Mills
Glossop, Derbyshire SK13 8HT
Tel: 01457 891 909
foundations@cel.co.uk
www.cel.co.uk/foundations

Crossroads Association of
Crossroads Care Attendant
Schemes Ltd
10 Regent Place
Rugby
Warwickshire CV21 2PN
Tel: 01788 573 653

Crossroads (Scotland) Care
Attendant Schemes
24 George Square
Glasgow G2 1 EG
Tel: 0141 226 3793
enquiries@crossroads-scot.k-
web.co.uk

Crossroads (Wales) Care Assistant
Schemes
3rd Floor, 49 Charles Street
Cardiff CF10 2GD
Tel: (029) 2022 2282
eirian@crossroads-
wales.demon.co.uk

Deafness

British Deaf Association
1–3 Worship Street
London EC2A 2AB
Tel: 020 7588 3520
Textphone: 020 7588 3529
info@bda.org.uk
www.bda.org.uk

British Deaf Sports Council
7 Bridge Street
Otley, West Yorkshire LS21 1 BQ
Tel: 01943 850214/850081

Council for the Advancement of
Communication with Deaf People
(CACDP)
Durham University Science Park
Block 4, Stockton Road
Durham DH1 3UZ
Tel: 0191 383 1155
Textphone: 0191 383 7915
durham@cacdp.demon.co.uk
www.cacdp.demon.co.uk

Deafblind UK
100 Bridge Street
Peterborough PE1 1DY
Tel: 01733 358 100
Textphone: 01733 358 858
Helpline: 0800 132 320
info@deafblind.org.uk
www.deafblind.org.uk

FYD (Friends for Young Deaf
People)
East Court Mansion
College Lane
East Grinstead
West Sussex RH19 3LT
Tel: 01342 323 444
Textphone: 01342 312 639
fyd.egho@charity.vfree.com
www.fyd.org.uk

Hearing Concern
7–11 Armstrong Road
London W3 7JL
Tel: 020 8743 1110
Textphone: 020 8742 9151
Helpline: 0845 074 4600
hearingconcern@hearingconcern.
com
www.hearingconcern.com

National Deaf Children's Society
National Office
15 Dufferin Street
London EC1Y 8UR
Tel/Textphone: 020 7490 8656
Helpline (10am–5pm Mon–Fri):
020 7250 0123
ndcs@ndcs.org.uk
www.ndcs.org.uk

RAD (Royal Association in Aid of
Deaf People)
Colchester Centre for Deaf People
Walsingham Road
Colchester, Essex C02 7BP
Tel: 01206 509 509
Textphone:01206 577 090
info@royaldeaf.org.uk
www.royaldeaf.org.uk

Royal National Institute for Deaf
People (RNID)
19–23 Featherstone Street
London EC1Y 8SL
Tel: 020 7296 8000
Voicephone helpline: 0808 808 0123
Textphone helpline: 0808 808 9099
helpline@rnid.org.uk
www.rnid.org.uk

Scottish Association of Sign
Language Interpreters (SASLI)
54 Queen Street
Edinburgh EH2 3NS
Tel/Textphone: 0131 225 9995
mail@sasli.org.uk
www.sasli.org.uk

SENSE (The National Deafblind
Rubella Association)
11–13 Clifton Terrace
London N4 3SR
Tel: 020 7272 7774
Textphone:020 7272 9648
enquiries@sense.org.uk
www.sense.org.uk

SENSE Cymru
Shand House
20 Newport Road
Cardiff CF2 1DB
Tel: (029) 2045 7641

SENSE Scotland
5th Floor
45 Finnieston Street
Clydeway Centre
Glasgow G3 8GU
Tel: 0141 564 2444
Textphone: 0141 564 2442
admin@sensescotland.org.uk

Sign Campaigning for Mental
Health & Deafness
13 Station Road
Beaconsfield
Bucks HP9 1YP
Tel: 01494 816 777
info@signcharity.org.uk
www.signcharity.org.uk

Talking Newspaper Enterprises Ltd
National Recording Centre
Heathfield, Sussex TN21 8DB
Tel: 01435 866 102
info@tnauk.org.uk
www.tnauk.org.uk

Teletec International United
(telephones for the deaf)
Sunningdale House
49 Caldecotte Lake Drive
Caldecotte Business Park
Milton Keynes MK7 8LF
Tel: 01908 270 003
Textphone: 01908 270 005
www.teletec.co.uk

The LINK Centre for Deafened
People
19 Hartfield Road
Eastbourne
East Sussex BN21 2AR
Tel: 01323 638 230
Textphone: 01323 739 998
linkcentr@dircon.co.uk

Wales Council for the Deaf
Glenview House
Courthouse Street
Pontypridd Rhondda
Cynon Taff CF37 1JY
Tel: 01443 485 687
Textphone: 01443 485 686
wcdeaf@freenet.co.uk

Diabetes

British Diabetic Association
10 Queen Anne Street
London W1G 9LH
Tel: 020 7323 1531
Helpline: 020 7636 6112
info@diabetes.org.uk
www.diabetes.org.uk

Insulin Dependent Diabetes Trust
PO Box 294
Northampton NN1 4XS
Tel: 01604 721 325
enquiries@iddtinternational.org
wwwiddtinternational.org

Disablement

AA (Automobile Association)
Disability helpline: 0800 262 050

Ability UK
29 Crawford Street
London WIH 1PL
Tel: 020 7724 0473
admin@ability-uk.org
www.ability-uk.org

AbilityNet
PO Box 94
Warwick CV34 5WS
Tel: 01926 312 847
National Freephone &Advice
Helpline: 0800 269 545
www.abilitynet.co.uk

Artificial Limbs and Appliances
Centres (ALAC):
Rookwood Hospital
Fairwater Road
Liandaff, Cardiff CF5 2YN
Hospital Telephone:
(029) 2056 6281
Centre Telephone:
(029) 2055 5677 / 2031 3905

Banstead Mobility Centre
Damson Way
Fountain Drive
Carshalton, Surrey SMS 4NR
Tel: 020 8770 1151
info@mobility-qe.com
www.qefd.org/mobilitycentre

BCODP Limited (British Council
of Disabled People)
Litchurch Plaza
Litchurch Lane
Derby DE24 8AA
Tel: 01332 295 551
Textphone: 01332 295 288/581
Info Line: 01332 298 288
bcodp@bcodp.org.uk
www.bcodp.org.uk

British Paralympic Association
Room 14, Impact House
2 Edridge Road
Croydon, Surrey CR9 1 PJ
Tel: 020 8681 9655
info@paralympics.org.uk
www.paralympics.org.uk

British Wheelchair Sports
Foundation
Cuttman Road
Stoke Mandeville, Bucks HP21 9PP
Tel: 01296 395 995
wheelpower@dial.pipex.com
www.britishwheelchairsports.org

BT (British Telecom Age and
Disability Unit)
Freephone: 0800 671 504
Textphone: 0800 243 123
www.bt.com

Contact a Family (for families of
disabled children)
170 Tottenham Court Road
London W1T 7HA
Tel: 020 7383 3555
info@cafamily.org.uk
www.cafamily.org.uk

Council for Disabled Children
National Children's Bureau
8 Wakley Street
London EC1V 7QE
Tel: 020 7843 6061/6058
www.ncb.org.uk

Disability Information Trust
Mary Madborough Centre
Nuffield Orthopaedic Centre
Headington, Oxford OX3 7LD
Tel: 01865 227 592

Disability Scotland
Princes House
5 Shandwick Place
Edinburgh EH2 4RG
Tel: 0131 229 8632

Disability Sport England (DSE)
The Mary Glen Haig Suite
13–27 Brunswick Place
London N1 6DX
Tel: 020 7490 4919
info@dse.org.uk
www.britsport.com

Disability Wales/Anabledd Cymru
'Llys Ifor'
Crescent Road
Caerphilly
Mid Glamorgan CF83 1XL
Tel: (029) 2088 7325

Disabled Drivers Association
National HQ
Ashwellthorpe
Norwich NR16 1EX
Tel: 01508 489 449
ddahq@aol.com
www.dda.org.uk

Disabled Living Foundation
380–384 Harrow Road
London W9 2HU
Tel: 020 7289 6111
Helpline: 0870 603 9177
dlfinfo@dlf.org.uk
www.dlf.org.uk

Disabled Drivers Motor Club Ltd
Cottingham Way
Thrapston
Northamptonshire NN14 4PL
Tel: 01832 734 724
dddmc@ukonline.co.uk
web.ukonline.co.uk/ddmc

Employment Opportunities for
People with Disabilities
123 Minories
London EC3N 1NT
Tel: 020 7481 2727
eopps.holondon@care4free.net

GLAD (Greater London Action on
Disabled People)
33 Brixton Road
London SW9 7AA
Tel: 020 7346 5800
Textphone: 020 7346 5811
Information Line: 0207346 5819
(1:30–4:30pm Mon, Wed, Fri)
glad@btinternet.com
www.disabilitynet.co.uk/groups/glad

Kidsactive (formerly HAPA)
(Play for Disabled Children with
Disabilities and Special Needs)
Pryor's Bank
Bishop's Park, London SW6 3LA
Tel: 020 7736 4443
Textphone: 020 7384 2596
Information Line: 020 7731 1435

ICAN (Invalid Children's Aid
Nationwide)
4 Deyers Buildings
London EC1 NQP
Tel: 0870 010 4066
ican@ican.org.uk
www.ican.org.uk

Independent Living (1993) Fund
PO Box 183
Nottingham NG8 3RD
Tel: 0115 942 8191/2
funds@ilf.org.uk

John Grooms Association for
Disabled People
50 Scrutton Street
London EC2A 4XQ
Tel: 020 7452 2000
jgadp@globalnet.org.uk
www.johngrooms.org.uk

Lady Hoare Trust (for children
with arthritis and limb disabilities)
1st Floor, 89 Albert Embankment
London SE1 7TP
Tel: 020 7820 9989
info@lhtchildren.org.uk

L'Arche
10 Briggate
Silsden
Keighley
West Yorkshire BD20 93T
Tel: 01535 656 186
info@larche.org.uk

Liberator Ltd (appliances for
disabled people)
Whitegates
Swinstead
Lincolnshire NG33 4PA
Tel: 01476 550 391
staff@liberator.co.uk
query@liberator.co.uk
www.liberator.co.uk

Phab (physically handicapped and
able bodied) – Making More of
Life Together
Summit House
Wandle Road
Croydon CRO 1DF
Tel: 020 8667 9443
phab@ukonline.co.uk
web.ukonline.co.uk/phab

RADAR (The Royal Association for
Disability and Rehabilitation)
12 City Forum
250 City Road
London EC1V 8AF
Tel: 020 7250 3222
Textphone: 020 7250 4119
radar@radar.org.uk
www.radar.org.uk

Riding for the Disabled Association
Lavinia Norfolk House
Avenue 'R'
National Agricultural Centre
Stoneleigh Park
Warwickshire CV8 2LY
Tel: (024) 7669 6510
rdahq@riding-for-disabled.org.uk
www.riding-for-disabled.org.uk

Shaftesbury Society (for physically
disabled young people under 22)
16 Kingston Road
London SW19 1JZ
Tel: 020 8239 5555
info@shaftesburysoc.org.uk
www.shaftesburysoc.org.uk

Shape London (provides access to
the arts for disabled and older
people)
LVS Resource Centre
356 Holloway Road
London N7 6PA
Tel/Textphone: 020 7700 8139
maggie.woolley@shape-uk.co.uk

SKILL (National Bureau for
Students with Disabilities)
Chapter House
18–20 Crucifix Lane
London SE1 3JW
Tel: 020 7450 0620
Info line: 0800 328 5050
Info text Tel: 0800 068 2422
info@skill.org.uk
www.skill.org.uk

SPOD
(Association to Aid Sexual &
Personal Relationships of People
with a Disability)
286 Camden Road
London N7 0BJ
Tel: 020 7607 8851
spoduk@aol.com

STEPS: The National Association
for Children with Lower Limb
Abnormalities
Lymm Court
11 Eagle Brow
Lymm
Cheshire WA13 0LP
Tel: 01925 757 525
info@steps-charity.org.uk
www.steps-charity.org.uk

Thalidomide Society
19 Central Avenue
Pinner
Middlesex HA5 5BT
Tel: 020 8868 5309

The Stroke Association
123–127 Whitecross Street
London EC1Y 8JJ
Tel: 020 7490 7999
stroke@stroke.org.uk
www.stroke.org.uk

Voluntary Organisations Disability
Group
30 Millbank
London SW1 P 4QD
Tel: 020 7802 8200

Wellbeing
(health and disability information)
27 Sussex Place
Regent's Park
London NW1 45P
Tel: 020 7262 5337
wellbeing@rcog.org.uk
www.wellbeing.demon.co.uk

Winged Fellowship
(holidays for disabled people)
Angel House
20–32 Pentonville Road
London N 1 9XD
Tel: 020 7833 2594
admin@wft.org.uk
www.wft.org.uk

Down's Syndrome

Down's Syndrome Association
155 Mitcham Road
Tooting
London SW17 9PG
Tel: 020 8682 4001
www.dsa-uk.com

Elizabeth Fitzroy Homes
(for the mentally handicapped)
Caxton House, Lower Street
Haslemere, Surrey GU27 2PE
Tel: 01428 656 766

ENABLE (Scottish Society for the
Mentally Handicapped)
6th Floor, 7 Buchanan Street
Glasgow Gl 3HL
Tel: 0141 226 4541

Eating disorders

British Nutrition Foundation
High Holborn House
52–54 High Holborn
London WC1V 6RQ
Tel: 020 7404 6504
postbox@nutrition.org.uk
www.nutrition.org.uk

Eating Disorders Association
Wensum House
103 Prince of Wales Road
Norwich NR1 1DW
Tel: 01603 619 090
Adult Helpline: 01603 621 414
Youth Helpline: 01603 765 050
info@edauk.com
www.edauk.com

Obesity Advice
Tel: 0800 731 7138

The Women's Nutritional Advisory
Service
PO Box 268
Lewes
East Sussex BN7 1QN
Tel: 01273 487 366
wnas@wnas.org.uk
www.wnas.org.uk

Growth disorders

Children Living with Inherited
Metabolic Diseases (CLIMB)
(formerly RTMDC)
The Quadrangle
Crewe Hall
Weston Road
Crewe CW1 6UR
Tel: 01270 250 221

The Pituitary Foundation
PO Box 1944
Bristol BS99 2UB
Tel: 0117 927 3355
helpline@pitpat.demon.co.uk

Restricted Growth Association
PO Box 8919
Birmingham B27 6DQ
Tel: 0121 707 4328
rga1@talk21.com

Heart problems

Action Heart
Wellesley House
117 Wellington Road
Dudley DY1 1UB
Tel: 01384 230 222

Arterial Health Foundation
PO Box 8
Atherton
Manchester M46 9FY
Tel: 0942 683378
or
Flat 20
Harmont House
20 Harley Street
London W1N 1AL
Tel: 020 7935 6604
www.chelation.co.uk

Useful Addresses

British Heart Foundation
14 Fitzhardinge Street
London W1H 6DH
Tel: 020 7935 0185
Heartline:0990 200 656
www.bhf.org.uk

Cardiomyopathy Association
40 The Metro Centre
Tolpits Lane
Watord WD1 8SB
Tel: 01923 249 977
cmaassoc@aol.com

Incontinence

British Kidney Patient
Association
Bordon
Hants GU35 9JZ
Tel: 01420 472 021

Enuresis Resource and Information
Centre (ERIC)
34 Old School House
Britannia Road
Kingswood
Bristol BS15 2DB
Tel: 0117 960 3060
enuresis@compuserve.com
www.eric.org.uk

Incontinent and Stoma Children
(NASCPS)
51 Anderson Drive
Valley View Park
Darvel
Ayrshire KA17 0DE
Tel: 01560 322 024
john@stoma.freeserve.co.uk

National Kidney Federation
6 Stanley Street
Worksop
Notts S81 7HX
Tel: 01909 487 795
naf@kidney.org.uk
www.kidney.org.uk

The Continence Foundation
307 Hatton Square
16 Baldwin Gardens
London EC1N 7RJ
Tel: 020 7831 9831
continence.foundation@dial.
pipex.com
www.continence-foundation.
org.uk

Learning difficulties

British Institute of Learning
Difficulties (BILD)
Wolverhampson Road
Kidderminster
Worcestershire
DY10 3PP
Tel: 01562 850 251
bild@bild.demon.co.uk

Camphill Village Trust (for
mentally handicapped adults)
19 South Road
Stourbridge
West Midlands
DY8 3YA
Tel: 01384 372 122

CARE (for mentally handicapped
people)
(Cottage and Rural Enterprises Ltd)
9 Weir Road
Kibworth
Leicestershire LE8 0LQ
Tel: 0116 279 3225
carecentral@freeuk.com

Elizabeth Fitzroy Homes
(for the mentally handicapped)
Caxton House
Lower Street
Haslemere
Surrey GU27 2PE
Tel: 01428 656 766

ENABLE
(Scottish Society for the Mentally
Handicapped)
6th Floor, 7 Buchanan Street
Glasgow Gl 3HL
Tel: 0141 226 4541

Family Fund Trust
(aid for handicapped children)
PO Box 50
York YO1 9ZX
Tel: 01904 621 115
info@familyfundtrust.org.uk
www.familyfundtrust.org.uk

Keycomm
(Lothian Communication
Technology Service)
St Giles Centre
40 Broomhouse Crescent
Edinburgh EH11 3UB
Tel: 0131 443 6775
djans@keycomm.demon.co.uk

KIDS
(for families with children with
developmental or learning
problems)
6 Aztec Row
Berners Road
London N1 0PW
Tel: 020 7359 3635
nat.off@kids-online.org.uk
www.kids-online.org.uk

Leonard Cheshire Foundation (for
severely mentally handicapped
adults)
30 Millbank
London SW1P 4QD
Tel: 020 7802 8200
www.leonardcheshire.org.uk
MacIntyre Care (education and
care for people with learning
disabilities)
602 South Seventh Street
Milton Keynes
Bucks MK9 2JA
Tel: 01908 230100

Makaton Vocabulary Development
Project
31 Firwood Drive
Camberley
Surrey GU15 3QD
Tel: 01276 61390

MENCAP Royal Society for
Mentally Handicapped Children
and Adults
MENCAP National Centre
123 Golden Lane
London EC1Y 0RT
Tel: 020 7454 0454
www.mencap.org.uk

National Development
Team for People with
Learning Disabilities
Albion Wharf
Albion Street
Manchester
Ml 5LN
Tel: 0161 228 7055
office@ndt.org.uk
www.ndt.org.uk

Paget Gorman Society
(for language skills)
2 Dowlands Bungalows
Dowlands Lane
Smalifield Horley
Surrey RH6 9SD
Tel: 0134 284 2308
prup@compuserve.com

Pre-School Learning Alliance
69 Kings Road
London WC1X 9LL
Tel: 020 7833 0991
pla@pre-school.org.uk

Rathbone (for children
and young people with
learning difficulties)
4th Floor
Churchgate House
56 Oxford Street
Manchester Ml 6EU
Tel: 0161 236 5358

Scottish Sports Association for
People with a Disability
FIPRE
Viewfield Road
Glenrothes
Fife KY6 1RB
Tel: 01592 415 700

SCOVO
(The Standing Conference
of Voluntary Organisations
for People with a Learning
Disability in Wales)
5 Dock Chambers
Bute Street
Cardiff CF10 5AG
Tel: 029 2049 2443
cardiff2@scovo.demon.co.uk

Sheffield Speech & Language
Therapy Agency
Fulwood House
Old Fulwood Road
Sheffield
South Yorkshire S10 3TH
Tel: 0114 271 6765
The Signalong Group (language
for carers of people with learning
disabilities)
The Communication and
Language Centre
North Pondside
Historic Dockyard
Chatham
Kent ME4 4TY
Tel: 01634 819 915
signalong@tesco.net

United Kingdom Sports Association
for People with Learning Disability
(UKSAPLD) Solecast House
13–27 Brunswick Place
London Nl 6DX
Tel: 020 7354 1030

United Response (charity housing
for young adults with learning
disabilities)
113–123 Upper Richmond Road,
London SW15 2TL
Tel: 020 8246 5200
Textphone:020 8785 1706
info@united-response.co.uk
www.united-response.co.uk

Values Into Action (campaign for
rights of people with learning
difficulties)
Oxford House
Derbyshire Street

London E2 6HG
Tel: 020 7729 5436
general@viauk.org
www.viauk.org

Young Minds (charity providing a
parent's information service
and publications on children's
mental health)
102–108 Clerkenwell Road
London EC1M 5SA
Tel: 020 7336 8445
Parents' Information Service:
0800 018 2138
enquiries@youngminds.org.uk
www.youngminds.org.uk

Liver problems

The British Liver Trust
182 High Street
Guildford
Surrey GU1 3HW

Children's Liver Disease
Foundation
AXA Equity & Law House
36 Great Charles Street
Queensway
Birmingham B3 3JY
Tel: 0121 212 3839
info@childliverdisease.org
www.childliverdisease.org

Meningitis

Meningitis Research
Foundation
Midland Way
Thornbury
Bristol BS35 2BS
Tel: 01454 281 811
Helpline: 0808 800 3344
info@meningitis.org
www.meningitis.org
National Meningitis Trust
Fern House
Bath Road
Stroud
Gloucestershire GL5 3TJ
Tel: 01453 768 000
support@meningitis-trust.org.uk
www.meningitis-trust.org.uk

Men's health

Impotence Association
PO Box 10296
London SW17 9WH
Tel: 020 8767 7791
theia@btinternet.com
www.impotence.org.uk

Men's Health Matters
Blythe Hall
100 Blythe Road
London W14 0HB
Tel: 020 8995 4448
Medical Advisory Service:
020 8994 9874
(6–9pm, Tues & Thurs)

Men's Health Trust
PO Box 195
Bury St Edmunds
Suffolk IP31 3NQ
Please send SAE

Prostate Help Association (PHA)
Langworth
Lincoln LN3 5DF
Please send SAE

Prostate Research Campaign
36 The Drive, Northwood
Middlesex HA6 1HP
Tel: 01923 824 278

Neurological problems

Action for Dysphasic Adults
1 Royal Street
London SE1 7LL
Tel: 020 7261 9572
www.speakability.org.uk

Action for ME
PO Box 1302
Wells, Somerset BA5 1YE
Tel: 01749 670 799
(10am–12pm, 2–4pm)
Pre-recorded Advice
Tel: 08911 22976
(24-hour ME information line)

ADD Information Services
(ADDISS)
PO Box 340
Edgware
Middlesex HA8 9HL
Tel: 020 8906 9068
info@addiss.co.uk
www.addiss.co.uk

ADD–ADHD Family Support
Group
1a The High Street
Dilton Marsh
Westbury, Wiltshire BA13 4DL
Tel: 01373 826045
Helpline: 01380 726 710

AFASIC
(Unlocking Speech and Language)
69–85 Old Street
London EC1V 9HX
Tel: 020 7841 8900
Helpline: 0845 355 5577
info@afasic.org.uk
www.afasic.org.uk

Alzheimer Scotland
– Action on Dementia
22 Drumsheugh Gardens
Edinburgh EH3 7RN
Tel: 0131 243 1453
Helpline: 0808 808 3000
(24 hour freephone)
alzheimer@alzscot.org
www.alzscot.org

Alzheimer's Disease Society
Gordon House
10 Greencoat Place
London SW1P 1PH
Tel: 020 7306 0606
Helpline: 0845 300 0336
info@alzheimers.org.uk
www.alzheimers.org.uk

Association of Youth with ME
Box No 605
Milton Keynes MK2 2XD
Tel: 01908 373 300
info@ayme.org.uk
www.ayme.org.uk

Association for Spina Bifida and
Hydrocephalus (ASBAH)
ASBAH House
42 Park Road
Peterborough PE1 2UQ
Tel: 01733 555 988
postmaster@asbah.demon.co.uk
www.asbah.demon.co.uk

Ataxia (Friedrich's Ataxia Group)
10 Winchester House
Kenington Park, 11 Cranmer Road
London SW9 6EJ
Tel: 020 7820 3900
office@ataxia.org.uk
www.ataxia.org.uk

Ataxia-Telangiectasia Society
IARC – Rothamsted
Harpenden
Herts ALS 23Q
Tel: 01582 760 733
Helpline/Family Counsellor:
0131 667 4065
atcharity@aol.com

British Dyslexia Association
98 London Road
Reading RG1 5AU
Tel: 0 1 18 966 2677
Helpline: 0118 966 8271
admin@bda-dyslexia.demon.
co.uk
www.bda-dyslexia.org.uk

British Epilepsy Association
(BEA)
New Anstey Houe
Gateway Drive
Yeadon Leeds
West Yorkshire LS19 7XY
Tel: 0113 210 8800
Helpline: 0808 800 5050
epilepsy@bea.org.uk
www.epilepsy.org.uk

Cerebral Palsy Helpline
PO Box 833
Milton Keynes MK12 5NY
Helpline: 0808 800 3333
cphelpline@scope.org.uk
www.scope.org.uk

David Lewis Organisation
(for epilepsy)
Mill Lane
Warford, near Alderley Edge
Cheshire SK9 7UD
Tel: 01565 640 000
enquiries@davidlewis.org.uk

Dyspraxia Foundation
8 West Alley
Hitchin
Herts SG5 1EG
Tel: 01462 454 986
dyspraxiafoundation@hotmail.
com
www.emmbrook.demon.co.uk/dysp
rax/homepage.htm

Dystonia Society
46–47 Britton Street
London EC1M 5NA
Tel: 020 7490 5671

Guillain Barr Support Group UK
(GBS Support Group)
Lincolnshire County
Council Offices
Eastgate, Sleaford
Lincolnshire NG34 7EB
Tel: 01529 304615
Helpline: 0800 374 803
admin@gbs.org.uk
www.gbs.org.uk

Headway (National Head Injuries
Association)
4 King Edward Court
Nottingham NG1 1EW
Tel: 0115 9240800
enquiries@headway.org.uk
www.headway.org.uk

Huntington's Disease Association
108 Battersea High Street
London SW11 3HP
Tel: 020 7223 7000
susanwatkin@hda.org.uk
www.hda.org.uk

Méniére's Society
98 Maybury Road
Woking
Surrey GU21 5HX
Tel: 01483 740 597
info@menieres.co.uk

Motor Neurone Disease
Association
David Niven House
10–15 Notre Dame Mews
Northampton NN1 2PR
Tel: 01604 250 505
Helpline: 0845 762 6262
enquiries@mndassociation.org
www.mndassociation.org

Multiple Sclerosis Society
MS National Centre
372 Edgware Road
London NW2 6ND
Tel: 020 8438 0700
Helpline: 0808 800 8000
www.mssociety.org.uk

Myalgic Encephalomyelitis (ME)
Association
4 Corringham Road
Stanford-le-Hope
Essex SS17 0AH
Tel: 01375 642 466
Enquiries Line: 01375 361 013
(1.30–4pm)
enquiries@meassocation.org.uk
www.meassociation.org.uk

Myasthenia Gravis Association
Keynes House
Chester Park, Alfreton Road
Derby DE21 4AS
Tel: 01332 290 219
Helpline: 0800 919 922
www.crabby.demon.co.uk/mga/

Narcolepsy Association
2 Bishop's Close
Hurstpierpoint
Hassocks
West Sussex BN6 9XU
Tel: 01322 863 056

National Society for Epilepsy
Chalfont St Peter
Gerrards Cross
Bucks SL9 0RJ
Tel: 01494 601 300
Helpline: 01494 601 400
(10am–4pm)
www.epilepsynse.org.uk

Neurofibromatosis Association
82 London Road
Kingston on Thames
Surrey KT2 6PX
Tel: 020 8547 1636
Textphone
020 8392 0184
nfa@zetnet.co.uk
www.nfa-uk.org.uk

Neurological Alliance
41 Frewin Road
London SW18 3LR
Tel: 020 8875 0282

Parkinson's Disease Society
215 Vauxhall Bridge Road
London SW1 VIEJ
Tel: 020 7931 8080
Helpline: 0808 800 0303

Parkinson's Disease Society –
Scotland
Tel: 0141 332 3343

Parkinson's Disease Society –
Wales
c/o Interlink
Maritime Offices
Woodland Terrace
Maesycoed
Pontypridd CF37 1DZ
Tel: 01443 404916
pds-wales@parkinsons.org.uk

Progressive Supranuclear
Palsy (PSP) Europe
Association
The Old Rectory
Wappenham
Towcester
Northants NN12 8SQ
Tel: 01327 860 299
psp.eur@virgin.net
www.pspeur.org

Rett Syndrome Association UK
113 Friern Barnet Road
London Nll 3EU
Tel: 020 8361 5161
info@rettsyndrome.org.uk
www.rettsyndrome.org.uk

Scottish Motor Neurone Disease
Association
76 Firhill Road
Glasgow G20 7BA
Tel: 0141 945 1077
info@scotmnd.sol.co.uk
www.scotmnd.org.uk

Spinal Injuries Association
Newpoint House
76 St James's Lane
London N10 3DF
Tel: 020 8444 2121
Helpline: 020 8883 4296
sia@spinal.co.uk
www.spinal.co.uk

The Stroke Association
123–127 Whitecross Street
London EC1Y 8JJ
Tel: 020 7566 0300
Information Service:
0845 30 33 100
stroke@stroke.org.uk
www.stroke.org.uk

The Tourette's Syndrome (UK)
Association
PO Box 26149
Dunfermline KY12 9WT
Tel: (01892) 669151

Tuberous Sclerosis Association
Little Barnsley Farm
Catshill
Bromsgrove
Worcs B61 0NQ
Tel: 01527 871 898
secretary@tuberous-sclerosis.
com

Migraine

British Migraine Association
178a High Road
West Byfleet
Surrey KT14 7ED
Tel: 01932 352 468
Helpline:01932 352 468
info@migraine.org.uk
www.migraine.org.uk

The Migraine Trust
45 Great Ormond Street
London WC1N 3HZ
Tel: 020 7831 4818
www.migrainetrust.org

Useful Addresses

Pain

National Back Pain Association
16 Elm Tree Road
Teddington, Middlesex TW11 8ST
Tel: 020 89775474
back/pain@compuserve.com
www.backpain.org

Pain Association Scotland
Cramond House
Cramond Glebe Road
Edinburgh EH4 6NS
Tel: 0131 312 7955
pain_association_scotland@compuserve.com
www.painassociation.com

Pain Society
9 Bedford Square
London WC1B 3RE
painsoc@compuserve.com
www.staff.ncl.ac.uk/r.j.hayes/painsoc.html

Pregnancy

Action on Pre-Eclampsia
31–33 College Road
Harrow, Middlesex HA1 1E3
Tel: 020 8427 4217
info@apec.org.uk
www.apec.org.uk

British Pregnancy Advisory Service
(BPAS)
Head Office
Austy Manor
Wootton Wawen
Solihull
West Midlands B95 6BX
Telephone for general
information: 01564 793225
To make an appointment for a
consultation at a local centre for
abortion, vasectomy, sterilisation or
vasectomy/sterilisation reversal call:
Actionline: (lo-call) 08457 30 40 30
– open 7 days a week
calm@bpas.org
www.bpas.org.uk

Family Planning Association
2–12 Pentonville Road
London N1 9FP
Tel: 020 7837 5432
Helpline:020 7837 4044
www.fpa.org.uk

ISSUE (National Fertility
Association)
114 Lichfield Street
Walsall WS1 1SX
Tel: 01922 722 888
webmaster@issue.co.uk
www.issue.co.uk

LIFE (help group for anyone
pregnant and NOT considering
abortion)
Life House
1A Newbold Terrace
Leamington Spa
Warwickshire CV32 4EA
Tel: 01926 421 587
National Helpline: 01926 311 511
info@lifeuk.org
www.lifeuk.org

Miscarriage Association
Clayton Hospital
Northgate
Wakefield
West Yorkshire WF1 3JS
Tel: 01924 200 799
www.miscarriageassociation.org.uk

National Childbirth Trust
(Parent Ability)
Alexandra House
Oldham Terrace
London W3 6NH
Tel: 020 8992 2616
Enquiries: 020 8992 8637
www.nct-online.org

Stillbirth and Neonatal Death
Society (SANDS)
28 Portland Place
London W1N 4DE
Tel: 020 7436 7940
support@uk-sands.org
www.uk-sands.org

Psychiatric problems

Depression Alliance
35 Westminster Bridge Road
London SE1 7JB
Tel: 020 7633 0557
information@depressionalliance.org
www.depressionalliance.org

Ex-Services Mental Welfare Society
– Combat Stress
Head Office, Tyrwhitt House
Oak Lawn Road
Leatherhead
Surrey KT22 0BX
Tel: 01372 841 600
contactus@combatstress.org.uk
www.combatstress.com

First Steps to Freedom (practical
help to people who suffer from
phobias, OCD, general anxiety,
panic attacks, anorexia and
bulimia, and those who wish to
come off tranquillisers)
7 Avon Court
Park Road
Kenilworth
Warwickshire CV8 2GX
Tel: 01926 864473
Helpline: 01926 851608
firststepstofreedom@compuserve.com
ljh@firststeps.demon.co.uk
www.firststeps.demon.co.uk

Manic Depression Fellowship
21 St George's Road
London SE1 6ES
Tel: 020 7793 2600
mdf@mdf.org.uk
www.mdf.org.uk

MIND (National Association for
Mental Health)
Granta House
15-19 Broadway
Stratford
London E15 4BQ
Tel: 020 8519 2122
Helpline: 020 8522 1728
contact@mind.org.uk
www.mind.org.uk

National Phobics Society
407 Wilbraham Road
Manchester M21 0UT
Tel: 0161 227 9898

National Schizophrenia Fellowship
28 Castle Street
Kingston-upon-Thames
Surrey KT1 1SS
Tel: 020 8547 3937
Helpline:020 8974 6814
info@nsf.org.uk
www.nsf.org.uk

SANE (Schizophrenia A National
Emergency)
1st Floor
Cityside House
40 Adler Street
London E1 1EE
Tel: 020 7375 1002
Saneline: 0845 767 8000
sane@saneline.org.uk

Schizophrenia Association
of Great Britain
Bryn Hyfryd
The Crescent
Bangor
Gwynedd LL57 2AG
Tel: 01248 354 048
sagb@btinternet.com
www.btinternet.com/~sagb

Scottish Association for Mental
Health
Cumbrae House
15 Carlton Court
Glasgow GS 93P
Tel: 0141 568 7000
enquire@samh.org.uk
www.samh.org.uk

Skin and hair problems

Acne Support Group
PO Box 230
Hayes
Middlesex UB4 9HW
Tel: 020 8561 6868
Alison@the-asg.demon.co.uk
www.m2w3.com/acne

British Skin Foundation
19 Fitzroy Square
London W1T 6EH
Tel: 020 7383 0266
admin@bad.org.uk
www.bad.org.uk

British Allergy Foundation
Deepdene House
30 Bellegrove Road
Welling
Kent DA16 3PY
Tel: 020 8303 8525
Helpline: 020 8303 8583
baf@nascr.net
www.allergyfoundation.com

DEBRA
(Dystrophic Epidermolysis Bullosa
Research Association)
DEBRA House
13 Wellington Business Park
Duke's Ride
Crowthrone
Berks RG45 6LS
Tel: 01344 771 961
debra.uk@btinternet.com
www.debra.org

Ehlers-Danlos Syndrome Support
Group
PO Box 335
Farnham
Surrey GU10 1XJ
Tel: 01252 690 940
directa@ehlers-danlos.org

Hairline International
The Alopecia Patients' Society
Lyons Court
1668 High Street
Knowle
West Midlands B93 0LY
Tel: 01564 775281
www.hairlineinternational.co.uk

Herpes Viruses Association
(SPHERE) and Shingles Suppport
Society
41 North Road
London N7 9DP
Tel: 020 7607 9661
Helpline: 020 7609 9061
(24 hour access)
herpes.virusesassociation@virgin.net
www.herpes.org.uk

Lupus UK
St James's House
Eastern Road
Romford
Essex RM1 3NH
Tel: 01708 731 251

National Eczema Society
163 Eversholt Street
London NW9 1BU
Tel: 020 7388 4097
Helpline: 0870 241 3604
www.eczema.org

Neurofibromatosis Association
82 London Road
Kingston upon Thames
Surrey KT2 6PX
Tel: 020 8547 1636
Minicom: 020 8392 0184
(Monday–Friday: 9am–5pm)
nfa@zetnet.co.uk
www.users.zetnet.co.uk/neurofibromatosis

Pemphigus Vulgaris Network
Flat C
261 St German's Road
London SE23 1RJ
(Affiliated to The National
Pemphigus Foundation, Atrium
Plaza, Suite 203, 828 San Pablo
Avenue, CA, USA 94706)
www.pemphigus.org

Psoriasis Arthropathy Alliance
PO Box 111
St Albans AL2 33Q
Tel: 01923 672 837
info@paalliance.org
www.paalliance.org

Psoriasis Association
7 Milton Street
Northampton NN2 7JG
Tel: 01604 711 129
mail@psoriasis.demon.co.uk

Raynaud's and Scleroderma
Association
112 Crewe Road
Alsager
Cheshire ST7 2JA
Tel: 01270 872776
webmaster@raynauds.demon.co.uk
www.raynauds.demon.co.uk

Vitiligo Society
125 Kennington Road
London SE11 6SF
Tel: 020 7840 0855
ali@vitiligosociety.org.uk
www.vitiligosociety.org.uk

Women's health

Women's Health
52 Featherstone Street
London EC1Y 8RT
Tel: 020 7251 6333
Helpline: 020 7251 6580

Women's Health Concern
93 Upper Richmond Road
London SW15
Tel: 020 8780 3007

Miscellaneous

Aid for Children with
Tracheotomies (ACT)
215a Perry Street
Billericay, Essex CM12 0NZ
Tel: 02920 755 932
actuk@aol.com

Barnardo's
Tanners Lane
Barkingside
Ilford, Essex IG6 1QG
Tel: 020 8550 8822
Call Centre: 0845 769 7967
www.barnardos.org.uk

Barnardo's Scotland
235 Corstorphine Road
Edinburgh EH12 7AR
Tel: 0131 334 9893
www.barnardos.org.uk

Behcet's Syndrome Society
Answerphone: 01488 71116

Benefit Enquiry Line for People
with Disabilities (BELL)
Tel: 0800 882 200
Textphone: 0800 243 355

Birth Defects Foundation
Central Office
Martindale
Cannock
Staffordshire WS11 2XN
Tel: 01543 468 888
Family Helpline: 01543 468 400
enquiries@birthdefects.co.uk
www.birthdefects.co.uk

BLISS (for parents whose child was
or is in a special care baby unit)
2nd Floor
Camelford House
87–89 Albert Embankment
London SE1 7TP
Tel: 020 7820 9471
Parent Support Line: 0500 618 140
info@bliss.org.uk
www.bliss.org.uk

British Dyslexia Association
98 London Road
Reading RG1 5AU
Tel: 0118 966 2677
Helpline: 0118 966 8271
info@dyslexiahelp-
bda.demon.co.uk
www.bda-dyslexia.org.uk

British Lung Foundation
78 Hatton Garden
London EC1N 8JR
Tel: 020 7831 5831
blf@britishlungfoundation.com
www.lunguk.org

British Polio Fellowship
Ground Floor
Unit A, Eagle Office Centre
The Runway
South Ruislip, Middlesex HA4 6SE
Tel: 020 8842 1898
Helpline: 0800 018 0586
british.polio@dial.pipex.com

British Red Cross Society
9 Grosvenor Crescent
London SW1X 7EJ
Tel: 020 7235 5454
info@redcross.org.uk
www.redcross.org.uk

British Sjogren's Syndrome
Association (BSSA)
Unit 1, Manor Workshops
Nailsea Wall Lane
West End
Nailsea, Bristol BS48 4DD
Tel: 01275 854 215

British Snoring and Sleep Apnoea
Association
1 Dunne Cross Close
Reigate
Surrey RH2 9DE
Tel: 01249 701 010
www.britishsnoring.co.uk

British Stammering Association
15 Old Ford Road
Bethnal Green
London E2 9PJ
Tel: 020 8983 1003
Helpline: 0845 603 2001
mail@stammering.org
www.stammering.org

Childline
Freepost 1111
London N1 1QW
Children Requiring Counselling:
0800 1111

Couple Counselling Scotland
40 North Castle Street
EH2 3BN
Tel: 0131 225 5006
enquiries@couplecounselling.org
www.couplecounselling.org

Cruse Bereavement Care
Cruse House
126 Sheen Road
Richmond
Surrey TW9 1UR
Tel: 020 8940 4818
Helpline: 0870 167 1677
Telephone Counselling Helpline:
0845 758 5565
info@crusebereavementcare.org.uk

Cystic Fibrosis Trust
11 London Road
Bromley
Kent BR1 1BY
Tel: 020 8464 7211
enquiries@cstrust.org.uk

Family Planning Association
2–12 Pentonville Road
London N1 9FP
Tel: 020 7837 5432
Helpline:020 7837 4044
www.fpa.org.uk

Foundation for the Study of Infant
Deaths (Cot Death Research and
Support)
Artillery House
11–19 Artillery Row
London SW1P 1RT
Tel: 020 7222 8001
Helpline: 020 7233 2090
fsid@sids.org.uk
www.sids.org.uk/fsid

Genetic Interest Group
Unit 4D, Leroy House
436 Essex Road
London N1 3QP
Tel: 020 7704 3141
mail@gig.org.uk
www.gig.org.uk

The Haemophilia Society
Chesterfield House
385 Euston Road
London NW1 3AU
Tel: 020 7380 0600
Helpline: 0800 018 6068
info@haemophilia.org.uk
www.haemophilia.org.uk

Hyperactive Children's Support
Group
63 Arydle Road
Little Hampton
West Sussex P019 2LD
Tel: 01903 725 182

Interstitial Cystitis Support
Group
76 High Street
Stony Stratford
Buckinghamshire MK11 1AH
Tel: 01908 569 169

La Leche League
(Breastfeeding help and
information)
BM 3424
London WC1N 3XX
Tel: 020 7242 1278

Lymphoedema Support
Network
St Lukes Crypt
Sydney Street
London SW3 6NH
Tel: 020 7351 4480
adminlsn@lymphoedema.
freeserve.co.uk
www.lymphoedema.org/lsn

Marfan Association UK
Rochester House
5 Aldershot Road
Fleet
Hants GU13 9NG
Tel: 01252 810 472
Answerphone: 01252 617 320
marfan@tiny.co.uk
www.marfan.org.uk

Muscular Dystrophy Group
of Great Britain & Northern
Ireland
7/11 Prescott Place
London SW4 6BS
Tel: 020 7720 8055
www.muscular-dystrophy.org

National Association of Citizens
Advice Bureaux
115–123 Pentonville road
London N1 9LZ
Tel: 020 7833 2181
www.nacab.org.uk

National Asthma Campaign
Providence House
Providence Place
London N1 0NT
Tel: 020 7226 2260
Helpline:08457 010 203
www.asthma.org.uk

National Autistic Society
393 City Road
London EC1V 1NE
Tel: 020 7833 2299
Helpline: 0870 600 8585
nas@nas.org.uk
www.oneworld.org/autism_uk

NSPCC
(National Society for the
Prevention of Cruelty to
Children)
42 Curtain Road
London EC2A 3NH
Tel: 020 7825 2500
Child Protection Helpline:
08088 005 000

Raynaud's and Scleroderma
Association
112 Crewe Road
Alsager
Cheshire ST7 2JA
Tel: 01270 872776
webmaster@raynauds.demon.
co.uk
www.raynauds.demon.co.uk

St John Ambulance Brigade
1 Grosvenor Crescent
London SW1X 7EF
Tel: 020 7235 5231
postmaster@nhq.sja.org.uk
www.sja.org.uk

Save the Children Fund
17 Grove Lane
London SE5 8RD
Tel: 020 7703 5400
www.savethechildren.org.uk

The Sickle Cell Society
54 Station Road
Harlesden
London NW10 4UA
Tel: 020 8961 4006
sicklecellsoc@btinternet.com
www.sicklecellsociety.org

Tissue Viability Society
Glanville Centre
Salisbury District Hospital
Salisbury SP2 8BJ
Tel: 01722 336262 ext. 4057
tvs@dial.pipex.com
www.tvs.org.uk

Toxic Shock Syndrome
Information Service (TSSIS)
PO Box 450
Godalming
Surrey GU7 1GR
Tel: 01483 418 561
www.tssis.com

UK Thalassaemia Society
19 The Broadway
Southgate Circus
London N14 6PH
Tel: 020 8882 0011
Recorded Information Line:
0800 7311 109
office@ukts.org
www.ukts.org

Wound Care Society
PO Box 170
Huntingdon
Cambridgeshire PE18 7PL
Tel: 01480 434401

Index

Index

Index

Index

A RAPID ACTION GUIDE

When seconds count

• Every emergency demands urgent action. But sometimes the urgency is so pressing that seconds can mean the difference between minor and major damage or injury – in some cases, between life and death.

• This first 'Rapid action' section of *What to do in an emergency* is a guide to help you to cope with emergencies of the specially urgent kind that can occur in and around the home.

• The instructions give only the essential information needed for taking immediate action. Additional details about all of the emergencies dealt with here are given in the main sections of the book.

Someone who has stopped breathing will probably suffer brain damage after about three minutes. The kiss of life puts air into the lungs until the casualty can breathe again.

THE KISS OF LIFE

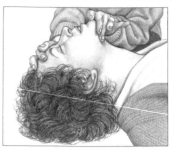

1 With one hand on the forehead, tilt the head backwards, and with the other hand lift the chin to open the airway.

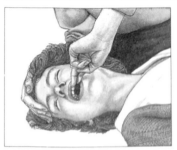

2 Remove obvious obstructions from the face. With the head to the side, quickly clear the mouth of any foreign material.

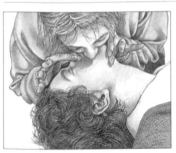

3 Check for pulse at neck (see page 52), pinch the nose closed with your fingers and blow in deeply. (For babies and small children, cover both nose and mouth and breathe gently.)

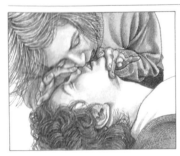

4 After each breath, turn your head to watch the chest fall. When it does, breathe into the mouth again and continue at 10 breaths per minute. (For babies and small children, breathe slightly more quickly than your normal rate.)

5 When breathing begins, put the casualty into the recovery position like this (see page 31).

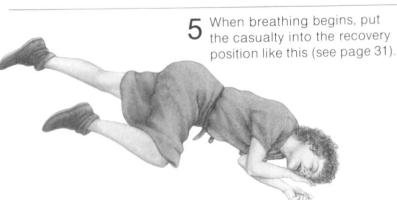

BLEEDING

Even if you cannot stop the bleeding altogether, reducing the flow of blood may be enough to save life.

Large foreign body in skin ▶

Bleeding that will not stop ▶

Bleeding from nose, ear or mouth ▶

If a deep cut causes blood to flow

1 Lay the casualty down. Remove clothing from around the wound if you can, without wasting time.

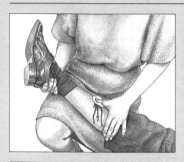

2 If there is no foreign object in the wound, press down hard on it with any clean, absorbent material, or your bare hands. If possible, raise the wound above the level of the heart to slow the flow of blood.

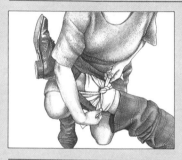

3 Maintain the pressure for up to ten minutes. While doing so, place an absorbent pad, such as the inside of a clean, folded handkerchief or pillowcase, over the wound, and bandage it firmly in place with a scarf or piece of clean linen.

4 If blood seeps through the dressing, do not remove it. Put another on top.

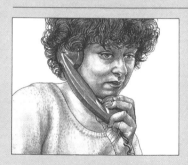

5 Telephone 999 and ask for an ambulance, or take the casualty to the Accident and Emergency Department at your local hospital.

If the wound is large

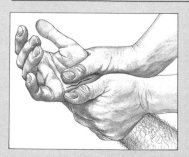

Squeeze the sides of the wound together gently but firmly, and maintain the pressure for up to ten minutes. If possible, raise the wound above the level of the heart. Continue as for a deep cut (step 3 above).

If there is a large foreign body in the skin

1 Squeeze the edges of the wound together around the foreign body.

- *DO NOT TRY TO REMOVE IT, AS IT MAY BE PLUGGING THE WOUND.*

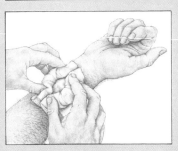

2 Put a piece of clean cloth over the wound. Then put thick pads of clean material either side of the wound, preferably higher than the object, to prevent pressure on it (see page 58).

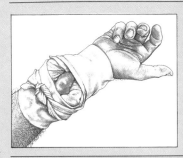

3 Bandage it with diagonally applied strips of material that do not go over the foreign body.

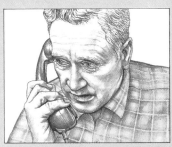

4 Telephone 999 and ask for an ambulance, or take the casualty to the Accident and Emergency Department of your local hospital.

If the bleeding will not stop

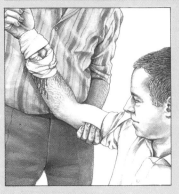

1 **A severely bleeding arm**
As a last resort, press your fingers between the muscles on the underside of the upper arm. This will compress the brachial artery, which roughly follows the seam of the sleeve. Press up and in, pushing the artery against the bone.

- *DO NOT MAINTAIN PRESSURE FOR LONGER THAN 10 MINUTES; YOU MAY CAUSE IRREPARABLE DAMAGE TO THE LIMB.*

- *DO NOT APPLY A TOURNIQUET.*

SEE NEXT PAGE

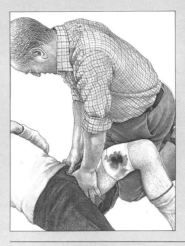

A severely bleeding leg
As a last resort, lay the casualty down with the injured leg bent. Press down in the centre of the fold of the groin with both thumbs, one on top of the other, against the rim of the pelvis. This will compress the femoral artery.

- *DO NOT MAINTAIN PRESSURE FOR LONGER THAN 10 MINUTES; YOU MAY CAUSE IRREPARABLE DAMAGE TO THE LIMB.*

- *DO NOT APPLY A TOURNIQUET.*

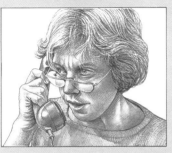

2 Tell someone to telephone 999 and ask for an ambulance.

If an injured person bleeds from nose, ear or mouth

1 This can indicate severe injury to the head or chest. Put the casualty in a half-sitting position, with the head inclined towards the injured side, to allow the blood to drain.

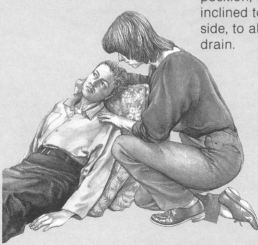

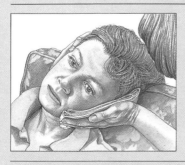

2 Cover the bleeding point, but do not apply pressure.

SEE NEXT PAGE

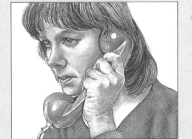

3 Telephone 999 and ask for an ambulance.

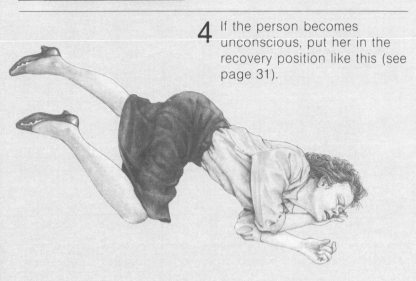

4 If the person becomes unconscious, put her in the recovery position like this (see page 31).

BURNS AND SCALDS

Many burns need medical attention because of the risk of
infection and shock. A young child or a sick or old person
should always be taken to a doctor.

If the burn or scald is smaller than a 10p piece

*Large burns and
scalds* ▶

1 If possible, remove rings,
watch or constricting clothing
before the area starts to swell.

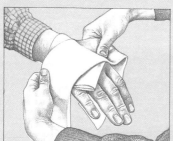

2 **Is it very painful?**
If so, the burn is probably
superficial. Put it under slow-
running cold water for ten
minutes, or longer if pain
continues.
Cover the burn with clean,
non-fluffy material. A sterile
dressing is best, but the inside
of a folded handkerchief,
bound on with cloth, will do.

Is it peeling or charred?
If the skin looks grey, and is
peeling or charred and not
very painful, the burn may be
deep and serious. Cover it
(see above) and take the
patient to the doctor or to the
Accident and Emergency
Department of a hospital.

- *DO NOT USE PLASTERS.*
- *DO NOT APPLY FAT, OINTMENT
  OR LOTION.*
- *DO NOT BREAK A BLISTER OR
  TOUCH THE BURN.*

If the burn or scald is larger than a 10p piece

1 If possible, remove rings,
watch or constricting clothing
before the area starts to swell.

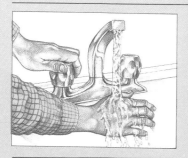

2 Cool the burn by running it
under a cold tap for at least
ten minutes, or longer if the
pain continues. Cool a large
area with a damp, clean cloth,
but do not waste time before
getting medical help.

SEE NEXT PAGE

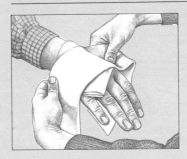

3 Cover the burn with clean, non-fluffy material. A sterile dressing is best, but the inside of a clean folded handkerchief, bound on with a scarf or other cloth, will do.

4 See your doctor or go to the Accident and Emergency Department of your local hospital.

- *DO NOT USE PLASTERS.*
- *DO NOT APPLY FAT, OINTMENT OR LOTION.*
- *DO NOT BREAK BLISTERS OR TOUCH THE BURN.*

If the burn or scald covers a large area of the body

A person who receives burns over a large area of the body, such as an arm, thigh, lower leg or chest, is likely to suffer shock, and needs urgent hospital treatment.

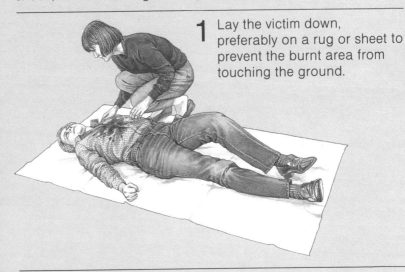

1 Lay the victim down, preferably on a rug or sheet to prevent the burnt area from touching the ground.

2 Cool the burnt area with cold liquid for at least 10 minutes.

If possible, remove any rings, watch, shoes or constrictive clothing before the area begins to swell.

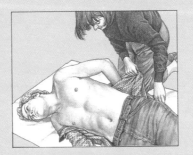

Carefully remove clothing soaked in boiling liquid when it has cooled.

SEE NEXT PAGE

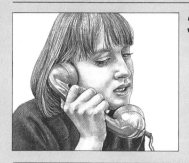

3 Ring 999 and ask for an ambulance, or arrange to take the victim to the Accident and Emergency Department of your local hospital.

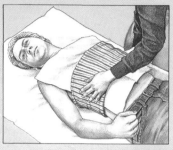

4 Cover the burn with clean, non-fluffy material, such as a freshly washed pillowcase. Fix it in place with a scarf or a piece of clean cloth.

- *DO NOT APPLY FAT, OINTMENT OR LOTION.*
- *DO NOT TOUCH THE BURN.*

For burns to the face, make a mask from a clean pillowcase by cutting holes for nose, mouth and eyes.

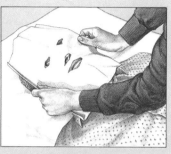

- *DO NOT APPLY FAT, OINTMENT OR LOTION.*
- *DO NOT TOUCH THE BURN.*

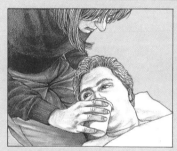

5 If mouth and throat are scalded and the victim is conscious, give sips of cold water to reduce swelling.

6 If a person with burns on the front becomes unconscious, put him in this recovery position. Turn the head to one side and tilt it back to open the airway. Raise the opposite side of the body by supporting it on a large cushion.

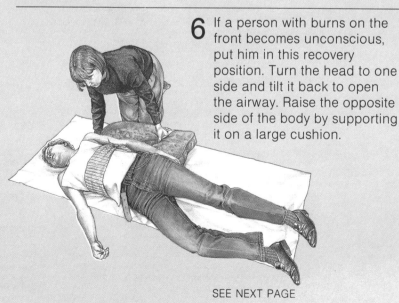

SEE NEXT PAGE

BURNS AND SCALDS

A person with burns on the back should be placed in the normal recovery position like this (see page 31).

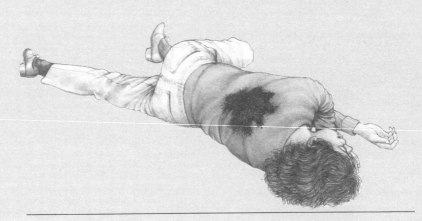

BURNS AND SCALDS

BURST PIPE OR TANK

When water pours through a bedroom ceiling, it is probably coming from a burst pipe in the loft, or a corroded cold-water storage tank.

If water pours through the ceiling

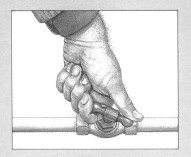

1 Turn off the main stop tap. It is probably under the kitchen sink or in the cellar. In a bungalow it may be in the airing cupboard. This will stop water entering the cold-water storage tank.

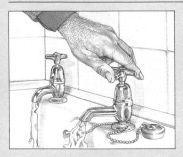

2 Open all the taps in the house to drain the cold-water storage tank. When the water stops flowing from the taps, the flow from the leak will have stopped, or will stop shortly afterwards.

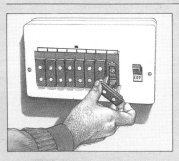

3 If water is running down a light fitting, switch off the light and remove the appropriate fuse from the main fuse box.

- *DO NOT REPLACE IT UNTIL EVERYTHING HAS DRIED OUT.*

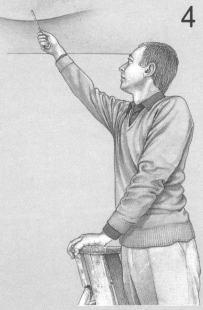

4 If the ceiling plaster is bulging, put a washing-up bowl beneath the bulge and pierce the plaster with a screwdriver or chisel. Stand out of the way, and have spare buckets ready. This will limit ceiling damage to one area.

SEE NEXT PAGE

5 Switch off a gas or oil-fired boiler, or an immersion heater. Damp down a solid-fuel boiler, but there is no need to extinguish it as the hot-water cylinder will not have emptied.

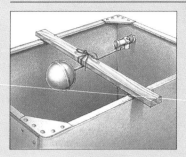

6 Find the source of the leak. If it was from a pipe supplied by the cold-water tank (see page 159), or if the tank itself was leaking, tie up the ball valve in the tank to stop it filling up again.

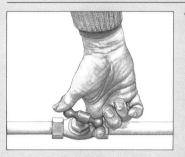

7 If you have tied up the ball valve, turn on the main stop tap. You now have cold water in the kitchen tap. And the lavatory cistern can be filled with a bucket.

8 Contact a plumber.

9 If possible, make an emergency repair to the burst pipe (see page 160).

If the victim becomes unconscious

1 Start the kiss of life (turn to page 2).

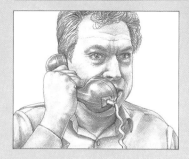

2 If a third person is present, tell him to telephone 999 and ask for an ambulance. If you are on your own, do not stop the kiss of life until normal breathing resumes.

3 If the kiss of life does not inflate the lungs with the first two breaths, roll the victim onto the side nearest to you, with the chest against your thigh and head well back. Give up to four slaps on the back.

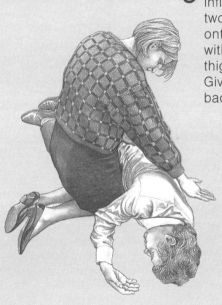

CHOKING

4 Look in the mouth to see if the blockage has become dislodged. If it has, hook it out with a finger.

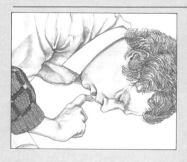

5 If not, turn the victim onto his back and tilt the head well back. Straddle the victim's thighs, or kneel alongside. Put the heel of one hand between the navel and the bottom of the breastbone.

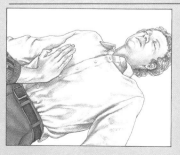

SEE NEXT PAGE

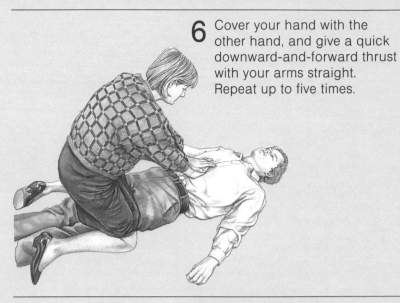

6 Cover your hand with the other hand, and give a quick downward-and-forward thrust with your arms straight. Repeat up to five times.

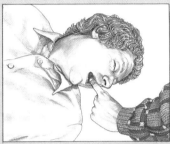

7 Check the mouth to see if the blockage has been dislodged. If it has, hook it out with a finger.

8 If not, resume the kiss of life.

9 If the lungs do not expand after the first two breaths, repeat steps 3 to 7 (see previous page).

DRUG OVERDOSE

An overdose of any drug (either an addictive drug or an ordinary medicine) is serious and requires urgent medical treatment. Symptoms of drug overdose include abnormal dilation or contraction of the pupils of the eyes, vomiting, difficulty in breathing, unconsciousness, sweating and hallucinations.

If a person takes a deliberate or accidental overdose

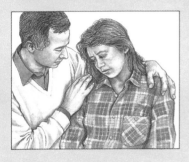

1 Ask the casualty what has happened. Obtain any information about the drug that you can as soon as possible. The casualty may become unconscious at any time.

- *DO NOT TRY TO INDUCE VOMITING. IT WASTES TIME AND MAY BE HARMFUL.*

2 If the person is unconscious, put her in the recovery position like this (see page 31).

Alcohol poisoning ▶

DRUG OVERDOSE

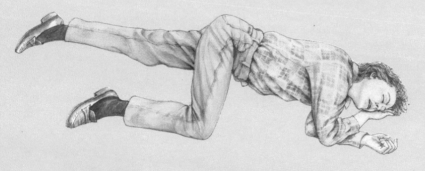

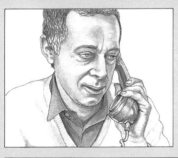

3 Telephone 999 and ask for an ambulance.

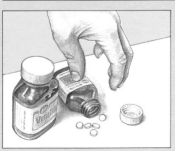

4 Collect a sample of vomit and any bottles or pill containers that are near the casualty. Send them to hospital with her as evidence to assist treatment.

If a person becomes unconscious from alcohol poisoning

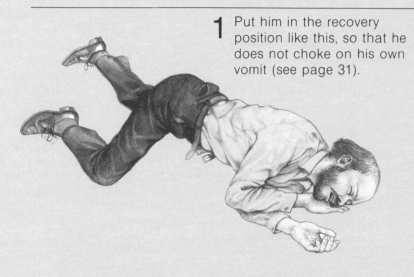

1 Put him in the recovery position like this, so that he does not choke on his own vomit (see page 31).

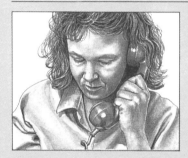

2 Telephone 999 and ask for an ambulance.

DRUG OVERDOSE

ELECTRIC SHOCK

If someone receives an electric shock at home or at work, cut off the source of electricity before doing anything else.

How to deal with an electrical injury

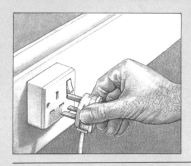

1 Stop the current by switching off at the socket or pulling out the plug. If you cannot reach the socket, switch off at the main fuse box.

- *DO NOT USE THE SWITCH ON THE APPLIANCE. A FAULTY SWITCH MAY BE THE CAUSE OF THE ACCIDENT.*

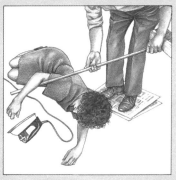

2 If there is no way to switch off, stand on dry insulating material, such as a thick layer of newspaper, a rubber mat or a wooden box, and push the victim's limbs away from the source with a broom or wooden chair.

- *DO NOT USE ANYTHING THAT IS DAMP OR MADE OF METAL.*

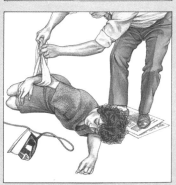

Alternatively, loop a rope, a pair of tights or any dry fabric around the victim's feet or under the arms, and pull her free.

- *DO NOT TOUCH THE VICTIM WITH YOUR HANDS.*
- *DO NOT USE ANYTHING WET, SUCH AS A DAMP TOWEL.*

3 If the victim is unconscious, and breathing, put her in the recovery position like this (see page 31)

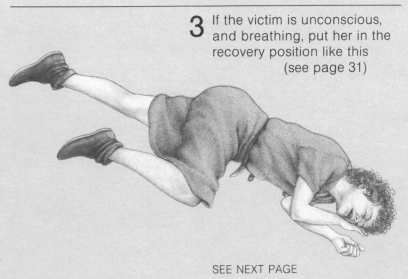

SEE NEXT PAGE

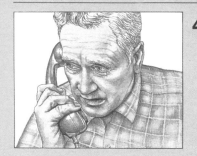

4 If the victim has been unconscious, has suffered burns or is feeling poorly, telephone 999 and ask for an ambulance, or drive her to the Accident and Emergency Department of your local hospital.
Tell the hospital how long she was in contact with the electricity.

**ELECTRIC
SHOCK**

FIRE

When fire has taken hold in a house, get out fast. Smoke from plastic-foam upholstery can kill in less than two minutes.

If a chip pan or frying pan catches fire

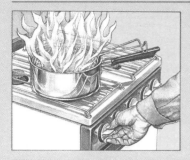

1 Turn off the heat on the stove.

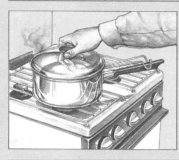

2 Cover the pan with a large lid or plate, or with a damp towel or a fire blanket.

- *DO NOT MOVE THE PAN.*
- *DO NOT THROW WATER ON IT.*
- *DO NOT LIFT THE LID OFF A CHIP PAN FOR HALF AN HOUR, EVEN IF THE FLAMES SEEM TO HAVE DIED DOWN.*

If an electrical appliance or fitting catches fire

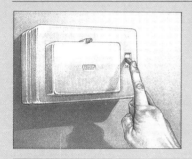

1 Switch off at the main fuse box.

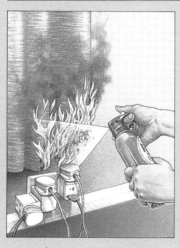

2 Extinguish the fire with water or a fire extinguisher, EXCEPT for a TV or computer fire (see next page).

- *DO NOT THROW WATER ON A BURNING APPLIANCE OR FITTING WHEN THE ELECTRICITY IS STILL TURNED ON.*
- *DO NOT TOUCH ANY SWITCH ON A BURNING APPLIANCE OR FITTING.*

TV set on fire ▶

Oil heater on fire ▶

Foam furniture on fire ▶

Clothing on fire ▶

Smell of burning at night ▶

Trapped on upper floor ▶

FIRE

If a TV or computer catches fire

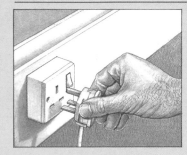

1 Pull out the plug or switch off at the main fuse box.

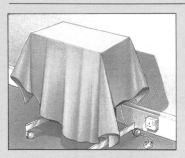

2 Smother the fire with a blanket or rug or a fire blanket.

- *DO NOT USE WATER OR A FIRE EXTINGUISHER, BECAUSE RESIDUAL ELECTRICITY MAY REMAIN IN THE SET.*

If an oil heater catches fire

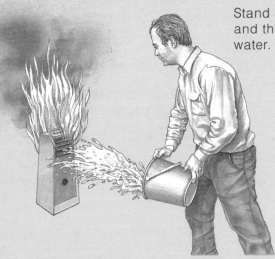

Stand at least 6ft (2m) away, and throw on buckets of water. If doing so is likely to knock the heater over, smother the fire with a water-soaked blanket instead.

If a foam sofa or armchair catches fire

Burning plastic foam gives off choking black smoke that can overcome you in one minute. Do not try to put out the fire.

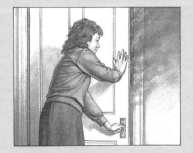

1 Get out of the room and close the door to prevent the smoke from spreading.

SEE NEXT PAGE

FIRE

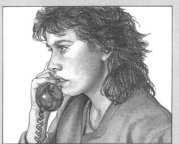

2 Telephone 999 and ask for the fire brigade.

If a person's clothes catch fire

1 Prevent the victim from rushing about in a panic; the movement will fan the flames.

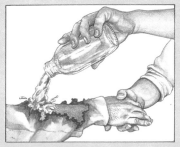

2 Lay the victim down to prevent the flames from rising up to the head, and douse the fire with water or other non-flammable liquid (in a kitchen a bottle of milk might be nearest to hand).

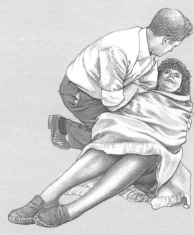

Alternatively, wrap her tightly in a coat, curtain, blanket (not the cellular type) or other thick fabric, and simultaneously lay her on the ground.

- *DO NOT USE NYLON OR MAN-MADE MATERIAL TO SMOTHER THE FLAMES.*
- *DO NOT ROLL THE VICTIM ALONG THE GROUND. IT CAN BRING THE FLAMES INTO CONTACT WITH UNHARMED PARTS OF THE BODY.*

3 Treat the victim according to the extent of the burns (see pages 7, 8, 9 and 10).

If you smell burning at night

1 Alert everyone in the house.

2 If the fire is too big to deal with safely, get everyone outside. If you think the fire is well alight in a closed room, do not open the door to find out.

SEE NEXT PAGE

Trapped on upper floor ▶

FIRE

23

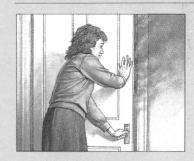

3 Shut all doors behind you to restrict the spread of flames and smoke.

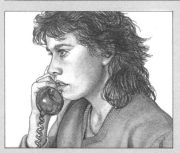

4 Go to the nearest telephone, dial 999 and ask for the Fire Brigade.

- *DO NOT GO BACK INSIDE.*

If you are trapped on an upper floor

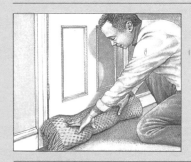

1 Go to a room at the front of the house, close the door and block up cracks with bedding or clothes.

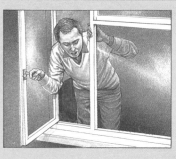

2 Open the window and call for help.

- *DO NOT JUMP OUT OF THE WINDOW, EXCEPT AS A LAST RESORT.*

FIRE

GAS LEAK

Your first priority must be to cut off the flow of gas.

If there is a strong smell of gas

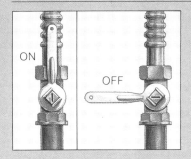

1 Turn off the main gas tap next to the meter.

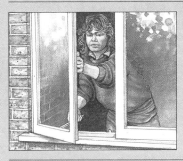

2 Open doors and windows.

3 Put out cigarettes or naked flames. Do not operate electric switches.

4 Put unconscious person in open air and in recovery position (see page 31).

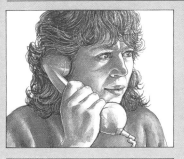

5 Telephone 999 and ask for an ambulance.
Telephone your local area gas office immediately – day or night. Find it under 'Gas' in the phone book.

- *DO NOT TRY TO TRACE THE LEAK WITH A NAKED FLAME (MATCH OR LIGHTER).*
- *DO NOT ENTER A ROOM OR AREA WHERE THE SMELL OF GAS IS ESPECIALLY STRONG. THE BUILD-UP OF FUMES MAY OVERPOWER YOU.*

GAS OFFICE

Tel. ....

If there is a slight smell of gas

1 Trace the source immediately. Often the pilot light on a cooker or gas fire has gone out, or a burner on the cooker has blown out in a draught.
SEE NEXT PAGE

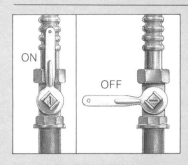

2 Turn off the pilot light or burner. If the pilot light does not have a tap, turn off the main gas tap next to the meter.

3 Put out cigarettes; extinguish naked flames; switch off any electric fire in the room.

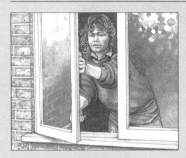

4 Open doors and windows to let the gas disperse. Wait for the smell to go.

5 Relight the pilot light or burner.

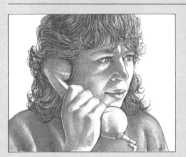

6 If the smell persists or returns, telephone your local area gas office immediately – day or night. Find it under 'Gas' in the phone book.

- *DO NOT ATTEMPT REPAIRS YOURSELF.*

GAS OFFICE

Tel. ....

GAS LEAK

POISONING

A house contains many substances, such as bleach, insecticides and paint stripper, that are highly dangerous to children. Get medical help quickly if a child swallows one.

If a child swallows a household chemical

1 If the victim is conscious, try to discover what has been swallowed. Remember that he may become unconscious at any time.

- *DO NOT INDUCE VOMITING. IT WASTES TIME AND MAY BE HARMFUL.*

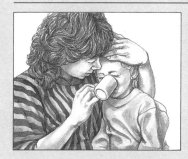

2 If the victim is conscious and has swallowed something that burns, such as bleach, cleaning fluid or paint stripper, give water or milk to sip.

3 If the victim is unconscious, place him in the recovery position like this (see page 31).

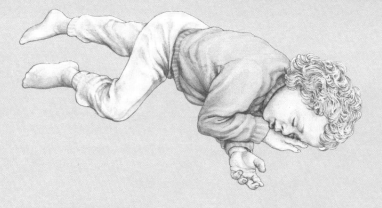

Plant poisoning ▶

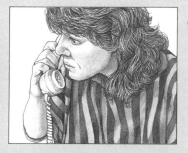

4 Telephone 999 and ask for an ambulance.

SEE NEXT PAGE

POISONING

27

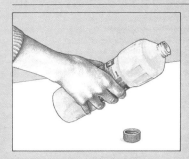

5 Give the ambulance men the poison container or a sample of vomit as evidence to assist treatment.

If a child eats a poisonous plant

The most common poisonous plants are the seeds and berries of laburnum and deadly or woody nightshade, green potatoes and death cap fungus. Symptoms of poisoning include vomiting, diarrhoea and stomach pains.

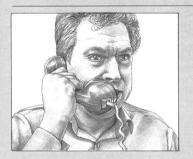

Telephone your doctor or take the child to the Accident and Emergency Department of your local hospital. Alternatively, telephone 999 and ask for an ambulance. If possible, give a sample of the plant to the hospital or ambulance men to help treatment.

POISONING

STROKE OR HEART ATTACK

STROKE SYMPTOMS There may be headache, paralysis down one side of the body, or difficulty swallowing and speaking. Possibly confusion and loss of consciousness.

HEART ATTACK SYMPTOMS Sudden crushing pain in the chest, often spreading to arms, neck and jaw. Possibly breathlessness.

Dealing with a possible stroke or heart attack

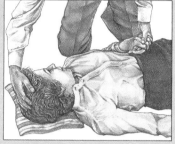

1 Suspected stroke
If the patient is conscious, lay her down with head and shoulders slightly raised and supported with a pillow. Place the head on one side to allow saliva to drain from the mouth.

Suspected heart attack
If the patient is conscious, place him in a half-sitting position, with head and shoulders supported with pillows or cushions, and another cushion under the knees.

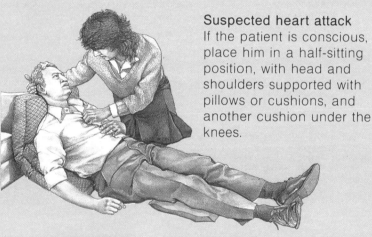

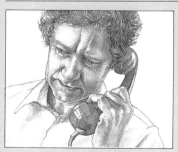

2 Call the patient's doctor, or telephone 999 and ask for an ambulance.

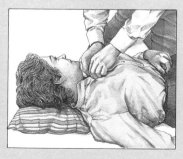

3 Loosen clothing around neck, chest and waist to help circulation and breathing.

- *DO NOT GIVE THE PATIENT ANYTHING TO EAT OR DRINK.*
- *DO NOT ALLOW A HEART-ATTACK PATIENT TO MOVE UNNECESSARILY; IT WILL PUT EXTRA STRAIN ON THE HEART.*

SEE NEXT PAGE

STROKE OR HEART ATTACK

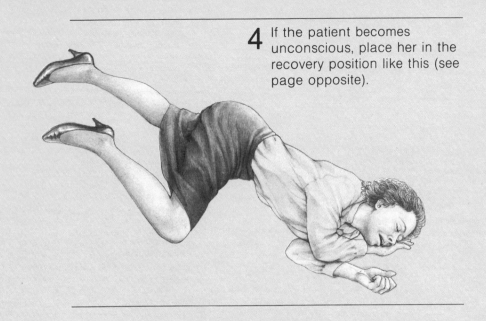

4 If the patient becomes unconscious, place her in the recovery position like this (see page opposite).

**STROKE OR
HEART ATTACK**

UNCONSCIOUS PERSON

Unless you suspect a fracture of the spine or neck, turn an unconscious, but breathing, casualty to the recovery position. This will prevent blood, saliva or the tongue from blocking the windpipe. The recovery position is a priority treatment.

Putting an unconscious casualty in the recovery position

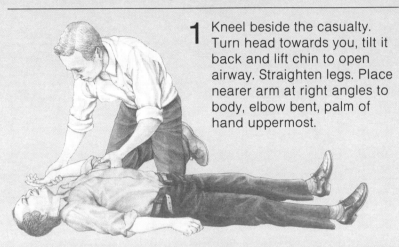

1 Kneel beside the casualty. Turn head towards you, tilt it back and lift chin to open airway. Straighten legs. Place nearer arm at right angles to body, elbow bent, palm of hand uppermost.

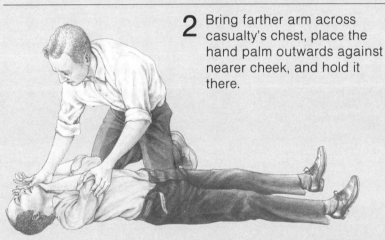

2 Bring farther arm across casualty's chest, place the hand palm outwards against nearer cheek, and hold it there.

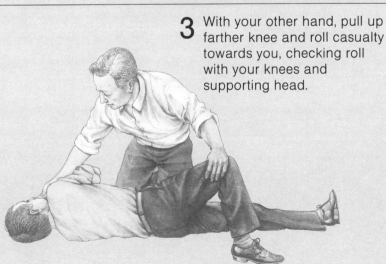

3 With your other hand, pull up farther knee and roll casualty towards you, checking roll with your knees and supporting head.

Turning a heavy person ▶

If an arm or leg is broken ▶

SEE NEXT PAGE

UNCONSCIOUS PERSON

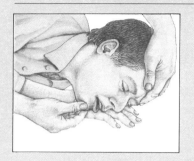

4 Tilt the chin forward to straighten the throat. This keeps the airway open, allowing the casualty to breathe freely. Adjust hand so that head is well supported.

5 Adjust uppermost leg to keep thigh and knee at right angles, and casualty propped securely. Check breathing and pulse regularly.

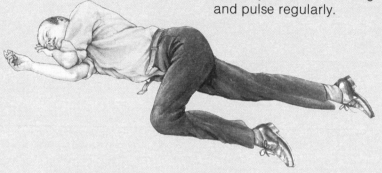

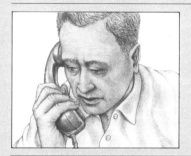

6 Telephone 999 and ask for an ambulance.

If the casualty is heavy

To roll casualty, grip clothing at the hip with one hand while pulling at knee with the other. If possible, get another person to support casualty's head while you turn the body.

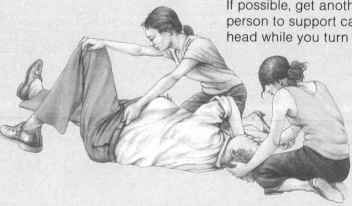

Alternatively, the helper can kneel facing you and push the casualty while you pull.

UNCONSCIOUS PERSON

If an arm or a leg is broken

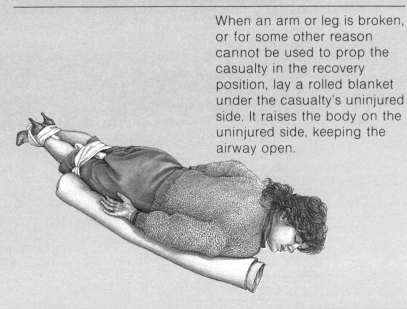

When an arm or leg is broken, or for some other reason cannot be used to prop the casualty in the recovery position, lay a rolled blanket under the casualty's uninjured side. It raises the body on the uninjured side, keeping the airway open.

WHAT TO DO IN AN EMERGENCY

was edited and designed by
The Reader's Digest Association Limited
London

Editor
Tony Scott
Art Editor
Neal V. Martin

First Edition
Copyright © 1986
The Reader's Digest Association Limited
Berkeley Square House
Berkeley Square
London W1X 6AB

Reprinted with amendments 1994

Copyright © 1986
Reader's Digest Association
Far East Limited

Philippines Copyright © 1986
Reader's Digest Association
Far East Limited

Printed in Belgium

ISBN 0 276 42085 3

EMERGENCY

READER'S DIGEST

WHAT TO DO IN AN EMERGENCY

PUBLISHED BY THE READER'S DIGEST ASSOCIATION LIMITED
LONDON · NEW YORK · MONTREAL · SYDNEY · CAPE TOWN

Contributors

WRITERS

Dr George Birdwood, MA, MB, ChB, MIL

Ted Clements
Chief Examiner
Institute of Advanced Motorists

Frank Eaglestone, Barrister, LLB, FCII, FCIArb
Insurance consultant
Co-editor, *Insurance Law Reports*

Fred Fearnley
Former survival and safety instructor
Special Air Service

Dr Max M. Glatt, DSc, MD, FRCP, FRCPsych, DPM
Medical Director, Addictive Disease Unit,
Charter Clinic, London;
Former Chairman, Medical Council on
Alcoholism

Anthony Greenbank
Author, *The Survival Handbook*;
Former Outward Bound instructor at Eskdale,
Cumbria, and Marble, Colorado, USA

Marcus Jacobson, MSc, CEng, FIMechE, FIMI
Former Chief Engineer
The Automobile Association

Dr Harvey Marcovitch, MA, MB, BChir, MRCP,
DObst.RCOG, DCH
Consultant Paediatrician
Horton General Hospital, Banbury

Dr Frank Preston, VRD, MBChB, DA, FFOM
Director Medical Services
British Airways

Tom Sanders, DLC
Water Safety Adviser
Royal Society for the Prevention of Accidents

Major Bertram Seymour
Former Chief Safety Officer
RCA Limited

Mike Stockman, MRCVS
Past President, British Veterinary Association;
Chairman, Breed Standards Committee
The Kennel Club

Superintendent Brian Turner,
Co-ordinator, Metropolitan Police Crime
Prevention Service
Scotland Yard

CONSULTANTS

Commander William Anderson, RN
Training manager
Royal Yachting Association

Dr Basil Booth, BSc, PhD
Former UK representative on UNESCO
Volcanic Hazards Committee

Malcolm Conway
Civil Aviation Authority

Dr James Cox, MD, BS, MRCGP, DObst.RCOG
General Practitioner
Caldbeck, Cumbria

Eric Franklin
Knotting Consultant to The Scout Association;
President, International Guild of Knot-Tyers

Geoff Good
Principal Coach
British Canoe Union

Dr Mark Harries, MB, MRCP
Consultant physician
Northwick Park Hospital and Clinical
Research Centre, Middlesex;
Medical Officer, British Olympic team, 1984;
Medical Adviser, Surf Lifesaving Association
and British Surfing Association;
Member of UK Resuscitation Council

Pippa Isbell
Association of British Travel Agents

Angela Large
Senior National Development Officer
Royal Life Saving Society

Dr W. Donald Mackenzie, MB, ChB, MFOM
Principal Medical Officer (Overseas)
British Airways

Contents

When emergency strikes

BE PREPARED

The time to read this book is *before* an emergency strikes, so that, forewarned, you know what to do as soon as danger threatens. Just as the middle of a darkening moor is no place to begin learning how to use a map and compass, the middle of a crisis is no time to begin discovering how to deal with it.

Safety experts also stress that, in any crisis, thinking is as crucial as doing. First assess the situation quickly, they say – then act. The experts identify three major rules to bear in mind: do not panic; improvise; and weigh the risks.

How this book is organised

WHAT TO DO IN AN EMERGENCY aims to cover all the crises that you are likely to run into. The first two sections – *When seconds count* and *First aid and medical emergencies* – are arranged alphabetically. In other sections, the information is arranged thematically: crises affecting swimmers, for example, are grouped separately from boating crises in the section called *Emergencies in the water*.

Within each section, there are also reassuring tips on ways of staying out of trouble, and real-life stories about people who have survived the most terrifying dangers by using their knowledge and their wits.

DO NOT PANIC

In any crisis, staying calm is the most important rule of all. Panic can turn a problem into a tragedy; and staying calm can do more than any other single factor to save a life – yours or someone else's.

A swimmer caught in weeds underwater can untangle himself with his hands if he keeps his head. If, in panic, he lunges blindly for the surface, he may pull the weeds tighter – and drown. Panic destroys judgment and paralyses the muscles.

Knowledge is one antidote to it. The best cure, though, is an unshakable determination not to give way to it. Keep telling yourself that panic will only make things worse.

IMPROVISE

No emergency is quite like any other. Treating a bad cut at home when you have a first aid kit to hand and an ambulance only a telephone call away is very different from trying to cope with the same problem when you are out camping far from help.

In any situation, if you do not have exactly what you need, be prepared to make do with whatever is to hand. Look around for possible substitutes. Keep looking until you find one.

A life buoy and rope, for example, are the best equipment for helping someone who has fallen into water. But if there is no life buoy nearby, a child's rubber ring, a couple of towels knotted together or even a pair of trousers can save a life, too.

WEIGH THE RISKS

Sometimes in a crisis there is no absolutely safe way out. There may be no choice but to take one risk in order to avoid a greater one. If your brakes fail on a steep hill, for instance, you may have to drive deliberately into a hedge – and risk wrecking your car – in order to avoid risking your life in an uncontrollable crash at the bottom.

In any emergency, only you, the person on the spot, can weigh the dangers of each possible course of action against the advantages, and pick the best.

To do that successfully requires clear knowledge and a cool head. This book will help you to achieve both.

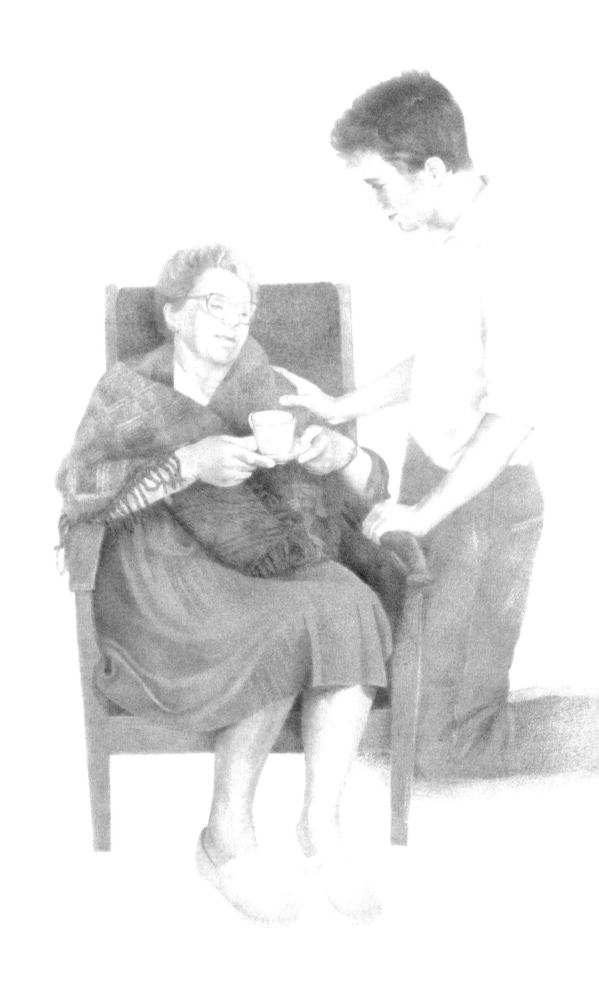

First aid and medical emergencies

What you need in a first aid kit

A home first aid kit is mainly intended for minor injuries that you can treat yourself, but it should also be equipped to deal with more serious injuries until the victim gets professional medical help. It should be kept in a well-sealed plastic box, such as an old ice-cream container. Put the box on the top shelf of the hall cupboard or some other place out of the reach of children. Do not keep first aid materials in unsealed containers in the bathroom or kitchen; they may deteriorate in the damp air. When you go on family holidays, take the kit with you.

Write the address and telephone number of your doctor and the address of the Accident and Emergency Department of your local hospital on a piece of paper and fix it to the inside of the first aid box. Tape it to the underside of the lid, for instance.

Do not keep old medicines left over from a previous illness. Flush them down the lavatory or return them to the chemist.

First aid kits can be bought ready-made from chemists, but you can make up your own from the items shown here, and at the same time become familiar with what your kit contains.

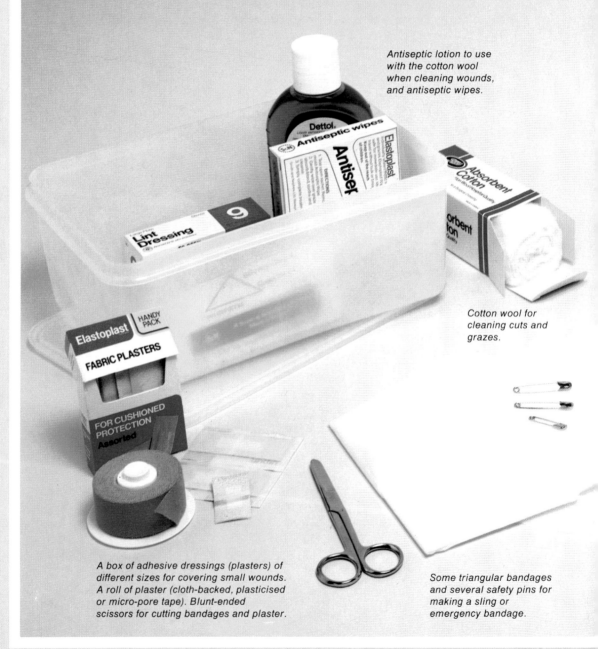

Antiseptic lotion to use with the cotton wool when cleaning wounds, and antiseptic wipes.

Cotton wool for cleaning cuts and grazes.

A box of adhesive dressings (plasters) of different sizes for covering small wounds. A roll of plaster (cloth-backed, plasticised or micro-pore tape). Blunt-ended scissors for cutting bandages and plaster.

Some triangular bandages and several safety pins for making a sling or emergency bandage.

A kit for hikers

On country walks – particularly in remote areas – take a small first aid kit which includes a foil blanket (also called a space blanket). The blanket can be wrapped around a casualty to preserve warmth in freezing temperatures.

The kit should also contain a triangular bandage, a crepe bandage for ankle injuries, some sterile dressings, adhesive dressings and a packet of antiseptic wipes for cleaning a wound when no water is available. Store the kit in a small plastic box.

How to improvise a dressing

If you have to treat a wound when no first aid kit is available, you can improvise dressings and bandages from a range of materials.
• For a dressing, take a clean handkerchief and fold it inside out so that the side that was protected from dirt can be placed on the wound. For a larger dressing, use a clean pillowcase or towel in the same way.
• Another way is to strip the wrapping off a packet of paper handkerchiefs and put the pad on the wound. Alternatively, discard the first few sheets of a toilet roll, then make a pad.

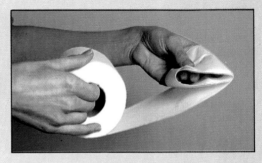

MAKING A TOILET-PAPER DRESSING *Wind toilet paper round your fingers to make a pad. Put its bottom, untouched side on the wound.*

• Do not put fluffy material such as cotton wool directly onto a wound because the fibres will become embedded in it.
• Whatever you make the dressing from, avoid touching the surface that will be in contact with the wound. Otherwise, dirt on your fingers could introduce infection.
• An improvised dressing can be bandaged on with any piece of reasonably clean material, such as a scarf, tie or old linen.

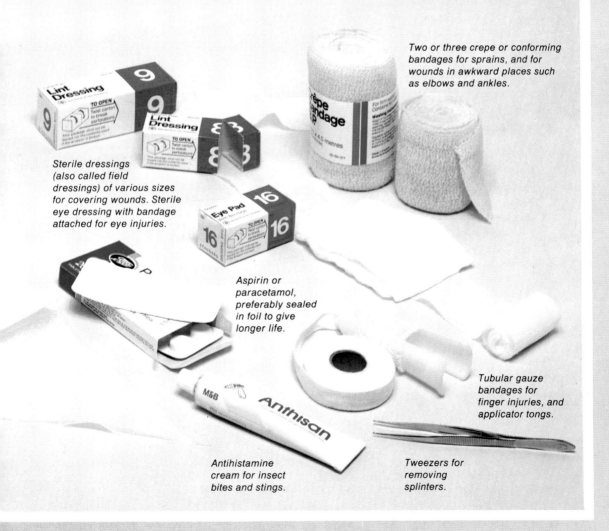

Two or three crepe or conforming bandages for sprains, and for wounds in awkward places such as elbows and ankles.

Sterile dressings (also called field dressings) of various sizes for covering wounds. Sterile eye dressing with bandage attached for eye injuries.

Aspirin or paracetamol, preferably sealed in foil to give longer life.

Tubular gauze bandages for finger injuries, and applicator tongs.

Antihistamine cream for insect bites and stings.

Tweezers for removing splinters.

Abdominal injuries

A car accident, a fall or a stab wound can cause serious injuries to vital organs inside the abdomen – the lower two-thirds of the trunk.

The abdomen contains organs such as the bladder, intestines and womb which are richly supplied with blood. An injury which damages the blood vessels can be as dangerous as one that affects the organs themselves.

Often the wound is clearly visible, and sometimes an organ may even be protruding.

If the wound runs lengthways on the body, lay the casualty flat on the back with the feet slightly raised on a cushion or folded jacket. If the wound runs across the body, lay the casualty on the back with the knees bent and the head and shoulders raised on a folded jacket or cushion. These two positions will help to hold the wound closed.

Treating the wound
Gently remove the clothing from around the wound, taking care not to cough, sneeze or even breathe on it, as it may become infected.

Put a dressing or a folded piece of clean linen over the wound to staunch the bleeding, and tie it in place with a bandage or scarf.

Cover the casualty with a coat or blanket, leaving the arms outside. Call for an ambulance, but do not leave the casualty alone.

Loosen any tight clothing – at the neck and

CASUALTY WITH A WOUND LENGTHWAYS TO THE BODY

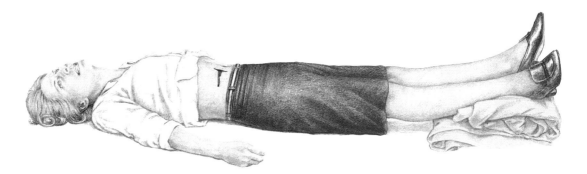

If the wound is running lengthways to the body, lay the casualty flat on her back with the feet slightly raised on a folded blanket, jacket or other convenient support. Do not raise the head off the ground. This position tenses the muscles of the abdomen and helps to close the wound.

CASUALTY WITH A WOUND ACROSS THE BODY

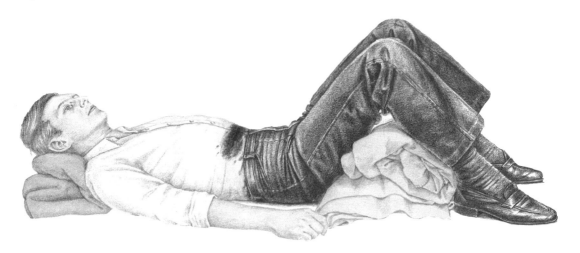

If the wound runs across the abdomen, lay the casualty on his back, with folded coats or blankets under the shoulders. Bend the knees and support them, too, with anything to hand. This position relaxes the abdominal muscles and helps to keep the wound closed.

waist, for example – to assist breathing and help blood circulation.

Do not offer anything to eat or drink, as the casualty may need a general anaesthetic at the hospital. If he complains of thirst, moisten his lips with water.

If the casualty becomes unconscious, carefully support the abdomen and gently turn him into the recovery position (see page 136).

If the casualty coughs or vomits, support the wound by pressing gently on the dressing to prevent internal organs from protruding.

If internal organs are already protruding from the wound, do not try to push them back or touch them.

Internal injuries of the abdomen

In some accidents there may be no external signs of injury, but the casualty may be bleeding internally.

All suspected cases of internal bleeding should be examined by a doctor as soon as possible. The warning signs are:
- Pain and tenderness in the abdomen.
- Tightening of the abdomen.
- Bruises and abrasions.
- Nausea and vomiting.
- Muscular spasms.
- Paleness, cold clammy skin and sometimes sweat on the forehead.
- Faintness.

HOW TO BANDAGE AN ABDOMINAL WOUND

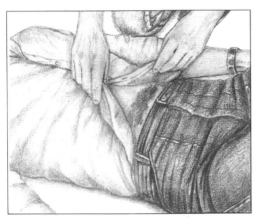

1 *Gently remove the casualty's clothing from around the wound to expose it for treatment. Do not cough, sneeze or breathe on the wound, as that may cause it to become infected. Do not touch the wound with your hands.*

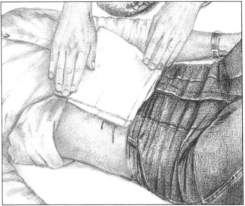

2 *Cover the wound and any protruding organs lightly with a large dressing, ideally a sterile dressing with bandage attached. Alternatively, use a piece of clean linen refolded so that the inside of the fold is now facing out.*

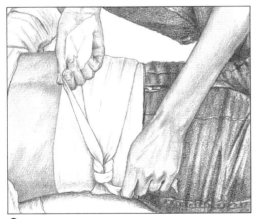

3 *Fix the dressing in place with a bandage, so that it covers, but does not press down on, the wound. Tie the knot away from the wound so that it does not press on the injury, either. If you cannot get a bandage under the casualty's back, secure the dressing with plaster.*

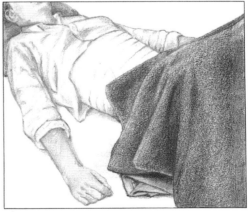

4 *Keep the casualty warm by covering him with a blanket or coat, leaving his arms outside so that you can check his pulse without disturbing him. Make sure that an ambulance has been called, but do not leave the casualty alone. Reassure him that help is on its way.*

Amputation

A finger, toe or major limb which has been severed in an accident can sometimes be sewn back on by microsurgery.

But do not waste time preserving the limb until you have taken care of the casualty, whose life is the first priority.

Do not try to restore the severed limb yourself – by binding it in place with surgical tape, for example. You will only cause the casualty great pain, and damage the tissues, which will make surgery more difficult.

What you should do
• Lay the casualty down and put a pad of gauze or clean linen, such as the inside of a clean, folded handkerchief, on the stump, and fix it in place with a bandage. A scarf will do.
• Immobilise an injured arm by bandaging it to the chest. If a leg is injured, bandage it to the other leg.
• Reassure the injured person and encourage him to keep still, then telephone 999 and ask for an ambulance.
• Once you have dealt with the casualty, try to find the severed limb. Wrap it in clean linen, such as a handkerchief or a pillowcase, and put it in a plastic bag.
• Keep it cool, if possible by packing ice around the plastic bag. Do not let the ice come in direct contact with the limb.
• Give the limb to the ambulance men, or doctor, to go to hospital with the casualty.

Animal bites

Bites from animals can introduce germs from the animal's mouth into the wound, possibly causing infection. There is a similar risk with human bites.

The area of any bite should be thoroughly washed, and if the skin has been broken the victim should see a doctor. Serious wounds should be treated at the Accident and Emergency Department of a hospital.

Report dog bites to the police, as failure to keep a dog under proper control is a legal offence.

CLEANING AND DRESSING A BITE

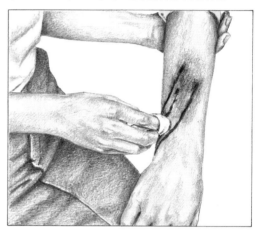

1 *Wash the area thoroughly with soap and warm water, or a mild antiseptic. Dry gently, wiping down and away from the wound. Cover with a clean dressing.*

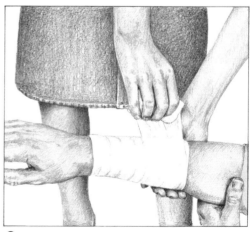

2 *Hold the dressing in place with a clean bandage or plaster. Take the victim to a doctor, because injections against tetanus or a course of antibiotics may be required.*

Ankle injuries

The ankle is the joint that most often suffers sprains – the stretching or tearing of a ligament linking the bones.

A sprain may be caused by twisting the foot as you walk or run. It causes pain in the joint, which becomes worse if it is moved, and the joint swells up.

The injury may take up to 14 days to heal, depending on the severity. For treatment, see *Sprains and strains*, page 132.

A serious sprain can be hard to distinguish from a fracture. So if there is any doubt, and the casualty cannot support himself on the ankle, assume that a bone is broken.

Treating a fractured ankle

A fracture of the ankle can follow a fall or a stumble that makes the ankle bend excessively, or it can be caused by falling on the foot from a height. The warning signs are:
• Immediate pain, which is often severe.
• The ankle soon becomes swollen or bruised.
• Pain when moving the ankle.
• It may be difficult or impossible to stand on the injured leg.

If you suspect a fractured ankle, apply a cold compress to limit the swelling, and see a doctor as soon as possible.

Make the cold compress by soaking a small towel or other material in cold water, wringing it out and wrapping it around the ankle. Or tie up some ice cubes in a plastic bag, wrap them in a cloth and crush them with a hammer. Then apply the compress to the ankle.

Appendicitis

Spasms of pain in the abdomen may be the first sign of appendicitis. The pain is caused by inflammation of the appendix, a short tube, closed at one end, that projects from the junction of the small and large intestines.

Appendicitis can occur if the open end of the appendix is blocked by fragments of hard waste matter, or if the appendix becomes kinked. As a result, infection sets in and the walls of the appendix become inflamed and swollen.

If the condition is left untreated, it may subside, only to recur – a condition known as chronic appendicitis.

If the condition is acute, however, the pain increases until the appendix finally bursts, spreading the infection through the area immediately around it, or throughout the intestine. This is a surgical emergency, requiring prompt treatment. For this reason, a doctor should be seen as early as possible in cases of suspected appendicitis, especially in children or old people.

The symptoms can take between 4 and 48 hours to develop. Because they are extremely variable, the condition can be difficult to diagnose. Call the doctor immediately if the pain gets worse, becomes continuous, or keeps the sufferer awake – and call him in any case if the pain lasts longer than four hours.

The danger signs
• Recurring spasms of pain. At first they may be felt near the navel, but sometimes in the lower right side of the abdomen.
• After a few hours, there is a constant severe aching in the lower right side of the abdomen.
• The lower right side of the abdomen is tender to the touch. The pain becomes more severe if the sufferer moves; it may interfere with sleep.
• The sufferer feels sick and may vomit. Often there is constipation, although the bowels may move normally, or even be loose.
• Food and drink are usually refused.
• It may hurt to walk, or to pass urine.
• The breath may smell foul.
• Body temperature generally rises to 39°C (102°F) in adults, and can be even higher in children. But sometimes it is only slightly raised.

What you can do to help
• Keep the sufferer lying still with a hot-water bottle wrapped in a towel on the abdomen.
• Rinse the mouth with sips of water, but do not give food or drink.
• Do not administer laxatives.

First aid and medical emergencies

Artificial respiration: the kiss of life

A person who has stopped breathing will die within minutes. After as little as three minutes without oxygen the brain can suffer irreversible damage. So it is urgent to get air into the lungs as quickly as possible. To tell if breathing has stopped, put your ear beside the casualty's mouth and nose and look along the chest. If he or she is breathing, you should be able to hear and feel it, and to see the chest moving.

When breathing stops, the lips, cheeks and ear lobes take on a bluish-grey tinge. Breathing may stop merely because the airway has become blocked for one of three reasons: the head may have fallen forward, making the airway narrower; the tongue may have slipped back in the throat, covering the airway; vomit or saliva may have collected at the back of the throat, blocking the airway.

• Your first step, therefore, must be to open the airway. Tilt the casualty's head backwards, push the chin up and clear out any obstruction in the mouth with your fingers.

• This may be enough to cause breathing to start spontaneously. In that case, turn the casualty over into the recovery position (see page 136) and call for an ambulance.

Breathing for a casualty

• If the casualty does not begin to breathe when the airway is opened, check neck pulse (see page 52). If there is a pulse, begin mouth-to-mouth respiration (the kiss of life) immediately.

• Pinch the nose shut, and seal your lips around the open mouth. Blow a full breath into the casualty's mouth, making the chest rise. Then remove your mouth and watch the casualty's chest fall.

• If there is no pulse, start external chest compression – but only if you have been trained in the technique (see page 52).

• Continue mouth-to-mouth respiration 10 times per minute – one breath about every six seconds.

• Once the casualty is breathing, turn him or her over into the recovery position (see page 136), *unless* you suspect a broken neck or back. Keep listening to the breathing: if it falters, restart artificial respiration.

Babies and small children

• When giving the kiss of life to a baby or a small child, seal your lips around both the mouth and nose, because the area is so small.

• Give the breaths more quickly than your normal breathing rate. For a small child, breathe more gently than you normally would. For a baby, deliver the air with gentle puffs.

If mouth-to-mouth is not possible

• Occasionally it is not possible to use a casualty's mouth for artificial respiration – perhaps because of mouth injuries. In such a case breathe into the nose, holding the mouth shut as you do so.

CLEARING THE PASSAGE FOR AIR

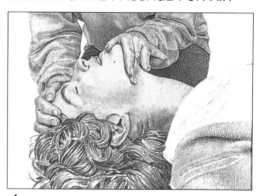

1 *Tilt the head back by lifting with one hand under the chin and pressing down with the other on the forehead. This opens the airway.*

MOUTH-TO-MOUTH RESPIRATION

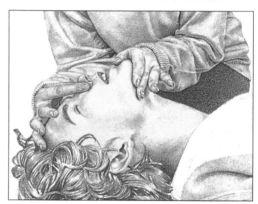

1 *Ensure that the head and chin are tilted well upwards, so that the casualty's airway remains open. Check for pulse (see page 52). Pinch the nose shut with your finger and thumb.*

MOUTH-TO-NOSE RESPIRATION

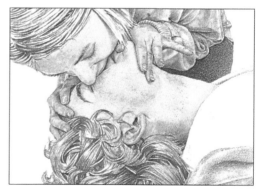

Tilt the head and chin well upwards, holding the mouth shut with one hand. Seal your lips around the nose, and breathe into the casualty in the same way as for the kiss of life.

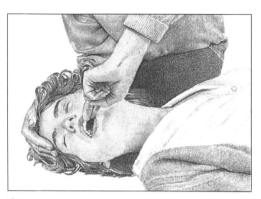

2 *If the casualty does not begin breathing, turn the head to the side and clear the mouth by sweeping inside it with two fingers.*

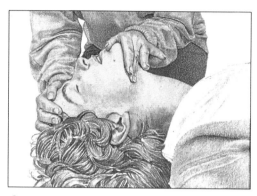

3 *Having cleared the mouth of debris, re-open the airway, tilting the head back by lifting chin and pressing forehead.*

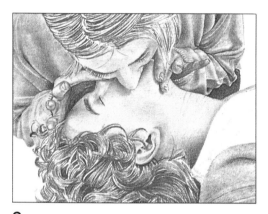

2 *Seal your lips around the open mouth and deliver two full breaths. Then remove your mouth and check the neck pulse (see* Has the heart stopped beating? page 52*).*

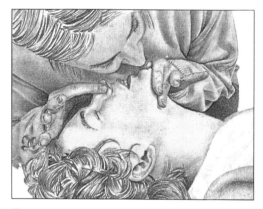

3 *Watch the chest fall. Replace your mouth and begin breathing into the casualty 10 times a minute (every six seconds). Keep going until she starts breathing again.*

GIVING ARTIFICIAL RESPIRATION TO A BABY
Clear the airway and hold the baby with its head tilted back. Cover both nose and mouth with your mouth and puff in gently, making the chest rise. Remove your mouth and watch the chest fall. Then continue the puffs, slightly faster than you would normally breathe yourself.

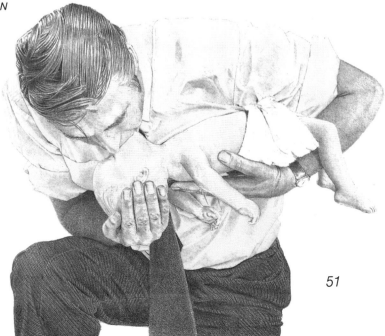

Artificial respiration: external chest compression

WARNING – THIS TECHNIQUE IS ONLY FOR PEOPLE TRAINED IN FIRST AID. IT IS DANGEROUS IF ATTEMPTED WITHOUT TRAINING.

If a casualty's heart stops beating, blood will no longer be pumped to the brain, and mouth-to-mouth respiration will be useless by itself. Brain damage will begin within minutes.

Squeezing the casualty's heart between the breastbone and the spine will make it work like a hand pump, forcing the blood around the circulatory system. If the brain continues to receive blood, the heart may spontaneously resume beating.

External chest compression is always used with mouth-to-mouth respiration (the kiss of life) to provide the blood with oxygen.

But chest compression can be a dangerous technique. The heart is sensitive, and if it is compressed while still beating faintly it may stop completely.

Compression should be used only by a person trained in first aid – and only after he or she has established conclusively that the casualty's heartbeat has stopped.

Consequently the information on these two pages is intended only as a memory aid for trained people. The technique should not be attempted without training, and should never be practised on a healthy person.

Compressing the casualty's chest
Compression is carried out on the lower half of the breastbone. The heel of the hand should be centred on a point two finger-widths up from the bottom of the breastbone.
• The pressure you apply should depress the chest of an adult by 1½-2in (35-50mm), and should be repeated at the rate of 80 per minute. If you are on your own, you should give 15 compressions, then inflate the lungs twice by mouth-to-mouth respiration.

HAS THE HEART STOPPED BEATING?

The only reliable way to discover if the heart has stopped beating is to feel the pulse of one of the carotid arteries in the casualty's neck to either side of the Adam's apple.

Feel the neck pulse. If there is no pulse; give two breaths of mouth-to-mouth respiration, then begin external chest compression at the rate of 15 compressions to two breaths.

If the casualty's colour improves, check the pulse again. If it is present, check the breathing. If the pulse is still absent, continue chest compression.

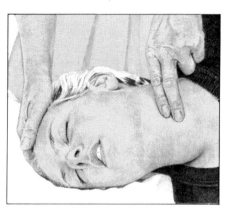

To feel the pulse of the carotid artery, place your fingers firmly in the hollow of the neck between the Adam's apple and the muscle at the side.

CHEST COMPRESSION ON AN ADULT

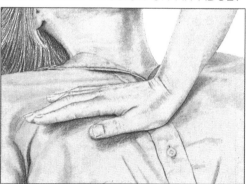

1 Place the heel of one hand on the casualty's chest, two finger-widths up from the bottom of the breastbone. Keep your thumb and fingers raised, so that they do not press on the ribs.

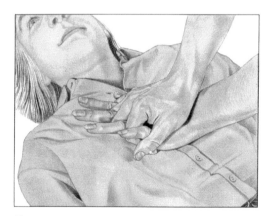

2 Keep the heel of your hand in place and put your other hand over it, fingers interlocked. Press down 1¾in (40mm), keeping your thumbs and fingers raised. Let the chest rise again.

• If two trained people are giving artificial respiration together, the sequence is five compressions to one inflation.

• If necessary, continue the sequence until medical help arrives.

• When you detect a neck pulse, stop compression, but continue mouth-to-mouth respiration until breathing starts. Keep checking the pulse. If it stops, restart compression.

Treating children and babies

• Use one hand only to compress the chest of a child under ten.

• The depth of the compression should be 1-1$\frac{1}{2}$in (25-35mm), and the speed a little greater – 100 times a minute.

• Give chest compression to a baby using two fingers only. The depth of compression must be no more than $\frac{1}{2}$-1in (13-25mm), and the speed 100 times a minute.

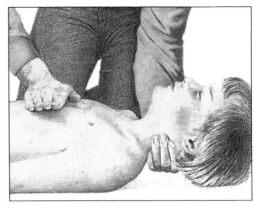

COMPRESSION ON A YOUNG CHILD
Press down the lower breastbone 1-1$\frac{1}{2}$in (25-35mm) at a slightly faster rate than an adult's pulse. Give five presses, then one lung inflation using mouth-to-mouth respiration.

COMPRESSION ON A BABY

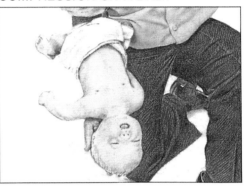

1 *Support the baby along one arm with your hand cradling its head, which should be slightly tilted down. You can also give mouth-to-mouth respiration in this position.*

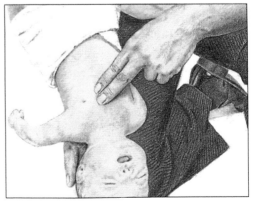

2 *Press down the middle of the breastbone $\frac{1}{2}$-1in (13-25mm), using two fingers only. Give five presses, then one lung inflation using mouth-to-mouth respiration.*

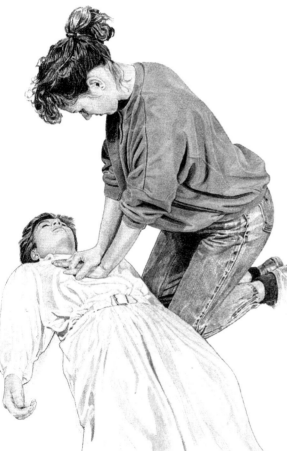

3 *Give 15 presses at normal pulse rate, then inflate the lungs twice by mouth-to-mouth respiration. Repeat the sequence four times a minute.*

Asphyxiation

A person suffering from asphyxiation (lack of oxygen in the blood) may die unless first aid is given promptly. Nerve cells in the brain can die after only three minutes without oxygen.

Common causes of asphyxiation
• Blockage of the airway by food, blood, vomit or broken teeth, or by the tongue falling to the back of the throat. Such blockages can occur with an unconscious person.
• Compression of the chest or damage to the lungs – possibly in a road accident.
• Gas poisoning – possibly from carbon monoxide given off by a car exhaust in a confined space.
• Electrical accidents.
• Suffocation – possibly from a plastic bag being placed over the head.
• Strangulation – possibly from attempted suicide by hanging.
• A severe attack of asthma or bronchitis.

Warning signs
• Breathing is difficult, and may become noisy and eventually stop altogether.
• The face turns blue, and the veins on the head and neck are swollen.
• The casualty gradually loses consciousness and may have fits.

What you should do
• If a person is suffocating because his mouth and nose have become blocked, remove the cause. If, for example, a plastic bag covers his head, tear it.
• Check for danger to yourself and to the casualty. If there is a continuing threat – from escaping gas, for example – stop it at the source or drag the casualty clear.
• If the casualty has been strangled, quickly cut or untie the cord or other material around the neck. If possible, keep the knot intact as possible evidence for the police.
• Check that the casualty is breathing. If not, clear the airway (see page 50).
• If breathing does not start, give mouth-to-mouth respiration (see page 50).
• If you suspect that the airway is blocked by food, treat for choking (see page 82).
• Once breathing is normal, turn the casualty into the recovery position (see page 136).
• Call for an ambulance but do not leave the casualty alone. Keep a careful watch on breathing, and give artificial respiration again if it falters.

Asthmatic attack

Most asthma attacks, while distressing, do not threaten life. However, a few particularly serious attacks are fatal each year.

During an asthmatic attack the muscles around the air tubes go into a spasm, impeding breathing. At the same time, the walls of the air tubes swell, and the tubes are further blocked by thick, tenacious mucus.

Warning signs of a severe attack
• Noisy, wheezy breathing.
• Pale or bluish-grey complexion.
• Beads of sweat on the forehead.
• An anxious expression.
• In a prolonged attack, mental confusion because of lack of oxygen.
• The victim struggles for breath, and is often

HOW TO HELP DURING AN ATTACK

1 *If possible, sit an asthma sufferer in an upright chair drawn close to a table or the back of another chair on which he can rest his forearms. His back should be fairly straight, and his elbows spread out.*

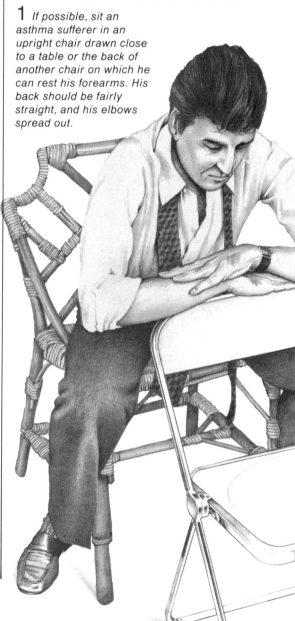

found sitting hunched up grasping the chair arms, a table-top or other support.

What you can do

• Most asthmatic attacks occur at night, often when the sufferer is in bed. In this case, open the window to provide fresh air and prop up the sufferer in bed with pillows.
• Even though the window is open, keep the room warm.
• Call the doctor for all but the mildest attack. Reassure the sufferer, telling him that expert help is on the way.
• If you have to take an asthma victim to hospital, transport him sitting up in the front passenger seat rather than lying down in the back.

Causes of asthma attacks

• Respiratory infection may cause inflammation of the air tubes.
• Allergy to various substances, including house-dust mites, animal fur or feathers, pollen and some foods.
• Night-time attacks in children are often associated with house-dust mites, down pillows or pets sleeping in the bedroom.
• Anxiety or excitement seems to bring on attacks in some people.

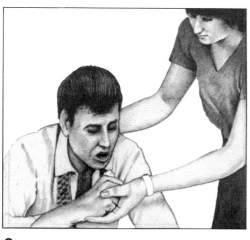

2 *If the sufferer has an inhaler, help him to use it. If he has an oxygen cylinder at home, give him oxygen only if you have been taught how to use it.*

Back or neck injuries

Mishandling a person whose back or neck is broken can cause permanent paralysis or even death.

A casualty with a suspected broken back or neck should be moved only if he is in immediate danger – in a burning building, for example. Otherwise leave him where he is. Any moving should be left to ambulancemen who have the right equipment.

Before you even touch an injured person, look for possible clues. For example, if he is lying at the foot of a ladder or a flight of stairs, it is possible he has suffered a back or neck injury.

Warning signs

• Loss of feeling and movement below the injured area, or a sensation of having been cut in half.
• Pain at the site of injury.
• A tingling sensation or pins and needles in the hands and feet (denotes neck injury).
• Inability to move fingers, wrists, toes or ankles when asked to do so, with no symptoms of a broken arm or leg.
• Inability to feel pain when the skin is gently nipped.
• Difficulty in breathing.

What you should do

• Tell the casualty to lie still.
• Cover him with a blanket and comfort him as much as possible. Do not raise the casualty's head or try to rest it on anything. Keep his head supported to prevent movement. Call for an ambulance.
• If the casualty is unconscious, and lying on his back, do not turn him over into the recovery position. Leave him face up, and clear his mouth of any obstructions to breathing with your fingers.
• Watch his breathing carefully. If it stops, begin mouth-to-mouth respiration (see page 50) immediately, even though tilting the head risks further damage to the spine. Be as careful and gentle as you can.

Bandages

In medical emergencies, bandages have three different uses. They keep a dressing in place over a wound, preventing dirt and germs from entering; they maintain pressure on a wound, controlling and absorbing bleeding; and they can be used to support or immobilise an injured part of the body (see *Slings*, page 121, and *Splints*, page 127).

Bandages are usually made of calico or gauze, but in an emergency they can be improvised from sheets, pillowcases, stockings, scarves or any other suitable material.

If no bandage is available, a dressing can be secured with strips of adhesive plaster.

Dressings, which are used to absorb blood and prevent infection, are usually a pad of cotton wool covered with gauze. Fluffy material such as cotton wool should not go directly on a wound because the fibres will stick.

In an emergency, a dressing can be made from a pad of any clean, dry, absorbent material. The inside of a folded handkerchief, a towel or pillowcase – even a pad of paper tissues or toilet paper – can all be used (see *How to improvise a dressing*, page 45).

Sterile dressings with a bandage attached, and sealed in a protective wrapping, can be bought from chemists. They are also known as field dressings, and will keep indefinitely in a family medicine cabinet.

Two other widely used types of bandage are the roller bandage, which varies in width from 1 to 6in (25 to 150mm), and the triangular bandage, with three sides about 3ft (1m) long.

APPLYING THE BANDAGE TO A WOUND

1 *Start by putting the end of the bandage on the limb and making a firm turn to hold it in place. Apply the outer surface to the skin so that you can unroll it easily. Bandage a limb in the position in which it is to remain.*

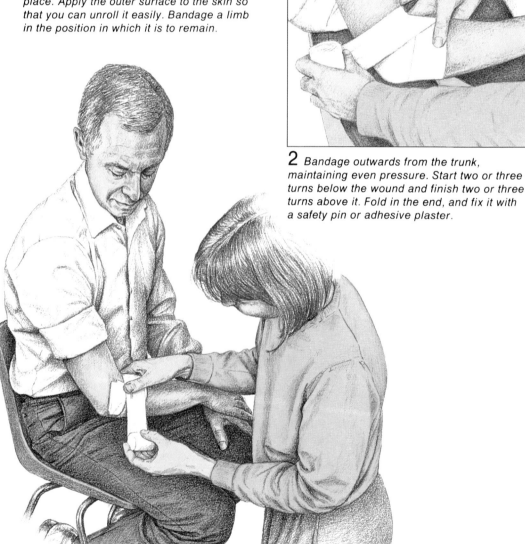

2 *Bandage outwards from the trunk, maintaining even pressure. Start two or three turns below the wound and finish two or three turns above it. Fold in the end, and fix it with a safety pin or adhesive plaster.*

How to use a roller bandage

Traditional roller bandages are made from non-stretch, open-weave gauze and are difficult to apply. Crepe, elasticated and 'conforming' bandages are easier to put on, and because they follow the contours of the body the pressure they exert on the wound is more evenly distributed.

Roller bandages can be bought in different widths for different purposes: a 1in (25mm) bandage for fingers and toes; 2in (50mm) for hands; $2\frac{1}{2}$in (65mm) for arms; 3 or $3\frac{1}{2}$in (75 or 90mm) for legs; and 4 or 6in (100 or 150mm) for the trunk.

Is the bandage too tight?

It is easy to bind a bandage so tightly that it interferes with the casualty's nerves or blood circulation. After applying a bandage, and again ten minutes later, check for the following warning signals.

• The casualty has a tingling feeling in the fingers or toes, or loses feeling altogether.

• The fingers or toes are very cold.

• The casualty is unable to move the fingers or toes.

• The beds of the fingernails or toenails are unusually pale or blue.

• The pulse of an injured arm is weak compared to the other arm, or completely absent.

If any of these danger signs occur, remove the bandage and apply it again more loosely.

Other types of bandage

Triangular bandages can be bought from chemists or they can be made by cutting a piece of

FINISHING OFF A BANDAGE WITH A KNOT

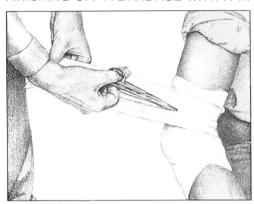

1 *If you do not have a safety pin or adhesive plaster, leave a piece of bandage free. The length will depend on the thickness of the area being bandaged. Cut the end of the bandage in half lengthways.*

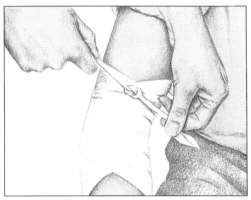

3 *Take the two ends around the limb again and tie them off, preferably with a reef knot (right end over left end, then left end over right). Once again, make sure that the knot does not press on the wound. Tuck in the ends.*

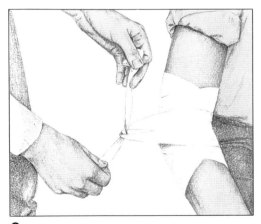

2 *Tie the two strips together with a single knot, pulling fairly tight at the bottom of the cut. This knot will stop the cut tearing further when you tie off the bandage. Make sure that the knot does not press on the wound.*

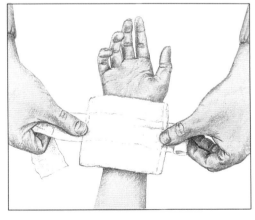

BANDAGE WITH DRESSING ATTACHED
A bandage and dressing combined, sealed in a wrapping, can be bought at chemists under the name of sterile dressing. The dressing is bound onto the wound, using the bandage.

linen or calico, about 3ft (1m) square, in half diagonally.

Unfolded, triangular bandages can be used as slings (see page 121).

They can also be folded into a broad bandage suitable for strapping up a broken limb, or into a narrow bandage for holding a dressing in place over a wound.

A built-up dressing can be used for a wound which contains a foreign object, or to protect an open fracture when a broken bone is jutting from the wound.

Seamless tubular bandages are easier to apply than conventional bandages, because they do not need to be tied.

Tubular bandages resemble stockings without feet, and they are available from chemists in various sizes to fit different parts of the body. They are all supplied with applicator tongs to slip them on over a dressing.

MAKING A BUILT-UP DRESSING

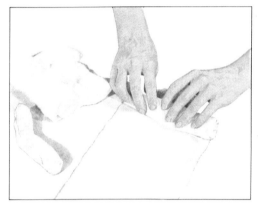

1 *Put a clean cloth, loosely, over the wound. Make two curved pads by rolling cotton wool or other material in a clean cloth, if possible making the pads higher than the foreign body.*

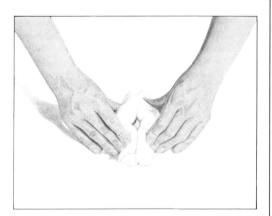

2 *Place pads around the foreign body, bandage them on with diagonal strips of material. If the foreign body is higher than the pads, do not cross the bandage over it.*

IMPROVISING WITH A TRIANGULAR BANDAGE

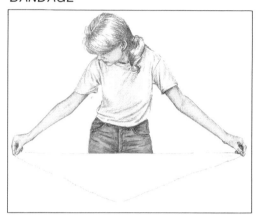

1 *To make a broad or narrow bandage in an emergency, spread the triangular bandage out on a flat, clean surface.*

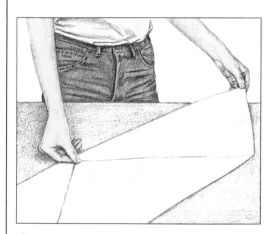

2 *Fold the apex of the triangle to the centre of the base, and then fold it once more in the same direction. This makes a broad bandage.*

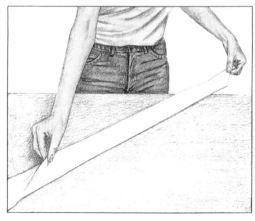

3 *To make a narrow bandage, fold a third time in the same direction. It can then be used like a roller bandage to bind wounds.*

PUTTING A TUBULAR BANDAGE ON A FINGER

Black eye

A blow to the eye socket and eyelid causes internal bleeding which colours the skin dark blue or black and produces a swelling.

Immediate treatment involves cold compresses. Do not put raw steak on a black eye; it is ineffective and wasteful.

There is always a possibility of damage to the eye itself or to the head, so have the injury examined by a doctor.

What you should do

• Put a cold compress over the eye to limit the swelling and relieve the pain. To make the compress, put crushed ice or ice cubes into a plastic bag, add some salt to encourage the ice to melt, seal the bag and wrap it in a cloth. Alternatively, soak a small towel in cold or iced water and wring it out.

• Cool the eye for at least 30 minutes, replacing the compress if it becomes warm.

• Take the casualty to a doctor as soon as possible to check that there is no serious damage to the eye or a fracture of the skull. A blow which is violent enough to blacken the eye may cause either.

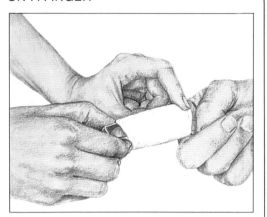

1 Cut a piece of tubular bandage 2½ times as long as the finger. Put the applicator over the finger and slide the bandage over the tongs.

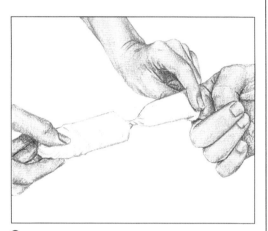

2 Slip the applicator off the finger, together with one end of the bandage. Turn the tongs so that the bandage is slightly twisted.

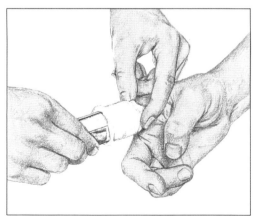

3 Push the tongs gently back down the finger, sliding the bandage off them as you go and leaving the finger covered with two layers.

Bleeding

Although bleeding can be alarming and dramatic, most cases are not fatal, provided the injury is treated promptly.

Bleeding can usually be stopped by pressing down on the wound, which slows the flow of blood and allows clotting to take place. If there is a foreign object, such as a piece of glass, in the wound, apply the pressure alongside it. Pressure must be maintained for up to 10 minutes.

The clotting process can be assisted by raising the injured area, which also slows the flow of blood. If severe bleeding continues, it may be possible to stop it by pressing on the appropriate artery. But this is a last resort only (see page 62).

Detecting bleeding in the dark

Usually bleeding is obvious, but after an accident – particularly in the dark – a casualty's position may conceal a serious wound. In this situation feel all over and under the body for patches of sticky dampness, and assume they are blood until you are sure that they are not.

Other warning signs of severe bleeding are:
- Pale skin which is moist and cold to touch.
- Profuse sweating.
- Fast but weak pulse (the normal adult pulse rate is 60-80 per minute).
- Casualty complains of thirst.
- Casualty's vision becomes blurred and he feels faint and giddy.
- Breathing becomes shallow, with yawning and sighing.
- Casualty becomes restless and talkative.

A large foreign object in the wound

If a large object, such as a piece of glass, is embedded in a wound, do not try to remove it. You may make the injury worse. Moreover, the object may be plugging the wound, helping to restrict the bleeding.

Control the bleeding by pressing the sides of the wound together around the object. Then bind up the wound, using a built-up dressing (see page 58) to keep pressure off the object.

Telephone for an ambulance, as the casualty will need hospital treatment.

HOW TO STOP SEVERE BLEEDING

1 *Lay the casualty down. Remove clothing from around the wound if you can without wasting time or causing distress. Press down hard on the wound with any absorbent material or your bare hands, unless something is embedded in it.*

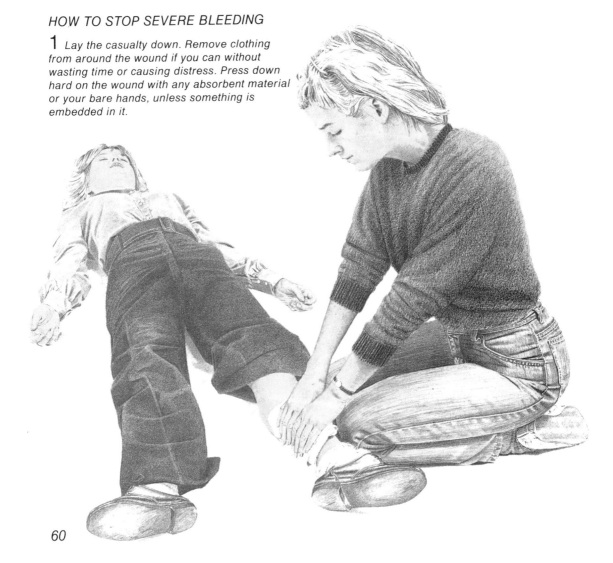

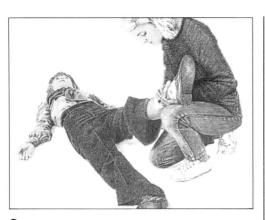

2 *If possible, raise the wounded area above the level of the heart to reduce the flow of blood. When the bleeding stops, put on an absorbent dressing, such as the inside of a clean, folded handkerchief.*

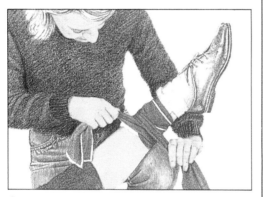

3 *If the blood seeps through the dressing, do not remove it. Put another dressing on top. Tie the dressing in place with a bandage or other material. Keep the casualty as still as possible and do not give food or drink.*

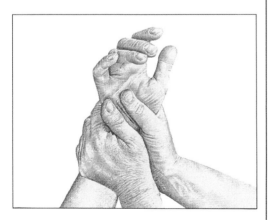

A LARGE WOUND
Squeeze the sides of a large wound together gently but firmly, and maintain the pressure for up to 10 minutes. Then treat as above and call an ambulance.

IF SOMETHING IS EMBEDDED

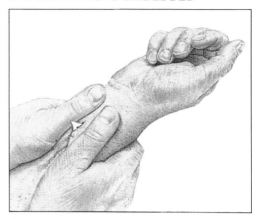

1 *To stop the bleeding, squeeze the edges of the wound together for up to 10 minutes. Do not try to remove the object.*

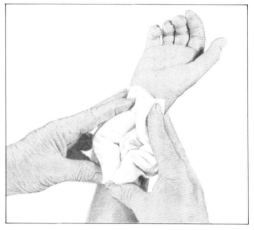

2 *Put a clean cloth, loosely, over the wound. Then put built-up pads of clean material each side of, and preferably higher than, the object to prevent pressure on it.*

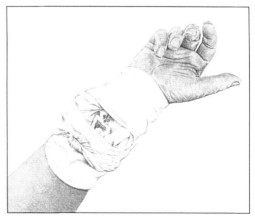

3 *Bandage the wound with diagonally applied strips of material that do not go over the object. Get the casualty to hospital.*

Stopping blood flow at a pressure point

If severe bleeding from an arm or leg cannot be stopped by direct pressure on the wound, or if direct pressure cannot be applied successfully, it may be possible to stop the bleeding by pressing on a pressure point.

Pressure points are places where an artery can be pressed against an underlying bone to prevent the blood flowing past. Use a pressure point to reduce severe bleeding only while a dressing is being prepared. Never maintain the pressure for more than 10 minutes, otherwise the tissues may be permanently damaged and the limb may have to be amputated.

There are two main pressure points. One is on the inner side of the arm where the brachial artery can be pressed against the bone. The other is high inside the thigh, where the femoral artery can be pressed against the pelvis.

When a varicose vein bursts

If a varicose vein in the leg bursts or is injured, severe blood loss can occur rapidly. The bleeding must be stopped as quickly as possible and the casualty taken to hospital.

• Lay the casualty down and press on the wound with a cloth pad, such as the inside of a folded handkerchief. If no pad is available, press with your bare fingers.
• Raise the leg onto your thigh and maintain the pressure for up to 10 minutes to stop the bleeding.
• Put a dressing on the wound and tie it firmly in place with a bandage or piece of material.
• If bleeding continues, lay further dressings and bandages over the first.
• Tell the patient to rest, and prop up the leg with pillows or on a chair seat.
• Call for an ambulance.

When blood flows from nose, mouth or ear

If an injured person bleeds from the nose, mouth or ear, he may be suffering from a severe internal injury to the head or chest.

A fractured skull may cause blood to trickle from the nose or ear. An injury to the lungs, caused by a fractured rib, may cause the casualty to cough up blood from the mouth.

Telephone for an ambulance as quickly as possible, and in the meantime place the casualty in a half-sitting position with the head tilted towards the side from which the blood is coming.

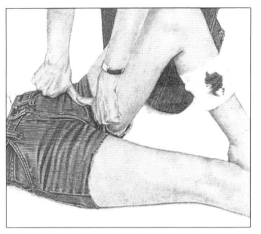

THE FEMORAL PRESSURE POINT
Lay the victim down and bend the injured leg at the knee. Press down firmly in the centre of the fold of the groin with both thumbs, one on top of the other, against the rim of the pelvis. Do not press for longer than 10 minutes.

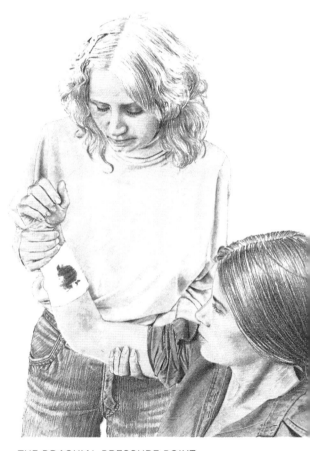

THE BRACHIAL PRESSURE POINT
Hold the casualty's arm at right angles to the body. The brachial artery runs along the inner side of the upper arm. To control bleeding from the lower arm, put one hand under the upper arm and press your fingers against the bone.

BLOOD FROM NOSE, MOUTH OR EAR

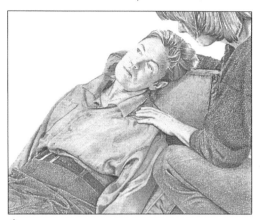

1 *Prop the casualty up in a half-sitting position, with the head tilted towards the side from which the blood is coming.*

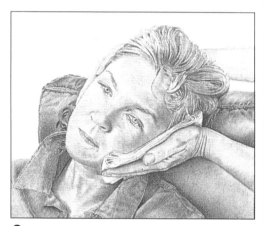

2 *Cover the bleeding point with a pad of clean material or cotton wool, but do not apply pressure. Telephone for an ambulance.*

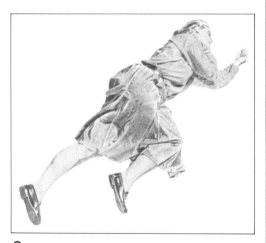

3 *If the casualty becomes unconscious before the ambulance arrives, put her in the recovery position like this (see page 136).*

Blindness

Sudden blindness can occur in one or both eyes for a number of reasons, some much less serious than others.

Migraine

The most common cause is migraine, which can produce bright spots or zigzag lines in the vision, preventing the victim from seeing properly. The disturbances of the vision are seen with both eyes. The sight will return to normal in 30 minutes or less, and a severe headache is likely to follow.

After the first attack, see your doctor. Once the condition has been diagnosed it should not be necessary to see the doctor after subsequent attacks.

Snow blindness

People who spend long periods in the snow risk snow blindness if they do not protect their eyes with dark glasses. The ultraviolet rays from bright sunlight reflected from the snow inflame the cornea, causing loss of vision.

Cover the victim's eyes with improvised pads and get medical help as quickly as possible. With prompt treatment, normal vision should return in a day or two.

Circulation problems in the eye

High blood pressure and diabetes can bring about haemorrhages or clots in the blood vessels of the eye. These clots can cause sudden, painless loss of vision – either partial or total – in one eye.

The victim should rest in a chair with eyes closed until medical help is obtained. The doctor will almost certainly arrange emergency admission to an eye hospital.

Detached retina

A sudden painless loss or change of vision, sometimes preceded by flashing lights, can be the main symptom of a detached retina.

Alternatively, the victim may have the sensation of a curtain coming across the field of vision.

Get medical help immediately. With prompt treatment, the eyesight can be successfully restored.

Acute glaucoma

Severe pain in and around the eye, with blurring of the vision, can indicate glaucoma, a rare but serious eye ailment. It occurs most often in elderly people, particularly women.

The main attack is often preceded by blurring of the vision and discomfort in the eye, which is better after sleep.

Attacks often occur in the evening, and can be caused by excitement.

Call for a doctor immediately and keep the patient in a well-lit room until help arrives. Treatment with drugs and possibly surgery can lessen the damaging effects on the vision.

First aid and medical emergencies

Blisters

Blisters caused by burns or friction to the skin usually heal within a week, whether they burst or not. A severe blister, affecting more than the outer layer of skin, will also heal completely but may leave a scar.

To burst or not to burst?

Do not burst a blister deliberately unless the taut skin is causing acute discomfort. Opening the skin increases the risk of infection.

If you decide to do so, observe scrupulous conditions of cleanliness.

• Wash the blistered area, and your hands, thoroughly.

• Pass a fine needle through a flame and let it cool for a moment. Do not wipe off any soot and do not touch the point.

• Hold the needle flat on the skin and press the point gently but firmly into the blister, just enough to burst it.

• Remove the needle and make a second puncture on the opposite side of the blister.

• Remove the needle and press gently on the blister with a clean piece of cotton wool.

• Wipe, and apply an adhesive dressing.

If a blister bursts by itself, expose it to the air as much as possible in hygienic conditions, but keep it covered with a bandage if there is a risk of dirt getting in.

See your doctor if a blister becomes infected, with a swollen, tender or inflamed area around it, or if blisters occur without any obvious cause. Multiple blisters are a symptom of several diseases, including shingles, chickenpox and impetigo.

How to avoid blisters

Blisters can be avoided by taking a few simple precautions.

• Take care when cooking or ironing. Cooks, for example, often receive burns on the arm when the oven door swings closed as they remove cooked food.

• Wear protective gloves for any heavy manual work to which you are not accustomed.

• Only buy shoes that fit well, and break them in with short periods of wear.

• For country walks, wear comfortable boots or shoes, with two pairs of socks to reduce friction on the feet. They can be a thin cotton pair next to the skin, with a thicker pair of woollen oversocks.

Boils

Most boils burst within a week of starting, but if the infection goes very deep it may take two weeks for the boil to 'come to a head'. The process can be speeded up by applying hot cloths or magnesium-sulphate poultices to the boil.

While waiting for the boil to burst, try to rest the affected area, and move it as little as possible. This allows the body's defences to work, and reduces the chance of the infection spreading below the skin.

Take paracetamol or aspirin to relieve the pain. Do not apply creams or antiseptics to the skin; they will not penetrate and so will not help to cure the boil.

When the boil bursts, cover it with a clean, dry dressing to prevent infection entering the wound.

Why do they occur?

Boils tend to occur in hairy parts of the body and areas where friction takes place, such as the nostrils, armpits, back of the neck and between the legs and buttocks.

They are caused by infection from bacteria, particularly in people with low resistance due to excessive tiredness, poor nutrition, diabetes mellitus or a blood disorder.

The bacteria create pockets of infection in the skin, often around a hair follicle. The follicle and surrounding cells in the skin are killed by the bacteria and form pus, which increases (or 'comes to a head') until it bursts through the skin and escapes.

A collection of boils, forming in several hair follicles, is called a carbuncle. The pocket of pus may be extensive, and can spread below the skin until two or more heads form and burst.

Boils tend to spread between members of a household, and sufferers should use their own towels and if possible sterilise underwear and handkerchiefs in boiling water or disinfectant while the boil is discharging.

It should be necessary to see a doctor only:

• If the boil is very painful.

• If the inflammation around the boil spreads without coming to a head.

• If the boil does not discharge pus, although a head has developed.

• If a person has many boils at the same time, or a sequence of infections.

The doctor may cut into the boil to release the pressure and ease the pain. Antibiotics may be prescribed to prevent the spread of infection. And tests may be made to discover any disease that is lowering resistance to infection.

To avoid boils in the future, eat a balanced diet and obtain plenty of rest to build up the body's resistance to infection. Control diabetes or any other disorders.

Bruises

Bruises are the visual sign of bleeding beneath the skin, usually as the result of a blow. Blood seeps into the tissues, causing swelling, soreness and discoloration.

The bruise is usually red or pink to start with, turning bluish and then greenish-yellow. These colour changes are caused by the gradual degeneration of the components of the blood as the bruise starts to heal.

Before treating a bruise check that there are no other injuries, particularly fractures.

Apply a cold compress to the bruised area to help to limit the swelling. The compress can be a small towel soaked in cold water and wrung out, or crushed ice cubes tied up in a plastic bag and wrapped in a cloth.

The cooling process slows down the blood flow. Apply the compress as soon as possible and keep it on for at least 30 minutes. Alternatively, instead of using a compress, hold the bruised area under a running cold tap.

A particularly severe blow can result in the outline of clothing becoming imprinted in the bruise. This is known as pattern bruising. If it should occur, see a doctor as the impact may have damaged internal organs.

See a doctor also:
• If the pain is severe, or if there is difficulty in moving the bruised part 24 hours later.
• If bruises occur without any apparent reason.
• If the lower leg is bruised in an elderly person or a person suffering from poor circulation.
• If the vision is disturbed as the result of a black eye (see page 59).

TREATING A BRUISED ARM

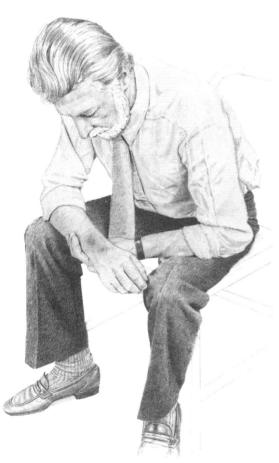

1 *Put the casualty in a comfortable position and get him to support the injured part before and during treatment. This helps to reduce the bleeding within the tissues.*

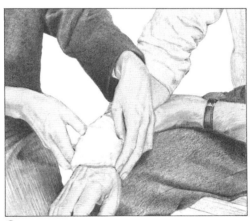

2 *Apply a cold compress at once to help to minimise the swelling. If necessary, fix the compress in place with a stretch bandage, winding from below the injury to above it.*

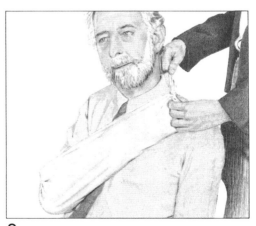

3 *Support a bruised arm with a sling (see page 121). If a leg is bruised, lay the casualty down and prop up the leg on a pillow. For bruises on the trunk, lay him down with pillows below head and shoulders.*

Burns and scalds

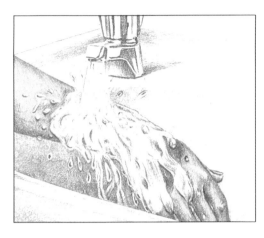

TREATING A MINOR BURN
A superficial burn smaller than a 10p piece can be treated by flooding it with cold water for at least ten minutes, or immersing it in any cold harmless liquid, such as milk or beer.

The seriousness of a burn or scald depends on how deep it is and how large an area it covers. All but minor burns and scalds are potentially serious and should be seen by a doctor. The treatment for burns and scalds is identical.

Do not put fat, ointment or lotion on a burn. It will have to be removed by hospital staff before they can give treatment, and may be a source of infection.

Do not apply any plasters, do not touch a burn and do not break any blisters. And do not remove anything that is sticking to a burn.

The first action in treating a casualty is to remove him from the source of heat. If the source is electrical, pull out the plug or switch off the power, taking care not to injure yourself.

If the burn is caused by a dry chemical, such as caustic soda or quicklime, brush away as much as you can with a duster or soft brush, taking care to protect your own hands. Remove contaminated clothing and check that the casualty is not lying on any of the chemical. For

REMOVING BURNT CLOTHING
When approaching a person with burning clothing, hold a blanket, rug or coat in front of you for protection. Wrap the material around him and lay him on the floor, burnt side uppermost. When the fire is extinguished, remove any hot clothing that can be taken off easily, but leave fragments that have stuck to the skin.

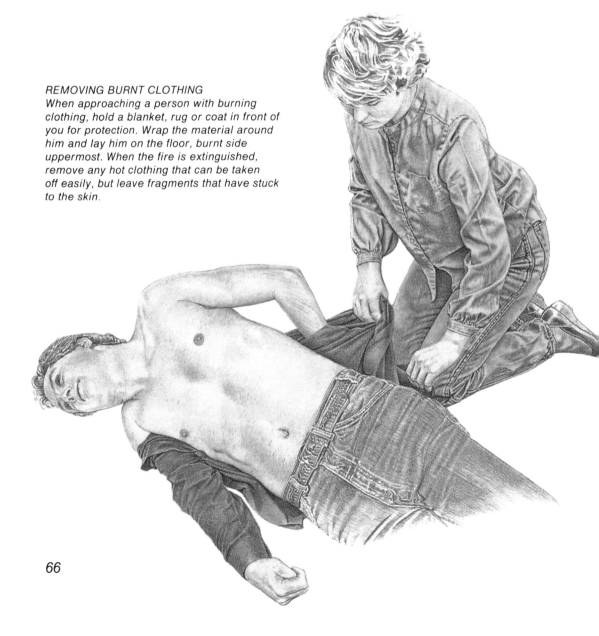

burns and scalds in the mouth, give the casualty ice cubes or ice cream to suck.

Treating a minor burn

If the burn is extremely painful it will probably be superficial, affecting only the outer layers of skin. It will be red, swollen and possibly blistered.

If a burn of this sort is smaller than a 10p piece, hold it under a slow-running cold-water tap or put it in cold water for at least ten minutes to cool the skin. If no water is available, use some other cold liquid, such as milk or beer.

Remove rings, watch or tight clothing before the area starts to swell, and finally cover it with a dressing of non-fluffy material.

Larger superficial burns

If a superficial burn is larger than a 10p piece, see a doctor or go to a hospital Accident and Emergency Department, because there is a danger of infection. Cool the burn in cold water and cover it with a clean dressing, but do not waste time before getting medical help.

Dealing with deep burns

If a burnt area of skin appears grey and is peeling or charred, the burn may be deep. It may not be particularly painful, as the nerves will have been damaged.

Whatever the size of a deep burn, first cool it with water. Cover it with a clean, non-fluffy dressing and get medical help at once, because there is a strong risk of infection.

Widespread burns

Burns covering a large area of the body, such as an arm, a thigh or the chest, are medical emergencies which must be treated in hospital as quickly as possible with minimum interference to the damaged skin.

Remove rings, watch or tight clothing before the area starts to swell. Cool the area with water, which will also extinguish any burning material. Dial 999 and ask for an ambulance urgently.

While waiting for the ambulance, cover the burn with clean, non-fluffy material, such as a freshly washed pillowcase. Fix it in place with a scarf or piece of clean cloth.

If the casualty is unconscious but breathing, put him in the recovery position (see page 136), before calling for an ambulance.

When a person's clothes catch fire

A person with burning clothes should be laid flat to prevent the flames rising to the head. Then douse the fire with water or any non-flammable liquid such as milk or beer (but *not* alcoholic spirits such as whisky or gin).

If no liquid is available, wrap the casualty in thick, non-synthetic material, such as a rug, blanket or woollen coat, to smother the flames.

If your own clothes catch fire, wrap yourself in thick material and lie down.

DEEP OR WIDESPREAD BURNS

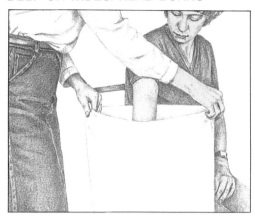

1 *Prevent infection by covering the burnt area with a clean dressing, such as a clean handkerchief or pillowcase. Hold it in place with a soft towel or other material.*

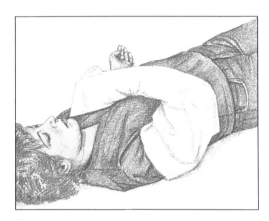

2 *If the burn is widespread, lay the casualty down and treat for shock (see page 120). Call an ambulance as soon as possible.*

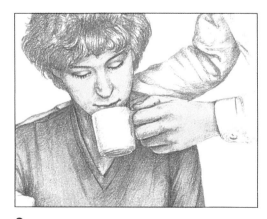

3 *When mouth and throat are scalded or burned, reassure the casualty and give sips of cold water to reduce swelling. Ice cubes may be given to suck. Ensure the airway is not obstructed.*

Chest injuries

Car accidents are the most common cause of chest injuries, particularly among drivers and passengers not wearing seat belts.

The other main causes are stab wounds and crushing by a heavy weight.

Serious chest injuries divide into two types, depending on whether the chest wall has been punctured.

'Sucking' wounds

If the chest wall has been penetrated by a sharp instrument, or by a fractured rib, the injury is known as a 'sucking' wound. As the casualty breathes, air is sucked into the chest through the wound, rather than down the airway, so that the lung does not inflate.

The lung on the uninjured side can also be affected, and the casualty can be in danger of dying from asphyxiation because of an inability to get enough air into the lungs.

Symptoms of a 'sucking' wound include:
- Pain in the chest.
- Difficulty in breathing.
- Blueness of the mouth and skin.
- Bubbles of blood-stained liquid emerging from the wound as the casualty breathes out.
- The sound of air being sucked through the wound as the casualty breathes in.

It is essential to seal the wound as quickly as possible so that the casualty can breathe.

Begin by placing the palm of your hand over the injury to provide immediate relief. Then, if

HOW TO TREAT A 'SUCKING' WOUND

1 *Rest the casualty in a comfortable position. Make him sit up and lean him towards the injured side. Leaning the casualty towards the injured side prevents blood draining across inside the chest and lessens the risk of the uninjured lung becoming affected. Lean him on cushions or against your knee. Slacken belt or waistband.*

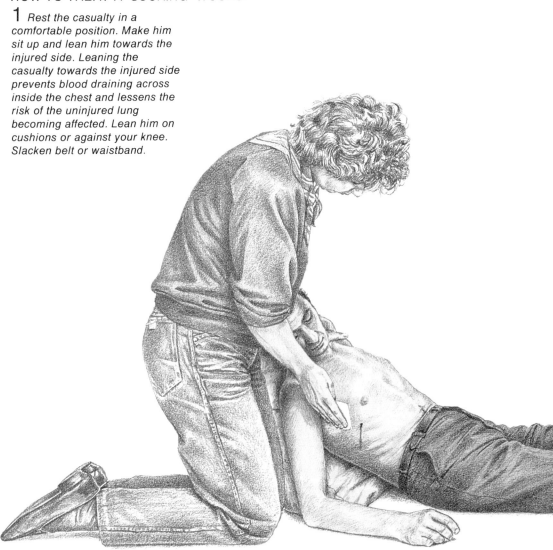

possible, apply a dressing and create an airtight seal by covering the dressing.

For the covering, use a piece of polythene, or plastic film of the type used to wrap up food, or kitchen foil, and seal the edges with adhesive tape or plaster.

Tell someone to dial 999 and ask for an ambulance.

Complicated fracture of the rib cage

A fractured rib may damage internal organs, such as the lungs, without penetrating through to the outside of the chest.

This will cause bleeding inside the chest. The casualty will then cough up red, frothy blood.

Other symptoms include:

- Bruising and bleeding from the chest.
- Pain which may become worse if the casualty coughs.
- Shallow breathing.
- A tight feeling in the chest. If several ribs are fractured, you may also be able to hear a crackling noise, which is caused by the bone ends rubbing together.

Ask someone to call for an ambulance as soon as possible, and if possible put the arm on the injured side in a triangular sling to support the fractured ribs.

Crushed chest

If the rib cage is fractured in several places – as can happen when the chest has been crushed by

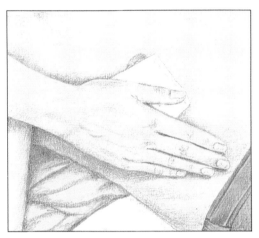

2 *Seal the puncture wound in the chest immediately with your hand – and a clean folded handkerchief if possible. Do not press hard if you suspect fractured ribs.*

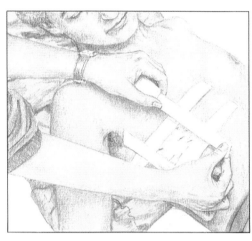

3 *To make a more permanent seal, cover the handkerchief with a sheet of polythene, plastic film or kitchen foil, securing it with plaster or any available adhesive tape to make it airtight.*

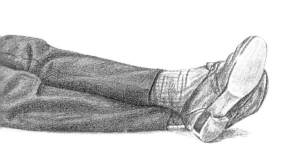

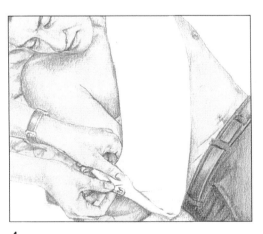

4 *While waiting for an ambulance, put the arm on the injured side across the chest to support the damaged area. Keep the arm in place with a triangular sling (see overleaf). Make the casualty as comfortable as possible.*

a heavy weight – a condition known as paradox-ical breathing may occur.

The fractured ribs will be sucked in when the casualty breathes in, and pushed out as he breathes out. This is the reverse of the normal chest movement and can cause extreme diffi-culty in breathing.

A patient in this condition should be treated as for a complicated fracture of the rib cage.

TREATING A COMPLICATED FRACTURE OF THE RIB CAGE

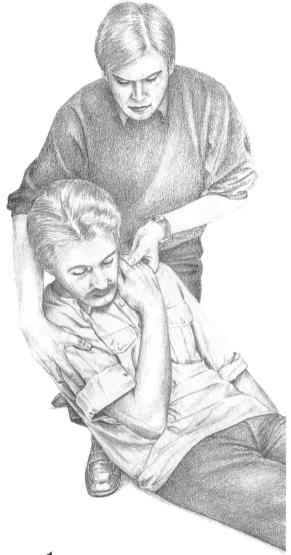

1 *Rest the casualty in a comfortable position. Make him sit up and lean him towards the injured side to help to drain blood and fluid away from the uninjured lung. Move the arm on the injured side diagonally across the chest, so that the hand rests on the opposite shoulder. The arm is now ready for a triangular sling.*

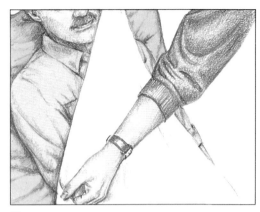

2 *Put one end of the base of the sling over the shoulder on the uninjured side, with the point extended beyond the elbow. The sling should hang over the arm.*

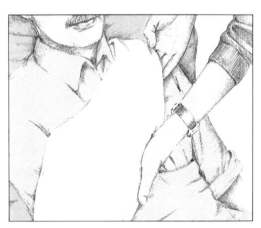

3 *Tuck the base under the hand, forearm and elbow. Bring the lower end up and around the back. Tie the ends together just above the collarbone on the uninjured side.*

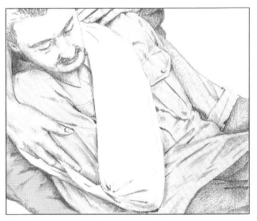

4 *Fold the point of the sling at the elbow and fasten it with a pin or tape, or twist then tuck it in. Get the casualty to support the sling with the other hand if possible.*

Chest pain

Pain in the chest may be clearly related to breathing or quite unrelated to it.

In either case, the pain can be a danger signal of a serious condition – in the lungs or the heart – and should not be ignored.

Pain related to breathing

Painful breathing can be caused by chest injuries, which are usually obvious (see *Chest injuries*, page 68, and *Rib fractures*, page 120). It can also indicate a disorder of the lungs or their lining (the pleura), or of the bones, muscles or skin of the chest.

The pain forces the sufferer to take short and often rapid breaths. There is often a cough as well.

See a doctor as soon as possible if there is:
- Severe pain.
- Breathlessness.
- High temperature.
- Blood-stained spit.

Pain not related to breathing

Chest pain that is not associated with breathing may have a clear connection with exertion or with eating.

Pain brought on by exertion usually feels 'crushing', and may radiate to the neck, shoulders or arms. It passes off with rest. It is usually a symptom of a heart disorder, and is known as cardiac or anginal pain.

If the pain is associated with eating it may be caused by a problem in the digestive system such as indigestion or duodenal ulcer.

See a doctor immediately if:
- There is paleness of the skin and sweating.
- A heart condition is suspected – either because the patient has already suffered a heart attack or because the pain fits the description of cardiac or anginal pain given above (see also *Heart attack*, page 105).
- The pain is not improved after an hour's rest.

Treat indigestion by resting in a chair and taking a proprietary antacid or half a teaspoon of bicarbonate of soda in a glass of water.

Chickenpox

A highly irritating rash which starts on the body and spreads to the arms, legs, face and head heralds an attack of chickenpox.

The rash begins as raised pink spots which change to watery blisters. These then burst or shrivel up, and crust over to form scabs. The spots appear in crops over about four days, so that all stages of the rash may be on the body at the same time.

The patient has a raised temperature and may feel quite ill for three or four days.

What you should do

Most cases of chickenpox do not require medical attention, and can be treated at home.
- Keep the rash clean and dry by having a quick shower every day and patting the skin dry.
- Apply calamine lotion to the rash twice daily to ease the itching.
- Do not pick the spots, or they will leave little pockmarks.
- Drink plenty of liquid. It does not matter if the patient refuses food during the illness.
- Rest, and take painkillers in recommended doses to help to reduce fever and discomfort.
- There is no need to isolate an infected child from your other children, as it is better to have the infection in childhood than in adult life. But keep the patient away from children being treated for serious diseases such as leukaemia, because chickenpox could be fatal to them.
- Try to avoid spreading the infection to babies under six months and to women in late pregnancy. If a woman has the disease within a few days before giving birth, the baby may have chickenpox and be quite ill. But chickenpox in earlier pregnancy does not affect the unborn child.
- Avoid spreading the infection to elderly people. They may otherwise develop shingles, a painful and sometimes long-lasting disease.

When to see the doctor

Chickenpox can be complicated by infected blisters and by pneumonia and encephalitis, which are rare but serious. See your doctor if:
- The patient has a high fever, is vomiting or is coughing excessively.
- There is some alteration in the patient's state of consciousness, or if he develops a severe headache or becomes confused.
- The eyes themselves (not simply the eyelids) are affected.
- The spots become inflamed.

Chickenpox patients are infectious from about four days before the rash appears until all the blisters have formed scabs. The scabs disappear about a fortnight after they begin to form.

Chickenpox is mainly a disease of childhood, but it occasionally affects adults. It occurs in sporadic epidemics and quickly spreads in schools. One attack ensures immunity to further attacks, but the virus may lie dormant in the body and cause shingles in later life.

First aid and medical emergencies

Childbirth

Most babies are born without difficulty. So your most important task in coping with an emergency delivery is to stay calm and reassure the mother and anyone else present.

Normally it is a criminal offence in Britain for anyone other than a doctor or midwife to supervise childbirth. But an unqualified person may have to take charge in an emergency, and the law recognises this. Before doing so, however, every effort should be made to contact a doctor or midwife – dial 999 if necessary.

There are three distinct stages in labour:

Stage 1 lasts for several hours – up to 14 hours in a first pregnancy, less in later births.

During this stage the muscles of the body of the uterus begin to contract, opening up the neck of the uterus (the cervix) to let the baby's head pass through. The contractions cause pain in the back and lower abdomen, and at first they occur about every 30 minutes. Blood may seep from the vagina at the start. Gradually the contractions become more frequent.

A watery fluid runs from the vagina. This is 'the breaking of the waters' – the release of fluid which has surrounded the baby in the womb.

Stage 2, during which the baby is actually born, lasts between 15 minutes and an hour. The contractions become stronger and the mother feels an urge to bear down.

Stage 3 happens after the birth, and is vital to the health of the mother. The placenta, or afterbirth, to which the umbilical cord is attached, is expelled after further contractions.

What you should do to prepare

Between contractions, or before labour starts, try to make the following preparations (you may have to improvise):

• Line the bottom of a cot with a folded blanket, shawl or towel. Fold another blanket ready for when the baby is born. You do not need a pillow. If there is no cot, use a drawer or a cardboard box.

• Prepare a bed or a large clean surface such as a table for the mother to lie on. Gather pillows or cushions for her to lean on. Spread a plastic sheet or newspaper over the surface and cover it with a clean sheet or towel.

• Fold a blanket in three from top to bottom to cover the mother's top during delivery. Wrap the blanket in a clean sheet if possible.

• Prepare three or four more clean towels and several pieces of cloth or sheeting, if available; also a sanitary towel for the mother to use after the birth, and a nappy for the baby.

• Keep the room comfortably warm: newborn babies can lose heat very rapidly.

• Have a large towel ready to wrap around the baby after birth, and a blanket or warm garment for the mother if she gets cold.

• Have a large bowl, such as a washing-up bowl, ready for the mother to sit on to deliver the placenta, a smaller bowl to put it in later, and another in case she vomits.

Cleanliness is essential

• Wash your hands and scrub your nails under running water before assisting, and as often as necessary during the birth. Do not dry them on a towel. Shake them as dry as possible.

• Keep anyone with an open cut or infection away from the mother and baby.

• Make sure that bedding, towels, cloths and swabbing materials are as clean as possible. When they become soiled, discard them and get fresh ones if you can.

DELIVERING THE BABY

1 *Tell the mother to lie in whatever position is the most comfortable, with her knees bent. Support her shoulders with pillows and cushions. When the baby's head first appears, put a clean towel or cloth under the mother's buttocks and a clean towel or sheet on the bed between her legs.*

How you can help a mother during labour

• Give the mother occasional small drinks of milk or water, but nothing to eat. The body's digestive system shuts down during labour, so food will not be digested anyway.

• As the contractions become more frequent or if the waters break, tell her to lie on the bed (or other prepared surface) in the position most comfortable for her.

• If the pains are bad, it may help if she shifts about, or breathes deeply with each contraction, and does not hold her breath.

• If she complains of tingling fingers or a trembling sensation when she does this, she is taking in too much oxygen. Cup your hands loosely over her mouth and nose during the contraction so that she re-breathes some of her own air. The tingling sensation should stop.

• During this first stage, encourage her to relax as far as possible between and during the contractions, and not to bear down.

As the second stage of labour begins, the mother will feel an unmistakable urge to bear down. By this time the contractions may be coming every two or three minutes, and the birth is imminent – though it may still take up to an hour to complete.

• Encourage her to hold her breath and bear down hard with each contraction, and to relax between contractions in order to conserve her energy.

• Tell her to grip her thighs behind her knees, and pull her legs at the same time as she is bearing down.

Delivering the baby

Your first sight of the baby will usually be the top of its head, and it will usually become visible at the height of a contraction.

Between contractions the head may slip back

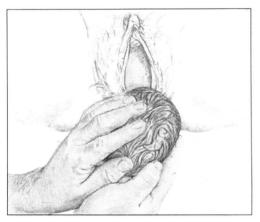

2 *When the baby's head is fully out, support it with clean, cupped hands. If a caul, or membrane, covers the baby's face, remove it gently but quickly.*

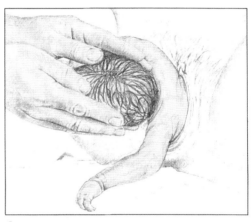

3 *As the shoulders emerge, support them gently but do not pull. One shoulder appears first. The second will follow easily if you gently raise the baby's head. Do not pull it.*

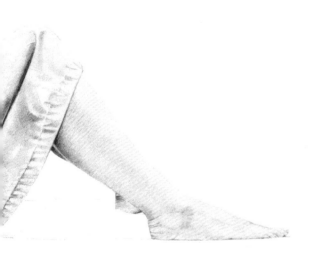

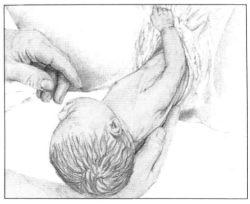

4 *The rest of the baby will be born without difficulty. Support the body with one hand. When it is fully born, wipe away any mucus or blood from the mouth with a clean cloth.*

out of sight at first. This is normal.

Tell the mother to stop bearing down, and to pant in quick breaths to prevent the baby being thrust out too forcefully.

Once the shoulders are out, the rest of the baby will be born without difficulty.

After the birth

When you are sure the baby is breathing, raise it to the mother's thighs or stomach. Encourage her to breast-feed her baby if she feels like doing so.

Some 5 to 15 minutes after the birth has occurred, the uterus will contract again to expel the placenta.

• When these contractions start, place a bowl between the mother's legs. It will take between 5

and 20 minutes for the placenta to be pushed out.

• Do not pull the umbilical cord to speed delivery of the placenta – it will deliver itself.

• When the placenta is fully out, put it aside in the bowl, to show the doctor or midwife later.

• Do not cut the cord – the midwife or doctor will do this later.

• Wash the mother, fix a sanitary pad or an improvised pad in place and give her fresh clothes if possible.

• Tidy up the room. If the mother wants something to eat or drink, she can now have it.

• If the mother is asleep, lay the baby in a cot on its side (to drain any remaining mucus from the lungs) and with the head low (to ensure a good flow of blood to the brain).

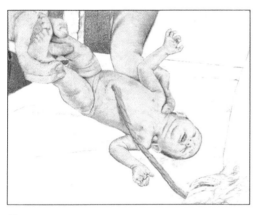

5 *If the baby does not breathe immediately, hold it with the head lower than the body to drain any mucus. Do not slap the baby. If necessary, blow hard on its chest.*

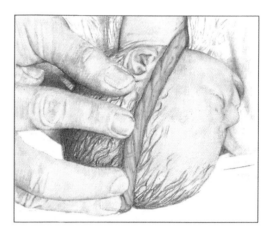

CORD AROUND THE NECK
If the baby appears with the cord loosely around the neck, just hook a finger around the cord and ease it gently over the baby's head. Do not pull the baby or the cord.

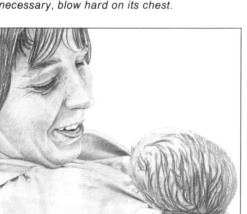

6 *Wrap the baby warmly. It will lose heat rapidly if left uncovered, particularly from the top of the head. Give the baby to the mother and wrap her warmly in blankets. Wait for the placenta to appear; do not pull on the cord to speed delivery, as it will normally deliver itself. Do not cut the cord. If the placenta does not appear, get medical help.*

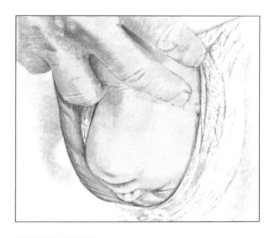

BREECH BIRTH
If the baby's bottom appears first, do not worry. Support it as it emerges, but do not pull. When the shoulders are out, ease the body up so that the mouth is clear to breathe.

First aid and medical emergencies

Unusual deliveries

Most babies emerge head first and face down.

• In a small number of cases, the baby may appear with the umbilical cord loosely around its neck. Hook a finger round the cord and ease it gently over the baby's head.

• In a very small number of cases, the baby may appear bottom first (breech birth). Support but do not pull the baby as it emerges. When the shoulders are out, hold the baby under them and ease the body up so that the mouth is clear to breathe.

If the baby does not breathe

A baby usually begins to breathe within a few seconds of birth.

• If it does not, hold it with the head down and blow hard on its chest. If it still does not breathe, open its mouth and clear out any mucus with your little finger. Clear the nose with a cloth, and lay the baby on one side with the head slightly lower than the body.

• Flick the bottom of the baby's feet sharply with your index finger to stimulate it into breathing. The child should breathe after a few taps. Do not smack the baby's bottom.

• If the baby fails to respond, give the kiss of life (see page 50), using very gentle puffs.

If the placenta fails to appear

Should the placenta not be expelled, or if it looks as though only part of the placenta has been expelled, get medical help as soon as possible.

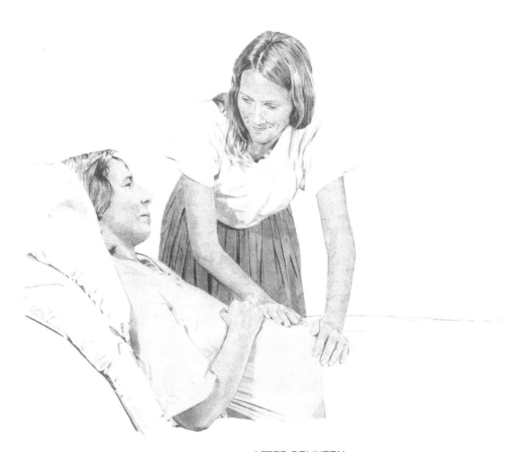

AFTER DELIVERY
Between 5 and 15 minutes after the baby has been born, the uterus will contract to deliver the placenta. When the contractions begin, put a bowl between the mother's legs. Delivery will take between 5 and 20 minutes. Do not pull on the cord. Slight bleeding is normal. If it is more profuse, call for medical help. Gently massage the mother's abdomen: this should stop the bleeding, and help the uterus to contract and harden. Do not cut the cord: the doctor or midwife will do this later. Put the placenta aside to show them.

Childhood illnesses

If you are worried that your child may be dangerously ill, ask yourself the following five questions first of all. If the answer to any of them is 'yes', contact a doctor or go to the Accident and Emergency Department of a hospital without delay.

1 Is the child not fully conscious or unnaturally drowsy?
2 Has the child's colour become *and stayed* very pale?
3 Is there blueness around the face or lips?
4 Does the child have serious difficulty in breathing?
5 Is there a rash that looks like bleeding under the skin, and which does not go pale when you press firmly?

If other symptoms are more prominent, their causes may, or may not, be dangerous. Use the charts on the following six pages to discover the best course of action. Begin by choosing the most appropriate major symptom, which is listed in capital letters at the head of each chart. Then start at the additional symptom in the red box and follow the arrows, answering each question either 'yes' or 'no', to find the likely cause of the symptoms. Where paracetamol is recommended, follow the directions on the packet.

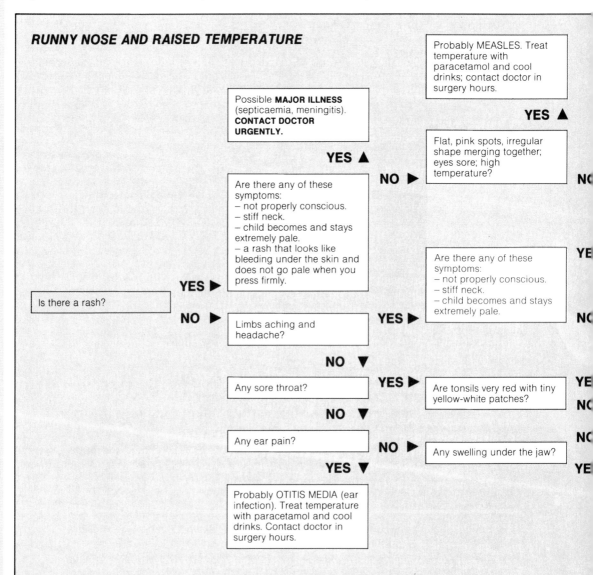

RUNNY NOSE AND RAISED TEMPERATURE

Probably MEASLES. Treat temperature with paracetamol and cool drinks; contact doctor in surgery hours.

YES ▲

Possible **MAJOR ILLNESS** (septicaemia, meningitis). **CONTACT DOCTOR URGENTLY.**

YES ▲

NO ►

Flat, pink spots, irregular shape merging together; eyes sore; high temperature?

NO

Are there any of these symptoms:
– not properly conscious.
– stiff neck.
– child becomes and stays extremely pale.
– a rash that looks like bleeding under the skin and does not go pale when you press firmly.

YES ►

Is there a rash?

NO ►

Limbs aching and headache?

YES ►

Are there any of these symptoms:
– not properly conscious.
– stiff neck.
– child becomes and stays extremely pale.

YE

NO

NO ▼

Any sore throat?

YES ►

Are tonsils very red with tiny yellow-white patches?

YE

NO

NO ▼

Any ear pain?

NO ►

Any swelling under the jaw?

NO

YE

YES ▼

Probably OTITIS MEDIA (ear infection). Treat temperature with paracetamol and cool drinks. Contact doctor in surgery hours.

DIARRHOEA

Are there any of the following symptoms: listlessness, sunken eyes, very dry mouth, not properly conscious?

YES ▶ Possible **MAJOR ILLNESS** (gastroenteritis with dehydration, meningitis, septicaemia). **CONTACT DOCTOR URGENTLY.**

NO ▶ Is there sore throat, ear pain or aching limbs and headache?

NO ▶ Probably GASTROENTERITIS without dehydration. Give plenty to drink – fruit juice, squash, clear soup, water, but not milk. Contact doctor if no improvement in 6–8 hours, or immediately if signs of dehydration appear (see first question).

YES ▶ Could be TONSILLITIS, EAR INFECTION or FLU. Treat temperature with paracetamol and cool drinks. Contact doctor in surgery hours.

Probably RUBELLA (GERMAN MEASLES). Treat as for measles and keep patient away from women in early pregnancy.

YES ▲

Tiny pink spots starting on face; tiny lumps behind ears; not very ill?

NO ▶ Raised blisters appearing in crops. High temperature?

NO ▶ Rash on face *only*?

YES ▼

Probably IMPETIGO. Make appointment with doctor for same or next day. Avoid contagion by reserving a flannel, towel etc for affected child.

YES ▼

Probably CHICKENPOX. Treat as for measles. Use calamine on skin.

Probable **MAJOR ILLNESS** (meningitis, septicaemia). **CONTACT DOCTOR URGENTLY.**

Possibly FLU. Give paracetamol and cool drinks Call doctor in surgery hours.

Probably TONSILLITIS. Treat temperature with paracetamol and cool drinks, and call doctor.

Probably COMMON.COLD. Treat temperature with para-cetamol and cool drinks.

Probably MUMPS. Contact doctor in surgery hours; treat temperature with para-cetamol and cool drinks.

JERKY MOVEMENTS OF LIMBS

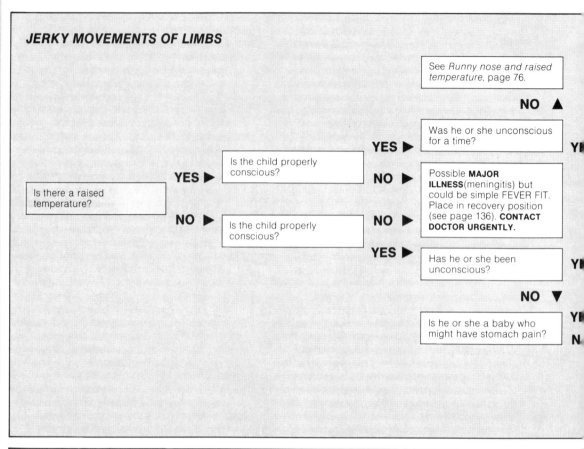

See *Runny nose and raised temperature*, page 76.

NO ▲

Was he or she unconscious for a time?

YES ▶ | Y

Is there a raised temperature?

YES ▶ Is the child properly conscious?

NO ▶ Is the child properly conscious?

NO ▶

Possible **MAJOR ILLNESS**(meningitis) but could be simple FEVER FIT. Place in recovery position (see page 136). **CONTACT DOCTOR URGENTLY.**

YES ▶ Has he or she been unconscious?

NO ▼

Is he or she a baby who might have stomach pain?

ABNORMAL BREATHING

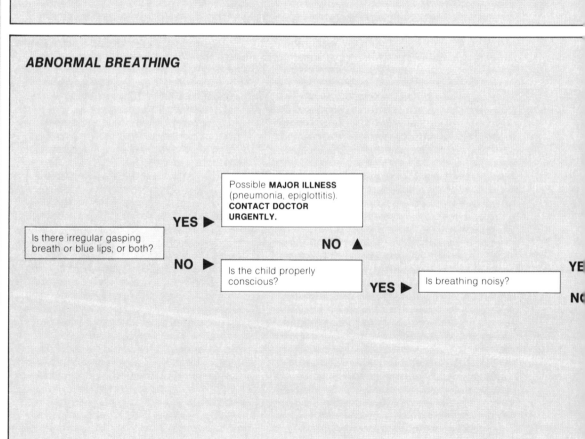

Possible **MAJOR ILLNESS** (pneumonia, epiglottitis). **CONTACT DOCTOR URGENTLY.**

NO ▲

Is there irregular gasping breath or blue lips, or both?

YES ▶

NO ▶ Is the child properly conscious?

YES ▶ Is breathing noisy?

▶ Probably FEVER FIT. Remove clothes; sponge body down with lukewarm water; give paracetamol. If this is the child's first attack, **CONTACT DOCTOR URGENTLY**. But if the child has had attacks before, and the symptoms are unchanged, contact doctor in surgery hours.

▶ Possibly CONVULSIONS. If this is the child's first attack, **CONTACT DOCTOR URGENTLY**. But if the child has had attacks before, and the symptoms are unchanged, contact doctor in surgery hours.

▶ Is there diarrhoea or vomiting?

YES ▶

NO ▶

▶ Probably not serious; wait and see.

Probably GASTROENTERITIS. Is there listlessness, sunken eyes, very dry mouth?

YES ▶ Possible **MAJOR ILLNESS** (dehydration). **CONTACT DOCTOR URGENTLY**.

NO ▶ Give plenty to drink (not milk). Contact doctor if no improvement in 6–8 hours.

Probably COLIC. Give usual medicine; try rocking or cuddling. If very upset discuss with doctor or health visitor at next convenient surgery.

Probably ASTHMA. Use your regular asthma medicine and contact doctor without delay unless the wheezing is mild only.

YES ▲

Musical note to breathing with rapid breathing and/or cough? Has the child had this before?

NO ▶ Probably BRONCHITIS. Contact doctor during day unless you are very worried; then you should not delay.

NO ▲

▶ Hoarse sound with ringing or 'cow-like' cough?

YES ▶ Does the child look very ill?

YES ▶ Could be **MAJOR ILLNESS** (epiglottitis). **CONTACT DOCTOR URGENTLY**.

NO ▶ Probably CROUP. Nurse in steamy room and contact doctor if no better in 2 hours.

▶ Very rapid breathing with high temperature and/or chest pain?

YES ▶ Probably **MAJOR ILLNESS** (pneumonia). **CONTACT DOCTOR URGENTLY**.

NO ▶ Severe paroxysms of coughing, which may cause vomiting or going blue in the face, indicate WHOOPING COUGH. See doctor in surgery hours.

STOMACH PAIN

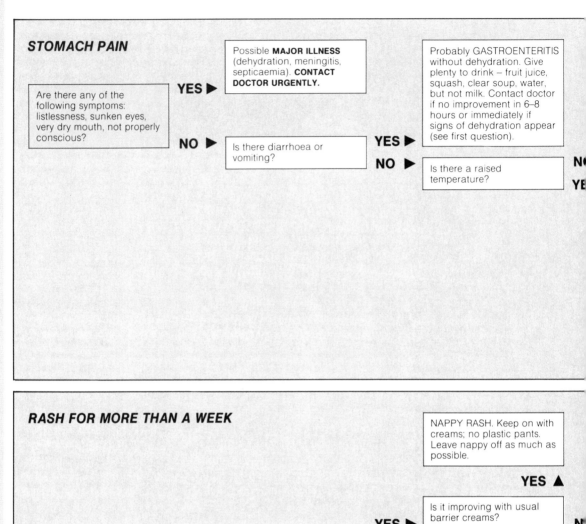

Are there any of the following symptoms: listlessness, sunken eyes, very dry mouth, not properly conscious?

YES ▶ Possible **MAJOR ILLNESS** (dehydration, meningitis, septicaemia). **CONTACT DOCTOR URGENTLY.**

NO ▶ Is there diarrhoea or vomiting?

YES ▶ Probably GASTROENTERITIS without dehydration. Give plenty to drink – fruit juice, squash, clear soup, water, but not milk. Contact doctor if no improvement in 6–8 hours or immediately if signs of dehydration appear (see first question).

NO ▶ Is there a raised temperature?

N
YE

RASH FOR MORE THAN A WEEK

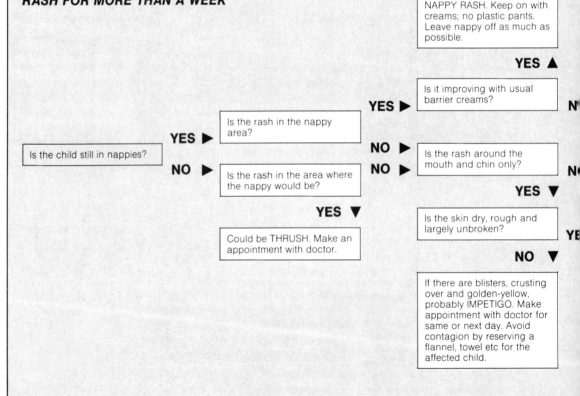

Is the child still in nappies?

YES ▶ Is the rash in the nappy area?

NO ▶ Is the rash in the area where the nappy would be?

YES ▶ Is it improving with usual barrier creams?

YES ▲ NAPPY RASH. Keep on with creams; no plastic pants. Leave nappy off as much as possible.

N

NO ▶ Is the rash around the mouth and chin only?

N

YES ▼ Is the skin dry, rough and largely unbroken?

YE

NO ▼ If there are blisters, crusting over and golden-yellow, probably IMPETIGO. Make appointment with doctor for same or next day. Avoid contagion by reserving a flannel, towel etc for the affected child.

YES ▼ Could be THRUSH. Make an appointment with doctor.

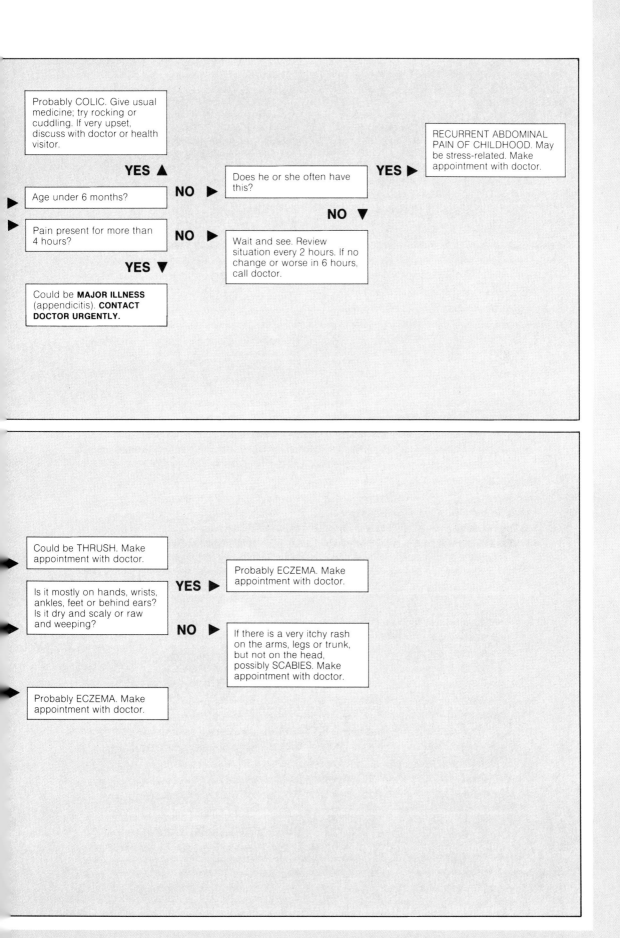

Probably COLIC. Give usual medicine; try rocking or cuddling. If very upset, discuss with doctor or health visitor.

YES ▲

Age under 6 months?

NO ▶

Does he or she often have this?

YES ▶

RECURRENT ABDOMINAL PAIN OF CHILDHOOD. May be stress-related. Make appointment with doctor.

NO ▼

Pain present for more than 4 hours?

NO ▶

Wait and see. Review situation every 2 hours. If no change or worse in 6 hours, call doctor.

YES ▼

Could be **MAJOR ILLNESS** (appendicitis). **CONTACT DOCTOR URGENTLY.**

Could be THRUSH. Make appointment with doctor.

Is it mostly on hands, wrists, ankles, feet or behind ears? Is it dry and scaly or raw and weeping?

YES ▶

Probably ECZEMA. Make appointment with doctor.

NO ▶

If there is a very itchy rash on the arms, legs or trunk, but not on the head, possibly SCABIES. Make appointment with doctor.

Probably ECZEMA. Make appointment with doctor.

Choking

A piece of food or some other object stuck in the airway will cause choking. In severe cases the victim cannot breathe at all, and if left untreated will die within minutes. It is vital, therefore, to act promptly.

Suspect choking if a person who is unconscious and not breathing is found anywhere near an eating area. However, choking can happen away from eating areas when the victim has been eating sweets, chewing gum or peanuts. Peanuts are a common cause of choking in young children, and should not be given to them.

Children can also choke on toys which they put in their mouths, and adults can choke on dislodged false teeth.

When choking occurs, the casualty may have a fit of coughing, his face turns blue and the veins on the head and neck are swollen.

He will instinctively make violent efforts to breathe, but the harder he tries to breathe in, the more firmly lodged the obstruction will become. Instant action is vital.

Treating a conscious casualty
• First, remove food or loose false teeth from the mouth and encourage the casualty to cough. It may be enough to dislodge the obstruction.
• If this fails, help the casualty to bend over with his or her head lower than the chest. He or she can be either sitting or standing.
• Slap him between the shoulder blades firmly with the heel of the hand up to five times. Each slap should be strong enough to induce an involuntary cough.
• When the casualty begins to breathe again, get him to sit quietly and take sips of water until he is fully recovered.

Small children and babies
• If the casualty is a child under about seven, encourage him to cough. If this fails to dislodge

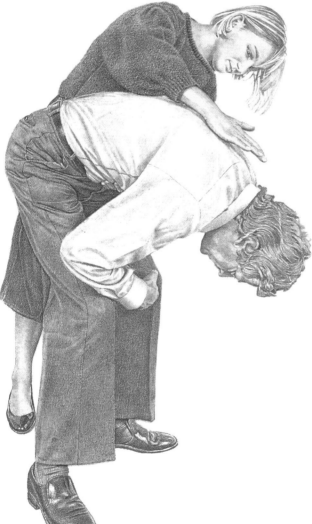

BACK-SLAPS FOR AN ADULT
Bend the casualty over with his head lower than his chest so that gravity will help the obstruction to become dislodged. This can be done with the casualty either standing or sitting. Slap him between the shoulder blades forcefully up to five times, using the heel of the hand.

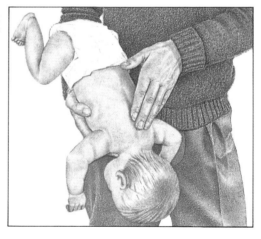

BACK-SLAPS FOR A BABY
Lay the baby along your forearm with his head downwards, and with the chest and head supported by your hand. Give up to five slaps between the shoulder blades with your fingers, using much less force than for an adult.

the obstruction, lay him over your knees with his head down.

• Support the chest with one hand while you slap him smartly between the shoulder blades with the heel of the other hand. Do this up to five times.

• Each of your slaps should be strong enough on its own to dislodge the obstruction.

• If a baby is choking, lay him along your forearm with his head downwards. Support the head and chest with your hand.

• Slap him smartly between the shoulder blades up to five times with the fingers of your other

hand, using much less force than for an adult.

• Be extremely careful when removing anything from a baby's mouth. Put your finger into his mouth only if you can actually see the object. Take care not to push it farther down the throat, making the condition worse.

Abdominal thrusts

If the casualty still cannot breathe, administer abdominal thrusts. This is a dangerous technique, which can damage the liver and other internal organs. But it may dislodge the obstruction and restore the casualty's breathing, even

ABDOMINAL THRUST ON A CONSCIOUS ADULT

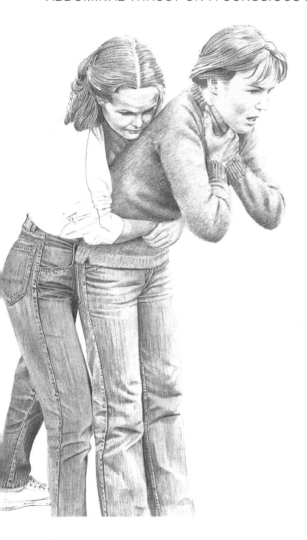

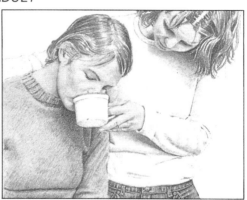

2 *When the throat is clear, reassure the casualty. Rest her in a comfortable position and give her frequent sips of water. Adults should sip half a cup of water over ten minutes.*

1 *Stand behind the casualty. Put your arms around her waist, clenching the fist of one hand. Place the thumb knuckle against the stomach (above the navel and below the rib cage). Hold the fist with your other hand and give three or four quick, strong pulls diagonally upwards and towards you.*

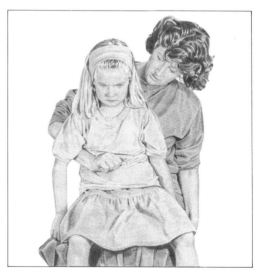

ABDOMINAL THRUST ON A CHILD
If you have been trained to apply it to children, sit the child on your lap and perform abdominal thrust as for an adult, but use only one hand. Do not use abdominal thrust on a baby.

if internal injuries have to be treated in hospital later.

• Stand or kneel behind the casualty. Clench your fist and put it, thumb inwards, over the stomach between the navel and the bottom of the breastbone.

• Hold your fist with the other hand and pull both hands towards you with a quick upward-and-inward thrust from the elbows. You are trying to pull the upper abdomen against the bottom of the lungs to drive out the remaining air and force out the obstruction.

• Repeat up to five times.

• Even if the thrusts are successful, the casualty may be winded by the force and unable to breathe for a few moments.

• Check in her mouth to see if the obstruction has come up. If so, remove it.

• Abdominal thrusts can be performed on a child seated on your lap, but use only one hand to administer the thrusts.

• A baby should be held or laid on his front, with head low and airway open and chest and head supported. Slap between his shoulder blades up to five times, using much less force than for an adult.

An unconscious casualty

If the casualty becomes unconscious, the muscles of the throat may relax sufficiently to

ABDOMINAL THRUST ON AN UNCONSCIOUS ADULT

1 *Turn the casualty face up. Kneel astride her hips, or alongside, and put the heel of one hand between the navel and the bottom of the breastbone. Cover one hand with the other, and give a quick downward-and-forward thrust with your arms straight. Repeat up to five times.*

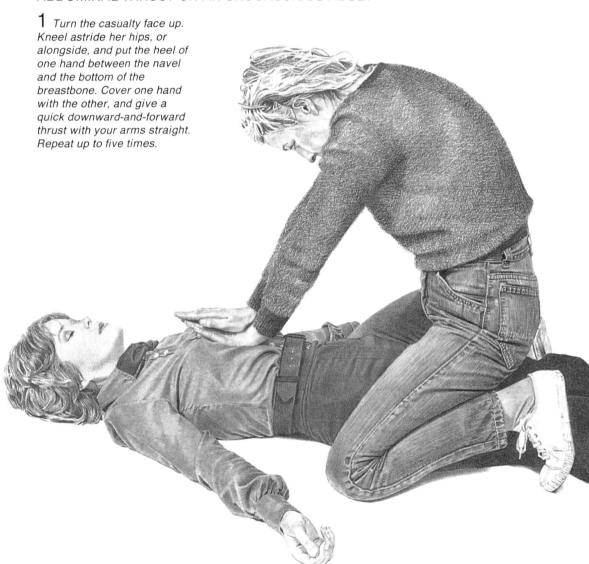

allow air to get past the obstruction. So begin mouth-to-mouth respiration to force air into the lungs (see page 50).

• If a third person is present, tell him to telephone 999 and ask for an ambulance. If you are on your own, do not stop mouth-to-mouth respiration until normal breathing resumes.

• If, however, the lungs do not inflate with the first two breaths, roll the casualty onto the side nearest you, with the chest against your thigh and the head well back. Give up to four hard slaps on the back.

• Look in the mouth to see if the obstruction has become dislodged. If it has, hook it out with a finger.

• If not, turn the casualty onto her back and tilt the head well back. Straddle the casualty's thighs, or kneel alongside. Put the heel of one hand between the navel and the bottom of the breastbone. Cover your hand with the other hand, and give a quick downward-and-forward thrust with your arms straight. Repeat the thrust up to five times.

• Check the mouth to see if the obstruction has been dislodged. If it has, hook it out with a finger.

• If not, resume mouth-to-mouth respiration. If the lungs again do not expand after the first two breaths, repeat the sequence of back-slaps, thrusts and mouth-to-mouth respiration.

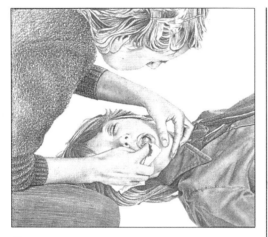

2 With your finger, clear the casualty's mouth of any object that has been expelled by the abdominal thrusts. Once her breathing has returned to normal, put the casualty into the recovery position (see page 136).

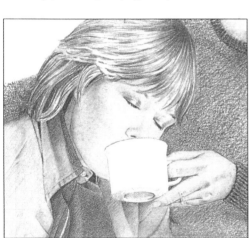

3 Telephone 999 and ask for an ambulance. If the casualty becomes fully conscious before the ambulance arrives, get her to sit up, supporting her if necessary, and give her some water to sip.

TWO METHODS OF SELF-HELP

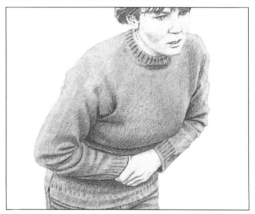

1 Someone choking can perform abdominal thrusts on herself. Clench a fist and place it, thumb side against the stomach, slightly above the navel. With the other hand, jerk it firmly inwards and upwards several times.

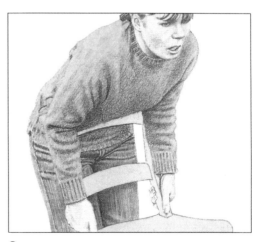

2 Alternatively, lean over the back of a chair, supporting yourself by holding on to the sides with your hands. With the top sticking into you just above the navel, pull yourself downwards and forwards onto it three or four times.

Concussion

A blow to the head or a heavy fall onto the feet can shake and disturb the brain, causing concussion. There is usually a brief period of unconsciousness, but it may be so short that it goes unnoticed.

If the casualty is unconscious for any length of time, his breathing may be shallow, his face pale and his skin cold and moist.

After the spell of unconsciousness – however brief – the casualty may suffer from nausea and vomiting and may remember nothing about the incident.

Anyone suffering these symptoms should see a doctor for examination in case a more serious condition called compression should develop.

While a person is unconscious, treat as described on page 136.

If a person feels very weak after a blow to the head, treat for shock (see page 120).

Recognising and treating compression

Any pressure on the brain – either from blood or fluid, or from a fracture of the skull – can cause the more serious condition of compression, which may develop up to 48 hours after the casualty appears to have recovered from concussion.

• The casualty's alertness and level of consciousness fall.
• There may be weakness or paralysis of one side of the body.
• Breathing may become noisy.
• The face may be flushed, and the casualty's temperature high.
• The pulse may be slow.
• The pupils of the eyes (the dark parts) may be unequal in size.

Usually most of these symptoms occur, but the absence of any of them does not mean that compression is not present.

Telephone 999 and ask for an ambulance. If the casualty is unconscious, treat as described on page 136.

Cramp

The sudden, involuntary spasm of muscles known as cramp causes acute pain, but it is usually dangerous only if a swimmer is affected (see *If you get into difficulties while swimming*, page 234). Cramp may be caused by chilling during or after exercise such as swimming, by poor muscular coordination during exercise, or by loss of salt through severe sweating, vomiting or diarrhoea. It can also occur during sleep for no apparent reason.

The spasm is generally relieved by stretching the affected muscles. This can be done by the sufferer, but it is often easier if another person can help gently to force the limb straight.

Cramp in the hand

• Straighten your fingers, using gentle force if necessary.
• Spread your fingers and press down on the outstretched tips.
• Massage the affected muscles as you stretch them.

Cramp in the calf

• Straighten your leg and stand up.
• Press down on your heel and toes alternately. Lean forward slightly to stretch the calf muscles.
• Massage the muscles as you stretch them.

Cramp in the foot

• Stand on the ball of the foot so that your toes are forced up. Alternatively, sit down and pull

HELPING A CRAMP VICTIM
To relieve cramp in the calf, the foot or the thigh, lay the victim down, straighten the knee and toes, and press the foot firmly up towards the shin. Massage the affected muscles.

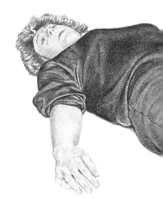

your toes up towards the shin with your hand.
• Massage the muscles as you stretch them.

Cramp in the thigh

• Sit on the floor and straighten the leg. Then bear down at the knee to stretch the thigh muscles. If there is someone to help, get him to raise your leg by the heel and press down on the knee with the other hand.
• Massage the muscles.

If cramp persists

Cramp caused by loss of salt from the body – through sweating, vomiting or diarrhoea – can persist for some time. It is often felt as a gripping pain in the stomach.

To treat it, drink plenty of slightly salted water. Use half a teaspoon of salt to a pint of water (about a teaspoon to 1 litre).

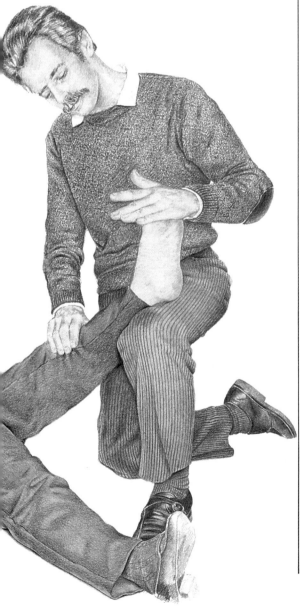

Crush injuries

Someone who has been trapped for more than a few minutes under a heavy weight, such as fallen masonry or a car, may suffer severe internal damage, even if there is little external sign of injury. Without treatment the damage can lead to shock, kidney failure and death.

The warning signs

• Redness, swelling, bruising or blistering of the trapped part.
• Numbness or tingling.
• Continued swelling and hardening of the injured tissue.
• Shock – symptoms can include pallid clammy skin, dizziness, fainting, blurred vision, nausea, vomiting, thirst, anxiety and restlessness.

What you should do

• If the casualty has been trapped for more than 10 minutes, do not try to release him.
• If the casualty has been trapped for less than 10 minutes, quickly release him, and treat for injuries and shock.
• If the casualty is unconscious, place him in the recovery position when released (see page 136).
• Get medical attention as quickly as possible. Make sure that the doctor or ambulance attendant is told that there may be crush injuries. Tell him how long the crushing lasted.
• Treat severe injuries as far as possible while the casualty is still trapped.

Minor crushing – what to do

• If fingers, hand or foot are crushed for a short time only, hold the injured part under cold running water.
• Show the injured part to a doctor in case it is fractured.

Crying baby

Normal babies generally cry only when they are hungry, angry, lonely, uncomfortable or in pain, and the crying will stop when you put right whatever is upsetting them.

It takes time for a new parent to learn what the different sorts of crying mean. The only way to find out is by discovering what stops it. There are some babies, however, who cry for no obvious reason.

What you should do
- Consult the chart and see if you can find a remedy.
- If you are feeling jumpy and nervous yourself, remember that this can affect the baby.
- Find some way to keep calm.
- Be sure to get enough rest. Perhaps you can persuade your partner to help out more than usual. Alternatively, get help from relatives,

ELEVEN REASONS WHY A BABY CRIES

Reason	Evidence
Hunger	Some hours since feed, or last feed not large enough.
Thirst	Hot weather. Baby feverish or sweating.
Passing urine	A sudden shriek.
Discomfort	Nappy rash, eczema, wet nappy, cold fingers and toes.
Colic	Restless, draws up legs, sudden cry, then relaxes. Passes a lot of wind.
Loneliness and boredom	Cries when he is alone, stops when you come in.
Habit	Usually cries at night. Stops when you come in.
Teething	May cause crying but less often than most people think.
Tiredness	Has missed a nap. A particular sort of moaning cry.
Personality	No other cause found.
Illness	Off feeds. Feverish. Signs of cold. Pulls at ear. Vomiting, diarrhoea. Pain is suggested if crying is severe, fails to stop when baby is picked up and comforted, or is accompanied by pale skin or drawing up of legs.

friends or neighbours. Your rest should come before housework or entertaining.

• If you feel desperate and unable to cope, seek the help of your health visitor or your local infant welfare clinic.

• If your worries are about housing, money or the state of your marriage, get advice from a social worker who can be contacted at your local council's social services department.

Remedy

Offer a feed.

Offer water or breast milk.

Change nappy.

Treat or remove discomfort.

Carry baby over shoulder. Rock in cradle. Take for a drive. Check hole in teat if bottle-fed. Consult doctor or health visitor.

Keep him with you. Prop him up so that he can see you or other members of the family.

Let him cry for a few minutes before going in; he may go to sleep again. Lift him out and hold him for a few minutes; perhaps sing a lullaby. You may decide to take him to bed with you, but this can start a habit that may be difficult to break.

Look for some other cause first. Consult a doctor if severe.

Try to get the baby to settle to sleep.

Consult doctor if worried.

See pages 76–81.

Cuts

Minor cuts do not need medical help unless infection has set in or the wound was caused by a dirty or rusty object.

The amount of blood lost and the extent of the injury usually show whether the wound is serious, but puncture or stab wounds are deceptive because the surface damage may be small. Get medical help for a puncture wound after giving first aid (see *Stab wounds*, page 133).

When treating a minor cut, first stop the bleeding by pressing on the wound with a piece of clean cloth. Then clean the skin around it with gauze or cotton swabs and lukewarm water with soap or a mild antiseptic. Wipe outwards and away from the cut and make sure the water you are using does not run into it. Use each swab once and then change to a fresh one.

If the bleeding is severe, see page 60.

HOW TO TREAT A CUT

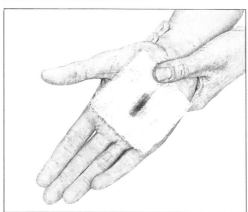

1 *Press a clean piece of cloth on the cut, or around the edges if a foreign body is in it. When bleeding stops, take the pad away and remove any foreign bodies that come out easily.*

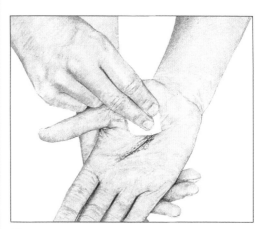

2 *Gently wipe the wound outwards with a swab soaked in warm, soapy water. Renew the swabs frequently. Dry around the wound with a new swab. Apply a plaster or bandage.*

Diabetic coma

A diabetic who appears to be drunk may be suffering from low blood sugar, a condition known as hypoglycaemia. It is brought on by taking too much insulin or eating too little food. It can also occur after exercise has burnt up the sugar in the blood.

Low blood sugar affects the brain and leads to coma. In some very rare cases, death could possibly follow in as little as 20 minutes after the onset of coma.

The condition can be distinguished from drunkenness by the person's breath, which will have no smell of alcohol.

Low blood sugar can lead to rapid deterioration in the diabetic, with the following symptoms:
• Pale appearance, with sweating, rapid pulse, shallow breathing and possibly trembling.
• Confused state, sometimes resembling drunkenness.
• Faintness, leading to unconsciousness in 15 to 20 minutes.

What you can do
If a diabetic collapse comes on quickly, you can assume that the patient needs sugar. If he is conscious, give him three or four teaspoons of sugar, some cake or biscuits, honey, jam, chocolate, or a sweet soft drink.
• If the patient is unconscious, put him in the recovery position (see page 136), then telephone 999 and ask for an ambulance.

The opposite condition of too much sugar in the blood (hyperglycaemia) can also eventually lead to coma, but it comes on much more slowly, and the diabetic will usually become aware of it and treat himself by taking insulin. If he does not take insulin, the symptoms will be:
• Flushed appearance with dry skin.
• Deep, sighing breathing, with the breath smelling of acetone (pear drops).
• Eventually unconsciousness.

If the person becomes unconscious, put him in the recovery position (see page 136) and get immediate medical attention.

What the patient can do
A person who is subject to hypoglycaemic attacks should carry a card or wear a bracelet giving his condition and emergency instructions. This can avoid the danger of being mistaken for being drunk when, in fact, all he really needs is some sugar.

A diabetic on insulin should avoid driving or using dangerous machinery unless he has had some food in the previous two hours. Consequently, regular mealtimes are important.

Dislocated joints

A bone that is wrenched out of place at a joint is said to be dislocated. The injury is usually accompanied by torn ligaments (a sprain) and sometimes by a fracture.

The symptoms may include severe pain, swelling and bruising, deformity of the joint and difficulty in moving the joint. Never try to push a dislocated bone back into place, but treat it as though it were broken.

In a case of dislocation, always assume there might be a fracture as well – the symptoms are similar (see page 98).

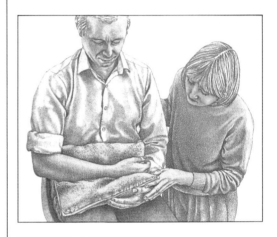

TREATING A DISLOCATION
Put the casualty into the most comfortable position possible, and support the dislocated joint with pillows or a rolled blanket. Telephone 999 and ask for an ambulance. If the dislocation is in the arm, you may be able to support it with an arm sling (see page 121).

Drowning

Death by drowning happens because, as the victim struggles for breath, water enters the airway. The water causes a spasm of the epiglottis, a cartilage flap at the back of the tongue, and this spasm blocks the air supply. Quick action can still save a victim's life.

Each year in Britain there are nearly 1000 deaths from drowning. Two-thirds occur in fresh water, because it is impossible to provide the same rescue facilities on rivers, lakes and canals as are available on holiday beaches. Most of the victims are able to swim, and most drown within 10yds (9m) of land.

Assume that anyone you see in the water fully clothed is a potential victim, and be ready to help. A swimmer who develops cramp or becomes exhausted is less easy to recognise. If he is having breathing problems, he may be unable to draw attention by shouting, and if he raises an arm to wave he may sink.

Warning signs

• As he gets more tired, the victim's body tends to sink until it is vertical and only his head shows above the water.
• The victim's strokes become erratic and his movement through the water appears jerky or simply stops.
• The victim's face – particularly the lips and ears – become congested and may turn a bluish-purple colour.

Rescuing a drowning person

For methods of getting a drowning person out of the water in a variety of different situations, see pages 231 and 240.

REVIVING A DROWNING PERSON

1 *If the drowning person has stopped breathing, start mouth-to-mouth respiration as quickly as possible (see page 50). Begin while still in the water if necessary – as soon as you can stand up or sooner if you are a strong swimmer. Remove any debris from the mouth with your index finger, tilt the head back and begin breathing into the mouth. Either press your cheek against the victim's nose to stop air escaping, or pinch the nose between finger and thumb. Move towards land between breaths. Once out of the water, continue artificial respiration, or begin if it is not already under way.*

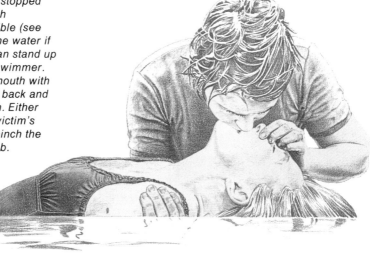

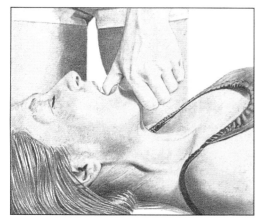

2 *Victims of drowning sometimes swallow water, which is brought up with food during artificial respiration. Turn the head to one side and regularly clear the mouth of any debris.*

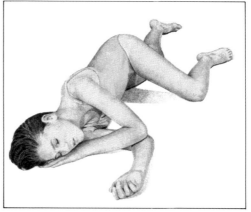

3 *Once breathing has re-started, turn the victim into the recovery position (see page 136). Cover her and treat any injuries. Get medical help as soon as possible.*

Drug overdose

Anyone who takes an overdose of a drug needs immediate medical attention. This applies to an overdose of a prescribed medicine as much as an addictive drug such as heroin.

A drug overdose is likely to cause a stronger than normal reaction in a person who suffers from asthma, kidney disease or hypersensitivity to certain medicines.

While waiting for medical help to arrive, gather any information you can about the drug by talking to the casualty, collecting pill bottles or taking samples of vomit.

Generally, do not try to induce vomiting. Inducing vomiting is worth doing only if you know that the overdose has been caused by barbiturates or tranquillisers. For details of how to treat overdoses of either of these drugs, see *Barbiturates*, page 358.

Do not try to keep the casualty awake by giving him black coffee or walking him about. Physical activity will only speed up the absorption of the drug into the body.

How to recognise an overdose

Symptoms depend on the size of the overdose and the type of drug, but they can include any of the following:
- Vomiting.
- Difficulty in breathing.
- Unconsciousness.
- Sweating.
- Hallucinations.
- Dilation or contraction of the pupils of the eyes (the dark parts).

What you should do

- Ask the casualty what has happened. Obtain any information about the drug as soon as possible, because the casualty may become unconscious at any time.
- If the casualty is unconscious, put him in the recovery position (see page 136).
- Telephone 999 and ask for an ambulance.
- Collect a sample of vomit and any bottle, pill container, hypodermic syringe or glue container that is near the casualty. Send them to hospital with him as evidence to assist treatment.

Alcohol poisoning

If a person collapses unconscious after drinking a large amount of alcohol, put him in the recovery position so that he does not choke on his vomit (see page 136).

Then telephone 999 and ask for an ambulance (see also *Spotting and coping with a drink problem*, page 350).

Ear injuries

Damage to the middle or inner ear can be caused by injuries to the head, loud noise, explosions, or probing in the ear – to remove a foreign body, for example.

The most serious injury to the ear itself is a perforated eardrum, but bleeding from the ear or discharge of watery, straw-coloured fluid can be a sign of a fractured skull (see page 102).

Symptoms of ear injury

- Severe earache.
- Dizziness and loss of balance.
- Deafness in one ear following an injury.
- Headache.
- Possible unconsciousness.
- Discharge of blood or watery fluid.

What you can do

- If the casualty is conscious, stop him from hitting the side of his head to try to restore hearing; this will only make the damage worse.
- Sit the casualty up with his head tilted over on the injured side so that blood or fluid can drain out.
- Cover the injured ear with a piece of clean cotton or gauze as protection. Bandage it lightly in place. Get medical attention.
- Do not attempt to plug the ear. This can cause a build-up of pressure in the middle ear.
- If the casualty is unconscious but breathing, place him in the recovery position with the injured ear downwards and a clean pad underneath it (see page 136). Get medical attention.
- If the casualty's breathing stops, begin artificial respiration (see page 50).

Foreign body in the ear

Children often push objects into their ears. This usually causes no more than temporary deafness, but if the object is pushed hard and deep into the ear the eardrum may be perforated.

The symptoms are variable:
- There may be no symptoms at all, just the knowledge that something is in the ear.
- Discharge from the ear.
- Pain or buzzing in the ear.
- Deafness on the affected side.

Do not attempt to remove a foreign body. If there are no symptoms, get medical attention in 24 hours. Go sooner if there are symptoms.

Insect in the ear

If an insect crawls or flies into a child's ear its buzzing can sound frighteningly loud.
- Calm and comfort the child.
- Stop him from putting a finger in the ear. If the insect has a sting, this may provoke an attack.
- Hold his head still with the ear angled towards the ground. The insect may crawl out.
- If, after a minute or two, it has not come out, gently flood the ear with tepid water.
- If all attempts fail, or if it stings while inside, get medical help.

Electric shock

Electricity can kill or produce a wide range of injuries, including severe burns and asphyxiation. The extent of the injuries it will cause depends on three main factors: the strength of the charge; how long the victim was exposed to it; and how well he was insulated – by wearing rubber-soled shoes, say, or standing on a dry wooden floor.

• Never touch the victim of an electrical accident until you are certain you are not risking a shock yourself. If the casualty is still touching the source of the electricity – such as an electric drill that has gone 'live' – cut off the power first. Switch off the appliance at the socket and pull out the plug. If the plug itself is causing the trouble, wrench it free by the flex or turn off the power at the main fuse box.

• If you cannot turn off the electricity, and the casualty is still in contact with it, move him away using a piece of wood or fabric, which do not conduct electricity. Use a broom handle to lever the casualty away, or loop a dry towel around an arm or leg and pull him free.

• Because water is an excellent conductor of electricity, use only dry wood or cloth, and preferably stand on insulating material such as a rubber mat or a folded newspaper.

High-voltage electricity

Electricity from high-voltage sources, such as power lines, overhead railway cables and some industrial equipment, can give a fatal shock up to 20yds (18m) away. Stay clear until you can get an expert to cut off the power. Railway stations and many pylons and substations display an emergency telephone number.

When lightning strikes

Another form of high-voltage electricity is lightning, which can do anything from merely stunning the victim to killing him (see *If you are caught in a lightning storm*, page 298).

HOW TO RESCUE A VICTIM OF ELECTRIC SHOCK

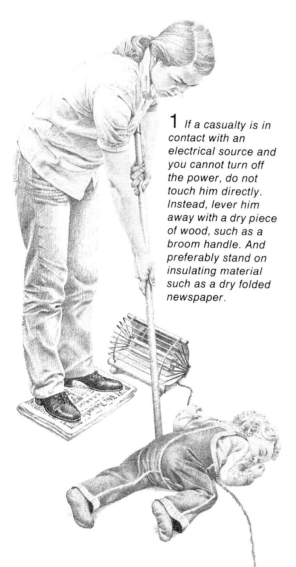

1 *If a casualty is in contact with an electrical source and you cannot turn off the power, do not touch him directly. Instead, lever him away with a dry piece of wood, such as a broom handle. And preferably stand on insulating material such as a dry folded newspaper.*

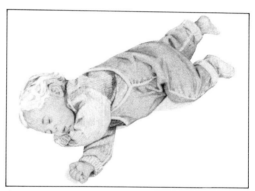

2 *If the casualty is unconscious, put him in the recovery position (see page 136). Dial 999 and ask for an ambulance. Cut off the power to the electrical source, but do not touch it.*

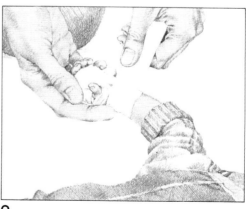

3 *Treat burns by cooling them with cold water. Then cover them with a dressing, such as the inside of a folded handkerchief, and secure it with a piece of clean cloth (see page 66).*

Epileptic fit

A major epileptic fit, also called *grand mal*, involves unconsciousness, convulsions and noisy breathing. Sufferers from epilepsy often carry an identifying card or bracelet which may reveal how long attacks normally last.

A series of fits, without the casualty regaining consciousness in between, is called *status epilepticus,* and is a serious condition which requires hospital treatment.

A minor epileptic fit, also called *petit mal*, usually involves only momentary inattention or confusion without loss of consciousness. Make sure that the sufferer is not in danger (from traffic, for example) and stay with him until he is once more quite alert.

The warning signs
• A sufferer from major epilepsy sometimes experiences a few seconds' warning of an attack. The warning may involve seeing flashing lights, or a sensation of noise, taste or smell.
• Loss of consciousness occurs.
• The limbs and neck stiffen for a few seconds; then the whole body is overcome by rhythmic and often violent twitching.
• The casualty may bite his tongue, froth at the mouth or urinate involuntarily.
• Finally the muscles will relax and the casualty may remain unconscious for some minutes.
• When consciousness returns, the casualty may be drowsy and confused for as much as an hour.

What you can do
• Do not try to restrain a victim of a major epileptic attack. Try only to stop him from hurting himself.
• If he is about to fall, catch him and lay him gently on the ground, or cushion his fall.
• Clear a space around him. Remove furniture and other objects that he may bump into.
• If possible, loosen clothing around the neck and place something soft under the head.
• Do not put anything in the mouth or try to force it open.
• When convulsions end, place the casualty in the recovery position (see page 136), and wait for him to regain consciousness. Do not leave him alone until he is fully recovered.
• Do not give him anything to drink until you are sure that he is quite alert.
• Call an ambulance only if the casualty has a series of fits without regaining consciousness in between, if he injures himself or if he takes longer than 15 minutes to regain consciousness.

Eye injuries

The most common injury to the eye is a small object, such as an eyelash or a piece of grit, lodged in it. Other injuries can be caused by corrosive chemicals or sharp objects, such as flying fragments of glass or metal.

Injury can also occur if contact lenses get displaced or stuck to the eyeball. If you have any difficulty with a contact lens, get medical help rather than risk hurting the eye.

Foreign body in the eye
If a person has something in his eye, tell him not to rub it. Turn the casualty's face up to the light. With your thumb and forefinger, push the eyelids away from the eyeball. Ask the casualty to look left, right, up and down while you look for the object.

REMOVING GRIT FROM THE EYE

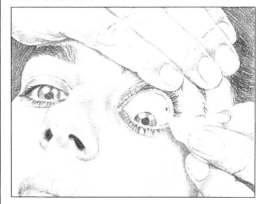

1 *Tilt the head back, and gently raise the eyelid with your finger (or draw down the bottom eyelid). Lift off the piece of grit or eyelash with the corner of a clean handkerchief.*

TREATING CHEMICAL BURNS

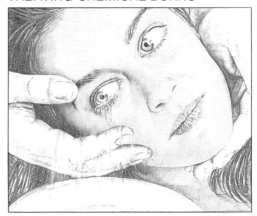

1 *Tilt the casualty's head, with the injured eye downwards. Flood the open eye with gently running water from a tap or jug for at least ten minutes. Or splash water onto it from a basin.*

Do not attempt to remove anything if it is on the pupil or iris (the black or coloured parts of the eye), or if it is sticking firmly to the eye. Leave the object and cover the eye with a clean, non-fluffy pad, such as the inside of a clean, folded handkerchief. Bandage it loosely in place and get medical help.

If you can see the object, try to wash it out. Tilt the casualty's head to the injured side, and gently run cold or lukewarm water over the eye from a tap or jug. Alternatively, get the casualty to blink his eyes underwater.

If no water is available, or flushing is not effective, try to lift the object off the eye with a moistened piece of clean gauze or the corner of a clean handkerchief.

If you are still unsuccessful, see a doctor.

Chemical burns to the eye

If chemicals – either liquid or solid – get into the eye, flood the eye with water immediately as they can cause serious damage.

You may need to force the eyelids open if they are shut tight in a spasm of pain.

Object impaled in the eye

Do not attempt to remove any object which is embedded in the eye, because you might cause irreparable damage. First, protect the eye, taking great care not to touch it or apply any pressure, by covering it with a paper or plastic cup. Then put a bandage over both eyes so that the casualty is not tempted to move them.

Telephone 999 and ask for an ambulance. Reassure the person while you wait for it.

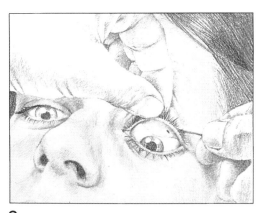

2 *If the grit is on the underside of the eyelid, press down the lid with a matchstick and pull up the lid against the matchstick with your finger and thumb.*

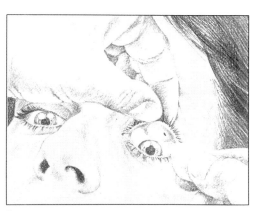

3 *Remove the grit with the corner of a clean handkerchief. Replace the lid by pulling down gently on the lashes. The same treatment can be used for the bottom lid.*

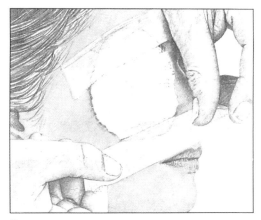

2 *When you have thoroughly flushed the chemical from the eye, dry the face and put a clean dressing lightly over the eye. Get the casualty to hospital as soon as possible.*

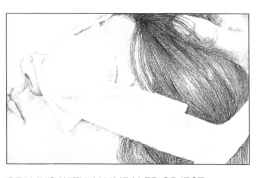

DEALING WITH AN IMPALED OBJECT
Do not try to remove any embedded or impaled object from the eye. Instead, cut a hole in a piece of clean cloth and put it over the eye. Place a paper or plastic cup over the cloth and hold it in place with a bandage. Cover the uninjured eye with the bandage as well. Call an ambulance.

Fainting

If the blood supply to the brain is suddenly and temporarily reduced, a person may faint. Fainting is usually the result of the victim being in a hot, stuffy atmosphere.

But an emotional stimulus, such as an unpleasant sight, a fright or bad news, can also cause fainting. So can a drop in blood sugar due to missed meals or dieting, or standing still for long periods of time.

Sometimes there may be a more serious cause such as illness or injury, in which case a doctor should be consulted.

Someone who is standing still for a long time can reduce the risk of fainting by rocking gently from the heels to the balls of the feet.

The warning signs
- A person who is about to faint becomes pale or greenish-white. He may yawn frequently, showing that he is lacking oxygen.
- The skin is cold and clammy.
- Beads of sweat appear on the face, neck and hands.

What you can do
If someone says he is about to faint, tell him to sit down. Loosen tight clothing at the neck and waist, and put his head down to his knees.

A person who actually faints should have the feet raised above the level of the head to increase the blood circulation to the brain.

Recovery from a faint is usually rapid and complete, but check for any injury that may have been received during a fall. If the fall resulted in a blow to the head that was hard enough to

cause a cut or wound, the casualty should see a doctor, because there is risk of a fractured skull or concussion (see page 86).

Do not give the casualty anything to eat or drink until full consciousness returns, and then only sips of cold water. Do not give the casualty any alcohol, such as brandy. It lowers the rate of the body's vital activities, and may make the condition worse.

If you are in any doubt about the casualty's condition, get medical advice.

TREATING SOMEONE WHO FAINTS
Lay an unconscious casualty on her back with her legs raised above the level of her head. Hold the legs up, or prop them on a chair or anything suitable. Loosen clothing at the neck, chest and waist, and ensure that the casualty gets plenty of fresh air. If she is indoors, open the windows; outside, protect her from the sun. She should recover after a few minutes, but tell her to stay seated for a few minutes more.

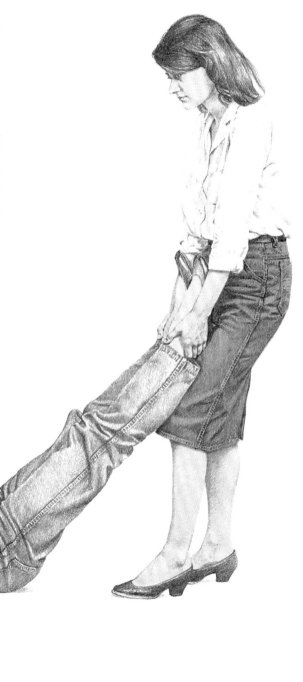

Flu

Epidemics of influenza (commonly called flu) occur during most winters. The illness is a virus infection, which spreads rapidly through an area for two or three weeks and then quickly subsides.

Flu leads to high temperature and aching muscles, and can be an emergency if it strikes a person with heart disease, chronic lung disease or diabetes, or someone over 65. The doctor should be called to a patient in any of these categories.

The warning signs
- Headache.
- Aching muscles and back.
- High temperature with the sensation of feeling cold.
- Sweating.
- General weakness.
- Coughing, and pain behind the breastbone which is made worse by coughing.
- Nasal catarrh and sneezing.

What you can do
- Put the patient to bed.
- Give extra fluids to replace losses caused by fever.
- Give painkillers in the doses recommended on the packet.
- To help ease coughing and chest pain, give hot lemon-and-honey drinks or a proprietary cough mixture.
- Do not allow the patient to return to work or school until the main symptoms are over – usually in about three days. It will increase the risk of bringing on pneumonia, and will spread the disease.

How long will it last?
The worst of the illness will be over in two or three days, but aching muscles, headache and fever may persist for a week.

General weakness may continue for a few weeks more, possibly accompanied by a period of depression.

Preventing an attack of flu
Each year a vaccine is produced against the viruses that are expected to cause flu in the following winter. Anyone over 65, and sufferers from heart disease, lung disease or diabetes, should be immunised in September or October. But if an epidemic is caused by a new strain of virus, immunisation may not be effective.

Food poisoning

Severe vomiting and diarrhoea, usually with pain in the abdomen, are the main symptoms of food poisoning (also called gastroenteritis).

Two main types of bacteria cause the ailment. Staphylococcal bacteria multiply in reheated or half-cooked food and produce severe vomiting from two to eight hours after the food is eaten.

Salmonella bacteria usually come from food handlers, flies or unhygienic cooking utensils. The bacteria multiply in the victim's bowel, and the symptoms begin with severe diarrhoea after 12 to 36 hours.

What you should do
- Give the patient sips of water. Do not give food or milk drinks. The stomach is trying to get rid of an irritant; do not irritate it any more. Let it rest.
- A medicine containing antidiarrhoeal and pain-killing drugs may be given to an adult.
- After the stomach has begun to settle for a few hours, give the patient dry biscuits, jelly, blancmange or clear soup. Avoid tea or coffee, or acid drinks such as lemon or orange; they may cause irritation, and vomiting could recur.
- Most attacks of food poisoning settle after two or three days, and the patient can be put back on a fuller, non-irritating diet.
- Call the doctor if there is abdominal pain, blood in the faeces, other unexpected symptoms, or if the symptoms are severe and last longer than three days.

How to avoid food poisoning
- Avoid any creamy foods, processed meat or fish which have been left too long at room temperature. The time depends on the air temperature, but in summer all such foods should be kept in a refrigerator.
- Avoid food which you suspect has been unhygienically prepared. This is especially important in hot climates.
- When heating up cold meat, make sure that it is thoroughly re-cooked.
- Discard any containers of food whose contents show signs of spoiling.

First aid and medical emergencies

Fractures

A fracture is a cracked or broken bone. It can be caused by direct force, as when a car hits a person on the thigh, or by indirect force, as when a person falls on an outstretched hand and breaks the collarbone at the top of the arm.

There are three main types of fracture. A closed fracture leaves the skin unbroken, although it may be heavily bruised. An open, or compound, fracture either has a bone protruding through the skin or a deep gash leading down to the bone. In either case germs may enter the wound, causing serious infection. A greenstick fracture, most common in children, involves a bone splitting as it bends.

The warning signs

• Often, the casualty will have heard or felt the bone break. There may be the feeling of broken bone ends grating together, which can sometimes be heard.
• The casualty may not be able to use the injured part of the body, and will feel pain when he does.
• The area around the break may be tender to the touch, swollen or bruised.
• A limb may be in an unnatural position or deformed when compared to the uninjured side.

What you should do

All doubtful cases of injured bones should be considered as fractures. The principles of treatment are the same in all cases.

TREATING AN OPEN FRACTURE OF THE LEG

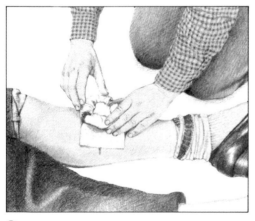

1 *If the ambulance is going to take more than half an hour, or if you have to carry the casualty, you must protect the wound and immobilise the leg. First gently remove clothing from the area of the fracture.*

2 *Cover the wound with a piece of clean non-fluffy cloth (not cotton wool). Then make a built-up dressing (see page 58) and put it around the protruding bone.*

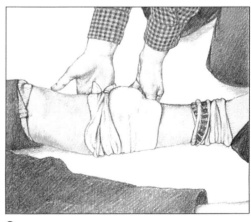

3 *Put a bandage around the leg, over the ring-pad. Try to get a helper to support the leg carefully as you do so. The pad will reduce pressure on the wound.*

Frostbite

- Do not move the casualty unless it is absolutely necessary.
- Telephone 999 and ask for an ambulance.
- Deal with any severe bleeding (see page 60), unconsciousness (see page 136) or difficulty in breathing (see page 50) before doing anything to the fracture.
- Put the casualty in the most comfortable position possible, and provide support for the injured limb with a rolled-up blanket or coat, or with cushions.
- Do not move the fractured part unnecessarily.
- To limit the dangers of shock, see page 120.
- If it is essential to move the casualty – and time allows – immobilise the injured limb by bandaging it to an uninjured part of the body.

Supporting a fractured leg

Tie a fractured leg to the other leg (see page 127), using scarves, neckties or any other piece of material, preferably something that is at least a few inches wide. This will support the leg until an ambulance arrives. If you need to improvise a stretcher, see page 115.

If a knee is broken, it will be extremely painful and may be bent in an unnatural way. Do not try to force it straight. Lay the casualty down with the leg in the most comfortable position.

Then put a cushion or folded jacket under the knee, and other soft supports such as rolled-up coats or rugs around the leg for further support. Call an ambulance.

Treating a broken arm

Support a broken arm in an arm sling (see page 121). Secure the arm to the chest by tying a broad bandage around the body, passing over the arm. Then take the casualty to hospital.

Never use force to bend a broken arm. If it will not bend, strap it to the body (see page 127) and wait for an ambulance.

In freezing weather, exposed parts of the body, such as the nose, ears, cheeks and chin, may develop frostbite as the skin cools and the blood vessels become constricted, cutting off the blood supply. The hands and feet can also become frostbitten, even when they are enclosed in gloves and boots. In severe cases, gangrene may develop unless the affected part is warmed up and the circulation restored.

The warning signs

- The affected part of the body feels cold and stiff, with a prickling pain.
- The skin becomes hard, and turns blue or white.
- The area becomes numb, and the feeling of cold and pain disappears.

What you should do

- If possible, get the casualty into shelter.
- Remove clothing from the frostbitten area; take off rings and watch from an affected hand.
- Warm the area with skin-to-skin contact. The casualty can put a frostbitten foot into your armpit, for instance. Cover ears, nose or cheeks with warm hands.
- Do not warm the area with dry or radiant heat. Slow thawing is essential.
- Do not rub or massage the frostbitten area.
- When warmth returns, wrap a frostbitten foot or hand in a towel or other cloth, and then cover that with a blanket or sleeping bag.
- To relieve swelling and pain, raise the affected area above the level of the casualty's chest.
- As the area thaws, it may become blue and develop blood-filled blisters. Do not break the blisters or apply any medication.
- Telephone 999 and ask for an ambulance, or get the casualty to the Accident and Emergency Department of a hospital.

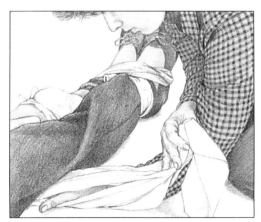

4 *Immobilise the leg by tying the two legs together with bandages, putting padding between the ankles and knees. Tie below, then above the fracture – but not on it.*

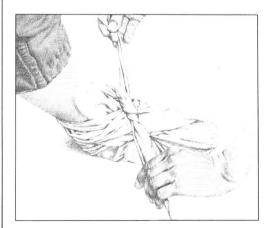

THAWING A FROSTBITTEN FOOT
When feeling begins to return, wrap the foot in a triangular bandage, towel or sweater, then cover it again with a sleeping bag or jacket.

Gas poisoning

The use of natural, non-toxic gas in the home has greatly reduced the number of deaths from accidental gassing. But there are many other danger sources, including propane and butane gases which are widely used in industry, ammonia which is used in refrigeration plants, the fumes given off by burning polyurethane foam found in furniture, and carbon monoxide from car exhaust fumes.

The warning signs
- The casualty may suffer from unsound judgment and may be difficult and uncooperative.
- The casualty may be confused, stupefied or unconscious.

What you should do
Whatever the cause of gassing, the treatment is always the same: try to cut off the source of gas and get the casualty into the open air.

If possible, before attempting a rescue tell someone else to call expert help, such as the fire brigade. Do not attempt a rescue if you are likely to become a casualty yourself.

RESCUING AN UNCONSCIOUS VICTIM

1 *Try to cut off the source of the gas, but be careful not to place yourself in danger. Take a few deep breaths of clean air, then drag the casualty into the open air. Pass your arms under the casualty's armpits and link them across the chest, grasping one of your wrists.*

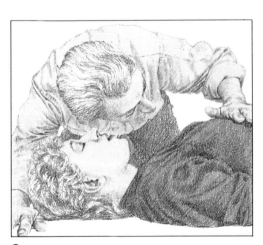

2 *Listen for casualty's breathing. Check the rise and fall of her chest. If she is not breathing and there is a pulse (see page 52), give artificial respiration (see page 50).*

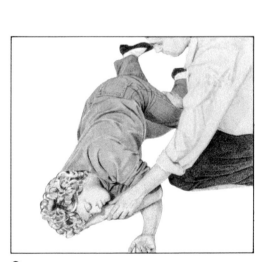

3 *Once she is breathing normally again, turn her into the recovery position (see page 136). Call an ambulance. Continue to check her breathing until help arrives.*

German measles

The main danger of German measles, known medically as rubella, is that it may affect an unborn child if contracted by a woman in early pregnancy. About 25 per cent of babies whose mothers get German measles in the first 16 weeks of pregnancy are born deaf or blind – sometimes with heart disease as well – or are stillborn. The risk is as high as 60 per cent in very early pregnancy.

The disease, which is otherwise not serious, is spread by contact with someone who has already been infected.

The warning signs

- The patient may feel unwell for a few days without any obvious symptoms.
- A rash of tiny pink, slightly raised spots then appears behind the ears or on the face, spreading downwards to the rest of the body.
- The glands become swollen, particularly behind the ears. The joints may swell and become painful, sometimes severely so, especially in young women.

Duration of the disease

The patient is infectious to others from five days before and until four days after the rash appears. The rash lasts from one to five days, but the joint pains may last for up to 14 days.

What you should do

A patient with German measles should be kept away from pregnant women, and should stay indoors for four days from the onset of the rash. If necessary, painkillers can be given.

You should consult your doctor if the joint pains become severe or if the patient develops a high temperature, a severe and persistent headache or becomes drowsy.

A woman who is in contact with German measles in early pregnancy, and does not know if she is immune, should also see her doctor. Blood tests will confirm whether she has been infected. If so, the doctor may ask the patient if she wishes to terminate her pregnancy, rather than risk having a child with deformities.

Developing immunity

German measles is very serious in pregnant women, so children should obtain immunity by catching the disease – you cannot get it twice.

Immunisation is now routinely offered to babies at 12 to 18 months, and to girls at puberty if they have not had the disease.

Women of child-bearing age who have not already had German measles, and who may wish to become pregnant, should be immunised. Pregnancy should be avoided for at least three months after the injection, as immunisation might affect the unborn child during this period.

Older women who do not know if they have had the disease can have a blood test. And immunisation after childbirth is usually offered to women who have no immunity.

Grazes

Minor grazes of the sort usually suffered by children rarely need medical attention. But if dirt or grit is embedded in the wound, there is a risk of infection, and the casualty should see a doctor.

What you should do

- Wash your hands before treating the wound.
- Clean the area around the graze with a clean gauze or cotton swab which has been dipped in lukewarm soapy water.
- Wipe outwards, away from the wound.
- Carefully remove any loose dirt or gravel, either by washing or with tweezers.
- Dry the area with a clean swab.
- Cover a small graze with an adhesive dressing (plaster) and a large graze with a sterile dressing. If you do not have a sterile dressing, dress the wound with a clean, folded handkerchief turned inside out so that the untouched side is on the wound. Fix it in place with a bandage or sticking plaster.
- Do not cough on the injury or on the dressing. You could introduce infection.
- Do not dress the wound with cotton wool, because the fibres will stick to it.
- See a doctor straight away if the wound is very dirty or if it was caused by a rusty object. The casualty may need a tetanus injection or a course of antibiotics.
- If pus starts to ooze from the wound later, or the wound becomes sore and inflamed, see a doctor about it.

First aid and medical emergencies

Gunshot wounds

Most gunshot wounds are caused by shotguns, which are widely used in field sports. But all types of firearms – even airguns – are potentially dangerous.

In all types of gunshot accidents the pellet or bullet may leave two wounds – one at the point of entry into the body and another, larger one, at the point of exit.

When treating a gunshot wound, check both the point of entry and the other side of the casualty's body for an exit wound. The casualty may be aware only of the entry wound.

If there is no exit wound, the pellet has either deflected off the body, leaving a wound similar in appearance to an entry wound, or it is lodged inside.

A bullet will cause a great deal of tissue damage, and it may hit and splinter a bone. All gunshot wounds require expert medical attention urgently.

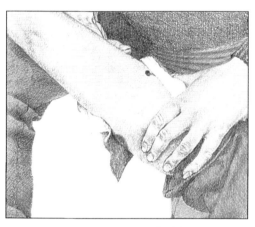

FIRST AID FOR A BULLET WOUND
Cover the wound with a clean pad or your bare hands to stop the bleeding. If there are entry and exit wounds, cover both. Once the bleeding has slowed, dress and bandage the wound (see page 56) and get medical help.

Head and face injuries

Any head injury which is severe enough to cause bleeding or a bruise could also fracture the skull or cause concussion (see page 86). So anyone who has suffered a head injury should be taken to a doctor or to the Accident and Emergency Department of a hospital for examination – even if, superficially, the injury does not appear to be serious.

Head injuries are common in road accidents, but they are also caused by falls – off a ladder or down a flight of stairs, for example. Old people are particularly prone to falls.

Sports are also a source of head injuries, particularly rugby. In cricket and hockey, the

HOW TO BANDAGE A SCALP INJURY

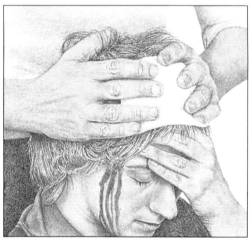

1 *Gently feel the skull around the wound. If part of it seems to move, suspect a fracture and do not press on it. Otherwise, press a clean pad on the wound to stop the bleeding.*

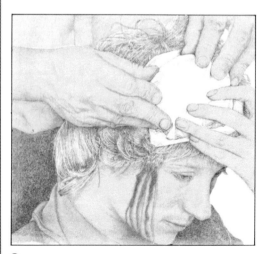

2 *Put a fresh cloth pad over the first. If you suspect a fracture, or if something is embedded, put the dressing on lightly, with a built-up dressing over it (see page 58).*

players may be hit on the head by the ball. Golfers, too, can be at risk.

Brain damage can occur without any obvious sign, except perhaps for brief unconsciousness. In elderly people, particularly, any slight knock to the head may cause internal bleeding which, if it is not recognised and treated, can result in permanent damage.

The warning signs

If you suspect that someone may have suffered a blow to the head, look for any or all of the following symptoms:

• The eye pupils (the black parts) may be unequal in size, and the casualty may have double vision and noisy breathing.
• Cuts, bruises and swellings on the scalp, face or jaw.
• Headache.
• Confusion or drowsiness, which may be followed by unconsciousness.
• Loss of memory of events before or at the time of the accident.
• Weak pulse and shallow breathing.

Bleeding scalp and face injuries

An injury to the scalp may bleed profusely because the scalp has a rich supply of blood.

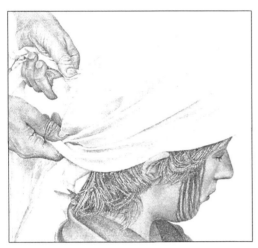

3 *Secure the dressing with a triangular bandage. Put the long edge across the forehead and the point at the neck. Bring the two ends around to the neck and cross them.*

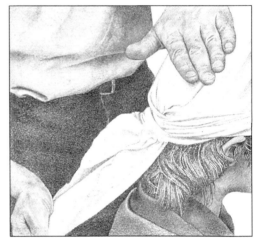

5 *Gently place one hand on the bandage to stop it slipping. With the other, draw the point downwards, parallel with the back of the neck, so that the bandage is snugly over the scalp.*

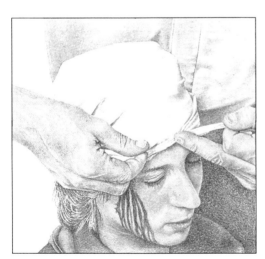

4 *Bring the two ends around to the forehead and tie them together, securing the bandage. Keep the casualty's head as steady as possible while you put the bandage on.*

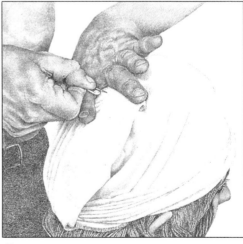

6 *Bring the point of the bandage up to the crown and fix it lightly in place with a safety pin or adhesive tape. Alternatively, tuck the point into the edge of the bandage at the front.*

Because the skin is stretched tight over the head, the wound may also gape open and look much more serious than it really is.

However, there is always the danger of a fracture to the skull, and the casualty should be examined by a doctor or at the Accident and Emergency Department of a hospital. In the meantime, control the bleeding by holding your hand or a cloth pad, such as the inside of a clean, folded handkerchief, on the wound.

A wound on the face will also bleed profusely, and may look much worse than it really is. But if it is deep, take the casualty to hospital because the wound may need to be stitched. If the wound followed a blow to the head, also get medical treatment at once.

A broken jaw

A person who has suffered a broken jaw will often have a wound inside the mouth. The casualty may have difficulty in speaking and there may be an excessive flow of saliva, often tinged with blood, and broken teeth. Usually only one side of the jaw will be broken.

Put a bandage under the casualty's chin and tie it in place on top of the head to support the jaw while you get the casualty to hospital. Do not tie the bandage too tightly.

TREATING A BLEEDING FACE

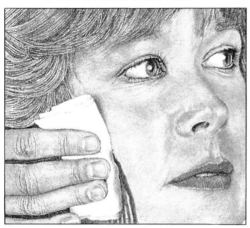

1 *A cut face may produce such severe bleeding that the wound may look worse than it really is. Press the inside of a clean, folded handkerchief, or a pad of paper tissues, against the wound. Do not use cotton wool.*

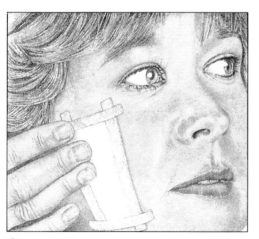

2 *When the bleeding slows (which may take 15 minutes), put a fresh handkerchief or pad on the wound – on top of the old one – and fix it in place with sticking plaster. If blood seeps through, put another pad on top.*

SUPPORTING A BROKEN JAW

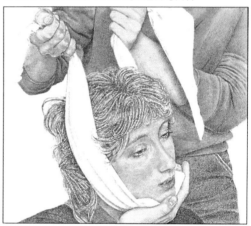

1 *If the jaw is broken or dislocated, make sure first that the mouth is clear of blood and broken teeth to avoid the risk of choking. Then put a pad of cloth under the point of the chin, and get the casualty to hold it in place.*

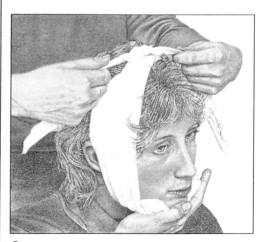

2 *Put a bandage or scarf over the pad, bring the ends to the top of the head, and tie them together in a reef knot. The bandage should be tight enough to support the jaw, but not so tight that the teeth are clenched.*

Heart attack

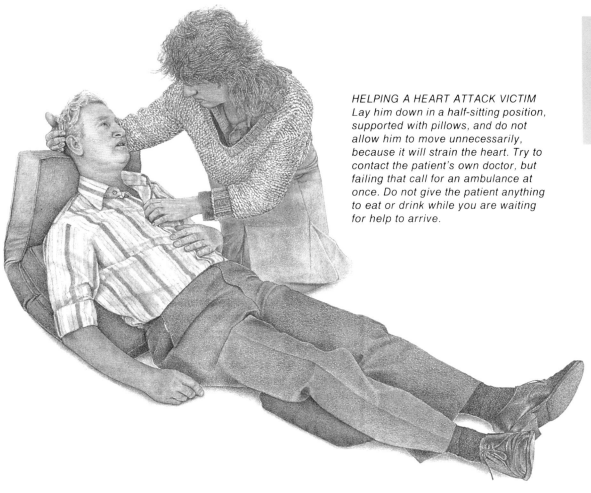

*HELPING A HEART ATTACK VICTIM
Lay him down in a half-sitting position, supported with pillows, and do not allow him to move unnecessarily, because it will strain the heart. Try to contact the patient's own doctor, but failing that call for an ambulance at once. Do not give the patient anything to eat or drink while you are waiting for help to arrive.*

Severe, crushing pain in the chest, often spreading to one or both arms, the neck and the jaw, is the main symptom of a heart attack. It comes on suddenly and, unlike anginal pain, is not related to exertion. It does not pass off if the patient keeps still.

The patient may also become breathless and sweat profusely. He may suffer sudden giddiness, causing him to sit down or lean against something for support.

During the weeks before an attack, the patient may have experienced unusual tiredness, shortness of breath and unaccustomed indigestion.

What you should do

- If the patient is conscious, put him in a half-sitting position, with head and shoulders supported with pillows, and knees bent.
- If possible, contact the patient's own doctor, as there may be a history of heart disease. If his doctor is not obtainable, telephone 999 and ask for an ambulance, and make it clear to the ambulance service that you suspect a heart attack.
- Loosen the patient's clothing around the neck, chest and waist to help circulation and ease his breathing.

- Do not give the patient anything to eat or drink, except an aspirin to chew slowly.
- Do not allow him to move unnecessarily; it will put extra strain on the heart.
- If the patient becomes unconscious, put him in the recovery position (see page 136).

Preventing heart attacks

Most heart attacks are caused by a blood clot in one of the arteries supplying blood to the heart muscle. The process is known medically as coronary thrombosis.

The likelihood of coronary thrombosis is increased by smoking, obesity, diabetes, raised blood pressure, lack of exercise, faulty diet and a family history of heart attacks.

The following five rules will help you to avoid a heart attack:

- Stay within your ideal weight for height.
- If you smoke, give it up.
- Take regular exercise.
- Eat only modest amounts of meat from chickens, cows, sheep and pigs, as the fat from the meat may be deposited in the arteries, interfering with the flow of blood.
- If you suffer from diabetes or high blood pressure, follow your doctor's advice carefully.

Heat exhaustion and heat stroke

People who exert themselves during a summer holiday in a hot climate, or long-distance runners on a warm day, may suffer from heat exhaustion, or from an even worse condition known as heat stroke.

Both conditions can lead to unconsciousness and they both require medical treatment.

The body can become overwhelmed by heat when its mechanism for keeping cool breaks down. Usually it cools itself in three ways:
• It produces sweat which evaporates and cools the skin – just as water that seeps through an unglazed jug will cool the remaining water when it evaporates off the outside.
• The capillaries of the skin enlarge and carry more blood to the surface, where it loses its heat. This produces the flushed look a hot person often has.
• Breathing increases, carrying surplus heat from the lungs.

The effects of heat exhaustion
Profuse sweating on a hot day leads to an excessive loss of moisture and salt, which is contained in sweat.

This brings on muscle cramps in the legs and body, and weakness – although the sweating prevents the body's temperature from rising. If the fluid and salt are not replaced, the condition will get worse and the casualty will collapse.

Other symptoms of heat exhaustion are dizziness, headache and nausea. The temperature stays normal and the skin feels cold and moist. The face looks pale.

The breathing is fast and shallow, and the pulse is fast and weak.

The condition can be made worse if the sufferer has had a stomach upset with diarrhoea or vomiting, causing even greater loss of fluid.
• To treat heat exhaustion, lay the casualty in a cool place, preferably indoors, and give cold, salted water to drink.
• If the casualty becomes unconscious, put him or her in the recovery position (see page 136) and get medical help.

TREATING HEAT EXHAUSTION

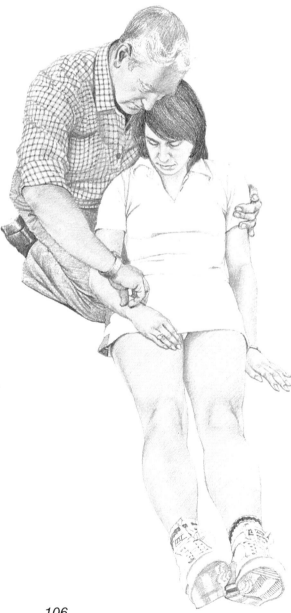

1 *Put the casualty in a cool place, preferably indoors. Remove any heavy clothing. If she is suffering from heat exhaustion, her pulse will be fast and weak. Check her temperature; if it is higher than normal she may be suffering from heat stroke. If she becomes unconscious, put her in the recovery position (see page 136).*

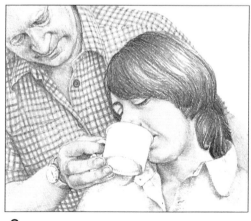

2 *If the casualty is conscious, give her a cup of weakly salted water every ten minutes. Use a quarter of a teaspoon of salt to each cup. Add fruit juice to improve the taste.*

Heat stroke: how to treat it

When humidity, as well as temperature, is very high, sweat is less able to cool the body as it cannot evaporate into the already moisture-laden air. It takes from three to six weeks to adjust to these conditions, and a person may suffer heat stroke before he has acclimatised.

Heat stroke may occur suddenly, with the body temperature rising to 40°C (104°F). The casualty's skin feels hot and may be dry. He may complain of headache, dizziness and nausea. As the condition worsens, he may become confused and lapse into unconsciousness.

TREATING HEAT STROKE

Treatment for heat stroke must be given quickly or the casualty may die. Babies and old people are particularly at risk.

• Move the casualty to a cool place. Remove the clothing and cover the body with a wet sheet. Keep it wet with cold water, and fan the casualty until the body temperature drops to 38°C (100°F).

• Call a doctor or ambulance as soon as possible. If the casualty becomes unconscious, put him in the recovery position (see page 136), and continue the cooling treatment.

How to deal with prickly heat

An intensely irritating skin rash, which may develop in hot, humid weather, is known as prickly heat. It is caused by swelling of the skin cells because of excessive sweating, and mostly affects babies and fat people. Pimples or small blisters appear, particularly in the skin creases and where clothing has been tight.

There is no quick remedy, but some relief will be gained by wearing loose clothing and lying under a fan during the heat of the day. Have frequent baths in cool water, using little soap, and apply calamine lotion to the affected area.

It may be necessary to see a doctor if the irritation becomes too severe to bear, or if the sufferer becomes weak and lethargic.

The skin will rapidly return to normal when you return to a cool climate.

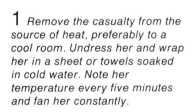

1 *Remove the casualty from the source of heat, preferably to a cool room. Undress her and wrap her in a sheet or towels soaked in cold water. Note her temperature every five minutes and fan her constantly.*

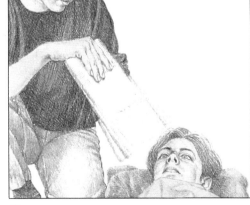

2 *When the casualty's temperature is down to 38°C (100°F), replace the wet sheet with a dry one. Continue fanning. If her temperature rises again, restart the cooling treatment.*

Hiccups

Most attacks of hiccups are over in 10 to 20 minutes, but occasionally attacks can last for days, causing distress and interfering with sleep. Persistent hiccups suggest some abdominal disorder requiring medical treatment.

Most hiccups are caused by irritation of the diaphragm – a muscular partition which separates the chest cavity from the abdomen. This occurs when the sufferer has overfilled the stomach with a large amount of food or drink, especially hot drinks. The diaphragm then goes into repeated and involuntary spasms.

What can be done to stop hiccups
Carbon dioxide gas – one of the products of breathing – inhibits hiccups. Simply holding the breath several times will cause carbon dioxide to build up in the body, and the hiccups may stop without further treatment.

Breathing in and out of a paper bag works in the same way. But *do not* use a plastic bag. It can mould itself to the mouth and nose, and obstruct breathing altogether.

Most other household remedies work by making the sufferer hold his breath. Drinking water slowly, sucking ice or pulling on the tongue are all ways of building up carbon dioxide.

If the hiccups last more than a day, the sufferer should see a doctor, who may prescribe sedatives or arrange a supply of 5 per cent carbon dioxide to be inhaled. The doctor may also examine the patient for kidney, liver, lung or abdominal disorders which could be causing the hiccups, although such disorders are rare.

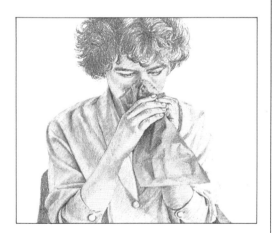

ONE WAY OF STOPPING HICCUPS
Breathing in and out of a paper bag builds up carbon dioxide in the body, which can bring the spasms of the diaphragm to a stop. But on no account use a plastic bag.

Hypothermia

If a baby in a cold room begins to look bright red, becomes lethargic and refuses food, it may have hypothermia, a serious condition in which the body's temperature drops below normal.

Unless the drop in temperature is reversed the baby may die in a few hours.

Old people are also at risk. At first they may complain of the cold. If these warnings go unnoticed or are ignored, the condition will grow worse until the victim becomes mentally confused and tired, with stiff muscles. Uncontrollable shivering may also occur or speech may be slurred.

Eventually the victim becomes unconscious, suffers brain damage and then dies.

(For hypothermia in outdoor conditions, see *Exposure: the silent killer*, page 301.)

How hypothermia sets in
Hypothermia begins when the body's temperature drops below about 35°C (95°F) from the normal level of 37°C (98.6°F).

With babies, the cause of hypothermia is usually a cold bedroom at night. Premature babies and babies which are suffering from illness are the most susceptible.

One problem in recognising the condition is that the red colour of the skin that develops may be mistaken for a healthy glow.

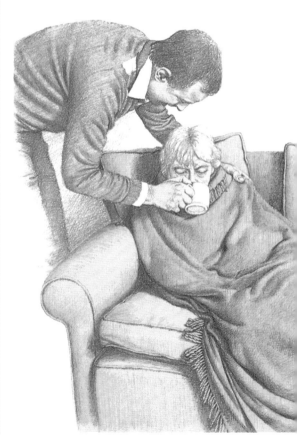

With old people, hypothermia usually results from inadequate food, clothing and heating in winter. Their resistance to cold will also be lessened if they are taking drugs or alcohol.

What you should do

If you suspect that someone is suffering from hypothermia, feel his or her skin. It will be abnormally cold to the touch if the condition has set in. You must take action to prevent the condition from getting worse, and you must call an ambulance to get the victim to hospital.

• If a blanket or rug is readily available, wrap it around the victim, covering the body but not the face. If possible, heat the room.

• Lay him down. If he is unconscious, put him in the recovery position (see page 136).

• If possible, increase the temperature of the room, or move the victim to a warmer room.

• Telephone 999 and ask for an ambulance.

• While waiting for the ambulance, give the victim – if conscious – hot, sweet drinks such as milk or hot chocolate. Do not give alcohol.

• Do not massage the victim's limbs or suggest that he takes exercise. This will only take blood away from the body's vital organs.

• If the ambulance is delayed, wrap a hot-water bottle in a towel or cloth and put it on the victim's trunk, not on the arms or legs.

Hysteria

A fit of hysterics is usually caused by an emotional upset or mental stress. The attack may resemble an epileptic fit, but is more dramatised and is 'staged' to gain sympathy and attention. It will continue as long as there is an audience.

In an adult, hysterics take longer to develop than an epileptic fit and may vary from temporary loss of control, when the person shouts or screams, to a noisy display or arm waving, tearing at clothes and hair, and rolling on the ground in an apparent frenzy.

Although genuinely distressed, sufferers take care not to hurt themselves. They may, for example, 'collapse' into a fairly safe position. They may also move weakly to suggest illness.

What you should do

• Be gentle but firm. Reassure and try to calm the person.

• Ask relatives and onlookers to leave the area.

• Do not slap a hysterical person on the face as it may cause psychological harm. In the case of a person with a weak heart, the shock could even be fatal.

• When the attack has subsided, suggest that the person sees a doctor.

First aid and
medical emergencies

TREATING AN ELDERLY
VICTIM OF HYPOTHERMIA
An elderly person living alone may become a victim of hypothermia because she has run out of fuel during winter. So it may not be possible to take quick action to heat the room. First, call an ambulance, as it is imperative to get her to hospital quickly. Then wrap her in a blanket and – if she is conscious – give her a hot drink. A hot-water bottle, wrapped in a towel, could also be placed against her trunk. Do not place it against her limbs, because it will draw blood away from the body's vital organs in the torso.

Insect stings and bites

Stings and bites from bees, wasps and ants can be painful but are not usually dangerous. It is only an allergic reaction, or a sting or bite in the throat or mouth, that can endanger life.

If the victim has been stung by a bee, the sting will probably be left embedded in the skin. Remove it by scraping with a fingernail, taking care not to squeeze the poison bag, which will only pump more poison into the skin.

Wasps and ants do not leave stings behind.

Dealing with an allergic reaction

A massive allergic reaction to a sting (or to a drug such as cocaine) is known as anaphylactic shock. It occurs within a few seconds or minutes, and the casualty will become very weak and feel sick. His chest will feel tight and he will have difficulty breathing. He may be sneezing and his face may swell up. Less often, he may become unconscious, and may stop breathing.
• Telephone 999 and ask for an ambulance.
• Reassure the casualty that help is on the way.
• Lay him on his back. Raise the feet on a cushion or folded coat. Keep his head low and turn it to one side in case he vomits.
• Keep the casualty warm with a blanket or rug.
• Loosen tight clothing around the neck and waist to help with breathing.
• Do not give the casualty anything to eat or drink. Do not allow him to smoke, either – it may make breathing more difficult.
• If the casualty becomes unconscious, or vomiting seems likely, or breathing becomes very difficult, put him in the recovery position (see page 136).

Stings to the mouth or throat

A sting to the mouth or throat can cause the throat to swell rapidly, blocking the airway.
• Give the victim an ice cube or some ice cream to suck, or cold water to drink, to lessen the swelling.
• If breathing stops, start artificial respiration immediately (see page 50).
• Telephone 999 and ask for an ambulance or take the victim at once to the Accident and Emergency Department of a hospital.

Blood-sucking ticks

Ticks are spider-like creatures which suck the blood of animals and humans by clinging to the skin with beak-like mouths. They are active in spring and summer, and may attach themselves to farmworkers or children who play in woods and grassy areas. Their bodies swell up to hold the blood they feed on.

Do not try to pull a tick out. Touch it with a lit cigarette or match and it will fall off. Alternatively, cover it with machine oil or cooking oil to close its breathing pores. It may fall off at once; if not, leave the oil for half an hour and then remove the tick carefully with tweezers.

Wash the area with soap and water and apply antihistamine cream.

TREATING BEE, WASP OR ANT STINGS

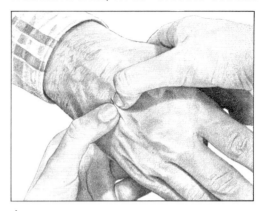

1 *Scrape out a bee sting with a fingernail, but take care not to squeeze the poison bag, because that will just pump more poison into the skin. Wasps and ants do not leave stings.*

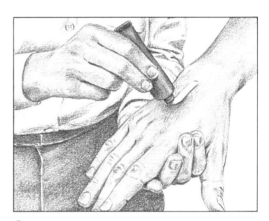

2 *Apply antihistamine cream to any sting. Or use a solution of 1 teaspoon of bicarbonate of soda in a tumbler of water for bee stings, a weak ammonia solution for wasps and ants.*

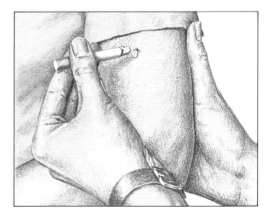

TREATING TICK BITES
Apply the glowing end of a cigarette, or a burning match, to the tick's body; this will make the tick fall off. Do not pull it out, as it may leave its head behind, causing infection.

Measles

The most obvious symptom of measles is the rash of brownish-pink, slightly raised spots which starts behind the ears and spreads in blotches over the whole body.

But before the rash breaks out, a dry, irritating cough generally occurs and the patient develops a high temperature. The cough can occur up to four days before the rash starts. The eyes can also be sore and red, or 'heavy', for a few days before the rash.

What you should do

• Put the patient – usually a child – to bed and give cool drinks to bring the temperature down. It does not matter if the child does not want to eat, as long as plenty of fluids are taken.
• Notify your doctor.
• Keep the child quiet and resting while there is a high temperature and illness. Many children prefer the room darkened because their eyes feel sore.
• If necessary, give temperature-reducing drugs, such as paracetamol, in the recommended doses.
• The disease is likely to last five to seven days after the rash first appears.

Complications that can occur

Most victims of measles recover completely, but there can be serious complications of the ears, lungs and brain.

Consequently the doctor may check the child for otitis media (an ear infection which can cause severe earache and deafness), pneumonia and encephalitis (a rare disease of the brain which causes headache, confusion or unconsciousness, an aching neck and fever).

If one of these diseases occurs, a course of antibiotics will probably be prescribed. Because measles is caused by a virus, antibiotics are of no use against the measles itself.

Because of the serious complications of measles, attempts are being made to eradicate the disease by immunisation. All children are offered immunisation at between 12 and 18 months of age. This is combined with mumps and rubella (German measles) immunisation in a vaccine called MMR. Although the campaign has greatly reduced the number of cases and the complications, measles is still one of the commonest diseases in the world.

Someone who has had the disease cannot catch it a second time.

Miscarriage

At the first sign of a miscarriage the woman should go to bed immediately. Rest is essential if the pregnancy is to be saved.

Three warning signs occur in succession if the miscarriage takes its full course.
• In the early stages the commonest symptom is loss of blood from the vagina. If the embryo has not been dislodged, this stage is known medically as a 'threatened abortion', and the pregnancy may still be saved.
• If the condition becomes worse, pains like small labour pains may come and go at regular intervals. This is a sign that the threatened miscarriage may have become inevitable.
• The bleeding may also increase at this stage.

What can be done

• Notify the doctor at the first signs and put the patient to bed.
• If the miscarriage passes into the inevitable stage, the doctor may send the patient to hospital.
• In hospital she may have an evacuation of the uterus, under anaesthetic, to remove any placenta or membrane left behind after the embryo has been lost.

How common are miscarriages?

Medical research has shown that probably about one-third of all pregnancies miscarry within four weeks of conception. In many cases the woman never knows that she has been pregnant; the miscarriage occurs about four weeks after her last menstrual period, and so passes unrecognised. In other cases miscarriages may occur a week or so later, and she just thinks that she has had a late period.

Miscarriages may be nature's way of ending a pregnancy that is in some way likely to be unsatisfactory.

Avoiding another miscarriage

If a woman has already had a miscarriage, she should discuss with her obstetrician how best to safeguard a new pregnancy as soon as she is aware of it. She may be advised to avoid strenuous work, certain sports or vigorous sexual intercourse. However, these activities pose no danger to most pregnant women.

First aid and medical emergencies

111

Moving an injured person

Injured people should be moved only if they are in immediate danger, or if they have to be taken to where medical help is available. This may occur if you have to move a casualty off a busy road, get him out of a burning house, or carry him to safety after a climbing accident.

Otherwise, leave the casualty undisturbed and carry out first aid while someone else calls for an ambulance.

If moving is essential, take care not to injure yourself. Back injuries are easily suffered when moving heavy weights, so keep your backbone straight, your head up, and use the stronger parts of your body to do the lifting – the thigh muscles, the hip and the shoulder. Keep the weight as close as possible to your body.

If other people are on the scene, ask someone to help you. It is always easier for two people to lift a weight than one.

It is usually best for an accident victim to be taken to hospital in an ambulance, but if he is suffering from only minor injuries to the arms or hands, he can be taken in a car.

Moving a casualty by yourself
If the person is only slightly injured and is able to stand, get him to put one arm around your shoulder. Supported in this way, he can be moved fairly easily. This is a useful method of moving a person with a sprained ankle.

An unconscious person can be dragged to safety in one of two ways. You can hold him under the shoulders and drag him backwards in a crouching or squatting position. Or you can tie his wrists together, put your head through the arms and crawl on all fours, dragging him with you. Either of these methods could be used to drag an unconscious person from a burning building or a gas-filled room.

When you have someone to help you
One of the simplest ways for two people to move a casualty is to carry him on a chair, with one person holding the back of the chair and the other holding the front legs.

This is a useful way of carrying an injured person down a flight of stairs. But first make sure that the staircase and passage are clear of obstructions, or any hazards such as loose rugs or children's toys.

A disabled person in a wheelchair can be carried in a similar way. First, put the wheel-

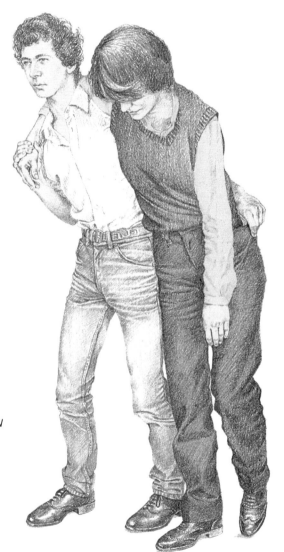

HELPING A CONSCIOUS PERSON
Stand close to the casualty on the injured side, unless the wound is to the hand, arm or shoulder. In that case, support from the uninjured side. Put your arm around her waist and grip the clothing at the hip. Get her to put her arm around your neck and grasp her hand. Take her weight with your body and move forwards with slow, short steps.

chair's brakes on, and get the casualty to sit well back in the chair. Then stand to one side of the chair, with your helper on the other side facing you. Lift the chair together, holding the fixed parts. Do not hold the wheels, as they might turn, and be careful of the arm rests and side supports, as they might be removable.

A casualty who cannot walk but can use his hands can be carried by two people using a 'four-handed seat'. The two helpers each grip their left wrist with their right hand, and then grip the other person's right wrist with their free hand. The casualty puts an arm around each helper's neck and sits on the 'seat'. The two helpers stand up straight and start walking with the outside foot.

MOVING AN UNCONSCIOUS PERSON

1 *Use this method if you have a fairly long way to go or if the casualty is heavy. Check the breathing but do not start artificial respiration until you are clear of danger. Turn the casualty face up and cross the arms at the wrists.*

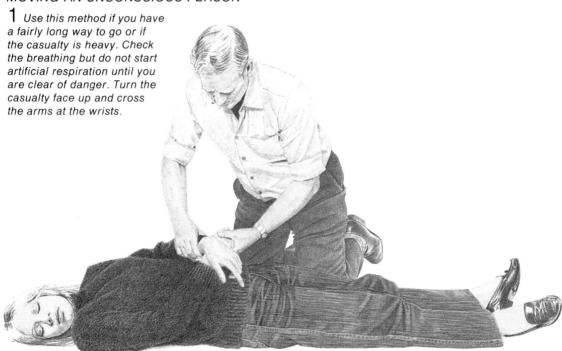

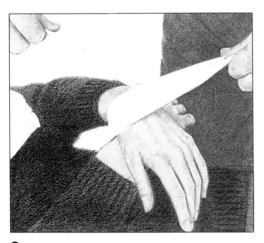

2 *Use a belt, scarf or bandage to tie the wrists together. Wind the material around the wrists tightly, but not so tightly as to impede circulation. Tie the ends with a reef knot, and check quickly with your fingers that the knot is completely secure.*

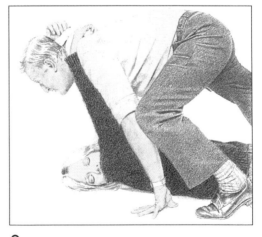

3 *Kneel astride the casualty and slip your head through the wrists so they are resting on your shoulders at the base of your neck. Push yourself up into a crouch, and work forwards to safety, using your arms to take the weight. Keep the casualty's head off the ground.*

Making an improvised stretcher

Two people can move an injured person a long distance by making an improvised stretcher out of two or more coats with their sleeves turned inside out and a pair of poles, such as broomsticks, pushed through the sleeves.

To get the person onto the stretcher, one of the stretcher bearers should roll the casualty gently onto the uninjured side. While he is doing that, the other bearer should put the open stretcher flat against the casualty's back. Then the stretcher, with the casualty on it, can be rolled back gently onto the ground.

If the casualty is unconscious, put the open stretcher against his front so that he is carried in the recovery position (see page 136).

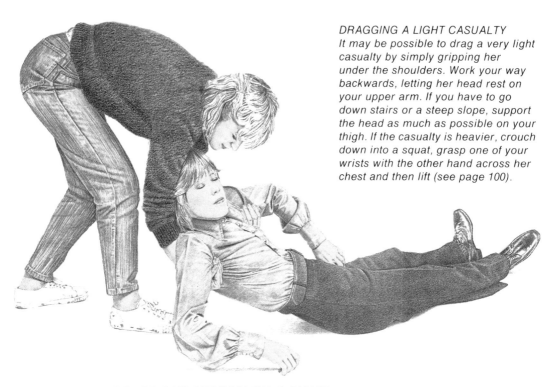

DRAGGING A LIGHT CASUALTY
It may be possible to drag a very light casualty by simply gripping her under the shoulders. Work your way backwards, letting her head rest on your upper arm. If you have to go down stairs or a steep slope, support the head as much as possible on your thigh. If the casualty is heavier, crouch down into a squat, grasp one of your wrists with the other hand across her chest and then lift (see page 100).

CARRYING A CONSCIOUS PERSON ON A CHAIR

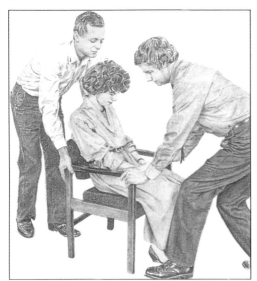

1 *Check that the chair is strong enough to take the weight. Sit the casualty well back in it, and stand in front with the other helper behind. Tilt the chair backwards as you lift it.*

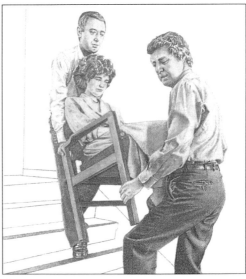

2 *Carry the chair with the casualty facing forwards, so that you go down stairs with the bearer at the front backing down. On wide stairs, the bearers can hold the sides instead.*

IMPROVISING A STRETCHER

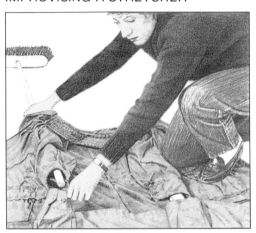

1 Take two or three coats or jackets, and turn the sleeves inside out. Pass a strong pole through one of the sleeves of each jacket, and a second pole through the other sleeves.

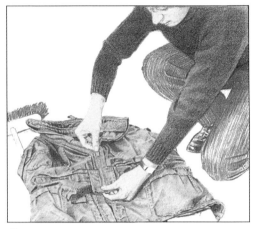

2 Zip or button up the jackets to create the stretcher. If possible, get an uninjured person to lie on the stretcher first, and lift it to make sure that it can take the weight.

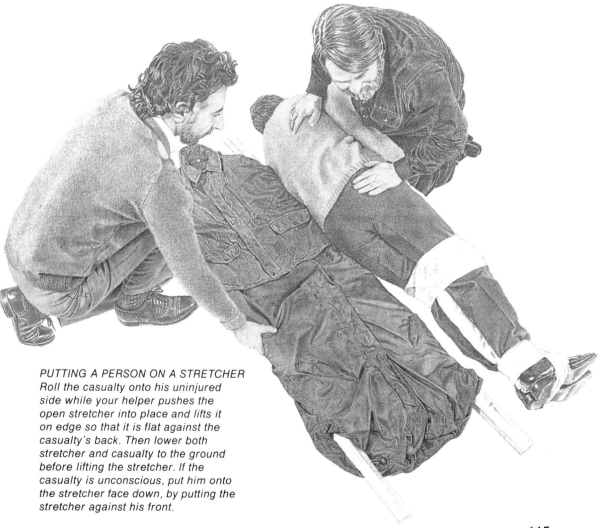

PUTTING A PERSON ON A STRETCHER
Roll the casualty onto his uninjured side while your helper pushes the open stretcher into place and lifts it on edge so that it is flat against the casualty's back. Then lower both stretcher and casualty to the ground before lifting the stretcher. If the casualty is unconscious, put him onto the stretcher face down, by putting the stretcher against his front.

Mumps

The most obvious sign of mumps is a large swelling on one side of the face. It is caused by a saliva-producing gland swelling up in front of the ear and over the angle of the jaw.

A day or two later the gland on the opposite side of the face may also swell. Other saliva-producing glands under the tongue and under the jaw may also be affected.

The patient may also suffer earache and pain when eating.

Mumps is a common infection, mostly affecting children over the age of two, and occurs in epidemics every three or four years. But it can also attack older people, and may cause inflammation of the testicles in men, inflammation of the ovaries in women, and inflammation of the pancreas in both sexes, producing pain in the abdomen.

What you should do
- Keep the patient at rest for a few days.
- If chewing is painful, offer soups and drinks.
- If a testicle is swollen or sore, support the scrotum with a pillow or bandage. A towel beneath the testicles, with the ends draped over the thighs, may help. Leave pyjama trousers off and give a mild painkiller such as paracetamol in recommended doses.

When you should call the doctor
- If the testicles are swollen or sore.
- If there is severe or persistent earache.
- If there is severe or persistent pain in the abdomen – the lower part of the trunk.
- If there is severe headache, with a stiff neck.
- If the patient finds light uncomfortable.

The doctor may examine the patient for an ear infection known as otitis media, for inflammation of the testicles (orchitis), for inflammation of the membranes surrounding the brain (meningitis) or, rarely, of the brain itself (encephalitis).

How long is the patient infectious?
Sufferers are infectious for about six days before the glands begin to swell, and remain infectious for a further two weeks.

Where possible, the patient should be kept away from others at risk of catching the disease, especially adult men and older boys who have never had mumps. There is a tiny risk that if their testicles are affected, their future fertility may be at risk.

An attack of mumps almost always confers life-long immunity. Vaccination against mumps is offered to all children aged between 12 and 18 months.

Nose injuries

The nose's function as an opening to the body and its prominent position on the face make it subject to a variety of problems.

Nosebleeds
Bleeding from the nose may be the result of blowing too hard, sneezing, picking, air-pressure changes or high blood pressure. Occasionally blood disorders may be the cause, and sometimes there may be no apparent cause for a nosebleed at all.

If blood mixed with a straw-coloured fluid trickles from the nose of an unconscious person, suspect a fracture of the skull (see page 102).

For a normal nosebleed, sit in a chair with your head slightly forward and pinch the nostrils together for at least 10 minutes.

Loosen any tight clothing around the neck.

Spit out any blood that goes down the back of the nose. It is preferable to spit it out as swallowed blood may make you feel sick, so have a bowl close by.

After 10 minutes, release the nostrils gradually. If the bleeding has stopped, sit quietly for a while, and do not blow your nose for at least three hours.

If the bleeding starts up again, squeeze the nostrils for a further 10 minutes.

If the bleeding still continues, see a doctor or go to the Accident and Emergency Department of your local hospital.

You should also see a doctor if you lose so much blood that you become pale or dizzy.

Broken nose
The bones at the bridge of the nose may be broken by an injury, often in a traffic accident. There is then a danger that a deformity of the nose may become permanent, as happens with some boxers.

The symptoms of a broken nose are:
- Severe pain.
- Irregular shape.
- Severe nosebleed.

If a broken nose is suspected, you should take the casualty to a doctor or to the Accident and Emergency Department of your local hospital.

Bleeding can often be stopped with gauze packed into the nostrils.

If there is no deformity causing an obstruction of the nose, treatment is usually unnecessary, apart from an X-ray. The fracture will take about two weeks to heal.

A deformed nose can be corrected by an operation under general anaesthetic.

Foreign body in the nose
Small children often push objects, such as pebbles or beads, into their nostrils. A smooth object may stick harmlessly in the nose, but something jagged can easily cause damage to the inside of the nose and make it bleed.

You should suspect that something is lodged in the nose if:

- A child is playing with its nose.
- One nostril is obstructed, and possibly bleeding.
- The child complains of discomfort or pain in the nose.

Do not try to remove the object yourself; you may make the problem worse.

Take the child to your doctor or to the Accident and Emergency Department of your local hospital, where the object will be removed gently with forceps, or under a general anaesthetic.

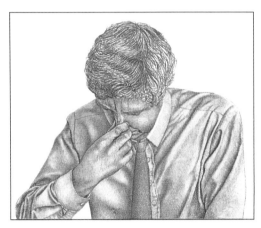

STOPPING A NOSEBLEED
Sit down with your head slightly forward to prevent blood running down into your throat. Hold the nostrils together for 10 minutes. If, after that, the bleeding continues, repeat for a further 10 minutes.

Poisoning

Many cases of poisoning occur when a person – often a child – drinks some household or garden chemical.

A child may take bleach, cleaning fluid, rat poison or paint stripper, and gardeners sometimes drink insecticides or weedkillers that they have made up and kept in a soft-drink bottle.

Some plants in Britain are also poisonous. The most common are the seeds and berries of laburnum and deadly or woody nightshade, 'green' potatoes and death cap fungus.

The warning signs
A person who has taken poison is likely to show some of the following symptoms:
- Stomach pain.
- Retching or vomiting.
- Diarrhoea.
- Delirium and convulsions.
- Burns around the mouth if the poison was corrosive, and severe pain in the mouth, gullet and stomach.
- Difficulty in breathing.
- Unconsciousness.

What you should do
- If the victim is conscious, try to find out what he has swallowed. Remember that he may become unconscious at any time.
- Look around for any container or the remains of a poisonous plant that might be a clue.
- Do not try to induce vomiting. It wastes time and may be harmful.
- If the victim is conscious and has swallowed something that burns, such as bleach, give him about a pint of water or milk to drink slowly to dilute the poison in his stomach.
- If the victim is unconscious, place him in the recovery position (see page 136).
- Call an ambulance. Give the ambulance men the container or a sample of vomit to help them to identify the poison.
- If the victim's breathing stops, begin artificial respiration (see page 50). Take care not to get any of the poison on your own mouth. Clean the victim's mouth, or use the mouth-to-nose technique.

How to avoid poisoning
A great number of substances found around the house – in the kitchen, bathroom, workroom and garden shed – are poisonous and may be drunk or eaten by an inquisitive toddler.

Apparently innocent things, including liquid soap, some cosmetics and fire lighters, are poisonous. And others invite a child to pick them up and put them in his mouth; some dangerous medicines look like sweets, and some spot weedkillers can be held and licked like ice cream.

Keep all dangerous chemicals out of the reach of small children, and never store unused weedkillers and insecticides in soft-drink bottles where they may be picked up by either children or unwary adults.

Pulse and breathing

The pulse rate plays an important part in diagnosing some injuries which may have no very obvious symptoms.

A rapid or weak pulse is often associated with shock, internal bleeding and heat exhaustion. Occasionally, a rapid or irregular pulse, occurring while a person is at rest, may be a symptom of serious heart disorder.

A slow pulse can occur if the body cools down to an unnatural degree, as happens to a victim of hypothermia.

The pulse measures the rate at which the heart beats, and this varies throughout life. In a baby's first weeks it may beat 140 times a minute, but by the age of ten the rate will have dropped to an average of 90 a minute. A man, awake but at rest, has a pulse rate between 60 and 80 a minute, with an average of 72. A woman's average rate is slightly higher – 78 to 82 a minute.

An elderly person may have a rate of only 60 a minute, and a sleeping adult of either sex has a rate of 60 to 65.

In times of extreme activity the pulse rate of an adult can go up to 140 a minute.

Each pulse beat is caused by a wave of blood pressure driven along the arteries by the pumping action of the heart. The pulse is most easily detected at two places on the body – the inside of the wrist, just below the thumb joint, and in the hollow of the throat just below the angle of the jaw.

When you take a pulse, note whether it is fast or slow, strong or weak, regular or irregular. Accurate taking of the pulse requires practice, and may be difficult even then. Practise on yourself or a member of your family from time to time so that, if an emergency arises suddenly, you will be able to find the pulse in the wrist or throat without having to hunt for it.

The breathing rate

Respiration – the process of breathing – is closely linked to heartbeat. A person breathes to absorb oxygen from the air into the blood. The oxygen is then circulated to all parts of the

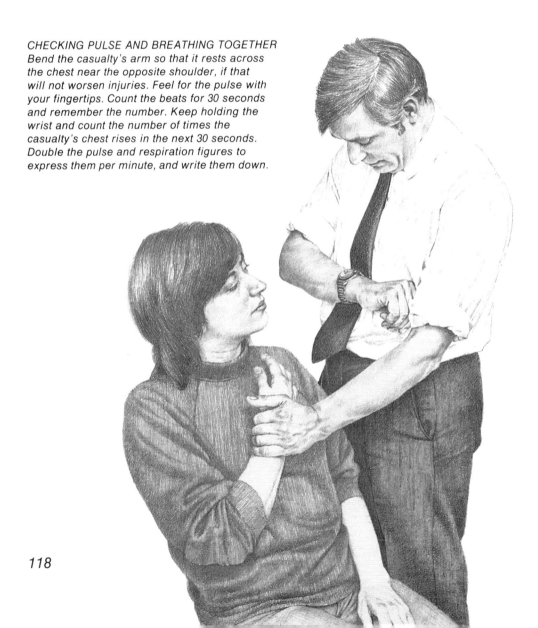

CHECKING PULSE AND BREATHING TOGETHER
Bend the casualty's arm so that it rests across the chest near the opposite shoulder, if that will not worsen injuries. Feel for the pulse with your fingertips. Count the beats for 30 seconds and remember the number. Keep holding the wrist and count the number of times the casualty's chest rises in the next 30 seconds. Double the pulse and respiration figures to express them per minute, and write them down.

body by the regular, pumping action of the heart. Children breathe an average of 20 to 30 times a minute, and adults an average of 12 to 16 times a minute. This increases during exercise and when a person is injured or under stress.

When measuring the breathing rate, count only the number of times the chest rises. Many people unknowingly alter their breathing rate if they are aware it is being checked. So, if the casualty is conscious, measure the rate, without telling him, while you hold his wrist.

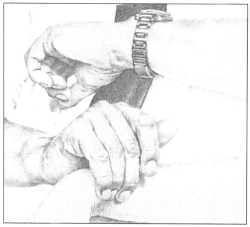

TAKING THE PULSE AT THE WRIST
The wrist pulse can be felt just below the base of the thumb, in the hollow between two bones. Place three fingers on the pulse and press slightly. Do not use your thumb as it has a pulse of its own. Count the beats for half a minute and double the number.

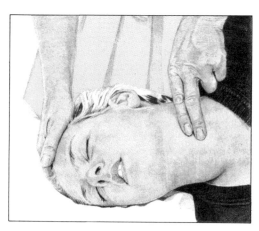

TAKING THE PULSE AT THE THROAT
The throat pulse can be felt in the hollow of the neck, to one side of the Adam's apple and below the angle of the jaw. Place two fingers on the pulse and press slightly. Count the beats for half a minute and double the number. Either side of the throat can be used.

Rabies

Holidaymakers in almost any foreign country run a risk of getting rabies if they are bitten by an animal there.

Rabies is a dangerous infectious disease caused by a virus carried by animals, particularly dogs and foxes. It is also known as hydrophobia (meaning 'fear of water'), because this fear is one of its symptoms.

The virus is transmitted to humans through the bite of an infected animal, and travels from the bite to the brain.

The nearer the bite is to the brain (on the face or neck, for example) the less far the virus has to travel and the quicker the treatment must be to prevent the disease.

The time between the bite and the onset of symptoms can range from ten days to more than a year, but is usually between 20 and 90 days. Before the symptoms begin, the bite usually heals but remains red and inflamed.

Once the symptoms have developed, treatment is ineffective and the patient usually dies within four days.

Rabies occurs in most parts of the world, except Britain, Scandinavia, Australia, Japan and Antarctica, and about 15,000 cases are reported each year.

What you should do
• See a local doctor immediately if you are bitten by an animal in any country where rabies may be present.
• Unless the animal can be proved to be free of rabies by a medical examination, the victim must have a course of injections *before* the symptoms appear.
• If possible, isolate the animal, but take care not to endanger yourself or others. If it escapes, notify the police immediately.

Symptoms of rabies
• Fever, headache, sore throat and muscle pains are followed by pain or numbness at the site of the healed bite.
• One or two days later the patient becomes restless and agitated.
• Confusion and hallucinations develop.
• Muscle spasms, stiffness of the neck and back, convulsions and areas of paralysis may also develop.
• Excess saliva and difficulty in swallowing produce foaming at the mouth.
• Painful throat spasms develop, with a reaction of terror on trying to swallow liquids.

Rib fractures

A hard blow to the chest, or a heavy fall, can fracture a rib, causing a sharp chest pain when the casualty breathes deeply or coughs.

A casualty who has only a simple rib fracture can be taken to hospital in a car, preferably in the back seat.

But there may be a serious chest injury if:
• The casualty is unable to breathe properly, and seems to be suffocating.
• Red frothy blood comes from his mouth.
• He becomes restless and thirsty.

If the casualty shows any of these symptoms, call an ambulance at once (see also *Chest injuries*, page 68).

Recognising a simple rib fracture

A person with a simple rib fracture will feel extremely tender around the site of the injury. The area will swell. Pain will increase with movement, including deep breathing or coughing. And there may be a crackling sound from the ribs.

But he is not likely to feel ill and will have no difficulty in breathing, even though the breaths may be shallow to avoid pain.
• Treat a fractured rib by putting the arm on the injured side in an arm sling (see facing page), and then taking the casualty to the Accident and Emergency Department of your local hospital.

Shock

Some injuries can cause the casualty to become generally weak – or even unconscious – in a condition known as shock, or traumatic shock.

The condition arises because the blood supply, carrying oxygen to all parts of the body, slows down. This may be because the heartbeat has become weak – from extreme pain or distress, say – or because serious bleeding, vomiting, diarrhoea or widespread burns have reduced the amount of body fluid, so that there is not enough blood to supply all the cells.

Shock may be immediate – as when someone receives bad news – or it may develop over two or three hours. And it can kill. It is not the same as the feeling of horror that occurs after an injury or other unpleasant experience, from which the victim may recover quickly.

The warning signs

Faced with the lack of adequate blood supply, the body reacts by concentrating the remaining supply on the vital organs – the heart, brain and kidneys. The less important areas, such as the muscles and skin, go without adequate blood, and the casualty weakens and becomes pale.

The condition also produces other effects:
• Faintness and giddiness.
• A feeling of anxiousness and restlessness.
• Nausea and perhaps vomiting.
• Thirst.
• Sweating.
• Shallow, rapid breathing, with yawning and sighing.
• A weak pulse which is fast and may be irregular.

What you should do

• Lay the casualty down with the head low, and treat any obvious injury or condition which may be causing the shock.
• Comfort and reassure the casualty.
• Loosen clothing at the neck, chest and waist to assist breathing and blood circulation.
• Ask someone to call an ambulance.
• If possible, raise the legs on a folded coat or cushion to direct the blood to the brain.
• Keep the casualty warm with a coat or blanket. But do not use a hot-water bottle, as it will bring the blood to the skin and away from the vital organs.
• If the casualty complains of thirst, moisten his lips, but do not give him anything to drink or eat, as it may cause delay in giving an anaesthetic in hospital.
• Do not move the casualty unnecessarily. It will increase the shock.
• Do not allow the casualty to smoke, as it may hinder breathing.
• If breathing becomes difficult, if the casualty seems about to vomit, or if he becomes unconscious, put him in the recovery position (see page 136).
• If breathing stops, begin artificial respiration immediately (see page 50).

Slings

Once an injury to a hand, arm or chest has been treated, put a sling on the casualty to give the damaged area support.

Slings are normally made from a triangular bandage – a piece of calico that can be bought ready-made from a chemist. But you can make your own with any piece of material about a yard (1m) square, either cut or folded diagonally. Alternatively, there are a number of ways in which you can improvise a sling.

When to use an arm sling

For a wound on the arm, and for some rib injuries, a conventional arm sling is usually used. But it is effective only if the casualty can stand or sit. It supports the forearm across the chest, with the hand slightly higher than the elbow and the fingers exposed.

When to use an elevation sling

A hand that must be raised to control bleeding

MAKING AN ARM SLING

1 *Get the casualty to support the injured arm with his hand. Place an open triangular bandage between the chest and forearm, its point stretching well beyond the elbow. Take the upper end over the shoulder on the uninjured side, around the back of the neck to the front of the injured side.*

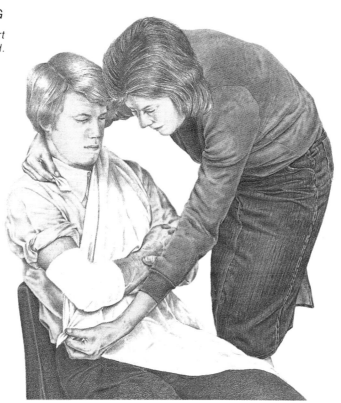

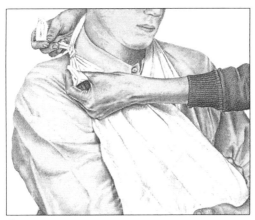

2 *Take the lower end of the bandage up over the hand and forearm and tie it in the hollow just above the collarbone. The tips of the fingers should just protrude from the sling.*

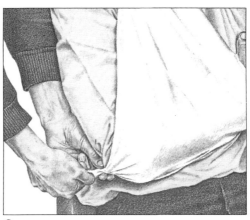

3 *Pin the point near the elbow, or twist and tuck it in. If the arm was bandaged before the sling went on, check that the nail beds are not turning blue. If they are, loosen the bandage.*

can be supported in an elevation sling. This sling is also used for complicated chest injuries or a broken collarbone. And it will support an arm for a casualty who cannot stand or sit.

Improvising a sling
If no triangular bandage is available, and you cannot make one, there are several ways to improvise a sling. Good support can be given, for example, by turning up the bottom edge of the casualty's jacket and pinning it firmly to the jacket at chest level. The arm will be well supported inside the fold.

Alternatively, suspend the injured arm from a belt, tie or scarf which is tied around the casualty's neck.

The sleeve of the injured arm can be pinned to the front of the jacket, or the casualty's hand can be pushed inside the fastened jacket at chest level, supported by a button or zip.

IMPROVISING A SLING

1 *If you do not have a triangular bandage, improvise a sling from a narrow scarf, tie or roller bandage. Wrap the strip of cloth once around the casualty's wrist on the injured arm, or make a loop round the wrist.*

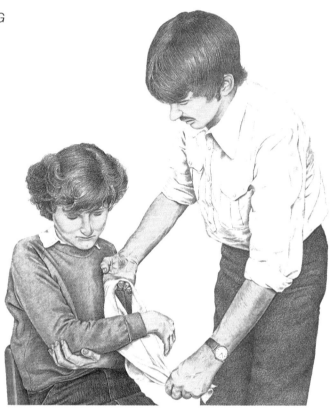

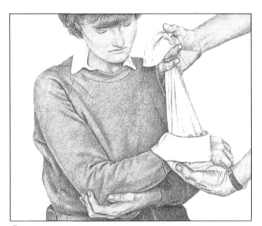

2 *Put one end of the sling over the casualty's shoulder on the uninjured side. Then bring the other end across the chest and around the casualty's neck to the uninjured shoulder.*

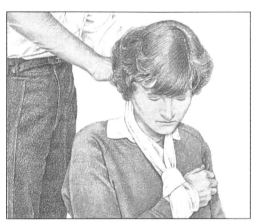

3 *Tie the ends in the hollow above the collarbone on the uninjured side. The hand should normally be just above elbow level, but at shoulder level for hand or forearm wounds.*

MAKING AN ELEVATION SLING

1 *Raise the injured arm – or the arm on the injured side, in the case of a chest injury – so that the hand rests on the opposite shoulder. If possible, get the casualty to hold it in place while you make the sling.*

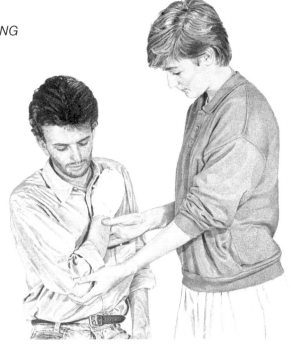

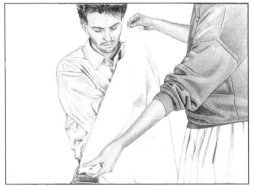

2 *Put one end of the base of the sling over the casualty's shoulder on the uninjured side, with the point extended well beyond the elbow. The sling should then be hanging over the arm.*

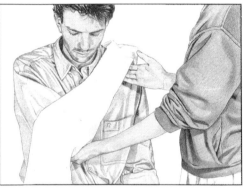

3 *Gently push the base of the sling under the hand, forearm and elbow of the injured arm, so that the lower end of the base is hanging free below the elbow.*

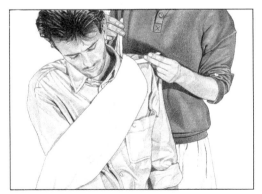

4 *Bring the lower end around the casualty's back on the injured side. Join the two ends of the sling together at the shoulder on the uninjured side, and tie them together.*

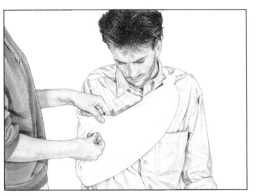

5 *Fold in the point and fasten it with a pin, or twist and tuck it in. If the arm has been bandaged, check that the nail beds are not turning blue. If they are, loosen the bandage.*

Slipped disc

A disc is a shock-absorbing layer between each of the vertebrae in the spine. A slipped disc is caused by the gradual degeneration and softening of these discs after the age of 25.

When a disc slips, its soft core protrudes from its fibrous casing and presses on one of the nerves leading from the spinal cord. This causes pain, which can be severe.

Warning signs

Most slipped discs occur in the lower back and the pain is usually felt there first. The pain may also spread down around the buttocks and hips and along one or both legs.

The pain often starts suddenly just after you have lifted something heavy or have straightened up after bending. But sometimes it comes on gradually or only becomes severe after several mild attacks.

The pain may be made worse by bending, getting up after sitting, coughing or straining. It is easier when lying flat, standing or walking.

The lower leg and the outer foot may also become numb.

What you should do

• Lie down on a firm flat bed which does not sag. If necessary, get somebody to put a wide board the full length of the bed under the mattress. Alternatively, get him to put the mattress on the floor. On no account try to move anything heavy yourself.
• Take painkillers, such as aspirin or paracetamol, in recommended doses.
• A hot-water bottle or heat lamp applied to the painful area may give relief.
• If the pain is not relieved after a day or two of rest, call the doctor. The doctor may confirm the diagnosis with X-rays, and perhaps arrange physiotherapy. Some cases may require immobilisation in a plaster jacket or corset.

Manipulation may help but can be dangerous, and should be considered only after an X-ray and discussion with the doctor.

Many mild attacks get better in a few days and never recur. About 75 per cent of more severe attacks recur within five years, but may then get better.

Avoiding a slipped disc

The risk of a slipped disc can be reduced by keeping the back straight and bending at the knees when lifting, and holding the weight close to you. Particularly avoid lifting and twisting at the same time. These precautions are especially important to people who have already suffered a slipped disc.

Smoke inhalation

If someone is being suffocated by smoke in a burning building, get him out as quickly as possible. But do not go into a burning building without telling someone, or if it will place you in danger.

Protect yourself by tying a towel or piece of thick cloth – preferably wet – around your nose and mouth. As you move through the building, keep low, and reduce the fire risk by closing windows and doors behind you (see *Rescuing someone from a fire*, page 148).

Inhaled smoke can irritate the throat, causing it to contract in a sudden spasm and close the airway. So someone found in a smoke-filled room may be unconscious and his breathing may have stopped.

Smoke from plastic foam in upholstered chairs and sofas is highly poisonous and can kill within two minutes.

What you should do

• Drag the victim away from the smoke (see page 113).
• Once clear of danger, if the victim is unconscious but breathing normally, put him in the recovery position (see page 136).
• If breathing has stopped or is very difficult, begin mouth-to-mouth respiration as soon as possible (see page 50).
• Get someone to telephone 999 and ask for an ambulance.

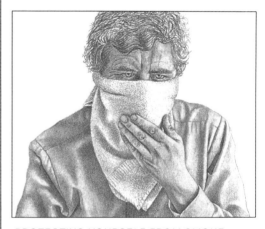

PROTECTING YOURSELF FROM SMOKE
Cover your mouth and nose with a piece of thick, wet cloth before entering a smoke-filled room. Keep close to the floor where the air should be clear, as hot, smoky air will rise.

Snakebite

Britain's one venomous snake, the adder, has a bite that is rarely fatal, but needs hospital treatment. Fear induced by the bite can sometimes cause more harm than the bite itself.

The victim of a snakebite should remain still and keep the area of the bite below the level of the heart. Movement will increase the circulation of blood around the body and so speed up the rate at which the venom is absorbed.

The victim should, if possible, be carried to an ambulance or car and taken to hospital.

In hot countries, where there are many venomous snakes, you should try to identify the species by remembering its size, colouring and skin pattern. This will help the doctor to decide if an anti-venom serum should be given. In Britain, a bite may come from a pet snake. The snake's owner should be able to tell the hospital which species it belongs to.

Warning signs
- Sharp pain and swelling around the bite.
- One or two small puncture wounds.
- The victim's vision may become disturbed.
- Nausea and possibly vomiting.
- Breathing may become difficult.

When a serious condition develops
- If the victim becomes unconscious, but is breathing normally, put her in the recovery position (see page 136) until help arrives.
- If breathing stops, begin mouth-to-mouth respiration immediately (see page 50).
- If the victim has been extremely frightened and then becomes weak, with skin that is pale and grey, she may be suffering from shock. Treat as described on page 120.
- Do not try to suck the venom out of the bite or cut the wound to let out blood. Both actions will increase blood circulation around the bite.
- Do not apply a tourniquet. It can cause serious damage to the limb.

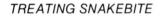

TREATING SNAKEBITE

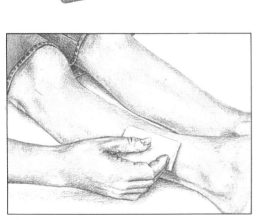

1 *Rest the victim in a comfortable position, and reassure her that a snakebite in Britain is unlikely to be serious. Even in tropical countries deaths from snakebite poison are rare. A greater danger comes from fear which may bring on shock.*

2 *Remove venom from around the bite by wiping outwards from the wound. Do not raise the injured limb. Apply a pad or sterile dressing to the wound and keep the limb still.*

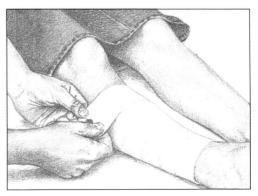

3 *Bandage the wound firmly if possible, with a crepe or two-way stretch bandage. Get someone to call 999 or the local emergency service. Try not to leave the victim alone.*

Splinters

Splinters of wood, metal or glass embedded in the skin can cause infection if they are not carefully, and cleanly, removed.

Do not try to remove a very large splinter, or one that is buried below the surface of the skin. In either case go to your doctor or to the Accident and Emergency Department of your local hospital.

Small, visible splinters can usually be removed with tweezers, but maintain hygienic conditions. If your hands are dirty, wash them before starting. Do not cough or sneeze on the wound, as germs may penetrate and infect it.

Sterilise the tweezers by passing the ends through a flame from a match, cigarette lighter or gas ring. Let them cool for a few moments but do not wipe off any soot, or touch the ends of the tweezers.

Do not probe the wound to get to the splinter. If it is deeply embedded, get medical help. Otherwise you may only push the splinter farther in, making it even harder to remove.

THE RISK OF TETANUS

A piece of splinter left in a wound, or a dirty splinter even if it has been removed, may lead to tetanus. This is a dangerous infection which causes acute muscle contractions, particularly in the jaw, giving the disease its other name of lockjaw.

Puncture wounds, burns, animal bites and road and agricultural accidents all carry a risk of tetanus. So anyone who suffers such a wound and who has not had a tetanus inoculation in the past five years should see a doctor to get a booster injection.

A person who contracts tetanus at first feels unwell and may have stiffness and pain in the jaw, difficulty in swallowing, raised temperature, headache and sweating.

Stiffness of other muscles may occur, in which case there may be painful arching of the back and drawing down of the neck. Sudden muscle contractions may be brought on by noise or by touching the patient.

If you suspect tetanus, take the patient to the Accident and Emergency Department of your local hospital immediately.

Immunisation is the surest prevention for tetanus. Children are given three routine injections in their first year, with boosters on starting and leaving school. A routine booster is recommended every ten years (or five years for people working close to animals or the soil).

REMOVING A SPLINTER

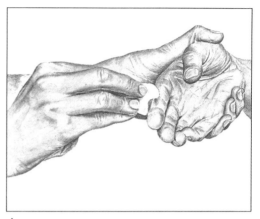

1 *Wash the skin around the splinter with warm, soapy water. Wipe downwards and outwards from the wound to avoid carrying dirt to it. Pat the skin dry with a clean towel.*

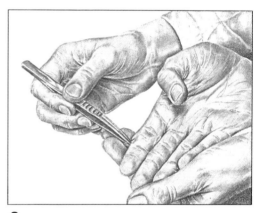

2 *Sterilise a pair of tweezers, then pull out the splinter directly in line with the way it went in. A magnifying glass may help. If it will not come out, get medical help.*

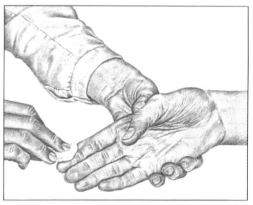

3 *When the splinter has been removed, wash the wound with a mild antiseptic and dry gently. Cover it with a plaster or sterile dressing. If it swells or becomes painful, get medical help.*

Splints

A person with a fractured bone should not be moved unless it is absolutely necessary (see page 112).

But if the ambulance is delayed, or you have to take the person to hospital yourself, the injured limb should be immobilised. The simplest way is to secure it to an uninjured part of the body with bandages – a technique known as body splinting.

To immobilise an arm, put it in a sling and then bandage it against the chest. A broken leg can be bandaged to the other leg, provided that plenty of padding is put between the ankles and knees to prevent chafing.

If the injured person has to be carried to safety, the fractured limb can be given greater support with a rigid splint, such as a tightly rolled blanket, a walking stick or a plank.

Any splint must be long enough to extend well beyond the joints above and below the fracture.

Do not remove clothes to apply a splint, and if possible add extra padding between splint and limb to make the casualty as comfortable as possible.

SECURING A FRACTURED ARM

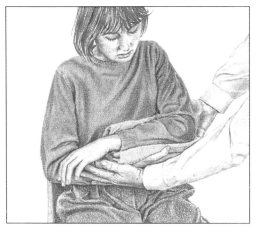

1 *If the arm will bend easily, place it across the chest and put some padding between the site of the fracture and the body. Do not bend the arm by force.*

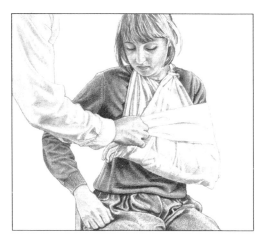

2 *Put on an arm sling (see page 121), and then strap the arm to the body with a piece of wide material around arm and chest. Tie off the strap on the uninjured side.*

SECURING AN ARM THAT WILL NOT BEND

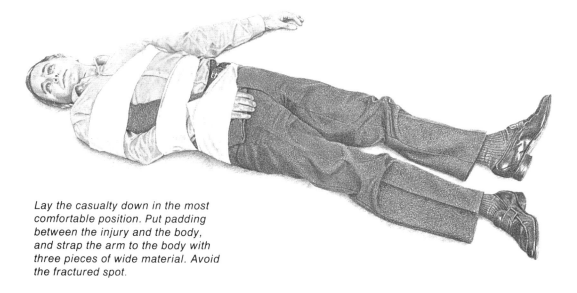

Lay the casualty down in the most comfortable position. Put padding between the injury and the body, and strap the arm to the body with three pieces of wide material. Avoid the fractured spot.

SPLINTING A FRACTURED ELBOW

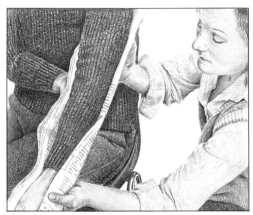

1 *If the elbow has been fractured, sit the casualty down and keep the arm straight. Fold a newspaper and place it along the arm.*

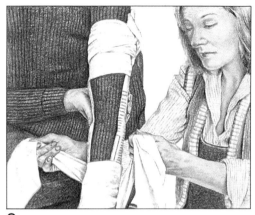

2 *Get the casualty to support the splint, and tie it in place with two bandages, one at the top of the splint and the other at the bottom.*

SECURING A FRACTURED LEG WITH BANDAGES

1 *A broken leg is most easily immobilised by bandaging it to the other leg. Move the uninjured leg to it, and put padding between the legs, especially at the knees and ankles.*

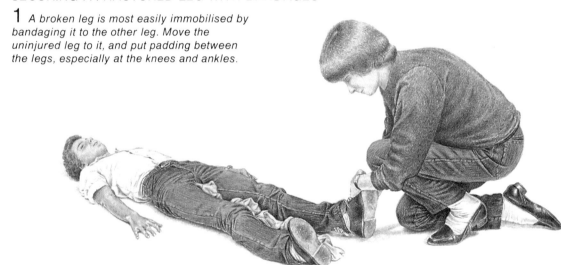

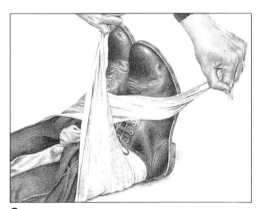

2 *Tie the feet together with a scarf or necktie in a figure of eight. Knot it on the outer edge of the shoe on the uninjured leg.*

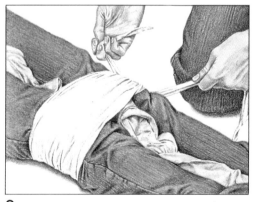

3 *Tie the knees together with a wide piece of material knotted on the uninjured side. Tie extra bandages above and below the fracture.*

A BLANKET SPLINT FOR A FRACTURED LEG

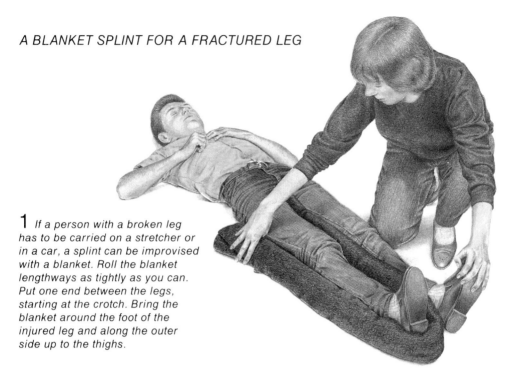

1 *If a person with a broken leg has to be carried on a stretcher or in a car, a splint can be improvised with a blanket. Roll the blanket lengthways as tightly as you can. Put one end between the legs, starting at the crotch. Bring the blanket around the foot of the injured leg and along the outer side up to the thighs.*

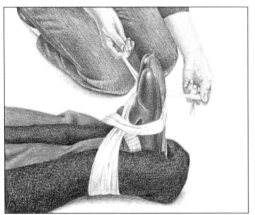

2 *Tie the feet and ankles together with a bandage or other piece of material in a figure of eight. Use a reef knot to tie it off.*

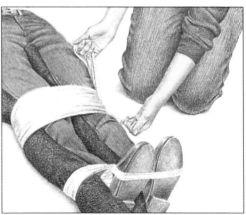

3 *Tie a wide piece of material around the casualty's knees, and knot the ends together on the uninjured side, again using a reef knot.*

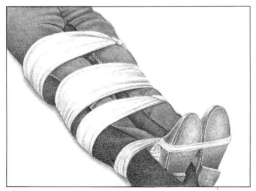

4 *Tie a third and fourth bandage above and below the site of the fracture.*

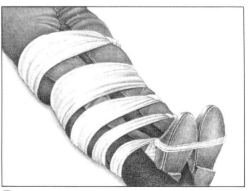

5 *Tie a fifth bandage around the thigh or calf, avoiding the fracture.*

129

Sports injuries

Two of the most common types of sports injuries are pulled muscles and sprained joints. The damage is similar in each case – tissue in the muscle or joint is torn and internal bleeding occurs, causing swelling and pain.

When one of these injuries occurs you should stop playing immediately, and rest. If you can use the injured part again in five minutes without pain, then it is safe to play on. But if the pain persists, you need treatment.

It is always possible that a bone has been broken, in which case go to the Accident and Emergency Department of the local hospital (see page 98). Suspect a broken bone if:
• The swollen part cannot be used.
• The swelling develops within minutes.
• The pain continues to be severe.

Treating a damaged muscle or joint

If the pain is not too severe and the swelling develops slowly it is usually safe to treat the injury without expert help.
• Put a cold compress on the injured area. Make the compress by putting ice cubes in a plastic bag and crushing them with a hammer or brick. Wrap the bag in a towel before applying it. Alternatively, use a cloth soaked in cold water and wrung out. The cold will cause the blood vessels to narrow and reduce bleeding.
• Bind the compress onto the injured part with a bandage and leave it for 20 to 30 minutes. The pressure also helps to close the blood vessels and slow the bleeding. But take care not to tie the bandage so tight as to cut off the circulation. If the person's fingers or toes become cold or tingle, loosen the bandage.
• At the same time, raise the injured area above the level of the heart for 30 minutes to an hour. This also slows the bleeding. Keep the limb raised as much as possible for the next 24 hours.
• If necessary, take aspirin or paracetamol in recommended doses to reduce pain the first night after an injury. But painkillers should never be used so that you can go on playing. Pain is a valuable warning sign.
• When the injured area has been free of pain for at least ten days, light exercise can be started again.
• If recovery is very slow, or if the problem recurs frequently, see your doctor.

When muscles stiffen up

The reason why muscles stiffen up is not fully understood, but a probable cause is that many small tears occur in the muscles. Also, during exercise pressure builds up inside the blood vessels in the muscles. Some of the fluid in which the blood cells are carried seeps out into the muscle fibres and builds up the pressure there, causing stiffness.

The best treatment is gentle exercise – easy swimming, for example – which helps the fluid to be reabsorbed. Careful warming up reduces stiffness, and so does 'winding down'. After hard exercise do not stop immediately; have a period of gentle exercise. Avoid wallowing in a hot bath after exercise. A quick shower and a brisk rub-down are much better.

Long-lasting injuries from overuse

Regular exercise often involves the repeated use of the same part of the body, and this can lead to the gradual development of painful injuries such as tennis elbow, golfer's shoulder and footballer's ankle.

To begin with, one part of the body aches towards the end of exercise or for a little while afterwards. Then, as the damage increases, the pain lasts longer after exercise and may occur at other times, perhaps when in bed. This type of injury needs expert attention. The first step is a period of rest, but if that does not help, see your doctor. You may be referred to a physiotherapist if you have pain in muscles or joints, or to a chiropodist for aching feet and heels.

How to avoid sports injuries

Many sports injuries can be prevented altogether by careful preparation, which includes proper training for the sport and warming up immediately before a game.

Take lessons to learn the correct way of doing

HOW DANGEROUS IS YOUR SPORT?

The most dangerous sport widely played in Britain is rugby. It has a higher rate of injury than soccer, and a greater number of broken bones and injuries to the face. Soccer injuries usually affect the legs.

In cricket and hockey, a major cause of injury is the hard ball hitting a player on the head. In squash, tennis and badminton, pulled muscles and sprains are the most common injuries, but eye injuries are also common in squash.

Most deaths in sport result from injuries to the head and spine – when being thrown from a motorcycle or falling while rock climbing, for example.

The following list gives the rate of injuries per 100 players each year in 16 sports.

Rugby	4.9	Squash	2.0
Skiing	4.9	Tennis	2.0
Soccer	3.2	Fencing	1.8
Gymnastics	2.9	Badminton	1.4
Hockey	2.9	Cycling	1.4
Cricket	2.4	Basketball	1.4
Judo	2.1	Golf	0.5
Rowing	2.1	Swimming	0.3

things from the very beginning. Faults in technique which may cause injury, such as an awkward golf swing, only get more difficult to eradicate as time goes on. To keep fit and avoid stiffening up, take exercise regularly, not in one burst on a Saturday afternoon.

Using the right kit and equipment also cuts down the risk of injury. This is particularly important in sports such as skiing and rock climbing, but in almost every form of exercise problems can be reduced if you wear the right shoes – broad enough tennis shoes, for example, or jogging shoes with well-padded heels that prevent you from jarring the spine.

DO'S AND DON'TS ABOUT SPORTS INJURIES

An unconscious player	DO roll an unconscious player into the recovery position (page 136).	DON'T lay an unconscious person flat on his face.
	DO remove foreign material (chewing gum, broken dentures, broken teeth, grass) from the mouth to prevent choking.	
Damaged bones	DO support the injured area with padding, a splint or bandage.	DON'T attempt to manipulate a fractured bone or dislocation.
Injuries to the face	DO sit a player upright and press a cold pad to a black eye – which results from bleeding into the soft tissue around the eyeball.	DON'T waste time and money on applying a raw steak to a black eye. This is no more effective than using a cold pad.
	DO treat a nosebleed by squeezing the soft part of the nose between finger and thumb and breathing through your mouth for 15 minutes.	DON'T continue with the treatment if the nosebleed lasts for more than 30 minutes. Either contact your doctor or go to a hospital.
	DO splash water with your hand on your eye if you get dirt or mud in it.	DON'T add antiseptic to the water used on the affected eye.
Cuts and abrasions	DO thoroughly clean and disinfect an abrasion caused by the skin being scraped along a hard surface, such as the ground.	DON'T forget to protect yourself against tetanus (lockjaw) – which can arise from a simple scratch – with an antitetanus injection. Booster injections should be given every ten years.
	DO see a doctor if particles of dirt remain in the abrasion after cleaning. A partly cleaned abrasion can result in an ugly scar – especially if the face is affected.	DON'T use old creams or harsh disinfectants on wounds; they can infect the cut or destroy tissues.
Caring for the feet	DO wash and carefully dry your feet immediately after sport to prevent athlete's foot – a fungus that affects sweaty skin.	DON'T soak your feet in very hot water.
Stiff muscles	DO take a quick warm shower or bath – followed by a cold shower or dip – to ease stiffness. Gentle exercise also helps.	DON'T wallow in hot water after sport or exercise.
		DON'T sit around 'resting'.

Sprains and strains

Injuries to the joints and muscles – known as sprains and strains – are common and can be extremely painful.

A sprain occurs in a joint when a ligament – the flexible tissue that holds the bones together – is wrenched or torn. A strain occurs when a muscle is overstretched or torn.

Treatment for both injuries includes a cold compress, raising the injured limb and firm bandaging. All three techniques are aimed at restricting internal bleeding from the damaged tissues.

To make a cold compress, put some ice cubes into a plastic bag, knot the opening of the bag and crush the ice with a hammer or brick. Then wrap the bag of ice in a towel and apply it to

the injury. Leave it in place for 20 to 30 minutes. If no ice is available, soak a small towel or some other piece of cloth in cold water and squeeze out the excess, then wrap the towel round the injured area. Keep the towel cold by re-wetting it as necessary.

A cold compress works by chilling and constricting the blood vessels around the injury, thus limiting the swelling caused by internal bleeding. To be effective, though, the compress needs to be applied within about 30 minutes.

After about 30 minutes, most of the swelling will already have taken place and the compress will no longer be of much help. In these circumstances raise the limb and bandage it firmly for support instead.

TREATING A SPRAINED ANKLE

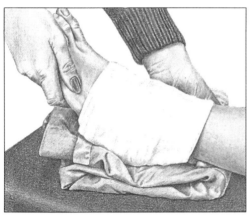

1 *Remove the shoe and raise the foot above the level of the heart. If the sprain has occurred within the past 15 to 30 minutes, apply a cold compress to the injured joint and bandage it in place for 20 to 30 minutes.*

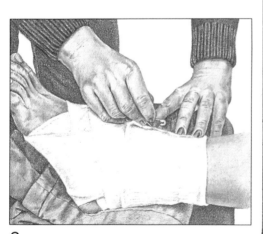

2 *After removing the compress, bandage the joint firmly. For an ankle joint, make one turn around the ankle, then go over the instep, under the foot, back across the instep and around the ankle again several times.*

TREATING A STRAINED MUSCLE

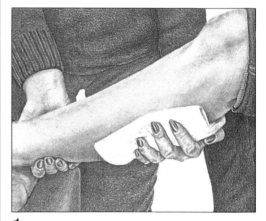

1 *Put the casualty in the most comfortable possible position, with the injured limb above the level of the heart. Apply a cold compress to the strained muscle, and bandage it in place for 20 to 30 minutes.*

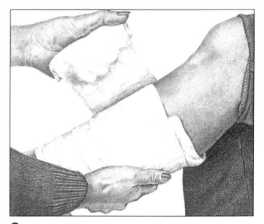

2 *Remove the compress and bandage the area firmly, but not so tightly as to stop circulation. The muscle may swell, causing pain if the bandage is too tight. Support a strained arm in an arm sling (see page 121).*

A sprained joint

The ankle is the joint most often affected by sprains, but the wrist, elbow, knee, hip and shoulder can also suffer.

A severe sprain can be extremely painful and is hard to distinguish from a fractured bone. If you are in any doubt, treat the injury as a fracture and get medical help (see *Fractures*, page 98, and *Splints*, page 127).

An ankle sprain occurs when a foot turns suddenly while walking or running – one of the reasons why boots (which help to support the ankle joints) are recommended for people walking in rough, stony country.

If a wrist, elbow or shoulder is sprained, support it in an arm sling after treatment with both a cold compress and firm bandaging (see *Bandages*, page 56, and *Slings*, page 121).

There are three main symptoms of sprains:
• Pain when moving the joint.
• Swelling of the joint, followed later by discoloration of the skin.
• Tenderness of the area over the torn ligament.

A strained muscle

A muscle may become overstretched or torn by sudden, unaccustomed exertion, perhaps when lifting a heavy weight. It can also be torn during a fall. If the injury occurs while playing sport it is known as a 'pulled muscle', and usually affects the calf or thigh (see page 130).

The main symptoms are:
• Sudden, sharp pain in the muscle.
• Stiffness or cramp developing in the muscle.
• Swelling of the area.
• Possibly discoloration of the skin.

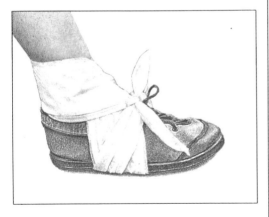

SUPPORTING AN ANKLE IN AN EMERGENCY
If you sprain an ankle during a country walk, leave your shoe and sock on, and bind a figure-of-eight bandage over the shoe or boot. This may give enough support to get you home.

Stab wounds

A nail sticking out of a piece of wood, or any other sharp object such as a bicycle spoke or needle, can cause a potentially serious wound.

On the surface the wound may look so small as not to be worth worrying about, but it may go deep into the flesh, carrying dirt or germs with it. If the wound becomes infected, the infection can spread to other parts of the body, causing serious illness and even death.

A stab wound can also cause serious internal injury to blood vessels and nerves.

Treat all stab wounds as serious. Stop any bleeding, dress the wound and take the casualty to your doctor or to the Accident and Emergency Department of your local hospital.

If the object which caused the wound remains embedded in the flesh, do not try to remove it. It could be helping to plug the wound, and pulling it out could make the bleeding much worse. Instead, cover the object with a ring-pad (see page 58) or the bottom half of a paper cup, so that it will not be forced deeper by the dressing while the casualty is being taken to hospital.

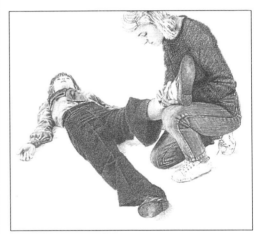

DEALING WITH A STAB WOUND
Stop any bleeding by pressing around the wound with a clean pad, or your bare hands. Do not try to remove any object embedded in the wound. Raise the injured area above the level of the heart to help to stem the bleeding. Bandage the wound and get medical help.

Stroke

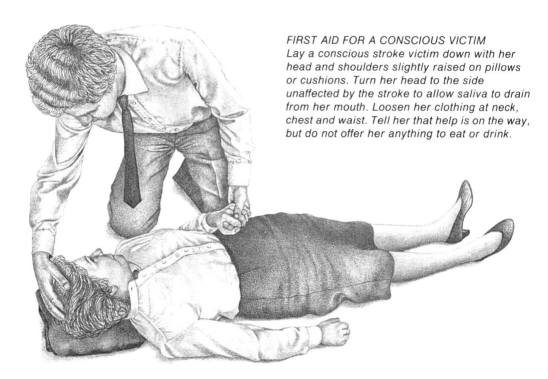

FIRST AID FOR A CONSCIOUS VICTIM
Lay a conscious stroke victim down with her head and shoulders slightly raised on pillows or cushions. Turn her head to the side unaffected by the stroke to allow saliva to drain from her mouth. Loosen her clothing at neck, chest and waist. Tell her that help is on the way, but do not offer her anything to eat or drink.

A person suffering a stroke may become weak or paralysed down one side of the body, including the face, arm and leg.

Alternatively, the victim may have difficulty in speaking or swallowing, with only slight weakness in the limbs.

The victim may also suffer confusion, drowsiness and involuntary urination. The symptoms can resemble drunkenness.

A severe stroke will cause unconsciousness.

What you should do

• If the victim is conscious, lay him or her down, with head and shoulders slightly raised on pillows or cushions.
• Turn her head to one side to allow saliva to drain from the mouth.
• Call the patient's doctor, or telephone 999 and ask for an ambulance.
• Loosen clothing around the patient's neck, chest and waist to help blood circulation and breathing.
• Do not give her anything to eat or drink.
• If the patient becomes unconscious, put her in the recovery position (see page 136).

The after-effects of a stroke

A person who suffers a stroke that paralyses the right side of the body may also be unable to speak, write, read or understand speech.

If the paralysis is on the left, the person may lose the awareness of the left half of the body.

Recovery from a stroke may be complete, with little risk of recurrence; but more usually – especially in elderly patients – the arm and, to a lesser extent, the leg on the affected side of the body will remain disabled.

A massive stroke, particularly in an older patient, is grave; but if the patient survives the first month, a considerable amount of activity can often be restored.

The hospital will arrange a course of physiotherapy aimed at restoring the patient to as much activity as possible so that he or she can return home.

Relatives, with the help of their family doctor, district nurses and hospital out-patient treatment, can make a large contribution to recovery. In the early days they can learn how to exercise the patient's affected limbs to prevent the muscles and joints from becoming stiff.

They can also help by speaking slowly or repeating things that seem not to be understood. They should listen carefully if speech is poor, and spend time talking to the patient, looking at pictures or photographs and encouraging him in his former interests.

Many areas have day hospitals which the patient can attend to ease the burden on relatives and at the same time receive additional therapeutic help.

Hospitals and local authority social services departments can provide aids for use in the home, including special beds, hoists and walking frames. Ask hospital social workers and the local council about which aids are most appropriate. To reduce the risk of further strokes, the patient should stop smoking, watch his or her weight and follow any treatment prescribed for high blood pressure.

Sunburn

If sunburn is very severe and distressing, take the patient to a doctor who may prescribe a cream to give relief.

See a doctor also if the patient has a headache, nausea or a high temperature, because he may be suffering from heat stroke as well as sunburn (see page 106).

If the sunburn is out of all proportion to the time the skin was exposed to the sun, the patient may be suffering from a condition called photosensitivity, which can be brought on by some medicines. The patient should see his doctor, who may prescribe an alternative medicine.

Treating mild sunburn

The symptoms of sunburn can range from skin that turns pink and feels rather hot to skin that becomes red, swollen, blistered and extremely painful.

Reasonably mild sunburn can be treated at home without seeing a doctor.

• Keep the skin cool with calamine lotion or cold compresses. Make the compress by soaking a towel or other cloth in cold water and squeezing out the excess. Or put ice cubes in a plastic bag, knot the opening of the bag and crush the ice with a hammer or brick. Wrap the bag in a cloth before putting it on the skin.

• Antihistamine creams are rarely worth using; they have little effect.

• Leave blistered skin exposed to the air.

• Take aspirin or paracetamol to relieve the pain.

• Avoid clothes that rub the sore area.

• Do not allow further exposure to the sun until the symptoms have disappeared.

How to avoid sunburn

Sunburn is caused by the ultraviolet rays of the sun. Fair-skinned people, who have little pigment in the skin, burn more easily than people with dark skin.

• To prevent sunburn, avoid overexposure to the sun on the first day of a holiday, particularly if you are fair skinned. Expose the skin for only 30 minutes the first day, increasing by 30 minutes each day until you have developed a suntan which will give protection.

• Remember that light cloud does not stop the sun's rays from burning.

• Use a suntan lotion or cream for protection. Most of them wash off easily, so put more on after swimming. Even if you do not swim they need to be renewed every two hours. Filter-type sun-screens may contain substances that cause skin reactions, so follow the instructions on the container.

• Keep small children covered with a shirt for most of the time during the first days of a holiday. Increase their exposure gradually.

• Remember that you can be burnt even while feeling cool in the water.

• Do not expect artificial skin-tanning creams to give protection.

Tooth injuries

All injuries to the teeth should be checked as soon as possible by a dentist or hospital dental department. If there are serious injuries to the mouth, the immediate aim is to ensure that the victim can breathe properly.

• Clear broken teeth and blood from the mouth with your fingers.

• If the casualty is conscious and has no other serious injuries, sit him in a chair with his head tilted forwards over a bowl or basin.

• Telephone 999 and ask for an ambulance, or drive the casualty to your local hospital. He should travel sitting up, leaning over the bowl.

• Never allow a person who is bleeding from the mouth to lie on his back, because he may choke on the blood.

When a tooth has been knocked out

If a tooth is knocked out completely, there may be profuse bleeding from the socket.

• Make a pad slightly larger than the socket from sterile gauze or other clean material. The pad should project slightly above the level of the surrounding teeth.

• Get the casualty to put it over the socket and bite on it firmly for 10 minutes, spitting out any blood that leaks through.

• If the bleeding does not stop, repeat for another 10 minutes.

• If the bleeding still does not stop, telephone your dentist and ask for emergency treatment, or go to your local hospital.

Saving a knocked-out tooth

It is sometimes possible to save a tooth that has been knocked out of its socket.

The roots must be kept moist with saliva, so suck a piece of clean gauze or cloth until it is thoroughly damp, or get the casualty to do so. Wrap the tooth in the gauze and put it in a matchbox or other container to take to the hospital or dentist.

If you get toothache

If you develop toothache at night or during a weekend when you cannot contact your dentist, look in the Yellow Pages of a telephone directory for a dentist who operates an emergency service (though fees for such services can be high). Alternatively, ask the Accident and Emergency department of a hospital if they know a dentist who can help, or ask the nearest police station or chemist.

• While you are waiting for a dentist, relieve the pain by dabbing a little oil of cloves (available from chemists) on the sore area, and by taking painkillers such as aspirin in recommended doses.

• Try also holding in your mouth a mouthful of ice-cold water or a mouthful of hot, salty water (one teaspoon of salt in a glass of water). Hold the water in your mouth for at least five minutes, spitting it out and renewing it as necessary, and repeat the treatment every 2–3 hours.

Unconsciousness

A person who has become unconscious is in danger of choking to death if he or she is left lying face up.

Vomit, blood or saliva may block the top of the windpipe, or the base of the tongue may slide back over the windpipe.

Normal reflexes do not work properly when people become unconscious. So they may not cough or turn over if something blocks their airway, as they would do automatically if they were asleep.

If an unconscious person is breathing normally, put her in the recovery position. This is a life-saving technique and takes priority over other treatment. An exception is if you suspect that the casualty has back or neck injuries, in which case she should not be moved at all (see page 55).

If the casualty is particularly heavy, it may be necessary to get someone else to help you by pushing while you pull.

If an unconscious person has to be carried on a stretcher, or if she is in a confined space, a modified version of the recovery position is used. In this case a rolled blanket is used to prop up one side of the body, rather than a bent arm and leg.

If the unconscious person is not breathing, you must begin artificial respiration immediately (see page 50). In any case get someone

IS THE CASUALTY BREATHING?

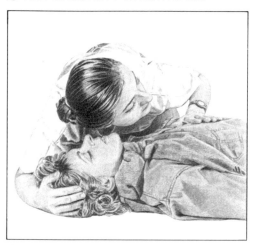

1 *Put your ear to the casualty's nose and mouth and listen for the sound of breathing. Watch the chest to see if it rises and falls, or rest your hand lightly on it to feel for movement.*

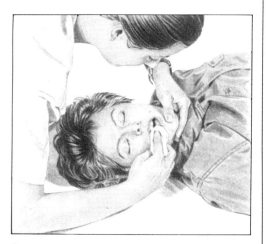

2 *If the casualty is not breathing but a neck pulse is present (see page 52), start artificial respiration (see page 50). If she is breathing, clear the mouth of foreign matter.*

THE RECOVERY POSITION

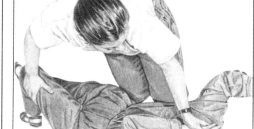

1 *Kneel beside the casualty. Tilt her head back and lift her chin to open the airway. Straighten her legs. Place casualty's nearer arm at right angles to body, elbow bent, palm of hand uppermost.*

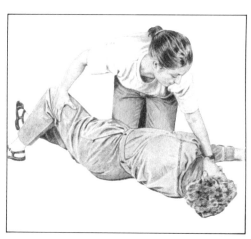

2 *Bring the arm farthest from you across the casualty's chest. Place the hand, with the palm outwards, against the casualty's nearest cheek, and hold it there.*

to telephone 999 and ask for an ambulance or, if nobody is available, do it yourself at the first opportunity. Anyone who has been unconscious, even for a short time, should receive immediate medical treatment.

Handle any serious wound gently while arranging the casualty. Once in the recovery position, the casualty can be helped by having clothing at the neck, chest and waist loosened. Injuries can be treated while you wait for expert help to arrive.

Do not leave an unconscious person alone, and do not give her anything to eat or drink, even if she regains consciousness (see also *What to do if someone collapses*, page 207).

Three stages of unconsciousness

Unconsciousness is not always total insensibility. There are three stages, and a person may go through all three or remain in one. The three stages are:

• Drowsiness, in which the victim is easily roused for a few moments, but then passes back into a sleep-like state. She may be able to give reasonably coherent answers to questions you ask her about her condition.

• Stupor, in which the victim does not react to questions easily or does so incoherently, giving the impression of being drunk.

• Coma, in which the victim cannot be roused at all, and is motionless and silent.

WHILE YOU WAIT FOR HELP

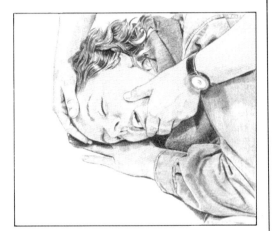

3 *With your other hand, pull on casualty's further knee, keeping her foot flat on the ground. Roll casualty towards you and onto her side, preventing her rolling too far with your knees and supporting her head.*

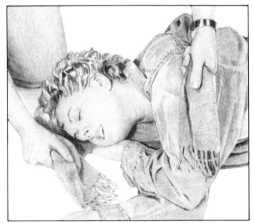

1 *Once the casualty is safely in the recovery position, loosen any tight clothing at the neck, chest and waist to assist breathing and blood circulation. Provide fresh air by opening a window or door.*

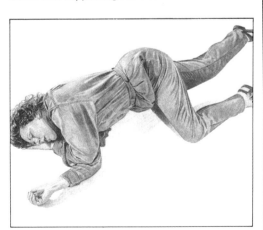

4 *Again tilt casualty's head back to ensure airway is clear. Adjust hand so that head is well supported. Adjust uppermost leg to keep thigh and knee at right angles. Check breathing and pulse regularly.*

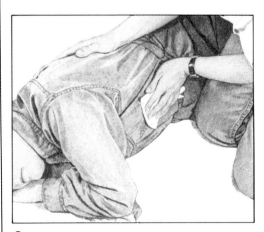

2 *Check for any other injuries and stop any bleeding (see page 60). Get someone to telephone for an ambulance. Then check to see if the casualty is carrying a treatment card – for diabetes, for example.*

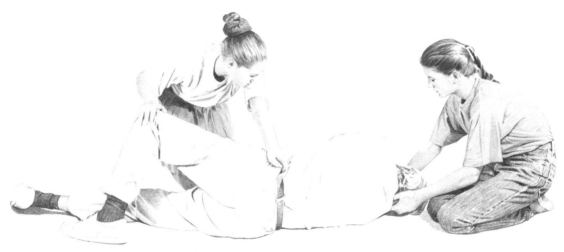

HOW TO TURN A HEAVY PERSON
Use both arms to do the turning, by gripping the unconscious
person at the hip with one hand while pulling up his knee with the other
(above). If possible get someone else to support the head while you
turn the casualty. Alternatively, get the other person to kneel on the far
side of the casualty facing you (below) and to push while you pull.

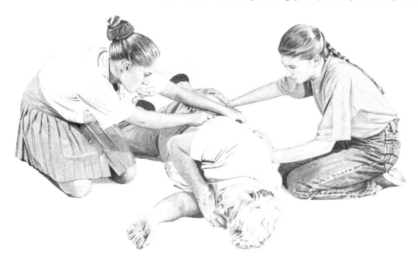

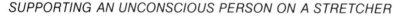

SUPPORTING AN UNCONSCIOUS PERSON ON A STRETCHER

Use a modified version of the recovery position
if you are carrying an unconscious person on
a stretcher or if she is in some other confined
space. Put a rolled blanket or coat under the
side towards which the casualty is facing.

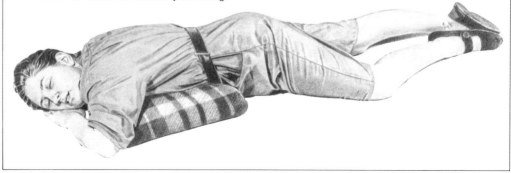

Vertigo

An unpleasant feeling of giddiness, as though the patient's head is moving when it is actually still, usually has a cause related to the ear.

The giddiness may be accompanied by nausea and deafness, and also by flickering of the eyes – a condition called nystagmus.

Vertigo can arise from several different medical conditions.
- An injury to the head.
- Ménière's disease and labyrinthitis, two ailments that disturb the hearing and also the balance of the inner ear.
- High blood pressure.
- A blockage of the blood vessels leading to the brain.
- Travel sickness.
- Overbreathing – a condition in which the patient breathes harder and faster than normal, usually brought on by pain, anxiety or sudden changes of mood.

What you should do
The patient should lie down quietly and rest until the attack ends. The length of an attack can range from seconds to hours.

Consult a doctor if:
- The attacks recur.
- There is severe vomiting.
- Deafness develops.

The doctor may prescribe drugs to relieve the symptoms, but even without treatment a person with recurring vertigo may recover spontaneously after several months.

Some elderly people suffer from vertigo without a treatable cause being found.

Positional vertigo, which is felt when the head is in certain positions, may continue to occur.

Whooping cough

A child who has a cold with a runny nose and bouts of excessive coughing may be in the early stages of whooping cough.

As the disease develops the cough will become worse, mainly at night. A few days after the cold begins, the 'whoop' will start – a sudden noisy intake of breath at the end of a coughing spasm. Vomiting may also occur after the coughing.

What you should do
Whooping cough is a serious disease that can lead to pneumonia and to severe dehydration if fluid loss from the vomiting is not controlled. So notify your doctor as soon as you suspect that a child has the disease.

The doctor may prescribe antibiotics for the patient and also for other children in the family. These do not cure whooping cough, but may prevent it from spreading to other people. In severe cases the patient will be sent to hospital for treatment.

While nursing the patient at home, provide extra drinks to make up for fluid lost by vomiting.

Proprietary cough medicines from the chemist may help the cough.

Do not expose the patient to cigarette smoke – it will make the cough worse.

Whooping cough may last for a period ranging from three weeks to as long as four months.

How to prevent whooping cough
The disease is caused by bacteria which are spread by droplets in the air breathed out by an infected child.

Because whooping cough is more dangerous than the risks of immunisation, all children should have a course of three injections (usually with diphtheria and tetanus vaccine) in the first year of life.

Because of a rare chance of brain damage, however, immunisation may be risky under a number of circumstances:
- If the child has fits or epilepsy.
- If there is a history of epilepsy in brothers, sisters or parents.
- If the child has a disorder of the nervous system or is known to have suffered brain damage at birth.
- If there is a feverish illness at the time of the proposed injection.
- If there has been a severe reaction to a previous dose of the vaccine.

In all these cases – or if you are in any doubt – consult your doctor before the child is immunised.

First aid and medical emergencies

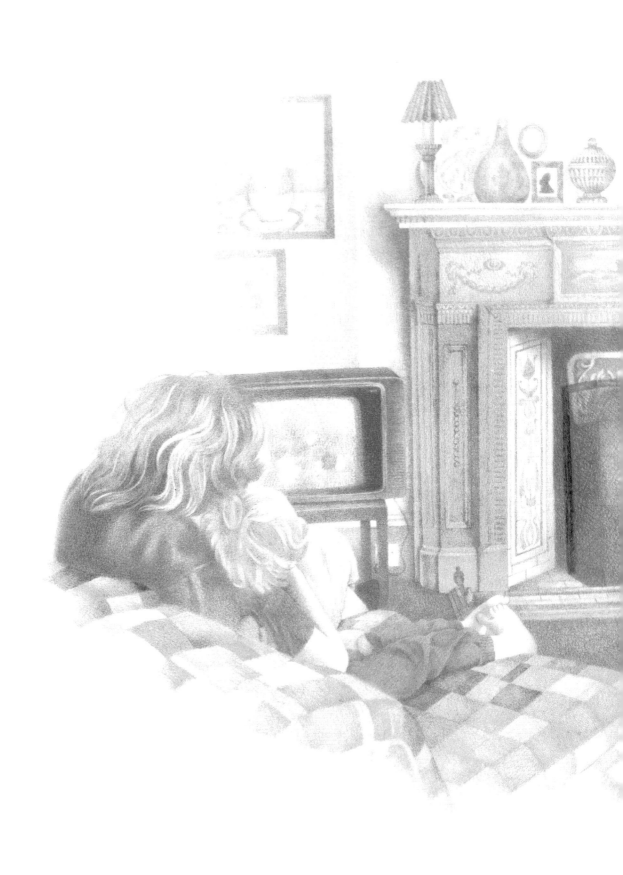

In the home and at work

If you are trapped in a blazing house

Once a fire takes hold, there is only one completely safe place to be – outside. If you are trapped inside, getting out is the priority.

Planning an escape route

If a fire should occur in your home, you have a better chance of escaping quickly if you have worked out the best route from each room beforehand. If you have not done this, take a moment to decide the best way out, unless this is obvious.

• If you cannot get down the stairs, for instance, consider which upstairs room is the easiest to get out of. Which has the largest windows? Which window is closest to the ground, and which has the clearest drop and the softest ground beneath it? Are there any balconies or garage roofs which might make it easier to reach the ground safely?

• Consider, too, which windows can be opened. It is more difficult to climb out through a window you have had to break, and it is more difficult to break a double-glazed window than a single-glazed one.

How to get out

• Try to find a safe way past the blaze to a ground-floor door or window. Firemen follow three cardinal rules when they move through a burning building: test all doors; close doors and windows; and stay low.

• Feel each door before opening it. Do not open it if it is hot, or if smoke is seeping around the edges. In a large or unfamiliar building, you can test doors quickly by touching the knob briefly with the back of your hand. The metal knob conducts heat faster than the panelling.

• Use the back of the hand for safety – heat on the back will make you jerk it away instinctively.

• If the door is cool, crouch behind it, open it a crack and glance out before deciding whether to go through. Put your foot against the back of the door to prevent it being opened by pressure from hot gases. If there are flames beyond, flinging the door wide could create a draught and cause a lethal surge in the fire's intensity.

• Close doors behind you and also close any open windows, if possible. This will help to slow the spread of fire. Open doors and windows feed air to the flames and allow them an easier passage from room to room.

• Stay low. Smoke fills a room from the ceiling down. Near the floor the air should be easier to breathe, and it should be easier to see.

When you have got out

• Once you have got outside and are safely clear of the building, check that everyone is accounted for. Stop anyone going back into the building to rescue possessions.

• Send someone to a neighbour's house or a phone box to dial 999 for the fire brigade, if that has not been done already.

• Remember when calling to give the exact

MOVING SAFELY FROM ROOM TO ROOM

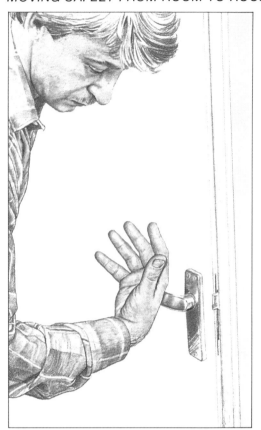

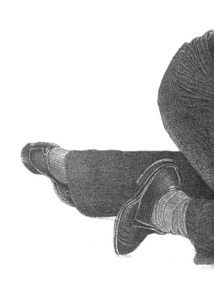

1 *As you move through rooms on your way out, test each door for heat by touching the handle or knob briefly. Use the back of the hand for safety – heat on the back will make you jerk it away instinctively, and avoid burns.*

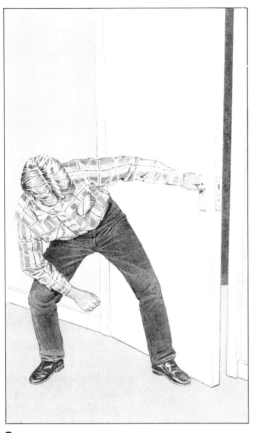

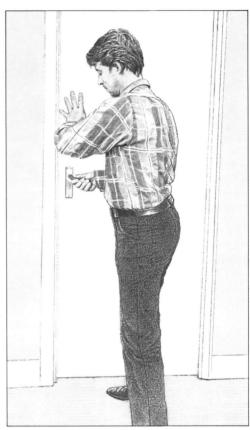

In the home and at work

2 *If the handle is cool, crouch behind the door and brace your foot against it before opening it a crack to peep through. Your foot will stop the door being forced wide open by the pressure of any hot gases on the other side.*

3 *Once through the door, take the time to close it firmly behind you. This will help to slow the spread of fire, fumes and smoke. Open doors (or windows) create draughts that feed air to the flames, intensifying the blaze.*

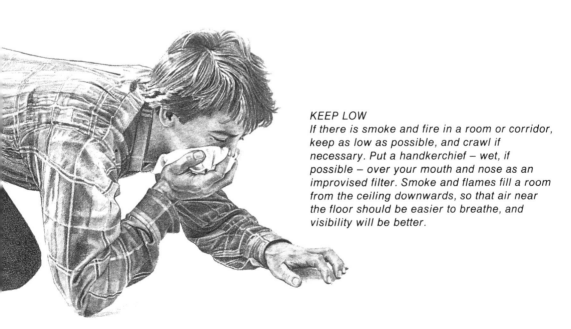

KEEP LOW
If there is smoke and fire in a room or corridor, keep as low as possible, and crawl if necessary. Put a handkerchief – wet, if possible – over your mouth and nose as an improvised filter. Smoke and flames fill a room from the ceiling downwards, so that air near the floor should be easier to breathe, and visibility will be better.

address and location of the blaze – in a moment of stress it is easy to forget such vital details, and that could delay the arrival of help.

If the exit is blocked

• Try to reach a window or balcony. Open the window. If there is a balcony get onto it and close the window behind you.

• If you are on the ground floor, jump out.

• If you are not on the ground floor and the drop is not too far and onto soft ground – a flowerbed, for example – hang out of the window with fully outstretched arms to lessen the distance you have to fall. It may be safer to risk a sprain, or even a broken bone, than to wait for rescue.

• Just before you drop, let go with one hand and use that arm and your legs to push yourself away from the wall as you fall.

• Do not jump out of an upstairs window except as a last resort. Instead, use anything to hand – knotted sheets, for example – to reach the ground or at least get closer to it before dropping. Anchor the rope to a solid piece of furniture inside the room.

• If you have to break a window to get out, use a chair or kick it out. If you have to use your hands, wrap something round your fist to protect it, or use an elbow if you are wearing something with sleeves.

• Knock out jagged pieces of glass around the edge, or throw a blanket or clothing over them, before climbing through.

• If there is no safe way down, shut the door of the room, open the window, then wave and shout to attract attention.

• On a balcony, shut the window behind you.

• If there is no balcony, try to keep the blaze out of the room while waiting for help. A building rarely collapses in a fire, so if you succeed you stand a good chance of surviving.

• Douse the walls and door between you and

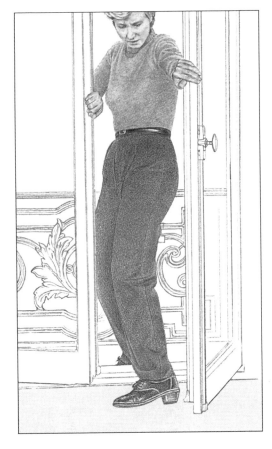

GET OUT ONTO A BALCONY
If you are trapped by fire on an upstairs floor and you can get out onto a balcony, do so. Close the door into the room before you go. Once outside, shut the window firmly behind you and shout for help. Try to remain calm while you are waiting to be rescued.

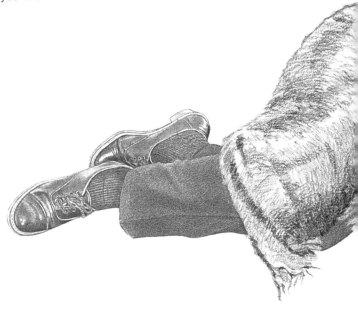

WHEN YOU ARE TRAPPED IN AN UPSTAIRS ROOM

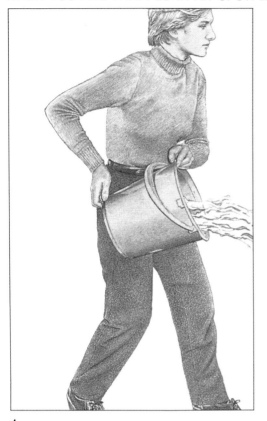

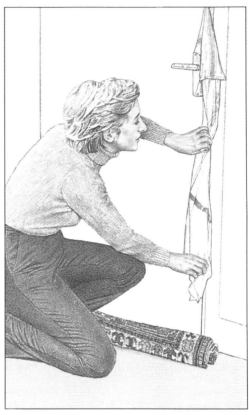

In the home
and at work

1 *If you cannot get onto a balcony, try to keep the blaze out of the room. If you can reach a tap, douse the walls and door with buckets of water. If you do not have a bucket, improvise with a saucepan, vase or any large container.*

2 *Stop smoke and fumes from entering the room by stuffing the cracks between the door and door frame with cloths – curtains, if necessary. Wet them first, if possible, and put a rolled-up carpet or blanket against the bottom.*

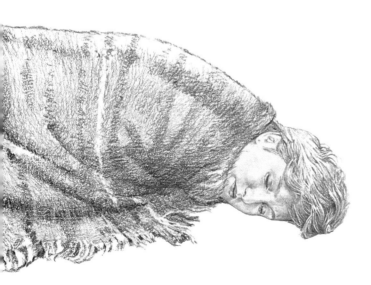

*IF YOUR CLOTHES
CATCH FIRE
Do not panic and run if your clothes catch fire. You will only fan the flames. Drop to the floor at once and smother the flames by rolling slowly – not quickly – over and over. Wrap yourself in a blanket or carpet, if you can.*

the flames with water. This will delay or prevent the spread of fire.

• Stuff cloths – wet, if possible – into the cracks around the door to stop smoke and fumes getting in. Smoke is a far bigger killer than the flames themselves – for every two people burnt to death in fires, five lose their lives through being asphyxiated by smoke or toxic fumes.

Escaping from a high-rise building

Just as you should plan in advance your escape route from a house fire, you should also know what to do to escape a fire in a block of flats or hotel.

• Never use a lift in a fire – you could be trapped if the power fails, or the doors could open on the floor that is ablaze, killing all inside.

• In many hotels a fire escape map is displayed in each room or corridor. Make a point of studying it when you arrive – there may not be time in an emergency.

• Make a mental picture of the halls and stairs between your room and the exit.

• Try the stairway door – if it is locked, have it opened.

• If a fire starts, make your way out as quickly as possible, testing each door before opening it and closing it behind you. Most doors take about half an hour to burn through, and make excellent fire shields.

• Always take your key with you, in case you are forced back into your room.

• As you go, alert others by banging on doors and shouting 'Fire!' Set off a fire alarm if there is one.

• If the stairway is blocked by flames or smoke, do not try to run through. Return to your room, or try to reach a floor which is not affected by the blaze. If necessary, walk up to the roof, then stand on the windward side of the building, with any smoke or flames being blown away from you, until firemen reach you.

• If you get trapped in your room and are too high to shout for help, wave a sheet, pillowcase or towel from the window to attract attention on the ground.

• If there is a telephone in your room, use it to call for help – the line may be open even if the fire has cut off the building's power supply.

When clothing catches fire

Clothing set ablaze through standing too near an unguarded fire or radiant heater is a common cause of serious burns – especially to children.

• Act instantly to smother the flames.

• If the clothing is your own, cross your arms over your chest, so that your hands touch your shoulders. This helps to keep the flames away from your face.

• Drop to the floor and roll over and over slowly.

• If possible, wrap yourself in a rug, wool blanket, coat or heavy curtains.

• If someone else's clothing is alight, get the victim onto the floor – trip him if necessary.

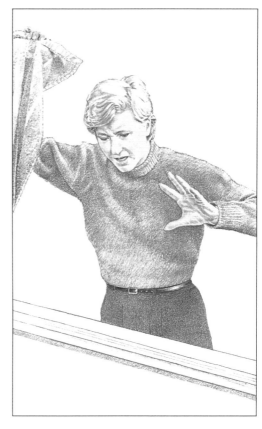

SIGNALLING FOR HELP
If you are trapped in a high-rise building too far from the ground for your voice to be heard, attract attention by waving something from the window. Use the largest and most brightly coloured piece of cloth you can find – a towel, say, a sheet, a rug or a curtain. Keep waving it until you are spotted by someone on the ground. You are unlikely to have to wait long for rescue. High-rise buildings are almost always in densely populated areas where a fire is likely to be noticed quickly and a fire station is likely to be within a few minutes' drive.

• Smother the fire with a fire blanket, rug, wool blanket, coat or heavy curtains.

• Throw water over the victim to help to cool him as well as extinguish the flames. Avoid using a fire extinguisher because it will not cool him, and any chemicals in it could cause difficulties when the burns are treated.

• When the fire is out, do not try to pull clothing away from the victim's skin.

• Call for medical help (dial 999 if necessary) and treat the victim for shock (see page 120).

Using a rope ladder

In a house, a rope ladder stored on an upper floor is a valuable (and relatively cheap) piece of safety equipment.

Ideally it should have built-in stanchions so

that it stands away from the wall in use, leaving room for hands and toes.

A traditional rope ladder is difficult to use if you try to climb up or down it as you would a rigid ladder – facing the rungs.

Used that way, the ladder will hug the wall of the building unless there is someone at the bottom to hold it away.

However, if it is the only type available there is a simple, effective technique used by sailors and mountaineers.

• Climb down the *side* rope of the ladder, placing one foot across the rung at the front of the ladder, and the other foot across the next rung at the back, splaying your feet with your toes pointing outwards.

• Your shoulder and hip will hold the ladder away from the wall, allowing plenty of room for hands and feet to grip.

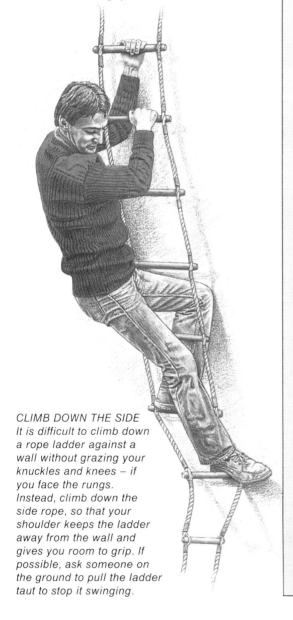

CLIMB DOWN THE SIDE
It is difficult to climb down a rope ladder against a wall without grazing your knuckles and knees – if you face the rungs. Instead, climb down the side rope, so that your shoulder keeps the ladder away from the wall and gives you room to grip. If possible, ask someone on the ground to pull the ladder taut to stop it swinging.

FIRE IN THE HOME: THE DANGER POINTS

Every year in Britain, more than 54,000 homes are damaged in fires that are started by accident.

Each year about 600 people die in fires in the home, and another 10,000 are burnt – many seriously.

More than 48,000 of these fires – almost 90 per cent – can be traced to one of ten major causes:

COOKERS are the largest single cause of domestic fires – nearly 25,000, or 46 per cent of the total – and the fires are often started by blazing chip pans.

Electric cookers are involved in around 16,800 blazes each year, gas cookers in another 7200.

HEATERS cause nearly 5000 blazes a year, usually because they are knocked over accidentally or are left too close to furniture.

Electric heaters account for about 1500 of these fires, gas heaters for 1600, solid-fuel burners for 1000 and liquefied petroleum gas (LPG) for 300.

SMOKERS leaving lighted cigarettes around start over 6000 fires a year. Particularly dangerous is the fire started by a cigarette left on an upholstered chair or settee. It can roll down the back or side of the seat and the upholstery can smoulder slowly, giving off poisonous fumes while the people in the house are asleep.

MATCHES are involved in starting about 3000 blazes. Often they are left too close to fires or are lit by children who are playing with them.

ELECTRICAL WIRING is the cause of over 3000 fires. The blazes are commonly started by old circuits, incorrect fuses or overloaded power sockets.

ELECTRIC BLANKETS trigger 1200 fires, usually because the insulation around the elements has been cracked by folding the blankets too tightly or because they have been creased.

BLOW TORCHES AND LAMPS, often those used by home handymen, account for some 1100 fires a year.

WASHING MACHINES are the source of 1900 fires a year.

CHIMNEY FIRES which spread outside the flue, commonly because of a build-up of soot inside the chimney, set nearly 1100 homes ablaze.

CANDLES and other naked lights such as tapers are the source of around 1200 fires each year.

In the home and at work

Rescuing someone from a fire

Getting someone out of a burning building calls for specialised knowledge and equipment and is highly dangerous. Safety experts say it should always be left to the fire brigade.

If, however, you are in a situation where you have to rescue someone – a child, say – who has been trapped or overcome by smoke, there are just two priorities: do not add yourself to the casualty list; and act quickly. Get the victim outside as fast as possible, regardless of his or her injuries.

- Always call the fire brigade (by dialling 999) before attempting any rescue yourself.
- Do not go into a building that is burning fiercely or in danger of collapse.
- Do not go into a building which you suspect may be filled with poisonous fumes. Some modern furniture gives off deadly gases when it burns. If some of this furniture is likely to be in the building, wait for firemen to arrive with breathing equipment.
- Before you go in, tie a rope round your waist and get somebody outside the building to hold it. If you get lost in the smoke you will be able to retrace your steps by following the rope, or if you are overcome by fumes you can be pulled to safety.
- Arrange a system of signals with the person outside. It is usually best to establish that you will keep a tension on the rope all the time by pulling it gently. If the rope slackens you will be pulled out.
- Tie a wet handkerchief or scarf over your mouth and nose. This will keep out the smoke but cannot protect you from poisonous fumes.
- If you have a blanket or coat to hand, carry it with you or drape it round your shoulders. It may be useful for wrapping up the casualty or for protecting both of you from the heat.
- As you go into and through the building, test each door before you go through it by touching the knob with the back of your hand. If the knob is hot, do not enter.
- Do not go forward if there is any danger of your escape route being cut off.
- If the door is cool, hold the handle firmly when opening it so that the door cannot be sucked wide open by any hot gases inside. If it opens outwards, crouch behind it and put your foot against the back to stop it bursting open.
- Take several deep breaths. Open the door a crack and wait for any hot air to be released, then go in (see *If you are trapped in a blazing house*, page 142).

HOW TO DO A FIREMAN'S LIFT

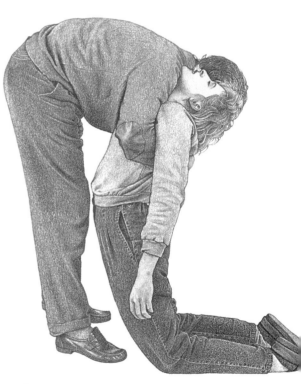

1 *Get the casualty onto her feet. If she is unconscious, lay her face down with her head at your feet. With your arms under her armpits, raise her to her knees, then to her feet.*

HANGING ON – 60 FEET UP
The ability to improvise is vital even for professional rescuers, who have specialised equipment to cope with most situations. On February 27, 1983, it saved the life of a teenage girl.

In the early hours of that morning, Leading Fireman Jeff Yates hung head-down out of a flat window, 60ft (18m) above ground, supported only by his colleague Keith Summerfield who was clinging to Jeff's legs. Hanging by her hands from a narrow ledge outside the next window in the Sheffield block of flats was 19-year-old Dawn Lipscombe. She had been trapped by flames but was beyond the reach of the firemen's ladders. Jeff's improvised trapeze act was the only way to get to her.

Suddenly, as Jeff was trying to reach Dawn, her window exploded. Glass splinters and flames sprayed outwards. Dawn let go of her ledge and flung herself sideways through the air. Jeff grabbed for her arms – and held on. For a few seconds the pair swung in the air until Keith finally managed to pull them both to safety. The unorthodox rescue technique had worked. Dawn was shocked but unhurt.

• Keep low as you go into a smoke-filled room. If necessary, crawl along the floor.

• Once you find the casualty, drag or carry her to safety as quickly as possible. Do not give first aid until you are both out of danger (see *Moving an injured person*, page 112).

Fireman's lift

If you have to negotiate stairs or manage many doors, you may find it easier to carry a casualty with the fireman's lift shown below, which leaves you with one hand free, than to drag her.

• Get the casualty onto her feet, facing you.

• Then put her across your shoulder.

• If you have to go down stairs while you are carrying someone in a fireman's lift, look down them first to see if there are any hazards, then go down backwards.

BUS-STOP RESCUE

Thick smoke and flames blocked the Glassford family's escape from their first-floor flat in Hamilton, Strathclyde. The fire had started at 6am on March 11, 1983, when a frying pan flared up as 17-year-old Thomas was cooking breakfast. It swiftly took hold, trapping Thomas, his parents and his six brothers and sisters.

But just in time, bus driver Jim Beaton saw the children screaming from the windows. He drove his bus up to the building, and he and a passenger helped the family out onto the bus roof.

A fire officer later said that Jim had 'almost certainly saved nine lives' by his quick thinking – and by his use of the bus as an improvised rescue platform.

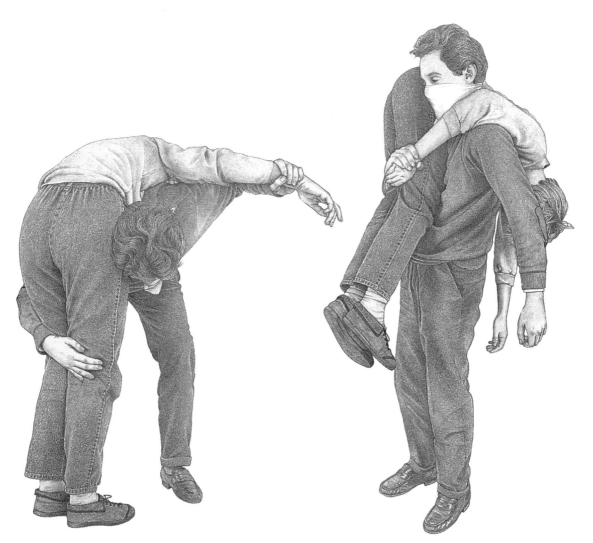

2 *Once she is on her feet, hold her right wrist with your left hand. Bend down, with knees bent, and put your head beside her right hip. Let her fall across your right shoulder.*

3 *Stand up carefully, keeping your back as straight as possible. Transfer her right wrist to your right hand, so leaving your left hand free to open doors and hold banisters.*

149

Fighting a fire

If fire breaks out, whatever the cause, the first thing to do is to make sure that nobody is in danger. Only then should you consider attempting to put out a small fire, such as a hearth-rug blaze. If the fire is large, fierce or spreading – or if it looks as though it might become so – do not try to fight it at all. Get out of the house and call the fire brigade at once by dialling 999.

Smoke is often more dangerous than the flames themselves. Many of the 600 people who die in fires each year in British homes are killed by smoke, not by flames.
• Do not put yourself at risk.
• Stand well back from the flames. Keep out of the smoke.
• Stand on the side of the fire nearest to your escape route so that you cannot be cut off.
• Do not try to drag burning objects away from the fire. This will only spread the flames.
• Work from the outside of the fire towards the centre. Use water, sand, heavy blankets and rugs to smother the flames, or use a fire extinguisher. (See *Protecting your home against fire*, page 152.)
• These general guidelines apply to all fires. In addition, however, safety experts recommend specific courses of action to deal with particular types of fire.

Chip pan

Fires in chip pans start when the cooking oil gets too hot and bursts into flame. If you see smoke coming off the oil, it means that the oil is about to ignite.
• Turn off the heat immediately.
• Do not move the pan. If you try to rush it out of the house, the air will cause the flames to flare up fiercely.
• Do not use water on the flames. It will spread the fire explosively.
• Smother the flames. Do not go looking for something; pick up whatever is to hand. Use a special fire blanket if you have one, or any thick cloth (wet if possible). A lid, plate or chopping board will also do as long as it is larger than the top of the pan.
• Hold the cloth or lid in front of you to shield your face as you place it over the chip pan.
• Once the fire is out, keep the pan covered until the oil is quite cool (wait at least 30 minutes). Otherwise it might burst into flames again.
• If you are unable to put the fire out, close all doors and windows, get out of the room and call the fire brigade.

Hearth rug

• If the flames are small, try to stamp them out or smother them with a wet cloth or mat.
• Otherwise, throw water over the flames.

Sofa or armchair

Most modern furniture, upholstered with foam, plastic or other synthetic materials, burns very quickly, giving off thick smoke and poisonous

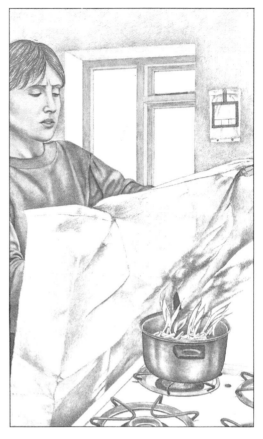

HOW TO PUT OUT A BLAZING CHIP PAN
Leave the pan where it is. Turn off the heat and cover it with a fire blanket. Hold the blanket up to guard your face as you approach.

fumes which can overcome you in one minute, and kill you in less than two.
• Do not try to put out the fire.
• Get everybody out of the room immediately.
• Close the door.
• Call the fire brigade – even if the fire appears to be out.
• Do not try to take a burning piece of furniture (of any kind) outside – even if it is only smouldering. The fresh air could cause it to flare up.

Television set or computer

Parts of a television set can get very hot. As a result, a fire can break out even after the set has been switched off and unplugged. If a set burns it gives off fierce flames and poisonous fumes. The tube behind the screen may also explode. The same risks apply to home computers. Fires in TV sets and computers should be handled in the same way.
• If a peculiar smell, like burning rubber or plastic, comes from the set or the computer, or you see even a trace of smoke, unplug it immediately. Do not use it again until a specialist engineer has examined it.

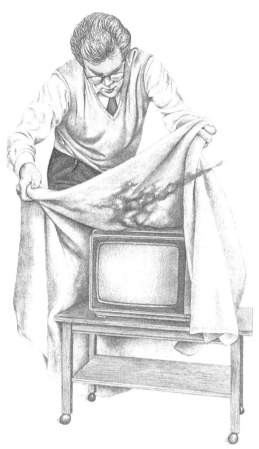

HOW TO SMOTHER A TV FIRE
Throw a fire blanket over a TV or computer
that bursts into flame. Approach the set from
behind in case the screen explodes in the heat.

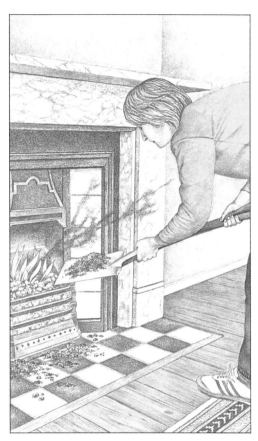

HOW TO DAMP DOWN A CHIMNEY FIRE
Cut off the heat that has set the flue ablaze
by putting out the fire in the grate. One quick
way to do this is to shovel on garden soil.

• If smoke or flames begin to pour out, unplug the set at once or switch off at the mains. Then cover the machine with a fire blanket, or a wet rug or towel. This will help to contain the flames and fumes, and will protect you from flying glass if the screen explodes.
• Call the fire brigade.
• Do not throw water on a TV set or computer, or use a fire extinguisher of any kind – even after the machine has been switched off. The sudden cooling could cause the tube to burst. There may also be residual electricity remaining in the machine, and throwing water on it could give you an electric shock.
• Do not look under the blanket. Keep well away until the fire brigade has dealt with it.

Chimney
Chimneys – even those serving some central-heating systems – can catch fire if soot and dirt are allowed to collect in them over a period of years. And fires in them can, if unchecked, threaten the rest of the house.
• Call the fire brigade. The fire may penetrate cracks in the flue and spread to other parts of the building. Move carpets and furniture away from the fireplace.
• Close doors and windows in the room.
• Shovel earth from the garden onto the grate or pour soapy water over the fire. Detergent in the water helps it to cling to the coals and smother the flames. The resulting steam will also help to put out the fire in the chimney.
• Once the fire in the grate is out, put a wire-mesh spark guard in front to prevent hot soot falling out of the flue into the room.
• Check other rooms through which the chimney passes. If the walls against the chimney are very hot, move the furniture away from them.
• When the fire has been extinguished, have the chimney swept. Regular sweeping – at least once a year – is the best precaution against chimney fires.

Electric blanket
• Unplug the blanket. But do not lift off the bedclothes – this will let air in and may turn a smouldering bed into a blaze.
• Call the fire brigade.
• Drench the bed with water.

151

PROTECTING YOUR HOME AGAINST FIRE

• Unplug electric appliances such as TV sets and heaters when they are not in use. This is safer than just switching them off.

• Before leaving the house or going to bed, close all doors and windows in empty rooms.

• Provide deep ashtrays in all rooms where people might smoke. (See *Fire in the home: the danger points*, page 147.)

• Keep matches well away from children, preferably in a locked cupboard.

• Do not air or dry clothes round a convector heater or against a radiant fire, or put them on a storage heater.

• Keep furniture, curtains and bedding well away from fires and heaters.

• Keep paraffin heaters away from doors. They could get knocked over. Never move or fill a paraffin heater while it is alight.

• Surround open fires with a fireguard. The guard should cover the entire fireplace, not just the fire.

• Do not put a mirror over the fireplace. It tends to encourage people to get too close to the fire.

• Never overfill chip pans. Oil and fat expand when heated, and they could overflow onto the burner and catch fire (see also *Danger points – room by room*, page 164).

Fire extinguishers

The simplest and most useful firefighting equipment for the home is a fire blanket and a bucket of water, kept in the kitchen. A portable fire extinguisher can be useful as long as it can be reached quickly by someone who knows how to use it properly. Some safety experts discourage fire extinguishers in the home, however, because they feel that the presence of an extinguisher may give a false sense of security and may make people careless about fire precautions.

If you are in doubt about what size of extinguisher to buy, choose one larger than you think you might need. The smallest useful extinguisher for home use is one with a capacity of about 3lb (1.5kg). And even this is sufficient only for a small fire. Aerosol extinguishers do not usually last long enough to put out more than a very small fire.

The most suitable general-purpose extinguisher for the home is the dry-powder type. It is the least dangerous to use, but makes a mess.

There are five different types of fire extinguisher. Each type is marked by a special colour. The extinguisher may be of one colour only or may be mostly red with the coding colour clearly displayed. The five types are: water (red); dry powder (blue); carbon dioxide (black); foam (cream, buff or white); and a vaporising-liquid type containing chemicals known as halon or BCF (green).

• WATER Use on burning wood, paper or cloth. Do not use on electrical fires where the apparatus is still switched on, or on flammable liquids such as petrol, spirits, oil or cooking fat. Do not use on a TV fire, even if the set has been switched off.

• DRY POWDER Use on flammable liquids or electrical equipment.

• CARBON DIOXIDE Use on almost all types of large fire, including electrical fires. But it is not suitable for oil-burning stoves or small fires.

• FOAM Use on flammable liquids.

• VAPORISING LIQUID Use on all large fires including electrical fires. But it should not be used in confined spaces because it gives off poisonous fumes.

If you have to tackle a fire with an extinguisher, make sure it is suitable for the fire concerned. Switch off the current if electrical equipment is involved. Crouch to keep clear of the smoke, and move the extinguisher from side to side with a sweeping movement. Aim it at the base of the flames and work steadily in from the edge.

Foam extinguishers should be aimed so that the foam drops onto burning liquid. If the foam is directed straight into the liquid under pressure it will be driven beneath the surface and be ineffective.

Learn how to use the extinguisher in advance. Otherwise, when fire breaks out, you could waste valuable minutes reading the instructions.

Keep extinguishers regularly maintained, otherwise they will deteriorate. The supplier will be able to advise you on how often your extinguisher needs checking.

Fire alarms

Domestic fire alarm systems should carry the British Standards Institution kitemark and the code number BS 5446.

Most systems are battery-powered, so that they will still work even if the mains electricity is cut off by a fire.

If you buy a battery-powered system, check that it is fitted with a device to warn when the battery is running low.

Get expert advice from the local fire brigade about where to place the detectors that trigger the alarm system, and about how many you need for your particular home.

If you smell gas or suspect a leak

Natural gas is not poisonous. But it can be dangerous because, when mixed with air in a proportion of between 5 per cent and 15 per cent, it is explosive. The gas has no smell of its own. But a smell is added to it deliberately, before it is piped to homes, to alert house-holders to leaks.

• If you smell gas or suspect (even with no smell) that gas is leaking from an appliance such as a cooker, put out cigarettes and any naked flames – a candle, say – at once.

• Turn off any electric fire in the room. But do not turn any other electric lights or appliances either on *or off*.

• Do not even allow the doorbell to be used. Operating a switch in either direction is likely to cause a spark which could ignite the gas.

• Open doors and windows to let the gas out, and leave them open until the leak has been stopped.

• Check that no gas taps have been left on accidentally, and that no pilot light has gone out. If no gas appliances are on, there is probably a leak. Turn the supply off at the meter at once.

• Telephone the British Gas emergency service, which operates 24 hours a day, every day of the year. The telephone number is shown under 'Gas' in the telephone directory.

• Do not attempt to repair any appliances or pipes, or allow anyone else to do so. Repairs must by law be left to a trained gas engineer – such as one who has been authorised by British Gas or the Council for Registered Gas Installers (CORGI).

• Stay out of the house until the source of the leak has been found and cured, and the smell of gas has cleared.

• If you think there is a gas leak at work or in the street, report it to British Gas at once.

When the gas has cleared

British Gas will check suspected gas leaks and make simple repairs free of charge. The company makes no charge for the first 30 minutes' work, nor for parts and materials up to the value of £2.50. The repairs of parts of the system belonging to British Gas – those which are on the supply side of the gas meter in your home – are paid for by British Gas.

• Once the leak has been repaired, make sure that you have turned off all gas taps on appliances.

• Then relight any pilot lights.

If the gas supply fails

The gas supply may be affected by causes outside the home – a burst gas main, say, or a sharp drop in pressure.

• If the gas pressure does drop sharply (so that the flames on a gas cooker or gas fire become much smaller than usual), or the supply stops altogether so that the flames go out, turn off all gas appliances, turn off the supply at the meter or emergency control and notify British Gas at once.

• Do not attempt to use the supply again until someone from British Gas has advised you that it is safe to do so.

If you think the meter is faulty

If you suspect that your gas meter is at fault – if, for example, it appears to be running when no gas is being used – ask your local British Gas district to test it.

• If the gas engineer discovers a meter fault, there is no fee for the test, and any payments the fault has affected will be adjusted.

• If, however, the meter is found to be accurate, you will be charged a test fee.

Living safely with gas

On average, there are some 40 serious gas explosions every year in Britain and about ten people a year die in such explosions. Most of these accidents happen because people have interfered with appliances or pipework – either deliberately (such as by tampering with the

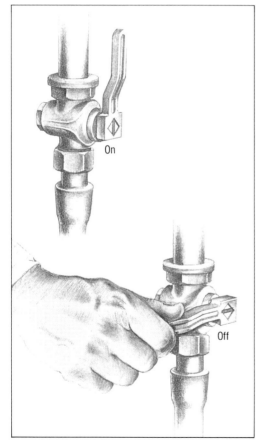

HOW TO TURN GAS OFF AT THE MAINS
Some main gas valves have built-in handles, others detachable handles. On either type, the supply is on when the mark on the pivot points along the pipe, off when it points across.

meter), or by accident. All repairs must, by law, be carried out by a competent person – they are not suitable tasks for the DIY enthusiast to undertake.

• Make sure you know where the main gas tap is in your home, and how to turn it off. If the tap is stiff to turn, do not force it. Call your local British Gas district; they will loosen it for you free of charge.

• Many of the accidents caused by faulty appliances involve secondhand equipment. If you buy such equipment make sure you get a guarantee and a copy of the user instructions, and get it installed by a qualified gas fitter.

• Get all gas appliances serviced regularly – central heating, water heaters and fires at least once a year, other appliances at least once every two years.

• If you know, or are warned, that a gas appliance or installation in your home is faulty, you must get it repaired. It is illegal to continue to use it, or to allow others to do so.

• Never block ventilators in a room where there are gas appliances. Gas needs a supply of fresh air while it is burning. If the fresh air supply is interrupted, the gas may not burn properly, and the poisonous gas carbon monoxide may be produced.

• Watch out for signs that the gas is not burning properly and is producing carbon monoxide. This could happen if a chimney or flue becomes blocked, cutting off the necessary air supply. Danger signs are staining soot or discoloration around the fire or water heater, and the appliance may burn with a yellow or orange flame. If you notice any of these danger signs, or if sitting in the room gives you a headache or makes you feel sick, weak or tired, turn off the appliance at once and get it checked. (Modern appliances often have built-in ventilation – they must be fitted to an outside wall, and they take in fresh air from outside. These are known as 'balanced-flue' or 'roomsealed' types.)

• If you use an older style of water heater (not a balanced-flue type), open the bathroom window while you run the water, turn the heater off before you get into the bath, and do not run more hot water while you are in the bath.

• Do not run an unflued sink water heater for more than five minutes at a time – it is not designed to fill a bath or washing machine, or to provide hot water for a shower.

• If you move house, get British Gas to disconnect your appliances and make the gas supply safe. It is against the law to leave unsealed or improperly capped gas points. Leave the instructions for any appliances you are not taking with you, for whoever is moving in.

• Authorised British Gas employees have a legal right of entry to any premises supplied with gas in order to inspect installations and appliances in the interests of safety. All such employees carry an identity card giving their name, photograph and signature, and will willingly show the card on request.

USING BOTTLED GAS

Bottled gas – the fuel sold in canisters for use by campers, in caravans, on boats, in heated greenhouses and in the home – is usually either propane (sold in red canisters) or butane (sold in blue or green canisters). Both fuels are forms of liquefied petroleum gas (LPG).

In use, both gases are effectively the same. But because they operate at different pressures, it is important to use the correct regulator valve for each fuel. Never switch from one gas to the other without also changing the regulator.

• Unlike natural gas, both gases are heavier than air. For this reason, canisters should always be stored outside, above ground level and away from drains if they are to be left for any length of time. This applies whether they are full or empty.

• Keep the canister upright, with the valve uppermost, whether it is in use or not.

• If a canister has to be left in a confined space – a caravan or boat, say – ventilate the area thoroughly before turning it on, before lighting any naked flame (even a cigarette) and before switching on any electrical equipment (because a spark could ignite leaked gas and cause an explosion).

• In particular, make sure that you ventilate thoroughly the bottom of the space – the bilges on a boat, say, or a cellar – to get rid of any gas that has collected there.

• Check gas hoses regularly for leaks by rubbing soapy water over them. Any leaks will be marked by erupting bubbles. Never use a naked flame to check for leaks.

• If you find any leaks, or if the hose is becoming worn, replace it. Do not try to repair it.

• When fitting connections, tighten them with a spanner. Finger pressure is not enough to ensure a gas-tight seal.

• Change canisters well away from any open flame or intense heat, preferably outdoors.

• Open the valve slowly when you want to turn the gas on.

• Ventilate any room where gas-burning appliances are in use.

Using electricity safely

The two major electrical hazards are shocks and fire. Any electrical wire gets warm in use. The thinner the wire, or the greater the amount of current it is carrying, the hotter it gets. Fuses are designed to cut off the power long before this heat builds up to the point where insulation could melt or a fire could start.

By following the guidelines suggested here, you can minimise the risks of starting a fire or suffering an electric shock (for details of first aid treatment, see page 93). You can also save yourself the inconvenience of being plunged into darkness by a blown fuse.

• When connecting an appliance to a plug, check that each wire goes to the correct terminal. Electric flexes always contain two or three separate wires. There is always a live and a neutral wire, and often an earth wire as well. The three wires are coloured in either of the following combinations:

Live	Neutral	Earth
Brown	Blue	Yellow/Green
Red	Black	Green

Red, black and green are the colours of older wiring.

• Never put wires directly into a socket – always fit a plug. Never pull a plug out by the cable; you could pull the wires loose.

• Do not overload a socket. For example, a three-bar fire and a 1kW electric iron together take more than 16 amps – which is too much for a standard 13 amp household socket. Turn at least one bar of the fire off if you have to use the same socket for the iron.

• If you have more than one appliance on a socket, check the total load by adding up the current each appliance uses. A two-bar fire, for instance, rated at 2kW (8 amps) and a television rated at 500 watts (2 amps) will – if they are both on together – use 10 amps, safely inside the 13 amp capacity of a standard household socket (see *Facts about fuses*, page 156).

• Check flexes and connectors regularly, especially where the appliance is moved or gets hot, such as a kettle. Terminal screws (in the back of a kettle, for instance) can work loose with heat.

• Check regularly plugs and flexes which are constantly being moved, such as those to food mixers and hair dryers.

• Drop flexes to ceiling lights become hot in use and the insulation tends to become brittle with age and may crack. Change the flexes if they become brittle.

• Switch the lights off at the mains before checking the flexes and before cleaning with a damp cloth. Otherwise water could seep into the cracks and give you a severe shock.

• Do not plug any appliance into a lighting point. It could overload the circuit or blow a fuse.

• The cord-grip in a plug – usually a piece of hard material just inside the hole where the wire goes into the plug – must grip the outer sheath of the wire securely. If you can see the inner wires, the grip needs to be refitted.

• Always unplug appliances before working on them or making any adjustments, and after use. Unplug a light, too, before replacing a bulb.

• Unplug an electric kettle before you fill it at the tap.

• Never take a hair dryer, heater or any appliance operated by the mains into the bathroom.

• Fit rubber plugs to appliances that receive hard wear. They chip and crack less easily than plastic plugs.

• Use a flex connector to join cables together, or, ideally, buy a longer length. Never join wires by twisting them together and insulating them with tape.

• All appliances used out of doors should have the flex plugged into a residual current circuit breaker (RCCB) at the circuit socket.

• Buy a 30 milliamp RCCB for outdoor tools. This cuts the power off at once if a damaged flex, a faulty tool or a loose connection creates a risk of electric shock.

• Use an orange flex on appliances which are used outdoors. The colour is easier to see.

• Never use an extension flex which is thinner than the flex attached to the appliance. A thinner flex will probably overheat.

• When using an extension flex fitted to a reel, pull out the entire length when it is in use. Wire warms up when current passes through it – the smaller the wire or the larger the appliance, the more heat is generated. If the flex is left on the

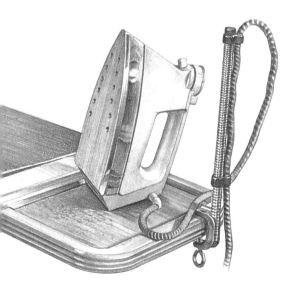

HOW TO PROTECT THE FLEX ON AN IRON
A lead-holder attached to the flex of an iron and secured to the ironing board will prevent the flex from chafing against the board and thus wearing through more quickly.

In the home and at work

reel, the heat cannot escape so easily, and it can build up to a point where the insulation melts, causing a short circuit.

Facts about fuses

The vast majority of houses are wired on a ring-main system, with each circuit supplying a number of plug sockets. Each circuit has its own fuse in the fuse box, and each plug is also fused. Modern plugs always have rectangular pins; round-pin plugs are almost invariably part of an older, pre-1947 'radial' wiring system, in which each plug socket has its own separate circuit. A house with these sockets may need rewiring: consult an electrician.

The box on this page (see *Fuse ratings*) shows what fuse you should fit in the plug for each of the named appliances. Using a much larger fuse than necessary carries the risk of causing a whole ring-main circuit to fail rather than a single appliance. There is also an increased risk of fire if the flex becomes overloaded.

To calculate the appropriate fuse for any electrical appliance, look for the manufacturer's plate or label – usually on the back or bottom of the appliance.

The plate will show how much power the appliance uses, expressed in watts (W) or kilowatts (kW). One kilowatt equals 1000 watts. Divide the figure, in watts, by 250 and the result is the minimum size of fuse necessary in amps. An appliance using 1.5kW (1500 watts), for instance, needs at least a 6 amp fuse (1500 ÷ 250) – or, in practice, a 13 amp fuse.

FUSE RATINGS

Appliance	Rating
Cooker 6kW shower	30 amps
3kW immersion heater Storage heater	15 amps
Appliances rated at 720 watts and above including: Dishwasher 3kW fire Freezer Kettle Refrigerator Spin/tumble drier Television (colour) Toaster Vacuum cleaner Washing machine	13 amps
Appliances rated at under 720 watts including: Electric blanket Clock Extractor fan Food processor/mixer/blender Hair drier Hi-fi stereo system/radio Home computer Iron Shaver Standard or table lamp Tape recorder Television (black and white)	3 amps

---

THREE TYPES OF FUSE

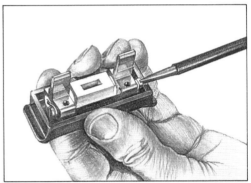

1 *Older types of fuse box are commonly fitted with fuses containing a length of wire attached to screw terminals. Always replace a burnt-out fuse with wire of the same rating.*

HOW TO FIT A PLUG

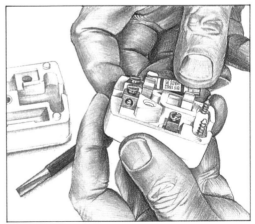

1 *Check that the fuse is the correct rating for the appliance (most plugs are sold with 13 amp fuses). Remove 2in (50mm) of the flex's outer sheath, and bare about ¼in (6mm) of each wire.*

How to change a fuse in a fuse box

- Turn off the mains supply at the main switch.
- Open the fuse box. Pull out fuses until you find the one that has blown. Look for loose wires or signs of scorching. Mark the fuses so that you know which one controls which circuit.
- If fuse wire is used, remove the old wire. Wind new wire of the same rating around one screw and tighten the screw. Take the wire across the bridge (or through the channel in an enclosed fuse) and twist it clockwise round the second screw, leaving a little slack. Tighten this screw and cut off the surplus wire.
- Always fit the correct fuse wire for the circuit. If in doubt, consult your electricity company or electrician.
- If the fuses are cartridge types, check each one with a circuit-tester. There may be no visible marks on the failed fuse. Alternatively, take the base off a metal-cased torch, turn on the torch and hold the fuse so that it touches the base of the battery and the metal case. If the torch bulb does not light, the fuse is broken. Replace it with a cartridge of the correct amperage.
- If your fuse box has trip-switches, which are designed to turn themselves off automatically when the circuit becomes overloaded, there is no need to repair or replace anything. Switch off some of the appliances on the circuit, then reset the trip (usually by button or switch).
- If a fuse blows repeatedly, or if a trip-switch will not stay on when you reset it, telephone an electrical contractor or the electricity company's emergency service for help.

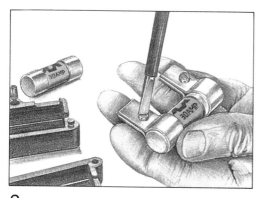

2 *Fuse-box cartridge fuses are coded by size and colour. White (the smallest) are for 5 amp circuits; then come blue (15 amps), yellow (20 amps), red (30 amps) and green (45 amps).*

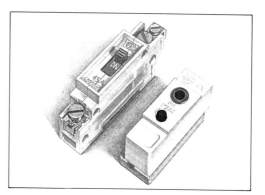

3 *Trip-switch fuses are small circuit-breakers which are fitted to many new fuse boxes. They have a built-in switch or button which turns itself off if the circuit becomes overloaded.*

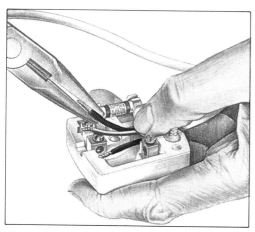

2 *Push the wires under the cord-grip. Use pliers if necessary to manoeuvre them into place. In a modern plug, the earth is the longer top pin; the live wire should go to the fused pin.*

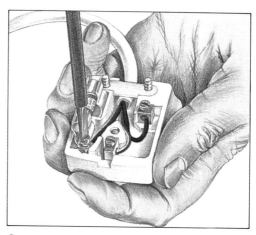

3 *Tighten the terminals with a screwdriver, making sure that there are no loose strands. Tighten the cord-grip screws so that they clamp the outer sheath, and refit the cover.*

When the power supply fails

During industrial disputes and during times of exceptional demand – in the middle of a particularly harsh winter, for instance – power cuts can cause considerable inconvenience, especially if they are unexpected. Normally they do not last long unless you live in a rural area remote from a local electricity substation.

It is possible to minimise the inconvenience, and the risk of accidents during a cut, by taking a few simple precautions.

● Switch off all electrical appliances except those that are normally on all the time, such as refrigerators and central-heating thermostats. When the power is restored after the cut, there will be an initial surge of current and, if a lot of appliances are on, the surge may be great enough to blow a fuse. More important, appliances such as heaters could become fire hazards if they are left on and forgotten, and the power comes back on late at night.

● As an extra precaution, make a point of unplugging the appliances at the sockets. Move the leads out of the way as well so that nobody can trip over them in the dark.

● Leave at least one light switched on so that you know when power is restored.

● Avoid opening a freezer, even a chest type. Food will generally keep safely for at least 12 hours with the power off. The fuller the freezer, the longer it will stay cold – up to 48 hours in safety, for instance, for a completely full freezer that is left unopened.

● Pack blankets and crumpled newspaper under and around the freezer's base to prevent heat rising in the appliance.

● No special action is needed for central heating – most systems are electrically controlled and will just not operate during a power cut.

● Use hot water carefully during a power cut. Although the water should stay hot for some time if the tank is well lagged, cold water is fed into the tank every time you draw off some of the hot.

● Use vacuum flasks to store spare water for hot drinks.

● If the failure is unexpected, telephone the local electricity company to tell them the power is off – it helps the company to identify an affected area quickly. They may be able to tell you when the supply will be restored. The telephone has its own power supply and will not be affected by the cut.

When power is restored

● Reset electric clocks and timers, including the central-heating timeswitch, after the cut.

● Remove any insulation that you have put round the base of your refrigerator or freezer. Make sure, particularly, that you uncover the vent or grille (normally on the back or side) through which surplus heat is discharged.

● Check that food in a freezer has not started to thaw. If it has, raw food can be cooked and refrozen (do not refreeze it raw). Precooked food

that has begun to thaw should be reheated and eaten at once, or thrown away.

● After checking the freezer, do not reopen it for six hours after a long power cut, to give time for the temperature inside to be lowered to a safe level again.

● If further cuts are expected, set freezer and refrigerator controls to maximum to extend the time that food will stay safely frozen.

Preparing for a power cut

Often there is some warning – either through a notice from the local electricity company or via newspapers, radio and TV – of impending power cuts. If there is, try to be ready for a cut well ahead of time.

● Keep a small torch by your bed, and a larger electric lantern in the kitchen.

● Fit these lamps with long-life batteries, and check them regularly.

● If you have to use candles, keep them away from anything that might catch fire, such as curtains. Stand candles in holders that cannot be easily knocked over.

● Try to set up alternative heating in at least one room: a gas fire, for example, a paraffin heater, a coal fire or a wood-burning stove.

● In an all-electric house, consider buying a camping stove for emergency cooking and heating during power cuts.

● Check your home insurance policy for the cover given for the loss of food in your freezer. Different policies give various forms of cover.

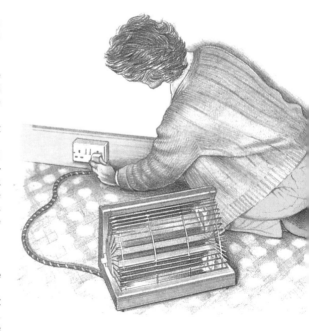

HEATER SAFETY IN A POWER CUT
If your power supply fails, turn off all electric fires and heaters. Pull all the plugs out at the sockets. Then tidy the flexes away so that you cannot trip over them in the dark.

Plumbing: emergency repairs

A flood in the home – from a blocked drain or a burst pipe – can be controlled or stopped before it does serious damage without waiting for a plumber to arrive.

But taking effective action calls for a cool head, speed and some preparation. It is therefore important to think ahead.

You need to know where to find stopcocks and shut-off valves inside and outside the house. If you do not know, find them and note their position for when an emergency arises. They are usually in or near the positions shown in the diagram below, but there are considerable variations even in modern houses. Once you

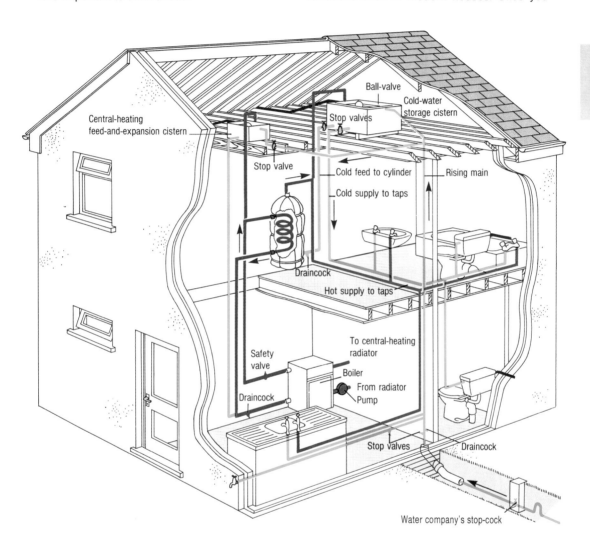

HOW THE WATER PIPES ARE LAID OUT IN A MODERN HOUSE
This is a typical modern plumbing layout. Exactly where the pipes run varies from house to house. But the principles are the same in all houses of any age. The supply enters the house via the rising main, which carries the water to a cistern in the loft. Only the kitchen cold tap, and sometimes a garden tap or a washing machine, are fed directly from the main. Lavatories, other cold taps and the hot-water cylinder are fed from the cistern.

A spiral tube inside the cylinder (often backed up by an electric immersion heater) heats the water. The tube is kept hot by water circulating through it from the boiler. The water inside the tube, like the water in any central-

heating radiators, is quite separate from the water which comes out of the taps, so that tap water cannot be contaminated by any anti-corrosion chemicals in the heating system.

To stop a leak from a cold-water or hot-water pipe, turn off the stop valve on the rising main (usually in the kitchen) and turn on all the taps. To shut off a leak from a hot-water pipe alone, turn off the valve on the pipe leading from the loft cistern to the hot-water cylinder.

In some flats, there is no cold-water cistern. Instead, lavatories and all cold taps are fed directly from the rising main; hot taps are fed from a mains-fed heater. Stop leaks by turning off the rising main and running the taps.

HOW TO DEAL WITH A LEAK

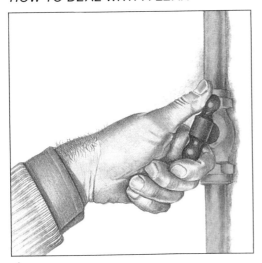

1 *Turn off the valve at the rising main. The valve is usually in the kitchen. Turn on all the taps and flush the lavatories. Do not waste time at this stage looking for the leak.*

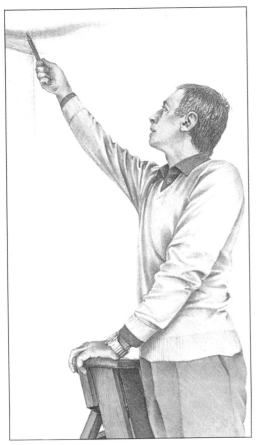

2 *If the leaking water has collected above a ceiling, forming a bulge in the plaster, put a bucket or any container below the bulge, and pierce the bulge with a large screwdriver.*

have identified the valves, it might be helpful to label each one so that you can be sure of identifying them quickly in an emergency.

If any valves are stuck, free them with a penetrating lubricant. Check them regularly.

Never leave any tap or valve full on for too long – it can easily become jammed. Once you have opened it fully, turn it back about half a turn and leave it in that position.

Emergency repairs will also be quicker and simpler if you keep the following items in the house: proprietary pipe repair tape; glass fibre tape and epoxy resin putty; plumber's tape (used to seal threaded pipe joints); a drain plunger; and a tin of radiator seal.

If water leaks through a ceiling

If water starts to drip through a ceiling, the most probable cause (other than a leaking roof) is a burst pipe or tank in the loft.

• The priority is to reduce the amount of water in the tank as quickly as possible to stop water flooding the house. Do not waste time at this stage looking for the cause.

• Turn off the main stop valve on the rising main in the house – the valve is usually under the kitchen sink or in the larder.

• Flush all lavatories and turn on all taps in the house except the kitchen cold tap, which is fed directly from the rising main.

• Leave the taps running and keep flushing the lavatories until the pipes and tank are empty, and the taps dry up.

• If you see a distinct bulge in the ceiling at the site of the leak, it means that a pool of water has collected over the spot.

• To stop the weight of water bringing down the ceiling, puncture the centre of the bulge with a large screwdriver and let the water drain out

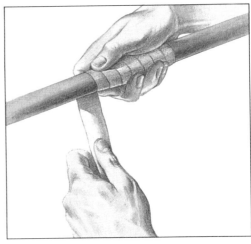

3 *Track down the source of the leak, which will probably be in the loft. When you find it, wait until it stops dripping, then bind the hole with pipe repair tape. Call a plumber.*

into a bucket or any other available container.
• Once water stops flowing from the leak, go up into the loft and find the source of the leak. Take care to step only on the joists if the loft floor is not boarded – otherwise your foot will almost certainly go through the plaster ceiling and you could be seriously hurt.
• Repair the pipe or tank temporarily with glass fibre tape and epoxy resin putty, or with pipe repair tape. You will then be able to turn the water on again. If you cannot repair the leak, leave the water off.
• Call a plumber (consult the Yellow Pages of a telephone directory) to make permanent repairs.
• If the leak is through a hole in the roof, make a temporary repair with a sheet of plastic (see *Storms and high winds*, page 172).

If a pipe bursts
Water expands when it freezes, and if the water is trapped inside a pipe, the expansion can be strong enough to burst the pipe.
  If you find a burst and frozen pipe, aim to make a temporary repair *before* it thaws out and the leak causes damage.
• Bind the damaged section of pipe with pipe repair tape, following the maker's instructions on the packet. Properly used, repair tape will withstand mains pressure.
• Alternatively, repair the break with glass fibre tape and epoxy resin putty.
• Once the seal is in place, thaw out the pipe with gentle heat – use a hot-water bottle or a piece of rag soaked in hot water.
• Have the pipe repaired later by a plumber.
• If the damaged pipe has already thawed and water is pouring out, try to cut off the water supply to the pipe.
• Turn off the nearest stop valve, if there is one, or run the taps that are fed by the pipe to reduce water pressure inside.
• When the leak stops or slows, bind the damaged section with pipe repair tape or repair the damage with glass fibre tape and epoxy resin putty.
• If the damage is extensive, it may be necessary to turn off the water supply to the house completely by shutting off the rising main. Wrap the pipe with a towel to confine the water and lead it into a bucket. Call a plumber.

If a joint leaks
If a pipe leaks at a joint, the repair needed depends on the type of joint. There are two types: compression joints and capillary joints.
• Compression joints, where the pipes are threaded and held together by nuts, can be made watertight by tightening the nut slightly with a spanner.
• Alternatively, shut off the water supply to the pipes, unscrew the nuts and wrap the threaded areas with several turns of plumber's tape. Then reassemble the joint.

• Capillary joints, where the pipes are sealed by a sleeve of metal soldered to them, may have to be remade by a plumber.
• On either type of joint you can also make a temporary repair.
• Turn off the nearest stop valve and run taps to reduce the water pressure inside.
• Bind the joint with pipe repair tape or seal it with epoxy resin putty.

If a radiator leaks
A large leak from a radiator can often be cured by draining the radiator and plugging the hole with epoxy resin putty.
  But a pinhole leak which allows water to weep out slowly is best dealt with by a proprietary liquid radiator seal.
• Add the seal to the small central-heating cistern in the loft – you should recognise it from the instructions given with the seal.
• Again following the instructions, open the draincock near the boiler so that water in this feed-and-expansion cistern flows into the system. The seal will then find its own way to the leak, on the same principle as the sealants used to mend car radiators.
• Either type of leak often means that the radiator is heavily corroded inside – and that other radiators in the system are also affected. So the only long-term answer is to drain the whole central-heating system and install a corrosion inhibitor. Consult a central-heating firm (local ones will be listed in the Yellow Pages).

If a central-heating pipe leaks
• If possible, put a container under the leak to catch as much of the water as possible.
• Switch off the central heating at the control panel. Shovel out the coal from a solid-fuel boiler so that the boiler pipes do not overheat when they are drained.
• Tie up the ball valve in the central-heating

IF WATER REACHES ELECTRICAL WIRING

Water conducts electricity so there is danger of shocks, short circuits and possibly fire if water from a leak runs along electrical wiring.
  If this happens, or there is a risk of it, switch off the main electricity supply at once. The switch is usually near the main fuse box.
  Alternatively, isolate the circuit concerned by removing the relevant fuse.
  If any wiring or electrical components have become wet, make sure they are thoroughly dry before switching on again.

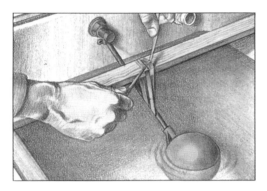

HOW TO SHUT OFF A BALL VALVE
To stop a central-heating tank filling up when you drain the system, lay a board across the tank and tie the valve's float arm up to it. You can use the same technique to stop a cold-water storage cistern filling up if you cannot find the stop valve on the rising main, or if the valve is stuck and you cannot turn it off.

cistern. It is probably in the loft, and is the smaller of the two cold-water storage tanks.
• Attach a garden hose to the draincock, which is usually beside the boiler.
• Run the hose to a nearby sink, or push it out of the kitchen door. Open the draincock with a spanner or pliers, and let the water run out of the central-heating circuit until water stops flowing from the leak. When the leak stops, close the draincock.
• Call a plumber or the people who service your central heating to repair the leak.

How to stop a cistern dripping
If a lavatory cistern drips water, particularly in cold weather, the problem is probably condensation – not a leak.

Moisture in the air is condensing on the cold outer surface of the cistern and dripping onto the floor, or trickling down the flush pipe between cistern and lavatory.
• The best cure is to keep the lavatory slightly warmer. Leave the door open so that warmer air from other parts of the house enters, or install a small radiator or tubular electric heater along the wall.

If water leaks under the bath
The commonest sources of bath leaks are the overflow outlet and the plughole.
• Try replacing the rubber gasket between the waste pipe and bath.
• Alternatively, try tightening the securing nut on the plughole joint very slightly – over-tightening can make the leak worse.

If a basin overflows
Floods in bathrooms and bedrooms are most often caused by leaving the plug in a basin with a tap running.
• If the overflow outlet is blocked, fill the sink so that the overflow outlet is underwater, then try to force out the obstruction with a drain plunger.
• Alternatively, push a curtain wire down the outlet and try to clear the blockage.
• Once the water starts to drain away, flush more water down the outlet – with caustic soda or a proprietary drain cleaner if necessary – to clear any remaining debris.

If a drain or pipe is blocked
• Turn off any taps that drain into the blocked section.
• Feel with your hand at the upper opening of the drain or waste pipe, and clear any obstructions you find. Outside drains, for example, can become choked with fallen leaves or silt.

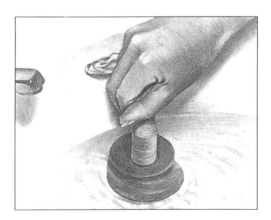

HOW TO CLEAR A BLOCKED DRAIN
Partly fill the sink, and use a drain plunger to free the blockage. Stuff a wet cloth in the overflow outlet if necessary to stop water spurting out of it while you pump the plunger.

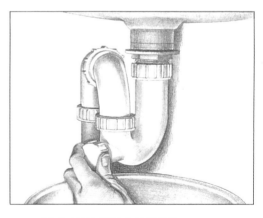

HOW TO CLEAN OUT A U-TUBE
If plunging does not work on a blocked sink or basin, put a bucket under the U-tube. Undo the drain valve, or take the whole U-tube apart and clean it out thoroughly by hand.

In the home
and at work

• On a waste pipe from a sink or basin, if there is no obvious obstruction, seal the overflow with a wet rag and use a drain plunger to try to force the blockage free.

• Once the water starts to flow, flush more water through to clear any remaining debris.

• If plunging fails on a kitchen sink or basin, put a bucket under the U-bend beneath the sink, disconnect the U-tube trap and clean it out. On modern plastic fittings, finger pressure may be enough to unscrew the trap. If you use a wrench, be gentle with it.

• If none of these methods works, it means that the obstruction is lodged farther along the pipe.

• Shift the obstruction with a plumber's snake – a stiff but flexible wire – if the pipe itself is blocked. If the drain is blocked, use drain rods. Both items of equipment can usually be rented from tool hire shops.

• If this does not work, or if you cannot get hold of the equipment, call a plumber.

If the lavatory will not flush

• If the mechanism in a lavatory cistern goes wrong for some reason, it is usually a job for a plumber.

• You can, nevertheless, go on using the lavatory until the plumber comes. Fill a bucket and pour the water into the lavatory pan – not the cistern – after each use. It will have the same effect as if the flush was working.

If a lavatory or drain is blocked

• Do not use or flush a lavatory if the pan or the sewage pipe beyond is blocked. You could create a health hazard if the sewage overflows, and you will certainly make the job of clearing it more difficult.

• Try first to clear the blockage with a large drain plunger. Do not, however, use the plunger with too much force or you could crack the lavatory pan.

• If plunging does not work, try to find the site of the blockage.

• Lift each drain manhole in turn. If there is stagnant water under the manhole, it means the blockage is farther down the pipe. If there is no water under the manhole, it means that the blockage is farther up the pipe.

• When you find the area of the blockage, explore the drain with a long stick. You may be able to dislodge the obstruction.

• If you cannot reach or shift the blockage with a stick, consider borrowing or hiring a set of drain rods or a plumber's snake (both are usually available from hire shops).

• If you use drain rods, be careful to twist the rods only in a clockwise direction as you work the rods into – and out of – the drain. If you twist them in the other direction, you are likely to unscrew the rods and leave the head deep inside the drain.

• Once the backed-up water begins to flow again, flush hot water or a chemical drain cleaner through the pipes to clear away any remaining debris. If you cannot clear the blockage yourself, call a plumber.

If your pipes are noisy

If water pipes start to make a banging or hammering noise, it may mean that there is an airlock somewhere in the plumbing system. Clearing such an airlock is a job for a plumber.

More commonly, however, the noise is caused by vibration in the ball valve which keeps your cold-water storage cistern topped up. And this can be put right without the expense of calling in a plumber.

• Check the cause of the noise by examining the cistern at the top of the house (it is usually the larger of the two tanks in the loft).

• If the ball valve is bouncing up and down on the surface of the water, releasing intermittent jets of water and creating the noise, try to slow down its movement by fitting a brake or damper of some sort.

• Hardware shops and plumbers' merchants sell an L-shaped piece which clips onto the arm of the valve and hangs underwater, acting like a brake on the arm.

• Alternatively, you can improvise a simple brake yourself with some stiff galvanised wire (such as a wire coat hanger) and a plastic cup.

• Make a loop in one end of the wire, big enough to hold the cup firmly. If necessary, pierce the wire through the side of the cup to anchor it.

• Wind the other end of the wire around the valve arm so that the cup is held upright underwater. The cup will then act as a brake, damping down the vibration and stopping the noise.

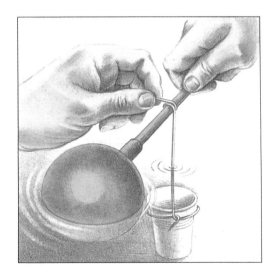

HOW TO QUIETEN NOISY PIPES
A damper made out of a plastic cup and wire will stop the vibrations on a ball valve which are often the cause of banging pipes. Hang the cup underwater below the float arm.

Danger points – room by room

Your own home is the most dangerous place on earth. More accidents happen there than anywhere else. Each year in Britain, around 5000 people are killed in accidents at home – almost as many as die on the roads – and another 3 million are hurt badly enough to need some form of medical treatment. Most accidents happen in the evenings or at weekends when people are usually at home. And there are 15 per cent more accidents in summer than in winter. Many of these extra accidents happen outdoors in the garden or in the garage. Just over half of all home accidents happen in the kitchen, the living room and dining room (often the same), and the garden.

Despite the grim statistics, there is much you can do to make your home safer, and so reduce the risks to yourself and your family. A room-by-room check of the accident black spots shown on these pages could prevent a hazard becoming a tragedy. Special additional precautions are needed if there are young children or elderly people in the house.

There are also safety devices on the market, such as smoke-detector kits, which can be installed by any home handyman. The smoke detectors will warn of fire before it gets out of control, giving valuable time in which to fight the blaze or to escape.

Kitchen

Of the 3 million or so accidents in British homes each year – and this figure does not include those minor accidents whose victims treat their injuries themselves – about one in six happen in the kitchen.
- Keep the shelving in your kitchen within easy reach, or have a sturdy stepladder to reach high shelves.
- Store dangerous liquids, such as bleach and disinfectant, well out of reach of children and preferably in a locked cupboard. Do not keep dangerous liquids in food containers or store them with food.
- Keep knives out of reach of children.
- Turn pan handles away from the edge of the stove when cooking. You – or a child – could catch them and tip them over.
- If there is a toddler in the house, do not use tablecloths which hang over the edge of the table. He might pull it, and whatever is on it, onto his head.
- Never leave chip pans or other deep-fry pans

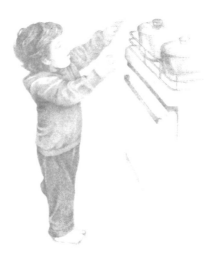

Ways to keep a cooker safe
Consider fitting a guard rail to your cooker, especially if there are young children about. Turn pan handles away from the edge, too.

USING A MICROWAVE OVEN

Modern microwave ovens are very safe in use. Early fears that they might be dangerous to cooks have been shown to have no foundation. The ovens are designed so that they cannot function unless the door is closed. All activity stops instantly when the door opens. If any microwaves were to leak, the strongest effect would be within 2in (50mm) of the oven. At arm's length the effect would be reduced to one hundredth of the strength. Microwaves are not like X-rays; the effect of many small doses is not cumulative or dangerous.

Do not turn the cooker on when it is empty, as this could damage it. Do not use metal cooking utensils – this could cause a fire.

If your oven suddenly begins to take longer than usual to cook food, the door seal may be dirty or damaged, and the microwaves may be leaking. Keep the door sealing faces clean, and call the service engineer if the seals are cracked or otherwise damaged. Do not use do-it-yourself radiation testers such as circuit-testing screwdrivers, as they are not a reliable way of measuring radiation. Get a microwave oven serviced regularly. Do not attempt to do any repairs yourself.

unattended, and do not fill them more than a third full with fat or oil.

• When using a deep-fry pan, have the lid, a fire blanket, a baking tray or a large damp towel handy to smother any fire. Never try to douse the flames with water (see *Fighting a fire*, page 150). Consider using chips that can be cooked in the oven to remove the need for deep-fry cooking altogether.

• When using a pressure cooker, follow the maker's instructions about how much water to put in, and time the cooking carefully so that the cooker does not boil dry.

• Wipe up any grease that spills on the floor immediately. Glue down the edges of any floor tiles that lift, to stop people tripping over them.

• Never use a thin or wet oven cloth.

• Make sure that all burners in a gas oven are alight before closing the door. If you have turned the heat right down, close the door slowly so as not to blow the flame out.

• Do not hang cloths or plastic bags above gas burners.

• Do not set burners so high that the flames come up the sides of cooking pans. The extra heat is wasted, and the flames may melt the handles or make them painfully hot.

• Keep plastic carrier bags and food bags away from young children. Pulled over the head in play, they can suffocate.

• Keep the doors of wall-mounted kitchen units closed whenever possible. Their sharp corners can be dangerous, particularly if they are near eye level.

• Lock potential hiding places for young children such as the freezer, broom cupboard, washing machine or tumble drier. A toddler could get trapped inside.

• Put a baby's bouncing chair on the floor – never on a work-top or table. It may shift as the baby bounces, and topple off the edge.

• Before removing the connector from a kettle

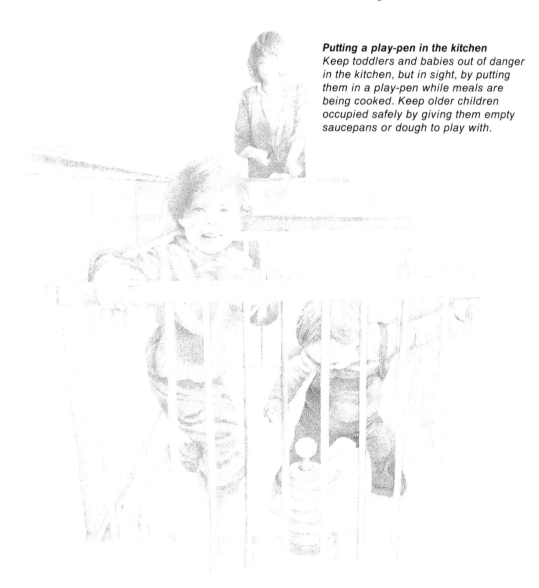

Putting a play-pen in the kitchen
Keep toddlers and babies out of danger in the kitchen, but in sight, by putting them in a play-pen while meals are being cooked. Keep older children occupied safely by giving them empty saucepans or dough to play with.

or other appliance with a removable lead, switch off or unplug at the wall socket. If a 'live' connector falls into a liquid – washing-up water, say – the resultant short circuit may cause the plug fuse to explode, often with sufficient violence to blow the plug to pieces.

• If a live connector does fall into water, turn off the power and unplug it before pulling it out of the water by the cord. If you put your hands in the water while the power is still on, you could get a severe electric shock.

• If a plug, lead or connector becomes wet, turn off the power and dry the plug thoroughly before attempting to use it.

• Turn the iron off if you are called away when ironing. When you have finished with it, leave it to cool out of reach of young children.

Bathroom and lavatory

About one accident in 23 in British homes happens in the bathroom – and one of the largest single causes is people falling when in the bath.

• If your bath or the base of your shower is smooth, use an internal bath mat which grips with suction cups. This will prevent you slipping.

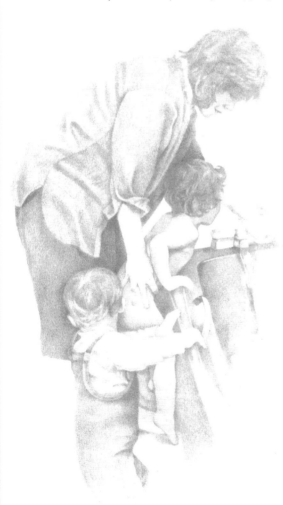

Cold water before hot
Always run the cold water into a bath first, then add the hot, in case a child falls in accidentally. Children can die from being scalded in very hot baths.

THE CURE THAT KILLED

Drinking water is a valuable on-the-spot first aid treatment for anyone who swallows a poisonous substance of any kind – a household cleaner, for instance, such as bleach. The water helps to dilute the poison and thus lessen its effects. The patient should drink as much water as he comfortably can without making himself sick. For an average adult, this may be 2-4 pints (about 1-2 litres). For a child, it could be less than·1 pint (about half a litre).

Drunk quickly in very large quantities, however, water can itself be poisonous.

In October 1982, a 40-year-old housewife from Hayes, London, accidentally swallowed some bleach that had been left in a cup to remove a stain. A hospital she rang advised her by telephone to drink water to minimise any risk, but in panic she took the remedy too far.

She drank water in enormous quantities, gulping it from a plastic bucket. 'She literally drank gallons,' a coroner later reported, 'and, despite making herself sick, continued to drink.'

Eventually the woman had a fit, collapsed and died from brain damage caused by water intoxication. At the inquest, doctors reported that the bleach had done her no harm at all.

• Fit a grab handle on the wall above the bath. This is particularly valuable for older people or for anyone who feels dizzy when getting up from a hot bath.

• If you have a shower unit, fit a thermostat to it to guard against scalding. Or consider buying

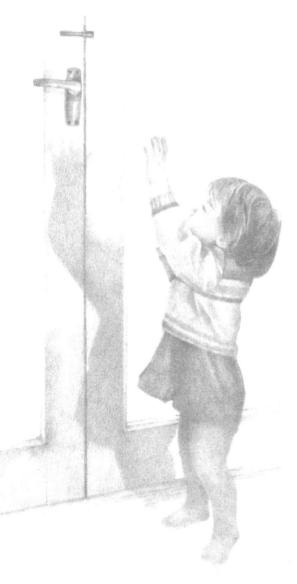

can condense inside the casing and make it 'live' – exposing you to a severe shock if you touch it. A battery-powered radio is, however, safe, because the voltage it uses is not high enough to be dangerous.

• Mop up water that spills on the floor to avoid the risk of you – or someone else – slipping on it. For the same reason, if you use a bath mat on the floor, make sure it has a non-slip backing.

• Never leave young children alone in the bath. If you have to leave the room, take them with you, wrapped in a towel to keep them warm.

• If you put a bolt on the inside of your bathroom or lavatory door, fit it high enough so that young children cannot reach it and lock themselves in. Remove the keys for the same reason.

• Never mix bleach or any bleach-based cleaner with other lavatory cleaners. The mixture can give off a poisonous gas.

• Store medicines well out of reach of children in a cabinet that can be locked.

• Do not transfer medicines from child-proof containers to ordinary ones.

• Dispose of old medicines safely. Either flush them down the lavatory, or return them to the chemist. Do not throw them away with the household rubbish.

Living room and dining area

More than one in five accidents happen in the living room or dining room – making these the most dangerous places indoors.

• Make sure that power points are not overloaded. If you have more appliances than you have points for, have extra sockets fitted.

• Check that flexes for lamps and other

Put door knobs out of reach
Fit handles high up to stop toddlers letting themselves out of the house or into a cupboard with medicines or chemicals. Add a higher bolt to stop them reaching the handle from a chair.

a shower head which has a thermostat built in for the purpose.

• By law, bathroom lights, heaters and any other electrical appliances must be controlled either by switches outside the bathroom, or by a cord-operated ceiling switch, so that it is impossible to touch water and the switch simultaneously. Electric shaver points are the only exception, because they use a special socket with an isolating transformer.

• Do not use mains electric appliances, such as a mains radio, in the bathroom. Water vapour

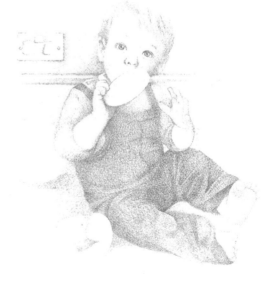

Cover plug sockets
Fit plastic safety plugs to power sockets when they are not in use, to cover up the holes and stop small children electrocuting themselves.

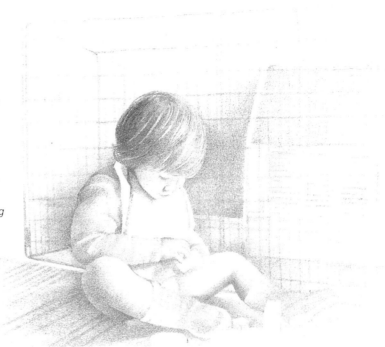

**Fix a fireguard
round every fire**
*Sturdy guards should be
fixed around all radiant
electric and gas fires, and
around open fires, and
attached to the wall with
fastenings that a child
cannot undo. They should
cover the whole fireplace,
not just the fire, and stand
far enough away from the
fire to stop a child reaching
it with bits of paper poked
through the wire.*

appliances do not trail across the floor where
people could trip over them. Do not run flexes
under the carpet – they may overheat and you
will not be able to see if they become worn.
• Fix rugs to the floor. Repair worn rugs or
carpets. Use non-slip polish on wooden floors.
• Do not balance ashtrays on armchairs or
sofas. A lot of modern upholstered furniture
contains foam plastic which gives off toxic fumes
and dense smoke if it catches fire. The smoke
and fumes, which can kill, are often more
dangerous than the flames themselves.
• Before going out or to bed, make sure that
cigarette ends are out and that fires are damped

down or thoroughly contained behind a
fireguard.
• Unplug electrical appliances at the wall at
night – especially the television set. Exceptions
to this are clocks, timers and video recorders,
which are designed for continuous operation.
• Ensure that all electrical appliances are protected by appropriate fuses – see the table on
page 156.

Bedroom
About one accident in nine happens in a
bedroom. Many involve poisoning, falls from
bunk beds or burns from sun lamps.

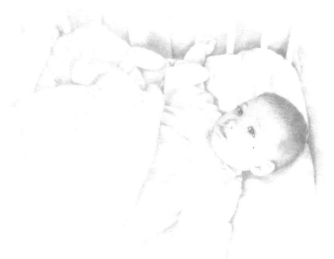

No pillows for a baby
*Babies under 12 months old
should never be given a
pillow. Because they cannot
easily turn over, they could
suffocate on it. If you decide
to give an older baby a pillow,
in or out of a cot, consider
using a safety pillow which
has air holes built into it.
Pillows of this type are
available from baby
equipment shops – as are
safety mattresses, which are
designed on the same lines.*

• Have your electric blanket checked for safety every year, and check its lead for brittleness and cracks every few months.

• Do not leave an electric underblanket switched on when the bed is occupied. It can overheat and set fire to the mattress and bedding. If the blanket is very badly worn, it could electrocute you.

• Make sure that the bulb in your bedside light is within the wattage range of the shade – too powerful a bulb can overheat the shade and create a fire hazard.

• Do not cover a shade with cloth or paper to cut down the brightness – this too can be a fire risk. Use a weaker bulb or a darker shade, or fit a dimmer switch.

• Moving about in the dark can be dangerous: keep a small torch, fitted with long-life batteries, by your bedside. Make sure that there are no trailing flexes or furniture for you to trip over.

• For the same reason, consider having a telephone socket fitted beside your bed, and plugging your phone in there at night. This is particularly valuable for elderly people who – if they become ill or have an accident – may not be able to reach the phone downstairs.

• Do not smoke in bed.

• Fit safety locks to windows in rooms for children. Do not position furniture that a child could climb on under a window.

Loft

• Fit some form of sturdy floorboarding between the hatch and water tank, so that you can stand safely.

• If the loft is unfloored, tread only on the joists – the ceiling between the joists will not bear the lightest foot.

• Make sure that the joists are strong enough if you plan to make any regular use of the loft – for storage, for example. A rough rule is to measure the unsupported length of the joists in feet, halve it and add 1, and that gives you the depth in inches the joists should be. A joist across a span of 12ft needs to be at least 7in deep if it is to be used in this way. If in doubt, get professional advice from an architect or a reliable local builder.

• If you plan to make any extensive use of your loft, bear in mind that you must have adequate ventilation and light, and the floor may need to be strengthened. Local council planning departments can advise on the detailed building regulations, which can vary from place to place.

• Fit a lighting point near the water tank so that you can see what you are doing if you have to work there.

• Make sure that all tanks and pipes are fully insulated to guard against the risk of their freezing up and bursting during a cold winter. If the loft floor is itself insulated, run the insulation

Switch off at night
Do not go to sleep with an electric underblanket switched on. Make a point of switching it off when you get into bed. With the extra heat of your body, an electric blanket can overheat if it is left on all night, and set fire to the mattress and bedding. A very badly worn blanket could also give you a severe electric shock.

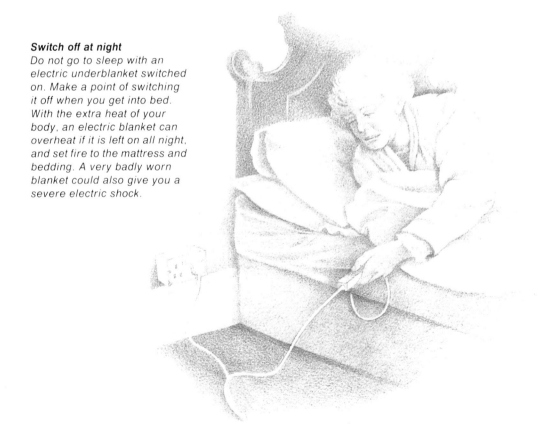

over the top of the tank and leave a gap in the insulation underneath to allow some warmth to rise from the house.
• Use either a properly fitted loft ladder or extending steps to gain access to the loft. Do not try to jump up from the top of an ordinary pair of steps.

Stairs and landings
One in nine home accidents are falls from stairs – and about a fifth of these falls involve children under five.
• Stair and landing carpets should be in good condition and firmly fastened – people may trip on loose or worn carpet.
• There should be at least one firm, continuous handrail on the staircase. If there are old people in the house, fit one on each side. Ensure that stairs are well lit, with two-way switches so that lights can be put on from either floor.
• Replace horizontal rails on a staircase or banister with vertical rails (close together so that a child cannot stick his head through them) or board them over.
• Consider fitting boards to the back of each tread on an open-riser staircase so that the gap is too narrow for a child to put his head through.
• Fit safety gates at the top and bottom of the staircase to prevent toddlers falling down the stairs or climbing them without supervision.
• Do not put a glass door at the bottom of a staircase – anyone falling into it could break it and suffer cuts on top of other injuries.
• Never put or leave loose objects on the stairs – if you tread on them you will almost certainly stumble, and may fall.

Garden
Gardens and other areas outside, such as garages, are the most dangerous places of all. They account for more than 750,000 accidents a year in Britain – between a quarter and a third of the total.
• Keep the garden path in good repair. Ensure that there are no loose or uneven stones on which people may trip.
• Do not leave tools such as rakes lying about.
• If you have young children, enclose or cover any garden pond or water butt. A child can drown in even a very shallow pool.
• Do not let a child use a lawn mower. If you are using a mower, keep children away.
• Never light a bonfire with paraffin or petrol. Keep a bonfire under control.
• If children are likely to play in your garden, check that there are no poisonous trees or

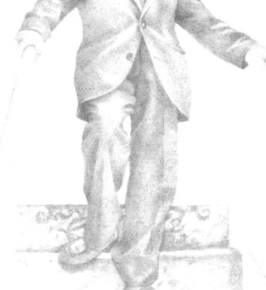

Making stairs safe
Old people should have two firm, continuous handrails to help them on the stairs. Keep the stairs well lit; dark areas can cause an elderly person to misjudge a step – and fall. The very young are also at risk on stairs. Every year, about 60,000 toddlers in Britain are injured on them – and some die. To cut this risk, fit safety gates top and bottom. Teach toddlers to climb down backwards, on all fours.

plants such as laburnum, deadly nightshade, yew or privet. The berries of all these plants can be dangerous to children.

• Keep garden gates locked or bolted high up so that young children cannot open them and run out into the street.

Doors

• When the house is unoccupied, or at night, keep all internal doors closed. In the event of fire breaking out, this will help to slow the spread of the flames.

• Fit safety locks on external doors so that young children cannot run outside.

• Glass doors should be fitted with safety glass – either toughened or laminated. Ordinary glass can shatter into lethal shards. If this is not possible, cover the glass with clear plastic film, available from DIY shops; it will prevent the glass from shattering if it breaks.

• If the glass in a door is clear, stick coloured tape or transfers onto the glass so that it is clearly visible when the door is closed.

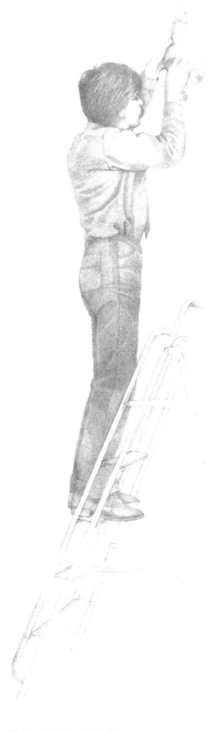

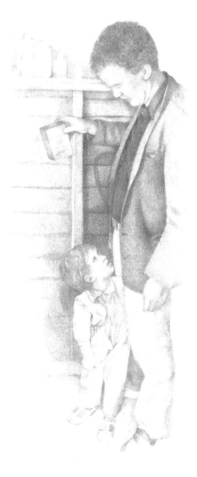

Where to store poisonous substances
Many DIY and household products, including turpentine, some glues, and oven cleaners, are poisonous. Lock them away out of reach of children. Do not leave them under the sink.

Take steps to be safe
Use a stepladder if you have to climb when working around the house. Even to change a bulb, take the time to set up a ladder. Do not be tempted to take shortcuts by standing on a chair or stool. They are less stable than a stepladder, and you have nothing to hold onto if you lose your balance.

Storms and high winds

Strong winds – even those well below hurricane force – can cause considerable damage, ripping tiles from roofs, dislodging chimney stacks and tearing down power cables and telephone wires. However, most well-constructed houses in good repair suffer little damage until winds reach speeds of about 47mph (75km/h).

On the Beaufort Scale this is Force 9 – a strong gale. Television weather maps usually show predicted wind direction and speed. The direction is shown by a black arrow with the speed marked in miles per hour.

Preparing for a storm

• Move indoors anything outside – such as garden tools or toys – that might blow about. This includes children's slides, unless they are very securely fixed.

• Secure dustbin lids and the lids of fuel bunkers with rope or wire. Make sure cloches, cold-frame lids and greenhouse windows are securely fastened.

• Close windows and doors tightly, especially those on the side facing the wind. If the storm is likely to be particularly severe, consider reinforcing the inside of windows with boards or heavy furniture. If the windows have external shutters, close them.

• Put candles, matches and torches close to hand in case the electricity is cut off. If you have camping equipment – a stove, say, or a gas lamp – get it out and keep it handy.

• Have buckets ready in case the roof starts to leak, and boarding, hammer and nails to shore up any window that is blown in.

• If you are expecting a thunderstorm, unplug electrical appliances where possible, including standard or table lamps. If you have an outside or attic TV aerial, unplug it at the wall socket if there is one, or else at the back of the set.

• If your home is prone to flooding in heavy rain, improvise sandbags – strong plastic bags, for instance, filled with any sand, soil or gravel to hand. Use the bags to line the bottoms of doors and low windows (see *What to do if you are caught in a flood*, page 331).

If a window is blown in

Wind and rain can wreak havoc in a room with a broken window.

• Move valuable objects, and anything else that can be shifted, to another room.

• Block the window with boarding or heavy furniture.

• Do not touch any electrical switches or appliances if you are wet or standing in water.

If tiles are blown off the roof

• Do not go outside to inspect the damage until the storm has eased. More tiles may come spinning off the roof onto you.

• If water starts coming through the roof, move everything from rooms likely to be flooded.

• Put buckets or bowls under the drips.

• If you can get access to the attic directly beneath the leaking area, place the buckets there. Set them on joists or on boards across the joists – not on the ceiling itself. Otherwise, the weight of the water or water splashing over the edge of the bucket may weaken the plaster and bring the ceiling down.

Leaks from outside

If a leak through the ceiling becomes apparent during heavy rain, it is probably coming through from outside. Remember, though, that the point from which the water drips is unlikely to be directly below where it is getting in.

• Go up into the loft and find the source by tracking the path the water has taken to its highest point.

• If the leak is through damaged or missing tiles or slates, or through a hole in the roofing felt, call a roofing specialist or builder (consult *Yellow Pages*) and have the tiles, slates or roofing felt replaced.

• If there is a delay, you can make a temporary repair with a sheet of strong plastic.

• Return to the loft and slide the top edge of the sheet of plastic up as far as possible under the tiles above the hole. Tuck it up tightly.

• Tuck the sides of the sheet tightly under the edges of the tiles on either side of the hole.

• Push the bottom edge of the sheet out through the hole and over the tiles below the hole, so that water is directed farther down the roof, where the tiles are sound.

• Try to allow at least 12in (300mm) overlap beyond the damaged area on all four edges of the sheet, and fix the sheet in place with

PATCHING A HOLE IN THE ROOF

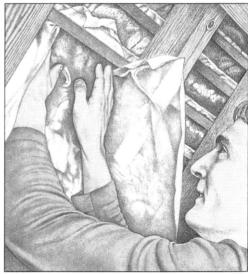

1 *Cut a sheet of plastic at least 12in (300mm) larger than the hole on all four sides. Slide the top edge between the roof battens and the tiles.*

HOW TO AVOID STORM DAMAGE

• Check that guttering and drains are kept clear of leaves and debris.

• Have a builder check tiles, aerial fixings and chimney pointing regularly. Make sure that windows and doors fit properly, and that the catches and locks are not loose.

• If you live in an exposed position, consider having a lightning conductor fitted.

• If there are any large old trees in your garden that could fall on the house, have them looked over by a tree surgeon.

• Cut back any branches on trees or shrubs that might flap against windows in a storm.

• Check that neighbours' trees are safe, too. If any appear to be dangerous, report their condition to the owner in writing. This will strengthen your position later if a tree does fall and you want to claim compensation from the neighbour or his insurance company.

• After a storm, check around the house for any signs of damage – loose or fallen tiles, for instance – and get them repaired.

• After a snowstorm, make a point also of checking in your attic to see whether snow has been driven in under the tiles or slates.

• If snow has got in, dig it out while it is still frozen, and take it outside at once. Otherwise, when it melts it could cause considerable damage in the house – even bringing down an entire ceiling, for example.

---

waterproof tape, or by tying its corners to the rafters with wire, or by tacking it to rafters.

• If the hole is large, the plastic may also need to be supported from below by a length of wood nailed to the rafters.

• Catch any remaining drips in a bucket and have the roof repaired properly later.

If a chimney pot is blown off

Rubble and tiles may come down the chimney if a chimney pot is blown off. The falling pot will probably damage the roof as well on its way down, letting water into the attic.

• Put out any fires caused by the scattering of a fire in the grate.

• Prevent debris from pouring down the chimney onto the carpet by blocking the fireplace with boards or the fireguard.

• When the debris has stopped falling, seal the base of the chimney with cardboard, bits of wood and newspaper to keep out the rain.

• Do the same in other rooms with fireplaces served by the same chimney stack in case other pots on the stack have been weakened.

• Check in the attic for leaks.

• Call a builder after the storm ends.

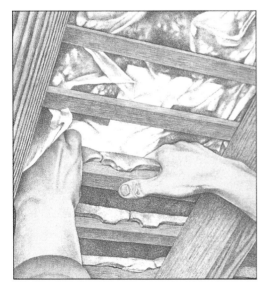

2 *Tuck the sheet's sides between battens and tiles on either side and then push the bottom out through the hole and over the tiles below.*

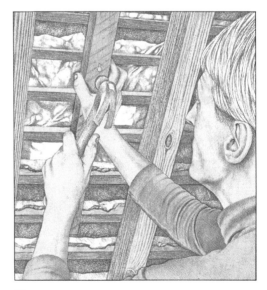

3 *Fix the sheet in place with tape, wire or nails. Nail a length of wood if necessary to the battens above and below to support it.*

COPING WITH THE COLD

Draught-proofing and insulation are the two most effective ways of keeping a house warmer during severe winters. Most DIY shops stock strips of metal and foam with which doors and windows can be lined to cut down the loss of heat through draughts.

Insulating a house – through double glazing, or by filling the cavities in the walls with a material such as plastic foam – is a more expensive and specialised job, best done during the summer when the specialist firms involved are likely to be less busy.

Walking on snow and ice
Falling over on hard ice or snow can be extremely dangerous, particularly for young children (who have less strength in their necks and so are more likely to damage their heads if they fall) and for the elderly (because their bones are more brittle).

It is possible, though, to cut the risk of falling by adopting some of the techniques used by skiers and mountaineers.
• Wear shoes or boots with a deep tread to improve your grip.
• On the flat, walk with your legs more apart than usual – rather like the gait of a sailor – and take smaller steps than usual.
• Avoid walking on icy patches at all, if possible. But if you cannot avoid a patch of ice, try to find a handhold to help you across – a garden wall, say.
• On slopes, walk with your toes pointing inwards. On each step, stamp your foot down firmly and at a slight angle so that the outside edge of your shoe digs into the snow and forms a small step.
• On steep downward slopes, bend your knees as well. It helps to improve your grip.

How to cut heating costs
Elderly people, particularly, need to keep warm in winter to avoid the risk of hypothermia (a potentially fatal loss of body heat). Each winter, more than 350 pensioners in Britain die of hypothermia. Nearly 60,000 other elderly people die each year of diseases such as pneumonia, chronic bronchitis and flu – all diseases to which the body is much more vulnerable in the cold.

To help pensioners on a tight budget, welfare organisations recommend these tips on how to keep warm economically:
• Wear several layers of clothing. Several thin layers are warmer than one thick one.
• Wear a night cap at night – and gloves and socks too, if necessary.
• Buy a small thermometer to hang on the wall, and keep an eye on it; elderly people often do not realise how cold they are. The ideal temperature for an elderly person's living room is 21°C (70°F).
• Stick kitchen foil, shiny side out, to the wall behind radiators to reflect heat into the room. This is particularly valuable where the radiator is against an outside wall.
• Fix small shelves above radiators to push warm air towards the centre of the room.
• Hang a heavy curtain inside the front door to make the hall warmer, and a small piece of carpet over the letter box.
• As an economical substitute for double glazing, attach plastic sheeting to the inside of windows. Fix it with masking tape, double-sided tape, a wooden frame or magnetic strips. But make sure the sheeting is easily detachable in case of fire.
• Try to cook complete meals in the oven all at once to save on fuel bills. Use a bowl instead of running hot water for washing your hands or dishes. Rinse dishes in cold water.
• Eating properly helps the body to keep itself warmer. Have a bowl of hot porridge for breakfast to give yourself a warm start to the day; and try to eat fish, eggs, cheese, meat, potatoes and green vegetables regularly. Eat at least one good meal a day.

Getting financial help
Nearly a million pensioners in Britain do not claim all the government and council benefits they are entitled to. Councils sometimes offer grants to help to pay for loft insulation, for instance, and for lagging water tanks. Gas and electricity boards have budget schemes to help to spread the cost of fuel bills through the year, and financial help with heating bills is available to pensioners who qualify for supplementary benefit from the Department of Social Security.

To check on what you – or an elderly relative or neighbour – are entitled to, contact your local Citizens Advice Bureau (listed in the phone book under 'C') or your nearest Age Concern Group (listed in the phone book either under 'A' or under 'Old People's Welfare'). If no local group is listed, write to the organisation's national headquarters: Age Concern England, Astral House, 1268 London Road, London SW16 4EJ.

Alternatively, contact your local council, your gas and electricity boards, and the DSS direct. Even if you have applied for these grants and benefits before, and been turned down, check again because the qualifying thresholds change frequently.

Working at a height

About 30,000 accidents a year in British homes involve ladders of various kinds, or scaffolding.

The safest way to work at a height in any situation – up a ladder, say, or in a tree – is to follow the 'three holds' principle used by mountaineers and rock climbers. Always make sure that you have at least three secure holds: two foot-holds and one hand-hold, or one foot-hold and two hand-holds. Do not leave any of the holds until your free hand or foot is secure on a hold to replace it.

• Check ladders or steps before use for cracked or rotten rungs or loose joints. If a stepladder or extension ladder has ropes, make sure they are in good condition.

• Varnish wooden ladders to protect them, but do not paint them. Paint could conceal developing cracks or weak spots in the wood.

• When you use a ladder, set it up so that its base is between a quarter and one-third of its height away from the object it rests against. The base of a 20ft (6m) ladder should be 5-7ft (1.5-2m) away from the wall or tree it is propped on. Any closer, and you risk pulling the ladder over backwards when you climb it; any farther, and you risk the base sliding outwards.

• On soft ground, rest the foot of the ladder on a wide board. Nail a batten firmly to the board to stop the ladder slipping off.

• On hard ground, lay something heavy – bricks or a bag of cement – against the foot. If possible, have someone hold the foot of the ladder steady as well.

• Do not hang out sideways to reach the work – when painting, for example. Move the ladder to suit the work.

• Make sure the top of the ladder is at least three rungs higher than the highest point you want to reach, so that the top is always within reach of your hands.

In the home and at work

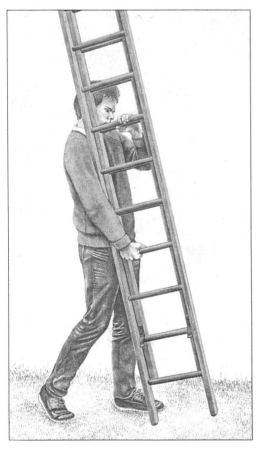

THE SAFE WAY TO CARRY A LADDER
Carry a ladder vertically to avoid accidentally hitting anyone behind you. Bend your knees slightly and, with one hand, grip the rung just below waist level. With the other hand, grip the rung at eye level. Rest the ladder against your shoulder and straighten up. Keep the ladder steady with the upper hand.

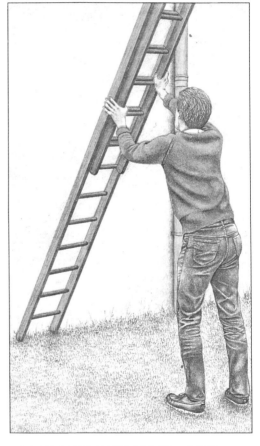

HOW TO RAISE AN EXTENDED LADDER
Extend the ladder while it is still on the ground and wedge its foot against the wall. Lift the top over your head and push the ladder up by moving forwards and working your hands down it. When the top is against the wall, pull the bottom out until it is at least a quarter of the ladder's length away from the wall.

- Do not climb a ladder while carrying a heavy load in one hand. Tie the load to a rope, carry the end of the rope up the ladder, then haul the load up once you are in position.
- For roof work, use a roofing ladder or crawling board which hooks over the ridge. Never rely on the gutter for support; it may break.
- Do not lean any ladder against guttering either – use a stay to hold it clear.
- For jobs requiring a lot of sideways movement, such as replacing gutters or pointing, hire a scaffold platform or use two stepladders with one or more planks laid across their rungs.
- Use the rungs rather than the top to improve the platform's stability and to give you something to grab hold of if you lose your balance. For extra security, you can suspend two handrails – made, for example, from thin bits of metal piping – between higher rungs or the tops of the ladders.
- Lash the planks to the rungs and to one side of the ladders to stop them slipping.
- If the planks have not been used for some time, test each one's strength at ground level first by putting a large block under each end and standing in the middle. Jump up and down on the plank. If it sags worryingly or creaks, do not use it.

THREE WAYS TO STEADY A LADDER

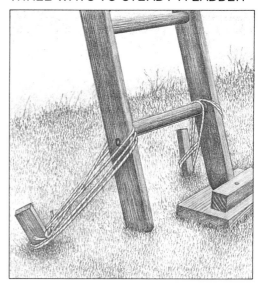

1 *Secure the foot of a ladder by tying it to stakes. On uneven ground, level the ladder up by putting a wide board with a batten nailed to it under one side of the ladder. On soft ground, put the board under both sides.*

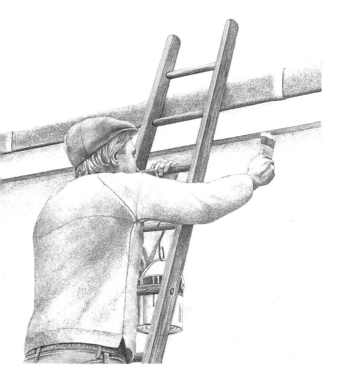

SAFETY ON A LADDER
Hold onto the ladder's rungs, not the sides; if you slip, you are less likely to lose your grip. While you work, hook your paint can or tool bag onto a rung so that you always have one hand free to hold on. Never hang out sideways to work. Move the ladder instead.

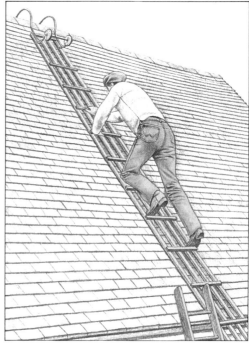

WHEN TO USE A ROOFING LADDER
Never rely on guttering to support you for roof work; it is not strong enough. A roofing ladder, though – available from most DIY hire shops – will bear your weight. Push the ladder up the roof on the wheels at its top. Then turn it over and hook it over the ridge.

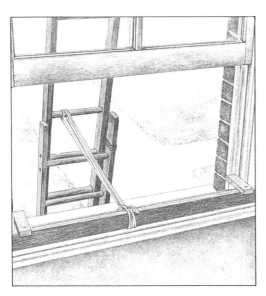

2 *Another way to hold a ladder steady is to anchor it by passing some rope around a rung and tying it to a wooden batten secured behind a window frame or letterbox. Nail pieces of wood to the batten to stop it sliding sideways.*

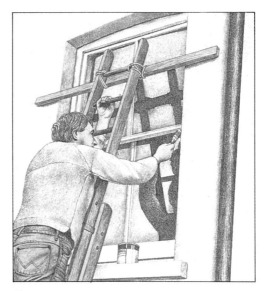

3 *If you have to lean a ladder against a window, lash a strong wooden batten, longer than the window is wide, to the top of the ladder. When you put the ladder up, rest the batten on the wall on either side of the window.*

IMPROVISING A PLATFORM
If you have to move sideways a lot while working, make a platform by suspending one or more planks between stepladders. Lash the plank both to the rungs at each end and to one side of each ladder to stop it from shifting around either lengthways or sideways.

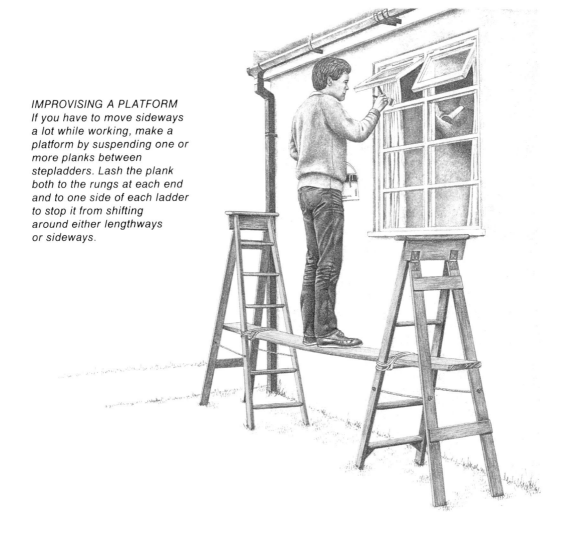

Do's and don'ts of using tools

Tools are safe as long as they are used and stored correctly, and kept in good condition and well out of the reach of children.

Yet about 210,000 people have to get hospital treatment every year in Britain as a result of DIY accidents.

Around 75,000 of these accidents are caused by or involve the use of hand tools, ranging from circular saws and blowtorches to screwdrivers, knives, pliers and hammers.

The other 135,000 or so accidents involve the equipment or materials used with tools or in DIY work generally, such as ladders, nails, screws, planks, and bricks.

Anyone who plans to use tools, especially power tools, for DIY work in the home should make himself or herself familiar beforehand with the positions of concealed water pipes and electric cables. The effort required to draw up a detailed plan is much less than the risk involved in cutting a wire accidentally or the trouble of repairing a hidden pipe.

Hand tools

• Keep sharp-edged tools sheathed and out of the reach of children when not in use, preferably under lock and key.
• Keep tools sharp – blunt tools are dangerous because they require more force to use and thus are more likely to slip.
• Protect the sharp ends of tools such as chisels and bradawls when carrying them in a toolbox. Cover them with fitted plastic covers, wrap them with several layers of cloth or push old bottle corks onto the blades or points.
• Similarly, cover the blades of saws, axes and similar tools when carrying them about.
• Make sure hammer heads are firmly attached to their handles. If necessary, replace the wedges.
• The metal head of a cold chisel roughens when the tool is struck, and sharp fragments may fly off in use. Grind or file these rough edges away regularly.
• Make sure that the material you are working on – a piece of wood or metal, say – is firmly held in a vice or by clamps so that both hands are free to manipulate the tools.
• In the garden, never leave a rake or fork lying down with the prongs up. If you tread on the prongs the handle can fly up and strike you in the face.
• Keep sharp-edged garden tools such as shears, secateurs and billhooks well away from your fingers and legs while in use.

Power tools

• Keep power tools unplugged except when in use, so that they cannot be started accidentally.
• For the same reason, unplug power tools before changing accessories, cleaning, adjusting or lubricating.
• With petrol-driven tools, remove the lead from the spark plug before working on them to remove any chance of the motor starting up by accident. Otherwise, a motor mower, for example, may spring into life when the blades are turned by hand.
• Wear protective goggles when sparks or chips are liable to fly – when using a grinding wheel, say, or an electric saw. Wear them too when working on bricks or concrete with a cold chisel or a hammer drill.
• Tie back long hair and avoid wearing loose clothing – both may become caught in revolving machinery.
• Do not defeat the makers' efforts to keep power tools safe by, for example, tying back the guard on a circular saw.
• Do not use electric tools outdoors in the rain – the wet may cause a short circuit and give you a severe shock.
• When using extension leads, plug into the house power socket last so that there are no unguarded live socket ends lying around. For the same reason, disconnect at the house socket

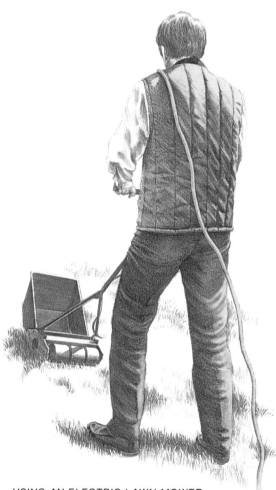

USING AN ELECTRIC LAWN MOWER
Hang an electric mower's cable over one shoulder to keep it behind you, and make sure there is nothing it could catch on. If you are on a slope, mow across it – not up and down.

first when the work is finished. Check cables, extension leads and connectors regularly for signs of wear or cracked insulation.

• Never use taped joints on loose power cables indoors or out – they may pull apart and are not waterproof. Use purpose-made waterproof connectors instead.

• When using a mains-powered hedge trimmer, lawn mower or grass trimmer, keep the cable behind you. Make sure the cable has a clear run so that it does not become snagged while you are working.

• Push a mower away from you – never pull it – and mow across slopes, not up them. That way there is less risk of the mower running over your foot.

• When using mowers and trimmers, always wear stout shoes and trousers. Wear goggles when using trimmers – they can throw up small stones and dust.

• Remember that the blade of an electric mower carries on spinning for several seconds after the power is switched off. Unplug it before clearing debris from around the blade.

• Hold electric mower trigger switches on by hand – never tie them down.

• Consider buying a circuit breaker (one type is called a residual current circuit breaker – RCCB) for use with electrical equipment. Circuit breakers are designed to cut off the mains power if there is a short circuit or the user gets an electric shock.

• Look out for a symbol showing two squares, one inside the other, when buying electrically powered tools. It means that the tool is doubly insulated.

Using a chain saw

• Apply the saw to the top of the work you are cutting. Do not cut from underneath – unless you are cutting a piece of wood supported at both ends. Otherwise the weight of the wood will tend to close the cut, gripping the saw.

• Cut using the part of the saw closest to the motor end. If you use the tip, you may lose control of the saw.

• Do not carry the saw about with the engine running, even if the blade is disengaged.

• Keep the chain at the correct tension, or it may fly off and cause a serious accident.

• Sharpen the teeth frequently, preferably every time you use the saw. Blunt teeth may make you use too much pressure.

• Before refilling the tank of a petrol-driven saw, make sure the engine is cold, or petrol spilt onto it may ignite.

• If you have a can of petrol with you, keep it well away from the saw. The exhaust will occasionally emit sparks.

• Wear sensible clothing: thick trousers and stout shoes (preferably with reinforced toecaps), and no loose sleeves. Wear goggles to protect your eyes against chips and sawdust.

• Always work in a clear area, so that there are

no twigs or brambles to catch the blade or the trigger. Hold the saw with both hands.

• If you have an assistant, make sure he or she keeps at least 10yds (9m) away, out of range of any flying chips.

• Always disconnect the spark-plug lead or mains lead before cleaning or adjusting the saw. Have the saw serviced regularly and the cutting chain checked for signs of wear.

Hiring tools from hire shops

Specialised power tools – such as jack hammers, cultivators, disc cutters and belt sanders – can be hired by the day from hire shops. This is a convenient way of getting the use of expensive tools that you need only occasionally. But do not forget that many of these tools are potentially dangerous.

Do not even attempt to use them unless you know exactly how to handle them. Get the hire shop to give you clear instructions and preferably a demonstration, too.

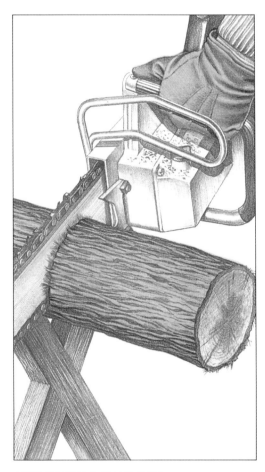

HOW TO USE A CHAIN SAW
Saw from the top downwards to cut the
unsupported end off a log. Cut with the part
of the blade closest to the motor. That way it
is easier to hold the saw steady.

How to remove stains

The best way to remove a stain depends on what has been spilt and what it has been spilt on. But one rule applies to any stain anywhere: try to deal with it quickly, before it dries. Once dry, most stains become more difficult to remove.

Remember, too, that many stain-removing agents are poisonous, flammable or both (see chart, this page).

Read carefully any instructions on proprietary preparations. Never store them in unmarked bottles, and keep them out of the reach of children. Work out of doors if possible, or in a well-ventilated place.

• The first step in treating a stain is to blot, lightly scrape or vacuum the material in order to clear as much of the stain as possible before further treatment.

• For grease stains, shake on plenty of talcum powder, powdered starch or a similar absorbent agent. When the worst of the grease has been absorbed, brush clear.

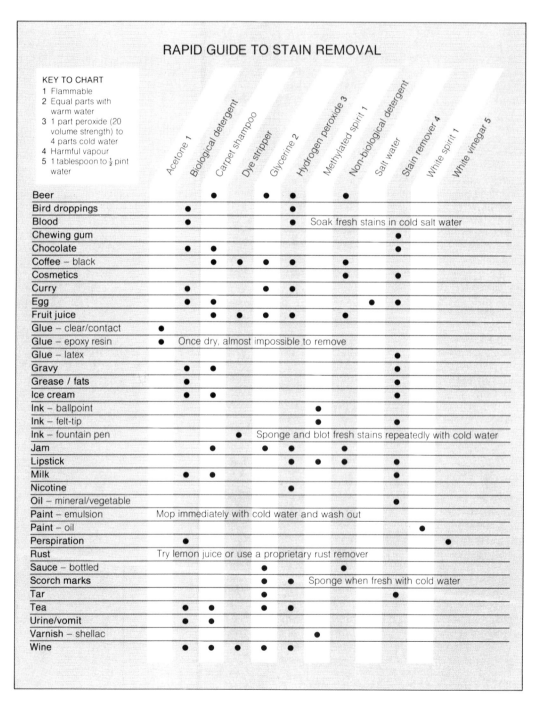

RAPID GUIDE TO STAIN REMOVAL

KEY TO CHART
1. Flammable
2. Equal parts with warm water
3. 1 part peroxide (20 volume strength) to 4 parts cold water
4. Harmful vapour
5. 1 tablespoon to ½ pint water

	Acetone 1	Biological detergent	Carpet shampoo	Dye stripper	Glycerine 2	Hydrogen peroxide 3	Methylated spirit 1	Non-biological detergent	Salt water	Stain remover 4	White spirit 1	White vinegar 5
Beer		●		●	●	●						
Bird droppings	●					●						
Blood	●					●	Soak fresh stains in cold salt water					
Chewing gum										●		
Chocolate	●	●								●		
Coffee – black		●	●	●	●			●				
Cosmetics								●		●		
Curry	●			●	●							
Egg	●	●							●	●		
Fruit juice		●	●	●	●			●				
Glue – clear/contact	●											
Glue – epoxy resin	●	Once dry, almost impossible to remove										
Glue – latex										●		
Gravy	●	●								●		
Grease / fats	●									●		
Ice cream	●	●								●		
Ink – ballpoint							●					
Ink – felt-tip							●			●		
Ink – fountain pen			●	Sponge and blot fresh stains repeatedly with cold water								
Jam		●		●	●		●					
Lipstick					●		●	●		●		
Milk	●	●								●		
Nicotine						●						
Oil – mineral/vegetable										●		
Paint – emulsion	Mop immediately with cold water and wash out											
Paint – oil											●	
Perspiration		●										●
Rust	Try lemon juice or use a proprietary rust remover											
Sauce – bottled				●				●				
Scorch marks				●		●	Sponge when fresh with cold water					
Tar				●						●		
Tea	●	●			●	●						
Urine/vomit	●	●										
Varnish – shellac							●					
Wine		●	●	●	●	●						

- For other stains, sponge or rinse through with cold or lukewarm water – never hot water, which could fix the stain.
- Blot carpets or upholstery frequently, while you work on getting out the worst of the stain, to avoid overwetting them.
- What you should do next to complete the job depends upon what caused the stain, and what will dissolve it (see chart).
- Not all stains can be removed. If in doubt, and for delicate and valuable articles, just blot the stain and do not attempt any further treatment at home. Instead, seek advice from a professional cleaning firm.
- In general, stains on suede and leather, waterproof fabrics or rich materials such as velvets should be left to a professional.
- With other fabrics and surfaces, start with the mildest treatment and test first on a hidden area. Some solvents can damage certain materials, such as rayon.
- Use a white absorbent pad for applying solvents. Where possible, work from the underside of the stain, holding another pad on the top side to absorb it.
- Dab at the stain. Rubbing can spread the mark and damage the surface. Work inwards from the edge to avoid spreading the stain.
- If a stain has become dried, try to soften it. Rub in some glycerine solution (equal amounts of glycerine and warm water) and leave it for an hour. Then sponge with cold water.
- Once the substance has been loosened, treat it as a freshly made stain.

Emergency alternatives

If you find in an emergency that you do not have the substances mentioned in the chart, there are other ways, using more common household items, to get rid of some stains.

- If somebody spills wine, for example, on your carpet, flush it out immediately with a soda siphon or by sponging with warm water.
- If you get wine on a washable fabric – a tablecloth, say – immediately sprinkle it with salt to stop the stain spreading. Then, as soon as possible afterwards, stretch the stained area over a bowl and pour hot water through the fabric. If it is red wine, you can also pour white wine over the stain; this will make it easier to remove.
- If a pet or a baby urinates on your carpet, immediately give the area a good squirt with a soda siphon. Blot up the soda water. Then sponge with warm water with a few drops of antiseptic added.
- Use lemon juice for tea and coffee stains on washable fabrics. Rub the juice into the stained area and then wash the fabric in warm soapy water.
- If you get chewing gum on your clothes, put the article of clothing in a plastic bag and leave it in a freezer until the gum has hardened. You will then be able to pick it off easily.

Trapped in a lift

When a lift breaks down with people trapped inside, the greatest danger is from panic.
- Stay calm and try to reassure anyone who shows signs of panic.
- Explain that you and they are not in danger, that help can be summoned in several ways, and that there is no possibility of the lift falling out of control down the shaft.
- Tell the others in the lift that automatic brakes, usually fitted under the floor of the lift, prevent this happening by clamping onto the steel guide rails that run down each side of the lift shaft. The brakes will work even if there is a power cut and the lights go out.
- Use the alarm button or the telephone inside the lift to call for help.
- If there is no alarm system, bang on the doors and shout. Use a shoe to bang with, if your hand hurts.
- Once you contact someone outside, explain what has happened and ask him to get expert help at once.
- If there is no lift engineer immediately available, lift rescues are often handled by the fire brigade. Tell your contact to dial 999. Firemen will usually winch the lift up or down to the nearest floor, then open the doors. Manual overrides enable them to do this even when the power supply has been cut off.
- Never try to escape from the lift without help from an expert outside.
- Do not even try to force the inner lift doors open. Even if you managed to do so, it is most unlikely that you would be able to reach and open the outer doors onto a landing, let alone climb out safely. There is also the danger that you might slip on the oil and grease that accumulates on the outside of a lift. Having shoes with a good grip or bare feet is no guarantee that you would be able to balance steadily.
- Do not be tempted, either, to climb out of any hatch there may be in the lift's ceiling. When a lift hatch is opened, an electrical contact prevents the lift from moving. But if the open hatch falls shut by accident the lift could move without warning, throwing you off balance. In the darkness of the shaft, you could also trip over the lift cables or slip on grease and fall off the roof of the lift.

If you cannot raise the alarm

It is very rare for calls for help to go unanswered for long, particularly in a block of flats where there are other people within earshot. But in an office block late at night or at the start of a weekend, it may happen that nobody passes near the lift for hours – or even days.
- The safest course in this situation is to stay put, stay calm and wait. You may get hungry, thirsty and hot – but you will survive.
- Listen for a caretaker and try to attract his attention. If that fails, wait for the building to open again, then bang on the doors and shout for help.

In the home and at work

Intruders in your home

The vast majority of people who are likely to visit your home are law-abiding citizens. But it is worth being cautious always, just in case the visitor is a thief or a confidence trickster.

If a stranger calls at your door
• Use a peephole to vet anyone who knocks at your door and keep the chain on the door if it is someone you do not know.
• Never let in strangers until you have checked their credentials.
• If the caller gives you a telephone number to ring, check it in the directory yourself – it may be that of an accomplice. Ask the caller to wait outside, with the door closed and the chain on, while you make the call.
• If you are still in doubt about the caller's identity, ring 999 and explain your suspicions. Suspect anybody who protests at your caution.
• If in any doubt, refuse entry politely but firmly.
• Always be fully clothed before opening the door. Close the door on a stranger before going for your purse or to make a phone call.
• If you live in a block of flats, do not automatically 'buzz open' the main door if a stranger calls your apartment on the intercom with a plausible excuse.
• Do not hold the door open for a stranger whose arrival coincides with your departure.

If you return to see signs of a break-in
• If you notice or suspect that somebody is inside your home when you arrive at the gate – you see movement, perhaps, or notice an open door – avoid entering the house at all.
• If you have driven in by car, back out of the drive again and drive off. The intruder may think you were just turning round.
• If you are on foot, walk on down the pavement.
• Go to a neighbour's house at once and call the police. Follow the same drill if you find strangers outside your house.

If you get indoors to find a prowler inside
• If possible, go to a neighbour's house and call the police.
• Do not, the police advise, give any impression that you intend to fight over money or possessions – you may get hurt. Try not to anger or provoke him.
• Memorise the intruder's appearance.
• Call the police as soon as the intruder has gone.

If you wake up to hear a burglar in the house
• If you wake at night to hear an intruder downstairs – or if you hear someone trying to break in – put all the lights on and make a lot of noise by moving about. Most burglars will choose to flee empty-handed rather than risk coming face to face with their intended victim.
• Do not go downstairs. Dial the police from your bedroom if possible. Find something that

IMPROVISING WINDOW LOCKS WHEN LEAVING YOUR HOME EMPTY

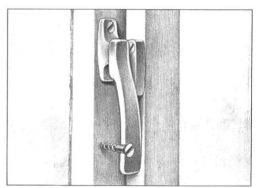

1 A screw makes an effective lock. Sink it about 1in (25mm) into the wood beside the catch.

USING A PLASTIC BLOCK-JOINT

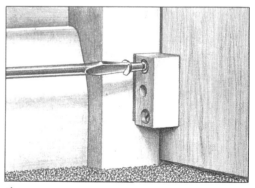

1 To make an inexpensive lock that can be left in place, fit block-joints in the angle between a door or window, and its frame.

DOWN A KNOTTED SHEET AT 76
Tied up, gagged and blindfolded by armed, masked burglars, and locked in a first-floor bedroom of their Wiltshire home with the phone wires cut, two elderly ladies seemed helpless on the night of October 23, 1984.

But 76-year-old Miss Dorothy Watson never thought of giving up. Instead, like others who have survived crises, she made use of inner strengths: courage and a cool head.

She managed to untie herself, and knotted sheets into a rope. She then climbed down the sheets to fetch help for her 86-year-old friend, Miss Beatrice Knatchbull. Miss Watson fell when still about 10ft (3m) from the ground and broke her ankle. In spite of the pain, she crawled to a neighbour to raise the alarm. Miss Knatchbull was later rescued unhurt.

Two men were later charged with the robbery.

you can use as a weapon – a comb, say, a vase, knitting needle or a bunch of keys – but plan to use it only if you cannot avoid a fight (see *If you are attacked in the street*, page 336).

• If you are on your own, call out loudly to an imaginary male companion: 'Harry, there's someone in the house.'

• Look out of your window after you hear the intruder leave and try to note what he looks like, what direction he heads in and what car, if any, he gets into. Then call the police.

How to give a description to the police

Anyone who contacts the police to report a crime – an intruder, say, or someone behaving suspiciously near his or a neighbour's home – may need to give a description of the person he has seen, or of the person's vehicle. This is a checklist of details useful to police:

• Male/female
• Colour of skin
• Complexion
• Height
• Hair (colour, length, straight/curly, receding)
• Build
• Age
• Eye colour
• Glasses
• Face (long, thin, round, clean-shaven, moustache, beard)
• Marks (scars, tattoos)
• Mouth (narrow/wide)
• Dress (description of clothing)
• Any other distinguishing features (mannerisms, say, such as a limp or a stutter)

If you see a suspicious vehicle, try to note these details:

• Car/van/lorry/motorcycle
• Colour
• Registration number
• Other details (damage marks, any company name on it and so on)
• Make/model
• Body type (saloon/estate car, number of doors, soft top)
• Direction it was travelling

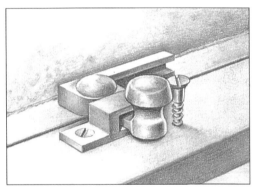

2 *On a sash window, put the screw in vertically to prevent the catch being moved from outside.*

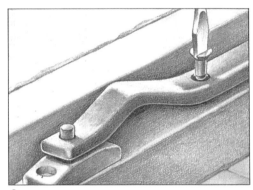

3 *For extra security, put another screw through one of the holes in a window stay-bar.*

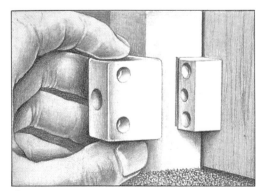

2 *Screw one half of the joint to the door, the other half to the door frame. On long windows, use two joints top and bottom.*

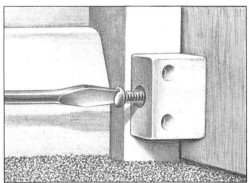

3 *Once the two halves are in position, they can be left there. To undo the lock, simply remove the bolt that holds the halves together.*

PROTECTING YOUR HOME

If you are going away or leaving the house for a period, the central rule is: do not advertise your absence.

• Cancel deliveries of milk and newspapers.

• Consider hiring a telephone answering service, so that your telephone gives no clue that you are absent. If you have a telephone answering machine, word your announcement as though you were merely away for an hour or two.

• Fit timeswitches (available from DIY shops) to turn your lights on at night.

• Consider using screws to make improvised locks for windows and internal doors (see pictures, pages 182-183). Fit the screws tight up against window catches to stop them being moved. Alternatively, sink the screw into a convenient part of the frame, and tie the catch to it with wire.

• Ask a neighbour to keep an eye on the house – to collect mail and other material left in the letterbox, to mow the lawn, sweep up leaves, leave footprints in the snow and generally make the house look lived in. Offer to do the same for the neighbour.

• If you are going away for only a short period, consider leaving your car locked outside. It may fool a prowling thief into thinking that the house is occupied. But if you will be away for a long holiday, remember that a dusty car may itself become an indication that the house is empty.

• Tell the local police station that you will be away. The police will then make a point of keeping an eye on the property.

How to deter burglars

Each year, around 1,360,000 buildings are burgled in Britain – an average of more than 150 every hour of the day and night. Burglaries of homes make up more than half the total. A skilled professional burglar will always find a way into a house if he wants to – and has the time. But eight out of ten burglaries are committed by unskilled and often young opportunists who are looking for easy pickings. You may deter both kinds of thieves by offering stiff resistance in the form of security devices. If a burglar has to make a lot of noise or spend a lot of time breaking in, he is likely to give up and look for an easier target elsewhere.

• Remember that windows are as vulnerable as doors. So consider fitting window locks to all windows that are on the ground floor or can be reached by an easy climb.

• Make sure that all security devices on doors and windows are fitted with strong screws or bolts. Small ones can be wrenched out of the wood by a firm shove or kick.

• The main value of burglar alarms is to deter amateur thieves. Ask local police for advice about the best type to fit.

• Do not put your name on your key ring. That way if you lose your house keys nobody will know which house they belong to (you can use a post code marking to identify them if they are handed in to the police).

• Keys should not be carried in a handbag. If it is stolen, letters or documents also in the bag could tell the thief your address.

Neighbourhood Watch: how it works

Neighbourhood Watch, Home Watch, Crime Alert and other similar schemes, which now operate in many parts of Britain, were first introduced in 1982 by the police in Cheshire. Their primary aim is to stem the rising tide of burglaries around the country by encouraging people to keep an eye out for suspicious activities near their homes – by being, in other words, good neighbours.

Police say that neighbourhoods which have joined the schemes – and announced the fact publicly by putting up stickers visible from the street – may have considerably lower crime rates than similar areas which have not joined.

The schemes do not encourage people to have a go themselves if they see anyone behaving suspiciously. But the schemes do encourage householders to phone the police at once by dialling 999, or to contact their street coordinator.

As a further deterrent to thieves, police also recommend that you should mark anything valuable you own – car, bicycle, furniture, household appliances and so on – with an indelible identification. The identification, they suggest, should show your post code, along with the number of your house or flat or the first two letters of your name.

The marking can be done at home by using a do-it-yourself engraving tool or stamp, or an invisible marker (available from many hardware shops) whose ink shows up only under ultraviolet light. The presence of the marks should be advertised through stickers placed in the windows of your house.

Stickers, leaflets and detailed advice about the police Property Marking scheme, about how to join or set up a local Neighbourhood Watch, and about ways of making your home more secure, are available free of charge from the Crime Prevention Officer at your nearest police station.

Caring for a sick or injured animal

There are more pet dogs and cats in Britain than there are people in the whole of Greater London. Around the country, there are 7.3 million dogs and about 6.9 million cats – compared with fewer than 7 million people in the capital. In addition, there are some 550,000 domesticated horses, including 11,500 which are involved in racing.

If a pet animal becomes seriously ill or is seriously injured in an accident, the safest course is to take it to a vet as soon as possible. But you can do much to alleviate its distress before you get there by using the first aid advice given here.

In some circumstances, swift action can save the pet's life. When a cat or dog gives birth, on the other hand, the best course is to leave the mother alone, and to call a vet only if the birth seems to be going wrong.

The section that begins on these pages describes the commonest emergencies that arise with a pet dog, cat or horse, and explains how to cope with each. It also explains what to do if a swarm of bees or a colony of wasps invades your home, and how you can help an injured bird or wild animal.

How to handle an injured cat or dog

Any dog or cat which has been injured is almost certain to be in pain. As a result, even the most loving, placid pet is liable to bite or scratch, or to run off, if it is given the chance. The priority, therefore, is to get the animal under control and into a safe, escape-proof place where you can examine its injuries.
- Approach the animal slowly and carefully, talking soothingly as you do.
- If it is a dog, have with you a rope, string or bandage fastened into a noose at one end.
- Drop the noose over the dog's head and draw it tight on the neck. Lead the dog to a safe place.
- If the dog is unable to stand, slide it onto an improvised stretcher – a large blanket or towel. Get someone to help you to lift the blanket by the corners and carry the dog to a safe place.
- In the case of a cat, grasp it by the scruff of

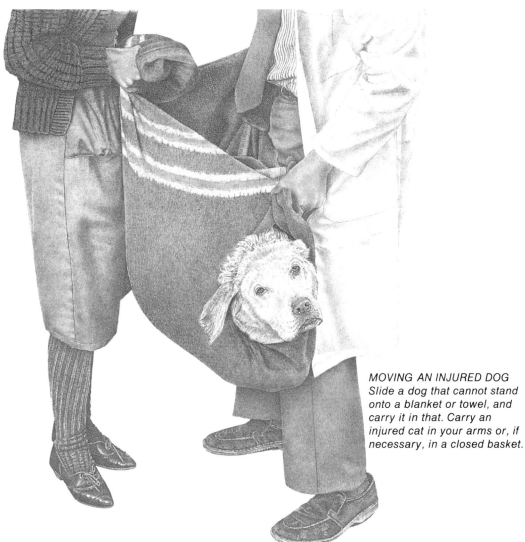

MOVING AN INJURED DOG
Slide a dog that cannot stand onto a blanket or towel, and carry it in that. Carry an injured cat in your arms or, if necessary, in a closed basket.

the neck with one hand and support its bottom with the other.

• Take it – in a closed basket, if necessary – to a safe place.

Preparing for treatment

• Before you start to examine a cat's or dog's injuries, get it onto a smooth surface such as a table or, if it is a heavy dog, on a slippery floor such as lino.

• Get someone else to help you to hold the animal – the slippery surface will stop it getting a grip and lessen its ability to escape.

• Put a collar on the animal to give yourself an easy handhold.

• Grip the animal firmly. Better still, get a helper to hold the animal so that you have both hands free to tend the injury.

• With a dog, tie a handkerchief or bandage firmly round its muzzle as well, so that it cannot open its mouth to bite.

Treating the injury

The principles of giving first aid to animals are much the same as they are for humans. Do what you can to stop the injury getting any worse, and then get professional help. This means taking the animal to a vet as soon as possible.

The commonest serious injuries are bleeding or a broken leg.

How to stop bleeding

• If an animal is bleeding badly, cover the wound with a clean pad – a piece of gauze or a handkerchief – and bind it on firmly with a bandage. If you cannot bandage the wound, hold the pad firmly in place by hand.

• If the wound is on a leg, and pressure does not stop the bleeding, apply a tourniquet above the wound. A bandage tightened by twisting a stick is effective. Tighten the tourniquet only until the bleeding stops, and relax it every 10-15 minutes to avoid the risk of gangrene.

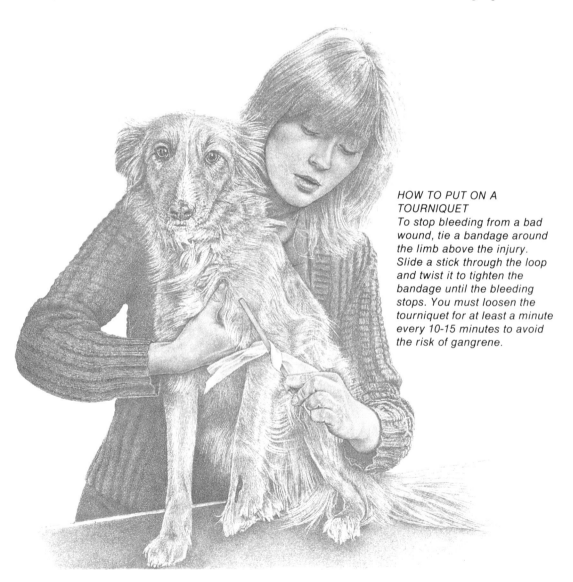

HOW TO PUT ON A TOURNIQUET
To stop bleeding from a bad wound, tie a bandage around the limb above the injury. Slide a stick through the loop and twist it to tighten the bandage until the bleeding stops. You must loosen the tourniquet for at least a minute every 10-15 minutes to avoid the risk of gangrene.

• Get the animal to a vet at once. If possible, have someone phone the surgery to alert the staff that an emergency case is on the way.

How to treat a broken leg

If a leg is lying at an awkward angle, it may mean that a bone is broken.
• Stop any bleeding.
• Ease the leg into as comfortable a position as possible. Warn whoever is holding the animal before you move the leg. The pain may make the animal try to bite or scratch.
• Straighten the leg gently into a more normal position. Then splint it by bandaging it gently but firmly to a piece of wood or hardboard of roughly the same shape as the leg.
• Take the animal to a vet.

Giving medicine to a cat or dog

Whenever you have to give pills or any other kind of medicine to a pet, prepare in much the same way as you would when examining a pet for injuries. Put a cat or small dog on a smooth-topped table. Put a large dog on a smooth floor with its back to a wall. Ask someone else to help you to hold the animal still.

Giving pills

• With a cat, grasp its head from behind with one hand and tilt the head up. Use the other hand to open the mouth by pressing down on the front of the lower jaw. Push the pill to the back of the tongue, then close the mouth and hold it shut until you see the cat swallowing. Rub the throat if necessary to encourage swallowing.
• With a dog, use one hand to hold it across the top of its muzzle just in front of the eyes, and push your thumb into the side of its mouth. Push up on the roof of its mouth. Use the middle

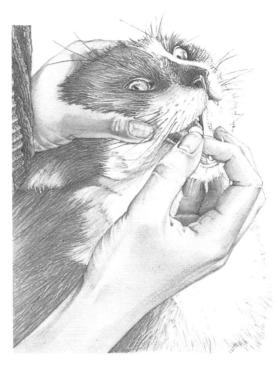

HOW TO GIVE A CAT A PILL
Tilt the cat's head well up with one hand, and with the other press down on the lower jaw to open its mouth. Push the pill to the back of the tongue, then close the mouth. Hold it shut until the cat swallows.

finger of the other hand to hold down the front of the lower jaw while you push the pill to the back of the tongue. Close the mouth and hold the jaws shut until the pill is swallowed. Rub the throat if necessary to encourage this.

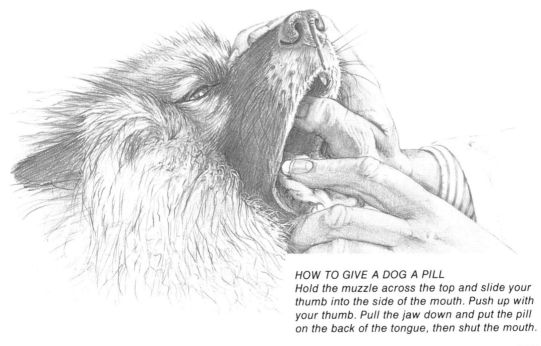

HOW TO GIVE A DOG A PILL
Hold the muzzle across the top and slide your thumb into the side of the mouth. Push up with your thumb. Pull the jaw down and put the pill on the back of the tongue, then shut the mouth.

Giving liquid medicine
• Buy a disposable plastic syringe without a needle. They are available from vets and most chemists.
• Load the medicine into the syringe.
• Hold the animal firmly and calm it by talking gently to it.
• With a cat, push the nozzle into the side of the mouth behind the large canine teeth and trickle the liquid in slowly. Hold the mouth up while you do this so that the medicine does not dribble out.
• With a dog, push the nozzle in where the lips meet at the side of the mouth. Pull the cheek back with one finger and hold the mouth up while you trickle the liquid in slowly.

Giving eye drops or eye ointment
• With both a cat and a dog, ask someone to hold the animal's head steady, or – if you are confident you will not be clawed or bitten – hold it steady against your body.
• Use two fingers above and below the eye to open the lids, and apply the drop or ointment directly onto the eyeball.

Giving ear drops or ear ointment
• With either pet, hold the ear flap with one hand to expose the ear canal and administer the medicine directly into the ear.
• Once the medicine is in, massage the base of the ear gently to ensure that the medicine gets well down into the ear.

• Never try to clean out the inner part of the ear canal of a cat or dog. You will damage the ear no matter how gentle you are, and the animal will resent the pain you cause.

When an animal has a fit
Fits are not uncommon in dogs; they are rarer in cats. They can have any of a number of causes, including brain tumours and epilepsy. With either animal, the basic principle of treatment is not to interfere more than necessary.
• Make sure the pet is not in danger – from knocking things over, for example.
• Try to keep it quiet and cool. Draw the curtains in the room to reduce the light.
• Get it to a vet as soon as you can, but do not try to move it while it is still convulsing.
• Take care when you do move it. An animal that is ill is more likely to bite or scratch unexpectedly.

If your cat or dog is poisoned
Ordinary vomiting and bad diarrhoea in pets are only rarely signs of poisoning. The usual symptoms of genuine poisoning are persistent vomiting and diarrhoea, often combined with shivering tremors or convulsions, leading later to coma.
• If your pet is already in a coma, get veterinary help at once.
• If your pet is still conscious and you know that it has swallowed a corrosive poison, such as acid or caustic soda, wash the mouth out

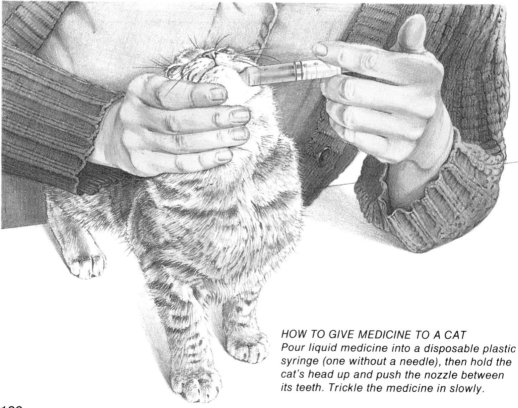

HOW TO GIVE MEDICINE TO A CAT
Pour liquid medicine into a disposable plastic syringe (one without a needle), then hold the cat's head up and push the nozzle between its teeth. Trickle the medicine in slowly.

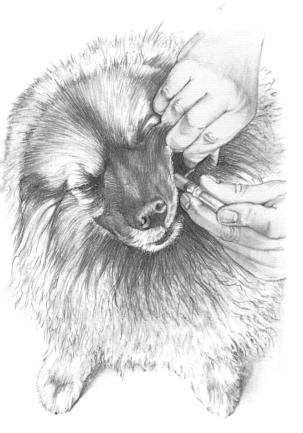

HOW TO GIVE MEDICINE TO A DOG
Use a syringe for a dog, in much the same way as for a cat. But instead of pushing the nozzle between its teeth, slide it alongside the teeth, so that the medicine trickles into its cheek.

rapidly with milk or water. If you have a syringe handy, use that to wash the mouth out. Otherwise hold the animal's mouth open and pour in the liquid from a jug or cup.
• After washing the mouth out, give the animal plenty of milk or water to drink. The aim is to dilute the poison without causing vomiting – because vomiting up a corrosive poison will burn the mouth and throat for a second time.
• Follow up the drink with a 'stodgy' meal of bread and water or porridge.
• If you are certain that the animal has swallowed a non-corrosive poison, make it vomit as soon as possible.
• The best way to make a pet vomit is to feed it a crystal of washing soda – anything from a hazelnut-sized piece for a cat to a walnut-sized piece for a large dog. Do not dissolve the crystal first. Just give it to the animal in the same way you would give it a pill. The washing soda will make it sick in about five minutes.
• If washing soda is not available, use a solution of 1 part of mustard powder in 20 parts of water.
• With either type of poisoning, take the animal to a vet and take with you labels or samples of the poison.

• If you are not sure what type of poison is involved, treat the animal as if it had swallowed a corrosive poison.

Dealing with a choking animal
The priority in treating a choking animal is the same as for a choking human: speed.
• If there is something tight around the neck, remove it at once.
• If something is lodged in the mouth or throat – a bone, say – hold the animal's mouth open and pull the obstruction out. Use a bar such as a spoon handle to stop the jaws closing while you work. Push the bar to the back of the animal's mouth and between the teeth like a gag.
• If a ball gets stuck in a dog's throat, the obstruction tends to make the dog salivate profusely, which makes the ball slippery and difficult to get hold of.
• Open the mouth wide and try to get a finger behind the ball. Alternatively, put the fingers of both hands on the outside of the dog's cheeks as far back as you can and press forward from behind the ball.
• If the dog is choking on a sharp stick which has pierced its mouth or the back of its throat, pull the stick free.
• Keep the dog warm, do not let it eat or drink and get it to a vet as fast as possible.

Treating a limp
If a cat or dog develops a limp for which there is no obvious cause, examine the injured leg gently (see *How to handle an injured cat or dog*, page 185).
• Feel the limb from the paw upwards, looking for swelling, heat and pain.
• Look for cuts too, especially in the pads of

In the home and at work

CHOKING – AVOIDING RISKS

• If your cat wears a collar, make sure it has an elasticated section.
• Never leave a choke chain on an unattended dog.
• If your dog enjoys chasing a ball, use one that is far too big for it to swallow. Never use a small, solid, hard rubber ball.
• If you throw sticks for a dog, use one with blunt ends. A sharp one can land end-on in the ground and a running dog can impale itself.
• Never give any animal cooked bones to chew. They can splinter and cause the animal to choke or to cut itself severely. Pork and chicken bones are particularly dangerous – even if they have not been cooked. The only safe bones for an animal are raw beef bones.

the feet, and for splinters, grit and thorns. Clean any cuts in cold water.

• Remove any foreign bodies you find, if you can do so easily. If you cannot remove them easily, get veterinary help.

• Bending and straightening the leg may reveal painful areas and help you to find the cause of the problem. But again, if you cannot find the cause easily, take the animal to a vet.

• If a cat or dog develops a limp, particularly if part of the affected leg is swollen, the chances are that it has been bitten in a fight. This is much more likely to happen to a cat than a dog.

• Bathe the swollen area in water which is as hot as your hand can tolerate. Put a little salt or Epsom salts in the water.

• After bathing the area, contact a vet.

• If a septic wound is obvious, apply a warm poultice to reduce inflammation, especially if there is any delay in getting to the vet.

• Make the poultice from hot kaolin paste – available from chemists – spread on a bandage. Or squeeze out cotton wool or a flannel in water as hot as you can stand, then bandage the hot pad over the wound.

Removing a barb from a paw

Barbed objects such as fish-hooks that become embedded in the skin of a cat or dog need special treatment, to avoid making the injury worse when the barb is removed.

• Get the animal to a safe, escape-proof place before you start trying to treat it (see *How to handle an injured cat or dog*, page 185).

• Cut the hook free from any fishing line it is attached to.

• If the hook will not pull out easily, push it through until the barb is exposed.

• Cut off the barb with the wire-cutting section of a pair of pliers.

• Remove the rest of the hook by pulling the shank back out through the original incision.

• Clean the wound, cover it with a clean dressing and consult a vet.

• Do not try to remove a hook that has pierced a particularly sensitive part of the body such as the lips or eyes. Treatment of these areas may require an anaesthetic and is best left to a vet.

If a dog gets heat stroke

Never leave a dog in a car on a hot day. It can quite rapidly become seriously overheated, to the point of collapse.

• If a dog is obviously in distress, get it at once into a cool place and soak it in cold water, using towels or sponges. Wrap cold, wet towels round its head and body as well.

• If possible, put it in a bath or paddling pool – but do not do this if the dog is unconscious.

• If you have small lumps of ice handy, push them up the dog's bottom.

• Get the dog to a vet as soon as possible. Keep it cool on the journey by wrapping it in more wet towels. Use more ice if you have any.

If your cat or dog is bitten

A pet that has been bitten or scratched in a fight may have several small wounds which are not easily visible through the fur.

• Use your fingers to find the site of the injury.

• Clip away the fur around the wound, but do not pull the hair away if it seems to be part of a scab or clot. You may start the wound bleeding again.

• Clean the wound with warm water containing a little salt or Epsom salts.

• Cover and bandage the wound if it looks serious.

• Have the injuries checked by a vet. Bites and scratches suffered in a fight may go septic without treatment.

• With cats particularly, the first evidence of a bite may be an abscess, which often develops behind a tiny wound. You may notice the swelling, or the cat may become listless and off its food. The cat will need antibiotics – get it to a vet for treatment as soon as possible. If there is any delay, bathe the swelling with warm water to reduce the inflammation.

How to stop a dogfight

• Intervene in a dogfight only if it looks serious. Most dogs will, in ordinary circumstances, stop fighting of their own accord fairly quickly.

• If you do decide to intervene, take care not to get bitten yourself.

• Make a loud noise, such as a shrill whistle. Alternatively, throw a bucket of water over both contestants or turn a hose on them.

• If there is someone else available to help, ask the helper to move in behind one of the dogs at the same time as you move in behind the other.

• Grab the dog by the collar, if it is wearing one, or the scruff of the neck.

• Do not pull the dogs apart because this will worsen any wounds – if one has its teeth in the other, say. Instead, hit the dog in the side of the chest to make it let go, then pull it away.

• Once the dogs have been parted, keep a firm grip on them to make sure that they do not start fighting again.

If cats fight

• Stop a cat fight by chasing the combatants and shouting and shooing at them. Cat fights rarely last long.

• Do not try to get hold of a fighting cat – you are very likely to be scratched or bitten.

If a pet is stung

Cats and dogs often chase wasps and bees. So when they are stung, it is often on or around the face.

• If the sting is on the skin, rub on a proprietary cream such as Waspeze. It is as effective on animals as on humans. Do not use a cream of this kind near the eyes or mouth, however.

• If the sting is inside the mouth, get the animal

HOW TO GET A HOOK OUT OF A PAW

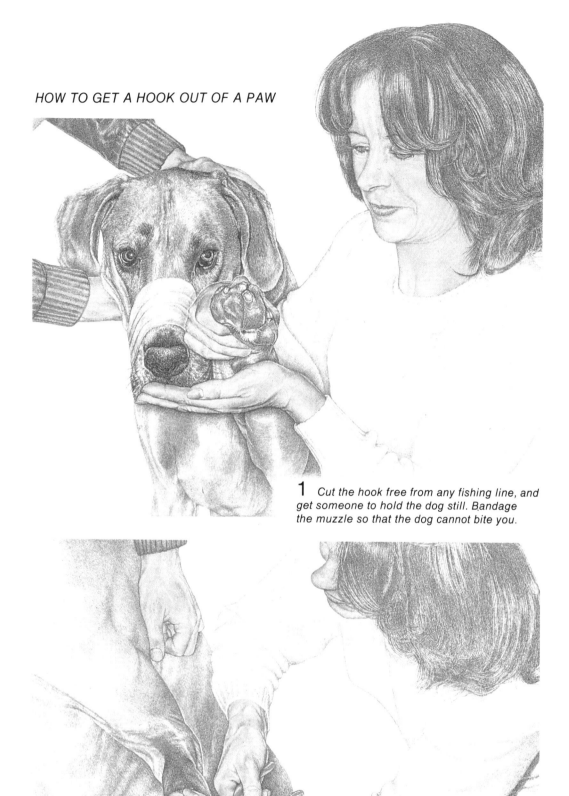

1 *Cut the hook free from any fishing line, and get someone to hold the dog still. Bandage the muzzle so that the dog cannot bite you.*

2 *If the hook will not pull free easily, push it through until the barb is exposed. Cut the barb off with a pair of pliers, then pull the shank back and out. Dress the wound and see a vet.*

191

to a vet at once. A sting in the mouth is much more serious because the swelling could block the animal's airway and choke it.

Coping with wasps or bees

• If your home is invaded by a swarm of bees or a colony of wasps, do not try to hold them back with pesticide sprays.

• Retreat quickly, closing all doors and windows between you and the swarm.

• Get expert help at once.

• If the problem is wasps, telephone the local council's Health Department, which will normally clear the colony free of charge or for a small fee. Alternatively, contact a local pest-control firm, who will usually provide treatment within 24 hours, but will charge a higher fee. Most firms are listed in the Yellow Pages under 'Pest and Vermin Control Services'.

• If the problem is bees, contact the police, the local council or the nearest Citizens Advice Bureau. They will put you in touch with a local beekeeper who will remove the swarm.

• If you are attacked by bees or wasps – and this is likely to happen only if a nearby colony has been disturbed for some reason – the safest course depends on where you are.

• If you are in a garden, retreat indoors quickly but calmly, closing doors and windows behind you. Stay inside until the insects disperse, which they will do within a few minutes.

• If you are in open country away from any building, plunge into the nearest patch of dense undergrowth or bushes. Keep going until you leave the insects behind. This will usually happen within 50yds (45m) because the insects will be disorientated by the moving branches. When you are clear, wait until the insects disperse.

• A swarm of bees on its way to found a new colony will not normally attack a person. If you are in the path of a swarm, move out of its way, or lie flat and cover yourself with a coat in case any bees settle on you.

Caring for an injured bird or wild animal

If you come across an injured bird, a helpless fledgling, or a wild animal such as a rabbit that is obviously hurt, there is little you can do by way of first aid without knowing what the problem is. And that requires expert help.

• If the creature is young and helpless but apparently uninjured, do not interfere unless you are certain it has been abandoned. If the mother is about she will help and feed it, but if you handle it she may be frightened away.

• If you can catch an injured wild creature without hurting it, take it to a vet. You will not usually be expected to pay a fee.

• If you cannot catch it easily, tell the Royal Society for the Prevention of Cruelty to Animals or the police. The nearest RSPCA office will be listed in the telephone directory under 'RSPCA'. Alternatively, contact the society's head office in West Sussex on Horsham (0403) 264181.

Handling a sick or injured horse

Like any animal in pain, a horse is likely to become vicious and turn on even a person who knows it well. So get it under control first.

• Approach the horse quietly with a halter, talking to it steadily and looking at it all the time. Let it see you coming. Slip the halter on and hold the rope firmly. But do not wind the rope round your hand. If the horse jerks back, it could give you a painful rope burn.

• If further restraint is necessary, use one hand to hold it round the soft tip of its muzzle.

• If someone else is with you, ask him to hold the horse by an uninjured foreleg and bend it to lift it off the ground. This will help to immobilise the animal. Once the horse is under control, examine it for injuries.

• If the horse is standing on three legs, it may mean that it has gone lame or that the leg is broken – if the leg is at an awkward angle or badly swollen, say. Do not move the horse unless it is in danger of further injury (on a road, for example). Get veterinary help at once.

• If the horse is lying down and cannot get up, leave it alone and get veterinary help.

• If the horse is lying down and thrashing about, try to restrain it from causing itself further injury. Get hold of its head and lie on it to hold it still. But stay well away from the forefeet. Get veterinary help at once.

Dealing with a horse that has gone lame

Lameness in a horse usually happens when the lower part of the leg or the foot is damaged in some way and the tissues inside the hoof swell up. The rigid hoof constricts the swollen tissues, causing considerable pain.

• If you are riding a horse that goes lame (you can tell because the animal's gait becomes awkward and lopsided as it tries to guard the painful foot), dismount at once.

• Pick up the foot of the affected leg and examine it for injuries. A nail may have penetrated the sole, or a stone may have caught in the hoof.

• Remove any foreign body you find, then lead the horse home.

• Once you get there, pack a hot poultice round the foot and call a vet. Make the poultice from hot kaolin paste – available from chemists – spread on a bandage; or use a cloth pad that has been squeezed out in hot water.

• If you find nothing in the foot, feel the rest of the leg for areas which feel hot or swollen or which seem to cause the horse pain. Whether or not you can find the source of the trouble, call a vet. Rest the horse until the vet arrives.

If a horse is caught on barbed wire

• Restrain the horse and hold it firmly to stop it tearing itself away from the wire and making its injuries worse.

• Restrict its movement by lifting its foreleg as well, if you can.

• Ease the barbed wire free, making all your

movements slow so as not to startle or hurt the horse. Once the horse is free, clean any cuts with warm water containing a mild antiseptic (the same antiseptics that work on people work on horses, too).

• Ask a vet to come and look the horse over. Horses are highly susceptible to tetanus, and even minor cuts can easily become infected.

Treating a horse for colic

Colic in a horse is abdominal pain usually resulting from it eating or being fed something other than its natural diet of grass and vegetation. The pain can often be violent.

The symptoms of internal pain are: restlessness; pawing and scraping at the ground; looking round at the flanks; getting up and down frequently; rolling; sweating; and rapid breathing. In addition, a horse suffering from colic may strain as it tries to defecate without success, or with very limited success.

• Once you have the horse under control, get it walking gently and try to keep it on the move.

• Try to stop it rolling on the ground. Rolling could lead to the intestines being twisted, and could seriously worsen the horse's condition.

• Call a vet. Keep the horse on its feet and moving until the vet arrives.

If fire breaks out in a stable

• Dial 999 and ask for the fire brigade, or get someone else to make the call.

• Open the stable door and chase the horse out, if you can do so without getting burnt yourself. Do not wait for it to bolt out – it will probably be too terrified to move and may need a prod with a pitchfork.

• Shut the door once the horse is out. A horse panic-stricken by the flames may well try to get back into its stall unless you prevent it by shutting the door.

• Let the horse or horses run free if necessary while you clear the rest of the stable.

• Once all the animals are safe, fight the blaze as best you can until firemen arrive (see *Fighting a fire*, page 150).

In the home and at work

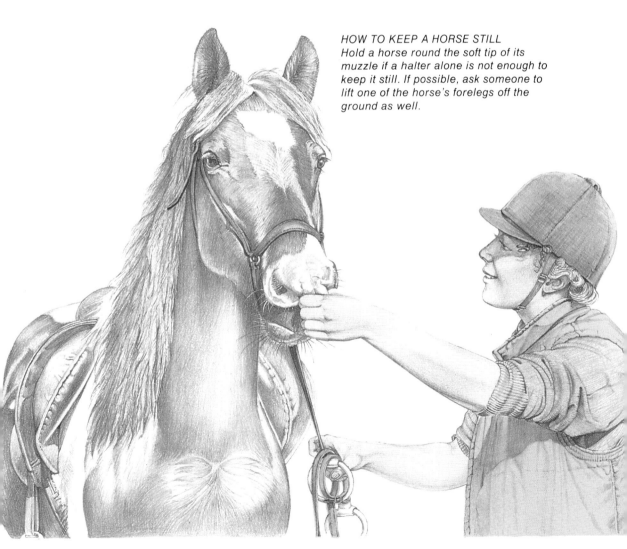

HOW TO KEEP A HORSE STILL
Hold a horse round the soft tip of its muzzle if a halter alone is not enough to keep it still. If possible, ask someone to lift one of the horse's forelegs off the ground as well.

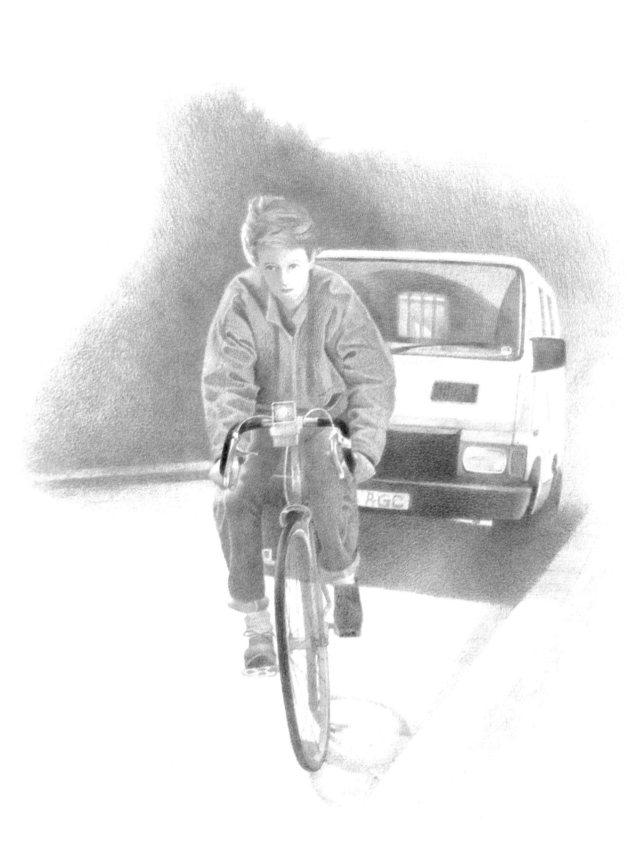

Emergencies on the road

At the scene of an accident

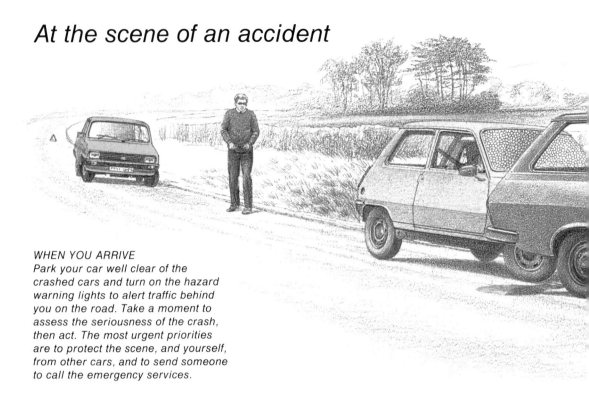

WHEN YOU ARRIVE
Park your car well clear of the crashed cars and turn on the hazard warning lights to alert traffic behind you on the road. Take a moment to assess the seriousness of the crash, then act. The most urgent priorities are to protect the scene, and yourself, from other cars, and to send someone to call the emergency services.

If you are the first on the scene of a crash, do not dash headlong from your car to the aid of an injured person – you or your car may be struck by another vehicle and add to the disaster.

For this reason, the first thing to do at the scene of any accident is to protect the area from other traffic.

Once you have warned other traffic, the priorities, in order, are: send for the police; immobilise the crashed vehicles; and help anyone who has been injured.

Warn other traffic

• Park your car well away from the accident – behind it, if possible. Turn on your hazard warning lights. At night, train your headlights on the wrecked vehicles as well.

• Leave your car with its front wheels turned towards the kerb so that if another car runs into yours, your car will be pushed off the road, not into you or the crashed vehicles.

• If one of the crashed vehicles is on fire, keep clear. Its petrol tank could explode without warning.

• Take charge of the accident scene if no one else has done so. If someone is already in charge, make yourself useful to him.

• Warn approaching traffic in both directions. If other traffic is coming up behind you, flag it down, keeping well to the side of the road; at night use a torch or light-coloured scarf. Ask someone to stop traffic coming the other way.

• Put a warning triangle, if one is available, about 100yds (90m) behind the wrecked vehicles, towards the nearside edge of the road. Ideally, put another the same distance in the opposite direction.

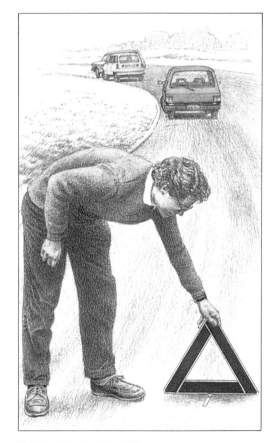

WARN OTHER TRAFFIC
Put a red warning triangle about 100 yds (90m) behind the crashed cars, and, ideally, another the same distance ahead. Flag down the first car and send the driver to call the police.

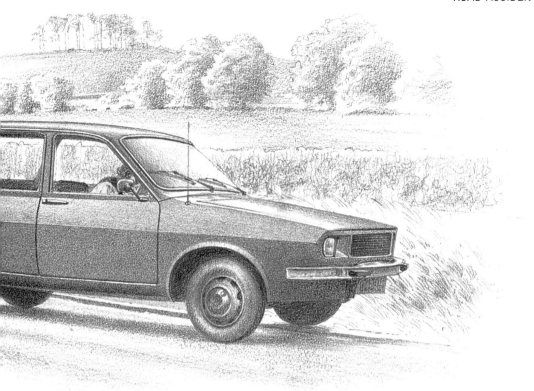

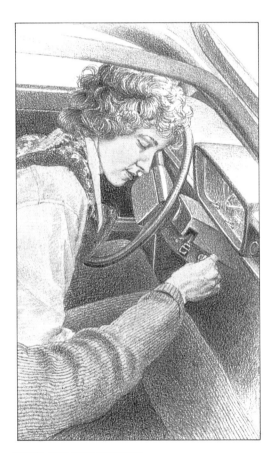

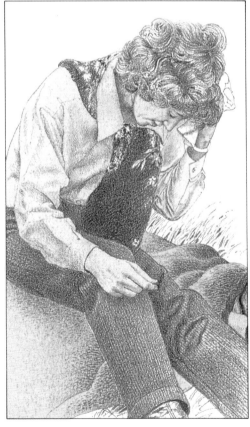

TURN OFF THE IGNITION
*Switch off the engines of all the crashed cars
to cut the risk of fire, and put the handbrakes
on. But leave the keys in the ignition in case
the cars have to be moved later.*

START SELF-HELP TREATMENT
*See if the casualty can help herself, and show
her what to do. She can, for instance, stem
bleeding by pressing a clean handkerchief over
a wound. Tell her that help is on the way.*

197

Send for the police

• Check the number of vehicles involved, and the number of victims, noting whether anyone is trapped.

• Ask a passing driver or anyone living nearby to make a 999 call at the nearest telephone. Tell him how many people are injured or trapped. It does not matter if more than one person makes a call.

• If you make the call yourself on a public or private telephone, dial 999. Do not put any coins in a coin box.

• When the operator answers, ask for the police, who will alert other services.

• Tell the police you are reporting an accident, and give the telephone number in case you are cut off.

• Describe the accident location as exactly as you can. Say how many vehicles are involved, whether any vehicle is on fire, how many people are injured and whether anyone is trapped.

• Answer any other questions, and do not hang up until the operator tells you to.

Immobilise the crashed vehicles

• Switch off the ignition of each vehicle, but leave the key in the ignition in case the steering locks – the vehicle may have to be moved later.

• Check that the handbrake of each car is on. If it is not, put it on.

• Do not smoke, and warn others not to – even away from the cars. There may be petrol running in the gutter or leaking across the road from a ruptured fuel tank.

Help the injured

• Do not move anyone unless he is in immediate danger – if there is a car on fire close by, for example, or if he is lying in leaking petrol which you think might catch fire. If you move an injured person, you risk aggravating his injuries; that risk is worth taking only to protect him from a greater risk.

• Do not attempt to pick out glass from face or body wounds. If the glass is plugging the wound, you could make the bleeding worse by pulling it out.

BREAD OF LIFE
For six days in July 1983, Peter Marsh lay trapped under his crashed motorcycle. His leg was broken, he had no food or water and the standing crop in the Cambridgeshire cornfield where he had landed hid him from passers-by. To obtain some sustenance, he sucked juices from the stalks and grasses around him.

Marsh, who was 42, was discovered when police were called to another accident close by. His broken leg was badly infected, he was covered in insect bites and he was delirious and severely sunburnt. But thanks, in part, to the stalks he had chewed, he was alive.

TRAGEDY OF A CRASH HERO
Hampshire publican John Dodd did not hesitate when he came to the scene of an accident in the winter of 1981. He ran to help. But he overlooked the first rule of rescue on the road: make sure that the area is safe.

He was driving in snow along the Kingston bypass near London when he saw a car that had crashed into the central reservation and was blocking the fast lane. Sitting in the car was a woman driver, who was paralysed by fear and shock. 'I didn't think about it,' Dodd said later. 'I just went to help.'

Although he succeeded in getting the woman out of the car and behind the crash barriers on the central reservation, Dodd was himself hit by another car while he was trying to move the crashed car out of the way.

He suffered a broken leg that left him with a permanent limp, and was unconscious for three days as a result of head injuries. Even after his recovery from the immediate injuries, he suffered from headaches and loss of concentration to the extent that he had to give up the tenancy of his public house in Droxford.

Three years after the accident, in December 1984, he won £65,000 damages in the High Court from the motorist whose vehicle ran into him. But Dodd, by this time working as a weighbridge clerk, commented: 'The money can't give me back what I have lost.'

• Check that each casualty can breathe freely. Loosen tight clothing round the neck.

• Do not give anyone anything to eat or drink. Hot, sweet tea is appropriate only for someone who has had an emotional fright. It should not be given to anyone who has been injured or who is suffering from the serious clinical condition known as shock (see page 120).

• See if the casualty can treat himself and show him what to do. He can stem blood coming from an arm or leg by gripping the wound with his hand, or by pressing on it with a clean handkerchief or tissue.

Treatment priorities

• Treat casualties in any accident – on the road or anywhere else (a bomb blast, say) – in the following order:

1. Unconscious and not breathing (see *Artificial respiration*, page 50).
2. Bleeding severely (see page 60).
3. Unconscious but breathing (see page 136).

• Then search the scene in case someone has left or been thrown from a crashed vehicle and is wandering around in shock – or has collapsed at a distance. Persuade anyone wandering around in a state of shock to lie down.

• Cover each injured person lightly with a rug or coat.

• Reassure them that help is on the way. Tell

them that any missing friend, relative or pet is being taken care of – even if at that stage you are not sure. The priority is to keep each casualty safe and as calm as possible until the emergency services reach the scene.

• If possible, do not leave the casualties alone after you have treated them. Get someone – a passer-by, say, or another motorist – to stay with each casualty until help arrives.

At the scene of a motorway crash

Because of the volume of traffic on motorways, the road can quickly get blocked if motorists stop at the scene of a crash, and the resulting traffic jam can delay the arrival of police and ambulance services.

For this reason, and because of the extra risks for rescuers caused by the speed of traffic, safety experts recommend that motorists should not stop at the scene of a motorway accident unless it is absolutely necessary – if, for example, someone is lying injured in the path of traffic, or struggling to get out of a car on fire.

• Go to the nearest emergency telephone and call for help. Emergency telephones are 1 mile (1.6km) apart, and there are marker posts at intervals by the hard shoulder giving the direction of the nearest.

• To make a call from an emergency telephone on the motorway, simply pick up the handset (there is no dial). This will automatically connect you to the motorway police control room.

• Give the letter and number on the side of the phone box, which pinpoints its location.

• Briefly describe the accident, the number of vehicles involved, and the number injured.

• Do not hang up until told to do so by the police operator. Some older types of phone work in one direction only, so the operator cannot call you back. On newer types he can call you back.

Emergencies on the road

ACCIDENTS: WHERE, WHEN AND WHY THEY HAPPEN

On average, there are around 2 million accidents on British roads each year. About 310,000 people are injured in them, and well over 4000 people die.

Nearly a third of those who are killed or injured are young people of between 15 and 24, three-fifths of them car drivers. About one-sixth of the accident victims are pedestrians – often children or the elderly. More than a tenth are motorcyclists.

Most accidents happen in built-up areas – three times as many as on country roads and more than 25 times as many as on motorways. But motorway accidents and crashes on country roads are more often serious because of the higher speeds involved.

More accidents occur in summer and autumn – when driving conditions are usually good but there is more traffic – than in winter and spring. And four-fifths take place when the weather is good.

Each week, too, there is a regular pattern to the toll on the roads.

The commonest times for an accident are: weekday rush hours; late evenings around pub closing times between Thursday and Sunday; Saturday shopping hours; and Sunday afternoons between 2pm and 4pm, when many people go out for a spin or are coming back from a lunchtime drink.

The accident blackspots

Most accidents need not happen. They are caused by errors of judgment or sheer carelessness much more often than by mechanical failure. These are the ten most common road situations that can turn a car trip into a tragedy.

DRIVING STRAIGHT About 120,000 accidents happen each year when drivers are on a perfectly ordinary stretch of road. The most common cause is the manoeuvring of other drivers; others are careless, dangerous or drunken driving, ignoring traffic signals – or, less commonly, mechanical faults such as defective brakes or steering.

TURNING RIGHT About 30,000 accidents are caused each year by motorists misjudging a right turn or crashing into someone who is turning right.

OVERTAKING About 13,000 accidents are caused by drivers overtaking other vehicles dangerously.

PARKED CARS Badly parked cars, and people getting out of them carelessly, are responsible for more than 9000 accidents.

TURNING LEFT Drivers turning left and swinging too wide as they do so, or turning into the path of a cyclist, cause more than 8000 accidents each year.

STOPPING Sudden, unexpected stops by the motorist in front bring about nearly 8000 crashes.

MOVING OFF Nearly 3000 accidents happen because a motorist pulls out carelessly into traffic or bumps into the car in front in a slow-moving queue.

U-TURNS They are responsible for almost 2000 accidents a year.

REVERSING Around 2500 accidents a year happen when a driver backs into something or someone.

If you are involved in an accident

A traffic accident may involve only your vehicle and damage to property, such as a lamppost. Or it may involve other vehicles and perhaps injury to people or animals. Whatever the involvement, there are certain steps the law requires you to take and others that are advisable for insurance purposes.

Try to keep cool and note down essential information, even though you will probably be feeling shocked and flustered by the incident.

At the scene

• Stop as soon as you safely can. You must stop even if your vehicle is undamaged but you have been indirectly involved – if, for example, one car collided with another after swerving to avoid you.

• Whatever the circumstances, do not become involved in arguments with other drivers or onlookers about what happened. Particularly, do not make any statement admitting liability. If you think you may have been at fault, it is wisest to say as little as possible.

• If anyone is seriously injured, dial 999 and ask for the police, who will alert other emergency services. Otherwise there is no need to call the police unless there is a serious traffic obstruction.

• Before any vehicles are moved, make a sketch plan or note of their position in the road and in relation to the other vehicles involved. Note, for example, if any car has crossed the central white line. If any car has skidded, make an estimate of the length of skid marks.

• Examine your vehicle and the others involved and make a note of the damage each has sustained. Look, too, at the condition of the other cars. Were all their lights working at the time, for instance, and were their tyres in good condition?

• If anyone has been injured, you must also produce a motor insurance certificate on the spot. If you cannot, report the accident to the police within 24 hours.

• Give your name and address and the registration number of your car to other motorists involved and to anyone else who has reasonable grounds for asking, such as the owners of any damaged property. If you are not the owner of the car you are driving, give the owner's name and address as well.

• Collect the same information from other motorists involved. If anyone refuses, write down his car registration number (the owner can be traced through the number).

• If the police have not been called, try to find an independent witness (not someone travelling in your car) who is willing to make a statement about the incident to your insurance company. Take his name and address.

After the accident

• If the accident involved serious damage to a vehicle or property, or if a traffic sign was damaged, you must either give your name and address to anyone with reasonable grounds for requiring them, or report the accident to the police as soon as possible – certainly within 24 hours.

• If you hit and damage an unoccupied car, report it to the police. If you fail to do so and are eventually traced, you could face not only a claim for repair of the damage you caused, but also criminal charges as a hit-and-run driver.

• Tell your insurance company of the accident within 24 hours, whether or not you or anyone else will be making a claim on your policy.

• Ask the company at the same time to send you an accident report and claim form.

• Ask a garage to give you a written estimate of the cost of repairs to your car, but do not get any repairs done at once if you plan to claim the cost from an insurance company. The

MAKING A SKETCH OF THE ACCIDENT
A sketch of the accident scene, made on the spot, will be useful in any later court case and for making an insurance claim. Show the road layout and the cars' positions. Mark where any witness was standing. Add the compass points, too (get them from a map if necessary); official reports often refer to them.

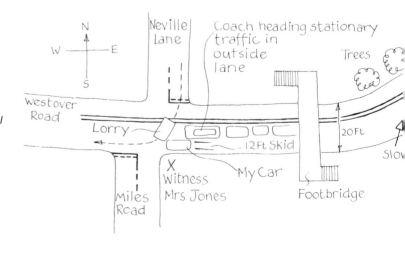

insurers will probably want the damage inspected first by an engineer.
• Send any bills or letters you get from other motorists involved to your insurance company. Do not write to or contact the other motorists or their insurers.
• Let your insurance company know if you receive a Notice of Intended Prosecution from the police. This should arrive within 14 days of the accident unless you were warned at the time that you would be charged.

If you have an accident abroad
The legal requirements about what to do if you are involved in an accident vary in detail from country to country, even within Europe. Nevertheless, if you follow these general guidelines, you will be doing at least as much as the law requires in any country.
• Stop at the scene of the accident.
• Warn approaching traffic of the obstruction by setting up a red warning triangle at least 100 yds (90m) from the scene – ideally use two, one in each direction.
• Call the police, or ask a passing motorist to call them. Even if this is not obligatory under local laws, it is always advisable.
• Help anyone who has been injured (see *At the scene of an accident*, page 196). Call an ambulance if necessary.
• Generally, do not move the car or cars from the positions in which they have come to rest. But if they are seriously obstructing other traffic, mark the positions on the road and get the details confirmed by independent witnesses before moving them.
• Do not leave the scene of the accident until the police arrive, unless there is an overriding reason for doing so. If you think there is such a reason, explain it to the police by telephoning them, and get their permission before leaving.

• Give your name and address, and any other details requested, to others involved in the accident. Collect the same details from them.
• Cooperate with the police when they arrive. Answer their questions as fully as you can, but avoid saying anything which could be construed as an admission of liability.
• Make notes or a sketch plan of the accident to help you fill in your insurance company's accident form later. If you have a camera, back the notes up by taking photographs of the cars and the scene. Try particularly to show any factors which might have helped to cause the accident – a concealed road sign, for instance. Take close-up pictures of the damage, too; they may be useful evidence if you want to claim compensation from the other driver or from your insurance company.
• Report the accident to the insurance company or bureau whose address is given on the back of your Green Card or frontier insurance certificate. Telephone as soon as possible, and follow up your call with a letter – within 24 hours, if possible.
• If you have additional insurance cover through a British company or motoring organisation, report the accident to the British insurer as well. The policy will tell you how soon after the accident you should let the firm know. If the time limit is short, make the first contact by phone and follow it up with a letter.
• Some insurance policies – such as the Automobile Association's Five-Star Service and the Travellers Bond Foreign Touring Service of the Royal Automobile Club – cover the costs of repairs to your car, medical expenses and a variety of other costs which may arise after an accident. If your policy is of this type, ask the insurer about where and how to get the repairs done, and about how medical bills will be settled (see also *Seeing a doctor overseas*, page 288).

Emergencies on the road

HOW TO AVOID A HEAD-ON COLLISION

If you see another vehicle coming towards you on the wrong side of the road, whose driver seems to be either unwilling or unable to get out of your way, you must act quickly and coolly to avoid a head-on collision. Head-on collisions are the most dangerous of all road accidents.
• As soon as you see the hazard, sound your horn or flash your headlights as an early warning of your presence.
• Brake firmly but not violently. Otherwise the car may start to skid and you could lose steering control.
• As you reduce speed, scan the road ahead to see if there is anywhere to get out of the

way safely – a verge, say, or a side turning.
• Start to pull left, but do not commit yourself until you see which way the other car is going. There is a danger that both of you could pull onto your nearside verge and collide there.
• As soon as you see which way the other vehicle is swerving, turn away from it – even if this means side-swiping another car on the road. This type of accident is far less likely to kill you and your passengers than a head-on smash.
• If a collision is unavoidable, try to scrape the side of the other vehicle rather than meet it head on.

Defensive driving

The best way to avoid an accident is to be alert to what might cause one – to develop your powers of observation so that you can see danger coming and react to it in time. The principle of the technique known as defensive driving is to be prepared for the unexpected by observation and anticipation. These pages show how to apply the principle in practice.

Other motorists – watch for:

• Taxi ahead – it may slow down and move to the left with little warning. Keep an eye open for someone hailing it from the kerb.

• Learner stopped on a hill – do not get too close. He may roll back when starting off.

• Bus ahead – beware of people running to catch it. If it has a rear platform with people on it, the bus is probably about to stop. Watch out for people jumping off.

• Motorcyclists at a road junction ahead – if you see two ready to come out and one emerges safely, watch for the other. Will he follow?

• Pedal cyclist ahead – if he glances over his

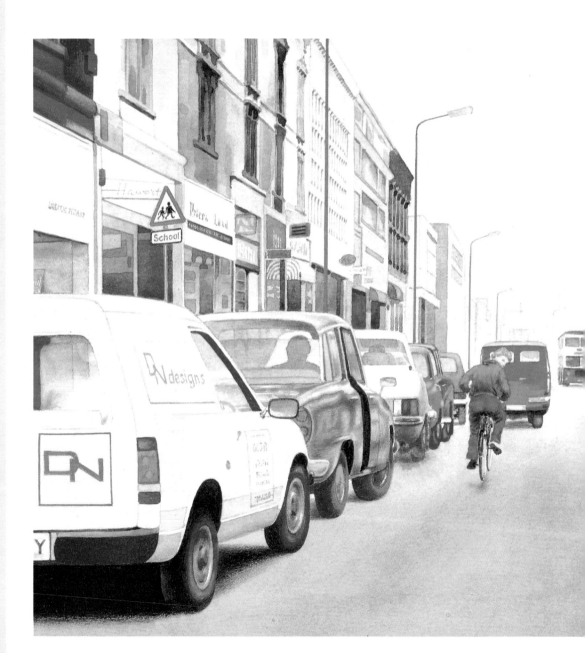

shoulder he is probably preparing to pull out to the right, and may hesitate and wobble. Watch his movements.

• Turning signal on a car ahead – never rely on the driver doing as he has signalled. He may have forgotten to cancel a previous signal, or may change his mind.

• Turning signal on a car to your right – if you are waiting to emerge from a side road onto a main road, never assume that it is safe to pull out just because an oncoming driver is signalling left. Wait until he slows down and is obviously going to turn.

• Brake lights coming on ahead – touch your own to warn traffic behind. There may be an accident or obstruction ahead.

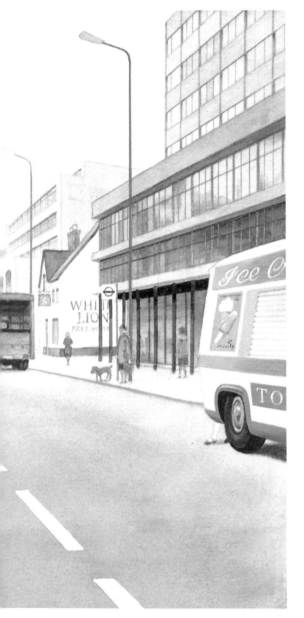

• Headlamp flashed as signal – never assume another driver means: 'You go ahead, I will wait.' He may mean: 'I'm going ahead. You wait.' Such a signal is easily misinterpreted and could lead to an accident. Headlamp-flashing should be used only to let another driver know you are there.

• Siren sounding on police car, ambulance or fire engine – if you do not know where the sound is coming from, slow down and keep to the side of the road. Do not move across a road junction until you are certain you will not be in the path of the emergency vehicle.

• Headlamp dazzle – if a car approaches with headlamps on full beam, do not look at them directly. Look slightly to the nearside. Do not retaliate by switching your own headlamps to full beam. This is offensive rather than defensive driving and could cause an accident.

• Slow vehicle ahead very close behind another – the rear vehicle is probably being towed, even if it is not displaying a towing notice. Be careful about overtaking.

• Moving out from a side road onto a main road – watch for cycles and motorcycles near the kerb as well as for cars. A cyclist or motorcyclist is easy to overlook if you are trying to nose out of a side road in heavy traffic.

Approaching a parked car – watch for:

• People inside – the door may be opened.

• Flashing indicator – the car may pull out into your path.

• Wisps of smoke from the exhaust – the car may be about to move off.

• Feet under vehicles – a child may run into the road.

• An ice-cream van – there are bound to be children around it, and they may dart across the road to or from it without warning.

Roadside signs – watch for:

• Bus stops – people may run across the road from the right.

• School signs – children may run across the road, especially in the morning between 8.30

How to make use of clues
Be alert, as you drive, to clues which can warn of potential danger. There are six such clues in this urban street scene. The slightly open door on the parked car may mean that the driver is about to get out – and he may not have noticed you. The smoke from the exhaust and the lit brake light on the parked car beyond both mean that it may be about to pull out, perhaps without indicating. The cyclist is looking over his shoulder; he may be about to swing across the road. There are feet visible below the van on the right; a child may be about to dash into the street. And the loose dog on the pavement farther down the street may run across your path without warning.

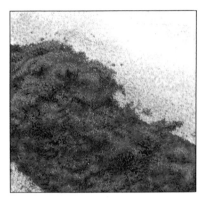

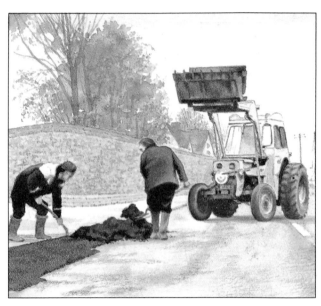

Debris from roadworks
A loose pile of sand or tar by the side of the road (above) may be a warning of roadworks ahead. Look out for workmen and machinery which may be blocking the road around the next corner (right).

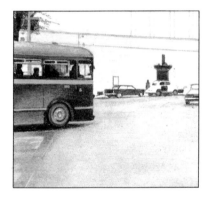

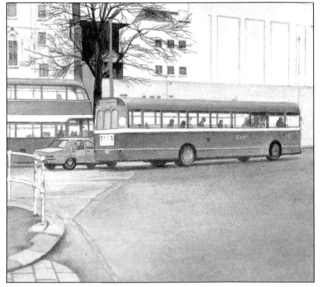

Vehicles emerging from a turn
Watch out for cars and buses moving out of a side road. In a town, others could be queuing behind the first, and one or more of them – fed up, perhaps, with waiting – could try to slip out as well, blocking your path.

and 9.30 and in the afternoon between 3.30 and 4.30. But look out for a lone child near the school at any time of day.
• Zebra crossings – scan the pavement on both sides to see if anyone is preparing to cross.
• Garage or pub forecourt – vehicles are likely to pull in and out without signalling, especially late at night.
• Red traffic light – stop. Before starting off again, watch the cross traffic and pedestrians, in case someone tries to rush through at the last minute.
• Amber traffic light – be decisive. Slow down and stop unless you are almost at the lights. If you are almost at the lights, accelerate through; otherwise traffic behind may run into you.
• Green traffic light – do not treat it as an open

door; it may change. Reduce speed as you approach, and look right and left to make sure that nothing is coming through.
• Roadworks sign – prepare to slow down or stop; the roadworks may be some distance ahead round a bend, or masked by parked cars.
• Road-narrows sign – get into the continuing lane in good time, and watch for other drivers cutting across.

Making use of clues – watch for:
• Mud or hay on a country road – there may be a slow-moving tractor ahead.
• Droppings on a country road – there may be horses, cattle or sheep ahead.
• Telegraph poles – in country areas, the line of poles ahead of you can sometimes alert you

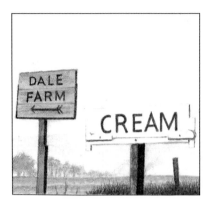

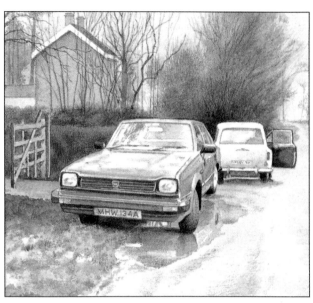

Farm-produce shops
Slow down whenever you see a sign advertising a farm shop or a roadside stall. Cars ahead may be backed up waiting to get into a narrow turning, or they may be carelessly parked along the verge

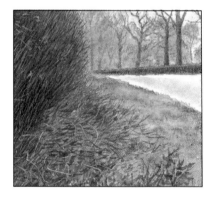

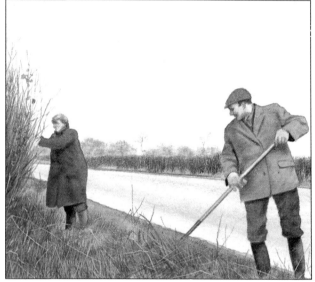

Hedge or grass clippings
Freshly mown grass, or a newly trimmed hedge – with or without loose clippings – indicates that a road gang or a hedge-clipping tractor may be working on the road ahead. Slow down until you are sure.

to bends in the road that may be masked by hedges. Do not rely on them, however; the lines sometimes cut across fields, rather than go round them, and so can mislead you.
• County boundary sign – the road surface is likely to change, and at night the street lighting ahead may be different.
• Shop-window reflections – in built-up areas, make full use of reflections in windows and on shiny vehicles. They can help you to see round bends, round corners at awkward junctions, and to see how close you are to the car behind when parking on the street.
• Builders' or rubbish skips (large metal containers) – note their position during the day in case you are returning at night. They may not be lit after dark.

Approaching animals – watch for:
• Dog not on lead – it may wander into the road or run across, especially if there is another dog (or a cat) on the other side.
• Cat crouching on footpath watching traffic – it may be intending to cross the road, and may dash in front of your car, relying on speed to get across.
• Horses ahead – slow down and give them plenty of room as you pass. Do not toot your horn or accelerate hard, or they may shy into your car.
• Herd of cattle or flock of sheep ahead – stop until they have gone round you or off the road. Do not sound your horn or rev your engine. If you startle them, they may blunder into your car and damage it.

What to do if you hit an animal

If you suddenly find an animal in your path – a pet, a straying farm animal or a wild animal – there may be no time to avoid it. In heavy traffic or bad weather, there may be no choice but to hit it rather than to swerve and risk a serious accident.

• Pull over to the side of the road and stop as soon as you can after the impact. Find out whether the animal is dead or injured.

• If it is injured, try to restrain it so that its injuries can be treated (see *Caring for a sick or injured animal*, page 185).

• Whether the animal is dead or injured, and whatever type of animal it is, call the police.

• If the animal is a pet or a farm animal, go to the nearest house or farmhouse as well and try to find the owner.

• If the animal is injured and small enough to handle, consider taking it to a vet at once. Tell the police if you plan to leave the scene of the accident to do this.

• Tell the vet that you have informed the police about the accident. In such a case, the vet will sometimes not charge you for treating the animal, but will instead claim his fee from a fund administered by the police.

PET-OWNERS AND THE LAW

Anyone who owns or looks after a pet has a legal duty to try to make sure that it does not hurt anyone or damage their property. If it does – if it bites someone, for example, or if it runs in front of a car and causes an accident – you could be sued for compensation by the victim.

In ordinary circumstances you will not be liable for the cost of any damage or injury your pet causes, unless it can be shown that you were in some way to blame – if, for instance, you let your dog run loose in a busy street.

If, however, you own or look after what the law calls a dangerous animal – a poisonous snake, for example, or an alligator – then the courts may hold you responsible for any accident it causes, even if you are not, in the ordinary sense, to blame.

This responsibility is known in law as 'strict liability'.

In practice, owners of cats are rarely held to be responsible for damage done by their pets because the law recognises that cats are very difficult to control.

• If your pet has a habit of chasing passers-by, cyclists or cars, keep it well fenced in so that it cannot run into the street.

• Keep your dog on a lead in crowded places and in a field of livestock.

• Train your dog properly. A local vet will probably be able to tell you about nearby training classes. The Kennel Club – whose head office is at 1 Clarges Street, London W1; telephone 071-493 6651 – also has details of training classes around the country.

• Keep children and strangers away from a bitch with a litter. She may be unusually aggressive.

• If your dog has already bitten somebody, take extra care to keep it under control. If it bites somebody again, the courts could order you to have the dog destroyed.

• Consider taking out insurance against your pet doing harm if you do not already have it. Most household insurance policies include such cover as a matter of course.

Motorists and the law on animals
Although it is always advisable to call the police if you hit an animal on the road – because they can help to arrange treatment or for the body to be removed, and can help to trace the owner – it is not always obligatory to do so.

This is because your legal duties as a motorist if you run over an animal on the road depend on what animal it is.

• If you injure a horse, cow, bull, ass, mule, sheep, pig, dog or goat, you must stop at the scene of the accident and give your name and address and the car's registration number to anyone involved in the accident who has reasonable grounds for asking for them – the owner of the animal, for instance.

• If there is no one else present – if you have knocked over a straying animal, for example – you must report the accident to the police within 24 hours.

• You are not legally obliged to stop or to report the accident to police if you run over any other animal – including a cat.

• If you accidentally kill a wild animal it is not an offence – even if the animal is a protected species, such as the otter.

• If you accidentally injure a wild animal – even a protected species – you may keep it, but only until it can fend for itself. Then it must be released.

• Alternatively, if a wild animal is too badly hurt to recover, the law allows you to kill it humanely. In these circumstances, the humane way is the quickest way available.

• The law does not, however, allow an unqualified person to kill a farm animal or pet in these circumstances.

What to do if someone collapses

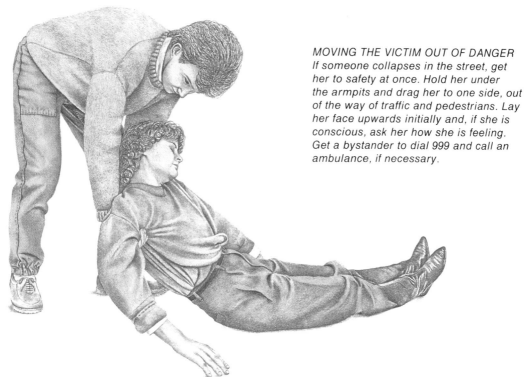

MOVING THE VICTIM OUT OF DANGER
If someone collapses in the street, get her to safety at once. Hold her under the armpits and drag her to one side, out of the way of traffic and pedestrians. Lay her face upwards initially and, if she is conscious, ask her how she is feeling. Get a bystander to dial 999 and call an ambulance, if necessary.

Emergencies on the road

A person may collapse in the street for any of a number of reasons. The most common cause is fainting (see page 96).

Less often the cause may be an epileptic fit (see page 94). More rarely still, it could be a heart attack (see page 105) or a stroke (see page 134).

Whatever the cause, the priority is always the same: move the victim to a safe place out of the way of traffic.

• Watch out for traffic as you approach the victim, and flag down cars if necessary.
• Lift or drag the victim to the side of the road.
• Once out of immediate danger, lay the victim down on his or her back.
• If the victim is conscious, ask her to describe her symptoms. If necessary, call an ambulance, or get a passer-by to do so.
• If she is unconscious, put one hand under her neck, the other on her forehead and tilt her head well back. This will open her airway.
• Check that the victim is breathing. Rest one hand on her chest to feel for movement; watch for movement as well.
• Put your ear near her mouth so that you can hear and feel her breath.

If the victim is breathing
• Someone who is unconscious but is breathing normally should be turned into the recovery position until she comes round (see page 136). Do not make a fainting victim sit up unless she feels she wants to.
• Send a bystander to dial 999 for an ambulance. Ask him to return afterwards to confirm

that he has done so. Anyone who has been unconscious, even for a short time, should have immediate medical treatment.

If the victim is not breathing
• If the victim's breathing stops, use a finger to clear her mouth of any blood or vomit.
• If there is still no breathing, check neck pulse (see page 52).
• If there is a pulse, begin artificial respiration (see page 50).
• If you cannot detect a pulse, give chest compression as well if you have been trained in the technique (see page 52).
• Once the casualty is breathing, loosen her clothing at the neck, chest and waist.
• Turn her into the recovery position.
• Stay with her until an ambulance comes. Do not give her anything to eat or drink – you could make hospital treatment more difficult.

Helping the victim of an epileptic fit
• If the victim is having an epileptic fit, do not try to push anything into his or her mouth.
• Simply restrain her gently. Muscle spasms – twitching or convulsing limbs – and the breath-holding often associated with fits rarely last more than a minute.
• Once the fit passes, the victim may fall into a deep sleep. Use a finger to clear any blood, mucus or vomit from her mouth.
• If she is breathing normally, turn her into the recovery position.
• Get someone to call an ambulance. Stay with the casualty until help arrives.

207

Controlling a skid

A car skids because the tyres lose their grip and begin to slide over the road surface instead of rolling along it. What to do to control a skid depends on which tyres are skidding and whether or not the car has front-wheel drive. The 'natural' reaction – jamming the brakes on hard – is the worst thing you can do.

How to stop a rear-wheel skid
In a rear-wheel skid the back of the car slides sideways and the vehicle begins to swing round back to front. This usually happens when you drive too fast round a bend or corner, but can occur if you brake harshly on an uneven surface or a steeply cambered road. It is most likely to happen in a car with front-wheel drive.

Whether the car has front-wheel or rear-wheel drive, the action to take is the same.
• Take your foot off the accelerator or brake. Do not push in the clutch pedal or grip the steering wheel hard.
• Turn the steering wheel in the direction the back of the car is sliding (turn right if it is sliding to the right, for example). Do not turn it too far or you may start a second skid in the opposite direction.
• When all four wheels are back in line, accelerate gently.

How to stop a front-wheel skid
In a front-wheel skid, the front of the car keeps straight on, even though you have turned the steering wheel to right or left.

Front-wheel skids usually happen when the driver accelerates too harshly round a bend. What to do depends on whether the car has rear-wheel or front-wheel drive.
IN A CAR WITH REAR-WHEEL DRIVE Take your foot off the accelerator. Do not apply the brake or push in the clutch pedal.
• Turn the steering wheel so that the front wheels are straightened – pointing again in the direction the car is moving. Do not turn it too far or you could cause the rear wheels to skid.
• Once the front wheels are gripping again, accelerate gently and steer in the direction you wish to go.
IN A CAR WITH FRONT-WHEEL DRIVE Ease off the accelerator smoothly, but maintain enough pressure on the pedal to keep the car in motion. If you decelerate too fast the rear wheels may skid as well.
• Do not touch the clutch or brake pedals, and do not straighten the steering wheel.
• Continue steering smoothly in the direction you want to turn, but do not turn the wheel violently or too far.
• As the car moves back on course, straighten the wheels and accelerate gently.

How to stop a four-wheel skid
In a four-wheel skid – which usually happens during hard braking – the wheels lock and the car slides forward not seeming to lose speed. It may skid in a more or less straight line, or off to the side if the road is steeply cambered.

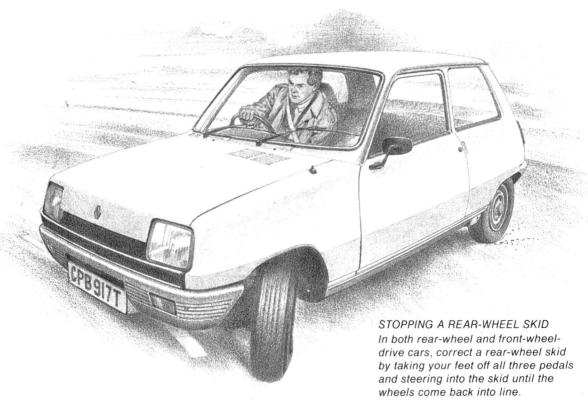

STOPPING A REAR-WHEEL SKID
In both rear-wheel and front-wheel-drive cars, correct a rear-wheel skid by taking your feet off all three pedals and steering into the skid until the wheels come back into line.

• To control a four-wheel skid, ease off on the brake pedal until the wheels start to roll again. Do not push in the clutch pedal.

• Once steering control is restored, straighten the wheels.

• Reapply the brakes by repeatedly pushing them on and off with a pumping action – a technique known as cadence braking – to avoid locking the wheels again.

How to avoid skidding

A car is most likely to skid when it is driven too fast for the road conditions and the driver is forced to alter course or speed abruptly. This results in a sudden redistribution of the car's weight – it may be thrown forward or to one side – so that weight is lifted from some of the tyres to the extent that they lose their grip on the road (their area of contact with the road surface is only the size of an average man's shoe). Tyres will also lose their grip if the wheels lock during hard braking, or if the wheels spin during harsh acceleration.

Following a few commonsense rules will cut the chances of your being involved in a skid.

• Make sure your car has good all-round vision before you drive. Misty glass can prevent you from seeing a hazard in good time.

• Drive smoothly and steadily.

• Read the road ahead and adjust speed in good time to avoid hazards (see *Defensive driving*, page 202).

• Make allowances for road conditions. Braking distances are greater in wet weather, and on a slippery or icy surface may be much longer than normal (see box, this page).

• Keep a lookout as you drive for slippery areas such as ice, mud, wet leaves, patches of dry dust or loose gravel.

• Be particularly careful in damp weather after a long dry spell. Oil and rubber-dust deposits on the road surface are extremely slippery when blended with mist or water.

• Try to anticipate the actions of other drivers. Keep well clear of those who appear to be uncertain or rash.

• Make sure your car is in good condition. Worn tyres, worn dampers and badly aligned steering all increase the risk of skidding. The legal minimum tread depth in Britain is 1mm, but for safety it should be at least 2mm, preferably 3mm or more, for at least three-quarters of the width all round the tyre.

Learning to control a skid

About half the vehicles which are involved in serious accidents on snowy or icy roads in Britain were skidding before impact. Drivers may lose control in a skid because they do not recognise what is happening, so do not respond smoothly or quickly enough.

A good way to become familiar with the sensation of different types of skid is to practise skidding deliberately on a skid pan – an area with a surface designed to give minimum tyre grip. The local council or the police should be able to tell you where the nearest skid pan is, and how to join courses which use it.

HOW LONG IT TAKES TO STOP AT 50MPH

This chart shows how road conditions and tyres can radically affect the distance a car takes to stop from 50mph (80km/h). On a dry or damp road, or on ice, tread depth makes little difference. But in the wet, it is crucial.

At higher speeds, the differences between good and bad tyres become even more marked. At 70mph (110km/h) on a wet road, a tyre with 5mm of tread depth can stop a car in little more than half the distance it takes for a tyre whose tread depth is at the 1mm legal minimum.

Damp roads – such as occur in misty conditions – are even more dangerous than wet roads, largely because light moisture combines with the rubber dust and oil on the road to create a slippery film. Heavy rain washes the film away.

Road condition	Tyre condition	Reaction distance	Braking distance
Dry	Tread depth 1mm or more	50ft (15m)	106ft (32m)
Wet (2mm of water)	Tread depth 5mm	50ft (15m)	120ft (37m)
Wet (2mm of water)	Tread depth 1mm	50ft (15m)	145ft (44m)
Damp	Tread depth 1mm or more	50ft (15m)	172ft (52m)
Black ice	Tread depth 1mm or more	50ft (15m)	625ft (191m)

Brake failure at speed

If the brakes fail when you try to stop a car at speed – perhaps on the approach to a crossroads – your only option is to slow down using the engine and possibly the terrain, such as a steep upward slope or a thick hedge.

• Apply the handbrake smoothly and at the same time pump the footbrake in the hope that brake pressure will be restored.

• Keep a firm grip on the steering wheel while you do this, because using the handbrake at speed may lock the rear wheels and cause a skid (see page 208).

• Do not switch off the engine, because you will then be unable to use its power as a brake by changing down to a lower gear. Moreover, the car will take a long time to roll to a stop from high speed. In addition, on cars with power-assisted brakes, the brakes will not work properly with the engine switched off.

• With manual gears, change down to third gear as the handbrake slows the car, and keep changing down as soon as you can. Attempting to change too quickly will throw the car about. To engage lower gears at speed, try double-declutching (see box, this page).

• With automatic transmission, move the lever into L (low lock) or 2 (second gear) as soon as you are slow enough. In most cars, this is likely to be at about 20mph (30km/h).

• If you cannot slow down or stop fast enough to avoid a collision, try to run the car up a slope or bank.

• Mounting the kerb, if it is safe to do so, and scraping the car along a hedge or fence will also slow it down. You may be able to drive straight into a hedge to stop, but you risk hitting a concealed tree or fence post – or someone unseen on the other side.

If the handbrake fails on a steep hill

If the handbrake fails when you stop on your way up a steep hill, starting off again is difficult in a car with manual gears because, with your left foot on the clutch, you cannot move your right foot from the brake to the accelerator without the car rolling backwards.

• Swivel your right foot so that your toe remains on the footbrake while you place your heel on the accelerator.

• As you release the clutch pedal, ease your right toe off the footbrake and press your heel down on the accelerator. This should allow you to hold the car until you move forwards and can release the brake completely.

• If you cannot stop the car rolling backwards, turn the steering wheel so that the car backs into the kerb and does not crash into any other vehicles behind you.

WHY BRAKES FAIL

Complete brake failure is rare because modern cars have two separate circuits of hydraulic fluid operating the brakes. If one circuit is damaged, the other can operate the brakes on its own, although less effectively. Nevertheless, water, driving habits or inadequate maintenance can all cause brakes to become dangerously unreliable.

Brakes may become temporarily ineffective after driving through floods (see page 220) because the discs or shoes get wet.

They may also fail temporarily on a steep descent or after prolonged use because the fluid gets hot and may partially vaporise; if this happens, the pedal feels spongy when it is depressed.

Repeated pumping of the brakes usually restores pressure in these circumstances. Use a low gear on a long or steep descent and brake gently to lessen the chances of the brakes overheating.

Sometimes hard braking causes the brake pads to get so hot that they temporarily lose their stopping power. When this happens, the pedal does not feel spongy, and the brakes will work again after a short stop to let them cool off.

How to double-declutch

Changing down a gear enables you to use the engine as a brake, but changing down at high speed puts considerable extra strain on the gearbox.

On a manual gearbox, it is possible to minimise this strain and to make changing down at speed easier by using the technique known as double-declutching. Its purpose is to match the speed of the road wheels with the speed of the engine in the new gear and so make it easier for the cogs inside the gearbox to engage. To double-declutch down through the gears:

• Take your foot off the accelerator.
• Press in the clutch pedal.
• Move the gear lever to neutral.
• Release the clutch pedal.
• Give the accelerator a quick burst, then remove your foot.
• Press in the clutch pedal.
• Move the gear lever into the lower gear.
• Gently release the clutch.

With an automatic gearbox, double-declutching is impossible. The only option is to move the gear lever into a lower gear and risk some mechanical damage.

When a tyre bursts

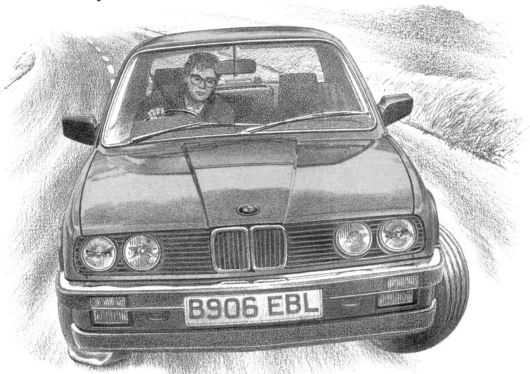

HOW TO STAY IN CONTROL
If a front tyre bursts, counter the pull towards
the side of the burst tyre by turning the steering
wheel smoothly in the opposite direction. Once
you are back on course, slow gently to a halt.

A burst tyre may be caused by a fault in the tyre structure, but it is much more likely to be caused by a puncture.

A punctured tyre does not always burst; it may deflate, giving the driver the impression he is travelling over something bumpy like cobbles, but the steering is affected in the same way as a burst. The main concern is to avoid slewing into other traffic.

If a front tyre bursts or deflates, the car pulls strongly to one side (the side on which the tyre has burst).

If a rear tyre bursts or deflates, the back end of the car may slide to one side.

• If a front tyre bursts, avoid braking if possible – let the car roll to a stop – and turn the steering wheel smoothly and gently to counter the sideways pull and keep the car on course.

• If a rear tyre bursts, brake gently – not suddenly or fiercely – and keep a firm grip on the steering wheel to keep the car on course.

• Do not change gear.

• Signal left, if you can, and steer the car to the side of the road to pull up.

• If you are on the outside lane of a motorway, it may be safer to pull onto the central reservation if possible.

• Try to stop on hard ground rather than a soft verge, because you will need a firm base for changing the wheel.

AVOIDING TYRE TROUBLE

Punctures occur when a sharp object such as a nail or screw lying in the road pierces the tyre wall. They tend to occur more in wet weather, probably because the water lubricates the screw or nail and helps it to penetrate. Many punctures are unavoidable, but some might be prevented by regular checking.

• Check tyres regularly for embedded stones, nails or other objects that might result in a puncture, and remove them.

• If anything is piercing the casing, change the wheel and get the tyre repaired.

• Check also for cuts, cracks or bulges in the sidewalls that might cause tyre failure, and get damaged or worn tyres renewed or repaired. A tyre that develops a bulge affects the car in the same way as a puncture, but there may be more warning that it is failing – such as a repeated slapping sound against the road.

• Always maintain tyres at the pressure recommended by the tyre manufacturer.

Driving through fog

In foggy conditions, being seen – particularly by drivers behind you – is as important as seeing. When fog is forecast, make sure all lamp glass on your car, front and rear, is clean and bright. The film of dust and dirt that collects on a lamp from road spray can cut the light intensity of the beam by half.

• By day or night, drive through fog with dipped headlights. Sidelights are not bright enough and full-beam headlights will reflect from fog particles and may dazzle you.

• Use fog lights if they are fitted. A single fog lamp must be used in conjunction with headlights, otherwise your car may be mistaken for a motorcycle.

• Switch on the windscreen wipers to keep the windscreen clear, and operate the washer as necessary. Use the demister to keep warm air blowing onto the inside of the screen.

• Keep your speed low. You should be able to stop within your range of vision, which could limit you to 5mph (8km/h).

• Drive with your window open. You may hear something coming, or hear a warning toot from a horn, even if you cannot see another vehicle. You need to glean every scrap of information in order to avoid obstacles and other traffic.

• Do not hunch over the wheel and peer forward. You will see better if you sit relaxed in your normal driving position.

• Try to drive in line with the nearside kerb or verge; if you have a passenger, ask him to keep you informed of your distance from the roadside.

• Alternatively, use the reflective studs in the middle of the road as a guide. But do not drive on the central line, or you may collide with vehicles coming the other way.

• Avoid getting too close to the vehicle in front. With vision restricted, you will not be able to anticipate it making an emergency stop You therefore need more reaction time before braking than in normal conditions.

• Remember that fog makes road surfaces even more slippery than rain. So braking distances will be greater, too (see *How long it takes to stop at 50mph*, page 209).

• Beware of blindly following red lights in front; if the driver ahead gets into trouble, you could follow him into it. Plot your own course.

• Do not overtake unless you are sure it is safe to do so. When you are behind another vehicle, especially a large one, it pushes the fog aside and gives you the impression that the fog is thinner than it actually is.

• If you do have to overtake, or pass a stationary car, give plenty of warning by sounding your horn and flashing your headlights.

• Turn right with extreme care. Signal in plenty of time, and put your head out of the window to look and listen for oncoming traffic before you make the turn.

• If a large vehicle is going in your direction, follow behind it at a safe distance. In a high cab the driver has a better view of the road and may be able to see above the worst of low-lying fog.

• When you have to stop in fog, try to park off the road. If you are forced to stop on the carriageway or a motorway hard shoulder, switch on the car hazard lights.

• For a lengthy stay, put out a warning triangle as well. It should be 100yds (90m) behind the car towards the nearside edge of the road – 150yds (135m) behind the car if you are on a motorway hard shoulder.

THE HAZARDS OF FOG

Most fog occurs in the highly populated lowlands of central England and Wales, where the average amount is from 5 to 20 days a year; air pollution from factories, power stations and domestic heating increases its density. In patchy, swirling fog, the uncertain visibility and the unnatural quietness (fog particles muffle sound) strain a driver's senses and soon bring on fatigue. Sometimes, too, drivers do not slow down in fog, where they would in heavy rain or snow.

Research suggests that with vision restricted and landmarks blotted out, drivers lose all sensation of speed, especially on motorways. In addition, because fog distorts distances, other vehicles may seem to be farther away than they really are. It may also be that the stress of the conditions makes drivers want to forge ahead in the hope that the fog will be thinner farther on.

Many drivers drive too close to the vehicle in front in fog, probably in the belief that it is safest to keep in sight of the tail lights of the vehicle ahead as a guide to direction.

This can be dangerous because it leaves insufficient time for reaction and braking if the car in front stops, and this is what leads to multiple pile-ups.

If, for example, a driver travelling at 50mph (80km/h) sees an obstacle ahead, it might take him as much as three-quarters of a second to react and begin braking. In that time he will have travelled about 55ft (16.5m). If all the drivers travelling behind are driving at the same speed and have the same reaction time, the tenth driver in the chain will travel some 550ft (165m) after the first driver sees the obstacle before reacting. So unless each car is at least 55ft (16.5m) apart – about five car lengths – and has reasonably efficient brakes, a string of collisions is inevitable.

When the windscreen shatters at speed

Most standard windscreens are made of glass which has been toughened so that it does not break easily. If it does shatter, however, it makes a crazed pattern of small pieces that can obscure vision. Zone-toughened screens break so that larger pieces remain immediately in front of the driver, giving him enough vision to stop safely.

• If your windscreen shatters, do not follow the natural impulse to punch out an area of the glass with your fist as you drive. You risk cutting your hand or arm badly, or having a splinter blown into your eye.

• Instead, lean forward. It will help you to see more clearly through the shattered glass. Pull in and stop as soon as it is safe to do so.

• Stuff rag or paper tissues into the demister slots on top of the dashboard and spread news-paper or cloth over the car bonnet. Pad your hand with a glove or cloth, get back inside the car and push the glass outwards onto the paper.

• Remove as much of the glass as possible, otherwise it may fall out while you are driving.

• If you have any adhesive tape, such as mask-ing tape, put a strip right round the windscreen so as to cover the grooved rubber flange which held the glass, and thus prevent fragments being blown into your face.

• If you have no tape, wear sunglasses to guard your eyes. Alternatively, pull the rubber flange off the car completely.

• Wrap up the glass in the newspaper. Dust any fragments off the top of the dashboard before removing the stuffing from the slots. Take the glass home to the dustbin – do not leave it at the roadside.

• Fit a temporary windscreen, if you have one.

Emergency screens are usually wrapped round the front door jambs so that they are held in place when the doors are shut.

• If you do not have a temporary screen, drive slowly and carefully to the nearest garage.

• Alternatively, you can get an emergency windscreen fitted at the roadside by a specialist firm (these firms are usually listed in the Yellow Pages of the telephone directory). If you call one, check whether there is an extra charge for attendance; at night this could be expensive.

• If you suspect that glass fragments may have fallen through the heater vents, do not use the demister until the system has been cleaned. You may be able to clear it yourself by uncoup-ling the hoses and sucking out the bits of glass with a vacuum cleaner.

Cutting the risks

A windscreen usually shatters because it has been hit by a stone flung into the air by the tyre of another car. There is no way of avoiding a stone, but there are ways to cut the risks.

• Consider fitting laminated safety glass to your car. The glass – which is usually tinted – will not shatter, no matter how hard it is hit. It may crack or chip, however, and eventually need replacement.

• On a newly surfaced road with loose chip-pings, keep your speed low and keep a more generous distance than usual between you and the vehicle in front.

• Consider taking out insurance to cover wind-screen damage, if your policy does not already include it. Ideally, the insurance should cover the whole cost of replacement, with no excess and no loss of your no-claim bonus.

Emergencies on the road

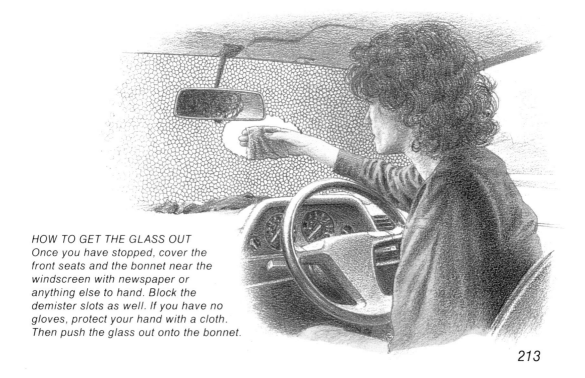

HOW TO GET THE GLASS OUT
Once you have stopped, cover the front seats and the bonnet near the windscreen with newspaper or anything else to hand. Block the demister slots as well. If you have no gloves, protect your hand with a cloth. Then push the glass out onto the bonnet.

If you feel drowsy at the wheel

If you find yourself beginning to nod off while driving, you must make an urgent effort to revive yourself until you can stop the car safely and wake yourself up.

Danger signs

Cruising for long periods in a warm car – particularly on a wide straight road such as a motorway – can be more hazardous than negotiating busy urban streets. With little to do, you can be tempted to daydream and let your attention wander dangerously. And the road sliding unvaryingly past the windscreen can exert a hypnotic effect powerful enough to put you into a mental state not unlike a trance.

Since fatigue builds up only gradually, judging – in yourself or someone else – when it has reached a dangerous level can be very difficult. These are the symptoms to watch for. If you notice any of them, take action at once.
- Continual yawning.
- Eyes feel heavy and are difficult to keep open.
- Difficulty in concentrating, especially on a monotonous stretch of road.
- Suddenly realising that you have no recollection of the last few miles you have travelled.
- A spasmodic jerk of the body, recalling you from the brink of sleep.
- The car begins to wander off course and you have to correct the steering hurriedly.
- You have to take rapid action to avoid a hazard you had not noticed.
- You start at a shadow, reacting to an imagined hazard.

Reviving yourself at the wheel

- If you do find yourself becoming drowsy, pull off the road to a safe parking place as soon as possible. Do not stop on a motorway hard shoulder, however – it is only for emergencies such as breakdowns.
- In the meantime, slow down.
- Direct the dashboard air vents onto your face. The blast of cold air will help to wake you up.
- Lick your finger and dampen your forehead and your eyelids – particularly at the inner corner of each eye. Let the air blow onto your face to cool it.
- Take a deep breath, purse your lips, and then breathe out again very slowly.
- Encourage passengers to chat with you.
- Wind down the window if the road is quiet and the weather dry. On a motorway or a busy road, however, let in blasts of fresh air only for short spells, because the extra noise increases fatigue.
- Play the radio or taped music only if it is something you will respond to positively. Some sounds can send you to sleep; others can irritate you and increase tiredness.

HOW TO STAY WIDE AWAKE ON A JOURNEY

- Do not drink alcohol or take drugs shortly before starting.
- Do not eat a heavy meal immediately before a journey; the process of digestion encourages sleep.
- Before a long journey, eat a light meal and take a rest. Do not set off on an empty stomach. You need to be comfortable to concentrate well.
- If you intend to drive through the night, make sure you have at least three hours of sleep first.
- Adjust the seat if necessary to ensure that you have a comfortable driving position before you set off.
- Avoid wearing tight clothes. When you sit for long periods, the stomach and ankles tend to swell up.
- If you are driving in bright sunshine, wear sunglasses. Glare puts extra strain on the eyes, and adds to fatigue. But do not wear night driving glasses or any other tinted glasses after dark; although they help to cut the dazzle of oncoming headlights, they restrict your ability to see dimly lit objects.
- Make sure the car is well ventilated.

- In heavy traffic, take advantage of hold-ups by exercising your limbs gently. For example, curl your toes, rotate your wrists and stretch your shoulders and neck. This helps the blood circulation and relieves boredom or frustration.
- On a long journey, alternate the driving with someone else, if possible.
- Suck boiled sweets occasionally for refreshment while you are driving.
- Make regular stops on a long run – never drive for more than three hours without a break.
- If you are driving abroad, take breaks more frequently than normal. Driving on the right and interpreting unfamiliar signs demand extra concentration and so will tire you more quickly.
- When you stop for a break, take a short nap if you feel you need it. But always get out of the car and go for a stroll to exercise cramped limbs and pep up circulation. A hot drink is also beneficial.
- On a brief stop, try taking your shoes and socks off for a while. Relaxing and cooling the feet seems to help to clear the head.

Fire in your car

A car fire must be put out very quickly because of the danger of the petrol tank exploding if the petrol vapour should ignite. As with any fire, the way to extinguish it quickly is to cut off its air and fuel supply.

• As soon as you notice smoke or flames, switch off the ignition but leave the key in position to avoid locking the steering.
• If the car is moving, coast to the side of the road if possible and stop.
• Get all passengers out and away from the vehicle.
• Disconnect the battery if you can, by pulling the wires off the terminals. But if the fire is under the bonnet do not open it wide, as air will increase the flames.
• If you do not have a fire extinguisher, try to smother the flames with a blanket, car rug or any thick material.
• If this is not successful, dial 999 and call the fire brigade.

Using a fire extinguisher
• If the fire is under the bonnet, lift the lid just enough to direct the extinguisher through it.
• Direct the extinguisher at the base of the flames and work methodically from side to side and from the edge inwards.
• Do not leave a patch uncovered, otherwise the flames may spring up again.

FITTING A FIRE EXTINGUISHER IN YOUR CAR

Every year, about 25,000 cars in Britain are damaged or destroyed by fire. Over one-third of the fires are caused by faults in the wiring, and a quarter by petrol under the bonnet catching fire. Others result mainly from collisions or are started by cigarettes.

An aerosol extinguisher of at least 3lb (1.4kg) capacity is effective for putting out most car fires. The extinguisher should be either of the type known as dry powder or one containing a liquid gas known as BCF (see *Protecting your home against fire*, page 152). Both can be safely used on electrical equipment. BCF fumes are, however, toxic in a confined space, so the car should be well ventilated once the fire has been put out.

A car fire extinguisher needs to be mounted in an easily accessible place, such as on the dashboard or in the driver's footwell – not in the boot.

Get it checked once a year by the manufacturer to ensure that the filling is kept up to capacity.

Stuck on a level crossing

Your chances of surviving a crash with a train are minimal. If your car stalls or breaks down on a level crossing, therefore, the priority is to protect yourself and your passengers – not the car. Even if the train driver can see you, he is unlikely to be able to stop in time. A train moving at 125mph (200km/h) takes up to a mile (1.6km) to stop.

• Get everyone out of the car and off the crossing as quickly as possible.
• Telephone the signal box immediately. The driver and passengers in an approaching train could be injured in an accident as well – and the sooner you can alert the signalman, the more chance he has of stopping any trains before they reach the crossing. There is an emergency telephone at most level crossings.
• Do not waste time trying to move the car before warning the signalman.
• Try to move the car off the crossing only if the signalman tells you that there is no train approaching.
• If the engine will not start, take off the handbrake, put the gear lever into neutral and try to push the car clear of the tracks.
• In a car with a manual gearbox, you can also use the starter motor to move it. Put the car in first gear with the handbrake off and your foot off the clutch, and turn the ignition key. The car will lurch forward as the starter motor turns.
• If you succeed in moving the car, let the signalman know immediately.

If the barriers come down
• If the alarms start to sound, the lights flash or the barriers come down while the car is still on the crossing, get everyone right away from the tracks. A derailed train or the wreckage from a crash can travel hundreds of yards from the point of impact.
• Abandon the car and everything in it. The train might be at the crossing within a matter of seconds – especially on a modern automatic type of level crossing.

Safety on crossings
There are about 9200 level crossings in Britain, and each year they are the scene of around 70 accidents, which cost the lives of up to 20 people. Motoring experts recommend four rules for crossing a railway line safely.
• Approach at a moderate speed.
• At an open level crossing – one with no barriers, attendant or warning lights – treat the crossing as if it were a major road. Stop, look both ways and listen carefully before you cross, to make quite sure that no train is approaching.
• Do not drive nose to tail over a crossing. Start to cross only when you can see that the road on the other side is clear.
• Do not stop on a level crossing for any reason. If you are already on the crossing when the lights start to flash or the alarms sound, carry on over.

Emergencies on the road

Stuck in snow

If you are forced to stop in snow or on ice, it is often difficult to start off again because the tyres cannot grip the surface. It is particularly easy to get stuck if you stop while driving up a hill.

The techniques described here for getting out of snow also apply to getting out of mud or sand.

If you get stuck on hard snow or ice

• Do not accelerate hard in an attempt to pull away. The spinning of the wheels will compact the snow and make gripping even more difficult; snow may also become packed into the tyre treads, lowering their gripping ability.

• Ensure that the wheels are straight so that the treads are in the best position for gripping the surface.

• Find something to pack under the driving wheels to improve their grip, such as sand, grit, sacking or twigs.

• To lessen the risk of wheel spin, start in

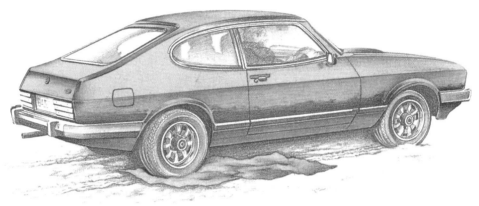

GETTING UNSTUCK
Give a stuck car's driving wheels something to grip by packing sacking, say, in front of them.

DRIVING ON SNOW AND ICE

• Make sure that tyres are inflated to the recommended pressures. Underinflated tyres do not give as good a grip. Radial-ply tyres, which have wide grooves, may grip snow better if they are inflated to a slightly higher pressure than normal.

• Keep your speed low because it takes much longer to pull up than on a normal surface. On ice, the braking distance can be ten times longer than normal.

• Drive in as high a gear as possible for the low speed. High gear reduces the amount of torque on the wheels, and so reduces the chance of wheel spin.

• Stay well behind the vehicle in front to give yourself plenty of room for braking.

• Use the brakes and accelerator very gently.

• Do not brake and steer at the same time.

• Brake with a pumping motion to avoid wheel lock. The brake lights flashing on and off also give a good warning to a car behind.

• Do not use the gears to slow the car. This could result in the wheels locking and causing a skid.

• Try to avoid stopping or changing gear on

a hill. If necessary wait at the bottom until you can climb without interruption.

• Descend a steep hill very slowly in low gear, and use the brakes very gently and cautiously.

• In a country area, if snow is widespread use snow chains or snow traction clamps to improve tyre grip.

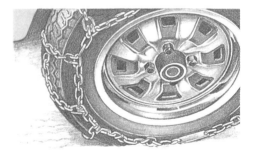

GETTING A GRIP ON ICE OR SNOW
Snow chains fitted around a car's tyres help to improve the tyres' grip on icy or snowbound roads.

second gear so that there is less torque (turning effort) applied to the wheels.

• Press the accelerator gently, just enough to move the car forward slowly, and slip the clutch as necessary to keep the engine revving.

• If there are any passengers in the car, they may be able to help by pushing the car forwards as you drive off. Tell them to stand at the sides – so that the car does not roll or slide into them – but well away from the driving wheels or they will be sprayed with dirt, snow and packing material.

• Once the car gets moving, do not stop to pick up passengers or gear until you have reached a firmer, level surface.

Getting out of deep snow

• It is sometimes possible to drive out of snow about 12in (300mm) or so deep by moving the car backwards and forwards to build up a track – a technique known as rocking.

• Try to move forward a few inches by engaging first gear and then revving gently, slipping the clutch as necessary to avoid stalling.

• While the car is as far forward as it will go, quickly engage reverse and move slowly backwards for a few inches.

• Repeat the backwards and forwards movements until you can mount the piled up snow and drive out of the trough.

• If this method fails, the alternative is to dig the snow away from in front of all four wheels, and use the techniques recommended above for moving off on hard snow or ice.

If you are trapped in a snowbound car

Driving is usually impossible in a blizzard, or if snow becomes deeper than about 12in (300mm). In a snowbound car, the main things to concentrate on are keeping warm and keeping awake.

• Stay in the car; it will give you shelter. Do not try to walk for help – you risk falling into a snowdrift or getting lost in a blizzard, and could die of exposure only a few yards from a building.

• Before the snow gets too deep, try to clear the area round the exhaust tailpipe. Otherwise poisonous fumes are likely to enter the car when you run the engine to use the heater.

• If you have a separate boot, take anything you need from it into the seating area. Look for an implement that you can use to make an air channel should the car become completely buried – a wheelbrace, for example.

• Keep warm by wrapping yourself up in clothing, rugs, blankets, sacking or carpet. Wrap your head up as well.

• Newspaper wrapped round limbs or stuffed into clothing helps to conserve body heat; it can also be used to improvise a hat.

• Run the engine and heater to help you to warm up for only about ten minutes every hour. Do not run them constantly; not only will the warmth make you drowsy, but you need to conserve fuel in case you are trapped for a long time. There is also a higher risk of exhaust fumes entering the car.

• Keep awake. If you doze off, you are more likely to succumb to frostbite or hypothermia (excessive loss of body heat). Or you could suffocate if the car became buried by snow.

• Open a window to let in air occasionally. Use a window on the side away from drifting snow.

• Avoid drinking alcohol in the hope that it will warm you up. It dilates the blood vessels and so encourages the loss of body heat. It may also make you sleepy.

• Exercising gently from time to time will help you to keep awake and keep your blood circulating. For example, stretch or wriggle your toes, fingers, knees, shoulders and neck.

• Do not attempt violent exercise, as this will increase your need for oxygen, use up your body heat and make you tired.

• Do not keep the radio or car lights on constantly, or you may drain the battery.

• If the car gets completely buried by snow, open a window and poke an air channel through the snow. Use an implement such as an umbrella or wheelbrace if necessary. Keep the channel clear.

• If a number of cars are snowbound together, join forces with the other occupants. Sitting together in one vehicle generates warmth, boosts morale and helps you to keep awake.

SURVIVAL PACK

When motoring in snowy weather – especially in Scotland, northern England or the West Country – make sure the car is well equipped to keep you moving on a slippery surface and to keep you warm and occupied if you break down or become snowbound in cold, icy conditions. This is a list of useful equipment to keep in the car.

• Shovel.
• Sacking or bag of grit.
• Snow chains or traction clamps.
• Wellington boots.
• Extra clothing, rugs and blankets.
• Torch and spare batteries.

If you are going on a long journey – especially at night – in conditions where you anticipate you might be held up, consider taking some additional items:

• A hot drink in a flask.
• Emergency high-energy rations such as chocolate, biscuits or boiled sweets.
• Something to pass the time – for example, a novel, a battery-powered tape player or radio, a quiz book, a book of crosswords or pencil and paper.

Escaping from a car underwater

IF IT SINKS BEFORE YOU CAN GET OUT

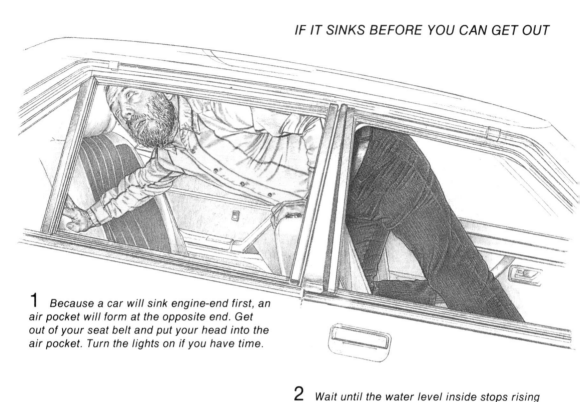

1 *Because a car will sink engine-end first, an air pocket will form at the opposite end. Get out of your seat belt and put your head into the air pocket. Turn the lights on if you have time.*

2 *Wait until the water level inside stops rising (until then it may be impossible to open a door). Take a deep breath, open a door or window and swim out. Breathe out slowly as you rise.*

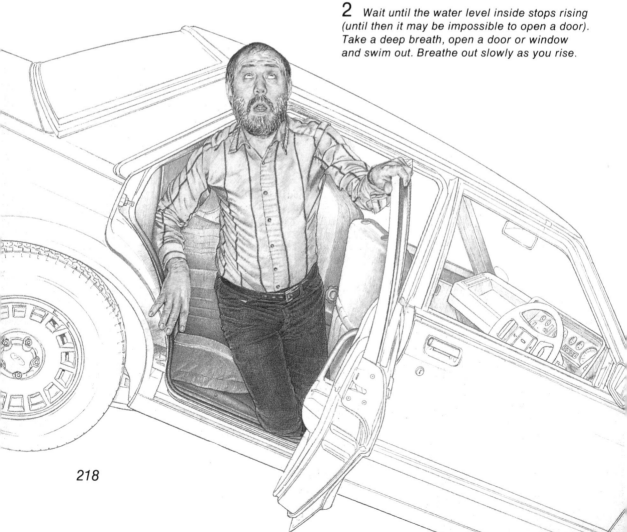

If your car plunges into deep water, you may be able to escape through a door or window before it sinks – usually within a minute or so. But even if the car sinks with you inside, you can still escape because it may take 30 minutes or more to fill up with water. Precisely how long it takes depends on whether the windows are open, how well sealed the car is and how deep the water is. The deeper the car sinks, the higher is the pressure of the surrounding water and the faster it will force its way in.

How to get out of a sunken car

• A car will sink engine-end first, and a pocket of air will form inside at the opposite end near the roof. Use this pocket of air to escape.

• Release your seat belt.

• If there is time, turn the headlights and interior lights on. They will enable you to see better and will help rescuers to find the vehicle.

• Place yourself so that you can put your head into the air pocket and breathe. In a front-engined car, climb into the back seat.

• Close any open windows and ventilation ducts, if there is time, to retain air in the car.

• As the car settles, water will find its way in through cracks and holes until the pressure inside and outside the car equalises. Keep calm and wait until the pressures equalise – when the water level inside stops rising. Until then it will be extremely difficult to open a door – and failure to do so might lead to panic, which could be fatal.

• When the level stops rising, take a deep breath, open a window or door and swim out.

• As you swim to the surface, allow air to bubble slowly out of your mouth. Because the air pocket in the car was under pressure, the air in your lungs will be as well – and will expand as you rise. If the excess is not allowed to escape, it could damage your lungs.

LIFE-SAVING BUBBLE
When Kenneth Hope's car plunged into the river at Mark in Somerset in November 1982, it turned over, trapping him inside. He crawled into the boot of the car where there was a large enough air pocket to keep him alive until he was rescued by emergency services several hours later.

He was suffering from exposure because of the chilly water, but was otherwise unharmed.

Emergencies on the road

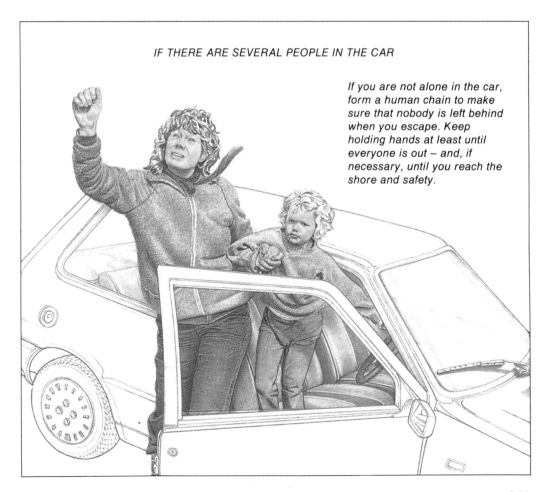

IF THERE ARE SEVERAL PEOPLE IN THE CAR

If you are not alone in the car, form a human chain to make sure that nobody is left behind when you escape. Keep holding hands at least until everyone is out – and, if necessary, until you reach the shore and safety.

Driving through floodwater

Flooding is likely on many low-lying roads after heavy rain, and some roads have fords that are quite deep in wet weather.

• If you see a sheet of water ahead, slow down.

• If the water is obviously not very deep – other traffic may be going through, for example – there is no need to stop and check the depth. Wait until the car in front is clear of the water, then drive through slowly.

• Stop if you are uncertain of the depth. It is not advisable to drive on if the water level is higher than the bottom edge of the cooling-fan blades, because they will send a fine spray of water over the engine and could short-circuit the spark-plug leads or crack the hot engine block. In most cars, the blades are 10-12in (250-300mm) above the ground – about as high as the centre of the road wheels.

• Enter the water on the crown of a cambered road so that you keep to the shallowest part.

• Drive slowly in first or second gear – on an automatic in L (low lock) or 1 (first gear) – so that as little water as possible is splashed on the engine. But do not let the engine stall.

• To keep the engine revs high at low speed with a manual gearbox, apply steady pressure on the accelerator (keep it about half depressed) and at the same time slip the clutch by pushing the clutch pedal a little way down.

• Avoid changing gear. If you alter the engine speed there is a risk of water being sucked back through the exhaust.

• As soon as you drive out of the water, test the brakes. They are likely to be soaked and useless. To dry them out, drive slowly with your left foot pressing lightly on the brake pedal. Do not pick up speed until you have tested the brakes several times and are sure they are pulling evenly on all wheels.

HOW FLOODWATER CAN DAMAGE YOUR CAR

If you drive through even quite shallow water at speed, the car will throw up a considerable wave. The wave can be heavy enough to obscure your vision, and the water may wrench the front wheels to one side so that you lose steering control.

The surge of water may also swamp the engine compartment, damaging the electrics and causing the engine to stall. If this happens, you will either have to push the car out or wait for a tow.

If the engine stalls, water may be sucked back through the exhaust into the cylinders. This could damage the pistons, connecting-rods and crankshaft, and although the damage might not become apparent for another 100 miles (160km) or so, the repairs would be expensive.

Where the risk is greatest

Flooding is most likely: on roads beside rivers and lakes; in dips on undulating roads; on roads liable to subsidence (this is sometimes signposted); under bridges, where the road often dips; and where roadside fences and buildings ahead seem unnaturally low.

After heavy rain, keep an eye out for flood warning signs. Look out, too, for depth marker posts which are usually set up at fords and other places where flooding happens regularly.

HOW TO KEEP THE ENGINE GOING
Drive slowly but keep the engine revs high. The flow of exhaust gases will then stop water entering the tailpipe and stalling the engine.

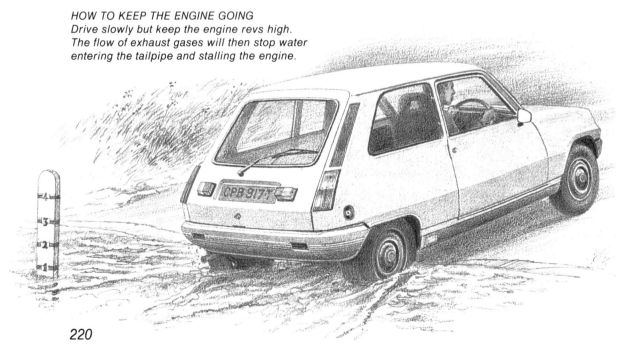

Emergency repairs

When a car breaks down miles from help, there may be little or nothing you can do about it unless you happen to be carrying the necessary spare parts.

But some common causes of breakdown can be repaired temporarily on the spot with little more than ingenuity, and others can be dealt with merely by know-how.

All the methods described here have been used successfully by motorists in an emergency to get them home or to a garage.

If the fan belt breaks

If the ignition light comes on while you are driving, indicating that the generator is not charging the battery, the reason may be a broken drive belt or fan belt.

• This should not happen if the belt is regularly checked during the car's normal servicing. Check it at least once a year, and replace it as a matter of course every five years – even if it is showing no signs of wear. And carry a spare fan belt in the car.

• Do not be tempted, if the fan belt breaks, to improvise one from string, nylon tights or cord. These substitutes are often recommended, but they do not work properly.

• Modern fan belts work under much greater tension than the belts on older cars. This means that the substitutes are likely to break within a minute or two. And the broken pieces can cause expensive damage – by getting tangled up in the timing mechanism, for instance.

• If you do not have a proper replacement fan belt – or if you do not have the tools necessary to fit it – get to a telephone and call a motoring organisation or a garage for help.

• If getting to a telephone is impossible, you can, in an emergency, drive on without the belt.

• If you decide to do this, wait first of all for the engine to cool off – a process which usually takes about half an hour. Remove any loose pieces of belt from the engine compartment while you are waiting.

• After that period, drive on – keeping the engine speed as low as possible by getting into a high gear quickly – for no more than 3 miles (5km). If you drive any farther than this, you risk overheating the engine and causing expensive damage.

• Then stop and let the engine cool off again for half an hour. Repeat the process until you reach a garage.

• One good way to extend the driving range of the engine between stops is by turning the car heater to maximum. The heater will draw more heat from the engine, preventing the engine from overheating so quickly even if you get uncomfortably warm, and allowing you to drive a few extra miles before stopping.

• During the journey, the battery will not be getting topped up. So keep all the car's electrical systems turned off as much as possible. Otherwise you will in time drain the battery, and

without electrical power for the spark the engine will not work.

• In many modern cars, the fan that cools the engine is driven by an electric motor, not a fan belt. If your car is one of these, the ignition light coming on and staying on as a steady bright red probably means that the belt which drives the alternator (the modern equivalent of a generator) is broken. If this is the case, the engine will not overheat if you drive on without the belt. But you will, in time, drain the battery.

• Stop and remove any loose pieces of belt from the engine. Turn off all unnecessary electrical systems – including the heater fan and any radio – so as to preserve the battery's charge for as long as possible.

• Drive on to the nearest telephone or garage and get the belt replaced.

• At night, a fully charged battery will usually keep the engine going, with the headlights on, for at least an hour – although the lights will become progressively dimmer. During the day, if no lights or other electrical systems are being used, a fully charged battery will keep the engine going for several hours.

• If the ignition light comes on only intermittently or dimly, the reason is not a broken fan belt. Usually, it means that the engine is turning over too slowly. Rev up the engine a little and the light should go out.

If the petrol gets low

If the petrol gauge reads very low, you may, by careful driving, be able to conserve fuel long enough to reach a filling station.

• Drive smoothly, but not fast, in top gear – normally about 25-30mph (40-50km/h). Do not, however, use an overdrive or a fifth gear.

• Avoid stopping and starting if you can. Anticipate conditions ahead so that you can slow down as much as possible simply by taking your foot off the accelerator. The more the accelerator is pressed, the more petrol is consumed.

• Try to approach traffic lights at such a speed that you can cruise through without stopping. If you have to stop and start again, get into top gear smoothly and as early as practicable.

• When approaching a hill, gently build up speed beforehand. Do not stay in top gear too long as you go up the slope so that you lose speed and have to increase acceleration. Instead, change down so that you can keep going in a lower gear without having to press hard on the accelerator.

• Coasting down hills in neutral with the engine switched off is not recommended, both because it limits your control of the car and because, in the absence of the help provided by the engine vacuum, you may need to press twice as hard on the brake pedal to achieve the same braking effect. On automatic cars, it can lead to the gearbox overheating. On cars with power brakes and power steering, the effort required to operate the brakes and steering will be alarmingly increased. On a car with a steering lock, you could lock the steering as well.

• Try to avoid driving until the petrol runs out completely, because dirt and moisture from the tank bottom will be dredged through the fuel system and probably cause a blockage.

• If the petrol does run out, the engine is likely to splutter and falter a little before it finally stops. Pull off the road if this happens.

• If you are stranded on a motorway, pull onto the hard shoulder and use the nearest emergency telephone to call for assistance.

• On other roads, call out a garage or motoring organisation for help, but you may find somewhere to buy a can of petrol as quickly as you can find a telephone.

• It may be difficult to pour petrol into your tank from the can. If necessary, improvise a funnel from a rolled-up newspaper or magazine.

If the windscreen wipers fail

If the windscreen wipers break down in rain and you cannot put the fault right, you may be able – on older cars – to improvise a way of operating them manually.

• The fault may be that the drive cable from the wiper motor has broken. If it has not, disconnect the cable anyway – it is usually under the dashboard or bonnet near the base of the wipers. Otherwise the arms will be too stiff to pull.

• Tie a piece of string or flex to the wiper arm on the driver's side and stretch it through the open driver's window. An alternative could be a scarf or belt.

• Tie another string from the driver's wiper to the passenger-side arm and run it through the passenger window into the car.

• Ask the front passenger to pull the wipers back and forth across the windscreen by hand as needed to clear it. A driver alone should not attempt this, because it would limit his control of the steering.

• Alternatively, improvise a return spring such as linked elastic bands or a pair of braces from one of the wiper arms. Retain it against the jamb of the closed door on the same side. This may make the arms easier to operate manually by a driver alone, because he only has to pull one string. Again, though, it is safer for a passenger to operate the arms so that the driver has both hands free for steering.

• On a modern car, it may be difficult, if not impossible, to disconnect the wiper arms from the motor without an array of tools and considerable time. In these circumstances, abandon any idea of operating the arms manually.

• Either wait for the rain to stop; or, if you have to continue your journey for some overriding reason, drive on very slowly without the wipers, stopping as often as necessary to clear the windscreen by hand. Get the wipers mended as soon as possible. Driving a car with faulty wipers is against the law.

If you lose the wheel nuts

• If you lose the nuts on a wheel, perhaps while changing a wheel at night, remove one nut from each of the other three wheels, and use them

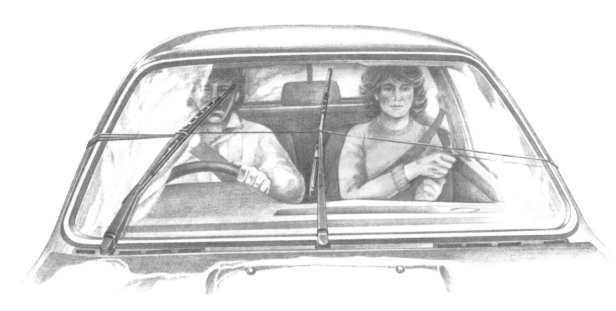

HOW TO WORK BROKEN WIPERS BY HAND
On older cars, disconnect the cable that drives the wipers, and tie something elastic such as a pair of braces to the driver's wiper. Clamp the other end in the door. Tie string between the arms and run it through the passenger's window. If the wipers are stiff, though, as they often are on newer cars, do not force them. Wait until the rain stops, or do without.

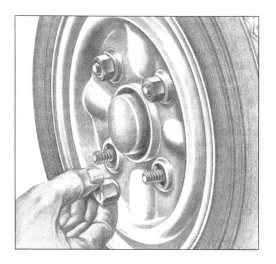

SHARING OUT WHEEL NUTS
If you lose some wheel nuts while changing a wheel, share out the remaining nuts so that there are at least three on each wheel. Put any extra nuts on the front wheels, not the back.

as replacements, so that you have three nuts on each wheel.
• Drive on smoothly – braking gradually and using only gentle acceleration – at no more than 30mph (50km/h), to lessen the strain on the remaining nuts.
• Get a full set of nuts on each wheel as soon as possible.
• If the wheel has only three nuts (or bolts) to start with, it is still possible to borrow from the other wheels. But it is not advisable unless you have no alternative, because the strain on the remaining two nuts is greater than with three on a four-nut wheel, or four on a five-nut wheel.
• If you lose only some of the wheel nuts so that you have a total of, say, 14 nuts between the four wheels, put the extra nuts on the front wheels rather than the back, because the front wheels have to take the additional strain of the steering. Also, in many modern cars, the drive is through the front wheels.

If the engine is flooded with petrol
If you use too much choke or pump the throttle when trying to start the car, the points of the spark plugs can become soaked with petrol, and the engine will not fire.
   Similarly, if the car stalls when you stop at a road junction shortly after setting off, and will not start again, overuse of the choke has probably fouled the spark plugs.
• If the engine has a manual choke, push it right in to increase the flow of air to the cylinders.
• Slowly press the accelerator to the floor and hold it there. This also increases the airflow.
• With the accelerator held down, turn the starter for a few seconds. This should blast the plug ends dry and clear over-rich mixture from

the combustion cylinders. The engine should then fire.
• If it does not fire, wait for about ten minutes and then repeat the operation.

If the engine fades out because of vapour lock
Petrol sometimes vaporises in a car's fuel line if it gets very hot – and the restricted fuel supply will cause the engine to misfire or cut out altogether.
   Such a vapour lock might occur on an older car after a long drive at high speed, or in a lengthy traffic jam, or in unusually hot weather. It may also happen if you are driving at high altitudes – across the Alps, say – where the lower atmospheric pressure reduces the boiling point of liquids, including water and petrol.
• Park safely in the shade and wait for the engine to cool and the fuel to condense. This will probably take at least half an hour. Then start up again.
• If the trouble recurs, get the car checked.

Suspected fuel faults in cars with fuel injection or engine management systems should be investigated by a garage.

If the accelerator jams
If the accelerator stays down when you ease off it while driving, the return spring near the pedal or the carburettor may be broken. This means the engine will continue at high revs – it will not slow down automatically.
• Try to hook your toe under the accelerator pedal and raise it. This will slow down the revs and stop the engine racing.
• Signal left and check in the mirror whether it is safe to pull over and stop the car.

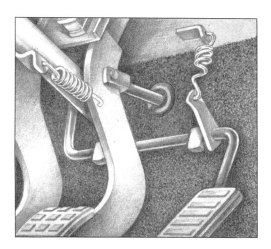

WHEN A THROTTLE SPRING BREAKS
Shape the larger part of the broken spring by hand to form a new spring, if possible. If you cannot improvise a spring, slip your foot under the pedal and lift it to slow the engine.

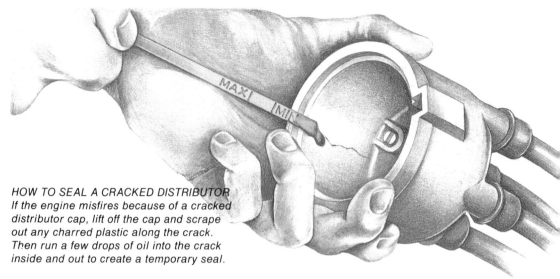

HOW TO SEAL A CRACKED DISTRIBUTOR
If the engine misfires because of a cracked
distributor cap, lift off the cap and scrape
out any charred plastic along the crack.
Then run a few drops of oil into the crack
inside and out to create a temporary seal.

• If it is, switch off the ignition and brake to a stop. Be careful not to turn the key so far that it engages any steering lock on the car.
• If you cannot pull over and switch off immediately – if you are on the outside lane of a motorway, for example – keep going until you can, braking if necessary.
• Remember, though, that the car's braking power will be below normal because of the counter-effect of the high engine power.
• Once you have stopped, you may be able to repair the return spring temporarily by unwinding part of the spring, forming the end into a new hook shape, and refixing it.
• If not, improvise a temporary spring using strong rubber bands, for example, or a piece of elastic.
• Fix the ends of the improvised spring in position with something that will not melt, such as wire, because the fixed point of the spring is often close to the exhaust pipe.
• Drive smoothly and slowly – no faster than 30mph (50km/h) – to a garage to get a new spring fitted. Do not jab the accelerator, or you will put too much strain on the temporary spring and probably break it.

If the distributor cap is cracked
A hairline crack may develop in the distributor cap because of damage or old age. This gives the high-tension current to the spark plugs an easy alternative path, so the engine becomes difficult to start or misfires.
• Lift off the cap and look inside for a telltale blackened track burnt into the plastic along the line of the crack by the escaping current.
• Scrape away as much of the burnt plastic as possible with something sharp, such as a small screwdriver or a nail file.
• Seal the crack with nail varnish, if you have any to hand, or run a small amount of oil from the end of the dipstick into it.

• If it is a bad crack, put the sealant on both sides – inside and outside the cap.
• Have a new distributor cap fitted as soon as possible.

Suspected ignition faults in cars with electronic ignition or engine management systems should be investigated by a garage.

If a fuse blows and you have no spare
If one part of the car's electrical system fails but others do not – if, for example, the lights go out but the brake lights and indicators work – the reason is most likely a blown fuse.
• Open the fuse box. The car handbook will tell you where it is – usually under the bonnet near the bulkhead or inside the car under the dashboard. Sometimes there is a spare fuse supplied in the box. Locate the burned-out fuse.
• If possible, transfer a fuse of the same rating from a circuit you can temporarily manage without to the position of the blown one – for example, the fuse covering the rear window heater. In most fuse boxes there is an indication of which fuse covers which circuit.
• If the fuse you have transferred blows as well, there is a short circuit in the system – perhaps a chafed wire or a faulty switch. Try to find it and rectify it.
• If you cannot discover the fault, either drive on if possible – without using the faulty circuit – or call out a garage or motoring organisation. Do not try to drive on by replacing the blown fuse with a temporary fuse that is too strong for the circuit: you risk starting a fire.
• If you can discover and cure the fault, it is possible, in an emergency, to make a temporary substitute fuse by wrapping fuse wire round the core of the blown one. If the fuse is a rectangular type, push the wire between the connectors.
• Use 13 amp household fuse wire if you have

any in the car. If you have no fuse wire, abandon the idea of making a substitute. Never bridge a fuse with ordinary wire, or with some other piece of metal such as a paper clip.

• In addition, engineers do not recommend using a layer of silver foil from a cigarette or chocolate packet wrapped round the fuse holder – a method sometimes suggested as a last resort. This is because you run a high risk of damaging a major component or setting the car on fire.

Thawing a frozen door lock

If you cannot get the door key in the lock on a frosty or snowy morning – or if it will not turn when inserted – the lock is probably frozen. To free it, use one of the following methods:

• Heat the end of the key with a match or lighter, then put the key in the lock. Repeat the process several times until the lock turns freely. Do not force it.

• If the weather is not too cold, hold your bare hand over the lock for a few seconds – body heat is often enough to melt the ice in the lock. Alternatively, warm the end of the key in your mouth for a few seconds.

• Squirt a few drops of lighter fuel or antifreeze into the lock, but take care not to get it on the paintwork. Using a de-icer spray is not recommended because you cannot avoid spraying it on the surrounding paintwork, and it may damage the surface.

• To prevent the lock freezing in future, put one or two drops of light oil on the end of the key and work it round the lock so that it coats the interior. This will help to stop the lock interior getting wet. Repeat the procedure regularly, particularly during the winter.

SPARE PARTS FOR EVERYDAY MOTORING

Carrying a few spares of the parts most likely to fail, as well as some tools and a few repair aids, can save any motorist hours of trouble.

• Generator drive belt (or fan belt) – a replacement of the type used for your make of car. Emergency fan belts are also available, but are not recommended. They do not last long and may be awkward to fit.

• Fuses – one or two of each type of fuse used in your make of car.

• Light bulbs – packaged sets are available for different makes.

• Spark plug – one of the type suitable for your car. You do not need to carry a complete set, because it is rare for all to fail at once.

• High-tension lead – a length of heavily insulated lead of the type used between the coil, distributor cap and spark plugs. Carry a length equal to the longest HT lead in your car, and any tools necessary to fit it.

• Duplicate ignition key – keep it in a magnetic box, which can be fixed to the outside of the car in a concealed spot.

• Emergency windscreen – a clear plastic screen packed in a cardboard holder.

• Can of fuel – useful if you are journeying in a remote area. The can should be of metal and clearly marked with the word 'Petrol'. Storage cans can be bought with built-in pouring spouts. Replace the petrol every three months or so. Petrol deteriorates in time, so that after a few months 4-star petrol will degrade to 2-star quality.

• Tools – a straight-bladed and a cross-headed screwdriver; a circuit tester; spanners of the sizes most common on your car; and a spanner for removing spark plugs.

Useful extras

• Torch.

• Radiator sealant.

• Water-repellent lubricant.

• Exhaust bandage and sealing cement.

• PTFE plumbers' tape – useful for packing out worn screw threads.

• Strong adhesive tape.

• PVC insulating tape.

• Tyre inflators – proprietary get-you-home tyre seals that contain compressed air and sealant. They are suitable for a flat tyre caused by a puncture and handy if you have difficulty in changing a wheel. But if there is any damage to the tyre structure, they may make the tyre difficult to repair later, and garages may be reluctant to handle them.

• Magnet – for retrieving small metal parts dropped into inaccessible areas.

• A coil of baling wire – soft, galvanised iron wire suitable for innumerable small repairs such as fashioning a temporary exhaust hanger.

• Jump leads – useful for obtaining a start from another car if your battery is flat. They are not safe to use, though, if your car has fully electronic ignition and fuel-injection equipment; check in your handbook to see if your car is of this type. When using jump leads, always connect the two batteries positive terminal to positive terminal (+ to +) and negative to negative (− to −). Connect the negative lead (usually coloured black) first, and disconnect it last.

• Tow rope.

• A length of cord.

• A packet of strong elastic bands.

Menaced by a hitchhiker

More often than not, someone thumbing a lift is quite harmless and intent only on being helped on his way. But there is always a risk that he is planning to rob you, and even if not, there have been cases of hitchhikers slashing the back seat or doing other damage. Police crime prevention experts advise motorists never to give a lift to a stranger.

• If a hitchhiker you have picked up threatens you with a weapon, do as you are told and drive on. Do not attempt to struggle with him.

• Look for the first opportunity to get out of the situation. The police suggest that, if possible, you stop the car at a place where there are a lot of people about – a bus station, say – and attract attention by yelling and screaming.

• Another way is to stall the car deliberately at busy traffic lights and pretend it will not re-start. With the build-up of other traffic and irate drivers, the attacker may run off, or you may manage to get away from the car.

• If you cannot shake off the attacker, hand over money, car keys or other possessions if ordered to do so.

• As soon as the hitchhiker leaves or you escape, write down all you can remember about the incident – where and when it happened, what the hitchhiker looked like, and what was said. Sign and date what you have written, and take it to the police; it will be powerful evidence if the hitchhiker is later caught and prosecuted.

If a girl tries to blackmail you

• If, as a male driver, you give a lift to a girl who threatens to rip her blouse and scream 'rape' if you do not give her money, remain calm. Make no attempt to touch her or argue with her.

• Drive straight to the nearest police station, flag down a passing police car or stop where there is a large crowd.

• Tell someone what is happening and ask him or her to call the police.

If you are flagged down at night

There is a possibility that what appears to be an accident or someone in need of help is a ruse to stop a car driver and rob him. This is most likely to happen to a motorist who is known to be carrying money and who regularly uses a particular route.

• As you approach the person flagging you down, lock all doors from the inside.

• Slow down and change to a low gear so that you can accelerate away if necessary.

• Turn your headlights to full beam to light up the scene so that you can assess the situation.

• If you slow to a stop, do not turn off the engine or get out of the car until you are satisfied that the situation is genuine. Be ready to drive off quickly.

• If you are not sure whether the situation is genuine, drive on and call the police from the nearest telephone.

Safety on two wheels

More than 70,000 motorcyclists are injured on British roads every year. Motorcyclists make up about one in five of all road accident casualties and they are about eight times more likely to be involved in a crash than a car driver. The commonest motorcycle accident is a collision with a motorist turning onto a major road, and it happens because the car driver simply fails to see the machine in time – even in daylight on an urban road.

The same circumstances account for most bicycle accidents as well. Four out of five of the 20,000 serious cycling accidents in Britain each year happen within a few yards of a junction.

For this reason the most important safety rule for motorcyclists and cyclists is: be visible.

On a motorcycle

• Make sure you can be seen. Wear brightly coloured clothing, or a fluorescent sash or waistcoat.

• Keep the headlight on constantly while riding, even during the day. But do not assume that the headlight alone will make you conspicuous. On smaller machines, particularly – 250cc and under – the light is not powerful enough to be very bright.

• Before overtaking, flash your headlight to make sure the driver has seen you. If you have been riding behind the offside edge of the car, his view of you may have been masked.

• Do not overtake on the inside. The car driver may not see you and could pull over towards the kerb or turn left in front of you.

• If the car in front of you turns left, beware of another vehicle pulling out across your path from the same side road. The driver may not have seen you behind the turning car.

• When motorcyclists ride in a group, the one in front should take up the best position on the road. Those behind should be staggered to right and left so that they have as much vision and braking space as possible.

• For a safe braking distance in dry weather, road safety experts recommend keeping as far behind the vehicle in front as you can travel in two seconds, which means allowing about 1yd for each 1mph (2m for every 3km/h). You can measure the distance using a roadside marker such as a postbox. You should be able to say: 'Only a fool forgets the two-second rule' (which takes about two seconds to repeat) in the time between the vehicle in front passing the marker, and passing it yourself.

• In wet weather, braking distances may be doubled, so you need a four-second gap between your machine and a vehicle ahead.

• If you want to brake when riding upright on a firm, dry surface, the safest and most effective way is to pull more firmly on the front brake than on the rear brake.

• On a firm but wet surface, put even pressure on both front and rear brakes.

• When riding with the machine leaning to one

side, when turning, or when riding on a poor surface such as loose chippings, avoid using the front brake at all.

On a bicycle
• Wear brightly coloured clothing, and a fluorescent sash and arm or leg bands.
• At night, make sure your lights are on. You must, by law, have working front and back lights and a rear reflector.
• Slow down when you approach a turning and look out for vehicles coming unexpectedly across your path. Be ready to brake suddenly.
• Keep at least 1yd (1m) from the kerb – to give yourself space to swerve into if a passing car comes too close. Give parked cars a wide berth; a driver getting out might not see you.
• Remember that a bicycle is a road vehicle like any other. It is just as illegal for a cyclist to cross against a red light or to go the wrong way up a one-way street as it would be for a driver.

PROTECTIVE CLOTHING: WHAT TO WEAR ON A MOTORCYCLE

• Your safety helmet, which is required by law, should conform to the British Standards Institution specification 5361 (1976) or 2495HP (1977).
• Wear goggles or a visor, whether part of the helmet or not. The law does not require you to wear them, but if you do, it requires them to conform to BS4110.
• A well-fitting, two-piece windproof suit (jacket and leggings) is convenient for normal use on a motorcycle. Leather gives the best protection from abrasions if you fall from the machine and slide on the road, but it will not keep out the cold and wet for long. For riding long distances or in very wet or cold weather, wear a one-piece waxed cotton stormsuit over your normal riding gear.
• Protect your hands with gloves whatever the weather. In summer wear thin, unlined leather. In cold weather, wear leather lined with silk or lambswool. Alternatively, you can buy heated gloves that have a small wire heating element along each thumb and finger. The elements are powered from the motorcycle battery and are quickly detachable.
• Wear strong, waterproof boots. When you buy them, make sure there is room for extra socks in cold weather. Zip-up boots are easy to fit, but in cold weather they may lose more heat than lace-up or strap-up types; a rear zip may also let in the rain.

If police stop you

The police can stop any motorist and question him – whether or not they suspect him of an offence. But they are not entitled to delay him for longer than he reasonably consents to stay, unless they make an arrest or have some other authority, such as a search warrant.
• You are not obliged to stop if you are flagged down by a civilian, even if he is a plain-clothes police officer, because you have no way of knowing whether he is a policeman or a thief.
• If a uniformed policeman stops you, give your name and address when asked. If you are genuinely in a hurry – rushing to see someone seriously ill in hospital, say – explain your haste and ask to give the details later.
• If the policeman does not agree to this, though, he can insist on taking your name and address on the spot anyway.
• You are not obliged to carry any motoring documents such as a driving licence with you. But if you have them, show them if asked. It will save you time. If you do not show them, or if you do not have them on you, the police can insist in any case that you produce them at a police station within seven days.
• You must obey a policeman if he asks you to move your vehicle. Otherwise you can be prosecuted for obstructing the police – regardless of whether or not you were blocking the road and regardless of whether or not you were legally parked.
• If the police are looking for a stolen car, they may ask questions about your car, such as the registration number or the make of the tyres. Answer the questions as best you can – you will be helping to confirm that the car is yours.
• Be polite and cooperative, but do not answer any questions that you think might incriminate you. You are under no legal obligation to do so.
• If the police say they are going to arrest you, they must give you the reason for the arrest. Do not resist, even if you are innocent, otherwise you could be charged with resisting arrest or obstructing the police. And you could be convicted of that even if the courts find you not guilty of the charge for which you were arrested.
• Make a note of the reason you are given for the arrest – it could help your defence later – and when you reach the police station, ask to contact a solicitor.

If you are asked to take a breath test
• Only an officer in uniform can ask you to take a breath test.
• If you are asked to take the test, you must comply. If you refuse to take the test, you will be arrested and are liable to be fined, jailed or to lose your licence – regardless of whether or not you were over the limit.
• If the breath test proves positive, you will be taken to a police station for further tests.

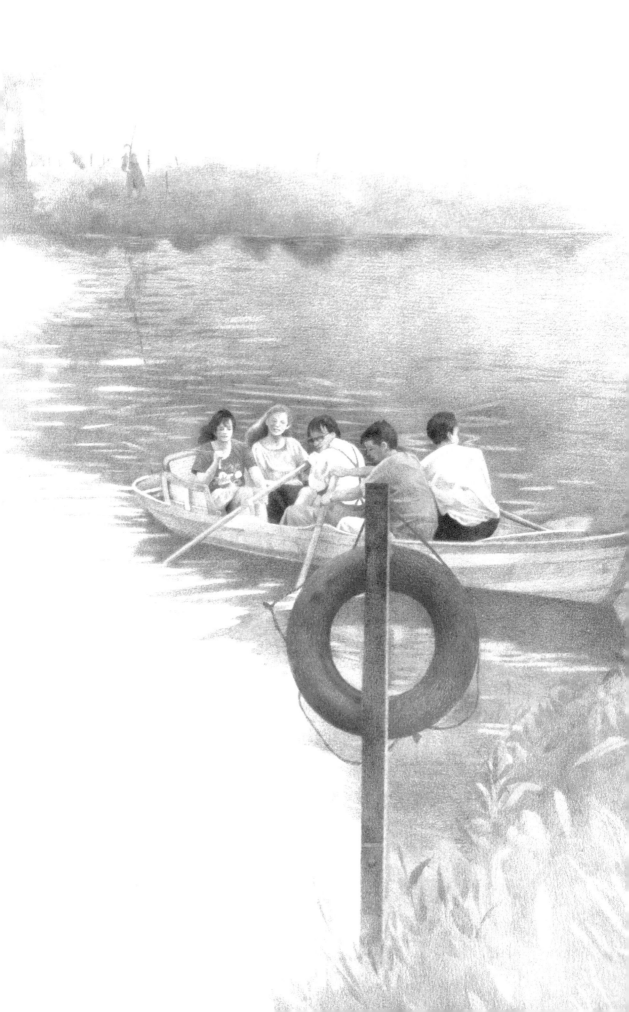

Emergencies in the water

If you fall into a river, lake or canal

Shock and cold are the biggest hazards in British waters. Inland waters are often very cold, and cold quickly saps the strength of even a good swimmer. Concentrate your efforts on getting out as fast as possible.

Deep, steady breathing will help to calm you. Keep your strokes slow and steady as you swim or tread water. Apart from these unavoidable movements, move as little as possible to slow up heat loss.

• As you fall, try to hold your breath, pinch your nose and avoid swallowing water. Once in the water, try to stand up; many canals and rivers are not very deep.

• If the water is too deep for standing and you cannot reach the bank at once, keep afloat by treading water. See if there is any floating debris at hand to cling to. If there is, use it.

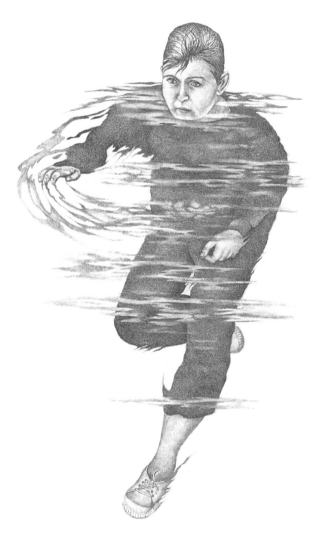

TREADING WATER
One way to stay afloat is to tread water. Pedal with your legs as if you were cycling, and scull your hands back and forth in the water. Leave your clothes on; they help to keep you warm.

• Do not remove any clothing; you need it to keep warm. Air trapped between clothing layers may also aid buoyancy. But do discard heavy shoes and anything heavy in your pockets.

• Remove wellington boots if you are wearing them – they will fill with water and weigh you down. But do not discard them. If you cannot swim, you may be able to use the boots as air cushions to help to keep you afloat; turn them upside down, empty them of water and hold them under your arms.

• If you can swim, make for the nearest suitable bank. If there is a current, do not waste strength fighting it. Go with the flow and swim diagonally across it to work your way to a bank. If the river curves, head for the inside of the curve where the water is likely to be shallower and the current less powerful.

• If you cannot swim, call for help but avoid tiring yourself by screaming frantically. Stay calm and cooperate with anyone who is trying to rescue you. If he has swum to your aid, relax and leave him to take charge. Do not cling to a rescuer, or you may both drown.

• If the side is steep and you find it difficult to get out, look for a handhold while you choose the most likely escape point. Work towards it by edging from one handhold to another. If necessary, remain clinging to a good handhold and breathe deeply in between calls for help.

How to tread water
To keep your head above water without swimming, kick your legs as if you were cycling and continually paddle with your arms to add support and balance.

Alternative methods of kicking are with both legs brought up, knees outwards, and pushed down together (like breast stroke when swimming); or keep your legs straight and use a fast, beating movement of each leg alternately below the knee, as in the crawl stroke.

AVOIDING AN ACCIDENT

About three out of four of the people who drown in Britain each year die in inland waters, not in the sea. Many of the casualties are people who did not intend going into the water – they fell in while fishing, walking, playing, boating or cycling.

• Be cautious when alongside water. Banks are often wet and slippery, or may crumble underfoot.

• Never disregard danger notices. Do not be over-confident because you can swim. Swimming in cold water is very different from swimming in a pool.

• Do not go fishing on your own.

Rescuing someone from a river, lake or canal

Water-safety experts use a four-word rhyme to summarise the safest ways of getting to someone who has fallen in the water. It is: reach, throw, wade, row.

Never get into the water yourself unless there is no alternative and you are a strong swimmer. The shock of the cold water, the possibility of injury from submerged obstacles, and the risk of being pulled under by a panicking victim could put you in danger as well.

Reach

• If the person is not far from reach, give him encouragement while you find something to stretch out to him, such as a stout stick, a rope, or a piece of clothing.
• Lie on your front at the water's edge and anchor yourself in some way if possible. Hook your ankle round a post, or get someone to hold you. Tell the person in the water to grasp the stick or rope. Then haul him in steadily.

Throw

• If the person is out of reach, throw something, such as a life buoy or a child's rubber ring, to help him to keep afloat while you get help.

Wade

• If you decide to wade out to get nearer to the person in trouble, first test the temperature of the water and note any currents.
• Test the bottom with a stick before each step forward. There could be submerged obstacles or sudden changes of depth.

Row

• If a boat is available and you have the skill to manage it, use it to get near to the person, but take care not to get too close. Otherwise the weight of the boat may push him under, knock him out or injure him. To lessen the risk of capsizing the boat as you haul him aboard, bring him in over the stern.
• If no other method is possible and you are a good swimmer, swim out with something buoyant such as a life buoy or tyre, preferably with

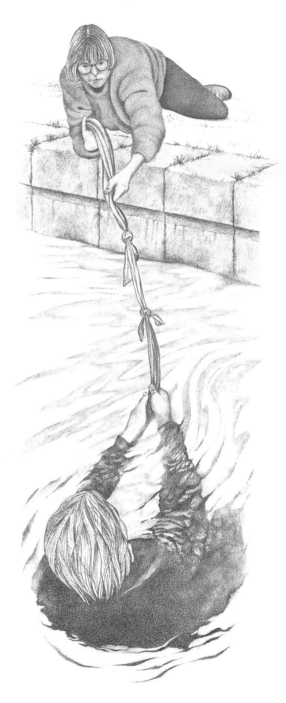

USING AN IMPROVISED ROPE
Reach from the bank using anything to hand. Tie pairs of trousers, jackets, scarves or towels together to make an improvised rope.

IT'S NEVER TOO LATE
Brian Miller's face was blue. He wasn't breathing and his heart was still. The teenager had been that way for 35 minutes. Yet his four friends went on working to revive him, blowing air into his lungs and pumping his chest to force blood round his body.

Brian had been pulled from the Nacimiento River in California after he fell into tumbling rapids and became trapped underwater against rocks. His friends – led by the youngest, 15-year-old Peter Anderson – had been trained to give artificial respiration (the kiss of life) and chest compression. They had gone to work on him at once. And that afternoon, March 29, 1983, not one forgot the teacher's insistence on never giving up.

Five minutes later – 40 minutes after Brian had been dragged seemingly lifeless from the water – his arm twitched, and he started to breathe again. After a spell in hospital, he made a complete recovery.

231

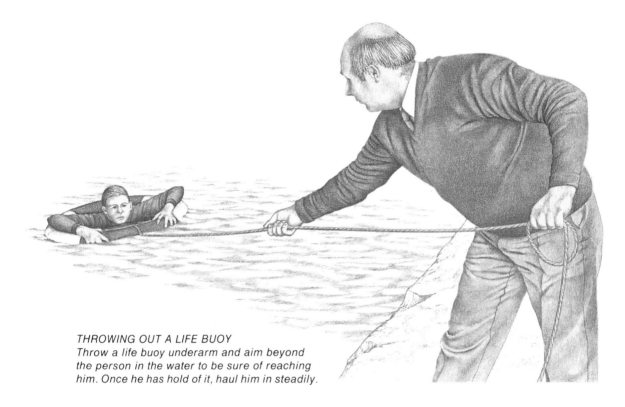

THROWING OUT A LIFE BUOY
Throw a life buoy underarm and aim beyond
the person in the water to be sure of reaching
him. Once he has hold of it, haul him in steadily.

a line attached to the shore (see also *How to deal with a panicking swimmer*, page 240).
• Keep your clothing on to combat the cold, but discard heavy shoes and anything heavy in your pockets before you enter the water.
• Tell the person to hold on to the life buoy, then tow it back. But let go if he attempts to climb on it or to grab hold of you directly.

If someone falls into a canal lock
• Never get into a canal lock to rescue someone while the lock is filling or emptying. The turbulence caused by the open sluices or valves can make it impossible for even the strongest of swimmers to stay afloat.
• If someone falls in in these circumstances, shut the sluices before you go into the water.
• If there is a boat in the lock, ask the skipper to stop his engine.
• Whatever the situation, make sure, before you go in, that there is a ladder for you to get out by; and throw in at least one life buoy with a line made fast to the lock's side.

Getting the victim ashore
• In a river, if there is a strong current, it may be difficult to haul the person straight to the bank. Instead, move downstream and haul him diagonally across the current. If there is a bend, aim for the inside bank where the water will be shallower and the current less powerful.
• If the side is steep, as in a canal lock or some gravel pits, try to tow the person to something he can grasp – a chain, say.

• Lifting a person out where the side is steep is very difficult on your own. Keep him from submerging by tying a line round him under the armpits. Tell him firmly and clearly why you are doing this; the cold and shock may have made him confused.
• Climb out of the water, holding the other end of the line; then tow him to a better landing point, or secure him while you get help.

KEEPING CHILDREN SAFE

• Keep a watchful eye on children playing near water, especially children under five – they can drown within a few minutes even in quite shallow water.
• Rivers, canals and gravel pits are not the only dangers for children. Other dangers include water butts, water tanks and garden pools. Make sure that butts and tanks are covered; where there are toddlers, cover garden ponds with a grid which is strong enough to support a child.
• Be prepared for accidents by getting expert instruction on artificial respiration and life-saving techniques.
• When near waterways, make sure you know where to find life-saving equipment and the nearest telephone.

Cut off by the tide

If you visit a bay, cove or islet and are unable to return because the water has risen and cut you off, it may be more than 12 hours before the tide retreats far enough for you to walk back by the same route. This is the average time between one low water and the next.

• Do not climb any higher than necessary to get out of the reach of the tide, and do not attempt to scale cliffs. If you get stuck, or fall and injure yourself, you will make rescue more difficult.

• When out of the reach of the water, wait for help. Keep a lookout, and wave a shirt or

WARNING FLAGS AT THE BEACH

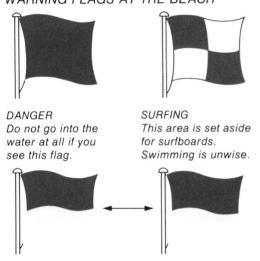

DANGER
Do not go into the water at all if you see this flag.

SURFING
This area is set aside for surfboards. Swimming is unwise.

PATROLLED BEACH
The stretch of beach between two red and yellow flags like this is supervised by lifeguards.

something similar if you see anyone who can help or can call the rescue services.

• If you are marooned on a sandbank, shout and wave for help. If you are some way from the beach, it is usually better to stay where you are and await rescue than to attempt to wade ashore, because there may be currents or deep channels between you and the beach.

SIX HOURS ON A SEASIDE CLIFF

Seven schoolboys and their three instructors huddled together in the dark on two small cliff ledges above the Bristol Channel. All were shivering. Two were wet as well after falling into the water earlier.

The schoolboys – all 11 or 12 years old – were on an adventure course on the North Devon coast and they had set out with their instructors on the morning of March 28, 1983, to explore caves in Combe Martin Bay near Ilfracombe. Rounding a headland near the bay that afternoon, an instructor and one of the boys had fallen into a deep rock pool. By the time the pair had been rescued by the rest of the party, a spring tide had risen, blocking their way out. Trapped, they scrambled up the cliff to the ledges beyond the reach of the waves.

At dusk, the course organisers raised the alarm and at about 10pm the group were spotted by the Ilfracombe lifeboat. They were rescued – cold but unhurt – after six hours on the cliff. A course organiser said later: 'The party just got a bit behind schedule.'

But rescue experts point out that even such a small detail can matter. Coupled with the afternoon rock pool accident, the delay was enough to put ten lives at risk.

Emergencies in the water

KEEPING ABOVE THE WAVES

An average of about one person a day in Britain has to be rescued by coastguards after being cut off by the tide. Each year, another 250 or so people have to be rescued from cliffs, where many take refuge after being cut off. The highest tides in Britain occur in estuaries. On the River Severn around Avonmouth and Cardiff, for example, the water can rise 40-50ft (13-15m). For most of Britain, the average distance between high and low water is about 13-16ft (3-4m).

Most resorts have two tides a day, with each high water about 12 hours 25 minutes after the one before. Southampton and the Solent, however, have four tides a day – a peculiarity caused by the sheltering effect of the Isle of Wight. Generally, high tide occurs

50 minutes later each day. The highest tides are spring tides, which occur every two weeks at about the time of a new moon or full moon. The lowest tides (neap tides) occur when the moon is half full – a week either side of a full moon.

• To avoid the risk of getting cut off, check the times of high tide before setting out. The time is often displayed on the beach; if not, look in a local newspaper or check with a tourist office.

• Use the tide table to estimate when the rising water will reach any part of your route off the beach. Allow a generous safety margin on top of your estimate. Weather conditions, currents and land configuration can all affect the predicted time.

If you get into difficulties while swimming

Cramp, exhaustion and strong currents are the commonest problems facing swimmers. Cramp and exhaustion can both be caused by cold.

If you get cramp
- Stop swimming. Turn on your back and float.
- Stretch the cramped muscle. If the cramp is at the front of your leg, point your toes and straighten the leg. If the cramp is in your calf or the back of your thigh, turn your toes upwards and straighten the leg. Use your hands if necessary to pull your foot upwards.
- When the cramp goes, swim to shore using a different stroke. If you must use the same stroke, keep alert in case the cramp returns.

If you become exhausted
- Swim ashore as soon as you begin to feel cold or tired. If you are too far out, or are too exhausted to reach the shore at once, turn on your back and float to conserve your strength.
- Raise one arm, keep it straight, and move it from side to side as a distress signal.
- When someone comes to help you, relax and let him take control. Do not try to cling to him.
- If nobody comes, float until you feel better, then make for the shore.

Caught in a current
- Do not try to swim against a current.
- If you are swimming in a river, swim diagonally across it to land farther downstream. If the river bends, aim for the bank on the inside edge. The current will be at its weakest there.
- On the coast, waves piling into the beach can trap water behind offshore sandbanks. The sandbanks may be completely submerged at some or all stages of the tide. Gaps in the sandbanks then become outlets for the water, generating rip tides which may be invisible from the beach. Rip tides can flow out to sea at 4-5mph (6-8km/h) – impossible to swim against. But they usually dissipate within a short distance of the gap.
- If you are caught in a rip tide, let the current take you, then strike vigorously across it parallel to the beach. Once you are free of the current, turn back towards the beach.

If you get caught in waterweeds
- Unless you are carrying a knife with which to hack away weeds, try to kick yourself free.
- If kicking fails, try to roll the weeds from your limbs as if rolling down a sock. Duck your head under the water when you do this so that you can see what you are doing.
- Once free of the weeds, swim with a shallow kick until you are clear of them.

How cold water affects a swimmer
When you plunge into cold water, the first few seconds are taken up by huge, involuntary gasps (doctors call this hyperventilation), followed by anything up to several minutes of increased blood pressure and faster heartbeats as your body responds to the shock. At this time,

---

DO'S AND DON'TS OF SAFE SWIMMING

The highest proportion of drownings in Britain – more than one-third – occurs among men aged between 15 and 35, who are often the strongest swimmers. They die usually because they have ignored the safety rules recommended by experts.
- Never swim on an empty stomach or just after a heavy meal. Doing either can cause painful and disabling cramp. Allow at least an hour for your meal to digest.
- Test the water temperature before you get in. Do not swim if it is too cold.
- Always swim in a group, not by yourself.
- Look out for red flags or markers. They indicate areas unsafe for swimming. Flags or markers in other colours denote patrolled areas, surfing areas and so on (see *Warning flags at the beach*, page 233).
- Do not swim in water-filled gravel or sand pits, or in flooded quarries. They are cold and often deep with steeply shelving sides that may be impossible to climb out of. There may also be submerged obstacles.

- Never dive into water unless you are sure that the water is deep enough – at least 10ft (3m) – and free from underwater hazards such as weeds, rocks or other obstacles. Climb down or wade in if you can, but if you have to jump, do so feet first.
- Swim parallel to the shore and keep within easy reach of standing depth. Unless you are a strong swimmer, do not go out of your depth at sea at all. Wade out, then swim back.
- Watch for underwater hazards. Their presence is sometimes, but not always, indicated by visible breaks in the usual pattern of waves or currents.
- Keep an eye on a shore mark so that you can see if you are being carried out to sea or along the beach. Do not swim out with a current. You may not be able to swim back.
- Do not swim in the sea using inflatable swimming aids. You may be carried out of your depth without realising it – and be unable to get back.

there is a high risk of breathing water into your lungs and drowning. Hyperventilation also reduces the amount of carbon dioxide in the blood, and this can lead to cramp.

Loss of body heat is very fast in water. Even with a water temperature of around 20°C (68°F) it can exceed the body's capacity to produce heat. The body reacts to cold-water immersion by forming a cold outer shell to insulate the inner core, and the consequent cooling of muscles and nerves in the arms, legs and outer trunk weakens movement and reduces coordination. Even a good swimmer may drown quickly under these circumstances, and in water below 10°C (50°F), swimming ability commonly fails in less than 15 minutes.

The length of time you can hold your breath underwater is also severely affected by the tem-

perature. In cold water it is likely to be only one-third as long as in a heated swimming pool; in water below 15°C (60°F) the average time is about 15-25 seconds.

In an indoor swimming pool the water temperature is generally between 26 and 29°C (80 and 84°F), but the sea around Britain's coasts averages only 7-10°C (45-50°F) in the south, with short-lived summer temperatures of 15°C (60°F). In the north-east it is generally about 3°C (5°F) lower. Inland waters such as rivers, lakes and streams are even colder.

If you have to swim in cold water, it is best to get in gradually, keeping your head well above water until the initial shock is over, and to try to control your breathing consciously. Wear a wetsuit as well, if possible. It will lessen the effects of the cold on your body.

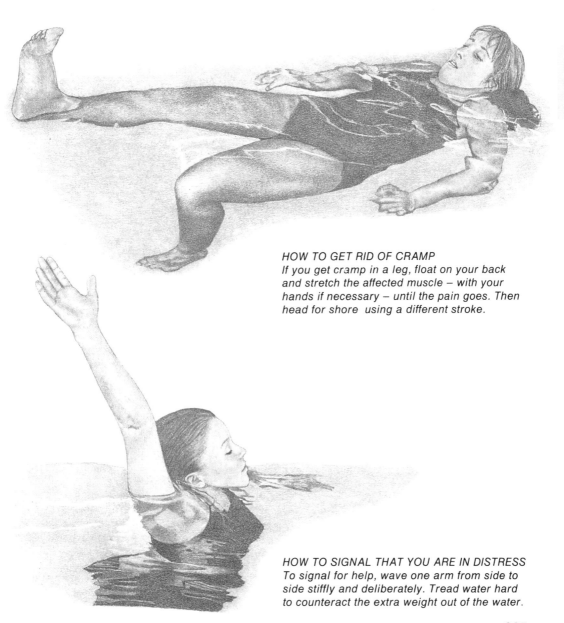

Emergencies in the water

HOW TO GET RID OF CRAMP
If you get cramp in a leg, float on your back and stretch the affected muscle – with your hands if necessary – until the pain goes. Then head for shore using a different stroke.

HOW TO SIGNAL THAT YOU ARE IN DISTRESS
To signal for help, wave one arm from side to side stiffly and deliberately. Tread water hard to counteract the extra weight out of the water.

Getting out of trouble in surf

The continuous pounding of heavy breakers soon saps the energy of an inexperienced swimmer, and can be hazardous even for a strong and proficient swimmer. Do not be tempted to swim in heavy surf if your swimming ability and experience do not go beyond swimming in a pool or in sheltered water.

How to swim ashore through surf

• Use the waves to get ashore. Between waves rest and wait, then swim vigorously shorewards as each wave crest approaches and keep kicking to get the maximum ride forward.
• To increase the forward motion, use a technique known as bodysurfing. Just as the wave catches you, stiffen your body. Hold your head up with chin thrust forward. Either hold your arms straight in front of your head, or back beneath your body, to make your body into a living surfboard.
• When the wave has gone past, tread water, and watch over your shoulder for the next wave.
• Once you are able to stand up, brace yourself against the strong pull of the water as it flows backwards between the waves. If necessary, crouch and hold onto the bottom.

How to get out onto rocks

• Time your landing so that you go ashore just behind the crest of a wave, to avoid being hurled against the rocks.
• Quickly get a good handhold on a rock so that you are not pulled back into the water as the wave falls back.

BODYSURFING TO GET ASHORE

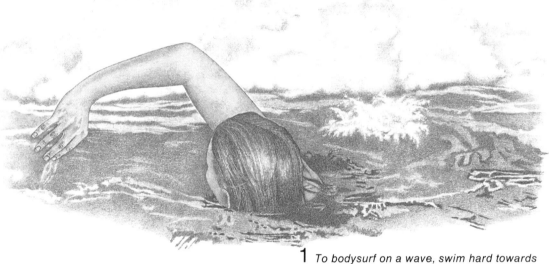

1 *To bodysurf on a wave, swim hard towards the shore as the wave crest approaches. Watch it over your shoulder as you go.*

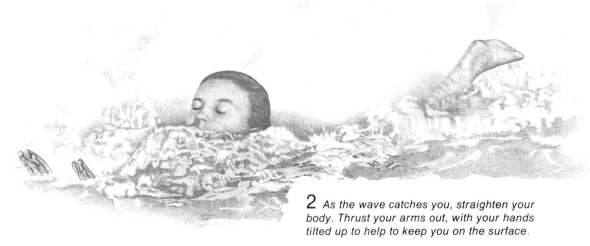

2 *As the wave catches you, straighten your body. Thrust your arms out, with your hands tilted up to help to keep you on the surface.*

- Hold on while the wave recedes.
- Scramble up the rocks as quickly as you can before the next wave reaches you.

How to cope with turbulent breakers

Waves become turbulent and thus difficult to swim through only after they get close to the shore and break. Before then, the easiest way to swim seawards past a wave – or to hold your position while the wave passes you – is to jump, float or swim over its crest.

Once the wave has broken, however, the water forms a turbulent tube, rolling over and over as it foams towards the beach.

Any swimmer caught in this turbulence can be tumbled helplessly, losing his sense of up and down, being unable to breathe, and risk-ing – in shallow water – being hurled against the bottom and stunned.

A wave's turbulence usually affects only the upper layers of the water. So a swimmer who wants to get past the wave without being caught in the turbulence needs to get below it.

- As the wave approaches, dive well below the surface. The heavier the surf, the deeper you will need to dive.
- If necessary, dive right to the seabed and hold on by digging your hands into the sand while the wave passes overhead. It is often possible to feel the turbulent water skim your back as it passes.
- When the wave has gone by, gather your legs beneath you and push back to the surface. Watch for the next wave as soon as you emerge.

SWIMMING OUT THROUGH LARGE WAVES

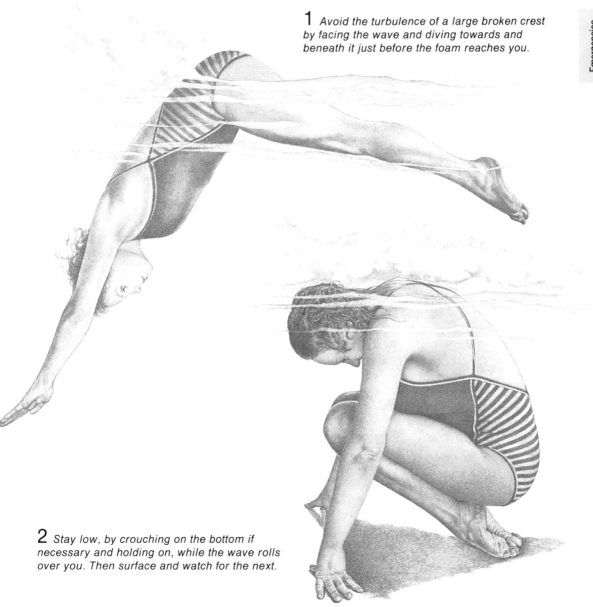

1 *Avoid the turbulence of a large broken crest by facing the wave and diving towards and beneath it just before the foam reaches you.*

2 *Stay low, by crouching on the bottom if necessary and holding on, while the wave rolls over you. Then surface and watch for the next.*

Snorkelling: what to do if things go wrong

With a face mask, a breathing tube (snorkel) and a pair of flippers, a swimmer can breathe with his face below the surface and so watch the underwater world without interruption. But difficulties can arise, particularly in open water. All need prompt, calm action.

If water fills the tube

An unexpected wave or a careless dip of the head can send water down the breathing tube without warning.

- If this happens, do not breathe in. Make sure that the end of the tube is above water.

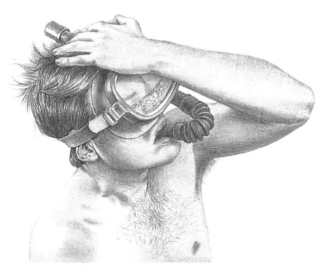

HOW TO CLEAR THE MASK UNDERWATER
Tilt your head back, hold the top of the mask and breathe out slowly through your nose. The air will force the water out of the bottom.

- Tilt your head up so that water can flow more easily from the tube.
- Blow out forcefully to expel the water.

If water leaks into the mask

- On the surface, one easy way to clear water from a mask is to lift your head above the water and pull the mask away from your face with your hands to drain it. Tread water with your legs while you do this.
- To clear the mask while you are still below the surface – during a dive, say – tilt your head well back until you are looking upwards towards the surface.
- Press the top of the mask firmly against your forehead.
- Breathe out slowly through your nose. This will fill the mask with air and force water out of the bottom. Stop breathing out as soon as the mask is clear, to retain the maximum amount of air in your lungs.

How good a swimmer you need to be

Because of the extra swimming ability needed to go snorkelling in safety, the British Sub-Aqua Club recommends that no one should take up the sport until he or she can:

- Swim 200m (220yds) freestyle (except backstroke) without a stop.
- Swim 100m (110yds) backstroke.
- Swim 50m (55yds) freestyle wearing a 10lb (4.5kg) weight belt.
- Float on his back for five minutes, using hands and legs if desired.
- Tread water with his hands above water and using legs alone for one minute.
- Recover six objects in succession from the deep end of a swimming pool with only one dive for each object.

CHOOSING THE RIGHT EQUIPMENT

- Ask if the snorkel you buy meets the safety requirements of British Standard BS4532. Equipment made by a reputable manufacturer normally does, although it may not be so marked. Cheap equipment often does not.
- The best tube is a simple J shape, 12-14in (300-350mm) long with an internal diameter of 0.6-0.8in (15-20mm). Longer or narrower tubes are harder to breathe through. Do not buy a tube with air valves – these often look like table-tennis balls. If a valve jams it can cut off the air supply.
- The mask should be fitted with toughened safety glass – not Perspex, which is less strong and mists up more easily.
- The mask should cover nose and eyes only and should have a 'compensator' – a shaped nose-piece. It allows you to hold your nose through the mask, if necessary, and thus to clear your ears during a dive.
- Test that the mask fits by holding it against your face without putting on the straps. Breathe in through your nose. A well-fitting mask will stick to your face.
- The breathing tube should be separate from the mask. A built-in tube is dangerous because it can let water into the mask. It is also more difficult to clear.
- If you plan to snorkel in places where there could be weeds underwater, buy a diver's knife with a serrated edge (see *If you get into difficulties while swimming*, page 234).
- Buy buoyant flippers. They are less easily lost in the water.

Menaced by a shark

Each year there are about 50 shark attacks on humans around the world. Most of the attacks take place in tropical waters. But three out of five of the victims survive.

Two of the largest species of shark – the basking shark, which grows as long as 45ft (14m), and the gigantic whale shark, reputed to reach up to 60ft (18m) – are harmless plankton-feeders. All other shark species, however – and there are some 250 of them around the world – should be treated as dangerous.

If you see a shark near someone else

• Call a warning to anyone in the water if you spot a shark nearby.
• Make a noise – it may frighten the shark away. If you are in a boat, start the engine or bang on the hull.
• Help those in the water to get ashore or aboard a boat as quickly as possible.

If you are in the water

• Do not try to swim away fast if a shark approaches you. You cannot outswim a shark, and the frantic movement may simply add to the danger by attracting its attention.
• If you are spear-fishing, release at once any fish you have speared. Blood in the water tends to attract sharks.
• Make a noise in an attempt to frighten the shark away. Shout into the water, for example, or beat on diving tanks if you have them.
• Swim slowly back to the boat or to the shore. Swim backwards if necessary. Keep facing the shark all the time as you go, preferably under-water, to reduce the chances of being attacked from beneath or behind.
• A shark attack is often preceded by a nudge. If this happens, strike the shark as hard as you can with your fists, feet or any object to hand in order to startle it and drive it off.

LESSENING THE CHANCES OF AN ATTACK

Along Britain's coasts there is little danger of swimmers or skin divers being attacked by sharks, although the blue shark – which is dangerous to man – migrates from the Atlantic to Britain's south-west coast in summer. Usually, however, it keeps to deep water, far from beaches.

Most Continental waters are also reasonably safe from sharks, but swimmers and divers in the Adriatic or Aegean seas – off the coast of Italy and off Yugoslavia and Greece – should keep a watch for them.

Most attacks occur in or near the tropics, in water warmer than 21°C (70°F). The most dangerous places include New Zealand, eastern Australia, South Africa, the West Indies, Mexico, and the coasts of California and Florida in the USA.

Wreck survivors in warm waters on the open ocean are also at risk.

Sharks are unpredictable, and there is no reliable way of telling when they will, or will not, attack. Nevertheless, shark experts do recommend some ways of reducing the risk of an attack.

• In areas where there may be sharks, keep away from dark and murky water; sharks seem particularly adept at detecting prey in these conditions.
• Do not swim too far from shore or near deep channels. Sharks rarely swim into water that is shallow enough for a man to wade in.
• Do not swim at dusk or at night, when sharks are more likely to be looking for food.
• Do not swim or skin dive alone. Having another person close by helps you to keep an all-round lookout, and may deter a shark.
• Do not go into the water if you have a cut or scratch. Blood may attract a shark.
• Do not carry captured fish if you are spear-fishing. Put them in a boat.
• Where there are known to be sharks, make and carry what the French oceanographer Jacques-Yves Cousteau calls a shark billy – a stout stick about as thick as a broom handle and 3ft (1m) long, with a loop for the wrist at one end and a circle of small nails, points outward, at the other end.
• Jab the billy firmly into the snout of any shark that comes within reach. The nail points prevent the stick sliding off the shark's skin and help to keep him away from your body without wounding or angering him. A shark billy rarely drives a shark off completely, however; it only keeps it at bay.
• If you see sharks in the area where you are swimming or skin diving and you are close to shore or a boat, leave the water as quickly as possible.
• But remember that you are in most danger as you leave the water. For this reason, try to time your exit so that any shark is well out of striking range when you climb out.
• Clothing or a diver's wetsuit appears to give some protection from sharks. A naked person seems to be more liable to attack than a clothed one.
• Be careful if you have a partial suntan, with white areas exposed while swimming. Areas of light and shade also seem to attract sharks and make an attack more likely.

How to deal with a panicking swimmer

A person in difficulties in the water is often panic-stricken and will cling with the strength of desperation to anything that offers a safe hold – including someone trying to help him. Never swim to the aid of a swimmer in distress if there is any other way of reaching him – from the shore, say, or from a boat (see *Rescuing someone from a river, lake or canal*, page 231).

Even trained life savers are taught to go into the water only as a last resort. An untrained rescuer runs a still greater risk of losing his own life in the attempt to save another's.

• If you decide that you have to swim to the rescue, try to stay out of the swimmer's reach. If, however, you need to get close to him – because he does not respond to your instructions, say – and he suddenly tries to grab you,

avoid his grasp by reversing immediately into backstroke and swimming vigorously out of his reach.

• Once at a safe distance, offer him one end of a piece of clothing, a towel or one side of a lifebuoy and tell him to hold on to that. Tow him to the shore by holding the other end.

• If he tries to pull himself towards you, let go of your end and swim out of his reach.

• If you have no choice but to make contact with the swimmer, approach him from behind.

• Grasp him firmly and support him in the water. Calm him down by talking, and tow him to shore using one of the techniques shown on the pages overleaf.

• Keep an eye on him as you swim and keep talking, if you can, to calm him.

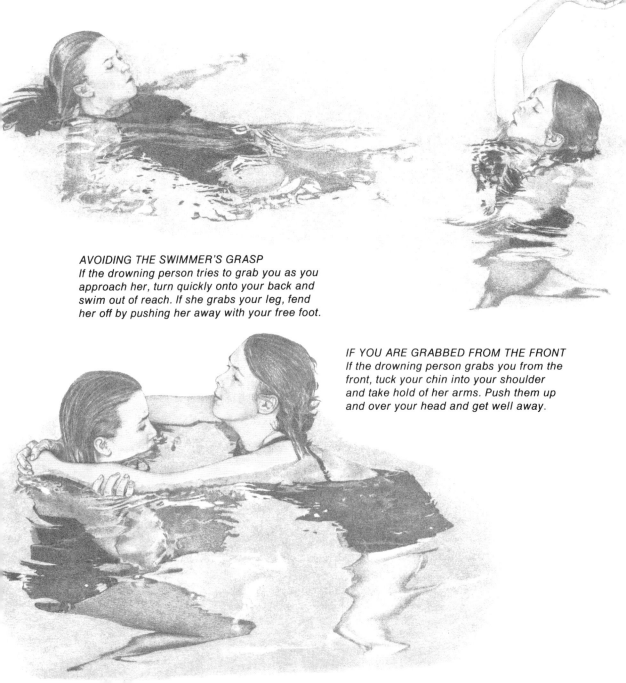

AVOIDING THE SWIMMER'S GRASP
If the drowning person tries to grab you as you approach her, turn quickly onto your back and swim out of reach. If she grabs your leg, fend her off by pushing her away with your free foot.

IF YOU ARE GRABBED FROM THE FRONT
If the drowning person grabs you from the front, tuck your chin into your shoulder and take hold of her arms. Push them up and over your head and get well away.

Breaking a hold
- If a panicking swimmer grabs you, break free at once. If he grasps your leg, push it down into the water and thrust against his shoulder with your free foot.
- If he clutches you from the front round your head and shoulders, tuck your chin down into your shoulder, grasp him under the arms and push him up and away.
- If he grasps you from behind round your head and shoulders, lower your chin to protect your throat. Then grasp him by the wrist of his uppermost arm and pull down, at the same time pushing up his elbow with your other hand. In this way you both break his clutch and keep hold of him.
- As a last resort, take a deep breath and allow yourself to be pushed underwater. The aim of most panicking swimmers is to stay on the surface. Swim downwards until he lets go, then return to the surface out of his reach and grab him from behind.

Helping an unconscious or panicky person
- Tow an unconscious person by the chin from behind. Use a side stroke and keep your towing arm straight so that your legs are clear of the victim and you can look forwards regularly to see where you are going. Make sure you keep his face out of the water.
- If he is conscious but panic-stricken and needs firm control, grasp him under the chin, draw him close (ear to ear) and clamp his shoulder firmly with your elbow. If necessary,

IF YOU ARE GRABBED FROM BEHIND

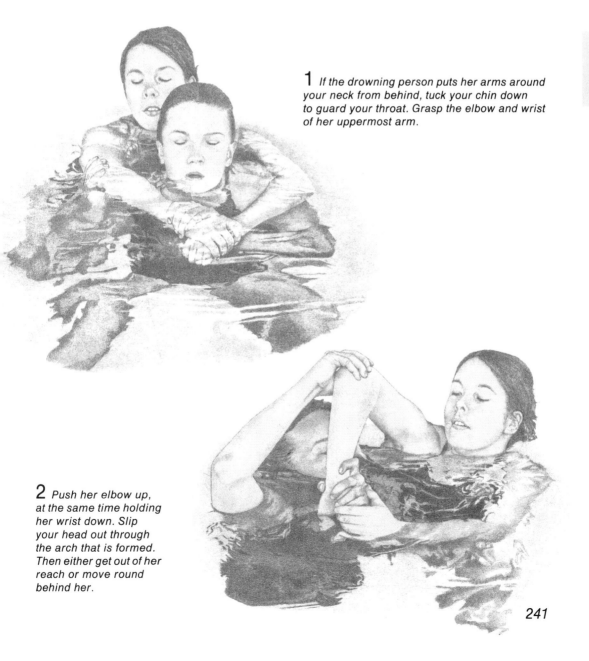

1 *If the drowning person puts her arms around your neck from behind, tuck your chin down to guard your throat. Grasp the elbow and wrist of her uppermost arm.*

2 *Push her elbow up, at the same time holding her wrist down. Slip your head out through the arch that is formed. Then either get out of her reach or move round behind her.*

restrain him with your other arm as well. Tell him to stop struggling. Keep talking to him to try to keep him calm while you swim.
• In rough water, it is better to tow the person by holding him across the chest. This enables you to swim on your side, breathe more easily, and see where you are going.

Helping a swimmer with cramp
• Support him in the water while he tries to relieve the cramp by stretching the muscles.
• If the cramp does not go, tell him to lie on his back and tow him ashore using one of the life-saving techniques shown here.
• Once ashore, wrap him in a coat, towel or blanket. Stretch the affected muscle gently and massage it to relieve the cramp.

SAFETY FIRST

The central rules for a rescuer – recommended by the Royal Life Saving Society – are to stay out of the water if you can, and to avoid making direct physical contact with the victim if you can.

Specialised training in all the techniques shown here, and others, is available through swimming clubs or from the Royal Life Saving Society at Mountbatten House, Studley, Warwickshire B80 7NN; telephone Studley (0527) 853943.

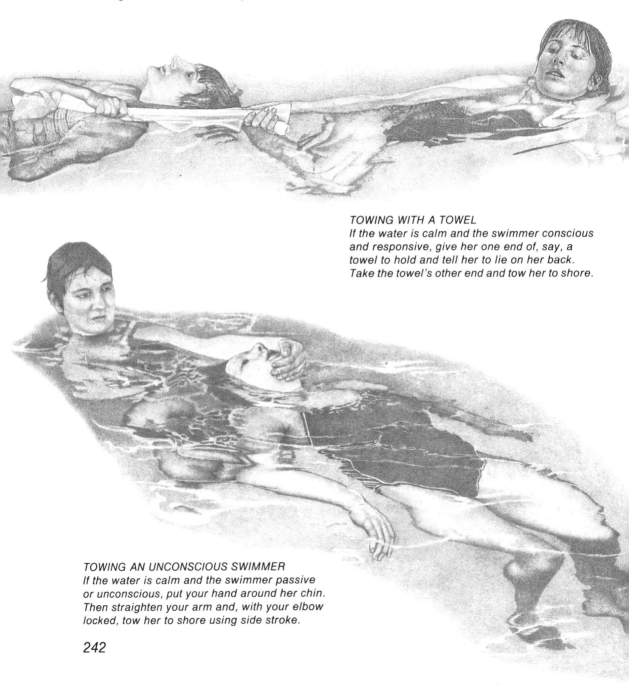

TOWING WITH A TOWEL
If the water is calm and the swimmer conscious and responsive, give her one end of, say, a towel to hold and tell her to lie on her back. Take the towel's other end and tow her to shore.

TOWING AN UNCONSCIOUS SWIMMER
If the water is calm and the swimmer passive or unconscious, put your hand around her chin. Then straighten your arm and, with your elbow locked, tow her to shore using side stroke.

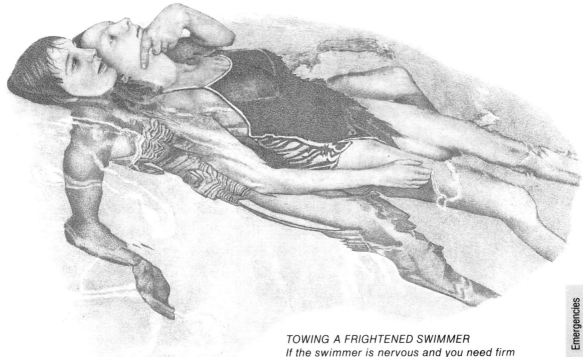

TOWING A FRIGHTENED SWIMMER
*If the swimmer is nervous and you need firm
control, take her by the chin and pull her, face
upwards, until her head is by yours. Grip her
shoulder with your elbow and make for shore.*

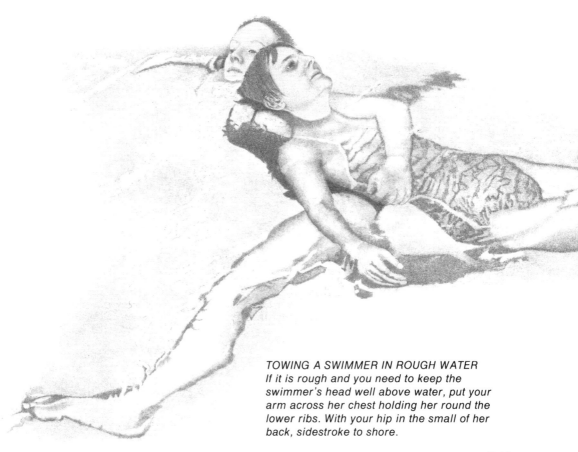

TOWING A SWIMMER IN ROUGH WATER
*If it is rough and you need to keep the
swimmer's head well above water, put your
arm across her chest holding her round the
lower ribs. With your hip in the small of her
back, sidestroke to shore.*

If you fall through thin ice

Inland waters in Britain do sometimes freeze solidly enough to be used safely as skating rinks. The country's changeable island climate, however, means that it is not possible to predict with any certainty when any particular patch of water will freeze up to this degree, nor how long it will stay solid.

The biggest danger for anyone who goes onto a frozen patch of water is not an inability to swim; clothes contain enough air, initially at least, to help to keep afloat anyone who falls in. The biggest peril is the shock of the cold water, which can paralyse the muscles and render even the strongest of swimmers helpless in a matter of a few minutes.

- Do not wait to be rescued. Get yourself out if you can. Cold will quickly sap your strength.
- Keep afloat by treading water – kick your legs as if you were cycling and continually paddle with your arms. Breathe deeply and slowly. It helps to prevent panic.
- Break the ice around you – moving generally towards the bank – until you find some that seems strong enough to hold you.
- Extend your arms forward onto the stronger ice and kick your legs behind you to bring your body up so that it is almost level.
- Keep kicking to drive your body forward, and pull at the same time until you are out of the water. If the ice cracks under you, keep flat and keep edging forward.
- When you reach ice that is firm enough to take your weight, roll away from the broken area towards the bank.
- Once safely on firm ground make for shelter and warmth. Keep moving to stay warm. If dry clothes are available, put them on. Otherwise, keep your wet clothes on until you reach somewhere warm.

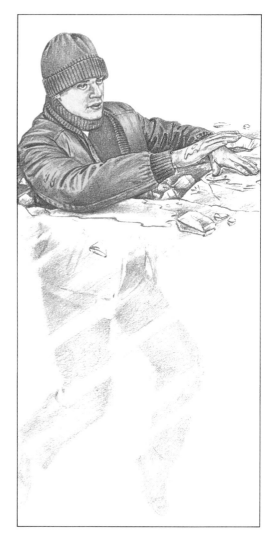

TREADING WATER TO KEEP AFLOAT
If you cannot get out at once, tread water to keep your head and neck out of the water, and to stop yourself getting trapped under the ice.

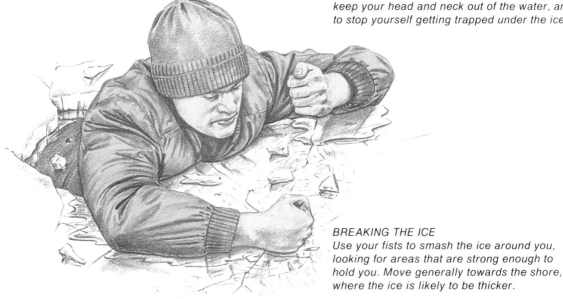

BREAKING THE ICE
Use your fists to smash the ice around you, looking for areas that are strong enough to hold you. Move generally towards the shore, where the ice is likely to be thicker.

EDGING YOUR WAY TO SAFETY

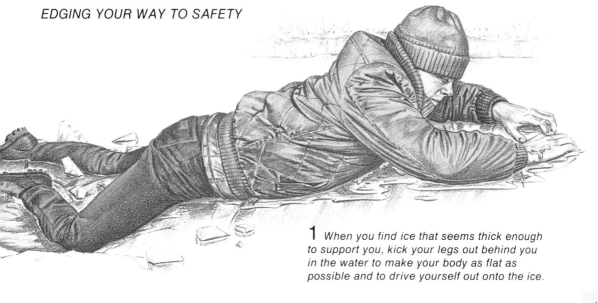

1 *When you find ice that seems thick enough to support you, kick your legs out behind you in the water to make your body as flat as possible and to drive yourself out onto the ice.*

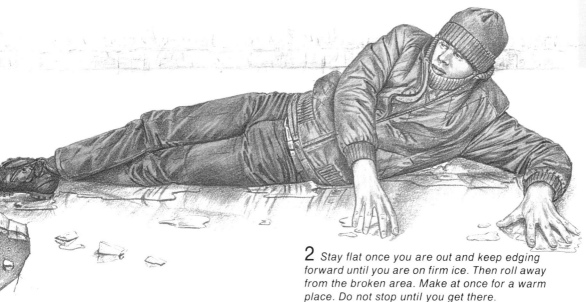

2 *Stay flat once you are out and keep edging forward until you are on firm ice. Then roll away from the broken area. Make at once for a warm place. Do not stop until you get there.*

Emergencies in the water

DANGER – THIN ICE

• Never venture onto ice without first testing its strength. Find a firm handhold on the bank while you stamp with one foot at the edge in several places. Throw the largest stone you can find into the middle of the water area.

• Ice over shallow water is usually the safest. Ice over flowing water or underwater vegetation is weaker because the water is relatively warmer.

• Ice is not uniformly thick over a whole stretch of water. It gets thinner towards the centre. Ice also weakens as the sun's warmth builds up during the morning and early afternoon, and if the weather gets warmer.

• Never allow children onto ice without the supervision of a responsible adult. Do not allow a child onto any ice if the water below is deeper than the height of the child's waist.

• Make sure that rescue equipment is available – a light ladder, say, a strong rope, or a pole with a looped line attached. Take it with you if necessary.

245

If someone falls through the ice

A person who falls through ice into a pond or river – even someone who is ordinarily a competent swimmer – can drown within minutes. Even if the person can keep a head above water, the shock affects breathing and the cold can paralyse the limbs (see *Drowning – the perils of the cold*, page 251). For rescuers, therefore, the priority is speed.

Helping a conscious victim

• Stay off the ice yourself unless there is no other way of reaching the victim and there is someone else to pull you back if you fall in.

• Slide a stick, with a rope attached, across the ice towards the victim. If necessary, make a rope from sweaters or scarves.

• If you cannot reach the victim from the shore, lie flat on the ice so that your weight is widely distributed.

• Slide forward cautiously, pushing the stick in front of you, until it is within the victim's reach. Do not go any farther than absolutely necessary. Ice generally gets thinner towards the centre of a river or pond.

• Tell the victim to stretch her arms forward on top of the ice and kick back to keep her body as level in the water as possible. This will lessen

the chance of her being pulled under the ice by any current, and make it easier for her to get out onto the ice.

• Tell her to grasp the stick or rope with one hand and break the ice in front with the other until the ice is strong enough to support her. Pull on the other end to help her haul herself out of the water.

• Tell her to kick her legs as if she were swimming and to slide forward onto the ice. Do not hold her directly or let her hold you, unless you are well anchored. Otherwise she could pull you into the water.

• Once she is on the ice, tell her to lie flat. Pull her in.

• Another way to help a conscious victim is to stretch a rope from bank to bank – of a pond, say – across the spot where he or she has fallen in. Tell her to grab hold of the rope and haul herself in, hand over hand.

Forming a human chain

• If there are several people to help and there is no other way to reach the victim, form a human chain.

• The first person should lie flat on the ice and slide towards the victim. The next should lie flat

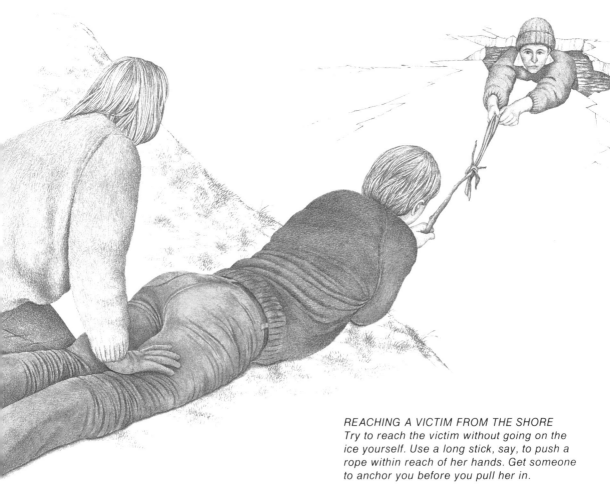

REACHING A VICTIM FROM THE SHORE
Try to reach the victim without going on the ice yourself. Use a long stick, say, to push a rope within reach of her hands. Get someone to anchor you before you pull her in.

and hold the ankles of the person in front, and so on until the chain is long enough to reach from a safe position on shore to the victim.

Using a ladder on ice

• The easiest way to rescue somebody who has fallen through ice is by using a light ladder.
• Lie on the ice with the ladder flat in front of you and push it towards the victim.
• Tell the victim to pull herself onto the ladder and lie flat. Pull the ladder back.

If the victim is too weak to hold on to a rope

• To help a weakening victim, attach a looped rope to the end of a pole or light ladder.
• Slide the pole across the ice until the loop is within reach of the person in the water. Tell her to put the loop over her head and shoulders and under her arms. Then pull her in.
• If you cannot pull her in, tie the other end of the rope to a tree or post on the bank to support her in the water while you get help.
• If you have no rope or pole, slide over the ice at full length, grab the victim's arms or clothing and try to pull her out onto the ice.
• If this is impossible, hold her so that she does not slip beneath the water. Shout for help.

Once back on shore

• As soon as the victim is out of danger, check that she is breathing. If not, begin artificial respiration at once (see page 50).
• If the victim is breathing, wrap dry clothes or blankets over her own wet clothes and move her to a warm sheltered place. If she is unconscious, put her in the recovery position (see page 136) and move her on a stretcher.
• Once in shelter, take off her wet clothes and wrap her in any dry clothes, blankets or a sleeping bag (see *Hypothermia*, page 108).

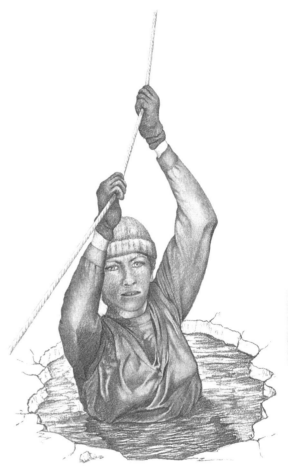

HAULING ON A ROPE OVERHEAD
On a narrow stretch of ice, hang a rope from bank to bank. Tell the victim to haul herself hand over hand to the bank, if necessary breaking the ice with her feet as she goes.

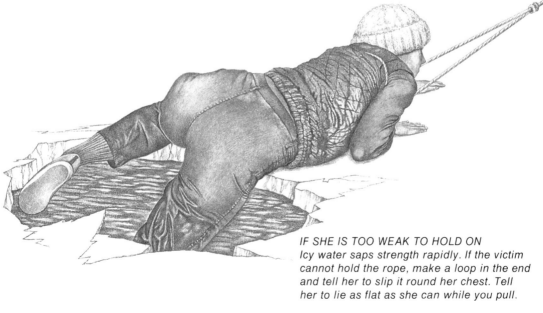

IF SHE IS TOO WEAK TO HOLD ON
Icy water saps strength rapidly. If the victim cannot hold the rope, make a loop in the end and tell her to slip it round her chest. Tell her to lie as flat as she can while you pull.

Emergencies in the water

If you fall overboard

Falling into water unexpectedly can cause shock (see page 120). Cold water also saps the strength quickly, leading to loss of coordination, confusion and exhaustion.

• Call out to alert other crew members as soon as you feel yourself start to fall.

• Once in the water, inflate your life jacket (unless it is a permanently buoyant type). It will automatically bring you back to the surface.

• If you are wearing a life jacket, keep warm by adopting a foetal position with your knees drawn up to your chest (see picture, page 276).

• Raise one arm so that you can be seen from the boat more easily. Even though you may well lose sight of the boat before it turns – particularly in rough water or at sea – other crew members will be able to pinpoint your position more easily by your arm.

• If you are not wearing a life jacket, remove heavy boots or shoes and any heavy objects from your pockets, but do not remove clothing, especially in cold water. Even soaked through, it will help to conserve vital body heat.

• Tread water if necessary to stay afloat, but otherwise conserve heat by moving as little as possible. Float on your back if you can.

• Do not try to swim after the boat whether or not you are wearing a life jacket. You will make little progress wearing clothes, and the effort will quickly exhaust you.

Ways of keeping afloat without a life jacket

• In cold water, continue to float on your back if you can, or tread water while you are waiting for the boat to return. Breathe slowly and move as little as possible; both will help to conserve energy and body heat.

• In warm water, use the drownproofing technique (see box, opposite).

• Alternatively, in warm water use a piece of clothing to construct a makeshift float. Remove trousers or slacks and knot each ankle. Hold the waistband open behind your head, the legs pointing away from you, then whip the trousers over your head into the water in front of you. Air will be trapped in the trouser legs.

• Pull the waistband down against your chest, and float in the crotch, with the legs under your arms like a child's water wings.

• A polo-neck sweater can be used in much the same way. Remove it by bunching it up under your arms, then pulling it over your head in one movement.

• Knot the neck and both wrists, and flick it over your head to fill it with air. Hold the sweater open waist-down underwater with the sleeves under your arms and the knotted neck against your chest.

Getting into a life buoy

• If someone on board throws you a ring life buoy, do not duck dive and try to come up inside it. Putting your head underwater will only make you colder and tire you more quickly. Instead, stay on the surface.

• Grasp the life buoy, bend your head and lift its near edge over your head and one arm.

• Work your other arm through the life buoy so that it supports you under both armpits and across your chest.

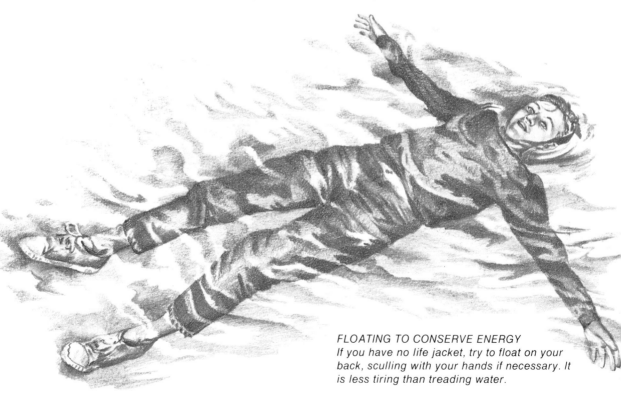

FLOATING TO CONSERVE ENERGY
If you have no life jacket, try to float on your back, sculling with your hands if necessary. It is less tiring than treading water.

HOW TO IMPROVISE A FLOAT

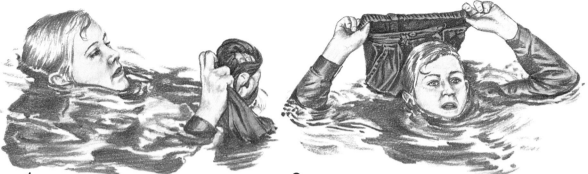

1 *Clothing can be used to make an improvised float. To make one out of a pair of trousers, take them off and tie a knot in each ankle.*

2 *Hold the trousers behind your head with the waistband open, then whip them forwards and down so that you trap air in the trouser legs.*

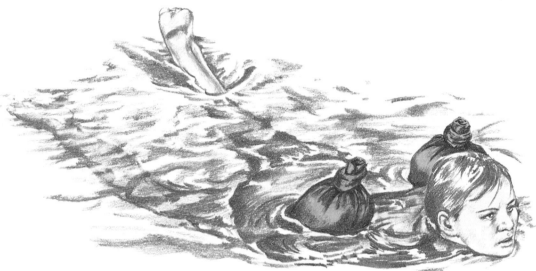

3 *Tuck the legs under your arms and float in the crotch of the trousers. Air will probably leak out slowly through the fabric, so repeat the process as necessary. Use this technique only in warm water. In cold water, keep your clothes on to help to conserve your body heat.*

Emergencies in the water

DROWNPROOFING – A TECHNIQUE FOR SURVIVAL

In warm water, one of the easiest ways to stay afloat for an extended period without a life jacket is to use a technique known as drownproofing.

• Take a deep breath, relax, and hang in the water with your face under the surface and arms forward – as if lying over a barrel.

• To breathe again, breathe out underwater, pull down with your arms and lift your head until your mouth is just clear of the water.

• Take a deep breath, and continue alternately relaxing and breathing.

In warm water, this technique allows a swimmer to stay afloat with very little effort for hours, or even days. It works because the totally submerged human body with a lungful of air is slightly lighter than the same volume of water – and so will float naturally. Keeping part of the body constantly above the surface requires more effort and is more tiring.

Drownproofing should not be used in cold water – such as open water in and around Britain – because immersing the head speeds up the rate at which the body loses heat. It is better in cold water to float on your back, using the hands if necessary, or to tread water slowly, so that your face and most of your head stays out of the water.

Man overboard

When someone falls overboard from a motor boat or sailing dinghy, the priorities for action can be summed up in eight words: turn; shout; throw; watch; and approach to leeward.

• Start turning the boat as soon as you notice the accident.

• If there are other crew aboard, shout: 'Man overboard.'

• Throw a life buoy, or anything else that will float, to the person in the water. Make allowance for the wind when you throw.

• Keep watching the person in the water, or get someone else aboard to do so. If you lose sight of him, especially in rough water or at sea, it may be difficult to find him again.

• Steer the boat so that you approach from downwind of him. That way, there will be no danger of the boat being blown over him.

• Slacken any wire or rope guard rails around the deck so that they do not make it more difficult to get the person back on board.

• On a sailing dinghy, turn the boat into the wind as you come alongside and let the sails flap so that the boat stops. On a motor boat, stop the engine.

• Help the person in. In calm water, lift him over the stern (stop any propeller first). In rough water, though, bring him in over the side. Otherwise the drag of his body on the stern may swing the boat broadside to the wind and waves, and could cause a capsize.

• If the person's weight or exhaustion make pulling him aboard by hand impossible, tie a bowline in a piece of rope and put the loop over his head and under his arms.

• Get another member of the crew to hold the person while you tie the knot, both to keep his head above water and to stop him floating away from the boat.

• Hoist him aboard. If necessary, attach the rope to a halyard (the tackle used for hoisting the sails) to give yourself extra leverage.

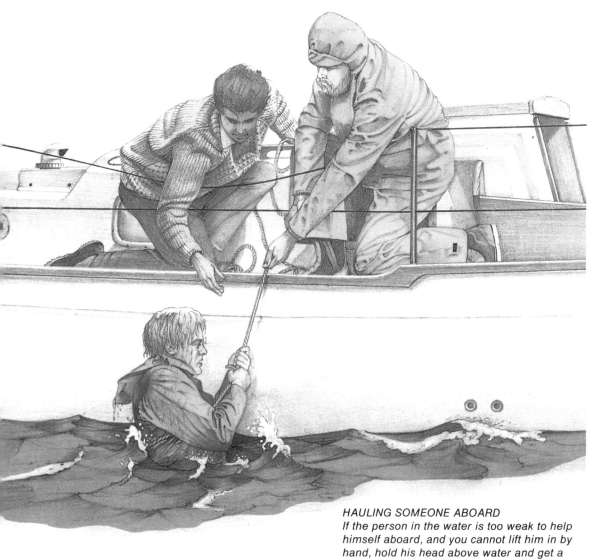

HAULING SOMEONE ABOARD
If the person in the water is too weak to help himself aboard, and you cannot lift him in by hand, hold his head above water and get a loop of rope under his arms. Then haul him up.

HOW TO MAKE A BOWLINE KNOT

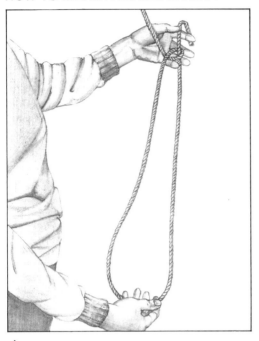

1 *To make a rope loop which will not slip, twist a small ring in the rope about 4ft (1.2m) from one end, and pass the end through it.*

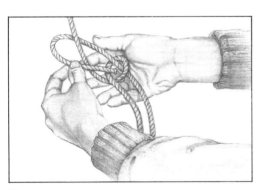

2 *Take the end round behind the rope and slip it back through the same ring.*

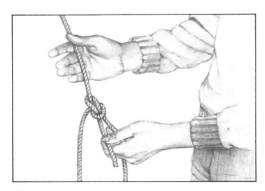

3 *Pull the rope tight to form the completed bowline knot.*

DROWNING – THE PERILS OF THE COLD

Nearly 1000 people drown in Britain each year, and many of them die not because they cannot swim, but because of the cold.

In 1984, doctors at the Institute of Naval Medicine in Gosport, Hampshire, tested the strength-sapping effects of cold water on ten volunteers, all capable of swimming fully clothed in warm water for at least ten minutes.

The swimmers went fully clothed into water at a temperature which is typical of British inland waters in winter: 5°C (41°F). Seven of the ten foundered after between two and seven minutes, and had to be helped out. Even the three who stayed afloat were exhausted by the experience.

The test's most striking result was that those who breathed slowly and deeply lasted longest. Those who breathed fastest failed. The doctors recommend that if you fall into cold water and decide to swim to safety, you should not start swimming at once. Instead, wait – moving as little as possible – until your breathing is under control. Provided you do not panic, your breathing will slow down naturally after four to five minutes.

If you are wearing a life jacket, hug your knees in a posture known as HELP while you wait (see picture, page 276).

When cold water can be a life-saver

At ordinary swimming pool temperatures, a swimmer will die after seven minutes underwater. He will become unconscious long before that, but he can be revived with the kiss of life. At very low temperatures, however, he can survive much longer, even if he appears to be dead.

Early in 1984, a four-year-old boy named Jimmy Tontlewicz was under ice and water for 20 minutes in Lake Michigan, USA, before he was pulled out by divers. The rescuers thought he was dead, but doctors at a nearby hospital were able to revive him.

The boy lived because the icy water had lowered his body temperature to less than 30°C (86°F) – 7°C (12.6°F) lower than normal – slowing his metabolism and reducing his brain's need for oxygen.

The message for rescuers is clear, doctors believe. Keep trying to resuscitate a victim of drowning until medical help arrives. Even when all apparent signs of life have ended, the effort could save the victim's life.

Emergencies
in the water

Safety for windsurfers

The fast-growing sport of windsurfing has its dangers as well as its thrills. But following a few commonsense rules should keep you or get you out of trouble.

• Wear a life jacket or buoyancy aid and, on all but the hottest days, a wetsuit or drysuit.

• Do not windsurf at dusk, at night, or when visibility is poor. Never put out to sea in an offshore wind (one blowing away from the beach). The land and any buildings act as a windbreak, and by the time you feel the wind's true strength, it may be too late to get back to shore safely.

• Do not windsurf in places where there are no other people about. But do keep clear of others using the water.

• Carry a towline, in case you need to be pulled back to shore. Tie the sail rig to the board, so that you will not lose it if the foot of the mast jumps out of its housing.

• Always swim towards the board if you fall off, and stay with it if you get into trouble. If you start feeling tired, or the weather is too much for you, head for shore *before* you get exhausted and while you still have some energy.

What to do if you get into trouble

There are two recognised ways for a windsurfer in trouble to signal for help. Whichever you use, the first step is to lower the mast and sail into the water.

• Kneel on the board and raise both arms above your head as if in surrender.

• Alternatively, stand on the board. Hold on with one hand to the uphaul line (used to pull the mast up) for stability. Wave the other arm stiffly and vigorously from down by your side to above your head, and back. Some windsurfers carry a small red flag, or a red cloth, strapped to the ankle, to make the SOS message plain. Distress flares can be carried, too.

• If you are out of sight of possible rescuers and unable to sail back to shore, lower the mast and sail into the water and sit astride the board.

• Remove the foot of the mast from its housing. Hold the outer end of the wishbone – the end of the boom away from the mast – and lay the mast alongside the board in the water. Untie the sail from the wishbone and swing the wishbone up to the top of the mast.

• Roll the sail tightly towards the mast, removing the battens as you come to them and folding them into the sail.

• Lash the rolled-up sail and wishbone to the mast with the uphaul line and lay them lengthways on the board. Tie them to the board, too.

• Lie face down on the board, with your shoulders across a narrow section near the front, and paddle back to shore.

• If the wind, tide or current is against you, aim diagonally across it, not directly into it.

• If the sail rig gets seriously in your way as you paddle, roll it overboard and abandon it; it is not worth risking your life for.

Righting a capsized dingh

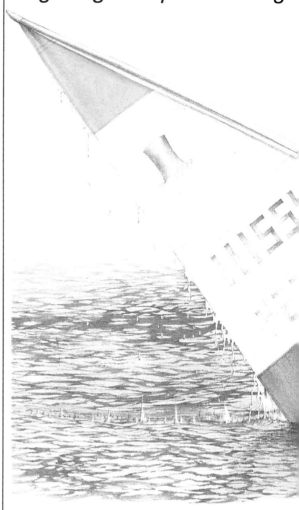

A squall, a freak wave or a mistake in manoeuvring can tip a small dinghy over with little warning, throwing the crew into the water. Whatever the cause, the action to take is the same. The techniques described here are not difficult, but they do need some practice. Try them out several times by capsizing a boat deliberately in calm water close to the shore.

• Get clear of any entangling ropes or sails, and make sure that any other crew members are clear too.

• If the hull turns completely upside down, trapping you underneath, take a deep breath in the air space that will be left under the hull, then swim out underwater.

• Do not leave the boat, even if you cannot get it back upright. It will stay afloat indefinitely, and rescuers will be able to spot the hull more easily than they will see a swimmer.

• If the boat is completely upside down, a partial vacuum will be formed under the hull, sucking the boat against the water surface and making it difficult to turn onto its side. Pull down or climb onto one corner of the stern to break the vacuum, then roll the boat onto its side.

• Free the sheets – the ropes used to set the angle of the sails – so that the sails can swing

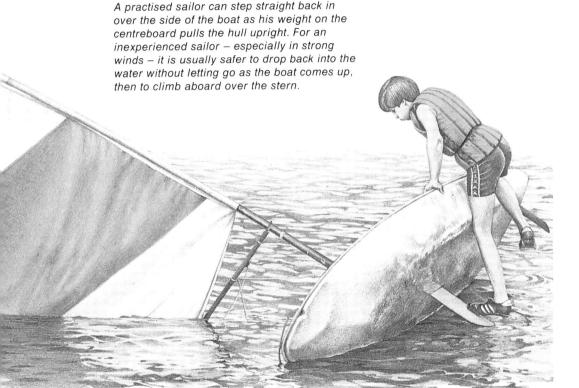

GETTING BACK ON BOARD
A practised sailor can step straight back in over the side of the boat as his weight on the centreboard pulls the hull upright. For an inexperienced sailor – especially in strong winds – it is usually safer to drop back into the water without letting go as the boat comes up, then to climb aboard over the stern.

freely. Otherwise the wind will fill them as the boat comes upright, and may tip it over again.

• Check that the rudder and tiller are secure and not tangled in the ropes.

• Make sure that the centreboard is fully down, then climb onto it, keeping your feet close to the hull to avoid breaking the centreboard off.

• If it is difficult to get onto the board, ask a crew member to throw one of the jib (front sail) sheets over the hull, and use the rope to pull yourself up.

• Once on the board, hold the side of the boat – the gunwale – or the jib sheet, and lean back, pressing with your feet against the centreboard. Your weight should pull the boat back upright.

• An agile sailor can climb in over the side directly from the centreboard as the boat rolls upright, but there is a risk that he could pull the boat over again on top of him, unless there is someone else in the boat to balance it. If you have not practised this technique, pull yourself round to the stern instead, and climb in there.

• If the weight of water on the sails prevents the boat from coming upright, lower the sails and try again.

• If there is more than one person in the boat, ask one of them to swim into the cockpit while the boat is on its side and to lie along the inside of the hull. He or she will be scooped up into the boat when you pull it upright, and can help to stabilise it while you climb in. The crew may also need to bail out the boat partially to improve its buoyancy before you get back in.

HOW TO AVOID A CAPSIZE

If the force of the wind threatens to tip your dinghy over – in any sailing situation – let go of the sheets (the ropes from the sails) so that the sails flap freely.

At the same time, steer into the wind (if you are sitting on the windward side of the boat, this means pushing the tiller away from you) and move quickly into the centre of the boat to balance it.

Whatever the situation, steering into the wind and letting the sails flap freely will end the sideways pressure on the boat and allow it to come upright again.

Avoiding collisions at sea

There are a number of internationally recognised 'rules of the road' on the water to stop boats colliding with each other. The rules are contained in detail in the International Regulations for Preventing Collisions at Sea (1972), available from Her Majesty's Stationery Office at 49 High Holborn, London WC1. These are the main rules:
• When two sailing boats are on a collision course, the one with the wind to port (coming from the left-hand side of the boat, looking forwards) must keep out of the way. If two sailing boats have the wind on the same side, the boat upwind must give way.
• Power boats must give way to sailing craft if they can, but a large power boat following a narrow channel may not be able to do so. In this case, the sailing boat should keep clear. All boats should give way to fishing boats, which have right of way while fishing.
• If a sailing boat is using its engine it is treated as a power craft, and must give way to boats under sail.
• Power boats approaching each other end on (or nearly end on) should both turn to starboard (to the right). If power boats are crossing each other's course, the one that sees the other on its starboard (right-hand) side must keep out of the way.
    When there is a risk of collision, boats can also signal their intentions to other nearby boats by means of a whistle or siren. One short blast means: I am altering course to starboard. Two short blasts mean: I am altering course to port. Three short blasts mean: My engines are going astern.

If a sailing boat crosses your path
If you are in a sailing boat with the wind coming from the left-hand (port) side of your boat, you must give way to a sailing boat which is crossing your path on the opposite (starboard) tack. Steer your boat behind the other's stern to be sure of missing it.

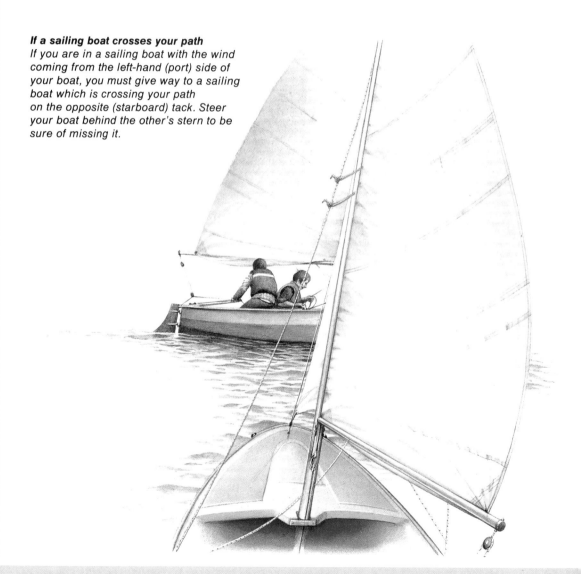

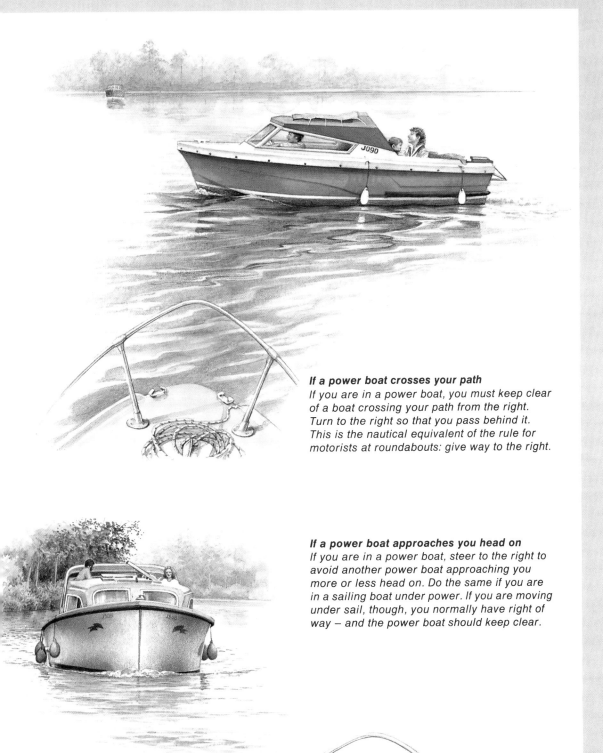

If a power boat crosses your path
If you are in a power boat, you must keep clear of a boat crossing your path from the right. Turn to the right so that you pass behind it. This is the nautical equivalent of the rule for motorists at roundabouts: give way to the right.

If a power boat approaches you head on
If you are in a power boat, steer to the right to avoid another power boat approaching you more or less head on. Do the same if you are in a sailing boat under power. If you are moving under sail, though, you normally have right of way — and the power boat should keep clear.

Running aground

A grounded boat must be freed quickly – provided that its hull has not been holed or damaged below the waterline. What to do depends to some extent on the wind direction, the type of keel and – in coastal waters – the state of the tide. If the tide is rising, the boat must be prevented from being driven farther aground. If it is falling, the boat must be moved off fast or it will be left high and dry. The easiest route off is usually the same as the route on.

• On a lee shore (with the wind blowing shorewards) or in a rising tide, drop all sails at once or turn the boat into the wind and let go an anchor to prevent the boat being driven farther aground. On a weather shore (with the wind blowing away from the shore) set the sails so that the wind helps to swing the bow towards deeper water.

• At the same time that you trim the sails, start the engine, applying moderate power in reverse. Your own wake rolling under the stern may free the boat.

Using a kedge anchor

• If these actions do not free the boat, try to haul it into deeper water by means of a kedge anchor – a light anchor with a chain and rope attached.

• Secure the end of the rope to a winch or run it through a pulley on the boat.

• Coil the rest of the rope and the chain in a dinghy or rowing boat and suspend the anchor over its stern. This saves you having to lift it over the side.

• Row away from the stuck boat into deeper water, paying out the rope as you go, then drop

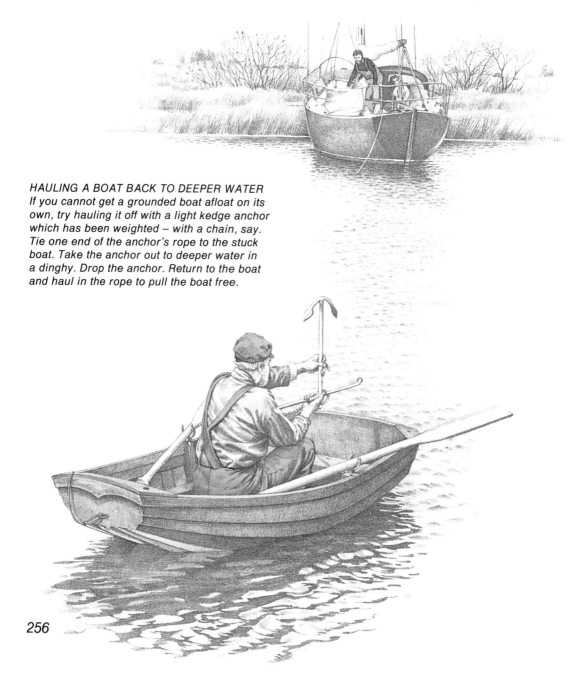

HAULING A BOAT BACK TO DEEPER WATER
If you cannot get a grounded boat afloat on its own, try hauling it off with a light kedge anchor which has been weighted – with a chain, say. Tie one end of the anchor's rope to the stuck boat. Take the anchor out to deeper water in a dinghy. Drop the anchor. Return to the boat and haul in the rope to pull the boat free.

the anchor. Once the kedge anchor is firmly gripped on the bottom, return to the boat and pull in the rope to haul the boat free.

• If necessary, shift heavy weights onto the dinghy to lighten the load on the stuck boat.

Using the weight of the crew

• Another method of freeing a boat is to get the crew to rock it from side to side. This may break the suction of mud on the keel.

• If the rocking does not work and the boat does not have twin keels (known as bilge keels), it may be possible to free it by using the weight of the crew to heel, or tilt, it to one side; somebody can sit on the end of the boom if necessary. This will help to loosen the keel from mud or sand and may lift it sufficiently to free it.

• In a boat with a full single keel, which is

TILTING THE BOAT FREE

You can sometimes free a stuck boat by getting one or more people to sit on the end of the boom and then swinging the boom out. This will tilt the boat and loosen the keel, and it may lift the keel enough to set the boat free. The boat can then be hauled off with a kedge anchor (see opposite).

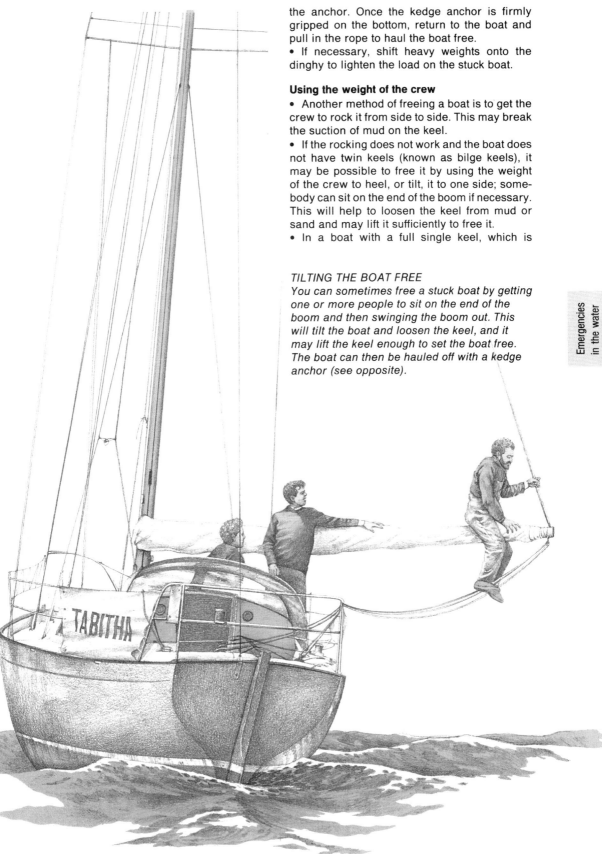

Emergencies in the water

257

normally deeper towards the stern, try moving all the crew well forward. This may weigh down the bows sufficiently to free the keel.

Leaving the boat high and dry

• If getting off proves impossible, prepare the boat for being left aground until you can get more help or until the next high tide. Normally, a boat will refloat as long after low water as the period before low water that it ran aground.

If a boat runs aground at the height of a spring tide (a high tide occurring near the time of a new or full moon) it could be about two weeks before the water reaches the same level again.

• Leave the kedge anchor in position and put out the main anchor as well.

• A boat with a single keel will heel onto one side as the tide recedes. Make sure it lies with

the keel towards deep water by weighting the deck – with an anchor chain, say – on the side towards the shallows. This will protect the superstructure from waves when the tide returns.

• As the water level drops, wedge sailbags, fenders and other padding under the leaning hull to prevent it being damaged as the returning waves pound it against the ground.

• Secure all loose gear on board. Shut off fuel and water supplies to prevent spillage. Close all seacocks and plug tank ventilator pipes. If possible, offload batteries onto a dinghy to avoid the risk of acid spilling from them.

• Pump out the bilge so that there is no waste water to weigh the boat down or to affect its balance while it is righting. Batten and seal all hatches to prevent seawater entering.

• If you can stay on board till the tide returns,

WAITING FOR THE NEXT TIDE
If you cannot get a boat afloat, leave it until the next tide. First, though, put out the anchors. If the boat has a single keel, weight it – with a chain, say – towards the shallows, so that it comes to rest with the keel towards deep water. Put fenders and other padding under the leaning hull to protect it. Secure loose gear. Shut off all pipes and pump out the bilge.

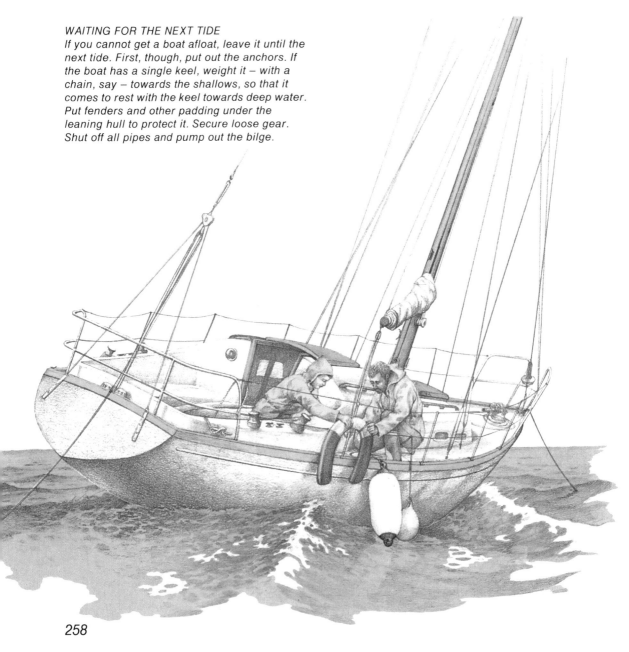

fill bags, pillow cases and buckets with sand. Store them on the boat until it begins to float, then empty them overboard. This will minimise the pounding the boat gets as the water rises.
• Alternatively, a deep-keeled boat can be kept upright by rigging beaching legs (props that fit under the hull on each side). If you have no ready-made props, improvise with a boom or spinnaker pole lashed to the boat's rigging.
• As a last resort, if there is heavy surf and a hard bottom, scuttling the boat will prevent it being pounded to pieces as the tide rises. To do this, leave the anchors in position, move out as much gear as possible, and open the seacocks so that the boat settles on the bottom.
• Later, as the water deepens again, close the seacocks and pump the boat out so that it rises with the tide and floats free.

TIPS FOR STAYING AFLOAT

• Bear in mind the state of the tide and the time of low water. Study charts of the area. Never sail too close to a lee shore.
• Be aware of any change of motion in the boat – such as a shorter rise and fall – that might indicate shallow water. If you are in any doubt, sound the depth with a lead and line.
• Bear in mind, too, the depth and shape of your keel. You may not be able to sail as close to the shore as other boats of apparently similar size.

PROPPING UP THE BOAT
If you have no beaching legs, use a boom as a prop. Tilt the boat with weights towards the shallows. Remove the boom and rest one end on the seabed on the shallow side. On mud or sand, put a plank underneath to stop it sinking in. Then lash the boom to the shrouds both at its top and at deck level. Stop the boom slipping by tying the top to a strong deck fitting.

Emergencies in the water

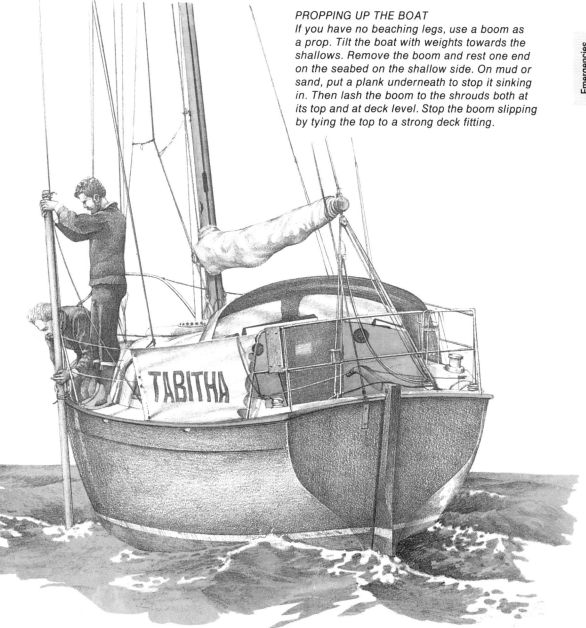

Dealing with a hole or leak

Colliding with a rock, a floating log or another boat can all put a hole in the hull of a small boat. But a hole need not mean that the boat will sink at once, or even at all.

Plugging a large hole

• On a sailing boat, if there is a hole on or near the waterline, sail the boat on a suitable tack to heel it over slightly and raise the hole from the water. On a sailing boat or motor boat, re-arrange movable equipment and the crew's position for the same purpose.

• If the hole is below the waterline, use the bilge pump or bail out by hand to control the water level while you make emergency repairs inside and outside the hull.

• Plug the hole first from the inside with any suitable material, such as sailbags, cushions or mattresses. Wedge the plugging in place with something solid, such as a table or seating boards. Alternatively, use a damage-control device (see box, this page).

• Then, if you have no purpose-built device, make what sailors call a collision mat. The idea is to spread the mat – which could be a tarpaulin or a spare sail – across the hole on the outside of the hull so that water pressure helps to hold it in place.

• If the hull is so shaped that canvas will not lie flat against it, wrap the tarpaulin or sail round a foam mattress or cushion, which is more likely to shape itself to the hull. Then use the bundle as a mat.

• To move the mat into position, tie chains or ropes to each corner. Then tie two or three corners of the mat to fittings on the damaged side of the boat.

• Loop the remaining rope or ropes over the front of the boat and work them along under the hull until the mat is pulled tight over the hole. Tie the ropes to fittings on the undamaged side of the boat. Then make for shore at once.

Repairing a small leak

• If a boat starts shipping water slowly, it may be difficult to find the source of the leak. So make a systematic check of the likely places where water could get into the boat.

• Check all seacocks – the valves that prevent a back-flow of water in any pipe that goes through the hull. Seacocks are usually built into the galley, toilet, engine intake and exhaust, bilge pump and cockpit drains.

• Check any fittings which pass through the hull, such as the rudder shaft.

• Check the stuffing box – the greased stuffing compressed round the propeller shaft where it goes through the hull.

• Check the water tank or tanks.

• Check seams in the hull.

• Once you find the leak, plug it firmly with caulking cotton (cotton fibre and sealant), greased rags, underwater resin, towels or any other similar material.

• Make permanent repairs as soon as possible when you get back to shore.

HOW TO USE A DAMAGE-CONTROL DEVICE

Specialist boating shops usually sell purpose-built damage-control devices. The devices, which resemble umbrellas, are designed to be used at sea to plug a hole in a hull until more permanent repairs can be made when the boat gets back to port.

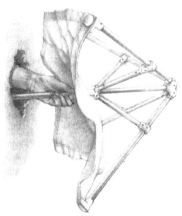

1 *Close the device and push it out through the hole. Then open it like an umbrella.*

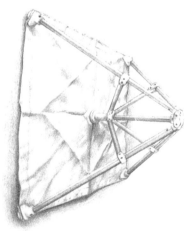

2 *Pull it back against the hull to seal the hole. Tie the handle to a fitting inside.*

TWO WAYS TO PLUG A HOLE IN A BOAT

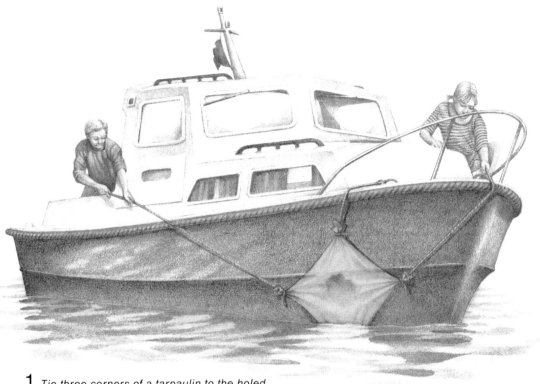

1 *Tie three corners of a tarpaulin to the holed side. Loop the remaining rope under the bow and tie it to the other side. Adjust the ropes' lengths to position the tarpaulin over the hole.*

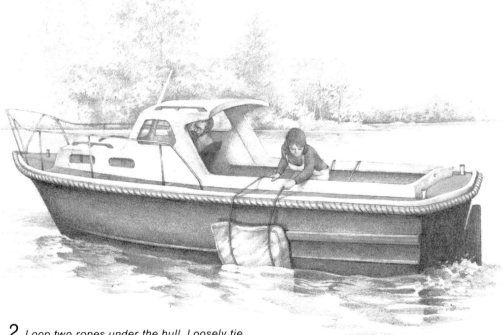

2 *Loop two ropes under the hull. Loosely tie them to fittings. Slide a mattress into place under the rope straps, then pull them tight.*

Emergencies in the water

Fire on board

Because the fittings in most family-size sailing boats and power boats are largely made out of wood, and because the boats often contain fuel tanks and gas cylinders in a fairly small space, a fire, once started, can spread at alarming speed. If you are away from land at the time, there may be no easy escape route, either.

For these reasons, fast decisive action is imperative if a fire breaks out on board.

- Shout 'Fire' to raise the alarm.
- If the engine is running, turn it off.
- Throw burning equipment such as mattresses overboard. Do not, however, try to move a burning chip pan (see *Fighting a fire*, page 150).
- Never throw water on burning petrol or gas. It spreads the blaze, sometimes explosively. Instead, use a fire extinguisher containing dry powder or foam.
- In a sailing boat, if the wind is light, drop the sails; if the wind is strong, minimise its ability to fan the flames by sailing downwind.
- If the fire is below decks, make sure everyone is out, then stop air reaching it by closing doors, hatches and ventilators. Fight the blaze from above or from somewhere where you can retreat easily if necessary.
- If you cannot extinguish the fire quickly, evacuate the area or abandon ship if necessary.
- After the fire is out, damp down the area thoroughly with water.

GUARDING AGAINST A BLAZE

Most fires in boats are caused by sparks or naked flames igniting petrol or gas leaks or accumulations of petrol vapour (likely to collect where there are drip trays, spills, or loose caps on an engine or fuel tank).

You can cut the risk of fire on board, however, by following a few commonsense rules.

- Make sure that bilges (the space between hull and floor in a boat) and engine spaces have ventilation hoses that reach right to the bottom. Petrol vapour and bottled gases are all heavier than air, and so will accumulate at the lowest levels. Each fuel tank should have a vent pipe to disperse petrol vapour; the pipe should go out through the hull and be covered with wire gauze. You can also buy equipment for the automatic detection of petrol vapour or gas in bilges or cabins. Ask at a chandler's for information.
- Before starting a petrol engine, open all doors and vents and allow air to circulate for at least five minutes.
- Fit carburettors with drip trays (covered with wire gauze to prevent anything being

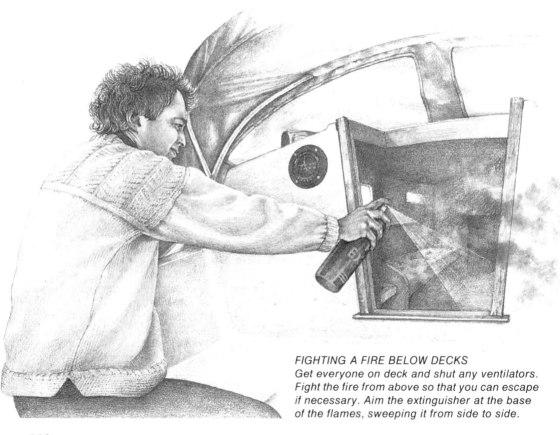

FIGHTING A FIRE BELOW DECKS
Get everyone on deck and shut any ventilators. Fight the fire from above so that you can escape if necessary. Aim the extinguisher at the base of the flames, sweeping it from side to side.

dropped in), and clean the trays before starting the engine. That way you will minimise the chances of leaking fuel collecting in the bottom of the boat.

• Fit flame traps in the air intakes.

• Check wiring and plugs regularly and replace faulty parts. Make sure that connectors have the correct fuse; a fuse with too large a capacity will allow cables to overheat.

• Ensure that generators and all switches are as far as possible above the bilges to minimise the chance of water causing short circuits.

• Do not strike matches, smoke, or use a kerosene or any other open-flame lamp inside the engine space. Anywhere on board, use only safety matches. Other types of matches, and also cigarette lighters, can spark if they are rubbed accidentally or dropped.

• Cover batteries so that tools cannot fall on the terminals and cause a spark.

• Avoid overfilling petrol tanks – leave some space for the fuel to expand. Check for leakages regularly. The top of the filler pipe should reach to the open deck so that any spillages will run overboard and not down to the bilges. Do not use petrol for cleaning. Instead, use clean cotton rags – and dispose of them, and all other rubbish, regularly.

Fire-fighting equipment

• Carry one fire extinguisher of at least 3lb (1.5kg) capacity, containing dry powder, carbon dioxide or foam. Extinguishers containing a chemical known as halon or BCF (bromochlorodofluoromethane) are less appropriate for a boat because they give off poisonous fumes which are dangerous in a confined space. Carry two extinguishers if there is a galley on board. Keep them in a place accessible from the open deck so that a fire can be fought from a safe position (see *Protecting your home against fire*, page 152; *Using bottled gas*, page 154).

• Carry a fire blanket and keep it near the galley. Never leave a cooking stove unattended while it is in use.

• Keep two bailer buckets with lanyards on deck for hauling up seawater.

Emergencies in the water

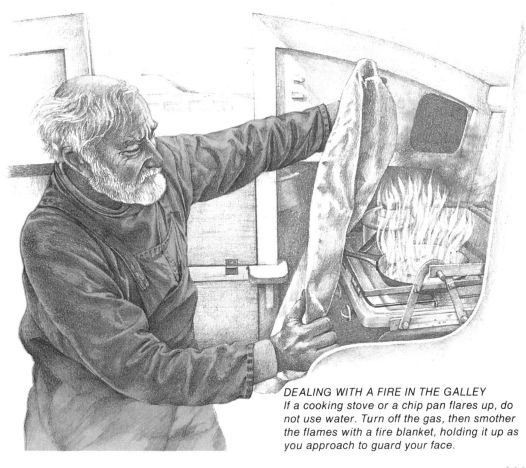

DEALING WITH A FIRE IN THE GALLEY
If a cooking stove or a chip pan flares up, do not use water. Turn off the gas, then smother the flames with a fire blanket, holding it up as you approach to guard your face.

263

Deciding what to do in heavy weather at sea

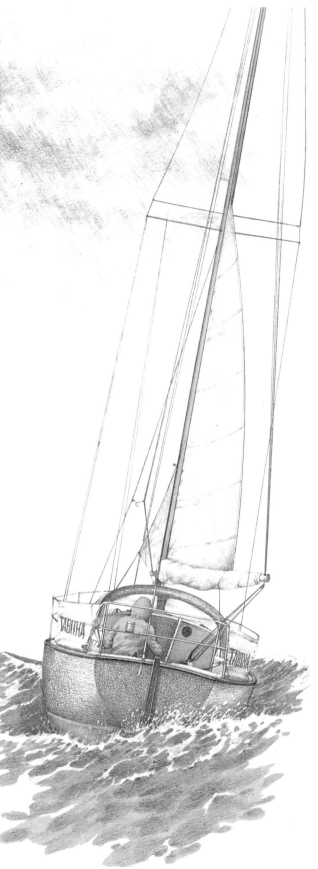

If the sea gets very rough while you are out in a sailing boat or motor boat, you have to decide whether to continue on course (under reduced power or sail so that you can keep control of the craft), head for port as fast as possible, heave to (stop moving), or run before the storm.

If in doubt, it is usually safer to stay at sea rather than to head for harbour and risk being swept and battered against the shore.

Whatever your decision, the boat needs to be rigged for stormy conditions (see *Caught in a storm*, page 270).

Rough seas are no place for the novice, though. Before you contemplate taking any boat into the open sea yourself, learn about the problems and risks at first hand by crewing for experienced sailors and boat-owners. Local yacht and boat clubs can often put you in touch with knowledgeable skippers. The clubs may also run training courses.

Continuing on course

Carrying on under reduced sail or power is a viable option if the wind is blowing in a direction suitable for the course you want to follow. If the wind is unfavourable, take other action.

Heading for port

Running for shelter is worth considering if the wind is right and the weather is worsening slowly enough for you to be able to beat it to a port or other refuge (such as the sheltered side of a headland). Remember, however, that heavy seas will slow you down.

• A motor boat or a sailing boat with an engine is likely to be able to head for port faster than a boat travelling under sail alone. But first check how much fuel is in the tank – refuelling from a petrol can may be impossible in rough water.

Heaving to

• Stopping at sea without anchoring – what sailors call heaving to – is safe only if you are well away from a lee shore: one the wind is blowing towards. But even a boat which is hove to still drifts slightly with wind and current. It could drift at 2 knots (just over 2mph) or more, and a storm could last up to 30 hours.

• The advantage of heaving to is that the boat's motion in the water is more comfortable for those on board. Also, little effort is required from the crew once the boat has been prepared.

• The disadvantages are that the boat will move gradually across the wind and downwind, which

HOW TO HEAVE TO
To hold a boat more or less in position at sea, pull the front sail to the upwind side of the boat and keep steering into the wind. The boat will then sail a roughly crescent-shaped course: forwards until it is almost nose-on to the wind, then back and sideways again as the wind pushes more on the front sail.

could carry it into more dangerous waters, and there is constant strain on the sails and rigging.
• There is also a risk of the boat being swung broadside to the waves and capsizing. This is more likely with a shallow, unballasted hull such as a flat-bottomed centre-board vessel.
• If you decide to heave to, the aim in effect is to sail the boat into the wind at the same speed that the wind is blowing it downwind.
• Back the front sail (the jib) – that is, set it so that the wind is pushing it backwards. It then counterbalances the forward thrust of the mainsail.
• Reduce the area of the mainsail so that little sail is exposed to the wind.
• Lash or hold the tiller or wheel to keep the boat pointing towards the wind.

Running before the storm

• Sailing downwind in a storm is a viable option only if you have plenty of sea room – that is, if you are far enough from land not to be blown onto rocks or the shore. You can reduce sails to a jib only if necessary, or run with bare poles.
• The advantages are that the boat remains under control and manoeuvrable, and the strain and wear on sails and rigging is kept to a minimum.
• The disadvantages are that the crew must be on the alert, with someone constantly at the helm to keep the boat pointing downwind; and the cockpit is exposed to the seas.
• There is also a risk that the following waves will break over the stern. This can be offset by trailing ropes behind the boat, looping the very long ones, so that the waves break on the ropes, and their force is diminished. The drag of the ropes also helps to slow down the boat, making it easier to control. In addition, it helps to keep the stern into the wind, lessening the chance that the boat will swing sideways to the waves and capsize.
• As a last resort, if you are well clear of land and shipping lanes, lower all sails, stow everything securely, shut all hatches and retreat below decks until the weather eases.

Emergencies in the water

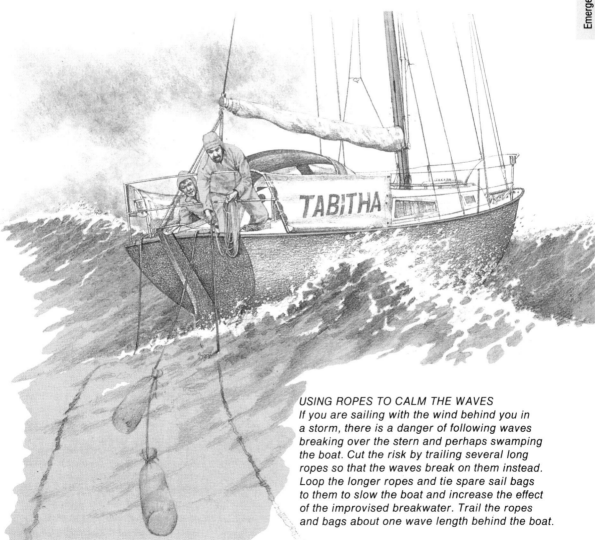

USING ROPES TO CALM THE WAVES
If you are sailing with the wind behind you in a storm, there is a danger of following waves breaking over the stern and perhaps swamping the boat. Cut the risk by trailing several long ropes so that the waves break on them instead. Loop the longer ropes and tie spare sail bags to them to slow the boat and increase the effect of the improvised breakwater. Trail the ropes and bags about one wave length behind the boat.

Wind and weather

Around Britain's coasts, bad weather never arrives suddenly or unexpectedly. There are always warnings, such as changes in wind and clouds and falling barometric pressure – and the more abrupt the drop in a barometer's reading, the more severe the bad weather is likely to be. All the same, the weather at sea may be quite different from weather on land. So listen to shipping forecasts before planning to put to sea.

Weather forecasts for small-boat users are broadcast on BBC Radio 3 FM (90.2–92.4mHz) at 6.55am daily, and local forecasts are often posted outside a harbourmaster's office. Gale warnings are broadcast on BBC Radio 4 long wave 1515m/198kHz and FM 92.4–94.6mHz and also by coastal radio stations on frequencies listed in the British Telecom publication *Notice to Ship Wireless Stations*. If there are storm or gale warnings, stay in port. A small boat is unsafe at sea in winds of Force 4 and upwards, when waves are likely to be at least 3ft (1m) high.

Bad-weather signs

The pictures opposite show the visible clues a sailor or a hiker should watch for. All of them indicate that bad weather is on the way.

Other bad-weather clues can only be felt, not seen, or become apparent only over a period of time. These are the main ones:

TEN WEEKS IN A LIFE RAFT
Playful dorado fish kept yacht designer Steven Callahan alive when he was shipwrecked in mid-Atlantic in 1982. Swimming around his tiny life raft and following it as it drifted across the ocean, the dorados became his only food. The 29-year-old American speared them from the raft and ate them raw.

Solar stills – part of his survival kit on the raft – provided him with 3 pints of water a day (a little over 1.5 litres), just enough to live on.

The dorados also helped in his rescue. As he drifted near the Caribbean Leeward Islands, the fish attracted flocks of birds – which were spotted by a fishing boat. When the boat picked up Callahan on April 21, 1982, he was 3 stone (20kg) lighter than normal but remarkably fit after 76 days adrift.

Four years earlier, in 1978, two middle-aged Americans were washed out to sea during a fishing trip after the motor on their boat broke down. They survived the blistering heat of the Gulf of California by making their own still to turn seawater into fresh.

The two men improvised a stove by burning a mixture of petrol and oil from their broken-down outboard motor in two open tins. After their matches ran out, they lit the stove by sparking wires from the motor's battery against a petrol-soaked piece of cardboard.

They used the stove to boil seawater in a jerry-can. The steam condensed as it passed through a hose stuffed in the neck of the can, and trickled into a plastic bottle. The two men were found by a US Coastguard plane after a week and a half in their open boat – hungry but otherwise unhurt.

• The wind changes suddenly after several days of constant direction.
• The wind increases in the afternoon or evening.

Some weather signs indicate the approach of severe weather: a storm or gale. Mares'-tail clouds, and a copper-coloured sunset or sunrise are both danger signals. So are a number of other clues:
• A rapidly falling or unsteady barometer.
• Increasing humidity.
• A heavy but inexplicable swell at sea.

HOW TO READ A BAROMETER

The barometer most commonly used by sailors is the aneroid type shown below. Aneroid means 'without air'.

The pointer moves as air pressure squeezes a vacuum-filled metal bellows inside. The words on the dial – 'Fair', 'Stormy', 'Rain' and so on – are more traditional than useful. What matters more is a *change* in the reading. Generally, a drop in pressure indicates a storm is on the way. Steady or rising pressure usually means fair weather ahead.

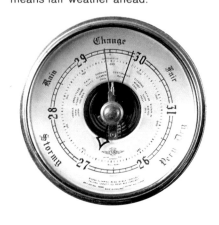

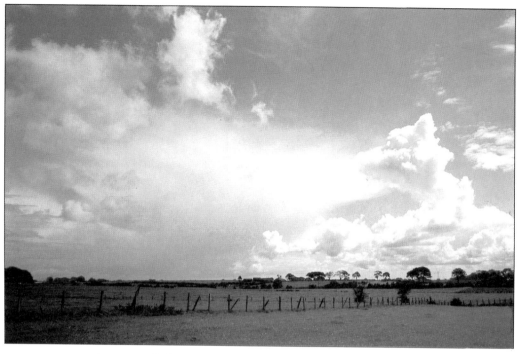

MESSAGE IN THE SKY *Large, anvil-shaped and often fuzzy-edged expanses of cloud, such as that in the centre of this picture, mark the* approach of more blustery weather. The change will probably bring showers, and may build into a thunderstorm.

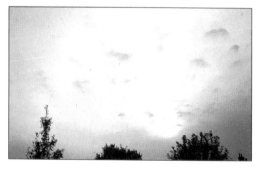

ICE HALO *A halo round the moon, formed when light is refracted by ice crystals, signals rain, or perhaps a storm, within 36 hours.*

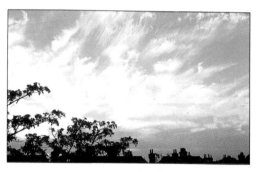

OUTRIDERS OF A GALE *Mares'-tail clouds – high wispy streaks across the sky – are often a warning of high winds on the way.*

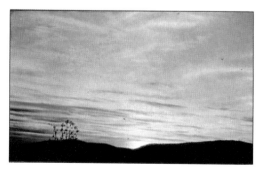

COPPER SUN *A copper-coloured sunset or sunrise is a warning of a gale or storm. A yellowish sunset indicates rain and wind.*

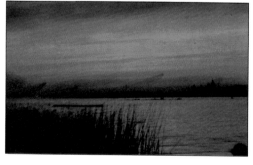

RED SKY AT MORNING *If the sunrise is red, or clear but with a red tinge, the weather is likely to take a turn for the worse soon.*

The wind and the sea

The Beaufort wind scale, devised in 1805 by the British admiral Sir Francis Beaufort (1774-1857), is still widely used in shipping forecasts and by sailors. It enables sailors to estimate the strength of the wind simply by observing its effects and without the need for precise measuring instruments. The scale begins at Force 0, when the wind is less than 1mph and the sea is flat calm, and rises to Force 12, a hurricane. The chart below shows how to judge the wind on land and sea, and gives the probable maximum wave height for each wind force. Average wave heights are lower.

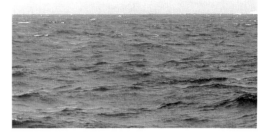

FORCE THREE *A touch of foam on some crests and a few white horses mark a Force 3 wind – what sailors call a gentle breeze..*

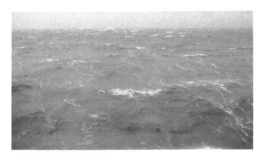

FORCE FIVE *A wind of Force 5 or above can be hazardous even for experienced sailors.*

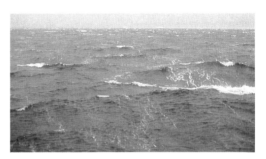

FORCE SIX *In a strong breeze, the waves can be anything from 8 to 13ft (2.5-4m) high.*

THE BEAUFORT SCALE ON LAND AND AT SEA

FORCE ONE: LIGHT AIR

Land: Smoke drifts slightly – but the wind is not enough to move a wind vane.
Sea: Tiny ripples shaped like fish scales form on the sea's surface. No foam crests.

Maximum wind speed: 3mph (5km/h).
Probable maximum wave height: Nil.

FORCE TWO: LIGHT BREEZE

Land: Breeze felt on the face. Wind vanes move and leaves rustle.
Sea: Small wavelets form. Crests are pronounced and have a glassy appearance, but they do not break into foam.
Maximum wind speed: 7mph (11km/h).
Probable maximum wave height: 1ft (0.3m).

FORCE THREE: GENTLE BREEZE

Land: Leaves and small twigs in constant motion. The breeze extends a light flag.
Sea: Large wavelets form. Crests begin to break into foam and there are occasional white horses.

Maximum wind speed: 12mph (19km/h).
Probable maximum wave height: 3ft (1m).

FORCE FOUR: MODERATE BREEZE

Land: The wind raises dust and loose paper and moves small branches on trees.
Sea: Small waves form and some begin to join together to make longer lines of waves. There are frequent white horses.
Maximum wind speed: 18mph (29km/h).
Probable maximum wave height: 5ft (1.5m).

FORCE FIVE: FRESH BREEZE

Land: Small trees sway, if they are in leaf. Crested wavelets form on inland waters.
Sea: Moderate-sized waves form into long lines. There are many white horses and some spray.

Maximum wind speed: 24mph (39km/h).
Probable maximum wave height: 8ft (2.5m).

FORCE SIX: STRONG BREEZE

Land: Large branches move. Telegraph wires whistle. Umbrellas used only with difficulty.
Sea: Some large waves, extensive white foam crests and some spray.

Maximum wind speed: 31mph (50km/h).
Probable maximum wave height: 13ft (4m).

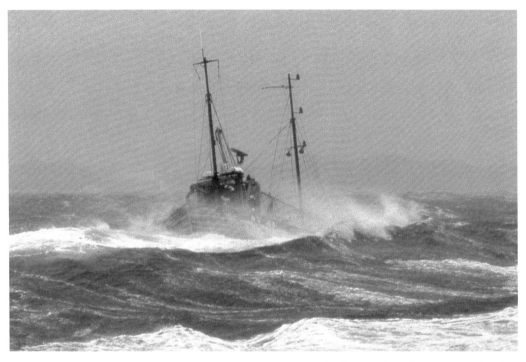

FORCE NINE *The hull of a 60ft (18m) fishing boat is almost concealed by waves and driving* *spray as it plunges through a strong gale off the Outer Hebrides in Scotland.*

FORCE SEVEN: NEAR GALE

Land: Whole trees in motion. Inconvenience felt when walking against the wind.
Sea: Sea heaped up. White foam from breaking waves blows out in streaks with the wind.

Maximum wind speed: 38mph (61km/h).
Probable maximum wave height: 20ft (6m).

FORCE EIGHT: GALE

Land: The wind generally impedes progress. Twigs break off trees.
Sea: Waves are long and moderately high. Spray, or spindrift, blows from their crests. Foam blown in clearly defined streaks.
Maximum wind speed: 46mph (74km/h).
Probable maximum wave height: 25ft (7.5m).

FORCE NINE: STRONG GALE

Land: Slight structural damage – chimney pots and slates are blown off.
Sea: Waves are high, their crests toppling, tumbling and rolling over. There are dense white streaks of foam and spray reduces visibility.
Maximum wind speed: 54mph (87km/h).
Probable maximum wave height: 33ft (9.75m).

FORCE TEN: STORM

Land: Rare in inland Britain. Considerable structural damage and trees uprooted.
Sea: High waves, with long overhanging crests, tumble heavily, shock-like. Sea surface appears white. Visibility poor.
Maximum wind speed: 63mph (101km/h).
Probable maximum wave height: 42ft (12.5m).

FORCE ELEVEN: VIOLENT STORM

Land: Widespread damage caused.

Sea: Exceptionally high waves, sometimes concealing small and medium-sized ships. Crests blown into froth. Foam everywhere. Visibility poor.
Maximum wind speed: 72mph (116km/h).
Probable maximum wave height: 53ft (16m).

FORCE TWELVE: HURRICANE

Land: Mostly confined to the tropics. Widespread damage caused.
Sea: The whole of the sea's surface is white with driving spray. Foam and spray fill the air and visibility is bad.
Maximum wind speed: Over 72mph (116km/h).
Probable maximum wave height: Unlimited.

Caught in a storm

The safest strategy for a small boat caught in a storm is to reduce power in order to steady the vessel and make it easier to control, and to secure everything movable.

In a sailing boat
• Reduce the sail area. Lash down deck gear.
• In stormy weather, it is usually safest to sail as nearly into the wind as possible – provided that this course does not take you into dangerous waters (see *Deciding what to do in heavy weather at sea*, page 264).

• Check the security of lifelines and jackstays (lines to which safety harnesses are clipped). Put on a life jacket if you are not already wearing one. Strap on a safety harness, too.
• Pump the bilge dry and check that the cockpit drains are clear. Close all other hatches, seacocks, ventilators and exhausts.
• Start the engine (if there is one) to check that it is working. Then shut it down to conserve fuel in case you need it later.

In a motor boat
• Head for the nearest shelter.
• Get passengers to squat as low as possible to improve the boat's stability.
• Head into the waves if possible, keeping speed low (to cut down spray and water from the waves). But keep up sufficient speed to maintain full steering power.
• If the engine fails, ride at anchor or put out a sea anchor – a cone-shaped canvas bag that

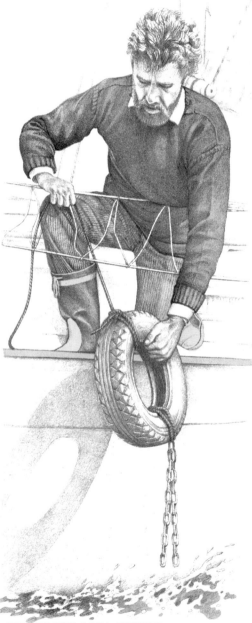

HOW TO USE A SEA ANCHOR
A sea anchor acts as a drag on a boat, keeping whichever end it is tied to pointing into the wind. It is usually trailed from the front.

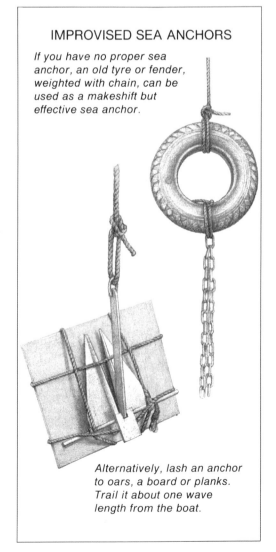

IMPROVISED SEA ANCHORS

If you have no proper sea anchor, an old tyre or fender, weighted with chain, can be used as a makeshift but effective sea anchor.

Alternatively, lash an anchor to oars, a board or planks. Trail it about one wave length from the boat.

will help to keep the front pointing into the wind.
• Avoid letting the boat swing sideways on to the waves. They could swamp or overturn it.

SAVED BY A CHILD'S CHATTER

On May 3, 1981, the Jeffery family – Les, a 37-year-old airport firefighter, his wife Virginia, son Darren, his 12-year-old daughter Tracy-Leigh and a family friend, Stewart Greenough – set out on a cruise off the east coast of Australia in their 47ft (14m) yacht Jedda.

Seven days later, in the early hours of the morning, battered by storm-force winds, they were forced to abandon ship. Roped together, the five tried to transfer from the Jedda to a rescuing oil tanker. But as the ships rolled, they were tossed into the water and pulled right under the tanker by the undertow.

The rope broke and Darren and Stewart were swept away. Their bodies were found later.

When Tracy-Leigh surfaced she found herself still tied to her mother and father. Her father was injured and her mother was floating face down – dead. In the darkness the tanker lost sight of the bobbing figures.

Tracy-Leigh knew that once her father lost consciousness he would drown in the huge waves. His only chance was to stay awake, so she talked to him – chattering about anything and everything. As she talked, she clung to her mother's life jacket because her own had been torn away against the tanker's hull.

Her talking worked. By the time a helicopter found them at dawn six hours later, she was exhausted – but her father was still alive.

Plotting a storm path

Storms are spirals of strong wind whirling around a low-pressure centre. In the Northern Hemisphere, the wind always blows in an anti-

---

WAYS OF SIGNALLING FOR HELP

The internationally recognised distress signal Mayday (which comes from the French phrase M'aidez, meaning 'Help me') should be used only when you are in grave and imminent danger and require immediate assistance. If you urgently need help but are not in imminent danger, use the signal Pan Pan (from the French panne, meaning 'breakdown'). Pan Pan is also the correct signal for man overboard.

Under the International Convention for the Safety of Life at Sea, there are a number of other recognised ways of calling for help. A ship's captain who sees any of these distress signals is legally obliged to respond to them.
• Gun or other explosive signal fired at intervals of about a minute.
• Continuous sounding of a fog signal, such as a foghorn.
• Rockets or shells throwing red stars fired one at a time at short intervals.
• Morse Code SOS (three dots, three dashes, three dots) transmitted by any means available.
• International Code flags NC (flag N above flag C), or a square flag with above or below it anything resembling a ball.
• Flames on a vessel (for example, burning tar, oily rags).
• Red parachute flare or red hand flare.
• Orange-coloured smoke.
• Slowly raising and lowering outstretched arms.

An additional sign – a piece of orange canvas with a black square and circle – can be used to attract the attention of aircraft. The British Merchant Navy's Red Ensign flown upside down has been used as a distress signal, but it is not internationally recognised under the convention.

Making a Mayday call

To call for help by radio, tune your transmitter to the international distress frequency: Channel 16 VHF or 2182kHz MF.
• Repeat the word 'Mayday' three times.
• Give the name of the craft three times.
• Repeat 'Mayday' once more.
• Repeat the name of the vessel once and then give its position, a brief description of the emergency and the help needed. Say 'over' at the end of the message.
• Listen for an acknowledgment before putting out the distress call again.

The phonetic alphabet

Phonetic alphabets use specific words to identify individual letters, in order to help to clarify a radio message. This is a widely used and internationally recognised list.

Alpha	Juliet	Sierra
Bravo	Kilo	Tango
Charlie	Lima	Uniform
Delta	Mike	Victor
Echo	November	Whisky
Foxtrot	Oscar	X-ray
Golf	Papa	Yankee
Hotel	Quebec	Zulu
India	Romeo	

clockwise direction around the storm centre. In addition the storm as a whole moves like a wandering top across the planet's surface at up to 25mph (40km/h).

If you are facing into the wind, the centre of a Northern Hemisphere storm is to your right. With your back to the centre of an approaching storm, the storm's fiercest weather is always to your right.

As the storm passes over, the direction of the wind changes. Sailors use the term 'veering' for a wind that shifts in a clockwise direction round the compass (N-E-S-W). A wind is said to be 'backing' if it shifts anti-clockwise around the compass (N-W-S-E).

You can roughly plot your position in relation to the storm centre and thus predict the likely weather by noting these changes in wind direction and keeping an eye on a barometer (see *How to read a barometer*, page 266). The barometric pressure falls as you get closer to a storm centre, and rises as you get towards the fringes. The faster the changes, the stronger the storm or the closer you are to the path of the storm centre.

The pictures on the right show how barometric pressure and wind direction change as a storm passes over three boats, all of which are sailing parallel to the storm path.

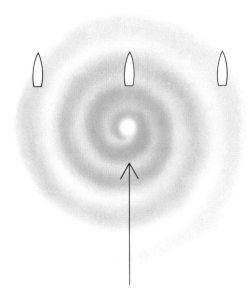

ANATOMY OF A STORM
In a full-blown storm, winds of more than 54mph (87km/h) whirl anti-clockwise around a relatively calm eye. In addition, the eye moves across the surface at anything up to 25mph (40km/h). The boats on this diagram are not to scale; a large storm can be 100 miles (160km) across, and gales can sweep out 50 miles (80km) beyond its fringes.

LEFT OF THE STORM CENTRE

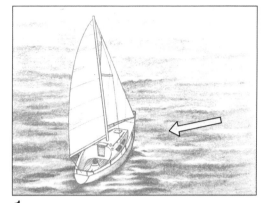

1 *A wind 'backing' anti-clockwise round the compass and a falling barometer mean you are left of the centre. Worse weather is coming.*

IN THE PATH OF THE STORM CENTRE

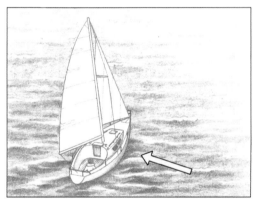

1 *As a storm overtakes a boat in front of the central 'eye', the barometer drops, but wind direction is steady. Weather worsens rapidly.*

RIGHT OF THE STORM CENTRE

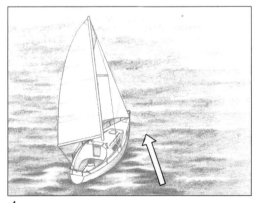

1 *A wind 'veering' clockwise round the compass and a falling barometer mean that you are in front of and to the right of the centre.*

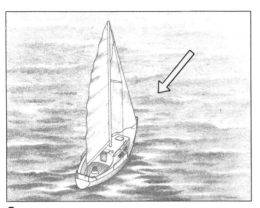

2 *Abreast and left of the storm centre, the barometer is steady and low, and the wind continues to back. The weather is at its worst.*

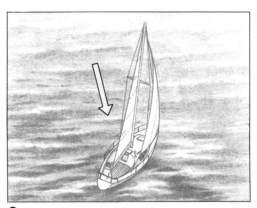

3 *A rising barometer means that the storm is moving away. The wind will go on backing, but the weather will gradually improve.*

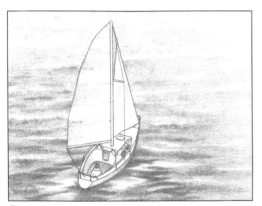

2 *In the eye, the barometer is low and steady, and the wind drops away. But high winds will return soon – from the opposite direction.*

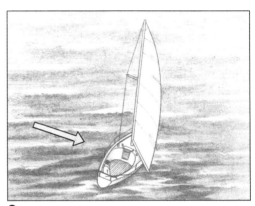

3 *A rising barometer means better weather is on the way. The wind, having reversed its direction, remains steady, but will ease soon.*

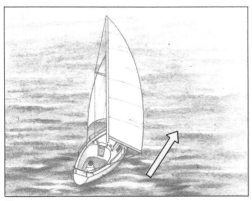

2 *Abreast and right of the centre, the barometer is low and steady, but the wind continues to veer. The weather is at its fiercest.*

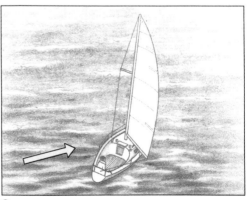

3 *As the storm moves away, the wind goes on veering and the barometer starts to rise. Better weather is on the way.*

Emergencies in the water

Abandoning ship

A small boat − even one that is badly holed − may take at least five minutes to sink. This gives you time to dress warmly, send out a distress signal and prepare to take to a life raft or the water. Do not abandon ship unless there is obviously no other course open to you. The greatest hazard you have to combat is the cold.

• Put on as many layers of warm, woolly clothing as possible, including a hat − and wear a final layer of waterproof clothing.

• Wear socks and light shoes as well to help to keep your feet warm.

• Put on a life jacket over the top of your clothes.

• Take with you personal and ship's papers and money, in a waterproof bag if possible.

• Send out a distress signal by radio, giving your position; or fire a distress flare or rocket (see *Ways of signalling for help*, page 271).

• Leave the boat from well forward or well aft of the mast to avoid being struck by spars or rigging if the boat heels over.

Taking to a life raft

• If you decide to take to a life raft, make sure that it has a line tied securely to the boat before you throw it overboard.

CHOOSING A LIFE JACKET

Not even a good swimmer can keep afloat in cold, rough seas for long without a life jacket. A life jacket for leisure use of a type approved by the British Standards Institution should carry the institution's kite mark and be marked with the number BS3595. A life jacket of this standard has 35lb (16kg) of buoyancy when inflated and will turn even an unconscious person to float face upwards within five seconds of entering the water.

There are three main types of life jackets: those that have to be blown up, either by mouth or by gas (a cylinder with a quick-release cord); those that are partly inflatable and partly made of permanently buoyant material; and those made wholly of permanently buoyant material.

Anti-splash hoods that can be fitted to most types of life jacket are now available. They protect the head from being swamped by splash and spray, which can drown anyone in a life jacket in even mildly choppy seas. The clear plastic hood is in a package that hooks to the jacket ties. It can be unrolled in the water and pulled over the head.

Inflatable life jackets are suitable for adults who swim well. Adults who cannot swim well should have partly inflatable types which provide at least some buoyancy while they inflate; and children (who are less buoyant than adults) should wear permanent-buoyancy types. A child should get used to putting on his own life jacket and to floating in it.

Waistcoat-type buoyancy aids are handier for good swimmers boating in sheltered or inland waters.

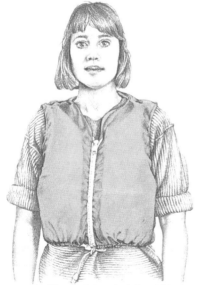

BUOYANCY AID *The waistcoat-style aid is less bulky than a life jacket but not so buoyant.*

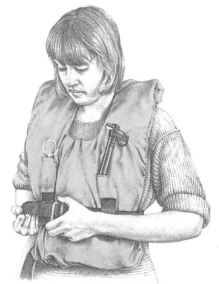

LIFE JACKET *A good life jacket will keep even an unconscious person floating face upwards.*

- If the life raft is an inflatable type, it will usually be fitted with an operating line to open the gas cylinder which inflates it. The line also acts as a mooring rope.
- Secure the operating line to the boat, throw the raft container overboard, then pull the line to inflate the raft.
- Board the raft as quickly as possible. The first aboard should be a strong, fit man to help in children or injured or weaker people.
- When everyone is aboard the raft, cut the line. On most inflatable rafts there is a covered-in area, and near its entrance is a safety knife. The knife is specially designed so that it can be used to cut the line without running the risk of causing accidental damage to the raft.
- Do not take off wet clothing. It will give some protection against heat loss.
- Unless you are within easy reach of shore, put out a sea anchor – a cone-shaped canvas bag that acts as a drag in the water. A sea anchor is often part of a life raft's equipment. It helps to keep the raft stable in heavy seas and helps to stop it drifting (see *Caught in a storm*, page 270).
- Try to stay as near to the wreck or its last position as possible. Rescuers will concentrate their search around the boat's last known position, and so you will have a better chance of being spotted and rescued quickly.
- Bail out any water in the raft bottom.
- Arrange a rota of lookouts to watch for rescuers. But keep the raft entrance closed as much as possible to keep warmth in.
- If the floor of the raft is inflatable, keep it topped up with air to provide insulation against

the cold water below. Take anti-seasickness tablets as soon as possible on the raft. Seasickness is common in survival craft and hastens the onset of cold and exhaustion.

If you have to jump into the water
- If there is no time to climb into a life raft and you have to jump straight into the water, go to the windward side – the side facing into the wind – so that the boat will not drift into you once you are in the water.
- Hold your life jacket down and away from your chin by crossing your arms over your chest. Cover your nose and mouth with one hand to keep the water out.
- Look straight ahead and jump feet first with your legs straight and together. Do not look down or you may fall forwards and land flat in the water, which is painful and could wind you.
- Your life jacket will bring you up to float at the surface within seconds. If you have an anti-splash hood on the jacket, unroll it and fasten it over your head (see box, opposite).
- Get well clear of the side of the vessel, especially if it is a large one. If you do not, you run the risk of being sucked under as it sinks.

Survival in the water
- Do not try to swim for the shore unless land is very near, because you will quickly become exhausted. The shore is often farther away than it looks, and rescuers are more likely to see the wreckage than to spot a lone swimmer.
- If you can, cling to floating wreckage with as much of your body out of the water as possible to cut down heat loss. The greatest loss of body

---

PROVISIONS FOR A LIFE RAFT

What you need on a life raft depends to some extent on the circumstances. If you are not far from shore, for example, you do not need to take food.

Most life rafts come supplied with survival packs on board. But before you go out to sea, make sure that the pack on your life raft has everything you are likely to need if you get into trouble. This is a list of the most important pieces of equipment:
Knife
Waterproof torch
Distress signals (flare pack)
Bailer bucket
First aid kit
Anti-seasickness tablets
Oars/paddles
Sea anchor and rope
Water and drinking cup
Length of buoyant rope – about 100ft (30m) –

with life buoy or rescue-quoit attached, for throwing to survivors in the water.

Coastguard Yacht and Boat Safety Scheme
When a small sailing boat or power boat is lost or in distress at sea, help may be delayed because no one knows anything about the boat. The Coastguard Yacht and Boat Safety Scheme aims to provide rescue services with the necessary information about small boats in their area.

All the sailor has to do is fill in and return to the coastguards a special postcard giving details of where he normally sails and in what sort of boat. The postcards are available from Coastguard Stations and most harbour offices and yacht clubs. Then, if the boat is overdue and a friend or relative ashore notifies the coastguards, they will have an idea where to look and what to look for.

heat is from the head, the neck, the armpits and the sides of the chest, and the groin.

• Stay in a group if there are several of you, to improve your chances of being spotted.

• If you are in a group of three or more in the water (all wearing life jackets), huddle close together for warmth with arms around each other's shoulders.

• Keep body movements to a minimum to preserve heat. If there is a child, sandwich him in the middle of the group, because children lose body heat faster than adults.

• If you are not in a group (and are wearing a life jacket), conserve body heat by sitting in the water, bringing your knees up and hugging them firmly to your chest. You do not need to paddle; the life jacket will keep you afloat. This is known as the Heat Escape Lessening Position (HELP), because it exposes as little of the body as possible to the water. In water of 10°C (50°F) – a typical sea temperature in British coastal waters – the average survival time before death from hypothermia is two and a half to three hours. Using the HELP position can enable you to survive for an hour or so longer, giving yourself more time to be found by rescuers.

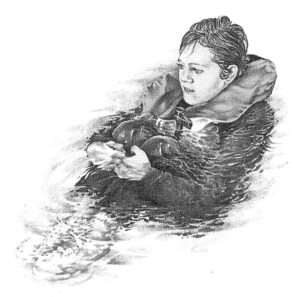

THE 'HELP' POSITION
The Heat Escape Lessening Position enables you to survive longer in cold water. Bring your knees up and hug them to your chest. Trust the life jacket to keep you afloat.

ADRIFT IN A SMALL BOAT

Anyone adrift in a small boat – a canopied life raft or an open boat – for any length of time has three crucial needs: protection from the weather; a supply of water; and some means of attracting attention.

Food is less important. Exposure to extreme heat or cold can kill much more quickly than starvation. A person can live for four weeks or so without food – but only days without fresh water.

• Try to limit your boat's movement through the water to make it easier for rescuers to find it.

• To help to keep your boat 'parked' in the water, turn the front into the wind and trail a sea anchor about one wave length away on the side from which the wind is blowing (see *Caught in a storm*, page 270).

• To conserve supplies, do not drink any water for the first 24 hours. Your supply of body fluid will still be adequate.

• After that, unless there is plenty of water from heavy rain, ration water to about 1¾ pints (1 litre) a day for each person aboard (more if possible in high temperatures). Drink it in small quantities throughout the course of the day.

• Send out distress signals at regular intervals. When using rockets or flares, fire them in groups of two, firing the second in the pair a few seconds after the first goes out. The first may be ignored, but the second will confirm the signal and may help to give rescuers a bearing. But use the flares sparingly, so that you keep a supply for use when help is in sight.

• In hot weather, keep as cool as possible. Shade your body, if you can. Avoid unnecessary movement. And soak your clothing in seawater during the day; this minimises the loss of body fluid through perspiration. Allow clothing to dry before nightfall, when it is likely to be much cooler.

• In cold weather, keep warm by huddling together and by regularly moving limbs, especially fingers and toes, to maintain blood circulation. Wrap up in as much clothing and blankets as possible.

• Collect rainwater or water that condenses on any cold surfaces on the craft – morning dew, for instance.

• Do not drink seawater, or use it to ease parched lips. Its salt content is three times greater than the amount the body can cope with, and it can cause death.

• If necessary, alleviate thirst by sucking a small object such as a button.

• Do not eat unless you have some water to drink with the food. Digestive processes use up precious body fluid.

When a canoe capsizes

A kayak (a covered-in canoe which is propelled with a double-bladed paddle) may have a small or large cockpit for the canoeist to sit in. In types with a small cockpit, canoeists often wear a soft, elasticated spray cover – or spray deck – which fits over the lip of the cockpit and keeps it watertight. There is a strap on the front of the spray cover which releases the cover from the cockpit lip when the strap is pulled.

• If you are thrown out when a large-cockpit canoe overturns, immediately grasp the boat and work your way along to one end, where it is easier to hold on.

• If you are trapped in your seat by a spray cover and you cannot right the canoe at once with your paddle, lean forward underwater and pull the spray-cover strap. Get out with a for-ward roll. If necessary, help yourself out by pushing against the boat just behind your hips.

• Once you are out, work your way along to the end of the hull. Hold onto it.

• Hang onto your paddle as well if you can.

• Do not try to right the canoe, but swim with it downstream across any current to the shore.

• If the land is too far, or you do not think you can reach it, stay with the canoe and wait for rescue. The boat will support you in the water.

Canoeing through surf

Canoeing off a beach calls for strength and a skill that can be learnt only by practice, starting in easy conditions. If you are caught in surf by accident, the golden rule is never to let the canoe get broadside to the waves.

Never launch a canoe into surf near rocks, swimmers, or a rip tide where there is a strong current moving out from the shore.

• If you are canoeing seawards, paddle firmly to maintain enough speed to be able to steer, and travel as far forward as possible between

---

CANOEING IN SAFETY

• Do not use a canoe unless you can swim at least 55yds (50m) wearing light clothing. Before setting out, pack extra buoyancy – in the form of special canoe air bags or empty plastic containers – into the ends.

• Always wear a life jacket or buoyancy aid – a buoyant waistcoat designed to allow maximum freedom of movement.

• Learn how to canoe safely at a club or on a course. Many canoe clubs in Britain organise proficiency tests designed by the British Canoe Union. The tests include dealing with a capsize.

• The union – whose head office is at John Dutteridge House, Ardbolton Lane, West Bridgford, Nottingham NG2 5AS, telephone Nottingham (0602) 821100 – has details of local canoe clubs and training courses, and prepares canoeing maps.

---

waves to get beyond the breakers. Meet each wave head on. At the same time lean back away from the crest and press your knees up against the deck to lift the bow over the wave.

• If you are heading for the shore and you do not have experience of riding waves, face into them – turning round between waves if necessary. Keep the bow pointing into the waves and paddle towards them as they break to keep the canoe straight.

• Between breakers, paddle shorewards or let the canoe drift backwards.

Emercencies in the water

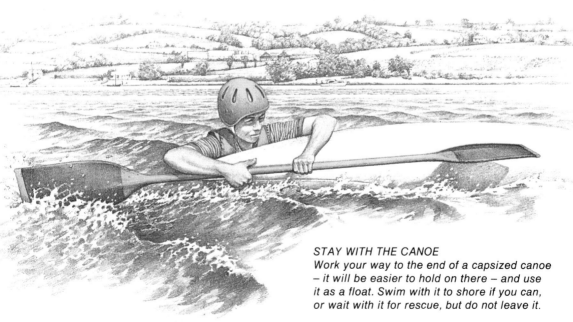

STAY WITH THE CANOE
Work your way to the end of a capsized canoe
– it will be easier to hold on there – and use
it as a float. Swim with it to shore if you can,
or wait with it for rescue, but do not leave it.

Canoeing: if you are caught in rapids

The noise of falling water and possibly a narrowing of the river are signs that you are approaching rapids. A white line of foam or spray may also be visible, or the water may appear to end unnaturally short of the horizon.

• Beach the canoe well before the start of the rapids, then walk along the bank and try to work out a safe route through them. If there is no safe route through, carry the boat round.

• If you are accidentally caught in the rapids, paddle firmly either forwards or backwards so that your speed is faster or slower than the water. This will help you to retain control of your course. If you let the water take you at its own speed, you will have no control.

• Areas of white, disturbed water and spray indicate rocks, fallen trees or other obstacles, which may or may not be visible. Avoid them.

• Aim for areas of darker, smoother water between disturbed, white-water patches. The channel will be deeper and safer there.

• If the canoe is swung right round by the current, do not try to turn it back again or you may be carried sideways and hit an obstacle. Continue through the rapids backwards, watching over your shoulder.

• Take bends on the outside if possible. The water is deepest there and flows faster, but be careful not to get swept against trees or banks.

• If the canoe slews round and is caught sideways against a rock, do not let it tilt upstream, or water will flood the cockpit.

• Throw your weight against the rock or obstruction to tilt the boat towards it. Hold the rock and use it to lever yourself and the canoe into a position where you can go forwards. (Take care not to let go of your paddle.)

• If this does not work, get out of the canoe quickly. Hang onto the rock and wait for rescue.

If you are swept over a weir

Weirs are perilous in the extreme, even for canoeists wearing full life jackets. Beginners should avoid them. Even if you are experienced, avoid a weir unless you are with others who have shot it before and who know what to do in an emergency. Never approach a weir where there are warning signs such as notices, cones or a boom. Stop well upstream and carry the canoe round it.

The reason for the danger is that water falling over a weir rolls back on itself after it hits the bottom, creating an endlessly circulating current – a spinning cylinder of water trapped by foaming breakers known as stopper waves. A swimmer or a boat caught in this deadly turbulence is tumbled over and over, and is constantly thrown back against the weir.

• If you are in a boat which gets trapped or capsized at the foot of a weir, abandon it.

• Dive down and away from the weir, *beneath* the turbulence.

• Swim underwater until you are well clear of the turbulence (you will be able to feel the swirling currents ease as you swim), then surface and make for the bank.

PLANNING YOUR ROUTE

Never canoe down a river or any other waterway until you have studied it on a map and noted any steep descents (where rapids are likely) and any weirs.

On specialist canoeing maps, such as those prepared by the British Canoe Union (see *Useful addresses*, page 385), rivers are graded according to an international coding system for rough water. The grades appear as the letters RW (Rough Water) or WW (Wild or White Water), followed by a number in Roman numerals. Grades I, II and III are easy, medium and difficult respectively. Grades IV-VI are taxing even for experts.

Always canoe in a group. Go through moderate rapids in single file, far enough apart to avoid collisions and for each canoeist to pick his own route. Severe rapids should be left to experienced canoeists, and then shot by one group member at a time, with the most experienced going first.

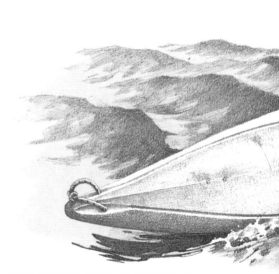

HOW TO GET PAST AN OBSTACLE
If the current sweeps you against a rock, lean downstream to keep water out of the cockpit and push the boat round it with your hands.

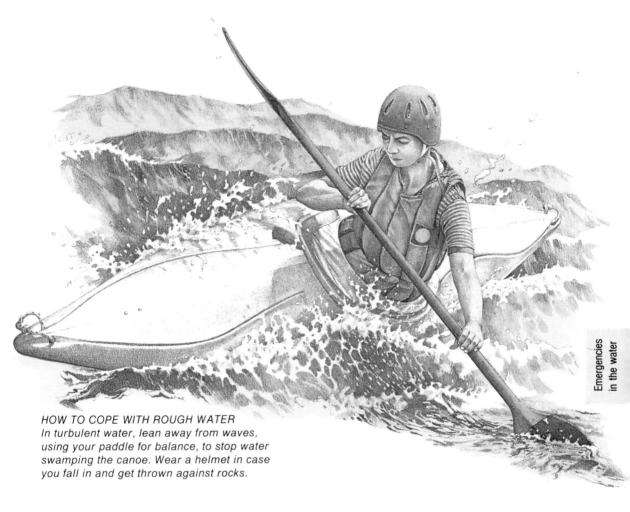

HOW TO COPE WITH ROUGH WATER
In turbulent water, lean away from waves, using your paddle for balance, to stop water swamping the canoe. Wear a helmet in case you fall in and get thrown against rocks.

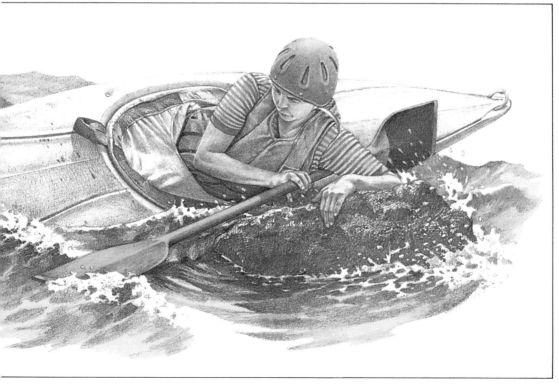

Emergencies on holiday and in the country

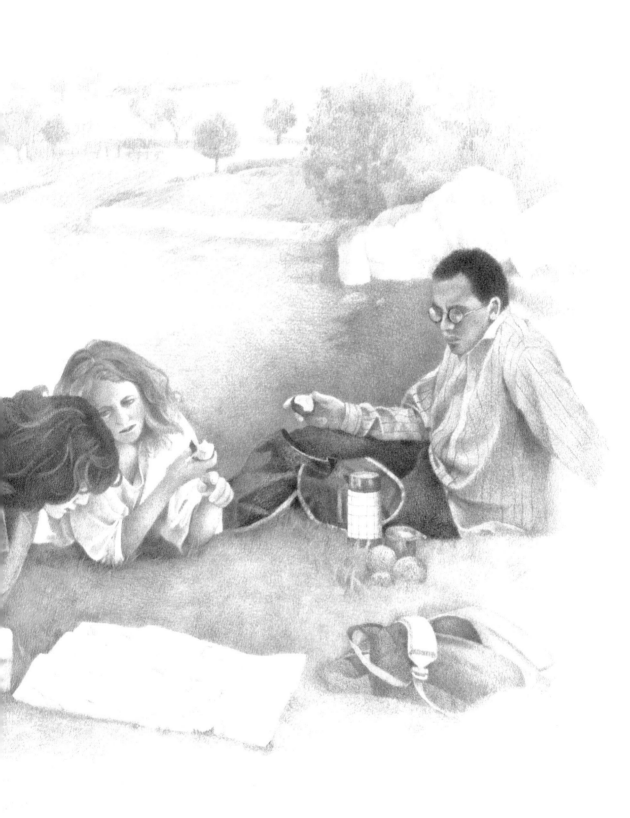

Travelling abroad

Air travel and holiday companies have brought some of the most exotic parts of the world within reach of millions of British holidaymakers.

But long-distance travel – particularly to tropical or Third World countries – carries special risks and problems as well.

You may, for instance, need to arrange visas or special immunisation against tropical diseases. You may need to take with you medicines that are freely available in Britain but almost unobtainable in the country you plan to visit.

It is worth thinking, too, about how you should take your spending money – as cash or travellers' cheques, for example – about which currency you should take, and about whether it makes sense to take notes and cheques in small denominations rather than large ones.

Once you arrive you may also, depending on where you are, have to take precautions against heat or altitude sickness, and to take care about what you eat and drink.

All these risks and difficulties are most likely to arise in tropical or Third World countries, not in the West. But some travel problems, such as the collapse of a holiday firm or travel agent, can affect holidaymakers anywhere (see *If your holiday firm goes out of business*, page 286).

Visas
● Check with the airline or travel agent at the time you book your flight whether you need a visa for the country you plan to visit.
● If you do need a visa, contact the country's embassy or consulate in Britain to find out how to get it. Alternatively, ask a travel agent to make the application for you. Many countries charge a fee for the visa and you may have to supply one or more passport-type photographs with your application.
● Allow extra time if you need more than one visa. Your passport will have to go to each embassy or consulate in turn to be stamped with the visa, and some countries can take several weeks to process the application.
● If you plan to visit countries which are politically hostile to each other – Israel and some of the Arab states, for instance – you may save yourself unpleasantness at the frontier by making sure that visas or entry stamps for the opposing countries do not appear in the same passport.
● In circumstances like these, it is sometimes possible to arrange for one or both of the visas to be stamped on separate sheets of paper which can be clipped to your passport and removed after the visit. Ask the consulates or embassies concerned whether they will agree to do this.
● Alternatively, contact the Passport Office in London and ask for a second passport valid only for one or other of the opposing countries. You can then take both passports with you and show one at each border.
● If the offending visa or stamp is the result of

an earlier trip, it is also possible simply to surrender your old passport – regardless of how long it has to run – and buy a new one.

Immunisation
● Find out from the airline or travel agent what the immunisation rules are in the country you are visiting. Airlines have an interest in keeping you up to date about the rules because they have to fly you home at their expense if you do not have all the right jabs.
● Consult a doctor about immunisation as well. Whatever the formal regulations, it may be medically advisable to get other jabs too, because people who live in a temperate climate such as Britain's have no natural immunity to diseases prevalent in the tropics and subtropics.
● Check up on immunisation at least three weeks before you travel. For immunisation against some diseases you will have to be given two injections at least a week apart and, if you need protection from several diseases, it may not be possible or medically desirable to have all the jabs at once.
● It is usually simplest to get immunised at an official immunisation centre. Your doctor can help you to find the nearest one. The advantage is that the centre can issue you with an officially stamped and internationally accepted certificate on the spot. If your doctor gives you the jab, the certificate has to be taken to the Health Department of the local town hall for stamping.
● Immunisation may be advisable against any or all of a number of diseases. The main ones are: cholera; hepatitis; poliomyelitis; typhoid; and yellow fever. Smallpox vaccination is no longer necessary for any foreign travel because the World Health Organisation has declared the whole world to be free of the disease.
CHOLERA The vaccine gives limited protection. The course is two injections 7-14 days apart.
HEPATITIS (jaundice) Injections of gamma globulin give limited protection against the disease, which is common in many tropical countries.
POLIOMYELITIS (infantile paralysis) The disease is still common in many parts of the Middle East and North Africa. The vaccine is usually dripped onto a sugar lump which is eaten.
TYPHOID Immunisation is advisable for all travellers going to the Mediterranean coastlands, Asia or the tropics, and is effective for a year. It takes the form of a single injection if time is short, or two injections at least 14 days apart.
YELLOW FEVER The disease, which is confined to the equatorial regions of Africa and the northern, tropical parts of South America, is spread by mosquitoes. Immunisation against the disease consists of a single injection which is effective for ten years.

Malaria
Travellers in tropical areas are particularly at risk from malaria, which is spread by mosquitoes. There is no system of immunisation, but

preventive medicines provide some protection.
• Contact a hospital for tropical diseases, an immunisation centre or an airline medical department and ask them for advice on which medicine to use. You usually have to start taking the medicine some days before entering a malarial area, and to keep taking it for some time after you have left it.
• Also get medical advice on a suitable insect repellent to reduce the risk of being bitten.
• Apply insect repellent in the evening, and put on a long-sleeved shirt and long trousers after dark, because malarial mosquitoes fly at night.
• If possible, stay only in air-conditioned hotels. Mosquitoes dislike cool places. If this is not possible, sleep under a mosquito net, and spray your room with insecticide before going to bed.
• If there is an electric fan in your bedroom, leave it on all night – mosquitoes also dislike draughts.

Medicines
• If you need to take medicines regularly, take a sufficient supply with you to last the entire holiday. Many drugs are unobtainable – or enormously expensive – in other countries.
• Consider taking pain-killing medicines, such as aspirin, and antidiarrhoeal medicines with you for the same reason.

Money
• If you become ill while you are out of Britain, you may have to pay on the spot for medical treatment, even if you have medical insurance and even in European countries which have social security arrangements with Britain. Take extra money to cover this possibility (see *Seeing a doctor overseas*, page 288).
• Carry minimum amounts of cash on you. Women should carry nothing of value in a handbag. It can easily be snatched.
• Instead, keep passports, air tickets and travel documents, travellers' cheques and other money in a hotel safe.
• If you have to carry valuables on you, use a money belt. Keep a note of your passport number, and its date and place of issue. It will speed up the process of getting a new passport from the nearest British consulate if the passport is lost or stolen abroad.
• Credit cards are now widely accepted in many countries. But keep a separate note of each number so that you can tell the company at once – by phone or fax – if you lose it (see *Lost credit card, cheque book or cheque card*, page 383).
• If you take money in the form of travellers' cheques, get them from a company which has offices in the country you are visiting and which will guarantee to replace them quickly – within a day or so – if they are lost or stolen.
• Buy insurance against the risk of your cash being lost or stolen; but remember that British insurance companies will usually refund the lost money only after you get home. You will not be able to replace it during the holiday.
• Get advice from a travel agent or airline about which currency is most easily negotiated. In some countries, cash and travellers' cheques in US dollars, German marks or Japanese yen are more readily accepted than sterling.
• During the holiday, shop around for the best

DIARRHOEA AND DYSENTERY

Despite taking precautions you may come down with traveller's diarrhoea – also called Montezuma's Revenge, Rangoon Runs, Aztec Two-Step, Delhi Belly and other names, depending on where you catch it. It generally lasts only two or three days and is often accompanied by vomiting, abdominal cramps and sweating. You can usually treat it successfully yourself.
• Drink bottled water in sufficient quantities to replace lost body fluid. Add a teaspoon of salt to each pint of water. Do not take any food or milk drinks.
• Take antidiarrhoeal medicines.
• When the vomiting and diarrhoea have settled for a few hours, start to eat bland food such as dry biscuits, jelly, blancmange and clear soup. Avoid tea, coffee and acid drinks such as fruit juice because they will further irritate the stomach lining.

Dysentery
Traveller's diarrhoea usually causes only a few days' discomfort and inconvenience. Dysentery is a much more serious cause of diarrhoea. There are two forms, one caused by bacteria and one caused by an amoeba. The amoebic form is more serious and very rare in Britain, but the symptoms of both kinds of dysentery are the same: severe diarrhoea and vomiting; stools often streaked with blood, pus or mucus; and gripping pains, tenderness and swelling in the abdomen. The symptoms usually appear 6–48 hours after eating infected food.
• See a doctor if: the symptoms are severe, persistent or getting rapidly worse; the disease was contracted in a country where amoebic dysentery is known to occur; or blood or mucus occur in the stools. Otherwise, treat as for traveller's diarrhoea.

rate of exchange. Hotels often give poor rates compared with banks, for instance. Some gift shops will also accept payment in foreign currency at better-than-usual rates.

• Aim to buy any international travel tickets you need – particularly air tickets – before you leave Britain. Immigration authorities in many Third World countries insist on travellers having a ticket to take them out of the country. If, on arrival, you do not have a return or onward ticket, you may have to pay a hefty deposit – which is sometimes difficult to reclaim later – or you may have to buy a ticket on the spot. In some countries, foreigners have to pay for such tickets in foreign currency at exchange rates which are much worse than usual.

• If you are visiting a country with a high rate of inflation, such as Russia or some South American countries, take your money in small-denomination banknotes. Exchange rates in these countries can change on a daily basis, so converting only small amounts into the local currency each day can make your money go significantly further.

• Many Third World nations have strict regulations governing how much of their local currency can be taken into or out of their country. Check with the country's embassy or consulate in Britain.

• Towards the end of your holiday, run down the amount of local cash you are carrying. It may not be possible or permissible to change local currency back into sterling before you leave, and the currency may have little value once you get back to Britain.

Clothing

• In hot and humid climates, clothes should absorb sweat, be loose-fitting, and reflect the heat. They should, therefore, be lightweight and light in colour.

• Cotton is the best material for hot-weather clothing. It is capable of absorbing 50 per cent of its weight in water. Avoid drip-dry clothes and those made of man-made fibres, particularly next to the skin. They have little ability to absorb sweat. As a result, sweat stays on the skin, encouraging prickly heat (see page 107).

• Take a lightweight hat and sunglasses for protection against hot sunshine and glare. In areas where snakes are likely, wear boots, not open sandals.

How to treat travel sickness

Seasickness, car sickness, air sickness – all are the same affliction, and about nine out of ten people suffer from it at some time or other. The symptoms include nausea, vomiting, sweating, faintness, pallor and diarrhoea.

Travel sickness occurs when the movement of a vehicle disturbs the relationship between what the eye sees and what the balance mechanism in the ear feels. The eye adjusts to the motion but the ear does not.

• If you feel sick, put your head back and hold it still. Lie flat, if you can, without a pillow.
• Take travel sickness pills.
• Get some fresh air – go up on deck if you are on a boat, or keep the car window open and make regular stops.
• Take small amounts of fluid regularly to avoid dehydration. Try also to eat small amounts of food regularly, even if you are vomiting.
• Stay away from smokers – particularly if you are a non-smoker. The smell may otherwise make you feel more queasy.

Food and drink

Numerous tropical and subtropical diseases are transmitted by food and drink which have been infected by bacteria, or contaminated by flies

---

PREVENTING TRAVEL SICKNESS

The most effective way to avoid feeling sick on a journey is to use travel sickness pills. The first one usually needs to be taken about 30 minutes before setting out. The pills may cause drowsiness, impair driving performance and enhance the effects of alcohol. Do not drive or operate machinery until the effects have worn off. This may take from four to six hours.

Travel sickness pills usually contain either hyoscine or an antihistamine. Hyoscine is the more effective but it can cause a dry mouth and constipation.

Antihistamines (such as cinnarizine, cyclizine and phenergan) are not quite as effective but have milder side-effects. The name of the active ingredient in the pills is given on the packet. If you have any health problems – particularly urinary or eye disorders – or are taking medicines, consult your doctor before taking travel sickness pills.

Several other techniques can also help to alleviate or avoid the miseries of travel sickness – whether or not you have taken a travel sickness pill.

• Do not have a large meal or alcohol before setting out.
• Eat small, easily digested meals before and during the journey.
• Keep occupied. This will keep your mind off feeling sick. But do not attempt to read or write during a car journey.
• Look out of the front of the car. Watching to the side at objects flashing past windows can make nausea worse.
• Look at the horizon, not at objects close by. This helps to keep the head still and lessens feelings of queasiness.

---

or unhygienic handling. The diseases include cholera, hepatitis and dysentery.

If you have any doubt at all about the cleanliness of the food and drink you buy or are offered, you can minimise the risks of infection by following a few guidelines.

• Avoid milk and tap water, unless they have been thoroughly boiled. Black tea or coffee, for instance, is likely to be safe to drink.

• Avoid unbottled cold drinks, ice cream and ice for the same reason. Freezing does not kill bacterial contamination – it merely suspends it until the ice melts. Bottled cold drinks are, however, usually safe.

• Avoid uncooked foods such as salads, locally prepared mayonnaise, raw vegetables and peeled fruit. All may have been washed in contaminated water, or made with contaminated milk, or contaminated by handling. Fruit you peel yourself, however, is safe to eat.

• Avoid eating in fly-blown restaurants. If flies are hovering thickly about the tables, the kitchen is likely to be much worse.

Altitude sickness – how to treat it

Climbing too high or too quickly in the mountains, or travelling in an unpressurised aircraft, can cause altitude sickness because of the reduced level of oxygen in the air.

The signs of a mild attack are breathlessness, palpitations, headache, loss of appetite and insomnia.

The symptoms of severe altitude sickness – which can cause serious lung damage if left untreated – are dizziness, nausea, vomiting, convulsions, severe thirst, weakness, drowsiness, blurred vision and hearing difficulties.

People usually begin to be affected on mountains over 10,000ft (3000m), but the symptoms can occur at as low as 6500ft (2000m).

• If you get a mild attack of altitude sickness, avoid all strenuous exercise until you become acclimatised. Go to bed and rest. The symptoms usually disappear on their own in 24-48 hours.

• If the symptoms do not ease in that time, or if they are severe, get medical help.

• Take a few breaths from an oxygen canister, if one is available. It will give immediate relief in a mild attack, and will be of some help even in a severe attack.

• If no medical help is available and severe symptoms persist, the only solution is to descend to a lower altitude at once. The symptoms will ease automatically as you lose height.

• Spend several days at a lower altitude before attempting to climb once more. Ascend in easy stages, getting acclimatised at each level before going higher.

When the sun is an enemy

Too much direct exposure to the sun can cause painful burns, especially to fair-skinned or freckled people. Darker skins respond more readily to sunlight than fair skins, by producing

---

HOW TO AVOID SUNBURN

• Avoid the sun as much as possible if your skin is very fair or freckled.

• Keep small children well covered.

• Use sun-tan cream or lotion applied frequently. Remember, though, that artificial tan preparations which simply colour the skin may not protect you. Consult the chemist when buying.

• Limit your time in the sun to no more than half an hour on the first day, an hour on the second, adding 30 minutes on succeeding days.

• Take care when sailing, swimming or skiing – you can still get burnt even when you are feeling cool.

• Protect your skin in cloudy weather – most of the ultraviolet rays in sunlight can penetrate clouds.

• Men should not use aftershave.

• The main defences against heat exhaustion and heat stroke are to wear a hat that shades the back of the neck, and to drink plenty of water. In extreme conditions, take salt tablets as well.

---

a brown pigment (melanin) which screens out harmful rays. Freckled skins are particularly prone to solar burns because their melanin does not spread evenly.

Too much heat – in or out of direct sunlight – can induce heat exhaustion or heat cramp, and a more dangerous condition, heat stroke, which can kill (see *Heat exhaustion and heat stroke*, page 106).

Particular care is needed when visiting countries hotter than Britain, and in mountains, where thin air offers less protection against the sun's rays than the more absorbent atmosphere at lower levels.

In minor cases of sunburn, the skin reddens for three or four days with little discomfort, then tans. In more severe cases, the reddened skin becomes painful and tender, the tissues swelling up after a few hours.

Within 48 hours, when the condition is at its worst, the skin may blister and perhaps crust. Finally, a few days later, it peels.

This sequence of discomforts results from the body's complex reaction to the ultraviolet rays in sunlight, as the skin releases potent chemicals that include histamine, prostaglandins, kinins and serotonin.

A sun-tan preparation offers some protection – but keep applying it. Severe cases need treatment (see page 135). Complete recovery – even from severe sunburn – is normal within 30 to 60 days.

Emergencies on holiday and in the country

If your holiday firm goes out of business

Holidaymakers travelling on package tours from Britain are very unlikely to be stranded abroad for more than a day or so if the holiday firm they book with goes out of business during the holiday. Rescue schemes, financed by holiday firms and administered by the Association of British Travel Agents (ABTA) or the Civil Aviation Authority (CAA), protect most holidaymakers against this risk.

The ABTA scheme covers all holiday firms which are members of the association – whether they carry passengers by air, sea or land. The CAA scheme covers holiday firms to which the authority has issued an Air Travel Organiser's Licence (ATOL), but which are not ABTA members.

By law, any holiday firm offering air tickets on a charter basis must have an ATOL. Each ATOL has a number, and the holiday firm should quote its ATOL number in its publicity material. You can check whether your holiday firm has an ATOL by telephoning the CAA at its head office in London on 071-379 7311.

ABTA members should also display the association's symbol in their publicity material. You can check whether the firm is a member by telephoning the association's head office in London on 071-637 2444.

There is, in addition, a third rescue scheme, run by a group of the smaller British tour operators – the Association of Independent Tour Operators (AITO). They can be contacted on 081-744 9280. All of these schemes try to ensure that people already on holiday can continue with no disruption.

• If you are in any doubt whether the company you plan to use is covered by one of the rescue schemes, check with ABTA, AITO or the CAA before you part with any money – not afterwards.

• If you book a holiday which does not involve air travel, make sure that the firm you use is a member of ABTA or AITO. Otherwise you will not be protected and will need to buy insurance to guard against the risk of the firm's collapse.

• If your holiday firm collapses before you leave, contact ABTA if it is an ABTA member or the CAA if it has an ATOL, or AITO. The CAA will give you a refund. ABTA will offer you a refund.

• If your holiday firm is covered by one of the rescue schemes and it collapses while you are on holiday, there should be no need for you to do anything yourself. The holiday firm's local representative, or officials from the rescue scheme, will normally make the necessary arrangements and keep you informed.

• Nonetheless, take extra money on holiday with you. Even if you are protected by one of the rescue schemes or are fully insured, you may have to pay certain bills on the spot and claim the money back later. Your hotel, for example, may demand money for your room and meals – even though you have already paid the holiday firm.

• Keep receipts for all expenses you incur. If you have to organise any journey on your own, keep all booking documents and ticket stubs. You will need them to claim a refund.

• If your holiday firm was not covered by a rescue scheme, you can claim compensation from the collapsed firm. But there is likely to be a long wait, and you are very unlikely to get all your money back.

• Another way to cover yourself against the costs of a broken holiday is through insurance. Some holiday firms include cover for these expenses as part of a standard insurance package which is offered to holidaymakers. The insurance policy will explain exactly what costs are covered. Alternatively, get advice from an insurance broker, your travel agent or from one or more insurance companies.

If your travel agent goes out of business

The Association of British Travel Agents (ABTA) also administers a scheme designed to protect holidaymakers if the travel agent they book through goes out of business before they travel.

If, for example, you have already paid for an airline ticket but have not received the ticket from the travel agent before it goes out of business, ABTA will make sure you get the ticket or a refund. This scheme, though, covers only agents who are ABTA members.

• Make sure that the agent you use is a member of ABTA. The scheme does not protect you if a non-member goes out of business between the time you pay him and the time the holiday firm confirms your booking. If the agent does go out of business during this period you are very unlikely to get your money back.

• Once the holiday firm's confirmation comes through, however, the collapse of the travel agent will not affect your holiday – regardless of whether the agent was a member of ABTA.

• Travel agents who are members of ABTA should have a sign in their office saying so. But you can check by telephoning ABTA on 071-637 2444. If in doubt, contact ABTA before handing over any money.

If your airline goes out of business

If you travel overseas with a holiday firm, the firm remains responsible for looking after you, should any airline it uses go out of business. It is the holiday firm's responsibility to find a replacement airline or to compensate you if it cannot. If you have bought your ticket direct from the airline, however, you may have to find some other way of reaching your destination. You are very unlikely to get the full cost of your ticket back from the failed airline.

• Take your ticket to another airline flying the route you want to travel, and ask the airline to book you onto one of its flights. Airlines which are members of the International Air Transport Association (IATA) will usually accept tickets issued by other member airlines, and may

SYMBOLS OF SECURITY

Look out for these symbols at your travel agent and on holiday brochures.

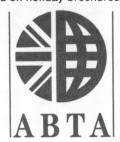

You will be protected if an ABTA member goes out of business.

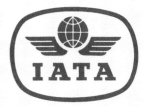

International Air Transport Association airlines may help IATA ticket-holders.

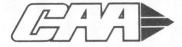

The Civil Aviation Authority will get you home if your firm has an ATOL licence.

accept tickets from non-member airlines as well. But they are not obliged to.

• If you cannot persuade another airline to accept your existing ticket, you will probably have to pay for a new ticket yourself. If you are insured against this possibility, though, you will be able to claim the cost of the new ticket back from the insurance company later.

If you miss your plane

If you arrive at the airport and discover that you have missed your plane, go immediately to the airline check-in desk for help. Whether you will be able to get on another flight depends on what type of ticket you have.

If you have paid the full normal fare, the ticket will be valid for a year and will not restrict you to a specific flight.

A charter, special excursion or cheap ticket is likely to have conditions attached to it. Restrictions such as 'Valid only for flights and dates shown' will be written on the ticket.

• Show your ticket to the person at the check-

in desk and explain what has happened. Ask to be put on the next available flight.

• If you have an unrestricted ticket, the airline is obliged to put you on the first flight with seats available, possibly with another airline.

• If the next few flights are fully booked, ask for a connecting flight to another airport and get a flight to your destination from there.

• If you have bought a cheap ticket, the airline company may be willing to find you an alternative flight, but is not obliged to.

• The only reliable way to avoid the risk of missing a flight and perhaps having to buy a new ticket is to give yourself plenty of time to reach the airport.

If you make your own holiday arrangements

If you arrange a foreign holiday as an individual – booking directly with a foreign hotel, say – and the hotel goes out of business, there are no official schemes to help you to get back to Britain or to help you to get your money back.

You could sue the foreign company for compensation, but it would probably not be worth doing unless the sum involved was very large.

The only reliable way to guard against the risk is to book through a travel agent which is a member of ABTA.

If your journey is held up

If bad weather, technical faults or industrial disputes delay your journey, in Britain or overseas, the airline, ferry company or coach firm you have booked with will often provide refreshments and even overnight accommodation during the delay.

But airlines, ferry companies and coach firms are not obliged to look after passengers during a delay. So if you are held up for days because of a dock strike, you cannot claim compensation from the ferry company. You can only claim under an insurance policy – if you have one that covers such risks.

On a package holiday – where you have booked with a holiday firm rather than directly with a transport company – the same principles apply. The holiday firm will usually look after holidaymakers held up at docks or airports. But it is not obliged to unless its booking conditions contain a promise to do so.

If the booking conditions do not contain such a promise, consider buying insurance to cover the costs of delays. Many holiday firms include this cover in their standard package.

Emergencies on holiday and in the country

Seeing a doctor overseas

Medical treatment abroad can be extremely expensive – especially in the USA. The safest way to guard against the expense of an accident or illness is to buy medical insurance. In some countries, however, it is possible to get some treatment free or at reduced rates.

Major bills – for a stay in hospital, say – may be settled by the insurance company direct. Smaller bills, however, for a visit to a doctor or a dentist, or for medicine, will usually have to be paid on the spot, and the money reclaimed after you get back to Britain.

Getting free or cheap treatment

Britain has health agreements with a number of countries, under which UK citizens and residents are entitled to free or cheap medical treatment – and, sometimes, dental treatment.

The main countries are other members of the Common Market. Other countries which in 1993 were offering free or cheap treatment under similar agreements were: Australia; Austria; Bulgaria; the Channel Islands; Czech Republic; Finland; Hong Kong; Hungary; Iceland; Isle of Man; Malta; New Zealand; Norway; Poland; Romania; Russia; Sweden; and a number of British Dependent Territories including Anguilla and the Falkland Islands.

The agreements do not, however, cover the cost of getting you home if you are ill, nor do they cover non-medical costs, such as repairs to your car after a crash or making alternative travel arrangements. You can guard against these expenses by buying insurance.

The details of the entitlements vary from country to country. In Germany, for instance, medical and dental treatment are normally free, but you have to pay for treatment in hospital. In Norway, by contrast, treatment in hospital as an in-patient is normally free, but you have to pay for medical and dental treatment.

The entitlements also change from time to time depending on the policy of the government involved. Whatever the detailed rules, however, the initial steps to take are the same.

• At least a month before you travel, ask the nearest office of the Department of Health for a copy of the leaflet T4, *Health Advice for Travellers*. The office's address will be in your local telephone directory, listed under 'Health'. The leaflet explains in detail what you are entitled to in each country, and how you can claim it. The claiming procedure varies from country to country.

• In some countries, the only evidence you need to establish your entitlement to free or cheap treatment is a passport. In other countries, however, you may need to show a driving licence, a National Health Service medical card, or a special certificate known as an E111.

• If you need an E111 – the leaflet makes clear whether you do or not in the country or countries you are visiting – fill out the application form which is inside the leaflet and send the form to the DSS. The countries for which UK citizens needed an E111 in 1993 were: Belgium; France; Germany; Greece; Italy; Luxembourg; and the Netherlands. But since international agreements can change at any time, it is always worth checking with the DSS.

• Take the E111 and the leaflet with you on your holiday.

• In some countries you have to pay the bill and claim a refund before you return to Britain. The leaflet and the E111 explain how to claim a refund in each country. In many countries, though, you will not get all the money back. In Belgium and France, for example, the refund amounts to only about three-quarters of what you pay.

• If you do not have enough money with you to pay the bill, contact your bank in Britain by phone or telegram, or go to a local bank and make contact from there.

• If you cannot raise the money from your bank, contact the nearest British consulate for assistance.

Medical insurance

Insurance against medical emergencies abroad can be bought through travel agents and motoring organisations, or direct from insurance firms. It is often included in a package covering cancellation and lost or stolen baggage and money. The policy will make clear which risks are covered, and for how much.

Some travel insurance packages now include unlimited medical cover for little more than the standard premium. This option may be attractive to holidaymakers such as motorists and skiers, who run extra risks, or to people travelling to countries such as the United States and Canada, where medical costs are much higher than in Western Europe.

• Make a copy of the policy or certificate to leave at home, and take the original with you on holiday as evidence that you are covered (a photostat copy may not be acceptable). Show it to the hospital or doctor you see, if you want to delay paying the bill until you get home.

• How much cover to buy depends in part on your age and medical condition. For Europe, cover of about £2 million will be adequate for most people. The premium for this amount for a fortnight is likely to amount to between £15 and £20.

• For North America cover of about £5 million (which, for two weeks, is likely to cost between £60 and £70) should usually be adequate.

• Check when you buy the policy how soon you have to notify the company if you need to make a claim. The policy may require you to phone or send a telegram as soon as possible – not when you get home.

• If you have to pay on the spot, get a receipt and send it to the insurance company with your claim form when you get home (see *Making an insurance claim*, page 381).

Aboard a crashing train or plane

Train and plane crashes often seem more terrifying than a car crash because they involve such large numbers of people.

In fact, your chances of being injured in a train or plane are far smaller than your chances of being hurt in a road accident.

If your train crashes

There is unlikely to be much warning before a train crash, but you might feel the emergency brakes go on, and in the seconds before final impact you may be able to take up a safer position.

• Get clear of windows and doors. Throw yourself to the floor, if necessary. Hang on to anything fixed to prevent yourself being thrown out of the carriage.

• Brace yourself against anything solid.

• Tuck your chin down onto your chest. This will help to protect your neck against the risk of whiplash injury.

• If you are sitting with your back to the engine, away from windows and doors, stay put.

• If you are not sitting with your back to the engine, away from windows and doors, move into this position if you can, but do not risk being caught unsupported when the impact comes.

• Do not try to jump out of the train, even if it careers for some distance off the tracks. While you remain in the train, the compartment will absorb some of the crash impact. If you jump out, your body hitting the tracks will receive the full force. There may also be a danger from a live rail or other hazards – broken equipment, for example. A broken train battery could create a pool of acid which would be indistinguishable from a rain puddle.

• Once the train has come to rest, assess the situation. In a busy area, or if the train is trapped in a tunnel, it may be best to stay put until official

---

RESCUE ON THE 5.54

Three people died when a London commuter train crashed into the side of a goods train outside Wembley on the evening of October 11, 1984. All three died because they were thrown through or against the broken windows of the first carriage, and crushed as it rolled.

Army Staff Sergeant Peter Kemp was saved from going the same way by the strength of 38-year-old Warrant Officer Colin 'Slim' Cheetham of the Royal Signals.

Staff Sergeant Kemp, then 39, escaped with cuts and cracked ribs. 'The carriage rolled over to the left and was dragged along the line,' he said later.

'The carriage window broke and all I could see was the railway line. Slim got behind me and got his arm under my tummy and was pulling me away from the window.'

A man in the same carriage who fell onto the window was killed.

---

help comes. Wandering about outside the train may expose you to further dangers, particularly since you are likely to be in a state of shock after a crash.

• If there is a live rail, do not get out of the train until you are told by rail staff that the current has been turned off.

• The most modern long-distance carriages have double-thickness glass which is unlikely to break even if the carriage turns over. If you need to get through the window – if the exits at either end of the coach are blocked, for example – break out using the hammers which are kept in red boxes at each end of the coach.

• Once you are outside, call the emergency services. If you are near a set of signals, there is often a telephone at the base of them. Use it to call the signal box. If there is a public call box or a house nearby, contact the emergency services by dialling 999.

If a train door swings open

Leaning out of a moving train to close a door is extremely dangerous – trains coming in the opposite direction pass within inches. A sudden jolt could also throw you out of the train.

• If you find a door open on a moving train, do not try to shut the door.

• Move well away from the open doorway, and get others to do the same.

• Notify a guard, or, if this is not possible, pull the communication cord. Do not take any other action until the train has stopped. Let the train staff deal with the problem. They will want to check the door lock.

If your plane crashes

Being frightened of flying is a common and understandable problem among air passengers. Doctors believe that the fear is often related to the fear of being helpless if things go wrong, or the fear of being in a confined space. Ask your doctor's advice if the fear is serious. Otherwise, keep reminding yourself that air travel is safer than motoring.

The riskiest part of any journey by air is the beginning and the end; six out of ten plane crashes happen on takeoff or landing.

So listen carefully when the cabin crew brief you on emergency procedures at the start of the flight, and make yourself familiar with safety features such as exits before the plane leaves the ground.

• Identify the nearest emergency exit to your seat. Memorise its position and how to open it – the instructions will be on the door. In the aftermath of a crash, you might have to find and open it in thick smoke.

• Read the emergency procedures card in the seat pocket in front.

• In the event of an emergency, follow the instructions of the cabin crew. They are highly trained in emergency procedures.

• If instructed, remove any spectacles, dentures

and high-heeled shoes you are wearing. Also remove sharp objects such as pens and pencils from your pockets.

• If there is smoke in the aircraft, protect your nose and mouth with a handkerchief. Wet the handkerchief, if possible. Keep near the floor when moving to the emergency exit.

• Escape slides inflate automatically when the door is opened. Jump onto the slide in a seated position.

• When you reach the ground, move well away from the aircraft. Do not attempt to go back for personal belongings.

• If you or someone else has been injured, tell one of the crew. They are trained in first aid, and have the equipment necessary for dealing with casualties.

• While waiting for outside help to arrive, try to keep up morale by chatting to and comforting other passengers.

HOW TO STAY COMFORTABLE IN THE AIR

• Choose your flight schedule carefully. If you are travelling east or west across time zones, plan to arrive early in the evening by local clocks so that you can get to bed shortly after arrival.

• Plan to arrive early at the airport and give yourself plenty of time to get there. More heart attacks occur at airports than during flight. This is due chiefly to passengers panicking on late arrival (see *If you miss your plane*, page 287).

• If you have a choice of seats, try to get as far forward in the plane as possible. The ride will be more comfortable there, which is why first-class compartments are always at the front. Noise and vibration tend to be worst near the tail. There is no evidence, though, that where you sit makes any difference to your safety in the event of a crash.

• Wear casual, loose-fitting clothes and shoes for the flight. Sitting upright for long hours may cause stomach, ankles and feet to swell, and make tight clothes uncomfortable.

• Carry a comfortable sweater to slip on or off. Temperatures may change even on a short flight. On a longer flight, climatic conditions may vary enormously. When it is winter in England, for instance, it is high summer in Australia. Think about climatic changes at refuelling stops, and dress appropriately for the weather. Make a note of the local time at these stops; a desert airport at night can be surprisingly chilly. Take a sponge bag, too, so that you can freshen up en route.

• Avoid smoking, or, if you are a compulsive smoker, cut it down. Smokers are more affected by high altitudes than non-smokers, because tobacco smoke hinders the body's ability to absorb oxygen. In flight, the oxygen level in the air inside the plane – which is usually pressurised to the equivalent of an altitude of 6000-7000ft (1830-2130m) – is lower than when on the ground.

• If you experience popping in the ears, do not worry. It is perfectly normal and occurs as air in the middle ear adjusts to the air pressure in the cabin. To clear your ears on the ascent, swallow; on the descent, shut your mouth, hold your nose and try to blow out gently. Try to avoid flying if you have a heavy cold or sinus problems, but if you have to fly, use a nasal decongestant.

• Make a point of drinking plenty of liquid during a long flight. Aim to consume 4-5 pints (2-3 litres) of liquid every 24 hours. At high altitudes, the aircraft cabin air is extremely dry, and you lose fluid which must be replaced if you are to avoid increased fatigue and dehydration. The best drinks are water and fruit squashes.

• Avoid alcohol, because it dehydrates the body. Coffee and tea also tend to dehydrate, so drink them sparingly.

• Aircraft meals help to relieve the boredom of a long international flight. But try to time your meals so that they conform to your normal eating pattern. For example, if your internal clock says it is 2am, it is best to avoid a meal because your gastrointestinal system has largely shut down for the night. If you do want something, drink water or a fruit squash.

• Sleep as much as you can on a long flight. Even dozing or taking short naps will help to minimise jet lag – the disorientation caused by crossing several time zones.

• Travel sickness (see page 284) is rarely experienced today on large jet aircraft. They rapidly penetrate bad weather and cruise high above it, so the effects of motion and acceleration are minimal.

• If you are prone to travel sickness, try to get a seat away from the windows and in the centre of the aircraft, where there is the least motion.

• If you use travel-sickness pills, take the first dose 30 minutes before takeoff, and others at recommended intervals thereafter. Remember, though, that some pills, such as antihistamines, cause drowsiness; they should be avoided if you plan to drive at the end of the flight.

Coping with a caravan tyre puncture

A caravan tyre may puncture when you are miles from a telephone. If you have no spare and no tyre inflators (see *Spare parts for everyday motoring*, page 225), you may be tempted to leave the caravan and seek help – leaving it vulnerable to thieves or vandals.

But there is a way to make an emergency repair on the spot.
• Jack up the caravan under its axle.
• Remove the wheel and undo the tyre valve to let the air out. Then stand on the tyre and tread out any air left in it (jumping on it will help).
• Use a jack handle or tyre lever to prise one edge of the tyre over the wheel rim.
• Having exposed the inside of the tyre, pack in any soft vegetation to hand – for example, grass, straw, bracken, heather, leaves or sea-weed. Stand the wheel upright to check that the vegetation is packed solidly.
• Refit the tyre to the rim. To get the last part of the bead back over the rim, unhook the caravan and lay the wheel flat, in front and just to the side of the car. Drive across the edge of the tyre just behind the unfitted bead. Be careful not to drive over the metal rim of the tyre; you could crush it. Then refit the wheel.
• Hook up the caravan and drive slowly to the nearest telephone or garage to arrange a proper repair. Check the state of the tyre frequently and, if necessary, pack it with more vegetation.

SITING A CARAVAN SAFELY

On most caravan sites, pitches are allocated when you book in. But on some you are allowed to choose a pitch in an allotted field, and if you get a landowner's permission, you may be able to camp 'wild' on his property. Take care in choosing your site.
• Ask local people what direction the prevailing wind blows from, and look for firm, flat ground sheltered from it. Listen to local radio weather forecasts as well.
• Farm buildings, natural banks and thick hedgerows will all help to break the wind. Avoid tall trees, however – they could themselves be blown over in high winds.
• Avoid any area that looks prone to flooding – riverside meadowlands, for example.
• On sloping ground, use the corner steadies to adjust the height from front to rear and make the van as level as possible. Chock up the wheels to prevent the caravan rolling.
• If you park across the slope, dig a trench, if necessary, to lower the higher wheel. This is safer than jacking up the lower wheel because it keeps the caravan's centre of gravity nearer the ground and thus improves its stability.
• Check whether the clearance underneath the caravan affects the positioning of the waste-water container. If it does, you may have to dig a space for the container or turn the caravan round.
• Replace soil and turf before leaving.

Securing a caravan against theft
Protecting a caravan against theft is more like guarding a house than guarding a car.
• Fit secure locks and an efficient alarm system. Display conspicuously a sign warning that the caravan is fitted with an alarm – even if you do not in fact have one.
• Make sure that any gas cylinders are secure by locking their container. If they have no container, chain and padlock them to their carrier or fixing clamps.
• Lock the towbar into a cover (known as a hitchlock) so that the caravan cannot be towed away. If the cover has a padlock, make sure the padlock has an enclosed shackle so that it cannot be cut through.
• Make sure the corner legs cannot be raised, either by padlocking the steel collars that enclose the heads of the threaded rods or by locking each leg, using what is known as a 'steady' clamp.
• Whenever you leave the caravan, lay out a table set for a meal with plates, cups, cutlery, bread and so on. This will suggest an imminent return to any potential burglar.
• If you are leaving the caravan for a short period, hang washing on the line and leave a radio playing inside.
• Consider fitting a timeswitch or electronic trigger to turn the caravan lights on if it is unoccupied after dark.
• When you go away on day trips, ask a neighbour or the site warden to keep an eye on the caravan for you.
• If you plan to stay at one site for some time, get locking wheel nuts fitted, or use wheel clamps. Clamps also help to make the wheel into a stable, rigid support.
• Consider having each of the caravan windows etched or engraved with your postcode and the number of your house (or the first two letters of its name). This will make the caravan easier to identify if it is stolen, and may discourage a thief. The Caravan Club or a local police station should be able to advise on where to get the marking done. The Caravan Club's information office is at East Grinstead House, East Grinstead, West Sussex RH19 1UA; telephone (0342) 326944.

Emergencies on holiday and in the country

Righting an overturned caravan

If high winds topple a caravan onto its side, the safest course is to get expert help from a garage or motoring organisation. But it is possible to get the caravan back up on your own.

To use the technique, you need three fairly strong adults and at least 60ft (18m) of stout rope such as that used by climbers. You also need to practise the pulley knot shown here. It uses the rope to make a series of loops which act like pulleys, giving you extra leverage. Once you have mastered the knot, however, you can use it in any situation to move much heavier weights than you could otherwise handle: to help to free a car stuck in mud, for example.

• Remove as much equipment as possible from the caravan, and put it in the car. If the door is inaccessible, get into the caravan through an end window. Turn off any gas cylinders and disconnect the electricity as well.

• Raise the corner legs, or 'steadies', on the lower side. Put a block against the lower wheel, too, to stop it slipping. Lower the upper steadies slightly – not fully – so that they will make a three-point touchdown with the wheel.

• Tie the middle of the rope securely to the upper axle or a nearby part of the chassis. Then make the pulley knot shown here. Put the loop at the end of the knot round a sturdy stake driven into the ground at an angle.

• Throw the rope's other end over the caravan and wind it twice round a second stake to make a lowering line.

• Pull slowly and carefully on the free end of the rope. Ask at least two adults to pay out the lowering line gradually at the same time. Use as many adults as are available.

• Alternatively, you may be able to use the car either to help to pull the caravan up or in place of one of the stakes. Attach or loop the rope round the car's towing bracket.

• As the caravan comes upright, do not let it drop the last few feet; you could damage the axle and sub-frame. Let it down carefully.

HOW TO MAKE A PULLEY KNOT

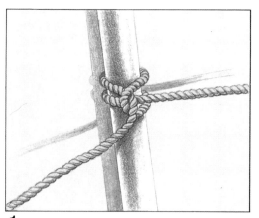

1 *Attach the middle of the rope firmly to the caravan's axle or chassis. Throw one end over the caravan to make the lowering line.*

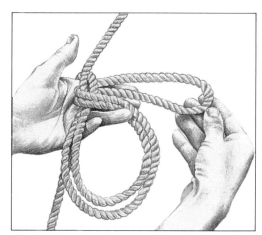

2 *Make a fold in the other rope about 2ft (600mm) from the fixing point, and bring the doubled section across and behind the rope.*

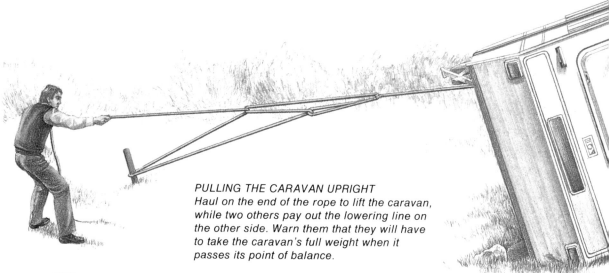

PULLING THE CARAVAN UPRIGHT
Haul on the end of the rope to lift the caravan, while two others pay out the lowering line on the other side. Warn them that they will have to take the caravan's full weight when it passes its point of balance.

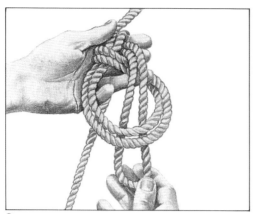

3 *Bring the end of the folded section round the rope and push it through the loop to make a figure-of-eight pattern.*

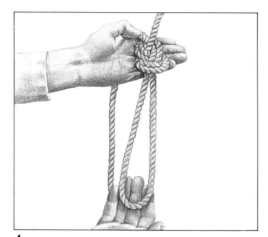

4 *Pull the figure-of-eight tight. This figure-of-eight is safer than a simple half-hitch because it will not shift under strain.*

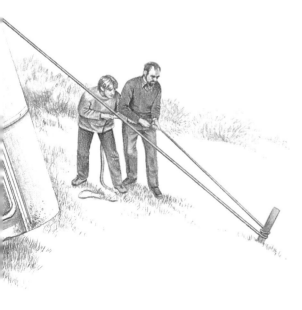

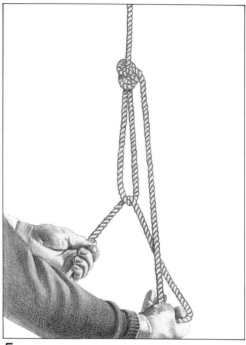

5 *Take a second fold in the rope and slip it through the loop to make a second loop. In use, the two loops act like pulleys, effectively more than doubling your strength.*

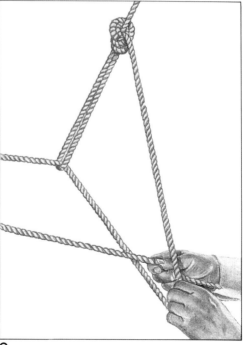

6 *Hook the rope's free end round a stout stake in the ground about 10-15ft (3-5m) from the caravan. Bring the end back to and through the second loop to complete the pulley knot.*

Camping out

Modern tents are compact, strong and light. But they can be as vulnerable as any other shelter – to wind, rain, snow and fire.

If you are caught in a burning tent

• Get out fast if your tent catches fire. As you go, beware of pieces of burning fabric – brush them off if they fall on you, and smother the flames with clothes or a sleeping bag. They will not be damaged if this is done decisively.

• Once outside, collapse the tent poles and, if necessary, the main guy ropes. Then stamp out the flames, if possible, or grab the tent by the end away from the fire, and pull it clear of your equipment inside.

• If the fire is too fierce to approach, though, let it burn. Equipment can be replaced; your life cannot.

• If the cause of the fire is a blazing stove in the doorway, push or kick it clear before getting out and collapsing the tent.

• When the fire in the tent is out, pour water over the area round the stove to stop undergrowth catching fire.

• Try to keep the fire away from any foam rubber or plastic mat being used as a sleeping pad. Many of these materials give off poisonous fumes when they burn.

If the tent leaks

• If rain or melting snow finds its way into the tent, try to block up the holes by pressing warm candle wax or sticky tape onto the fabric from the inside or outside. Alternatively, run a finger down the inside of the tent from the site of the leak to divert the drips.

• If the leaks persist, protect clothes and sleeping bags with a waterproof anorak or a sheet of

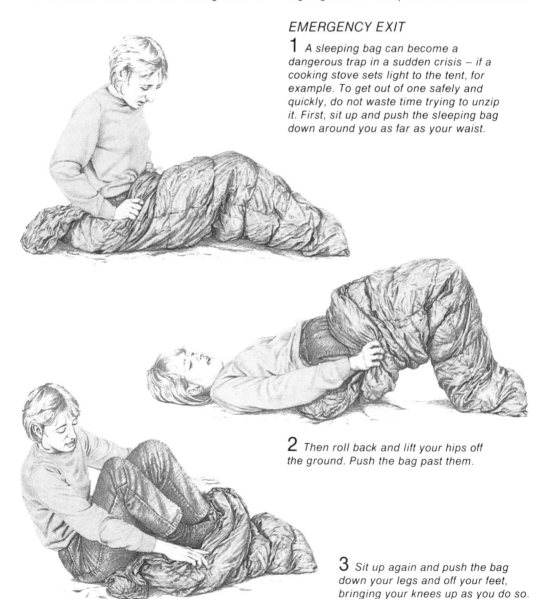

EMERGENCY EXIT

1 *A sleeping bag can become a dangerous trap in a sudden crisis – if a cooking stove sets light to the tent, for example. To get out of one safely and quickly, do not waste time trying to unzip it. First, sit up and push the sleeping bag down around you as far as your waist.*

2 *Then roll back and lift your hips off the ground. Push the bag past them.*

3 *Sit up again and push the bag down your legs and off your feet, bringing your knees up as you do so.*

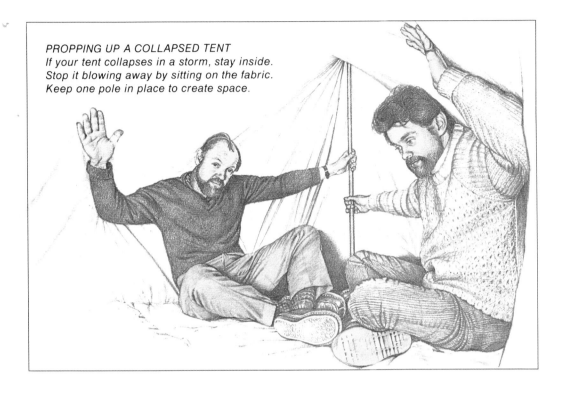

PROPPING UP A COLLAPSED TENT
If your tent collapses in a storm, stay inside.
Stop it blowing away by sitting on the fabric.
Keep one pole in place to create space.

plastic. If you have a survival bag – a large plastic bag – climb inside it with your sleeping bag to keep dry and warm.

If the tent is flooded

The safest course of action in a flood depends on what your sleeping bag is made of. A down-filled bag loses its insulation properties if it gets soaked. The safest course then is to abandon tent and bag, and make for somewhere dry.

• If there is no shelter nearby, make a platform – of branches, say – and sit out the night in your driest clothes.

• In very cold weather, preserve body heat by not using the sleeves of the top one or two layers of clothes. Instead, button or zip the clothes up; then work them down over your head and body. Fold your arms under the cocoon, tucking your hands into your armpits.

• Sleeping bags which are filled with synthetic material retain warmth even when wet. The safest course then is to prevent any further water coming in – perhaps by digging a channel around the tent to divert the flow. Mop out the tent, wring out the bag and stay put.

If the tent blows down

• Repitching a collapsed tent in high winds is very difficult. In severe weather, if there is no other shelter – a car, say – stay inside the tent.

• Use the weight of your body on the edges of the tent or on the sewn-in groundsheet to stop the tent being blown away.

• Make some space inside by propping up the fabric with a backpack or one of the tent poles.

PITCHING CAMP

Setting up a campsite carefully can minimise the risk of things going wrong.

• Pick a site on firm, flat ground away from river banks and dried-up watercourses.

• Pick a spot that is sheltered from the wind. Test the site for concealed stones by lying down on the ground.

• Pitch the tent so that its doorway faces away from the wind. Pull the fabric and guy ropes drum-tight; on modern tents, there is no need to slacken ropes in rain.

• If rain is expected, dig channels under the edge of the tent roof and across any slope above the tent to carry water away.

• When high winds are likely, rest heavy stones on the pegs and flaps.

• Always keep some ventilation – especially if, in bad weather, you decide to do your cooking inside. If you start to feel drowsy, or a stove burns with a yellow flame rather than a blue one, it may mean that there is insufficient oxygen. Get out into the open at once.

• Anchor a stove to the ground with tent pegs to stabilise it while it is in use. When it is not being used, store it and any fuel containers away from the tent. Do your cooking outside if at all possible.

If you are threatened by a dangerous animal

Fierce dogs and angry bulls are the two most hazardous animals you are likely to meet in the British countryside. Both need to be treated with the utmost caution.

Be alert for danger from bulls. On average, two people die every year because of attacks by bulls, and 18 people are injured.

In most parts of Britain, farmers are not allowed to keep a bull in a field which is crossed by a public footpath.

Bulls that are less than ten months old, however, or ones that are not of a recognised dairy breed (such as Ayrshire or Guernsey), may be kept in such a field if they are with a group of heifers. A cow with a calf can also be very dangerous. Keep well away from all cattle.

If you are chased by a bull

• There are few circumstances in which it is wise to run from a bull. If the creature is a long way off, sudden movements will only excite its attention. Contrary to popular belief, bulls are not particularly enraged by the colour red – it is movement, not colour, which provokes them. Research suggests that bulls probably cannot distinguish very well between colours. So make for safety at a controlled pace, with your eye on the animal all the time.

• If the bull is close and starts to give chase, do not turn your back and run. The farmers' rule is simple: 'Never turn your back to a bull.' Instead, make quickly for safety, but keep your eye on the bull all the time.

• Try discarding an item of clothing: this may distract the bull long enough for you to make extra ground. But do not flap things at the bull or wave your arms.

• If you cannot reach and get over a wall or fence before the bull catches up with you, stop and face the danger. Do not square up to the bull in a threatening manner. Instead, be prepared to dodge to one side at the last moment. This is not as difficult as it might sound. A bull is an unwieldy animal, and once it has built up momentum in a charge it cannot easily change direction or come to a halt.

• Once you have dodged out of the bull's path, continue to make as quickly as you can for safety. But make sure that you keep your eye on the bull – and be prepared to dodge out of its way again.

If you are threatened by a fierce dog

• If you are menaced by an angry dog, do not look it in the eye. The dog will probably interpret this as a threatening gesture and it may become more aggressive as a result.

• Do not make any other kind of gesture which could suggest to the dog that you intend to kick or strike it.

• Stand still and order the dog off in a commanding tone of voice. Try shouting 'Leave!' or 'Stay!', for example.

• Alternatively, try to calm the dog by talking to it in quiet, soothing and friendly tones.

• Try both the commanding and calming approaches, if necessary, to see which of the two brings the better response.

• If the dog persists in coming at you, try to grasp it by the neck. Then push it backwards towards and through any door or gate which can be firmly closed.

• Do not grasp the dog by its tail. It will whip round and bite your hand.

• If the dog clearly intends to bite, offer it a forearm. If you are able to, cover your arm with a sweater or jacket. Then push your forearm down hard towards the animal's throat. This should weaken its grip. Keep pushing till it lets go. Do not try to pull your arm away from the dog's mouth. Its grip is very strong and by pulling you will cause a nasty, lacerated wound in your arm instead of a clean one.

• If you have been bitten by a dog, wash the wound carefully with soap and water, cleaning away all saliva. Seek medical attention quickly so that an anti-tetanus injection can be administered. (See also *Animal bites*, page 48.)

DOGS – STAYING OUT OF DANGER

Every year in Britain, more than 200,000 people are treated in hospital after being bitten by a dog.

You may meet a strange dog anywhere on holiday or in the countryside. In particular, be prepared for sudden barking if a footpath takes you through a farmyard. Farm dogs are not necessarily as fierce as they sound, but, like any other unknown animal, should be treated with respect.

Keep away from places where guard dogs are kept, and let your family know about the danger. A trained guard dog is a creature that has been reared to deter intruders. Some guard dogs are well disciplined. Many more are not, however, and all guard dogs are dangerous to strangers.

It is never wise to approach any strange dog, still less to try to touch it. Do not encourage children to do so either – in the false belief that children should be actively friendly to unknown animals. One happy experience with a stray dog may lead to a less happy one – with a creature that bites.

What to do if you encounter a snake

Most snakes are timid creatures which will attack only when startled or cornered. The adder, or viper, the only poisonous snake native to Britain, will usually hurry away before you get near it. Even if you are bitten, the bites rarely prove fatal. There have been barely a dozen deaths from snakebites in Britain during the past 60 years.

• If you see any snake, stop at once and move quickly to at least 20ft (6m) from it.

• If you do get bitten, clean the wound and bandage it firmly. Keep the injured limb low (see *Snakebite*, page 125).

Where snakes live

Snakes are cold-blooded, and most live in tropical or subtropical parts of the world. There are no snakes near the Poles. Snakes in cooler regions – including Britain – hibernate during the winter.

In Britain there are only two common snakes: the adder; and the grass snake. Adders live in almost any dry place, but they prefer sandy heathland or rough common.

Outside Britain, although many of the snakes encountered are harmless, all should be treated with extreme caution. If you go walking in areas where snakes are likely, keep to paths and wear lightweight boots (not sandals) to protect your feet and ankles – the commonest target of a striking snake.

HOW TO AVOID INSECT BITES

If you are stung by an insect in the British countryside, the consequences are unlikely to be serious. However, a sting may cause an allergic reaction, and a bee or wasp sting inside the mouth is dangerous to anyone. For first aid, see *Insect stings and bites*, page 110.

• To minimise the chance of getting bitten by insects such as mosquitoes and midges, use a repellent cream. One of the best active ingredients is diethyl toluamide, which is available from chemists as a gel, a stick or a spray.

• Apply the repellent all over the body. Also apply it to bedsheets or clothing, as appropriate. Repellents are washed off the skin in time by perspiration, but they last longer when applied to material.

• Avoid camping at the edge of a river, lake or stream. Waterside campsites are particularly prone to constant attack by midges in summer.

• Avoid hillside bracken beds, which house sheep ticks and a swarm of other insects. Stay on paths in such areas.

ADDERS AND GRASS SNAKES: HOW TO TELL THE DIFFERENCE

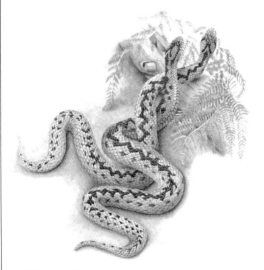

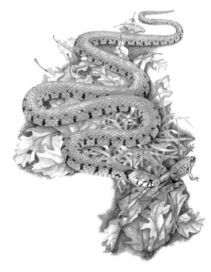

Adders, which are most often seen in spring, have dark zigzag markings, and grow to about 18-24in (450-600mm) long. Females are usually duller and browner than the males shown here.

Grass snakes, which live in damp grass and near slow-moving water, have no V-shaped marks on their heads. They are Britain's largest snakes, growing to 30-42in (0.75-1.1m). Despite their size, they are harmless.

If you are caught in a lightning storm

When lightning comes to earth, it tends to strike the highest point around and to travel to earth along the line of least resistance.

Tall, isolated trees and buildings are particularly vulnerable. But people can be targets too, either because they are themselves the tallest object in the area, or because they are in contact with, or close to, something struck by lightning.

Every year in Britain, two or three people are killed by lightning.

- If your skin tingles and you feel your hair stand on end during a thunderstorm, it means that a lightning strike may be imminent.
- If you are in an open area, drop to the ground at once and lie flat. This lessens the risk that you will be struck.
- If you are near tall objects, such as trees or boulders, get away from them quickly if you can.
- Make for low, level ground and lie flat.
- If you cannot get away from tall objects, sit on something dry with your feet together. Keep your feet on the insulating material and off the ground. It is important that the material you sit on should be dry. Wet objects provide no insulation and thus no advantage because water is a good conductor of electricity.
- Hug your knees to your chest with both arms and tuck your head – the most vulnerable part of your body – well down.
- Do not put down a hand to steady yourself. This will make double contact with the ground and expose you to greater risks.

If someone is struck by lightning

A lightning strike is not necessarily fatal. Many people have escaped with only shock and minor burns.

Lightning is most likely to kill if it strikes the head and passes through the torso on its way to earth. In such circumstances it is more likely to cause heart failure or asphyxiation.

Lightning may also cause severe burns, broken bones – because of muscular spasms caused by the shock – and cuts.

In addition, the victim's clothing may catch fire and metal ornaments or watch straps may melt.

- If the victim's clothing is on fire, lay him down on the ground at once to keep the flames away from his face. Otherwise he could die from lack of air or from burns caused by breathing in the flames.
- If necessary – if, say, he is panicking and not responding to your instructions – trip him up or knock him over, taking care as you do this not to get burnt yourself.
- Put out the flames quickly by dousing them with water or wrapping the person in a heavy coat or blanket.
- Treat as for electric shock (see page 93).
- Get medical attention immediately – even if the victim appears to be unhurt.
- Reassure him and keep him warm and comfortable until help arrives.

SAFETY DURING A THUNDERSTORM

Your chances of getting struck by lightning during a thunderstorm are extremely small. Nevertheless, lightning is not entirely predictable and it is worth taking precautions to cut the risk still further.

- Get off high ground, such as the brow of a hill, and away from tall trees.
- Do not take cover in cave mouths, rockface overhangs or recesses under boulders. They create spark gaps across which lightning can arc on its way to earth, striking anyone there. A deep cave is, however, safe; go right to the back.
- Keep well away from metal fences and other metal objects. Lightning does not have to strike directly to kill. Subsidiary flashes can arc out sideways from the main spark across several yards. In addition, the enormously high temperature of the bolt heats the air along its path explosively, causing shock waves. At a distance, these shock waves are audible as thunder. But close to, they are powerful enough to crush the lungs.
- If you are swimming or in a small boat, make for the shore at once. If you are in a larger boat, the crew should go below deck and the helmsman should avoid touching anything metal.
- Never fly a kite, ride a bicycle or ride a horse in a thunderstorm.
- If you are driving, stay in your car. It is one of the safest places to be. If lightning does strike, it will flash over the surface of the vehicle – which is virtually a metal cage – and run harmlessly to earth.
- In general, buildings offer good protection, but avoid isolated barns and huts.
- At home, unplug the TV at both the power socket and the aerial.
- Outdoors, rubber-soled shoes or wellington boots may offer some protection but they are no guarantee of safety.
- The traditional beliefs that you should close your windows and stay away from a fireplace during a thunderstorm are of only limited value. Closing windows is potentially useful only against ball lightning – a phenomenon so rare that nothing reliable is known about it. Ordinary lightning would not come through an open window anyway. Staying away from a fireplace was of more importance in the days of inglenooks when it was possible to sit directly under the chimney – and thus be in danger from falling debris if lightning demolished the stack.

Poisoned by a crop-sprayer

Crop-spraying with pesticides and fertilisers usually takes place on farms in spring and autumn. In Britain it is mostly done by tractor, but occasionally planes or helicopters are used.

Even in light winds, spray and dust can sometimes drift out of the field being sprayed and pose a threat to nearby workers, ramblers and picnickers. Many of the chemicals used by farmers are poisonous or corrosive if they are inhaled, and some can poison simply through contact with the skin.

• If you see a tractor or plane spraying, move well away from the area.

• Do not let dogs run on fields which are being sprayed with pesticide or sprinkled with fertiliser. They may pick up the chemicals on their paws, or swallow them.

• If the spray or dust falls on you or someone else, assume – for the sake of safety – that the spray is poisonous.

• Get out of the spraying area.

• Send someone for medical help immediately. Tell the doctor or ambulanceman the name of the pesticide being used – if you know it – or what crop is being sprayed. This will help doctors to decide which is the most appropriate treatment.

• If you do not know what chemical is involved, tell the doctor where the field is. With the help of local police, he will be able to find out quickly who owns the field and which pesticide or fertiliser was being used.

• Remove any contaminated clothing, and wash thoroughly any areas of skin that have been exposed to the chemicals. Use soap and water if possible.

• If chemicals have entered the eyes, flush them with clean water, under a running tap if possible, for at least ten minutes.

• Keep warm by wrapping up in a clean blanket or coat.

• If you have not been exposed to the spray yourself but are helping someone who has been, put gloves on before you touch any piece of his contaminated clothing. Otherwise the chemicals will get onto your skin too. If you do not have any gloves, wrap your hands loosely with, say, a jersey.

• If the person who has been sprayed loses consciousness, place him in the recovery position (see page 136).

• If he stops breathing, apply artificial respiration, the kiss of life (see page 50). If his face has been exposed to the spray, clean the area around his mouth and nose thoroughly first, and protect your mouth with a handkerchief.

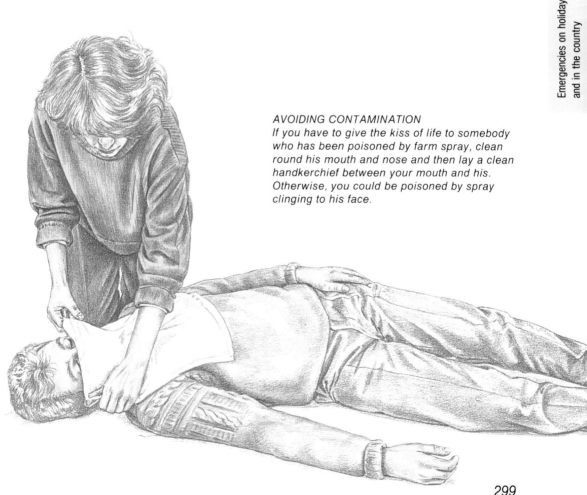

AVOIDING CONTAMINATION
If you have to give the kiss of life to somebody who has been poisoned by farm spray, clean round his mouth and nose and then lay a clean handkerchief between your mouth and his. Otherwise, you could be poisoned by spray clinging to his face.

Emergencies on holiday
and in the country

299

Trapped in a bog or quicksand

Hazardous bogs, marshes and quicksands are found on both high ground and low. And they can be lethal to the unsuspecting walker. The principle of surviving is the same whichever you fall into: spread your body weight as widely as possible, and move very slowly.

• As soon as you realise that you are stuck, fall as gently as you can onto your back, spreading your arms wide as you drop. Spreading your weight in this way will enable you effectively to float on the surface.

• If you are wearing a pack or cape, leave it on. It may improve your buoyancy. If you have a stick, get it underneath you.

• Make all your movements – including getting your feet back to the surface – deliberate and *extremely* slow. You have to allow time for the mud or sand to flow around your limbs as you move. Quick movements only create pockets of vacuum in the mud or sand, which will tend to suck you deeper.

• If you are with a companion, lie still. Wait until he or she throws you a line, or holds out a pole to you. Use long, firm pulls to haul yourself out. Frantic jerks will be less effective and will tire you more quickly.

• If you are alone, stay on your back and use your arms and legs as paddles with a breast-stroke movement to propel yourself very slowly towards the edge.

• Use roots or large clumps of grass, if there are any, to pull yourself along.

• Do not hurry. It may take an hour or more to cover only a few feet in safety. If you need to rest, spread your arms and legs wide, and lie still. You will float.

DANGER SIGNS

A bog is an area of wet, spongy ground in marsh or moorland terrain. Some of the worst bogs in Britain are in parts of the New Forest and Dartmoor. Beware of flat, black expanses with no vegetation.

Beware too of bright green expanses covered with sphagnum moss. This is a treacherous vegetation which sometimes spreads like a carpet over a lethal mire.

If you have to cross boggy terrain, always keep to the highest ground where taller trees or bushes grow. Tread where possible on tussocks of heather – they indicate drier ground. If you are in any doubt about which way to go, throw heavy stones ahead of you as well to check the firmness of the ground. At the edge of a doubtful patch, try also stamping hard. If the ground ahead quivers, the patch is probably waterlogged; avoid it.

A quicksand is a bed of loose, wet sand which will swallow up any heavy weight. It is often difficult to spot, for a firm crust may cover the fluid below. The golden beaches of Morecambe Bay in Lancashire conceal notorious quicksands.

When exploring any unfrequented beach or unknown sandy area, carry a stick or pole as a probe, and toss stones ahead of you to test the ground.

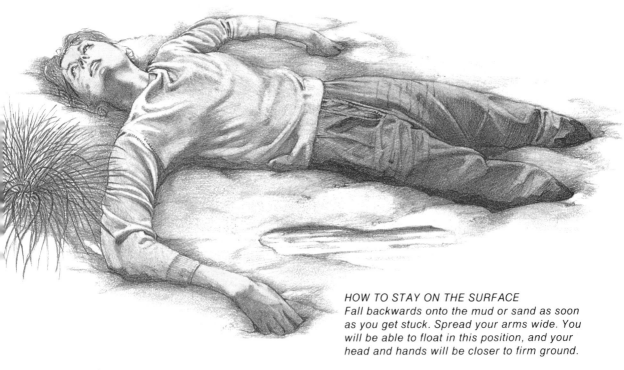

HOW TO STAY ON THE SURFACE
Fall backwards onto the mud or sand as soon as you get stuck. Spread your arms wide. You will be able to float in this position, and your head and hands will be closer to firm ground.

Exposure: the silent killer

Anyone who is exposed to the cold without adequate protection may suffer from a drop in the body's normal temperature, which can be fatal if left untreated. Doctors call the condition exposure or hypothermia.

It is blamed for the deaths of about five people a year on Britain's hills. But mountain rescue experts say that exposure could be the indirect cause of many more deaths because it saps the victim's strength and clouds his judgment, increasing the chances of some other accident, such as a fall.

Most cases occur in the summer, when hill-walkers are least likely to be well prepared for sudden, biting winds and rain. The severity of the condition varies with age and general health. But exposure can kill even a vigorous healthy person in less than four hours.

Warning signs

Apathy and listlessness are usually the first signs of falling body temperature. Other symptoms are: abnormally cold skin; stumbling; shivering; cramps; slurred speech; abnormal vision; and erratic behaviour or irritability.

What to do

• If you notice any of the warning signs in yourself, change into dry clothes if your clothes are wet. Cover your head, face and neck as well as your body to minimise further heat loss. About 50 per cent of the heat lost by the body escapes through the head and neck.
• Find shelter quickly, and get into a sleeping bag or a plastic survival bag – a bag large enough to enclose a person completely.
• Consume warm, sweet drinks and food.

How to help a casualty

• If you notice the symptoms of exposure in somebody else, do not force him or her to keep moving or to walk quickly.
• Stop. Place the casualty in a sleeping bag – with a companion for extra warmth.
• If the symptoms are severe, leave the casualty's clothes on, even if they are wet. Changing clothes in these circumstances costs too much body heat for safety.
• Protect the casualty against the weather with a tent, a plastic sheet or any makeshift shelter. Use clothes, grass or anything else available to insulate the sleeping bag from the ground.
• If the casualty is conscious, give him warm drinks and food.
• Do not offer alcohol or massage: both tend to dilate the blood vessels near the skin. This draws body heat away from deeper organs at a time when it is crucial to warm the core of the body, not the surface.
• If the casualty loses consciousness, put him in the recovery position (see page 136). Never give an unconscious person anything to eat or drink. It could choke him.
• Once the worst symptoms have passed, treat the casualty as a stretcher case. Even if he appears fully recovered, do not move him without covering his head, neck and face.
• If you reach a house and the victim is conscious, put him in a warm, but not hot, bath. Keep the water at a temperature that is comfortable to the elbow.
• When the casualty begins to sweat, dry him, put him in a warm bed and keep him rested.
• Do not put an unconscious person in a bath. Instead, once you are indoors, take off any wet clothes he is wearing and put him in a warm bed. Place hot-water bottles (wrapped thickly in towels to avoid burning him) around his torso.

HOW TO AVOID EXPOSURE

• Get a good night's rest before spending a day in the hills. Victims of exposure often admit to having felt off-colour on the morning of the incident. Common causes are arduous overnight travelling – and drinking sprees – before setting out.
• Eat a good breakfast with plenty of fluids before you leave. Eat high-energy snacks such as chocolate frequently during the day.
• Always carry a plastic survival bag – a bag large enough to hold a person inside a sleeping bag – inside your rucksack.
• Wear warm clothing that gives full protection against the wind. Outer clothing should be fully waterproofed. Do not rely on jeans or showerproof anoraks – they are totally inadequate in severe weather.
• Carry a spare set of dry clothing.
• When walking, take off excess clothing if you get hot. It is important not to get soaked in sweat, because water draws warmth from the body faster than air.
• Never carry more weight than you can comfortably bear. In cold weather, it will make you more vulnerable to fatigue and exposure. For the same reason, go at a comfortable pace.
• Be alert to the risk of exposure in windy conditions even when the air temperature out of the wind is comfortable. As a rule of thumb to calculate this 'wind chill factor', subtract 1°F from the temperature for every 1mph of wind speed (1°C for every 3km/h). A strong breeze of about 30mph (48km/h) in an air temperature of about 60°F (15°C), for example, will have the same chilling effect as if there were no wind and the temperature was down at a freezing 30°F (−1°C). Use the Beaufort scale to estimate the wind speed (see *The wind and the sea*, page 268).

Emergencies on holiday and in the country

What to do if you get lost

What you should do if you get lost in the country depends largely on the circumstances. At night or in cold weather, the priority is to find warmth and shelter. On a sunny day, the priority is likely to be to find a main road or a telephone.

If you get lost on a clear day
- Once you suspect you are lost, stop and take stock of your situation. Going on blindly may only make the situation worse.
- If you have a map, check the key so that you know what its symbols stand for. You will probably have at least a rough idea of where you are.
- Look around you for landmarks that match the map.
- Try to find on the map the last position you were sure of, and try to trace your route since then by remembering any buildings, streams or other landmarks you have passed.
- Examine the contour lines on the map to get an idea of the shape of the ground in the area where you are lost. Widely spaced contour lines (which join places of equal height) indicate gentle slopes. An absence of contour lines indicates a plain or a broad ridge. Contours bending in a loop usually mark the spur of a hill or a valley.
- Check the scale of the map, too. It is usually given as a ratio figure – 1:50,000, say. This means that 1cm on the map equals 50,000cm (0.5km) on the ground. On this scale, 1¼in on the map equals 1 mile.
- Use a finger as a rough distance guide if you have no pen and paper. The index finger of most adults measures about 1in (25mm or

2.5cm) from its tip to the first joint. All Ordnance Survey maps are also marked with a grid of squares. On the 1:50,000 maps commonly used by walkers, each square represents an area of 1km by 1km. On smaller-scale maps, such as those often used by motorists, each square represents an area of 10km by 10km.
- Turn the map until the symbols on it are lined up with the landmarks they represent. Decide on the direction you want to travel to reach a main road or settlement.
- Check that there is nothing – a cliff, say, or a wide river – to bar the way to your chosen destination. If there is, work out a way to get round it.
- Look on the map and on the ground for a landmark to aim for. Check your progress on the map by watching out for more landmarks on either side of your path as you walk (see *How to use a map and compass*, page 306).

If you have no map
It is still possible to find your way to safety even if you have no map and no compass.
- Consider first retracing your steps to the last main road you passed.
- If going back is not practicable, look around you. If you can see a road – or something that indicates its presence, such as a building or telephone wires – head for the road.
- If you can orientate yourself by any landmarks, so that you know at least roughly where you are, aim for the nearest road, path, railway line or stream which you know will lead you to safety.

HOW TO CALL FOR HELP IN THE WILD

People on foot in open country are extremely difficult to spot from a distance or from the air. But there are a number of ways of improving your chances of being found.
- The internationally recognised mountain distress signal is six whistle blasts or torch flashes a minute, then a minute's pause – repeated as often as necessary.
- If you have wood and matches, light one or more fires. Once the fire is well alight, add damp wood or grass to make plenty of smoke.
- Wear brightly coloured clothing and a brightly coloured hat.
- Lay objects on the ground – branches, stones or clothing – to form the words HELP or SOS. Make the letters as large as possible – at least 20ft (6m) long. If there is snow on the ground, tread out trenches in snowdrifts to form the same words.
- In addition, wave a large flag made out

of the most brightly coloured clothing you have.
- If you are being rescued by helicopter – on a mountain, say – let off a flare if you have one or light a small smoky fire near the pick-up point when the helicopter approaches. The smoke will show the pilot the direction of the wind, and help him to hold his position accurately while he is hovering.

Using a home-made heliograph
Heliographs – devices which use reflected sunlight to flash messages from one person to another – have been used by military signallers since the time of the ancient Greeks. They are easy to make at home before you travel – though they can be improvised on the spot – and, on a clear day, can attract attention from a distance of several miles. This is how to make and use one.
- You need a flat sheet of metal which is bright enough to show a reflection on both sides. A tin

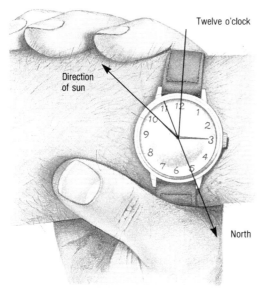

HOW TO FIND NORTH WITH A WATCH
Point the hour hand at the sun (ignore the minute hand). South in the Northern Hemisphere is halfway between the hour hand and the 12.

• Ideally, head for a feature, such as a road or stream, which you know cuts squarely across your line of travel. That way, you will still be able to find it even if you stray slightly off course.
• If no reliable landmarks are visible, decide what direction to head in, then orientate yourself by using the sun.
• The sun rises in the east and sets in the west.

At midday it will be due south in the Northern Hemisphere, and due north if you are in the Southern Hemisphere.
• If the sun is obscured by clouds, check its position by holding a nail file or knife blade on edge on a glossy surface such as a plastic credit card or a thumbnail. Turn the file until you see a faint shadow. The sun will be opposite it.
• If you are in Britain and you have a watch with hands, set it by Greenwich Mean Time (put it back an hour in summer). Elsewhere in the world, leave it on local time.
• Point the hour hand at the sun, and divide the angle between the hour hand and 12 o'clock in half with an imaginary line. If it is 4pm, for instance, the line will pass through 2 o'clock. The imaginary line will point due south in the Northern Hemisphere, due north in the Southern Hemisphere. In the Southern Hemisphere, point the figure 12 at the sun, and north is between the hour hand and the 12.
• If the clouds are too dense to find the sun, look for moss on trees and rocks. Since moss grows best in the shade, the most luxuriant growth will be on the north or north-east side in the Northern Hemisphere, on the south or south-east side in the Southern Hemisphere. This will give you a rough idea of your bearings. But confirm your direction from the sun as soon as there is a break in the clouds.
• If you have to stay put for a time, you can work out your bearings by placing a stick upright on flat ground. Mark the tip of the stick's shadow on the ground every hour or so. A line drawn through the marks will point due east and west.

Emergencies on holiday and in the country

lid rubbed clean will work, or a piece of tin foil.
• Make a small hole through the centre of the lid. Look through the hole until you can see the person or place you want to signal to.
• Now, holding the lid steady, look at the reflection of your own face in the back of the lid. You will see a spot of light on your reflected face from the sunlight shining through the hole.
• Tilt the lid until the spot of light in the reflection disappears into the hole. When it does, the flash is on target.
• Rock the lid slowly to generate a series of flashes. A series will be more readily noticeable than a constant beam, which could be dismissed as a chance reflection from water or a discarded piece of glass.
• Time the flashes, if possible, to match the international mountain distress signal – six flashes in one minute, followed by a minute's pause, followed by another six flashes in the next minute, and so on.

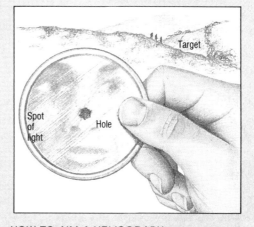

HOW TO AIM A HELIOGRAPH
Sight through the central hole on your target. Then tilt the lid so that the spot of light on your reflected face vanishes into the hole.

If you are caught in bad weather

• If you have survival equipment, such as a plastic survival bag – a plastic bag or a tube large enough to sit inside with your whole body and head protected – consider staying where you are and sitting out the bad weather.

• If you have no survival equipment and the weather turns bad with driving rain or high winds, the priority is to get down from high ground. It does not matter if you arrive in the wrong valley – so long as you do it in one piece.

• Check for danger spots on a map, if you have one. Steep-sided crags, for instance, are shown by hachures (knuckle-shaped marks). Plot a route around them.

• Use the direction of flow in streams to tell you which way leads downhill. But do not follow streams too closely; on hills, water sometimes carves deep ravines that could be dangerously steep. Instead, keep the stream within earshot and aim to follow its line.

• Avoid areas in a depression where there are tufts of spiky, light green grass. Tufts of this kind often indicate a bog or swamp.

• As you come down the hill, watch out for places that might offer or lead to shelter – a farmhouse, say, or a track. Make for them.

If you are lost in mist or fog

• If mist closes in, line a map up with a compass and decide which direction to go in.

• Sight along the bearing you want to follow, using a straight-edge or a compass, and pick out some visible marker along the line – a rock, say, or a branch or fern.

• Walk to the marker, then use your compass again to identify another marker in the same direction.

• Repeat the procedure until you walk out of the mist.

• If you have no map or compass, stay put until the mist clears.

Caught in a whiteout

When the light reflected by snow is the same colour as the sky, the landscape loses all form. It has no horizon, no height, no depth and no shadows. Climbers and explorers call this weather condition a whiteout.

• Stop and wait for the whiteout to pass if you can. In a blizzard, find a snowdrift, scoop out a depression in the snow and burrow into it for shelter (see *How to make a snow-hole shelter*, page 317). Alternatively, enlarge the depression that often forms in snow around the base of a tree and shelter in that.

• If you have a plastic survival bag, sit inside it. Use a pad – a rucksack, say, or branches – to insulate your body from the cold ground.

• Put on as many layers of clothing as you can. Take your arms out of the sleeves of the top jacket or anorak. Button or zip it up, then work it down over your head and body like a tube.

• Cross your arms underneath the jacket and

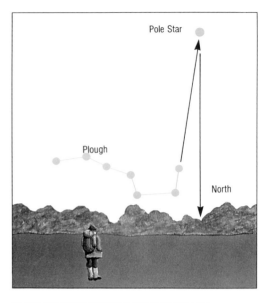

HOW TO FIND NORTH BY THE STARS
Look for the Plough, which can be at any angle in the sky. Its end stars point at the relatively faint Pole Star, which marks true north.

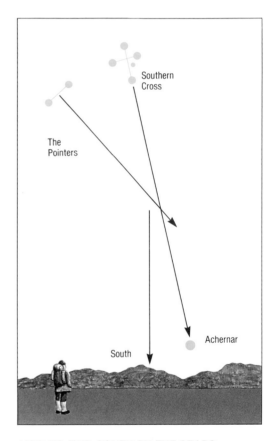

HOW TO FIND SOUTH BY THE STARS
Draw a line through the Southern Cross and three times its length. Due south is slightly to one side of the end of the line. Use Achernar and the Pointers to help to pinpoint the spot.

tuck your hands into your armpits to help to conserve warmth.

• If you have to move during a whiteout, use a map and compass to find your way. Toss snowballs ahead of you as you walk. Watching where they land and how they roll when they do will show you the direction of any slope. If they vanish altogether, it means you could be on the edge of a cliff.

Lost at night

• If there is a moon, moonlit grass or snow can give good visibility. In these circumstances, try to reach a road or any house or barn.

• If you have no compass, use the stars as a guide. In the Northern Hemisphere, Polaris, the Pole Star, which can be found using the constellation of the Plough, is always due north. In the Southern Hemisphere, the Southern Cross points towards the south, though not precisely.

• Another way of finding the Pole, in either hemisphere, is by using the constellation Orion. A line drawn between the middle star of Orion's belt and the centre of his head points due north (above his head) and south (below his feet).

• If visibility is too poor to travel by and you are on a mountain, find what shelter you can in the lee of a wall or rocks, and get inside a plastic survival bag if you have one.

• Members of a group can help each other to stay warm, even if they do not have survival bags, by sitting or lying huddled together. The middle position is the warmest, so change over from time to time.

If a child gets lost

An adventurous toddler or child, absorbed in his exploration of a beach, a picnic spot, a hillside or a funfair, can easily get lost.

• At the start of the outing, impress on the child the dangers of wandering out of sight. But fix some prominent place where you can meet should he or she nevertheless get lost.

• As soon as you notice the child's absence, make a quick search of the area where he or she was last seen.

• Go to the prearranged meeting place. If possible, have somebody wait there while you look around.

• If there is a public address system – as there often is at a funfair, say – find the people in charge of it and ask them to describe the missing child over the air.

• If all this fails, phone the police as soon as possible. Be ready with a detailed description of the child – his name, height, age, colouring, and what he was wearing.

• Once you contact the police, stay where you have arranged to meet them – even if there is a delay before they arrive.

HOW TO STAY OUT OF TROUBLE

Anyone who ventures into rough country on foot can minimise the risks of getting lost or stranded by following a few simple guidelines.

• Tell someone where you are going and when you expect to arrive. Check in when you do arrive, so that your contact does not call out rescue services unnecessarily.

• Estimate how long your journey will take. A fit adult can reckon to walk over open country at about 2½mph (4km/h), not counting rest stops.

• Add 30 minutes to your estimate for each 1000ft to be climbed along the route (50 minutes for each 500m).

• Telephone for a local weather report before you go, and dress accordingly.

• Walk in groups of at least four people. Then if one person is hurt – with a sprained ankle, say – another can stay with him while the other two go for help.

• If you have little experience of walking in open country, consider joining a walking club. The Ramblers' Association – whose headquarters are at 1/5 Wandsworth Rd, London SW8 2LJ; telephone 01-582 6826 – can provide information about clubs and groups near you, and give you their addresses.

What to take with you

• Carry a plastic survival bag – a large plastic tube or bag big enough to envelop completely a person in a sleeping bag.

• Carry or wear: a waterproof (not just showerproof) anorak and waterproof trousers; stout, comfortable boots; a spare sweater; and a warm hat and gloves. Also carry: food, including chocolate and dried fruit; an up-to-date large-scale map of the area and a compass; matches; a first aid kit; whistle and torch; and pencil and paper.

• In addition, take a first aid kit which includes a foil space blanket (see *What you need in a first aid kit*, page 44).

• For extended journeys, take a more comprehensive survival kit as well (see *Individual survival pack*, page 321).

• If your plans change for any reason after you set out, telephone those expecting you if at all possible. If necessary, contact the police and make sure that the emergency services are not alerted unnecessarily.

How to use a map and compass

With an accurate map and a compass, plus a pencil and a straight-edge (a ruler, say, a cigarette packet or the edge of a walker's compass), it is possible to navigate with a fair degree of precision across even totally unfamiliar country. And if you get lost, you can – provided there are two or three identifiable landmarks in sight – rediscover fairly quickly where you are.

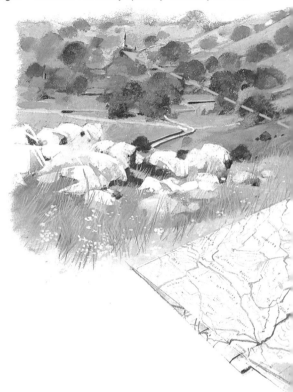

Finding your position on the map

• Fold the map flat so that the arrows on it which identify north are visible. Large-scale maps (1:50,000 or larger) of the kind used by walkers normally have two arrows. One shows true north (the direction indicated by the Pole Star); the other shows magnetic north (the direction to which a compass points). The grid lines on Ordnance Survey maps are closely though not exactly aligned with true north.

• Lay the compass on the map, and turn the map until the compass needle and the arrow pointing to magnetic north are aligned.

• Once the map is lined up, look around you for clear landmarks – a church, say, or a known peak. Find the same landmark on the map.

• Lay the straight-edge on the map so that it touches the landmark symbol. Sight along the edge and turn it – *without turning the map* – until it points directly at the corresponding landmark on the ground. Draw a line along the straight-edge from the map landmark back towards the position of your eye.

• Repeat the procedure with a second landmark. Your position is approximately where the two lines on the map cross. Use a third landmark, if one is visible, as a check.

• Once you have worked out where you are, use the map to work out where you want to go. Lay the straight-edge along your intended line of travel and – again without turning the map – sight along the edge at the landscape ahead.

• Choose some easily recognisable feature along the line and use it as a beacon. When you reach it, use the map to replot your line of travel – avoiding any obstacles such as cliffs and bogs – then pick another marker to walk to.

• Whenever you use a compass, make sure it is well away from metal, which could affect it, and away from the magnetic fields generated by electric current, such as in pylon cables.

• It is possible to use a compass instead of a straight-edge to measure the direction, or bearing, of each landmark from your position, and to use a straight-edge only to draw the lines on the map. But it is easier, and just as accurate, to use a straight-edge for both jobs.

• If you use the compass method, remember to draw each line in the *opposite* direction from the bearing you measure. If one landmark is, say, exactly NE of you, draw the line SW from the corresponding spot on the map. To calculate a 'back-bearing' in this way, add 180 degrees to the bearing if it is less than 180 degrees; subtract 180 degrees if it is more.

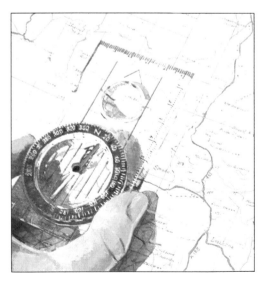

Lining up the map with a compass
Find on the map the arrow showing the direction of magnetic north – it is usually on the top edge or the side. Turn the map until the arrow and the compass needle are exactly in line.

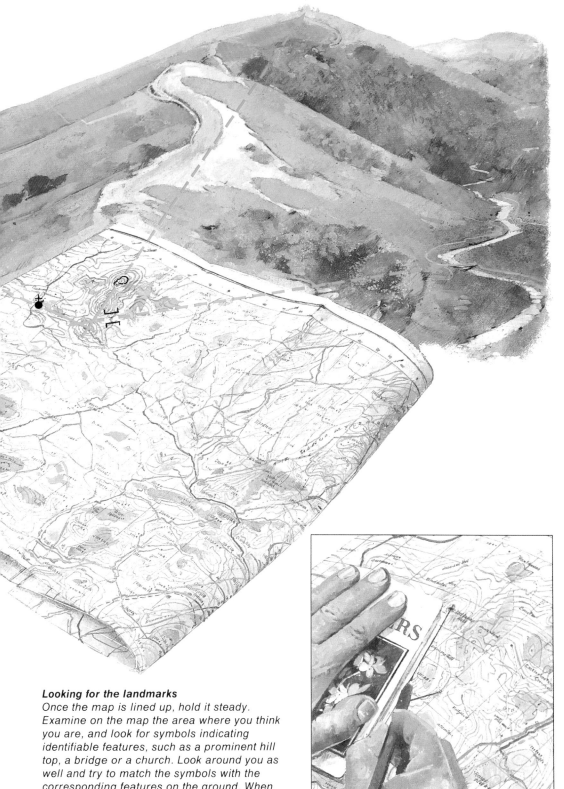

Looking for the landmarks

Once the map is lined up, hold it steady. Examine on the map the area where you think you are, and look for symbols indicating identifiable features, such as a prominent hill top, a bridge or a church. Look around you as well and try to match the symbols with the corresponding features on the ground. When you find a match, sight across the map so that the symbol and its real counterpart are in line. Your position is somewhere along that line. Repeat the process with other landmarks and your position is where the lines meet: somewhere in the triangle they usually form.

Using a straight-edge

Any straight-edged object can be used as a sighting instrument. Look along it the way a golfer sights along a putter, or hold it and the map up to eye level without turning the map.

Skiing: coping with an accident

Ski resorts are well equipped to cope with accidents. If you break a leg on a well-used slope, emergency services are unlikely to be far away. But if you go skiing alone far from the normal routes, a broken leg may threaten your life unless you can reach shelter on your own.

• If you do break a leg, stop any bleeding by making bandages from torn strips of cloth. Use shirt-sleeves or underclothing. But do not use an outer garment; you must keep warm.

• Apply snow to the wound to reduce swelling.

• Put splints on either side of the leg, tying them above and below the fracture (see *Splints*, page 127). The task may be painful, but it must be done: tackle it with patience and determination. For splints, use ski sticks or any branches available.

• Do not try to walk across the snow. You are likely to sink in and do more damage. Instead, lie flat on your stomach on one or both skis and propel yourself with your hands.

• Follow a zigzag or diagonal path downhill, heading for anywhere help may be available.

• The best way to avoid the risk of having to find your own way to safety with a serious injury is never to ski alone. If you do plan a trip away from well-used routes, even with companions, consider setting your ski bindings looser than usual. It is easier to put a ski back on if you fall than to deal with a badly twisted ankle or a broken leg.

How to help an injured companion

• If a companion breaks a leg on a remote slope, apply emergency first aid (see page 98).

• Make an improvised litter using skis, ski sticks, and jackets or scarves (see page 115). Do not use the casualty's jacket for this purpose; he needs to be kept warm.

• Tow the litter slowly and carefully – on foot unless you are an expert skier. Head for the nearest well-used route.

ALONE WITH A BROKEN LEG
In August 1984, a 33-year-old Dutch maths teacher, Ton Peters, spent five days on a Scottish hillside with a broken leg. He missed his footing as he walked on Beinn nan Aighenan, above Glen Kinglass, and fell 40ft (12m) into a ravine, breaking his leg high up on the thigh. Realising that he was extremely unlikely to be found, he resolved to stay put until the pain in his leg had subsided, then try to climb out.

An experienced hill-walker, Ton was well equipped to survive. In his rucksack he had food for more than a week, pain-killing tablets, a tent, sleeping bag and a portable sleeping mat. He reckons the mat saved his life. Once he had dragged himself to a rock ledge, he was able to cover himself with the tent and sleeping bag (he could not put the tent up) and to lie on the mat. Without the mat to insulate him from the cold ground, he believes he would have died.

On the fourth night after Ton's fall, rain triggered a flash flood which swept all his gear away and washed him off his ledge. From his new position, Ton was later able to climb out of the ravine. In the morning, after a night of shivering agony in the open, he saw a car pull up at a house below. He shouted, waved his red anorak – and was spotted.

In hospital later, he said: 'If someone had told me before that I could endure all this and still live, I wouldn't have believed him. The main point is that you should never give up. You are stronger than you think.' There was one piece of equipment which Ton did not have: a whistle.

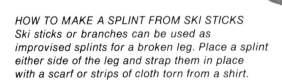

HOW TO MAKE A SPLINT FROM SKI STICKS
Ski sticks or branches can be used as improvised splints for a broken leg. Place a splint either side of the leg and strap them in place with a scarf or strips of cloth torn from a shirt.

If he had had one, he might have attracted attention much sooner – and his ordeal might not have come so close to costing him his life.

If you lose your skis

• Skis spread your body weight over the snow. If you lose them in a fall, but are unhurt, do not make for home simply by walking across the slopes. Walking through deep, soft snow will quickly exhaust you. If possible, improvise snow shoes. They spread your weight, and help to save energy too.

• Find two bushy pine branches, the thicker the needles the better. Place them on the snow with the natural curve down at the centre, rising forward and behind. The wider end of the branch should be towards the front and the stem behind your heel.

• Strap the branch onto your foot using improvised binding. Strips of cloth, laces or soft pine twigs will all serve for binding.

• Move downhill with care, and cross slopes diagonally or following a zigzag course. Use your ski sticks for support as you walk.

If your bindings break

Ski bindings can snap, making conventional skiing impossible. If this should happen, you can still get down a slope safely – and more quickly than would be possible on foot – by making an improvised hobbyhorse.

• Bind your skis together, using strips of cloth for lashing, and tie the ski sticks across the back end of the skis.

• Sit astride the skis with the tips behind you. Hold onto the ski sticks and lift them.

• Follow a zigzag path down the slope, controlling your descent with your feet.

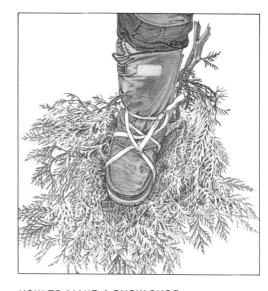

HOW TO MAKE A SNOW SHOE
If you have to walk through soft snow, make improvised snow shoes by tying bushy branches, stems backwards, to your feet.

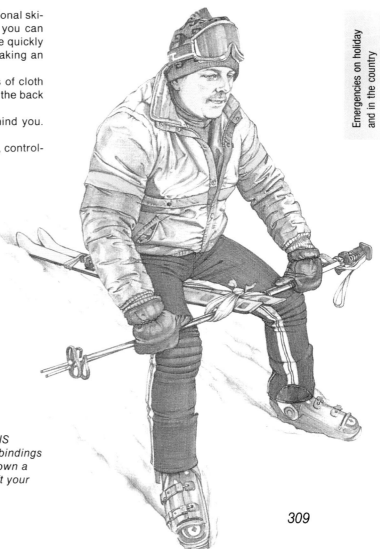

Emergencies on holiday and in the country

HOW TO TOBOGGAN ON BROKEN SKIS
On firm snow, make skis with broken bindings into a hobbyhorse to help you to get down a slope more easily. Sit well back and lift your toes so that you plane over the snow.

Crisis underground

Exploring caves can be extremely dangerous for the casual or ill-equipped. On average, cave rescue organisations in Britain are called out to help cavers in trouble about 50 times a year, and between two and three people die every year in Britain as a result of potholing accidents.

Mine workings are particularly dangerous because they often contain unmarked vertical shafts, whose entrances can easily be mistaken for deep shadows on the floor of a tunnel. Miners also used to store waste rock on timber platforms in the ceilings of tunnels. When the timbers rot, the rock can be left jammed precariously overhead and can be dislodged without warning by noise or an unwary hand. Old mines may also contain dangerous or even lethal con-

centrations of foul air or poisonous or explosive gases. Because of these hazards, never explore a man-made hole in the ground, or any hole which looks man-made.

If you get lost in a cave system
• If you think you might be lost, stop at once. Try to work out where you might have gone wrong.
• Calculate the time you have spent underground so that you can estimate roughly how long it ought to take you to get back.
• Mark where you are. Scrape a mark in mud on the floor or pile rocks to make a small cairn. If this is impossible, scratch on the wall with a knife or make a mark with soot from a candle flame.
• Try to retrace your steps.
• Keep looking back to recognise passages. A passage viewed from one direction on the way into a cave system can look very different on the way out.
• Leave markers as you go.
• Rest often to save energy. Switch your light off whenever you stop, to prolong the life of the batteries. Warming the batteries against your body will also make them last longer.
• If your path takes you deeper into unfamiliar territory, return to the last point you were sure of by following your markers, and try another route. Keep trying until you find the right one. Even in a honeycomb of passages you will gradually narrow the options.
• Shout, or blow a whistle, if you hear sounds that may be other people in the cave.

If you get stuck in a passage
• Relax completely. Taut muscles and fast, panicky breathing inflate your body and make escape more difficult. Go limp.

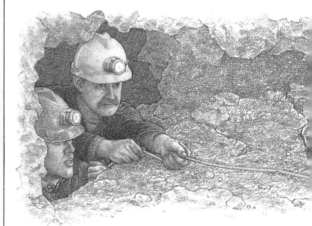

HOW TO GET OUT OF A TIGHT SPOT
If you get stuck underground and can find nothing to hold on to, get your companions to tie a loop in one end of a line. Put your foot in the loop and bend your leg. Tell the others to pull the line taut and anchor it, then push your leg down hard and heave your way out.

SAFE CAVING

• The only safe way to go caving or potholing is with experienced and properly equipped cavers, usually members of a specialist club. Public libraries often have lists of local caving clubs. Alternatively, contact the National Caving Association or the British Cave Research Association. Neither has a permanent head office, but a library should be able to help you to find their current addresses.
• Never go caving with fewer than four in a group. If there is an accident, one can stay behind with the injured person while two go for help.
• If you leave markers such as cairns on the way in as a precaution, remove them on the way out. Follow the cavers' rule: Take nothing but photographs – leave nothing but footprints.
• Tell someone of your plans so that help can be raised quickly if necessary.
• If you have to raise the alarm, dial 999 and ask the police to put you in touch with the local Cave Rescue Organisation.
• Check weather reports before you go. Rain can flood some caves very quickly.
• Wear warm clothing covered by a boiler suit – caves are chilly, muddy and usually damp all year round. Wear strong lace-up boots or wellingtons, and a plastic safety helmet.
• Take with you: a headlamp with a battery that will last longer than the trip is expected to take; spare batteries and spare lights or candles and matches; high-energy food – such as chocolate, glucose, fudge or raisins – and water; a map of the cave system; a first aid kit; a whistle; a watch with a luminous dial; and strong climbing rope.

- Once you are breathing normally, try to wriggle out slowly. Tackle the task patiently, keeping as relaxed as possible.
- Use your whole body. It is often easier to push your way out with your legs than to pull with your arms.

If your light goes out

Inside a cave system, the blackness is total. And without light it is easy to become completely disorientated.

- Stop immediately. Crouch down and put one hand on the ground directly in front of your feet, the other hand directly behind you.
- Keep your hands still and turn round, using your hands as markers, so that you are facing towards the way out Do not turn any more or wander about.
- Sit down and wait for at least ten minutes to let your eyes adjust as much as possible to the dark. If you are not far from the entrance, a glimmer of light may become visible as your eyes adapt.
- While you are waiting, try to recall the caves and passages you came through.
- If there is a glimmer of light from the opening, crawl towards it slowly, on hands and knees, testing the ground in front of you as you go. Keep feeling in front of your face and body, too, to check for projecting rocks and boulders.
- If there is no light at all but the route you took was straightforward – few bends, no passages branching off, a floor without hazards – retrace your steps on all fours, keeping the route in your mind's eye. Feel your way along the wall of the cave.
- If you have come through a hazardous or complicated system, wait for somebody to come and rescue you. Your chances of finding your own way out safely are minimal.

A STONE'S THROW FROM SURVIVAL
Twenty times, a hundred times, a thousand times, Larry Ritchey threw a stone tied to a rope up into the patch of light that was his only chance of escape. Each time, it fell back.

Ritchey, a 35-year-old salesman, had been walking in the Cascade Mountains of the north-western USA one November weekend in 1982. Suddenly, as he picked his way through deep snow, the ground gave way beneath him. He plunged 14ft (4.3m) into a subterranean stream flowing through a cavern about 10ft (3m) wide. The stillness of the air showed that there was no exit to the surface via the stream. And the rock walls were sheer. There was no chance of scrambling out.

Ritchey tied the stone to the end of his 30ft (9m) climbing rope and tossed it up through the hole in the cavern ceiling in the hope that it would catch on something. Again and again he threw, working his way round and round the lip of the hole. Three times the stone seemed to hold fast and then pulled loose as he tried to climb. But he never gave up, even after five days of failure. By the end of the fifth day he had no more food, the water was rising about him, and he was showing signs of hypothermia.

At last the stone caught again. This time it held. Ritchey hauled himself painfully back to the surface. He trudged and staggered 10 miles (16km) to a road and flagged down a car.

A search had been organised once Ritchey was overdue, but his shouts would never have been heard over the crashing of the stream, even had the rescuers come near him. What had saved his life was his own endurance – and the adage he had kept repeating to himself: 'If at first you don't succeed . . . .'

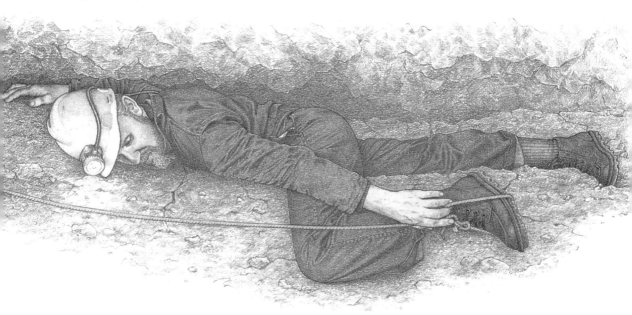

Emergencies on holiday
and in the country

Survival in the wild

An injury, a breakdown, bad weather or sheer bad luck can turn an adventurous expedition into a fight for life. It can happen anywhere: on a moor or mountain, in a tropical rain forest or a barren desert. Wherever it happens, there are four immediate priorities. In order of importance they are: shelter; a signal; water; and food.

The ten pages that begin here describe how survival experts cope with these priorities in a variety of circumstances. All the techniques mentioned have been used in real-life emergencies and are part of the survival training used by such organisations as the Special Air Service (SAS). Some, however, are themselves hazardous and should be used only when their risks are outweighed by other dangers.

The first steps

• Wherever you are, the first step is to get out of the cold, heat, wind or rain so that you can make plans with thought and care.

• Next, let others know where you are by setting up a conspicuous signal. Use anything to hand for this. Spread out bright clothing that contrasts with the environment. Light a fire to make a smoke signal. Use a whistle if you have one. The internationally recognised distress signal is six blasts in a minute – then a minute's pause followed by another six and so on. Improvise mirrors to reflect the sun, or, at night, flash lights. There is no point in foraging for food and water before this task is done. Search parties may be in the vicinity already – and may miss you if no signal is set up.

• Finding water is more vital than finding food. An average person can survive for only a few days without water – and then only in a temperate climate. During the time spent finding and improving a shelter, setting up a signal and so on, you will have used up a significant amount of body fluid, which has to be replaced.

• Finally, find food. Under average conditions, an adult male can survive for at least a week without food before serious physical deterioration sets in.

• Nevertheless, start foraging early. Where necessary, test nearby vegetation for edible foods (see *The edibility test*, page 316).

Making and using a fire

Survival in the wild may depend on your ability to light a fire. Warmth, cooking, boiling water, drying clothes, signalling, warding off insects – all are essential needs. On any excursion into remote or difficult terrain it is vital to take an adequate supply of matches or a lighter. Waterproof matches are available; otherwise carry ordinary matches in a waterproof container.

Finding dry tinder and kindling

• Tinder must be bone-dry. Sources of tinder include dry grasses, stems, straw, leaves, twigs, bark fragments and splinters of wood. In wet weather, look especially under the bases of trees and under rock overhangs for the driest material.

• Even in wet weather, birch bark peeled from a tree makes good tinder since it contains highly inflammable oils. The resinous pitch in pine knots has the same inflammable properties.

• Where no natural dry tinder can be found, shred fragments of clothing. Tufts of cotton wool,

---

PREPARING FOR A JOURNEY IN THE WILD

No amount of preparation can remove all the risks from a journey through remote or rugged country. But preparation can considerably lessen the chances of things going wrong, and improve your chances of survival if they do.

• Learn to use a map and compass until you can navigate with confidence.

• Before setting out, inform relatives, friends or the police of your route, departure time, estimated time of arrival, and the number in your party. They can raise the alarm if you are held up. Never travel alone.

• Talk over your plans with people familiar with the area you are going to. They will often be able to give you valuable advice about local conditions.

• Wear clean, loose-fitting clothes that protect you against the weather. What you wear will depend on the climate.

• Wear next to the skin fabrics that will absorb sweat. In general cotton and wool are better than man-made fibres, but synthetic 'thermal' material is also good. Cotton is good in warm climates because of its sweat-absorbing properties, but it is not suitable for cold weather because it dries out slowly.

• In warm climates wear lightweight trousers. For cooler conditions the best clothing is breeches – made of tweed, corduroy or special synthetic fabric – and long socks. Do not wear jeans. When the fabric is wet it loses all its heat-retaining properties.

• Wear one or two pairs of wool socks. They absorb sweat and cushion the feet.

• Roughly 50 per cent of the heat that escapes from the body is lost from the head and hands. Wear a hat and gloves to help to conserve it in cold weather.

• Carry a survival kit (see pages 320-321)

unravelled bandages from a first aid kit and fluff from pockets all serve as valuable tinder.

• Blow gently on glowing tinder, and add bits of kindling sparingly as it ignites. Remember that split branches burn better than whole ones. Stack fuel loosely so that the air continues to circulate as you build the fire. Once the fire is going, add whatever wood is to hand.

Lighting a fire with a car battery

If you are stranded in a car but have no matches, there are two main ways that you can use the car to get a fire going. Never be tempted, however, to use petrol to light a fire or to keep one going. Petrol burns explosively, and the flames or the blast can kill.

• If the car has a cigar lighter, twist a piece of paper into a spill, or use a piece of dry, frayed cloth or dry bark (birch bark is best).

• When the cigar lighter is red-hot, pull it out and touch it to the spill to light it. Then use the spill like a match to light the fire.

• Alternatively, if the car has no built-in lighter, use the car battery to light a fire.

• Disconnect the battery and remove it from the vehicle. Keep the battery upright when you lift it out to avoid splashing any acid onto yourself.

• Take two pieces of inessential wiring – from

HOW TO USE A BATTERY TO LIGHT A FIRE

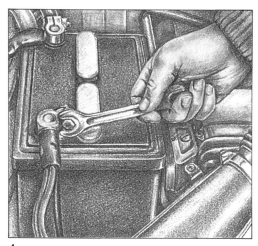

1 *Disconnect the terminals on the battery, and lift it out of the car. Take care not to touch both terminals at once with the spanner.*

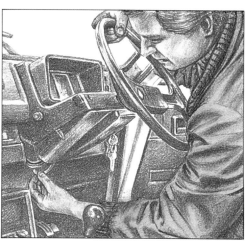

2 *If you have no spare wire or jump leads, take out two pieces of insulated wire – the longer the better.*

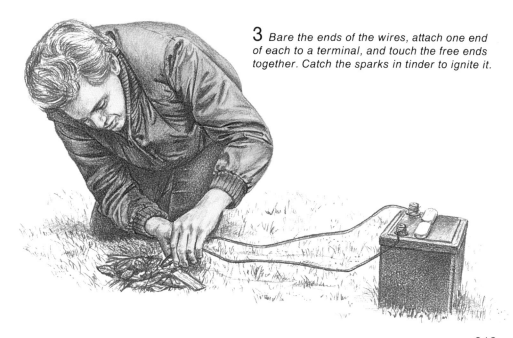

3 *Bare the ends of the wires, attach one end of each to a terminal, and touch the free ends together. Catch the sparks in tinder to ignite it.*

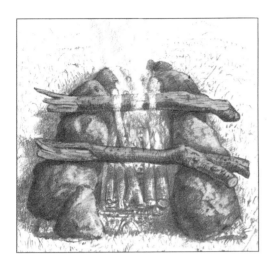

HOW A HUNTSMAN'S FIRE WORKS
The fireplace's funnel shape, which can be made out of logs, stones, earth or turf, acts like a natural flue. Use green logs or a metal grille to support cooking pans over the embers.

an interior light cable, say. Or use jump leads.
• Connect one wire or lead to each terminal. Then, carefully, touch the free ends together and catch the sparks in a pile of dry tinder.

How to build a fire
Before you light any fire, clear the ground around it of anything that might burn, and have something handy to put it out if necessary: water, perhaps, or branches to beat it out.

One particularly effective and simple fire is a type sometimes called a huntsman's fire. It makes an excellent cooking fire.
• Use logs, earth or stones to form a funnel shape about 12–18in (300–450mm) long. The wider end should point directly into the wind and be about 12in (300mm) across. The narrow end, pointing away from the prevailing wind, should be about 3–4in (75–100mm) across.
• Light the fire at the wider end.
• The hottest part of the fire will be a little downwind of the embers. So by moving pans towards or away from the narrow end, you can control the cooking temperature fairly precisely.
• Another way to make the funnel is to slice through the turf with a knife and roll back the turf on either side of the cut. The turf then forms the walls of the funnel, and the grass can be rolled back into place later, when you leave.

MAROONED IN AN ALASKAN WINTER
The Wortman family – 53-year-old Elmo, a disabled carpenter, and his three children – were on their way home from a visit to the dentist on February 13, 1979, when they were shipwrecked on the hostile coast of Alaska.

The family, who had travelled by boat to the nearest dentist, across the border in Canada, were washed up on a bleak snow-covered island, injured and without food or shelter. They had with them matches, protected in glass bottles by Elmo in the last moments before the boat went down. With these, they were able to start a fire. Using salvage from the boat, the children – Cindy, 16, Randy, 15, and Jena Lynn, 12 – built a shelter. They rested two poles on a pair of large rocks and draped over them a sail, covering top, back and floor. The opening faced the fire to keep the crude shelter warm.

The Wortmans ate clams, mussels and seaweed scavenged from the shore.

With logs and some of the salvage from the boat – electrical wire, rubber tubing and plywood – they later improvised a raft, and managed to reach a trapper's cabin on a neighbouring island. From there, all were rescued on March 10 – weak and frostbitten but alive.

Keeping a fire going through the night
• To keep a wood fire burning overnight, reduce the draught of air by banking around the edges with earth or stones. Add slow-burning hardwoods or green logs.
• For maximum warmth at night, lie between the fire and any natural barrier such as a bank, rock wall or big log. This will reflect the heat back at parts of the body not facing the fire.
• If necessary, improvise a heat-reflector by rolling boulders or logs into position.
• Huddle together with any companions for extra warmth and to conserve heat.

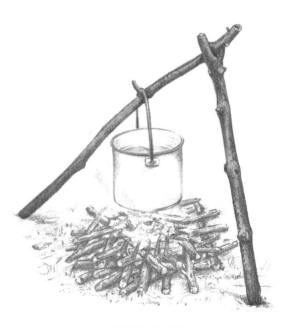

HOW TO HOLD A POT IN PLACE
Stick a forked branch firmly into the ground, and prop another stick against it to hold a cooking pot securely in place over a fire.

Cooking in the wild

• Cook on glowing embers, not on flames.

• Cook all food – especially meat and fish – thoroughly before eating. This is particularly important in hot and humid countries where bacteria thrive. Cooking destroys harmful bacteria, and also neutralises some poisons.

• Boiling is usually the safest method of preparing food for eating. Boiling will also soften tough meat.

• If you are in doubt about whether any particular species of animal or plant is safe to eat, use the edibility test (see page 316).

How to cope with stomach upsets

You may succumb to severe stomach pains in the wild. Common causes are eating a poisonous plant, or drinking contaminated water.

• If you think that food or water is the cause of the pain, and you have no medicines for it, try to make yourself sick. Either put a finger down your throat or drink clean salt water.

• Alternatively, eat some carbon or chalk. Either is capable of absorbing poisons. Chalk may be available from nearby rocks; carbon can be any piece of charred wood from a fire.

• Crush the pieces and eat one or two tablespoons of the powdered chalk or carbon. Wash the powder down with plenty of clean drinking water.

If you suspect that water is contaminated

• Dirty or contaminated water should be boiled. To be completely safe, the water should be boiled for ten minutes. Alternatively, it can be purified chemically (see *Potassium permanganate – the all-purpose aid*, page 320).

• Filtering water will not purify it, but it will often improve the water's appearance and taste.

• If no proper filters are available, you can make your own equipment. For the container, use a canvas bag, a polythene bag, a large tin, a knotted shirt sleeve – or even a sock.

• Fill the bottom of the container with a layer of fine gravel. Above it place alternate layers of crushed carbon and sand – as many as will fit. Make each layer about 1in (25mm) thick. If no sand is available, use fine gravel instead.

• Make small holes in the container's base. Pour the water through, catching it in a cup.

• If you decide to filter the water, do the filtering before you boil or treat it chemically – not afterwards. The filter may otherwise contaminate the water again.

Using snow or ice

Where there is snow, there is water. But snow needs to be melted before consumption. Never eat raw snow. Because of the air it contains, raw snow causes diarrhoea and dehydration.

In general, ice is more valuable than snow, because it takes 50 per cent less fuel to melt it. When heating snow, much fuel is wasted warming the air trapped among the flakes.

Surviving in the jungle

Getting stranded in jungle is, in some ways, less of an ordeal than fighting to survive in other environments. Food and water, for example, are usually plentiful. And trees

HOW TO FILTER WATER

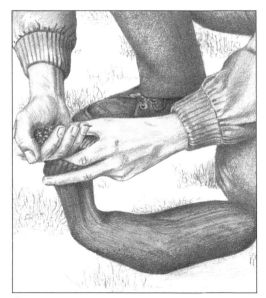

1 *Any tubular container with holes at the bottom – a clean sock, say – can make a filter. Put 1in (25mm) of gravel in the bottom.*

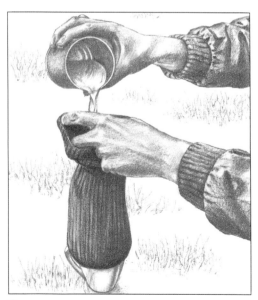

2 *Add layers, alternately, of sand and carbon (crushed burnt wood), then pour the water through. Boil the water afterwards to purify it.*

offer both fuel for fires and protection against the elements.

The worst enemy is generally anxiety: you cannot afford to be squeamish about anything that walks, crawls, swims or flies.

• Use what natural shelter you can find, or build a simple lean-to off the ground.

• When building a shelter, bamboo is an invaluable plant and found widely in tropical rain forests. It has innumerable additional advantages. You can make anything from a spear to a full-scale raft with bamboo. The canes can be used as firewood, and the tender shoots are both edible and nutritious.

• Filter and boil all water. Cook all food. Germs, like the vegetation, thrive in humid forests. When collecting food, beware of any brightly coloured plants, especially red and orange ones. They are often poisonous.

• Wash yourself whenever possible to discourage insects and prevent skin infections.

• Wash your clothes every day to stop sweat from rotting the fabric.

• Use fire to get rid of bugs, midges and other insects. Use an insect repellent, too – it also helps to ward off leeches.

• When travelling through thick jungle, movement is bound to be slow. Do not try to rush. It often helps to move backwards – if you get tangled in climbing vines, say.

• To find your way out of the jungle, locate any flow of water and head downstream. Follow a spring to a stream, a stream to a river, and a river to the sea if necessary.

• Sooner or later you will almost certainly come across other human beings, for waterways are the main lines of communication in tropical rain forests.

TWENTY-EIGHT YEARS IN THE JUNGLE
One night in January 1972, two hunters on the Pacific island of Guam came across a mysterious figure. He was wearing trousers and jacket made of tree and bark fibre, and he was heavily bearded. Brought in at gunpoint, he turned out to be Shoichi Yokoi, a former sergeant in the Japanese army. He had been hiding out in the jungle for 28 years – ever since the end of the Second World War.

Yokoi had fled into the jungle when US

THE EDIBILITY TEST

If you are stranded in remote country, you may be forced to live off the land, and that will mean trying to survive mostly by eating plants. The range of poisonous and non-poisonous plants is vast, and you may get confused trying to remember the different species. In an emergency, it is possible to find out which is which by using yourself as a cautious guinea pig.

Do not try this technique at home, however, and particularly do not encourage children to try it. Use it only in an emergency when the risk of making yourself ill is outweighed by the risk of starving.

• One person should test only one plant at a time, and each plant should be tested by only one person. And remember that just because you see birds or animals eating a plant, it does not mean that the plant is safe for humans.

• Choose a species which seems to grow plentifully in the area. But do not experiment with fungi. Unless you know that a fungus is edible, make no attempt to eat it or to prepare it for eating. Even boiling fungi does not always remove dangerous toxins.

• Having selected a plant, look for the colour of the sap by squeezing the leaf or stem between your fingers.

• Discard any plant that has a creamy or milky sap – it is probably poisonous. (An important exception to this rule is the dandelion: the whole plant is edible and nutritious. It also helps to stop diarrhoea.)

• Rub the juices or sap around the tender parts on the inside of your bottom lip. At the same time, place a small piece of the plant – fingernail-size or smaller – on the tip of your tongue. Wait for 4-5 minutes. If you detect any stinging, burning or putrid sensation, discard the plant.

• If you detect none of these sensations, take a larger piece of the plant, roughly 2in (50mm) square. Chew it and swallow it. Wait for two hours. If you experience any stomach upset or feeling of nausea, discard the plant – it is probably poisonous.

• If you detect none of these symptoms, take a larger portion of the plant, roughly 6in (150mm) square, chew and swallow it, and wait a further two hours. If you feel no ill effects, the plant is probably safe to eat.

• Having identified the plant as probably safe, boil it and throw away the juices. Then, as a final precaution, boil it again before eating.

• As the days pass, repeat the test with other plants – trying out roots, fruits, berries and flowers as well as leaves and stems – so that you build up, in time, a varied diet.

troops recaptured the island in 1944. Fearing capture, he had burnt his service uniform and improvised clothing with the materials to hand. For shelter he dug out a cave in a bamboo thicket and left it only at night.

Through the entire period he survived on a diet of nuts, breadfruit, mangoes, papaya, fish, shrimps, snails, rats and frogs. When discovered by the hunters he was on his way to a river to set his traps for fish.

Yokoi was in good physical health (though bewildered by the world of TVs and space travel to which he was returned). His largely salt-free diet had, however, left him slightly anaemic. Salt is present in roasted meat, but not in boiled food. In an emergency, it can be obtained by boiling sea water and collecting the salt crystals left behind.

Surviving in the mountains

• Look for shelter in caves and overhangs. Besides offering protection from the elements, they almost always contain some water or moisture. But avoid them during a thunderstorm. They are dangerous if lightning strikes.

• Avoid any area which threatens landslide or avalanche, such as a scree slope.

• If you are trapped in a remote valley, the higher ground to either side may be safer than the basin.

• Use spare clothes or a bright groundsheet to mark your position.

• Try to attract attention by using a whistle or by calling out – sound travels far in mountains. Give the international distress signal – six blasts a minute, then a minute's pause, followed by another six and so on. This is more likely to be noticed than random shouts.

How to make a snow-hole shelter

• If you are in snow, and bad weather or fading light prevents you from travelling for the time being, you can make your own shelter in the form of a snow hole.

• Use natural snow cavities where possible. The heavily snow-laden branches of a tree, for example, may provide a promising shelter which needs little extra work. Otherwise, dig into the side of a drift.

• Test the drift for depth: about 5-6ft (1.5-1.8m) is best.

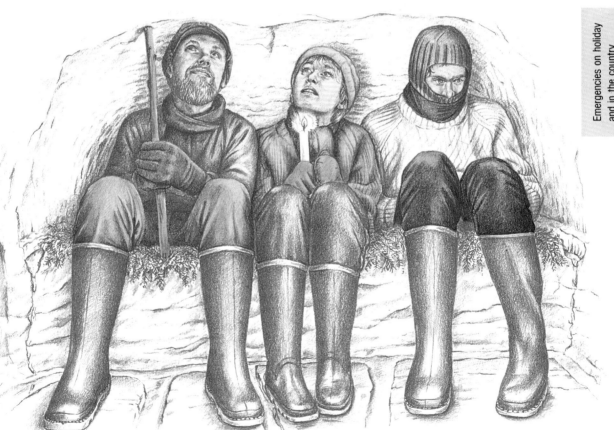

USING A SNOW HOLE FOR SHELTER
Once you have dug a snow hole, get inside and block the entrance tunnel. Keep a stick or pole handy to poke ventilation shafts through the roof, and keep them open. Burn a candle if you have one. Put heather or branches on the bench to insulate yourself from the snow.

- Once you have found a suitable spot, mark your position conspicuously. Dig out a small entrance low down, tunnel in about 2ft (600mm) and scoop out a cavity. It should be large enough to hold you in a sitting position. If there are more than three of you, it may be necessary to dig more than one hole, but otherwise share. Company and additional body warmth will make the ordeal easier to endure.
- Dig with a shovel or an ice-axe, or improvise using cooking pans, for example, or branches. Your hands alone will not be enough.
- Pierce an air shaft through the roof with a stick for ventilation. You may need more than one shaft if several people are in the hole. Keep the stick handy to clear the shaft in case it gets blocked by snow.
- Shape a rough bench for yourself within the cavity. Scoop out a small trench where the bench meets the back and side walls. This will prevent any melting snow from flooding your seat. Line the bench with bushy branches.
- Scoop out a well in the floor in front of your feet. Cold air travels downwards, and the well will help to ensure that the chilliest air collects below the level of your body.
- Once the snow hole is ready, get inside, block up the entrance and stay put until morning or until the weather clears and you can move on.
- Avoid falling asleep in a snow-hole shelter unless you are properly equipped with a sleeping bag and plastic survival bag. Keep your spirits up by singing, telling yourself stories – whatever it takes to keep you alert.
- Light a candle, if you have one. It will provide warmth and help to keep your spirits up.

BOYS AGAINST A BLIZZARD
Training, preparation and a determination to stay alive saved the lives of three teenage American climbers who became trapped on Mount Hood in Oregon by a terrifying blizzard. Once Gary Schneider and Matt Meacham, both 16, and 18-year-old Randy Knapp realised they could go no farther during their New Year hike in 1976, they dug a snow hole and settled in to wait out the storm. They were well equipped and had plenty of food, and they kept wriggling their toes and rubbing their feet to keep the circulation going.

They were rescued after two weeks when the storm died away. Each had lost about 2 stone (13kg) in weight, and Randy and Matt had minor frostbite. But all were well enough to go back to school within a couple of weeks.

Surviving in the desert
The vital need in a desert is to avoid dehydration. If you are stranded in a car, use its shelter to keep cool during the heat of the day. If you are on foot, find whatever shade you can – in a cave, say, or in the shadow of rocks.
- Improvise a headdress – a hat with a handkerchief, say, hanging from the back of it – to protect your head and the back of your neck from the sun. It is important to cover the back of the neck as well as the head to guard against heat stroke (see page 106).
- Set up a signal for rescue parties (see page 312), then take cover from the sun. Keep to the shade throughout the day. Move only at night.
- If you are stranded in a car, never leave it and try to walk out. Stay with the vehicle.
- An adult in the shade can make do on 4 pints (2.25 litres) of water a day. Try to drink in the early morning and evening. Drinking during the heat of the day can lead to excessive perspiration and loss of body salts.
- To obtain drinking water, collect water in a solar still or use a dew trap.
- Look, too, for a natural source of water in the beds of dried-up streams or rivers. Dig in damp

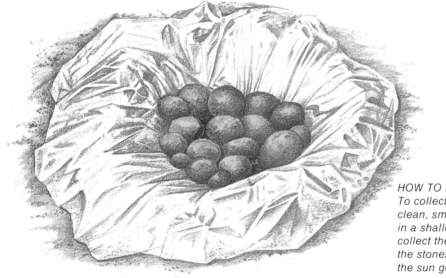

HOW TO MAKE A DEW TRAP
To collect dew in the desert, pile clean, smooth stones on plastic in a shallow hole. Each morning, collect the dew that drains from the stones into the plastic before the sun gets up and evaporates it.

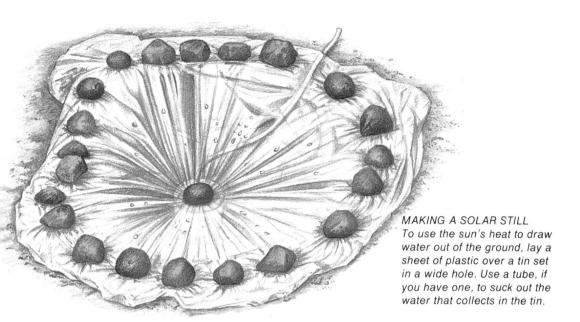

MAKING A SOLAR STILL
To use the sun's heat to draw water out of the ground, lay a sheet of plastic over a tin set in a wide hole. Use a tube, if you have one, to suck out the water that collects in the tin.

patches or around the bases of plants. There may be moisture underground.

• Watch also the behaviour of wildlife. Wherever there are insects, flies, animals and birds, there is moisture somewhere nearby.

• For food, look for any vegetation around. Most desert plants have some edible part to them (see *The edibility test*, page 316).

Making a dew trap

During the night, water collects on shiny surfaces such as windows and metal, or on smooth stones and pebbles. The dew can be collected by wiping the surfaces with a cloth early in the morning and wringing it out into a container. It can also be collected in a dew trap.

• Dig a shallow hole and line it with plastic sheeting or some other non-absorbent material.

• Pile clean, smooth stones onto the sheet. The dew which collects on the stones will drain into the plastic sheeting.

• Early in the morning – before the sun evaporates the dew – remove the stones and collect the water.

• Sterilise the water before drinking it. The stones may be contaminated.

How to make a solar still

Another way to collect water in the desert is to suck it out of the ground with a solar still. A well-constructed still will collect up to $3\frac{1}{2}$ pints (2 litres) of water a day.

• Dig a hole at least 3ft (900mm) across.

• Place a clean can, or any other container with a wide neck, centrally in the bottom of the hole.

• If there are any leaves or shrubs near, put them loosely in the base of the hole. This will increase the water yield.

• Spread a sheet of plastic over the hole and anchor it round the edge with stones or other heavy objects. Place a stone in the centre of the plastic so that its lowest point is right over the container, but not touching it. Condensation will collect on the underside of the plastic, trickle down the sheet and drip into the can.

• If you have a length of plastic tubing, place one end in the can and the other on the surface, protruding from under the sheeting. You will then be able to suck the water from the can without disturbing the still.

• There is no need to sterilise water from a solar still as long as the can and the plastic are clean. The process of collecting the water distils it and so makes it safe to drink.

Surviving on moorland

Wet, cold weather is the particular hazard of open moorland. If you get damp and chilled, you run the risk of exposure, so look for dry shelter immediately (see *Exposure: the silent killer*, page 301).

• Seek out places where animals are taking refuge from the elements – such as woods, copses, caves, overhangs and banks by streams. Try to share the shelter with them, or move them on and use the space yourself. Moorland sheep and cattle pens are also good for getting out of the wind.

• Collect rain or melt snow or ice for drinking water. But do not venture out unnecessarily in heavy rain, mist or snow.

• When conditions clear, head for the nearest place of safety (see *What to do if you get lost*, page 302).

SURVIVORS ON THE MOOR
In April 1981, five cadets from the Air Training Corps on a weekend exercise survived two days and nights of freak blizzards on Dartmoor.

Richard Stubbs, aged 16, his brother Russell, Roger Pheasant and Daren Green, all 14, and Stephen King, 15, ran into trouble on the Saturday afternoon as weather conditions worsened across the moor.

All five of them huddled into their single two-man tent, which they had pitched in a sheltered river valley. With just one sleeping bag between them, and only a single day's rations, they sang and told jokes to keep cheerful as the blizzard roared outside.

Temperatures were so low that the peas froze in the whistles of the rescue party called out to look for the teenagers after they failed to reach a checkpoint.

When the blizzard finally eased 50 hours later on Monday morning, the teenagers set off back, and were met, only 2 miles (3km) from the main road, by members of the 200-strong rescue team. The five teenagers were suffering from exposure and mild hypothermia but were otherwise unharmed. Inspector Rachel James, of Okehampton police, who was in charge of the rescue operation, said afterwards: 'The boys did everything right. They survived through sheer guts and determination.'

Potassium permanganate – the all-purpose aid

Potassium permanganate – a chemical normally sold as small purple crystals – is one of the most versatile items in any survival kit. It can be used to purify water, disinfect a wound, start a fire or signal distress.

• To purify water, add three or four crystals of potassium permanganate to 1 litre of water. Leave for 30 minutes. The chemical will stain the water slightly but the water will then be safe to drink or cook with.

• To clean cuts and abrasions, or treat fungal

MOTORIST'S SURVIVAL KIT

A survival kit – kept in the boot of the car, or under the back seat – is a valuable piece of equipment for any motorist preparing for a long journey in remote country.

The contents suggested here are not expensive to assemble: many of the items can be old or used materials from everyday life. You may never need to use the kit at all – but on the one occasion when you do, it could prove absolutely invaluable.

The clear polythene bag can serve as the container for the kit. It is important that the bag should be clear, because in an emergency you will not want to waste valuable time rummaging through an opaque container for a small item which is needed immediately.

Item	Uses
Large, clear polythene bag	Keeping things dry and together; shelter; flotation aid; cordage (when torn into strips); solar still; water container; emergency windscreen.
Nylon washing line at least 16ft (5m) long	Tow rope; lashing.
Blanket	Warmth; stretcher; cordage or bandages if torn into strips.
Sweater and socks (in various colours)	Warmth; improvised filters; distress signals.
Flexible water can	Water container; flotation aid.
Tins of food	Nourishment; cooking utensils (when empty); signalling (using metal lid as mirror – see box, page 302).
Waterproof matches	Firelighting.
Potassium permanganate	Disinfectant; firelighting (see text above).

infections, dissolve permanganate crystals in a glass of water one by one. Stop adding the crystals as soon as the water turns purple. Bathe the wound in the solution.

• To start a fire, take 1 part of sugar and 2 parts of potassium permanganate. Mix them dry and grind them together between two pieces of dry kindling. If the conditions are sufficiently dry, the kindling will burst into flames.

• As an alternative method of starting a fire, take a dessertspoon of potassium permanganate crystals and place it in a newspaper. Add a few drops of antifreeze and squeeze the newspaper into a ball. The chemical reaction will produce a flame within 30 seconds.

• To signal distress in snowy terrain, sprinkle potassium permanganate dissolved in water onto the snow. It will stain the snow a vivid purple as a marker for search parties.

• Mixing permanganate in water will also act as a temporary dye marker to help rescuers to spot you if you are adrift in a small boat.

THE ORDEAL OF SVERRE BØRNES
On October 17, 1982, during a storm off the Norwegian coast, the engine of Sverre Børnes's 16ft (5m) boat failed. Børnes, a 35-year-old engineer, was on a weekend trip to his island cabin, and had planned to do some hunting along the way. He managed to steer into a rock to stop being swept out to sea, but his boat sank, stranding him.

He salvaged his hunting rifle, and a tarpaulin which became his only shelter. For food, he scavenged limpets and seaweed. He also shot a seagull, which he plucked and ate raw.

Børnes's right foot had been badly cut as he scrambled ashore. Terrified that it would turn gangrenous from the cold and wet, he spent days pounding it with his fist to keep the circulation going – and saved it.

He was rescued after ten days – $1\frac{1}{2}$ stone (10kg) lighter, but otherwise fit and well.

INDIVIDUAL SURVIVAL PACK

Even a pocket-sized personal survival kit can carry enough equipment to stop a problem becoming a crisis. It should be carried as a back-up kit and separately from a rucksack – in an anorak pocket, say. Then, if you get parted from your gear for any reason, you can use it to find your way back to safety – or to stay alive until rescuers find you.

Item	Uses
Empty tin with lid (such as a tobacco tin)	Container for survival pack; cooking utensil; signalling device (when used as a mirror – see box, page 302).
Small compass	Direction finding.
Waterproof matches	Firelighting.
Small, square candle	Light; warmth; firelighting aid.
Cotton wool	Swab; packing; tinder.
Knife	Cutting; opening tins; cooking.
Thin nylon line	Repair of equipment; ties for shelter.
Foil space blanket	Warmth; shelter.
Potassium permanganate	Disinfectant; firelighting (see page 320).
Whistle	Signalling.

Emergencies on holiday and in the country

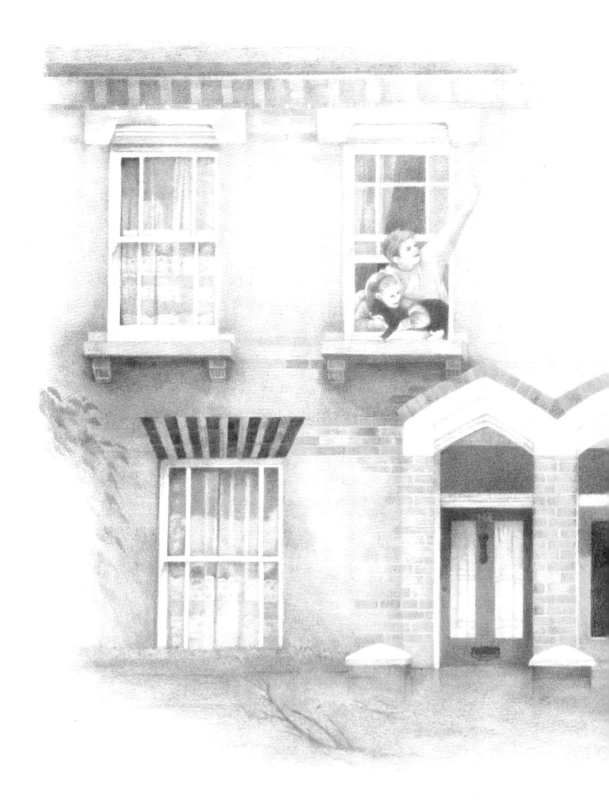

Natural disasters

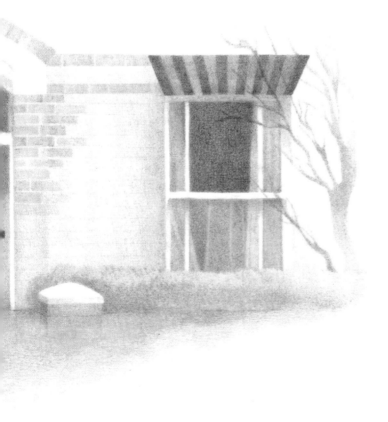

Caught in an avalanche

A snow slope that starts to slide may come down slowly like a flow of wet concrete, sometimes halted by obstacles in its path.

Alternatively, it may hurtle down the mountainside as a 'slab' avalanche of broken chunks, preceded by a mighty blast of air.

In either case, the priority is the same: get out of its path.

• Assess the situation. Your first instinct may be to run downhill, but the avalanche is travelling downhill too – and it may be moving at as much as 100mph (160km/h).

• It is usually safer to head to the side. You may be able to get out of the path of the avalanche, or to reach higher ground.

• Get rid of any encumbrances such as a rucksack, skis and ski poles. They will make it more difficult for you to move if the snow engulfs you.

• Do not try to escape by skiing unless you are on the very edge of the avalanche's path where a sprint will see you clear.

• If you cannot escape and the avalanche overtakes you, clamp your mouth tightly shut and hold your breath. This will prevent snow from entering your throat and lungs, and so minimise the risk of suffocation.

• Hang on to the downhill side of any fixed object – a rock pinnacle, for example. Even if you are engulfed for a time, the avalanche may eventually flow past and come to rest farther down, leaving you free.

• If you are swept downhill, fight to stay on top of the avalanche. Swim *against* the tide and towards the nearest side, using breast stroke, dog paddle or back stroke.

• While swimming, you may need to use your arms to fend off rocks and snow slabs, but above all keep fighting for the surface.

If you are buried by an avalanche

• Summon every effort to break out immediately the avalanche begins to slow up, because avalanche debris begins to set hard within minutes of coming to rest.

• Wrap both arms around your head to create as much of a breathing space as possible.

• To find out which way up you are, collect saliva in your mouth and dribble it from your lips. If the spit travels towards your nose, for example, you will know you are upside down.

• When you know which direction to aim for, try to break out of the snow.

• If you cannot break out, conserve your oxygen by moving as little as possible and breathing slowly. It is possible to survive under snow for some time until rescuers reach the scene.

SAFETY IN AVALANCHE COUNTRY

• When skiing or walking in mountainous areas, listen regularly to weather reports. Conditions can change very suddenly and it is better to cancel or cut short a planned excursion than to endanger your life and the lives of your rescuers.

• Never venture onto a mountain slope soon after a heavy snowfall. Avalanches often happen after successive falls of snow have built up in layers. The upper layers may then become unstable, and the weight of a single skier – or even the vibrations of a shout – may be enough to trigger a slide.

• Be particularly careful during intervals of warm weather or once a general thaw has set in during the spring.

• Be alert for the first signs of an avalanche: sounds of cracking ice; snowballs rolling down the hill; a dull roaring sound; or clouds of white dust farther up the hill.

• Obey all warning notices and avoid crossing risky slopes.

• If you have to cross a dangerous slope, do not go alone. Travel in a party and cross one at a time so that there is always someone to go for help.

• Continue to cross singly until all are safely over. Just because one person negotiates the slope successfully, it does not mean that the slope is safe.

• On long ski tours or walks in high hills, always take a professional guide. Touring parties should work to a timetable so that the alarm can be raised quickly if they do not reach their destination.

Precautions against avalanches

Helicopters, dogs and mountain rescue teams provide emergency services in areas where avalanches are common. For skiers and walkers, there are specific aids that may save life if disaster strikes.

• An avalanche bleeper is a small, portable electronic device which sends out a signal enabling rescue parties to locate victims buried in the snow immediately.

• Avalanche cords are thin, red or orange nylon lines which are easily seen against snow. They are 60-100ft (18-30m) long. Tie one round your waist and trail it behind if you have to cross any slope that looks remotely hazardous. The cords are sometimes crimped at intervals with arrowed metal tags to show the direction of the victim and the depth at which he is buried. Make sure you tie the correct end around your waist.

Escaping a volcanic eruption

Whether dormant or active, a volcano may erupt without warning. In a violent cataclysm, clouds of ash darken the sky, shattered rocks hail from above and molten lava floods down the slopes. Clouds of poisonous gas may also be released from the crater or from fissures on the flanks of the mountain.

A volcanic eruption is a catastrophe on such a large scale that it may seem impossible that any action one person could take would make any difference. Luck, of course, plays a large part in determining who survives and who does not, but decisive action may tip the balance of luck in your favour.

• If you are near a volcano and you notice any of the symptoms of an imminent eruption (see box, this page), leave at once. Travel is likely to be much more difficult – because of panicking refugees and the breakdown of services – if or when an eruption begins.

• If you are caught in an eruption, leave the area immediately.

• Use any transport available. Be prepared, though, for wheels to stick in deepening ash. You may have to abandon the vehicle. If necessary, run, heading where possible for the nearest road out of the area.

• If you are threatened by lava flows, climb to high ground.

• Try to protect your head. Flying rocks are a serious hazard, and a hard hat or crash helmet is ideal. However, any kind of headgear, padded out with newspaper, will provide useful protection.

• Improvise a mask against toxic fumes, using whatever material is to hand. A wet scarf or handkerchief over nose and mouth will help to filter out dust and gases.

• Put on close-fitting goggles, such as swimming goggles, if you have them, to protect your eyes.

• Wear the thickest clothing possible for protection.

• In some areas of volcanic activity there are shelters designated for emergency use. If there is none near you, avoid taking cover in buildings unless you are under imminent threat from advancing lava. Though walls may survive the impact of flying debris, roofs are likely to be crushed.

• If you find yourself in the path of what scientists call a *nuée ardente* (glowing cloud) – a red hot cloud of dust and gases which can roll down the side of the volcano at more than 100mph (160km/h) – there are only two known means of survival.

• The best way is to take cover in a strong, brick underground shelter. Alternatively, jump into a river and hold your breath underwater. A small *nuée ardente* normally passes over in less than 30 seconds.

• If a period of calm follows an eruption, continue your escape from the area. Further – and more violent – eruptions may follow.

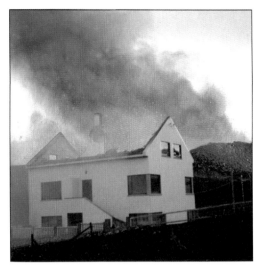

FIRE AND ICE *Ash and rocks caved in the roof of this house during an eruption which partly buried a fishing port on the island of Heimaey off Iceland in 1973.*

WARNING SIGNS

A volcanic eruption may occur anywhere where the earth's surface is deeply fissured. There is an especially well-defined volcanic belt around the Pacific, but many volcanoes exist elsewhere. Vesuvius near Naples, Etna in Sicily and Hekla in Iceland are European examples. Most volcanoes are in areas which are also prone to earthquakes.

Some volcanoes are constantly rumbling, but even a volcano dormant for centuries may suddenly burst into life. The warning signs ahead of a major eruption may last for weeks, and can include:

• Increasing seismic activity, ranging from barely noticeable tremors to substantial earthquakes.

• Loud rumbling noises from the volcano or the ground.

• The smell of sulphur coming from local rivers. The water may also feel warm.

• A cloud of steam hovering over the mountain top.

• Falls of acidic rain, which may sting unprotected skin.

• Fine pumice dust hanging in the sky like heavy talcum powder.

• Periodic emissions of hot ash and gases from the volcano's throat.

If any of these symptoms occur from a nearby volcano, the safest course is to leave the area at once.

How to stay safe in a hurricane

Hurricanes are the world's largest and wildest storms. Racing winds of up to 190mph (300km/h) can destroy houses, tear down power lines and uproot trees.

Hurricanes – known in some parts of the world as typhoons and cyclones – also bring torrential rain and may cause tidal waves which crash inland, washing out roads and flooding large areas. You are unlikely to be caught entirely unawares by a hurricane. In a high-risk area, warning broadcasts and steadily increasing winds will give time to make preparations.

• When a hurricane is imminent, keep well away from the shore, rivers, and any low-lying areas which may be swept by storm tides. Head for high ground. Try to get as high above the possible flood level as you can.

• If you have access to a car, top it up with petrol and drive at once out of the danger area. Aim to get out of the storm's predicted path or well inland – hurricanes weaken as they pass over land.

• If a hurricane strikes before you can escape, stay indoors. The wind and rain make travel extremely dangerous, if not impossible, once the storm begins.

• Take shelter in the largest and most solidly constructed building available. The safest place is usually under the stairs or in a cellar.

• Take with you stocks of food and drinking water. Avoid foods that need cooking, refrigeration or dilution. Supplies of power and water may be disrupted for days.

• Lock doors and windows securely. Close any window shutters. Put bands of sticky tape across windows in a star pattern to reduce the risk of flying glass if the wind shatters the panes. Keep well away from all windows – even if they are taped, pieces of glass can still fly about.

• If you are caught on high or open ground as the winds reach hurricane force, lie flat on the ground. Crawl on your stomach into the lee of anything – a boulder, a belt of trees or an outcrop of rock – which will break the full force of the wind. If you are sheltering close to trees, however, take care in case there are falling branches or the trees are in danger of being uprooted.

• Shortly after the winds reach their fiercest, there may be a period of calm. This occurs as the central 'eye' of the hurricane passes overhead, bringing a patch of clear sky and respite from the winds.

• Stay in a sheltered spot. In less than an hour the hurricane will resume, this time with the winds blowing from the opposite direction.

• If you are sheltering behind a rock or trees when the 'eye' reaches you, move to the other side during the period of calm.

What to do if a tornado strikes

Tornadoes are whirling funnels of air which descend from the base of a storm cloud. They are usually about 80-160ft (25-50m) across.

Where the funnel touches the ground it causes great destruction.

The winds in the funnel may be spinning at more than 200mph (320km/h). But the tornado itself moves forward at about 30-40mph (50-65km/h), so the storm is over in minutes.

Tornadoes most often strike over the prairies of North America, but occasionally small tornadoes occur in Britain.

• Buildings in the path of a tornado can explode, because the normal air pressure inside is much higher than the exceptionally low pressure in the storm's centre.

• If your house is in a tornado's path, open all the doors and windows on the side away from the approaching storm to help to equalise the air pressure inside and out.

• Keep the windows and doors tightly closed on the side from which the tornado is approaching. If the wind gets in, it may lift off the roof or blow out the walls.

• Take other precautions as for hurricanes.

WHERE HURRICANES HAPPEN

Hurricanes form over tropical and sub-tropical seas. Winds swept in from the Atlantic may reach close to hurricane force on mountain tops in Britain, but true hurricanes are almost unknown in this country. The storms go under different names in different parts of the world: typhoons in the Pacific, cyclones in Australia and hurricanes in the Atlantic. But they are all essentially the same.

Around the calm 'eye', winds race at 75-190mph (120-300km/h), and the area they cover is an average of 100 miles (160km) across. Outside the spinning mass of air, gale-force winds – over 40mph (65km/h) – may sweep an area four times as great.

The most violent hurricanes tend to occur in well-defined regions: the south-west Indian Ocean; the Bay of Bengal; the Arabian Sea; off the north coast of Australia; in the West Indies and Gulf of Mexico; and in the west Pacific.

Hurricanes are also common in the south-eastern and southern United States. There the hurricane season lasts roughly from June to October, and as soon as the weather bureau issues an alert, a comprehensive disaster organisation goes into action. The hurricane is located and its movement forecast. Threatened areas are identified and the inhabitants are warned in repeated radio and television broadcasts.

Earthquake!

An earthquake is unlike a hurricane or flood in that no reliable advance warning can be given, although small tremors in an area prone to earthquakes may be a sign that a larger shock is coming. The immediate risk during a quake is from falling debris.

• If you are indoors when tremors begin, do not rush out into the streets.

• Take cover beneath a strong desk, table or bed. If no heavy furniture is available, stand in a doorway – the frame will provide some protection.

• Keep away from windows. The vibrations of the shock or movement in the building could shatter them.

• If you are outdoors when the earthquake strikes, keep away from tall buildings, trees, power lines and any other high structure which might collapse.

• Run into an open space as far from any high structure as possible. If there is no such space, take cover in a doorway.

• Do not take refuge in cellars, subways or underground tunnels. The exits could become blocked by debris, or the tunnels themselves could cave in.

• If you are in a car, stop the vehicle and dive for the floor, crouching below seat level if possible. If you are in an open area and the earthquake is severe enough to throw you off balance, lie flat.

• When the initial tremor is over, stay put. Several further tremors may follow the first one at unpredictable intervals. Wait until police or rescue teams give the all clear.

• In the aftermath of a major earthquake, fires may start from overturned cookers and broken power lines, and pollution could result from shattered sewage pipes. Water is likely to be in short supply, too, or cut off entirely because of broken mains. Check your own home for signs of damage, and listen to radio or TV broadcasts for official instructions and warnings.

• If you have to go outside, keep well away from houses or any other structures which may have been weakened by the shocks. They could collapse without warning.

Earthquake zones

Certain areas of the world are more prone to earthquakes than others. The main areas are: the Pacific coast of North and South America; Japan; South-east Asia; Indonesia; the east coast of China; central Asia; and a band which stretches across the Mediterranean from Italy to Iran.

But there is nowhere in the world that is entirely safe. Even the United Kingdom has experienced earthquakes, though the tremors have been small compared with those in other parts of the world. In many of the cities in very unstable areas, such as Tokyo and San Francisco, modern buildings are constructed on earthquake-resistant rafts.

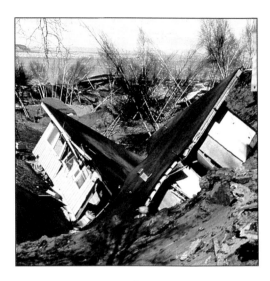

WHEN THE EARTH MOVED *A bungalow, crumpled and half swallowed by the earth, and trees tipped at crazy angles, testify to the force of a quake which devastated the city of Anchorage, Alaska, on Good Friday 1964. The earthquake measured 8.6 on the Richter scale.*

SHAKING BRITAIN

It has been estimated that more than 1000 earthquakes have taken place in Britain since the first known tremors in AD 103. And some have been serious enough to cause deaths.

In 1382 the bell tower at Canterbury Cathedral in Kent was demolished, and in 1580 a quake centred on the Strait of Dover killed people as far away as London and Belgium. The city of Swansea has been damaged by earthquakes four times since 1700. London had two more small but damaging quakes in 1750.

The worst calamity of modern times was the great Colchester earthquake of 1884. Occurring at 9.18am on April 22, it shattered more than 1200 buildings. Church steeples tottered in East Anglia, many people were made homeless and three were killed.

In April 1984, the worst tremor in Britain since 1884 rocked Newtown in central Wales, shaking houses, cracking walls and overturning furniture. Measuring 3.3 on the Richter scale, the quake was felt over an area of 400 square miles (1030 square kilometres). The next month a tremor measuring 2.7 was felt over most of Leicestershire, Nottinghamshire and parts of Lincolnshire.

Natural disasters

Trapped in a forest fire

A forest fire can spread at enormous speed, defying every attempt to contain it. In a large blaze, burning leaves and twigs, blown ahead of the flames, can enable the fire to leapfrog across the countryside faster than a galloping horse, and to jump even wide natural barriers such as rivers and roads. So, before you try to outrun the fire, quickly assess the situation. There may be better courses of action.

• Aim for a road or a river – these are the best escape routes. Otherwise, head for a ploughed field or an expanse of rocky scree – anywhere which has little vegetation. If possible, aim diagonally away from the fire to try to get out of its path.

• If the flames block your escape route, get into the middle of the largest open area you can reach.

• Avoid dry bracken beds and other areas of dead vegetation – they may be tinder-dry and practically explode on contact with the flames.

• If you are in a car, stay in it. The risks of the petrol tank exploding are less than the risks of being burnt by the fire's fierce heat or suffocated by smoke.

• If you are on foot, get as low as you can when the flames come close. Thick smoke and lack of oxygen can suffocate.

• If the ground is soft enough, scrape a hole and lie in that. If there is a stream or pond, wade or swim to the centre.

• Cover your head and body with a blanket or coat, wet if possible, to protect your skin from the hot air.

• Stamp out nearby sparks or smother smouldering clothes after the main fire front has passed.

• Once the main fire has gone past you, look for a way out upwind through areas where the blaze has died away.

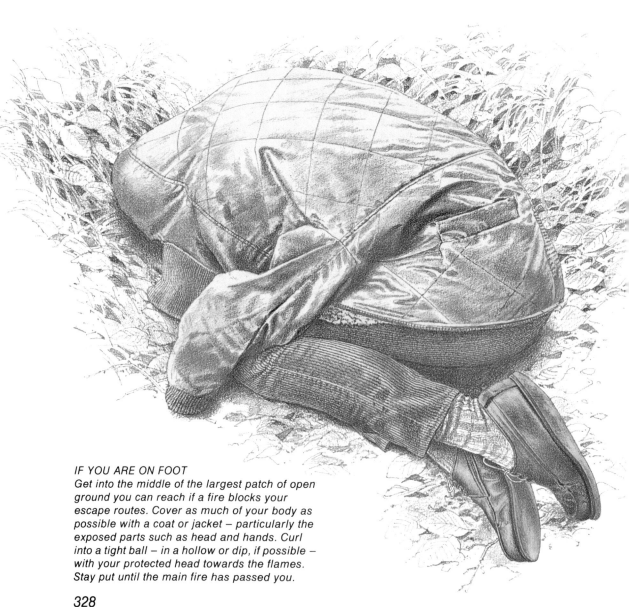

IF YOU ARE ON FOOT
Get into the middle of the largest patch of open ground you can reach if a fire blocks your escape routes. Cover as much of your body as possible with a coat or jacket – particularly the exposed parts such as head and hands. Curl into a tight ball – in a hollow or dip, if possible – with your protected head towards the flames. Stay put until the main fire has passed you.

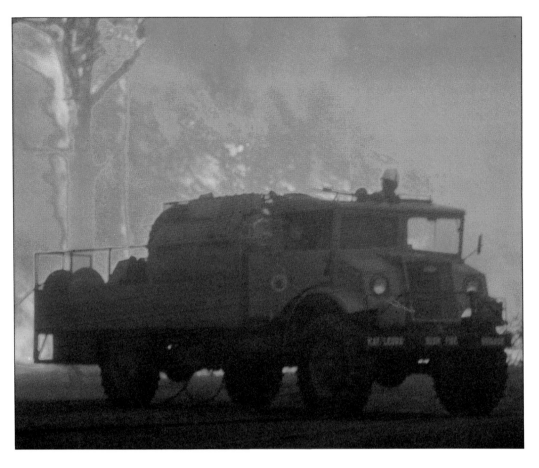

TOWERING INFERNO *Silhouetted against a wall of flame, an Australian fire-fighter guides a water tanker during a bushfire that raged through the Blue Mountains, west of Sydney,* *in November 1968. Vehicles are one of the safest places to be in a forest fire. Despite the risk of the petrol tank exploding, you are much safer inside a car than on foot.*

WHEN FIRE RISKS ARE HIGH

Forests are most vulnerable to fire when dead vegetation dries out. Most forest fires occur in plantations of conifers where the forest floor is always carpeted with dead wood rich in flammable resin. Fires can start even during a winter frost, when moisture evaporates into the dry atmosphere. In Britain the worst period is usually late spring and early summer. But a long, dry summer can extend the period of maximum fire hazard. So-called forest fires can also blaze on heath and peaty moorland.

• *Never* discard cigarettes, cigars or pipe tobacco unless they are totally extinguished. Careless smokers are the main cause of forest fires – the tiniest fragment of glowing ash can set acres of woodland ablaze.

• Keep picnic stoves well away from any vegetation in summer. Fires can start on roadside verges as easily as anywhere else. Use stoves only in designated picnic areas.

• Keep alert when farmers burn fields of dead vegetation such as stubble or heather. The fires are usually carefully controlled by the use of firebreaks (broad paths of empty ground across which flames cannot travel). But accidents do happen. If you see a field burning dangerously close to the edge of a forest, keep away and raise the alarm.

• If you see any uncontrolled fire burning in the countryside, find the nearest telephone. Dial 999 and tell the police where you are and what you have seen. If no telephone is immediately to hand, you may be able to locate one by following telephone lines to a farm or house.

How to cope with a small fire

If a small patch of dried grass or heather catches fire, you may be able to smother it. Fire beaters are often kept at strategic points in forests, and along forest boundaries. They look like brooms or long-handled rubber-bladed shovels, and are for public use in an emergency.

• If you are in a group of people, send two of them for help before setting to work on the fire.

• Lift the beater and press down hard on the burning vegetation to smother the flames. Do not wave the beater quickly. It will only fan the flames and spread sparks.

• Work with the wind behind you, moving inwards from the fire's edges, so that you are not caught in the path of the flames if the fire flares up.

• A branch, a sack or a picnic blanket can also be used as an improvised beater to help to smother the flames.

• Work as hard as you can to contain the fire, always shovelling ash and debris inwards.

• If the fire becomes uncontrollable, make immediately for safety. Move upwind so that you stay out of the fire's path, and raise the alarm as quickly as possible.

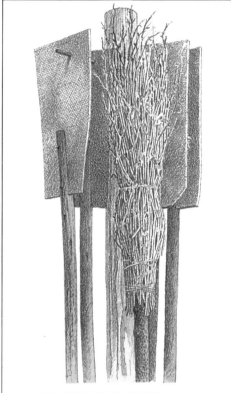

FIREFIGHTING EQUIPMENT
Emergency beaters are kept at strategic points in woods owned by the Forestry Commission. There are two main types: a birch broom; and a spade-shaped beater with a rubber blade.

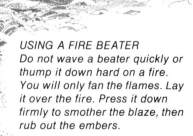

USING A FIRE BEATER
Do not wave a beater quickly or thump it down hard on a fire. You will only fan the flames. Lay it over the fire. Press it down firmly to smother the blaze, then rub out the embers.

What to do if you are caught in a flood

Major floods tend to occur in river valleys, on coastlands and in other low-lying regions. If you live in an area prone to flooding, keep alert during and after storms and periods of prolonged rainfall. Many areas have a system of flood warnings which may include notices or boards informing of the degree of flood alert, and siren signals. Learn the system in your area. Contact the police in good time when danger threatens. They will advise you on what action to take.

• If a flood threatens your home, turn off gas and electricity at the mains at once to lessen the risk of fire from flooded wiring.

• If you have time, take up carpets and collect all valuables, putting them on an upper floor for safety.

• If there is no time to spare, place valuables for safety on any raised surface such as a table, cupboard or shelf.

• To keep water out of your home, first block all gaps under the outside doors. This is best done by lining the *outer* edge of the threshold with sandbags. The police may have provided bags. If not you can make your own. Ideally, the bags should measure 6in (150mm) round by 12in (300mm) long, but you can improvise by using any plastic bags filled with soil, sand or gravel. If nothing else is available, pack the cracks tightly with old carpets or blankets.

• Sandbag ground-floor windowsills on the outside in the same way if the water seems likely to rise that far.

• If the flood water continues to rise, take any food in the house upstairs. If you live in an isolated area it may be two or three days before anyone can reach you. The essentials are drinking water, food, warm clothing and materials for heating water. If you have no portable stove, candles can be used as heaters. Take a gas-filled cigarette lighter or dry matches with you.

• In a very severe flood, you may be forced onto the roof and have to improvise a raft for escape. As the waters rise, gather up any equipment which can be used to signal for help, such as a torch, whistle, flags, bright coloured sheets or blankets, oily rags (for flares) and a mirror.

• Before going outside for any reason, eat and drink as much as you can to build up your energy reserves. Put on your warmest clothing and footwear – they will help to preserve body heat even if you are immersed in water.

• Take ropes or sheets to tie yourself to the chimney-stack, to prevent you from slipping down the roof.

• To improvise a raft, assemble whatever buoyant materials are to hand: an air bed, wooden beams, chests, planks or even a wardrobe. If you have no rope for lashing a raft together, use bedsheets.

• Use the raft only as a last resort, and test it to see that it floats before climbing aboard. Take some sort of paddle with you, and your signalling equipment.

KEEPING WATER OUT OF THE HOME

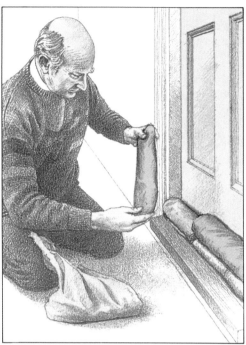

1 To stop water getting into a house, lay sandbags along the outside thresholds of the doors. If necessary, improvise by rolling up plastic shopping bags partly filled with soil.

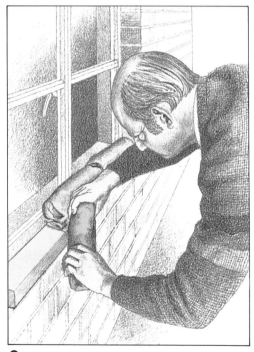

2 If the flood seems likely to rise as far as the windows, pack more bags along the sills outside. If you run out of bags, pack any gaps tightly with strips of old carpet or blankets.

Natural disasters

How to cross a flooded river

If you are trapped by a river in flood, take the utmost care when attempting a crossing. Even a small stream, swollen by fast-flowing water, may be strong enough to sweep you away.

• Make absolutely sure that the crossing is necessary before starting. It may be possible to make a detour to a bridge or to go upstream where the river may divide into smaller tributaries which are easier to negotiate.

• Remove your socks, then put your boots or shoes back on to give you a firm footing on the stream bed. Once across, you will be able to empty your footwear of water and replace your socks to help to keep your feet warm and dry.

• If you are carrying a rucksack, adjust it so that it rides high on your back. Do not discard the contents. The weight will provide stabilising ballast when you cross. As a precaution, however, undo the waist strap so that you can jettison the pack quickly in an emergency.

• Use a walking stick, or any other strong staff available. A staff about 6ft (1.8m) long is best. It will act as a third leg for stability, and you can also use it to probe for depth. Hold it on your upstream side so that the current does not tug the base away from you.

• Aim either straight across or diagonally downstream. But walk sideways, facing upstream so that your knees are braced against the current. If you face downstream, your knees may fold under the pressure of water from behind.

• Sidestep through the water, shuffling one foot at a time and moving each leg only when you are sure that the other is firmly planted.

• Do not cross your legs as you sidestep – you may lose balance.

Crossing with a rope

The safest way to cross a flooded river, if you are not alone, is with a rope.

• One person should cross the river holding

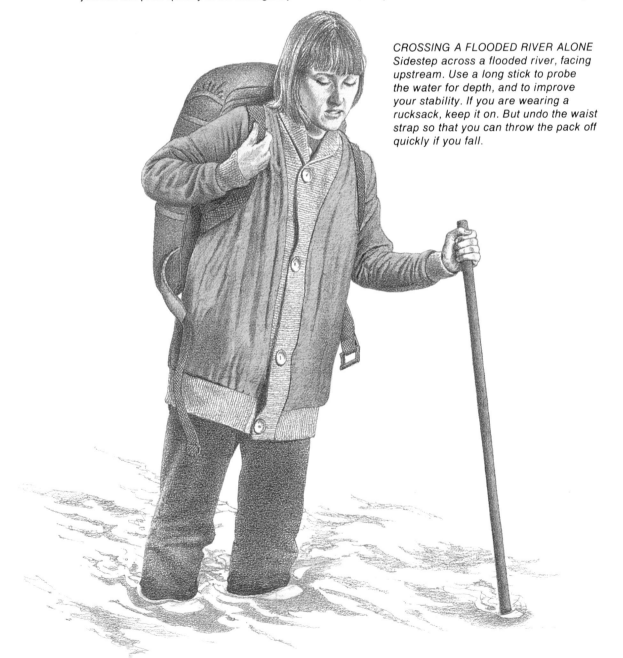

CROSSING A FLOODED RIVER ALONE
Sidestep across a flooded river, facing upstream. Use a long stick to probe the water for depth, and to improve your stability. If you are wearing a rucksack, keep it on. But undo the waist strap so that you can throw the pack off quickly if you fall.

one end of the rope. If the rope is long enough, he should tie it around his body. His companions should secure the other end of the rope by tying it to a tree or rock. If this is not possible, hold the rope so that if the first person slips he can be pulled back.

• When the first person reaches the far bank he should secure his end of the rope.

• The others should cross one by one, holding onto the rope with one hand and using a staff to steady themselves.

• If the rope is not long enough to cross the river, the group should tie themselves together in a line. Each should have a staff. Only one person should move at a time. While he is moving, the others should be braced against the current in case he slips.

Crossing in a group

Three or more people who have no rope can help each other by crossing in a group.

• Form a file, one behind the other, in a direct line down the current, all facing upstream. Each person should hold the waist or shoulders of the one in front. First, the leader takes a small step sideways, then the second, then the third and so on. While one person is moving, the others should be braced in case he slips.

• Alternatively, the whole file can move as one person. Everyone behind the leader should hold the person in front, and all take a step sideways at the same time.

• Three people can also cross with linked arms. The middle person faces upstream, and the other two face each other sideways on to the current. Only one person moves at a time.

Choosing a crossing point

• Look for a section where the river has broadened out. The flow should be slower and shallower there.

• Avoid crossing at a bend. Although the current may be slow and the river shallow on the inside of the bend, the water will be deeper and more powerful towards the outside bank.

• Large rocks and boulders can provide valuable handholds as you wade past them. But do not try to use them as stepping stones – the surface may be slippery or the base unsteady.

• Avoid crossing near submerged trees, high or slippery banks, and above rapids or weirs.

• Avoid stretches where a stream approaches a lake or valley basin. In flood, the stream will deepen and flow most powerfully here. It is best to head upstream until you come to a point where the flow is divided.

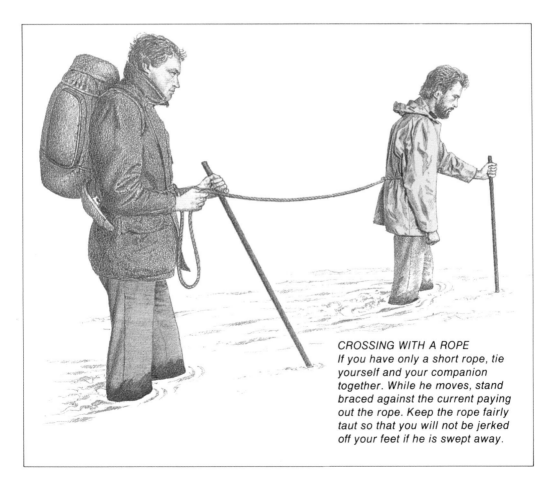

CROSSING WITH A ROPE
If you have only a short rope, tie yourself and your companion together. While he moves, stand braced against the current paying out the rope. Keep the rope fairly taut so that you will not be jerked off your feet if he is swept away.

Natural disasters

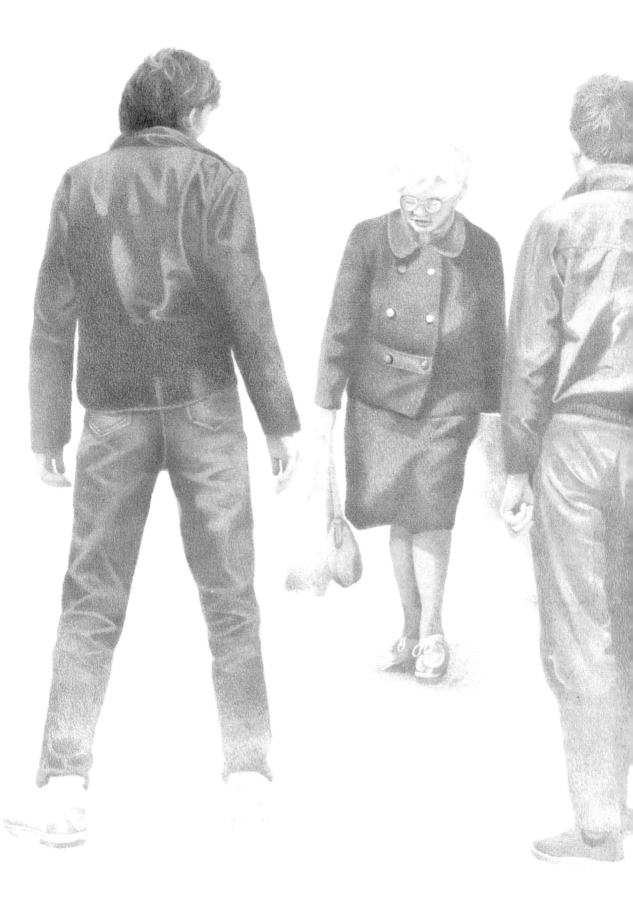

Crime

If you are attacked in the street

Escape if you can. Fight if you have to. These are the cardinal rules for dealing with an attacker. Precisely what you do depends on your strength, your confidence and your assessment of the assailant's intentions.

Faced with an armed mugger who wants your cash, it may be safer to hand it over rather than to risk getting seriously injured in a fight.

Faced with a potential killer and no way to escape, on the other hand, there may be nothing to lose by fighting. In each situation, take any opportunity to escape or disable your attacker. The techniques shown here need some practice, but not extensive training. All are dangerous – some are lethal. Never use them in earnest except in an emergency, and never use more than sufficient and reasonable force.

If you fight, never give a warning. Strike swiftly and as hard as you can. Be ready to repeat the blow or follow up with a different one. Scream or shout as you fight. Keep on until you can escape or your assailant collapses.

THE STOMACH JAB

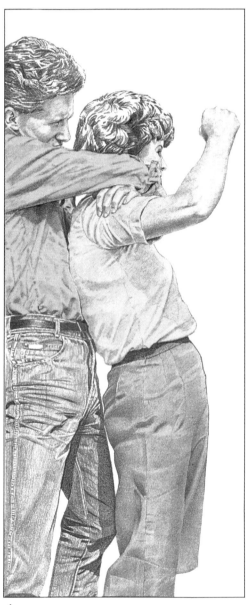

1 *If an assailant attacks you from behind, with his arms about your neck, the stomach jab is an effective deterrent. Twist your body slightly, clench your fist, and raise your arm. . . .*

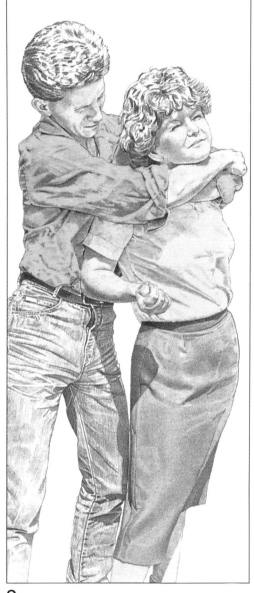

2 *Jab backwards with your elbow into the attacker's stomach as hard as you can, aiming to wind him. This should force him to relax his grip enough for you to break free.*

THE SCRAPE AND STAMP

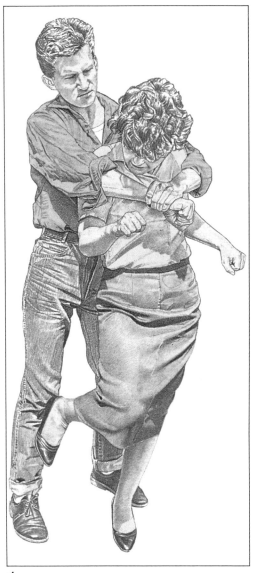

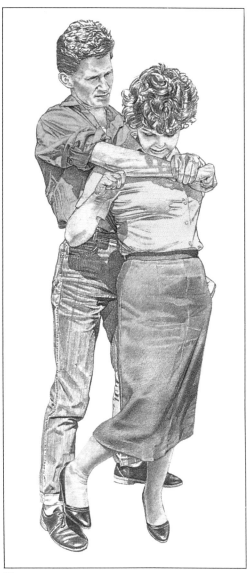

1 *If the stomach jab fails to break his grip, lift a foot and scrape the edge of your shoe down the front bony part of his shin. High-heeled shoes are particularly effective.*

2 *Stamp hard on the attacker's foot – a stiletto heel under the weight of an 8 stone (50kg) woman presses down with a force of more than three-quarters of a ton per square inch.*

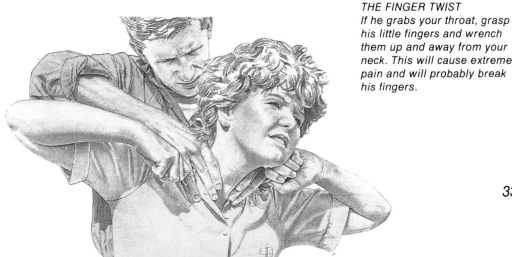

THE FINGER TWIST
If he grabs your throat, grasp his little fingers and wrench them up and away from your neck. This will cause extreme pain and will probably break his fingers.

Crime

337

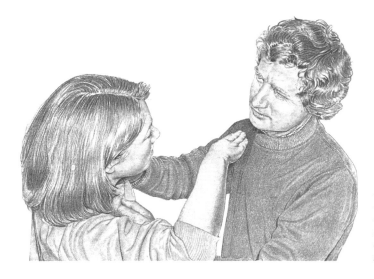

THE THROAT JAB
Hold the fingers of one hand rigidly straight and jab them into his throat, using either the ends of the fingers or the edge of your hand.

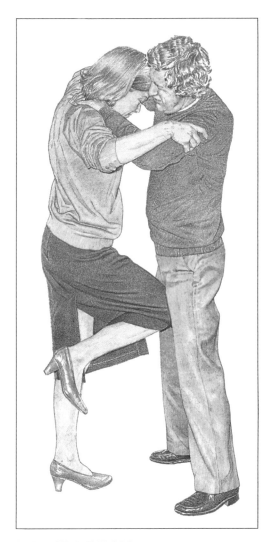

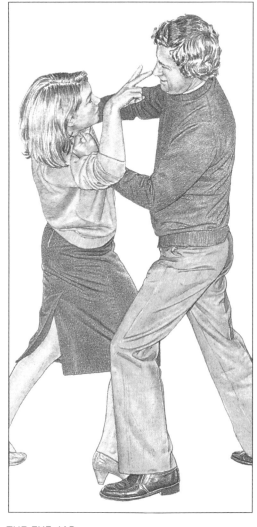

THE KNEE IN THE GROIN
Move in close and bring your knee up sharply into his groin. This will not work, though, if he is wearing a coat or if he twists away from you.

THE EYE JAB
Drop anything you are carrying to free your hands. Make a V with two fingers and poke them hard into the attacker's eyes.

338

How to escape

If you are approached by a suspicious-looking stranger, take evasive action early.

• Scream as loudly as you can.

• Run for the nearest well-lit street where other people are likely to be about.

• Alternatively, run to the nearest house that looks occupied and hammer on its door.

HOW TO AVOID A MUGGER

• Walk with friends if possible, and stay with them all the way to your front door.

• If you are dropped off at home by a car, ask the driver to wait until you are inside.

• Stay in well-lit streets at night, and avoid lonely alleys or waste ground.

• Walk on the street side of the pavement, or in the middle, so that an attacker lurking in a doorway or alley has farther to come to reach you.

• Walk with confidence, even if you do not feel it. An air of purposefulness is often enough to deter an attack.

• Carry a torch after dark. Flashed in an attacker's face, it could dazzle him and give you time to escape. Carry a personal attack alarm.

• On a familiar train route, try to sit in a carriage which will pull up near the exit at your station. You will save yourself a lonely and potentially dangerous walk along what may be a dimly lit platform. If you do not know where the exit is, sit near the middle of the train; that way, at worst, you will have to walk only half the length of the platform.

• On a road, walk facing the traffic. That way, a car cannot pull up behind you unobserved. Do not hitchhike.

• If you have a bag, hold it with the flap towards you, and in the hand or on the shoulder away from the road. Some muggers work on motorcycles or scooters, snatching handbags as they ride by.

• Carry a cheque book and cheque card separately. If you keep one in a bag, keep the other in a pocket.

• Keep your keys in your pocket, not in a briefcase or handbag. Then, if a mugger steals the bag, you can still get home.

• Do not put your name and address on keys. If they are stolen, they could be passed on to a burglar. Instead, attach to the key ring a tag marked with your postcode. The code will be useless to a thief, but will help to identify the keys if you lose them and they are later handed in to the police.

USING AN UMBRELLA

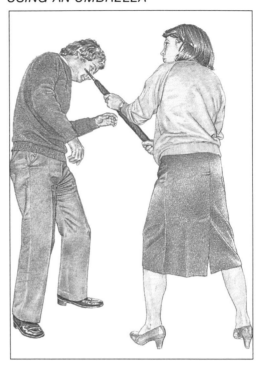

1 *An umbrella or a walking stick makes a powerful defence weapon. Hold it in both hands and jab its end hard into the attacker's face . . .*

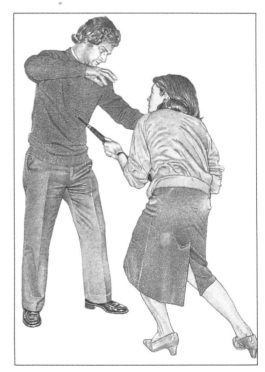

2 *. . . or stomach. If you have no weapon, feel for his testicles. Grasp and twist them violently. The pain can knock an attacker unconscious.*

Crime

If you are threatened with rape

On average in Britain, a rape takes place every six hours. More than 4000 rapes are reported around the country each year – and a much larger but unknown number of rapes and attempted rapes are thought to go unreported.

Scotland Yard experts recommend that anyone at home who thinks she might be in danger from a prowler should contact the police, via a 999 call, sooner rather than later (see *Intruders in your home*, page 182).

The police say they are always happy to help to allay people's genuine fears, even if the fears turn out to be unfounded.

If you are attacked by a mugger or a rapist, at home or in the street, police experts say that the best advice is to run away if you can, and to fight only if you have to (see *If you are attacked in the street*, page 336).

If you are followed in the street

• If you think you are being followed, cross over the street to check your suspicions. Listen or glance back to see if the other person crosses the street after you.
• If you decide that you are being followed, go into any place where there are other people – a launderette, say, or a pub. Alternatively, knock at the first house which appears to be occupied.
• Tell the occupants you believe you are being followed and ask to use their phone. Call the police and give them a description of the person who was following you.
• Avoid using a phone box on the street to call for help, particularly in a quiet road. You could be trapped in the box by an attacker.

If you are accosted

If you are approached by someone whose motives are plainly sinister, and you cannot get away at once, you can use any or all of a number of ways of dealing with him.

Which is best depends on the circumstances and on your own strength and confidence. None of the methods described here can guarantee your safety, but all have been used successfully by women to escape a would-be rapist.

• If you have time before the person accosts you, try to get some hard object in your hand – a comb, perhaps, a bunch of keys, or a can of spray.
• If you pick keys, dangle them between your fingers and close your hand over them so that the ends of the keys stick out from your fist.
• Keep your improvised weapon concealed until the attack starts. Then use the weapon – suddenly, without warning and as hard as you possibly can.
• Jab the end of the comb into his face or drag the teeth across underneath his nose. Scrape the keys across his face. Or spray into his eyes. At the same time, scream as loudly as you can.
• Keep using the weapon until the attacker lets go, then run to the nearest well-lit street or the nearest occupied house and get help.
• If you have no weapon, scream at the attacker to leave you alone. Use forceful language when you do this – as loud and forceful as possible.
• At the same time as you shout, use a personal alarm if you have one.

STAYING OUT OF DANGER

Most of the precautions you can take to avoid being attacked by a thief also apply to protecting yourself against the possibility of rape (see *How to avoid a mugger*, page 339).

If you live alone, though, or if you have to go out alone – particularly if you have to be out after dark – consider taking some additional precautions.

• Consider, for instance, buying a hand-held personal alarm. Carry it in your hand, not in your handbag where it may be difficult to reach in an emergency.
• If you live in a flat, use only your initials – not your full first name – on the tab beside your bell at the front door. That way, a stranger cannot tell whether a man or woman lives there.
• If you live alone, add another, fictitious name to the tab. A flat that appears to be shared is far less likely to be picked out as a target by a rapist or a thief.

• Fit a stout chain to the door, and a peep-hole viewer, and make a habit of using both to check visitors.
• Do not open your door unless you are certain that it is safe.
• Arrange with your friends to use a special pattern of rings or knocks as a recognition signal, but even then make sure of your visitor's identity before opening the door. A thief or a rapist might have overheard the signal and could be copying it.
• Gas and electricity companies will also agree to use a private codeword chosen by you to confirm the identity of meter readers. To arrange a codeword, contact your local gas or electricity office.
• If you are on your own when someone comes to the door, pretend that you have company. As you approach the door, call out loudly to your fictitious companion something like: 'Okay, Harry, I'll go.'

• As soon as you get away from the attacker, dial 999, ask for the police and give them a detailed description of him (see *How to give a description to the police*, page 183).

• If you are attacked, report the assault to the police as soon as possible. This will give them a chance to arrest your attacker, and could save someone else from being assaulted.

• The police will do all they can to help and reassure you. You can have a relative, friend or other person with you for support during the interview.

• Do not wash yourself or change the clothes you were wearing at the time of the assault. Doing so might destroy useful evidence.

• After reporting to the police you will be asked to agree to a medical examination. This will look for relevant evidence, and will be thorough. Whenever possible you will be offered the choice of a male or female doctor. The examination will take place in a special suite or doctor's surgery.

• The police will need a detailed statement of what happened to help their investigation, and for later use in court. If an arrest is made you may be asked to identify your attacker from a group of at least eight other people, or from a video film.

• Court proceedings can be stressful. Whenever possible the police will provide a specially trained officer to help you. Alternatively a Victim Support volunteer will accompany you. Police and volunteers will do all they can to make the experience easier for you.

• If you decide not to report the attack to the police, you should seek medical advice anyway. Your doctor or hospital will help. Consider getting advice and help from the nearest Rape Crisis Centre or Citizens Advice Bureau. The telephone numbers are in your local directory. Male victims may contact Survivors, a registered charity, on 071-833 3737.

Pestered by a drunk

A drunken stranger is more likely to be a nuisance than a danger. Nevertheless, the unpredictability of his behaviour and sudden switches in mood can be extremely frightening.

• Ignore a drunk, if possible, and keep out of his way. Do not invite his notice. On a train, for example, get off and move to another carriage as soon as you can – ideally before he notices you. In the street, cross to the other side of the road before you reach him.

• If avoidance is impossible, assess his mood and character. If he seems harmless and merely wants to chat, humour him until he goes away or until you are able to leave.

• Try not to appear embarrassed, because this may encourage him.

• In the street, do not stop; just say 'Goodnight' in response to his opening conversational gambit, and walk quickly by.

If he becomes aggressive

• Should he be either aggressive or maudlin, make a fuss and try to attract the attention of other people.

• Shout at him to go away, using language as forceful as you can make it. He is less likely to continue pestering someone fierce and firm than someone scared and submissive.

• If he is persistent and you are in a confined space such as a train, walk through the connecting doors between the carriages and find the guard.

If he attacks you

• If he makes a grab for you or attacks you, make as much noise as possible to attract other passengers.

• As a last resort, pull the communication handle – but only when the train reaches a station, not before. Pulling the handle will lock the doors on a tube train, but will quickly bring the guard along.

• Defend yourself if you have to. Hold him at bay by swinging something such as a handbag (see *If you are attacked in the street*, page 336).

Avoiding trouble on a train

• To cut down the risk of being pestered by someone on a train, always pick a carriage well occupied by both sexes. Avoid carriages where there is only one person – a man or a woman – or where there are groups of youths, such as football supporters.

• At night on a train, try to sit in a carriage which will stop near the exit at your destination. Drunks sometimes seek out railway stations, either in the hope of finding company or simply for shelter. Picking the right part of the train will save you a walk down what could be a lonely and shadowy platform.

• If you are not sure where the exit is on the platform at your destination, try to sit near the middle of the train. That way, you will at worst have to walk only half the length of the platform.

Crime

When a crowd turns ugly

Being part of a large, good-humoured crowd – at a public occasion, say, such as the New Year revel in Trafalgar Square, London – can be exhilarating. But if the mood of the crowd turns sour for any reason, anyone caught in the crush, as a participant or simply as a bystander, can be seriously hurt or even killed.

Danger is most likely to arise in situations where people's feelings become inflamed for some reason – at or after football matches, for instance, at protest meetings and demonstrations, and on picket lines. Panic, however, can turn any crowded place, such as a cinema or discotheque, into a potential death trap.

If you are on foot

• If you find yourself in the path of an obviously unruly or frightened crowd, walk away from it and get well out of its way. Do not run, though, because this may attract the crowd's attention.

• If you have no time to get right away from the scene before the crowd overtakes you, go into the nearest shop, knock at the door of the nearest house and ask for help, or tuck yourself into a convenient doorway.

• Stay put until the crowd has gone by.

• If you get caught up in the crowd, remember two overriding priorities: stay away from glass shop fronts; and stay on your feet. If you get pushed through a plate-glass window or trampled by the crowd, you are unlikely to escape without serious injury.

• Hang onto something fixed, such as a lamp post, if you can, and let the crowd surge on past you. Once the crowd clears, move calmly but briskly away from the scene.

• If you are swept along by the crush, create space for yourself by grasping one wrist in front of you with your other hand and bracing your elbows away from your sides. This will protect

IF YOU ARE SWEPT ALONG BY A CROWD

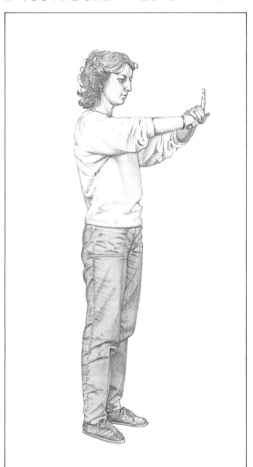

1 In a crush you cannot escape from, create space for yourself around your chest so that you can breathe. Grip one wrist with the other hand and brace your arms in front of you with your elbows well out to the sides.

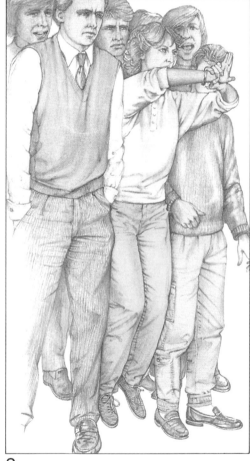

2 Stay on your feet and stay away from glass shop fronts for safety. If necessary, lift your feet off the ground so that your toes do not get trampled, allowing yourself to be supported by the people around you in the crowd.

you from being squeezed by the people around you, and possibly fainting from sheer inability to breathe. Bend forwards slightly at the waist at the same time to create extra room for your lungs to expand.

• If necessary, bend your knees as well and lift your feet completely off the ground to avoid getting your toes trodden on. The crush of people will support you.

• Be ready to put your feet down again as soon as the crowd begins to open up.

• If you are pushed to the ground, try to get against a wall.

• Roll yourself into a tight ball facing the wall with your hands clasped around the back of your neck. This will help to protect the most vulnerable parts of your body.

• Do not panic; a street crowd is likely to sweep on past you within a few seconds.

If you are in a car

• Never drive through a crowd, particularly if it is in an angry or hostile mood – or if it looks as though it could become hostile. You could be seriously injured if the mob turns on the car and breaks the windows or turns the car over.

• If you find yourself in the path of a crowd, do not stop to watch it. Turn into a side road, reverse or turn round, and drive away calmly.

• If you cannot get away from the approaching crowd altogether, park the car, lock it and leave it. Take shelter in a side street, a shop, a house or a doorway.

• If there is no time even to park the car, stop it – in the middle of the road if necessary – and turn the engine off.

• Lock all the doors and stay quiet inside the car until the crowd has gone by.

STAYING OUT OF TROUBLE

• At public events where there are large numbers of people, check the exits as you go in. But remember that the safest way out may not be the same as the way you came in. If a fire breaks out in a crowded place – in a football grandstand, say, or a disco – look around for alternative escape routes. At a football match, the safest place might be on the pitch, not trying to fight your way out through narrow turnstiles.

• Stay behind at the end for at least 15 minutes to allow the main crowd to disperse.

• After a football match, never wear a scarf which identifies the team you support. Tuck it out of sight on your way home. Otherwise you could be picked on by rival fans. Most injuries occur after a match, not before or during it.

IF YOU ARE PUSHED TO THE GROUND
Try to get beside a wall if you lose your balance and go down. Tuck yourself into a tight ball, facing the wall. Clamp your hands together around the back of your neck. Your fingers, back and legs may get hurt, but you will protect the most vulnerable parts of your body.

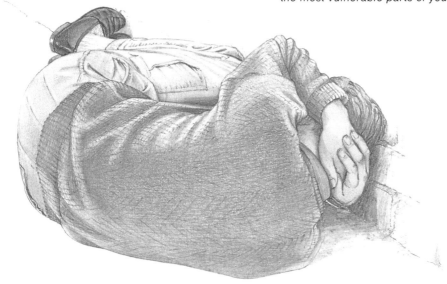

Crime

How to deal with an obscene telephone call

Obscene calls are unpleasant and may be upsetting, but they are extremely unlikely to lead to personal contact or a physical attack.

• Never give your number when answering the telephone, the police advise – just say 'Hello'. This is because, in most cases, nuisance callers do not bother to find specific numbers in a directory. Usually they ring a combination of numbers at random until a woman answers. As a result, they are unlikely to know your number, or to remember what they dialled, unless you remind them by saying it.

• If you have an answering machine, the recorded message should never give your name or telephone number, or say you are out or away from home. It should say simply that you cannot answer the phone at the moment.

• If you have not had a similar call before, ring off without making any reply as soon as you realise the nature of the call. Check with everyone else in your home to find out if it has happened before.

• If the calls become persistent, tell the police or BT. They work together to put an end to malicious calls of all kinds. They will discuss and agree with you the best action to take, which may include tracing calls. Almost all calls made in Britain can be traced.

If nuisance calls continue

• If the calls continue after you have informed the police or BT, do not engage in conversation with the caller. Put the handset down for a few minutes, then replace it. Also listen for clues that might help to track him down. For example, note whether you hear rapid pips – indicating that the call is from a pay-phone – or whether there is background noise such as machinery or traffic.

• If possible, while the call continues get someone to ring the police on another phone. The police may then be able to trace the call.

• If you find the calls disturbing, or are afraid your child might answer an obscene call, you can do a number of things that might solve the problem while the police investigate. Some options are listed below. To get detailed advice on the measures you can take, contact BT free of charge on 0800 666 700 at any time, or 0800 661 441 during office hours.

• Change your telephone number to reduce the chance of the same caller bothering you again. In 1993 the fee for changing a number was £30.50 plus VAT. But the fee is sometimes waived if the change is being made because of nuisance calls.

• Install a plug and socket system. In 1993 this cost from £10 plus VAT, depending on the number of plugs. When the phone is pulled out of the plug, the caller can still hear it ringing but you cannot hear it at your end. The caller will think that you are out or have decided not to answer, and may give up dialling.

• Do not simply leave your phone off the hook. This can create chaos at the local exchange and can cause faults on the line.

• If you make many more phone calls than you receive, arrange for the phone to be adjusted so that you can make only outgoing calls.

• Agree a code with friends and relatives who are likely to phone you. Ask them, for instance, to let the phone ring three times, hang up and dial again. Then you will be sure that you are not answering an unwanted call.

AVOIDING UNWELCOME CALLS

Obscene telephone calls are usually made by men who are on their own for long periods and who have access to a private telephone. They are rarely made from public call boxes, because the callers are usually secretive, and may call while indulging in some sexual aberration.

• If a caller asks you to confirm your number, do not do so; just ask what number is wanted. If it is not yours, do not give your number. Say: 'Sorry, wrong number', and ring off. If it is your number, do not give it to a stranger.

• If your children are likely to answer the phone, make sure they do not give the number. Obliterate it from the telephone dial if necessary.

• If you are uneasy about having your name and number published in the telephone directory, apply for an ex-directory number. You can then expect calls only from people to whom you have given your number. This does not prevent a random obscene call, but as long as you do not mention the number when answering, a repeat call is unlikely.

• If you are having a new phone put in, or if you simply ask for your existing number not to be listed in future editions of your telephone directory, an ex-directory number costs no more than an ordinary number. But if you want to change your existing number for an ex-directory one, you may have to pay for the change of number; in 1993 this fee was £30.50 plus VAT.

• If you are a woman and want your name put in the directory, make sure that the entry gives only your surname and your initials – and no Mrs, Miss or Ms either.

Caught up in a robbery

Every day in Britain, the number of robberies – thefts involving violence or the threat of it – continues to increase, and in about one in ten of them the robbers are armed. Their targets are most commonly places where valuable goods, such as jewellery, or large amounts of cash are stored or handled: banks, for instance, security vans, payroll offices or shops.

Burglary and housebreaking are far more common crimes. For details on how to cope with them, see *Intruders in your home*, page 182.

Most major robberies take place during the day, when the scene of the hold-up may be crowded with people. The thieves rely on speed and the terror they create to make their getaway.

If you are caught up in a robbery – at home, as a bystander when robbers burst in, as an employee of the firm that is being attacked, or, in rare cases, as a hostage – Scotland Yard crime prevention experts recommend that you should not 'have a go' at the raiders. Cash, they point out, can be replaced; life cannot.

What you can do, they say, is use your eyes and ears to help to ensure that police catch the thieves afterwards.

At home or in a shop

• If robbers – whether armed or not – burst into your house or into a shop where you are a customer, do not try to run away. By doing so, you make yourself the focus of the robbers' attention and could be killed or injured.
• Stay quiet. Do what you are told quickly and quietly. Do not argue.
• Make a mental note of everything you see and hear – including even the robbers' accents. Write it down as soon as possible, so that you do not forget details in the confusion after the raiders leave.
• Dial 999 as soon as you can after the raid, and pass on your information to the police (see *Making a 999 call*, inside back cover; *How to give a description to the police*, page 183).
• If you are on the street and notice a robbery taking place – through a shop window, say – but you are not in danger yourself, do not go inside.
• Dial 999 at once. Do not put down the phone once you have raised the alarm. Keep talking. If you are close to the scene, you may well be able to pass on to the police an immediate description of the getaway car and the direction it heads in when the robbers leave.
• If you cannot get to a phone, make written notes of what you have seen as soon as possible. Sign and date the notes – this makes them powerful evidence in any subsequent court trial.
• Take the notes to the nearest police station as soon as possible.

In an office

If the office, shop or factory where you work is raided by thieves, police recommend that you follow the same guidelines as those suggested for people who are caught up in a robbery at home or out shopping.
• Do not try to be a hero. Stay quiet and do what the robbers tell you. Observe, and make notes when the robbers have gone.
• Contact the police as soon as possible.

If you are taken hostage

The chance of your being taken hostage by robbers is very small. But it can happen.

The stress involved in being grabbed and threatened with instant death can be enough to drive every thought out of your head and create blind panic. But if you give way to panic, you only increase the danger you are in. Remember that anyone who takes a hostage does not intend to harm him or her. The intent is to use the *threat* of harm to force others to do what the robber wants.
• Do not struggle. Do not try to run away.
• Do what you are told.
• Remember everything you can about your captor – his approximate age, build, type of voice, appearance, clothes and so on.
• As soon as you are released, make a written note of what you recall and dial 999 at once.

GUARDING AN OFFICE

There are a number of precautions that can be taken in offices to prevent a raid. For high-risk targets, for instance, a silent alarm can be connected directly to a police station and triggered by a concealed button in the office. Reinforced doors and windows can make it difficult for thieves to get in.

Staff training can help as well. If, for instance, the cash-handling area is protected by a door that is kept locked from the inside, thieves may take a member of staff hostage to gain access. In this situation, a pre-arranged code – such as '*George*, can you let me in?' – could alert staff inside without arousing the thieves' suspicions. Police can then be contacted while other members of staff stall the thieves by, say, pretending that the mythical George has the key but he is not available for the moment.

Modern electronic locking systems can also have a code built in to warn staff and police of an attack.

A detailed security plan will depend on the size of the business being protected and the layout of the offices. Managers and staff can get free advice and help with training by contacting the Crime Prevention Officer at the nearest police station.

Crime

What to do if a bomb goes off

A terrorist bomb is one of the least predictable and most terrifying emergencies anyone can be involved in. Faced with the sights and sounds of dozens, perhaps scores, of injured people, it is easy to feel helpless. Nevertheless, your help could be invaluable. The advice here was compiled with the help of crime prevention experts from Scotland Yard.

• If you have a camera, use the whole of the film on taking photographs of the scene. Concentrate particularly on taking pictures of people leaving the scene immediately after the explosion. The pictures could help to identify a bomber.

• Do not, however, put your own safety at risk – from falling debris, say – while you are taking the photographs.

• Dial 999 and ask for the police. They will alert other emergency services.

• Give what help you can to the injured until the emergency services arrive and take over (see *Treatment priorities*, page 198).

• If you feel you cannot help at the scene, leave the area quietly. Try not to run; you could start a panic and add to the casualty toll.

• Make a note of everything you remember as soon after the incident as possible.

• Take your notes – and your film if you had a camera – to the nearest police station.

If you see a suspect package

• Do not, under any circumstances, touch a package or container that you think might be a bomb. Many terrorist bombs contain anti-tampering devices which can trigger an explosion as soon as the container is moved.

• Do not shout 'Bomb' or anything else that might cause panic.

• Move away from the package and encourage others to do the same.

• If you are on a moving train, do not pull the communication cord or handle. Stopping the train between stations only makes it more difficult for bomb disposal experts to reach the scene, and for passengers to get away to safety.

• Find the nearest person in authority and tell him of your suspicions. If you are on a train, find the guard, for instance; otherwise find a policeman, traffic warden or station porter. Alternatively, dial 999 from the nearest telephone and ask for the police.

• If you see someone placing a suspect package and making off, make a written note of what he looks like on anything handy (see *How to give a description to the police*, page 183).

• If you have a camera, take a picture of him – if you can do so safely – and of the package. Even a fuzzy back view of the bomber may help to identify him. And if the package later explodes, knowledge of what it looked like to start with could give police valuable clues in finding the terrorists who masterminded the operation.

• If you think the package might have been left by accident, call to the person: 'Is that yours?'

If he denies it, act on the assumption that the package is a bomb.

• Get well clear of the package and make sure that others do so too.

• Alert the police at once by dialling 999.

HOW TO RECOGNISE A LETTER BOMB

Letter bombs, like other types of terrorist bomb, are almost always disguised to look entirely harmless. Conversely, some hoax devices are deliberately designed to look like bombs in order to cause maximum panic. There is thus no reliable way of identifying a bomb.

Nevertheless, Scotland Yard experts do recommend looking for these warning signs among letters and parcels: any signs of wires or batteries; grease marks; or a smell of almonds.

More generally, they recommend that you look for the unusual. Is the package oddly bulky, for instance? Is it wrapped or sealed in an unusual way? If you are not expecting a package, do you know anyone living in the area where this one was postmarked?

If you find a suspect letter

• If you do come across a letter or package that arouses your suspicions, do not try to open it – letter bombs are designed to withstand postal handling and to explode on opening. Do not press, squeeze or prod it.

• Do not put it in another container. Do not put it in sand or water. Do not let anyone else do any of these things.

• Look for the name of the sender on the back. Phone the sender and check whether the package is genuine. If the package is not addressed to you, but to someone else in your home or office, ask the person to whom it is addressed if he or she is expecting a package.

• If these checks do not allay your suspicions, leave the package where you found it. Clear the room.

• Lock the door and keep the key so that nobody can walk unknowingly into the danger zone.

• If there are glass windows in the room, tell colleagues and passers-by outside to stay well clear of them to avoid being hit by flying glass if the bomb goes off.

• Contact your firm's security officer, if there is one, or the manager. Dial 999 and ask for the police.

If your plane is hijacked

Hijacking is not a common occurrence, but it does happen. In the five years to the end of 1992, an average of almost 20 aircraft a year were hijacked around the world. The planes affected varied from light craft to huge jumbo jets.

The most vulnerable airports are those with the poorest security – often in Third World countries. Hijackers can more easily smuggle in weapons and make their presence known after take-off, or shoot their way on board.

At the start of any hijack, the hijackers, the crew and the passengers are all likely to be in a highly charged, emotional and excitable state which can lead to violence.

• Do not be aggressive. Try to melt into the background. Otherwise you may be singled out and put yourself and others at risk.

• Hide or dispose of any possessions – such as military identification papers – which, if found, might arouse the hijackers' hostility.

• As time passes, the situation will improve. Experience has shown that a rapport gradually builds up between passengers and hijackers. You may be asked to help with meals, clearing up and attending to the needs of others.

• Accept the more relaxed mood – but do not argue with your captors' political views.

• The hijack may last for days, and you may have to fly through a wearisome series of airports as the hijackers seek political sanctuary. Be alert for evidence of tension among fellow passengers, and reassure them where possible.

• Make allowances, too, for any symptoms of stress among hijackers and crew.

Surviving the ordeal

• If you are confined in a grounded aircraft, problems of heating and cooling may arise, especially if the aircraft has no ground power. Desert areas, for example, are hot by day and cold by night. Under these conditions, it may be worth asking the hijackers if you can remove the aircraft emergency windows for ventilation by day, and replace them for warmth at night.

• At night, if the hijackers agree, distribute all available blankets and get everyone bedded down if possible.

• Be prepared for sanitation problems. The toilet arrangements on most aircraft are self-contained, chemical recirculation systems. They will quickly fill, become offensive, and may have to be drained by opening a valve outside the aircraft. Water for washing may be in short supply, or may not be available at all while the aircraft's engines are switched off.

• In the prolonged crisis of a hijacking, passengers may do unaccountable things. Some will become depressed and withdrawn. Others will become hyperactive, nervous and unpredictable. Children, however, may present fewer problems than anticipated – and can be a useful contact with your captors.

• Try to keep your mind occupied with things other than the hijacking. Crossword puzzles, packs of cards, books and magazines will all help. A vacant mind, obsessed with the situation's dangers, tends to panic and take rash action.

• Try to keep fit – this is essential to a healthy frame of mind. Opportunities for exercise may be limited, but take every opportunity to get sleep. Even cat-napping is beneficial. If you are deprived of sleep, you will not think straight.

• Take fluid whenever possible – it is more important than food. A healthy person can go without food for a month or more, but in high temperatures body fluid is lost quickly in the form of sweat and urine. While on the ground, an average individual not taking exercise needs at least 2 pints (a little over 1 litre) of water every day – at high altitudes 4-5 pints (2-3 litres) is needed daily. Do not drink alcohol, though, because it dehydrates the body.

• As any deadline given by the captors approaches, tension is bound to increase. Try to calm any passengers showing signs of hysteria.

• If the aircraft is attacked by rescuing forces, get down on the floor and stay there. Try to make yourself as small as possible; roll into a ball between the seats. There may be flashes of light, explosions, shooting and cries of terror. Do not stand up until given the all clear.

• When this happens, leave the aircraft as quickly as possible. It may have been wired with explosives, or fuel may be leaking from punctured tanks.

• Outside the aircraft the rescue services will meet all your needs, providing medical attention, clean clothing, washing facilities and – best of all – a bed. Accept their assistance. The Press may be asking for interviews, but the airline staff will protect you from their approaches if you wish.

After the hijack

• Be prepared to face difficulties in the days that follow the ending of the hijack. You will feel completely drained physically and mentally. The experience may leave deep mental scars which may take weeks or months to overcome.

• Be prepared especially for feelings of guilt. Some people may be disappointed with their own performance during the emergency. They may feel that they lacked bravery, panicked easily or behaved irrationally under stress. Others, however, may have surprised themselves by discovering unsuspected strengths of character.

• Because the cause of a hijack is usually faulty airport security, hijack victims cannot normally claim compensation for their ordeal from the airline they were flying with. It may also be impracticable to pursue a claim against the airport responsible. It is, however, possible to buy insurance against the risks of being hijacked, and the cover is often included in holiday insurance packages.

Crime

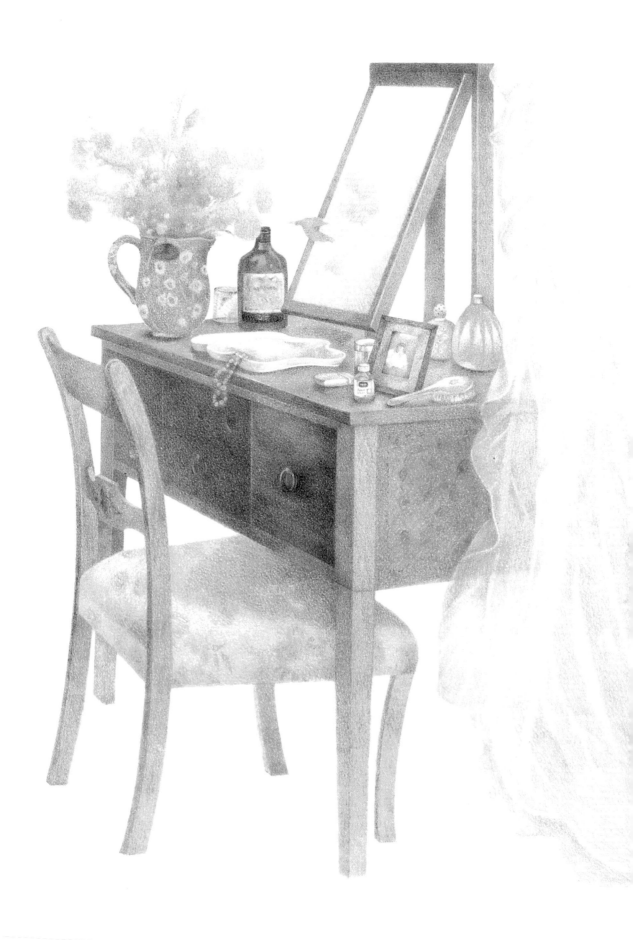

Drink and drugs

Spotting and coping with a drink problem

Though moderate and occasional drinking among friends is unlikely to prove harmful, alcohol *is* a drug.

Its damaging effects become more obvious when it is taken persistently or in excess.

Through abuse, alcohol can cause hallucinations as terrifying as those of LSD; like barbiturates, it can cause fits during withdrawal; and like heroin, it can induce coma and death.

Medically speaking, alcohol is a sedative with tranquillising and hypnotic effects. Though a drinker may experience some initial elation, alcohol depresses rather than stimulates the central nervous system.

For this reason it belongs to the most dangerous category of abused drugs – those most likely to kill through overdose (see *Drug abuse: the risks*, page 355).

Alcohol as a drug

WHAT THE DRINKER FEELS Mild consumption of alcohol tends to free the drinker from inhibitions, reducing tension and anxiety. The drinker may feel relaxed, confident, euphoric or inspired. Large amounts induce excitement, agitation, nausea and vomiting. The drinker may *feel* alert both mentally and physically, but become confused, walk unsteadily and have difficulty in speaking clearly.

WHAT OTHERS SEE Alcohol reduces restraints and responsibility. These effects are often more evident to others than to the drinker. He or she may become impulsive and over-talkative, behaving in a grandiose, offensive or sometimes violent manner.

Judgment and concentration are affected progressively as more drink is consumed. The drinker may stagger and slur his or her speech. Accidents are a serious risk.

OVERDOSE SYMPTOMS Do not automatically assume that because a person *appears* drunk, he is *drunk*.

Other conditions – including diabetes – can produce similar symptoms, and so can numerous other drugs (see page 356).

After excessive drinking, the drinker may lapse into a stupefied state, leading to coma. In severe cases, he may stop breathing or choke on his own vomit.

How to treat an overdose

• If the patient stops breathing, start artificial respiration at once (see page 50).
• If the patient is unconscious but still breathing, use your finger to clear any obstruction from the mouth and throat.
• Do not, however, try to induce him or her to vomit. Vomiting can kill an unconscious or comatose patient.
• Turn the patient onto his stomach, with his head facing sideways, in the recovery position (see page 136).
• Loosen his clothing and ensure that the airway is still clear. Be especially careful to check

---

DRINKING – THE LONG-TERM EFFECTS

Besides the immediate risks associated with drunkenness, alcohol can also cause long-term damage. The liver and the central nervous system are especially vulnerable. Liver damage results from the poisonous action of the drug, while mental deterioration appears to result from organic changes which alcohol causes in the brain.

• Heavy drinkers tend to develop a fatty liver. Most will recover fully if they give up drink. A minority, however, develop more dangerous liver complications such as hepatitis (inflammation) and cirrhosis (replacement of healthy cells by fibrous tissue). With abstinence, the liver may recover from hepatitis, but the damage done by cirrhosis is irreversible. The condition can kill – but abstinence will at least check the progress of the disease.

• Other physical disorders include gastritis (inflammation of the stomach lining), pancreatitis (inflammation of the pancreas) and anaemia (a reduction of the oxygen-carrying haemoglobin in the red blood cells).

• Damage to the central nervous system may lead to polyneuritis, which is also known as polyneuropathy. This is an inflammation of the nerves which may result in some degree of paralysis.

• The symptoms of brain damage may include loss of memory, pathological feelings of jealousy and persecution, delusions and hallucinations. Additionally, alcoholic dementia may occur. This is an irreversible deterioration of the intellect, with confusion, incoherence and numbed understanding resembling the symptoms of senile dementia. Heavy drinkers who escape these penalties are, however, no more likely than non-drinkers to lapse into senile dementia in old age.

• Women should drink modestly – or, if possible, not at all – during pregnancy. Little is known about the effects of alcohol on an unborn child, but experts believe that heavy drinking restricts growth and may also lead to mental retardation.

that the tongue has not fallen back to block the windpipe.

• Call an ambulance if the patient is unconscious or if he cannot be roused. Other danger signs include an uneven or slow pulse rate, pale colour and continued difficulty in breathing. If any of these occur, call an ambulance at once.

• Call an ambulance if the patient has sustained an injury, if he vomits persistently or if he remains in a state of excitement or agitation.

• Call an ambulance if the patient is a diabetic, or if you suspect that any drugs have been taken in combination with the alcohol.

Withdrawal symptoms

Alcohol is an addictive drug, and with heavy drinking over a long period the body develops a tolerance for large doses.

The drinker may lose all pleasurable effects from drinking, and may come to rely on alcohol simply to stay 'normal' – to cope with the minor stresses and anxieties of life.

Often, a serious alcoholic problem is not detected until supplies are cut off or drastically reduced. When this happens, a serious withdrawal crisis may result. The symptoms resemble those experienced by withdrawal from barbiturates and tranquillisers.

• An alcoholic may exhibit anxiety, sweating and shaking before the onset of a withdrawal crisis. So-called 'morning shakes', often experienced by alcoholics, are in fact withdrawal symptoms which usually occur after sleep and are relieved by the first drink of the day.

• Delirium tremens (often known as the DTs) is a particularly severe complication of alcohol withdrawal. Typically, it begins some two to four days after the last drink was taken and may follow a convulsion, or fit, 12 to 36 hours after the last drink.

• A patient suffering from delirium tremens begins trembling uncontrollably, and becomes feverish and intensely agitated. Vividly realistic hallucinations may occur. These are usually visual and often terrifying.

• Whether or not delirium tremens develops, the withdrawal crisis may last for three days or longer before stopping, often abruptly.

• The withdrawal crisis may be so intense that there is a serious risk of accidental injury, and of complications, such as pneumonia, setting in. For these reasons, a heavy drinker should *not* stop drinking suddenly without first seeking medical advice. Friends and relatives should encourage him or her to enter a hospital or specialist clinic for expert treatment.

How to deal with an alcoholic

There is no single cause of alcoholism. The disease may arise, for example, from a psychological problem.

But it can also arise from a particularly stressful occupation, or simply from the company of hard-drinking friends who may themselves be dependent on alcohol. Similarly, alcoholism may appear in a variety of forms. Some people go for long periods without touching a drop – then go on prolonged 'binges' in which they find it impossible to stop drinking.

Other people seldom get truly drunk, but they keep topping up with small quantities of alcohol from morning to night.

Whatever the cause or the pattern of drinking, remember that *you* cannot stop an alcoholic drinking. The drinker himself – or herself – must make the decision.

However, there are a number of things you can do to encourage positive thinking about the problem and assist the recovery process.

What not to do

• Do not start drinking yourself. Husbands and wives of chronic alcoholics are subject to the extra stress and tension of living with a drinker and sometimes they succumb to the same disease as their spouses.

• Do not put your own mental and physical well-being at risk. Make sure that you safeguard your health and constructive attitudes.

• Do not nag, lecture, preach or get involved in angry slanging matches. All hostile approaches tend to belittle the drinker. They may provoke violence, or drive the drinker deeper into a sense of personal worthlessness for which drink has already become the remedy.

• Do not try to bargain with the drinker's emotions in an effort to make him or her stop drinking. Do not, for example, ask the drinker to demonstrate love for you by giving up alcohol. Similarly, do not threaten to leave – unless you are prepared to carry out your threat.

• Do not throw away any bottles you may find hidden about the house. You risk provoking violence and destroying such bonds of trust as still exist. An alcoholic will usually find some means of obtaining further supplies. And if he cannot find more drink, the enforced abstinence may only precipitate a withdrawal crisis with which you are unable to cope.

• Do not try to cover up for the drinker's habit by protecting him from its consequences. This mistake often takes the form of paying debts run up by the drinker. If money is owed, let the alcoholic face the problem. By smoothing the path, you act only as an 'enabler', indirectly encouraging the drinking habit.

• Do not be misled by glib promises. If a resolution to give up drinking is made, make sure that it is backed up by definite action such as seeing the family doctor, joining Alcoholics Anonymous (see page 354), or both.

• Do not give up hope. Ultimately, most alcoholics who face up to their problem and accept qualified help do well. The addiction can be ended. Out of every three alcoholics, about one eventually recovers completely, and another can be greatly improved after treatment. So never be satisfied with doing nothing.

Drink and drugs

What you can do to help

- Recognise that alcoholism is a sickness. No good is served by considering it a sign of weak will or self-indulgence.
- Join Al-Anon (see page 354). This is a fellowship for the families and friends of drinkers. Learn as much as possible about the disease, and attend meetings regularly.
- Encourage the drinker to join Alcoholics Anonymous (AA). Make the suggestion with tact, and offer to go to open meetings with him – attendance carries no obligation, and he will not be asked for his full name.
- Leave literature such as AA pamphlets lying about the house. The drinker may resent lecturing, but may nevertheless look at leaflets when you are not there.

- If the drinker shows any interest in giving up, encourage him to see the family doctor. In some cases, an alcoholic may not have acknowledged the scale of the problem to himself. Often, there will be reluctance to see a doctor, but greater readiness to speak to an understanding clergyman. The church minister may then persuade the drinker to seek medical advice.
- Strongly encourage any hobbies or activities which interest the drinker, so long as they keep him away from alcohol. Try to steer him away from playing darts in a pub, for instance.
- If a crisis occurs, for example through overdue debts, let the drinker face the problem. If he asks you for help, suggest that he contacts Alcoholics Anonymous; the organisation is skilled at advising on specialised problems.

FOUR STAGES IN THE DEVELOPMENT OF AN ALCOHOLIC

Stage one –
the pre-alcoholic phase

Anyone who answers 'yes' to any of these questions – particularly question 4 – should make an effort to control his drinking habits, as they could lead to serious problems.

1 Does he drink to feel at ease on social occasions?
2 Does he drink to forget worry or anxiety?
3 Does he feel more efficient or confident in his work when he is drinking?
4 Does he need to drink more than he used to in the past to obtain the same effect?

Stage two –
the warning phase

The answer 'yes' to one or more of the following questions shows that the drinker is well on the road to alcoholism. He should cut down his intake sharply. Most people can manage to do this without outside help.

1 After a period of drinking during which he was not obviously drunk, does he find it difficult to remember things he said or did?
2 Does he drink surreptitiously or secretly?
3 If he thinks there will not be enough to drink at a party, does he 'top up' with alcohol beforehand?
4 Does he arrange appointments so that they do not interfere with the opening hours of pubs and bars?
5 Does he gulp his drink?
6 Does he look for work in jobs where there is easy access to alcohol?
7 Does he ever drive after he has had several drinks?

Stage three –
the crucial phase

Every 'yes' in answer to these questions is a warning that the drinker must cut down his intake drastically, or in certain cases stop drinking altogether. He may need encouragement to do so from his family or friends, or to seek medical advice. He is not necessarily yet a fully fledged alcoholic, but he will be unless he changes his habits immediately.

1 Does he continue to drink after initially deciding to have 'just one or two'?
2 Does he frequently suffer from hangovers?
3 Does the idea of 'a hair of the dog' as a remedy for a hangover appeal to him?
4 Does he suffer from morning shakes?
5 Does he have a drink first thing in the morning?
6 Does he neglect his meals because of his drinking?
7 Does he feel guilty about his drinking?
8 Does he prefer to drink alone?
9 Does he lose time from work because of drinking?
10 Does his drinking harm his family in any way?
11 Does he need to drink at a definite time each day?
12 Does he need to 'top up' with a drink every few hours?
13 Does he carry drink with him, for example, in his car or briefcase?
14 Does his drinking make him irritable?

Where to go for help with a drink problem

If you are trying to overcome a drink problem of your own, keep in touch with your doctor.

Remember, though, that a chronic alcoholic should on no account try to give up drinking suddenly without taking medical advice.

In a specialised treatment centre, you may be given vitamins and possibly anticonvulsants (to guard against fits).

Additionally, the family doctor may suggest tablets to cope with a drink problem.

• Accept medical advice, but keep strictly to the prescribed doses.

• Remember that as an alcoholic you may be prone to excess and to the dangerous belief that four tablets are better than one.

• Also remember that no tablets can 'cure' alcoholism. They offer only a temporary aid, not an alternative, to the help which organisations such as Alcoholics Anonymous can provide.

• Under certain conditions, the doctor may recommend alcohol-sensitising tablets, such as Antabuse or Abstem. These are deterrent drugs which, combined with alcohol, induce unpleasant effects such as headache, nausea, vomiting and breathing difficulties. They are available only on prescription.

• Psychotropic drugs (which alter the taker's mood) are occasionally recommended. They should, however, be avoided unless your doctor strongly advises them. Psychotropic drugs can themselves be addictive and they may prove harmful, by weakening your determination to stay off drink.

---

15 Has he become jealous of his wife since he started heavy drinking?
16 Does his drinking cause physical symptoms, such as stomach pains?
17 Does drinking make him restless, or prevent him from sleeping?
18 Does he need a drink to be able to sleep?
19 Does he lose self-control after drinking?
20 Does he show less initiative, ambition, concentration or efficiency than before?
21 Has his sexual desire decreased?
22 Is he particularly moody?
23 Has he become more isolated and lost friends?
24 Have his wife and children had to change their way of life – for example, by not going out, or not inviting guests – because of his drinking?
25 Has drinking made him harder to get on with, or otherwise changed his personality?
26 Does he tend to drink with people of a different background to his own, or in places where he hopes he will not meet friends and acquaintances?
27 Does drinking affect his peace of mind?
28 Does he feel resentful, self-pitying or that everyone is treating him unfairly?
29 Is drinking jeopardising his job or damaging his reputation?

Stage four – the chronic phase

The answer 'yes' to any one of the first three questions means that there is a strong likelihood that the drinker is an alcoholic. The answer 'yes' to any one of the last five questions means that he is an alcoholic. He needs help *now* or he may do himself irreversible mental or physical harm.

1 Has he ever seriously considered suicide when drinking?
2 Does he feel incapable of coping with life, whether or not he has been drinking?
3 Does he suffer from any of the following conditions, all of which (in the absence of any other cause) are complications of heavy drinking? Vomiting blood; passing blood in the stools; severe abdominal pains; unsteadiness of gait when not drinking; pain in the calves; epileptic-like fits; hallucinations (delirium tremens, or 'DTs'); or severe tremors or sweating at night.
4 Does he go on alcoholic 'binges', drinking for several days in succession?
5 Does he get obviously drunk on much less than in the past?
6 Is he unable to take any action unless he has fortified himself with a drink beforehand?
7 Does he feel unable to give up drinking, even though he has been warned it is going to kill him?
8 Does he return to uncontrolled, excessive drinking again and again, even though he has tried to cut it down or give it up altogether?

Drink and drugs

Staying on the wagon

If you discover yourself to be heavily dependent on drink, you may need specialist care to cope with withdrawal symptoms. Afterwards, friends, relatives and advisers can help you to stay off drink. But remember that, ultimately, the responsibility for recovery is yours.

• At all costs, stay away from the *first* drink. If you allow yourself one, others will almost certainly follow.

• Stay in close touch with a specialist organisation (see box, this page).

• Build up your own network of non-drinking friends whom you can contact whenever you feel the need for support.

• Keep in close touch with your doctor. The doctor may suggest special tablets (see page 353) to help to deter you from drinking.

• Do not let the prospect of keeping off drink for the rest of your life become an obsession. Tackle the problem a day at a time: the days will mount to weeks, months and years. In time, abstinence will become part of your daily life.

• Do not be discouraged if, for some time after giving up drink, you still experience occasional cravings. Feeling like a drink is not the same as having one. The longer you stay sober, the less you will be troubled by cravings.

• Try to fill the gap created by giving up drink. Keep busy, exploring any activities which interest you. Cultivate new friends and new hobbies.

• Look closely at your own emotional make-up. Certain attitudes may have led you into alcoholism, such as feelings of guilt, inadequacy or self-destructive urges. If you can acknowledge and overcome them, the urge to drink may greatly diminish. Professional help through analysis or therapy may be useful in this context.

• Do not give up hope. Alcoholics who *really* want to get better usually do so.

Things to avoid

• Keep away from pubs, bars and other drinking places. If you have drunk heavily for long, you most likely have particular haunts and drinking companions – avoid them at all costs.

• Avoid keeping drink in your home. Only when you are certain that you have conquered your problem should you risk keeping alcohol.

• Avoid stressful situations which have encouraged drinking in the past. Learn when to call 'HALT'. The letters of the word are a simple reminder of the states in which you are most vulnerable – when you are Hungry, Angry, Lonely, Tired or Thirsty.

SPECIALIST ORGANISATIONS THAT CAN HELP

ALCOHOL CONCERN
275 Grays Inn Road,
London WC1X 8QF (071-833 3471)
Alcohol Concern has information, education and advice centres throughout Britain. It replaces a number of earlier bodies including the National Council on Alcoholism, and the Alcohol Education Centre.

REGIONAL ALCOHOLISM UNITS
The National Health Service maintains some 35 rehabilitation units for alcoholics. The units provide specialised services for both inpatients and outpatients, as well as organising home visits and sometimes arranging for alcoholics to visit or stay in hostels and day centres. The units are distributed throughout the country. Addresses are available from the Department of Health. Ask your family doctor whether referral to a unit might be helpful.

MEDICAL COUNCIL ON ALCOHOLISM
1 St Andrew's Place,
London NW1 4LB (071-487 4445)
The council is a voluntary body set up to inform doctors about the problems of alcoholism. It can also advise alcoholics and their families on where to go for specialist help.

ALCOHOLICS ANONYMOUS
General Service Office, Po Box 1, Stonebow House, Stonebow, York YO1 2NJ (0904 644026)
The AA organisation will help anyone who has a drinking problem and who wants to do something about it. Its services include advice, support and the companionship of alcoholics who have stopped drinking. Closed meetings are held for alcoholics alone; open meetings are for families and friends as well. Centres are maintained throughout the country, and details can be obtained from the General Service Office.

AL-ANON FAMILY GROUPS UK AND EIRE
61 Great Dover Street,
London SE1 4YF (071-403 0888)
Al-Anon specialises in helping the families and friends of problem drinkers. Information about regional centres can be obtained from the London head office.

SALVATION ARMY
101 Queen Victoria Street,
London EC4P 4EP (071-236 5222)
The Salvation Army maintains hostels for homeless men and women throughout the country. Information can be obtained from the London headquarters.

Drug abuse: the risks

The abuse of any drug – including alcohol – may warp behaviour patterns, increase the risk of accidents and cause long-term distress among the user's friends and relatives. Most drug-related emergencies are caused by overdose, and in this area the greatest hazards arise from strong sedatives.

Sedatives are drugs which tend to induce sleep and damp down muscle activity. When taken in excess, they may slow the whole body system to the point where the user goes into a coma. In extreme cases, the drugs can kill by stopping the patient's breathing.

Even if a patient who is in a coma goes on breathing, he or she may choke to death on vomit, or suffocate because the tongue falls back and blocks the windpipe.

The drugs most likely to induce coma are: opiates such as heroin and morphine; strong tranquillisers; barbiturates; alcohol; and the inhaled fumes of solvents, glues, lighter fuel and similar volatile fluids.

Death through coma is less likely to result from the other main types of drugs abused. They include: stimulants such as cocaine and amphetamines; hallucinogens such as LSD; cannabis; and mild tranquillisers.

The risk of accidents

Whatever the risk of overdose and coma, all drugs are more or less intoxicating, depending on their strength and the dose taken. They can therefore seriously impair judgment and behaviour, creating risks of dangerous accidents on and off the roads.

An LSD user, for example, might imagine that he can fly – and might jump to his death from a window in that belief.

In people with disturbed personalities, heavy cannabis use may precipitate temporary psychiatric disorder, including disorientation.

Massive amphetamine stimulation causes a 'blocked' mental state in which the user loses his grip on reality and may commit crimes without regard for the consequences.

The risk of injection

Any drug injected by an addict carries serious risk to the user, in addition to the risks of the drug itself.

Unskilled injection may result in ulcers on the skin, collapsed veins or a potentially lethal internal blood clot (a thrombosis).

Addicts also often become victims of infectious diseases such as AIDS, septicaemia and hepatitis. The diseases are caused by handling hypodermics carelessly, sharing syringes or needles, or by using impure water to dilute the drug in the syringe.

In general, injection into a vein is the most dangerous way of taking any drug, because the whole dose acts immediately on the body. Amphetamines, for example, have only a moderately harmful effect if they are swallowed, because digestion spreads the effect of the dose over several hours. If the same dose of an amphetamine is injected, though, the intensity of the resulting 'hit' makes the drug as dangerous and addictive as heroin.

Heroin itself is the most potent of all the widely abused drugs. It is usually heated on silver foil and the fumes inhaled, but may be injected. The body develops a tolerance for larger doses. But if the addict goes off the drug for a time, the tolerance is lost. As a result, a single injection of the addict's former dose can kill.

The risk of impure drugs

The dangers of taking pure drugs are multiplied in practice because those which appear on the black market have often been adulterated with other substances in order to increase the supplier's profit.

The additives or impurities may themselves be poisonous or contaminated with disease organisms, or they may be quite unsuitable for the use to which the drug is put. For example, a desperate addict may inject impure heroin (suitable only for smoking) with unpredictable toxic effects. Equally, an additive may induce nausea and vomiting – with lethal consequences to a drowsy user.

A grim variety of junk products circulate on the black market and are passed off as pure drugs. Users generally have no way of knowing quite what it is they are taking, or how strong it is – or, as a result, what doses of the substance their body can tolerate.

The risk of mixing drugs

Users themselves may mix drugs into cocktails with disastrous consequences. For example, a sedative or alcohol may be taken to try to 'come down' from a stimulant.

But drugs – even those with opposite effects when taken singly – do not necessarily counteract each other when they are taken in quick succession.

In some circumstances, they can combine to increase intoxication – with unpredictable and possibly tragic results.

The margin of safety

Different drugs affect the body's chemistry in different ways. LSD, for example, rarely produces an overdose, probably because it acts like a trigger on the brain. Once the chemical trigger has been pulled, extra amounts have little effect. Taking two or three times the normal dose, therefore, may not significantly alter the user's experience.

With glues and solvents, however, there is a very narrow margin of safety between the dose the user needs to achieve a 'high', and a dose that could threaten his life. While a single dose may only intoxicate, a double dose could be enough to stop the breathing and kill.

Drink and drugs

Drug identification and emergency treatment

The ten-page section that begins here covers, in alphabetical order, all the drugs which are most commonly abused in Britain.

Each entry describes what an individual drug looks like, and illustrates its most common forms – which may be a form in which it is usually prescribed by doctors, or the form in which it is most often sold on the black market. The entry goes on to explain what it is commonly called by users (since a parent's first knowledge of a drug problem in the family may be a youngster's chance remark).

Each entry also explains what a user feels when he or she is 'high', what someone else might notice, and tells you how to recognise and treat an overdose. For first aid details on how to treat an overdose of an unknown drug, see page 92.

The size of a dose is no guarantee of immunity from an overdose because drugs do not always act on different individuals in the same way. A single aspirin may cause acute stomach pain in some people. Others are hypersensitive to cocaine and may collapse in life-threatening shock immediately after sniffing the powder. There is, therefore, no amount of any of these drugs that can be taken in complete safety.

Age, weight and general health also play a part in determining what effect a given dose will have. Other factors being equal, an older or less healthy person runs a greater risk of suffering from an overdose than a fit person in his late teens or early twenties.

Similarly, the bigger the user, the more diluted the dose becomes in his body. So someone who is physically large and heavy is likely to be less affected by a given dose (again, other things being equal) than someone who is small and slight.

How the drug is taken makes a difference, too. A dose that is injected has a far more dramatic effect – and thus carries a greater risk of overdose – than the same quantity sniffed, smoked or eaten.

Moreover, a user who buys drugs on the black market has no reliable way of knowing what he is getting, or how strong it is. The drug is likely to have been 'cut' – in other words, adulterated – to an unknown degree in order to boost the pusher's profit.

The additive may itself be poisonous, or it may be a cheaper drug whose effects may magnify the effects of the drug it has been mixed with, affecting in an unpredictable way the chances of an overdose (see *Drug abuse: the risks*, page 355).

EMERGENCY SYMPTOM SORTER

A person who has taken a drug overdose may be in no condition to identify the drug involved, or may be unwilling to admit to taking a drug at all. This list shows the major overdose symptoms and the drugs that are most likely to cause them. For more details and for how to treat the overdose, look under the entry for the appropriate drug. For more details on alcohol, and on how to treat an alcohol overdose, see page 350.

Symptom	Possible causes	Symptom	Possible causes
Apparent drunkenness	Amyl nitrite barbiturates glues tranquillisers	*Fast pulse and fever*	Amphetamines cocaine, ecstasy
		Flushed skin	Amyl nitrite
Coma	Alcohol barbiturates, ecstasy glues, heroin morphine methadone opium tranquillisers	*Hallucinations*	Cannabis, cocaine glues, LSD
		Hysterical outbursts	Amphetamines cocaine, LSD
		Severe headache	Amyl nitrite, ecstasy
Drowsiness	Barbiturates cannabis, ecstasy tranquillisers	*Terror*	LSD
		Twitching and fits	Amphetamines cocaine, ecstasy
Extreme restlessness	Amphetamines cocaine	*Violence*	Amphetamines, LSD

Amphetamines (and other stimulants)

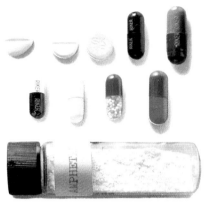

Amphetamine sulphate powder.
Pills and powder all about actual size

WHAT THEY LOOK LIKE As amphetamines are now hardly ever prescribed by doctors, most street supplies are in the form of a white powder, amphetamine sulphate, produced illegally. This is sold either as a loose powder, often adulterated with chalk or talcum, or made up into capsules. Very occasionally amphetamine pills find their way onto the black market.

TRADE NAMES Dexedrine.

WHAT THEY ARE CALLED Speed, pep pills and uppers are among the slang terms loosely used by drug-takers to cover the whole range of stimulant drugs. Amphetamine powder may be referred to as sulphate, sulph or whizz.

Black bombers, blues, and hundreds and thousands take their names from the appearance of specific capsules and tablets. Bennies and dexies are slang contractions of trade names. Similarly, 'sulphate' refers to amphetamine sulphate.

HOW THEY ARE TAKEN Tablets and capsules are swallowed. Amphetamine sulphate powder may be sniffed, swallowed or (more rarely) dissolved in water and injected.

WHAT THE TAKER FEELS The short-term effects include heightened mental and physical activity. Users may feel no need for sleep, and may lose their normal inhibitions.

The drugs cause dryness in the mouth, so users often feel a strong thirst.

Excessive or repeated doses result in a sense of detachment from reality, sometimes accompanied by delusions. As the stimulation wears off, a depressed reaction sets in. The 'hangover' may be severe and persistent, leading to craving for another dose. The drugs become habit-forming, and addicts often experience acute craving, depression and anxiety when supplies are cut off.

WHAT OTHERS SEE Moderate stimulation produces talkative, erratic and restless behaviour. The user may sound hoarse, and may drink much more than normal.

Larger doses 'block' an awareness of reality. The user may stop communicating with other people, and may become accident-prone. Users also lose awareness of the consequences of their actions and may commit crimes or become violent.

With the craving for renewed supplies, an addict may plead for money, and there may be evidence of pilfering at home.

OVERDOSE SYMPTOMS In an overstimulated or 'blocked out' state, there may be extreme restlessness, irrational acts, outbursts of frustration, hysteria and delusions.

Physical symptoms can include a faster-than-usual pulse rate, fast breathing, twitching and even fits. If persistent, the whole body temperature may rise.

How to treat an overdose

• Make sure that no more stimulants – or any other drugs – are taken.

• Keep the patient away from bright lights, loud noise and fast movement – all will intensify the crisis.

• Try to calm the patient and keep a constant watch on him or her to prevent accidents. With a violent patient, some physical restraint may be necessary.

• Seek medical advice by telephoning your doctor or a hospital. If the patient is taken to hospital, doctors may administer a stomach wash-out to remove any drugs not yet absorbed. In severe cases, the overdose takes several hours to wear off, and the doctor may give a sedative or tranquilliser.

Drink and drugs

Amyl nitrite

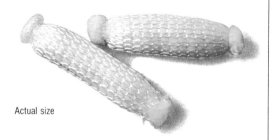

Actual size

WHAT IT LOOKS LIKE Amyl nitrite is a clear liquid contained in a small glass ampoule. The container is often sheathed in a cotton cocoon.

TRADE NAMES None.

WHAT IT IS CALLED Ammies, sniffers, snappers, amps and nitrite amps.

HOW IT IS TAKEN The glass ampoule is broken and the vapour sniffed directly, or the contents are spilt onto the cotton covering or a cloth and inhaled.

WHAT THE TAKER FEELS Users experience an intoxicated 'high'. Sometimes the drug is used to enhance sexual experience. Users may need several ampoules to obtain sufficient effect, and may suffer a pounding headache. Large doses produce hallucinations.

WHAT OTHERS SEE Users appear drunk, elated or confused. The skin is often flushed, and the user may complain of a headache. The liquid also has a distinctive ether-like smell which may linger about the user.

OVERDOSE SYMPTOMS An excessive dose results in intensified symptoms. The headache may cause anguish and the skin can appear brightly flushed.
Staggering, incoherence and other symptoms of intoxication all become worse.
In a very severe case, the user may suffer temporary collapse and may have difficulty in breathing.

How to treat an overdose
• Apply artificial respiration at once if the patient stops breathing (see page 50).
• If artificial respiration is necessary, get medical help at once.
• Otherwise, stay with the patient to prevent accidents happening while he is intoxicated.
• Wait for the drug's effects to wear off. They should do so within about 30 minutes, provided no other drugs are involved.

Barbiturates

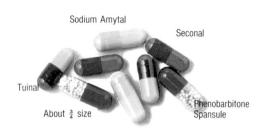

Sodium Amytal

Seconal

Tuinal

About ¾ size

Phenobarbitone Spansule

WHAT THEY LOOK LIKE Barbiturates are now rarely used as sleeping tablets, but occasionally reach the street market in tablet form or as capsules containing a white powder. Phenobarbitone, sometimes prescribed for epileptics, is a white tablet. Occasionally barbiturates are available on the black market as a loose white powder, which may be derived from anaesthetic drugs.

TRADE NAMES Sodium amytal (blue capsules), Amytal (white tablets), Seconal (orange capsules), Tuinal (half-orange, half-blue capsules). Ampoules of white powder are usually the anaesthetic thiopentone.

WHAT THEY ARE CALLED Barbs, downers and sleepers.
Specific capsules often get their names from their appearance: blues, bluebirds, yellows and yellowjackets, for instance.

HOW THEY ARE TAKEN Capsules and tablets are usually swallowed. Users often take them with alcohol – a combination which can prove fatal. The anaesthetic drugs thiopentone and ketamine may be injected.
Attempts are also made to inject powders extracted from capsules and tablets and dissolved in water, but most barbiturates are dangerously unsuitable for this use. The powder is caustic, only partially dissolves and may burn or cause serious ulcers.

WHAT THE TAKER FEELS The sensations felt by users who take even mild doses of barbiturates resemble drunkenness, but users are more prone to accidents and they progress more easily into drowsiness.
Barbiturates are addictive, and withdrawal symptoms include acute anxiety, headache, abdominal cramps, pains in the limbs and fits.

WHAT OTHERS SEE Users exhibit the typical symptoms of drunkenness, including slurred speech, stumbling, confusion and drowsiness.

OVERDOSE SYMPTOMS Heavy doses produce drowsiness deepening into semiconsciousness and coma. Breathing may stop, especially after the injection of a large dose.

How to treat an overdose

- Dial 999 and ask for an ambulance at once, stating clearly that you believe the emergency has been caused by an overdose of barbiturates.
- Provided the patient is conscious and cooperative, induce vomiting by putting your fingers down his or her throat.
- If the patient is not conscious or if he or she is not cooperative, however, do not try to make him or her vomit.
- Prevent any more drugs or alcohol being taken, and keep a close watch to prevent accidents.
- If the patient is comatose or unconscious but breathing, clear any obstruction from the mouth and put the patient in the recovery position (see page 136).
- If breathing has stopped, start artificial respiration immediately (see page 50).
- When medical help arrives, a stomach wash-out will be urgently needed to remove any unabsorbed drugs from the patient's body. The patient will need to be admitted to hospital.

Cannabis

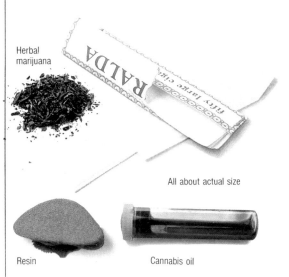

Herbal marijuana

All about actual size

Resin

Cannabis oil

WHAT IT LOOKS LIKE In herbal form, cannabis – which comes from the hemp plant, *Cannabis sativa* – resembles a coarse tobacco. The dried leaves are greenish-brown, often chopped up with stems, seeds and flower parts.

The sap of the plant is also dried to extract cannabis resin, which takes the form of a greenish, brownish or blackish block, stick or lump, or a coarse brown powder.

Very occasionally, the drug appears in liquid form, either as yellowish-brown cannabis oil, or as cannabis tincture (a practically obsolete medical preparation).

TRADE NAMES None.

WHAT IT IS CALLED The herbal form is often known as grass, pot, marijuana, Mary Jane, weed, bhang, dagga or ganja. Resin is commonly referred to as hash, hashish, dope or resin. Other slang terms – such as Thai sticks, Moroccan gold, Lebanese gold and Nepalese black – derive from the drug's place of origin and its colour.

Cannabis cigarettes are described as joints, spliffs or reefers. The butt of a used joint is often referred to as the roach.

HOW IT IS TAKEN Cannabis is usually smoked in joints (often made with larger-than-usual cigarette papers) or in pipes to produce an immediate effect. In herbal form, it may be smoked on its own. Alternatively, in any form, it may be mixed with tobacco.

Sometimes, powdered resin is added to cake mixtures, which are cooked and eaten. The drug's effects are then more delayed.

WHAT THE TAKER FEELS The effects depend on the mood and expectations of the user, and many people experience little on first use. Pleasurable effects include relaxation, feelings

Drink and drugs

of cheerfulness and contentment, and heightened appreciation of one's surroundings. Concentration and short-term memory are impaired, so driving may be hazardous and mental performance reduced. Using cannabis when anxious or depressed can intensify these feelings. With high doses disturbed vision or panic reactions may occur.

WHAT OTHERS SEE Evidence of cannabis smoking may be present in the form of discarded butts, cigarette papers or torn strips of cardboard (used to make improvised cigarette filters).

Additionally, cannabis smoke has a distinctive smell, resembling that of burnt grass or a garden bonfire.

The eyes of a user are often red. He or she may appear unusually relaxed and distant, mildly confused or prone to senseless laughter.

Judgment is impaired, and users may appear clumsy and accident-prone.

Cannabis rarely produces a hangover, but habitual users may become anxious and urgent in their search for more drugs when supplies are cut off.

OVERDOSE SYMPTOMS Large doses produce intensified symptoms of drowsiness, disorientation or hallucinations. The symptoms may cause distress, but are not normally life-threatening. Nevertheless, intoxication may create serious accident risks, especially if the user is driving or operating machinery. Large or repeated doses can also produce 'cannabis psychosis' – a state of mental disorder and delusion which may take several days to pass.

How to treat an overdose

• Restrain the user from taking any more cannabis. Try to calm and reassure him. Take care to prevent accidents, remembering that, in severe cases, his judgment may be impaired for several days.
• If the user has persistent delusions or his behaviour becomes severely disordered, seek medical or psychiatric advice.

Cocaine

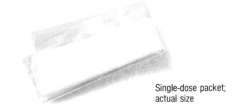

Single-dose packet;
actual size

WHAT IT LOOKS LIKE A fine white powder. On the black market it is often sold in individual doses, folded in small pieces of paper or plastic. Because pure cocaine is extremely expensive, most doses are heavily adulterated with inactive powders such as chalk or talc. Some doses may contain no cocaine at all, but consist of cheaper amphetamine, often mixed with lignocaine (a local anaesthetic).

'Crack', a more powerful and addictive form of cocaine, is made by 'cooking' it with water and baking soda.

TRADE NAMES None.

WHAT IT IS CALLED Coke, crack, snow, lady snow, C, big C, princess and sniff. Individual doses are referred to as snorts.

HOW IT IS TAKEN The powder is most commonly sniffed ('snorted'). Alternatively, it may be dissolved in water and injected into a vein, a practice known as mainlining. The drug may also be mixed with tobacco and smoked, a practice known as freebasing. Wads of coca leaves – whose effects are much weaker than the powder's – are chewed. 'Crack' is usually smoked.

WHAT THE TAKER FEELS The drug counters drowsiness and prevents sleep. Large doses may give rise to hallucinations.

A depressed reaction sets in as the effects of the drug wear off. Depression is relieved by a further dose, and so the drug becomes habit-forming.

WHAT OTHERS SEE The user's mood may visibly brighten and his behaviour may become more uninhibited. He may seem mildly intoxicated or become accident-prone. Behaviour can also become erratic and may extend to violent outbursts if the user is frustrated.

Physically, cocaine tends to dry out the lining of the nose, and some users develop sniffing as a nervous tic.

An intensely depressed hangover is often experienced on the morning after taking the drug. Cocaine addicts develop powerful cravings with severe withdrawal symptoms if supplies are cut off. Frantic drug-seeking behaviour may result, often leading to crime to raise money.

OVERDOSE SYMPTOMS A few individuals are hypersensitive to cocaine; even a small dose may cause sudden collapse through an allergic reaction known as anaphylactic shock.

In any individual, an overdose may produce hysteria, delusions, physical tremors, muscle twitching and fits. Pulse, breathing rate and body temperature may also rise.

How to treat an overdose

• If a user collapses suddenly, call a doctor or ambulance immediately. Urgent medical care will be needed to treat anaphylactic shock (see *Dealing with an allergic reaction*, page 110).

• Otherwise, an overdose is rarely life-threatening. Prevent any more drugs being taken and try to calm and reassure the patient. Keep him or her away from bright lights, loud noise or fast movement, and keep watch to prevent accidents.

• The effects decline spontaneously over a few hours. A stomach wash-out is not necessary unless other drugs have been taken. If the overdose symptoms persist for longer than a few hours, however, or if they are very severe, get medical help.

Glues, solvents and lighter fuel

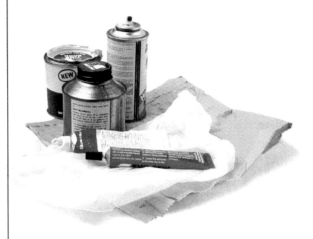

WHAT THEY LOOK LIKE Many household and industrial products are based on solvents which give off intoxicating vapour.

These freely available products include a wide range of glues, thinners, varnishes, paint strippers, spirits, dry-cleaning fluids, nail varnishes and nail-varnish removers. Petrol and lighter fuel have similar properties.

WHAT THEY ARE CALLED Glue, thinner, sniffer, spirit, evo and other contractions of familiar trade names.

HOW THEY ARE TAKEN Glues and solvents are either sniffed or inhaled by the mouth. Sometimes the vapours are obtained directly from the tube, tin or aerosol spray.

More often the vapours are inhaled from a plastic or paper bag into which the glue has been poured, or from a cloth which has been soaked in the fluid.

WHAT THE TAKER FEELS A rapid intoxication which relaxes and sedates like alcohol, and which may include hallucinations. Drowsiness or drunken stupor may follow.

WHAT OTHERS SEE Mild intoxication resembling drunkenness, with staggering and slurred speech. However, the use of solvents is often readily identified by their pervasive smell.

Spilt glue, impregnated cloth or discarded plastic bags are all signs that a product may have been abused.

OVERDOSE SYMPTOMS Severe intoxication may lead rapidly to coma. In severe cases, breathing may stop. This is a particular risk if the patient falls forward and continues to inhale vapour while unconscious. Some users have choked to death on their own vomit while unconscious.

Drink and drugs

How to treat an overdose

- Remove the source of the vapour at once.
- In a room, open doors and windows.
- Clear any obstruction from the patient's mouth, and apply artificial respiration at once if breathing stops (see page 50).
- If the patient is unconscious or comatose, put him or her in the recovery position at once (see page 136).
- Then dial 999 and call an ambulance.
- If the patient is conscious but disorientated, watch him closely. If his condition deteriorates or fails to improve within five minutes, call an ambulance.
- Keep watch to prevent accidents while the patient remains under the influence.
- Take special care to avoid fire risks. Many glues and solvents are flammable – or even explosive – as well as intoxicating. This is a special risk where petrol or lighter fuel have been used: even a sparking light switch could ignite the vapour.

Heroin and morphine

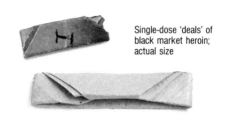

Single-dose 'deals' of black market heroin; actual size

WHAT THEY LOOK LIKE Heroin and morphine are usually sold in powdered form. Both are prepared from opium, and although the refined powder is white, it often appears brownish-yellow because of impurities. Heroin (a derivative of morphine) is the stronger of the two, and probably the most dangerous drug in illegal use. Both drugs are usually 'cut' (meaning adulterated) with an inactive powder for sale on the black market.

Less commonly, the drugs may be sold in solution in glass ampoules, or, very occasionally, as small white tablets.

TRADE NAMES None in general use.

WHAT THEY ARE CALLED H, horse, smack and shit are among the slang terms for heroin. Morphine is usually known as M or morph. An individual dose is referred to as a fix or a hit.

HOW THEY ARE TAKEN Heroin and morphine are usually smoked – a practice sometimes called 'chasing the dragon'. They may be swallowed, or taken by injection, with the powder dissolved in water. Addicts generally inject directly into a vein, a practice known as 'mainlining'. Alternatively, the drugs may be injected under the skin, a practice known as 'skin popping'.

WHAT THE TAKER FEELS Users of either drug lose touch with reality, and feel drowsy. Some people, however, experience only unpleasant effects after taking heroin.

Heroin and morphine are both addictive, and habitual users tend to stop feeling any pleasurable effects. The drugs become necessary simply to remain 'normal', or to escape from harrowing withdrawal symptoms.

WHAT OTHERS SEE Signs of intoxication are often slight. The user may seem merely withdrawn into a private world, and have tiny, 'pinpoint' pupils. Larger doses produce more marked drowsiness.

Scars of injection, known as 'tracks', may be visible on the user. These are commonly found on the inside of the forearms and the front of the elbows. There may also be ulcers, or the scars of healed ulcers.

Discarded syringes, needles and ampoules, or foil and tube (used for sniffing the smoke from the drug), may indicate that the drugs are being used. If supplies are threatened, the user is likely to exhibit acute withdrawal symptoms and to become frantic and violent. He or she may turn to crime in the search for more.

OVERDOSE SYMPTOMS Deep coma, in which the patient is breathing but cannot be woken. The pupils of the eyes are reduced to mere pinpoints. Breathing may also stop.

An overdose is a particular risk when an addict has been off drugs for some time: in hospital, for example, or in prison. A single injection within days of discharge can kill, because the body can no longer tolerate doses to which it was previously accustomed.

How to treat an overdose
• Dial 999 and call an ambulance at once.
• If breathing stops, immediately clear any obstruction from the mouth and throat and apply artificial respiration (see page 50).
• Continue until breathing restarts, or until medical help arrives.
• If the patient is breathing but unconscious, check that the airway is clear and place him or her in the recovery position (see page 136).

LSD, ecstasy and similar drugs

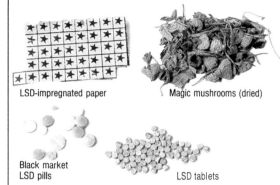

LSD-impregnated paper

Magic mushrooms (dried)

Black market LSD pills

LSD tablets

All about actual size

WHAT THEY LOOK LIKE LSD (lysergic acid diethylamide) is a synthetic chemical hallucinogen. It may be sold as tablets, capsules or colourless liquid. LSD liquid may be dropped onto sheets of paper or blotting paper to produce individual doses called microdots, often sold separately. LSD sugar lumps or biscuits are also sold.

Ecstasy is sold as tablets or capsules of varying colour. They often contain a mixture of drugs from the same family, sometimes adulterated with amphetamine or LSD, so potency varies widely.

Parts of dried plants such as the Mexican peyote cactus (containing mescalin), some fungi, and morning glory seeds may be sold for the mind-altering chemicals they contain.

TRADE NAMES None.

WHAT THEY ARE CALLED LSD is commonly called acid, and individual doses referred to as tabs (tablets). Similar synthetic chemicals are known by their abbreviated names, such as STP, DMT or PCP (also called angel dust). Hallucinogenic fungi are known as magic mushrooms, while mescalin portions may be called buttons.

Ecstasy and related drugs may be called E, XTC, Adam, Eve and GBH. Individual pills are known as love doves, New Yorkers or Phase 4, and also go under a bewildering variety of names related to their appearance, which changes frequently with new batches of drugs. Examples are Dennis the Menace (red and black capsules), or rhubarb and custard (red and yellow capsules).

HOW THEY ARE TAKEN Almost always swallowed. Very rarely, LSD may be injected.

WHAT THE TAKER FEELS On an LSD 'trip', senses are distorted and heightened, often with full-blown hallucinations. The user may experience the world as a highly coloured dream sequence lasting for several hours. On a 'bad trip', ter-

Drink and drugs

363

rifying imagery and visions can become nightmarish.

Ecstasy produces an initial euphoric 'rush' followed by calm, serenity, reduced hostility and increased empathy for other people – hence it is sometimes called 'the love drug'. It may give heightened perception and a 'mind-expanding' feeling without the hallucinations of LSD.

WHAT OTHERS SEE The effects vary widely according to the mixture of drugs taken and the potency. LSD users may seem to be in a daydream or trance, and detachment from reality is occasionally so strong that they believe they can fly or walk on water – with the obvious dangers. On a bad trip the user may become hysterical or react violently to imagined threats.

Ecstasy users may have wide pupils and often appear clumsy and uncoordinated. They may appear serene and content, but can become agitated and anxious if challenged.

OVERDOSE SYMPTOMS True overdoses are rare, although impure drugs and high doses of magic mushrooms may produce nausea, vomiting or physical collapse. High doses of LSD will prolong an experience and may produce persistent terrors on a bad trip.

Prolonged high doses of ecstasy can cause headaches, panic, confusion and insomnia. Occasionally hallucinations, liver damage and fits have occurred. In Britain a number of ecstasy takers have died after suffering convulsions, circulatory collapse and high temperature, afterwards lapsing into coma. Toxic effects do not seem to be related to the size of dose, and deaths have occurred after as little as one tablet, possibly because some people are abnormally susceptible, or because taking the drug while dancing energetically produced a form of heatstroke.

How to treat an overdose

• If there is any sign of fits, high temperature, difficulty in breathing or drowsiness, call an ambulance immediately.
• If the user is unconscious, clear any obstruction from the mouth and put him or her in the recovery position (see page 136).
• If takers become agitated, try to keep them calm. Do not show anger or antagonism. Keep them away from bright lights and loud noises.
• Do not allow the user to drive, and be wary of potential causes of accidents.
• If a bad trip lasts more than four hours, call a doctor to come to the patient. Do not take the patient to a surgery or hospital because of the risk of stirring up the horrors again.

Methadone

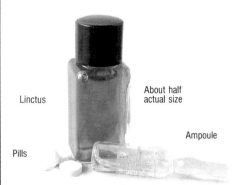

Linctus

About half actual size

Ampoule

Pills

WHAT IT LOOKS LIKE Small ampoules containing a clear solution. The drug may also be sold as a linctus or coloured syrup, or in the form of small white tablets.

TRADE NAME Physeptone.

WHAT IT IS CALLED Meth, phy or linctus.

HOW IT IS TAKEN The drug may be injected, either in a vein or under the skin. In drug clinics, it is widely used to treat heroin addiction since it may reduce heavy craving and dependence.

Linctus and tablets are swallowed. In clinics they are used to try to break the heroin-injection habit.

WHAT THE TAKER FEELS Methadone has effects similar to those of heroin and morphine. The effects last somewhat longer, however. Methadone itself is addictive, and may produce withdrawal symptoms.

WHAT OTHERS SEE The observable effects and signs of methadone abuse are the same as those of heroin and morphine abuse.

OVERDOSE SYMPTOMS The same as those of heroin and morphine.

How to treat an overdose

• Treat as for an overdose of heroin or morphine (see page 363).

Opium

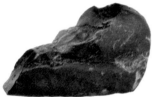

Actual size

WHAT IT LOOKS LIKE Raw opium (pictured above) appears in the form of blackish or brownish dried sap from the opium poppy. Refined opium is much paler in colour and often powdered. It was once widely used in medical preparations such as tinctures and cough linctus. But most have been phased out because of the dangers of creating dependency.

TRADE NAMES None.

WHAT IT IS CALLED Poppy.

HOW IT IS TAKEN Raw opium is generally smoked, in an opium pipe. It may also be swallowed. Refined opium may be smoked, swallowed or (in some forms) injected. All forms are addictive.

WHAT THE TAKER FEELS The effects are similar to those of heroin and morphine, which are both derived from opium. The sensations are generally milder, though.

WHAT OTHERS SEE Dreaminess, drowsiness and detachment may be evident, though less marked than in heroin or morphine users. Injection scars will not necessarily be present.

There may be evidence of smoking in the form of an opium pipe with a sweet, heady smell. Some experts, however, say that the smoke smells like burning old socks.

OVERDOSE SYMPTOMS An excessive dose may produce effects similar to those of heroin and morphine, but there is less risk that the patient will fall into a coma or stop breathing.

How to treat an overdose

• If the patient appears comatose – breathing, but incapable of being woken – treat as for heroin and morphine (see page 363).
• In milder cases, the patient can be allowed to recover on his own.
• Keep him under observation to ensure complete recovery, and to prevent any other drugs from being taken.

Tranquillisers

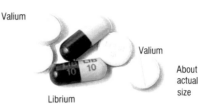

Valium

Valium

Librium

About actual size

WHAT THEY LOOK LIKE Tablets and capsules of various shapes and colours. Some are also sold as syrup or in ampoules.

TRADE NAMES Librium and Valium are known as 'mild' tranquillisers. In normal doses they tend to relieve stress without inducing sleep. The sleeping pill temezepam is increasingly sold on the black market. Largactil and Sparine are stronger tranquillisers, and are sometimes prescribed for mental disorders. They have a sedative effect, and may induce drowsiness even in a normal dose.

WHAT THEY ARE CALLED Like the stronger sedatives (see *Barbiturates*, page 358), tranquillisers are known as downers because they tend to relax than stimulate.

HOW THEY ARE TAKEN Tranquillisers are usually swallowed. The contents of gel-filled capsules of temezepam are often injected.

Drug users often take them in dangerous combinations with alcohol, or in order to 'come down' after taking stimulants. Occasionally, the drugs are injected.

WHAT THE TAKER FEELS An easing of mental agitation and emotional stress. The drugs are mildly intoxicating, but more strongly so – sometimes much more strongly so – when they are taken with alcohol.

WHAT OTHERS SEE The characteristic symptoms of mild drunkenness, which may include staggering and clumsiness. Large doses, or smaller ones taken with alcohol, lead to greater confusion, drowsiness, slurred speech and uncoordinated movements.

Habitual use of tranquillisers may create a dependency, so that users exhibit anxiety when supplies are cut off.

OVERDOSE SYMPTOMS Excessive doses may lead to coma, though this is less common than with barbiturates.

How to treat an overdose

• Treat as for an overdose of barbiturates (see page 359).

Drink and drugs

Coping with a teenager on drugs

Drug abuse may come to light before an emergency arises. Your suspicions may be aroused, for instance, by an unexpected change in a teenager's behaviour patterns or by his or her poor performance at school.

Faced with evidence of drug-taking, it is best not to overdramatise the situation. Bear three major aims in mind:
• Try to keep on good terms with the user, who will often be the only person able to tell you what is going on.
• Try to establish some firm facts about the drug or drugs being used. Are they smoked, swallowed, injected or inhaled? Do they stimulate or relax? For how long and how often have the substances been taken?
• Consult your family doctor, who may be able to advise on the most sensible policy for coping with the problem. If the situation is serious, your doctor may refer you to a drug clinic or to a hospital where specialists will advise on treatment.

How you can help

Drug abuse among teenagers is widespread in Britain. Sometimes a youngster succumbs to temptation simply to be 'one of the gang'. In this case, a full explanation of the dangers may be enough to stop him or her using drugs again.

Often, however, the problem has its roots in mental or emotional stress. All teenagers face difficulties in growing up, and drugs may appear to offer an easy solution to loneliness, depression or anxiety.
• Try to be sympathetic and talk problems over.
• Direct the youngster's attention towards making friends away from the drug scene, and towards interests and activities which will help to boost his or her confidence.
• Try to arrange something he or she can look forward to, so that he or she does not slip back into depression or anxiety.
• In cases of long-term addiction, expert help may be needed to cope with withdrawal symptoms. But the care and attention of friends and family remain essential. Even when 'cured' at a drug addiction clinic, many addicts return to their habit after release.
• With heroin, the statistics are alarmingly high: the great majority of addicts return to the drug after clinical treatment, and more die than achieve lasting cures. Few among the survivors can kick the habit for good without the support and understanding of those closest to them.

HEROIN – THE SCALE OF THE PROBLEM

Once confined to the back streets of a few big cities, black market heroin has become available across the length and breadth of Britain. There are about 25,000 known users of heroin and other opiates, but the true figure may be as much as five times higher than this.

On average, each addict takes about $1\frac{1}{2}$ gram (0.06oz) a week of adulterated heroin, and experts estimate that as much as 1.3 tons (1300kg) of the drug may be coming into Britain each year. The street value of the total is thought to be well over £100 million.

Street prices vary from around £100 per gram, but there are wide regional variations. Driven by the need to support the heroin habit, addicts may become involved in crimes ranging from petty pilfering to housebreaking, mugging and worse.

Drug traffickers eager for new clients sometimes offer teenagers and novice users impure heroin, suitable for smoking, at a cheap rate – or even free. Once initiated, the user may come to crave stronger doses – for which he will have to pay.

Withdrawal – the price of giving up

Habitual users of heroin and other addictive drugs (including morphine, barbiturates and alcohol) become physically dependent on them. Missing two or three doses may precipitate a severe withdrawal crisis known among addicts as 'cold turkey'. Addiction treatment clinics and certain hospitals – family doctors will recommend where to go – provide specialist care for patients during such a withdrawal crisis.

The symptoms may come on within hours of a user being deprived of supplies.
• Typically, the onset of a withdrawal crisis begins with symptoms similar to those of a head cold: running eyes and nose, for example. These are often accompanied by acute anxiety and frantic drug-seeking behaviour.
• Stomach cramps, limb pains, headache, vomiting and intense anguish are likely to follow. In some cases, there may be minor convulsions as well.
• In severe cases, the symptoms of a drug withdrawal crisis may include fits. This is a particular feature of withdrawal from barbiturates.
• The crisis takes two or three days to pass. Then the symptoms gradually decrease in intensity over a week or two. But the craving for the drug persists and may stay with the user for the rest of his life.

Drugs and the law

Many drugs prone to abuse are restricted by law. Britain's Misuse of Drugs Act 1971 makes it a criminal offence to be in unauthorised possession of what the law calls a 'controlled' drug. It is also illegal to produce, import or export controlled drugs, or to supply them to others. The main controlled drugs are heroin, morphine and other opiates; cocaine; amphetamine stimulants; LSD, mescalin and other hallucinogens; and cannabis.

The controlled drugs are further divided into three classes – Classes A, B and C – according to how dangerous they are judged to be.

Class A

Drugs in this category are considered to be the most dangerous. They include heroin, morphine and other opiates, cocaine, LSD, mescalin, injectable amphetamines and cannabinol (the refined, active constituent in cannabis).

Class B

Drugs in this category are less dangerous and include several amphetamines, herbal cannabis and cannabis resin.

Class C

Drugs in this category include several amphetamines.

What the penalties are

In Britain, for trafficking in Class A drugs, the maximum penalties are life imprisonment, an unlimited fine and seizure of the pusher's assets. Lesser penalties apply to simple possession, and to offences involving controlled drugs in Classes B and C. The proceeds of drug trafficking will be confiscated.

Similar laws exist in most countries. Drug trafficking has become one of the most profitable forms of organised crime all over the world, and severe deterrents are considered necessary. In some countries, drug offences carry the death penalty.

Evidence of possession

The Misuse of Drugs Act and similar laws abroad are directed mainly against criminal drug trafficking. But most of those charged with drug offences (around 25,000 each year in Britain) are in possession of small quantities for their own use.

Evidence of possession of a controlled drug is generally regarded as proof of guilt. The few exceptions involve cases where the defendant can prove that the drug was medically prescribed, or that he or she was totally unaware of possessing not only the drug, but also its container.

Simple possession may be dealt with leniently by the authorities, if the quantity is small. However, smuggling drugs – particularly those in Class A – usually attracts very severe penalties even if the defendant is an innocent courier who is merely carrying a parcel on behalf of a friend.

Search and arrest

The police and Customs and Excise officers have wide powers to search and arrest people for suspected drug offences. In the street, a person or a vehicle can be stopped and searched without a search warrant if officers have reasonable grounds for suspecting that the person or anyone in the vehicle is in unauthorised possession of a controlled drug.

However, the police do need a warrant to search private homes and other buildings, unless they are invited in to do so.

Customs officials have somewhat wider powers to search for drugs. They may search without a warrant not only at ports, airports and inside vehicles, ships and planes – but also inland and inside any building.

The courts can be asked to force a bank to disclose details of the accounts of someone suspected of drug trafficking.

If your home is used for drug offences

It is a criminal offence for a householder knowingly to permit the production, supply or unauthorised use of controlled drugs (including cannabis) on his premises.

It is not an offence, however, if these things happen without the householder's knowledge.

If you discover that drugs are being prepared, sold or used in your home or in any building you own, you are legally obliged to report the offence to the police. Failure to do so may result in your being charged as an accessory. It is also an offence to tip off a suspected trafficker.

Doctors, however, who treat victims of drug overdoses are not legally obliged to report their patients to the police, and they rarely do so.

If you discover a controlled drug in your home – or anywhere else – the law permits you to take possession of it to prevent an offence being committed.

You must, however, then hand it over to an authorised person, normally the police, or destroy it yourself without delay.

If a friend is charged with a drug offence

If someone close to you is charged with a drug offence, seek legal advice immediately. Ideally, contact a solicitor experienced in the field. Any local solicitor should be able to advise you on a suitable lawyer (see *Getting help with a legal problem*, page 370).

Not all drugs are controlled by the Misuse of Drugs Act, and possession may not constitute an offence. However, the law may change, which is one reason why expert advice is always necessary.

Additionally, there may be mitigating circumstances, and it is always essential for the defendant to know his or her rights.

Drink and drugs

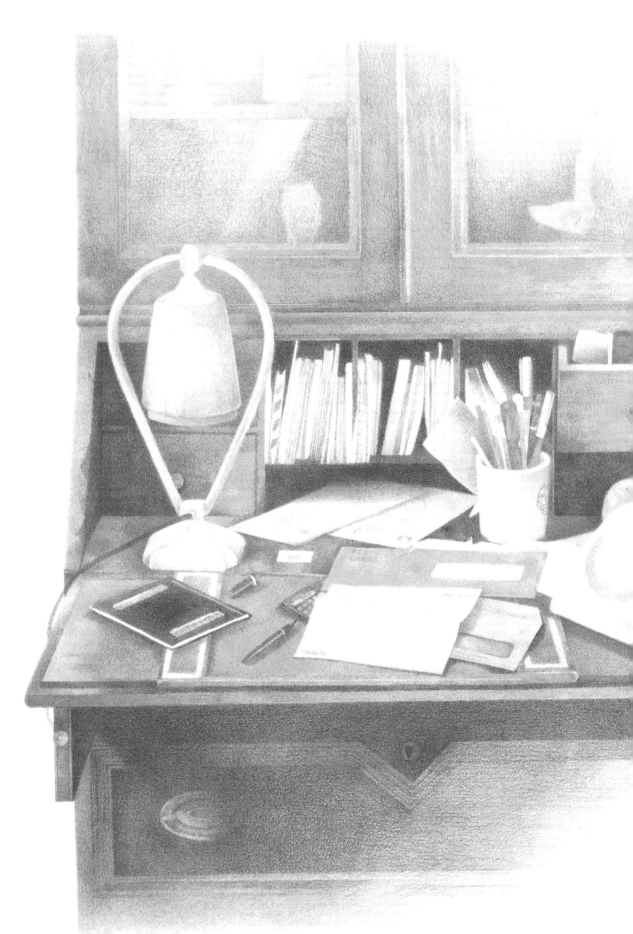

Legal and financial emergencies

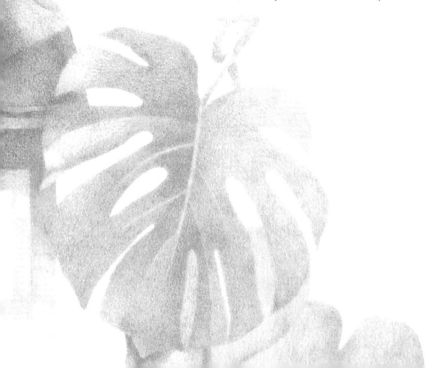

Getting help with a legal problem

There are three main sources of legal advice in Britain: Citizens Advice Bureaux (CAB); Law Centres; and solicitors.

Citizens Advice Bureaux

You can get free information and advice on a wide range of legal problems from local branches of the CAB, which is a national government-supported network of advice centres. Each bureau is staffed by trained volunteers who can help, for instance, with: divorce; disputes at work; disputes over property; social security questions; and consumer affairs.

• To find your nearest CAB, look in the local telephone directory or ask at a post office, public library or council office.

• You can telephone the bureau or call at the office. At some offices, a solicitor attends at regular times to give free advice.

• The CAB may also direct you to a legal advice centre, if there is one in the area. Legal advice centres – which are not connected with Law Centres – are independent charitable organisations which do not receive government funds.

Law Centres

There are about 50 Law Centres funded by central and local government in Britain. They offer free advice on legal problems, but only to people living within the districts they cover. Sometimes a Law Centre can also provide free representation in court. Each centre has at least one solicitor, and most centres have two.

Law Centres specialise in helping people who have problems over housing. Department of Social Security benefit claims, child care and immigration.

• If you do not know of a Law Centre near you, you can find out whether there is one in your area by contacting The Law Centres Federation at Duchess House, 18-19 Warren Street, London W1P 5DB (telephone 071-387 8570).

• Telephone your local centre to make an appointment. Alternatively, ask the staff at the centre whether and when it holds advice sessions – for advice sessions no appointment is usually necessary.

Finding a solicitor

At any stage in dealing with a legal problem of any kind – whether or not you have been to a CAB – you may decide that you need or want formal legal advice.

• If you do not know a solicitor already, ask a knowledgeable friend to recommend one. Your bank manager might also be able to advise you.

• Alternatively, ask the local CAB for a list of local solicitors and ask the bureau to recommend one who specialises in the sort of problem you face.

• If there is no CAB near your home, consult the Solicitors' Diary and Directory in a public library. This gives a list of solicitors, with the kind of work they specialise in.

• Alternatively, look in the Yellow Pages of a telephone directory under 'Solicitors'. Telephone one near you and find out whether he deals with your type of problem. If not, ask him to recommend other local solicitors.

• Telephone two or three firms, ask for estimates and compare them. Many solicitors will give an initial half-hour consultation for £5. Ask if they will do this – it is called the Fixed Fee Scheme. But remember that any later work may well cost much more.

• If you become dissatisfied with your solicitor or feel that he has not acted in your best interests, you can complain to The Law Society, the solicitors' professional body. For advice on how to make a complaint, contact the Solicitors Complaints Bureau, Victoria Court, 8 Dormer Place, Leamington Spa, Warwickshire CV32 5AE (telephone 0926 820082).

HOW TO GET LEGAL AID

If you need a solicitor's help but have a low income, it is possible to get legal aid to cover all or part of the costs – including the cost of having a solicitor or barrister to represent you in court.

• If you need advice, but no court action is involved, ask a solicitor for a £5 interview or ask for advice under the 'green form' scheme. Any solicitor will be able to advise you on whether you are eligible for help under the scheme, and on how to apply.

• If a court case is involved, you need a legal aid form.

• In a civil case, get the form from a CAB or any local solicitor. A solicitor can help you to fill in the form. When the form is completed, send it to the area office of the Legal Aid Board. The bureau or the solicitor will have the address.

• In a criminal case, get the form from the magistrates' court which is to hear the case. Fill it in and return it to the clerk of the court.

• Because legal aid is means-tested, you may still have to pay some of your legal costs even if your application is approved. In addition, if you win your case and are awarded damages, some or all of the money you win may have to be paid back to the legal aid fund.

• If you lose the case, you may have to pay damages to the other side on top of your contribution to your own costs. Ask your solicitor how much this is likely to be before you decide to go to court.

Helping police inquiries

Under the Police and Criminal Evidence Act 1984, the police cannot stop and search someone without reasonable suspicion that the person has committed a crime or is about to do so.

• If you are stopped and questioned by police, you are not usually obliged to answer, or even to give your name and address. But it is usually sensible to help. They may, for instance, be looking for witnesses of an accident or crime.

• You must give your name, address and date of birth if the inquiries involve a motoring case or are under the Official Secrets Acts.

• You can generally refuse to be searched, unless the police have a warrant. But this right to refuse does not apply if the police have reason to suspect that you have dangerous drugs, stolen goods, an offensive weapon or an implement that can be used for theft or burglary.

• If the police find anything that they think might be useful as evidence, they can confiscate it – though they may return it later.

• Before the police search you, they must identify themselves and tell you why they are searching you and what they are looking for. Then, or immediately afterwards, if you ask for it they must give you a note confirming these details in writing.

• If you are not sure whether the police are within their rights to search you, it is usually safer to allow the search anyway, and to complain later – through a solicitor, if necessary.

• You are not obliged to go to a police station unless you are arrested or unless the police want to continue the search.

• If you need a solicitor, telephone him if possible before going to the police station. If you do not know a solicitor, the police at the station will have a list of duty solicitors.

If a policeman comes to your home

A uniformed policeman who comes to your home should tell you his name and say why he wants to question you. An officer in plain clothes must show you his warrant card as well if you ask to see it.

• A warrant card is always in a sealed plastic case. It gives the policeman's name and rank, the name of his police force, and sometimes has a crest on it. It also has a photograph.

• Check that the photograph matches the person at the door. If you are not sure that he is a real policeman, telephone the station he is attached to for verification. Ask him to wait outside until you have made the call.

• You must let a policeman enter your house if he shows you a search warrant.

• Even if he has no warrant, you must also let him in if he says he wants to arrest someone inside, or if he says he wants to question someone he thinks is hiding inside.

• In other circumstances, you are not obliged to let a policeman into your house. If you do invite him in, you can ask him to leave at any time – and he must comply.

If you are arrested

If the police arrest you, they must tell you why they are doing so.

• Make a note of the reasons the police give you for your arrest. The note may help your solicitor later.

• Go quietly to the police station. If you do not, you can be charged with resisting arrest or obstructing a police officer. You can be jailed and fined for this offence even if you are later acquitted of the charge on which you were arrested. The police are entitled to use reasonable force, or handcuffs.

• Once you get to the police station, if you think you have been wrongly arrested, say so.

• You can refuse to answer questions. If you do reply, the police will note what you say and may repeat your words as evidence in court.

• You can ask for a copy of the Codes of Practice – which have replaced the old Judges' Rules. They say that, as soon as a police officer has grounds for believing that someone has committed a crime, the accused must be warned that he need not answer further questions.

• You can ask to see a solicitor. But if the offence is very serious the police may delay this for up to 36 hours if they think that it would lead to accomplices being alerted.

• However, nobody (except a suspected terrorist) can be held in a police station for more than 36 hours without the approval of a magistrates' court. This approval can be granted only after a hearing where both the suspect and his solicitor, if he wants one, are present.

At the police station

• The police may search anyone who has been arrested, and may take away items which are needed as evidence, or which could cause injury or damage. You will be asked to check a list of what is taken.

• If you make a voluntary statement, read it over carefully before signing it. Alter anything that is wrong or unclear.

• You can in some circumstances refuse to have your fingerprints taken. But the police can insist if, for example, an officer of the rank of superintendent or above has reasonable grounds for believing that your fingerprints will tend to confirm or disprove your involvement in an offence.

• You can refuse to attend an identity parade, and you can choose where you stand if you decide to attend one. If you want an identity parade, you can demand one.

Getting bail

• You must be given a copy of any charge against you. Once you are charged, the police will either release you on bail or keep you in custody until you appear before magistrates. Even if the police have refused to grant bail, you can ask the magistrates to overrule them.

• If you have no solicitor, ask the court to arrange one for you.

Legal and financial emergencies

If you are prosecuted

Unless you have been warned at the time of an incident that you will be charged, your first knowledge of an impending criminal prosecution will normally be when you receive a summons from the police.

The summons will contain details of the alleged offence, and tell you the time and place of the court hearing.

• Check that the details in the summons are correct. If there are mistakes, you may be able to get the charge dropped on technical grounds.

• Decide whether to plead guilty or not guilty. If you are innocent, you should always plead not guilty – even if (as in some driving offences) you can plead guilty by post without appearing in court.

• If in doubt, consult a solicitor (see *Getting help with a legal problem*, page 370). Do not be afraid to ring several – their charges and experience vary.

• If you decide to conduct your own defence without a solicitor, consult Stone's *Justices' Manual* (published by Butterworths) or some other legal reference book at a library. Stone's *Justice's Manual* gives the guidelines and penalties for the kinds of offences which are tried in magistrates' courts.

• Write down exactly what happened during the incident which led to the charge.

• If you are going to call witnesses, write down what they are going to say as well. You will need both these sets of notes when presenting your case.

• Visit the court beforehand and sit in on some of the trials being held there, so that you can get to know the procedure.

• If the case is at all complex, however, or if the maximum penalty you face is large, it is usually best to ask a solicitor to act for you.

• Consider, also, applying for legal aid (see *How to get legal aid,* page 370). You may be able to get enough aid to cover at least some and possibly all of the solicitor's fees.

If you are sued

Most civil disputes are settled by negotiations between the people involved in the dispute or their solicitors. If, however, the two sides cannot agree, the dispute can be referred to a court.

A civil dispute that goes to court may sometimes be heard by magistrates. More often, though, the case is dealt with by a county court or by the High Court.

Magistrates hear some actions over debts – non-payment of rates, for example – and disputes over the maintenance of wives and single parents.

County courts hear claims for debts and personal injury cases where the amount in dispute in not above £50,000, disputes involving landlords and tenants, undefended divorces, and disputes over hire-purchase transactions.

The High Court hears claims for higher damages for personal injury, breach of contract, debts of any amount, and libel and slander. It also hears defended divorces.

Whichever court hears the case, the person making the claim is called the plaintiff. The person he or she sues is called the defendant.

Most civil court cases begin with the plaintiff – or, more commonly, his solicitor – applying to the appropriate court for a summons or a writ. (The corresponding document in a divorce case is known as a petition.)

The summons or writ is likely to be your first formal notification that legal action has been started, but in most cases you will have been warned, through letters from the plaintiff, that the dispute could go to court.

If you do receive letters threatening legal action, and you dispute the claim, consider getting professional advice before legal action starts (see page 370).

Paying a solicitor to negotiate a settlement out of court may be cheaper than fighting the case in court – even if you win.

Receiving a summons

If someone claims you owe him money, he may serve a summons (called a default summons) on you, or get a court official to do it. The summons may be given to you personally, or it may be sent by registered post or recorded delivery. It will show the amount claimed, including court fees and solicitors' charges. The summons also contains a form which allows you to admit the claim, defend it or make a counter-claim of your own.

• If you agree that you owe the money and can pay at once, send or take the money to the court office. The court will pay the plaintiff and that will end the action.

• If you admit the debt but cannot pay it, fill in the admission section of the form and send it to the court. You can offer to pay by instalments, or give a date when you can pay.

• If you dispute the debt, fill in the defence section. If the plaintiff owes you money, use the counterclaim section too.

• If you are not sure how to fill in the form, the clerk at the court office which issued the summons will often be able to give you advice free of charge. Alternatively, consult a solicitor.
• If the action is in the county court and is by an amount under £1000, it will be dealt with by an informal procedure called Arbitration. Under this procedure, the case is normally heard in private and the formal rules of evidence need not apply – you can describe what someone else said, for example. Also, the loser does not have to pay the winner's legal costs.

Receiving a writ

If someone claims that he has been injured because of your negligence, he may issue a High Court writ against you. This could happen because of a car crash, for instance, or an accident at work.

The writ will say that an action is to be brought and give brief details of the reasons.

When you receive the writ, it is said to have been 'served'.
• With the writ will be a form for acknowledgment of service. Return the form to the court that issued the writ within 14 days.
• Consult a solicitor as soon as possible. You have 28 days from the date the writ was served to let the court know how you wish to answer the writ – by defending it, for instance, or by making a counterclaim of your own.
• If you are short of money, you may be able to claim legal aid. Ask your solicitor or a local Citizens Advice Bureau to help you to make the application (see *How to get legal aid*, page 370).

YOU AND THE LAW

Most people go through life without ever being involved in a court case. But the law still governs much of what we do. It is involved, for instance, when we take a job, get married, buy goods or drive a car. Knowledge of the law helps us to safeguard our rights and those of our families, and to protect our property.

There are two main branches: the criminal law and the civil law.
• Criminal law lays down penalties for breaking society's rules – from parking in the wrong place to murder.
• Civil law deals with disputes between individual members of society, businesses and organisations. It enables people to seek financial compensation or some other remedy from someone who may have been negligent, broken a contract, who may owe money or who may otherwise have acted unfairly.

If squatters move in

If you come home – from a holiday, say – to find that squatters have taken over a house you own, your legal rights depend on whether you live in the house or not.

Your rights are more extensive if you normally live in the house or if you intend to live in it (if, say, you have been working abroad and have just returned to Britain, or if you have just bought the house). Your rights are more limited if you do not normally live there (if, for example, it is a holiday home that you use for only a few weeks a year).

If you live in the house
• If you normally live in the house, show the squatters proof of this – a letter addressed to you there, for instance – and tell them to go.
• If they will not let you in, and insist on staying, call the police.
• You are entitled by law to use 'reasonable force' to enter your home or to eject squatters. What counts as reasonable, though, depends on the circumstances. And if you use what the courts regard as excessive force, you could be open to a charge of assault. For this reason, it is usually better to call in the police than to try to evict the squatters yourself.
• The police can evict squatters on the spot.
• Check your home insurance policy as soon as possible. Under most house and contents policies, it is possible to claim back from the insurance company the cost of temporary accommodation. In addition, it is usually possible to claim back the cost of any damage the squatters have done to your house or to your possessions inside it.
• The cover usually applies so long as the house had not been left empty for more than 30 days.
• If the policy documents are unreachable – perhaps because you left them in the house – contact the insurance broker or company which sold you the policy. They will usually have a copy of the documents. The policy may in any case require you to let the company know that you intend to make a claim.
• It is also possible to get the squatters evicted through the courts, and to sue them for the cost of your accommodation as well as for the cost of any damage they do. But since squatters are usually short of money and may be difficult to trace once they leave your home, this course is rarely worth pursuing.
• If you plan nevertheless to take court action – if your insurance policy does not cover the costs, say – get advice from a solicitor (see *Getting help with a legal problem*, page 370).

If the house is unoccupied
It is not a crime for squatters to move into an unoccupied house – such as an empty holiday home – unless they use violence to get into the premises, or unless they cause damage.

Provided the squatters do not use violence or

cause damage, they offend only the civil, not the criminal, law.

The police, therefore – who enforce only the criminal law – may often have no power to help. In addition, you do not, in these circumstances, have the right to use 'reasonable force' to eject the squatters.

• Ask the squatters to let you in, and tell them to leave.

• You can go in if they let you. But if they refuse, you are not entitled to force your way in.

• If they do refuse to let you in, wait until they go out – to go shopping, for instance. Then take possession. You are entitled to break in – by breaking a window, for example – if necessary.

• Stay out of sight while you are waiting. Otherwise the squatters may guess what you have in mind and make a point of leaving at least one person permanently in the house.

• If this tactic fails, get in touch with a solicitor. Ask him to apply to a county court for a possession order.

• Once the court order has been issued, a court official will evict the squatters – by force if necessary.

After the squatters leave

• Once you regain possession of the house, do not destroy any property the squatters have left behind. They are entitled to reclaim it – even after a number of years have elapsed.

• If their property becomes a nuisance, get a solicitor's advice on what to do with it.

If someone is evicted

People evicted from their home with nowhere to go should ask the local council's housing authority for help.

• The housing authority is legally obliged to provide accommodation for priority cases, such as pregnant women, families with children, and households where there is an elderly or handicapped person.

• The authority may send those evicted to a reception centre, give them a short-term lease on an empty house, or arrange a temporary stay in a guesthouse or hotel.

If the council refuses to help

Many councils classify tenants evicted for non-payment of rent as intentionally homeless, and may refuse to help for that reason.

• If the council refuses to help, those evicted should appeal to their local councillor or MP.

• If they have nowhere to store possessions, they should ask the housing authority to store them. It must do so, but may charge for it.

• If those evicted need money, they should ask their local Department of Health and Social Security office.

• Homeless people are as entitled to supplementary benefit as those who have a home. They should not be refused benefit because they have no fixed address.

Finding temporary accommodation

If evicted people have no friends or relatives with whom they can live, and the local council's housing department will not provide them with accommodation, a charitable organisation may be able to help.

Evicted people who find themselves without a roof over their head can contact Shelter at 88 Old Street, London EC1V 9AX (telephone 071-253 0202; emergency housing nightline freefone 0800 446441), or the Salvation Army at 101 Queen Victoria Street, London EC4P 4EP (telephone 071-236 5222). The Salvation Army runs hostels for the homeless all over Britain.

The London head offices of both organisations will also know of local housing aid centres where evicted people can stay. Alternatively, a Citizens Advice Bureau should be able to supply a list of hostels in the area.

If you lose your job

An employee can lose his or her job in two main ways: by being dismissed; or by being made redundant.

When somebody is dismissed

• An employee who is dismissed should write to his employer. In the letter, the employer should be asked to give his reasons for the dismissal in writing, unless he has already done so. The employer is obliged by law to reply within 14 days of receiving the request.

• If the employer does not reply, or if the employee is dissatisfied with the reasons given or with the way in which the dismissal has been handled, he should talk to a local Citizens Advice Bureau, a solicitor or a trade union official (see *Getting help with a legal problem*, page 370).

• Any of these will be able to tell him whether he has a claim for unfair or wrongful dismissal, or for redundancy. They will also be able to advise him on how to pursue the claim in an industrial tribunal or the courts.

When somebody is made redundant

• An employee who is made redundant should contact the personnel department of his firm as soon as possible.

• If he is dissatisfied with the redundancy pay the employer is offering, he should discuss it with the personnel department.

• If still dissatisfied, he should get advice from a Citizens Advice Bureau, a solicitor, or a trade union official. They may be able to negotiate more generous redundancy terms, and can advise him about whether it is worth taking the case to an industrial tribunal.

• The legal minimum for a redundancy payment depends on the employee's age and how long he has been employed by the firm. For each year of service he should get one and a half weeks' pay if he is over 41, one week's pay if he is between 22 and 41, and half a week's pay if he is between 18 and 22. Some employers offer larger redundancy payments than these, but they are not obliged to.

If you are injured at work

More than $1\frac{1}{2}$ million people are injured at work in Britain each year. The Health and Safety at Work Act 1974, and other measures which relate to specific industries, aim to limit this casualty toll and to protect the victims of industrial accidents.

The measures put a legal obligation on employers to provide: a safe place and system of work; safe plant and tools; and competent staff.

Anyone who is injured at work, or who becomes ill as a result of the work he does, can usually claim one or more of the state benefits administered by the Department of Health. He may also be able to sue his employer for a lump sum in compensation if he can show that the accident happened because the employer or a workmate was careless in some way.

If you get hurt

• If you are injured in any accident at work, report the accident to a supervisor at once.

• A factory, mine or quarry, or any company that employs ten or more people on the premises, must by law have an accident book.

• If there is such a book where you work, record the accident in it.

• If you are too badly injured to write, ask someone else to record the accident in the accident book for you.

• Later, when you are able, write to the firm saying what happened.

• Take signed statements from witnesses, or get a workmate to do so.

• Make a note of the witnesses' home addresses as well, in case they leave the firm and you need to contact them later.

• See your doctor, even if your injury has been treated by first aid staff at work and the accident seems minor. There may be complications later.

Claiming benefit

Most employees who are unable to work because of industrial injury are entitled to claim sick pay from their employers in exactly the same way as they would if they were off work through illness.

Sick pay lasts for up to 28 weeks. Many firms pay full wages during this period. Thereafter, an employee can normally claim invalidity benefit from the government.

• Claim sick pay by telling your employer that you are ill and providing him with whatever evidence he requires.

• If you are still unable to work after 28 weeks, you are entitled to claim invalidity benefit from the Department of Health. Your employer will give you the change-over form SSP1 so that you can claim.

• If you are not entitled to sick pay from your employer for some reason – the personnel department in your firm will tell you whether you are entitled – you can claim the state sickness benefit at once.

Legal and financial emergencies

- To claim sickness benefit, get a 'self-certification' form SC1 from the local DSS office. Fill it in and return it to the office. You do not need a doctor's certificate until you have been sick for more than seven days.
- If you are too ill to move, ask someone else to make the claim on your behalf. If you are claiming sickness benefit from the time of the accident, the claim should reach the social security office within six days of the accident; otherwise you may lose some benefit.
- You may qualify for other benefits as well, depending on the severity of the accident. If you lose a finger or toe, for instance, you can claim disablement benefit.
- If you are in doubt about what you are entitled to claim, ask the social security office for advice as soon as possible after the accident.
- Telephone or write to the office if you cannot get there yourself, or ask someone else to visit the office for you.

Going to court
You may be able to get compensation if your employer, or a workmate, has been negligent or your employer has broken safety rules. All employers are required to insure against this.
- If you think you have a case, talk to a union official or solicitor as soon as possible after the accident (see *Getting help with a legal problem*, page 370).

Trouble at the shops

Surrounded by goods in a crowded store, it can be easy to knock something off a shelf and break it. With modern packaging techniques, you may not discover that you have bought faulty goods until after you get home. In both these situations, the law tries to strike a fair balance between the rights of the shopper and the shopkeeper.

What to do if you break something
- If you knock something over in a shop, or drop it, through carelessness, you are legally responsible for any damage you cause. If you feel that it was clearly your fault, it is best to pay for the breakage if the manager of the shop asks you to do so. The manager is entitled to ask for the full amount of the retail price – not just the cost price to the shop.
- If the accident was not your fault – because the goods were badly stacked, say – you are not liable for any damage. If you feel that this is the case, do not pay.
- If the manager of the shop disagrees with you, he may decide to take you to court (see *If you are sued*, page 372). If he asks for your name and address, you should give it to him.
- Before leaving the shop, collect the names and addresses of any witnesses – in case you need them to give evidence in your support.

How to complain
When making a complaint – about faulty goods, for example, or bad service – be systematic, reasonable and persistent. Have clear in your mind the reasons for your complaint and what you want done about it.
- Make your first complaint to the person you have been dealing with – the salesman or waiter, for example. Do not get angry. Contact the person as soon as you can. Undue delay will weaken your position. If this approach fails, ask to see the manager or the person in charge. Make it clear at each stage what you want done to settle the matter.
- If you still get no results, make your complaint formally in writing. Address it to the manager or person in charge of the office, shop or organisation that you have been dealing with. Get the address from the telephone directory.
- Set out your complaint in full. Give any relevant names and dates. Enclose photocopies of any documents. Do not send the originals.
- Set a time within which you expect a reply – 14 days, say. Make it clear that if you receive no reply you will take matters further.
- Send the letter by recorded or registered delivery. The organisation will then not be able to deny receiving the letter. Keep a copy.
- If you receive no reply within the time you have set, write again enclosing a copy of your first letter. Make it clear that you are also sending a copy of the letter to someone higher up in the firm such as the area manager, managing director or chief executive. If you do not know the address, you may find it in the local library.

Alternatively, ring the firm and tell the switchboard operator that you have to write to the company. Ask for the name and address of the managing director, but do not say why you will be writing to him.

• If you still get no response, consider taking your complaint to the firm's trade association, or to the local council's health officer or trading standards officer. Alternatively, contact the nearest Citizens Advice Bureau.

• As a last resort, consider consulting a solicitor. But weigh up first whether the cost of going to law is more than you are likely to get if you win your case. If your claim is fairly small (less than £1000) you will have to pay your own legal costs whether you win or lose.

IF YOU ARE FALSELY ACCUSED OF SHOPLIFTING

Anyone who intentionally takes goods from a shop without paying for them is guilty of theft. But absent-mindedness in a busy supermarket can result in someone accidentally putting goods in the wrong basket, or forgetting to pay. Being falsely accused of shoplifting is distressing. The main thing is to stay calm.

• If the store detective or a member of the staff asks you to go to the manager's office, you are not obliged to do so. If you refuse, he may let you go – or arrest you.

• Do not resist if the store detective arrests you – even if you are innocent. Go with him to the manager's office.

• You do not have to answer any questions at any stage. Nor does the store detective have any right to search you or your bag without your permission.

• Once you are in the manager's office, ask to make a telephone call. Get in touch with a solicitor and follow his advice. If you do not know a solicitor, ask a friend or relative to come to the shop.

• Make the call out of earshot of the shop staff, if possible. Anything you say may be repeated as evidence if you are prosecuted.

• Wait until the solicitor, or your friend, arrives before saying anything. The only exception to this rule might be if you realise that you have made a mistake. You may try to explain what happened – but remember that what you say may be taken down and repeated in court.

• If the manager decides to prosecute you, he will call in the police. He must do this as soon as possible after your arrest (see *If you are prosecuted*, page 372).

If a child causes damage

Whether a parent has to pay for damage his child causes depends largely on the age of the child. If a three-year-old ran out into the road and caused a crash after his mother left the front door open, the courts might make the parents pay the costs of the accident.

If a 16-year-old did the same thing, the chances are that his parents would not be held responsible because the child could have been expected to know better.

Similarly, if parents gave their normally sensible 15-year-old son an airgun and instructed him fully on how to use the gun safely, the courts would be unlikely to hold them responsible if the boy accidentally injured someone with it.

On the other hand, if the boy was often reckless by nature and the parents had given him the airgun without any advice on how and where to use it, the parents might well have to pay compensation to the injured person.

In general, the courts follow the principle that parents are responsible for their child's actions only in so far as they can reasonably be expected to have control over the child.

• If your young child causes minor damage – such as breaking a neighbour's window with his football – offer to pay for the cost of the repairs on the spot.

• If your child causes major damage or injury – suppose, for example, he lights a bonfire which gets out of control – and it looks as though court action could follow, the safest course is not to do or say anything which could be interpreted as an admission of responsibility.

• Instead, get advice from a solicitor as soon as possible (see *Getting help with a legal problem*, page 370).

When somebody dies

Even if the last illness has been long and death expected, coping with the formalities of a death is distressing. However, all the officials involved will be sympathetic and anxious to make procedures as simple and painless as possible.

As soon as a person dies, the first step is always to call a doctor, unless one is there already. Under certain circumstances, the doctor – or sometimes the registrar – will be obliged to report the death to a coroner.

Over the following days, five further responsibilities usually have to be faced: notifying the next-of-kin; arranging the funeral; registering the death; sorting out the dead person's affairs; and claiming financial help from the state.

Calling in a doctor

• If the death occurs at home, call a doctor – ideally the one who treated the dead person during his last illness. The doctor will complete an official medical certificate of death, identifying the cause of death. If the death occurs in hospital, the hospital will arrange this for you.

• The doctor may give you either the medical certificate or a tear-off slip from it called the Notice to Informant. Keep the document safely. You will need it for registering the death.

• If the dead person wished to donate parts of his body to be used for transplants, consult the doctor or the hospital authorities immediately.

• About 1 in 5 deaths in Britain are reported to the coroner, usually because the dead person was not seen by a doctor in the 14 days before he died. In the vast majority of cases, the fact that the coroner is informed does not imply any suspicion of foul play. If a coroner becomes involved – the doctor will tell you whether he will or not – you do not have to register the death within any particular time limit.

• No death certificate can be issued, nor can a funeral take place, until the coroner gives his permission. If he decides that a post-mortem and perhaps an inquest are necessary, there may be a few days' delay. You need do nothing for the time being. Any arrangements will be made by the doctor or the coroner's office.

• When the coroner has satisfied himself as to the cause of death he will either register the death directly, or ask the next-of-kin to do so.

Notifying the next-of-kin

• Let any close relatives and friends know of the death. You may also wish to put a notice of the death in a newspaper. Instructions on how to do this usually appear next to the paper's births, marriages and deaths column.

• Contact the executors of the dead person's will, if you know who they are.

Arranging the funeral

A funeral is usually arranged by the dead person's executors or his relatives.

If the dead person expressed a particular wish about his funeral, this is usually respected.

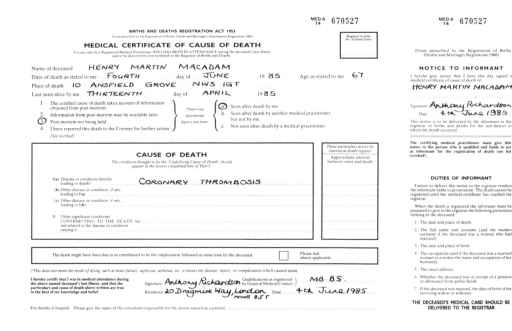

WHAT THE MEDICAL CERTIFICATE IS FOR
A doctor must fill in a certificate of the cause of death before the death can be registered. He will also sign the Notice to Informant (on the right of the certificate). This tells whoever is going to register the death what information he or she must give the registrar.

But the person organising the funeral is not legally obliged to follow the dead person's wishes, even if they are set out in the will.

• Call an undertaker. If you do not know of one, the doctor or hospital authorities may be able to suggest one to you. The undertaker will take the body away. Discuss with the undertaker what kind of funeral you would like him to organise and what the probable cost will be.

• If the body is to be cremated, a number of special forms have to be filled in. The undertaker will make the arrangements for you.

Registering the death

The person responsible for registering a death is specified by law (see box, page 380).

• Take the Notice to Informant – or the medical certificate of death, if the doctor has given it to you – to the local registrar of births, deaths and marriages. The doctor who completed the medical certificate will give you the address of the registrar. Otherwise it can be found in the telephone directory under 'Registration'.

• Take also the dead person's National Health Service medical card.

D. Cert.
R.B.D.

CAUTION—Any person who (1) falsifies any of the particulars on this certificate, or (2) uses a falsified certificate as true knowing it to be false, is liable to prosecution.

CERTIFIED COPY
Pursuant to the Births and

OF AN ENTRY
Deaths Registration Act 1953

DEATH		Entry No. *10*
Registration district *Hampstead* Sub-district *St. Pancras*		Administrative area *London Borough of Camden*

1. Date and place of death *Fourth June 1985*
10 Ansfield Grove, St. Pancras

2. Name and surname *Henry Martin MACADAM*

3. Sex *Male*

4. Maiden surname of woman who has married

5. Date and place of birth *7th September 1917*
Basingstoke, Hampshire

6. Occupation and usual address *Accountant (retired)*
10 Ansfield Grove, St. Pancras, NW3.

7. (a) Name and surname of informant *Agnes Dorothy Macadam*

(b) Qualification *Widow of the deceased present at the death*

(c) Usual address *10 Ansfield Grove, NW3*

8. Cause of death

Coronary thrombosis

Certified by Anthony Richardson MB. BS

9. I certify that the particulars given by me above are true to the best of my knowledge and belief.
Agnes Macadam
Signature of informant

10. Date of registration *Fifth June 1985*

11. Signature of registrar *P. Smithson Registrar*

OBTAINING A DEATH CERTIFICATE
Ask the registrar for at least one copy of the death certificate (which you will have to pay for). You will need it to claim under a life assurance policy. The registrar will give you a free certificate of registration. You will need that to claim death grant and widow's benefit.

• You must visit the registrar in person within five days of the death. If you are unable to do so – because you are ill, for example – you must inform the registrar of the death in writing within five days. You cannot delegate this duty to the person next in order of responsibility.

• When you write, send the registrar the Notice to Informant or the medical certificate of death. You should then go in person to complete the registration within 14 days of the death.

• When you register the death, the registrar will want to know the full name of the dead person, his place and date of birth, occupation, place and date of death, usual address, whether he was receiving a pension or allowance from public funds, and, if he was married, the age of the surviving spouse.

• The registrar will give you a certificate of registration of death and a disposal certificate.

• Take the disposal certificate to the undertaker. Until he has it, the funeral cannot take place.

• If you are responsible for winding up the dead person's affairs, get copies of the death certificate as well (available for a fee). You may need to send one to a solicitor, and you will need one to claim under a life assurance policy.

WHO MUST REGISTER THE DEATH?

The law not only insists that every death must be registered, it also specifies who must do the registering.

• If the death occurs in a house or hospital, the first available person on the following list is obliged to register the death. He or she cannot delegate this duty to someone in another category. In order of precedence, the people are:

1. A relative who was present at the death.
2. A relative who was present during the last illness.
3. A relative who lives nearby or is staying nearby.
4. Anyone present at the death.
5. Anyone living in the same house as the dead person.
6. The person arranging the funeral.

• If the death occurs anywhere other than in a house or hospital, one of the following people is obliged to register the death. In order, they are:

1. Any relative who knows any of the details that need to be registered.
2. Anyone present at the death.
3. Anyone who found or took charge of the body.
4. Anyone arranging the funeral.

Sorting out the dead person's affairs

The responsibility for sorting out the affairs of someone who has died usually lies with the executor of his will. The executor is usually the widow or widower, or a close friend or relative. In some cases, especially if there is a large or complicated estate, there may also be a professional executor such as a solicitor, accountant or bank.

• The first step for the executor to take after the death is to find the will. If it is not immediately to hand, check with the dead person's solicitor or bank. The will may have been given to them for safekeeping. The will is the executor's legal authority to act.

• If there is no will or no executor – because the named executors are dead, for example – the nearest relatives should apply to the local probate registry for what lawyers call 'letters of administration'. These give you the same authority and duties as an executor. A local Citizens Advice Bureau will have the address of the nearest probate registry.

• To apply, ask the probate registry or a registrar for a copy of the form PR48, entitled Personal Application for Probate or Letters of Administration. The form also sets out the duties of an executor.

• If the estate is complicated and if no professional executor has been named in the will, it may be wise to engage a solicitor to help. His fees can be deducted from the estate.

• Find out what assets the dead person had. You will need to examine his personal papers and consult his bank manager, accountant or solicitor.

• Contact all the organisations with which the dead person had dealings – such as banks, National Savings, building societies and insurance companies. They will tell you which of the dead person's assets can be used at once – such as joint bank accounts – and which are frozen until the dead person's affairs have been sorted out and formally wound up.

Claiming financial help from the state

When somebody dies, his or her dependants may need financial help. There are various government benefits which can be claimed. The main ones are: death grant; widow's benefit; and industrial death benefit.

• Contact the local office of the Department of Social Security. It will be able to tell you whether you are entitled to any of the benefits and how to claim them. Ask also for a copy of the leaflet What to do after a death (D49), which explains the benefits in detail.

If a Briton dies abroad

• Get in touch with the local British embassy or the consulate. The staff will advise on the local regulations for registering a death, and will help you to make arrangements for the funeral or for bringing the body back to Britain.

Making an insurance claim

If your home or car is damaged – by vandals or thieves, say, or simply by accident – and you decide to claim under your insurance, tell the insurance company as soon as possible.

Tell the company even if you are not sure that you want to make a claim – because you want to protect a no-claim bonus on a car, for instance. Otherwise you could lose the option of making a claim later.

Claiming on your home insurance
• Telephone the company as soon as possible after the loss or damage occurs, and tell the official you speak to what has happened. Find out the official's name and, at the same time, ask for a claim form.
• Get any emergency repairs done at once. Emergency repairs are those necessary to safeguard the property: covering a storm-damaged roof, say, or repairing a door that has been forced open by a burglar. There is no need to submit estimates for these repairs, or to wait for the company's approval.
• If you are in doubt about whether repairs you think necessary are urgent, telephone the company and discuss it with an official there. Again, get the official's name.
• Get at least two estimates for any non-urgent repairs. When the claim form arrives, fill it in with details of the damage and of any property that has been lost or stolen, attach the repair estimates and send it back to the company. Keep copies of everything you send. You do not normally have to submit proof of the value of stolen goods.
• If you do not hear from the company within a week, telephone. You may get approval over the phone to go ahead with the repairs. If you do, make a note of the official's name and ask him to send you a letter confirming what he has said. If not, ask the official when approval is likely to come through.

Claiming after a car accident
• If your car is damaged in an accident, tell the insurance company as soon as possible by telephone. Get the name of the person you speak to and ask for a claim form at the same time.
• Even if your car is undamaged and you decide you do not want to make a claim, report the incident to the company anyway in case someone else claims against you. A local council, for instance, might want to claim for damage to a bollard.
• Decide whether it is worth claiming under the insurance at all. The loss of all or part of a no-claim bonus may cost more than paying for the repairs yourself.
• Get at least two estimates for the repairs to your car. But do not get the repairs done at once. The company may want to inspect the damage first.
• When the claim form arrives, fill it in, attach the estimates and send it back to the company. If you are not sure whether you want to make a claim, mark the form 'For information only' and explain in a covering letter that you are not at present making a claim, but that you might change your mind later. Keep copies of everything you send.
• Contact the company if you hear nothing after a week. If the official you speak to says you can go ahead with the repairs, get his name and ask for a letter of confirmation.
• If you do decide to make a claim under your insurance policy, pass on to the company at once any letter or writ you receive from anyone else who was involved in the accident. Do not reply to it yourself.

What to do if your car is stolen
A motorist whose car is stolen should contact the police, as well as his insurance company, as soon as possible after he discovers the theft. Insurance companies usually insist on the theft being reported to the police.

In addition, if the car is leased, or if it is covered by a hire-purchase or credit agreement, inform the loan company involved.

You may not see your car again if it is stolen. Of the 600,000 cars reported missing in Britain each year, only about three-quarters are recovered – and most of those have been damaged by the thieves.
• If you see the theft being committed but are unable to stop the thieves yourself, dial 999 (or the foreign equivalent) at once and ask for the police. Do not put yourself at risk. If the theft has happened some time before, contact the nearest police station.
• Either way, tell the police your name and address, the car's make, colour and registration number – and the chassis and engine numbers, if you know them.
• Try to remember anything that makes the car easy to recognise, and tell the police about it. Details such as a large dent in the bodywork, a distinctive sticker in the window or an unusual aerial may help them to identify your car among all the others on the road.
• Once you have alerted the police, telephone your insurance company and ask for a claim form. If the theft happened in Britain, give the name of the police station handling it.
• Fill in the form with the same information that you have given the police and return it as soon as you can. If the theft took place abroad, attach a copy of the foreign police report.
• You will probably not hear from the insurance company for at least two or three weeks because many cars are recovered during this period. If your car is not found and there is no dispute over the claim, you should receive a cheque five or six weeks after you claim.
• If your car is found, you can claim for any damage done to it by the thieves in the same way as for damage caused in an accident.

When an insurance claim is disputed

If your insurance company delays payment on any claim you make, or if it offers less than you have asked for, you have the choice of accepting the company's decision – or fighting it.

• The first step, if you decide to fight, is to complain to the company in writing, stating clearly what you want. Keep a copy of the letter, and of any others you send.

• If the letter does not produce a satisfactory response, phone or write to the company and ask if it has any standard arrangement for arbitration over disputed claims.

Going to arbitration

Most companies use one of three agencies to handle disputed claims in order to avoid the delay and expense of going to court: the Insurance Ombudsman Bureau; the Personal Insurance Arbitration Service; or a department of Lloyd's of London.

• If the company's arrangement is with the Insurance Ombudsman Bureau, you must write to the chief executive of the insurance company asking for your claim to be reviewed before the Ombudsman will intervene. If you are still dissatisfied, contact the bureau at City Gate 1, 135 Park Street, London SE1 9EA (telephone 071-928 4488), and they will tell you what to do next.

• Under the bureau's scheme, disputes are decided by an independent party, whose services are free. You can choose to accept or reject his decision.

• If you accept the independent party's decision, the company is also obliged to accept, and to pay you what the solicitor recommends.

• If you reject the decision, you retain the right to take the company to court.

• If the arrangement is with the Personal Insurance Arbitration Service, the arbitration is handled by the Chartered Institute of Arbitrators at 24 Angel Gate, City Road, London EC1V 2RS (telephone 071-837 4483). The insurance company will explain how to apply for a hearing.

• Under the arbitration service scheme, which is free, the arbitrator's decision is legally binding. This means that you lose the option to sue the insurance company in the courts if you disagree with the decision.

• If the amount in dispute is large – and you risk losing a lot if the arbitrator's decision goes against you – get the advice of a solicitor before deciding to use the scheme.

• If your insurer is a Lloyd's syndicate, contact the Manager, Complaints and Advisory Department, Lloyd's of London, 51 Lime Street, London EC3M 7HA (telephone 071-623 7100). The department does not offer a formal arbitration service, but it will check to make sure that your claim has been properly dealt with. There is no fee for this service, and if you remain dissatisfied you retain the right to go to court, or to refer the matter to the Insurance Ombudsman.

• If your insurance company has no standard arbitration arrangement, write to the Association of British Insurers, Consumer Information Department, 51 Gresham Street, London EC2V 7HQ (telephone 071-600 3333).

The association will investigate on your behalf and may persuade the company to improve its offer. There is no fee for this help and you retain the right to sue the insurance company if you are still dissatisfied.

Using a loss assessor

If none of these steps produces a satisfactory settlement of your claim, consider employing an insurance expert known as a loss assessor, who will look into the claim and try to negotiate a more acceptable settlement.

• Before a claim is considered – especially if it is a large one – the insurance company will usually want to inspect the damage to check that the claim is reasonable. It may either send a member of its own staff to carry out the inspection or an independent adviser known as a loss adjuster.

• A loss assessor does the same work as a loss adjuster, but he acts on your behalf. Loss assessors are, however, expensive and it is generally worth employing one only if there is a substantial difference between the amount the insurance company is offering and the amount you have claimed.

• To find out the names and addresses of loss assessors in your area, contact the Institute of Public Loss Assessors, 14 Red Lion Street, Chesham, Buckinghamshire HP5 1HB; telephone Chesham (0494) 782342.

• If you do contact a loss assessor, check what his fees are likely to be before asking him to start work.

Going to court

• If you still cannot agree a satisfactory settlement of your claim, the only remaining option is to take the company to court.

• Get the advice of a solicitor before deciding to take this course (see *Getting help with a legal problem*, page 370).

Lost credit card, cheque book or cheque card

If you discover that your credit card, cheque book, cheque card or cash card is missing, telephone the credit card company or bank as soon as possible. Follow up the call with a letter. If you suspect theft, tell the police as well.

In most circumstances, provided you act quickly, you will not have to pay any bills a thief runs up on your account. And most home insurance policies will cover you against even this limited risk.

Because plastic money is now so common, central registration schemes such as Credit Card Sentinel and Card Protection Plan exist to help customers whose cards are lost or stolen.

Under the schemes, customers file details of all their cards – including cash cards, and account cards issued by shops – with a central registry, for a small annual fee. Then if any or all of a customer's cards are stolen, he needs to make only one phone call to the registry, which is open round the clock 365 days a year.

As soon as he has called, his responsibility for any bills run up by a thief ends, and the scheme's staff make sure that all the companies whose cards he holds are notified.

What you stand to lose on a stolen card

CREDIT CARD You will not have to pay more than £50 of the bills a thief runs up with your card. If you report the loss before the card is used, you will not have to pay anything.

CHEQUE BOOK Unless you have been careless – by signing blank cheques, say – you will not have to pay for any forged cheques a thief passes. The bank or the shop that accepts them will have to bear the loss.

GUARANTEE CARD You need not pay for any cash or goods a thief gets with your card.

DEBIT CARD (Switch or Visa Delta) The banks operate a system similar to that for credit cards, in that you are liable for bills only up to £50.

If your cash card is stolen

Legally, you can be made to pay back any sums a thief withdraws using your card, but only up to the time you report the loss and up to £50, unless the bank can prove gross negligence, such as writing your personal identification number on your card.

• Never keep a cash card and a note of your personal number (which does not appear on the card) together.

• Memorise your personal number if possible. If you must make a note of it, disguise it as something else – a telephone number, say.

• The same rules and precautions apply to a credit card used as a cash card.

If you damage a banknote

If you accidentally damage a banknote – by putting it through a washing machine after leaving it in a pocket, say, or by partially burning it – you may be able to get the note replaced.

• Take the remains of the note to a bank or post office and tell the staff you want a replacement. If the note is only slightly mutilated you may be able to exchange it then and there.

• If you cannot exchange it over the counter the bank or post office will ask you to fill out a form giving details of how the damage occurred, and will send the form – and the damaged note – to the Bank of England.

• If the Bank of England approves the application, it will send you a cheque through the post.

• Approval is not, however, automatic. The Bank of England may reject the application if the note is very badly mutilated. Alternatively – if, for example, only half the note has survived – the bank may delay replacing it for up to six months just in case the other half turns up.

IF YOU ARE ABROAD

• If you lose a credit card, cash card, cheque book or cheque card while you are abroad, telephone or cable the credit card company or bank as soon as possible.

• If the loss leaves you short of local currency, ask for an urgent transfer of cash to a convenient bank.

• Inform the local police of your loss and ask them for written confirmation that you have done so.

If you lose your passport

• If your passport is lost or stolen abroad, report the loss first to the local police. If you do not speak the local language, ask someone who does to come with you and help you to make the report.

• Ask the police for written confirmation that you have reported the loss. If they will not give you such a statement, make a note of the police station you visit and, if possible, the name of the officer you speak to.

• Once you have told the police, contact the nearest British consulate, embassy or High Commission. They can issue a replacement passport, or an emergency document to get you home. The police should be able to give you the consulate's address and telephone number. Alternatively, look in the telephone directory covering the nearest large town or the country's capital city.

• If you needed a visa for the country where you lose the passport, you will probably need to get a replacement visa stamped into a new passport. Ask the consulate whether this is necessary and, if so, how to apply.

Useful addresses

Advice on how to deal with or prevent particular emergencies is available from scores of organisations around Britain. The major ones are listed here.

Many of these organisations have branches or affiliated clubs throughout the country. In these cases, the head offices that are listed on these pages will be able to help you to get in touch with a local branch or club.

First aid and medical emergencies

BRITISH RED CROSS SOCIETY
9 Grosvenor Crescent, London SW1X 7EJ
Tel: 071-235 5454
Provides a wide range of services to the sick, elderly or handicapped. Runs courses in first aid, nursing and welfare services. Attends public events to provide first aid.

ST ANDREW'S AMBULANCE ASSOCIATION
St Andrew's House, Milton Street, Glasgow G4 0HR
Tel: 041-332 4031
Runs courses in Scotland on first aid, nursing and other welfare subjects. Attends public events to provide first aid.

ST JOHN AMBULANCE
1 Grosvenor Crescent, London SW1X 7EF
Tel: 071-235 5231
Runs courses throughout England and Wales on first aid, nursing and other welfare subjects. Members of the brigade also attend public events to provide first aid.

In the home and at work

AGE CONCERN ENGLAND
Astral House, 1268 London Road, London SW16 4EJ
Tel: 081-679 8000
Advises on the welfare of older people. Branches throughout Britain.

CONSUMERS' ASSOCIATION
2 Marylebone Road, London NW1 4DF
Tel: 071-486 5544
Publishes books and magazines with information and advice on consumer matters.

FIRE PROTECTION ASSOCIATION
140 Aldersgate Street, London EC1A 4HX
Tel: 071-606 3757
Advises on all aspects of fire and its prevention.

GOOD HOUSEKEEPING INSTITUTE
National Magazine House, 72 Broadwick Street, London W1V 2BP
Tel: 071-439 5000
Gives advice on household and consumer problems to readers of *Good Housekeeping* magazine.

THE KENNEL CLUB
1 Clarges Street, London W1Y 8AB
Tel: 071-493 6651
Keeps lists of local dog-training clubs.

MENCAP – The Royal Society for Mentally Handicapped Children and Adults
117-123 Golden Lane, London EC1Y 0RT
Tel: 071-454 0454
Offers a wide range of services to people with learning disabilities and their families. Local societies throughout the country.

NATIONAL SOCIETY FOR THE PREVENTION OF CRUELTY TO CHILDREN
67 Saffron Hill, London EC1N 8RS
Tel: 071-242 1626
Offers a 24-hour child protection helpline on freephone 0800 800500. Child protection teams and centres throughout England, Wales and Northern Ireland.

ROYAL COLLEGE OF VETERINARY SURGEONS
32 Belgrave Square, London SW1X 8QP
Tel: 071-235 4971
Has directory of all local vets in Britain.

ROYAL SCOTTISH SOCIETY FOR THE PREVENTION OF CRUELTY TO CHILDREN
Melville House, 41 Polwarth Terrace, Edinburgh EH11 1NU
Tel: EDINBURGH 337 8539
Advice and information.

ROYAL SOCIETY FOR THE PREVENTION OF ACCIDENTS
Cannon House, The Priory Queensway, Birmingham B4 6BS
Tel: 021-200 2461
Gives information on all aspects of safety.

ROYAL SOCIETY FOR THE PREVENTION OF CRUELTY TO ANIMALS
Causeway, Horsham, West Sussex RH12 1HG
Tel: HORSHAM 264181
Advises on animal welfare. Maintains animal hospitals and clinics and a network of inspectors throughout the country.

Emergencies on the road

AUTOMOBILE ASSOCIATION
Fanum House, Basingstoke, Hampshire RG21 2EA
Tel: BASINGSTOKE 20123
Operates a vehicle breakdown service for members, coming to the home and recovering vehicles broken down on the road. Offers touring and travel information and insurance benefits.

BRITISH MOTORCYCLISTS FEDERATION
129 Seaforth Avenue, Motspur Park, New Malden, Surrey KT3 6JU
Tel: 081-942 7914
Offers insurance benefits and information on all aspects of motorcycling. Runs a training scheme.

CYCLISTS' TOURING CLUB
Cotterell House, 69 Meadrow, Godalming, Surrey GU7 3HS
Tel: GODALMING 4177217
Advises members on all aspects of cycling. Offers free legal aid and insurance benefits.

Publishes information on cycle touring.

DISABLED DRIVERS' ASSOCIATION
Ashwellthorpe, Norwich NR16 1EX
Tel: FUNDENHALL 449
Offers disabled people information and advice on how to keep mobile. Local groups throughout the country.

EUROP ASSISTANCE LTD
252 High Street, Croydon, Surrey CR0 1NF
Tel: 081-680 1234
Operates a Europe-wide breakdown and recovery service and a worldwide medical emergency service. Representatives worldwide can help subscribers in motoring or medical emergencies.

INSTITUTE OF ADVANCED MOTORISTS
359 Chiswick High Road, London W4 4HS
Tel: 081-994 4403
Runs advanced driving tests. Local volunteer groups run training courses.

RAC MOTORING SERVICES
PO Box 700, Spectrum, Bond Street, Bristol BS99 1RB
Tel: BRISTOL 232444
Provides members with a vehicle breakdown service, both at members' homes and on the road. Offers touring and travel information and insurance benefits.

Emergencies in the water

BRITISH CANOE UNION
John Dudderidge House, Adbolton Lane, West Bridgford, Nottingham NG2 5AS
Tel: NOTTINGHAM 821100
Offers advice, guides to waterways, and insurance benefits to members. Affiliated clubs throughout the country. Many clubs run training courses.

BRITISH SUB-AQUA CLUB
Telford's Quay, Ellesmere Port, South Wirral, Cheshire L65 4FY
Tel: LIVERPOOL 357 1951
Branches throughout the country and overseas. Publishes

diving instruction manuals. Keeps lists of snorkelling and aqualung courses given by approved instructors.

BRITISH WATERWAYS
Willow Grange, Church Road, Watford WD1 3QA
Tel: WATFORD 226422
Administers over 2000 miles of canals and rivers in Britain. Sells maps and issues licences authorising craft to use its waterways.

ROYAL LIFE SAVING SOCIETY
Mountbatten House, Studley, Warwickshire B80 7NN
Tel: STUDLEY 853943
Branches throughout Britain. Runs courses in water safety, and rescue and resuscitation techniques. Provides lifeguard training for certain beaches and some inland waterways.

ROYAL YACHTING ASSOCIATION
RYA House, Romsey Road, Eastleigh, Hants SO5 4YA
Tel: EASTLEIGH 629962
Affiliated sailing clubs throughout Britain. Keeps lists of recognised training schools. Covers motor as well as sailing boats, and windsurfing.

Emergencies on holiday and in the country

ASSOCIATION OF BRITISH TRAVEL AGENTS
55-57 Newman Street, London W1P 4AH
Tel: 071-637 2444
Provides financial safeguards for holidaymakers who have booked package holidays through ABTA travel agents.

BRITISH CAVE RESCUE COUNCIL
c/o The Secretary, Mr Brian Boardman, 8 Yealand Avenue, Giggleswick, Settle, North Yorkshire BD24 0AY Keeps lists of local affiliated cave rescue organisations.

BRITISH MOUNTAINEERING COUNCIL
Crawford House, Precinct Centre, Booth Street East, Manchester M13 9RZ
Tel: 061-273 5835

Local climbing clubs throughout Britain. Runs training courses. Advises on equipment. Publishes guides and instruction manuals.

THE CAMPING AND CARAVANNING CLUB
Greenfields House, Westwood Way, Coventry, Warwickshire CV4 8JH
Tel: COVENTRY 694995
Runs campsites throughout Britain. Offers members breakdown and recovery services throughout Europe, and worldwide medical insurance cover.

THE CARAVAN CLUB
East Grinstead House, East Grinstead, W Sussex RH19 1UA
Tel: EAST GRINSTEAD 326944
Runs caravan sites throughout the country. Has a breakdown and recovery service for members. Advises on foreign touring.

CIVIL AVIATION AUTHORITY
CAA House, 45-59 Kingsway, London WC2B 6TE
Tel: 071-379 7311
Provides financial safeguards for holidaymakers who have booked package holidays through companies holding an Air Travel Organiser's Licence.

COUNTRYSIDE COMMISSION
Postal Sales, PO Box 124, Walgrave, Northamptonshire NN6 9TL
Tel: NORTHAMPTON 781848
Publishes information on long-distance footpaths and on the rights and responsibilities of visitors to the countryside.

THE RAMBLERS' ASSOCIATION
1-5 Wandsworth Road, London SW8 2XX
Tel: 071-582 6878
Provides information on all aspects of walking. Local groups throughout the country.

THE SKI CLUB OF GREAT BRITAIN
118 Easton Square, London SW1W 9AF
Tel: 071-245 1033
Provides information on ski resorts throughout the world. Representatives in many Alpine resorts. Advises on equipment and skiing courses.

THE YOUTH HOSTELS ASSOCIATION
Trevelyan House, St Stephen's Hill, St Albans, Hertfordshire AL1 2DY
Tel: ST ALBANS 855215
Runs hostels offering members cheap overnight accommodation throughout the world. Publishes handbook.

Natural disasters

FIRE AND EMERGENCY PLANNING DEPARTMENT
The Home Office, 50 Queen Anne's Gate, London SW1H 9AT
Tel: 071-273 3000
Offers information on civil defence. For advice on local civil defence arrangements – including flood warning and prevention – contact your local council.

Crime

CRIMINAL INJURIES COMPENSATION BOARD
Whittington House, 19-30 Alfred Place, London WC1E 7LG
Tel: 071-636 9501
Awards financial compensation to the victims of crimes of violence.

RAPE CRISIS CENTRE
PO Box 69, London WC1X 9NJ
Tel: 071-837 1600 or 021-766 5366 (Birmingham) or 031-556 9437 (Edinburgh) or 0222 373181 (Cardiff)
Counselling service Mon-Fri offering advice and help.

Drink and drugs

AL-ANON FAMILY GROUPS UK AND EIRE
61 Great Dover Street, London SE1 4YF
Tel: 071-403 0888
Specialises in helping the families and friends of problem drinkers. Groups throughout the country.

ALCOHOL CONCERN
275 Grays Inn Road, London WC1X 8QF
Tel: 071-833 3471
Runs information, education and advice centres on alcoholism throughout the country.

ALCOHOLICS ANONYMOUS
General Service Office, PO Box 1, Stonebow House, Stonebow, York YO1 2NJ
Tel: YORK 644026
Helps alcoholics who want to stop drinking. Centres throughout Britain. Offers the support and companionship of reformed alcoholics.

MEDICAL COUNCIL ON ALCOHOLISM
1 St Andrews Place, London NW1 4LB
Tel: 071-487 4445
Voluntary body helping to educate the medical profession on alcohol and alcoholism, and alcoholics and their families to find specialist care.

NARCOTICS ANONYMOUS
PO Box 1980, London N19 3LS
Tel: 071-498 9005
A fellowship of drug victims, modelled on Alcoholics Anonymous, whose members help each other to stay free of their addiction.

SALVATION ARMY
101 Queen Victoria Street, London EC4P 4EP
Tel: 071-236 5222
Maintains hostels for the homeless throughout the country.

THE SAMARITANS
Head Office, 10 The Grove, Slough, Berkshire SL1 1QF
Tel: SLOUGH 532713 (Office); 071-734 2800 (London 24-hour emergency line)
24-hour service listening to and befriending those in despair and with suicidal urges.

Legal and financial emergencies

ASSOCIATION OF BRITISH INSURERS
Consumer Information Department, 51 Gresham Street, London EC2V 7HQ
Tel: 071-600 3333
Advises and assists with insurance problems.

THE CHARTERED INSTITUTE OF ARBITRATORS
24 Angel Gate, City Road, London EC1V 2RS
Tel: 071-837 4483
Arranges binding arbitration to settle commercial and consumer disputes.

INSTITUTE OF PUBLIC LOSS ASSESSORS
14 Red Lion Street, Chesham, Buckinghamshire HP5 1HB
Tel: CHESHAM 782342
Keeps lists of experts who will help to settle disputed insurance claims.

INSURANCE OMBUDSMAN BUREAU
City Gate 1, 135 Park Street, London SE1 9EA
Tel: 071-928 4488
Investigates some disputes between individuals and insurance companies.

THE LAW CENTRES FEDERATION
Duchess House, 18-19 Warren Street, London W1P 5DB
Tel: 071-387 8570
Keeps lists of centres in some major cities and towns offering free legal assistance and advice.

LLOYD'S OF LONDON
Complaints and Advisory Department, Lloyd's of London, 51 Lime Street, London EC3M 7HA
Tel: 071-623 7100
Checks that a claim on a Lloyd's insurer has been dealt with properly.

SOLICITORS COMPLAINTS BUREAU
Victoria Court, 8 Dormer Place, Leamington Spa, Warwickshire CV32 5AE
Tel: LEAMINGTON SPA 820082
Deals with written complaints about solicitors.

Index

All about CHILDREN

All about ELECTRICITY

F

All about FIRE

In the home

Out of doors

Escaping from a fire
If you are trapped on an upper floor 145
action summary 24
How to rescue a victim of smoke
inhalation *124*
If a house is on fire **142-7**
Getting out of a blazing house *142-4*
If the exit is blocked *144-6*
Escaping from a high rise building 146
Using a rope ladder *146-7*
Rescuing someone from a fire **148-9**
How to do a fireman's lift **148-9**
Escaping from a sleeping bag *294*
Escaping from a forest fire **328-30**

Fire prevention
The causes of house fires 147
How to protect your home against fire 152
How to use fire extinguishers 152
Choosing a fire alarm 152
Preventing chip pan fires 164-5
How to use fireguards *168*
Guarding against fire on a boat 262-3

First aid for fire victims
How to treat burns **66-7**
first aid summary 7-10
Treating blisters caused by burns 64
Removing burnt clothing *66*
Treating chemical burns 66
Treating burns or scalds in the mouth 67
Treating electrical burns 93

G

gardens
safety measures 170-1
gas
appliances
safety with 154

All about GAS

All about MOTORING

Road accidents

Defensive driving

Problems on the move

O

P/Q

T

All about TRAVELLING

U

Acknowledgments

Many organisations and individuals gave assistance during the preparation of this book, and the publishers would like to thank them. They include:

Access; Age Concern England; David Andersen, Thomas Cook Ltd; Brian Apps, Banking Information Service; Andrew Bevan; British Gas Corporation; British Horse Society; British Telecom; British Veterinary Association; Clive de Bruyn, Essex County Beekeeping Instructor; Janice Cave, Royal Society for the Prevention of Accidents; Central Criminal Court, Old Bailey; Child Accident Prevention Trust; Community Medicine Department, University of Manchester; Consumer Safety Unit, Department of Trade; Thomas Cook Ltd, London; Mike Cuddihey, London Electricity Board; Department of Health and Social Security; Electricity Council; Forestry Commission; Ron Foster, Department of Health and Social Security; Guy's Hospital Dental School; Ray Hankey, Tour Operators' Study Group; HM Coastguard; Ingrid Holford; Home Office; Institute of Public Loss Assessors; Dick Kesby; The Law Society; Legal Office, City of London Police; Isobel McLean; Brian Morrison, Assistant Director, Home Safety, RoSPA; National Association of Lift Makers; Peter Newton; Northern Ireland Office, Belfast; Otis Elevator Company Ltd; Passport Office, London; Ramblers' Association; Registrar General of Births, Deaths and Marriages, London; Royal National Lifeboat Institution; Royal Society for the Prevention of Cruelty to Animals; Scottish Office, Edinburgh; Sealink UK Ltd; Bernard Shally, British Sub-Aqua Club; Brian Sims; Ski Club of Great Britain; Survival Aids Ltd, Cumbria; Tottenham Magistrates' Court; Captain O.M. Watts Ltd; Peta Watts; Norman Webb, British Dental Association; R. Wyatt, Bedwell Boatyard.

The publishers also acknowledge their indebtedness to the following books, which were consulted for reference:

AA Book of the Car (Drive Publications); *AA Car Maintenance Course* (Drive Publications); *Alcoholism*, Max Glatt (Hodder and Stoughton); *All about Motoring Breakdowns* (The Automobile Association); *The Boat* (Time-Life Books); *Boat handling* (Time-Life Books); *Book of Driving* (The Automobile Association); *Dealing with Household Emergencies* (Consumers' Association); *Dinghy Sailing*, Bob Bond and Steve Sleight (Pelham Books); *Emergencies in the Home*, ed. Stephen Lock (British Medical Association); *The Emergency Book*, ed. Jane Anthony (Macdonald and Jane's); *The Emergency Book*, Bradley Smith and Gus Stevens (Penguin); *First Aid Manual*, St John Ambulance Association, St Andrew's Ambulance Association and British Red Cross Society (Dorling Kindersley); *Human Nutrition and Dietetics*, Davidson and Passmore (E. & S. Livingstone Ltd); *Owning Dogs and Cats*, M.J.R. Stockman (J. Sainsbury PLC); *Oxford Companion to Sports and Games* (OUP); *Sailing, A Basic Guide*, Alain Gree (John Bartholomew and Son Ltd); *Scouting for Boys*, Robert Baden-Powell (The Scout Association); *Shark Attack*, H. David Baldridge (Everest Books Ltd); *Shark Attack*, V.M. Coppleson (Pacific Books); *The Shark: Splendid Savage of the Sea*, Jacques-Yves and Philippe Cousteau (Cassell); *The Small Boat Skipper's Handbook*, Geoff Lewis (Hollis & Carter); *Stay Alive in the Desert*, K.E.M. Melville (Roger Lascelles); *Under Way (A-Z guide to safe and successful seamanship)*, Bill Beavis (Lutterworth Press); *Waterwise*, Gordon Fairley (William Luscombe Publisher Ltd in association with Mitchell Beazley); *The Yachtsman's Weather Guide*, Ingrid Holford (Ward Lock); *The Young Specialist Looks at Marine Life*, W. de Haas and F. Knorr (Burke Books).

Picture credits

The photographs in this book were provided by the following photographers and agencies. Work commissioned by Reader's Digest is shown in *italics*.

Page 266 *Johan du Plessis*/Reader's Digest, South Africa; **267** *all* Professor R. Scorer; **268** *all* John Lythgoe/Planet Earth Pictures; **269** Jonathan T. Wright/Bruce Coleman Ltd; **325** S. Jonasson/Frank Lane Picture Agency Ltd; **327** S. McCutcheon/Frank Lane Picture Agency Ltd; **329** Jeff Cutting

Separations: Reprocolor Llovet S.A., Barcelona
Paper: Townsend Hook Paper Co. Ltd, Snodland
Printing & Binding: Fabrieken Brepols N.V., Belgium
40-069-5

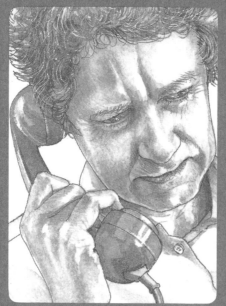

These panels are for you to write in the telephone numbers you might need in a crisis. Write the numbers large and in a strong colour – you might have to read them in poor light.

CITIZENS ADVICE BUREAU

....

COASTGUARD

....

CREDIT CARD COMPANIES

....

....

....

....

DENTIST

....

BANK

....

DOCTOR

....

CHURCH

....

ELECTRICITY

....

Making

- Before making the call, work out where you are, if possible. The operator will need to know this if he is to get help to you promptly. He will also ask for your telephone number. It will enable the emergency services to find you if you are cut off.

- Call 999. On a pay phone, do not put any coins in. In the dark, find the number on a push-button phone by feeling for the 9, which is the right-hand bottom button on the panel.